ANDERSON'S
PATHOLOGY

VOLUME TWO

ANDERSON'S PATHOLOGY

Edited by

JOHN M. KISSANE, M.D.

Professor of Pathology and of Pathology in Pediatrics,
Washington University School of Medicine;
Pathologist, Barnes and Affiliated Hospitals,
St. Louis Children's Hospital, St. Louis, Missouri

Former editions edited by

W.A.D. ANDERSON,
M.A., M.D., F.A.C.P., F.C.A.P., F.R.C.P.A. (Hon.)

Emeritus Professor of Pathology and Formerly Chairman
of the Department of Pathology,
University of Miami School of Medicine,
Miami, Florida

EIGHTH EDITION

with **2949** *illustrations and* 8 *color plates*

THE C. V. MOSBY COMPANY

ST. LOUIS • TORONTO • PRINCETON 1985

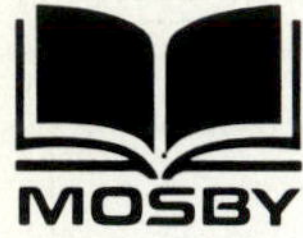

A TRADITION OF PUBLISHING EXCELLENCE

Editors: Rosa L. Kasper, Don E. Ladig
Assistant editor: Anne Gunter
Manuscript editor: Patricia Tannian
Design: Staff
Production: Carol O'Leary, Teresa Breckwoldt, Mary Stueck

Two Volumes

EIGHTH EDITION

Printed in the United States of America

The C.V. Mosby Company
11830 Westline Industrial Drive, St. Louis, Missouri 63146

Library of Congress Cataloging in Publication Data

Pathology (Saint Louis, Mo.)
Anderson's Pathology.

Rev. ed. of: Pathology / edited by W.A.D. Anderson, John M. Kissane. 7th ed. 1977.
Includes bibliographies and index.
1. Pathology. I. Anderson, W.A.D. (William Arnold Douglas), 1910- II. Kissane, John M., 1928- III. Title. IV. Title: Pathology. [DNLM: 1. Pathology. QZ 4 A5521]
RB111.P3 1984 616.07 84.9868
ISBN 0-8016-0191-6

TS/VH/VH 9 8 7 6 5 4 3 2 1 01/B/001

Contributors

ARTHUR C. ALLEN, M.D.

Professor of Pathology, State University of New York, Downstate Medical Center; Director of Laboratories, Jewish Hospital and Medical Center (currently Interfaith Medical Center), Brooklyn, New York

ROBERT E. ANDERSON, M.D.

Professor and Chairman, Department of Pathology, The University of New Mexico, Albuquerque, New Mexico

FREDERIC B. ASKIN, M.D.

Professor of Pathology, University of North Carolina School of Medicine; Director of Surgical Pathology, North Carolina Memorial Hospital, Chapel Hill, North Carolina

SAROJA BHARATI, M.D.

Chairperson, Department of Pathology, Deborah Heart and Lung Center, Browns Mills, New Jersey; Clinical Professor of Pathology, Temple University Medical School, Philadelphia, Pennsylvania; Clinical Professor of Pathology, The Pennsylvania State University, The Milton S. Hershey Medical Center, Hershey, Pennsylvania; Research Professor of Medicine, University of Illinois, Abraham Lincoln School of Medicine, Chicago, Illinois

CHAPMAN H. BINFORD, M.D.

Consultant to the Leprosy Registry, American Registry of Pathology; Formerly Chief, Special Mycobacterial Diseases Branch, Geographic Pathology Division, Armed Forces Institute of Pathology, Washington, D.C.

FRANCIS W. CHANDLER, D.V.M., Ph.D.

Chief, Experimental Pathology Branch, Center for Infectious Diseases, Centers for Disease Control, Atlanta, Georgia

JACOB L. CHASON, M.D.

Neuropathologist, Department of Pathology, Henry Ford Hospital; Clinical Professor of Pathology (Neuropathology), Wayne State University School of Medicine, Detroit, Michigan

MASAHIRO CHIGA, M.D.

Professor of Pathology, Departments of Pathology and Oncology, University of Kansas College of Health Sciences and Hospital, School of Medicine, Kansas City, Kansas

A.R.W. CLIMIE, M.D.

Chief of Pathology, Harper-Grace Hospitals; Associate Professor of Pathology, Wayne State University School of Medicine, Detroit, Michigan

JOSE COSTA, M.D.

Professor of Pathology, University of Lausanne, Lausanne, Switzerland; Formerly Chief, Pathologic Anatomy Branch, National Cancer Institute, National Institutes of Health, Bethesda, Maryland

CHARLES J. DAVIS, JR., M.D.

Associate Chairman, Department of Genitourinary Pathology, Armed Forces Institute of Pathology; Professor of Pathology, Uniformed Services, University of Health Sciences, Washington, D.C.

KATHERINE DeSCHRYVER-KECSKEMETI, M.D.

Associate Professor, Division of Surgical Pathology, Washington University School of Medicine, St. Louis, Missouri

GEORGE Th. DIAMANDOPOULOS, M.D.

Professor of Pathology, Department of Pathology, Harvard Medical School, Boston, Massachusetts

HUGH A. EDMONDSON, M.D.

Professor of Pathology, University of Southern California, School of Medicine, Los Angeles, California

ROBERT E. FECHNER, M.D.

Royster Professor of Pathology and Director, Division of Surgical Pathology, University of Virginia Medical Center, Charlottesville, Virginia

GERALD FINE, M.D.

Chief, Division of Anatomic Pathology, Department of Pathology, Henry Ford Hospital, Detroit, Michigan

KAARLE O. FRANSSILA, M.D., Ph.D.

Chief of Pathology Laboratory, Department of Radiotherapy and Oncology, Helsinki University Central Hospital, Helsinki, Finland

ROBERT J. GORLIN, D.D.S., M.S.

Regents' Professor and Chairman, Department of Oral Pathology and Genetics, and Professor, Departments of Pathology, Dermatology, Pediatrics, Obstetrics-Gynecology, and Otolaryngology, Schools of Dentistry and Medicine, University of Minnesota, Minneapolis, Minnesota

ROGERS C. GRIFFITH, M.D.

Assistant Professor of Pathology and Surgical Pathology, Washington University School of Medicine; Assistant Pathologist, Barnes and Affiliated Hospitals, St. Louis Children's Hospital, and The Jewish Hospital of St. Louis, St. Louis, Missouri

JOE W. GRISHAM, M.D.

Professor and Chairman, Department of Pathology, University of North Carolina, School of Medicine, Chapel Hill, North Carolina

PAUL GROSS, M.D.

Adjunct Professor, Department of Pathology, Medical University of South Carolina, Charleston, South Carolina

DONALD B. HACKEL, M.D.

Professor of Pathology, Department of Pathology, Duke University Medical School, Durham, North Carolina

GORDON R. HENNIGAR, M.D.

Professor and Chairman, Department of Pathology, Medical University of South Carolina, Charleston, South Carolina

CHARLES S. HIRSCH, M.D.

Director of Forensic Pathology, Hamilton County Coroner's Office; Professor of Pathology, University of Cincinnati College of Medicine, Cincinnati, Ohio

DAVID B. JONES, M.D.

Professor of Pathology, Department of Pathology, State University of New York, Upstate Medical Center, Syracuse, New York

HAN-SEOB KIM, M.D.

Associate Professor of Pathology, Baylor College of Medicine; Attending Pathologist, The Methodist Hospital; Attending Pathologist, Harris County Hospital District, Houston, Texas

JOHN M. KISSANE, M.D.

Professor of Pathology and of Pathology in Pediatrics, Washington University School of Medicine; Pathologist, Barnes and Affiliated Hospitals, St. Louis Children's Hospital, St. Louis, Missouri

FREDERICK T. KRAUS, M.D.

Director of Laboratory Medicine, St. John's Mercy Medical Center; Professor of Pathology (Visiting Staff), Washington University School of Medicine, St. Louis, Missouri

CHARLES KUHN III, M.D.

Professor of Pathology, Washington University School of Medicine, St. Louis, Missouri

MICHAEL L. KYRIAKOS, M.D.

Professor of Pathology, Washington University School of Medicine; Surgical Pathologist, Barnes Hospital; Consultant to St. Louis Children's Hospital and Shriner's Hospital for Crippled Children, St. Louis, Missouri

PAUL E. LACY, M.D.

Mallinkrodt Professor and Chairman, Department of Pathology, Washington University School of Medicine, St. Louis, Missouri

MAURICE LEV, M.D.

Director, Department of Pathology, Deborah Heart and Lung Center, Browns Mills, New Jersey; Clinical Professor of Pathology, Temple University Medical School, Philadelphia, Pennsylvania; Clinical Professor of Pathology, The Pennsylvania State University, The Milton S. Hershey Medical Center, Hershey, Pennsylvania

CHAN K. MA, M.D.

Staff Pathologist, Department of Pathology, Henry Ford Hospital, Detroit, Michigan

VINCENT T. MARCHESI, M.D.

Professor and Chairman, Department of Pathology, Yale University, School of Medicine, New Haven, Connecticut

MANUEL A. MARCIAL, M.D.

Research Fellow in Pathology, Department of Pathology, Brigham and Women's Hospital and Harvard Medical School, Boston, Massachusetts

RAÚL A. MARCIAL-ROJAS, M.D., J.D., M.P.H., M.P.A.

Professor of Pathology and Dean, School of Medicine, Universidad Central del Caribe, Cayey, Puerto Rico; Formerly Chairman, Department of Pathology, University of Puerto Rico, School of Medicine, San Juan, Puerto Rico

ROBERT W. McDIVITT, M.D.

Professor of Pathology, Washington University School of Medicine; Director of Anatomic Pathology, Jewish Hospital of St. Louis; Associate Pathologist, Barnes Hospital; Consultant, Children's Hospital of St. Louis, St. Louis, Missouri

WILLIAM A. MEISSNER, M.D.

Emeritus Professor of Pathology, New England Deaconess Hospital, Harvard Medical School, Boston, Massachusetts

F. KASH MOSTOFI, M.D.

Chairman, Department of Genitourinary Pathology, Armed Forces Institute of Pathology, Washington, D.C.; Professor of Pathology, Uniformed Services University of Health Sciences, Washington, D.C.; Associate Professor of Pathology, Johns Hopkins University, School of Medicine; Clinical Professor of Pathology, University of Maryland Medical School, Baltimore, Maryland; Clinical Professor of Pathology, Georgetown University School of Medicine, Washington, D.C.

WAYKIN NOPANITAYA, Ph.D.

Professor, Department of Pathology, Prince of Songkla University, Songkla, Head-Yai, Thailand

JAMES E. OERTEL, M.D.

Chairman, Department of Endocrine Pathology, Armed Forces Institute of Pathology, Washington, D.C.

ROBERT L. PETERS, M.D.

Professor of Pathology, University of Southern California, School of Medicine, Los Angeles, California; Chief Pathologist, Rancho Los Amigos Hospital, Downey, California

R.C.B. PUGH, M.D., F.R.C.S., F.R.C. Path.

Consulting Pathologist, St. Peter's Hospitals and Institute of Urology, London, England

ALAN S. RABSON, M.D.

Director, Division of Cancer Biology and Diagnosis, National Cancer Institute, Bethesda, Maryland

JUAN ROSAI, M.D.

Professor of Laboratory Medicine and Pathology and Director of Anatomic Pathology, University of Minnesota Medical School, Minneapolis, Minnesota

ARKADI M. RYWLIN, M.D.

Director, Department of Pathology and Laboratory Medicine, Mount Sinai Medical Center; Professor of Pathology, University of Miami School of Medicine, Miami, Florida

DANTE G. SCARPELLI, M.D., Ph.D.

Ernest J. and Hattie H. Magerstadt Professor and Chairman, Department of Pathology, Northwestern University Medical School; Chief of Service, Northwestern Memorial Hospital, Chicago, Illinois

THOMAS M. SCOTTI, M.D.

Formerly Professor of Pathology, University of Miami School of Medicine, Miami, Florida

STEWART SELL, M.D.

Professor and Chairman, Department of Pathology and Laboratory Medicine, University of Texas Health Science Center at Houston, Houston, Texas

HERSCHEL SIDRANSKY, M.D.

Professor and Chairman, Department of Pathology, The George Washington University Medical Center, Washington, D.C.

RUTH SILBERBERG, M.D.

Visiting Scientist, Department of Pathology, Hadassah Hebrew University School of Medicine, Jerusalem, Israel

MORTON E. SMITH, M.D.

Professor of Ophthalmology and Pathology, Washington University School of Medicine, St. Louis, Missouri

SHELDON C. SOMMERS, M.D.

Clinical Professor of Pathology, Columbia University College of Physicians and Surgeons, New York, New York; Clinical Professor of Pathology, University of Southern California, School of Medicine, Los Angeles, California

STEVEN L. TEITELBAUM, M.D.

Professor of Pathology, Washington University School of Medicine and The Jewish Hospital of St. Louis, St. Louis, Missouri

JACK L. TITUS, M.D., Ph.D.

Professor and The Moody Chairman, Department of Pathology, Baylor College of Medicine; Chief, Pathology Service, The Methodist Hospital; Pathologist-in-Chief, Harris County Hospital District, Houston, Texas

DAVID H. WALKER, M.D.

Associate Professor, Department of Pathology, University of North Carolina, School of Medicine; Associate Attending Pathologist, North Carolina Memorial Hospital, Chapel Hill, North Carolina

NANCY E. WARNER, M.D.

Hastings Professor of Pathology, University of Southern California, School of Medicine, Los Angeles, California

JOHN C. WATTS, M.D.

Attending Pathologist, Department of Anatomic Pathology, William Beaumont Hospital, Royal Oak, Michigan; Clinical Assistant Professor of Pathology, Wayne State University School of Medicine, Detroit, Michigan

ROSS E. ZUMWALT, M.D.

Associate Professor of Pathology, University of Cincinnati College of Medicine; Associate Pathologist, Hamilton County Coroner's Office, Cincinnati, Ohio

Preface to eighth edition

Readers and followers of this book will have noticed that this is the first edition in which Dr. W.A.D. Anderson ("Wad" to his innumerable friends) has not actively participated. He remains vigorous and active, however, and has offered welcome encouragement and advice. We all wish him well.

Since the preparation of the seventh edition, spectacular advances have occurred in the basic sciences and in clinical medicine, on which pathology depends and to which it contributes. Advances in immunopathology and hematopathology, to mention only two general areas, and in diseases of the breast and of somatic soft tissues, to mention only two organ systems, have compelled revision of the text.

My first responsibility as editor was to examine the organization of the book to see if major structural revision was in order. I have retained the initial presentation of mechanisms both as a didactically effective transition between the basic sciences and pathology and as a review for readers whose exposure to the basic sciences has not been recent. This section of the book is followed by considerations of diseases of the various organ systems. The emphasis throughout is on the mechanisms whereby normal phenomena and processes become disturbed, giving rise to diseases and lesions.

The seventh edition introduced a chapter on geographic pathology. Even by that time, however, the Jet Age had made geographic pathology an authentic subspecialty with a language and information base of its own. It deserves separate consideration without the duplication of language and concepts that its introduction in a primary pathology text would impose. Thus, with some regret, I decided to remove the chapter on geographic pathology and rely on contributors of organ-system chapters to include geographic factors in their discussions of the epidemiology of various disorders. This effort I believe has been effectively addressed in this edition.

I chose also not to include a separate chapter on venereal diseases. Such a chapter has, over several decades, come to include sociologic and public health considerations that transcend the mechanisms and morphologic expressions of the venereal diseases. These aspects are more appropriately dealt with in works directed to public health or preventive medicine than in a work on pathology. In this edition venereally transmitted diseases are considered along with other agent-mediated diseases.

In the preparation of this edition I have been fortunate in being able to recruit several new contributors. I welcome their contributions and at the same time express my appreciation to previous contributors.

Finally, I would like to express my gratitude to the generation of supporters of *Anderson's Pathology*. I hope the eighth edition continues to merit their support.

John M. Kissane

Preface to first edition

Pathology should form the basis of every physician's thinking about his patients. The study of the nature of disease, which constitutes pathology in the broad sense, has many facets. Any science or technique which contributes to our knowledge of the nature and constitution of disease belongs in the broad realm of pathology. Different aspects of a disease may be stressed by the geneticist, the cytologist, the biochemist, the clinical diagnostician, etc., and it is the difficult function of the pathologist to attempt to bring about a synthesis, and to present disease in as whole or as true an aspect as can be done with present knowledge. Pathologists often have been accused, and sometimes justly, of stressing the morphologic changes in disease to the neglect of functional effects. Nevertheless, pathologic anatomy and histology remain as an essential foundation of knowledge about disease, without which basis the concepts of many diseases are easily distorted.

In this volume is brought together the specialized knowledge of a number of pathologists in particular aspects or fields of pathology. A time-tested order of presentation is maintained, both because it has been found logical and effective in teaching medical students and because it facilitates study and reference by graduates. Although presented in an order and form to serve as a textbook, it is intended also to have sufficient comprehensiveness and completeness to be useful to the practicing or graduate physician. It is hoped that this book will be both a foundation and a useful tool for those who deal with the problems of disease.

For obvious reasons, the nature and effects of radiation have been given unusual relative prominence. The changing order of things, with increase of rapid, worldwide travel and communication, necessitates increased attention to certain viral, protozoal, parasitic, and other conditions often dismissed as "tropical," to bring them nearer their true relative importance. Also, given more than usual attention are diseases of the skin, of the organs of special senses, of the nervous system, and of the skeletal system. These are fields which often have not been given sufficient consideration in accordance with their true relative importance among diseases.

The Editor is highly appreciative of the spirit of the various contributors to this book. They are busy people, who, at the sacrifice of other duties and of leisure, freely cooperated in its production, uncomplainingly tolerated delays and difficulties, and were understanding in their willingness to work together for the good of the book as a whole. Particular thanks are due the directors of the Army Institute of Pathology and the American Registry of Pathology, for making available many illustrations. Dr. G.L. Duff, Strathcona Professor of Pathology, McGill University, Dr. H.A. Edmondson, Department of Pathology of the University of Southern California School of Medicine, Dr. J.S. Hirschboeck, Dean, and Dr. Harry Beckman, Professor of Pharmacology, Marquette University School of Medicine, all generously gave advice and assistance with certain parts.

To the members of the Department of Pathology and Bacteriology at Marquette University, the Editor wishes to express gratitude, both for tolerance and for assistance. Especially valuable has been the help of Dr. R.S. Haukohl, Dr. J.F. Kuzma, Dr. S.B. Pessin, and Dr. H. Everett. A large burden was assumed by the Editor's secretaries, Miss Charlotte Skacel and Miss Ann Cassady. Miss Patricia Blakeslee also assisted at various stages and with the index. To all of these the Editor's thanks, and also to the many others who at some time assisted by helpful and kindly acts, or by words of encouragement or interest.

W.A.D. Anderson

Contents

Color Plates

CHAPTER 24

Upper Respiratory Tract and Ear

ROBERT E. FECHNER

The upper respiratory tract comprises the nose, paranasal sinuses, nasopharynx, larynx, and middle ear with its adjacent mastoid air cells. These structures encounter innumerable airborne agents that are potentially infectious, allergenic, or carcinogenic. Many of the reactive processes and neoplasms provoked by these agents are unique to the upper airway. In addition, diseases that involve multiple systems, such as Wegener's granulomatosis or malignant lymphoma, sometimes have their initial manifestation in the upper respiratory tract. The upper airway may also be secondarily affected by systemic diseases of diverse pathogeneses. Rheumatoid arthritis can damage the small joints in the larynx; tuberculosis or fungal infections can involve the upper airway by hematogenous spread from the lungs; hypothyroidism can produce laryngeal myxedema with resultant alterations in the voice.

This chapter is divided according to the anatomic areas of the upper respiratory tract just listed. A concluding section includes diseases that involve multiple parts of the upper airway.

NOSE

Malformations

Choanal atresia or choanal stenosis results from a membrane, which may contain bone or cartilage, that completely or partially occludes the nose at its junction with the nasopharynx. The defect is probably a persistence of the bucconasal membrane that ordinarily disappears at the seventh week of fetal development. Newborn infants with choanal malformations experience respiratory distress because they instinctively breathe through the nose, and they can be asphyxiated while nursing. The condition occurs in about 1 of 7000 births; there is a familial tendency.[12] About one half of infants with choanal atresia have other anomalies.[5]

Absence of the external nose can occur in association with choanal atresia.[6] Partial or complete duplication of the nose may be accompanied by duplications of foregut structures or may occur as an isolated malformation.[10]

Brain tissue can be located in the subcutaneous tissue of the glabella, with or without an intranasal component. In some patients the brain tissue connects with the cranial cavity through a defect in the skull—a meningoencephalocele. In others there is no communication, and the inaccurate term "nasal glioma" is applied to this heterotopic tissue. Nasal gliomas are not neoplasms, and any growth is commensurate with the growth of the child. Glial tissue dominates, and ganglion cells are rare. Irregular bands of vascular fibrous tissue are intermixed.[7] Heterotopic brain tissue has also been found in the pharynx.[4]

Cysts of the nose are of two major types: dermoid and fissural. Dermoid cysts are developmental anomalies.[8] They are located beneath the skin at any point between the glabella and columella and are usually detected in childhood.[11] In addition to a cutaneous fistula, they can extend deep into the nasal septum or superiorly into the epidural space. The cysts are lined by squamous epithelium associated with hair follicles, sweat glands, and sebaceous glands in any combination.

Fissural cysts arise along the closure lines of the embryonic maxillary and globular processes and are often called nasolabial (nasoalveolar) or globulomaxillary, depending on the location. The cysts are lined mainly by squamous epithelium or columnar epithelium that may or may not be ciliated. Goblet cells are interspersed. Despite their presumed origin from entrapped embryonic epithelium, most do not appear until adulthood. Blacks have a predilection for these cysts.[9]

Skin

The skin of the nose is especially susceptible to solar damage and to inflammatory lesions that are centered in the sebaceous glands, for example, acne vulgaris. *Rhinophyma* is a term used for the hyperplastic glandular type of acne rosacea. Sebaceous glands are increased in number and size, the ducts are distended with keratinous debris, and dilated capillaries populate the dermis. This histologic complex is seen as an enlarged, lumpy, red nose. Although a variety of neoplasms have been reported in rhinophyma, there is no convincing evidence to indicate more than a chance association.[3]

NASAL CAVITY AND PARANASAL SINUSES

Infectious, allergic, and inflammatory processes

Acute rhinitis and sinusitis

The two most common causes of acute rhinitis are viral infections and allergic reactions. Mucosa reacting to an allergic insult is edematous and hyperemic with an inflammatory infiltrate rich in eosinophils.[58] In viral infections the virus replicates in the epithelial cells and the degenerating epithelial cells are exfoliated.[19] The stroma becomes hyperemic, edematous, and infiltrated with neutrophils, lymphocytes, and plasma cells. Serous or mucinous fluid exudes through the epithelium. Clinically, these changes are manifest as nasal stuffiness and rhinorrhea. If a bacterial infection is superimposed, neutrophils dominate the inflammatory infiltrate and are evident clinically as a thick, purulent discharge.

Similar reactions to allergens or infectious agents occur in the mucosa of the paranasal sinuses, thus readily occluding the ostia. Retention of the exudate adds a sensation of facial fullness or pain to the nasal symptoms.

Bacterial infections of the sinuses can lead to serious complications. Infection of the ethmoid air cells may spread into the orbital soft tissues and the meninges. Sphenoiditis can lead to retrobulbar neuritis. Frontal sinusitis can be followed by meningitis or osteomyelitis of the frontal bone.

Nasal polyps

Nasal polyps are enormous, localized enlargements of the lamina propria mucosa caused by edema, inflammation, and the proliferation of fibroblasts (Fig. 24-1). Abnormal mucous glands are formed in about half of the polyps. These glands are often distended with mucus and form cysts, which contribute further to the mass.[72] Polyps are covered with ciliated epithelium that may be slightly thickened and sometimes undergoes squamous metaplasia. A thick, subepithelial basal lamina is often conspicuous. Ulceration of the surface or infarction of the polyp can occur.

Nasal polyps are often called allergic polyps in patients with atopy. In the absence of atopy the polyps are usually attributed to infection. There are no constant histologic findings that permit this etiologic distinction. Eosinophils, traditionally viewed as a manifestation of allergic response, can be seen in polyps when no allergic basis can be identified clinically.

The pathogenesis of nasal polyps is not clearly understood. Polyps are uncommon before 20 years of age and are seen more frequently in asthmatics than in the general population.[66] It is likely that more than one mechanism exists, depending on different inciting factors and variables in the host's response. In some patients immunoglobulins have been found in polyps at a concentration higher than can be explained by passive diffusion.[21] Eosinophils are especially prominent in these polyps.

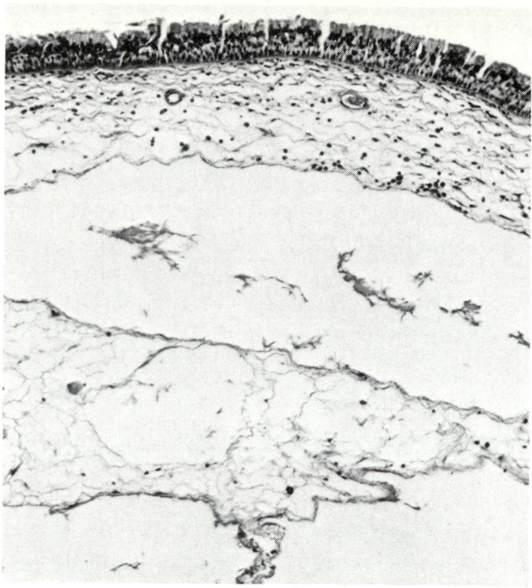

Fig. 24-1. Nasal polyp is edematous stroma with a few subepithelial inflammatory cells. It is covered with normal ciliated epithelium.

A nasal polyp in a person younger than 20 years of age signals the likelihood of cystic fibrosis. Polyps from these patients differ from typical nasal polyps in lacking basement membrane thickening and tissue eosinophilia. The mucus is also histochemically abnormal.[61]

Antrochoanal polyps arise from the mucosa of the maxillary sinus and enter the nasal cavity through a large accessory ostium near the middle meatus. Approximately 10% of normal individuals have an accessory ostium, which appears necessary for the development of the polyp. Within the nasal cavity the polyp protrudes posteriorly through the choana into the nasopharynx. In contrast to typical nasal polyps, approximately one third of the patients with antrochoanal polyps are younger than 20 years of age.[67] The lesions are almost always unilateral and are uncommonly associated with typical nasal polyps. Histologically, however, antrochoanal polyps are similar to nasal polyps except that basement membrane thickening and eosinophilia are less pronounced. Stromal cells with marked nuclear abnormalities may be seen in antrochoanal polyps, as well as in typical nasal polyps. They must not be mistaken for malignant cells.[25]

Mucocele and cholesterol granuloma

The epithelium of the paranasal sinuses secretes 1 to 2 liters of fluid daily as it humidifies the air. If the ostium of a sinus is blocked by inflamed mucosa, trauma, or an osteoma, the secretions accumulate. Two thirds of mucoceles are in the frontal sinus, and most of the remainder affect the anterior ethmoid sinus. The mucosal lining consists of normal or compressed ciliated epithelium that sometimes has squamous metaplasia. Mucus accumulates not only in the lumen but also in the lamina propria, where it can be phagocytosed by histiocytes (mucophages). The surrounding bone may be eroded.[60]

Hemorrhage into an obstructed sinus results in the accumulation of cholesterol from the breakdown of erythrocytes. The engulfment of cholesterol by histiocytes is termed cholesterol granuloma.[43]

Rhinosporidiosis

Rhinosporidium seeberi is presumably a fungus, but it has not been cultured on artificial media. The various forms of the organism include thick-walled sporangia that contain several thousand spores. The spores mature into trophocytes that have clear cytoplasm, possess a distinct outer membrane, and measure up to about 30 μm wide.[52] Rhinosporidiosis is typically manifested as a friable, nasal polyp, but the nasopharynx, larynx, and conjunctiva are sometimes affected. The organisms elicit a nonspecific inflammatory response of neutrophils, lymphocytes, and plasma cells. The disease is most common in India and Sri Lanka, but rare cases have occurred in lifelong urban residents of the United States.[55]

Rhinoscleroma

A gram-negative diplobacillus, *Klebsiella rhinoscleromatis*, induces a chronic inflammatory response that usually includes plasma cells and foamy histiocytes. The histiocytes, referred to as Mikulicz cells, contain organisms as well as undigested mucopolysaccharides.[46] The inflammation produces deforming, nodular mucosal masses that obstruct the nose, nasopharynx, middle ear, larynx, or lower respiratory tract. Rhinoscleroma is endemic in well-demarcated areas of Africa, Central and South America, Southern Asia, and Eastern Europe. Sporadic cases occur elsewhere, including the United States.[15]

Mucormycosis (phycomycosis)

Mucormycosis is an opportunistic infection by organisms of the order *Mucorales*. Nonseptate hyphae spread along nerves, across tissue planes, and into blood vessels.[71] The last results in thrombosis and infarction. There may be a neutrophilic infiltrate, or inflammation may be negligible. Complications include meningoencephalitis and cerebral infarction.[16]

Aspergillosis

Infections of the paranasal sinuses by *Aspergillus* can take several forms. Septate hyphae can grow within the sinus and form a mass (aspergilloma) that elicits little reaction. At other times there is an indolent inflammatory reaction. Finally, in an immunosuppressed patient the clinical course can be fulminant with spread into the orbit and cranial fossa in a manner identical to mucormycosis.[56]

Atrophic rhinitis

The nasal mucosa of a patient with atrophic rhinitis is dry, appears crusted, and emits a fetid odor. A loss of vascularity and seromucous glands contributes to the atrophy. The normal ciliated epithelium and mucous cells are replaced by squamous epithelium. In some patients there is a history of repeated infections that could explain the condition. Other patients yield no clues regarding the cause.[59]

Myospherulosis

Myospherulosis is an inflammatory and fibrous reaction that occurs after a surgical procedure on the nose or paranasal sinuses. If a hemostatic packing impregnated with antibiotic ointment is used postoperatively, the oil-based vehicle can produce a foreign body reaction. This is accompanied by a peculiar encystment of degenerating erythrocytes. The recrudescence of symptoms that necessitates reoperation may be caused, at least in part, by the foreign body reaction.[73]

Destructive midline processes and Wegener's granulomatosis

The often-used rubric "lethal midline granuloma" is not an acceptable pathologic diagnosis. It is a clinical designation referring to a patient with a destructive lesion of unknown etiology that involves the upper aerodigestive tract. Batsakis[14] has listed no fewer than 35 specific entities that can cause so-called lethal midline granuloma, including unusual infections, Wegener's granulomatosis, and neoplasms that are difficult to diagnosis such as lymphoma, lymphoepithelioma, or midline malignant reticulosis. To be sure, there is the rare patient with a destructive midline lesion that cannot be specifically diagnosed, even after exhaustive study. The term "lethal midline granuloma" can be applied clinically, but only as an admission of diagnostic failure. Some patients in this category have responded to radiation therapy.[31]

Wegener's granulomatosis is characterized by vasculitis and, usually, granulomatous inflammation (Fig. 24-2). Although the changes may be an immune response, the inciting agent(s) is unknown. Patients have nonspecific symptoms interpreted as "chronic sinusitis" or "chronic otitis media." Eventually there is ulceration of the mucosa, discharge, and destruction of subjacent structures such as nasal cartilage. At its fullest expression, Wegener's granulomatosis can attack virtually every organ, but the upper and lower respiratory tract and the kidneys are usually the most severely affected. Most patients respond to cyclophosphamide therapy.[53] Localized forms occasionally occur in either the upper respiratory tract or the lung.[30]

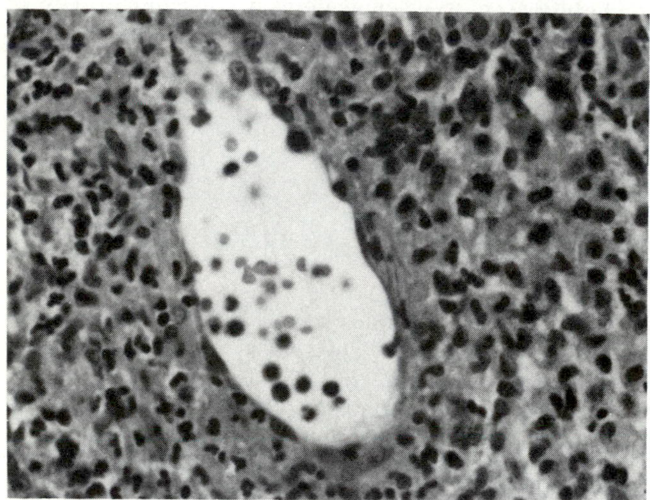

Fig. 24-2. Major alteration in Wegener's granulomatosis is acute inflammation and necrosis of vessel walls. Histiocytes are also seen (*right*).

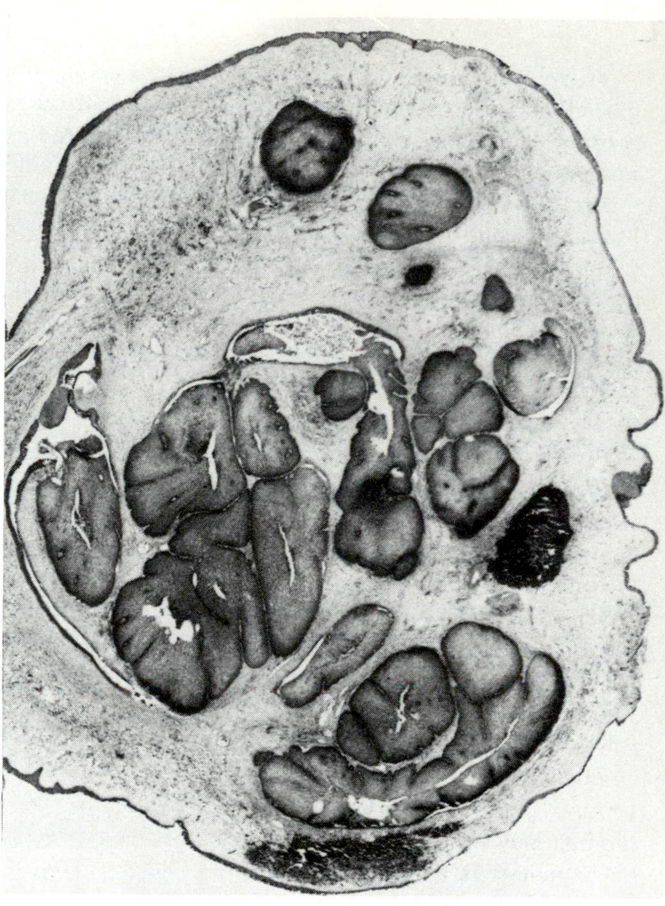

Fig. 24-4. Inverted papilloma has invaginations of intermediate epithelium into stroma. Lesion shown has normal ciliated epithelium on surface.

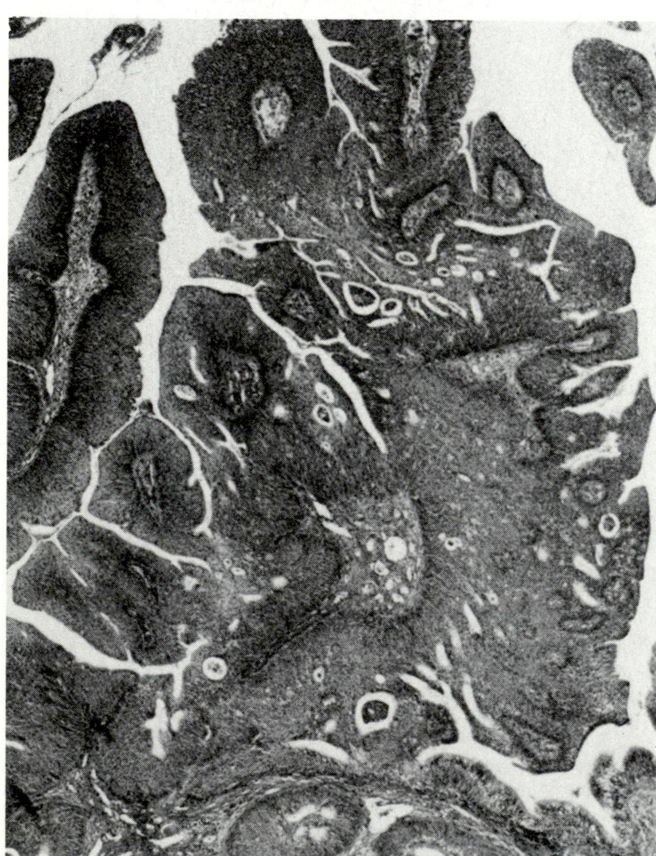

Fig. 24-3. Fungiform papilloma of nasal septum is lined predominantly by intermediate epithelium.

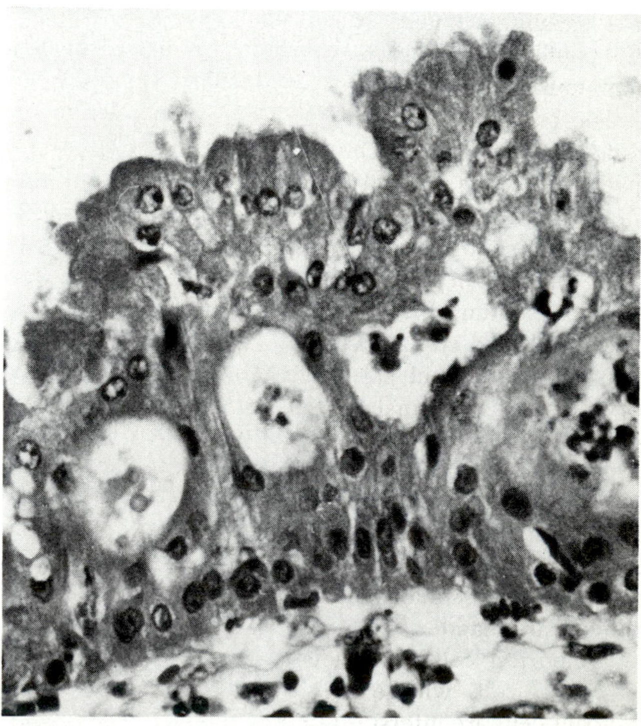

Fig. 24-5. Cylindrical cell papilloma has eosinophilic cells and spherical accumulations of mucus.

Vasculitis is a prerequisite for the diagnosis, whereas granulomas are of secondary importance and need not be present. Vascular changes range from a transmural inflammation of an otherwise intact vessel to necrosis of either a sector or a segment of a vessel. Thrombosis and luminal fibrous obliteration also occur. The granulomas, when present, are composed of mononuclear or multinucleated histiocytes. They may or may not be partly necrotic. Sometimes the only evidences of granuloma formation are small, poorly circumscribed collections of histiocytes.

Papillomas

Papillomas lined by normal or hyperkeratotic epidermis arise in the hair-bearing skin of the nasal vestibule. They are solitary and have no malignant potential.

Papillomas of the nasal cavity and paranasal sinuses have been given a bewildering number of names. The terms most widely employed are inverted papilloma, fungiform papilloma, and cylindrical cell papilloma. Sometimes they are collectively referred to as schneiderian papillomas. Although their cause is not known, they can be viewed as hyperplastic, reactive processes characterized by a proliferation of various epithelial types. Papillomas may erode bone but do not metastasize. They occur mainly in adults, especially middle-aged men. At least half recur locally unless major resections are performed to remove microscopic foci that extend beyond the grossly visible lesion.[20] Patients with fungiform papilloma are not at increased risk for malignancy, but about 5% of patients with inverted papilloma or cylindrical cell papilloma have synchronous or metachronous carcinoma, usually squamous. The carcinomas may be located in the papilloma per se or may arise at the site of a previous papilloma.[68]

The pattern seen with low-power microscopy distinguishes fungiform from inverted papillomas. Fungiform papilloma has an everted or exophytic configuration (Fig. 24-3); the inverted papilloma has invaginations or inversions of the epithelium into the underlying stroma (Fig. 24-4). Fungiform papillomas are nearly always located on the nasal septum. Inverted papillomas involve the lateral nasal wall, and often there is a paranasal sinus component. Both types of papillomas are lined with various combinations of normal ciliated epithelium, hyperplastic ciliated epithelium, mucous cells, squamous epithelium, or intermediate epithelium. The last derives its name because it is morphologically intermediate between normal columnar and normal squamous epithelium. It has also been called transitional epithelium, but this implies an unjustified relationship to transitional epithelium of the urinary bladder.[62]

Cylindrical cell papilloma has columnar or slightly polygonal cells with eosinophilic granular cytoplasm. Mucous cells are interspersed, and they may mimic fungal yeast forms when the mucus is inspissated (Fig. 24-5). The epithelium is arranged serpiginously over an edematous or loosely fibrous stroma.[48]

Benign lesions

Lobular capillary hemangioma (pyogenic granuloma)

Lobular capillary hemangioma has a distinctive lobular arrangement of capillaries in an edematous, fibroblastic stroma (Fig. 24-6).[57] The surface may be ulcerated and have an inflammatory cell infiltrate as well as superimposed reactive granulation tissue. The term "pyogenic granuloma" is often used for the ulcerated lesions. This is a misnomer because they are neither pyogenic infections

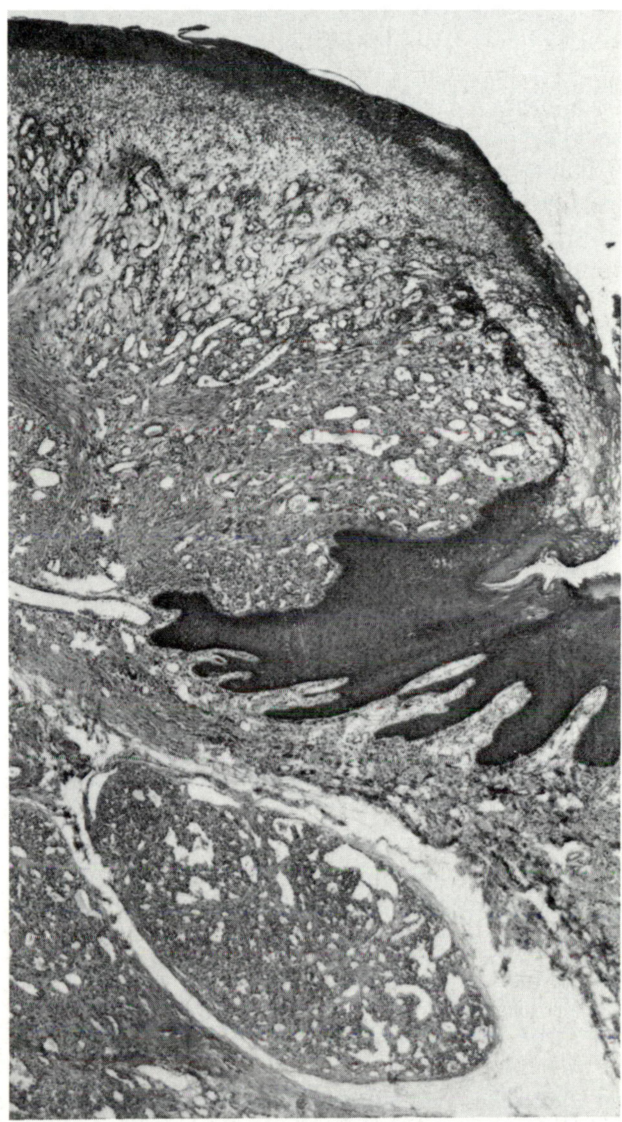

Fig. 24-6. Lobular capillary hemangioma (so-called pyogenic granuloma) has lobular pattern beneath epithelium. Lobular arrangement is lost in superficial, ulcerated portion. (From Fechner, R.E., Cooper, P.H., and Mills, S.E.: Arch. Otolaryngol. **107**:30, 1981. Copyright 1981, American Medical Association.)

nor granulomas. Patients range from 8 to 80 years of age. The lesions are rarely associated with trauma. Some have developed in pregnant women, which explains the appellation "pregnancy epulis" or "pregnancy tumor." Other types of hemangiomas, hemangiopericytoma and angiosarcoma, occur rarely in the nose.[24,34]

Miscellaneous lesions

Necrotizing sialometaplasia can be found in the glands of the nose or paranasal sinuses after surgery.[50] Any tumor arising in the mucosal glands or connective tissue eventually produces obstruction. Lesions include mixed tumors,[26] neural tumors,[63] and fibromatosis.[38] Meningiomas without intracranial connections arise in the nose and sinuses.[45] Osseous lesions that encroach on the airway include fibrous dysplasia and ossifying fibroma, osteoma, odontogenic tumors, and myxoma.[35,39]

Malignant neoplasms

Nasal cavity carcinoma

Squamous carcinomas constitute the majority of cancers arising in the nasal cavity. Most patients are men beyond 50 years of age who are smokers; only about 25% survive.[17] Occupational exposure in nickel refinery workers has been clearly related to nasal squamous cancer. Their neoplasms are concentrated on the anterior tip of the middle turbinate where the maximum air flow takes place.[13] Woodworkers are also at an increased risk for nasal squamous cancer.[44]

Adenocarcinoma is a rare tumor of the nasal mucosa but makes up a disproportionate number of carcinomas in woodworkers.[18,44] Specific carcinogens have not been identified. The tumors seldom metastasize but grow relentlessly and kill more than half of the patients. The microscopic pattern of the neoplasms in woodworkers as well as patients with other occupations often resembles that of colonic carcinoma.[49,65]

Paranasal sinus carcinoma

About 80% of cancers of the paranasal sinuses arise in the maxillary antrum, and most are squamous carcinoma. The patient often has a history of severe, chronic sinusitis. The diagnosis is rarely made when the squamous cancer is still confined to the mucosa. Almost invariably there is extension into surrounding bone, cheek, nose, palate, or orbit. About 75% of patients die of their tumor, usually because of local extension, although 10% have widespread metastases.[23]

Adenocarcinomas comprise about 5% of sinus cancers. Adenoid cystic carcinoma, the most common, has a 90% 10-year mortality.[70] Adenocarcinoma similar to the colonic-like cancer of the nasal fossa occurs in any sinus,[42] but it is especially frequent in the ethmoid sinuses of woodworkers.[44] Mucoepidermoid carcinomas and small cell ("oat cell") carcinomas also arise in the glands of the sinonasal region.[54] Approximately 8% of sinus malignancies are lymphomas, usually of histiocytic type.[69] Following radiation therapy, about 50% of patients survive.

Esthesioneuroblastoma (olfactory neuroblastoma)

The olfactory mucosa covers the superior one third of the nasal septum, the cribriform plate, and the superior turbinate. It has a mitotically active reserve cell layer from which esthesioneuroblastoma is probably derived. Clinically, there is a polypoid mass that may invade the paranasal sinuses or cranial vault. The tumors have diverse histologic patterns resulting from variable amounts of intercellular neurofibrillary material. Rosettes are formed in about 10%. If the tumor lacks these features, it is difficult to distinguish from other small cell malignancies such as rhabdomyosarcoma, undifferentiated carcinoma, or lymphoma. Ultrastructural examination is helpful if neuritic cell processes, neurofilaments, and neurotubules in association with dense core (neurosecretory) vesicles are found.[22]

Esthesioneuroblastoma occurs in all decades, with a peak incidence between the ages of 10 and 30 years. The course of the disease is capricious. Some patients die quickly with widespread metastases, whereas others live for several years before metastases or local recurrence develops. Occasionally, a patient may live with symptomatic disease for many years.[47] Approximately 50% of patients survive the disease, especially young patients with tumor confined to the nasal cavity. Small cell malignancies of the paranasal sinuses may secrete such peptides as calcitonin, ACTH, and MSH. Their relation, if any, to esthesioneuroblastomas remains to be determined.[51]

Malignant lymphoma and midline malignant reticulosis (polymorphic reticulosis)

Malignant lymphomas of conventional histologic types may appear initially in the nasal fossa, paranasal sinuses, or nasopharynx. Most patients subsequently manifest evidence of disseminated disease, although a few are cured by irradiation of the upper respiratory tract.[40]

Midline malignant reticulosis is a histologically distinctive lymphoproliferative disorder. The affected mucosa is thickened and ulcerated. Granulation tissue and inflammation may overlie the neoplastic component, and a deep biopsy is often necessary to reach the lesion. The lymphocytes are variable in size, and the nuclei are often hyperchromatic and convoluted, with prominent nucleoli. Many cells have abundant clear cytoplasm and sharply defined cell membranes (Fig. 24-7). Some cells have features of immunoblasts. The tumor often has a perivascular distribution with infiltration of vessel walls. This vascular invasion by abnormal cells must be differentiated from the inflammation of vessel walls seen in Wegener's granulomatosis.[32] The changes of midline malignant reticulosis are histologically similar, if not identical, to lymphomatoid granulomatosis. The two conditions probably represent the same process in different anatomic locations.[28,29]

Other malignant neoplasms

Malignant melanoma of the nasal cavity arises most often during the fourth to sixth decades of life. Survival is 7% at 10 years.[27,33] Soft tissue sarcomas are rare in the upper airway. Rhabdomyosarcoma is the most common (see discussion later in the chapter). A few cases of fibrosarcoma,[38] leiomyosarcoma,[37] malignant fibrous histiocytoma,[41] and synovial sarcoma[64] have been recorded. The most frequent malignant neoplasms of the facial bones are osteosarcoma and chondrosarcoma.[35,36]

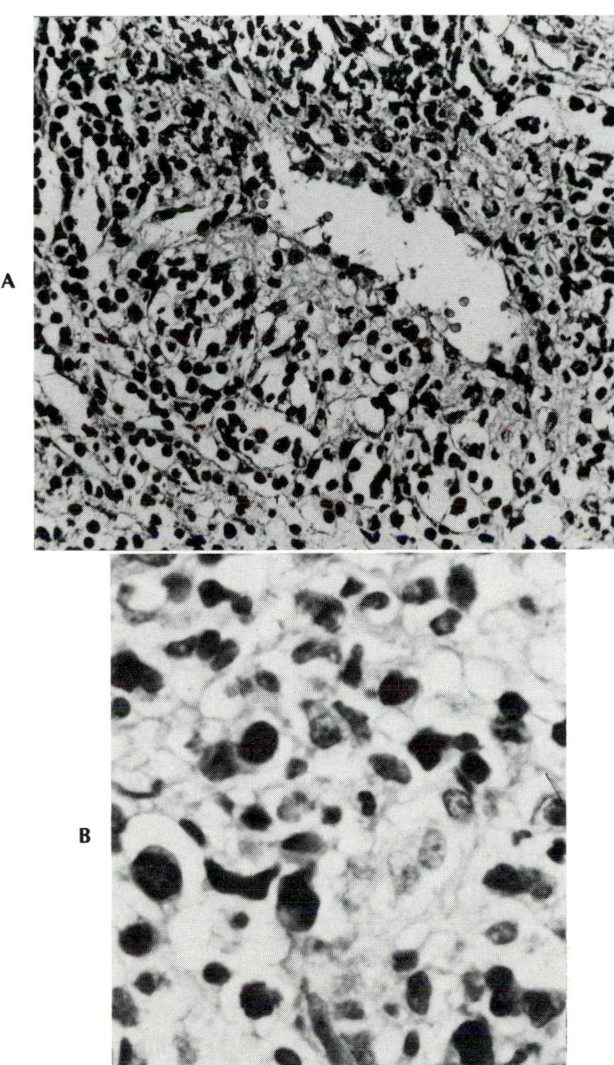

Fig. 24-7. Midline malignant reticulosis. A, Proliferating cells surround and invade vessel wall. B, Pleomorphic lymphocytes frequently have large quantity of clear cytoplasm. (A, From Fechner, R.E., and Lamppin, D.W.: Arch. Otolaryngol. 95:467, 1972. Copyright 1972, American Medical Association).

NASOPHARYNX

Angiofibroma

Angiofibromas arise in the nasopharynx or extreme posterior portion of the nasal cavity. They can grow into paranasal sinuses, cheek, orbit, or base of the skull, but they do not metastasize. With a few questionable exceptions, the lesion is confined to males.[82] Nearly all occur between 10 and 20 years of age, suggesting hormonal influences. In fact, the tumors contain testosterone receptor proteins.[80]

The angiofibroma is a gray, rubbery mass that completely belies its vascularity and the risk of exsanguination. Microscopically, a fibrous stroma contains innumerable, small vascular slits (Fig. 24-8). Ultrastructurally, the stromal cells are myofibroblasts, and their nuclei possess distinctive electron-dense inclusions of uncertain character.[85]

Nasopharyngeal carcinoma

In ascending order of frequency, three histologic types of nasopharyngeal carcinoma can be recognized: nonkeratinizing squamous carcinoma, keratinizing squamous carcinoma, and undifferentiated carcinoma. Many tumors from the first and last groups are called "transitional cell carcinoma," but because of its inconsistent application, that term should be abandoned. Another time-hallowed term, "lymphoepithelioma," is useful as long as it is recognized as only a histologic variant of undifferentiated carcinoma with numerous lymphocytes that surround and intermix with the cancer. The lymphocytes are a nonneoplastic reaction to the carcinoma.

The keratinizing and nonkeratinizing carcinomas are microscopically similar to the commonplace squamous

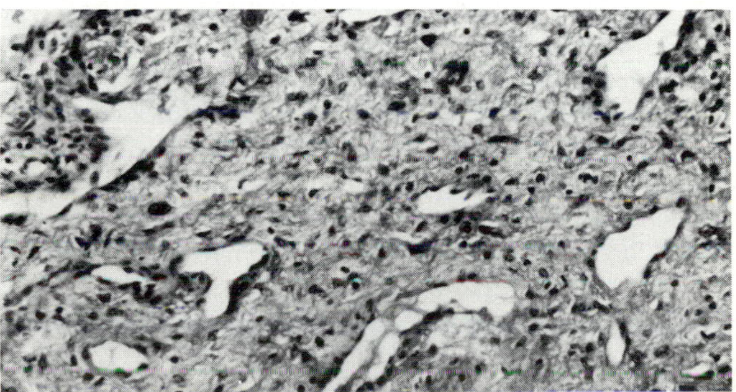

Fig. 24-8. Angiofibroma has capillaries scattered among myofibroblasts.

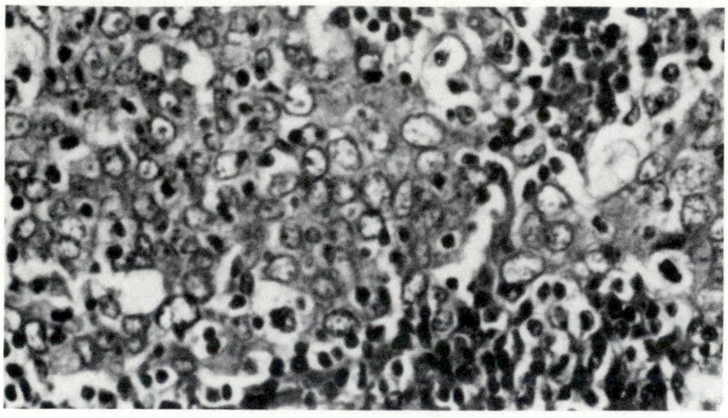

Fig. 24-9. Undifferentiated nasopharyngeal carcinoma is syncytium of cells with vesicular nuclei. This is lymphoepithelioma variant of undifferentiated carcinoma because of lymphocytic admixture.

carcinomas that arise in other sites. Conversely, undifferentiated carcinomas are characterized by cells with large vesicular nuclei, often arranged in a syncytium (Fig. 24-9). This carcinoma is frequently misdiagnosed as malignant lymphoma.[76] The keratinizing and nonkeratinizing carcinomas are almost invariably fatal; about 25% of patients with undifferentiated carcinomas survive after radiation therapy.[74]

About one third of nasopharyngeal carcinomas, especially undifferentiated carcinomas, are seen in teenagers and young adults. Many patients have no complaints referable to the nasopharynx. Palpable cervical lymph node metastases are the first sign of disease in half of the patients.

Genetic factors influence the risk of nasopharyngeal carcinoma. The Chinese are remarkably susceptible, especially before 45 years of age, and there is a significant association with the A2/sin HLA type.[84] Environmental factors are also important. Chinese immigrants to Hawaii and California have a decreased risk in succeeding generations that cannot be completely explained by genetic dilution.[78] In another study, all cases of nasopharyngeal carcinoma in American blacks were undifferentiated cancers.[75] Most occurred before 45 years of age, but specific genetic or environmental factors have not been elucidated. The association with tobacco usage is less well established in patients with nasopharyngeal cancer than in other respiratory tract cancers. A history of recurrent otitis media, sinusitis, or tonsillitis is significantly more common in patients with nasopharyngeal carcinoma.[81] Long-standing inflammatory changes might alter nasal architecture and air currents, focally increasing concentrations of carcinogens.

The role of the Epstein-Barr virus in nasopharyngeal cancer is unclear. High titers of antibody to the viral capsid are found in most patients with nonkeratinizing carcinoma or lymphoepithelioma.[83] The titers often rise as the tumor burden increases.

Miscellaneous lesions

Other lesions in the nasopharynx include congenital teratomas, teratocarcinomas,[79] soft tissue sarcomas,[38] and fibromatoses.[38] Chordomas, pituitary adenomas, and bone tumors arising in the base of the skull can protrude into the nasopharynx and mimic a primary carcinoma.[77]

LARYNX

Congenital malformations

The most common malformation is a dense fibrous tissue web that extends between the true cords. The web usually leaves an adequate airway and may not be diagnosed until the child begins to talk, or even until middle age.[131]

Laryngeal atresia or stenosis can occur in the subglottic region. These malformations are usually incompatible with life. Laryngeal clefts represent a failure of the posterior larynx and trachea to become separated from the esophagus. The mortality is high because of aspiration. Moreover, infants with laryngeal clefts frequently have other major congenital defects.[127]

Victims of the sudden infant death syndrome have an excess of laryngeal mucous glands. Whether this is a congenital or an acquired condition is uncertain.[109]

Allergic and infectious processes

The larynx can be the site of an allergic response. The edematous component of the reaction can lead to life-threatening airway obstruction.[150]

Acute laryngotracheobronchitis (croup) occurs almost exclusively during the first 3 years of life. Influenza A and B, parainfluenza, rhinovirus, and respiratory syncytial viruses are the most frequent causes. They damage the epithelium and excite an inflammatory infiltrate, edema, and congestion of the lamina propria. The stromal changes narrow or occlude the airway, especially in the subglottic area.[145] Viral infections can be localized to a portion of the larynx. Extensive ulceration and inflammatory exudate can mimic carcinoma.[134,139]

Infection confined to the epiglottis may be life threatening. *Haemophilus influenza* is the major cause. Acute epiglottitis usually affects infants and children but occasionally strikes adults. Regardless of the patient's age, emergency treatment is required to prevent asphyxiation.

Corynebacterium diphtheriae multiplies in the pharyngeal mucus and elaborates a toxin that produces epithelial necrosis. A fibrinous exudate containing a few mononuclear cells, nuclear and epithelial fragments, and bacteria accumulates on the damaged mucosa. The membrane can extend to the larynx and obstruct it.

Tubercle bacilli or fungi can involve the larynx as a part of disseminated disease. Indeed, laryngeal symptoms may be the initial manifestation. *Mycobacterium tuberculosis* usually, but not always, evokes a typical granulomatous inflammation.[147] By contrast, the granulomatous response to fungi is often absent, and the inflammation may consist of acute and chronic inflammatory cells with only a few mononuclear histiocytes intermixed. The organisms of *Histoplasma capsulatum* are apt to be imperceptible except on silver-methenamine stain.[96] One must think of fungal infection and perform the silver stain without the presence of granulomas to serve as a clue. Other fungi, such as *Cryptococcus*,[137] *Aspergillus*,[108] *Coccidiomyces*,[149] *Blastomyces*,[144] and *Candida*,[152] are usually visible on hematoxylin and eosin–stained sections.

Laryngeal papillomatosis (juvenile papillomatosis)

Laryngeal papillomas are tiny proliferations of squamous epithelium supported by a delicate fibrovascular tree. The disease is a nonneoplastic reaction, almost certainly to a virus of the papova group.[89] The offspring of mothers with genital condylomata acuminata seem to be at special risk.[136] A few papillomas cause hoarseness, but if hundreds are present, as is frequently the case, they can asphyxiate the patient. Sometimes there is progression of the disease down the trachea and bronchi. Papillomas of the larynx may deeply invade the mucosa but do not metastasize.[107] There are, however, a few examples of extensive bronchial papillomatosis that have been followed by metastasizing carcinomas.[138]

Papillomatosis is usually first diagnosed in children between 1 and 6 years of age, but adult onset also occurs. Careful removal is the most effective therapy, but there are nearly always one or more recurrences. About 25% of patients have no further episodes after 10 years of age, but approximately 20% have disease well into adulthood.[128]

Solitary squamous papilloma of the larynx is probably unrelated to papillomatosis. Solitary papillomas occur almost exclusively in adults and rarely recur. One must be certain that the squamous papilloma in an adult is not a papillary squamous carcinoma. Invasive squamous carcinoma sometimes has a papillary surface component. Many cases interpreted as papilloma evolving into invasive carcinoma were actually carcinomas from the start.[111]

Postintubation granulation tissue (intubation granuloma, pyogenic granuloma)

Endotracheal tubes invariably erode the epithelium.[105] Granulation tissue can form during the several days following the injury, resulting in a polypoid mass that is frequently referred to as intubation granuloma or pyogenic granuloma. These are misnomers because there is no granuloma formation.[106] Long-standing intubation can lead to fibrous stenosis of the subglottic area.[115]

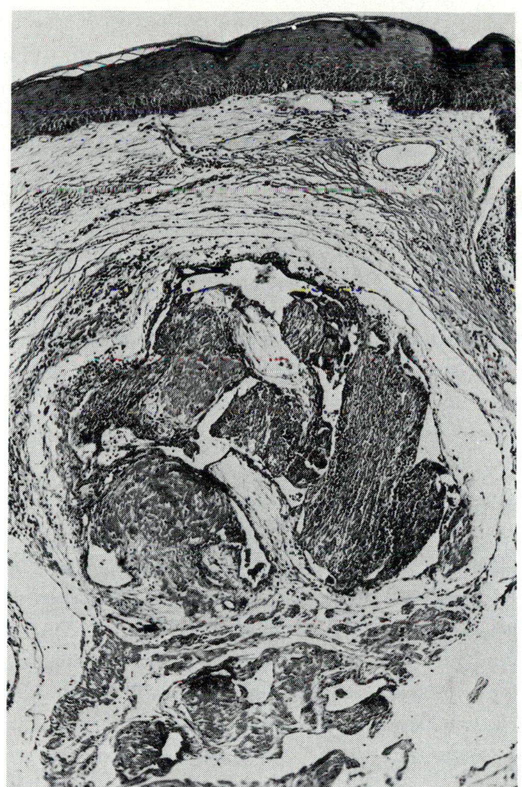

Fig. 24-10. Vocal nodule with edematous stroma, ectatic vessels, and fibrin deposits (*dark material*).

Vocal nodule and polyp

Vocal nodules are 1 to 2 mm bulges of Reinke's space at the junction of the anterior and middle thirds of the true cord. The cause is thought to be trauma from vocal abuse. This is reflected in such terms as screamer's node and preacher's node. Microscopically the nodules are extremely variable. Edema is usually prominent. Fibrous tissue may be sparse or dense. Newly formed, irregular, ectatic vascular channels are often numerous. There may be large deposits of fibrin that resemble amyloid (Fig. 24-10). A greatly thickened subepithelial basement membrane contributes to the mimicry of amyloid. The epithelium can be hyperplastic and slightly keratotic, but dysplastic changes are absent unless the patient is a smoker.

Vocal polyps have the same microscopic spectrum as vocal nodules. However, they involve the entire cord. There is usually a history of heavy smoking and sometimes vocal abuse.[143]

Amyloid

Amyloid forms symptomatic, nonulcerated masses of the larynx in adults. The amyloid is deposited within vessel walls and mucous glands and as amorphous masses. Plasma cells may be numerous or sparse. Laryngeal amyloidosis usually occurs in the absence of systemic amyloidosis.[117]

Cysts

Laryngeal cysts form by retention of secretions in the occluded ducts of the mucous glands. Hoarseness is the usual symptom, but rarely there may be respiratory embarrassment by large cysts arising from the saccule of the ventricle.[103] The cysts are lined by squamous or ciliated columnar epithelium, the normal types of duct epithelium.[88] Some cysts are lined by columnar cells with eosinophilic, granular cytoplasm (oncocytic cysts). The cytoplasmic appearance is caused by mitochondrial hyperplasia; hence the cells are true oncocytes.[119]

A laryngocele is an air-filled cyst that arises from the saccule of the ventricle. It can bulge into the supraglottic larynx or herniate beyond the larynx into the soft tissue of the neck. Laryngoceles may cause airway obstruction; they are also subject to infection (laryngopyocele).[97]

Keratosis and carcinoma in situ

Keratosis is found mainly in smokers and less often in those who abuse their voices. Microscopically a granular layer covered with keratin is present at the surface. The deeper epithelium may or may not have dysplastic nuclear changes. The patient who has keratosis without dysplasia is at a negligible risk of carcinoma although the keratosis may recur. On the other hand, patients with dysplastic cells have a small but increased risk of cancer. Cancer develops in about 3% of patients with keratosis, often several years later.[102] Moist keratin, whether covering a benign or a dysplastic lesion, causes a white patch called leukoplakia. The term "leukoplakia" should never be used to describe the microscopic findings.

It is imperative to differentiate carcinoma in situ from keratosis. Carcinoma in situ is the full-thickness replacement of epithelium by severely dysplastic cells. Carcinoma in situ is found in about 75% of larynges that have invasive carcinoma. As an isolated lesion, carcinoma in situ comprises only about 1% of laryngeal carcinoma, and it is almost always located on the true cord.[93] The presence of carcinoma in situ in a biopsy specimen should stimulate an intensive search for an associated invasive cancer, especially if the specimen is not from the true cord.

The meticulous autopsy studies by Auerbach, Hammond, and Garfinkel[90] suggest that dysplasia and even carcinoma in situ are reversible in cigarette smokers who quit smoking. Nearly 16% of smokers had carcinoma in situ and 99% had dysplasia. By contrast, none of the former cigarette smokers had carcinoma in situ and only 25% had mild dysplasia, a percentage similar to those who had never smoked.

Carcinoma

About 99% of laryngeal malignancies are squamous carcinomas that arise almost exclusively in cigarette, cigar, or pipe smokers. Smokers who are ethanol abusers are at even greater risk, especially for cancer of the epiglottis and false cord.[151] The role of radiation, including dental x rays, remains to be determined.[118]

The behavior of carcinomas of the larynx depends on the anatomic compartment of origin. Differences in access to lymphatics and routes of extension into the adjacent soft tissues influence the anatomic extent of tumor at the time of diagnosis. If the tumor is confined to the compartment of origin (and therefore is relatively small), the survival rate is around 90%. When there is extension into soft tissues, the rate is only 40%. If the invasion is sufficient to fix the larynx, that is, render it immobile on palpation, the survival rate is still lower. The presence of cervical lymph node metastases results in about a 40% survival rate. If the nodes are fixed, the rate is 20%.[141]

Two thirds of laryngeal cancers are in the glottis (true vocal cords and anterior commissure). The cord has minimal lymphatic drainage and, if the tumor is small and confined to the cord, more than 90% of patients are cured with radiation therapy or conservative laryngeal resection. Fixation of the cord, however, is evidence of extension into the vocalis muscle where lymphatics are more numerous. Between 8% and 15% of patients with glottic carcinoma have cervical node metastases.[141] One third of cancers are supraglottic tumors that involve the laryngeal surface of the epiglottis, the arytenoids, the false cords, or the ventricle. Between 30% and 40% have lymph node metastases when first seen.[123,141] The rare subglottic carcinoma arises inferior to the true cord. Lymph node metastases are found in about half of these patients, and the survival rate is correspondingly poor.[114] Transglottic carcinomas are either advanced glottic or supraglottic cancers that cross the ventricle and involve the other side. One third of these patients have lymph node involvement.[122] Carcinomas of the piriform sinus (properly a part of the hypopharynx rather than the larynx) have a poor prognosis, with fewer than one third of patients surviving. Most deaths occur within 2 years of the diagnosis.[130]

Death from laryngeal cancer is usually a result of uncontrolled local growth into vital structures such as the trachea or carotid artery. The patient's general status is also compromised by an inability to sustain adequate nutrition. Thirty percent to 60% of patients have distant metastases at the time of death, but most also have persistent growth of cancer in the neck.[86,132] Patients with carcinoma of the larynx are at high risk for primary carcinoma of the lung should they survive their laryngeal tumor.

Squamous carcinomas in the supraglottic and subglottic regions tend to be more poorly differentiated than glottic tumors.[100] In addition to the conventional criteria of cellular maturity and keratin formation, a number of features can be assessed in determining the degree of differentiation. Nuclear pleomorphism, mitotic rate, vascular invasion, inflammatory response, and patterns of infiltration are important in predicting the risk of recurrence or metastasis in tumors of the same clinical stage.[120,121]

Two special variants of squamous carcinoma, spindle cell and verrucous, deserve amplification. The nature of the elongated cells of spindle cell carcinoma ("pseudosarcoma") is controversial. Most of the cells are squamous, but sometimes they have features of mesenchymal cells.[126] It is possible that squamous cells can assume the appearance and function of myofibroblasts.[92] The tumor is often polypoid, and if there is a narrow base of attachment, the prognosis is favorable. Large infiltrative lesions, on the other hand, have the prognosis of conventional squamous carcinoma at the same clinical stage.[125]

Verrucous carcinoma is a nonmetastasizing, locally invasive neoplasm composed of squamous cells that lack cytologic features of malignancy.[148] The epithelium is markedly thickened and has an irregular (verrucoid) surface. The distinction between epithelial hyperplasia and verrucous carcinoma may be arbitrary.[140] Close communication between the clinician and the pathologist is imperative to arrive at the best diagnosis.

Most of the nonsquamous malignancies of the larynx arise from the mucous glands. The majority are poorly differentiated adenocarcinomas of no special type, and they are rarely curable.[142] Other tumors, such as mucoepidermoid and adenoid cystic carcinomas, have courses similar to their counterpart in the major salivary glands.[94,133]

Miscellaneous tumors

Granular cell tumors of the larynx occur predominantly during middle age and are concentrated in the posterior glottis. They are not related to smoking. Pseudoepitheliomatous hyperplasia of the squamous epithelium is often pronounced and can be mistaken for squamous carcinoma. Local excision is occasionally followed by recurrence, but metastases do not occur.[87]

Hemangiomas of the larynx are of two clinicopathologic types. The first is the congenital tumor located predominantly in the subglottic region and consisting of closely packed nodules of capillaries. The second is the cavernous hemangioma located in the vocal cords or supraglottic region of adults.[95]

Cartilaginous tumors of the larynx usually arise from the cricoid cartilage and project into the subglottic region. Regardless of whether the tumor appears microscopically benign (chondroma) or malignant (chondrosarcoma), metastases are rare.[116]

Additional benign lesions of the larynx include mixed tumor,[101] carcinoid,[129] lymphoid hyperplasia,[135] neurofibroma,[99] and paraganglioma.[112] Malignant lesions include small cell undifferentiated carcinoma,[124] primary malignant lymphoma,[91] lymphoepithelioma,[146] the ubiquitious malignant fibrous histiocytoma,[98] synovial sarcoma,[113] postradiation fibrosarcoma,[104] metastatic carcinoma,[110] and plasmacytoma.[184]

MIDDLE EAR

The middle ear and the pneumatized portions of the temporal bone (mastoid air cells) are an extension of the upper respiratory tract. The middle ear is lined by a single layer of flat epithelium that includes nonciliated cells, ciliated cells, and goblet cells. Following an allergic or bacterial infectious insult, there is a generalized hyperplasia of epithelium, and the proportion of ciliated and goblet cells increases.[162] Viral infections also produce histologic alterations; for example, Warthin-Finkeldey cells are seen in measles infections.[153]

Otitis media

There are three clinically and pathologically overlapping variants of otitis media: suppurative, serous, and mucoid.[158] The type depends on the exciting agent and the variable proportions of stromal, inflammatory, and epithelial changes. For example, a neutrophilic exudate dominates the reaction when there is bacterial invasion. *Diplococcus pneumoniae*, *Haemophilus influenzae*, and beta-hemolytic streptococci are the most common causes. Serous otitis media either follows an infection or is triggered as an allergic response. It is characterized by the accumulation of fluid in the middle ear, associated with alterations in the epithelium.[165]

Keratoma (cholesteatoma)

Keratoma is the accumulation of keratin in the middle ear or mastoid air cells. At least 95% of patients with keratoma have a history of acute or chronic otitis media. Squamous epithelium penetrates the damaged tympanic membrane from the external auditory canal. A small percentage of keratomas occur behind an intact membrane, however, and are presumably congenital in origin.[155] The rate of exfoliation of the keratin may be slow, requiring years of accumulation before creating symptoms. In the presence of infection it may develop rapidly. In addition to the presence of keratin, a keratoma often has a large component of histiocytes surrounding cholesterol crystals (hence the name *cholesteatoma*.) The cholesterol is derived from the degradation of keratin and degenerating erythrocytes if there has been hemorrhage. Keratoma incites resorption of bone and can lead to deafness by destroying the ossicles. The destruction may result from an active enzymatic process and not merely pressure erosion.[157] Keratoma differs from *cholesterol granuloma*. Hemorrhage into the middle ear, resulting from infection or allergic reaction, causes a histiocytic engulfment of cholesterol as the erythrocytes disintegrate. Squamous epithelium is absent.

Otosclerosis

Otosclerosis is an overgrowth of the temporal bone just anterior to the oval window. Fibrous fixation of the stapedial footplate occurs first and the footplate is subsequently replaced by sclerotic bone. Only the footplate is affected, and the footplate must be submitted if otosclerosis is to be diagnosed histologically. The cause is unknown but may be related to localized metabolic abnormalities.[154] The onset is during the second and third decades. The amount of hearing loss is related to the degree of immobilization of the stapedial footplate.

Tympanosclerosis

The inflamed mucosa of long-standing otitis media sometimes becomes densely fibrotic, hyalinized, calcified, or ossified. This stiffens the tympanic membrane and fixes the ossicles, producing a conductive hearing loss.[161]

Jugular paraganglioma (glomus jugulare tumor or glomus tympanicum tumor)

Glomus jugulare bodies are normally present at several sites within the middle ear and in the bulb of the jugular vein beneath the floor of the middle ear. In common parlance paragangliomas originating in the middle ear are called glomus tympanicum tumors, and those arising in the jugular bulb are called glomus jugulare tumors. Three fourths of the tumors are in women, and most occur between 25 and 65 years of age. Patients complain of hearing loss and pulsating tinnitus.

The tumor is composed of irregular nests of chief cells set in a highly vascular network.[164] The nests are not as sharply defined as the nests in carotid body tumors. The chief cells of the jugular paraganglioma are smaller and have denser nuclei than the cells of carotid body tumors.

Because of its location, complete removal of the tumor is usually impossible. The course may be rapid or prolonged, depending on the site of origin and direction of spread. Radiation can slow the growth by affecting vascular supply, although it does not eradicate the chief cells.[163] Approximately 15% of patients eventually die as a result of intracranial extension. Distant metastases are rare.[159]

Adenoma

Virtually all epithelial neoplasms of the middle ear are noninvasive adenomas that arise from the lining epithelium.[156] A few invasive tumors called adenocarcinoma have been reported but are probably extensions of cerumen gland adenocarcinomas.

Ectopic salivary gland tissue of the middle ear may reach a size that becomes symptomatic.[160] Salivary gland tumors, for example, mixed tumor, may arise from this ectopic tissue.[166]

EXTERNAL EAR

Aural (otic) polyp

Most aural polyps form as a result of chronic otitis media when the inflamed, hyperplastic mucosa of the middle ear perforates the tympanic membrane. Tumors arising in the middle ear such as rhabdomyosarcoma or paraganglioma can also induce an aural polyp when they extend into the external canal. The surface of the polyp is covered with pseudostratified columnar or squamous epithelium. The stroma may have cystic inclusions of middle ear epithelium, variable numbers of capillaries, and inflammatory cells.

"Malignant" external otitis

Infection by *Pseudomonas aeruginosa* produces necrotizing inflammation that begins in the auditory canal and can involve the external ear. The process can be lethal because of spread throughout the temporal bone and into the cranial cavity. Elderly diabetics are the usual victims.[168]

Cerumen gland tumors

The most common tumor of cerumen gland origin is adenoid cystic carcinoma that frequently grows intracranially or metastasizes. Other tumors resemble the apocrine epithelium of the normal cerumen gland. Based on cytologic features, these are divided into cerumen gland adenoma and cerumen gland adenocarcinoma. Both tumors tend to invade the temporal bone toward the cranial cavity. Compared to the adenoma, the adenocarcinoma is more aggressive locally and sometimes metastasizes. Mixed tumor, mucoepidermoid carcinoma, and sebaceous carcinoma occur rarely.[169]

Squamous cell carcinoma

Squamous cell carcinoma of the ear canal is extremely rare and occurs more frequently in women than in men. Causative factors are unclear, since solar damage cannot be implicated. A history of chronic external otitis is often obtained, but its role is questionable. Most lesions are poorly differentiated and deeply invasive. Seventy-five percent of patients are dead within 2 years, usually from uncontrollable growth into the cranial cavity.[170]

Auricle

Basal cell and squamous cell carcinomas of the auricle are common because of solar exposure.[167] Chondrodermatitis nodularis helicis is a painful lesion of the superior border of the helix that generally affects middle-aged and elderly men. The initial change is degeneration of the dermal collagen, possibly because of vascular insufficiency. The epidermis may be hyperkeratotic and is sometimes ulcerated.

The cartilage of the external ear may undergo cystic necrosis, resulting in a large, deforming cyst. This localized process is unrelated to relapsing polychondritis.[171]

TEMPORAL BONE

On rare occasions the temporal bone has been the site of nearly all of the benign and malignant neoplasms that arise elsewhere in bones.[174] Metastatic carcinoma can involve the temporal bone.[172] Eosinophilic granuloma (histiocytosis X) affects the temporal bone, either as a solitary focus or as part of widespread disease. It produces symptoms of intractable otitis media or mastoiditis.[176] Osteomas are nodules of bone that bulge into the external auditory canal. The subperiosteal trabeculae of new bone are a reactive process. Swimming in cold water is one stimulus.[175] Meningiomas can occur within the temporal bone (including the middle ear) without an apparent intracranial component.[173]

DISEASES OF DIVERSE SITES

Relapsing polychondritis

Polychondritis is a disease of young and middle-aged adults.[177] The cartilage of the ear, nose, eustachian tubes, larynx, and lower respiratory tract softens and collapses. Arthritis, ocular inflammation, inner ear disease, and aortitis are sometimes present. Lymphocytes and plasma cells infiltrate the degenerating cartilage. There is an almost complete loss of glucosaminoglycans. This is probably the result of accelerated destruction rather than a failure in biosynthesis.[185]

Rhabdomyosarcoma

Rhabdomyosarcomas arise in the nasal fossa, paranasal sinuses, orbit, larynx, middle ear, nasopharynx, external ear canal, or soft tissues of the face, usually in the first decade of life.[179,182] Mucosal tumors may be polypoid and are sometimes called botryoid sarcomas. (Botryoid means "grapelike" and refers only to the gross configuration.)

Rhabdomyosarcomas of the head are usually embryonal rhabdomyosarcomas and, less commonly, their subset, alveolar rhabdomyosarcoma. Pleomorphic (adult) rhabdomyosarcomas are extremely rare in the head. Embryonal tumors have essentially patternless arrangements of cells, often with a myxoid background. The alveolar tumors have fibrous septa that surround large aggregates of cells.[178] The cells of both types recapitulate, in a disorganized way, the early embryonic development of striated muscle. The cells can be round with scant cytoplasm or elongated with eosinophilic cytoplasm. Since the myoblast of the 7- to 9-week fetus is a primitive mesenchymal cell, it is not surprising that cross striations are rarely seen optically in rhabdomyosarcomas of the embryonal and alveolar types. Ultrastructurally, myofilaments are commonly present, but cross bands are few and poorly developed.[186]

Whether the tumor has an embryonal or alveolar pattern, combined treatment with surgery, radiotherapy, and chemotherapy results in long-term survival for about 70% of patients.[188] Death results either from uncontrolled local growth or from widespread metastases, especially to the lung.

Rhabdomyoma

Rhabdomyomas are benign tumors that are divided into adult and fetal forms depending on the degree of resemblance to mature muscle. The pharynx, larynx, and postauricular soft tissue are sites of predilection.[180,181] The tumors occur at any age, and they may recur if not totally excised. There is no relation to rhabdomyosarcoma.

Plasmacytoma

The majority of extramedullary plasmacytomas occur beyond 40 years of age as nonulcerated masses in the nasal cavity, sinuses, nasopharynx, middle ear, tonsils, or larynx.[183,187] The plasma cells have varying degrees of immaturity and pleomorphism. Most patients have either locally destructive tumors or plasma cell neoplasms that develop elsewhere, and multiple myeloma develops in many. A few patients, however, are cured by surgical excision or radiotherapy or both.[183]

If a lesion contains only mature plasma cells, it is unlikely to behave as an aggressive process. The diagnosis of a reactive lesion is reinforced by the presence of an admixture of lymphocytes and prominent capillary proliferation. This is sometimes called, rather inaccurately, plasma cell granuloma.

REFERENCES

General

1. Batsakis, J.G.: Tumors of the head and neck: clinical and pathological considerations, ed. 2, Baltimore, 1979, The Williams & Wilkins Co.
2. Schuknecht, H.F.: Pathology of the ear, Cambridge, Mass., 1974, Harvard University Press.

Nose

3. Broadbent, N.R.G., and Cort, D.F.: Squamous carcinoma in longstanding rhinophyma, Br. J. Plast. Surg. **30**:308, 1977.

4. Cohen, A.H., and Abt, A.B.: An unusual cause of neonatal respiratory obstruction: heterotopic pharyngeal brain tissue, J. Pediatr. **76**:119, 1970.
5. Evans, J.N.G., and Maclachlan, R.F.: Choanal atresia, J. Laryngol. Otol. **85**:903, 1971.
6. Gifford, G.H., Jr., Swanson, L., and MacCollum, D.W.: Congenital absence of the nose and anterior nasopharynx: report of two cases, Plast. Reconstr. Surg. **50**:5, 1972.
7. Gorenstein, A., et al.: Nasal gliomas, Arch. Otolaryngol. **106**:536, 1980.
8. Hoshaw, T.C., and Walike, J.W.: Dermoid cysts of the nose, Arch. Otolaryngol. **93**:487, 1971.
9. Karmody, C.S., and Gallagher, J.C.: Nasoalveolar cysts, Ann. Otol. Rhinol. Laryngol. **81**:278, 1972.
10. Mahindra, S., et al.: Lateral nasal proboscis, J. Laryngol. Otol. **87**:177, 1973.
11. Szalay, G.C., and Bledsoe, R.C.: Congenital dermoid cyst and fistula of the nose, Am. J. Dis. Child. **124**:392, 1972.
12. Weseman, C.M.: Management of choanal atresia in the newborn, Laryngoscope **83**:1160, 1973.

Nasal cavity and paranasal sinuses

13. Barton, R.T., and Hogetveit, A.C.: Nickel-related cancer of the respiratory tract, Cancer **45**:3061, 1980.
14. Batsakis, J.G.: Wegener's granulomatosis and midline (nonhealing) "granuloma," Head Neck Surg. **1**:213, 1979.
15. Berger, S.A., Pollock, A.A., and Richmond, A.S.: Isolation of *Klebsiella ozaenae* and *Klebsiella rhinoscleromatis* in a general hospital, Am. J. Clin. Pathol. **67**:499, 1977.
16. Blitzer, A., et al.: Patient survival factors in paranasal sinus mucormycosis, Laryngoscope **90**:635, 1980.
17. Bosch, A., Vallecillo, L., and Frias, Z.: Cancer of the nasal cavity, Cancer **37**:1458, 1976.
18. Brinton, L.A., et al.: A death certificate analysis of nasal cancer among furniture workers in North Carolina, Cancer Res. **37**:3473, 1977.
19. Bryan, M.P., and Bryan, W.T.K.: Cytologic and cytochemical aspects of ciliated epithelium in the differentiation of nasal inflammatory diseases, Acta Cytol. **13**:515, 1969.
20. Calceterra, T.C., Thompson, J.W., and Paglia, D.E.: Inverting papillomas of the nose and paranasal sinuses, Laryngoscope **90**:53, 1980.
21. Chandra, R.K., and Abrol, B.M.: Immunopathology of nasal polypi, J. Laryngol. Otol. **88**:1019, 1974.
22. Chaudhry, A.P., et al.: Olfactory neuroblastoma (esthesioneuroblastoma): a light and ultrastructural study of two cases, Cancer **44**:564, 1979.
23. Cheng, V.S.T., and Wang, C.C.: Carcinomas of the paranasal sinuses: a study of sixty-six cases, Cancer **49**:3038, 1977.
24. Compagno, J., and Hyams, V.J.: Hemangiopericytoma-like intranasal tumors: a clinicopathologic study of 23 cases, Am. J. Clin. Pathol. **66**:672, 1976.
25. Compagno, J., Hyams, V.J., and Lepore, M.L.: Nasal polyposis with stromal atypia: review and follow-up study of 14 cases, Arch. Pathol. Lab. Med. **100**:224, 1976.
26. Compagno, J., and Wong, R.T.: Intranasal mixed tumors (pleomorphic adenomas): a clinicopathologic study of 40 cases, Am. J. Clin. Pathol. **68**:213, 1977.
27. Cove, H.: Melanosis, melanocytic hyperplasia, and primary malignant melanoma of the nasal cavity, Cancer **44**:1424, 1979.
28. Crissman, J.D.: Midline malignant reticulosis and lymphomatoid granulomatosis: a case report, Arch. Pathol. Lab. Med. **103**:561, 1979.
29. DeRemee, R.A., Weiland, L.H., and McDonald, T.J.: Polymorphic reticulosis, lymphomatoid granulomatosis: two diseases or one? Mayo Clin. Proc. **53**:634, 1978.
30. DeRemee, R.A., et al.: Wegener's granulomatosis: anatomic correlates, a proposed classification, Mayo Clin. Proc. **51**:777, 1976.
31. Fauci, A.S., Johnson, R.E., and Wolff, S.M.: Radiation therapy of midline granuloma, Ann. Intern. Med. **84**:140, 1976.
32. Fechner, R.E., and Lamppin, D.W.: Midline malignant reticulosis: a clinicopathologic entity, Arch. Otolaryngol. **95**:467, 1972.
33. Freedman, H.M., et al.: Malignant melanoma of the nasal cavity and paranasal sinuses, Arch. Otolaryngol. **97**:322, 1973.
34. Fu, Y.-S., and Perzin, K.H.: Nonepithelial tumors of the nasal cavity, paranasal sinuses, and nasopharynx: a clinicopathologic study. I. General features and vascular tumors, Cancer **33**:1275, 1974.
35. Fu, Y.-S., and Perzin, K.H.: Nonepithelial tumors of the nasal cavity, paranasal sinuses, and nasopharynx: a clinicopathologic study. II. Osseous and fibro-osseous lesions, including osteoma, fibrous dysplasia, ossifying fibroma, osteoblastoma, giant cell tumor, and osteosarcoma, Cancer **33**:1289, 1974.
36. Fu, Y.-S., and Perzin, K.H.: Nonepithelial tumors of the nasal cavity, paranasal sinuses, and nasopharynx: a clinicopathologic study. III. Cartilaginous tumors (chondroma, chondrosarcoma), Cancer **34**:453, 1974.
37. Fu, Y.-S., and Perzin, K.H.: Nonepithelial tumors of the nasal cavity, paranasal sinuses, and nasopharynx: a clinicopathologic study. IV. Smooth muscle tumors (leiomyoma, leiomyosarcoma), Cancer **35**:1300, 1975.
38. Fu, Y.-S., and Perzin, K.H.: Nonepithelial tumors of the nasal cavity, paranasal sinuses, and nasopharynx: a clinicopathologic study. VI. Fibrous tissue tumors (fibroma, fibromatosis, fibrosarcoma), Cancer **37**:2912, 1976.
39. Fu, Y.-S., and Perzin, K.H.: Nonepithelial tumors of the nasal cavity, paranasal sinuses, and nasopharynx: a clinicopathologic study. VII. Myxomas, Cancer **39**:195, 1977.
40. Fu, Y.-S., and Perzin, K.H.: Nonepithelial tumors of the nasal cavity, paranasal sinuses and nasopharynx: a clinicopathologic study. X. Malignant lymphomas, Cancer **43**:611, 1979.
41. Fu, Y.-S., and Perzin, K.H.: Nonepithelial tumors of the nasal cavity, paranasal sinuses, and nasopharynx: a clinicopathologic study. XI. Fibrous histiocytomas, Cancer **45**:2616, 1980.
42. Gamez-Araujo, J.J., Ayala, A.G., and Guillamondegui, O.: Mucinous adenocarcinomas of nose and paranasal sinuses, Cancer **36**:110, 1975.
43. Graham, J., and Michaels, L.: Cholesterol granuloma of the maxillary antrum, Clin. Otolaryngol. **3**:155, 1978.
44. Hadfield, E.H.: A study of adenocarcinoma of the paranasal sinuses in woodworkers in the furniture industry, Ann. R. Coll. Surg. Engl. **46**:301, 1970.
45. Ho, K.-H.: Primary meningioma of the nasal cavity and paranasal sinuses, Cancer **46**:1442, 1980.
46. Hoffman, E.O., Loose, L.D., and Harkin, J.C.: The Mikulicz cell in rhinoscleroma: light, fluorescent, and electron microscopic studies, Am. J. Pathol. **73**:47, 1973.
47. Homzie, M.J., and Elkon, D.: Olfactory esthesioneuroblastoma—variables predictive of tumor control and recurrence, Cancer **46**:2509, 1980.
48. Hyams, V.J.: Papillomas of the nasal cavity and paranasal sinuses: a clinicopathological study of 315 cases, Ann. Otol. Rhinol. Laryngol. **80**:192, 1971.
49. Ironside, P., and Matthews, J.: Adenocarcinoma of the nose and paranasal sinuses in woodworkers in the state of Victoria, Australia, Cancer **36**:1115, 1975.
50. Johnston, W.H.: Necrotizing sialometaplasia involving the mucous glands of the nasal cavity, Hum. Pathol. **8**:589, 1977.
51. Kameya, T., et al.: Neuroendocrine carcinoma of the paranasal sinus: a morphological and endocrinological study, Cancer **45**:330, 1980.
52. Kannan-Kutty, M., and Teh, E.C.: *Rhinosporidium seeberi:* an ultrastructural study of endosporulation phase and trophocyte phase, Arch. Pathol. **99**:51, 1975.
53. Kornblut, A.D., et al.: Wegener's granulomatosis, Laryngoscope **90**:1453, 1980.
54. Koss, L.G., Spiro, R.H., and Hajdu, S.: Small cell (oat cell) carcinoma of minor salivary gland origin, Cancer **30**:737, 1972.
55. Lasser, A., and Smith, H.W.: Rhinosporidiosis, Arch. Otolaryngol. **102**:308, 1976.
56. McGill, T.J., Simpson, G., and Healy, G.B.: Fulminant aspergillosis of the nose and paranasal sinuses: a new clinical entity, Laryngoscope **90**:748, 1980.
57. Mills, S.E., Cooper, P.H., and Fechner, R.E.: Lobular capillary hemangioma: underlying lesion of pyogenic granuloma; a study of 73 cases from the oral and nasal mucous membranes, Am. J. Surg. Pathol. **4**:471, 1980.

58. Mygind, N.: Pathogenesis of allergic rhinitis, Acta Otolaryngol. **360**(suppl.):9, 1979.
59. Mygind, N., Thomsen, J., and Jorgensen, M.B.: Ultrastructure of the epithelium in atrophic rhinitis: transmission electron microscopic studies, Acta Otolaryngol. **78**:106, 1974.
60. Natvig, K., and Larsen, T.E.: Mucocele of paranasal sinuses: a retrospective clinical and histological study, J. Laryngol. Otol. **92**:1075, 1978.
61. Oppenheimer, E.H., and Rosenstein, B.J.: Differential pathology of nasal polyps in cystic fibrosis and atopy, Lab. Invest. **40**:445, 1979.
62. Ridolfi, R.L., et al.: Schneiderian papillomas: a clinicopathologic study of 30 cases, Am. J. Surg. Pathol. **1**:43, 1977.
63. Robitaille, Y., Seemayer, T.A., and El Deiry, A.: Peripheral nerve tumors involving paranasal sinuses: a case report and review of the literature, Cancer **35**:1254, 1975.
64. Roth, J.A., Enzinger, F.M., and Tannenbaum, M.: Synovial sarcoma of the neck: a followup study of 24 cases, Cancer **35**:1243, 1975.
65. Sanchez-Casis, G., Devine, K.D., and Weiland, L.H.: Nasal adenocarcinomas that closely simulate colonic carcinomas, Cancer **28**:714, 1971.
66. Settipane, G.A., and Chafee, F.H.: Nasal polyps in asthma and rhinitis: a review of 6,037 patients, J. Allergy Clin. Immunol. **59**:17, 1977.
67. Sirola, R.: Choanal polyps, Acta Otolaryngol. **61**:42, 1966.
68. Snyder, R.N., and Perzin, K.H.: Papillomatosis of nasal cavity and paranasal sinuses (inverted papilloma, squamous papilloma): a clinicopathologic study, Cancer **30**:668, 1972.
69. Sofferman, R.A., and Cummings, C.W.: Malignant lymphoma of the paranasal sinuses, Arch. Otolaryngol. **101**:287, 1975.
70. Spiro, R.H., Huvos, A.G., and Strong, E.W.: Adenoid cystic carcinoma of salivary origin: a clinicopathologic study of 242 cases, Am. J. Surg. **128**:512, 1974.
71. Straatsma, B.R., Zimmerman, L.E., and Gass, J.D.M.: Phycomycosis: a clinicopathologic study of fifty-one cases, Lab. Invest. **11**:963, 1962.
72. Tos, M., and Mogensen, C.: Mucous glands in nasal polyps, Arch. Otolaryngol. **103**:407, 1977.
73. Wheeler, T.M., Sessions, R.B., and McGavran, M.H.: Myospherulosis: a preventable iatrogenic nasal and paranasal entity, Arch. Otolaryngol. **106**:272, 1980.

Nasopharynx

74. Baker, S.R.: Nasopharyngeal carcinoma: clinical course and results of therapy, Head Neck Surg. **3**:8, 1980.
75. Easton, J.M., Levine, P.H., and Hyams, V.J.: Nasopharyngeal carcinoma in the United States: a pathologic study of 177 U.S. and 30 foreign cases, Arch. Otolaryngol. **106**:88, 1980.
76. Giffler, R.F., et al.: Lymphoepithelioma in cervical lymph nodes of children and young adults, Am. J. Surg. Pathol. **1**:293, 1977.
77. Heffelfinger, M.J., et al.: Chordomas and cartilaginous tumors at the skull base, Cancer **32**:410, 1973.
78. Henderson, B.E., et al.: Risk factors associated with nasopharyngeal carcinoma, N. Engl. J. Med. **295**:1101, 1976.
79. Hjertaas, R.J., Morrison, M.D., and Murray, R.B.: Teratomas of the nasopharynx, J. Otolaryngol. **8**:411, 1977.
80. Lee, D.A., et al.: Hormonal receptor determination in juvenile nasopharyngeal angiofibromas, Cancer **46**:547, 1980.
81. Lin, T.M., et al.: Interaction of factors associated with cancer of the nasopharynx, Cancer **44**:1419, 1979.
82. Neel, H.B., III, et al.: Juvenile angiofibroma: review of 120 cases, Am. J. Surg. **126**:547, 1973.
83. Neel, H.B., III, et al.: Anti-EBV serologic tests for nasopharyngeal carcinoma, Laryngoscope **90**:1981, 1980.
84. Rousch, G.C.: Epidemiology of cancer of the nose and paranasal sinuses: current concepts, Head Neck Surg. **2**:3, 1979.
85. Taxy, J.B.: Juvenile nasopharyngeal angiofibroma: an ultrastructural study, Cancer **39**:1044, 1977.

Larynx

86. Abramson, A.L., et al.: Distant metastases from carcinoma of the larynx, Laryngoscope **81**:1503, 1971.
87. Agarwal, R.K., Blitzer, A., and Perzin, K.H.: Granular cell tumors of the larynx, Otolaryngol. Head Neck Surg. **87**:807, 1979.
88. Altmeyer, V.L., and Fechner, R.E.: Multiple epiglottic cysts, Arch. Otolaryngol. **104**:673, 1978.
89. Arnold, W.: Tubular forms of papova viruses in human laryngeal papilloma, Arch. Otorhinolaryngol. **225**:15, 1979.
90. Auerbach, O., Hammond, E.C., and Garfinkel, L.: Histologic changes in the larynx in relation to smoking habits, Cancer **25**:92, 1970.
91. Babbitt, D.C., Yarington, C.T., Jr., and Yonders, A.J.: Malignant lymphoma of the larynx, J. Laryngol. Otol. **87**:807, 1973.
92. Battifora, H.: Spindle cell carcinoma: ultrastructural evidence of squamous origin and collagen production by the tumor cells, Cancer **37**:2275, 1976.
93. Bauer, W.C., and McGavran, M.H.: Carcinoma in situ and evaluation of epithelial changes in laryngopharyngeal biopsies, J.A.M.A. **221**:72, 1972.
94. Binder, W.J., et al.: Mucoepidermoid carcinoma of the larynx: a case report and review of the literature, Ann. Otol. Rhinol. Laryngol. **89**:103, 1980.
95. Bridger, G.P., Nassar, V.H., and Skinner, H.G.: Hemangioma in the adult larynx, Arch. Otolaryngol. **92**:493, 1970.
96. Calcaterra, T.C.: Orolaryngeal histoplasmosis, Laryngoscope **80**:111, 1970.
97. Canalis, R.F., Maxwell, D.S., and Hemenway, W.C.: Laryngocele—an updated review, J. Otolaryngol. **6**:191, 1977.
98. Canalis, R.F., et al.: Malignant fibrous xanthoma (xanthosarcoma) of the larynx, Arch. Otolaryngol. **101**:135, 1975.
99. Chang-Lo, M.: Laryngeal involvement in von Recklinghausen's disease: a case report and review of the literature, Laryngoscope **87**:435, 1977.
100. Chung, C.K., et al.: Histologic grading in the clinical evaluation of laryngeal carcinoma, Arch. Otolaryngol. **106**:623, 1980.
101. Cotelingam, J.D., Barnes, L., and Nixon, V.B.: Pleomorphic adenoma of the epiglottis, Arch. Otolaryngol. **103**:245, 1977.
102. Crissman, J.D.: Laryngeal keratosis and subsequent carcinoma, Head Neck Surg. **1**:386, 1979.
103. DeSanto, L.W., Devine, K.D., and Weiland, L.H.: Cysts of the larynx—classification, Laryngoscope **80**:145, 1970.
104. Donaldson, I.: Fibrosarcoma in a previously irradiated larynx, J. Laryngol. Otol. **92**:425, 1978.
105. Dubick, M.N., and Wright, B.D.: Comparison of laryngeal pathology following long-term oral and nasal endotracheal intubations, Anesth. Analg. **57**:663, 1978.
106. Fechner, R.E., Cooper, P.H., and Mills, S.E.: Pyogenic granuloma of the larynx and trachea: a causal and pathologic misnomer for granulation tissue, Arch. Otolaryngol. **107**:30, 1981.
107. Fechner, R.E., Goepfert, H., and Alford, B.R.: Invasive laryngeal papillomatosis, Arch. Otolaryngol. **99**:147, 1974.
108. Ferlito, A.: Primary aspergillosis of the larynx, J. Laryngol. Otol. **88**:1257, 1974.
109. Fink, B.R., and Beckwith, J.B.: Laryngeal mucous gland excess in victims of sudden infant death, Am. J. Dis. Child. **134**:144, 1980.
110. Freeland, A.P., Van Nostrand, A.W.P., and Jahn, F.F.: Metastases to the larynx, J. Otolaryngol. **8**:448, 1979.
111. Friedberg, S.A., Stagman, R., and Hass, G.M.: Papillary lesions of the larynx in adults: a pathologic study, Ann. Otol. Rhinol. Laryngol. **80**:683, 1971.
112. Gallivan, M.V.E., et al.: Laryngeal paraganglioma: case report with ultrastructural analysis and literature review, Am. J. Surg. Pathol. **3**:85, 1979.
113. Gatti, W.M., Strom, C.G., and Orfei, E.L.: Synovial sarcoma of the laryngopharynx, Arch. Otolaryngol. **101**:633, 1975.
114. Harrison, D.F.N.: The pathology and management of subglottic cancer, Ann. Otol. Rhinol. Laryngol. **80**:6, 1971.
115. Hawkins, D.B., and Luxford, W.M.: Laryngeal stenosis from endotracheal intubation: a review of 58 cases, Ann. Otol. Rhinol. Laryngol. **89**:454, 1980.
116. Hellquist, H., Olofsson, J., and Gröntoft, O.: Chondrosarcoma of the larynx, J. Laryngol. Otol. **93**:1037, 1979.
117. Hellquist, H., et al.: Amyloidosis of the larynx, Acta Otolaryngol. **88**:443, 1979.

118. Hinds, M.W., and Thomas, D.B.: Asbestos, dental x-rays, tobacco, and alcohol in the epidemiology of laryngeal cancer, Cancer **44**:1114, 1979.
119. Holm-Jensen, S., et al.: Oncocytic cysts of the larynx, Acta Otolaryngol. **83**:366, 1977.
120. Hordijk, G.L.: The high-risk group in early glottic carcinoma, Arch. Otolaryngol. **106**:621, 1980.
121. Jakobsson, P.A.: Histologic grading of malignancy and prognosis in glottic carcinoma of the larynx. In Alberti, P.W., and Bryce, D.P., editors: Centennenial conference on laryngeal cancer, New York, 1976, Appleton-Century-Crofts.
122. Kirchner, J.A., Cornog, J.L., Jr., and Holmes, R.E.: Transglottic cancer: its growth and spread within the larynx, Arch. Otolaryngol. **99**:247, 1974.
123. Kirchner, J.A., and Som, M.L.: Clinical and histologic observations on supraglottic cancer, Ann. Otol. Rhinol. Laryngol. **80**:638, 1971.
124. Kyriakos, M., Berlin, B.P., and DeSchryver-Kecskemeti, K.: Oat-cell carcinoma of the larynx, Arch. Otolaryngol. **104**:168, 1978.
125. Lambert, P.R., Ward, P.H., and Berci, G.: Pseudosarcoma of the larynx: a comprehensive analysis, Arch. Otolaryngol. **106**:700, 1980.
126. Lasser, K.H., et al.: "Pseudosarcoma" of the larynx, Am. J. Surg. Pathol. **3**:397, 1979.
127. Lim, T.A., Spanier, S.S., and Kohut, R.I.: Laryngeal clefts: a histopathologic study and review, Ann. Otol. Rhinol. Laryngol. **88**:837, 1979.
128. Majoros, M., Parkhill, E.M., and Devine, K.D.: Papilloma of the larynx in children: a clinicopathologic study, Am. J. Surg. **108**:470, 1964.
129. Markel, S.F., Magielski, J.E., and Beals, T.F.: Carcinoid tumor of the larynx, Arch. Otolaryngol. **106**:777, 1980.
130. Marks, J.E., et al.: Carcinoma of the pyriform sinus: an analysis of treatment results and patterns of failure, Cancer **41**:1008, 1978.
131. Montgomery, W.W., and Smith, S.A.: Congenital laryngeal defects in the adult, Ann. Otol. Rhinol. Laryngol. **85**:491, 1976.
132. O'Brien, P.H., et al.: Distant metastases in epidermoid cell carcinoma of the head and neck, Cancer **27**:304, 1971.
133. Olafsson, J., and van Nostrand, A.W.P.: Adenoid cystic carcinoma of the larynx: a report of four cases and review of the literature, Cancer **40**:1307, 1977.
134. Pahor, A.L.: Herpes zoster of the larynx—how common? J. Laryngol. Otol. **93**:93, 1979.
135. Pellettiere, E.V., II, Holinger, L.D., and Schild, J.A.: Lymphoid hyperplasia of larynx simulating neoplasia, Ann. Otol. Rhinol. Laryngol. **89**:65, 1980.
136. Quick, C.A., et al.: Relationship between condylomata and laryngeal papilloma: clinical and molecular virological evidence, Ann. Otol. Rhinol. Laryngol. **89**:467, 1980.
137. Reese, M.C., and Colclasure, J.B.: Cryptococcosis of the larynx, Arch. Otolaryngol. **101**:698, 1975.
138. Runckel, D., and Kessler, S.: Bronchogenic squamous carcinoma in nonirradiated juvenile laryngotracheal papillomatosis, Am. J. Surg. Pathol. **4**:293, 1980.
139. Schwenzfeier, C.W., and Fechner, R.E.: Herpes simplex of the epiglottis, Arch. Otolaryngol. **102**:374, 1976.
140. Shear, M., and Pindborg, J.J.: Verrucous hyperplasia of the oral mucosa, Cancer **46**:1855, 1980.
141. Smith, R.R., et al.: Revision of the clinical staging system for cancer of larynx, Cancer **31**:72, 1973.
142. Spiro, R.H., et al.: Mucus gland tumors of the larynx and laryngopharynx, Ann. Otol. Rhinol. Laryngol. **85**:498, 1976.
143. Strong, M.S., and Vaughan, C.W.: Vocal cord nodules and polyps—the role of surgical treatment, Laryngoscope **81**:911, 1971.
144. Suen, J.Y., et al.: Blastomycosis of the larynx, Ann. Otol. Rhinol. Laryngol. **89**:563, 1980.
145. Szpunar, J., et al.: Fibrinous laryngotracheal bronchitis in children, Arch. Otolaryngol. **93**:173, 1971.
146. Toker, C., and Peterson, D.W.: Lymphoepithelioma of the vocal cord, Arch. Otolaryngol. **104**:161, 1978.
147. Travis, L.W., Hybels, R.L., and Newman, M.H.: Tuberculosis of the larynx, Laryngoscope **86**:549, 1976.
148. Van Nostrand, A.W.P., and Olofsson, J.: Verrucous carcinoma of the larynx: a clinical and pathologic study of 10 cases, Cancer **30**:691, 1972.
149. Ward, P.H., et al.: Coccidiomycosis in the larynx of infants and adults, Ann. Otol. Rhinol. Laryngol. **86**:655, 1977.
150. Williams, R.I.: Allergic laryngitis, Ann. Otol. Rhinol. Laryngol. **81**:558, 1972.
151. Wynder, E.L., et al.: Environmental factors in cancer of the larynx: a second look, Cancer **38**:1591, 1976.
152. Yonkers, A.J.: Candidiasis of the larynx, Ann. Otol. Rhinol. Laryngol. **82**:812, 1973.

Middle ear

153. Borley, J.E., and Kapur, Y.P.: Histopathologic changes in the temporal bone resulting from measles infection, Arch. Otolaryngol. **103**:162, 1977.
154. Chevance, L.G., et al.: Otosclerosis: an electron microscopic and cytochemical study, Acta Otolaryngol. **272**(suppl.):1, 1970.
155. House, J.W., and Sheehy, J.L.: Cholesteatoma with intact tympanic membrane: a report of 41 cases, Laryngoscope **90**:70, 1980.
156. Hyams, V.J., and Michaels, L.: Benign adenomatous neoplasm (adenoma) of the middle ear, Clin. Otolaryngol. **1**:17, 1976.
157. Jahn, A.F., and Farkashidy, J.: New perspectives on the pathology of chronic otitis media, J. Otolaryngol. **9**:131, 1980.
158. Juhn, S.K., et al.: Pathogenesis of otitis media, Ann. Otol. Rhinol. Laryngol. **86**:481, 1977.
159. Rosenwasser, H.: Long-term results of therapy of glomus jugulare tumors, Arch. Otolaryngol. **97**:49, 1973.
160. Saeed, Y.M., and Bassis, M.L.: Mixed tumor of the middle ear: a case report, Arch. Otolaryngol. **93**:433, 1971.
161. Schiff, M., et al.: Tympanosclerosis: a theory of pathogenesis, Ann. Otol. Rhinol. Laryngol. **89**(suppl.):70, 1980.
162. Schimada, T., and Lim, D.J.: Distribution of ciliated cells in the human middle ear: electron and light microscopic observations, Ann. Otol. Rhinol. Laryngol. **81**:203, 1972.
163. Spector, G.J., Maisel, R.H., and Ogura, J.H.: Glomus jugulare tumors. II. A clinical pathologic analysis of the effects of radiotherapy, Ann. Otol. Rhinol. Laryngol. **83**:26, 1974.
164. Stiller, D., Katenkamp, D., and Küttner, K.: Jugular body tumors: hyperplasias or true neoplasms; light and electron microscopical investigations, Virchows Arch. (Pathol. Anat.) **365**:163, 1975.
165. Tos, M.: Middle ear epithelia in chronic secretory otitis, Arch. Otolaryngol. **106**:593, 1980.
166. Wine, C.J., and Metcalf, J.E.: Salivary gland choristoma of the middle ear and mastoid, Arch. Otolaryngol. **103**:435, 1977.

External ear canal and auricle

167. Bailin, P.L., et al.: Cutaneous carcinoma of the auricular and periauricular region, Arch. Otolaryngol. **106**:692, 1980.
168. Chandler, J.R.: Malignant external otitis: further considerations, Ann. Otol. Rhinol. Laryngol. **86**:417, 1977.
169. Dehner, L.P., and Chen, K.T.K.: Primary tumors of the external and middle ear: benign and malignant glandular neoplasms, Arch. Otolaryngol. **106**:13, 1980.
170. Johns, M.E., and Headington, J.T.: Squamous cell carcinoma of the external auditory canal: a clinicopathologic study of 20 cases, Arch. Otolaryngol. **100**:45, 1974.
171. Santos, V.V., Polisar, I.A., and Ruffy, M.L.: Bilateral pseudocysts of the auricle in a female, Ann. Otol. Rhinol. Laryngol. **83**:9, 1974.

Temporal bone

172. Hill, B.A., and Kohut, R.I.: Metastatic adenocarcinoma of the temporal bone, Arch. Otolaryngol. **102**:568, 1976.
173. Maniglia, A.J.: Intra and extracranial meningiomas involving the temporal bone, Laryngoscope **88**:12, 1978.
174. Naufal, P.M.: Primary sarcomas of the temporal bone, Arch. Otolaryngol. **98**:44, 1973.

175. Seftel, D.M.: Ear canal hyperostosis—surfer's ear, Arch. Otolaryngol. **103**:58, 1977.
176. Sweet, R.M., Kornblut, A.D., and Hyams, V.J.: Eosinophilic granuloma in the temporal bone, Laryngoscope **89**:1545, 1979.

Diseases of diverse sites

177. Arkin, C.F., and Masi, A.T.: Relapsing polychondritis: review of current status and case report, Semin. Arthritis Rheum. **5**:41, 1975.
178. Churg, A., and Ringus, J.: Ultrastructural observations on the histogenesis of alveolar rhabdomyosarcoma, Cancer **41**:1355, 1978.
179. Dehner, L.P., and Chen, K.T.K.: Primary tumors of the external and middle ear. III. A clinicopathologic study of embryonal rhabdomyosarcoma, Arch. Otolaryngol. **104**:399, 1978.
180. Dehner, L.P., Enzinger, F.M., and Font, R.L.: Fetal rhabdomyoma: an analysis of nine cases, Cancer **30**:160, 1972.
181. di Sant'Agnese, P.A., and Knowles, D.M., II: Extracardiac rhabdomyoma: a clinicopathologic study and review of the literature, Cancer **46**:780, 1980.
182. Fu, Y.-S., and Perzin, K.H.: Nonepithelial tumors of the nasal cavity, paranasal sinuses, and nasopharynx: a clinicopathologic study. V. Skeletal muscle tumors (rhabdomyoma and rhabdomyosarcoma), Cancer **37**:364, 1976.
183. Fu, Y.-S., and Perzin, K.H.: Nonepithelial tumors of the nasal cavity, paranasal sinuses, and nasopharynx: a clinicopathologic study. IX. Plasmacytomas, Cancer **42**:2399, 1978.
184. Gorenstein, A., et al.: Solitary extramedullary plasmacytoma of the larynx, Arch. Otolaryngol. **103**:159, 1977.
185. Kindblom, L.-G., et al.: Relapsing polychondritis: a clinical, pathologic-anatomic and histochemical study of 2 cases, Acta Pathol. Microbiol. Scand. **85**:656, 1977.
186. Morales, A.R., Fine, G., and Horn, R.C., Jr.: Rhabdomyosarcoma: an ultrastructural appraisal, Pathol. Annu. **7**:81, 1972.
187. Noorani, M.A.: Plasmacytoma of middle ear and upper respiratory tract, J. Laryngol. Otol. **85**:125, 1975.
188. Razek, A.A., et al.: Combined treatment modalities of rhabdomyosarcoma in children, Cancer **39**:2415, 1977.

CHAPTER 25 **Face, Lips, Tongue, Teeth, Oral Soft Tissues, Jaws, Salivary Glands, and Neck**

ROBERT J. GORLIN

FACE AND LIPS

Developmental anomalies including minor variations from normal

Facial clefts. Facial cleft, occurring in approximately 1 of every 800 births in whites, may exist as an isolated anomaly or in combination with other developmental disturbances (about 15% of clefts are so associated). Clefts have a racial predilection. They are most common in Native Americans (about 1 in 250) and least common in blacks (about 1 in 2500). Clefts in combination with other developmental disturbances may be so well known as to constitute a syndrome. Over 200 cleft syndromes are known[14]; only a few will be discussed here. Similarly, details of lateral and oblique facial clefts, cleft uvula, and microforms are left for comprehensive discussions elsewhere.[3,10]

Facial clefts arise from the failure of the ectomesenchyme to cross the junction of fusion of facial processes about the seventh week in utero. Thus cleft upper lip (harelip), the most common facial cleft, results from failure of fusion of the lower part of the median nasal (globular) process with the maxillary process. Unilateral cleft is about eight times more common than bilateral involvement. It is more common in males (about 60%) and on the left side (about 2:1). The degree of cleavage may vary from a slight notch at the lateral border of the philtrum to a complete separation extending into the nostril.

Commonly (in about 50% of cases), cleft lip is associated with cleft palate. When the cleft extends through the line of fusion between the primary and secondary palates, the area subsequently to be occupied by the developing lateral incisor frequently is disturbed. Supernumerary, impacted, or (most commonly) missing maxillary lateral incisors often are observed.

Cleft palate also may exist to varying degrees, ranging from bifid uvula to complete cleft. Not uncommonly, a submucous palatal cleft may remain undetected. Cleft palate unassociated with cleft lip (about 25%) is seen more commonly in females. Associated with abnormally small mandible (micrognathia) and tongue (microglossia) and posterior displacement of the tongue (glossoptosis), it is known as Pierre Robin syndrome. Cleft lip and cleft palate are commonly associated with chromosomal abnormalities; for example, cleft lip or cleft palate or both are seen in about 65% of infants with trisomy 13 and 4p-syndrome and in about 15% of the cases of trisomy 18.[2,3,13]

The tongue is cleft into two to four lobes in association with asymmetric cleft palate, pseudocleft of the upper lip, and digital anomalies in the orofaciodigital syndrome.[16]

Congenital lip pits. Congenital paramedian pits of the lower lip vary in size from small bilateral dimples on the vermilion border to large snoutlike structures in the midline (Fig. 25-1). Resulting fistulas are lined by stratified squamous epithelium and are connected at the base with the mucous glands of the lip by means of communicating ducts. Mucus may exude from the openings.

The pits may occur alone or in combination with cleft palate or cleft lip and agenesis of second premolars as part of a syndrome. Inheritance is autosomal dominant with variable expressivity.[18] An unrelated condition, commissural lip pits, is observed on one or both sides in up to 15% of those examined.[12]

Fordyce's granules. Fordyce's granules are collections of sebaceous glands symmetrically located on the lateral vermilion part of the upper lip and on the buccal mucosa of approximately 65% of adults. They increase in number during mature adult life. The most common oral mucosal sites are lateral to the angle of the mouth about Stensen's papilla and lateral to the anterior pillar of the fauces.[17]

TONGUE

Developmental anomalies

Aglossia, microglossia, and macroglossia. Aglossia and its modification, microglossia, are rare congenital anomalies. Often, severe hypoglossia is associated with other defects, especially diminution of the extremities (hypoglossia-hypodactylia syndrome). The tongue, although apparently absent, is present as a small nubbin located posteriorly in the mouth and consisting essentially of that part normally developed from the copula. Cleft palate and bony fusion of the jaws have been associated with aglossia and microglossia.[3]

The term *macroglossia* is rather nonspecific, referring only to the presence of an enlarged tongue. In cases observed at birth or in the neonatal period, the usual cause is lymphangioma or hemangiolymphangioma, although rarely there may be true muscular hypertrophy or enlargement caused by congenital neurofibromatosis. Enlargement of half the tongue occurs in congenital hemifacial hypertrophy. The tongue may protude from the mouth in trisomy 21 syndrome, congenital hypothyroidism, Hurler's syndrome, Beckwith-Wiedemann syndrome, glycogen storage disease type 2 (Pompe's disease), and many other conditions.[20]

Lingual thyroid gland. The presence of thyroid tissue within the tongue indicates arrested, partial, or incomplete embryologic descent of the gland. Approximately 10% of patients at autopsy have ectopic lingual thyroid tissue. Although the heterotopic tissue may occur anywhere along the normal path of the thyroglossal tract, the most frequent location is the base of the tongue at the foramen cecum. When superficial, the tissue is often raised, purplish, and crenulated and may be associated with hemorrhage. About 25% of patients are hypothyroid. The incidence appears to be about 1 in 3000 patients with thyroid disease. Grossly, the heterotopic nodule measures about 2 to 3 cm and resembles the normal thyroid gland, although encapsulation is often less well defined.[21]

Median rhomboid "glossitis." Median rhomboid "glossitis" is manifest as a roughly diamond-shaped reddish pattern on the dorsum of the tongue, immediately anterior to the circumvallate papillae. Occurring in somewhat less than 1% of individuals, it reportedly represents developmental failure of coverage of the tuberculum impar by the lateral tubercles of the tongue. *Candida albicans* infection has also been suggested as playing an etiologic role, but a cause-and-effect relationship has not been proved. It may arouse suspicion of malignant neoplasm in the minds of clinicians unaware of the nature of this condition.[19]

Fissured tongue. Fissured tongue occurs in about 5% of the population, with the frequency increasing with age. It is noted more commonly in trisomy 21, being present in about 30% of affected individuals, and is also part of the Melkersson-Rosenthal syndrome (upper facial edema, facial palsy, cheilitis granulomatosa, buccal mucosal plication).[94]

TEETH

Developmental anomalies

Anomalies of number. Rarely is there complete absence of teeth (anodontia) or noticeable suppression in tooth formation (oligodontia). More commonly, a mild reduction in number (hypodontia) is observed.[10,31] The third molars, and less commonly the maxillary lateral incisors and second premolars, are the teeth most likely to be missing. Irradiation of the jaws may injure or inhibit developing tooth buds. Supernumerary teeth occasionally are observed—most commonly mesiodens in the midline of the maxilla and extra molars posterior to the third molars.

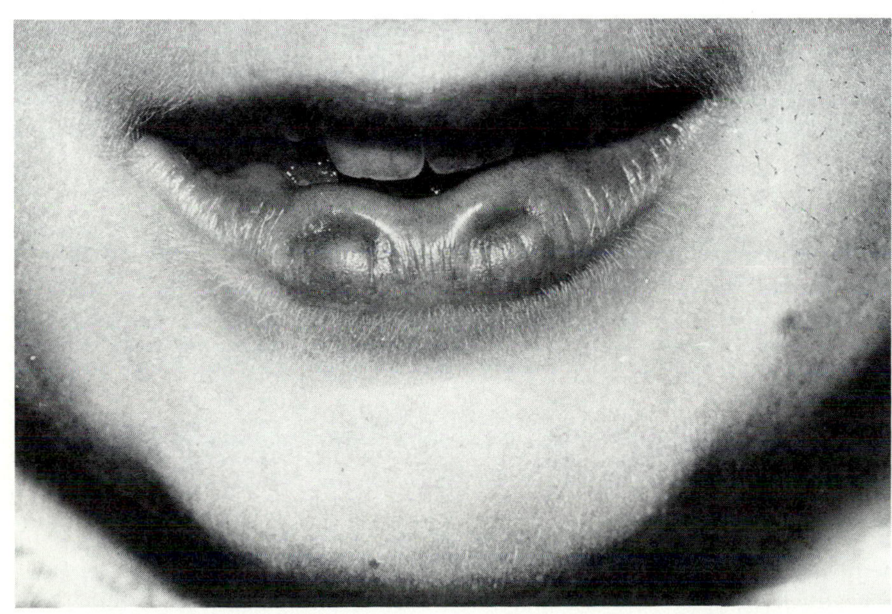

Fig. 25-1. Congenital lip pits (fistulas). Usually bilateral, frequently associated with facial clefts, and symmetrically situated on vermilion border of lower lip, fistulas represent failure of closure of evanescent sulci that appear in 10 to 14 mm embryo.

Anomalies of size. Rarely are all the teeth too large or too small. More frequently a single tooth is reduced in size (microdontia) or disproportionately enlarged (macrodontia).

Anomalies of shape. An anomaly called "dens invaginatus (dens in dente)" is manifest most commonly in the maxillary lateral permanent incisor.[10]

Anomalies of eruption. Rarely (1 in 2000 white infants) are teeth present at birth (natal teeth). This condition may occur idiopathically or occasionally in association with other anomalies (chondroectodermal dysplasia, pachyonychia congenita, oculomandibulodyscephaly) in the neonatal period. Delay in eruption may be related to physical obstruction (impaction), endocrine disturbances (cretinism), or a multitude of other causes (cleidocranial dysplasia, fibromatosis gingivae, and so on).[2,3,10]

Anomalies of dental pigmentation. The teeth may be discolored as a result of exogenous factors (usually chromogenic bacteria) or endogenous factors (usually altered blood pigments resulting from internal hemorrhage from trauma, congenital porphyria, erythroblastosis fetalis, and so on). Tetracyclines administered to the mother during the last trimester of pregnancy or to the infant are also incorporated in developing teeth, producing a yellow to gray color.[5,7,8] Their presence may be demonstrated by a noticeable yellow fluorescence under ultraviolet light.[10]

Premature loss of teeth. Premature loss of a tooth or teeth may be attributable to trauma, histiocytosis X, or various genetic disorders such as hypophosphatasia, cyclic or chronic neutropenia, or premature periodontoclasia with hyperkeratosis of palms and soles (Papillon-Lefèvre syndrome).[3]

Hereditary enamel defects. Hereditary enamel defects occur in about 1 in 16,000 children, affecting both dentitions. According to Witkop and Rao,[34] there appear to be at least 10 distinct types.

In the hereditary enamel dysplasias, the teeth are frequently brown and the enamel has a tendency to flake off, but the enamel varies in hardness and thickness according to the specific type. The underlying dentin and the root formation are entirely normal, in contrast to dentinogenesis imperfecta and dentin dysplasia.

Hereditary dentin defects. Only two dentin defects are considered here: dentinogenesis imperfecta (hereditary opalescent dentin) and radicular dentin dysplasia. Both are transmitted as autosomal dominant traits.[9,34]

Dentinogenesis imperfecta usually occurs as an isolated phenomenon (1 in 8000 individuals). A somewhat similar condition may occur as a component of osteogenesis imperfecta. Both deciduous and permanent teeth have an opalescent blue to brown color. Because of poor attachment at or near the dentinoenamel junction, the enamel fractures off. The roots are frequently thin and short and the canals obliterated. Microscopically, irregularly arranged dentinal tubules and defective matrix formation are noted.

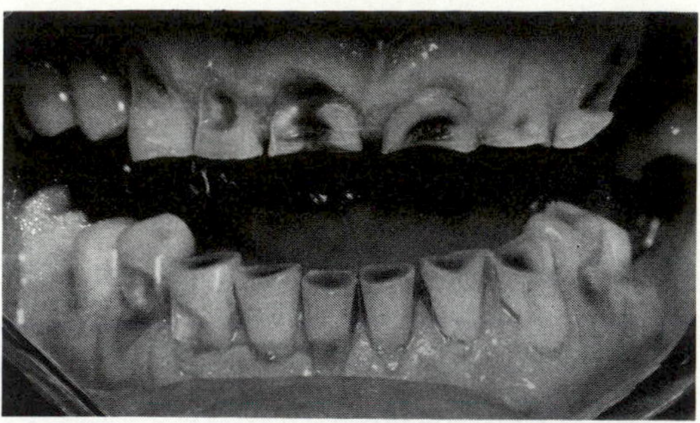

Fig. 25-2. Dental erosion. Characterized by smooth surface dissolution of enamel, especially at cervical portion, condition is of unknown etiology.

Radicular dentin dysplasia is characterized by rootless teeth, generally exhibiting an absence of pulp chambers and canals but normal-appearing crowns.[9] Many teeth exhibit large periapical radiolucencies, and a pathognomonic half moon–shaped pulp chamber may be seen on radiographic examination.

Other enamel disturbances. Nonhereditary enamel disturbances may affect either dentition, and they may be widespread or involve only a single tooth. The disturbance may be severe, causing deep pitted grooves, or so mild as to be manifest by only a small chalky spot. Defective enamel may result from injury to the enamel organ at any time from the earliest period of matrix formation to the last stage when calcification is taking place or may result from acquired abnormalities as in dental erosion (Fig. 25-2).

Nutritional deficiencies (of calcium, phosphorus, vitamin D), endocrine and related disorders (hypoparathyroidism, pseudohypoparathyroidism, hypophosphatasia, rickets), congenital syphilis, infection of the deciduous precursor (Turner's tooth), ingestion of excessive fluoride (in excess of 1.5 ppm), and many miscellaneous conditions can injure the developing ameloblast, producing enamel hypoplasia.[10]

Other dentin disturbances. In rickets the developing dentin is hypocalcified, with a wide margin of predentin analogous to the wide osteoid seams in forming bone.

Vitamin D–resistant rickets, an X-linked dominant trait, is associated with defective dentin formation and resultant periapical abscess development. Similar changes have been reported in a variety of related metabolic disorders.[10]

Diseases of teeth

Dental caries. Dental caries is a disease of the enamel, dentin, and cementum that produces progressive demineralization of the calcified component and eventual destruction of the organic component, with the forma-

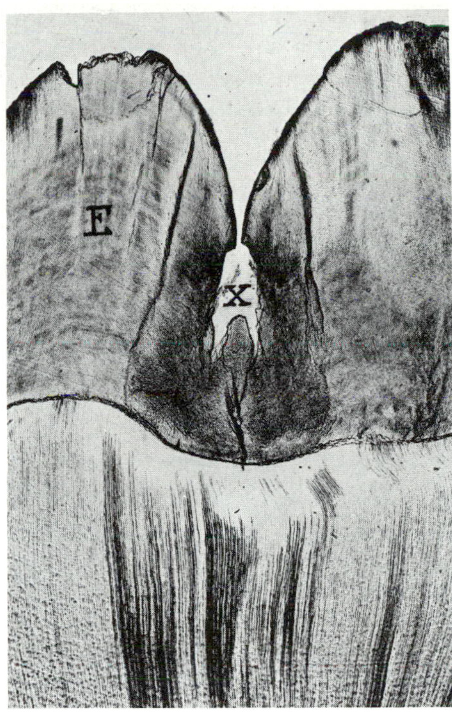

Fig. 25-3. Dental caries. Fissure lesion resulted in establishment of cavity, *X*, in enamel, *E*. Ground section of molar.

tion of a cavity in the tooth (Fig. 25-3). Microorganisms are present at all stages of the disease and, from the results of animal experiments, appear to be essential etiologic factors.[24,26,30] Specific strains of streptococci, especially *Streptococcus mutans* in its various serotypes, have been shown to induce dental caries in rats and hamsters. The etiologic process involves the metabolism of fermentable carbohydrates by these bacteria with the production of organic acids, which demineralize the tooth surface. Destruction of tooth structure by caries is easily differentiated from dental erosion and abrasion.

Tooth decay occurs or has occurred in the majority of individuals living in the United States, Canada, and Europe. Once a carious cavity has formed, the defect is permanent. The designation DMF (decayed, missing, filled) has proved useful in comparative studies of the frequency of dental caries, particularly in children and young adults.

Caries occurs in areas on tooth surfaces where saliva, food debris, and bacterial plaques accumulate. These areas are chiefly the pits and fissures, cervical part of the tooth, and interproximal surfaces. Surfaces that are cleansed by the excursion of food and the action of the tongue and cheeks are usually free of caries. If this process is disrupted (for example, by prosthetic appliances or lack of saliva), caries may develop rapidly.

The formation of bacterial plaques in areas of stagnation precedes cavity formation, especially in smooth dental surfaces. Acidogenic and aciduric bacteria, together with filamentous forms, are present in such plaques (Fig. 25-4).[26,32]

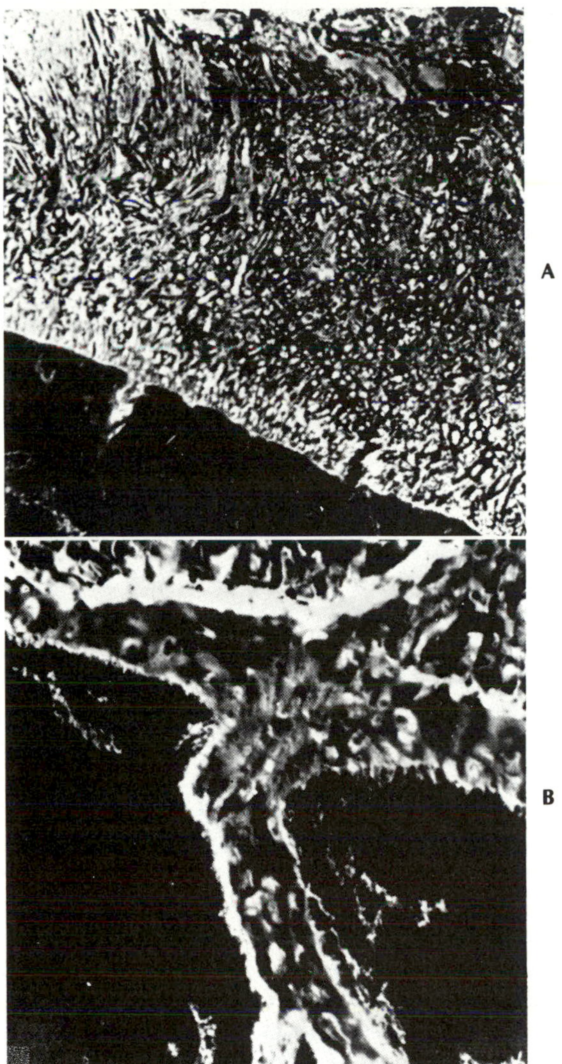

Fig. 25-4. A, Bacterial plaque isolated by acid flotation from clinically noncarious enamel. **B,** Mass of bacteria at enamel surface extending from plaque into lamella. (**A,** 2000×; **B,** 6000×; **A** and **B,** from Scott, D.B., and Albright, J.T.: Oral Surg. 7:64, 1954.)

Studies throughout the world have given striking evidence of the efficiency of fluoridation of communal water supplies in reducing the rate of tooth decay in children.[22] After the introduction of fluoride to the drinking water (1 ppm) the DMF rate has generally decreased over a period of years by more than 50%.[27] Partial control of tooth decay by this method constitutes an important public health achievement. Topical applications of fluoride solutions to tooth surfaces and brushing the teeth with dentifrices containing fluoride appear to be effective in further reducing susceptibility to dental caries.

Excessive amounts of fluoride cause a condition called

mottled enamel. It occurs in children who have consumed drinking water containing 1.5 ppm fluoride or more during the time when tooth enamel is being formed in the developing, unerupted teeth.

Pulp and periapical periodontal disease. The tooth, projecting into the oral cavity through the mucous membrane and extending deep into the jawbone, affords a surprisingly direct pathway for infection after exposure and infection of the dental pulp and after ulceration or breakdown of the epithelial attachments.

Carious destruction of dental hard tissues frequently produces pulpitis or inflammation of dental soft tissues, including, by way of extension, those surrounding the apex of the tooth. An alternative, yet equally dentally threatening, pathway exists through the gingival attachment (see following discussion concerning periodontal disease).

Inflammation of the dental pulp may be noninfective. Trauma to the tooth from a blow, which may or may not fracture the tooth, from dental operations, or from excessive thermal changes may also induce inflammation. This may be minimal with recovery, particularly in teeth with incompletely formed roots, or it may be severe leading to necrosis.

Pulpitis, regardless of the etiologic agent, may be acute or chronic. In acute pulpitis, pain is usually severe and increased by heat or cold. Pulpitis, acute or chronic, may be asymptomatic or accompanied by a mild fever and leukocytosis. Periapical tissues become involved by extension.

Acute alveolar or periapical abscess is usually the result of spread of suppurative infection from the tooth pulp through the root canals to the periodontal ligament about the tooth root apices. Drainage through the oral mucosa or to the adjacent skin of the face or neck may follow.

A more common sequela to dental pulp infection is the dental granuloma. Clinically, this may be completely symptomless. Radiographic examination frequently discloses an area of bone rarefaction about a tooth root apex, with a chronically infected or partially obliterated root canal. This area is usually spherical and well demarcated. Histologically, the tissue consists of fibrous connective tissue, often heavily infiltrated by lymphocytes and plasma cells, surounding necrotic tissue at the apex of the root canal foramen or within the pulp canal. Peripherally, loose and dense connective tissue merges into the surrounding bone, which may develop a definite cortical layer (Fig. 25-5).

Remnants of epithelium (rests of Malassez) are found in the periodontal ligament, surrounding the teeth. In granulomas this epithelium may proliferate. The root end may become surrounded by fluid with epithelium lining the surface, thus forming a cyst. The cyst may enlarge to a considerable size. Although epithelium is present in practically all granulomas and often proliferates to line small cystic cavities, the development of large cysts is relatively uncommon (see also section on odontogenic cysts).

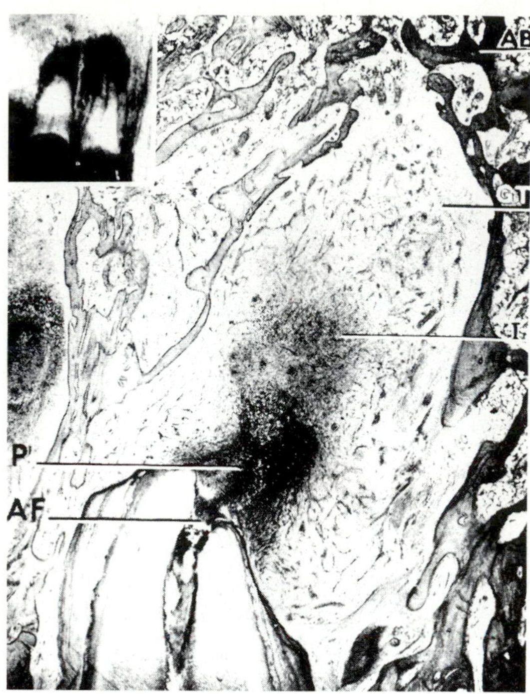

Fig. 25-5. Mesiodistal section through apex of maxillary first premolar with granuloma. *Inset,* Radiograph of specimen shows large areas of bone destruction around root ends of both maxillary premolars. *AB,* Alveolar bone; *AF,* apical foramen; *GT,* granulation tissue; *I,* dense cellular infiltration next to foramen; *P,* breaking down of tissue and formation of pus at foramen. (From Boyle, P.E., editor: Kronfeld's histopathology of the teeth and their surrounding structures, Philadelphia, 1955, Lea & Febiger.)

Periodontal disease. The inflammatory and degenerative processes that develop at the gingival margin and progress until the tooth-supporting structures are lost have much in common with periapical periodontal disease. In both instances, chronic asymptomatic infection by a variety of oral pathogens is usual, although episodes of acute suppuration may occur.

Strict anaerobes are primary etiologic agents, but the destructive process if thought to be mediated in large part by immunologic reactions of the host.[29,33] The tissue response involves a walling-off process with a pronounced chronic inflammatory cell infiltration. The proliferation of epithelium is always present in the marginal form of periodontal disease. It represents an attempt to cover the surface of the chronic ulcer that develops about the involved tooth root area (Figs. 25-6 and 25-7).[23,25,28]

The disease commonly begins as a gingivitis. Deposits of plaque and calculus on the tooth surfaces, impaction of food, decayed teeth, overhanging margins of dental res-

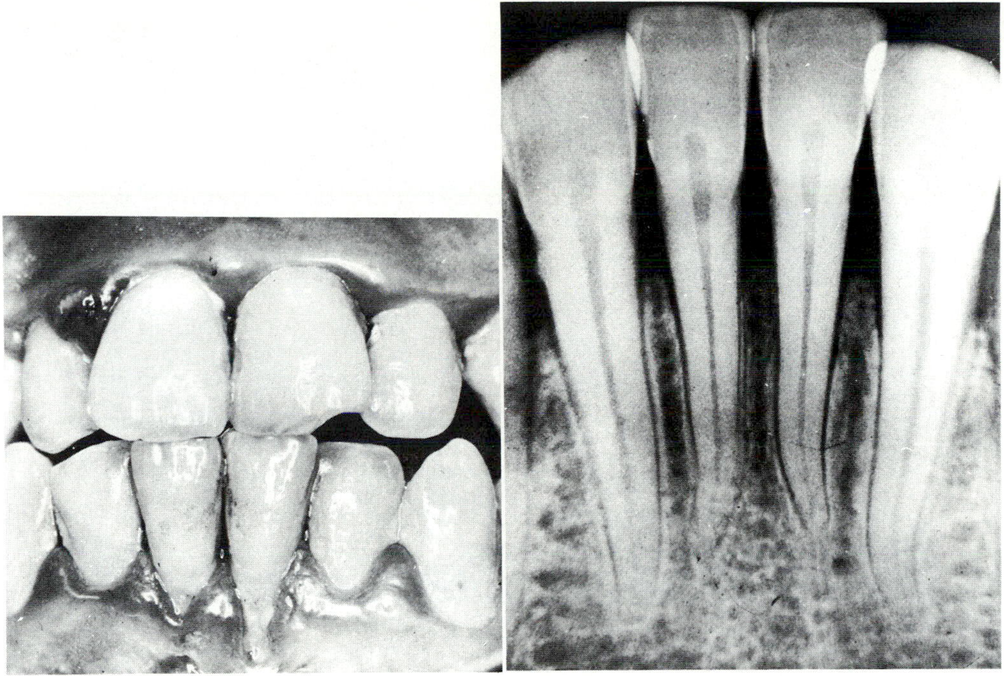

Fig. 25-6. Periodontitis. Edema, periodontal abscess, hemorrhage upon slight pressure, tissue recession with retraction of gingival margin, color change from light pink to deep red, loss of tissue in interdental area, horizontal bone loss, and widening of periodontal space. See Fig. 25-7.

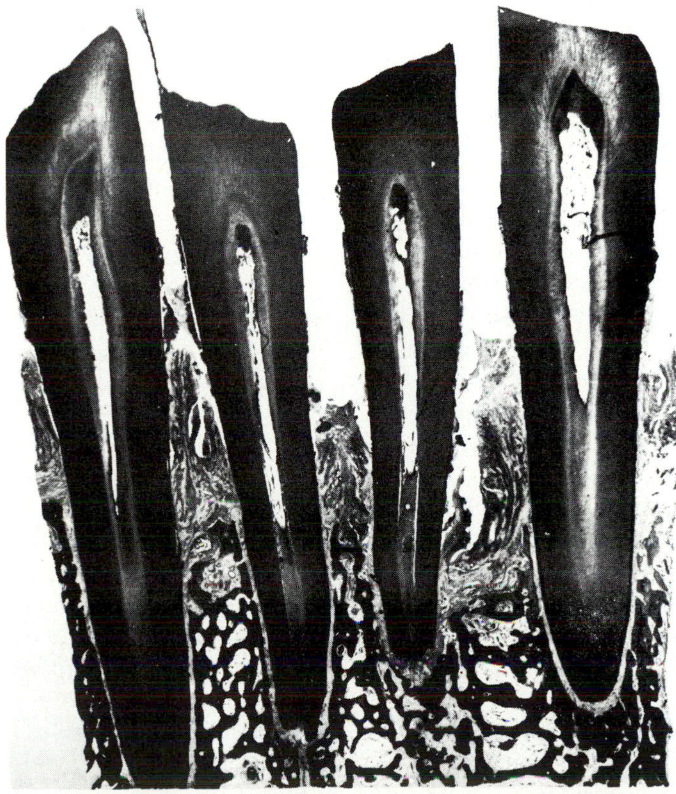

Fig. 25-7. Periodontitis (advanced). Mesiodistal section through mandibular incisors. Chronic inflammation of gingiva followed by proliferation of epithelium of gingival attachment along cementum, excessive osteoclastic resorption of interdental bone, and deep periodontal pocket formation between gingiva and surface of roots.

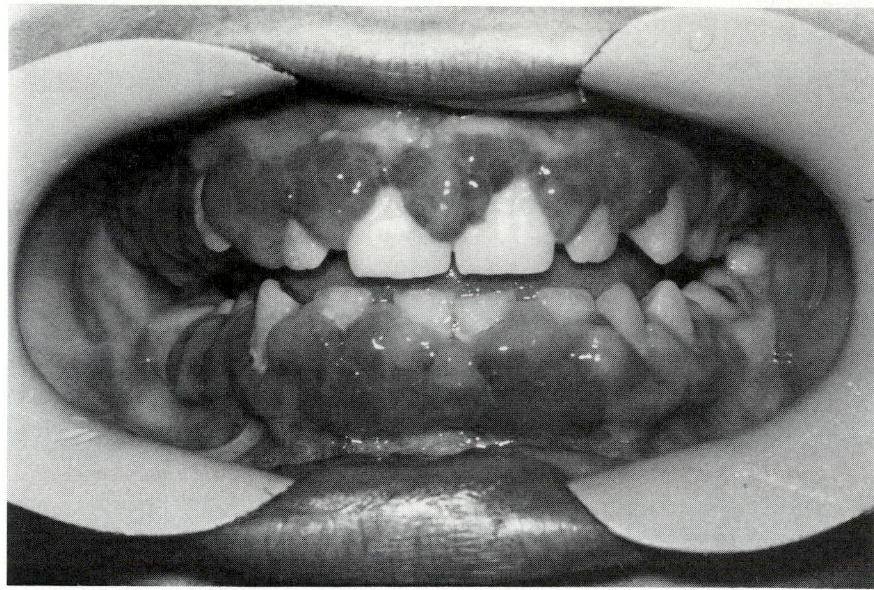

Fig. 25-8. Hyperplasia of gingiva associated with phenytoin (Dilantin).

torations, and ill-fitting dental appliances are among the predisposing factors. With progression, a pocket is established below the gingival margin, thus prolonging and promoting the inflammatory process, with progressive resorption of tooth-supporting structures. Proliferation of epithelium to line the pocket occurs concomitantly with the loss of tissue. A purulent discharge from periodontal pockets can be elicited by digital pressure in many adult patients and sometimes even in adolescents. Some individuals may show great resistance to the development of periodontal pockets despite adverse local factors, just as others have an extraordinary resistance to dental caries. Periodontal disease is more common in older individuals, and after middle age it becomes the chief cause of tooth loss.[25]

Pregnancy with its change in endocrine balance frequently is accompanied by gingivitis and hyperplastic inflammatory responses. Gingivitis may be somewhat more frequent during puberty.

Drug action may cause gingival response. The hyperplasia associated with the use of phenytoin (Dilantin) may be so extensive that the teeth are almost completely covered by gingival enlargement (Fig. 25-8).[25,42]

ORAL SOFT TISSUES

Mucocutaneous diseases

Although mucocutaneous disorders constitute a heterogeneous group, they are conveniently discussed together.

Lichen planus. Lichen planus usually appears as an irregular, lacelike whitening or keratosis of the buccal mucosa (Fig. 25-9), but other oral areas (gingiva, tongue, palate, and so on) also may be involved and the clinical appearance also may be bullous or erosive. Approximately one third of affected patients have only oral lesions. The other two thirds have only cutaneous or skin and oral manifestations. Mucosal surfaces of other body sites are much less frequently involved. The diagnosis may be suspected when the lacelike whitening of the surface of the buccal mucosa (Wickham striae) is seen. Lesions on the dorsum of the tongue are diffusely opaque. Biopsies and immunofluorescence of nonulcerated whitenings may be used in the diagnosis.[40,84,149,155,165]

The cause of lichen planus is not known. Patients are most frequently between 40 and 60 years of age. Oral lesions of the keratotic type of lichen planus are asymptomatic, but pain and discomfort have been observed with bullous or erosive types of the disease. Approximately half of the patients experience concurrent nervous stress and express anxiety or fear of having oral cancer. There may be an association between lichen planus and diabetes mellitus.

Pemphigus. Pemphigus, especially pemphigus vulgaris, characteristically involves the oral mucosa during its course and usually appears initially in this location.[140] The oral tissues are very red, friable, and pebbly (Fig. 25-10). Vesicle and bulla formation is observed, but the blisters do not remain intact for long periods in the mouth. Smear preparations, biopsies of oral sites, and immunofluorescence (to detect intercellular IgG deposits)[106,127,150] are most useful in establishing the diagnosis (Fig. 25-11). A similar picture may be seen following penicillamine therapy.[69]

Benign mucous membrane pemphigoid. Benign mu-

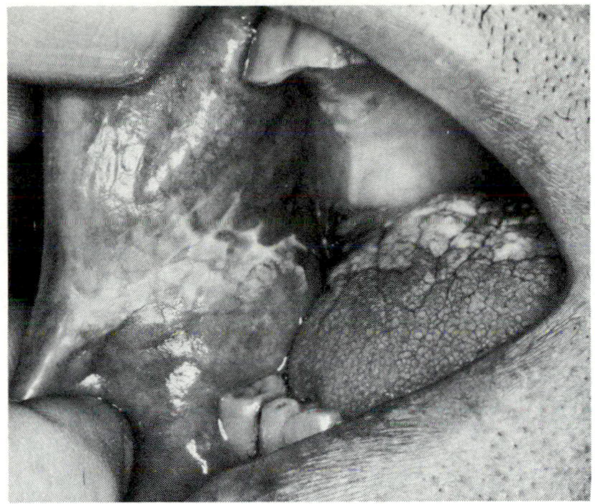

Fig. 25-9. Lichen planus of buccal mucosa. Dorsum of tongue is also involved. (Courtesy Jens O. Andreasen, Copenhagen.)

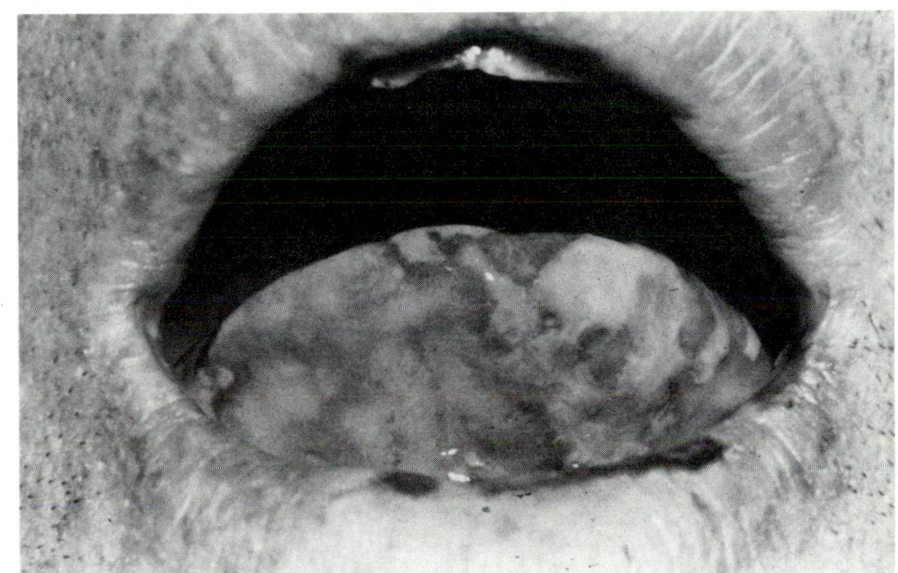

Fig. 25-10. Pemphigus involving lingual mucosa.

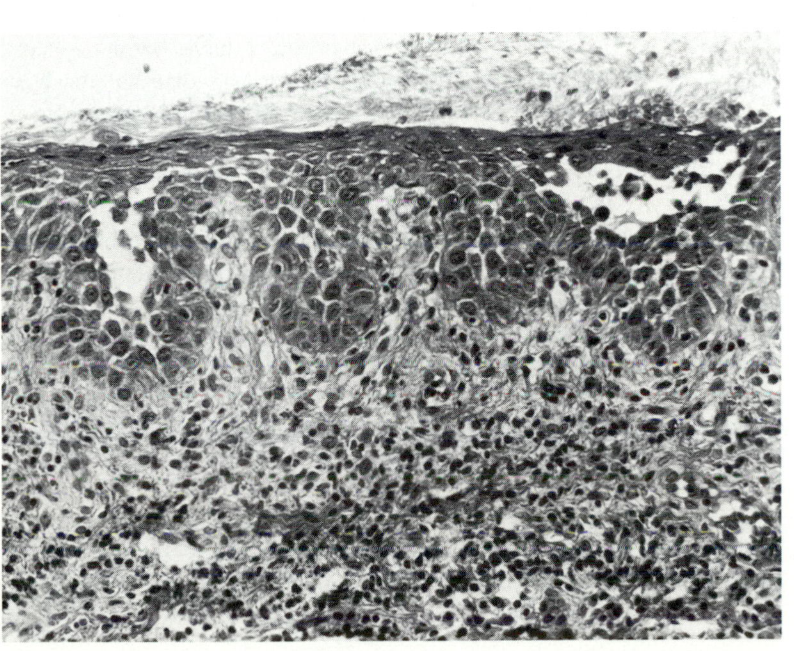

Fig. 25-11. Biopsy specimen of oral mucosa in pemphigus showing intraepithelial acantholysis.

cous membrane pemphigoid is a vesicular or bullous disease involving the oral mucosa. It occurs most often in older women. Conjunctival tissues are frequently affected, and the associated inflammation and scarring of this site are the most serious sequelae.[128] Microscopically vesicle formation occurs immediately below the epithelium, and biopsy specimens of the short-lived vesicles are helpful in establishing the diagnosis, as are immunofluorescence studies that show complement and IgG deposits in the basement membrane zone.

Erythema multiforme. Erythema multiforme is characterized by large, vesiculobullous or erosive, frequently hemorrhagic lesions of the lips, buccal mucosa, and tongue. Oral and facial tissues are involved in approximately 25% of the patients.

Stevens-Johnson syndrome is a term applied to clinically severe examples of erythema multiforme, especially when the conjunctiva, genitalia, and, often, lungs are involved. The disorder appears to be a reaction to various medications (penicillin, sulfa drugs, phenobarbital) and the herpes simplex virus.[54,112,125]

Epidermolysis bullosa. Oral tissues are involved in several genetic types of epidermolysis bullosa. Microstomia, after the scarring of buccal mucosa, and dental abnormalities are complications of the dystrophic forms of this disease.[38,86]

Other mucocutaneous diseases. Keratosis follicularis (Darier's disease), lupus erythematosus, and herpes zoster are additional examples of so-called mucocutaneous conditions with oral manifestations.[10,124,127]

Hyalinosis cutis et mucosae (Urbach-Wiethe syndrome) causes induration of the oral mucosa, especially that of the lips and the tongue, which becomes atrophic and bound down to the oral floor.[3,76] In primary amyloidosis, infiltration of the tongue may be associated with macroglossia. Deposits of secondary amyloid in the gingiva are not clinically manifested. Scleroderma and acrosclerosis occasionally (about 7% of cases) are associate with a widening of the periodontal ligament of the teeth.

Hairy tongue is associated with proliferation of saprophytic organisms that cause extrinsic staining of elongated filiform papillae. Although the etiology is unknown, hairy tongue may follow therapeutic use of antibiotics or radiation.[75] Benign migratory glossitis (geographic tongue), also of unknown etiology, is characterized by irregular superficial areas devoid of filiform papillae. It is more common in females and is seen in about 2% of the population.[10]

Oral and labial papillomatosis may be associated with the adult (malignant) form of acanthosis nigricans.[3] The oral lesions, in contrast to the cutaneous, are not pigmented.

Swelling of the lip and oral mucosa with facial palsy and plicated tongue is seen in the Melkersson-Rosenthal syndrome.[94]

Inflammatory disease

Acute herpetic gingivostomatitis. Acute herpetic gingivostomatitis is the most common manifestation of primary infection with the herpes simplex virus, type 1. It is frequently misdiagnosed as necrotizing ulcerative gingivitis or Vincent's stomatitis. Occurring clinically in less than 1% of the population, it is rarely if ever seen in a child under 1 year of age. It reaches its peak between the ages of 1 and 3 years, although it is also observed in older children and young adults. The incubation period is 4 to 8 days. The gingiva is red and swollen, is exquisitely tender, and bleeds easily. Numerous vesicles and bullae are present on the labial, lingual, and buccal mucosae.[56,71,88,122]

Microscopically the herpes simplex vesicle shows multinucleated giant cells having two to 15 nuclei per cell and eosinophilic inclusion bodies within the nuclei. Intraepithelial edema (ballooning degeneration) and intracellular edema are especially pronounced.

The herpes simplex virus may be identified by determination of neutralizing antibody titer, complement fixation, or specific skin test performed after the infection. There is a high incidence (70% to 90%) of neutralizing antibody in the adult population.

Recurrent herpes (cold sore, fever blister). Recurrent herpes simplex infections occur most frequently about the face and lips and tend to recur at the same site in about 30% of the population. The condition is characterized by groups of small, clear vesicles on an erythematous base. The recurrent lesions seem to be induced by such agents as sunshine, fever, mechanical trauma, menses, and allergy. Intraoral involvement is rare but may involve the hard palate and fixed gingiva with pinhead-sized, grouped ulcers.

Accidental vaccination. There have been several examples of accidental vaccination of the lip, gingiva, palate, buccal mucosa, and tongue, with erythema multiforme arising as a complication. Transfer of the vaccine to the orofacial area occurs by means of the fingers, towels, or clothing. Although the vaccinia virus differs from both the cowpox virus and the smallpox virus, because of its close relationship it offers cross immunity.[142]

Recurrent aphthae (canker sores). Although resembling the lesions of recurrent herpes, recurrent aphthae, which occur in about half of the population, are not caused by the herpes simplex virus.[71,87,121,148] The lesions are larger than those of recurrent herpes and occur on freely movable mucosa. Circinate superficial lesions are seen on the oral mucosa in Reiter's syndrome (arthritis, conjunctivitis, and urethritis).[3] The term *major aphthae* (Sutton's disease) refers to large chronic aphthae that scar.[10] Similar lesions are seen in Behçet's syndrome (orogenital ulceration and iridocyclitis).[3,87]

Infectious mononucleosis. Infectious mononucleosis may present pronounced oral signs.[46] In addition to inflammation of the oral pharynx and lymphadenopathy, about one third of patients exhibit a grayish or grayish green membrane resembling that of diphtheria or Vincent's angina over the throat or posterior buccal mucosa. The gingiva bleeds easily and becomes enlarged. Petechiae are common on the soft palate.

Hand-foot-and-mouth disease. Generally unrecognized, hand-foot-and-mouth disease is a self-limited, febrile disease caused by group A coxsackieviruses, principally type 16 and less often types 5 and 10, and echovirus, type 6.[50,51] It is manifest by many small vesicles or punched-out ulcers of the lips and buccal mucosa. The gingiva characteristically is spared, in contrast to herpetic stomatitis. Those affected are principally under 10 years of age. Cutaneous involvement is usually limited to the palms, soles, and ventral surfaces and sides of fingers and toes.

Agranulocytosis. Agranulocytosis often is manifest by ragged necrotic ulcers of the gingiva, palate, tonsils, or oropharynx.[1] Sialorrhea may be profuse. Drug sensitivity, especially to the barbiturates, chloramphenicol, antithyroid drugs, and the sulfonamides, is the best-known cause. Similar lesions are seen in cyclic neutropenia, an autosomal dominant disorder in which the neutrophils are decreased every 21 days.[10] Various autosomal recessive chronic neutropenias also result in oral ulceration and premature periodontal destruction. Cytotoxic agents employed in cancer chemotherapy produce severe oral ulceration.

Lethal granuloma (midline lethal granuloma). Probably a form of malignant reticulosis, lethal granuloma involves the palate, sinuses, and nasopharynx in a severe, progressive, ulcerative, destructive process.[119]

Wegener's granulomatosis. Considered to be a form of hypersensitivity, Wegener's granulomatosis, a possible variant of polyarteritis nodosa, may be heralded by multiple pyogenic granulomas of the interdental papillae of the gingiva.[68,141]

Crohn's disease. Oral lesions may occur in Crohn's disease. They are principally of three types. Most frequently involved is the buccal mucosa, which has a cobblestone appearance. In the mucobuccal fold are linear hypoplastic lesions and ulcers. Next most frequently involved are the lips, which may be diffusely swollen and indurated. Less frequently involved are the gingiva and alveolar mucosa. There the lesions are more granular and erythematous. The palate may be involved with multiple aphthous lesions. In contrast to intestinal lesions where there is no sexual predilection, oral lesions have at least a 4-to-1 male-to-female predilection.[47]

Eosinophilic ulcer of soft tissues. This lesion, albeit rare, is of sufficient interest for discussion. Most examples have involved the tongue of adults, although rarely other oral structures such as the gingiva or palate may be involved. It may be related to trauma of the tongue muscle.[115,147,161,163,174] It is not related to either the cutaneous facial eosinophilic granuloma or the eosinophilic granuloma of bone (histiocytosis X). There is marked (7-to-1) male predilection. The etiology is obscure and the lesion self-limiting.

Acute necrotizing ulcerative gingivitis (Vincent's disease, fusospirochetosis). Acute necrotizing ulcerative gingivitis is far less common than supposed. Often the term "trench mouth" is used as a catchall to include primary herpetic gingivostomatitis, herpangina, infectious mononucleosis, and similar oral manifestations of disease. This is especially true in children, for fusospirochetosis is extremely uncommon in childhood (except in Africa), afflicting instead young and middle-aged adults. The disease is almost exclusively limited to the interdental papillae and the free gingival margin, rarely extending to the faucial area (Vincent's angina). Necrosis and ulceration of one or more interdental gingival papillae, mild fever, fetid breath, malaise, and local discomfort characterize the condition. Predisposing conditions seem to allow penetration of the oral tissues by several symbiotic organisms normally inhabiting the mouth, among these a fusiform bacillus and an oral spirochete, *Borrelia vincentii*.[10]

Noma (cancrum oris, gangrenous stomatitis). Noma may occur as a complication of acute necrotizing gingivitis in children or, rarely, in adults debilitated by infectious disease or possibly malnourishment. It is rare except in the Far East and Africa. The process usually begins in a gingival ulceration and rapidly spreads to involve the cheeks, lips, and jawbones. The tissues become blackened and necrotic. Pneumonia and toxemia are common sequelae.

Syphilis. In both the prenatal and the acquired forms, syphilis may be manifest about the mouth.[77,117,118,133] In the acquired form, the primary lesion or chancre may appear on the lips or tongue, simulating a squamous cell carcinoma. The secondary stage is characterized by the mucous patch (a milky white, focal, superficial ulcer of the oral mucosa), sore throat, and occasionally a condyloma at the corner of the mouth (split papule). The hard palate may be perforated in the tertiary stage as a result of gumma formation. The tongue may be involved with a diffuse inflammatory process (syphilitic glossitis) that may predispose to the development of squamous cell carcinoma. Prenatal syphilis may be demonstrated by rhagades or radiating scars about the mouth and characteristic alteration in the form of the permanent teeth (Hutchinson's incisors and mulberry molars), in addition to the changes seen in the secondary and tertiary stages of acquired syphilis.

Gonorrhea. The variable clinical conditions associated with oral, tonsillar, or pharyngeal infection by the gram-negative intracellular diplococcus *Neisseria gonorrhoeae* are perhaps too poorly appreciated and diagnosed. Its identification, although rare, has been documented.[60,98] Generally acute, erythematous, and ulcerative with associated systemic symptoms, it may also be pseudomembranous or even vesicular in its manifestations. Burning and itching have been early subjective symptoms.[116]

Yaws. Yaws presents lesions somewhat similar to those of syphilis. The secondary papular lesions are commonly perioral. Tertiary lesions (gangosa) result in extensive destruction of the soft palate, hard palate, and nose.[10]

Granuloma inguinale. Oral lesions of granuloma inguinale are the most common extragenital (about 5% to 6%) manifestations of the disease.[134]

Actinomycosis. Actinomycosis of the cervicofacial type arises through invasion of oral mucous membranes or a tooth socket, spreading to involve the jawbones, musculature, and salivary glands. Multiple foci of suppuration lead into sinus tracts that drain to the cutaneous surface or oral mucosa, liberating pus containing the typical and diagnostic "sulfur granules" of *Actinomyces israelii*.[85]

Histoplasmosis. Oral lesions of histoplasmosis appear most frequently as nodular or ulcerated areas on the tongue or palate.[181]

Tuberculosis. Tuberculosis of the oral tissues is rare and usually is associated with advanced pulmonary disease. The typical lesion is an irregular, slowly enlarging, painful ulcer of the base of the tongue or palate.[81,132]

Other granulomatous infections

Many other fungal and tropical diseases have oral lesions—among them tropical sprue, leishmaniasis, scleroma, leprosy, and South American blastomycosis.[10,111,137]

Candidiasis (thrush). Candidiasis is a fungal disease occurring most often in debilitated persons, infants, or especially individuals who have been taking oral antibiotics. It also may be associated in the form of a syndrome with hypoparathyroidism, keratoconjunctivitis, and Addison's disease.[3,6] A chronic hyperplastic candidiasis is often present. It is characterized by a pseudoepitheliomatous hyperplasia, with fungal invasion and a noticeable chronic inflammatory reaction. The fungus may invade the oral mucosa, skin, female genitalia, or urinary tract. Since the fungus *Candida albicans* is a normal oral inhabitant, the diagnosis cannot be based on smear alone. The presence of hyphae is more significant diagnostically. The clinical appearance is that of numerous milk-white plaques—occasionally covering the entire oral mucosa—that are easily stripped off, leaving a bleeding surface because of penetration of the mycelia.[93,103] Overclosure of the jaws in the edentulous patient or in the patient with poorly constructed dentures commonly results in low-grade chronic infection at the corners of the mouth, attributable at least in part to candidal organisms.[48,55] This is called perlèche, or angular cheilitis.[138] Cheilosis caused by deficiency of one or more of the B complex vitamins is rare.

Childhood exanthematous diseases. The childhood exanthematous diseases frequently manifest oral lesions. Koplik's spots, one of the prodromal signs of measles, are pinhead-sized, bluish white spots surrounded by erythematous halos. They appear in the buccal or labial mucosa about 18 hours before the skin rash. Warthin-Finkeldey giant cells may be histologically observed in the tonsils or other oral lymphatic lesions (Fig. 25-12).[110]

Disturbances of pigmentation

Melanotic pigmentation. Melanin may occur in the oral mucosa and about the lips under both normal and pathologic conditions.[58,66,92] Racial pigmentation, especially of the gingiva, is the most common type and appears to be directly related to skin color. It is present not only in nearly all blacks but also in Orientals and those of Mediterranean background. Even 10% of Scandinavians may have oral melanotic pigmentation. Little melanin is present at birth. It is deposited largely during the first decade.

Chronic adrenocortical insufficiency (Addison's disease), hemochromatosis, and Albright's syndrome (polyostotic fibrous dysplasia and precocious puberty)[3] may be associated with pigmentation of the oral mucosa and the skin. Pigmentation also is seen in chronic steatorrhea and in the Peutz-Jeghers syndrome. The latter is characterized by gastrointestinal polyposis, mucocutaneous pigmentation, and autosomal dominant inheritance.[2,3] Palatal melanotic pigmentation may be seen after extensive use of various antimalarial drugs, such as amodia-

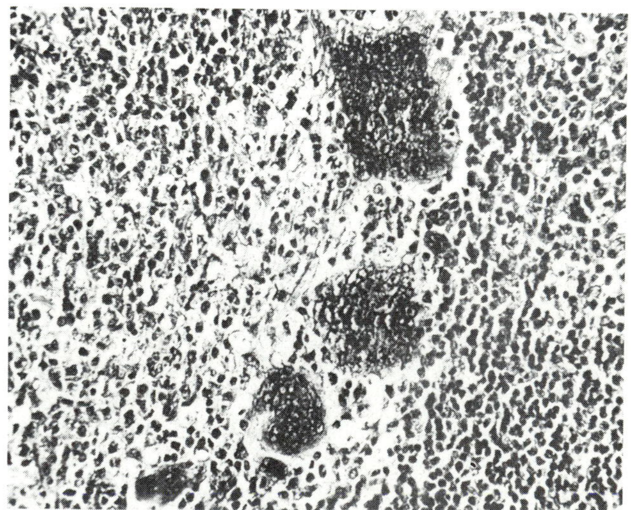

Fig. 25-12. Warthin-Finkeldey giant cells seen in lateral lingual tonsillar tissue during prodromal measles.

quin (Camoquin) or chloroquine. It also may be seen in patients with oral lichen planus ("melasmic" staining).

All types of melanotic nevi have been reported in oral tissues, as has malignant melanoma.

Nonmelanotic pigmentation. Nonmelanotic pigmentation usually is caused by heavy metals. Amalgam tattoo results from implantation of particles of filling material under the mucosa at the time of dental procedures.[52] Lead, bismuth, arsenic, and mercury intoxications may be associated with a deposit of the metallic sulfide in the inflamed gingival margin.

Tumors and tumorlike lesions

Benign tumors and tumorlike lesions of the oral soft tissues

Generalized or localized enlargement of the gingiva should arouse clinical suspicion of neoplastic disease. Enlarged gingival papillae, with bleeding on slight pressure, are found in vitamin C deficiency (scorbutic gingivitis). Clinically similar appearances may indicate the local infiltration of the gingiva with immature leukocytes characteristic of one variety or another of leukemia.

Phenytoin (Dilantin) frequently causes a striking enlargement of the gingiva associated with a dense overgrowth of fibrous tissue (Fig. 25-8).[42]

All gingival enlargements become traumatized during mastication and toothbrushing. Plasma cells, characteristically present in the gingiva in small numbers, may increase under inflammatory stimuli to simulate plasma cell myeloma or solitary plasmacytoma, but the presence of other inflammatory cells suggests plasma cell granuloma.[37]

Fibromatosis gingivae. Fibromatosis gingivae represents a proliferation of the entire gingiva. Inflammation is characteristically absent, since the gingiva is of normal color and hard texture. The normal eruption of teeth is prevented. Fibromatosis gingivae may rarely be associated with hypertrichosis, seizures, and mental retardation. An autosomal dominant genetic pattern is common. There are several other varieties.[3,179]

Papilloma. Papilloma is an arborescent growth consisting of numerous squamous epithelial fingerlike projections, each of which contains a well-vascularized, fibrous, connective tissue core.[35] Although it may be seen throughout the mouth, the soft palate, tongue, and lips are common sites. There is no sex or age predilection.[90]

Focal epithelial hyperplasia. This condition was first described by Heck as occurring on oral mucosal tissue of Navajo children and has since been observed in others, most prominently Greenlandic Eskimos.[131,158,166] It is usually a soft, nonulcerated white or reddish papule approximately 0.5 cm in diameter (Fig. 25-13). The lesions are frequently multiple, are probably of viral etiology, and have now been observed in the United States and other countries.

Fibroma. The most common benign growth on the oral mucous membrane is fibroma that occurs as a discrete, superficial, pedunculated mass. Such lesions appear to be nonneoplastic, arising as an exuberant response to physical trauma or other inflammatory agents. An example of this type of reaction is the so-called denture-injury tumor.[64] Some examples probably represent burnt-out pyogenic granulomas.[108] A cellular variant has been termed calcified fibroblastic granuloma.[39] Microscopically these fibromas are composed of collagenic fibrous connective tissue covered by keratinized or parakeratinized stratified squamous epithelium.

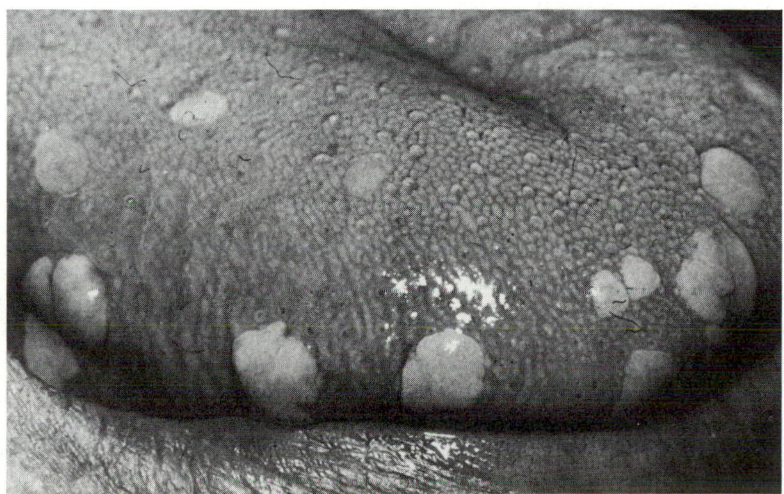

Fig. 25-13. Multiple lesions of focal epithelial hyperplasia on tongue. (From Praetorius-Clausen, F.: Pathol. Microbiol. **39:**204, 1973.)

Myxomatous degeneration, metaplastic bone formation, or fatty infiltration is noted in the connective tissue. Focal fibrous gingival masses may occur in tuberous sclerosis.

Lipoma. Although uncommon, lipoma occurs most frequently in the cheek, tongue, and oral floor. There is no sex or age predilection.[91,169]

Verruciform xanthoma. The verruciform xanthoma is often misdiagnosed as a papilloma. The most frequent site is the gingiva or alveolar ridge. About 75% of the patients are in the fifth to seventh decades of life. There may be a 3-to-2 female sex predilection. Microscopically the rough verrucous surface is covered by parakeratin, which forms invaginating crypts that extend deep into the epithelium. The latter exhibits acanthosis with uniform elongation of rete ridges. Numerous foamy xanthomatous cells fill the connective tissue papillae extending downward *only* to the tips of the rete ridges.[61,126]

Neuroma, neurilemoma, and neurofibroma. Neurilemoma and neurofibroma are also observed in oral environs, especially the tongue. Neurofibroma may occur as an isolated lesion or as part of neurofibromatosis.[3] The lesions of the latter condition may be of at least three types: discrete, diffuse, or plexiform.[167,180]

The traumatic neuroma occurs at the proximal end of crushed or severed peripheral nerves.[154] A history of extraction of teeth or prior soft tissue trauma is usually elicited. The lesion usually appears as a nodule having normal surface coloration. The most common sites are the mental foramen area, lower lip, and tongue, although any area of the oral mucosa may be involved. Although the lesion may occur at any age, about 65% of the patients are 45 years of age or older. There may be a slight female predilection. In approximately 50% there is pain associated with the lesion. The pain ranges from tenderness to severe constant pain. Rarely a trigeminal neuralgia–like paroxysmal pain may be triggered by pressure applied to the lesion. However, when patients are less than 20 years of age, the lower lip and buccal mucosa appear to be more frequently involved, probably reflecting tissue trauma suffered in accidents rather than dental extraction. Microscopically the traumatic neuroma consists of a nonencapsulated tangled mass of axons, Schwann cells, and endoneural and perineural cells in a dense collagenous matrix. Similar lesions may be noted in the tongue and lips in multiple endocrine adenomatosis, type 3 (multiple mucosal neuroma syndrome).[67,100]

Rhabdomyoma and leiomyoma. Intraoral rhabdomyoma is a relatively uncommon tumor of middle-aged to older men (male-to-female incidence 5:2). It arises most often in the oral floor, and less commonly in the tongue or soft palate.[173] Histologically the tumor is composed of large polyhedral skeletal muscle cells having occasional cross striations and granular eosinophilic cytoplasm, with glycogen-containing vacuoles and intracellular crystalline material, probably hypertrophic Z lines.[63,99]

Leiomyoma is also a rare oral tumor. Most oral examples arise from the tunica media of the walls of blood vessels. The most common sites are the tongue (especially the base), buccal mucosa, palate, and lower lip. There is a 2:1 male sex predilection. Most often the patient is 40 to 60 years of age. The tumors are nonulcerated, sessile, and asymptomatic; microscopically, they show numerous uniform stellate smooth muscle cells, often surrounding several dilated vascular channels. The cells appear to intertwine. Masson trichrome stain is used to demonstrate smooth muscle origin.[59]

Granular cell tumor (granular cell "myoblastoma"). First described by Abrikossof in 1926 and assumed initially to be of striated muscle origin, granular cell tumor has in recent years been the subject of considerable controversy. Many investigators believe it to be of neural origin, whereas others suggest that it represents not a true neoplasm but a special type of muscle degeneration. Histochemical and electron microscopic investigations have added support to the neural (Schwann cell) theory of origin.[49,80,120,136] Others have suggested the pericyte.[139]

Although having its origin in many tissues, especially the skin, about 30% arise in the tongue. There appears to be no age preference except for a possible variant that occurs at birth on the anterior alveolar ridges and has been called congenital epulis of the newborn. It occurs predominantly (8:1) in female infants and twice as often in the upper jaw as in the lower jaw.

Microscopically the tumor consists of large polyhedral cells with an acidophilic granular cytoplasm. Ultrastructural studies have demonstrated that the "granules" are lysosomal structures. The nucleus is small, somewhat pyknotic, and eccentrically placed. Pseudoepitheliomatous hyperplasia, characteristically absent in the congenital epulis, may be so pronounced in the tongue lesion that a diagnosis of squamous cell carcinoma is made (Fig. 25-14). Although the histologic features of this lesion are clear, its histogenesis is not.

Giant cell granuloma. The peripheral form of this lesion is similar to the central form discussed on p. 1020.

Hemangioma. Hemangioma of the oral mucous membranes is essentially similar to that of the skin and may occur in any area of the mouth with many appearances. Although it is most commonly of the capillary type, cavernous and mixed types also are seen. These often congenital lesions should not be confused with the exuberant overgrowth of granulation tissue designated as pyogenic granuloma,[108] which apparently arises as the result of trauma and nonspecific infection. The pyogenic granuloma is indistinguishable microscopically from the so-called pregnancy tumor that arises on the gingiva during the second trimester of gestation in approximately 10% of gravid females. Consisting of new capillaries, fibro-

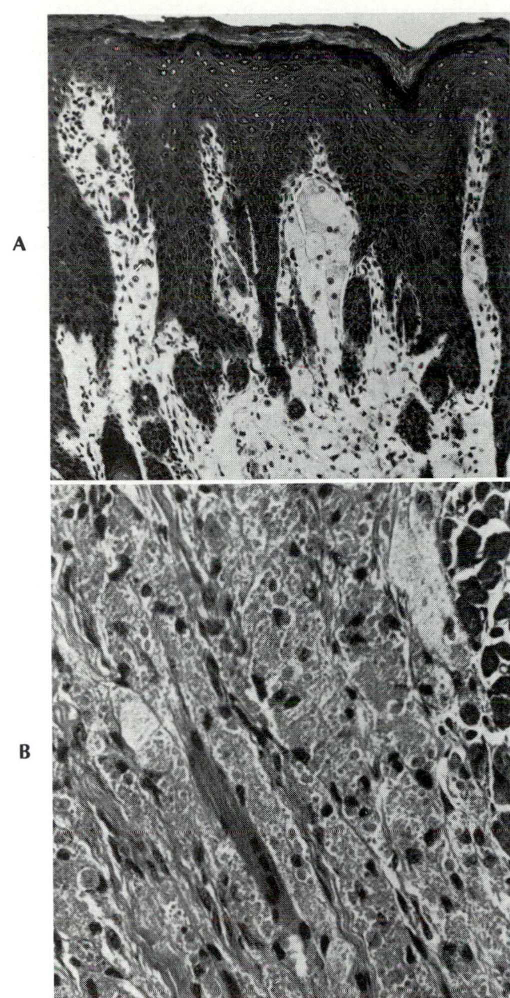

Fig. 25-14. Granular cell tumor (granular cell myoblastoma). Tongue and skin are two most frequent sites. **A,** Pseudoepitheliomatous proliferation may be pronounced, simulating squamous cell carcinoma. **B,** Tumor consists of sheet of large cells with granular eosinophilic cytoplasm and small hyperchromatic nuclei.

blasts, and polymorphonuclear neutrophils, these lesions frequently last long after termination of pregnancy, eventuating in a fibroma-like lesion.[41,48]

Hereditary hemorrhagic telangiectasia (Osler-Rendu-Weber disease). Hereditary hemorrhagic telangiectasia is manifest by numerous spiderlike angiomatoses of the lips and tongue. Nasal mucosal involvement results in frequent epistaxis. Usually noted at puberty, the condition has autosomal dominant inheritance. Microscopically the individual lesion is a superficial blood vessel surrounded by abnormal elastic fibers that permit dilatation.[2,3]

Encephalofacial angiomatosis (Sturge-Weber syndrome). Encephalofacial angiomatosis consists of superficial and deep-seated hemangiomas, usually of the upper two thirds or half of the face, associated with leptomeningeal angiomas, cerebral calcifications, seizures, glaucoma, and mental retardation. There are many clinical variations.[3]

Lymphangioma. The majority of lymphangiomas are found at birth in the head and neck region and may cause enlargement of the tongue (macroglossia) and the lip (macrocheilia). Cystic hygroma is a special type of lymphangioma occurring in the cervical region in the newborn.

Solitary plasmacytoma. Solitary plasmacytoma of the mouth occurs as a soft tissue lesion without bone involvement (especially about the tonsillar area and antrum) or as part of a generalized myeloma. About one third of the cases of solitary plasmacytoma eventuate in multiple myeloma.[102,130] There is a definite predilection for males (about 2:1). Rarely are they seen in individuals under 30 years of age. Grossly they are smooth, soft, and somewhat rubbery tumors. Microscopically they are indistinguishable from plasma cell myeloma. Differential diagnosis includes plasma cell granuloma.[37]

Osteoma and chondroma. Chondroma of the tongue usually occurs in the lateral border.[182] There is no marked sex predilection. Osteoma of the tongue occurs in the posterior dorsum near the foramen cecum.[105] There is a 3:1 female predilection. Peripheral ossifying fibroma is a relatively frequently encountered reactive gingival lesion. Some cases represent burnt-out "pyogenic" granulomas.[10]

Nevi. The intramucosal cellular nevus, pigmented or more often nonpigmented, is the most common nevus to occur on the oral mucosa.[172] Next most frequent is the intraoral blue nevus. Over 65% of the nevi arise in the mucosa of the hard palate, and another 25% in the lips. There does not appear to be a sex predilection. The compound nevus and junctional nevus are both rare.[53,83,89,151]

White lesions of oral mucosa

A change in color of the normally reddish oral mucosa to white constitutes one of the most frequently encountered oral abnormalities. Failure to recognize and identify the cause of this alteration can be a serious omission, since early squamous cell carcinoma may appear white.

The term "leukoplakia" has been used so differently by so many that it has come to signify only a white patch that does not rub away.[176]

Leukoedema. Leukoedema is a slight whitening of oral mucosa without dysplasia or abnormalities of keratinization.[113]

Hyperkeratoses. An increased retention and production of keratin by mucosal stratified squamous epithelium is the most frequent cause of white patches of the oral cavity. This is termed hyperkeratosis and may be associated with chronic mechanical irritation and other factors. Biopsy specimens of oral white patches may demonstrate cytologic and histologic alterations of a degree to warrant considerating the patch as a dysplasia. Specific alterations of dysplastic or "premalignant" character include dyskeratosis, abnormal nuclear shapes and size, and increased numbers of mitotic figures.[171] Most pathologists term such alterations epithelial dysplasia. The red counterpart is called erythroplakia.[146] Microscopic examination of oral white patches that do not resolve with conservative management within a short time (1 to 2 weeks) is indicated.

Snuffbox granuloma is a term denoting the white, leathery, oral patches seen in patients using snuff or intraoral tobacco. Patients using snuff have an increased incidence of oral carcinoma.[178] The microscopic findings are characteristic.[156]

Keratoacanthoma. Keratoacanthoma of the lip (usually the lower lip, with a 5:1 male predilection) appears to arise at the skin-mucosa junction of the lip. It is a painless exophytic crateriform lesion 1 to 2 cm in diameter. Several cutaneous examples have manifested a rapid onset, with a growth period of 6 to 10 weeks followed by spontaneous healing over 4 to 6 months. Most labial examples have been removed entirely and diagnosis has been made on microscopic criteria alone. Average age has been 60 years.[43,82,95]

Few examples of solitary intraoral keratoacanthoma have been documented. They have involved the anterior maxilla or hard palate. One must always be certain that the lesion is not well-differentiated squamous cell carcinoma or verrucous carcinoma, but the examples reviewed by Svirsky, Freedman, and Lumerman[159] seem to fulfill the clinical and microscopic criteria. Perhaps they arose from sebaceous glands.

Eruptive keratoacanthomas may rarely involve the oral mucosa as part of a generalized skin and mucosal dissemination. They heal within 6 to 8 weeks.[10,177]

Squamous acanthoma is a white, flat or elevated, sometimes granular, verrucous, and sessile or pedunculated oral lesion that results from trauma. Most patients are white middle-aged men. Microscopically there are confluence of enlarged rete ridges, mild pseudoepitheliomatous hyperplasia, and hyperorthokeratosis.[36]

Other white lesions. The white oral lesions of lichen planus were discussed previously (Fig. 25-9). Wickham's striae or lacelike patterns in this condition are characteristic. Several hereditary conditions feature whitening of the oral cavity. Hereditary benign intraepithelial dyskeratosis, white sponge nevus (leukokeratosis heredita), pachyonychia congenita, Darier's disease, and dyskeratosis congenita (Zinsser-Engman-Cole syndrome) are examples.[3]

Aspirin burns resulting from the unprescribed use of tablets as dental topical anesthetics or troches frequently are seen. Soft, focal, oral whitenings that peel away easily, leaving a raw, bleeding surface, occur in candidiasis.

Malignant tumors of oral cavity

Squamous cell carcinoma. Squamous cell carcinoma (epidermoid carcinoma) is the most common oral malignant neoplasm, and approximately 2% of deaths in the United States are currently attributed to it annually. Investigations in Minnesota indicated that among adults 45 years of age or older, 1 in every 1000 examined had this lesion of the lip or other oral structure.[168] Tobacco, whether smoked or in the form of snuff, and alcohol have been etiologically implicated for many years.[152] Chronic inflammation caused by poorly fitting prostheses, poor oral hygiene, or inadequate dental restorations probably is not an important etiologic factor. Approximately 10% of patients who have or have had an oral carcinoma will have another. Oral white patches are observed in association with squamous cell carcinoma in up to 75% of instances, and it is likely that many superficial malignancies evolve in this fashion.[160]

The clinical appearance of small or early examples of the malignancy may vary from white, thickened, or verrucous to soft, red, velvety, or ulcerative. Induration is also clinically suggestive of oral malignancy.

Squamous cell carcinomas of the lip or oral cavity generally are histologically well differentiated and occur most often in men 40 years of age or older.[104] The oral cavity offers epithelial neoplasms with as great a clinicopathologic diversity as any body part; however, metastasis most frequently occurs first in ipsilateral, submandibular, or cervical lymph nodes. The presence or absence of lymph node metastasis is an important index of the clinical stage of the disease. A sarcoidal reaction may be seen in regional cervical lymph nodes in perhaps 6% of cases of carcinoma of the tongue, parotid gland, and oral cavity, especially after radiotherapy, probably as a result of the necrotic products of the tumor.

Squamous cell carcinoma of lip. Squamous cell carcinoma of the lip is almost exclusively a male disease, with less than 3% of the cases occurring in women. It is rare in blacks. It originates most frequently in the sixth to eighth decades. Approximately 90% arise on the vermilion border of the lower lip, usually on one side of the midline. It appears as a painless, characteristically indurated, ulcerated or exophytic lesion. Usually, lip carcinoma is well differentiated (about 60%) and slow to metastasize to the submental and submandibular nodes. Prognosis is good whether the lesion is treated by radiation or by surgery, 5-year cure rates being about equal (80%). Carcinoma of the lip is more common in individuals of light complexion, especially those who, because of their occupation, receive an unusual amount of actinic radiation, such as farmers, sailors, and policemen. Some doubt has recently been expressed concerning the importance of the role of actinic radiation. About 6% have multiple lip carcinomas, either simultaneously or at intervals. Over 10% have at least one cancer of the skin, and over 3% have an oral, pharyngeal, laryngeal, or esophageal carcinoma.[170]

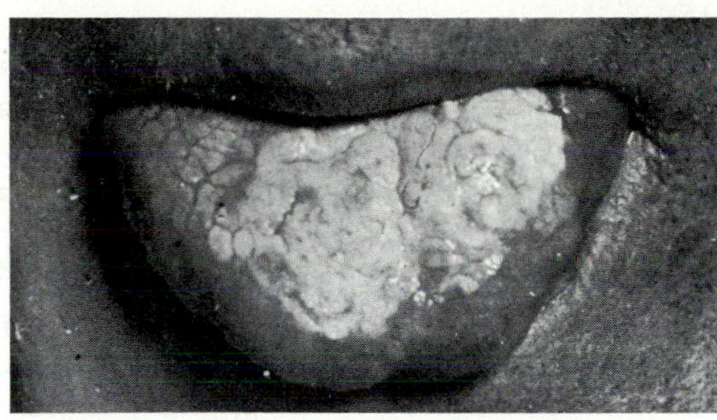

Fig. 25-15. Leathery and warty whitening (leukoplakia) of tongue associated with carcinoma of low-grade malignancy.

Early or premalignant alterations of lip epithelium appear as localized keratotic plaques that may resolve, only to reappear. Alternatively, malignant degeneration is indicated by diffuse, thin whitening of superficial portions of the vermilion border of the lip.

Squamous cell carcinoma of tongue. Squamous cell carcinoma of the tongue is the most frequent intraoral malignant lesion, comprising about half of the cases.[175] It is largely (about 85%) a male disease. Approximately 80% of the cases arise in the sixth to eighth decades. In Scandinavia, however, the disease is not rare in women and commonly is associated with Plummer-Vinson syndrome (atrophy of mucous membrane, iron deficency anemia, and dysphagia). The positive correlation between carcinoma of the tongue, especially of the dorsal surface, and syphilitic glossitis appears to be less significant than formerly supposed (Fig. 25-15).

The lateral border and ventral surfaces of the tongue are frequent sites of carcinoma (about 65%). Metastases, frequently bilateral (about 20%), are present in about 35% of the patients at the time of hospital admission. Contralateral metastasis occurs in less than 3%.

Survival figures indicate that the prognosis for patients with squamous cell carcinoma of the tongue is dependent on several factors. The small, early lesion of low-grade malignancy without evidence of metastasis or conspicuous local invasion may be successfully managed by surgery or radiotherapy. Approximately 60% of such patients live 5 years or more. This figure is reduced to 30% in instances where the tumor is anaplastic or has metastasized.[77]

Squamous cell carcinoma of floor of mouth. Squamous cell carcinoma of the floor of the mouth (about 15% of oral cases) is typically manifest as an indurated ulcer in the anterior portion about the openings of the sublingual and submandibular glands, with over 80% occurring in males.[45,101,123] The carcinoma invades rapidly, spreading to the submandibular lymph nodes (about 50%) and to the submandibular and sublingual salivary glands, tongue, and mandibular gingiva. The survival rate is about 70% with localized disease. If regional nodes are involved, this is reduced to about 25%. Although white patches are observed throughout the oral cavity in a variety of clinical circumstances, the white patch on the mouth floor, however subtle, should be thoroughly investigated. Early squamous cell carcinoma of the area may be overlooked if this is not done.

Squamous cell carcinoma of buccal mucosa. Squamous cell carcinoma of the buccal mucosa constitutes from one fourth to one third of all oral carcinomas. There is a male predilection. The peak incidence is at 60 to 70 years. The posterior part of the buccal mucosa is the area most commonly involved.[62] The disease varies in frequency in different geographic areas. In India and other countries in which betel nut and tobacco chewing are commonplace, buccal carcinomas are the major cancer. Abnormal keratinization is especially common in this group. Oral submucous fibrosis may be another premalignant mucosal alteration of the buccal mucosa. Progressive infiltrative growth, local recurrence after treatment, and local lymph node metastasis characterize squamous cell carcinoma originating in the cheeks. The 5-year survival figures vary, but approximately 40% of affected patients survive this period after diagnosis and adequate surgical treatment or radiotherapy. Patients rarely die of complications associated with distant metastasis. Rather, malnutrition, asphyxia, or pneumonia complicates local tumor growth and leads to death.

Squamous cell carcinoma of gingiva. Squamous cell carcinoma of the gingiva constitutes about 10% of oral malignancy and is more common in men than in women (about 2:1). It occurs most commonly on the mandibular gingiva, and its early clinical resemblance to more common inflammatory conditions in this location may lead to delayed diagnosis. Tobacco and syphilis are less clearly related etiologically to gingival carcinoma than to carcinomas of the tongue or cheek. Early involvement of contiguous structures, such as bone and lymph nodes, characterizes the tumor. The 5-year survival rate is about 35%.[57,107]

Squamous cell carcinoma of palate. Squamous cell carcinoma of the palate may be ulcerative or tumorous or both. The tumors are more often well differentiated and occur somewhat more frequently in men than in women. Although the lesions often are symptomless, patients may complain of a dental prosthesis that has become ill fitting. Pain may be a late clinical feature. Early involvement of underlying bone is a common feature. The soft palate is the more frequent site. Extension occurs most often to the tonsillar area. The 5-year survival rates range from about 50% with highly differentiated lesions to 25% with poorly differentiated ones.[73,135,143]

Verrucous carcinoma. An unusual form of epidermoid carcinoma most frequently involving the buccal mucosa and mandibular gingiva is verrucous carcinoma. It appears to be synonymous with oral florid papillomatosis. In the United States, in the middle South, it is commonly associated with the prolonged use of snuff placed in the gingivobuccal sulcus. It is characteristically associated with leukoplakia, growing into large, fungating, soft, papillary masses. Microscopic diagnosis may be difficult and delayed, for the tumor presents an unusually well-differentiated pattern. Multiple foci of atypical squamous epithelium may be noted in parts of the mucosa not involved by neoplasm. Although destruction may be extensive and recurrence frequent (about 75%), metastasis is unusual. Patients are especially prone to develop additional, sometimes less differentiated, oral carcinomas, especially after radiotherapy.[78,114,144]

Adenoid squamous cell carcinoma. Adenoid squamous cell carcinoma is an unusual variant of squamous cell carcinoma. Most examples have come from the head and neck. A few dozen cases have involved the vermilion of the lower lip, rarely the upper lip. Most of the patients were middle-aged to older men. None developed regional lymph node spread, but almost 40% had local recurrence. Presumably the lesion is preceded by solar keratosis with acantholysis. Characteristic microscopic changes include downward proliferation, with the deeper islands of tumor cells exhibiting adenoid or tubular configuration. The ductlike structures are lined with cuboidal cells, usually two layers thick. In the central portion the tumor masses exhibit acantholysis, shedding desquamated keratinized cells into the lumen. The adjacent stroma usually hosts a dense lymphocytic infiltrate.[97,162]

Spindle cell carcinoma (pseudosarcoma, carcinosarcoma). Spindle cell carcinoma occasionally is associated with an intramucosal or in situ squamous cell carcinoma of the mouth, oropharynx, or upper respiratory or alimentary tract. Bizarre, sarcoma-like proliferation of neoplastic cells results in bulky polypoid masses that may only faintly resemble carcinoma. In the mouth the lower lip, tongue, and alveolar ridge are most often involved. There probably is no sex predilection. Most of the patients have been in their sixth or seventh decade, female patients being somewhat older. The 5-year survival rate is about 35%.[70,96,109,157]

Carcinoma in situ. An occasional oral carcinoma, regardless of location, may demonstrate all cytologic features of malignant neoplasia yet fail to show any histologic evidence of invasion. The term *carcinoma in situ* has been used in this case. Considerable variability in the clinical appearance of carcinoma in situ has been noted. They may be white, red, or a mixture. The terms *bowenoid* (see Bowen's disease of skin, p. 1610), *erythroplastic* (see erythroplasia of Queyrat, pp. 814 and 1611), and *leukoplakia-like* are used to describe the variable clinical appearance. High-risk sites are the oral floor, tongue, and lips.[145,146]

Lymphoepithelial carcinoma. Lymphoepithelial carcinoma may be found in the faucial area and base of the tongue, as well as in the nasopharynx and nasal cavity. Since the primary lesion is frequently small and undiscovered, the first clinical sign is often regional adenopathy and dysphagia. The "lymphoepithelioma" consists of syncytial masses of large polyhedral cells with eosinophilic cytoplasm, a large nucleus, large eosinophilic nucleoli, and a stroma infiltrated by numerous small lymphocytes (Regaud type of lymphoepithelial carcinoma). The cells of the "transitional cell carcinoma" are large, poorly differentiated, and anaplastic (Schmincke type of lymphoepithelial carcinoma). Radiotherapy is employed for both neoplasms, with the survival rate approaching 30%.

Rhabdomyosarcoma. There are many forms of rhabdomyosarcoma, each of which represents some degree of mimicking of the developmental stage of skeletal muscle in its embryonal development, from a small primitive round cell to a spindle cell form to a multinucleate muscle fiber with characteristic striations.[1,4] The most differentiated is the pleomorphic rhabdomyosarcoma.[44,66] It is most often recognized because it contains numerous cells manifesting cross striations. Embryonal rhabdomyosarcoma mimics developing muscle in the 7- to 10-week fetus.[79] Round and spindle cells of small to moderate size having scant cytoplasm may erroneously lead to the diagnosis of lymphosarcoma, neuroblastoma, or retinoblastoma. However, careful examination of sections often reveals alveolar arrangement of rhabdomyoblasts or cells having a spindle form. The nucleus is elongated or ovoid, and bipolar cytoplasmic processes may be noted in which fibrils or even cross striations are present. Not uncommonly the cells are loosely arranged. Alveolar rhabdomyosarcoma, the name derived from the characteristic arrangement of its cells, produces an adenocarcinoma-like or pseudoglandular appearance.[74] The alveolar spaces contain lining cells that do not form a continuous surface but are irregularly spaced. Any one rhabdomyosarcoma commonly contains more than one of the patterns mentioned.

In children rhabdomyosarcoma occurs especially in the head and neck, the soft tissues of the neck, tongue, and palate being frequently involved. The tumor usually appears in this region during the first decade of life. At least half of the children are under 6 years of age. Rarely, congenital rhabdomyosarcomas have been reported. Histologically the embryonal or botryoid embryonal form is the most common type involving the oral mucous membrane. Rhabdomyosarcomas of the tongue have usually been of the adult pleomorphic type. The alveolar rhabdomyosarcoma is the least common form.

The 5-year survival rate for oral rhabdomyosarcoma is very poor, less than 10%. The 10-year survival rate is probably only 5%. Metastasis may occur by either blood or lymphatic spread.

Primary malignant melanoma. Primary malignant melanoma of the oral cavity constitutes only about 2% of all melanomas. There is no sex predilection. The peak incidence is in the sixth decade. Seldom has a case been reported in anyone under 20 years of age. Approximately 80% arise in the hard palate, alveolar ridge, or soft palate. Metastatic spread is common. The 5-year survival rate is less than 5%.[58,65,72,164]

Other malignant tumors. Kaposi sarcoma, liposarcoma, and alveolar soft tissue sarcoma have been reported but are uncommon. Kaposi sarcoma occurs in acquired immune deficiency syndrome (AIDS) and in other immunosuppressed states.[112a] Leukemic infiltration of the gingiva is frequently seen in affected patients.

JAWS

Developmental lesions

Exostoses (tori). Exostoses or bony protuberances are not uncommon about the mouth. The most frequent is torus palatinus, which occurs in the midline of the hard palate in about 25% of females and in 15% of males. Torus mandibularis is less frequent (about 7% of the population), generally bilateral (80%), and found on the lingual surface of the mandible, usually opposite the premolars.[237,270] Multiple exostoses are still less common and occur as small nodular outgrowths on the buccal surface of the maxilla and mandible, opposite the premolars and molars.[192]

Osteomatosis. Osteomatosis may be associated with polyposis and adenocarcinoma of the colon and multiple cutaneous and mesenteric fibromas and lipomas (Gardner's syndrome). Epidermoid inclusion cysts are scattered over the body. The syndrome is transmitted as an autosomal dominant trait.[205,241] Microscopically the bony growths consist of dense, irregular bone with well-marked haversian systems and fibrous medullary portions.

Melanotic neuroectodermal tumor of infancy. A tumor of the jaws, the melanotic neuroectodermal tumor, is a rare benign lesion of neural crest origin, largely restricted to the maxilla of infants.[194,245] At time of discovery of the tumor, the infant is nearly always under 6 months of age. There is no sex predilection. The local recurrence rate is about 15%. A few similar tumors have been reported in the shoulder, epididymis, mandible, calvaria, brain, and mediastinum. Borello and Gorlin[196] have demonstrated that a tumor elaborated vanillylmandelic acid, and neural crest origin appeared likely. Ultrastructural evidence supports this view.[227]

Grossly the tumor is often pigmented and well circumscribed, although no well-defined capsule is present. Microscopically the tumor consists of a fibrous connective tissue stroma in which tubules or spaces are present in large numbers (Fig. 25-16). The spaces are lined by a single layer of large cuboid cells with abundant cytoplasm in which are found numerous melanin granules. The spaces frequently are filled with many deeply staining neuroblast-like cells that are smaller than the duct cells and contain much less cytoplasm.

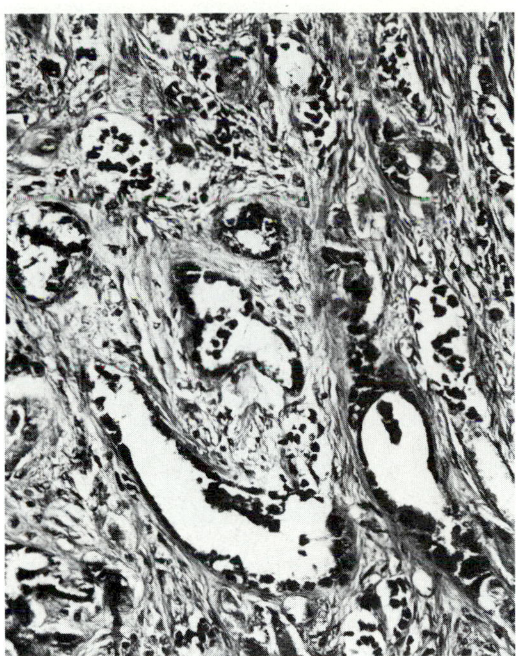

Fig. 25-16. Pigmented neuroectodermal tumor of infancy. This choristomatous lesion is composed of numerous tubules in fibrous connective tissue stroma. Tubules lined by large cuboid cells contain melanin. Within lumina are cells resembling neuroblasts.

Inflammatory and metabolic lesions

Acute suppurative osteomyelitis. Acute suppurative osteomyelitis of the jaws has become a relatively rare disease with the advent of antibiotics.[243,260] Usually because of infection of the marrow cavity with *Staphylococcus aureus* subsequent to jaw fracture or severe periapical disease, the process spreads, especially in the lower jaw, causing severe pain and facial cellulitis. When the resistance of the host is high or the virulence of the organism low, a chronic focal sclerosing osteomyelitis or condensing osteitis is seen.

Osteomyelitis of jaw of newborn infants. A distinct clinical entity, osteomyelitis of the jaw of the newborn infant almost exclusively involves the upper jaw.[257]

Garré's chronic sclerosing osteomyelitis with proliferative periosteitis. Garré's chronic sclerosing osteomyelitis with proliferative periosteitis is a nonsuppurating type seen most often in the lower jaw in children and young adults. There may be a slight female predilection. The usual inciting factor is an abscessed mandibular first permanent molar. Histopathologic changes consist of supracortical but subperiosteal proliferation of reactive new bone with prominent osteoblastic rimming. Associated fibrous connective tissues are variably infiltrated with chronic inflammatory cells.[211,242]

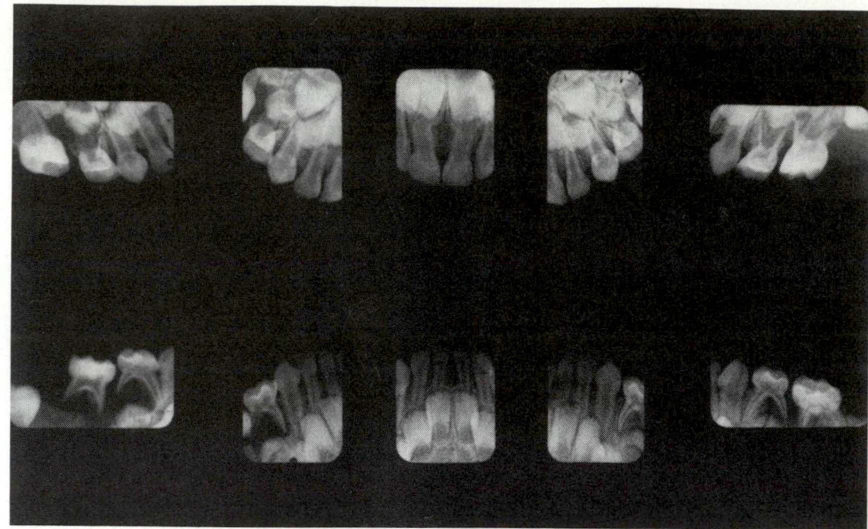

Fig. 25-17. Dental radiographs from patient with histiocytosis X. Molars appear to float in areas of bone loss.

Infantile cortical hyperostosis (Caffey's disease). Infantile cortical hyperostosis appears in infants, usually within the first 3 months of life, as a bilateral cortical thickening of the mandible.[193,214]

Osteoradionecrosis of the jaws. Osteoradionecrosis of the jaws, principally affecting the mandible, occurs after extensive therapeutic radiation in about 5% of patients. The severity seems to be proportional to the radiation dose, the presence of periodontal sepsis, the susceptibility of the host, and especially the presence of open mucosal wounds. When a patient is dentally healthy, there appears to be a low risk for osteoradionecrosis.[251]

Osteitis deformans (Paget's disease of bone). Osteitis deformans may involve the jaws, especially the maxilla, with progressive enlargement and displacement of teeth as part of the generalized disease.[233,250] This becomes especially apparent if the patient wears dentures. True giant cell tumors of the jaws or osteosarcoma may occasionally arise in Paget bone.[232,248]

Histiocytosis X (Letterer-Siwe disease, Hand-Schüller-Christian disease, eosinophilic granuloma). In histiocytosis X the jaws are sites of deposits of foamy histiocytes. It has been reported that 93% of patients had sore, swollen necrotic gingivae and 78% had loose, sore teeth that rapidly exfoliated (Fig. 25-17). The premolar-molar region of the mandible is more frequently involved than the maxilla. Loss of trabeculae, pseudocyst formation, and dental root resorption are typical radiographic findings.[226,264]

Giant cell granuloma. Giant cell "reparative" granuloma is a nonneoplastic lesion of unknown etiology that appears to be limited to the jaws.[185,186,218,239,267] Treatment consists of simple excision and curettage. Although resembling true giant cell tumor of bone, giant cell granuloma has certain properties and microscopic characteristics that separate it as a distinct entity. It constitutes about 3% of benign jaw tumors. It is found either centrally or peripherally, being about equally distributed. It is more common in the mandible (anterior to molars) and in females (2:1). Over 65% of the patients are less than 30 years of age. The radiographic appearance is not pathognomonic, being solitary, unilocular (70%), radiolucent, and sharply delineated. The lamina dura may be displaced but rarely are the cortical plates perforated. Grossly the tissue is usually reddish brown or black, depending on the amount of hemorrhage. Not uncommonly the surface is eroded or ulcerated.

Microscopically the giant cell granuloma consists of an admixture of multinucleated giant cells scattered in a very cellular stroma from which the giant cells probably are derived (Fig. 25-18). The stromal cell has a round or oval nucleus, small nucleolus, prominent nuclear membrane, and poorly delineated cytoplasmic boundaries. Nuclear pleomorphism, hyperchromatism, and increased mitotic activity are characteristically absent. Hemosiderin pigment, evidence of old hemorrhage, often is seen lying free or ingested by mononuclear phagocytes. Collagen production is quite common, whereas osteoid is present less often, and both are nearly always absent from the true giant cell tumor.

Microscopic differentiation should include true giant cell tumor (extremely rare in the jaws), cherubism, fibrous dysplasia, and aneurysmal bone cyst. The lesions of hyperparathyroidism, both primary and secondary, cannot be differentiated on a microscopic basis from central giant cell granuloma, and blood and urinary calcium levels always should be determined in the case of recurrence or multiple or satellite lesions.[235] Also suggestive

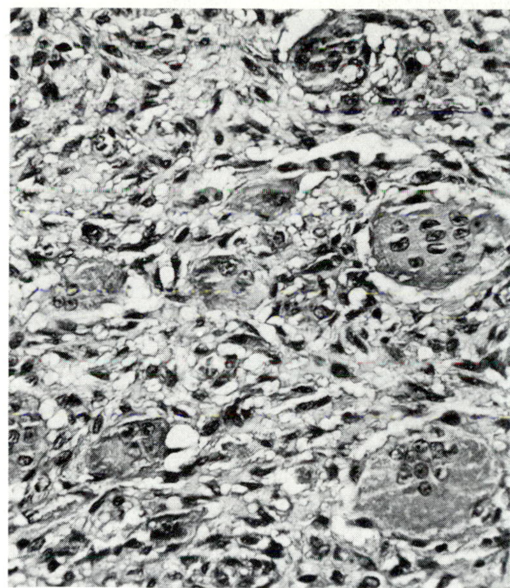

Fig. 25-18. Giant cell granuloma. Lesion is characterized by numerous multinucleated giant cells in fibrous cellular stroma from which giant cells are derived. Collagen, osteoid, or bone is formed.

of hyperparathyroidism is disappearance of the lamina dura about the teeth, but this is less common than is generally believed.

Tumors and tumorlike lesions

Fibro-osseous lesions. The term "benign fibro-osseous lesion" has been a catchall to include a wide variety of lesions: various forms of cementoma (discussed later), ossifying fibroma, cementifying fibroma, central fibroma, desmoplastic fibroma, and even fibrous dysplasia. The indiscriminate use of this term serves little purpose.[209,223,276] The clinician should be encouraged to provide the pathologist with all available information to aid in the specific diagnosis.

Fibrous dysplasia. The jaws may be involved in fibrous dysplasia of the monostotic or polyostotic types.[210,277] The monostotic form is the more common and seems to be more frequent in children and young adults. Clinically it is manifested by a painless swelling of the bone. Displacement of teeth may be present. Polyostotic fibrous dysplasia, in addition to manifestation in several or many bones, may be accompanied by melanotic pigmentation of the skin and oral mucosa and endocrine disturbances, including precocious puberty in girls (Albright's syndrome).[3]

Cherubism. Cherubism is an autosomal dominant disease essentially limited to the jawbones. It has been imprecisely referred to as familial fibrous dysplasia. This condition is characterized by bilateral enlargement of the jaws usually during the second or third year of life, especially in the mandibular molar and retromolar areas. Bony expansion increases for a few years and then tapers off, usually regressing by 20 years of age. If the maxilla is severely involved, a rim of sclera is exposed, giving rise to the cherubic facies.[275,278]

Microscopically the bony lesion consists of vascular and usually collagenic fibrous connective tissue, having an abundant admixture of perivascular osteoclastic giant cells. Not uncommonly fibrin is deposited around small capillaries. In rare cases the lesion cannot be differentiated from giant cell granuloma.

Malignant tumors metastatic to jaws. Malignant tumors metastatic to the jaws are uncommon; spread probably takes place through the vertebral system of veins. In a survey of 150 cases, there was an indication of the following order of frequency: carcinoma of breast, lung, kidney, large intestine, thyroid gland, prostate, and stomach.[188]

The tooth-bearing area of the body and the molar regions of the mandible are the most frequent sites, possibly because of greater arterial blood supply in these regions. In about half the cases, the oral metastasis is the first sign of the generalized cancer. Swelling, pain, and anesthesia are the most common symptoms (Fig. 25-19).

Osteosarcoma (osteogenic sarcoma). Approximately 10% of osteosarcomas occur in the jaws. The upper and lower jaws are equally involved, and there is no sex predilection. The 5-year survival rate is about 35%. Accessibility, which makes early treatment possible, and greater histopathologic differentiation likely contribute to the relatively more favorable prognosis of this malignant tumor in oral sites.[207,244] Some oral examples have arisen in Paget's disease or in fibrous dysplastic lesions that have been irradiated. The rare juxtacortical form has also been reported in the jaws.[199]

Chondrosarcoma. Less frequently encountered in the jaws than osteosarcoma, chondrosarcoma is also less aggressive. It usually does not metastasize but recurs and spreads locally. The 5-year survival rate is about 40%. The maxilla is more frequently involved than the mandible. Microscopically, chondrosarcoma and osteosarcoma may appear benign early in their development. Although both these entities may contain bone and cartilage, only the neoplastic cells of osteosarcoma produce osteoid.[189]

Mesenchymal chondrosarcoma is a rare tumor that sometimes occurs in facial bones. The tumor may involve soft tissue as well as bone. It occurs most commonly in the second and third decades of life. There is probably neither sex nor age predilection. The recurrence rate is approximately 50%. Microscopically the tumor is characterized by highly undifferentiated small round or oval cells coexisting with islands of well-differentiated cartilage, which in turn may exhibit calcification or metaplastic bone formation. The small cells often manifest an

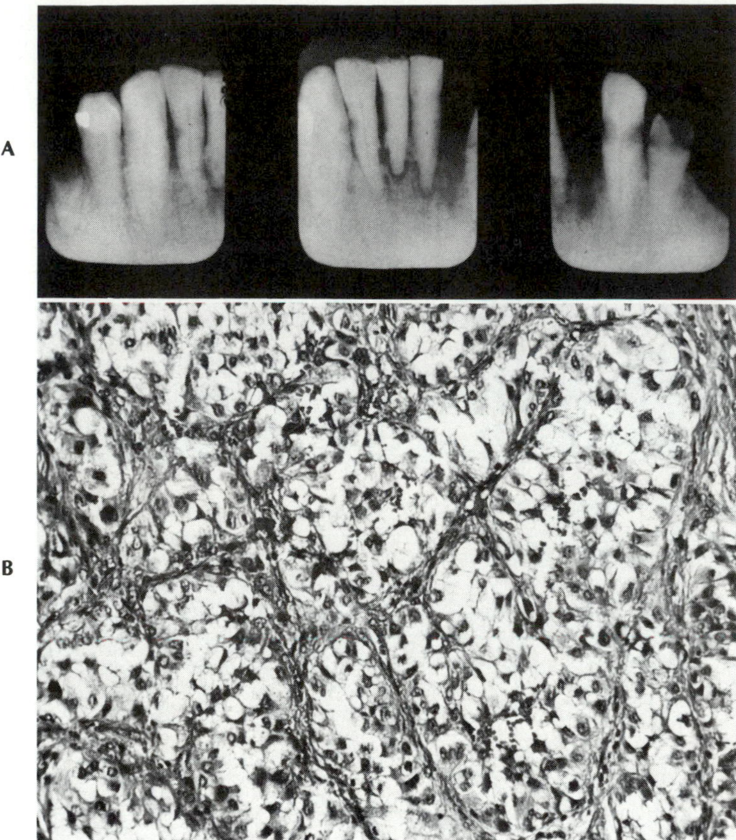

Fig. 25-19. Clinical radiographic, **A,** and histologic, **B,** appearance of metastatic adenocarcinoma of kidney. Similarity to inflammatory conditions of dental tissue in radiograph may be striking.

alveolar or a hemangiopericytoma-like organoid pattern.[261]

Fibrosarcoma. About 10% of fibrosarcomas arise in the jaws. They may originate in periosteal or central locations. The mandible is three times as often affected as the maxilla. Histopathologic interpretation and diagnosis are complicated by the numerous other fibrous or spindle cell neoplasms observed in the jawbones.[262]

Multiple myeloma and Ewing's sarcoma. In about 30% of cases of multiple myeloma there are associated jaw lesions.[291] In 15% of these cases the jaw lesion is the primary manifestation. Perhaps 10% of patients with multiple myeloma have amyloidosis, and some of these have macroglossia. Another oral manifestation is solitary plasmacytoma. Ewing's sarcoma may be initially manifest as a lesion of the jaws.[188a] Usually, jaw involvement is merely a part of the generalized disease.[204]

Malignant lymphoma. In contrast to most other primary malignancies of the jawbones, malignant lymphomas of the jaws occur more frequently in the maxilla.

Burkitt's lymphoma. There are two forms of Burkitt's lymphoma, African and American. An undifferentiated lymphosarcoma, the African Burkitt's lymphoma, has been described in the jaws (50% to 75%) and abdominal viscera of equatorial African children from 3 to 10 years of age (mean, 7 years), constituting about half of all malignant tumors in this age group.[252] There is a male predilection. Arising most often in the maxillary alveolar process, it produces gross distortion of the maxilla, mandible, and orbital areas.[240] It is destructive, effecting loss of deciduous molars. The process extends to involve the parotid gland, antrum, nasopharynx, and orbit. Rarely is there associated lymph node involvement. Abdominal involvement is common in older patients.

American Burkitt's lymphoma involves the jaws in only 5% of cases, and these are often older individuals. The mean age for this form to appear is about 11 years. In contrast to the African form, associated lymphadenopathy is common. Evidence suggests that the Epstein-Barr virus is usually immunologically associated with the African Burkitt's tumor but not with the American form.[183,190] Histologically there is no difference between the African and American forms.

Cysts

Cysts of the jaws and mouth usually are classified according to their odontogenic or nonodontogenic origin. However, a number of oral lesions called "cysts" on clinical or radiographic evidence alone do not fall within the definition of a pathologic, epithelium-lined cavity containing fluid or debris. The salivary gland retention cyst (mucocele), traumatic bone cyst, and static bone cyst are not epithelium lined. The following is a classification of cysts[10]:

A. Odontogenic cysts
   1. Dentigerous cyst
   2. Eruption cyst
   3. Gingival cyst of the newborn
   4. Lateral periodontal cyst and gingival cyst of the adult
   5. Keratinizing and calcifying odontogenic cyst (cystic keratinizing tumor)
   6. Radicular (periapical) cyst
   7. Odontogenic keratocysts
      a. Solitary (primordial) cyst
      b. Multiple keratocysts of jaws and nevoid basal cell carcinoma syndrome
B. Nonodontogenic and fissural cysts
   1. Nasoalveolar (nasolabial, Klestadt) cyst
   2. Nasopalatine (median anterior maxillary) cyst
   3. Anterior lingual cyst
   4. Dermoid and epidermoid cysts
   5. Palatal cyst of newborn infants
C. Cysts of neck, oral floor, and salivary glands
   1. Thyroglossal duct cyst
   2. Parathyroid cyst
   3. Thymic cyst
   4. Lymphoepithelial ("branchial cleft") cyst
   5. Oral cysts with gastric or intestinal epithelium
   6. Salivary gland cyst
   7. Mucocele and ranula
D. Pseudocysts of jaws
   1. Aneurysmal bone cyst
   2. Static (developmental, latent) bone cyst
   3. "Traumatic" (hemorrhagic, solitary) bone cyst

Odontogenic cyst

Periodontal cyst. The most common odontogenic cyst is the periodontal cyst. Most often it is observed at the apex of an erupted tooth (radicular type).[200] The origin of this cyst appears to be in the cystic degeneration of epithelialized granulomas that have resulted most frequently as sequelae to dental caries and pulpitis. The origin of the stratified squamous epithelium lining these cysts is the epithelial rests of Malassez, which lie in the periodontal ligament. They are derived from the Hertwig's root sheath. The walls of smaller cysts usually are infiltrated with chronic inflammatory cells.

Gingival cyst. Gingival cysts of the newborn, which are multiple as a rule, occur in the anterior jaws of infants and children.[255] They rupture and disappear within the first few weeks of life. They represent cystic degeneration of remnants of the dental lamina. Those situated on the lateral surface of the root of erupted teeth, usually mandibular premolars, have been called lateral periodontal cyst[281] and gingival cyst of the adult.[202] The latter involves soft tissue only, whereas the former is intrabony.

Dentigerous cyst. Cyst formation may be associated with unerupted teeth and originates from epithelium of the dental lamina or dental organ. The mandibular third molars and maxillary canines are most often involved. This cyst has significance because of the occasional massive resorption of involved jawbone that results from its unhampered expansion. Whereas the incidence of ameloblastomatous transformation within dentigerous cysts has not been precisely determined, the fact that such transformation does occur, further that ameloblastomas may appear cystic, and, finally, that histopathologic examination is required for these determinations render pathologic examination of such material prudent.[10] Carcinoma arising in dentigerous cysts has also been observed.[201]

Eruption cyst. A special type, occasionally bilateral, that does not involve bone, the eruption cyst is seen rarely in the gingiva overlying erupting deciduous canines or molars.[266]

Odontogenic keratocyst. Multiple odontogenic keratocysts of the jaws may be associated in the nevoid basal cell carcinoma syndrome, which has autosomal dominant inheritance.[208,221,258] Lamellar calcification of the dura is common. Various skeletal anomalies include splayed or bifid ribs and scoliosis. Medulloblastoma and bilateral calcified ovarian fibromas also may be part of the syndrome. Odontogenic keratocysts are often observed unassociated with the syndrome.[197] The recurrence rate is about 50%.

Keratinizing and calcifying odontogenic cyst. This odontogenic cyst (Fig. 25-20) is characterized by masses of "ghosts" or aberrantly keratinized epithelium intermixed with the cells lining the cystic cavity.[187] In about 35% of the cases a nontubular dentinoid substance has been noted in the connective tissue wall. About 25% of these cysts occur extraosseously. They should *not* be mistaken for ameloblastoma.

Nonodontogenic cysts

As the name implies, nonodontogenic cysts are not derived from the tissues of the developing tooth. Many have been classified as fissural or inclusion cysts, since they are believed to have their origin in epithelial rests in bone resulting from fusion of two or more embryologic processes.

Median anterior maxillary cyst (nasopalatine duct cyst, incisive canal cyst, cyst of palatine papilla). The most common nonodontogenic cyst is the median maxillary cyst, which arises from the epithelial remnants of the nasopalatine duct. It often is discovered in routine dental

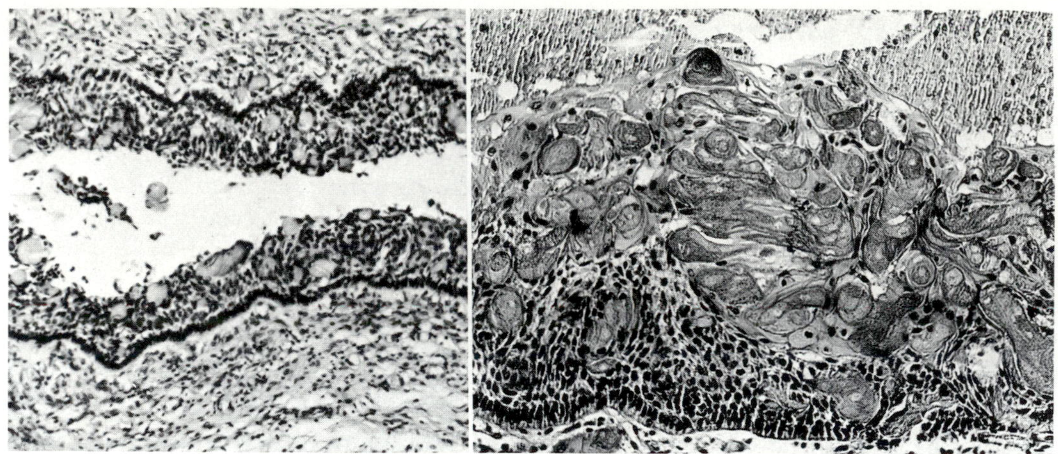

Fig. 25-20. Keratinizing and calcifying odontogenic cyst. Note pronounced basal layer with palisaded cells and large masses of partially keratinized "ghost" cells.

radiographs. It lies above and midway between the roots of the maxillary central incisors but may extend posteriorly.[184]

Globulomaxillary cyst. So-called globulomaxillary cyst has been described as intraosseous and located between the maxillary lateral incisor and canine; however, there is no reason to believe in its existence.[229] Nearly all examples are odontogenic keratocysts.

Nasoalveolar (nasolabial) and dermoid cysts. In contrast to the intraosseous cysts just mentioned, the nasoalveolar cyst and dermoid cyst are formed within soft tissue. The nasoalveolar cyst is formed at the junction of the median nasal, lateral nasal, and maxillary processes, being located at the ala of the nose and frequently extending into the nostril.[234] The dermoid cyst is especially common in the head and neck, with the floor of the mouth being the principal site. Dermoid cysts probably are derived from formation of enclaves of epithelial debris in the midline during closure of mandibular and other branchial arches.[253]

• • •

From the practical standpoint, few cysts of the jaws can be differentiated from one another on microscopic basis alone. Generally, radiographic evidence and further information such as history, clinical appearance, and evidence derived from tooth vitality tests are necessary to establish a definite diagnosis. However, the following hints may help. Gingival, periodontal, dentigerous, and fissural (nasopalatine, nasoalveolar, and so on) cysts usually are lined by nonkeratinizing, stratified squamous epithelium overlying dense fibrous connective tissue. The dermoid cyst, on the other hand, is lined by a keratinized stratified squamous epithelium plus skin appendages. The radicular, periodontal, and fissural cysts commonly show secondary chronic inflammatory infiltrate especially rich in plasma cells. This is seen far less frequently in dentigerous or gingival cysts. Fissural cysts of the maxilla not uncommonly are lined by ciliated columnar epithelium, at least in their superior part. The odontogenic keratocyst is lined by a thin layer of keratinized or parakeratinized epithelium. Mucous glands and congeries of blood vessels and nerves frequently are noted in the connective tissue wall of the nasopalatine cyst. The mandibular dentigerous cyst occasionally may be lined in part by goblet cells or have lymphoid follicles or epithelial cell rests beneath the lining in the cyst wall. These proliferated rests of Malassez are responsible occasionally for an incorrect diagnosis of ameloblastoma.

Traumatic bone cyst (solitary or unicameral bone cyst). The traumatic bone cyst is not a true cyst, nor does it have traumatic origin.[191] It is not lined by epithelium but by a thin membrane of connective tissue. Usually, no content is found other than a small amount of blood, serum, or granulation tissue laden with hemosiderin, macrophages, and a few foreign body giant cells.[191]

Static or latent bone cyst (Stafne's cyst). The static or latent bone cyst is not a cyst but is a developmental defect usually containing salivary gland tissue.[195] It is located on the inferior surface of the mandible just in front of the angle. It occurs in 1 in 250 persons.

Gastric or intestinal epithelium–lined cyst. The gastric or intestinal epithelium–lined cyst is rare. It has been observed almost exclusively in males. The most common location is in the anterior portion of the oral floor or body of the tongue. It corresponds to developmental abnormalities (duplications) seen elsewhere in the gastrointestinal tract.[220,225]

Odontogenic tumors

Odontogenic tumors of the jaws arising from tooth-forming tissues are uncommon. There has been an interest in them, however, and classifications have been relatively numerous since that of Broca in 1867. Since there is a certain necessary complexity, the World Health Organization adopted a classification that allows for evaluation of the numerous transition forms. The interested reader is referred to this work[11] and that of Vickers and Gorlin[10] and of others[219,268] for a comprehensive discussion of the subject.

The abbreviated classification that follows presents odontogenic tumors in a fashion that attempts simplification without sacrifice of histogenetic considerations. Moreover, it emphasizes clinical behavior in the traditional manner.

1. Benign
   a. Ameloblastoma
   b. Odontogenic adenomatoid tumor
   c. Calcifying epithelial odontogenic tumor
   d. Ameloblastic fibroma
   e. Odontomas
   f. Cementomas
   g. Myxoma/myxofibroma
2. Malignant
   a. Ameloblastic carcinoma (malignant ameloblastoma)
   b. Ameloblastic fibrosarcoma

Ameloblastoma. Ameloblastoma is the most common of epithelial odontogenic tumors. It is comparatively uncommon, reportedly comprising about 1% of tumors and cysts arising in the jaws. It may arise from the epithelial lining of a dentigerous cyst, the remnants of dental lamina and enamel organ, or the basal layer of the oral mucosa.

Ameloblastoma appears most commonly in the third to fifth decades.[217,246] No sex or racial predilection is noted. Over 80% occur in the mandible, and 70% of these arise in the molar-ramus area. Rarely an extraosseous example is discovered.

Because of its invasive property and tendency to recur, the ameloblastoma has been usually considered locally malignant but is benign. Distant metastases,[231] especially to the lungs, have been reported in rare instances, but factors such as aspiration and transplantation are considered significant in most.[10] Frankly carcinomatous neoplasms resembling dental organ epithelium are best considered ameloblastic carcinoma. Traditionally, ameloblastoma has been divided into solid and cystic types, but nearly all ameloblastomas demonstrate some cystic degeneration. Microscopically, many subtypes or patterns have been suggested: follicular, plexiform, acanthomatous, granular cell (Figs. 25-21 and 25-22), and vascular varieties. However, two or more types may occur within the same tumor, and there is no evidence that any subtype is more aggressive than any other.

The majority of ameloblastomas demonstrate one of the two predominant patterns, follicular or plexiform, the former being the more common. In the follicular type there is an attempt to mimic the dental organ epithelium. The outermost cells resemble those of the inner dental epithelium of the developing tooth follicle, that is, the ameloblastic layer. The cells are tall columnar, with polarization of the nuclei away from the basement membrane.[274] These stringent criteria have recently been challenged.[217] The central portion of the epithelial island is composed of a loose network of cells resembling stellate reticulum. Squamous metaplasia within the stellate reticulum gives rise to the acanthomatous type. The epithelial islands demonstrate no inductive influence on the collagenized connective tissue stroma. Enamel and dentin are never formed by the ameloblastoma. The plexiform pattern demonstrates irregular masses and interdigitating cords of epithelial cells with a minimum of stroma.

Odontogenic adenomatoid tumor. A benign lesion, the odontogenic adenomatoid tumor probably arises from the preameloblast or from the inner enamel epithelium.[206,236,256,269] It appears to be more common in females, arises somewhat more often in the anterior region of the upper jaw, and occurs most frequently in the second decade of life. Frequently it is associated with an unerupted canine. Although the tumor expands, it is not invasive and does not recur even after extremely conservative surgical therapy.

Microscopically the lesion consists of congeries of ductlike structures, lined by medium to tall columnar epithelium, in an extremely scant fibrous connective tissue stroma (Fig. 25-23). Small calcified deposits are often seen scattered throughout the epithelial tissue.

Calcifying epithelial odontogenic tumor. The calcifying epithelial odontogenic tumor is a relatively rare lesion. The tumor may be invasive and locally recurrent, behaving like an ameloblastoma. It seems to occur most commonly in the fourth and fifth decades. There is no sex predilection. About 65% of reported cases have arisen in the mandibular premolar-molar area in association with an embedded tooth.[215,238,273,278] There is a 10% to 15% recurrence rate.

Microscopically, the tumor is composed of polyhedral epithelial cells with scanty stroma. The closely packed cells frequently demonstrate nuclear pleomorphism. Intracellular degeneration results in numerous spherical spaces filled with eosinophilic homogeneous material that in time becomes calcified. Although this substance stains like amyloid, ultrastructural studies have shown that it represents some fibrillar proserine secreted by the tumor epithelium (Fig. 25-24).[254]

Ameloblastic fibroma. The ameloblastic fibroma is characterized by proliferation of both epithelial and mesenchymal elements in the absence of hard tooth structure (enamel or dentin). In contrast to ameloblastoma,

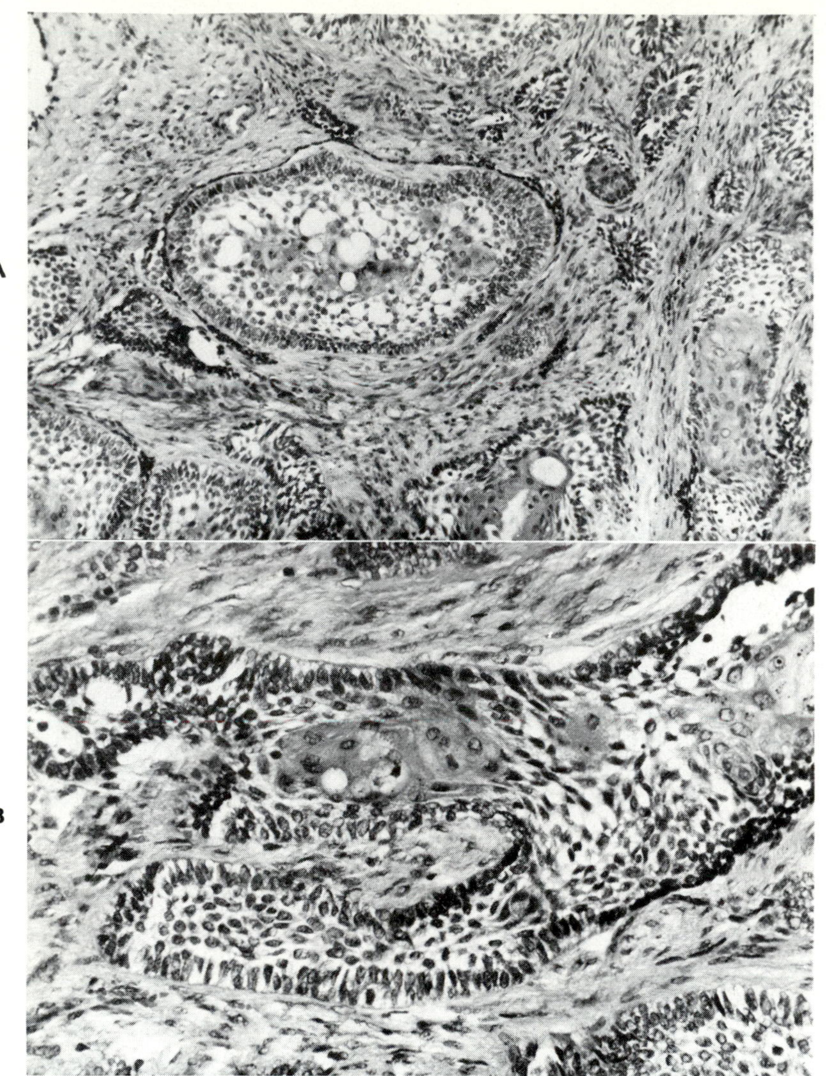

Fig. 25-21. Ameloblastoma. **A,** Numerous islands of odontogenic epithelium in mature fibrous connective tissue stroma. Note resemblance to developing dental epithelial enamel organ. Within stellate reticular area are sites of squamous metaplasia. **B,** Higher-power view showing tendency of nuclei to polarize away from basement membrane. (Courtesy J. Sciubba, New Hyde Park, N.Y.)

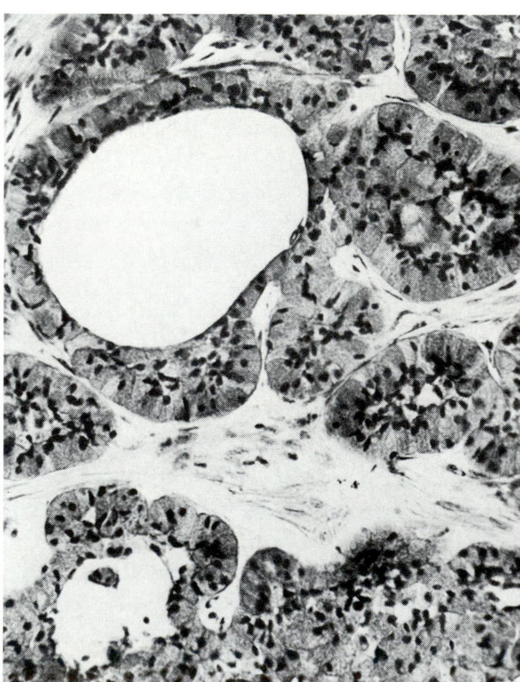

Fig. 25-22. Ameloblastoma exhibiting granular cell pattern. Occasionally, whole tumor may be composed of large granular cells with eosinophilic granular cytoplasm.

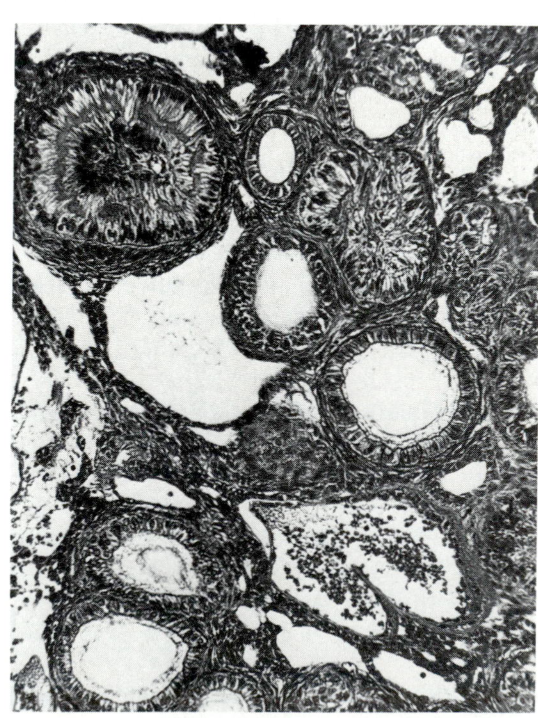

Fig. 25-23. Odontogenic adenomatoid tumor. Tumor consists of congeries of tubules and possibly arises from preameloblast.

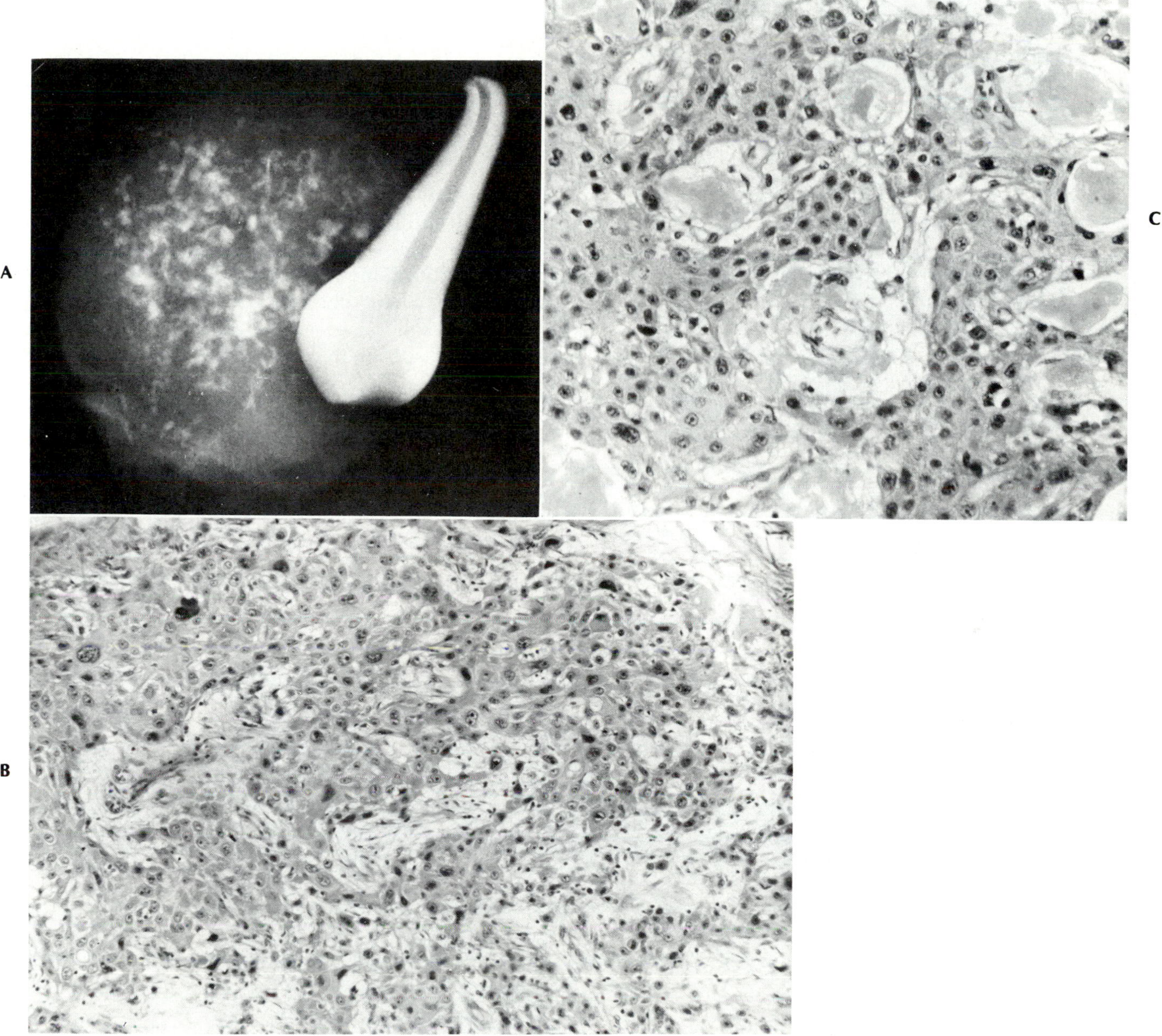

Fig. 25-24. Calcifying epithelial odontogenic tumor. **A,** Radiograph of upper canine tooth and tumor showing flecky calcification. **B,** Pleomorphic cells. **C,** Hyalinized amyloid-staining material. (Courtesy J. Sciubba, New Hyde Park, N.Y.)

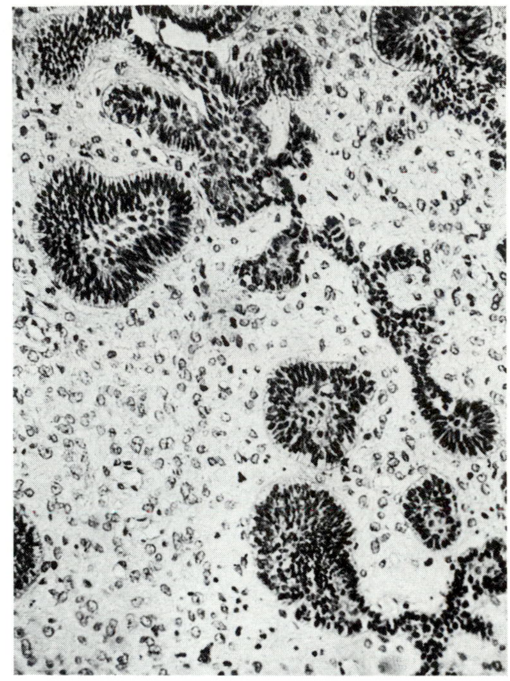

Fig. 25-25. Ameloblastic fibroma. Tumor consists of numerous islands of odontogenic epithelium in cellular mesenchymal matrix. This tumor is nonaggressive and must be differentiated from ameloblastomas, which lack mesenchymal matrix.

the tumor for which it is most commonly mistaken, the ameloblastic fibroma usually occurs in a young age group, rarely being seen in individuals over 21 years of age. Clinical behavior is entirely benign.[272]

Microscopically the ameloblastic fibroma is composed of strands and buds of epithelial cells in a very cellular connective tissue stroma (Fig. 25-25). The presence of this mesenchymal portion clearly differentiates this lesion from ameloblastoma. For the most part the cells composing the strands of epithelial cells are cuboid and are two cell layers thick. Occasionally a stellate reticulum is present. In contrast to ameloblastoma, simple curettage of the ameloblastic fibroma is usually adequate treatment.

Odontomas. Three subtypes or varieties of odontogenic tumors featuring production of calcified parts of teeth are usually considered: complex odontoma, in which enamel, dentin, cementum, and so on have not differentiated to the point at which an actual tooth can be recognized; compound odontoma, in which a tooth or teeth, regardless of size or fine form, can be discerned; and ameloblastic fibro-odontoma, in which the lesion looks like an ameloblastic fibroma with odontoma formation.[224,230,249]

Complex odontoma has been most frequently encountered in molar areas of the mandible and more often observed in female patients. Differentiation is poor, and a variety of calcified patterns are observed. The enamel, dentin, and cementum may be virtually unidentifiable.

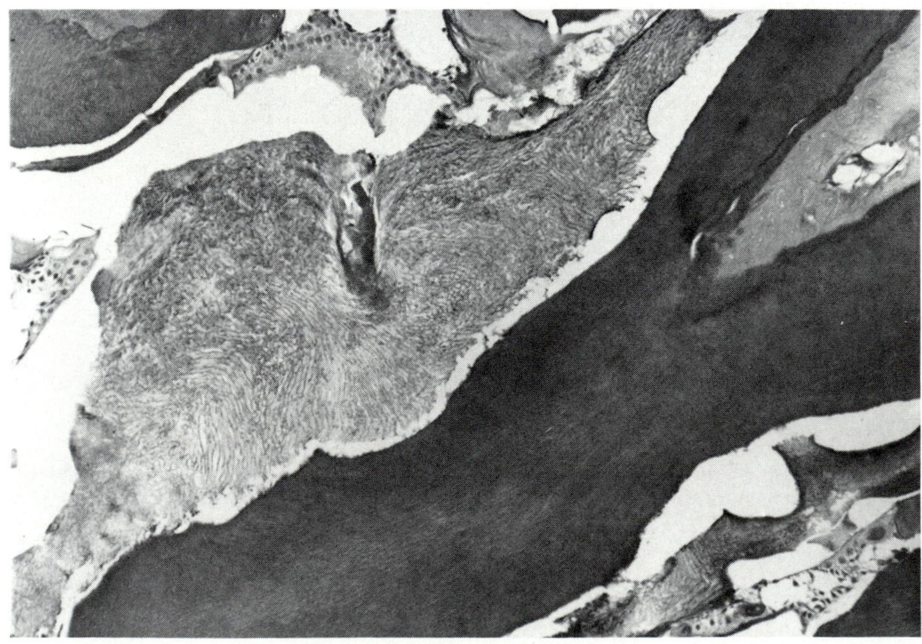

Fig. 25-26. Complex odontoma consists of unorganized mass of dentin, enamel, cementum, and pulpal tissue and occasional areas of enamel epithelium.

Although the tumors occasionally achieve considerable proportions, they are entirely benign. Growth and symptoms are slight. The tumors are frequently diagnosed after routine radiographic examinations (Fig. 25-26).

Compound odontoma presents a higher degree of differentiation than does complex odontoma, and the individual lesion characteristically consists of masses of small, misshapen teeth. Some may have as few as three teeth, whereas one lesion reported contained 2000 denticles. These odontomas behave in an entirely benign fashion. They are more commonly encountered in anterior regions of the jaws and in the maxilla more often than in the mandible.

Ameloblastic fibro-odontoma is much less frequent than either complex or compound odontoma. Although dental hard tissues such as enamel and dentin in the odontomas under discussion necessarily form through action of ameloblasts and odontoblasts, certain odontomas are encountered that possess a striking epithelial component. In these instances, the term *ameloblastic odontoma* has been employed. They may represent the simultaneous occurrence of an ameloblastoma and an odontoma.

Cementomas. Four, possibly five, apparently unrelated lesions of the jaws can be identified within this group characterized by benign neoplastic formation of cementum or cementum-like hard tissue within a cellular fibrous connective tissue.*

Cementoma or periapical fibrous dysplasia (periapical cemental dysplasia) has been the most frequently encountered, and estimates place the prevalence at 2 to 3 per 1000 individuals. Females, most often middle aged and black, are principally affected. Multiple mandibular teeth are usually involved by asymptomatic, small radiolucencies or, later, radiopacities that may be confused with dental inflammation. Treatment is not required.

Florid cemental dysplasia, much less frequently encountered, has been reported with varying terminology in middle-aged black women. Multiple areas of both jaws appear to be affected.

Diagnosis of the several fibrous, ossifying, or "cementifying" jaw lesions, such as the so-called true cementomas, cementoblastomas, cementifying fibromas, gigantiform cementomas, and fibrous dysplasias, represents a highly difficult exercise of pathology. In such instances, clinical history, radiographic examination, histopathologic tests, and, occasionally, blood chemistry studies are required.

Myxoma and myxofibroma, odontogenic fibroma. Myxoma of bone does not occur outside of the jaws. Most investigators believe that this lesion is of tooth germ origin (dental papilla) and have called it odontogenic myxoma. Some examples are associated with a small number of epithelial rests of Malassez. The odontogenic fibroma differs microscopically from the myxoma only by the presence of collagenic fibrous connective tissue and greater numbers of odontogenic epithelial rests.[212]

About 60% of odontogenic myxomas and fibromas occur during the second and third decades. The maxilla and mandible are equally affected. The tumors are slow growing. Bony expansion may be great, however, producing obvious facial deformity. Microscopically the myxoma consists of loose stellate cells with long, anastomosing cytoplasmic processes (Fig. 25-27). Occasionally an inactive strand of odontogenic epithelium is noted around the edge of the tumor.[222,228,279]

Malignant ameloblastoma (ameloblastic carcinoma). We have encountered four neoplasms, three maxillary and one mandibular, that besides possessing histologic criteria of ameloblastoma manifest malignant cytologic features such as numerous mitotic figures and clinical aggressiveness. Although malignant odontogenic neoplasms are relatively rare, this possibility cannot be excluded.

Ameloblastic fibrosarcoma. Ameloblastic fibrosarcoma is a rare lesion composed of islands or strands of odontogenic epithelium in a cell-rich mesenchymal stroma, the cells of which exhibit the histologic features of a fibrosarcoma. Approximately 25 cases have been documented. The mean age of presentation is about 30 years, although there is a wide range. There does not appear to be any sex predilection. Most have arisen in the molar-ramus area of the mandible. In most patients pain has preceded the swelling, which is an important diagnostic

Fig. 25-27. Odontogenic myxoma. Tumor consists of loose, embryonal connective tissue. Occasionally, strands of odontogenic epithelium are present.

*References 10, 198, 203, 213, 247, 265.

criterion that helps to differentiate this tumor from most other odontogenic tumors. Tooth extraction in an effort to relieve the pain may be followed by growth of the tumor from the socket. Microscopically the epithelium cannot be differentiated from that in ameloblastoma or an ameloblastic fibroma. However, the mesodermal component is highly cellular, consisting of spindle-shaped and polyhedral cells, many of which are bizarre, with hyperchromatic nuclei consistent with a diagnosis of fibrosarcoma. Mitotic activity is high, with frequent mitotic atypia. In recurrences the epithelial element is completely overgrown by the fibrosarcomatous portion. In no case has metastasis occurred. Death follows extensive local recurrence and extension.[259]

SALIVARY GLANDS

Development

Both the major and the minor salivary glands develop as buds of oral ectoderm, arising in much the same manner as teeth. The epithelial bud proliferates into the adjacent ectomesenchyme, enlarging at its most distal end to form alveoli, with the epithelial cords becoming hollow to form ducts. The parotid and submandibular gland anlagen first become apparent by the sixth fetal week (13 to 15 mm embryo), although acini are not developed until the fifth month in utero. During the eighth week (19 to 25 mm embryo), the buds of the sublingual gland become apparent. The minor salivary glands are initiated by the tenth week.

Labial glands arise as epithelial buds of the vestibular epithelial plate before the opening of the alveolabial sulcus. Buccal and molar glands arise at the same time, associated with the terminal portion of Stensen's duct. Retromolar glands develop in the fifth fetal month.

The major salivary glands are subject to many developmental anomalies. One or more lobes (rarely, whole glands) may be congenitally absent or aplastic. Total absence of all major glands also has been reported.[297,382,398] Accessory glands and glands ectopically placed within the mandible, tonsil, or neck have been noted.[322,372,381] Major salivary ducts may be congenitally atretic or, rarely, imperforate or duplicated.[317,328,361]

Structure and types

The salivary glands, both major and minor, are tubuloalveolar structures. Both the parotid and submandibular glands are well encapsulated, although the sublingual is not. The adult parotid gland is serous in type, whereas the submandibular and sublingual glands are mixed, the former being predominantly serous and the latter mucous. Minor salivary glands are widespread, being scattered over the lips, buccal mucosa, palate, and tongue. Pure serous glands are seen about the circumvallate papillae (glands of von Ebner); pure mucous glands are located in the palate and base of the tongue (Weber's glands). All others are of the mixed type.

Function

Saliva, the product largely of the major salivary glands, varies in quantity from 150 to 1300 ml per day (mean, 345 ml). The amount and the degree of viscosity depend on many factors (mechanical, chemical, and psychologic) but ultimately on the type of nerve stimulus received by the glands.

The secretory nerve fibers to the salivary glands are under both parasympathetic and sympathetic control. Sympathetic stimulation of the submandibular gland via the superior cervical ganglion, for example, evokes a secretion of thick viscous mucus, whereas parasympathetic stimulation via the chorda tympani elicits a copious, thin watery flow.

The saliva performs several known functions, the most important being lubrication for deglutition and speech. Both mucin, a glyoprotein elaborated by mucous glands, and the voluminous watery secretion of the parotid glands aid in this process. In cases of diminished flow (xerostomia), poor oral hygiene and increased dental decay are observed. Taste is altered greatly. Saliva has antibacterial properties and a high buffering capacity. It probably contributes little toward digestion, although it contains a salivary amylase (ptyalin) capable of transforming starch to maltose and of splitting glycogen.

Disturbances of salivary flow

Increased salivary flow (sialorrhea, ptyalism) can result from many causes. It is most commonly associated with acute inflammation of the oral cavity, such as herpetic or aphthous stomatitis, and with "teething." It is often seen in mentally retarded individuals, in severe schizophrenics, and in patients with neurologic disturbances with lenticular involvement. Mercury poisoning, acrodynia, pemphigus, pregnancy, rabies, epilepsy, nausea, and ill-fitting dentures all may be accompanied by an increased degree of salivation. Also, increased gastric secretion is accompanied by increased salivary flow.

Familial autonomic dysautonomia (Riley-Day syndrome). Familial autonomic dysautonomia is characterized by excessive perspiration, sialorrhea, erythematous blotching of the skin, defective lacrimation, wide blood pressure fluctuation, emotional instability, cold hands and feet, hyporeflexia, and absence of lingual fungiform and circumvallate papillae.[3] It is first manifested in infancy by impaired sucking and swallowing and an absence of tears. Growth is retarded, and the ability to sit, walk, and speak is delayed. The sialorrhea is especially noticeable during excitement. The disorder is inherited as an autosomal recessive trait and occurs almost exclusively in Jews of Ashkenazi extraction.[294]

Xerostomia. Decreased salivary flow, xerostomia, is also associated with many conditions. Rarely there is congenital absence of one or more major glands or ducts. Epidemic parotitis (mumps) and sarcoidosis (uveoparotitis) are associated with reduced flow. Sjögren syndrome patients exhibit xerostomia. Therapeutic radiation to the lateral cervical area commonly produces fibrotic changes after acinar destruction of the parotid glands. Megaloblastic anemias (pernicious anemia, anemia of pregnancy) are not uncommonly associated with decreased salivary output. The majority of cases of xerostomia appear to be medication related (tricyclic antidepressants, antihistamines, hypotensive drugs, and phenothiazines). Reduced salivary flow occurs with various disorders associated with fever or dehydration.

Enlargements

Enlargement of one or more salivary glands may be associated with sialorrhea, xerostomia, or normal salivary secretion. A single glandular enlargement may denote localized inflammation, cyst, or neoplasm. Bilateral enlargement may signify an inflammatory process, such as mumps or sarcoid, or a diffuse neoplastic infiltrate (leukemia or lymphoma), or it may be attributable to unknown factors related to malnutrition, alcoholic cirrhosis, or hormonal disturbance.

Cysts

Cysts of salivary gland origin fall in three categories: true cysts, ranulas, and mucoceles or mucus retention phenomena.

True cyst. The true cyst is usually small, 1 cm or less in diameter, and located within the body of the parotid or submandibular gland. It is lined by simple or stratified squamous epithelium.[295,329]

Ranula. Ranula is a term used rather loosely to indicate a thin-walled, cystic lesion located on the floor of the mouth.[300] It includes sublingual gland mucoceles and a deep burrowing lesion that frequently extends through the mylohyoid muscle. The so-called congenital ranula appears to represent the effect of atresia of the orifice of either the sublingual or submandibular ducts.[371]

Mucocele (mucus retention phenomenon). The extravasation mucocele is a cavity lined by granulation tissue containing an eosinophilic hyaline material (mucus) composed of a variable number of mucus-laden macrophages (Fig. 25-28). Trauma, chiefly mechanical, appears to be responsible for damage to the ducts of minor salivary glands, resulting in the spillage of mucus into the lamina propria and submucous tissue.[299,326] The site is most commonly the lower lip and less often the buccal mucosa or oral floor. There is no sex predilection; most cases are seen in children or young adults, probably reflecting the role of trauma. This mucus pool may be localized and surrounded by a wall of granulation tissue. The retention mucocele is lined by a single or double layer of oncocytic epithelium and probably represents cystic changes in an oncocyte-lined duct. It occurs most often in the oral floor and buccal mucosa of older patients.[384] It is much rarer than the extravasation type, constituting no more than 10% of all mucoceles. Mucocele of the glands near the

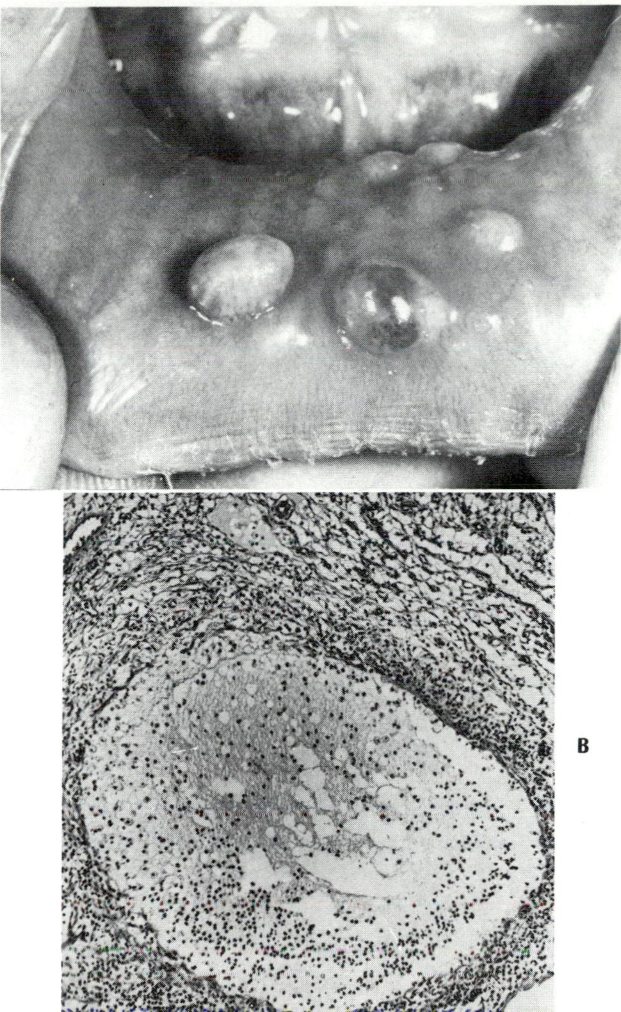

Fig. 25-28. Mucocele or minor salivary gland retention "cyst." **A,** Most commonly observed on lower lip, mucoceles are observed throughout oral cavity. They arise from spillage of mucus into surrounding connective tissue. **B,** Low-power photomicrograph showing extraductal mucus surrounded by inflammation. Note absence of epithelium.

ventral tip of the tongue is called cyst of Blandin-Nuhn. Mucocele of the maxillary sinus floor is not rare, being found in more than 1% of the population.[298]

Enlargements related to malnutrition, hormonal disturbances, and alcoholic cirrhosis (sialosis)

The relationship of parotid gland enlargement to malnutrition has been pointed out by many investigators.[310] Hypertrophy also has been noted in cases of alcoholism and cirrhosis. Enlargement of the submandibular glands also has been noted occasionally in these cases. It is well known that both alcohol consumption and restricted dietary intake contribute to hepatic cirrhosis. The enlargement may be associated with excessive salivation. Experimentally, parotid enlargement can be produced in

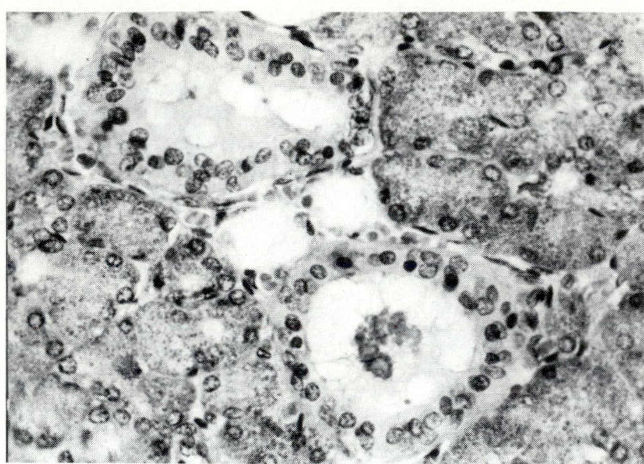

Fig. 25-29. Sialosis. Note granular alterations in acinar cells of parotid glands. Patient had severe alcoholism. (Courtesy G. Seifert, Hamburg, Germany.)

rats on a protein-free diet or by feeding proteolytic enzymes.

Parotid enlargement has also been reported in mental patients, patients with bulimia, and Native American hospital patients who were assumed to be receiving adequate diets.[282,347,348] The past dietary history was not known, however. Cases also have been cited in association with diabetes mellitus, pregnancy and lactation, thyroid disease, cardiospasm, and menopause. In association with diabetes, the parotid swelling may precede the elevation in blood glucose level by many months.

Microscopic changes consist of enlarged acinar cells exhibiting a granular pattern, a numerical increase in secretory granules, or a vacuolar alteration of the cytoplasm (Fig. 25-29). No inflammatory changes are observed. The pathogenesis is unknown but is probably related to an alteration in the autonomic nervous system.

Inflammatory diseases

Acute parotitis (secondary suppurative type). Acute parotitis is caused by ascent of microorganisms, usually *Staphylococcus aureus*, up Stensen's duct when salivary flow is reduced by inadequate fluid balance as a result of fever, diuretics, starvation, and so on. It occurs most often in neonates,[344] the elderly, or postoperative patients.[405] It may become recurrent, leading to scarring and chronic parotitis.[337]

Microscopically there are widespread destruction of acini and replacement with fibrous connective tissue. Plasma cell and lymphocytic infiltration is usually considerable. Ducts and acini are frequently dilated.

Acute submandibular adenitis. This acute disorder nearly always follows acute obstruction from a salivary duct stone.

Chronic submandibular adenitis. Chronic submandibular adenitis is often (40%) attributable to blockage by stricture or calculi (sialoliths). This, in turn, renders the gland susceptible to retrograde bacterial invasion.[378]

Sjögren's syndrome. Sjögren, in 1933, first described a syndrome consisting of keratoconjunctivitis sicca, pharyngolaryngitis sicca, rhinitis sicca, rheumatoid arthritis with (about 35%) or without parotid (occasionally submandibular) enlargement, and xerostomia. This syndrome subsequently was shown to accompany at times other disorders such as dermatomyositis, polyarteritis nodosa, systemic lupus erythematosus, chronic active hepatitis, primary biliary cirrhosis, purpura and hypergammaglobulinemia of Waldenström, scleroderma, Hashimoto's thyroiditis, Reiter's syndrome, and Behçet's syndrome.

The patient, usually a postmenopausal woman (about 90%), has red, burning eyes, photophobia, and lack of tears.[316] The disorder has also been reported in children. The saliva is thick and ropy. Dysphagia and dysphonia may be pronounced, and the oral mucosa, especially that of the tongue, is atrophic and shiny. There is angular cheilitis and cracking of the lips. Dental caries, usually at the neck of the teeth, becomes widespread as the disease progresses.[307,373]

Sjögren's syndrome is believed to be a chronic inflammatory disease of autoimmune etiology. It has been suggested that an antigen released from damaged acini coming into contact with lymphatic tissue (normally present with parotid gland) would result in the production of antibodies that in turn would damage more acinar epithelium, continuing the cycle. Arguing for the autoimmune nature of the disease are the following:

1. Associated rheumatoid arthritic changes in over 50%
2. Hypergammaglobulinemia
3. Rheumatoid factor in over 75%
4. Antithyroglobulin antibodies (about 35%) and antinuclear factors (about 65%)
5. Autoantibody reaction with salivary duct cytoplasm in over 50%
6. Association with other connective tissue disorders such as systemic lupus erythematosus, scleroderma, polymyositis, or polyarteritis

It has been suggested that there is impaired IgG autoantibody production.[356,392,400] Malignant lymphoma, principally reticulum cell sarcoma, may develop late in the course of the disease. Microscopically the changes were long recognized under the names *Mikulicz disease* or *benign lymphoepithelial lesion*. Initially there is a periductal mononuclear cell infiltrate consisting predominantly of small lymphocytes. Later, large lymphocytes and reticular cells appear. The acinar tissue is eventually totally replaced (Fig. 25-30). Epimyoepithelial islands arising from ductal proliferation are scattered throughout the tissue. Similar changes have been described in the lacrimal glands and the minor salivary glands of the lip and palate.[324,394,404]

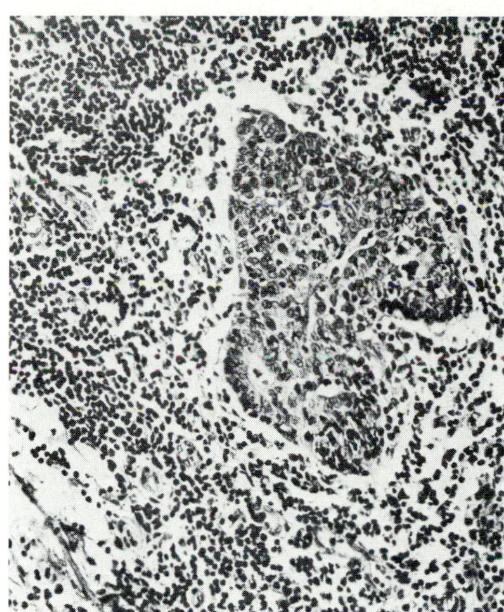

Fig. 25-30. Sjögren's syndrome (benign lymphoepithelial lesion). Acini are replaced by pronounced lymphocytic infiltrate. Differentiation from lymphosarcoma is made with difficulty.

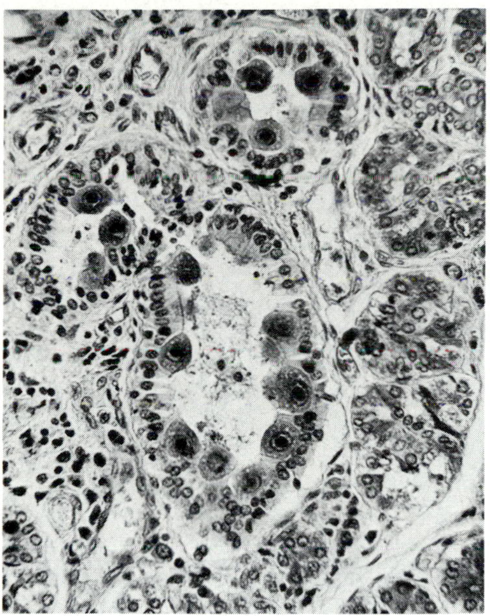

Fig. 25-31. Cytomegalic inclusion disease illustrating numerous, large, doubly contoured inclusion bodies within cytoplasm of duct cells of parotid gland. (Courtesy R. Marcial-Rojas, San Juan, Puerto Rico.)

Sialolithiasis. Sialolithiasis, the occurrence of salivary stones or calculus, is found most commonly in the submandibular gland or especially its duct. Involvement of the parotid gland is less common (estimated 4% to 21%). Calculus in the sublingual gland is relatively rare. For sialolithiasis of minor salivary glands, the two most common sites are the buccal mucosa and the upper lip. The disorder is not as rare as stated in most texts. For involvement of both major and minor glands there is a 2:1 male-to-female predilection. Most patients are middle aged.[335,368,369]

Although the etiology is unknown, theories have been advanced that salivary retention, with resultant precipitation of calcium salts, is the significant factor. Whether the retention is preceded by inflammation of the duct because of a foreign body, bacteria, or other factor is debatable.

Because of the intermittent obstruction of the duct system, inflammation of the proximal portion of the gland occurs. Contrast media may be employed to demonstrate tortuous dilatation of the principal ducts and the presence of strictures. There is atrophy of the acinar cells, with replacement by scar tissue and fat cells if the obstruction process continues.

Cytomegalic inclusion disease. Cytomegalic inclusion disease is a widespread viral disease that becomes clinically manifest in only a small percentage of the population.[402] It appears to be largely harmless ouside infancy but remains a risk to the fetus if first contracted by the mother during pregnancy.

Although initially believed to be limited to salivary and lacrimal glands, cytomegalic inclusion disease was subsequently shown to be generalized, producing a clinical picture resembling erythroblastosis or hepatitis in neonates and characterized by a train of events: mild jaundice, hepatosplenomegaly, bruising, and finally purpura. Interstitial pneumonitis, Addison's disease, or interstitial nephritis with hematuria also may occur. A high proportion of fatal cases have exhibited a peculiar laminar necrosis immediately beneath the ependyma of the brain. These areas become calcified and simulate congenital toxoplasmosis.

Microscopically the inclusions may be seen in the salivary glands, lacrimal glands, liver, kidney, lung, and so on. In the salivary gland the inclusions are round, highly refractile, homogeneous, eosinophilic bodies within the cytoplasm or nucleus of ductal cells (Fig. 25-31). These cells also may be seen with standard Wright's stain in gastric washings, subdural fluid, or sediment from freshly voided urine.

Epidemic parotitis (mumps). Epidemic parotitis is an acute, highly contagious viral disease. Despite the name, it is systemic, affecting many organs other than the parotid gland. It is probable that some degree of pancreatitis (and orchitis in men) occurs in nearly every case, but severe complication is rather uncommon. Oophoritis also may occur but is quite rare.

There is diffuse tender enlargement of one or both parotid glands, accompanied by mild fever. Less commonly, the submandibular and sublingual glands are involved and, very rarely, the lacrimal glands. Examination of the buccal mucosa during the active state usually will reveal an erythematous halo about the opening of Stensen's duct.

In adolescent and adult males, clinical orchitis (usually unilateral) is present in about 25%. Only rarely is sterility produced, however. Pancreatitis, manifested by epigastric pain and nausea, although not very common as a severe complication, is probably a constant factor, causing elevated serum amylase and lipase levels.

Microscopically in the parotid glands there are degenerative changes of the ductal epithelium, with infiltration of lymphocytes and macrophages about the ducts. The acini may undergo pressure atrophy.

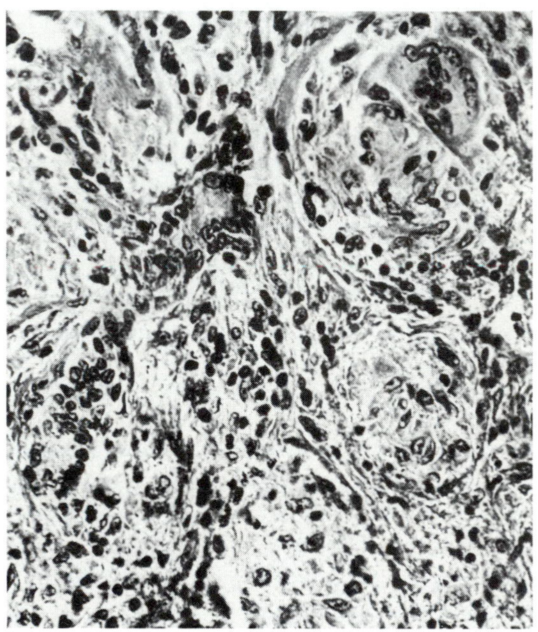

Fig. 25-32. Heerfordt's syndrome (uveoparotid fever) or sarcoidosis. Acini are replaced by multiple, usually discrete, sarcoidal granulomas. Lacrimal glands, as well as major salivary glands, are enlarged; this is associated with facial nerve paralysis.

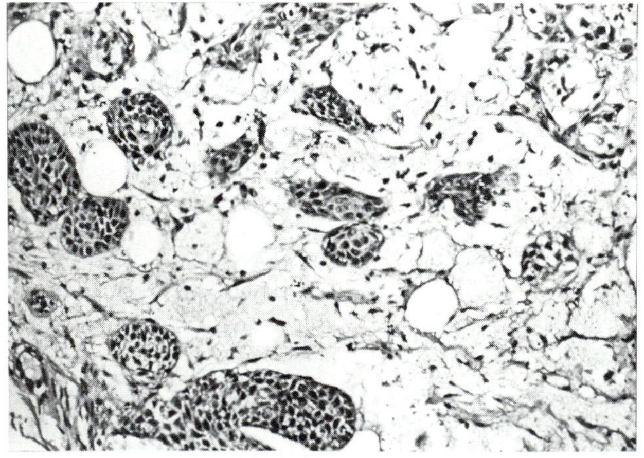

Fig. 25-33. Necrotizing sialometaplasia. Note acinar necrosis with mucus pooling and squamous metaplasia with lack of cellular atypia. (From Lynch, D.P., et al.: Oral Surg. **47**:63, 1979.)

Uveoparotid fever (Heerfordt's syndrome). Uveoparotid fever is a form of sarcoidosis originally described by Heerfordt in 1909. The syndrome consists of a triad of signs: parotid enlargement, uveitis, and facial paralysis. It usually is seen in the second and third decades and is decidedly more common in black women. It represents about 10% of the cases of sarcoidosis.

The parotid swelling, which is bilateral in over half of the cases, often is preceded by mild fever, lassitude, and anorexia. The swelling, in contrast to mumps, is not painful and is firm and nodular. Minor salivary glands may also be involved. The lacrimal glands occasionally are involved (Fig. 25-32). Ocular involvement, usually bilateral, may be severe and prolonged. Uveitis, iridocyclitis, and optic neuritis are not uncommon complications. Paralysis of the facial nerve occurs in about 25% of the patients with uveoparotid fever.[396]

Necrotizing sialometaplasia. This nonneoplastic self-healing inflammatory disorder of minor salivary glands may be confused clinically and microscopically with squamous cell carcinoma or mucoepidermoid carcinoma. The lesion is usually a single, rarely (15%) bilateral, elevated mass or crateriform ulcer, 1 to 2 cm in diameter, that most often involves the hard palate of adults. Rarely, lesions have been reported in the nasopharynx and parotid gland. There appears to be a 3:1 male sex predilection. The lesion heals spontaneously in 6 to 10 weeks. Characteristic microscopic features involve coagulative lobular necrosis of minor salivary glands, marked squamous metaplasia of mucous acini and ducts, pseudoepitheliomatous hyperplasia of the surrounding mucosa, maintenance of lobular morphology, and variable amounts of granulomatous tissue (Fig. 25-33). The squamous epithelium appears entirely benign. The basic lesion appears to be an infarct with subsequent ulceration and repair.[309,351,370]

Tumors (Table 25-1)

Hemangioma and lymphangioma. The hemangioma is the most common tumor of the parotid gland during the first year of life, usually appearing within the first 3 months (Fig. 25-34). It is occasionally noted at birth. It may also arise in the submandibular gland. Skin hemangiomas overlie the salivary gland tumor in about 40% of patients. There is a 3:1 female predilection.[321,365]

Histologically the hemangioma is composed of capillary vessels lined by two or more layers of endothelial cells. The vessel lumina are often obscured as a result of the marked cellularity. The hemangioma is never encapsulated but infiltrates the gland, replaces the acini, and leaves only the ductal elements. Spontaneous regression is usual, and recurrence following surgical resection is very rare.

Lymphangioma is an extremely rare congenital tumor related to cystic hygroma.[340,364]

Pleomorphic adenoma (mixed tumor). The benign pleomorphic adenoma is the most common tumor of the major (about 60% to 75%) and minor (about 50%) salivary glands. Conversely, about 93% arise in major glands, while 7% have their origin in minor glands.[308,342] The tumor occurs nine times as often in the parotid gland as in the submandibular gland. Only rarely is it found in the sublingual gland. There are a few reports of the tumor within the mandible or ear canal.

The pleomorphic adenoma occurs most frequently in the fourth to sixth decades, although some examples have been congenital.[343] It is found somewhat more commonly in women. It is rare in children.[332] The primary growth occurs as a painless, single, slow-growing, moderately firm, movable, smooth nodule or mass. Although usually single, multiple mixed tumors have been reported, arising in two independent sites within the same gland, bilaterally, or within the homolateral parotid and submandibular glands. In the parotid gland, about 90% arise in the tail of the superficial part, but about 10% have their origin in the deep portion and may appear in the tonsillar area.[353]

Numerous theories of origin have been postulated: mesenchymal, branchiogenic, embryonal gland anlagen, and adult epithelial or myoepithelial tissue. Of special interest are the histochemical studies, which support a theory of histogenesis from intercalated ducts. Two types of mucus have been demonstrated: (1) an epithelial type elaborated by glandular structures, and (2) a "mesenchymal" type found in myxomatous areas, apparently the product of myoepithelial cells.

Grossly the pleomorphic adenoma is rounded to bosselated.[312] Recurrent growths tend to be multilobulated. Although it appears to have a fibrous capsule, it is not truly encapsulated, a condition that has been responsible for its high rate of recurrence in the past.[354] Most tumors are from 2 to 5 cm in size, although some have attained gigantic proportions. The cut surface is usually solid, grayish white, and semitranslucent. Areas containing cartilage appear bluish. Secondary cyst formation or hemorrhage is rare.[397]

Microscopically the wide variety of patterns found,

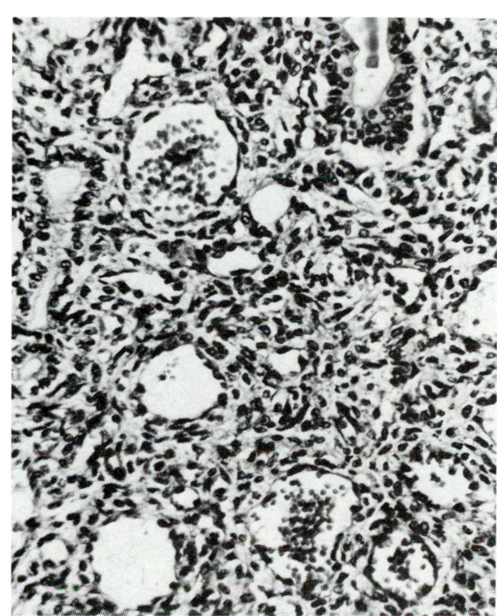

Fig. 25-34. Hemangioma of parotid gland, most common tumor of parotid gland in children under 1 year of age. Tumor is usually of capillary type, with few well-defined lumina.

Table 25-1. Tumors of major and minor salivary glands

Tumor type	Percent	
	Major	Minor
BENIGN		
Pleomorphic adenoma (mixed tumor)	60-75	45-55
Papillary cystadenoma lymphomatosum	6-8	—
Oxyphil granular cell adenoma (oncocytoma)	Rare	Rare
Papillary cystadenoma	Rare	2-3
Hemangioma	Rare except in infants	—
Miscellaneous (adenoma, lipoma, neurilemoma, neurofibroma, sebaceous adenoma, etc.)	Rare	Rare
MALIGNANT		
Carcinoma in pleomorphic adenoma (malignant mixed tumor)	2-3	2-3
Adenocarcinoma (includes "classic," trabecular, etc.)	1-2	10-18
Adenoid cystic carcinoma (cylindroma)	4-5	16-20
Mucoepidermoid carcinoma	2-4	10-12
Acinic cell carcinoma	2-3	Rare
Squamous cell carcinoma	1	?
Undifferentiated carcinoma	3-5	Rare
Miscellaneous (unclassified, oxyphil adenocarcinoma, melanoma, lymphoma, etc.)	Rare	1-2

both within the same tumor and in different tumors, may lead to considerable diagnostic confusion (Fig. 25-35). Myxoid areas occur in possibly 90%, whereas over one third exhibit such an area as a dominant feature. One half contain pseudocartilage. Squamous epithelial masses are seen in about 25%, and a pseudoadenoid arrangement of epithelial cells resembling adenoid cystic carcinoma is manifest in about 10% of the cases. Sebaceous glands or tyrosine crystals may be occasionally seen.[397]

A histologic feature in many pleomorphic adenomas is the presence of well-differentiated ductlike structures. Some tumors are composed entirely of these structures. These have been called basal cell adenomas and will be discussed separately. Other pleomorphic adenomas are composed almost entirely of mucoid pools, with only scant evidence of epithelial elements.

The epithelial cells vary in appearance from single-layered or double-layered high columnar to low cuboid. They correspond to inner duct lining cells and outer myoepithelial cells arranged in various tumors in varying proportions. Material found in the ductlike lumina in some cases resembles colloid and in others, mucin. The former has been called epithelial mucin, whereas the latter has been characterized as being of myoepithelial origin. This myoepithelial product may simulate cartilage. True cartilage and rarely even bone are observed in a

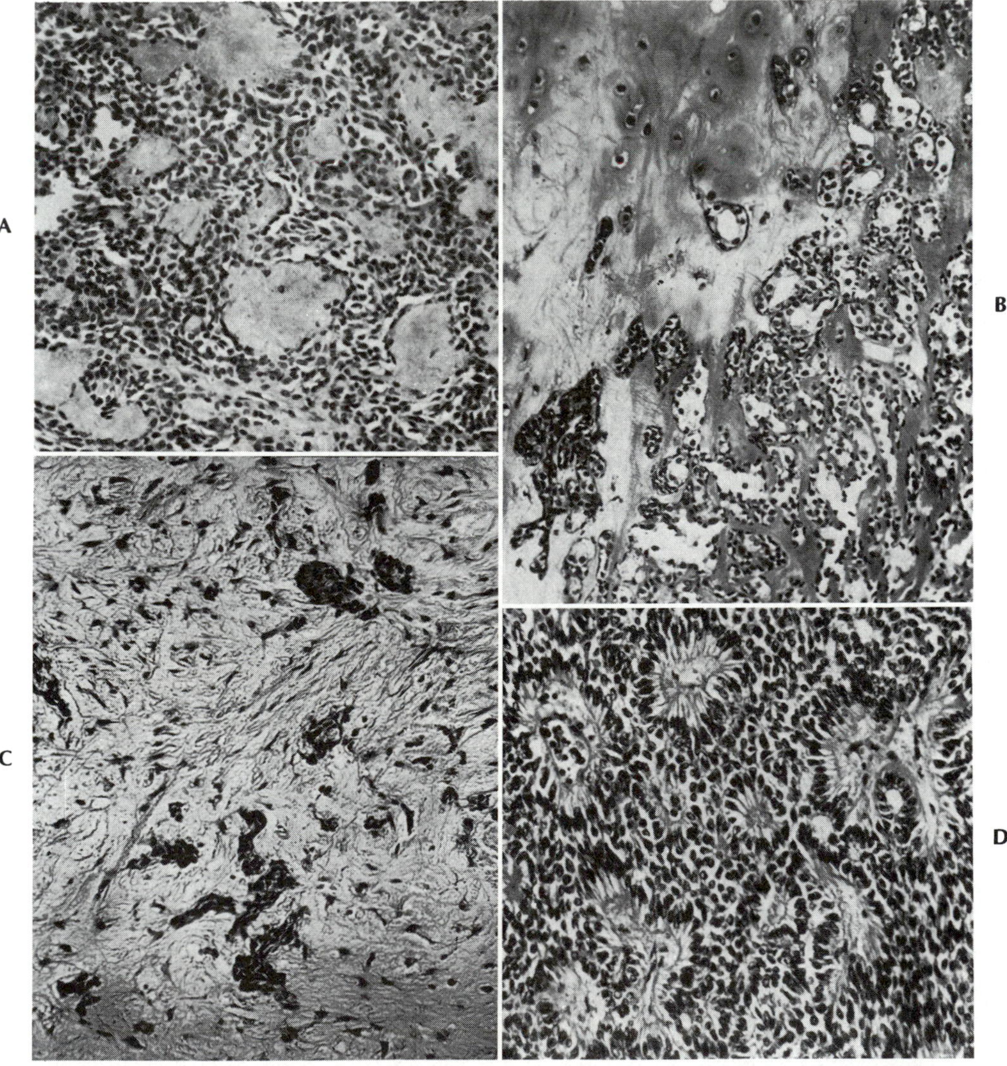

Fig. 25-35. Pleomorphic adenoma (mixed tumor). There is considerable variability of microscopic picture. **A,** Some tumors are exceedingly cellular, consisting of masses or sheets of small oval or rounded cells exhibiting little tendency to form ducts. **B,** Some tumors exhibit large masses of cartilage-like tissue. True cartilage is occasionally produced by metaplasia of fibrous connective tissue stroma. Numerous ductlike structures are manifest in this tumor. **C,** Certain tumors contain only few islands of epithelial cells in sea of loose mucoid matrix. **D,** Unusual variant of pleomorphic adenoma, so-called adenomyoepithelioma.

small percentage of these tumors. Calcification may be seen in old tumors. In some, islands of acidophilic granular cells (oncocytes) are noted. Cylindromatous areas may cause considerable difficulty in diagnosis, especially if the biopsy specimen is small. Fortunately, adenoid cystic carcinoma rarely if ever arises in mixed tumor.

Although several investigators have attempted to classify the mixed tumor into numerous subtypes on the basis of histologic pattern, clinical behavior is probably similar in all types. The local recurrence rate is low. Various investigators have estimated this to be in the range of none to 5%. Because there is seldom any change in histologic pattern with recurrence, poor encapsulation or pseudoencapsulation has been generally accepted as the responsible factor.[403]

Basal cell adenoma. Basal cell adenoma is a monomorphic benign tumor of salivary glands. Most often affected are the parotid gland and the minor glands of the hard palate and upper lip. The tumors are circumscribed nodules, harder than a mucocele. Patients are usually between 50 and 75 years of age. There is no sex predilection.[306,350,360] The basal cell adenoma has generally been grouped with pleomorphic adenoma from which it differs morphologically by the virtual absence of myoepithelial cells. Histologically it has been classified into trabecular-tubular, canalicular, and basaloid types (Fig. 25-36). The canalicular, the most common pattern and most often mistaken for adenoid cystic carcinoma, has characteristic small capillaries and venules in the microcystic areas of the tumor. Ultrastructural studies have generally suggested origin from the intercalated duct.[334,406] It may represent the benign analog of the adenoid cystic carcinoma.

The basal cell adenoma is most often mistaken for adenoid cystic carcinoma, but the former is usually encapsulated, grows in an expansile pattern, and is monolobular. Those occurring in the lips may be mistaken for eccrine spiradenomas, eccrine cylindromas, or trichoepitheliomas.

Myoepithelioma. Although there are myoepithelial cells in virtually all cases of pleomorphic adenoma, there are rare tumors of both major and minor salivary glands composed exclusively of myoepithelial cells. There are two types: the spindle and stellate myoepithelioma[346] and the plasmacytoid myoepithelioma.[362] It is conceivable that both types have a common histogenetic origin. Both are more frequently found in minor than in major salivary glands and tend to occur in young patients.[391] They may appear well circumscribed or locally invasive. Ultrastructural studies have been employed to differentiate the two types.[377] There also appears to be a clear cell variant[320,374] and a malignant variety.[305]

Sialadenoma papilliferum. Sialadenoma papilliferum, a rare benign exophytic salivary gland tumor first reported by Abrams and Finck[283] in 1969, arises in major or more often minor salivary glands of the palate. Most of the dozen documented cases have been in men in their sixth to eighth decades.[319,357]

Microscopically the tumor is pedunculated. Numerous dilated salivary ducts open onto the surface of the

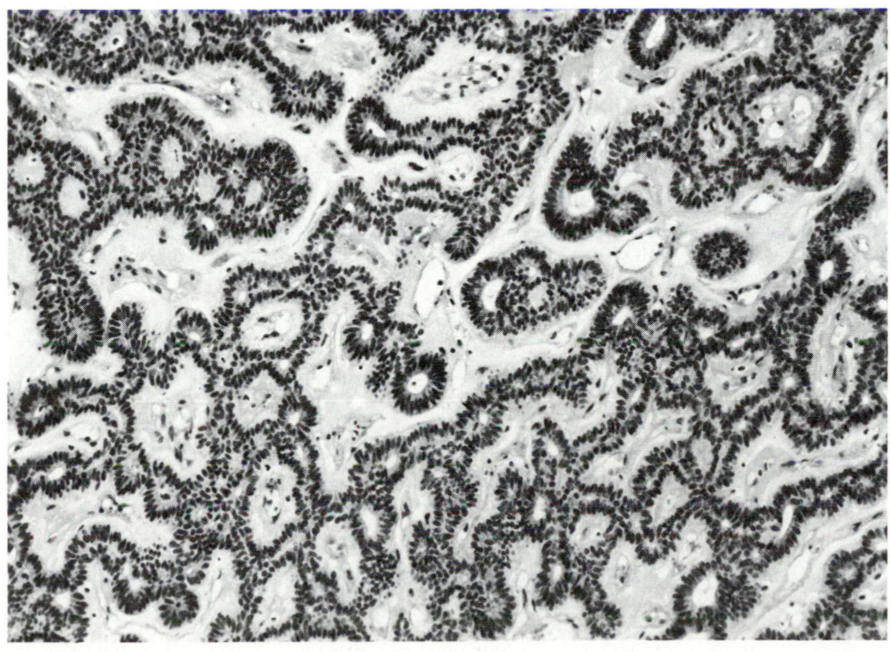

Fig. 25-36. Basal cell adenoma. Several patterns may be present: trabecular, tubular, canalicular, and basaloid. (From Klein, H.Z.: Arch. Pathol. **95**:94, 1973. Copyright 1973, American Medical Association.)

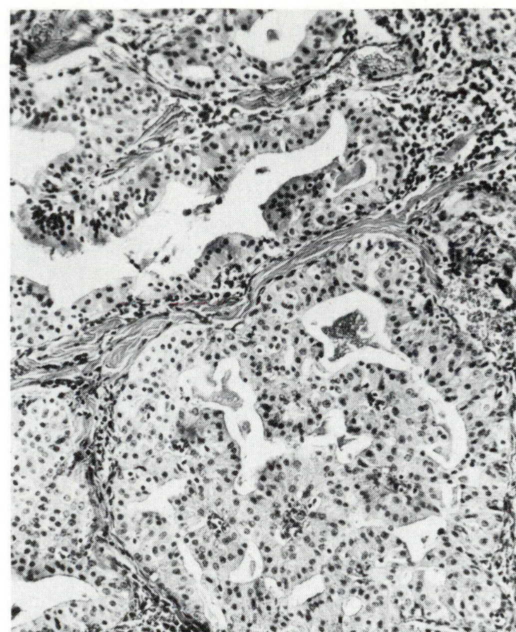

Fig. 25-37. Papillary cystadenoma. This tumor arises from neoplastic proliferation of ducts, being essentially a Warthin's tumor without lymphoid stroma.

tumor. The ducts appear to proliferate haphazardly, extending laterally under the mucosal surface. The ducts are lined with stratified squamous epithelium within the mucosa but are transformed into a double layer of luminal columnar and basilar cuboidal cells within the submucosal connective tissue. Both cell types exhibit abundant granular eosinophilic cytoplasm and oval vesicular nuclei. In the deeper parts of the tumor the duct lining manifests numerous papillary projections.

Papillary cystadenoma. Papillary cystadenoma is a rare tumor occurring most frequently in the parotid salivary gland and less commonly in the submandibular and minor salivary glands of the palate, buccal mucosa, and oral floor. Care must be exercised not to mistake the retention type of mucocele for a papillary cystadenoma.[338] Microscopically the tumor consists of glandlike spaces lined with tall columnar epithelium having eosinophilic cytoplasm. Mucin is commonly produced and may fill the glandlike spaces. A mucous cell variant has also been described (Fig. 25-37).

Papillary cystadenoma lymphomatosum (Warthin's tumor, adenolymphoma). Papillary cystadenoma lymphomatosum is a benign tumor of the parotid gland, arising most commonly in the lower portion of the gland overlying the angle of the mandible. It comprises from 6% to 10% of all parotid neoplasms. It chiefly affects men (5:1) from 40 to 70 years of age.[359] About 7% of the tumors occur bilaterally. The tumor may be superficial or deep to parotid fascia, or within the substance of the gland or occasionally posterior to it. Rarely, an extraparotid lesion is encountered. A malignant variant has been described.[339]

There have been numerous theories of the histogenesis of papillary cystadenoma lymphomatosum. One theory is that the tumor represents neoplastic proliferation of heterotopic salivary gland rests entrapped during growth and development in lymph nodes adjacent to or within the parotid gland. However, because the amount of lymphoid tissue is far greater than that of a small lymph node in which the tumor theoretically originated, there is current support for the hypothesis that the proliferating epithelial cells somehow cause the accumulation of lymphoid tissue and the differentiation of IgA plasma cells.[330]

Grossly, this well-encapsulated tumor is round or oval or often flattened. Its surface is usually smooth, occasionally lobulated, and commonly pinkish gray. The cut surface is studded with whitish nodules that correspond to the germinal centers. Irregular cystic spaces filled with serous or milky fluid and containing papillary projections are observed.

Microscopically the essential components of the neoplasm are epithelial parenchyma and lymphoid stroma. The parenchymatous tissue is composed of tubules and dilated cystic spaces into whose lumina project slender, fingerlike, papillary processes, giving the neoplasm its characteristic appearance (Fig. 25-38, *A* and *B*). The lining epithelium is composed of two rows of cells, an inner row of tall nonciliated columnar cells with oxyphilic granular cytoplasm and an outer layer of cuboid, polygonal, or rounded cells. The cell nuclei of the inner layer tend to be deeply stained and are evenly arranged toward the luminal end. The nuclei of the basal layer are round or vesicular, with a distinct nuclear membrane and one or two nucleoli. Occasionally a mucous or goblet cell or sebaceous differentiation is observed. Within the tubular and cystic spaces, a pink, granular, or, more often, homogeneous substance is seen, probably a product of the lining epithelial cells. A thin basement membrane separates the epithelium from the lymphoid stroma. When present in abundant quantities, the lymphoid stroma contains numerous germinal centers.

Electron microscopic studies have demonstrated that the epithelial cells are oncocytic (that is, essentially bags of mitochondria).[358] The mitochondria are of two types, the usual form and the giant form; the latter is two to three times the size of the former. The cristae of the giant form are in the shape of closely packed lamellae (Fig. 25-38, *C*).

Oncocytoma (oxyphilic adenoma). The oxyphilic adenoma is a rare benign tumor constituting less than 1% of neoplasms of the major salivary glands. Although a few examples have been reported in the submandibular gland, the minor salivary glands are not involved. One must differentiate oncocytic proliferation from true onco-

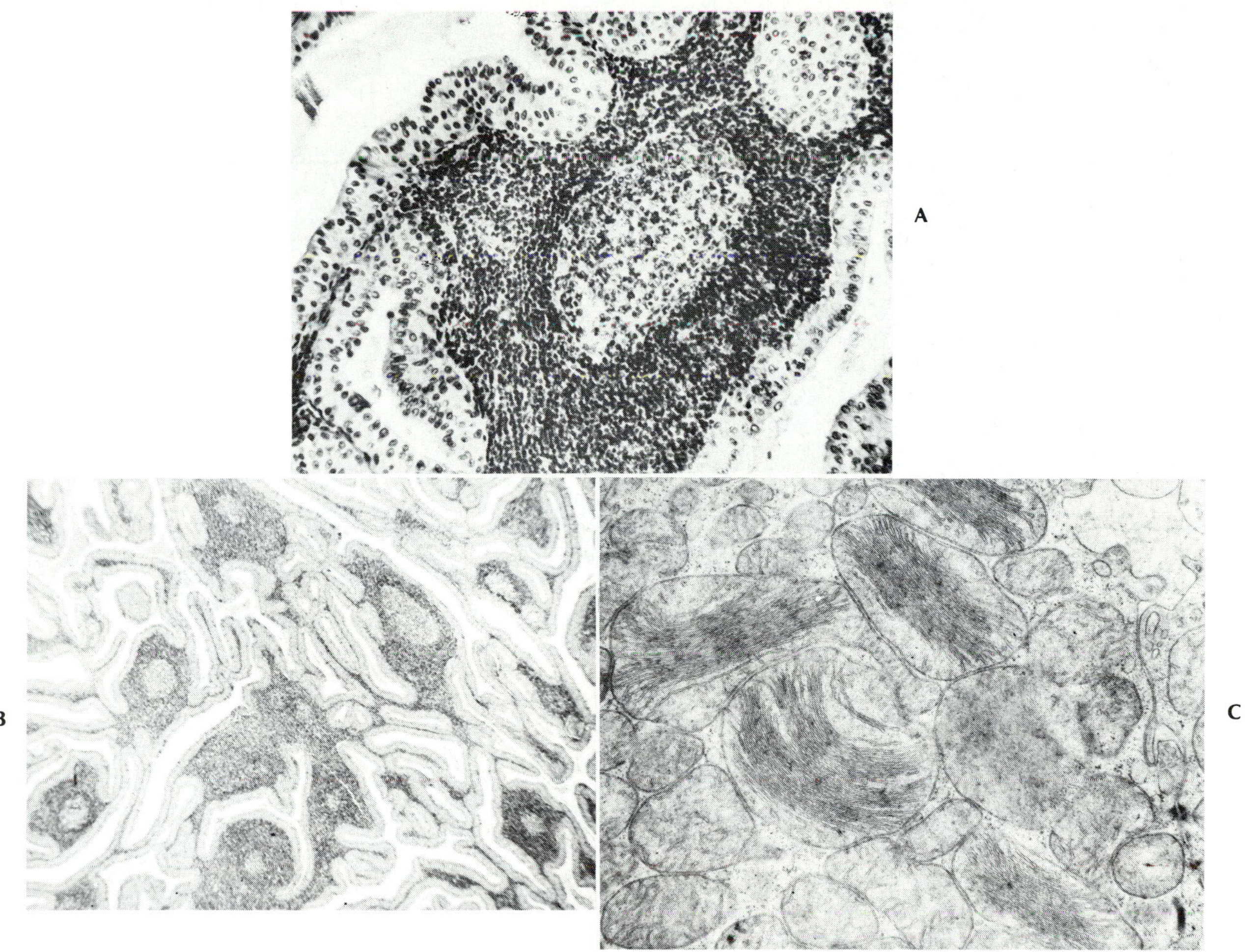

Fig. 25-38. Papillary cystadenoma lymphomatosum of parotid gland. **A,** Papillae extending into cavity contain lymphoid core covered by columnar epithelium. **B,** High magnification of area of **A** showing layer of columnar epithelium and lymphoid tissue. **C,** Admixture of normal and enlarged mitochondria. (**C,** From McGavran, M.H.: Virchows Arch. [Pathol. Anat.] **338:**195, 1965.)

cytomas.[291] The true tumors are slow growing, behaving rather like pleomorphic adenomas. Most patients are between 55 and 70 years of age. Bilateral examples have been reported, but it is not known whether these are hyperplasias or true tumors. There does not appear to be a marked sex predilection, but perhaps the true tumor is more common in women. Grossly the oncocytoma is well circumscribed, smooth surfaced, and rather firm. The cut surface is usually tan and is quite uniform in appearance.[323]

Microscopically, the cells are rather monotonous. They are pink, plump, and polyhedral. The nucleus is rounded and usually centrally located. Not uncommonly there are two or more nucleoli. The most common arrangement of the cells is in broad parallel columns, although acinar or tubular formations may be rarely present. A thin delicate connective tissue is present between the columns of cells. There are no lymphoid cells in the true oncocytoma (Fig. 25-39).

Origin from transformed duct and acinar cells is extremely likely, since the true oncocytoma resembles the oncocytes that occur in salivary glands.

Ultrastructural studies reveal that the cytoplasm is loaded with accumulations of mitochondria, which give rise to the oxyphilic staining.[287,336,375] Occasionally the mitochondria are larger than normal. Unlike normal mitochondria, however, mitochondria from the true oncocytoma produce only very small quantities of high-energy phosphate. There have been many attempts to differentiate oncocytic hyperplasia from true neoplasia.[291] It has been stated that, in the hypoplastic lesion, the cells have a nearly normal nuclear/cytoplasmic ratio, the nucleoli being inconspicuous, and that there is a normal polarity of the long axis of the cell to its basement membrane. True oncocytomas, in contrast, presumably have larger nuclei, increased nucleolar/cytoplasmic ratio

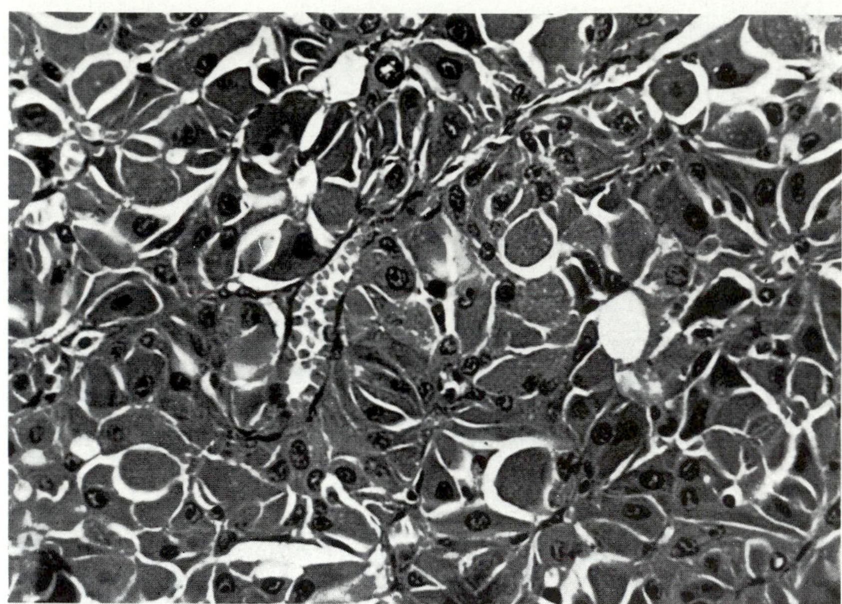

Fig. 25-39. Oxyphilic adenoma (oncocytoma) of parotid gland. Sheets and glandular formations of tall columnar cells with eosinophilic granular cytoplasm.

with prominent nucleoli, and, frequently, altered polarity.[376] I have never been able to substantiate these allegations. Recurrence is extremely rare and probably results from incomplete removal of the oncocytoma initially. The so-called malignant oncocytoma is extremely rare.[345,379] In 1977, Johns and co-workers[336] were willing to accept only 11 published cases. Microscopically, the histologic difference from benign oncocytoma is not great. Those that have metastasized have been found in regional lymph nodes.

Sebaceous lymphadenoma, sebaceous carcinoma, and sebaceous adenoma. Sebaceous lymphadenoma is the most common of these rare lesions. Less than a dozen examples had been documented by 1976. The tumor is composed of proliferated sebaceous glands in a matrix of normal-appearing lymphoid tissue, suggesting its development in an intraparotid or paraparotid lymph node (Fig. 25-40). One should be aware that it is not at all uncommon to observe sebaceous structures in normal parotid glands. According to one estimate, approximately one third of the adult population possesses these structures.[286,288,399]

Sebaceous carcinoma of the parotid gland is less common than sebaceous lymphadenoma. There are poorly defined margins and fingerlike invasion of adjacent structures. Focal areas of keratinization are common, as well as sites of necrosis. Not enough data exist concerning the frequency of recurrence or metastasis.[352,380]

Sebaceous adenoma is the least common salivary gland sebaceous cell lesion.[289] Only a few examples have been reported.

Mucoepidermoid carcinoma. Mucoepidermoid carcinoma is composed of epidermoid cells, mucus-secreting cells, and cells of intermediate type. Clear cells and columnar cells may also be present. The varied cell types suggest that the tumor arises from ductal epithelium with marked potential for varied differentiation and metaplasia. This concept has been supported by ultrastructural studies.[302] Squamous metaplasia is most common while mucous metaplasia occurs less often, but both types may commonly occur in conjunction.[327,333,389]

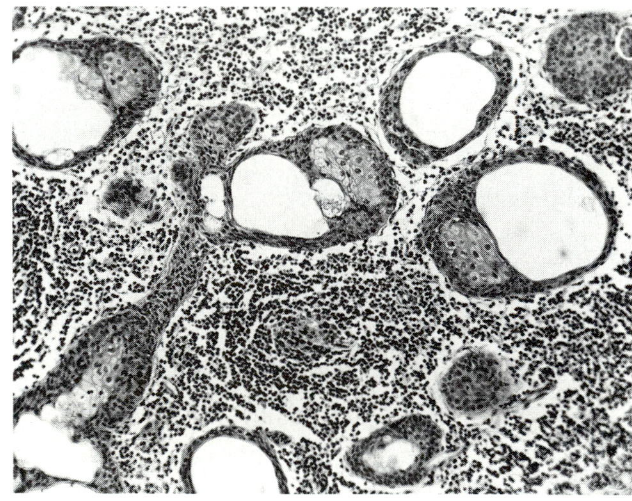

Fig. 25-40. Sebaceous lymphadenoma. Note proliferated sebaceous glands in matrix of normal-appearing lymphoid tissue.

About 5% to 10% of major salivary gland tumors and 10% of minor salivary gland tumors are mucoepidermoid carcinomas. Within the major salivary glands, 90% of these arise in the parotid salivary gland. In the minor salivary glands they occur most often in the palate, constituting about 25% of malignant tumors at that site.[315]

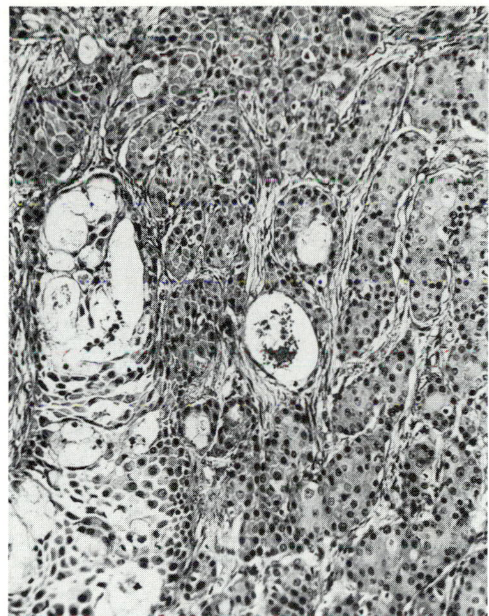

Fig. 25-41. Mucoepidermoid carcinoma of high-grade malignancy, strongly resembling squamous cell carcinoma. Careful search usually will reveal some cells that are producing mucus. Periodic acid–Schiff stain may aid in diagnosis.

Not uncommonly the tumor appears on the retromolar pad as a "mucocele." In several cases tumors have been reported within the body of the mandible and less often in the maxilla.[296] The tumor is usually painless, firm, nontender, and slow growing. Involvement of the facial nerve is exceedingly rare. There appears to be no sex predilection for tumors of the major and minor salivary glands, but there is a female sex predilection for intraosseous tumors. There does not seem to be an age predilection.

Grossly, mucoepidermoid tumors may be partially, but rarely completely, encapsulated. On cross section, cysts containing clear, rather mucoid fluid are often present. The tumor is generally grayish. Infiltration of adjacent tissues by the tumor is often noted.

Microscopically there is marked variability among mucoepidermoid carcinomas. Those with low-grade malignancy have an abundance of mucus-secreting cells, whereas the more anaplastic have few or no mucous cells and may be mistaken for squamous cell carcinoma (Fig. 25-41). A mucin stain such as Meyer's mucicarmine or Schiff's stain should be employed in all doubtful cases. Not uncommonly the squamous epithelial cell nests of low-grade malignant tumors become hydropic (clear cells). The presence of small cysts is very common in these well-differentiated tumors. The cysts become filled with mucus and commonly rupture. Even the well-differentiated tumor has the capacity to metastasize. Cystic arrangement is rare in the more malignant variety. Here the pattern is more nestlike or sheetlike, with mucous cells being uncommon in the primary tumor. However, metastasis from these tumors sometimes manifests mucous cells. Occasionally sebaceous cells or oncocytic cells are present.

The 5-year survival rate for well-differentiated tumors in either the parotid gland or the palate is 90% to 100%; for poorly differentiated tumors it is 40% and 20%, respectively. Metastasis occurs most often to the lymph nodes, bones, lungs, and brain.

Adenoid cystic carcinoma (cylindroma). Adenoid cystic carcinoma constitutes about 5% to 10% of parotid gland tumors, about 20% of submandibular and minor salivary gland tumors, and about 30% of malignant oral salivary gland tumors.[386] It also occurs in the lacrimal gland, nasopharynx, paranasal sinuses, and lower respiratory system.[311] Of adenoid cystic carcinomas, about 35% occur in the major salivary glands and 65% arise in minor glands. The most common oral sites are the palate, tongue, oral floor, and buccal mucosa. There appears to be a slight female predilection. Most patients are between 30 and 70 years of age, with a peak occurring in the sixth decade. The tumor is slow growing and of moderate to low-grade malignancy, but it is widely infiltrative. It is poorly encapsulated. Patients with tumors arising in a major salivary gland complain of associated pain in about 40% of the cases. Pain is less frequently (about 15%) a feature when it involves a minor salivary gland. In the palatal lesion, ulceration of the overlying mucosa is noted in about 15%. In the nasal cavity and paranasal sinuses, nasal airway obstruction and epistaxis are occasionally noted.[395]

The tumor is usually small (2 to 4 cm), firm, homogeneous, and grayish white in cross section. Microscopically, adenoid cystic carcinoma manifests varying patterns of small, darkly staining cells with scant cytoplasm (Fig. 25-42, *A*). The patterns most often exhibited are cribriform or sievelike, a solid pattern, or occasionally small, well-formed, ductal or tubular structures.[363] The cribriform pattern is characterized by nests of tumor cells with a Swiss cheese configuration. Some spaces contain mucicarmine-positive mucinous secretions of both epithelial and connective tissue origins.[301] A hyalinized fibrous tissue may also be present in the spaces, or a combination of mucinous and hyalinized material may be noted (Fig. 25-42, *B*). The tubular or trabecular pattern is characterized by elongated tubular structures having a central lumen. Depending on the plane of section, the tubules may appear long and thin, or on cross section round and glandular. In contrast to the cribriform units, the tubular structures are small and slender and demonstrate little stratification of cells. The so-called solid pattern consists of individual units of variable size completely filled with cells exhibiting new lumina. If enough sections are made, all three patterns can be observed in various examples of adenoid cystic carcinoma. Recurrences have been noted in approximately 60% of those with a predominantly tubular pattern, 90% of those with a cribri-

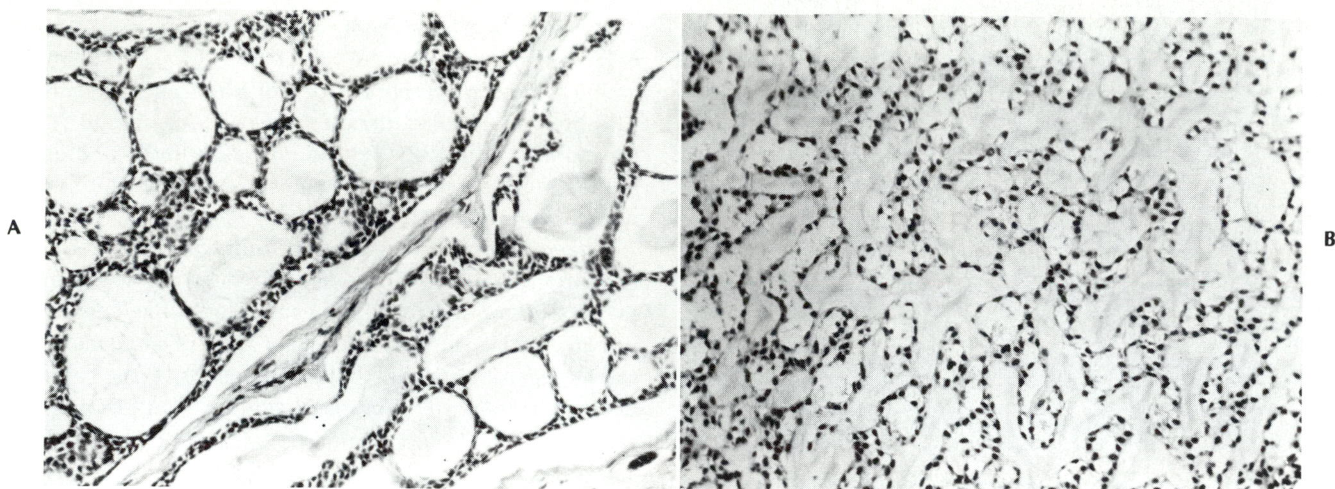

Fig. 25-42. Adenoid cystic carcinoma. **A,** Cribriform pattern. **B,** Hyaline or mucoid material with concomitant separation of tumor epithelium into strands.

form pattern, and 100% of those in which the neoplasm has been described as solid.[366] The overall salvage rate for patients with tumors of the major glands is about 50%, considerably better than the 30% for those with tumors of the minor salivary glands. Only 20% never appear to have recurrence of the tumor following initial therapy. Facial nerve involvement is common, invasion of perineural lymphatics being readily demonstrated in section in about half of the cases. This finding is correlated with poorer prognosis. Ultrastructural studies[301,355,393] have varied in their ability to demonstrate myoepithelial cells.

Acinic cell carcinoma (acinic cell tumor). Acinic cell carcinoma is a relatively rare tumor of salivary glands. It comprises about 2% to 3% of tumors of the parotid or about 10% to 20% of malignant parotid tumors. For every six examples that arise in the parotid gland, there is one in the submandibular gland and one in the oral minor salivary glands. There may be a slight female sex predilection.[367,388]

The tumor is usually firm and rounded. In the parotid gland it most often arises in the lateral portion or tail. It is well encapsulated in less than 15% of the cases. It is slow growing but has a tendency to recur, especially when poorly encapsulated. Local recurrence occurs in about 15% and is usually multiple. Metastasis occurs most frequently to the lymph nodes, lungs, bone, and brain. Survival rates for 5, 10, and 15 years are approximately 80%, 60%, and 45%, respectively.[290] A poor prognosis seems to be correlated with size of tumor, involvement of the deep lobe of the parotid, the amount of nuclear atypia and numbers of mitoses, and absence of a capsule. Somewhat less than 30% of the patients complain of pain, but facial nerve involvement is rare. The tumor occurs most commonly in the third and fourth decades in the major salivary glands, but in the minor salivary glands it is most often seen in the sixth decade; there is no sex predilection.[248,303] The palate, buccal mucosa, and tongue are most frequently involved, and the prognosis appears to be excellent. There has been a rare intraosseous example.

Grossly the tumor is often rubbery. On cut section the color is tan to yellow-gray, and cystic areas are noted in about 35% of the cases. Histologically, acinic cell carcinoma is composed of varying proportions of one or more of four cell types: acinic cells, intercalated duct cells, vacuolated cells, and nonspecific glandular cells.[285] The cells form large lobules with little intervening stroma. It has been suggested that the tumor arises from pluripotential duct cells, most likely the intercalated or terminal duct cells.

The acinic cells resemble polyhedral cells of normal acini and contain abundant, finely to coarsely granular cytoplasm exhibiting basophilia of variable intensity (Fig. 25-43). The nuclei are usually small and hyperchromatic. The vacuolated cells are characterized by one or two large vacuoles or by many small ones. The cells are often distended and appear to have coalesced into groups of small cysts separated by a syncytial network of cytoplasm producing a latticelike pattern. The nuclei are somewhat larger than those of acinic cells. Intercalated duct cells are smaller and cuboidal, exhibiting amphophilia and distinct borders. Occasionally these cells are arranged in a ductlike pattern. Nonspecific glandular cells cannot be clearly classified into any of the three aforementioned categories. They feature the most mitoses and nuclear atypia. Numerous mitoses are seen in about 10% of the specimens. Rarely, clear cells are seen that may represent acinic cells that have lost their granules or never had granules. Various growth patterns are seen: solid, micro-

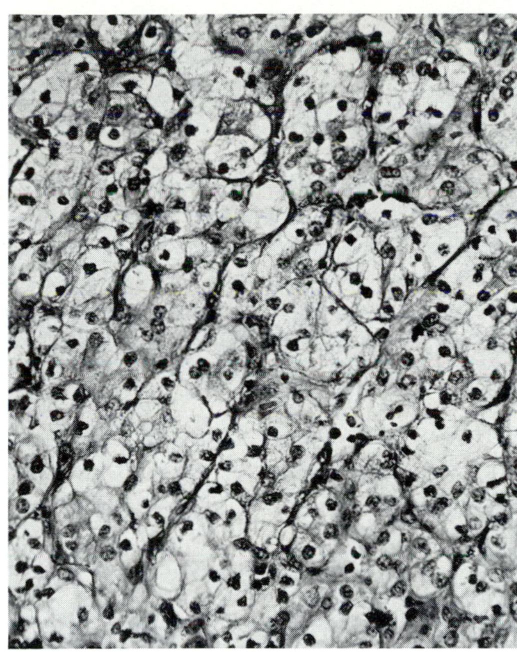

Fig. 25-43. Acinic cell carcinoma. Note hypernephroid appearance.

cystic, papillary cystic, and follicular. Stroma is usually sparse. Periodic acid–Schiff–positive material may be present, especially in microcystic areas. In tumors of the major glands a lymphoid stroma is occasionally present. This may represent origin in an intraparotid lymph node. A lymphoid stroma is never present in tumors of minor salivary gland origin. Some tumors greatly resemble adenocarcinoma (hypernephroma) of the kidney. Ultrastructural studies have demonstrated that the acinic cells resemble the serous acinar cells of normal glands; that is, they contain secretory granules and histochemically are identical to serous cells.[314,331]

Carcinoma in pleomorphic adenoma (malignant mixed tumor). By definition, this lesion is a binary combination of benign mixed tumor and a malignant neoplasm, most often a poorly differentiated adenocarcinoma. It may comprise as much as 2% to 5% of all mixed tumors. There may be a second type of malignant mixed tumor in which the lesion maintains the pattern of pleomorphic adenoma (epithelial tubules and nests in a myxoid or chondroid stroma), but the epithelial elements are all malignant. The tumor occurs in both major and minor salivary glands. In the major glands the tumor is usually poorly circumscribed. In the minor glands the tumor has infiltrating margins. Hemorrhage, necrosis, cystic degeneration, and irregular edges have been seen in about 25% of the cases and should alert the pathologist if these features are observed grossly in an otherwise benign mixed tumor. The microscopic features of the pleomorphic adenomatous portion of the tumor are in no way atypical. The malignant areas vary considerably from tumor to tumor. Some tumors exhibit considerable anaplasia, the cells having large and hyperchromatic nuclei and large nucleoli. Mitoses are often present. The cells may be organized into small nests or tubules or into large nests or sheets. The latter are more likely to exhibit necrotic foci. Perineural invasion and infiltration into adjacent salivary gland connective tissue or fat are noted in 60% to 80% of the cases.

There appears to be a 3:1 female sex predilection. Ages at time of diagnosis have ranged from 35 to 85 years, with a mean of 60 years. This is about 10 years older than the mean age for benign mixed tumor. There has been considerable debate concerning whether the malignant mixed tumor arises from the benign mixed tumor or is merely associated with it. Palatal neoplasms appear to have a better prognosis than those in a major salivary gland. Local recurrences have been noted to occur in about 40%. The 5-year survival rate is about 55%. Metastasis most often occurs to the lymph nodes, lungs, or bone.[313,349]

Primary squamous cell carcinoma. Primary squamous cell carcinoma is essentially limited to the parotid gland. It is a relatively rare tumor, probably representing about 1% of parotid neoplasms or about 5% to 10% of primary malignant tumors of the gland. Although studies done earlier indicated a higher frequency, this probably resulted from the erroneous assignment of mucoepidermoid tumors to this category. One must also avoid the error of mistaking metastases from squamous cell carcinoma to the parotid gland for squamous cell carcinoma of the skin of the head and neck. The tumor arises predominantly in males in the sixth or seventh decade. Most of the documented cases have been well or moderately differentiated carcinoma. Intercellular bridges and keratin pearl formation are often noted. The tumor commonly infiltrates the skin and involves the facial nerve early in its clinical course. Pain may be severe. Local recurrence and regional lymph node metastases have been noted in approximately 70%. There are insufficient data to indicate 5-year survivals.

Adenocarcinoma. Adenocarcinoma of the salivary glands does not differ from adenocarcinoma of other organs. The cells are arranged in ducts or tubules. The tumor cells infiltrate blood and lymphatic vessels and perineural spaces. Some tumor cells produce mucus, which may fill the lumen of the tubules or may spill into the stroma. One must be careful to distinguish those that produce mucus from mucoepidermoid carcinoma. In one variant the cells appear similar to oncocytes, leading to the diagnosis of malignant oncocytoma. Some adenocarcinomas appear to arise from pleomorphic adenomas.[292,403]

The incidence of adenocarcinoma is difficult to establish. In some studies it has been as high as 3% of parotid salivary gland tumors. There is no age or sex predilection. The tumor is usually firm and may be papillary or nonpapillary and mucus-secreting or non-mucus-secreting. The papillary is the predominant form. The papillary structures often project from the walls of cystic lumina. The 5-year survival rate appears to be about 40%. Prognosis, as in other cases of adenocarcinoma, depends on the degree of differentiation.[387,397]

Undifferentiated carcinoma. Undifferentiated carcinoma consists of sheets or cords of anaplastic epithelial cells surrounded by varying amounts of fibrous stroma. It constitutes about 3% to 5% of all salivary gland tumors. Although it occurs at any age, it is most common in the seventh and eighth decades of life. There is no sex predilection. The tumor is so undifferentiated that it cannot be otherwise classified. It is composed of compact cell masses that vary in size. Mitoses are frequently abundant. Necrosis sometimes occurs. Invasion of adjacent structures such as the auditory canal, paranasal sinuses, and mandible is common, as is local and widespread metastasis. With local recurrence there is often infiltration of overlying skin, adjacent muscle, or mucous membrane. About half of the patients die from tumor spread, even following removal of the primary tumor. The most common sites of metastasis are lung, bone, and liver. The 5-year survival rate is approximately 25%. The tumor appears to run a more malignant course in children than in adults. In contrast to adenoid cystic carcinoma, in which death occurs late, most fatalities from undifferentiated carcinoma occur during the first 5 years following diagnosis and treatment.[293,341,401]

Other tumors of salivary glands. Several other tumors having their origin in the stromal tissues of salivary glands have been described: lipoma, rhabdomyosarcoma, leiomyoma, neurofibroma, neurilemoma, leiomyosarcoma, xanthoma, lymphangioma, malignant hemangioendothelioma, and fibromatosis.

Tumors of oral minor salivary glands. Neoplasms of the oral minor salivary glands include all those that occur in the major salivary glands with the exception of adenolymphoma, sebaceous tumors, and hemangioma. The incidence of malignant salivary gland tumors is markedly higher in minor salivary glands than in the parotid. Tumors of the minor salivary glands represent approximately 15% of those that occur in the major glands. The palate is affected in approximately half of the cases. Although the incidence of malignant minor salivary gland tumors has varied remarkably with the series published, a reasonable assessment is that approximately half of minor salivary gland tumors are malignant. The pleomorphic adenoma is the most common benign tumor; the most common malignant tumors, in order of frequency, are the adenoid cystic carcinoma, mucoepidermoid carcinoma, and adenocarcinoma. In the palate, salivary gland tumors occur almost as frequently as squamous cell carcinomas. Benign tumors most often involve the soft palate and posterior hard palate, upper lip (upper lip/lower lip, 6:1), buccal mucosa, tongue, oral floor, and retromolar region. Malignant minor salivary gland tumors, however, involve the tongue far more frequently than the upper lip. Tumors of the buccal mucosa are more often benign.[318,383,390]

Benign tumors occur most frequently in the fourth and fifth decades. The malignant tumors are most common in the sixth decade. Pleomorphic adenoma in the oral cavity has an extremely low recurrence rate, approximately 5% to 7%. The mucoepidermoid carcinoma involves the minor salivary glands about twice as frequently as the major salivary glands. Approximately 40% arise in the palate and another 20% each within the jaw bone and oral floor. Adenoid cystic carcinoma involving the minor salivary glands occurs about twice as often in women and in a slightly older age group. Adenocarcinoma of the minor salivary glands also most frequently involves the palate, buccal mucosa, and tongue. Recurrences are common and metastasis is usual.

Submandibular salivary gland tumors. Tumors of the submandibular salivary gland are about one ninth as common as those in the parotid and one half as common as those of the minor salivary glands. Malignant tumors are more frequent than in the parotid salivary gland. About 50% are benign tumors, nearly all pleomorphic adenomas. Among the malignant tumors, adenoid cystic carcinoma accounts for 40%, mucoepidermoid carcinoma for about 15%, and adenocarcinoma 15%, and carcinoma in pleomorphic adenoma, squamous cell carcinoma, and undifferentiated carcinoma constitute about 10% each.[304,325,385]

Sublingual salivary gland tumors. The sublingual, the smallest of the major salivary glands, is rarely the site of a primary neoplasm, but most cases (almost 80%) have been malignant. This contrasts sharply with tumors of the other two major salivary glands: 35% are malignant in the parotid gland, and 50% in the submandibular gland. Adenoid cystic carcinoma and mucoepidermoid carcinoma each represent 40% of sublingual salivary gland neoplasms.

NECK

Tumors

Carotid body tumor. Carotid body tumor (chemodectoma) arises in the carotid bodies, small ovoid nodules situated on the medial aspect of the bifurcation of the common carotid arteries that mediate chemosensory reflexes sensing changes in pH and arterial oxygen tension. The carotid bodies are also involved in catecholamine storage. Histologically identical tumors are found in the aortic bodies, the glomus jugulare (paraganglion tympanicum), and the ganglion nodosum of the vagus nerve. All of these structures are derived from neural crest cells and migrate to areas about the vessels of the embryonic branchial arches.[415,419]

The tumor may become manifest at any age but rarely

before puberty.[422,424] There is a slight female predilection. About 5% are bilateral. In some cases there appears to be autosomal dominant inheritance.[426,433]

Microscopically the tumor is lobulated and thinly encapsulated or embedded in loose connective tissue. It consists of nests of rather large polyhedral cells grouped together in an alveolar or organoid pattern (Fig. 25-44). The cell nests are separated by loose connective tissue and a richly vascular stroma. The individual cells are of two types: (1) large cell, with a rounded vesicular nucleus and a pronounced nucleolus, and (2) a smaller cell with a darker nucleus (less numerous). Its cytoplasm is pale, eosinophilic, and frequently vacuolated, with indistinct cell boundaries. Rarely, bizarre hyperchromatic cells, active mitoses, and capsular invasion may be observed. Spread to regional nodes or even distant dissemination has been noted in about 5% of the cases but rarely results in death of the patient.

Cervical thymus. There have been several case reports in which the thymus has failed to descend and appears as a cervical mass.[432]

Benign symmetric lipomatosis. Benign symmetric lipomatosis, also called Madelung's disease or Launois-Bensaude syndrome, is characterized by slow, massive accumulation of fatty tissue in the cervical and supraclavicular regions, causing severe swelling about the neck and at times severe respiratory distress. There may be extensions of tonguelike projections of fatty tissue between the cervical and upper thoracic muscles, as well as a "buffalo hump" of fat over the cervical region. Involvement of the preauricular and postauricular regions may give the patient a chipmunk appearance. Similar masses may appear symmetrically in the axillae and groin.[418,430]

Benign symmetric lipomatosis appears in adult life, although onset in most patients is rather ill defined. Enlargement is intermittently progressive. In some patients, the size of the masses has remained relatively stationary for a long time and then increased rapidly within a few weeks. Not uncommonly the patient is an alcoholic. Microscopically the deposits appear to be normal, nonencapsulated, adipose tissue.

Fibromatosis colli. Fibromatosis colli (torticollis, wryneck) occurs both as a primary and as a secondary disease. Primary or congenital torticollis is manifest by a firm, fusiform swelling of the sternocleidomastoid muscle, especially in its lowest third, either at birth or within the first few weeks of life. The swelling usually increases for several weeks and then regresses, occasionally disappearing between the sixth and eighth months.[408,412]

Grossly the muscle is shortened, contracted, and fibrous. Clinically the chin becomes tilted upward and toward the unaffected side. If the disease is untreated, facial asymmetry results, with adaptive scoliosis of the lower cervical and upper thoracic spine, foreshortening of the skull, and flattening of the facial bones on the involved side. The etiology is unknown, but theories have implicated uterine malposition. Often (35% to 50%) it is associated with breech delivery.

Microscopically the muscle fibers are widely separated by dense, scarlike fibrous connective tissue (Fig. 25-45). It should be differentiated from desmoid tumor. Secondary torticollis is usually caused by a myositis that is attributed to a "chill." Occasionally it occurs after a tumor of

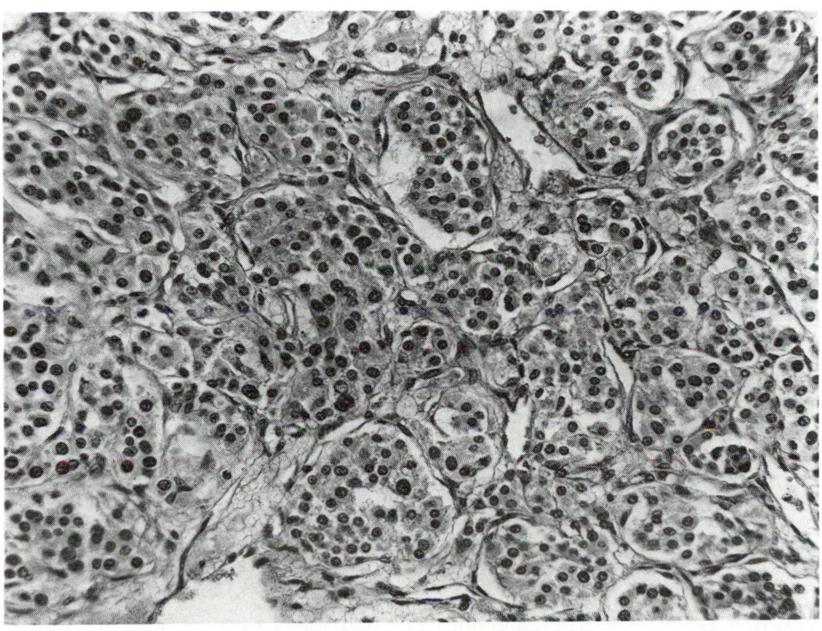

Fig. 25-44. Carotid body tumor. Note classic "cell-ball" pattern. (From Abell, M.R., et al.: Hum. Pathol. **1**:503, 1970.)

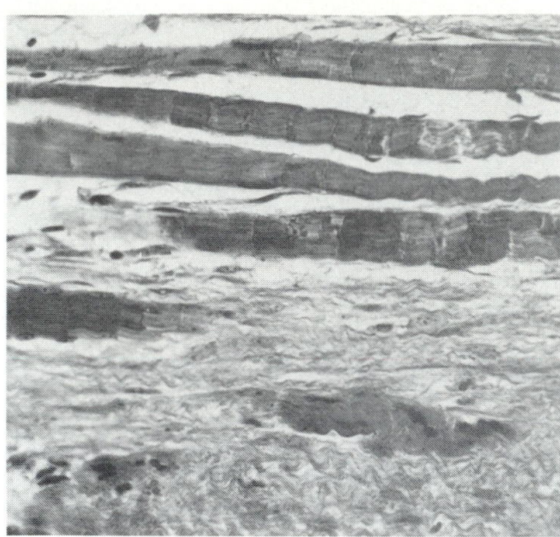

Fig. 25-45. Torticollis. Fibrous connective tissue replaces striated muscle fibers.

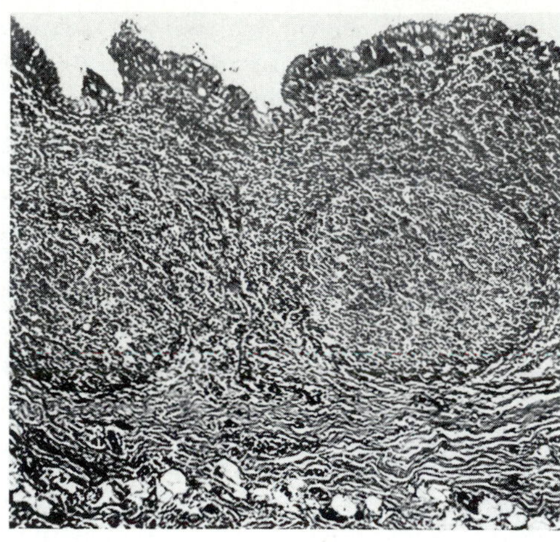

Fig. 25-46. Lymphoepithelial cyst lined by respiratory epithelium with lymphoid tissue in connective tissue wall.

the cervical cord, or it may be a hysterical manifestation.

Congenital teratoma of neck. Congenital cervical teratoma is relatively rare. There is argument for thyroid gland origin, but it is not entirely convincing. Some cervical teratomas assume massive dimensions. In over 40% of the patients the tumor is larger than 10 cm. A history of polyhydramnios is obtained in about half of this latter group. About 30% of the children are either stillborn or premature. Another third die of respiratory obstruction soon after birth. There is no sex predilection, but about half of the patients are black, suggesting increased incidence in this racial group. Grossly the mass is usually semicystic but may be solid or multiloculated and is nearly always encapsulated. Microscopically all three embryonal layers are represented. Fetal brain tissue is especially common (about 70%). Nearly all congenital cervical teratomas so far reported have been benign. Teratoma of the neck in adults, which is extremely rare, is always malignant.[413,427,429]

Cysts

Thyroglossal tract cyst. The thyroid gland arises in the region of the foramen cecum of the tongue and begins descent into the anterior neck around the third intrauterine week. If it persists in its original embryonal position, it is spoken of as lingual thyroid. Rarely, a strand of epithelium persists and connects the base of the tongue with the normally positioned thyroid gland. The thyroglossal tract cyst results from cystic degeneration of this tract. It is in the midline of the neck usually at or below the level of the hyoid bone, through which the tract usually passes. The cyst is lined by respiratory or stratified squamous epithelium, or by both types. In about 35% of the cases, the cyst may become infected and drain, becoming a thyroglossal tract fistula.[409,423]

Lymphoepithelial cyst. The lateral cervical cyst (branchial cyst) is located anterior to the sternocleidomastoid muscle near the angle of the mandible. The alleged association of these cysts or sinuses with squamous carcinoma appears unwarranted. Microscopically the cyst is lined by either stratified squamous or pseudostratified ciliated columnar epithelium (Fig. 25-46). Beneath the epithelium is abundant lymphoid tissue with germinal centers. The cysts are believed to arise from cystic degeneration of epithelium enclaved in cervical lymph nodes. The cyst usually becomes apparent during the third decade. Similar lesions may occur in the parotid gland or in the oral floor beneath the tongue.[407,410]

Parathyroid cyst. Microscopic cysts of the parathyroid glands are seen in at least 50% of normal persons. At autopsy about 2% have true cysts. Nevertheless, cysts large enough to produce clinical symptoms are rare.

The parathyroid cyst is solitary and slow growing and if large may cause dysphagia and displacement of the trachea to the contralateral side, producing hoarseness by pressure on the recurrent laryngeal nerve. In several instances, this symptom has led to a preoperative diagnosis of thyroid carcinoma. It is found anywhere in the lateral neck from the angle of the mandible deep to the sternocleidomastoid muscle to the mediastinum. Most of the patients are over 30 years of age, and a 3:1 female predilection is evident. About 60% of cysts occur on the left side.[411,421]

The cyst is usually very thin and filled with a clear, watery fluid. Microscopically it is lined by a somewhat flattened cuboid to low columnar epithelium. Within the collagenic connective tissue wall, one usually notes several types of parathyroid cells: water-clear cells, chief cells, and, occasionally, oxyphil cells. Not all three types are always present.

Cervical thymic cyst. Occasionally, remnants of thymus primordium are left in the neck, where they may remain undisturbed or, rarely, may undergo cystic alteration and subsequent enlargement. The cyst probably arises from degeneration of Hassall's corpuscles or from thyropharyngeal tubules. They occur clinically most often at about 7 years of age, and there appears to be a 2:1 male sex predilection. The cysts are usually elongated and may assume large proportions. They usually are located in the left (70%) lateral neck at the angle of the mandible just anterior to the sternocleidomastoid muscle.[416,420]

Microscopically the cysts are lined by stratified squamous epithelium and often contain a thick, reddish brown fluid. Rarely, cuboid epithelium is found. In the walls thymic structures (such as Hassall's corpuscles) may be identified. The cyst is well encapsulated and often exhibits cholesterol crystals among the connective tissue fibers.

Cystic hygroma. The cystic hygroma or diffuse lymphangioma is manifest as a rather poorly defined soft tissue mass in the neck, usually behind the sternocleidomastoid muscle. It is either present at birth (50%) or manifested within the first 2 years of life. About 15% extend to involve the axilla, mediastinum, cheek, tongue, or oral floor, about 15% resolve spontaneously, and about 30% become infected.[414,425] Microscopically the mass consists of numerous endothelium-lined lymphatic spaces of varied size in a loose connective tissue stroma.

Inflammatory disease

Ludwig's angina. Ludwig's angina is a severe, boardlike cellulitis of the neck involving all of the submandibular spaces. Before the advent of antibiotics this was a rare complication of periapical infection of the mandibular molars or extension from an acute osteomyelitis occurring after compound fracture of the mandible. Drainage of pus through the lingual plate of the mandible into one or more spaces and subsequent extension with pronounced edema of the glottis commonly resulted in death from severe toxemia and asphyxiation.[417,428]

REFERENCES

General

1. Batsakis, J.G.: Tumors of the head and neck, ed. 2, Baltimore, 1979, The Williams & Wilkins Co.
2. Goodman, R.M., and Gorlin, R.J.: Atlas of the face in genetic disorders, ed. 2, St. Louis, 1977, The C.V. Mosby Co.
3. Gorlin, R.J., Pindborg, J.J., and Cohen, M.M., Jr.: Syndromes of the head and neck, ed. 2, New York, 1976, McGraw-Hill Book Co.
4. Hajdu, S.I.: Pathology of soft tissue tumors, Philadelphia, 1979, W.B. Saunders Co.
5. Pindborg, J.J.: Pathology of the dental hard tissues, Philadelphia, 1970, W.B. Saunders Co.
6. Pindborg, J.J.: Atlas of diseases of the oral mucosa, ed. 3, Philadelphia, 1980, W.B. Saunders Co.
7. Pindborg, J.J., and Hjørting-Hansen, E.: Atlas of diseases of the jaws, Philadelphia, 1974, W.B. Saunders Co.
8. Shafer, W.G., Hine, M.K., and Levy, B.M.: Oral pathology, ed. 4, Philadelphia, 1983, W.B. Saunders Co.
9. Stewart, R.E., and Prescott, G.H., editors: Oral-facial genetics, St. Louis, 1976, The C.V. Mosby Co.
10. Waldron, C., and Gorlin, R.J., editors: Oral pathology, ed. 7, St. Louis, 1985, The C.V. Mosby Co.
11. World Health Organization: International histological classification of tumors. No. 5. Histological typing of odontogenic tumours, jaw cysts and allied lesions, Geneva, 1971, WHO.

Face and lips

12. Baker, W.R.: Pits of the lip commissures in Caucasoid males, Oral Surg. **21**:56, 1966.
13. Cohen, M.M., Jr.: Syndromes with cleft lip and cleft palate, Cleft Palate J. **15**:306, 1978.
14. Gorlin, R.J., Cervenka, J., and Pruzansky, S.: Facial clefting and its syndromes, Birth Defects **7**(7):3, 1971.
15. Melnick, M.: The etiology of cleft lip and cleft palate, New York, 1980, Alan R. Liss.
16. Melnick, M., and Shields, E.D.: Oral-facial-digital syndrome, type I: a phenotypic and genetic analysis, Oral Surg. **40**:599, 1975.
17. Sewerin, I.: The sebaceous glands in the vermilion border of the lip and in the oral mucosa, Acta Odontol. Scand. **33**:1, 1975.
18. Shprintzen, R.J., Goldberg, R.B., and Sidoti, E.J.: The penetrance and variable expression of the Van der Woude syndrome: implications for genetic counseling, Cleft Palate J. **17**:52, 1980.

Tongue

19. Baughman, R.A.: Median rhomboid glossitis: a developmental anomaly? Oral Surg. **31**:56, 1971.
20. Cohen, M.M., Jr., et al.: The Beckwith-Wiedemann syndrome: seven new cases, Am. J. Dis. Child. **112**:515, 1971.
21. Neinas, F.W.: Lingual thyroid: clinical characteristics in 15 cases, Ann. Intern. Med. **79**:205, 1973.

Teeth

22. Backer-Dircks, O.: The relation between the fluoridation of water and dental caries experience, Int. Dent. J. **17**:582, 1967.
23. Brandtzaeg, P.: Immunology of inflammatory periodontal lesions, Int. Dent. J. **23**:438, 1973.
24. Gibbons, R.J., and van Houte, J.: Dental caries, Annu. Rev. Med. **26**:121, 1975.
25. Goldman, H.M.: Periodontal disease. In Waldron, C., and Gorlin, R.J., editors: Oral pathology, ed. 7, St. Louis, 1985, The C.V. Mosby Co.
26. Hamada, S., and Slade, H.D.: Biology, immunology, and cariogenicity of *Streptococcus mutans*, Microbiol. Rev. **44**:331, 1980.
27. Horowitz, H.S.: A review of systemic and topical fluorides for the prevention of dental caries, Community Dent. Oral Epidemiol. **1**:104, 1973.
28. Lehner, T.: Cell-mediated immune responses in oral disease: a review, J. Oral Pathol. **1**:39, 1972.
29. Löe, H., Theilade, E., and Jensen, S.B.: Experimental gingivitis in man, J. Periodontol. **36**:177, 1965.
30. Scherp, H.W.: Dental caries: prospects for prevention, Science **173**:1199, 1971.
31. Schulze, C.: Developmental abnormalities of the teeth and jaws. In Gorlin, R.J., and Goldman, H.M., editors: Thoma's oral pathology, ed. 6, St. Louis, 1970, The C.V. Mosby Co.
32. Silverstone, L.: Dental caries. In Waldron, C., and Gorlin, R.J., editors: Oral pathology, ed. 7, St. Louis, 1985, The C.V. Mosby Co.
33. Socransky, S.S.: Relationship of bacteria to the etiology of periodontal disease, J. Dent. Res. **49**:203, 1970.
34. Witkop, C.J., Jr., and Rao, S.: Inherited defects in tooth structures, Birth Defects **7**(7):153, 1971.

Oral soft tissues

35. Abbey, L.M., Page, D.G., and Sawyer, D.R.: The clinical and histopathologic features of a series of 464 oral squamous cell papillomas, Oral Surg. **49**:419, 1980.

36. Abbey, L.M., Sawyer, D.R., and Syrop, H.M.: Oral squamous acanthoma, Oral Surg. **45**:255, 1978.
37. Acevedo, A., and Buhler, J.E.: Plasma cell granuloma of the gingiva, Oral Surg. **43**:196, 1977.
38. Album, M.M., et al.: Epidermolysis bullosa dystrophica polydysplastica, Oral Surg. **43**:859, 1977.
39. Anderson, L., Fejerskov, O., and Philipsen, H.P.: Calcified fibroblastic granuloma, J. Oral Surg. **31**:196, 1973.
40. Andreasen, J.O.: Oral lichen planus. I. A clinical evaluation of 115 cases, Oral Surg. **25**:31, 1968.
41. Angelopoulos, A.P.: Pyogenic granuloma of the oral cavity, J. Oral Surg. **29**:840, 1971.
42. Angelopoulos, A.P., and Goaz, P.W.: Incidence of diphenylhydantoin gingival hyperplasia, Oral Surg. **34**:898, 1972.
43. Azaz, B., and Lustmann, J.: Keratoacanthoma of the lower lip, Oral Surg. **38**:918, 1974.
44. Bale, P.M., and Reye, R.D.K.: Rhabdomyosarcoma in childhood, Pathology **7**:101, 1975.
45,. Ballard, B.R., et al.: Squamous-cell carcinoma of the floor of the mouth, Oral Surg. **45**:568, 1978.
46. Banks, P.: Infectious mononucleosis, Br. J. Oral Surg. **4**:227, 1967.
47. Bernstein, M.L., and McDonald, J.S.: Oral lesions in Crohn's disease: report of two cases and update of the literature, Oral Surg. **46**:234, 1978.
48. Bhaskar, S.N., Beasley, J.D., and Cutright, D.E.: Inflammatory papillary hyperplasia of the oral mucosa: report of 341 cases, J. Am. Dent. Assoc. **81**:949, 1970.
49. Blair, A.E., and Edwards, D.M.: Congenital epulis of the newborn, Oral Surg. **43**:687, 1977.
50. Boell, F., and Meier-Ewert, H.: Echo-6-Viren als Erreger des Hand-Fuss-Mund Exanthems, Hautarzt **28**:96, 1977.
51. Buchner, A.: Hand, foot and mouth disease, Oral Surg. **41**:333, 1976.
52. Buchner, A., and Hansen, L.S.: Amalgam pigmentation (amalgam tattoo) of the oral mucosa, Oral Surg. **49**:139, 1980.
53. Buchner, A., and Hansen, L.S.: Pigmented nevi of the oral cavity: a clinicopathologic study of 32 new cases and a review of 75 cases from the literature, Oral Surg. **49**:55, 1980.
54. Buchner, A., Lozada, F., and Silverman, S., Jr.: Histopathologic aspects of oral erythema multiforme, Oral Surg. **49**:221, 1980.
55. Budtz-Jørgensen, E., and Bertram, U.: Denture stomatitis, Acta Odontol. Scand. **28**:71, 1970.
56. Burns, J.C.: Diagnostic methods for herpes simplex infection: a review, Oral Surg. **50**:346, 1980.
57. Cady, B., and Catlin, D.: Epidermoid carcinoma of the gum: a 20-year survey, Cancer **23**:551, 1969.
58. Carlsson, G.O.: Pigmented lesions with special reference to the oral mucous membrane, Sven. Tandlak. Tidskr. **66(suppl. 3)**:1, 1973.
59. Cherick, H.M., Dunlap, D.L., and King, O.H.: Leiomyomas of the oral cavity, Oral Surg. **35**:54, 1973.
60. Chue, P.W.Y.: Gonorrhea—its natural history, oral manifestations, diagnosis, treatment and prevention, J. Am. Dent. Assoc. **90**:1297, 1975.
61. Cobb, C.M., Holt, R., and Denys, F.R.: Ultrastructural features of the verruciform xanthoma, J. Oral Pathol. **5**:42, 1976.
62. Conley, J., and Sadoyama, J.A.: Squamous cell cancer of the buccal mucosa, Arch. Otolaryngol. **97**:330, 1973.
63. Corio, R.L., and Lewis, D.M.: Intraoral rhabdomyoma, Oral Surg. **48**:525, 1979.
64. Cutright, D.E.: The histopathologic findings in 583 cases of epulis fissuratum, Oral Surg. **37**:401, 1974.
65. Dito, W.R., and Batsakis, J.G.: Intraoral, pharyngeal and nasopharyngeal rhabdomyosarcoma, Arch. Otolaryngol. **77**:123, 1963.
66. Dummett, C.O., and Barens, G.: Pigmentation of the oral tissues: a review of the literature, J. Periodontol. **38**:369, 1967.
67. Dyck, P., et al.: MEN 2B: phenotype recognition; neurologic features and their pathological basis, Ann. Neurol. **6**:302, 1979.
68. Edwards, M.B., and Buckerfield, J.P.: Wegener's granulomatosis: a case with primary mucocutaneous lesions, Oral Surg. **46**:53, 1978.
69. Eisenberg, E., et al.: Pemphigus-like mucosal lesions: a side effect of penicillamine therapy, Oral Surg. **51**:409, 1981.
70. Ellis, G.L., and Corio, R.L.: Spindle cell carcinoma of the oral cavity: a clinicopathologic assessment of fifty-nine cases, Oral Surg. **50**:523, 1980.
71. Embil, J.A., Stevens, R.G., and Manual, F.R.: Prevalence of recurrent herpes labialis and aphthous ulcers among young adults on six continents, Can. Med. Assoc. J. **113**:627, 1975.
72. Eneroth, C.M.: Malignant melanoma of the oral cavity, Int. J. Oral Surg. **4**:191, 1975.
73. Eneroth, C.M., Hjertman, L., and Moberger, G.: Squamous cell carcinomas of the palate, Acta Otolaryngol. **73**:418, 1972.
74. Enzinger, F.M., and Shiraki, M.: Alveolar rhabdomyosarcoma: an analysis of 110 cases, Cancer **24**:18, 1969.
75. Farman, A.G.: Hairy tongue (lingua villosa), J. Oral Med. **32**:85, 1977.
76. Finkelstein, M.W., Hammond, H.L., and Jones, R.B.: Hyalinosis cutis et mucosae, Oral Surg. **54**:49, 1982.
77. Fiumara, N.J., and Lessell, S.: Manifestations of late congenital syphilis, Arch. Dermatol. **102**:78, 1970.
78. Fonts, E.A., et al.: Verrucous squamous cell carcinoma of the oral cavity, Cancer **23**:152, 1969.
79. Fu, Y.-S., and Perzin, K.H.: Skeletal muscle tumors: rhabdomyoma and rhabdomyosarcoma, Cancer **37**:364, 1976.
80. Fuhr, A.H., and Krogh, P.H.J.: Congenital epulis of the newborn: centennial review of the literature and a report of a case, J. Oral Surg. **30**:30, 1972.
81. Fujibayashi, T., et al.: Tuberculosis of the tongue, Oral Surg. **47**:427, 1979.
82. Garrett, W.S., Ware, J.L., and Thorne, F.L.: Keratoacanthoma, Arch. Surg. **94**:853, 1968.
83. Giansanti, J.S., Drummond, J.F., and Sabes, W.R.: Intraoral melanocytic cellular nevi, Oral Surg. **44**:267, 1977.
84. Goldstein, B.H., and Katz, S.M.: Immunofluorescent findings in oral bullous lichen planus, J. Oral Med. **34**:8, 1979.
85. Goldstein, B.H., Sciubba, J.J., and Laskin, D.M.: Actinomycosis of the maxilla, J. Oral Surg. **30**:362, 1972.
86. Gorlin, R.J.: Epidermolysis bullosa, Oral Surg. **32**:760, 1971.
87. Graykowski, E., and Hooks, J.: Summary of workshop on recurrent aphthous stomatitis and Behçet syndrome, J. Am. Dent. Assoc. **97**:599, 1978.
88. Greenberg, M.S., Brightman, V.J., and Ship, I.I.: Clinical and laboratory differentiation of recurrent intraoral herpes simplex virus infections following fever, J. Dent. Res. **48**:385, 1969.
89. Haase, C.D., Zoutendam, G.L., and Bombas, O.F.: Intraoral blue (Jadassohn-Tieche) nevus, Oral Surg. **45**:755, 1978.
90. Haneke, E.: The Papillon-Lefèvre syndrome: keratosis palmoplantaris with periodontopathy, Hum. Genet. **51**:1, 1979.
91. Hatziotis, J.C.: Lipoma of the oral cavity, Oral Surg. **31**:511, 1971.
92. Hedin, C.A., and Larsson, A.: Physiology and pathology of melanin pigmentation with special reference to the oral mucosa, Swed. Dent. J. **2**:113, 1978.
93. Holmstrup, P., and Bessermann, M.: Clinical, therapeutic, and pathogenic aspects of chronic multifocal candidiasis, Oral Surg. **56**:388, 1983.
94. Hornstein, O.P.: Melkersson-Rosenthal syndrome: a neuromuco-cutaneous disease of complex origin, Curr. Probl. Dermatol. **5**:117, 1973.
95. Iverson, R.E., and Vistnes, L.M.: Keratoacanthoma is frequently a dangerous diagnosis, Am. J. Surg. **126**:359, 1973.
96. Jacobson, S., and Shear, M.: Verrucous carcinoma of the mouth, J. Oral Pathol. **1**:66, 1972.
97. Jacoway, J.R., Nelson, J.F., and Boyers, R.C.: Adenoid squamous-cell carcinoma (adenoacanthoma) of the oral labial mucosa, Oral Surg. **32**:444, 1971.
98. Jamsky, R.J., and Christen, A.G.: Oral gonococcal infections, Oral Surg. **53**:358, 1982.
99. Kay, S., Gerszten, E., and Dennison, S.M.: Light and electron microscopic study of a rhabdomyoma arising in the floor of the mouth, Cancer **23**:708, 1969.
100. Khari, M.R.A., et al.: Mucosal neuroma, pheochromocytoma and medullary thyroid carcinoma: multiple endocrine neoplasia, type 3, Medicine **54**:89, 1975.

101. Kolson, H., et al.: Epidermoid carcinoma of the floor of the mouth, Arch. Otolaryngol. **93**:280, 1971.
102. Kotner, L.M., and Wang, C.C.: Plasmacytoma of the upper air and food passages, Cancer **30**:414, 1972.
103. Kroll, J.J., Einbinder, J.M., and Merz, W.G.: Mucocutaneous candidiasis in a mother and son, Arch. Dermatol. **108**:259, 1973.
104. Krolls, S.O., and Hoffman, S.: Squamous cell carcinoma of the oral soft tissues: a statistical analysis of 14,253 cases by age, sex and race of patients, J. Am. Dent. Assoc. **92**:571, 1976.
105. Krolls, S.O., Jacoway, J.R., and Alexander, W.N.: Osseous choristomas (osteomas) of intraoral soft tissues, Oral Surg. **32**:588, 1971.
106. Laskaris, G., Sklavounou, A., and Bovopoulou, O.: Juvenile pemphigus vulgaris, Oral Surg. **51**:415, 1981.
107. Lee, E.S., and Wilson, J.S.P.: Carcinoma involving the lower alveolus, Br. J. Surg. **60**:85, 1973.
108. Leyden, J.J., and Master, G.H.: Oral cavity pyogenic granuloma, Arch. Dermatol. **108**:226, 1973.
109. Lichtiger, B., Mackay, B., and Tessmer, C.F.: Spindle cell variant of squamous carcinoma, Cancer **26**:1311, 1970.
110. Lightwood, R., and Nolan, R.: Epithelial giant cells in measles as an aid in diagnosis, J. Pediatr. **77**:59, 1970.
111. Limongelli, W.A., et al.: Disseminated South American blastomycosis (paracoccidiomycosis), J. Oral Surg. **36**:625, 1978.
112. Lozada, F., and Silverman, S., Jr.: Erythema multiforme, Oral Surg. **46**:628, 1978.
112a. Lozada, F., et al: Oral manifestations of tumor and opportunistic infections in the acquired immunodeficiency syndrome (AIDS): findings in 53 homosexual men with Kaposi's sarcoma, Oral Surg. **56**:491, 1983.
113. Martin, J.L., and Crump, E.P.: Leukoedema of the buccal mucosa in Negro children and youth, Oral Surg. **33**:49, 1972.
114. McCoy, J.M., and Waldron, C.A.: Verrucous carcinoma of the oral cavity, Oral Surg. **52**:623, 1981.
115. McDaniel, R.K., and Marano, P.D.: Reparative lesion of the tongue, Oral Surg. **45**:266, 1978.
116. Merchant, H.W., and Schuster, G.S.: Oral gonococcal infection, J. Am. Dent. Assoc. **95**:807, 1977.
117. Meyer, I., and Abbey, L.M.: The relationship of syphilis to primary carcinoma of the tongue, Oral Surg. **30**:678, 1970.
118. Meyer, I., and Shklar, G.: The oral manifestations of acquired syphilis: the study of 81 cases, Oral Surg. **23**:45, 1967.
119. Michaels, L., and Gregory, M.M.: Pathology of "non-healing (midline) granuloma," J. Clin. Pathol. **30**:317, 1977.
120. Miller, A.S., et al.: Oral granular cell tumors, Oral Surg. **44**:227, 1977.
121. Miller, M.F., Ship, I.I., and Ram, C.: A retrospective study of the prevalence and incidence of recurrent aphthous ulcerations in a professional population, 1958-1971, Oral Surg. **43**:532, 1977.
122. Muller, S.A.: Viral infections of the skin and mouth: a selected review, Oral Surg. **32**:752, 1971.
123. Nakissa, N., et al.: Carcinoma of the floor of the mouth, Cancer **42**:2914, 1978.
124. Nally, F.F., and Ross, I.H.: Herpes zoster of the oral and facial structures, Oral Surg. **32**:221, 1971.
125. Nazif, M., and Ranalli, D.N.: Stevens-Johnson syndrome, Oral Surg. **53**:263, 1982.
126. Neville, B.W., and Weathers, D.R.: Verruciform xanthoma, Oral Surg. **49**:429, 1980.
127. Nisengard, R.J., et al.: Diagnostic importance of immunofluorescence in oral bullous diseases and lupus erythematosus, Oral Surg. **40**:365, 1975.
128. Person, J.R., and Rogers, R.S.: Bullous and cicatricial pemphigoid: clinical, histopathologic and immunopathologic correlations, Mayo Clin. Proc. **52**:54, 1977.
129. Pindborg, J.J., Daftary, D.K., and Mehta, F.S.: A follow-up study of sixty-one oral dysplastic precancerous lesions in Indian villagers, Oral Surg. **43**:383, 1977.
130. Poole, A.G., and Marchetta, F.C.: Extramedullary plasmacytoma of the head and neck, Cancer **22**:14, 1968.
131. Praetorius-Clausen, F.: Geographical aspects of oral focal epithelial hyperplasia, Pathol. Microbiol. **39**:204, 1973.
132. Prahbu, S.R., Daftary, D.K., and Dholakia, H.M.: Tuberculosis of the tongue, J. Oral Surg. **36**:384, 1978.
133. Putkonen, T.: Dental changes in congenital syphilis, Acta Derm. Venereol. **42**:44, 1962.
134. Rao, M.S., et al.: Oral lesions in granuloma inguinale, J. Oral Surg. **34**:1112, 1976.
135. Ratzer, E.R., Schweitzer, R.G., and Frazell, E.C.: Epidermoid carcinoma of the palate, Am. J. Surg. **119**:294, 1970.
136. Regezi, J.A., Batsakis, J.G., and Courtney, R.M.: Granular cell tumor of the head and neck, J. Oral Surg. **37**:402, 1979.
137. Reichart, T.P.: Pathologic changes in the soft palate in lepromatous leprosy, Oral Surg. **38**:898, 1974.
138. Renner, R.P., et al.: The role of *C. albicans* in denture stomatitis, Oral Surg. **47**:323, 1979.
139. Rohrer, M.D., and Young, S.K.: Congenital epulis (gingival granular cell tumor): ultrastructural evidence of origin from pericytes, Oral Surg. **53**:56, 1982.
140. Rosenberg, F.R., Sanders, S., and Nelson, C.T.: Pemphigus: a 20-year review of 107 patients treated with corticosteroids, Arch. Dermatol. **112**:962, 1976.
141. Scott, J., and Finch, L.D.: Wegener's granulomatosis presenting as gingivitis, Oral Surg. **34**:920, 1972.
142. Scully, C.: Vaccinia of the lip, Br. Dent. J. **143**:57, 1977.
143. Seydel, H.G., and Scholl, H.: Carcinoma of the soft palate and uvula, Am. J. Roentgenol. **120**:603, 1974.
144. Shafer, W.G.: Verrucous carcinoma, Int. Dent. J. **22**:451, 1972.
145. Shafer, W.G.: Oral carcinoma in situ, Oral Surg. **39**:227, 1975.
146. Shafer, W.G., and Waldron, C.A.: Erythroplakia of the oral cavity, Cancer **36**:1021, 1975.
147. Shapiro, L., and Juhlin, E.A.: Eosinophilic ulcer of the tongue, Dermatologica **140**:242, 1970.
148. Ship, I.I.: Epidemiologic aspects of recurrent aphthous ulcerations, Oral Surg. **33**:400, 1972.
149. Shklar, G.: Lichen planus as an ulcerative disease, Oral Surg. **33**:376, 1972.
150. Shklar, G., and McCarthy, P.L.: Oral lesions of mucous membrane pemphigoid: a study of 85 cases, Arch. Otolaryngol. **93**:354, 1971.
151. Silverman, S., Greenspan, J.S., and Christie, T.M.: Junctional nevus of the oral mucosa, Oral Surg. **39**:259, 1975.
152. Silverman, S., Jr., and Griffith, M.: Smoking characteristics of patients with oral carcinoma and the risk for secondary oral primary carcinoma, J. Am. Dent. Assoc. **85**:637, 1972.
153. Silverman, S.J., and Griffith, M.: Studies on oral lichen planus. II. Follow-up on 200 patients: clinical characteristics and associated malignancy, Oral Surg. **37**:705, 1974.
154. Sist, T.C., and Greene, G.W.: Traumatic neuroma of the oral cavity, Oral Surg. **51**:394, 1981.
155. Smith, I.: Cancrum oris, J. Maxillofac. Surg. **7**:293, 1979.
156. Smith, J.F.: Snuff-dippers lesion: a ten-year follow-up, Arch. Otolaryngol. **101**:276, 1975.
157. Someren, A., Karcioglu, Z., and Clairmont, A.A.: Polypoid spindle cell carcinoma (pleomorphic carcinoma), Oral Surg. **42**:474, 1976.
158. Starink, T.M., and Woerdeman, M.J.: Focal epithelial hyperplasia of the oral mucosa, Br. J. Dermatol. **95**:375, 1977.
159. Svirsky, J.A., Freedman, P.D., and Lumerman, H.: Solitary intraoral keratoacanthoma, Oral Surg. **43**:116, 1977.
160. Szpak, C.A., Stone, M.J., and Frenkel, E.P.: Some observations concerning the demographic and geographic incidence of carcinoma of the lip and buccal cavity, Cancer **40**:343, 1977.
161. Tang, T.T., et al.: Ulcerative eosinophilic granuloma of the tongue: a light and electronmicroscopic study, Am. J. Clin. Pathol. **75**:420, 1981.
162. Tomich, C.E., and Hutton, C.E.: Adenoid squamous cell carcinoma of the lip, J. Oral Surg. **30**:592, 1972.
163. Tornes, K., and Bang, G.: Traumatic eosinophilic granuloma of the gingiva, Oral Surg. **38**:99, 1974.
164. Trodahl, J.N., and Sprague, W.G.: Benign and malignant melanocytic lesions of the oral mucosa: an analysis of 135 cases, Cancer **25**:812, 1970.
165. Tyldesley, W.R.: Oral lichen planus, Br. J. Oral Surg. **11**:187, 1974.

166. Van Wyk, C.F., Staz, J., and Farman, A.G.: Focal epithelial hyperplasia in a group of South Africans: its clinical and microscopic features, J. Oral Pathol. **6**:1, 1977.
167. Vickers, R.A.: Mesenchymal (soft tissue) tumors of the oral region. In Waldron, C., and Gorlin, R.J., editors: Oral pathology, ed. 7, St. Louis, 1985, The C.V. Mosby Co.
168. Vickers, R.A., Gorlin, R.J., and Lovestedt, S.A.: Minnesota oral cancer detection: 1957-1964 results, Northwest Dent. **44**:339, 1965.
169. Vindenes, H.: Lipomas of the oral cavity, Int. J. Oral Surg. **7**:162, 1978.
170. Waldron, C.A.: Oral epithelial tumors. In Waldron, C., and Gorlin, R.J., editors: Oral pathology, ed. 7, St. Louis, 1985, The C.V. Mosby Co.
171. Waldron, C.A., and Shafer, W.G.: Leukoplakia revisited: a clinicopathologic study of 3256 oral leukoplakias, Cancer **36**:1386, 1975.
172. Weathers, D.R.: Benign nevi of the oral mucosa, Arch. Dermatol. **99**:688, 1939.
173. Weitzner, S., Lockey, M.W., and Lockard, V.G.: Adult rhabdomyoma of soft palate, Oral Surg. **47**:70, 1979.
174. Welborn, J.F.: Eosinophilic granuloma of the tongue, J. Oral Surg. **24**:176, 1966.
175. Whitaker, L.A., Lehr, H.B., and Askovitz, S.I.: Cancer of the tongue, Plast. Reconstr. Surg. **30**:363, 1972.
176. WHO Collaborating Centre for Oral Precancerous Lesions: Definition of leukoplakia and related lesions: an aid to studies on oral precancer, Oral Surg. **46**:518, 1978.
177. Winkelmann, R.K., and Brown, J.: Generalized eruptive keratoacanthoma, Arch. Dermatol. **97**:617, 1968.
178. Winn, D.M., et al.: Snuff dipping and oral cancer among women in the southern United States, N. Engl. J. Med. **304**:745, 1981.
179. Witkop, C.J., Jr.: Heterogeneity in gingival fibromatosis, Birth Defects **7**:210, 1971.
180. Wright, B.A., and Jackson, D.: Neural tumors of the oral cavity, Oral Surg. **49**:509, 1980.
181. Young, L.L., et al.: Oral manifestations of histoplasmosis, Oral Surg. **33**:191, 1972.
182. Zegarelli, D.J.: Chondroma of the tongue, Oral Surg. **43**:738, 1977.

Jaws

183. Abaza, N.A., Iczkovitz, M.L., and Henefer, E.P.: American Burkitt's lymphoma manifested in a solitary mandibular lymph node, Oral Surg. **51**:121, 1981.
184. Abrams, A.M., Howell, F.V., and Bullock, W.K.: Nasopalatine cysts, Oral Surg. **16**:306, 1963.
185. Andersen, L., Fejerskov, O., and Philipsen, H.P.: Oral giant cell granulomas: a clinical and histological study of 129 new cases, Acta Pathol. Microbiol. Scand. [A] **81**:606, 1973.
186. Andersen, L., et al.: Oral giant cell granulomas: an enzyme histochemical and ultrastructural study, Acta Pathol. Microbiol. Scand. [A] **81**:617, 1973.
187. Anneroth, G., and Nordenram, Å.: Calcifying odontogenic cyst, Oral Surg. **39**:794, 1975.
188. Appenzeller, J., Weitzner, S., and Long, G.W.: Hepatocellular carcinoma metastatic to the mandible: report and review of the literature, J. Oral Surg. **29**:668, 1971.
188a. Arafat, A., Ellis, G.L., and Adrian, J.C.: Ewing's sarcoma of the jaws, Oral Surg. **55**:589, 1983.
189. Arlen, M., et al.: Chondrosarcoma of the head and neck, Am. J. Surg. **120**:456, 1970.
190. Arsinau, J.C., et al.: American Burkitt's lymphoma: a pathologic study of 30 cases, Am. J. Med. **58**:314, 1975.
191. Beasley, J.D.: Traumatic cyst of the jaws: report of 30 cases, J. Am. Dent. Assoc. **92**:145, 1976.
192. Blakemore, J.R., Eller, D.J., and Tomaro, A.J.: Maxillary exostoses, Oral Surg. **40**:200, 1975.
193. Blank, E.: Recurrent Caffey's cortical hyperostosis and persistent deformity, Pediatrics **55**:856, 1975.
194. Block, J.C., et al.: Pigmented neuroectodermal tumor of infancy, Oral Surg. **49**:279, 1980.
195. Boerger, W.G., Waite, D.E., and Carroll, G.W.: Idiopathic bone cavities of the mandible, J. Oral Surg. **30**:506, 1972.
196. Borello, E., and Gorlin, R.J.: Melanotic neuroectodermal tumor of infancy—a neoplasm of neural crest origin: report of a case with high urinary excretion of vanilmandelic acid, Cancer **19**:196, 1966.
197. Brannon, R.B.: The odontogenic keratocyst, Oral Surg. **42**:54, 1976; **43**:233, 1977.
198. Brannon, R.B., and Corio, R.: Benign cementoblastoma: clinicopathologic features of 50 cases. (In press.)
199. Bras, J.M., et al.: Juxtacortical osteogenic sarcoma of the jaws, Oral Sug. **50**:535, 1980.
200. Browne, R.M.: The pathogenesis of odontogenic cysts, J. Oral Pathol. **4**:31, 1976.
201. Browne, R.M., and Gough, N.G.: Malignant change in the epithelial lining of odontogenic cysts, Cancer **29**:1199, 1972.
202. Buchner, A., and Hansen, L.S.: The histomorphologic spectrum of the gingival cyst in the adult, Oral Surg. **48**:532, 1979.
203. Cannon, J.S., Keller, E.E., and Dahlin, D.C.: Gigantiform cementoma: report of two cases (mother and son), J. Oral Surg. **38**:65, 1980.
204. Carl, W., et al.: Ewing's sarcoma, Oral Surg. **31**:472, 1971.
205. Coli, R.D., et al.: Gardner's syndrome, Am. J. Dig. Dis. **15**:551, 1970.
206. Courtney, R.M., and Kerr, D.A.: The odontogenic adenomatoid tumor, Oral Surg. **39**:424, 1975.
207. Curtis, M.L., Elmore, J.S., and Sotercanos, G.C.: Osteosarcoma of the jaws, J. Oral Surg. **32**:125, 1974.
208. Donatsky, O., et al.: Clinical, radiologic, and histopathologic aspects of 13 cases of nevoid basal cell carcinoma syndrome, Int. J. Oral Surg. **5**:19, 1976.
209. Eversole, L.R., and Rovin, S.: Reactive lesions of the gingiva, J. Oral Pathol. **1**:30, 1972.
210. Eversole, L.R., Sabes, W.R., and Rovin, S.: Fibrous dysplasia: a nosologic problem in the diagnosis of fibro-osseous lesions of the jaws, J. Oral Pathol. **1**:189, 1972.
211. Eversole, L.R., et al.: Proliferative periostitis of Garré's: its differentiation from other neoperiostoses, J. Oral Surg. **37**:725, 1979.
212. Farman, A.G.: The peripheral odontogenic fibroma, Oral Surg. **40**:82, 1975.
213. Farman, A.G., et al.: Cementoblastoma, J. Oral Surg. **37**:198, 1979.
214. Finsterbush, A.A., and Rang, M.: Infantile cortical hyperostosis: followup of 29 cases, Acta Orthopaed. Scand. **46**:727, 1975.
215. Franklin, C.D., and Pindborg, J.J.: The calcifying epithelial odontogenic tumor, Oral Surg. **42**:753, 1976.
216. Gardner, D.G.: The central odontogenic fibroma: an attempt at clarification, Oral Surg. **50**:425, 1980.
217. Gardner, D.G.: Plexiform unicystic ameloblastoma: a diagnostic problem in dentigerous cysts, Cancer **47**:1358, 1981.
218. Giansanti, J.S., and Waldron, C.A.: Peripheral giant cell granuloma: review of 720 cases, J. Oral Surg. **27**:787, 1969.
219. Gorlin, R.J.: Odontogenic tumors. In Waldron, C., and Gorlin, R.J., editors: Oral pathology, ed. 7, St. Louis, 1982, The C.V. Mosby Co.
220. Gorlin, R.J., and Jirasek, J.E.: Oral cysts containing gastric or intestinal mucosa: unusual embryologic accident or heterotopia? J. Oral Surg. **28**:9, 1970.
221. Gorlin, R.J., and Sedano, H.O.: The multiple nevoid basal cell carcinoma syndrome revisited, Birth Defects **7**(8):140, 1971.
222. Gundlach, K., and Schulz, A.: Odontogenic myxoma, J. Oral Pathol. **6**:343, 1977.
223. Hamner, J.E., III, Scofield, H.H., and Cornyn, J.: Benign fibro-osseous jaw lesions of periodontal membrane origin—an analysis of 249 cases, Cancer **22**:861, 1968.
224. Hanna, R.J., Regezi, J.A., and Hayward, J.R.: Ameloblastic fibro-odontoma: light and electron microscopic observations, J. Oral Surg. **34**:820, 1976.
225. Harris, C.M., and Courtmanche, A.D.: Gastric mucosal cyst of the tongue, Plast. Reconstr. Surg. **54**:612, 1974.
226. Hartman, K.S.: Histiocytosis X: a review of 114 cases with oral involvement, Oral Surg. **49**:38, 1980.

227. Hayward, A.F., Fickling, B.W., and Lucas, R.B.: An electron microscope study of a pigmented tumour of the jaw of infants, Br. J. Cancer **23**:702, 1969.
228. Hendler, B.H., Abaza, N.A., and Quinn, P.: Odontogenic myxoma: surgical management and ultrastructural study, Oral Surg. **47**:203, 1979.
229. Hollinshead, M.R., and Schneider, L.C.: A histologic and embryologic analysis of so-called globulomaxillary cysts, Int. J. Oral Surg. **9**:281, 1980.
230. Hooker, S.: Ameloblastic odontoma: an analysis of twenty-six cases, Oral Surg. **24**:375, 1967.
231. Ikemura, I., et al.: Ameloblastoma of the mandible with metastasis to the lungs and lymph nodes, Cancer **29**:930, 1972.
232. Jacobs, T.P., et al.: Giant cell tumor in Paget's disease of bone: familial and geographical clustering, Cancer **44**:742, 1979.
233. Jolly, D.E., and Harris, T.B., Osteitis deformans—a case of late involvement of the maxilla, J. Oral Surg. **34**:54, 1979.
234. Karmody, C.S., and Gallagher, J.C.: Nasoalveolar cysts, Ann. Otol. Rhinol. Laryngol. **81**: 278, 1972.
235. Kennett, S., and Pollick, H.: Jaw lesions in familial hyperparathyroidism, Oral Surg. **31**: 502, 1971.
236. Khan, M.Y., et al.: Adenomatoid odontogenic tumor resembling a globulomaxillary cyst: light and electron microscopic studies, J. Oral Surg. **35**:739, 1977.
237. Kolas, S., and Halperin, V.: The occurrence of torus palatinus and torus mandibularis in 2,478 dental patients, Oral Surg. **6**:1134, 1953.
238. Krolls, S.O., and Pindborg, J.J.: Calcifying epithelial odontogenic tumor—a survey of 23 cases and discussion of histomorphologic variation, Arch. Pathol. **98**:206, 1974.
239. Leban, S.G., et al.: The giant cell lesion of the jaws: neoplastic or reparative? J. Oral Surg. **29**:398, 1971.
240. Lehner, T.: The jaws and teeth in Burkitt's tumour (African lymphoma), J. Pathol. Bacteriol. **88**:581, 1964.
241. Leppard, B., and Bussey, H.J.R.: Epidermoid cysts, polyposis coli, and Gardner's syndrome, Br. J. Surg. **62**:387, 1975.
242. Lichty, G., Langlais, R.P., and Aufdemorte, T.: Garré's ostemyelitis, Oral Surg. **50**:309, 1980.
243. Limongelli, W.A., Connaughton, B., and Williams, A.C.: Suppurative osteomyelitis of the mandible secondary to fracture, Oral Surg. **38**:850, 1974.
244. LiVolsi, V.A.: Osteogenic sarcoma of the maxilla, Arch. Otolaryngol. **103**:485, 1977.
245. Lopez, L., Jr.: Melanotic neuroectodermal tumor of infancy, J. Am. Dent. Assoc. **93**:1159, 1976.
246. Mehlisch, D.R., Dahlen, D.C., and Masson, J.K.: Ameloblastoma: a clinicopathologic report, J. Oral Surg. **30**:9, 1972.
247. Melrose, R.J., Abrams, A.M., and Mills, B.G.: Florid osseous dysplasia: a clinical-pathologic study of thirty-four cases, Oral Surg. **41**:62, 1976.
248. Miller, A.S., et al.: Giant cell tumor of the jaws associated with Paget disease of bone, Arch. Otolaryngol. **100**:233, 1974.
249. Miller, A.S., et al.: Ameloblastic fibroodontoma: report of seven cases, Oral Surg. **41**:354, 1976.
250. Murphy, J.B., Segelman, A., and Doku, C.: Osteitis deformans, Oral Surg. **46**:765, 1978.
251. Murray, G.C., Daly, T.E., and Zimmerman, S.O.: The relationship between dental disease and radiation necrosis of the mandible, Oral Surg. **49**:99, 1980.
252. Nkrumah, F.K., and Perkins, I.V.: Burkitt's lymphoma: a clinical study of 110 patients, Cancer **37**:671, 1976.
253. Oatis, G.W., et al.: Dermoid cyst of the floor of the mouth, Oral Surg. **39**:192, 1975.
254. Page, D.L., Weiss, S.W., and Eggelston, J.C.: Ultrastructural study of amyloid material in the calcifying epithelial odontogenic tumor, Cancer **36**:1426, 1975.
255. Peters, R.A., and Schock, R.K.: Oral cysts in newborn infants, Oral Surg. **32**: 10, 1977.
256. Philipsen, H.P., and Birn, H.: The adenomatoid odontogenic tumour, Acta Pathol. Microbiol. Scand. **75**:375, 1969.
257. Ramon, Y., et al.: Osteomyelitis of the maxilla in the newborn, Int. J. Oral Surg. **6**:90, 1977.
258. Rayner, C.R.W., Towers, J.F., and Wilson, J.S.P.: What is Gorlin's syndrome: the diagnosis and management of the basal cell nevus syndrome, based on a study of thirty-seven patients, Br. J. Plast. Surg. **30**:62, 1977.
259. Reichart, P.A., and Zobl, H.: Transformation of ameloblastic fibroma to fibrosarcoma, Int. J. Oral Surg. **7**:503, 1978.
260. Royer, R.Q., and Neiblung, H.E.: Osteomyelitis of the jaws, Semin. Roentgenol. **6**:391, 1971
261. Salvador, A.H., Beabout, J.W., and Dahlin, D.C.: Mesenchymal chondrosarcoma—observations in 30 new cases, Cancer **28**:605, 1971.
262. Saw, D.: Fibrosarcoma of maxilla, Oral Surg. **47**:164, 1979.
263. Schuchard, W.A., and Ponsky, J.L.: Familial polyposis and Gardner's syndrome, Surg. Gynecol. Obstet. **148**:97, 1979.
264. Sedano, H.O., Kuba, R., and Gorlin, R.J.: Autosomal dominant cemental dysplasia, Oral Surg. **54**:642, 1982.
265. Sedano, H.O., et al.: Histiocytosis X, Oral Surg. **27**:760, 1969.
266. Seward, M.H.: Eruption cyst: an analysis of its characteristic features, J. Oral Surg. **31**:31, 1973.
267. Smith, G.A., and Ward, P.H.: Giant cell lesions of the facial skeleton, Arch. Otolaryngol. **104**:186, 1978.
268. Spouge, J.D.: Odontogenic tumors: a unitarian concept, Oral Surg. **24**:392, 1967.
269. Spouge, J.D., and Spruyt, C.L.: Odontogenic tumors: histochemical comparison of the adenoameloblastoma and developing tooth, Oral Surg. **25**:447, 1968.
270. Summers, C.J.: Prevalance of tori, J. Oral Surg. **26**:718, 1968.
271. Tabachnick, T.T., and Levine, B.: Multiple myeloma involving the jaws and oral soft tissues, J. Oral Surg. **34**:931, 1976.
272. Trodahl, J.N.: Ameloblastic fibroma, Oral Surg. **33**:547, 1972.
273. Vickers, R.A., Dahlin, D.C., and Gorlin, R.J.: Amyloid-containing odontogenic tumors, Oral Surg. **20**:476, 1965.
274. Vickers, R.A., and Gorlin, R.J.: Ameloblastoma: delineation of early histopathologic features of neoplasia, Cancer **26**:699, 1970.
275. von Wowern, N.: Cherubism, Int. J. Oral Surg. **1**:240, 1972.
276. Waldron, C.A.: Fibro-osseous lesions of the jaws, J. Oral Surg. **28**:58, 1970.
277. Waldron, C.A., and Giansanti, J.S.: Fibrous dysplasia of the jaws, Oral Surg. **35**:190, 1973.
278. Wayman, J.B.: Cherubism: a report on three cases, Br. J. Oral Surg. **16**:47, 1974.
279. Wertheimer, F.W., Zielinski, R.J., and Wesley, R.K.: Extraosseous calcifying epithelial odontogenic tumor (Pindborg tumor), Int. J. Oral Surg. **6**:266, 1977.
280. White, D.K., et al.: Odontogenic myxoma: a clinical and ultrastructural study, Oral Surg. **39**:901, 1975.
281. Wysocki, G.P., et al.: Histogenesis of the lateral periodontal cyst and the gingival cyst of the adult, Oral Surg. **50**:327, 1980.

Salivary glands

282. Abelson, D.C., Mandel, I.D., and Karmiol, M.: Salivary studies in alcoholic cirrhosis, Oral Surg. **41**:186, 1976.
283. Abrams, A.M., and Finck, F.M.: Sialadenoma papilliferum: a previously unreported salivary gland tumor, Cancer **24**:1057, 1969.
284. Abrams, A.M., and Melrose, R.J.: Acinic cell tumors of minor salivary gland origin, Oral Surg. **46**:220, 1978.
285. Abrams, A.M., et al.: Acinic cell adenocarcinoma of the major salivary glands: a clinicopathologic study of 77 cases, Cancer **18**:1145, 1965.
286. Assor, D.: Sebaceous lymphadenoma of the parotid gland, Am. J. Clin. Pathol. **53**:100, 1970.
287. Balogh, K., Jr., and Roth, S.I.: Histochemical and electron microscopic studies of eosinophilic granular cells (oncocytes) in tumors of the parotid gland, Lab. Invest. **14**:310, 1965.
288. Baratz, M., Loewenthal, M., and Rozin, M.: Sebaceous lymphadenoma of the parotid gland, Arch. Pathol. Lab. Med. **100**:269, 1976.
289. Batsakis, J.G., Littler, E.R., and Leahy, M.S.: Sebaceous cell lesions of the head and neck, Arch. Otolaryngol. **95**:151, 1972.
290. Batsakis, J.G., et al.: Acinic cell carcinoma: a clinicopathologic study of thirty-five cases, J. Laryngol. Otol. **93**:325, 1979.

291. Blanck, C., Eneroth, C.M., and Jakobsson, P.Å.: Oncocytoma of the parotid gland: neoplasm or nodular hyperplasia? Cancer **25**:919, 1970.
292. Blanck, C., Eneroth, C.M., and Jakobsson, P.Å.: Mucus-producing adenopapillary (non-epidermoid) carcinoma of the parotid gland, Cancer **28**:676, 1971.
293. Blanck, C., et al.: Poorly differentiated solid parotid carcinoma, Acta Radiol. Oncol. Radiat. Phys. Biol. **13**:17, 1974.
294. Brant, P.W., and McKusick, V.A.: Familial dysautonomia: a report of genetic and clinical studies with a review of the literature, Medicine **49**:343, 1970.
295. Brennan, M.F., Gwynne, J.F., and Macbeth, W.A.: Simple parotid cysts, Aust. N.Z. J. Surg. **40**:15, 1970.
296. Browand, B.C., and Waldron, C.A.: Central mucoepidermoid tumors of the jaws: report of 9 cases and review of the literature, Oral Surg. **40**:631, 1975.
297. Caccamise, W.C., and Townes, P.L.: Congenital absence of the lacrimal puncta associated with alacrima and aptyalism, Am. J. Ophthalmol. **89**:62, 1980.
298. Casamassimo, P.S., and Lilly, G.E.: Mucosal cysts of the maxillary sinus: a clinical and radiographic study, Oral Surg. **50**:282, 1980.
299. Cataldo, E., and Mosadomi, A.: Mucoceles of the oral mucous membrane, Arch. Otolaryngol. **91**:360, 1970.
300. Catone, G.A., Merrill, R.G., and Henry, F.A.: Sublingual gland mucus-escape phenomenon—treatment by excision of sublingual gland, J. Oral Surg. **27**:774, 1969.
301. Chen, S.Y.: Adenoid cystic carcinoma of minor salivary gland: histochemical and electron microscopic studies of cystlike spaces, Oral Surg. **42**:606, 1976.
302. Chen, S.Y.: Ultrastructure of mucoepidermoid carcinoma in minor salivary glands, Oral Surg. **47**:247, 1979.
303. Chen, S.Y., et al.: Acinic cell adenocarcinoma of minor salivary glands, Cancer **42**:678, 1978.
304. Conley, J., Meyers, E., and Cole, R.: Analysis of 115 patients with tumors of the submandibular gland, Ann. Otol. Rhinol. Laryngol. **81**:323, 1972.
305. Crissman, J.D., Wirman, J.A., and Harris, A.: Malignant myoepithelioma of the parotid gland, Cancer **40**:3042, 1977.
306. Crumpler, C., Scharfenberg, J.C., and Reed, R.J.: Monomorphic adenomas of salivary glands: trabecular-tubular, canalicular and basaloid variants, Cancer **38**:193, 1976.
307. Daniels, T.E., et al.: The oral component of Sjögren's syndrome, Oral Surg. **39**:875, 1975.
308. Deppisch, L.M., and Toker, C.: Mixed tumors of the parotid gland: an ultrastructural study, Cancer **24**:174, 1969.
309. Donath, K.: Pathohistology of necrotizing sialometaplasia in parotid glands, Laryngol. Rhinol. **58**:70, 1979.
310. Donath, K.: Wangenschwellung bei Sialadenose, HNO **27**:113, 1979.
311. Eby, L.S., Johnson, D.C., and Baker, H.W.: Adenoid cystic carcinoma of the head and neck, Cancer **29**:1160, 1972.
312. Eneroth, C.M.: Salivary gland tumors in the parotid gland, submandibular gland and the palate region, Cancer **27**:1415, 1971.
313. Eneroth, C.M., Blanck, C., and Jakobsson, P.Å.: Carcinoma in pleomorphic adenoma of the parotid gland, Acta Otolaryngol. **66**:477, 1968.
314. Erlandson, R.A., and Tandler, B.; Ultrastructure of acinic cell carcinoma of the parotid glands, Arch. Pathol. **93**:130, 1972.
315. Eversole, L.R., Rovin, S., and Sabes, W.R.: Mucoepidermoid carcinoma of minor salivary glands: report of 17 cases with follow-up, J. Oral Surg. **30**:107, 1972.
316. Font, R.L., Yanoff, M., and Zimmerman, L.E.: Benign lymphoepithelial lesion of the lacrimal glands and its relationship to Sjögren's syndrome, Am. J. Clin. Pathol. **48**:365, 1967.
317. Foretich, E.A., Cardo, V.A., and Zambito, R.F.: Bilateral congenital absence of the submandibular duct orifices, J. Oral Surg. **31**:556, 1973.
318. Frable, W.J., and Elzay, R.P.: Tumors of minor salivary glands: a report of 73 cases, Cancer **25**:932, 1970.
319. Freedman, P.D., and Lumerman, H.: Sialadenoma papilliferum, Oral Surg. **45**:88, 1978.
320. Goldman, R.L., and Klein, H.Z.: Glycogen-rich adenoma of the parotid gland, Cancer **30**:749, 1972.
321. Goldman, R.L., and Perzik, S.L.: Infantile hemangioma of the parotid gland in children. a clinicopathological study of 15 cases, Arch. Otolaryngol. **90**:605, 1969.
322. Gorman, J.M., and O'Brien, F.V.: Salivary inclusion in the mandible, Br. Dent. J. **133**:69, 1972.
323. Gray, S.R., Cornog, J.L., Jr., and Seo, I.S.: Oncocytic neoplasms of salivary glands: a report of fifteen cases including two malignant oncocytomas, Cancer **38**:1306, 1976.
324. Greenspan, J.S., et al.: The histopathology of Sjögren's syndrome in labial salivary gland biopsies, Oral Surg. **37**:217, 1974.
325. Hanna, D.C., and Clairmont, A.A.: Submandibular gland tumors, Plast. Reconstr. Surg. **61**:198, 1978.
326. Harrison, J.D.: Salivary mucoceles, Oral Surg. **39**:268, 1975.
327. Healey, W.V., Perzin, K.H., and Smith, L.: Mucoepidermoid carcinoma of salivary gland origin: classification, clinical-pathologic correlation and results of treatment, Cancer **26**:368, 1970.
328. Hoggins, G.S., and Hutton, J.B.: Congenital sublingual cystic swellings due to imperforate salivary ducts, Oral Surg. **37**:370, 1974.
329. Hooper, R., Saxon, R., and Tropp, A.: Cysts of the parotid gland, J. Laryngol. Otol. **89**:427, 1975.
330. Hsu, S.M., Hsu, P.L., and Nayak, R.N.: Warthin's tumor: an immunohistochemical study of its lymphoid stroma, Hum. Pathol. **12**:251, 1981.
331. Hübner, G., Klein, J.H., and Kleinsasser, O.: Zur Feinstruktur und Genese der Azinuszelltumoren der Glandula Parotis, Virchows Arch. (Pathol. Anat.) **345**:1, 1968.
332. Jacques, D.A., Krolls, S.O., and Chambers, R.C.: Parotid tumors in children, Am. J. Surg. **132**:469, 1976.
333. Jakobsson, P.Å., Blanck, C., and Eneroth, C.M.: Mucoepidermoid carcinoma of the parotid gland, Cancer **22**:111, 1968.
334. Jao, W., Keh, P.C., and Swerdlow, M.: Ultrastructure of basal cell adenoma of parotid gland, Cancer **37**:1322, 1976.
335. Jensen, J.L., et al.: Minor salivary gland calculi: a clinicopathologic study of 47 new cases, Oral Surg. **47**:44, 1979.
336. Johns, M.E., Regezi, J.A., and Batsakis, J.G.: Oncocytic neoplasms of salivary glands: an ultrastructural study, Laryngoscope **87**:862, 1977.
337. Kaban, L.B., Donoff, R.B., and Guralnick, W.C.: Acute parotitis, J. Oral Surg. **31**:377, 1973.
338. Kerpel, S.M., Freedman, P.D., and Lumerman, H.: The papillary cystadenoma of minor salivary gland origin, Oral Surg. **46**:820, 1978.
339. Kessler, E., Koznizsky, I.L., and Schindel, J.: Malignant Warthin's tumor, Oral Surg. **43**:111, 1977.
340. Kornblut, A.D., Ilse, H., and Haubrich, J.: Parotid lymphangioma: a congenital tumor, ORL **35**:303, 1973.
341. Koss, L.G., Spiro, R.H., and Hajdu, S.: Small cell (oat cell) carcinoma of minor salivary gland origin, Cancer **30**:737, 1972.
342. Krolls, S.O., and Hicks, J.L.: Mixed tumors of the lower lip, Oral Surg. **35**:212, 1973.
343. Krolls, S.O., Trodahl, J.N., and Boyers, R.C.: Salivary gland lesions in children: a survey of 430 cases, Cancer **30**:145, 1972.
344. Leake, D., and Leake, R.: Neonatal suppurative parotitis, Pediatrics **46**:203, 1970.
345. Lee, S.C., and Roth, L.M.: Malignant oncocytoma of the parotid gland, Cancer **37**:1607, 1976.
346. Leifer, C., et al.: Myoepithelioma of the parotid gland, Arch. Pathol. **98**:312, 1974.
347. Levin, P.A., et al.: Benign parotid enlargement in bulimia, Ann. Intern. Med. **93**:827, 1980.
348. Levine, S.B., et al.: Asymptomatic parotid enlargement in Pima Indians: relationship to age, obesity and diabetes mellitus, Ann. Intern. Med. **73**:571, 1970.
349. LiVolsi, V.A., and Perzin, K.H.: Malignant mixed tumors arising in salivary glands, Cancer **39**:2209, 1977.
350. Luna, M.A., and Mackay, B.: Basal cell adenoma of the parotid gland, Cancer **37**:1615, 1976.
351. Lynch, D.P., Crago, C.A., and Martinez, M.O.: Necrotizing sialometaplasia, Oral Surg. **47**:63, 1979.
352. MacFarlane, J.K., Viloria, J.B., and Palmer, J.D.: Sebaceous cell carcinoma of the parotid gland, Am. J. Surg. **130**:499, 1975.
353. Main, J.H.P., et al.: Salivary gland tumors: review of 643 cases, J. Oral Pathol. **5**:88, 1976.

354. Malett, K.J., and Harrison, M.S.: The recurrence of salivary gland tumors, J. Laryngol. Otol. **85**:439, 1971.
355. Markert, J.: Zur Ultrastruktur des Cylindrom, Arch. Klin. Exp. Ohren Nasen Kehlkopfheilkd. **184**:496, 1965.
356. Martinez-Lavin, M., Vaughn, J.H., and Tan, E.M.: Autoantibodies and the spectrum of Sjögren's syndrome, Ann. Intern. Med. **91**:185, 1979.
357. McCoy, J.M., and Eckert, E.F., Jr.: Sialadenoma papilliferum, J. Oral Surg. **38**:691, 1980.
358. McGavran, M.H.: The ultrastructure of papillary cystadenoma lymphomatosum of the parotid gland, Virchows Arch. (Pathol. Anat.) **338**:195, 1965.
359. McGurk, F.M., Main, J.H.P., and Orr, J.A.: Adenolymphoma of the parotid gland, Br. J. Surg. **57**:321, 1970.
360. Mintz, G.A., Abrams, A.M., and Melrose, R.J.: Monomorphic adenomas of the major and minor salivary glands, Oral Surg. **53**:375, 1982.
361. Myerson, M., Crelin, E.S., and Smith, H.W.: Bilateral duplication of the submandibular ducts, Arch. Otolaryngol. **83**:488, 1966.
362. Nesland, J.M., Olafsson, J., and Sobrinho-Simões, M.: Plasmacytoid myoepithelioma of the palate: a case report with ultrastructural findings and review of the literature, J. Oral Pathol. **10**:14, 1981.
363. Nochomovitz, L.E., and Kahn, L.B.: Adenoid cystic carcinoma of the salivary gland and its histological variants, Oral Surg. **44**:394, 1977.
364. Noone, R.B., and Brown, H.J.: Cystic hygroma of the parotid gland, Am. J. Surg. **120**:404, 1970.
365. Nussbaum, M., Tan, S., and Som, M.L.: Hemangiomas of salivary glands, Laryngoscope **86**:1015, 1976.
366. Perzin, K.H., Gullane, P., and Clairmont, A.C.: Adenoid cystic carcinomas arising in salivary glands: a correlation of histologic features and clinical course, Cancer **42**:265, 1978.
367. Perzin, K.H., and LiVolsi, V.A.: Acinic cell carcinoma arising in salivary glands: a clinicopathologic study, Cancer **44**:1434, 1979.
368. Pullon, P.A., and Miller, A.L.: Sialolithiasis of accessory salivary glands: review of 55 cases, J. Oral Surg. **30**:832, 1972.
369. Rauch, S., and Gorlin, R.J.: Diseases of the salivary glands. In Gorlin, R.J., and Goldman, H.M., editors: Thoma's oral pathology, ed. 6, St. Louis, 1970, The C.V. Mosby Co.
370. Rauge, G.J., and Kessler, S.: Necrotizing sialometaplasia: a condition simulating malignancy, Arch. Dermatol. **115**:329, 1979.
371. Rees, R.T.: Congenital ranula, Br. Dent. J. **146**:345, 1979.
372. Samy, L.L., Girgis, I.H., and Wasef, S.A.: Ectopic salivary tissue in relation to the tonsil, Laryngoscope **82**:247, 1968.
373. Sapiro, S.M., and Eisenberg, E.: Sjögren's syndrome (sicca complex), Oral Surg. **45**:591, 1978.
374. Saskela, E., Tarkkanen, J., and Wartiovaara, J.: Parotid clear cell adenoma of possible myoepithelial origin, Cancer **30**:742, 1972.
375. Schulz, H.: Electron microscopy of oncocytomas and carcinoid tumors: recent results, Cancer Res. **44**:63, 1974.
376. Schwartz, I.S., and Feldman, M.: Diffuse multinodular oncocytoma ("oncocytosis") of the parotid gland, Cancer **23**:636, 1969.
377. Sciubba, J.J., and Goldstein, B.H.: Myoepithelioma: review of the literature and report of a case with ultrastructural confirmation, Oral Surg. **42**:328, 1976.
378. Seifert, G., and Donath, K.: On the pathogenesis of the Küttner tumor of the submandibular gland: analysis of 349 cases with chronic sialadenitis of the submandibular gland, HNO **25**:81, 1977.
379. Seifert, G., Heckmayr, M., and Donath, K.: Carcinome in Papillären Cystadenolymphomen der Parotis: Definition und Differentialdiagnose, Z. Krebsforsch. **90**:25, 1977.
380. Shulman, J., Waisman, J., and Morledge, D.: Sebaceous carcinoma of the parotid gland, Arch. Otolaryngol. **98**:417, 1973.
381. Singer, M.I., Applebaum, E.L., and Loy, K.D.: Heterotopic salivary tissue in the neck, Laryngoscope **89**:1772, 1979.
382. Smith, N.J.D., and Smith, P.B.: Congenital absence of major salivary glands, Br. Dent. J. **142**:259, 1977.
383. Soskolne, A., et al.: Minor salivary gland tumors: a survey of 64 cases, J. Oral Surg. **31**:528, 1973.
384. Southam, J.C.: Retention mucoceles of the oral mucosa, J. Oral Pathol. **3**:197, 1974.
385. Spiro, R.H., Hajdu, S.I., and Strong, E.W.: Tumors of the submaxillary gland, Am. J. Surg. **132**:463, 1976.
386. Spiro, R.H., Huvos, A.G., and Strong, E.W.: Adenoid cystic carcinoma of salivary origin, Am. J. Surg. **128**:512, 1974.
387. Spiro, R.H., Huvos, A.G., and Strong, E.W.: Cancer of the parotid gland: a clinicopathologic study of 288 primary cases, Am. J. Surg. **130**:452, 1975.
388. Spiro, R.H., Huvos, A.G., and Strong, E.W.: Acinic cell carcinoma of salivary gland origin, Cancer **41**:924, 1978.
389. Spiro, R.H., et al.: Mucoepidermoid carcinoma of salivary gland origin, Am. J. Surg. **136**:461, 1978.
390. Spiro, R.H., et al.: Tumors of minor salivary gland origin: a clinicopathologic study of 492 cases, Cancer **31**:117, 1973.
391. Stromeyer, F.W., et al.: Myoepithelioma of minor salivary gland origin, Arch. Pathol. **99**:242, 1975.
392. Talal, N., et al.: Blood and tissue lesions in Sjögren's syndrome, J. Clin. Invest. **53**:180, 1974.
393. Tandler, B.: Ultrastructure of adenoid cystic carcinoma of salivary gland origin, Lab. Invest. **24**:504, 1971.
394. Tarpley, T.M., Jr., Anderson, L.G., and White, C.L.: Minor salivary gland involvement in Sjögren's syndrome, Oral Surg. **37**:64, 1974.
395. Tarpley, T.M., Jr., and Giansanti, J.S.: Adenoid cystic carcinoma: analysis of fifty oral cases, Oral Surg. **41**:484, 1976.
396. Tarpley, T.M., Jr., et al.: Minor salivary gland involvement in sarcoidosis, Oral Surg. **33**:755, 1972.
397. Thackray, A.C., and Lucas, R.B.: Tumors of the major salivary glands. In Armed Forces Institute of Pathology: Atlas of tumor pathology, Fascicle 10, Series 2, Washington, D.C., 1974.
398. Vogel, C., and Reichart, P.: Aplasia der Glandulae parotides and submanibularis mit Atresie der Canaliculi lacrimales, Dtsch. Zahnaerztl. Z. **33**:415, 1978.
399. Wasan, S.M.: Sebaceous lymphadenoma of the parotid gland, Cancer **28**:1019, 1971.
400. Whaley, K., et al.: Sjögren's syndrome, Q. J. Med. **42**:279, 1973.
401. Wirman, J.A., and Battifora, H.A.: Small cell undifferentiated carcinoma of salivary gland origin: an ultrastructural study, Cancer **37**:1840, 1976.
402. Wong, T.W., and Warner, N.E.: Cytomegalic inclusion disease in adults, Arch. Pathol. **74**:403, 1962.
403. Woods, J.E., Chong, G.C., and Beahrs, O.H.: Experience with 1,360 primary parotid tumors, Am. J. Surg. **130**:460, 1975.
404. Yarington, C.T., Jr., and Zagibe, F.T.: The ultrastructure of the benign lymphoepithelial lesion, J. Laryngol. Otol. **83**:361, 1969.
405. Yonkers, A.J., Krous, H.F., and Yarington, C.T.: Surgical parotitis, Laryngoscope **82**:1239, 1972.
406. Youngberg, G., and Rao, M.S.: Ultrastructural features of monomorphic adenoma of the parotid gland, Oral Surg. **47**:458, 1979.

Neck

407. Acevedo, A., and Nelson, J.F.: Lymphoepithelial cysts of the oral cavity, Oral Surg. **31**:632, 1971.
408. Armstrong, D., et al.: Torticollis: an analysis of 271 cases, Plast. Reconstr. Surg. **35**:14, 1965.
409. Baughman, R.A.: Lingual thyroid and lingual thyroglossal duct remnants, Oral Surg. **34**:781, 1972.
410. Buchner, A., and Hansen, L.S.: Lymphoepithelial cysts of the oral cavity, Oral Surg. **50**:441, 1980.
411. Clark, O.H.: Parathyroid cysts, Am. J. Surg. **135**:395, 1978.
412. Clark, R.N.: Diagnosis and management of torticollis, Pediatr. Ann. **5**:43, 1976.
413. Devens, K., Holzmann, K., and Spier, J.: Teratomas in the cervical region, Z. Kinderchir. **30**:119, 1980.
414. Farman, A.G., et al.: Mandibulofacial aspects of the cervical cystic lymphangioma (cystic hygroma), Br. J. Oral Surg. **16**:125, 1978-9.
415. Glenner, G.G., and Grimley, P.M.: Tumors of the extra-adrenal paraganglion system (including chemoreceptors). In Armed

Forces Institute of Pathology: Atlas of tumor pathology, Fascicle 9, Series 2, Washington, D.C., 1973.
416. Guba, A.M., et al. Cervical presentation of thymic cysts, Am. J. Surg. **136**:430, 1978.
417. Holland, C.S.: The management of Ludwig's angina, Br. J. Oral Surg. **13**:153, 1975.
418. Hugo, N.E., and Conway, H.: Benign symmetrical lipomatosis, Plast. Reconstr. Surg. **37**:69, 1966.
419. Irons, G.B., Weiland, L.H., and Brown, W.L.: Paragangliomas of the neck: clinical and pathologic analysis of 116 cases, Surg. Clin. North Am. **57**:575, 1977.
420. Johnsen, N.J., and Bretlau, P.: Cervical thymic cysts, Acta Otolaryngol. **82**:143, 1976.
421. Lack, E.E., et al.: Paragangliomas of the head and neck region: a clinical study of 69 patients, Cancer **39**:397, 1977.
422. Lack, E.E., et al.: Cysts of the parathyroid gland: report of two cases and review of the literature, Am. Surg. **44**:376, 1978.
423. Macdonald, D.M.: Thyroglossal cysts and fistulae, Int. J. Oral Surg. **3**:342, 1974.
424. McGuirt, W.F., and Harker, L.A.: Carotid body tumors, Arch. Otolaryngol. **101**:58, 1975.
425. Ninh, T.N., and Ninh, T.X.: Cystic hygroma in children: a report of 126 cases, J. Pediatr. Surg. **9**:191, 1974.
426. Pratt, L.W.: Familial carotid body tumors, Arch. Otolaryngol. **97**:334, 1973.
427. Roediger, W.E., Spitz, L., and Schmaman, A.: Histogenesis of benign cervical teratomas, Teratology **10**:111, 1974.
428. Rosen, E.A., Schulman, R.H., and Shaw, A.S.: Ludwig's angina: a complication of a mandibular fracture, J. Oral Surg. **30**:196, 1972.
429. Rundle, F.W.: Cervical teratoma, J. Otolaryngol. **5**:513, 1976.
430. Schuler, F.A., Graham, J.K., and Horton, C.E.: Benign symmetrical lipomatosis (Madelung's disease), Plast. Reconstr. Surg. **57**:662, 1976.
431. Toto, P.D., Wortel, J.P., and Joseph, G.: Lymphoepithelial cysts and associated immunoglobulins, Oral Surg. **54**:59, 1982.
432. Tovi, R., and Mares, A.J.: The aberrant cervical thymus: embryology, pathology and clinical implications, Am. J. Surg. **136**:631, 1978.
433. Wilson, H.: Carotid body tumors: familial and bilateral, Ann. Surg. **171**:843, 1970.

CHAPTER 26 **Alimentary Tract**

GERALD FINE
CHAN K. MA

CONGENITAL ANOMALIES

Atresia

Most malformations of the alimentary tract are congenital and are related to the formation of the bowel lumen or bowel rotation.[78,128] Interruption in the continuity of the bowel lumen, which may be partial (stenosis) or complete (atresia), manifests itself in early infancy and is incompatible with life without prompt surgical correction. The sites commonly involved are the esophagus, small intestine, and anus.[57] Esophageal atresia is frequently associated with tracheoesophageal fistulas and occasionally with one or more of a variety of other malformations—anal atresia, vertebral defect, and renal dysplasia or agenesis (Vater association).[14] Webs of vascularized fibrous tissue covered by mucosa may be the cause of narrowing of the upper or lower portion of the esophagus (Fig. 26-1).[205] Those in the former site are more often seen in women and frequently are associated with atrophic glossitis, iron-deficiency anemia, and dysphagia (Plummer-Vinson syndrome). Intestinal atresia may be associated with meconium ileus (see discussion of cystic fibrosis, p. 1234), which some investigators have considered to be the cause of the atresia.[23] Faulty development of the hindgut, which is intimately related to the development of the cloacal septum, is frequently associated with fistulas between the rectum and urinary or genital tract or the perineum. Failure of the proctodeum to invaginate or of the anal plate to be absorbed results in imperforate rectum or anus.[126]

Heterotopia

Gastric mucous membrane may be found in the cervical esophagus[28,189] or associated with other malformations such as Meckel's diverticulum, duplications, or enteric cysts. Pancreatic tissue,[227] in the form of discrete nodules of acinar and ductal tissue and occasionally islets of Langerhans, occurs most commonly in the stomach[146] and duodenum and less frequently in the jejunum, Meckel's diverticulum, and appendix. Pulmonary tissue has been found in the terminal ileum.[142] The adenomyoma, an admixture of ducts and smooth muscle, is encountered in the stomach and gallbladder.

Duplications and enteric cysts

Duplications and enteric cysts are segments of gastrointestinal tube in apposition to any portion of the alimentary canal that may be completely independent of the adjacent normal intestine or share its lumen and mesentery and muscle coats. They develop in one of two ways—multicentric recanalization of the proliferated luminal gut epithelium or persistence, growth, and sequestration of diverticular buds of the developing intestine. The two are similar in makeup, but the cysts are more or less spherical and usually lack communica-

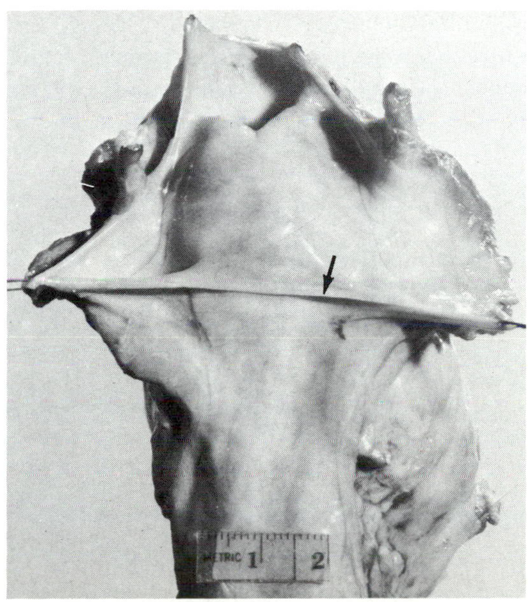

Fig. 26-1. Congenital esophogeal web. Esophagus has been opened posteriorly.

tion with the gut lumen. Duplications are most common in the region of the terminal ileum,[30] whereas cysts are most often intrathoracic and related to the esophagus. They may be lined by small intestinal, gastric, or even bronchial mucous membrane; if gastric, peptic ulceration with concomitant hemorrhage or perforation may occur.

Meckel's diverticulum

Meckel's diverticulum is a diverticulum on the antimesenteric aspect of the terminal ileum, 2.5 cm to 1.83 m proximal to the ileocecal valve, and possesses all the layers of small bowel (Fig. 26-2). It represents the most common of many possible residua of the omphalomesenteric duct; others are umbilical sinus, cyst between the ileum and umbilicus, and ileoumbilical fistula. Its mucosa is usually that of the small intestine, but in 25% of the cases gastric mucosa with or without pancreatic tissue may be present. It may be manifested clinically by peptic ulceration and hemorrhage, obstruction of its lumen, intussusception, or diverticulitis.[112,204,239]

Aganglionic megacolon (Hirschsprung's disease)[151]

Aganglionic megacolon is characterized by symptoms of partial or complete intestinal obstruction, usually from birth or very early in life, with great dilatation and hypertrophy of the colon. The underlying anatomic defect is a lack of ganglion cells in Auerbach's (myenteric) plexus and Meissner's (submucous) plexus in a narrowed, nonhypertrophied segment of intestine distal to the extremely dilated and hypertrophied colon, which is innervated normally (Plate 2, *A*). The aganglionic area usually does not extend higher than the sigmoid colon, but instances of involvement of the entire colon and even the small intestine occur. The diagnosis can be based on the failure to find ganglion cells in adequate rectal biopsy specimens. Surgical resection of the aganglionic segment relieves the condition. Adynamic bowel syndrome may simulate Hirschprung's disease clinically and roentgenographically, but there are no morphologic changes in the bowel ganglia.[117]

Pyloric stenosis

Congenital pyloric stenosis is gross narrowing of the pylorus as a result of an unexplained hypertrophy of the pyloric muscle, usually in male infants. It is manifested by vomiting with attendant dehydration and malnutrition.[20] Surgical relief is obtained by incision of the hypertrophied muscle. A similar condition is occasionally seen in adults and is usually associated with a gastric or duodenal ulcer.

Achalasia of esophagus

Loss of normal esophageal peristalsis and impaired relaxation of the lower esophageal sphincter result in progressive dysphagia and dilatation of the esophagus. Loss of ganglion cells in Auerbach's plexus is a consistent finding in the body of the esophagus; in the sphincter such cells have been reported to be normal in number, reduced, or absent. Alterations in the vagus nerves and their motor nuclei have also been implicated in the esophageal dysfunction, but some authors have considered these changes to be the result of the esophageal ganglion cell changes.[38,71]

Miscellaneous anomalies

A variety of anomalies of position may involve the gastrointestinal tract: the presence of portions of the tract in internal or external or diaphragmatic hernial sacs, malrotation or failure of descent of the intestine, transposition associated with transposition of other viscera, and variations in development or attachment of the mesentery. Any or all of these anomalies may be responsible for volvulus and intestinal obstruction.

Abnormal peritoneal bands also may produce obstruction. A congenitally short esophagus may be associated

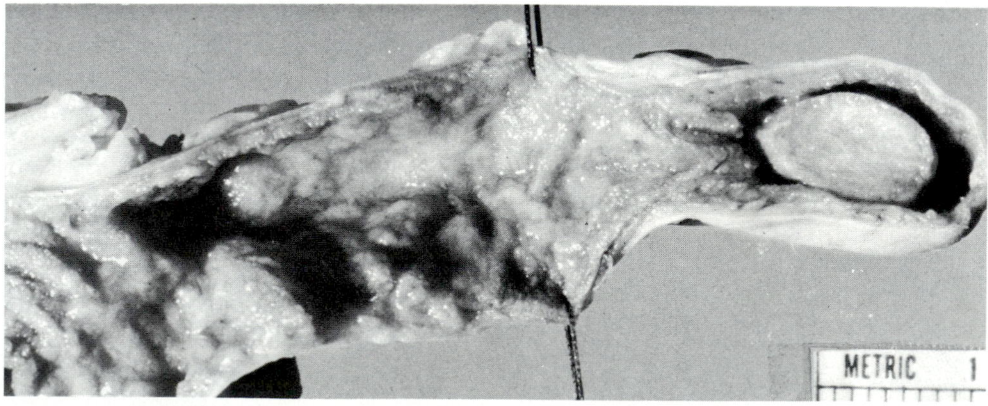

Fig. 26-2. Meckel's diverticulum. Note fruit pit in tip of diverticulum.

with herniation of a portion of gastric cardia into the thoracic cavity, so-called hiatus hernia (p. 1058).

Multilocular rectal cysts with variable epithelial lining—squamous, columnar with mucin, or transitional—presumably having their origin from the neurenteric canal or postanal gut, may be responsible for intestinal obstruction, abscesses, or fistulas.[76] Association of the cysts with a dimple of the anal mucous membrane in its posterior midline has been reported.

ACQUIRED MALFORMATIONS

Diverticula

Acquired diverticula of the gastrointestinal tract are for the most part "false" (pulsion diverticula), representing herniations of the mucous membrane and muscularis mucosae through weakened areas or defects in the muscularis propria. Their walls do not have all the layers of the segment of alimentary tract from which they arise but are composed of mucous membrane, muscularis mucosae, and areolar tissue (Fig. 26-3). They occur at the junction of the esophagus and hypopharynx (Zenker's diverticulum),[127] in the second portion of the duodenum, in the small intestine,[27,75] and in the appendix, but they are most common and clinically significant in the colon.[175] In the last site, they are frequently multiple and most prevalent in the descending and sigmoid colon. They occur on the convexity of the intestine opposite the mesenteric attachment and between the long muscle bands (taenias). Although numerous, they may be difficult to discern, being hidden externally by epiploic appendages and internally by muscle contraction, which diminishes their luminal orifice. Clinical manifestations may be acute or chronic and related to one or a combination of conditions, such as bowel spasm, diverticulitis, hemorrhage, fistulas, perforation, and intestinal obstruction.

The less commonly acquired diverticula, "true" (traction) diverticula, occur in the esophagus and first portion of the duodenum just distal to the pylorus. In both sites they are the result of inflammation and scarring; those in the esophagus are related to hilar and mediastinal lymph node disease, whereas those in the pylorus result from duodenal or pyloric ulcers.

Pneumatosis cystoides intestinalis[73]

In pneumatosis intestinalis, gas-filled cysts are found in the submucosa or wall of the small intestine, less fre-

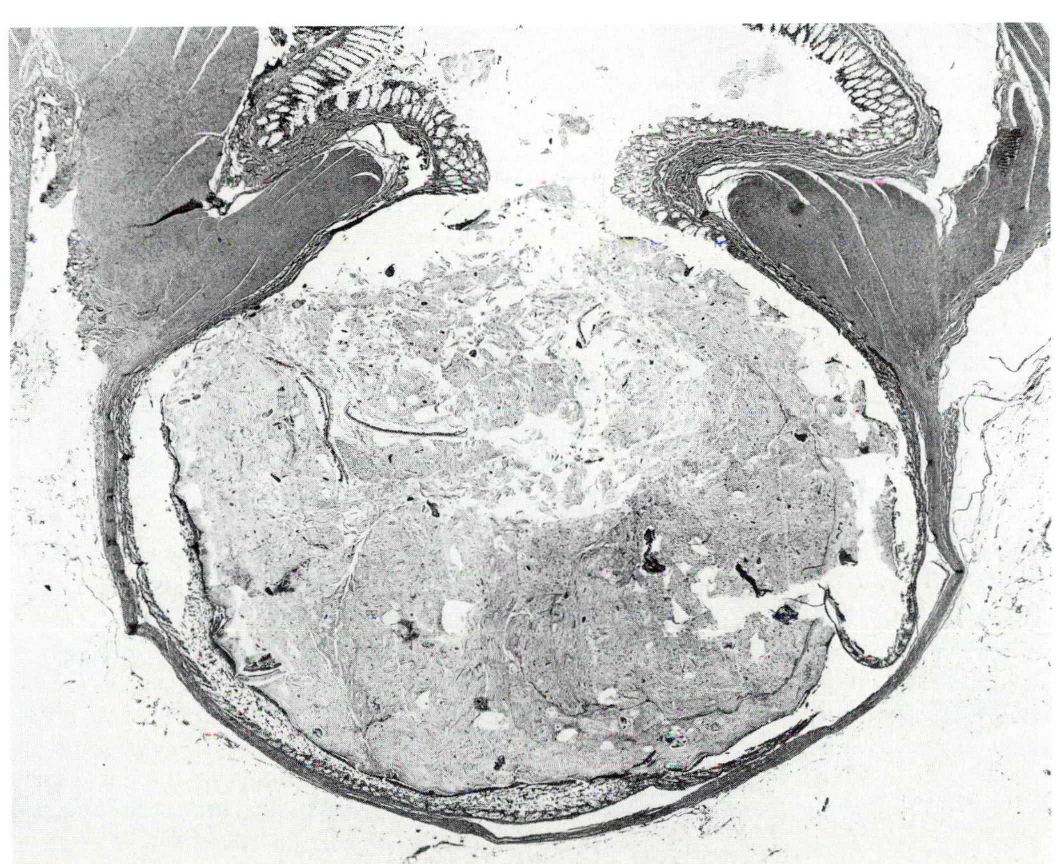

Fig. 26-3. Diverticulum of sigmoid colon, demonstrating hernia-like nature. Note fecal content. (17×.)

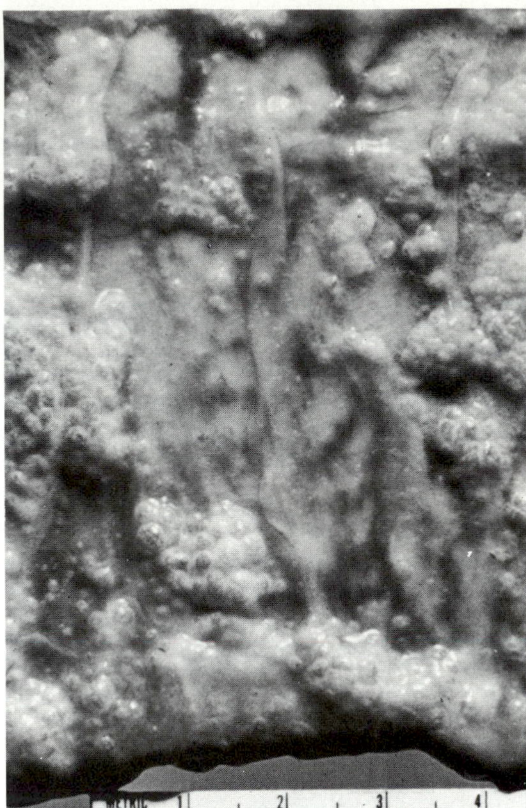

Fig. 26-4. Pneumatosis cystoides intestinalis.

quently in the colon, and rarely in the stomach and esophagus at necropsy (Fig. 26-4). The process is associated with gastric or duodenal ulcers, enterocolitis, or respiratory disease, notably asthma. It now appears that the condition can be explained on a mechanical basis in association with (1) obstruction with ulceration, (2) trauma from biopsy, sigmoidoscopic examination, and so on, or (3) respiratory disease with severe cough. In the last case it is postulated that pneumomediastinum occurs after pulmonary alveolar rupture, since the air then dissects retroperitoneally and reaches the intestine along the path of the mesenteric blood vessels.[125] The gas cysts range in diameter from a few millimeters to a centimeter or more and may be lined by flattened endothelium-like cells resembling lymphatic spaces of multinucleated giant cells, or they may have no visible lining.[209] The cysts do not communicate with the intestinal lumen or with each other. The symptoms of pneumatosis are generally nonspecific. Spontaneous resolution with roentgenographic clearing can and does occur.

Melanosis of colon

The mucous membrane of the colon and appendix may acquire a brown color because of the accumulation of brown granular pigment in phagocytes in the lamina propria. Although the pigment is referred to as melanin, its exact nature is unknown. The condition is not of clinical significance. One suggestion is that it is related to colonic stasis and the habitual use of anthracene laxatives.[72]

Endometriosis

Foci of endometrial glands and endometrial stroma may involve the colon,[221] usually the sigmoid or rectum, appendix, or small bowel. It may be responsible for obstructive symptoms, colic, and diarrhea, or even rectal bleeding. Obstruction is the result of fibrosis or muscle spasm, and cancer can be simulated both roentgenographically and at operation. Less commonly a decidual reaction associated with pregnancy may be found involving the serosa of the bowel.

MECHANICAL DISTURBANCES

Obstruction

The relative incidence of the various causes of intestinal obstruction varies, but hernias, adhesions, and neoplasms are the common causes. Other causes are volvulus, foreign objects, inflammatory disease, stricture, and external compression by tumors, cysts, enlarged viscera, and so on, as well as such congenital lesions as annular pancreas, meconium ileus, and the atresias, bands, and the like previously noted.

Hernia

Hernia is the protrusion of tissue, organ, or part of an organ through an abnormal opening in the wall of the body cavity in which it is normally confined. The majority of hernias are abdominal, resulting from herniation of abdominal contents through the internal or external inguinal rings, femoral ring, or defects in the abdominal wall resulting from trauma or improper healing after a surgical procedure.[148] Less common are internal hernias, wherein loops of intestine penetrate normally small peritoneal recesses, such as the fossa at the junction of the duodenum and jejunum. Diaphragmatic hernias are not a significant cause of intestinal obstruction. Herniation of abdominal viscera through congenital defects in the diaphragm is infrequent compared to hiatus hernia, which is the protrusion, often intermittent ("sliding" hernia), of a portion of the stomach and abdominal esophagus through the esophageal hiatus of the diaphragm into the thoracic cavity.[13,95,141] Symptoms in the latter—a disease of obese, middle-aged individuals—are related to the reflux of gastric secretions into the esophagus, with resultant so-called peptic esophagitis, ulceration, and hemorrhage. Herniation of the gastric cardia through the esophageal hiatus also may occur alongside the esophagus; this is called paraesophageal hernia.

Adhesions

In addition to congenital bands, peritoneal adhesions resulting from inflammation and after laparotomy may be

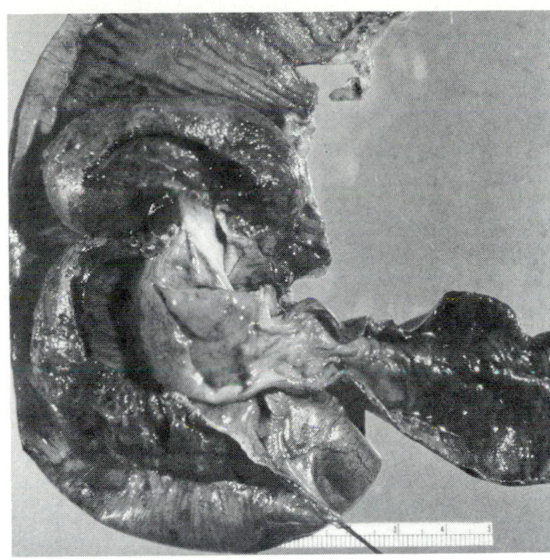

Fig. 26-5. Ileocecal intussusception with infarction.

responsible for intestinal obstruction, usually in the small intestine.

Neoplasms

Intestinal obstruction may result from primary or secondary bowel involvement by neoplasm. The most common obstructing primary tumors are the encircling carcinomas that occur in the left half of the colon where the intestinal content is semisolid.

Intussusception

Intussusception is the invagination of a segment of intestinal tract (the intussusceptum) into the immediately adjacent (almost always distal) intestine (the intussuscipiens). It is primarily a disease of infants and young children,[21] but it does occur in adults, in whom it may be initiated by a pedunculated benign or malignant primary tumor or a metastatic growth. In children it is more common in the ileocecal region, with the ileum telescoping into the colon and the ileocecal valve retaining its normal position (Fig. 26-5). Less common are ileoileal and colocolonic intussusception. Masses of lymphoid tissue, polyps, or the ileocecal valve itself may form the advancing head of the intussusception, or the lesion may be the result of uncoordinated muscle contractions of the bowel. Bowel obstruction or compromise of blood supply to the involved intestine requires surgical intervention if spontaneous correction does not occur. Multiple foci of intussusception, unassociated with any reaction, are seen occasionally at necropsy and are believed to be agonal.

Volvulus

Volvulus is the twisting of a loop (or loops) of intestine upon itself through 180 degrees or more, producing obstruction of both the intestine and the blood supply of the affected loop. Causative factors are usually long mesenteric attachment, redundant intestine, abnormal bands (congenital or acquired), or abnormal attachments of the intestine. The lesion is most common in the sigmoid colon and has a preponderance in men. Because strangulation occurs almost simultaneously with obstruction, operative treatment must be prompt to avoid death of the patient.

Obturation obstruction

A foreign body, exogenous or endogenous, large or small, may obstruct the intestinal lumen by inducing bowel spasm or becoming entrapped in areas of anatomic or pathologic narrowing of the intestinal lumen. Gallstone obstruction of the small intestine complicating cholecystogastric or cholecystoduodenal fistula, large-bowel obstruction by enteroliths, and appendiceal obstruction by fecaliths are examples of common endogenous obstruction. Almost any conceivable ingested foreign body may produce bowel obstruction.[171] Fruit pits and bezoars—masses of ingested hair (trichobezoars) or vegetable residues (phytobezoars), most notably persimmons—are worthy of mention. Parasites, particularly *Ascaris lumbricoides*, are also causes of intestinal obstruction.

Stricture

Intrinsic narrowing of the intestinal lumen may be the result of scarring in one or more of its layers as a result of chemical injury (for example, lye in the esophagus), peptic ulceration of the esophagus or duodenum, x-ray irradiation,[181] scarring at the sites of surgical anastomosis or intestinal resection, or scleroderma.

Adynamic (paralytic) ileus

The clinical picture of acute intestinal obstruction may occur in the absence of mechanical or organic obstruction as a result of paralysis of the musculature of a portion or all of the intestinal tract. Abdominal distension and accumulation of gas and fluid in the intestine may be extreme, producing the same effects as mechanical obstruction. It frequently occurs after laparotomy, usually in a mild form. It may be associated with intra-abdominal infection, trauma, or other disease (for example, ureteral stone) or systemic infection (for example, pneumonia in children).[173] Peritonitis resulting from acute appendicitis with perforation, perforated peptic ulcer, and so on is probably the most important single underlying cause. A related condition is acute dilatation of the stomach, which occasionally complicates surgery, usually abdominal.

Effects of intestinal obstruction

The systemic effects of bowel obstruction are variable in their severity, being dependent on the site involved and the degree of obstruction. They are related to fluid and electrolyte loss, distension with fluid and gas, and damage to the bowel wall and resulting permeability to bacteria and, potentially, peritonitis.[231] One or more of the following may be associated with the obstruction: dehydration, acidosis, alkalosis, hemoconcentration, decrease in intracellular fluid, and finally renal suppression. The bowel proximal to the obstruction shows varying degrees of dilatation and hypertrophy depending on the location and the completeness of the obstruction, as well as the duration.

Mallory-Weiss syndrome[51]

Any action that increases intra-abdominal pressure, but particularly bouts of repeated and forceful vomiting, may produce longitudinally oriented lacerations in the gastric cardia, distal esophagus, or esophagogastric junction, which may be the source of gastrointestinal hemorrhage. Alcoholism, aspirin ingestion, gastritis, and hiatus hernia have been commonly associated with the syndrome.[130]

VASCULAR DISTURBANCES

Esophageal varices

Elevated pressure in the portal venous system, most often the result of cirrhosis of the liver but at times caused by other lesions such as portal vein thrombosis, commonly results in esophageal varices.[11] The esophageal venous plexus receives blood from the gastric and coronary veins of the stomach, forming part of one of the routes by which portal venous blood may bypass the liver to reach the right atrium. As a result, the submucosal veins of the lower part of the esophagus, and sometimes of the upper part of the stomach as well, become greatly dilated, tortuous, and engorged. They are covered by a thin mucous membrane. The increased venous pressure, with or without inflammation or ulceration, often results in massive and frequently fatal hemorrhage.[135]

Ischemic bowel disease[172]

Compromise of the blood supply to the gastrointestinal tract may occur in a variety of ways and be responsible for a variety of bowel changes. The complex control of the mesenteric circulation[143] (cardiac, autonomic nervous system, peripheral collateral circulation, and peripheral autoregulation), coupled with the degree of local vascular disease, makes the bowel vulnerable to ischemia in a variety of ways. Abundant collateral blood supply to the stomach, duodenum, and rectum from extracoelomic vessels makes these sites less vulnerable than others to ischemia. Excluding strangulation, as discussed previously, the causes of bowel ischemia in order of decreasing frequency are sclerosis of the mesenteric arteries with or without associated thrombosis[225]; embolism (thrombotic, atherosclerotic plaques, or tumor); venous thrombosis, sometimes associated with contraceptive drugs[42]; hypotension generally associated with nonocclusive atheromatous disease,[191] which by itself has compromised the blood supply short of producing necrosis; and vascular diseases such as thromboangiitis obliterans and vasculitis of various types. The superior mesenteric vessels and consequently the jejunum and proximal part of the ileum are involved most frequently, although any part of the gastrointestinal tract may be affected.

Complete arterial occlusion results in full-thickness infarction of the bowel, which is usually anemic initially but with time becomes hemorrhagic. Venous occlusion preceding arterial blockage causes infarction that is hemorrhagic from its inception. The bowel becomes dusky and purple-red because of hemorrhage into the bowel wall and lumen and subsequent necrosis and inflammatory cell infiltration. The resulting paralysis of the bowel muscle produces an intestinal obstruction with its attendant physiologic alterations.

Reduction in blood flow to the intestine insufficient to produce a full-thickness infarct may result in a variety of nonspecific lesions (ischemic enteritis and colitis): ulceration, inflammation, cicatrization with stricture formation,[242] and "intestinal angina." The distinction between such lesions and those believed to be related to potassium ingestion is not always clear.[245]

Hemorrhoids

Hemorrhoids are varicosities of the hemorrhoidal vein—"internal" and covered by mucous membrane if of the superior hemorrhoidal plexus and "external" and covered by skin if of the inferior hemorrhoidal plexus. The former are the more important and the more troublesome. They result from increased venous pressure related to such causes as portal hypertension, cardiac failure, carcinoma of the rectum, or myomatous or pregnant uterus, but chronic constipation appears to be far more important in their pathogenesis.

The coincidence of hemorrhoids and rectal carcinoma is sufficiently great to make search for the latter mandatory in every patient with hemorrhoids.

Complications of hemorrhoids are thrombosis with associated inflammation, scarring, pain, and hemorrhage in the form of bright red blood passed by rectum. Organization of a thrombus may produce a histologic picture that may mimic the malignant hemangioendothelioma.

Gastrointestinal hemorrhage

Bleeding into the gastrointestinal tract may be the result of a wide variety of lesions and may be minimal, producing anemia, or massive and life threatening.[33] If the blood is eliminated orally or rectally soon after escaping from the vascular system, it is bright red, but if it is confined to the alimentary tract for a period of time before being eliminated, it is brown or black (coffee-ground vomitus and tarry stools—melena). The most important sources of massive hematemesis (vomiting of blood) are esophageal varices, gastric or duodenal (peptic) ulcers, and leiomyoma. Other tumors (benign or malignant), hiatus hernia, gastritis, and so on usually produce bleeding of lesser degree. Massive bleeding from the rectum or anus is less common than massive hematemesis. Hemorrhoids, diverticular disease, or the polyps of the Peutz-Jeghers syndrome may cause it. However, these lesions also may be associated with bleeding of small amount, as is commonly found in carcinoma of the large intestine and, less often, with other tumors, regional enteritis, ulcerative colitis, and anal fissure.[226] The lesions causing hematemesis are also associated with blood in the stool, which may be occult. Other potential causes of any type of gastrointestinal bleeding include hereditary telangiectasis (Rendu-Osler-Weber disease), other vascular malformations, any of the blood dyscrasias, and anticoagulant therapy.[74,210]

INFLAMMATIONS

Esophagitis

Esophageal inflammation most commonly results from secretion—reflux or peptic esophagitis—associated with hiatus hernia, achalasia, or scleroderma. Less common causes are corrosive substances (lye) and infectious agents—viral (herpes simplex and varicella) and fungous (*Candida*).[166] Scarring and stricture generally result from lye ingestion, prolonged gastric juice reflux, or neoplasms. Initially gastric juice produces basal cell hyperplasia of the esophageal epithelium, with elongation of the connective tissue papillae with or without neutrophilic infiltrates.[109] Persistent reflux leads to one or more complications—ulceration, stricture, or columnar epithelial metaplasia of the squamous mucosa (Barrett's esophagus),[178] in which there has been a 10% incidence of adenocarcinoma.[39,169]

Esophageal pseudodiverticulosis is a condition that roentgenographically mimics diverticula but that pathologically is dissimilar.[40] The x-ray changes are attributable to dilatation and tortuosity of the esophageal glands and their ducts, but there is no abnormal extension of mucosa beyond the confines of the esophageal submucosa.[139] The process appears to be the result of inflammation and obstruction of the increased number of esophageal glands and ducts, with dilatation and squamous metaplasia of their lining epithelium (Fig. 26-6).

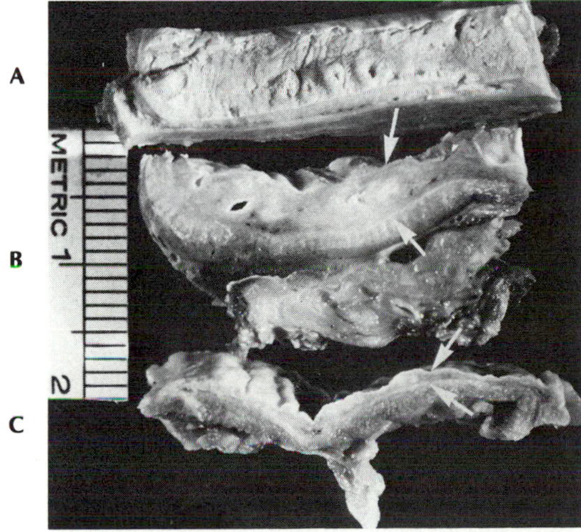

Fig. 26-6. A and **B,** Pseudodiverticulosis of esophagus. **C,** Normal esophagus. Ducts of esophageal glands are prominent in thickened submucosa *(arrows)* in pseudodiverticulosis, and their openings on mucosal surface are accentuated, **A.** (Courtesy Dr. Aaron Lupovitch, Detroit, Mich.)

Gastritis and gastroenteritis

The gastritis and gastroenteritis that are such common clinical complaints rarely come to the attention of the pathologist. They are the result of exogenous agents, such as ethanol, therapeutic drugs (salicylates and so on), irradiation, and corrosive agents, or endogenous agents, such as bacterial and viral agents involving the bowel or other organs and allergy. Phlegmonous gastritis,[49] usually of streptococcal origin, results from inflammation elsewhere in the body, such as osteomyelitis.

Inflammatory fibroid polyp and eosinophilic gastroenteritis

Inflammatory fibroid polyp and eosinophilic gastroenteritis manifest themselves as either a localized, fibrotic, polypoid, tumorlike mass (inflammatory fibroid polyp,[115] Fig. 26-7) or a diffuse infiltration throughout all coats of the gut wall.[114] Eosinophils are a prominent part of the histopathologic picture in both lesions, but blood eosinophilia and a history of allergy are associated only with the diffuse lesion. Sites of involvement in order of frequency include the stomach, jejunum, ileum, and cecum. The colon and rectum are rarely involved. No relationship between these conditions and histiocytosis X has been found.

Ulcers of stomach and duodenum

Ulcers, usually small and multiple and not penetrating the muscularis mucosae (erosions), are frequently encountered in the stomach as a terminal event in a variety of conditions.[90] Acute ulcers of the stomach or duodenum may be associated with extensive burns (Curling's ulcers, Fig. 26-8),[50,184] Cushing's disease, hypothalamic lesions, stress, or trauma; they may also be iatrogenic (resulting from corticosteroid therapy or gastric tubes). They may be fatal as a result of uncontrolled hemorrhage or spontaneous perforation and peritonitis.

Nonspecific ulcers in the small intestine have been

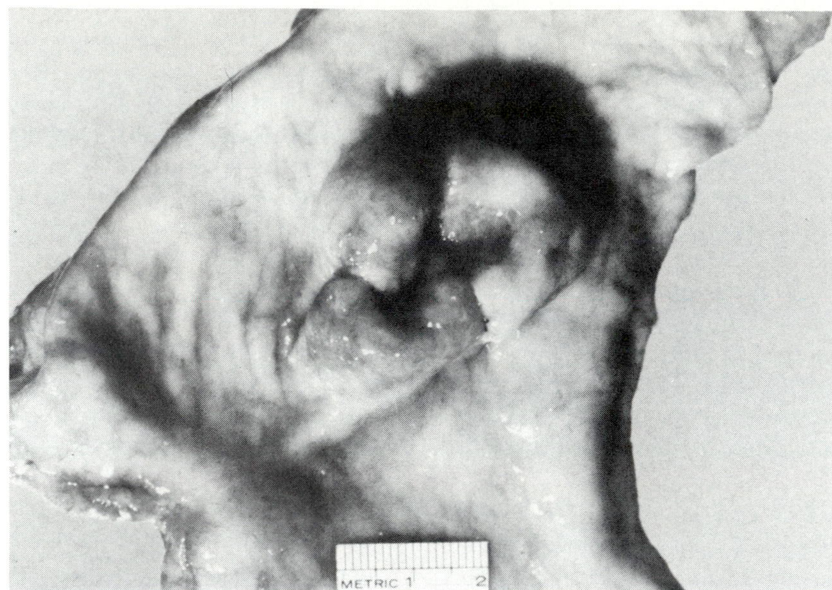

Fig. 26-7. Eosinophilic granuloma (inflammatory fibroid polyp) of stomach.

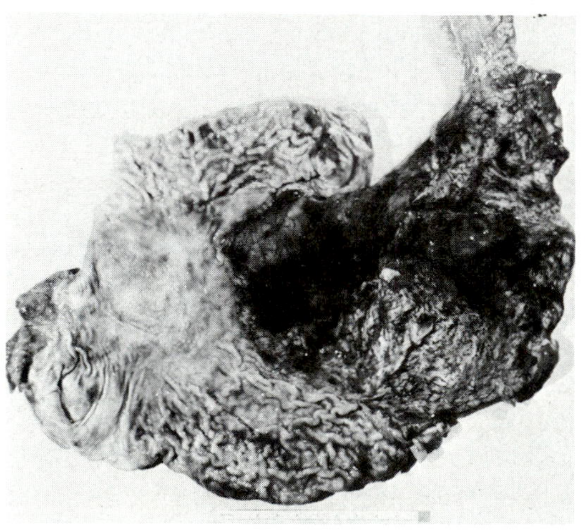

Fig. 26-8. Curling's ulcer of proximal part of stomach.

encountered with increasing frequency. They may be complicated by scarring and partial intestinal obstruction. Vascular changes and potassium, a known tissue irritant therapeutically employed in enteric-coated tablets, have been implicated in their pathogenesis.[237]

Peptic ulcer

Incidence and pathogenesis. Chronic ulcers having certain similarities and distinct differences occur in the stomach and duodenum, with a frequency of 2.5% and 1.4%, respectively, among men and women.[152] Duodenal ulcers are more common and more often found in young and middle-aged men of blood group O, particularly in nonsecretors. Gastric ulcers are more frequent at an older age, with a preponderance among blood group A. Duodenal ulcer has been associated with tension, stress, and anxiety, but this is by no means always the case and there is no agreement on the importance of stress in its pathogenesis.[79] Peptic ulcers occur only in the environment of acid gastric secretions: the stomach, duodenum, lower esophagus, jejunum just distal to the site of surgical gastroenteric anastomosis, and malformations containing gastric mucosa. The mucous membrane not accustomed to the acid-pepsin environment is the site involved. Thus gastric ulcers occur in the antrum, infrequently in the cardia, whereas the acid secretion is usually limited to the fundus.

Hypersecretion of gastric juice and emotional factors have been considered to be important in the pathogenesis of peptic ulcers. The gastroduodenal mucous membrane is protected against digestion of normal gastric secretions not only by its mucous coating but also by dilution and neutralization with swallowed food, saliva, and regurgitated duodenal fluids. Hypersecretion of hydrochloric acid into the fasting stomach at night is regarded by Dragstedt[65] as the cause of duodenal ulcer. This is considered to be the result of vagal stimulation and can be abolished by section of the vagus nerve. He regards the gastric ulcer also to be the result of increased hydrochloric acid secretion attributable to a humoral (gastrin) stimulation brought about by stasis of ingested food in an atonic stomach.[66]

Although hyperacidity is common among patients with peptic ulcers, hypoacidity is not uncommon with gastric ulcers, particularly those on the lesser curvature unassociated with ulcers in the duodenum or pylorus.[113,153] To explain the latter, it has been postulated that a number of factors singly or in combination—bile reflux, gastritis, and reduced mucus production by the gastric mucosa—may alter local tissue resistance to hydrochloric acid.[83,99,192]

Emotional factors responsible for vagal stimulation through the hypothalamus–anterior pituitary–adrenal cortex stress mechanism have been shown by Wolf[247] to affect gastric function. Cortisone, which may be the cause of ulcers, usually gastric, may also activate a preexisting ulcer and be responsible for perforation or hemorrhage.

Morbid anatomy and histology. Gastric ulcers most commonly occur on or near the lesser curvature of the stomach, usually within about 5 cm of the pylorus. They are more numerous on the posterior than the anterior wall. A few occur in the cardia, and a few seemingly straddle the pylorus, making it difficult to assign them definitely to either stomach or duodenum. Duodenal ulcers usually occur in the first centimeter or two distal to the pylorus on the anterior or posterior wall rather than laterally.

Although some gastric ulcers are large and irregular, the typical peptic ulcer is small (about 1 cm in the duodenum; 1 to 2.5 cm in the stomach). It is characteristically "punched out," with sharply defined margins, and has overhanging mucosa producing a flasklike appearance. Its edges are not raised, and the mucosal folds converging on the ulcer are distinct to its edge (Plate 2, *D*). Malignant gastric ulcers are generally bowl shaped, with margins that are usually sloped and generally without overhanging mucosa. The edges are raised and indurated, and the mucosal folds toward the crater are interrupted by nodular mucosal or submucosal thickenings (Plate 2, *E*).

Microscopically the bed of the ulcer is seen to be covered by fibrinous exudate containing fragmented leukocytes. Separating this from the scar tissue base is fibrotic granulation tissue with a plasma cell and lymphocytic infiltrate. Occasionally, eosinophils are prominent. The scar tissue is dense and avascular and occupies a full-thickness defect in the muscularis. Hypertrophic nerve bundles may be conspicuous, and in some cases a large artery, often thrombosed or sclerotic, may be seen. In some bleeding ulcers, such a vessel may be recognized on gross examination.

Many ulcers heal, and epithelium grows over the defect in a single layer. In time, glandlike structures may develop, but a completely normal mucous membrane is not regenerated. Because of the dense scar, the muscle does not regenerate, and evidence of the ulcer remains indefinitely.

Complications. The principal complications of peptic ulcer are hemorrhage, perforation, and obstruction. Which, if any, occurs is dependent in part on the location of the ulcer. Both gastric and duodenal ulcers are subject to massive hemorrhage. Duodenal ulcers are especially prone to perforation. Any ulcer, but especially those located posteriorly, may bleed in smaller amounts, producing melena or evidence of occult blood in the stool.

Anterior duodenal ulcers may perforate into the free peritoneal cavity, with resultant generalized peritonitis. Perforating posterior ulcers more often penetrate the pancreas, producing intractable pain. Posterior perforation also may occur into the lesser peritoneal sac, leading to localized peritonitis. The omentum or adhesions to adjacent organs also may serve to localize peritoneal inflammation. The peritonitis from perforated peptic ulcer is initially a chemical inflammation, but bacterial contamination soon follows.

Pyloric obstruction may be a complication of an ulcer, gastric or duodenal, situated near the pylorus. It usually results from a combination of cicatricial narrowing and spasm. The stomach becomes greatly dilated and hypertrophied.

The development of carcinoma has been referred to as one of the complications of peptic ulcer. It seems probable that carcinoma can develop in a preexisting ulcer, but it is equally probable that it is a rare event. It is extremely difficult to establish the occurrence of such a sequence of events in any particular case.

A complication of surgical treatment of ulcer is the development of a marginal (stomal) ulcer—peptic ulceration of the jejunum just distal to the site of anastomosis with the stomach after gastroenterostomy or gastric resection with gastrojejunostomy. Such ulcers may perforate. If perforation into the transverse colon takes place, gastrojejunocolic fistula is the result.

Inflammatory bowel disease

The term *inflammatory bowel disease* (IBD) includes regional enteritis (Crohn's disease [CD]) and ulcerative colitis (UC). Although they have many common features, most cases can be classified as either CD or UC on the basis of clinical, roentgenographic, and pathologic findings. The incidence of IBD is obscured because of inaccuracies in diagnosis. There is a preponderance in whites, especially Jews. Men and women are about equally affected, with a slightly greater incidence of UC in women. Both diseases can occur at any age but are more common in young adults, with a peak incidence at 20 to 30 years of age.

Etiology. Although much has been written regarding the etiology of IBD, it remains unknown. Search for infectious agents has not been fruitful, but injecting homogenates of UC or CD tissue into animals has produced pathologic changes in their bowel.[41,156] A genetic role has been considered important in view of a familial incidence and an association with ankylosing spondylitis, which is known to have genetic transmission. Psychogenic factors have been considered important in UC. More recently an immune-mediated mechanism for both diseases has been given much attention.[64,70,80,122]

Clinical features. The onset of both diseases may be acute or insidious; their course is protracted, manifested by exacerbations and remissions. Diarrhea and rectal bleeding occur in both diseases but are less frequent and severe in CD. Perirectal abscesses, fistulas, and bowel strictures are common in CD.

Ulcerative colitis

It is frequently stated that UC begins in the rectum or sigmoid and progresses to involve part or all of the colon. This is not universally accepted, and it is possible that the theory is based on the relative ease of establishing the diagnosis by proctoscopic examination. When the whole colon is examined, almost all of it is affected in the majority of cases. When a limited segment is involved, it is usually in the left half. It is probable that some of the instances of segmental distribution really represent regional enteritis or enterocolitis. The terminal ileum is involved in approximately one fourth of cases, almost always in direct continuity with colonic disease. The appearance of the colon varies greatly in different stages of the disease. Invariably there is hyperemia, and the mucosa is dark red or purplish red and velvety (Fig. 26-9). At first tiny erosions appear, later becoming deeper and coalescing to form linear ulcers, which have the appearance of longitudinal furrows distributed in the long axis of the colon. The ulcers are often undermining, partially freeing ragged remnants of mucous membrane. In occasional acutely progressing cases, the entire colon is extremely friable and bleeds freely. The muscle is thickened, apparently by contraction, and rigid, having lost all or part of its distensibility. This produces shortening as well as narrowing, and as the disease progresses, the colon increasingly resembles a garden hose. Inasmuch as chronic UC is a disease of remissions and exacerbations, periods of relative quiescence and healing alternate with periods of activity.

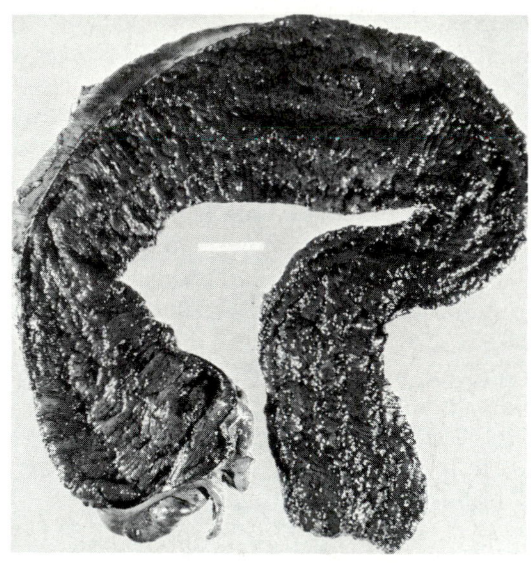

Fig. 26-9. Chronic ulcerative colitis.

The earliest histologic lesion in most cases is a crypt abscess, the accumulation of neutrophils in the crypts of Lieberkühn (Fig. 26-10). The abscesses tend to coalesce to form enlarging, shallow ulcers. Other usual changes of inflammation, that is, hyperemia, edema, hemorrhage, and, more deeply, accumulation of lymphocytes and plasma cells, are present. Frequently, eosinophils and basophils are present in impressive numbers. Some

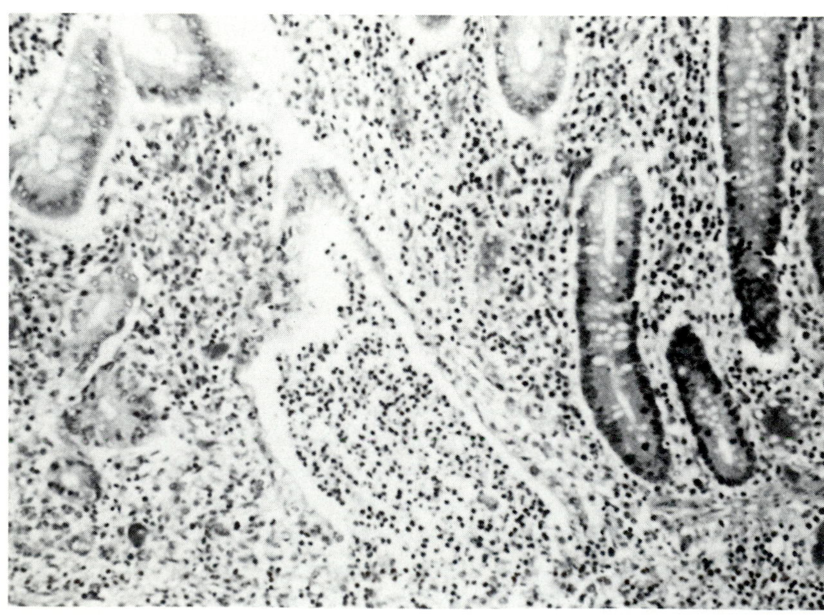

Fig. 26-10. Acute ulcerative colitis showing crypt abscess *(center)* and depletion of mucin production by epithelial cells. (63×.)

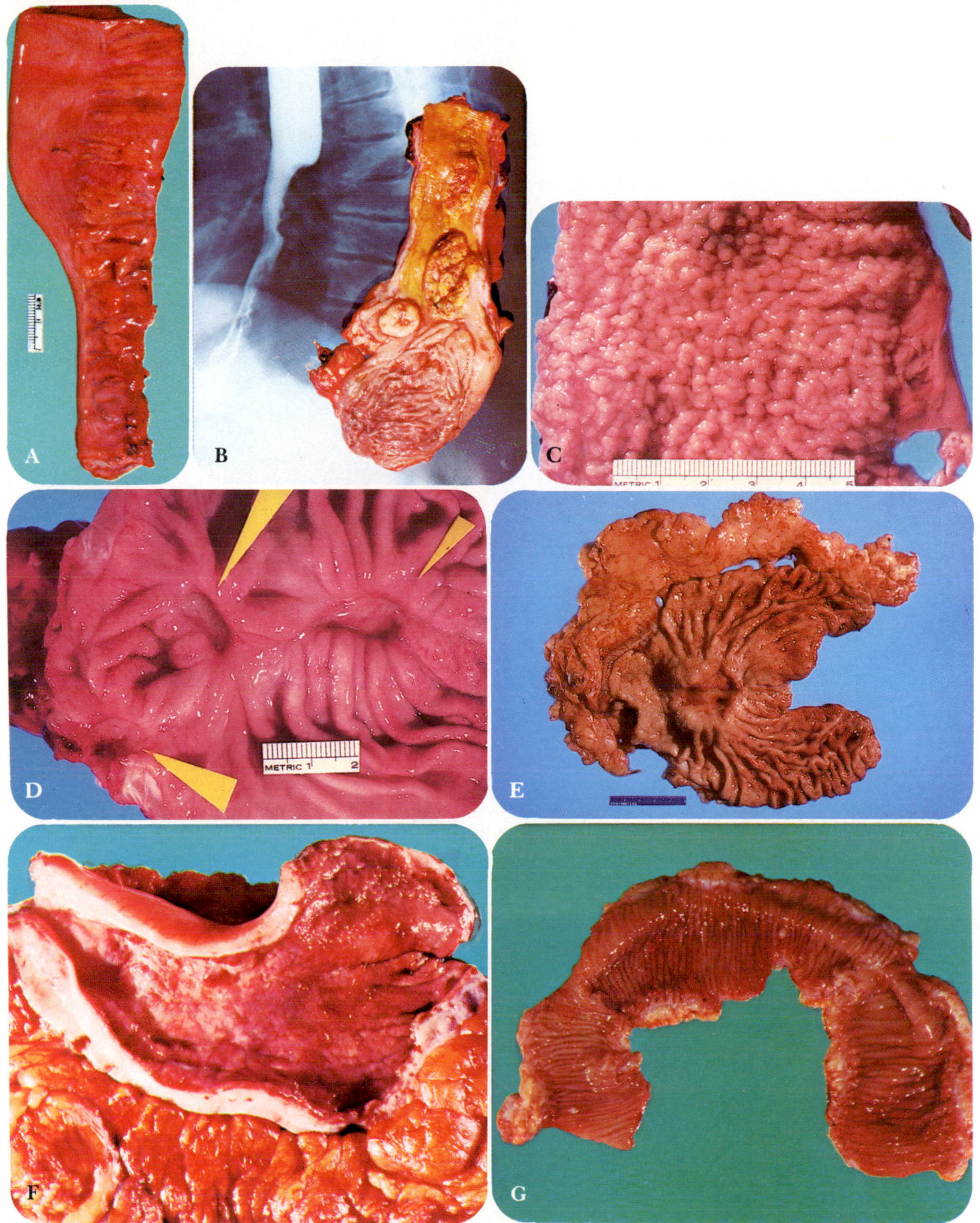

Plate 2

A, Congenital aganglionic megacolon (Hirschsprung's disease).

B, Multifocal epidermoid carcinoma of esophagus. Photograph of gross specimen superimposed on roentgenogram demonstrating lesion with aid of contrast medium.

C, Familial polyposis coli. Entire colon is carpeted by similar-appearing polyps.

D, Multiple gastric ulcers. Note mucosal folds converging on ulcer edge without interruption.

E, Malignant gastric ulcer. Mucosal folds are interrupted toward crater.

F, Carcinoma of stomach, linitis plastica type. Surgically resected specimen.

G, Multiple carcinoid tumors of ileum. Patient had lymph node and liver metastases and demonstrated carcinoid syndrome.

authors have emphasized vasculitis as an early feature, but this is striking only in occasional cases. UC is primarily a mucosal disease, with infrequent and usually limited involvement of the other layers, whereas regional enteritis is a disease of the submucosa and deeper tissues. Also, the inflammation of UC is not characteristically productive of abundant fibrous scar tissue. Granulomas with giant cells, so frequently found in regional enteritis, are only an occasional finding in UC. When the ulcers heal, they are covered by a single layer of epithelium. Although there is an attempt to re-form crypts, regeneration is not complete, and structural abnormalities persist. In the quiescent chronic stage, the mucosa remains red and granular. As noted in the discussion of regional enteritis, chronic UC is to be distinguished from granulomatus colitis.

Pseudopolyps are a frequent and striking finding in UC. They consist of polypoid masses of granulation tissue that include distorted, inflamed crypts, often with hyperplastic epithelium. In contrast to adenomatous polyps, they vary greatly in size and shape, may be long and pendulous, and show no clear distinction between stalk and main body of the polyp. True adenomatous polyps do occur, however, in association with these inflammatory pseudopolyps.

Crohn's disease

Unlike UC, Crohn's disease may involve any portion of the gastrointestinal tract, although it is most commonly found in the terminal ileum, often with extension into the cecum and sometimes into the ascending colon as well. In more than half of the cases, multiple areas of both small and large intestines are involved in segmental fashion; that is, lengths of normal intestine separate areas of disease (so-called skip areas). Changes may be limited to the colon segmentally or may involve the whole organ. Crohn's disease of the colon (granulomatosis colitis) is being recognized with greater frequency (Fig. 26-11). Anal lesions are often associated with lesions of the small and large bowel and may be the first manifestation of the disease. The inflammatory changes are nonspecific and more or less granulomatous. The mucosal surface has a red, nodular, cobblestone-like appearance, with multiple linear and serpiginous ulcerations often extending varying distances into the bowel wall. All coats of the diseased intestine are thickened—the mucosa by inflammatory infiltration, chiefly lymphocytes and plasma cells, the submucosa and subserosa by fibrosis, and the muscularis by hypertrophy (Fig. 26-12).

Histologically, irregular ulceration with a neutrophilic reaction is seen. Crypt abscesses are not as conspicuous as in UC. In the preserved mucous membrane, the glands are dilated, goblet cells are absent or decreased in number, and Paneth cells are more prominent than usual. Glands resembling Brunner's glands of the duodenum or pyloric glands are frequently seen. The muscularis mucosae is hypertrophied, and nerves in the involved segment are increased in number, size, and prominence. Lymphoid nodules are conspicuous in the submucosa and often in the subserosa as well (Fig. 26-13). Noncaseating tubercles composed of epithelioid cells, with occasional multinucleated giant cells, are conspicuous in

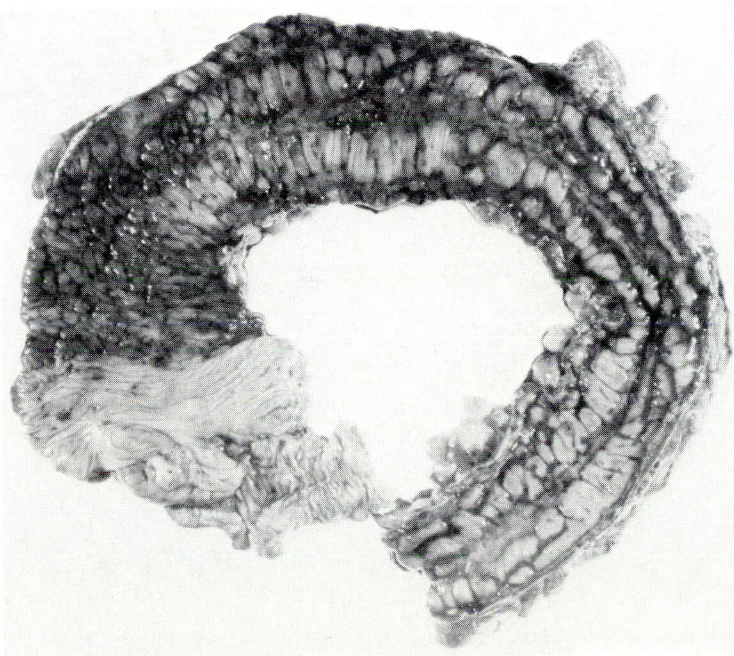

Fig. 26-11. Granulomatous colitis (Crohn's disease of colon) involving almost entire large bowel.

some areas. They gave rise to speculation of an etiologic identity with Boeck's sarcoid, an idea that has since been abandoned. It has been suggested that the recurrence rate is less in cases with granulomas.[86] Deep ulcers may give rise to sinus tracts and perforations, which usually are walled off by omentum or adhesions. Fistulas may complicate long-standing cases. They may be internal, involving other organs or other segments of intestine, or external, opening on the skin of the abdomen after surgical procedures. The lymph nodes are enlarged and usually show nonspecific inflammatory changes but may contain granulomas like those in the intestine.

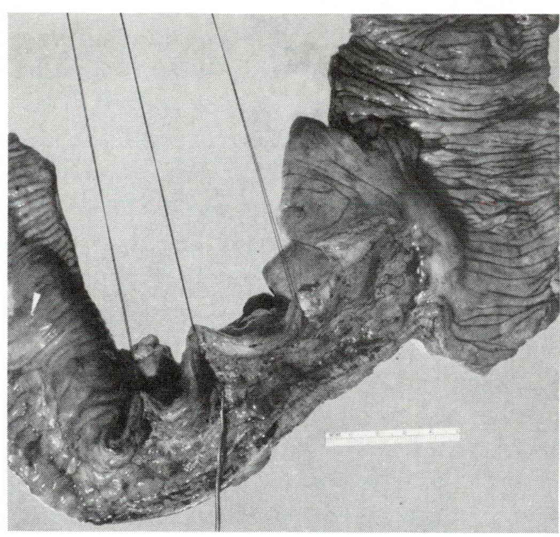

Fig. 26-12. Regional enteritis of terminal ileum. Note abrupt cessation of pathologic change at ileocecal valve.

Complications

Intestinal and extraintestinal complications occur frequently with CD and UC, some being common to both but with greater frequency in one. Bowel obstruction from stricture or adhesions, fistulas, or perforation is more frequent in CD. Acute toxic megacolon resulting in bowel perforation occurs in a small percentage of cases of IBD and is more common in UC. Carcinoma is a well-known complication of UC, the incidence being 3% to 5% of patients with long-standing disease.[161] Unlike bowel carcinoma unassociated with UC, the tumors are often multiple and uniformly distributed throughout the colon, tend to be flat and infiltrative, and histologically are of a higher-grade malignancy. The frequency of carcinoma in these patients has prompted repeated examinations for its early detection and treatment.[193,249] Carcinoma associated with CD occurs, but its frequency is not as great as with UC.[170,233,238]

Extraintestinal complications develop in a significant proportion of patients with IBD during the course of their disease. Among these are hepatobiliary tract abnormalities, that is, fatty metamorphosis, pericholangitis, primary sclerosing cholangitis, chronic active hepatitis, cirrhosis, and bile duct carcinoma[3,58,123]; arthritis; ankylosing spondylitis; erythema nodosum; pyoderma gangrenosum; and iritis.

Appendicitis

Acute appendicitis is uncommon at the extremes of age and is most frequently seen in older children and young adults.[45] The most important factor in its pathogenesis is obstruction of the lumen,[235] the most frequent cause being a fecalith, a molded mass of inspissated fecal

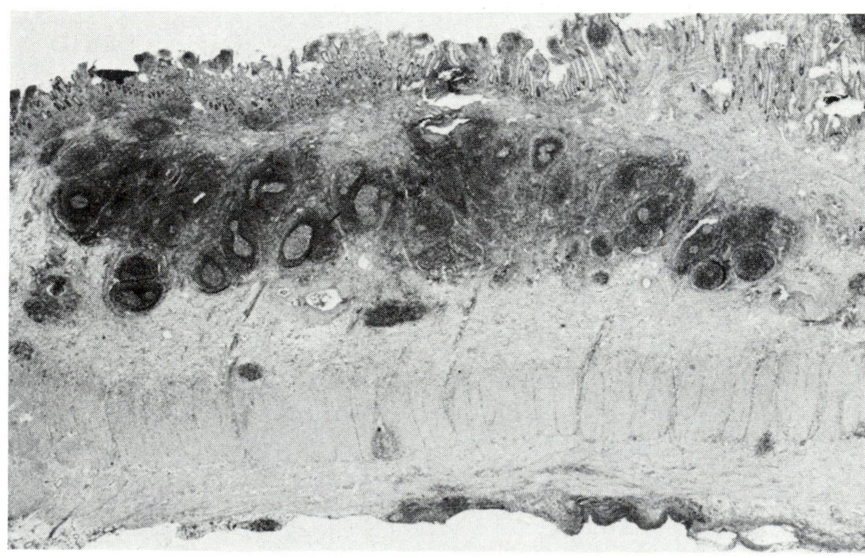

Fig. 26-13. Crohn's disease. Wall is thickened with conspicuous lymphoid nodules in the submucosa and subserosa. (75×.)

material that may develop rock-hard consistency. Fecaliths are found in at least three fourths of acutely inflamed appendices and in virtually all that are gangrenous. In youth the lymphoid tissue of the mucous membrane may become sufficiently hyperplastic, at times in association with systemic infection, to produce obstruction leading to appendicitis or to cause symptoms and signs indistinguishable from those of mild acute appendiceal inflammation. Other causes of obstruction are scars representing a residuum of previous attacks of appendicitis, tumors, external bands, adhesions, rarely masses of parasites[200] (especially pinworms), foreign bodies, and possibly spasm of the muscle at the base of the appendix. The immediate cause of acute appendicitis is bacterial infection from the intestinal lumen, although bacterial invasion from the bloodstream in systemic disease is possible. All species of bacteria common to the intestinal tract can be identified, and usually multiple organisms can be isolated from an individual case.[5]

Inflammation of limited extent may manifest itself grossly only by mild hyperemia. Microscopic examination[224] may show only small amounts of purulent exudate in the lumen, although careful study may reveal one or more foci of inflammation with ulceration of the mucosa. Many examples of focal appendicitis are not merely an early phase of diffuse inflammation but a milder form of the disease, perhaps dependent on temporary or incomplete obstruction by such mechanisms as lymphoid hyperplasia or muscle spasm. The inflammation may appear to be limited to the muscle coat or subserosa, or both, but careful search usually shows mucosal involvement.

Hyperemia and margination of leukocytes in the peripheral blood vessels of the appendix or even infiltration of polymorphonuclear leukocytes into the subserosal tissues may occur as a result of trauma during a surgical procedure, particularly if appendectomy is performed incidentally after a complex operation. Inflammatory change in the serosa and subserosa (periappendicitis) may be associated with disease primarily outside the appendix (such as salpingitis). At times a few neutrophilic leukocytes may be found in the lumen of an incidentally removed appendix without any evidence of inflammation of the appendiceal wall.

Diffuse acute appendicitis almost always occurs in an obstructed appendix. Increased intraluminal pressure compromises the blood supply, and thus the effects of ischemia and bacterial infection contribute to an anatomic picture that is dependent on the time when the appendix is removed. Degrees of ulceration of the mucous membrane, infiltration of leukocytes, and hemorrhagic necrosis result in a distended appendix whose vessels are engorged and whose surface is dulled by a fibrinopurulent exudate. Perforation[81] or sloughing of part or all of the appendix may result in peritonitis, which may be generalized, or walled off to form an appendiceal abscess. Infrequently encountered complications are pylephlebitis and liver abscess.

Not every instance of appendicitis follows this course. If tissue destruction is minimal, resolution or cicatrization occurs. Occasionally, true chronic inflammation of the appendix occurs, usually associated with fistula formation or a foreign body (intestinal content) after acute appendicitis with perforation. Otherwise true chronic appendicitis as a distinct entity does not exist.

Obliteration of part or all of the appendiceal lumen by a mixture of fibrous tissue, lymphocytes, lymphoid follicles, and nerve bundles is common. Although frequently referred to as obliterative appendicitis, there is no evidence that it is the result of inflammatory disease.

The appendix may be involved in diseases primarily affecting other portions of the gastrointestinal tract, such as regional enteritis, typhoid fever, and amebiasis, and in certain systemic diseases (for example, measles). In the prodromal stage of measles, characteristic Warthin-Finkeldey giant cells may be seen in the lymphoid tissue of the appendix, as well as in the lymphoid tissues of the rest of the body.[53]

Many parasites may be found in the appendix. *Enterobius vermicularis* is the parasite most often encountered and may be noted on gross and histologic examination.[200] Ordinarily they merely inhabit the appendix and have no relationship to appendiceal disease. On occasion, however, they may penetrate the wall and become the center of granulomatous inflammatory reaction.

Pseudomembranous enterocolitis

Pseudomembranous enterocolitis is a term used to describe an often lethal gastrointestinal lesion characterized by discrete, raised, yellow-green, adherent, sometime coalescing plaques separated by normal or edematous congested mucosa (Fig. 26-14). Any part of the intestinal tract may be involved, but the ileum and colon are more common. The pseudomembrane is composed of mucin, fibrin, nuclear debris, and neutrophils. The mucosa underlying the pseudomembrane may be partially or completely necrotic.[183]

Its occurrence in a variety of situations suggests that more than one cause may be involved. There has been an association with major surgical procedures (usually of the intestinal tract); ischemic cardiovascular disease; hypotension; staphylococcal infection; heavy metal poisoning; septicemia; uremia; colonic neoplasm with obstruction[93]; and a variety of antibiotics.[15] Studies indicate the toxin of *Clostridium difficile* to be the cause among the antibiotic group.[16,17,133]

Tuberculosis

Primary intestinal tuberculosis, ordinarily the result of ingestion of foods (especially dairy products) infected

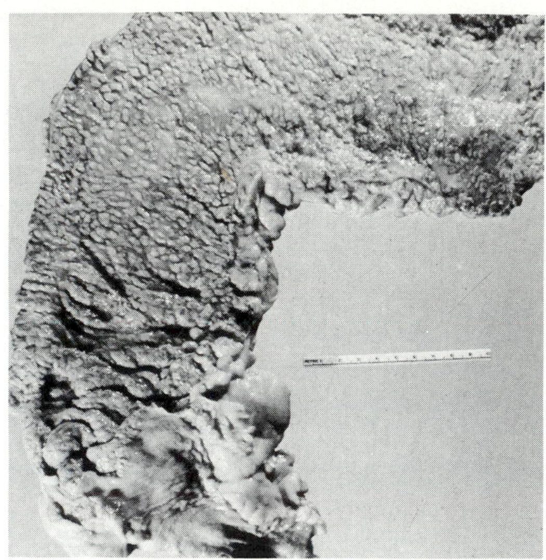

Fig. 26-14. Pseudomembranous enterocolitis.

with the bovine tubercle bacillus, has become rare in the United States. Tuberculosis of the gastrointestinal tract is almost invariably associated with advanced open pulmonary disease with discharge from the lung lesions, and subsequent swallowing, of large numbers of bacilli. In fatal pulmonary tuberculosis, gastrointestinal involvement is quite common, and in disseminated disease, gastrointestinal lesions may be widespread.[2]

The usual isolated gastrointestinal lesion involves the ileocecal or anal region.[48] Rarely the esophagus, stomach, or intestine may be involved. Differentiation must be made from other infrequently encountered granuloma-producing conditions—Boeck's sarcoid, syphilis, and fungal and parasitic infections—and the granulomas of talc and barium.

Necrotizing enterocolitis

Necrotizing enterocolitis is an inflammatory process that involves primarily the mucosa and submucosa or the entire wall of the terminal ileum and varying lengths of the colon, principally of premature infants within the first few days of life and less commonly full-term infants or children in the first 2 months of life. Air, either superficial in the bowel wall or in the peritoneum, is sometimes an accompaniment and in the latter site may be an aid in recognizing the condition by x-ray examination.[228] Factors considered important in the etiology of the condition are ischemia resulting from a Shwartzman-like reaction, shunting of blood from the involved areas as might occur with hypoxia and anoxia that is commonly seen in these infants, bacterial infections, and endotoxins. The disease is rapidly progressive and requires aggressive supportive therapy and surgical intervention in some instances if a cure is to be effected.

Fungal infections

Involvement of the gastrointestinal tract, in particular the esophagus and stomach, by fungi of the genus *Candida* is not an uncommon finding at necropsy in patients who had chronic debilitating diseases or received prolonged intensive antibiotic therapy. Other fungi, for example, *Mucor* and *Cryptococcus*, are rarely seen.

Intestinal histoplasmosis[195] may mimic tuberculosis in histopathologic detail, and its differentiation is made by demonstration of the causative organism either in microscopic sections or in cultures.It is most common in the ileocecal region, but widespread gastrointestinal lesions may be present as part of a generalized histoplasmosis.

When actinomycosis involves the gastrointestinal tract, it too shows predilection for the ileocecal region or appendix.[185]

Lymphopathia venereum

Lymphopathia (lymphogranuloma) venereum involving the anorectal region is a disease of male or female homosexuals.[94] Initially the perirectal fat is involved by chronic inflammatory change and fibrosis, rendering it very firm. The lymphatic lesions may suppurate and inflammation spreads to involve the rectal wall proper. Characteristically, stricture formation follows.

Parasitic infestations

Amebiasis. *Entamoeba histolytica* most frequently involves the cecal or rectal region and less commonly extensive segments of the large intestine.[120] In the earliest lesions there is a minimal mononuclear and eosinophilic leukocytic infiltration associated with the trophozoites penetrating the colonic epithelium.[176] This produces tiny, yellow, nodular elevations that eventuate in flask-shaped ulcerations. Organisms may be variable in number and difficult to identify without special staining procedures (Fig. 26-15). In advanced cases the mucosa may have a shaggy appearance with shreds of fibrin and tags of underlying mucous membrane attached to the margins of the ulcers. The colon may be greatly thickened, and there may be many adhesions to adjacent loops of intestine or to the mesentery. Amebic granulomas may develop.

Schistosomiasis. Ova of the parasite *Schistosoma mansoni* or *S. japonicum* in the mucosa and submocosa may excite a tubercle-like reaction and a polypoid adenomatoid hyperplasia of the mucous membrane of the colon or rectum.[60] Less often, adult worms may be found in the submucosal veins. Various other parasites that inhabit the intestinal tract are considered in Chapter 12.

Malakoplakia

A disease of unknown etiology[1] generally affecting the urinary tract has been reported in the appendix and

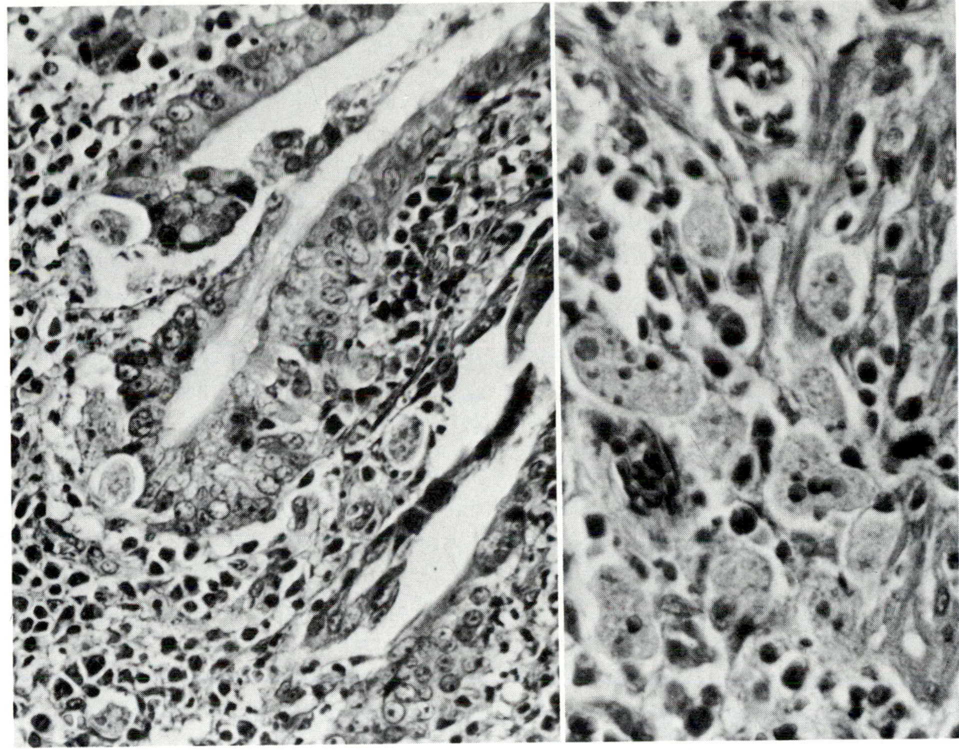

Fig. 26-15. Amebic colitis. Higher magnification demonstrates erythocyte ingestion by trophozoites.

colon.[198] The histopathologic condition is identical to that seen in the urinary tract—macrophages harboring calcium-containing Michaelis-Gutmann bodies and periodic acid–Schiff–positive granules.

Other causes of gastrointestinal inflammation

Radiation. Ionizing radiation given for treatment of cancer, usually of the female generative organs, may be responsible for inflammation in one or more focal areas of the small intestine or colon. Telangiectasia, edema and inflammatory cell infiltration of the submucosa, and necrosis of mucous membrane are early changes.[84] Chronic or delayed radiation injury may not manifest itself until many years after irradiation.[24] Radiation fibrosis, endarteritis, and vascular fibrosis may lead to bowel stricture or mucosal ulceration.

Drugs. Drugs used in therapy (aminopterin, 5-fluorouracil, lincomycin, clindamycin, and so on) have been associated with changes in the intestinal tract. Inflammation, usually mucosal and submucosal and accompanied by ulceration of the mucous membrane, is reponsible for a variety of gastrointestinal symptoms that subside after cessation of the drug.

Poisons. Mercury and arsenic may be responsible for nonspecific inflammation or necrosis in the colon, with the changes being less apparent and less extensive with arsenic. In addition, consumption of inorganic arsenical compounds such as Paris green may produce similar changes in the stomach and small intestine.[91]

Metabolites. Accumulation of metabolic products as occurs in patients dying of uremia may be responsible for changes ranging from minimal nonspecific inflammation to extensive necrotizing colitis. Some of the lesions may represent pseudomembranous enterocolitis or other specific infection.

Virus infections. Intestinal changes associated with viruses responsible for brief bouts of gastroenteritis are not encountered by the pathologist.[201] Rarely, one sees at necropsy inclusion bodies of varicella and herpes simplex in the esophageal epithelium and inclusions of the cytomegalic virus in the mucosa and granulation tissue of ulcers of the intestine.

Granuloma. Granulomatous inflammation characterized by tubercle formation is uncommon in the intestinal tract with the exception of that seen in Crohn's disease. It may occur anywhere in the gut but is more common in the ileocecal region. Diagnostic considerations include sarcoidosis, tuberculosis, Crohn's disease, syphilis, foreign body (food, barium, and so on), leprosy, fungi, and parasitic infestations. Since the histologic findings are not diagnostic unless a causative agent is identified, one must often rely heavily on clinical information and gross findings to distinguish granulomas. Even then, the various granulomas cannot always be differentiated.

ANORECTAL LESIONS

Stercoraceous (stercoral) ulcers[97] are irregular and involve the mucous membrane of the rectum and less often of the colon. They result from trauma caused by impacted, inspissated fecal masses. They may be associated with perforation and peritonitis or with hemorrhage.

Colitis cystica profunda may be diffuse and involve extensive areas of the large intestine, but it usually is confined to the rectum.[236] It is characterized by mucous cysts and glands lined by goblet cells in the submucosa. It is often associated with chronic inflammatory change and extraglandular accumulation of mucin. The condition may result from extension of surface epithelium along granulation tissue tracts after deep ulceration. Lesions with a similar appearance are infrequently encountered in the stomach.

The crypts of Morgagni have traditionally been implicated in the causation of most anorectal inflammatory disease, specifically perirectal abscesses and anorectal fistulas.[177] Corresponding to the columns in the sinuses of Morgagni is a circular band, 0.3 to 1.1 cm wide, of "transitional" or "cloacogenic" epithelium interposed between rectal and anal mucus membrane. This transitional epithelium, often including mucus-secreting cells, lines the sinuses of Morgagni and the anal ducts or glands that communicate with them. The distribution of the ducts and glands varies greatly. They may extend caudally penetrating the internal anal sphincter or cephalad beneath the rectal mucosa and may branch in complex fashion (Fig. 26-16). It is infection in the crypts of Morgagni and of these anal ducts that is responsible for the troublesome perianal and ischiorectal abscesses, which in turn are responsible for anal fistulas that may open internally in the region of the anorectal junction or externally on the perianal skin. Histologically, inflammation in this area is nonspecific, often with a foreign body reaction, no doubt because of contamination with fecal matter.

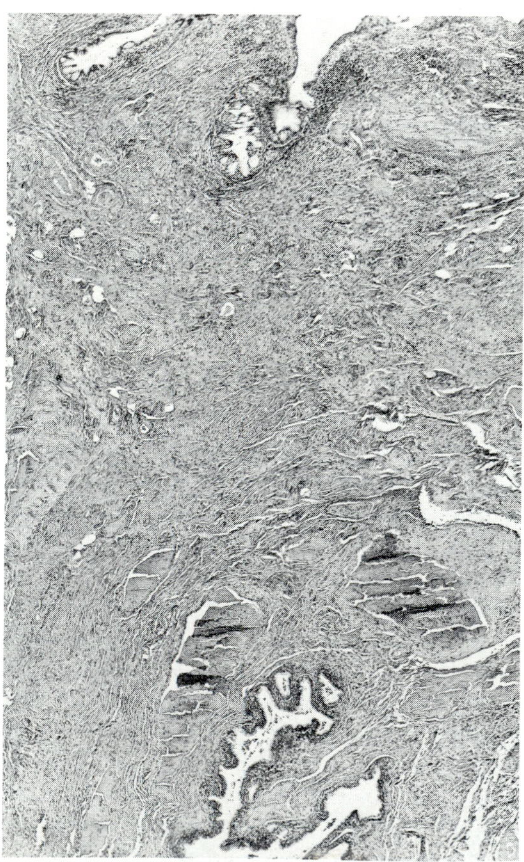

Fig. 26-16. Anal ducts. Small portion of epithelial lining of anal canal is visible above, and anal ducts occur both superficially and deep within muscle. (55×.)

Anal fissures are acute or chronic ulcers situated posteriorly in the anal canal just distal to the anorectal junction. These various anal, perianal, and anorectal lesions are insignificant in themselves, but they may be the source of great discomfort and disability.

DISEASES OF PERITONEUM, OMENTUM, RETROPERITONEUM, AND MESENTERY

Peritonitis

Inflammation of the peritoneum is an acute or chronic response, diffuse or localized, to a variety of agents—bacterial, chemical, viral, or foreign material.[106] The acute variety is most frequently encountered and is usually associated with inflammation of abdominal organs with or without perforation, for example, appendicitis, cholecystitis, intestinal infarction, diverticulitis, perforated peptic ulcer, and hemorrhage attributed to ruptured ectopic pregnancy. Less commonly encountered is the "primary" form caused by the pneumococcus or hemolytic streptococcus. The organisms causing acute peritonitis are numerous and most commonly include one or more of the normal flora of the gastrointestinal tract, usually *Escherichia coli*, *Proteus*, and *Enterococcus*, although *Bacteroides* and *Clostridium* are also important. Initially there are hyperemia, edema, and extravasation of red cells followed by exudation of leukocytes and fibrin, all of which account for the loss of the serous membrane's normal glistening sheen. To a limited extent the character of the peritoneal exudate depends on a particular dominant organism. Although it may be thin, watery, and only slightly turbid, it usually is frankly purulent or fibrinopurulent.

As the process progresses, the plastic exudate may cause adhesions between loops of intestine, omentum, and abdominal parietes forming abscesses in localized areas, rather than permitting general spread of the process. Such abscesses are most likely to develop in the lumbar gutters, the subphrenic space between the liver and diaphragm, the subhepatic area, and the pelvic cul-de-sac. After widespread peritonitis subsides, such focal accumulations of exudate may persist and require surgical drainage. Complications of acute peritonitis are adynamic or paralytic ileus and fibrous peritoneal adhesions.

Adhesions associated with inflammatory disease of the female pelvic organs, most importantly the fallopian tubes, are especially noteworthy. The causative infections are usually primarily of gonococcal etiology, but secondary superinfection is common. The disease is characterized by recurring episodes of acute but low-grade inflammation, and the resulting adhesions may become very dense and complicated, although generally limited to the pelvis.

Tuberculous peritonitis may occur as a manifestation of disseminated tuberculosis, miliary or otherwise, or in association with intestinal involvement. It also may be caused by disease of the female generative organs. The disease process is the same as in other parts of the body. It may produce widespread, dense adhesions.

A variety of irritants may be responsible for peritonitis—bile, hydrochloric acid, and other intestinal contents that gain access to the peritoneum as a result of rupture of a viscus (gallbladder, bile duct, duodenum, and so on), hemorrhage from an ectopic pregnancy or corpus luteum, and other foreign material such as *Lycopodium* spores and talc.

Bile may produce a profound initial systemic reaction in the host, but the nature of the resulting pathologic process is dependent on the source of the contaminating bile and the type and number of associated bacteria.[150]

Foreign body granulomas may result from *Lycopodium* spores and talc crystals—material used as dusting powders for surgical rubber gloves in the past.[77] The use of absorbable starch has eliminated such granulomas, but the starch does not appear to be completely innocuous. Instances of peritonitis and foreign body granuloma have been reported, presumably developing as the result of hypersensitivity to the starch.[211]

Infrequently, oily materials used in salpingography, parasites or their ova, barium sulfate administered for diagnostic roentgenographic study and escaping into the peritoneum as a result of perforation, and sclerosing agents used in the treatment of hernia may incite a foreign body reaction.

Periodic disease (familial Mediterranean fever, familial recurring polyserositis)

Periodic bouts of pain occur particularly in the abdomen, but they may also be noted in the chest and joints. During intervals between attacks, the patients are in excellent health. The disease is a genetic disorder of unknown etiology and pathogenesis affecting persons of Armenian, Arab, or Jewish ethnic origin, the last being predominantly the non-Ashkenazi Jews—the Sephardi and Iraqi ethnic groups.[212] Sterile exudates in the involved serous surfaces are minimal, consisting of focal collections of neutrophils, fibrin strands, and ecchymoses, and only rarely are fibrinous adhesions and scars produced despite the many attacks. Amyloid of the perireticular type, described in the kidneys, spleen, adrenals, pulmonary alveolar capillaries, and hepatic sinusoids but not in other organs, may result in the patient's death. Otherwise the course is a protracted one.

Ascites

Ascites is the condition of transudation of clear, low–specific gravity fluid into the peritoneal cavity. The protein content is less than 3%. Ascites is most commonly seen with cirrhosis of the liver but may result from other causes of hypertension in the portal venous system, such as thrombosis or cardiac decompensation, or from hypoalbuminemia. Chylous ascites, in which the fluid appears milky and has a high fat content, is related to obstruction of the thoracic duct, usually neoplastic.

Retroperitoneal lesions

The retroperitoneum is an ill-defined area that may share in the complications of diseases of the many organs that lie within it or impinge on it. Hemorrhage, infections, and extensions of neoplasms are the important complications and may be related to the urinary tract, retroperitoneal lymph nodes, and blood vessels, including the aorta and vena cava.

A number of possibly related conditions involve the mesenteric and retroperitoneal adipose tissue. At one end of the spectrum is a self-limited, chronic, productive inflammation of the mesentery, usually of the small intestine. This has been variously termed mesenteric panniculitis, lipogranuloma, and isolated lipodystrophy and likened to Weber-Christian disease.[174] It may produce a significant mass and may or may not be symptomatic. Retractile mesenteritis is a similar condition, distinguished by fibrosis and hyaline scarring and retraction of the mesentery, with distortion of intestinal loops producing episodes of pain, constipation, and obstruction.[223]

Idiopathic retroperitoneal fibrosis is a lesion characterized by dense fibrosis and a limited, nonspecific inflammatory reaction that frequently is manifested by ureteral obstruction.[157] The disease also occurs in the mediastinum. A similar lesion has been observed in association with methysergide therapy. It usually regresses after withdrawal of the drug.[202]

Torsion of omentum

Omental torsion, resulting from adhesions, tumors, and so on, or at times of unknown cause, may result in infarction and give rise to signs and symptoms simulating those of acute appendicitis but usually without vomiting.[6] Similarly, epiploic appendages may become infarcted. Fat necrosis of an appendage, presumably a late result, is not uncommon.

FUNCTIONAL STATES

Gastric atrophy (atrophic gastritis)

So-called atrophic gastritis is not properly classified as an inflammatory condition. The term is used by some as a synonym for gastric atrophy. Others consider the two to be different stages of the same pathologic process.

In atrophic gastritis the mucous membrane is greatly thinned, and the gastric glands are correspondingly shortened and also widely separated.[243] On inspection with the unassisted eye, the mucosa in advanced atrophy is smooth, is patently thinned, and has a waxy cast. The striking cellular changes in the gastric glands are two: (1) a decrease in number or, in the fully developed case, complete absence of parietal cells and (2) the occurrence, usually in the deeper part of the mucosa, of glands identical to those of the small intestine (Fig. 26-17, *C*). All cell types normally found in the glands of the small intestine may be represented. This change has been regarded as intestinal metaplasia by some and as heterotopia by others. The decrease or absence of parietal cells, which has been demonstrated to be associated with an autoan-

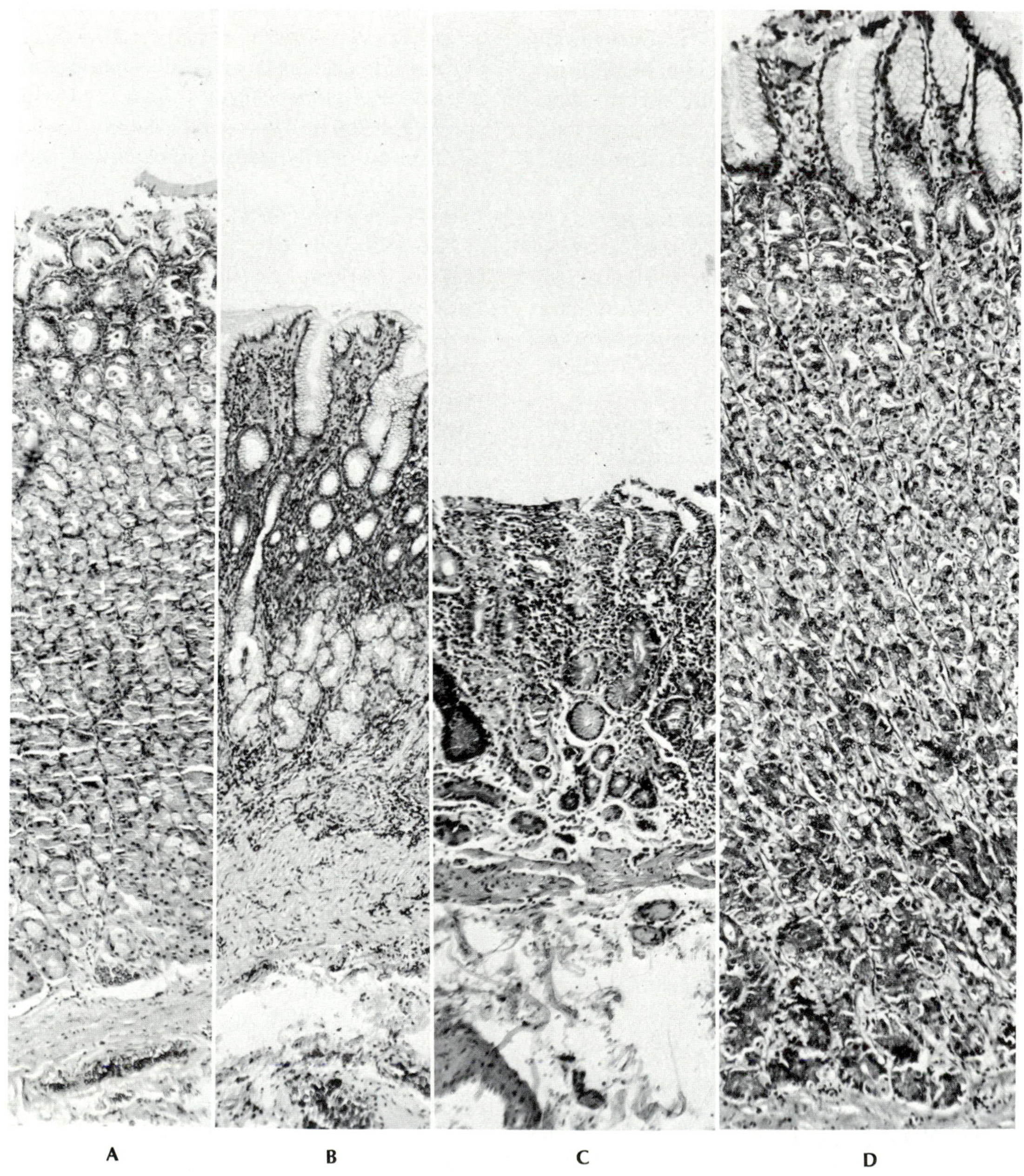

Fig. 26-17. **A** and **B**, Normal stomach. **A**, Fundus. **B**, Antrum. **C**, Atrophic gastritis. **D**, Gastric rugal hypertrophy. (**A** to **D**, 90×.)

tibody in a high percentage of patients with atrophic gastritis, accounts for deficient hydrochloric acid secretion or complete achlorhydria. Large numbers of lymphocytes and plasma cells are present in the lamina propria, but the increase may be more apparent than real. The changes described occur focally in many stomachs without overt disease. They are seen more often and in more widespread and advanced degree with increased age.

Atrophic gastritis commonly is associated with gastric carcinoma, but a postulated predisposing role has not been demonstrated. Advanced atrophy regularly accompanies polypoid carcinoma and adenomatous polyp. Indeed, the appearance of many of the latter and of some polypoid carcinomas strongly suggests origin from glands typical of the small intestine. Gastric atrophy, increased serum gastrin levels, and G-cell hyperplasia in the gastric antrum are frequently encountered in pernicious anemia,[134] a disease associated with achlorhydria and a high incidence of gastric carcinoma. Antibodies to parietal cells and intrinsic factor have been demonstrated in a proportion of patients with atrophic gastritis. These patients are predisposed to pernicious anemia, in contrast to those in whom the antibody cannot be demonstrated.[220] However, in general, it has been difficult to correlate the pathologic findings of atrophic gastritis with clinical disease or with roentgenographic or gastroscopic findings.

Hypertrophic gastropathy

Gastric rugal hypertrophy, called hypertrophic gastritis by some, is characterized by enlargement of the gastric mucosal folds in both length and breadth, producing thickening and convolution of the mucous membrane reminiscent of the appearance of the cerebral convolutions (Fig. 26-18). In some instances this appearance is not caused by mucosal thickening but by an increase in the submucosal connective tissue. The changes may be diffuse and pronounced or localized and of limited degree, sparing the antrum. Histologic and clinical differences have been observed in gastric rugal hypertrophy, permitting recognition of entities based on clinical and pathologic findings. Hyperchlorhydria (in some instances with extreme gastric hypersecretion), hypoproteinemia, hypochlorhydria and achlorhydria, and tumors or hyperplasias of multiple endocrine glands have been associated with gastric rugal hypertrophy. It is postulated that it is one manifestation of a syndrome consisting also of islet cell tumor, primary chief cell hyperplasia of parathyroid glands, and at times abnormalities of other endocrine glands, especially the adrenal cortex and pituitary, and having different modes of clinical expression.[159,163,167] The principal one is the Zollinger-Ellison syndrome, with intractable peptic ulcer often in an unusual location and islet cell tumor of the pancreas or duodenum.

Mucosal alterations in hypertrophic gastropathy may be of two types, both lacking in significant inflammatory cell infiltration, thus supporting the use of the term *gastropathy* rather than gastritis: (1) Glandular hyperplasia with increased parietal and chief cells and normal or reduced surface and foveolar mucous epithelium (Fig. 26-17, *D*), has been observed in the Zollinger-Ellision syndrome but may occur without clinical manifestations.[216] (2) In hyperplasia of the surface and foveolar

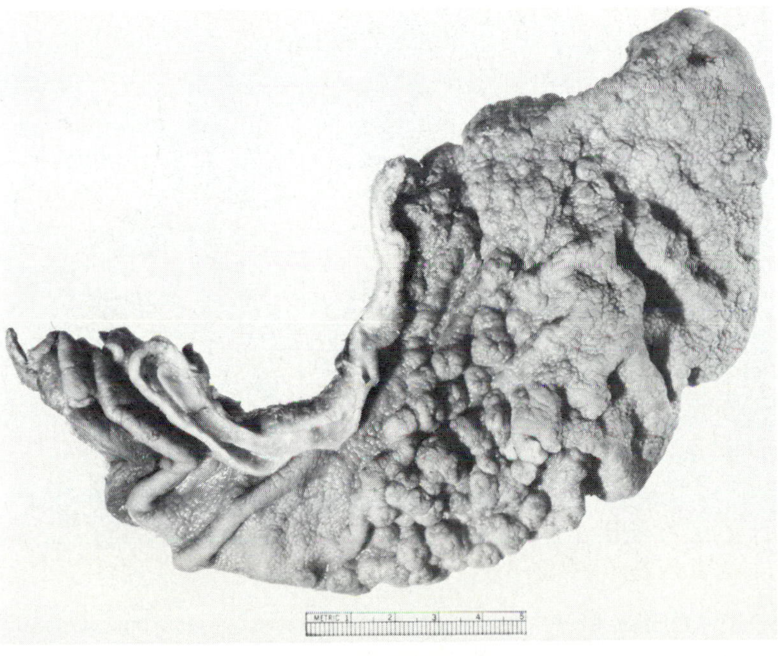

Fig. 26-18. Gastric rugal hypertrophy.

mucous cells with increased depth of the foveolae and other dilatation of the crypts, parietal and chief cells may be normal, atrophic, or hyperplastic. This change has been observed in Menetrier's disease, characterized by hypochlorhydria or achlorhydria and hypoproteinemia caused by albumin loss into the gastric juice.[55]

Malabsorption syndrome

The malabsorption syndrome is characterized by impaired intestinal absorption, especially of fats, and is manifested by diarrhea with bulky, foul stools, abdominal distension, and malnutrition with attendant vitamin deficiencies, all in varying degree. The clinical picture may be associated with a wide variety of underlying diseases, and the cases may be conveniently subdivided into primary and secondary groups. Among the numerous causes of secondary malabsorption are cystic fibrosis of the pancreas, chronic incomplete intestinal obstruction, surgical resection of significant segments of the gastrointestinal tract, infections (especially enteric), antibiotics, biliary tract disease, scleroderma, Whipple's disease, parasitic infestations, regional enteritis, diabetes, neoplasms (notably lymphoma), and possible allergy.

Celiac sprue (nontropical sprue)

The names given to primary malabsorption or steatorrhea are celiac disease in infants and children, nontropical sprue in adults, and tropical sprue. In the first two conditions there seems to be an identical, genetically controlled abnormality resulting in sensitivity to gluten (gluten-sensitive enteropathy [GSE]). Elimination of gluten from the diet usually relieves the symptoms, although it does not cure the underlying defect. Refractoriness to gluten withdrawal occurs in a small percentage of cases, some of which may be associated with collagen deposition in the subepithelial portion of the lamina propria.[240] The small intestine mucosa, of the upper jejunum in particular and to a lesser extent of the duodenum and ileum, has a flat surface partially or completely lacking in villi. The mucosal crypts appear elongated, dilated, and more widely spaced than normal. The surface epithelial cells are cuboid or low columnar with irregular nuclei (Fig. 26-19, *B*). Numerous plasma cells and lymphocytes and fewer eosinophils and neutrophils are present in the lamina propria. Two theories of pathogenesis for the mucosal changes have been suggested: (1) toxic effect on the mucosa by increased gluten resulting from an enzyme deficiency in intestinal mucosal cells, and (2) damage to mucosal cells by gluten-stimulated antibodies and lymphokines produced in the intestinal lymphoid tissue.[230] Clinical remissions and reversal of the bowel changes, although usually not complete, can be induced by a gluten-free diet. The pathologic changes are not specific for celiac disease or nontropical sprue and may be seen in tropical sprue, infectious gastroenteritis, giardiasis, and allergy to cow's milk and soybean protein.[180] A very small percentage of patients with GSE have IgA deficiency, with absence of plasma cells in the lamina propria.[7] An association between celiac sprue of

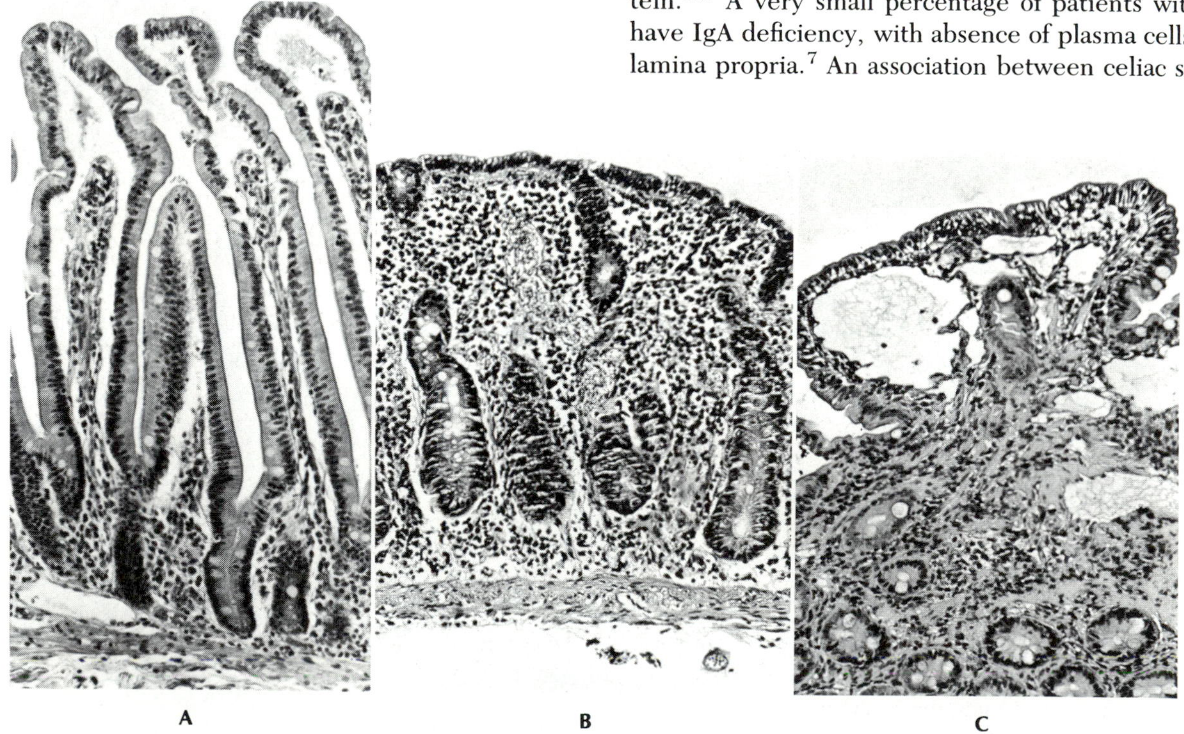

Fig. 26-19. A, Normal jejunum. **B,** Jejunum in nontropical sprue. **C,** Lymphangiectases of jejunum in protein-losing enteropathy. (**A** to **C,** 150×.)

long duration and intestinal lymphoma, esophageal and small bowel carcinoma, and dermatitis herpetiformis has been noted.[34]

Tropical sprue, endemic in the tropics and probably infectious in nature, is similar to celiac sprue in its clinical and morphologic expressions. The pathologic changes are usually not as noticeable and are reversible with broad-spectrum antibiotic and folic acid therapy, but they are unaffected by elimination of gluten from the diet. Macrocytic anemia is usually a feature of the disease.

Protein-losing enteropathy (exudative enteropathy)

In protein-losing enteropathy, which also may be associated with steatorrhea, large amounts of serum protein are lost in the intestine, and serum levels of both globulin and albumin are abnormally low. Like the malabsorption state, it may result from some specific gastroenteric disease state or congestive heart failure, or it may be idiopathic.[54,234]

Some of the gastrointestinal diseases that may be associated with considerable protein loss are gastric rugal hypertrophy, sprue, regional enteritis, and ulcerative colitis. Constrictive pericarditis is the most important underlying cardiac lesion. In some patients with "idiopathic" protein-losing enteropathy, dilatation of lymphatic channels (lymphangiectasia) in the intestinal mucosa and mesentery has been demonstrated (Fig. 26-19, *C*). Some of these latter patients have had systemic lymphatic abnormalities,[182] but in others no cause of lymphatic obstruction is found.

GASTROINTESTINAL MANIFESTATIONS OF SYSTEMIC DISEASE

The gastrointestinal tract may be the site of involvement in a number of diseases involving multiple organs. Such involvement may produce symptoms, which are the first manifestations of the disease, or it may be occult. In both situations biopsy of the intestinal tract may be helpful and an easily accessible means of establishing the diagnosis. Symptoms that may be present—diarrhea, steatorrhea, and those of malabsorption—may be unassociated with histologic changes in the gut or there may be degrees of villous mucosal atrophy. Gastrointestinal manifestations may be seen in a variety of endocrine diseases (diabetes, thyrotoxicosis, hyperparathyroidism, and hypoparathyroidism), skin diseases (dermatitis herpetiformis), pseudoxanthoma elasticum, Ehlers-Danlos syndrome, and mastocytosis.

Cystic fibrosis

The most important gastrointestinal manifestation is malabsorption with steatorrhea and azotorrhea, resulting from pancreatic achylia, and deficient secretion of the intestinal glands. Approximately 10% of patients have intestinal obstruction in the newborn period as the result of meconium ileus.[59] The abnormal accumulations of meconium distend the loops of intestine, which in one third of the cases rotate upon themselves producing a volvulus. Another complication is intestinal perforation in utero with the development of sterile peritonitis, so-called meconium peritonitis.[63] The escape of epithelial cells, mucus, and cellular debris usually stimulates a foreign body reaction, and calcification, visible roentgenographically, frequently takes place (see also p. 1234).

Progressive systemic sclerosis (scleroderma)

Although any portion of the intestinal tract may be involved, the esophagus is the most frequent site.[89] There is hyaline sclerosis of the submucosa with lymphocytic infiltration, as well as atrophy and fibrosis of the muscularis. The overlying mucous membrane may be thin and become ulcerated.[107] In the esophagus the rigidity of the wall may predispose the patient to regurgitation of acidic gastric juice from which there may be further complications.

Other collagen diseases, dermatomyositis and lupus erythematosus, may also involve the gastrointestinal tract, affecting the musculature in the former condition and blood vessels in both instances.

Whipple's disease (intestinal lipodystrophy)

Originally considered to be a disorder of intestinal function involving lipid metabolism, Whipple's disease is now recognized as a systemic disease.[19,206] Aggregates of large macrophages bearing intracytoplasmic sickle-shaped inclusions in the intestinal mucous membrane (Fig. 26-20, *A*) and mesenteric lymph nodes that react strongly with the periodic acid–Schiff stain dominate the microscopic picture, but similar deposits have also been described in virtually every organ of the body. Lipid deposits are striking in lymph nodes, especially those of the mesentery, but not in the other organs. Whipple's disease is generally a condition of adult white men and may be familial. The manifestations are diarrhea, gradual wasting, and migratory polyarthritis.[140] An infectious etiology has replaced the concept of a disorder of lipid metabolism. This is based on data generated from electron microscopic studies,[162,229] indicating that the "inclusions" are in fact bacilliform microorganisms (Fig. 26-20, *B* and *C*); bacterial cultures and production of the disease in rabbits[43]; and favorable response of the disease to antibiotic therapy. Host factors have also been suggested to be important in the pathogenesis of this disease, and immunologic defects have been described.[98,145]

Storage disease

Deposits of one of a number of substances seen in a variety of diseases—Tay-Sachs, Niemann-Pick, Fabry's,

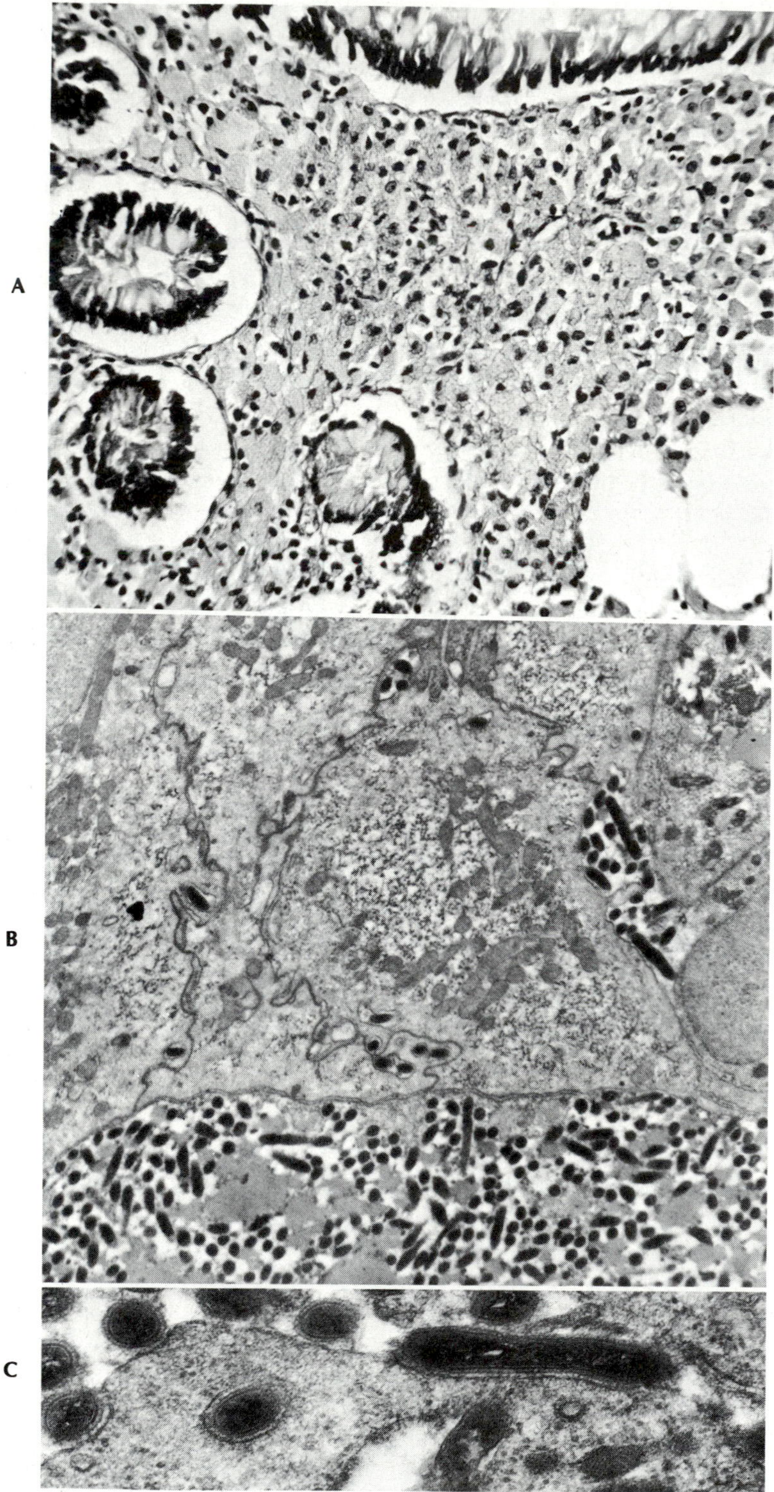

Fig. 26-20. Whipple's disease involving mucous membrane of small intestine. **A,** Pale macrophages in mucosa. **B,** Bacilliform bodies are extracellular. **C,** Encapsulated bodies are seen both intracellularly and extracellulary. (**A,** 300×; **B,** 8100×; **C,** 45,000×.)

Hurler's, Gaucher's glycogen storage, and metachromatic leukoencephalopathy—may be found in ganglion cells, histiocytes, or nerve fibers in the gut.

Tangier disease is an autosomal recessive inherited disease in which there is deposition of cholesterol esters in the reticuloendothelial system as well as in histiocytes of the mucous membrane of the pharynx and intestine.[12] The disorder is benign except for a possible predisposition to atherosclerosis.

Wolman's disease[138] is also inherited as an autosomal recessive disease in which cholesterol esters may be found deposited in histiocytes in the lamina propria of the intestine as well as in the reticuloendothelial system of the liver, spleen, lymph nodes, and bone marrow. Calcification of the adrenal glands is a common accompaniment. The central nervous system appears not to be involved. The patients reported have died before attaining 6 months of age.

Congenital beta-lipoprotein deficiency, an autosomal recessive disease, manifests itself in the intestinal tract by deposition of lipid droplets in the mucosal epithelial cells with practically no fat droplets in the lamina propria and submucosa.[61] It usually manifests itself within the first 2 years of life as a mild steatorrhea and neurologic symptoms resembling Friedreich's ataxia.

The frequent involvement of the intestinal tract in these storage diseases has made biopsy of the gut an easy approach to diagnosis.[31]

Rectal biopsy has also proved useful for obtaining diagnostic information in a large number of other disease entities—schistosomiasis, amyloidosis, amebiasis, Crohn's disease, Hirschsprung's disease, melanosis coli, ulcerative colitis, pneumatosis, hemochromatosis, and the changes produced by chemotherapeutic agents and antibiotics. The finding of colonic macrophages (muciphages),[9] however, must be carefully evaluated. The variation in interpretation given to them by different authors—early phase of Whipple's disease, ceroid-containing phages, and so on—appears to be in part the result of nonuniformity in the histochemical methods employed in their study. Recent investigations carried out on surgical and necropsy specimens indicate their frequent occurrence and lack of clinical significance.[137] It appears that they are unrelated to the many storage diseases cited previously and that they are the result of phagocytosis of mucin released from the goblet cells of the colonic mucous membrane.

NEOPLASMS

Adenomatous polyps, papillary adenomas, and miscellaneous polyps

Luminal projections of the gastrointestinal mucosa may result from a variety of neoplastic and nonneoplastic changes ultimately detected only by microscopic examination. Most commonly they are epithelial alterations, but they may result from submucosal mesenchymal lesions. The polypoid glandular neoplasms, adenomatous (tubular), papillary (villous), or mixed tubulopapillary, occur throughout the gastrointestinal tract from the stomach to the rectum, but are most frequent in the colon and rectum.[121] Their incidence increases after 30 years of age; estimates of incidence range as high as 25% to 50% in an autopsy population of the older age groups (60 to 80 years). In one fourth or more of cases, the polyps are multiple, frequently but not always limited to one part of the intestine. Approximately 75% of adenomatous polyps occur in the rectum and sigmoid colon, although their exact incidence in various segments of the large intestine varies from one reported series to another.

The earliest adenomatous change that can be recognized is the replacement of lining cells of the crypts, beginning at the base, by cells that are generally taller, more slender, and more deeply staining than the normal. They have hyperchromatic nuclei and lack vacuoles, indicative of mucin secretion (Fig. 26-21). Mitotic figures may be numerous. Proliferation progresses to the formation of epithelial tubular aggregates, grossly manifested as a lobulated, berrylike, tubular adenoma that is usually less than 2 cm in diameter and attached to the intestinal wall by a pedicle of varying length, composed of normal mucous membrane (Fig. 26-22). Villous adenomas are usually larger and sessile and have a papillary configuration (Fig. 26-23, *B*). The papillae consist of fingerlike projections with a core of lamina propria covered by epithelial cells (Fig. 26-23, *A*). Large villous adenomas have been recognized as the occasional cause of severe fluid and electrolyte loss producing electrolyte imbalance, which may threaten life.[241] The glandular changes are usually confined to the mucosa but on occasion may be seen in the fibrovascular stalk, sometimes associated with recent or old hemorrhage (Fig. 26-24). This has been regarded as pseudoinvasion, possibly resulting from twisting of the polyp's stalk.[168,186] These foci are not to be confused with invasive carcinoma, from which they differ in having benign cytologic characteristics. A number of polypoid epithelial lesions of the colon bear a resemblance to the adenomatous polyp and are commonly confused with it. Abnormal folds or minute elevations of the mucous membrane are sometimes mistaken for adenomas on proctoscopic or sigmoidoscopic examination. Rather frequently occurring polyps, best termed hyperplastic or metaplastic, are small, flat lesions composed of enlarged, regular glands with scalloped luminal borders showing excessive mucin secretion but lacking the neoplastic change and malignant potential of the adenomatous polyp described previously (Fig. 26-25). Another lesion that must be distinguished from the adenomatous polyp and that does not have any relationship to cancer is the juvenile polyp. Also referred to as a

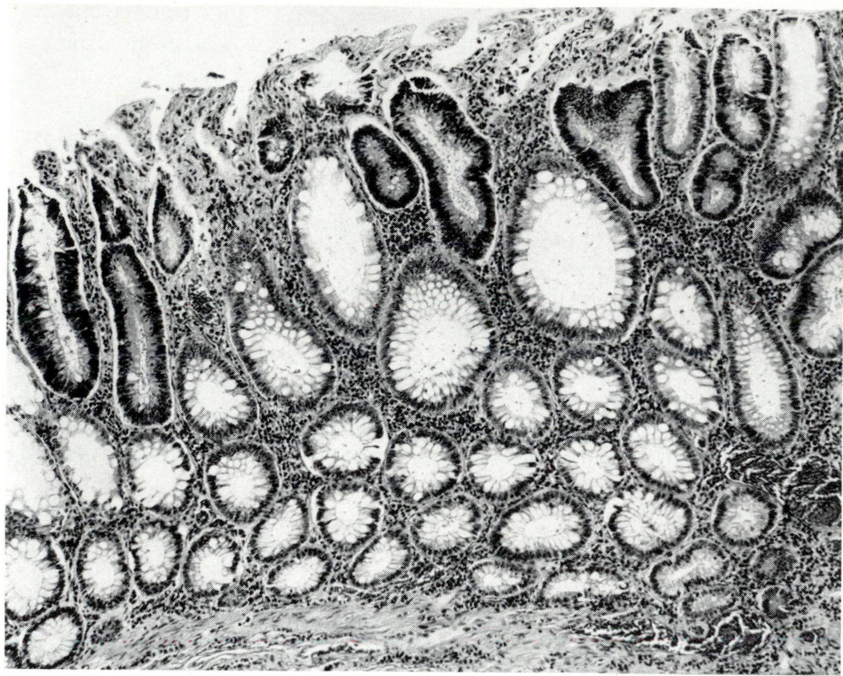

Fig. 26-21. Adenomatous (neoplastic) change in gland of colon *(upper part of field)* in contrast to normal glands. (115×.)

retention polyp, it is usually a single, smooth, rounded nodule, 1 to 3 cm in diameter (Fig. 26-26), composed of large, hyperplastic or cystic glands with an abundant, well-vascularized fibrous stroma infiltrated by inflammatory cells (Fig. 26-27). Multiple lesions in the gastrointestinal tract or colon alone, sometimes familial, have been reported.[36,196] The nodules are supported on a stalk of normal mucous membrane. Bleeding is the most frequent clinical manifestation. Juvenile polyp is a lesion of children, although similar polyps occasionally occur in adults.[149] They have been regarded as hamartomas or the result of inflammation.[194] Polypoid inflammatory or nonspecific granuloma-like nodules, inflammatory polyps, are occasionally seen as solitary lesions, but the inflammatory polyp or pseudopolyp is generally seen in chronic ulcerative colitis.

Polyps may be associated with other abnormalities. In Gardner's syndrome polyposis of the colon is associated with neoplasms of both bone and soft tissues elsewhere in the body—epidermoid cyst, fibroma, and osteomas (in the mandible and maxilla)—and sometimes with polyps in other portions in the gastrointestinal tract.

In the Cronkhite-Canada syndrome one finds multiple polyposis of the colon associated with ectodermal changes—alopecia, nail atrophy, and hyperpigmentation—as well as polyps in the stomach and small intestine. The polyps morphologically have the features of juvenile (retention) polyps. In Turcot's syndrome polyps of the colon are present with brain tumors.[232]

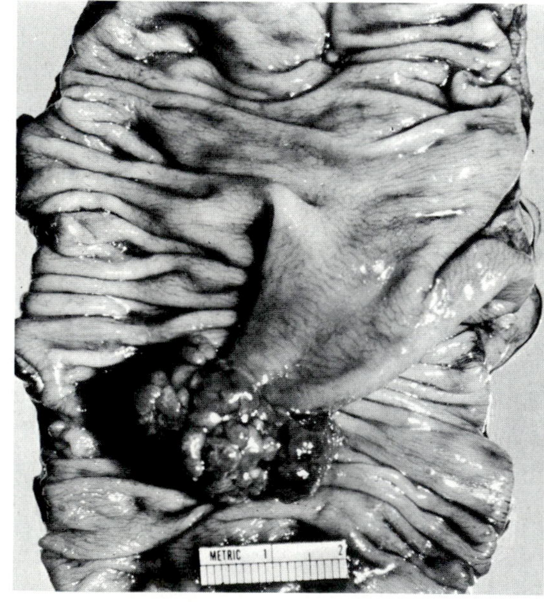

Fig. 26-22. Adenomatous polyp of colon.

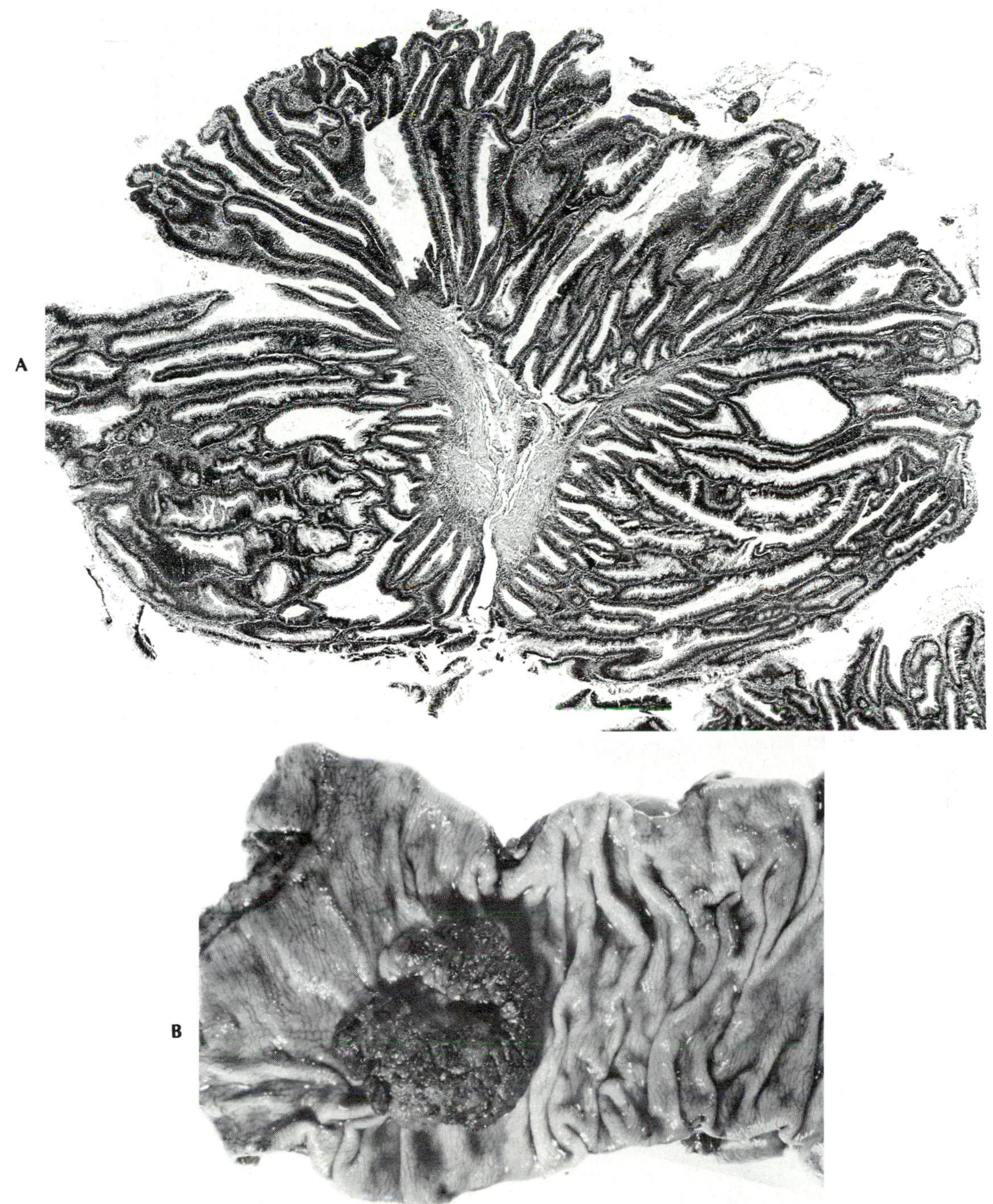

A

B

Fig. 26-23. A, Papillary (villous) adenoma of rectum. Papillary configuration readily apparent. **B,** Papillary adenoma of colon. (**A,** 25×.)

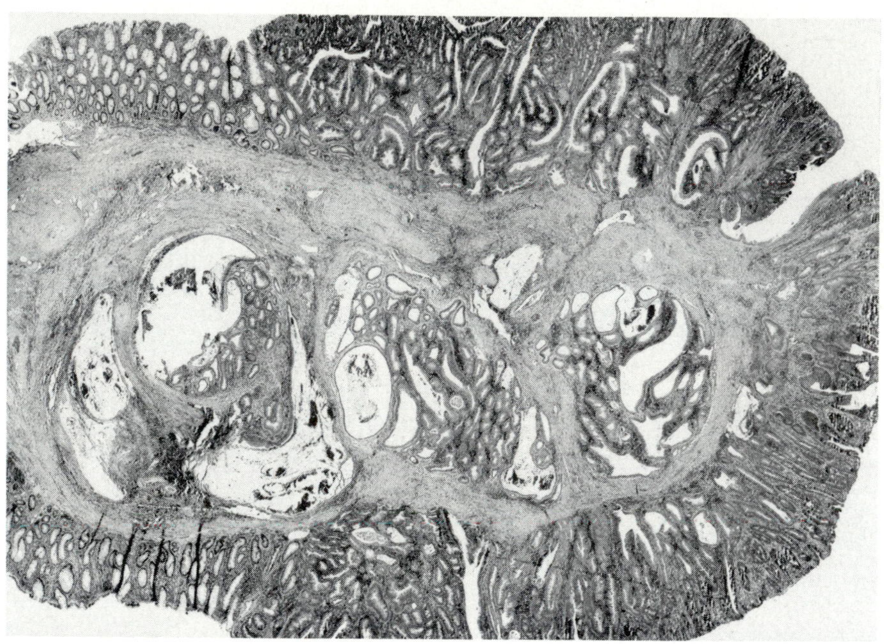

Fig. 26-24. Misplaced epithelium (pseudoinvasion) in tubular adenoma. (15×.)

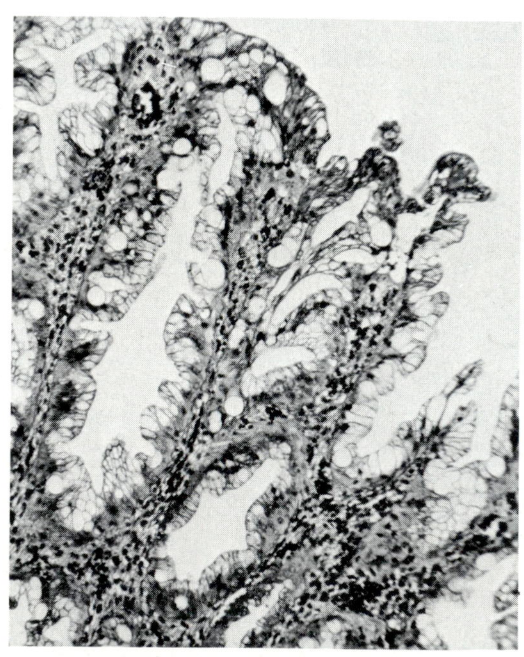

Fig. 26-25. Hyperplastic polyp of colon. (175×.)

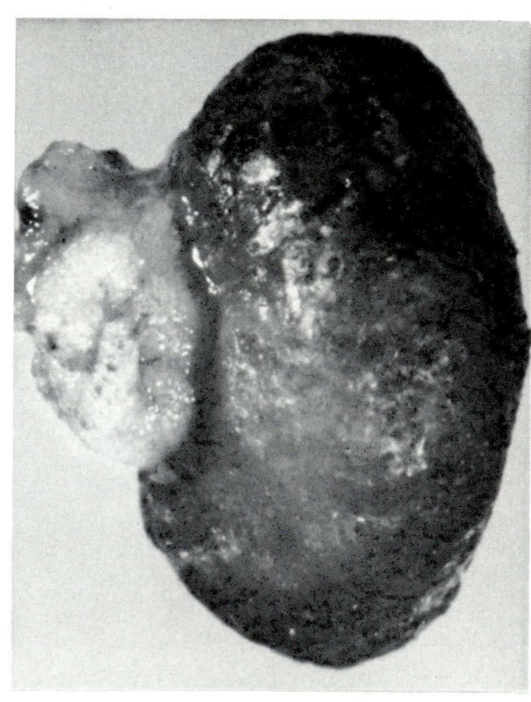

Fig. 26-26. Juvenile polyp of rectum.

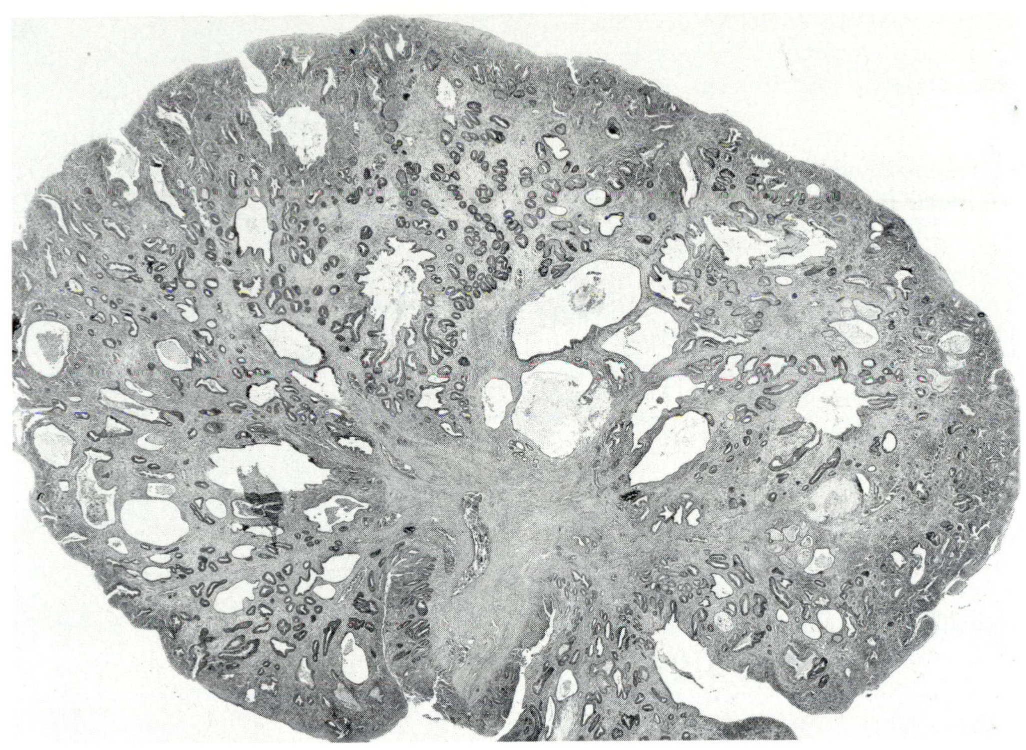

Fig. 26-27. Juvenile polyp of rectum. Cystic dilatation of glands and abundant stroma. (13×.)

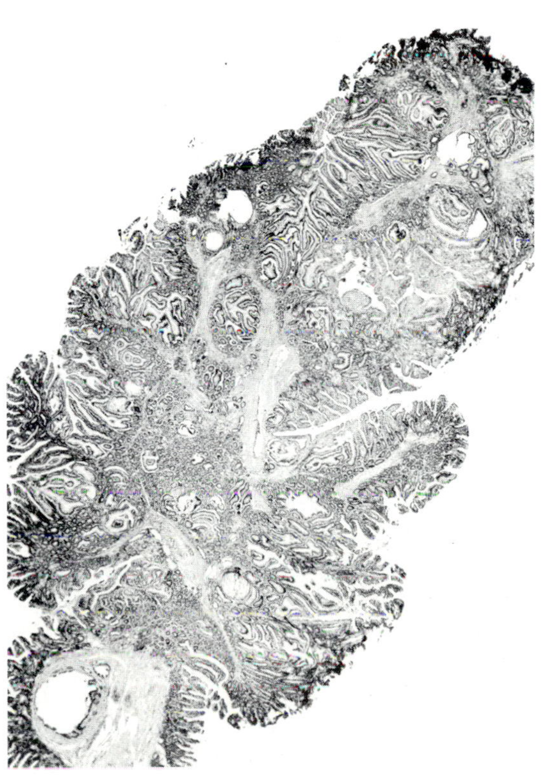

Fig. 26-28. Polyp of ileum from patient with Peutz-Jeghers syndrome. Note irregularities and variegated appearance. (16×; from Horn, R.C., Jr., Payne, W.A., and Fine, G.: Arch. Pathol. **76**:29, 1963.)

In the Peutz-Jeghers syndrome, melanin spots on the buccal mucosa, lips, and digits are associated with polyps occurring almost anywhere in the gastrointestinal tract but most commonly in the upper small intestine. The disease is transmitted as a simple mendelian dominant trait, but cases without a familial history have been recorded. The polyps differ from those generally found in the intestinal tract in that they are hamartomatous (that is, composed of normal-looking but irregularly arranged glands of any of the types normally occurring in the mucous membrane of origin) and may include bands of smooth muscle (Fig. 26-28). Thus parietal cells may be present in gastric polyps, Brunner's glands in duodenal lesions, and so on. The polyps of the large intestine are not always readily distinguishable from adenomatous polyps. The principal clinical manifestations of the Peutz-Jeghers syndrome are hemorrhage and intussusception. Instances of development of gastrointestinal carcinoma in patients with this syndrome have been documented, but progression of the Peutz-Jeghers polyps to cancer must be rare, as is the association of sex cord ovarian tumors with this syndrome.[62,105,203] Cytologic atypia is frequent but is apparently not significant.

In familial polyposis (Plate 2, *C*), the entire colon is studded with polyps, usually tiny and sessile. The disease is transmitted as an autosomal dominant trait and usually is manifested in childhood or adolescence. The incidence of carcinoma in this disease is so high and the cancers occur so often in young adults (or even adolescents) that total colectomy is generally regarded as the treatment of choice once the diagnosis has been established.

Relationship of adenomatous polyps and papillary adenomas to carcinoma of colon

Epidemiologic, histologic, and experimental studies support the concept of the precancerous nature of both tubular and villous adenomas, the incidence of malignant transformation being greater among the latter tumors.[132] The malignant potential of the colonic adenomas has been found to be related to size, histologic type (tubular or villous), and degree of epithelial dysplasia.[164]

GASTRIC POLYPS

Benign epithelial proliferations in the stomach are of three varieties: hyperplastic, adenomatous, and hamartomatous, in that order of frequency.[154] The hyperplastic polyp, which is small and pedunculated or sessile and smooth surfaced, is often multiple, occurs anywhere in the stomach, and represents approximately 75% to 95% of the polyps. Polyps are composed of the foveolar portion of the gland, dilated with mucin and lined by a mucin-producing epithelium with fewer parietal and chief cells or pyloric glands, depending on their location in the stomach (Fig. 26-29). They merge imperceptibly with the surrounding mucosa and are considered to be regenerative rather than neoplastic. They have no significant malignant potential, but carcinoma in other portions of the stomach is frequently associated with them. Adenomatous polyps, on the other hand, are not only commonly associated with carcinoma elsewhere in the stomach but are often the site of malignant transformation. They may be tubular or villous and are formed of poorly differentiated epithelium, resembling the colonic adenoma, and differing from the adjacent gastric mucosa, which may be atrophic with intestinal metaplasia. Despite the fact that some gastric cancers may arise in adenomatous polyps, not all polyps become invasive cancers and relatively few cancers can be traced to polyps as precursors. Hamartomatous polyps, composed of differentiated glandular or stromal cells normally present in the area of origin, are least frequently encountered. They and the adenomatous polyps may be associated with polyps in other portions of the gastrointestinal tract: hereditary Peutz-Jeghers syndrome, familial or juvenile polyposis, Gardner's syndrome, and nonhereditary Cronkhite-Canada syndrome.

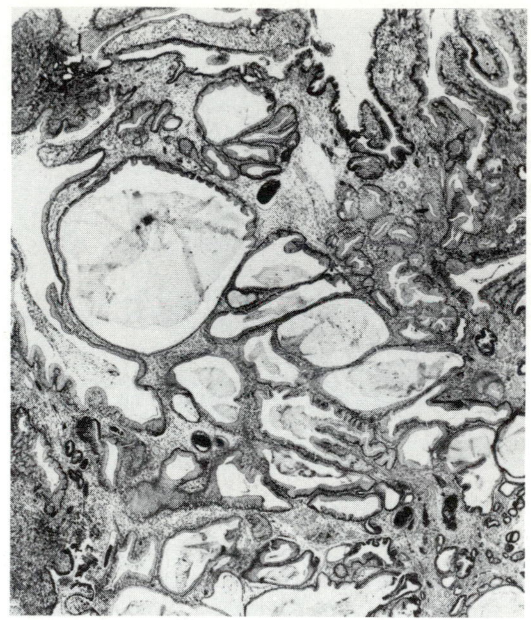

Fig. 26-29. Hyperplastic polyp of stomach. (15×.)

Carcinoma of the colon and rectum

Incidence. The incidence of cancer is higher in the colon and rectum than in any part of the body except the skin. Roughly three fourths of carcinomas of the large intestine occur in the rectum and sigmoid colon. Of the remainder, a majority arise in the cecum and ascending and descending colon, with the flexures and transverse colon being least often affected.

Histology and morbid anatomy. Generally they are well-differentiated tumors that reproduce the appearance of normal colonic glands more or less faithfully (Fig. 26-30). The usual cellular aberrations of neoplasia are generally obvious. Mucin production by tumors is variable, but tumors are sometimes capable of secreting very large amounts of mucin. Signet-ring cells (cells in which a large vacuole of mucin pushes the nucleus off to one side) may be conspicuous in some of these tumors (Fig. 26-31). In others, signet-ring cells may grow within the colonic wall without any readily apparent mucosal lesion, thus producing a linitis plastica type of growth.[207]

Distinct differences between the growth patterns of carcinoma of the right and left half of the colon can be observed. Those in the right colon are usually bulky and may show extensive necrosis because they outgrow their blood supply (Fig. 26-32, *A*). Occult bleeding is common, and the initial symptoms may be generalized weakness and anemia. In the more distal portions of the colon, the tumor frequently has a napkin-ring configuration (Fig. 26-32, *B*). Considerable fibrous tissue stroma accompanies the tumor and accounts for contraction and narrowing of the bowel lumen and thus a higher incidence of obstruction than carcinoma in the right side of the colon. Carcinomas of the rectum do not have a characteristic gross anatomic pattern. Bleeding is a common symptom. Many are discovered on routine proctoscopic or digital examination. Not uncommon in the rectum is the bulky "colloid" carcinoma, a varicolored mass with

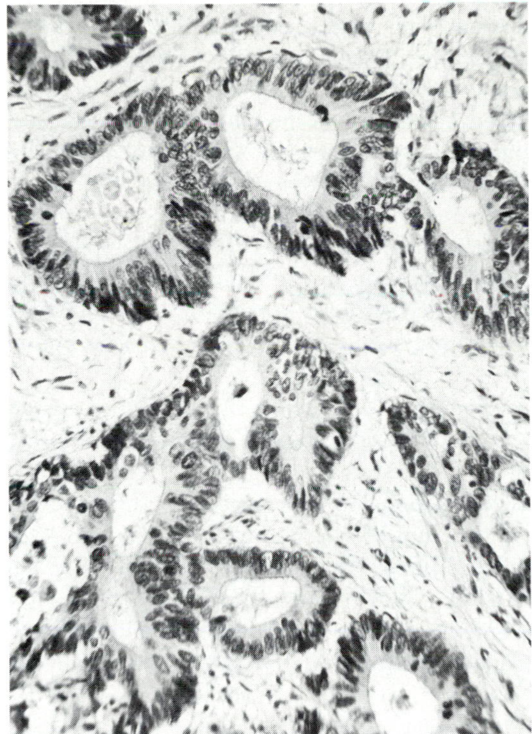

Fig. 26-30. Typical well-differentiated adenocarcinoma of colon. (300×.)

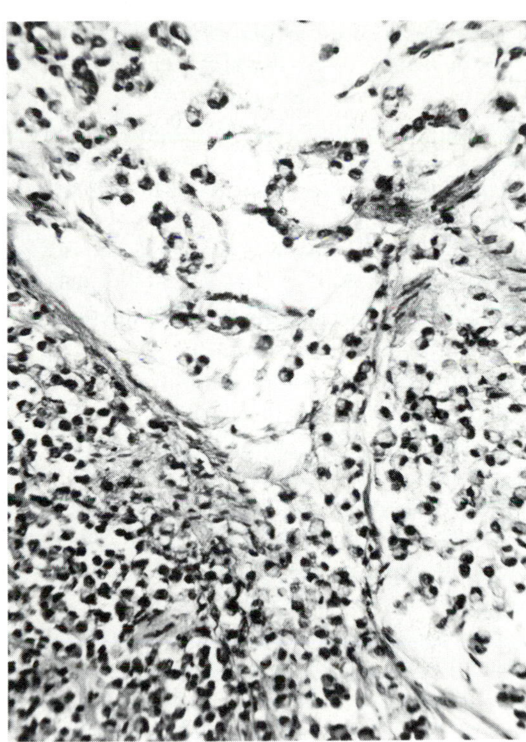

Fig. 26-31. Colloid (mucinous) carcinoma of cecum. Both patterns of pools of mucin and of sheets of individual signet-ring cells are seen. (300×.)

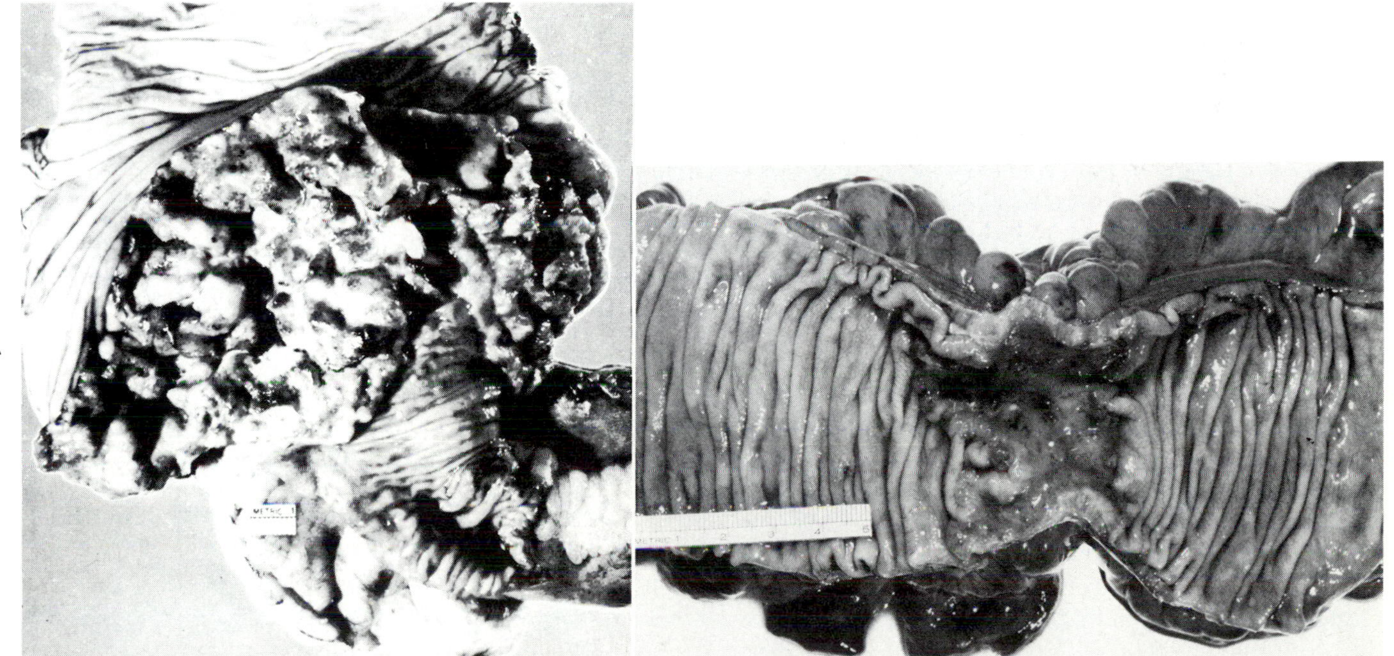

Fig. 26-32. A, Characteristic bulky, ulcerated carcinoma of right side of colon. Lesion in cecum. **B,** Characteristic constricting, "napkin-ring" carcinoma of left side of colon.

extensive ulceration. The smaller, more or less flat carcinomas that occur in the rectum and sigmoid colon commonly undermine the peripheral normal mucous membrane as they grow centrifugally. It is thus possible to obtain only overlying normal mucosa by a proctoscopic or a sigmoidoscopic biopsy, if the forceps bite is not deep enough.

Spread.[96] By the time the lesion is first observed, penetration of the muscular wall with involvement of the serosa and subserosa has usually occurred. Of greatest significance to the patient's longevity is spread via the lymphatics.[85] Extension is generally to anatomically predictable lymph nodes proximal to the growth. Knowledge of the anatomy of the lymphatic circulation and associated lymph nodes is the basis for properly planned surgical treatment of carcinoma in general, as well as specifically of carcinoma of the colon and rectum. Metastatic spread bypasses uninvolved nodes infrequently. In the laboratory the isolation of lymph nodes and demonstration of lymph node metastases are facilitated by clearing techniques.

Blood-vascular spread of colonic cancer is also highly significant.[160] Cancer cells have been found circulating in the bloodstream, but their significance remains incompletely understood. The finding of cancer cells in the circulating blood and the establishment of metastatic foci are not synonymous. In general, when venous invasion and blood-borne metastases are present, local growth and lymphatic spread are also extensive. However, striking examples are encountered of extensive venous dissemination of otherwise localized carcinomas and of locally far-advanced highly invasive tumors without significant lymphatic or venous spread.

The bulky tumors producing large amounts of mucin are prone to spread widely over the peritoneal surface and are in contrast to the usual carcinomas of the large intestine. This type of spread may result in the formation of a metastatic tumor mass palpable on rectal examination in the rectovesical or rectouterine space, the so-called rectal shelf. Implantation of cancer cells at the suture line of intestinal anastomosis or in the peritoneum is another mode of tumor spread.[213]

A number of classifications of colonic and rectal carcinoma, the most important of which are based on degree of differentiation and on the extent of spread both directly through the intestinal wall and via the lymphatics, as proposed by Dukes,[67,68] correlate reasonably well with the end results of surgical treatment. The 5-year survival rates after intestinal resection vary from 15% to 20% to better than 60% depending on the parts of the intestine involved and the extent of the disease at the time of diagnosis and treatment. The foregoing figures take into account only tumors not so far advanced as to be considered inoperable.

Carcinoma of the stomach

Incidence. The incidence of carcinoma of the stomach varies greatly in various parts of the world and among various peoples. It is known to be particularly frequent in Japan and is very rare among the Malay population of Java but not rare among the Chinese inhabitants of Java. In Iceland it accounts for 35% to 45% of all fatal cancers in males. This high incidence has been attributed to the consumption of considerable amounts of smoked fish and meat, particularly the former.[69] It thus appears that the geographic variation in the incidence of gastric carcinoma may depend, at least in part, on the dietary customs and resultant exposure to carcinogens. The incidence in women is about half that in men.

Classification. Most carcinomas of the stomach arise from the mucus-secreting cells. Differentiation is variable as to the extent and regularity of gland formation, mucus secretion, cytologic features, and so on, but in general they tend to be less well differentiated and less characteristic than the carcinomas of the colon and rectum (Fig. 26-33). The most common site of involvement is the antrum on or near the greater curvature. Ulcerative cancers in particular have a predilection for location in proximity to the greater curvature or to the pylorus.

Their association with a number of mucosal changes—atrophic gastritis, intestinal epithelial metaplasia, mucosal hypertrophy, peptic ulcer, and polyps—has been

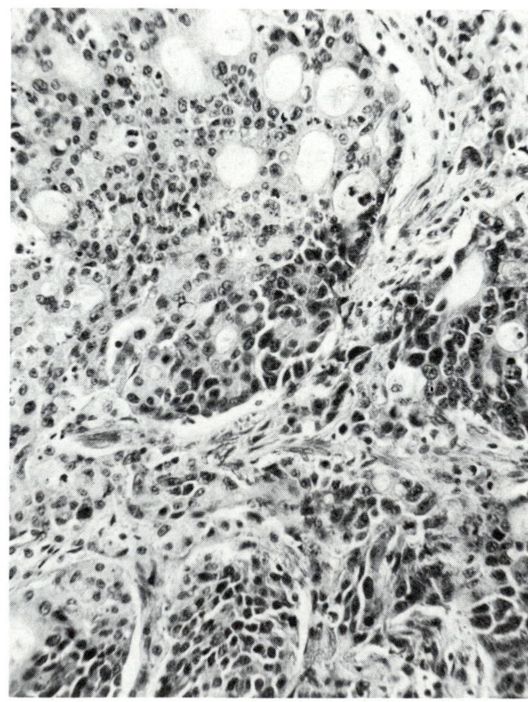

Fig. 26-33. Carcinoma of stomach showing limited degree of glandular differentiation. (300×.)

noted, but, except for the adenomatous polyp, a causal relationship is controversial.

Of the many classifications of gastric carcinoma, a large proportion lack the merit of clinical significance. An exception is that of Borrman. It is based upon the extensiveness of the lesion as judged by gross examination, showing a gradual gradation between the less malignant tumors that grow mainly within the lumen of the stomach and those prognostically less favorable, which are deeply invasive and penetrate the gastric wall. Stout's classification[217] is somewhat similar, being based upon direction of growth and the resultant gross configuration of the tumor. He recognized (1) a fungating or polypoid type, (2) an ulcerating type (ulcer cancer), (3) a superficial spreading type, and (4) a diffusely spreading type (linitis plastica).

Polypoid or fungating gastric carcinomas have a particularly favorable prognosis. An exception is the fungating carcinoma of the cardioesophageal junction, which is prone to become very extensive, both locally and in terms of lymph node spread, before giving rise to symptoms. Superficial spreading is also a relatively favorable type. Unfortunately these two forms of gastric carcinoma are relatively infrequent varieties. Linitis plastica type, equally or more rare, is hopeless in its outlook.

The various classifications and their clinical correlations support the concept that tumor growth by frank infiltration offers a greater and more immediate threat to the life of the host than does the gastric cancer that grows expansively, essentially pushing aside the host tissue.[155] Defects in the classification of gastric carcinomas arise in the fact that they often cannot be assigned to any of the categories, either because they are too far advanced to yield a clue to their initial gross configuration or because they show features of tumors of two or more growth types.

Morbid anatomy. Polypoid gastric carcinomas resemble adenomatous polyps except that they are usually larger and have a less delicate and often less distinct pedicle because of carcinomatous invasion. Hyperplastic polyps are commonly seen, and atrophic gastritis is always present in stomachs that are the site of polypoid carcinomas. Pernicious anemia may be associated. Polypoid carcinomas usually show good glandular differentiation, and the neoplastic glands very often resemble those of the small intestine.

The macroscopic differences between ulcer cancers and peptic ulcers have been described in the discussion of peptic ulcer (Plate 2, *D* and *E*). The old controversy over how many gastric cancers have their origin in peptic ulcers seems to have been largely resolved. Current opinion is that a small number of gastric carcinomas may arise in preexisting ulcers. Confirmation of such an occurrence must rest on demonstration of a characteristic peptic ulcer with cancer limited to one portion of its base or margin. Caution must be exercised not to misinterpret cytologically atypical, proliferative epithelial changes in the mucous membrane at the edge of an ulcer as malignant. A majority of ulcer cancers are malignant lesions from their inception, either because of primarily deeply penetrating growth or because of early peptic ulcerations of a small cancer. Ulcerative cancer has no specific histologic features.

The superficial spreading type is a distinctive variety of gastric carcinoma that spreads superficially in the mucosa or submucosa of the stomach forming a serpiginous lesion that may cover a large portion of the mucosal surface. Even without deeper penetration, lymph node metastases may take place. This type of tumor may be multicentric.[82,88]

In the linitis plastica or diffusely spreading type of carcinoma, the wall of the entire stomach is thickened, more or less uniformly, by neoplastic infiltration and new fibrous tissue production. The shrunken stomach with its relatively rigid wall has earned the descriptive term "leather-bottle stomach" (Plate 2, *F*). Characteristically the mucosa displays no focal lesion, although it may show thickening and irregularities, with flattening and distortion of its folds. Tumor infiltration involves all layers, but the submucosa and subserosa are chiefly affected. Lymphatic permeation is usual within the gastric wall proper, as well as into the adjacent omentum. Extension into the duodenum is generally sharply limited, although the subserosa may be involved to some extent. Histologically carcinomas of the linitis plastica type tend to be undifferentiated, and at times distinction from malignant lymphoma is difficult or impossible. If a tumor secretes mucin, this may be a helpful diagnostic feature. At times, mucin secretion may be abundant, and signet-ring cells may be the predominant cells. Desmoplasia often is pronounced and dominates the histologic picture, making recognition of cancer cells difficult. The prognosis is essentially hopeless in this variety of gastric cancer because of the extent of the disease by the time it is clinically recognized.[199] Occasionally, focal fibrotic thickening of the antrum, apparently of inflammatory nature, may simulate cancer clinically and on unassisted-eye inspection of the specimen.

The majority of gastric carcinomas, which do not meet the criteria of any one of these groups, are extremely variable in gross appearance and histologic pattern. Again, because they are usually far advanced before an opportunity for treatment is offered, the outlook is poor.

Spread. Direct spread and spread by way of the lymphatics are of foremost importance in dictating principles of surgical treatment and in assessing the individual patient's prognosis. Metastasis to lymph nodes along the greater and lesser curvatures of the stomach is frequent. Extension to the para-aortic and celiac lymph nodes is also often seen. Metastasis to the left supraclavicular lymph nodes by way of the thoracic duct may be an initial sign of gastric carcinoma, so-called Virchow's (Ewald's) node. Spread into the esophagus, especially submucosal, and to the mediastinal lymph nodes may be a feature. In occasional cases there may be permeation of pulmonary lymphatics and the bone marrow (with clinically unexplained anemia) as early manifestations of the disease.

Liver metastasis, common even in cases believed to be "early," results from invasion of the tributaries of the portal venous system.[104] Peritoneal spread and carcinomatosis occur, and gastric cancer is an important diagnostic consideration when a rectal shelf is demonstrated clinically. Carcinoma of the stomach, as well as other parts of the gastrointestinal tract, may metastasize early to the ovaries so that the ovarian tumor dominates the clinical picture, the so-called Krükenberg tumors. The typical Krükenberg tumor is characterized by signet-ring cancer cells with abundant fibrous tissue stroma.

Carcinoma of the esophagus

Among gastrointestinal cancer, epidermoid carcinoma of the esophagus ranks behind only carcinoma of the colon and rectum and carcinoma of the stomach in frequency. It is a disease of older age groups, affecting men more often than women.[35] Half of the cancers arise in the middle third of the esophagus, the remainder being approximately equally distributed between the upper and lower thirds. It is generally an ovoid growth with its long axis parallel to the long axis of the esophagus (Plate 2, *B*). Central ulceration of the elevated plaquelike growth undermines the peripheral mucous membrane. It may extend to involve the full circumference of the esophagus and commonly infiltrates the full thickness of the esophageal wall. Lymphatic spread and mediastinal invasion are frequent. As a result, carcinoma of the esophagus is generally well established when recognized, and the results of treatment, as measured in terms of 5-year survivals, are quite poor.[118]

Although epidermoid carcinomas are by far the most common in the esophagus, glandular carcinomas are occasionally seen. Although most of the adenocarcinomas are primary tumors of the gastric cardia with extension into the esophagus,[25] occasionally they originate in esophageal glands and may grow in an adenoid cystic pattern.

Carcinoma of the small intestine

Carcinoma of the small intestine is an infrequent primary malignant tumor[52] and when it occurs in the duodenum, one may have difficulty in distinguishing it from pancreatic carcinoma or carcinoma of the common bile duct secondarily infiltrating the duodenum.[214] With the exception of some of the periampullary carcinomas, many of which resemble the biliary duct system tumors morphologically, carcinomas of the small intestine are similar in appearance and behavior to those of the large intestine, although their clinical diagnosis may be more difficult and their evolutionary stage more advanced when they are diagnosed. An occasional carcinoma of the small intestine may originate in a papillary adenoma.[32]

Carcinoma of the anal region

A number of different epithelial tumors originate in the vicinity of the anus and anorectal junction. The epidermoid carcinoma arising from the squamous epithelium of the anal mucous membrane appears and behaves similarly to epidermoid carcinomas of other squamous epithelial mucous membranes. They spread freely by way of the rich perianal lymphatic plexuses to the lymph nodes of the groin.

The so-called basaloid tumors, which histologically resemble the common basal cell epitheliomas of the skin, presumably arise from the mucosa of the transitional or cloacogenic zone separating the rectal and anal mucous membranes. Although they may spread as the epidermoid carcinomas of the anus do, studies indicate a more favorable prognosis than that of the anal epidermoid carcinomas.[129]

Occasional epidermoid tumors in this area include some glandular elements or individual cells with mucin secretions—mucoepidermoid carcinomas.[165]

Anal duct carcinoma is an infrequent tumor, usually glandular and mucin secreting, that occurs in the anorectal area without apparent involvement of the anal skin or anal or rectal mucous membrane. It arises from anal glands or ducts and usually is not recognized as being malignant until some time has elapsed, often while treatment has been directed toward such conditions as fistula in ano.

Rarely, epidermoid carcinomas arise in the rectum without anatomic continuity with the anus. They also occur, but even more rarely, in the stomach as do mixed glandular and epidermoid tumors—adenoacanthomas.[29]

Malignant melanoma

Malignant melanomas have been encountered in many parts of the gastrointestinal tract, and with the exception of those primary in the anus and esophagus, they are considered to be metastatic. Unlike the metastases from carcinoma, they are infrequently accompanied by peritoneal spread. The appearance and behavior of the primary tumors do not differ from those of the corresponding skin lesions. Anal malignant melanomas may occur primarily as rectal lesions because anal sphincteric action may cause them to grow cephalad initially.

Establishment of the primary nature of gastrointestinal malignant melanomas rests on demonstration of junctional change, with the recognition of neoplastic proliferation in the area of the junction of epithelium and subepithelial stroma.[187]

Carcinoid tumor

Carcinoid (argentaffin) tumors are relatively uncommon neoplasms whose endocrine secretion may produce systemic effects. They are found throughout the gastrointestinal tract, from the stomach to the rectum, as well as in the gallbladder and in teratoid ovarian tumors. Morphologically and functionally identical tumors arise in the bronchial and tracheal mucous membranes. The cell of origin is believed to be the Kulchitsky cell, one of the cell types occurring in the crypts of Leiberkühn, characterized morphologically by the presence of cytoplasmic granules capable of reducing ammoniacal silver nitrate (argentaffin granules).

The origin of Kulchitsky cells—endodermal or neuroectodermal—is in dispute, but current data support the latter. It has been suggested that more than one cell type may be involved, since argentaffin granules are found frequently in the midgut carcinoids and rarely, if at all, in tumors of the bronchi, stomach, and hindgut.[144] Argyrophil granules, which stain with metallic silver after the addition of exogenous reducing agent, have a similar distribution pattern as do the argentaffin granules but are seen with greater frequency in tumors of the bronchi, stomach, and hindgut than are the argentaffin granules. The argentaffin cells secrete serotonin (5-hydroxytryptamine), a hormone also found in blood platelets and concerned with blood coagulation, probably through a vasoconstrictive action. Serotonin has also been shown to have a normal central nervous system function, and these facts, together with its pathologic role in the development of cardiovascular lesions and the "carcinoid syndrome," account for the widespread interest it has generated.

A variety of clinically evident endocrine dysfunctions have also been manifested by tumors with argyrophil cells from other sites (such as bronchus), lending support for the proposed name *neuroendocrine tumor* for these neoplasms.[92] Some carcinoids are grossly indistinguishable from carcinomas, but generally the lesions are small submucosal nodules or merely focal areas of submucosal thickening. Their yellow color has been emphasized, but many are actually gray or gray-white. Muscle hypertrophy is often considerable in the involved area, and this, together with the characteristic fibrosis and perhaps peritoneal adhesions, may produce kinking and partial obstruction (Plate 2, *G*).

Two histologic types of carcinoid tumors are recognized. The "classic" variety, composed of solid nests of uniform small cells with round or oval nuclei that are usually regular, is more commonly encountered. The less common histologic pattern is trabeculae of interanastomosing bands or ribbons of tumor cells. Rosettelike formation may occur with either type of tumor, and both patterns may be seen in some tumors (Fig. 26-34). Mucus-secreting cells may be found in either variety of tumor,[103] and in some instances when they are in great numbers, the diagnosis of mucus-producing carcinoma may be suggested.[100,101] The argentaffin granules when present appear to be concentrated at the periphery of the cell about one pole of the nucleus. The tumors tend to grow invasively and have the potential for metastasizing by way of lymphatics and bloodstream. However, even when metastases occur, it is not uncommon for a patient to live with essentially asymptomatic tumors for many years.

Carcinoid tumors occur more frequently in the appendix and rectum than elsewhere and are usually asymptomatic, being found during the course of proctoscopic examination or in the appendix removed surgically for acute inflammation or other reasons.[87] However, roughly 10% to 15% of rectal carcinoid tumors, usually those more than 2 cm in diameter, invade the muscularis propria and behave like rectal carcinomas, although perhaps progressing more slowly.[158] Occasionally, very small tumors may be associated with distant, even widespread, metastases. Carcinoid tumors that metastasize and prove fatal, as well as those associated with the "carcinoid syndrome," most often are encountered in the ileum and commonly are multiple. The carcinoid syndrome consists of diarrhea, a peculiar cyanotic flushing of the skin, and right-sided heart failure, the last being based on organic disease of the tricuspid or pulmonic valve. Almost invariably, extensive liver metastases are present in patients with the syndrome. In the usual functioning carcinoid tumor, 5-hydroxyindoleacetic acid (5-HIAA), a degradation product of 5-hydroxytryptamine (5-HT), can be demonstrated in the urine. The cardiac lesion consists of dense, fibrous endocardial thickening, the fibrous tissue apparently being deposited on the surface of the endocardium of the pulmonic valve, tricuspid valve, or endocardium of the auricle. Less commonly other chambers of the heart, the great vessels, and coronary sinus may be involved. As the result of these changes, functional pulmonary stenosis and tricuspid insufficiency may occur. Normally, serotonin is destroyed in the lungs by monoamine oxidase, accounting for the preponderance of right-sided cardiac disease.

The fibrosis seen in the heart and in the vicinity of the primary carcinoid tumor has been considered to be the result of release of histamine and mucopolysaccharides from mast cells, which in turn produce local edema, and fibrin deposition with organization of the latter resulting in fibrosis.[18]

Williams and Sandler[244] have subdivided carcinoid tumors into three groups: (1) those of the bronchus and

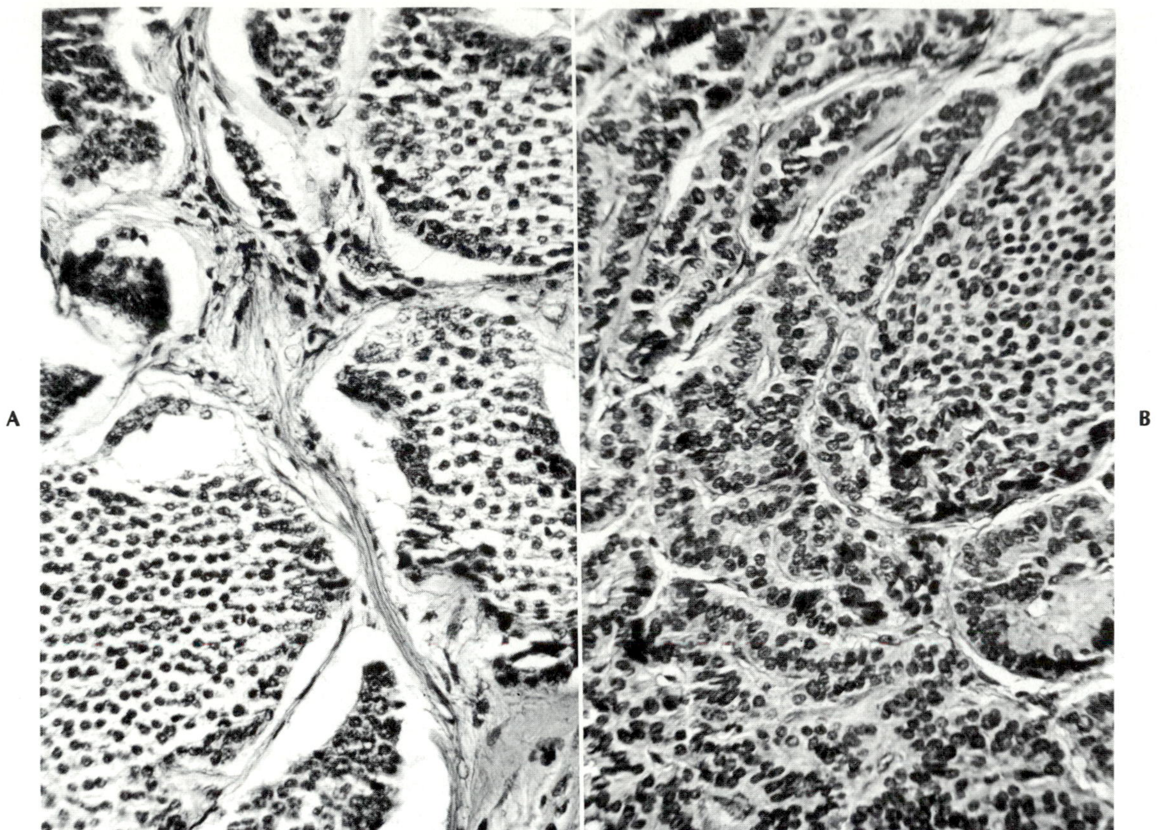

Fig. 26-34. Carcinoid (argentaffin) tumor. **A,** "Classic" pattern. **B,** Trabecular pattern. (**A** and **B,** 300×.)

stomach, arising from the foregut; (2) those of the jejunum, ileum, and cecum, arising from the midgut; and (3) those of the rectum, developing from the hindgut. They point out that those from the foregut are often of trabecular pattern and sometimes secrete 5-hydroxytryptophan, a precursor of serotonin, and store the latter poorly; those of midgut origin are the classic lesions morphologically, tinctorially (positive argentaffin reaction), and in the ability to store large amounts of serotonin; those of the hindgut are usually of trabecular pattern and lack secretory function. The syndrome, as well as 5-HIAA excretion, is more frequent with midgut tumors than those from the foregut and hindgut.

Neoplasms of smooth muscle

With the exception of the uterus, the muscle of gastrointestinal tract gives rise to more tumors of smooth muscle than any other organ or organ system of the body. As is true of the uterus, leiomyomas far outnumber leiomyosarcomas. They arise in any portion of the alimentary tract from the esophagus[26,37] to the rectum but are most common in the stomach.[22,208] The small intestine is next most frequently involved.[215] They may grow primarily into the gut lumen (Fig. 26-35), and in that part of the intestine supported on a mesentery, they may become pedunculated and form the head of an intussusception. They also may project primarily from the serosa and grow to a large size without producing gastrointestinal symptoms. Some tumors are dumbbell-shaped lesions projecting in both directions. It is common for gastrointestinal muscle tumors to ulcerate and undergo extensive central necrosis, accounting for the frequency of hematemesis (or melena). A small leiomyoma of the intestine may be the cryptic source of massive, even exsanguinating, hemorrhage.

These neoplasms are most frequently composed of interlacing bundles of fusiform cells with long processes and nuclei with blunted ends, often bearing a striking resemblance to normal smooth muscle. Less commonly they feature round or polygonal cells that are frequently vacuolated and sometimes associated with spindle cells more characteristic of smooth muscle. This pattern is now generally considered to represent an atypical growth pattern of smooth muscle tumors and is referred to as bizarre leiomyoma, leiomyoblastoma, and epithelioid leiomyoma.[8,222] Although they appear well delineated grossly, under the microscope no capsule is seen, and tumor muscle fibers usually can be seen to interdigitate with those of the muscularis propria or, occasionally, the muscularis mucosae. The histologic distinction

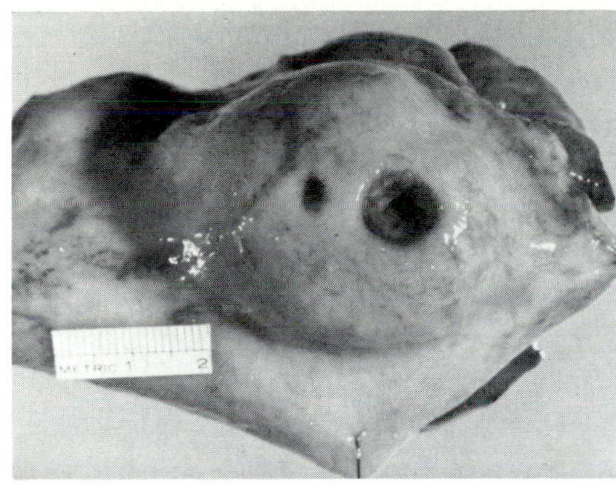

Fig. 26-35. Leiomyoma of stomach. Growth essentially endogastric.

between leiomyoma and leiomyosarcoma may be difficult regardless of the tumor's microscopic pattern; the atypical appearance of the leiomyoblastoma by itself is not indicative of malignancy. Occasional sarcomas appear very orderly and well differentiated, giving no hint of malignancy until metastasis occurs. More often, however, completely benign tumors show great cellularity and nuclear pleomorphism, even to the presence of bizarre giant cells. The presence of mitotic figures in appreciable numbers is generally a reliable indication of malignancy.[188]

Distant metastases of leiomyosarcomas are usually blood borne, but some display a tendency to spread over the peritoneal surface and some are only locally invasive.[4] Local invasion, particuarly of those arising in the retroperitoneum, makes complete removal and thus cure less likely.

Lymphoma

A benign lesion, often referred to as lymphoma of the rectum but also known as lymphoid polyp or rectal tonsil, is occasionally encountered on proctoscopic examination and removed as a "polyp." It is usually only a few millimeters in diameter but may reach a dimension as great as 1.5 cm. It can be recognized microscopically as benign by its excellent organization with "germinal centers" and its usual limitation to the mucosa and submucosa without invasion of the muscle coat. It is of significance only in differential diagnosis.[47] With this exception, the lymphomas of the gastrointestinal tract are malignant. Such malignant lymphomas may arise as primary, or apparently primary, gastrointestinal tumors or may be but one manifestation of generalized disease. The latter situation is more common, and all varieties of malignant lymphoma encountered in the lymphoid tissue of the body generally, may involve the alimentary tract. The same varieties also occur as "primary" lesions, but Hodgkin's disease and plasmacytoma are very rare.[56] Gastrointestinal lesions in generalized malignant lymphoma (including the leukemias) are of importance in themselves, and they may demand treatment when they are responsible for problems relative to gastrointestinal hemorrhage or obstruction. Malignant lymphomas readily perforate, occasionally at multiple sites, especially after radiotherapy.

"Primary" malignant lymphoma of the gastrointestinal tract is most often seen in the stomach, less commonly in the rectum, cecum, and ascending colon, and infrequently elsewhere.[10] Gastric malignant lymphomas usually simulate carcinoma in their clinical manifestations, and sometimes their gross pathologic appearance as well. However, many characteristically appear as flat, disclike or plateaulike elevations with rather sharply defined borders (Fig. 26-36, *A*). They are raised a few millimeters or a centimeter or so above the surrounding mucous membrane, and if they involve the antrum, their pyloric margin is abrupt. Frequently involvement is multifocal, and ulceration is usual, producing shallow, saucerlike lesions. In the intestine, involvement of submucosa rather than mucosa is a prominent feature, and again multicentric origin is frequent. As with carcinoid tumors, kinking and incomplete obstruction may bring the disease to the patient's attention (Fig. 26-36, *B*).

Lymphomas may be difficult to distinguish histologically from carcinoma, and at times they can be distinguished from inflammatory hyperplasia only with great difficulty (Fig. 26-36, *C*). In some cases the distinction from the latter requires observation of the clinical course over a period of years.

Although malignant lymphomas of the gastrointestinal tract have their greatest incidence in the same age range as carcinoma, they have a greater incidence during early ages, including childhood. Primary malignant lymphoma of the stomach, the most common malignant gastric tumor next to carcinoma, has a distinctly better prognosis than does carcinoma in terms of 5-year survival after surgical treatment.[116] On the other hand, so-called primary malignant lymphomas of the colon and rectum in the majority of instances prove to be manifestations of systemic disease, although the extraintestinal involvement may not be apparent at the time of recognition of the colonic or rectal lesion.

Occasional cases of multiple, polypoid, relatively well-differentiated and -organized lymphoid lesions of the gastrointestinal tract (so-called gastrointestinal pseudolymphomas) are encountered.[46] They are extremely difficult to differentiate from malignant lymphoma, and in some instances observation of the clinical course over a period of years is necessary for their distinction[110]

Miscellaneous rare tumors

Mucocele of the appendix is a cystic distension of the organ with thick, glairy mucus. Although there may be a

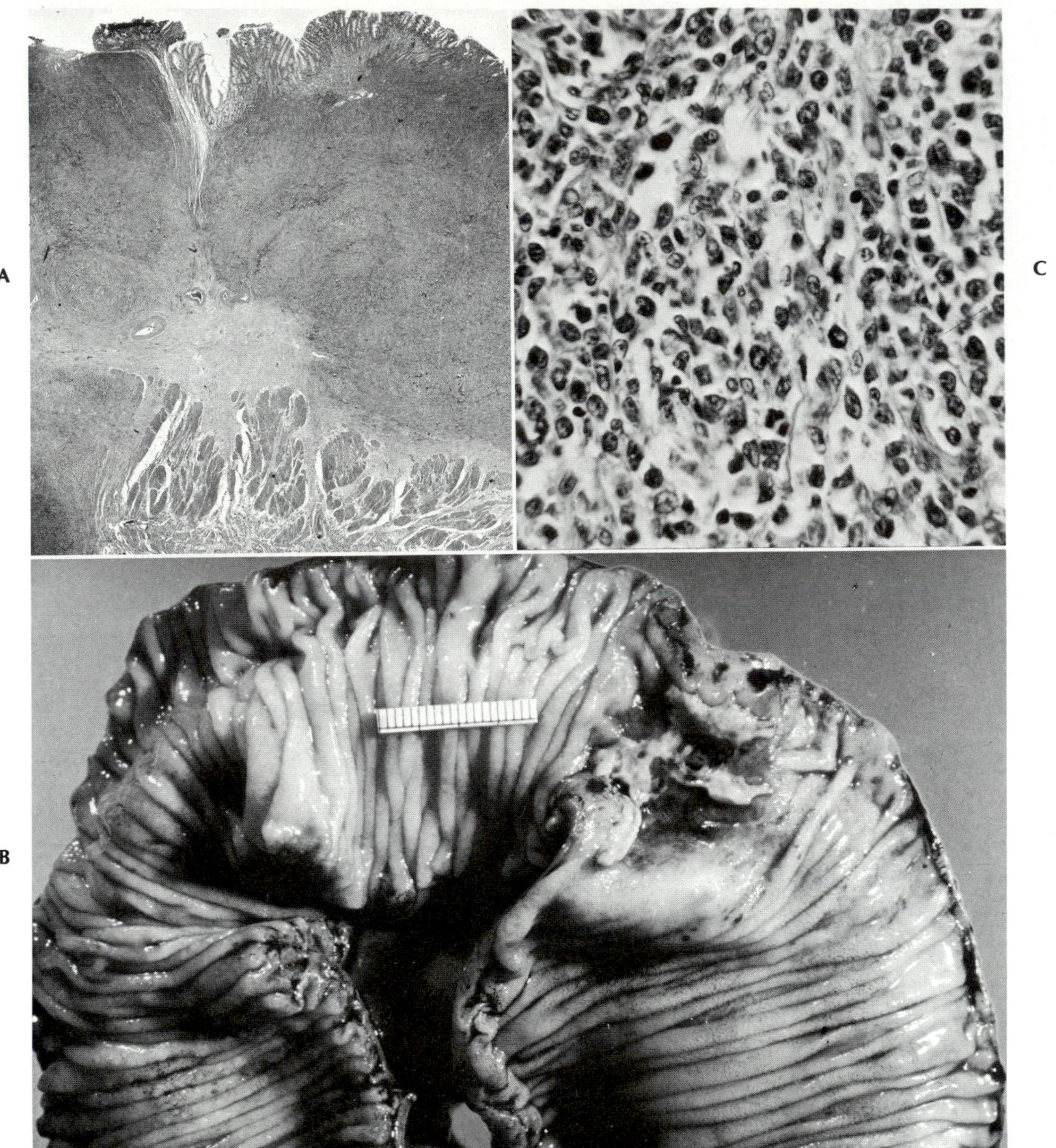

Fig. 26-36. A, Malignant lymphoma of stomach. Characteristic plateaulike elevation of mucosa and pronounced thickening of submucosa are well demonstrated. At left, muscle has been freely invaded. **B,** Malignant lymphoma of small intestine, with multiple sites of involvement. Note similarity to gross appearance of carcinoid tumor illustrated in Plate 2, *G.* **C,** Malignant lymphoma of stomach showing considerable pleomorphism. (**A,** 13×; **C,** 625×.)

cicatricial stricture proximal to the dilated portion, often there is not. The normal mucous membrane is replaced by focal or diffuse hyperplasia of the glands resembling those of the hyperplastic colonic polyp, a mucinous cystadenoma with epithelial atypia, or a mucinous cystadenocarcinoma.[102] In a number of cases there are associated mucinous ovarian tumors or carcinoma of the large bowel. Pseudomyxoma peritonei, spread of mucus-secreting cells over the peritoneal surfaces with accumulation of mucoid material in the peritoneal cavity, occurs in a variety of conditions. Most commonly it follows rupture of an appendiceal mucocele or mucinous ovarian tumor, but it may result from malignant mucinous tumors of other organs; in some instances the cause cannot be determined.[136] The behavior of pseudomyxoma peritonei is one of a locally infiltrating surface growth that generally cannot be eradicated.

Lipomas occasionally are encountered in various parts of the gastrointestinal tract, most often in the colon and rectum and particularly in the vicinity of the ileocecal

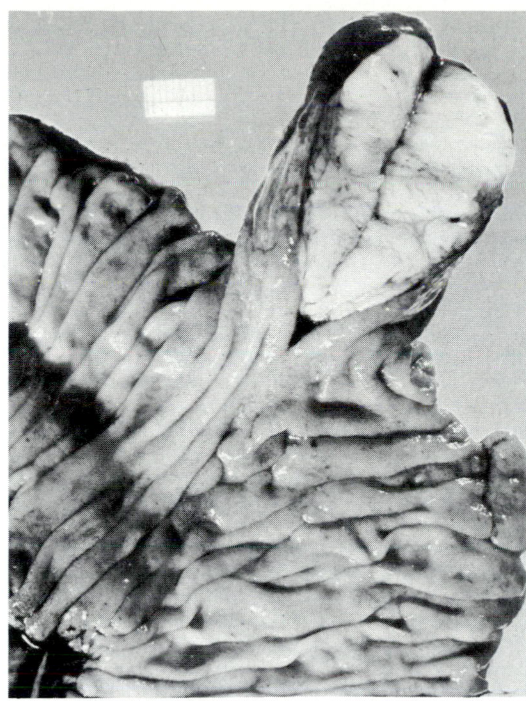

Fig. 26-37. Lipoma of jejunum.

valve, where appreciable submucosal adipose tissue is usually present.[197] They are submucosal, often superficially ulcerated, and may lead to an intussusception (Fig. 26-37). In instances of incipient intussusception, there may be puckering of the overlying serosa, and this, coupled with induration as the result of inflammation, accounts for their occasionally being mistaken for carcinoma at operation.

Vascular tumors, especially cavernous hemangiomas, have been reported as occurring in various parts of the gastrointestinal tract. Multiple hemangiomas may be seen as part of Osler-Weber-Rendu disease.[108] Lymphangiomas occur less frequently. Characteristic glomus tumors may form polypoid, sometimes painful, gastric tumors.[119] Rarely gastrointestinal lesions occur in Kaposi's sarcoma.

The gastrointestinal tract and mesentery may be involved by tumors of nerve origin—neurofibroma, neuroblastoma, ganglioneuroma and paraganglioma, teratoma, and choriocarcinoma.[124,179,190] Adenomas, or papillary cystadenomas, arise from the apocrine sweat glands in the region of the anus and may give rise to Paget's disease. Granular cell myoblastomas have been encountered in the stomach, rectum, and esophagus.[44]

Carcinosarcoma is a rare but spectacular tumor of the esophagus incorporating both epithelial growth (usually epidermoid) and a sarcomatous or sarcoma-like stroma, which may dominate the picture.[131] Many such tumors are polypoid. There is no agreement as to the nature of the stromal change—whether it is genuinely malignant or pseudosarcomatous.[147] The carcinosarcomas are distinctly less malignant than the much more common epidermoid carcinomas. Although they may be grossly simulated by the polypoid fibrovascular tumors occurring most commonly in the upper one third of the esophagus,[111] their malignant histologic features should serve adequately to distinguish the two growths. Metastases, which are relatively infrequent, may be carcinomatous, sarcomatous, or mixed.

Mesothelial cysts are encountered rarely in the mesentery or retroperitoneum. Of greater importance and slightly greater frequency are tumors arising from the serosal lining cells—mesotheliomas.[218] They may be solitary and fibrous, in which case they may be amenable to surgical removal,[219,248] but more often the peritoneal mesotheliomas, in contrast to most of those of the pleura, are diffuse and result in widespread adhesions.[246] They have a tubular pattern, forming multiple small spaces lined by mesothelium, and may secrete mucin. The histologic picture may closely simulate carcinoma. Rare peritoneal mesotheliomas may occur as multiple small papillary growths whose first discovery may be in a hernial sac. They may be difficult, if not impossible, to distinguish from mesothelial cell hyperplasia and metastatic carcinoma.

Metastatic tumors

Metastatic tumors, especially carcinoma, are common in the peritoneal cavity. Spread over the serosal surfaces to involve multiple organs and produce widespread adhesions is a frequent autopsy finding in disseminated cancer. The primary tumor may not be readily apparent without complete autopsy study; thus the distinction of metastatic carcinoma from diffuse mesothelioma is difficult, if not impossible.

REFERENCES

1. Abdou, N.I., et al.: Malakoplakia: evidence for monocytic lysosomal abnormality correctable by cholinergic agonist in vitro and in vivo, N. Engl. J. Med. **297**:1413, 1977.
2. Abrams, J.S., and Holden, W.D.: Tuberculosis of the gastrointestinal tract, Arch. Surg. **89**:282, 1964.
3. Akwari, O.E., et al.: Cancer of the bile ducts associated with ulcerative colitis, Ann. Surg. **181**:303, 1975.
4. Akwari, O.E., et al.: Leiomyosarcoma of the small and large bowel, Cancer **42**:1375, 1978.
5. Altemeier, W.A.: Bacterial flora of acute perforated appendicitis with peritonitis: bacteriologic study based upon 100 cases, Ann. Surg. **107**:517, 1938.
6. Altemeier, W.A., and Holzer, C.E.: Primary torsion of omentum, Surgery **20**:810, 1946.
7. Anderson, K.E., Finlayson, N.D.C., and Deschner, E.E.: Intractable malabsorption with a flat jejunal mucosa and selective IgA deficiency, Gastroenterology **67**:709, 1974.
8. Appleman, H.D., and Helwig, E.B.: Gastric epithelioid leiomyoma and leiomyosarcoma (leiomyoblastoma), Cancer **38**:708, 1976.
9. Azzopardi, J.G., and Evans, D.J.: Mucoprotein-containing histiocytes (muciphages) in the rectum, J. Clin. Pathol. **19**:368, 1966.

10. Azzopardi, J.G., and Menzies, T.: Primary malignant lymphoma of the alimentary tract, Br. J. Surg. **47**:358, 1960.
11. Baker, L.A., Smith, C., and Lieberman, G.: The natural history of esophageal varices; a study of 115 cirrhotic patients in whom varices were diagnosed prior to bleeding, Am. J. Med. **26**:228, 1959.
12. Bale, P.M., et al.: Pathology of Tangier disease, J. Clin. Pathol. **24**:609, 1971.
13. Barret, N.R.: Hiatus hernia: a review of some controversial points, J. Surg. **42**:231, 1954.
14. Barry, J.E., and Auldist, A.W.: The Vater association: one end of a spectrum of anomalies, Am. J. Dis. Child. **128**:769, 1974.
15. Bartlett, J.G.: Antibiotic-associated colitis, Clin. Gastroenterol. **8**:783, 1979.
16. Bartlett, J.G., et al.: Antibiotic-associated pseudomembranous colitis due to toxin-producing clostridia, N. Engl. J. Med. **298**:531, 1978.
17. Bartlett, J.G., et al.: Clinical and laboratory observations in *Clostridium difficile* colitis, Am. J. Clin. Nutr. **33**:2521, 1980.
18. Bates, H.R., Jr., and Clark, R.F.: Observations on the pathogenesis of carcinoid heart disease and the tanning of fluorescent fibrin by 5-hydroxytryptamine and ceruloplasmin, Am. J. Clin. Pathol. **39**:46, 1963.
19. Bayless, T.M., and Knox, D.L.: Whipple's disease: a multisystem infection, N. Engl. J. Med. **300**:920, 1979.
20. Benson, C.D., and Lloyd, J.R.: Infantile pyloric stenosis: a review of 1,120 cases, Am. J. Surg. **107**:429, 1964.
21. Benson, C.D., Lloyd, J.R., and Fischer, H.: Intussusception in infants and children: an analysis of 300 cases, Arch. Surg. **86**:745, 1963.
22. Berg, J., and McNeer, G.: Leiomyosarcoma of the stomach, Cancer **13**:25, 1960.
23. Bernstein, J., et al.: The occurrence of intestinal atresia in newborn with meconium ileus: the pathogenesis of an acquired anomaly, Am. J. Dis. Child. **99**:804, 1960.
24. Berthrong, M., and Fajardo, L.F.: Radiation injury in surgical pathology. II. Alimentary tract, Am. J. Surg. Pathol. **5**:153, 1981.
25. Block, G.E., and Lancaster, J.R.: Adenocarcinoma of the cardioesophageal junction, Arch. Surg. **88**:852, 1964.
26. Bogedain, W., Carpathios, J., and Najib, A.: Leiomyoma of the esophagus, Dis. Chest **44**:391, 1963.
27. Borow, M., Smith, M., Jr., and Soto, D., Jr.: Diverticular disease of the duodenum, Am. Surg. **33**:373, 1967.
28. Bosher, L.H., Jr., and Taylor, F.H.: Heterotopic gastric mucosa in esophagus with ulceration and stricture formation, J. Thorac. Surg. **21**:306, 1951.
29. Boswell, J.T., and Helwig, E.B.: Squamous cell carcinoma and adenoacanthoma of the stomach: a clinicopathologic study, Cancer **18**:181, 1965.
30. Bremer, J.L.: Diverticulas and duplications of the intestinal tract, Arch. Pathol. **38**:132, 1944.
31. Brett, E.M., and Berry, C.L.: Value of rectal biopsy in pediatric neurology: report of 165 biopsies, Br. Med. J. **2**:400, 1967.
32. Bridge, M.F., and Perzin, K.H.: Primary adenocarcinoma of the jejunum and ileum: a clinicopathologic study, Cancer **36**:1876, 1975.
33. Brief, D.K., and Botsford, T.W.: Primary bleeding from the small intestine in adult: the surgical management, J.A.M.A. **184**:18, 1963.
34. Brow, J.R., et al.: The small intestinal mucosa in dermatitis herpetiformis. I. Severity and distribution of the small intestinal lesion and associated malabsorption, Gastroenterology **60**:355, 1971.
35. Burgess, H.M., et al.: Cancer of the esophagus: a clinicopathological study, Surg. Clin. North Am. **31**:965, 1951.
36. Bussey, H.J.R.: Gastrointestinal polyposis, Gut **11**:970, 1970.
37. Camishion, R.C., Gibbon, J.H., Jr., and Templeton, J.Y., III: Leiomyosarcoma of the esophagus: review of the literature and report of 2 cases, Ann. Surg. **153**:951, 1961.
38. Cassella, R.R., et al.: Achalasia of esophagus: pathologic and etiologic consideration, Ann. Surg. **160**:474, 1964.
39. Castell, D.O., et al.: Dysphagia, Gastroenterology **76**:1015, 1979.
40. Castillo, S., et al.: Diffuse intramural esophageal pseudodiverticulosis: new cases and review, Gastroenterology **72**:541, 1977.
41. Cave, D.R., Mitchell, D.N., and Brooke, B.N.: Evidence of an agent transmissible from ulcerative colitis tissue, Lancet **1**:1311, 1976.
42. Civetta, J.M., and Kolodny, M.: Mesenteric venous thrombosis associated with oral contraceptives, Gastroenterology **58**:713, 1970.
43. Clancy, R.L., et al.: Isolation and characterization of an aetiological agent in Whipple's disease, Br. Med. J. **3**:568, 1975.
44. Cohen, R.S., and Cramm, R.E.: Granular cell myoblastoma: an unusual rectal neoplasm; report of a case, Dis. Colon Rectum **12**:120, 1969.
45. Collins, D.C.: A study of 50,000 specimens of human vermiform appendix, Surg. Gynecol. Obstet. **101**:437, 1955.
46. Cornes, J.S.: Multiple lymphomatous polyposis of the gastrointestinal tract, Cancer **14**:249, 1961.
47. Cornes, J.S., Wallace, M.H., and Morson, B.C.: Benign lymphomas of the rectum and anal canal: a study of 100 cases, J. Pathol. Bacteriol. **82**:371, 1961.
48. Cullen, J.H.: Intestinal tuberculosis: a clinical pathological study, Q. Bull. Sea View Hosp. **5**:143, 1940.
49. Cutler, E.C., and Harrison, J.H.: Phlegomonous gastritis, Surg. Gynecol. Obstet. **70**:234, 1940.
50. Czaja, A.J., McAlhany, J.C., and Pruitt, B.A., Jr.: Acute duodenitis and duodenal ulceration after burns: clinical and pathological characteristics, J.A.M.A. **232**:621, 1975.
51. Dagradi, A.E., et al.: The Mallory-Weiss syndrome and lesion: a study of 30 cases, Am. J. Dig. Dis. **11**:710, 1966.
52. Darling, R.C., and Welch, C.E.: Tumors of the small intestine, N. Engl. J. Med. **260**:397, 1959.
53. Davidsohn, I., and Mora, J.M.: Appendicitis in measles, Arch. Pathol. **14**:757, 1932.
54. Davidson, J.D., et al.: Protein-losing gastroenteropathy in congestive heart-failure, Lancet **1**:899, 1961.
55. Davis, J.M., Gray, G.F., and Thorbjarnarson, B.: Menetrier's disease: a clinicopathologic study of six cases, Ann. Surg. **185**:456, 1977.
56. Dawson, I.M.P., Cornes, J.S., and Morson, B.C.: Primary malignant lymphoid tumors of the intestinal tract: report of 37 cases with a study of factors influencing prognosis, Br. J. Surg. **49**:80, 1961.
57. DeLorimer, A.A., Fonkalsrud, E.W., and Hays, D.M.: Congenital atresia and stenosis of the jejunum and ileum, Surgery **65**:819, 1969.
58. Dew, M.J., Thompson, H., and Allan, R.N.: The spectrum of hepatic dysfunction in inflammatory bowel disease, Q. J. Med. **48**:113, 1979.
59. di Sant'Agnese, P.A., and Lepore, M.J.: Involvement of abdominal organs in cystic fibrosis of the pancreas, Gastroenterology **40**:64, 1961.
60. Dimmette, R.M., Elwi, A.M., and Sproat, H.F.: Relationship of schistosomiasis to polyposis and adenocarcinoma of large intestine, Am. J. Clin. Pathol. **26**:266, 1956.
61. Dobbins, W.O., III: An ultrastructural study of the intestinal mucosa in congenital beta-lipoprotein deficiency with particular emphasis upon the intestinal absorptive cell, Gastroenterology **50**:195, 1966.
62. Dodds, W.J., et al.: Peutz-Jeghers syndrome and gastrointestinal malignancy, Am. J. Roentgenol. **115**:374, 1972.
63. Donnison, A.B., Schwachman, H., and Gross, R.E.: A review of 164 children with meconium ileus seen at the Children's Hospital Medical Center, Boston, Pediatrics **37**:833, 1966.
64. Dopp, A.C., Mutchnik, M.G., and Goldstein, A.L.: Thymosin-dependent T-lymphocyte response in inflammatory bowel disease, Gastroenterology **79**:276, 1980.
65. Dragstedt, L.R.: Cause of peptic ulcer, J.A.M.A. **169**:203, 1959.
66. Dragstedt, L.R., and Woodward, E.R.: Gastric stasis: a cause of gastric ulcer, Scand. J. Gastroenterol. **6**(suppl.):243, 1970.
67. Dukes, C.E.: The classification of cancer of the rectum, J. Pathol. Bacteriol. **35**:323, 1932.
68. Dukes, C.E.: Cancer of the rectum: an analysis of 1,000 cases, J. Pathol. Bacteriol. **50**:527, 1940.

69. Dungal, N., and Sigurjonsson, J.: Gastric cancer and diet: a pilot study of dietary habits in two districts differing markedly in respect of mortality from gastric cancer, Br. J. Cancer **21**:270, 1967.
70. Eade, O.E., et al.: Lymphocyte subpopulations of intestinal mucosa in inflammatory bowel disease, Gut **21**:675, 1980.
71. Earlam, R.: Pathophysiology and clinical presentation of achalasia, Clin. Gastroenterol. **5**:73, 1976.
72. Ecker, J.A., and Dickson, D.R.: Melanosis proctocoli—the so-called "brown-bowel"—etiology and significance, Am. J. Gastroenterol. **39**:362, 1963.
73. Ecker, J.A., Williams, R.G., and Clay, K.L.: Pneumatosis cystoides intestinalis: bullous emphysema of the intestine; a review of the literature, Am. J. Gastroenterol. **56**:125, 1971.
74. Ecker, J.A., et al.: Gastrointestinal bleeding in hereditary hemorrhagic telangiectasia: review of the literature and report of a case with massive recurrent hemorrhage necessitating right colectomy, Am. J. Gastroenterol. **33**:411, 1960.
75. Edwards, H.C.: Diverticulosis of small intestine, Ann. Surg. **103**:230, 1936.
76. Edwards, M.: Multilocular retrorectal cystic disease: cysthamartoma; report of twelve cases, Dis. Colon Rectum **4**:103, 1961.
77. Eisman, B., Seelig, M.G., and Womack, N.A.: Talcum powder granuloma: frequent and serious postoperative complication, Ann. Surg, **126**:820, 1947.
78. Estrada, R.L.: Anomalies of intestinal rotation and fixation, Springfield, Ill., 1958, Charles C Thomas, Publisher.
79. Feldman, E.J., and Sabovich, K.A.: Stress and peptic ulcer disease, Gastroenterology **78**:1087, 1980.
80. Fiske, S.C., and Falchuk, M.: Impaired mixed-lymphocyte culture reactions in patients with inflammatory bowel disease, Gastroenterology **79**:682, 1980.
81. Fitz, R.H.: Perforating inflammation of the vermiform appendix, with special reference to its early diagnosis and treatment, Am. J. Med. Sci. **92**:321, 1886.
82. Friesen, G., Dockerty, M.B., and ReMine, W.H.: Superficial carcinoma of the stomach, Surgery **51**:300, 1962.
83. Gear, M.W.L., Truelove, S.C., and Whitehead, R.: Gastric ulcer and gastritis, Gut **12**:639, 1971.
84. Gelfand, M.D., et al.: Acute radiation proctitis in man: development of eosinophilic crypt abscesses, Gastroenterology **51**:401, 1968.
85. Gilchrist, R.K.: Lymphatic spread of carcinoma of the colon, Dis. Colon Rectum **2**:69, 1959.
86. Glass, R.E., and Baker, W.N.W.: Role of the granuloma in recurrent Crohn's disease, Gut **17**:75, 1976.
87. Godwin, J.D.: Carcinoid tumor: an analysis of 2,837 cases, Cancer **36**:560, 1975.
88. Golden, R., and Stout, A.P.: Superficial spreading carcinoma of the stomach, Am. J. Roentgenol. **59**:157, 1948.
89. Goldgraber, M.B., and Kirsner, J.B.: Scleroderma of the gastrointestinal tract: a review, Arch. Pathol. **64**:255, 1957.
90. Goldman, H., and Rosoff, C.B.: Pathogenesis of acute gastric stress ulcers, Am. J. Pathol. **52**:227, 1968.
91. Gonzales, T.A., et al.: Legal medicine, pathology and toxicology, ed. 2, New York, 1954, Appleton-Century-Crofts.
92. Gould, V.E.: Neuroendocrinomas and neuroendocrine carcinomas: APUD cell system neoplasms and their aberrant secretory activities, Pathol. Annu. **12**:33, 1977.
93. Goulston, S.J.M., and McGovern, V.J.: Pseudo-membranous colitis, Gut **6**:207, 1965.
94. Grace, A.W.: Anorectal lymphogranuloma venereum, J.A.M.A. **122**:74, 1943.
95. Grimes, O.F., and Stephens, B.H.: Surgical management of acquired short esophagus, Ann. Surg. **152**:743, 1960.
96. Grinnell, R.S.: The spread of carcinoma of the colon and the rectum, Cancer **3**:641, 1950.
97. Grinvalsky, H.T., and Bowerman, C.I.: Stercoraceous ulcers of the colon: relatively neglected medical and surgical problems, J.A.M.A. **171**:1941, 1959.
98. Groll, A., et al.: Immunological defect in Whipple's disease, Gastroenterology **63**:943, 1972.
99. Grossman, M.I., et al.: A new look at peptic ulcer, Ann. Intern. Med. **84**:57, 1976.
100. Hernandez, F.J., and Fernandez, B.B.: Mucus-secreting colonic carcinoid tumors: light and electron microscopic study of three cases, Dis. Colon Rectum **17**:387, 1974.
101. Hernandez, F.J., and Reid, J.D.: Mixed carcinoid and mucus-secreting intestinal tumor, Arch. Pathol. **88**:489, 1969.
102. Higa, E., et al.: Mucosal hyperplasia, mucinous cystadenoma and mucinous cystadenocarcinoma of the appendix: a re-evaluation of appendiceal "mucocele," Cancer **32**:1525, 1973.
103. Horn, R.C., Jr.: Carcinoid tumors of the colon and rectum, Cancer **2**:819, 1949.
104. Horn, R.C., Jr.: Carcinoma of stomach: autopsy findings in untreated cases, Gastroenterology **29**:515, 1955.
105. Horn, R.C., Jr., Payne, W.A., and Fine, G.: The Peutz-Jeghers syndrome (gastrointestinal polyposis with mucocutaneous pigmentation): report of a case terminating with disseminated gastrointestinal cancer, Arch. Pathol. **76**:29, 1963.
106. Horsley, J.S.: Peritonitis, Arch. Surg. **36**:190, 1938.
107. Hoskins, L.C., et al.: Functional and morphologic alterations of the gastrointestinal tract in progressive systemic sclerosis (scleroderma), Am. J. Med. **33**:459, 1962.
108. Hyun, B.H., Palumbo, V.N., and Null, R.H.: Hemangioma of the small intestine with gastrointestinal bleeding, J.A.M.A. **208**:1903, 1969.
109. Ismail-Beigi, F., Horton, P.F., and Pope, C.E., II: Histological consequences of gastroesophageal reflux in man, Gastroenterology **58**:163, 1970.
110. Jacobs, D.S.: Primary gastric malignant lymphoma and pseudolymphoma, Am. J. Clin. Pathol. **40**:379, 1963.
111. Jang, G.C., Clouse, M.E., and Fleischner, F.G.: Fibrovascular polyp—a benign intraluminal tumor of the esophagus, Radiology **92**:1196, 1969.
112. Johns, T.N.P., Wheeler, J.R., and Johns, F.S.: Meckel's diverticulum and Meckel's disease: a study of 154 cases, Ann. Surg. **150**:241, 1959.
113. Johnson, H.D.: Gastric ulcer: classification, blood group characteristics, secretion patterns and pathogenesis, Ann. Surg. **162**:996, 1965.
114. Johnstone, J.M., and Morson, B.C.: Eosinophilic gastroenteritis, Histopathology **2**:335, 1978.
115. Johnstone, J.M., and Morson, B.C.: Inflammatory fibroid polyp of the gastrointestinal tract, Histopathology **2**:349, 1978.
116. Joseph, J.I., and Lattes, R.: Gastric lymphosarcoma: clinicopathologic analysis of 71 cases and its relation to disseminated lymphosarcoma, Am. J. Clin. Pathol. **45**:653, 1966.
117. Kapila, L., Haberkorn, S., and Nixon, H.H.: Chronic adynamic bowel simulating Hirschsprung's disease, J. Pediatr. Surg. **10**:885, 1975.
118. Kay, S.: A 10-year appraisal of the treatment of squamous cell carcinoma of the esophagus, Surg. Gynecol. Obstet. **117**:167, 1963.
119. Kay, S., et al.: Glomus tumors of stomach, Cancer **4**:726, 1951.
120. Kean, B.H., Gilmore, H.R., Jr., and Van Stone, W.W.: Fatal amebiasis: report of 148 fatal cases from the Armed Forces Institute of Pathology, Ann. Intern. Med **44**:831, 1956.
121. Keeley, A.F., and Gottlieb, L.S.: Villous adenoma of the small bowel: an unusual lesion, Gastroenterology **57**:185, 1969.
122. Kemler, B.J., and Alpert, E.: Inflammatory bowel disease associated with circulating immune complexes, Gut **21**:195, 1980.
123. Kern, F., Jr.: Hepatobiliary disorders in inflammatory bowel disease, Prog. Liver Dis. **5**:575, 1976.
124. Kepes, J.J., and Zacharias, D.L.: Gangliocytic paragangliomas of the duodenum: a report of two cases with light and electron microscopic examination, Cancer **27**:61, 1971.
125. Keyting, W.S., et al.: Pneumatosis intestinalis: a new concept, Radiology **76**:733, 1961.
126. Kiesewetter, W.B., Turner, C.R., and Sieber, W.K.: Imperforate anus: review of a sixteen-year experience with 146 patients, Am. J. Surg. **107**:412, 1964.
127. King, B.T.: New concepts of etiology and treatment of diverticula of esophagus, Gynecol. Obstet. **85**:93, 1947.
128. Kissane, J.M.: Pathology of infancy and childhood, ed. 2, St. Louis, 1975, The C.V. Mosby Co.

129. Klotz, Jr., R.G., Pamukcoglu, T., and Souilliard, D.H.: Transitional cloacogenic carcinoma of the anal canal: clinicopathologic study of 373 cases, Cancer **20**:1727, 1967.
130. Knauer, C.M.: Mallory-Weiss syndrome: characterization of 75 Mallory-Weiss lacerations in 528 patients with upper gastrointestinal hemorrhage, Gastroenterology **71**:5, 1976.
131. Lane, N.: Pseudosarcoma (polypoid sarcoma-like masses) associated with squamous cell carcinoma of the mouth, fauces, and larynx, Cancer **10**:19, 1957.
132. Lane, N.: The precursor tissue of ordinary large bowel cancer, Cancer Res. **36**:2669, 1976.
133. Larson, H.E., Price, A.B., and Honour, P.: *Clostridium difficile* and the etiology of pseudomembranous colitis, Lancet **1**:1063, 1978.
134. Lewin, K.J., et al.: Gastric morphology and serum gastrin levels in pernicious anemia, Gut **17**:551, 1976.
135. Liebowitz, H.R.: Pathogenesis of esophageal varix rupture, J.A.M.A. **175**:874, 1961.
136. Limber, G.K., King, R.E., and Silverberg, S.G.: *Pseudomyxoma peritonaei:* a report of ten cases, Ann. Surg. **178**:587, 1973.
137. Lou, T.Y., Teplitz, C., and Thayer, W.R.: Ultrastructural morphogenesis of colonic PAS-positive macrophages ("colonic histiocytosis"), Hum. Pathol. **2**:421, 1971.
138. Lough, J., et al.: Wolman's disease: electron microscopic, histochemical, and biochemical studies, Arch. Pathol. **89**:103, 1970.
139. Lupovitch, A., and Tippins, R.: Esophageal intramural pseudodiverticulosis: a disease of adnexal gland, Radiology **113**:271, 1974.
140. Maizel, H., Ruffin, J.M., and Dobbins, W.O., III: Whipple's disease: a review of 19 patients from one hospital and a review of the literature since 1950, Medicine **49**:175, 1970.
141. Marchand, P.: The anatomy of esophageal hiatus of the diaphragm and the pathogenesis of hiatus herniation, J. Thorac. Surg. **37**:81, 1959.
142. Marsden, H.B., and Gilchrist, W.: Pulmonary heterotopia in the terminal ileum, J. Pathol. Bacteriol. **86**:532, 1963.
143. Marston, A.: Basic structure and function of the intestinal circulation, Clin. Gastroenterol. **1**:539, 1972.
144. Martin, E.D., and Potet, F.: Pathology of endocrine tumors of the GI tract, Clin. Gastroenterol. **3**:511, 1974.
145. Martin, F.F., et al.: Immunological alterations in patients with treated Whipple's disease, Gastroenterology **63**:6, 1972.
146. Martinez, N.S., et al.: Heterotopic pancreatic tissue involving the stomach, Ann. Surg. **147**:1, 1958.
147. Matsusaka, T., Watanabe, H., and Enjoji, M.: Pseudosarcoma and carcinosarcoma of the esophagus, Cancer **37**:1546, 1976.
148. Mayo, C.W., Stalker, L.K., and Miller, J.M.: Intra-abdominal hernia: review of 39 cases in which treatment was surgical, Ann. Surg. **114**:875, 1941.
149. Mazier, W.P., et al.: Juvenile polyps of the rectum, Dis. Colon Rectum **17**:523, 1974.
150. Means, R.L.: Bile peritonitis, Am. Surg. **30**:583, 1964.
151. Meir-Ruge, W.: Hirschsprung's disease: its etiology, pathogenesis and differential diagnosis, Curr. Top. Pathol. **59**:131, 1974.
152. Mendeloff, A.I., and Dunn, J.P.: Digestive disease, vital and health statistics monographs, Cambridge, Mass., 1971, Harvard University Press.
153. Menguy, R.: Pathophysiology of peptic ulcer, Am. J. Surg. **120**:282, 1970.
154. Ming, S.C.: The classification and significance of gastric polyps; International Academy of Pathology monograph. The gastrointestinal tract, Baltimore, 1977, The Williams & Wilkins Co.
155. Ming, S.C.: Gastric carcinoma: a pathological classification, Cancer **39**:2475, 1977.
156. Mitchell, D.N., Rees, R.J.W., and Goswami, K.K.A.: Transmissible agents from human sarcoid and Crohn's disease tissue, Lancet **2**:761, 1976.
157. Mitchison, M.J.: The pathology of idiopathic retroperitoneal fibrosis, J. Clin. Pathol. **23**:681, 1970.
158. Moertel, C.G., et al.: Life history of the carcinoid tumor of the small intestine, Cancer **14**:901, 1961.
159. Moldawer, M.: Multiple endocrine tumors and Zollinger-Ellison syndrome in families: one or two syndromes? A report of two families, Metabolism **11**:153, 1962.
160. Moore, G.E., and Sako, K.: The spread of carcinoma of the colon and rectum: a study of invasion of blood vessels, lymph nodes and the peritoneum by tumor cells, Dis. Colon Rectum **2**:92, 1959.
161. Morgan, C.N.: Malignancy in inflammatory disease of the large intestine, Cancer **28**:41, 1971.
162. Morningstar, W.A.: Whipple's disease: an example of the value of the electron microscope in diagnosis, follow-up, and correlation of a pathologic process, Hum. Pathol. **6**:443, 1975.
163. Morrison, A.B., Rawson, A.J., and Fitts, W.T., Jr.: The syndrome of refractory watery diarrhea and hypokalemia in patients with a non-insulin-secreting islet cell tumor: a further case study and review of the literature, Am. J. Med. **32**:119, 1962.
164. Morson, B.C.: Polyps and cancer of the large bowel, International Academy of Pathology monograph. The gastrointestinal tract, Baltimore, 1977, The Williams & Wilkins Co.
165. Morson, B.C., and Valkstadt, H.: Mucoepidermoid tumors of the anal canal, J. Clin. Pathol. **16**:200, 1963.
166. Moses, H.L., and Cheatham, W.J.: The frequency and significance of human herpetic esophagitis: an autopsy study, Lab. Invest. **12**:663, 1963.
167. Murphy, R.T., et al.: Peptic ulceration with associated endocrine tumors: collective review and report of a case, Am. J. Surg. **100**:764, 1960.
168. Muto, T., Bussey, H.J.R., and Morson, B.C.: Pseudocarcinomatous invasion in adenomatous polyps of the colon and rectum, J. Clin. Pathol. **26**:25, 1973.
169. Naef, A.P., Savary, M., and Ozzello, L.: Columnar-lined lower esophagus: an acquired lesion with malignant predisposition: report on 140 cases of Barrett's esophagus with 12 adenocarcinomas, J. Thorac. Cardiovasc. Surg. **70**:826, 1975.
170. Nesbit, R.R., et al.: Carcinoma of the small bowel: a complication of regional enteritis, Cancer **37**:2948, 1976.
171. Norberg, P.B.: Food as a cause of intestinal obstruction, Am. J. Surg. **104**:444, 1962.
172. Norris, H.T.: Ischemic bowel disease: its spectrum, International Academy of Pathology monograph. The gastrointestinal tract, Baltimore, 1977, The Williams & Wilkins Co.
173. Ochsner, A., and Gage, I.M.: Adynamic ileus, Am. J. Surg. **20**:378, 1933.
174. Ogden, W.W., Bradburn, D.M., and Rives, J.D.: Mesenteric panniculitis: review of 27 cases, Ann. Surg. **161**:864, 1965.
175. Painter, N.S., and Burkitt, D.P.: Diverticular disease of the colon: a 20th century problem, Clin. Gastroenterol. **4**:3, 1975.
176. Parathap, K., and Gilman, R.: The histiopathology of acute intestinal amebiasis: a rectal biopsy study, Am. J. Pathol. **60**:229, 1970.
177. Parks, A.G.: Pathogenesis and treatment of fistula-in-ano, Br. Med. J. **1**:463, 1961.
178. Paull, A., et al.: The histologic spectrum of Barrett's esophagus, N. Engl. J. Med. **295**:476, 1976.
179. Perea, V.D., and Gregory, L.J., Jr.: Neurofibromatosis of the stomach: report of a case associated with von Recklinghausen's disease and review of the literature, J.A.M.A. **182**:259, 1962.
180. Perera, D.R., Weinstein, W.M., and Rubin, C.E.: Small intestinal biopsy, Hum. Pathol. **6**:157, 1975.
181. Perkins, D.E., and Spjut, H.J.: Intestinal stenosis following radiation therapy, Am. J. Roentgenol. **88**:953, 1962.
182. Pomerantz, M., and Waldmann, T.A.: Systemic lymphatic abnormalities associated with gastrointestinal protein loss secondary to intestinal lymphangiectasia, Gastroenterology **45**:703, 1963.
183. Price, A.B., and Davies, D.R.: Pseudomembranous colitis, J. Clin. Pathol. **30**:1, 1977.
184. Pruitt, B.A., Jr., Foley, F.D., and Moncrief, J.A.: Curling's ulcer: a clinical-pathological study of 323 cases, Ann. Surg. **172**:523, 1970.
185. Putman, H.C., Jr., Dockerty, M.B., and Waugh, J.M.: Abdominal actinomycosis: analysis of 122 cases, Surgery **28**:781, 1950.
186. Qizilbash, A.H., Meghji, M., and Castelli, M.: Pseudocarcinomatous invasion in adenomas of the colon and rectum, Dis. Colon Rectum **23**:529, 1980.
187. Quan, S.H.Q., White, J.E., and Deddish, M.R.: Malignant melanoma of the anorectum, Dis. Colon Rectum **2**:275, 1959.
188. Ranchod, M., and Kempson, L.: Smooth muscle tumors of the gastrointestinal tract and retroperitoneum: a pathologic analysis of 100 cases, Cancer **39**:255, 1977.

189. Rector, L.E., and Connerley, M.L.: Aberrant mucosa in esophagus in infants and in children, Arch. Pathol. **31**:285, 1941.
190. Regan, J.F., and Cremin, J.H.: Chorionepithelioma of the stomach, Am. J. Surg. **100**:224, 1960.
191. Renton, C.J.C.: Non-occlusive intestinal infarction, Clin. Gastroenterol. **1**:655, 1972.
192. Rhodes, J., and Calcraft, B.: Aetiology of gastric ulcer with special reference to the roles of reflux and mucosal damage, Clin. Gastroenterol. **2**:227, 1973.
193. Riddell, R.H.: The precarcinomatous lesion of ulcerative colitis, International Academy of Pathology monograph. The gastrointestinal tract, Baltimore, 1977, The Williams & Wilkins Co.
194. Roth, S.I., and Helwig, E.B.: Juvenile polyps of the colon and rectum, Cancer **16**:468, 1963.
195. Rubin, H., et al.: The course and prognosis of histoplasmosis, Am. J. Med. **27**:278, 1959.
196. Sachatello, C.R., Pickren, J.W., and Grace, J.T., Jr.: Generalized juvenile gastrointestinal polyposis: a hereditary syndrome, Gastroenterology **58**:699, 1970.
197. Sahai, D.B., Palmer, J.S., and Hampson, L.G.: Submucosal lipomas of the large bowel, Can. J. Surg. **11**:23, 1968.
198. Sanusi, I.D., and Tio, F.O.: Gastrointestinal malakoplakia: report of a case and a review of the literature, Am. J. Gastroenterol. **62**:356, 1974.
199. Saphir, O., and Parker, M.L.: Linitis plastica type of carcinoma, Surg. Gynecol. Obstet. **76**:206, 1943.
200. Schenken, J.R., and Moss, E.S.: *Enterobius vermicularis* in appendix: report of study on 1,000 surgically removed appendices, Am. J. Clin. Pathol. **12**:509, 1942.
201. Schreiber, D.S., Trier, J.S., and Blacklow, N.R.: Recent advances in viral gastoenteritis, Gastroenterology **73**:174, 1977.
202. Schwartz, F.D., Dunea, G., and Kark, R.M.: Methysergide and retroperitoneal fibrosis, Am. Heart J. **72**:843, 1966.
203. Scully, R.E.: Sex cord tumor with annular tubules: a distinctive ovarian tumor of the Peutz-Jeghers syndrome, Cancer **25**:1107, 1970.
204. Seagram, C.G.F., et al.: Meckel's diverticulum: a 10-year review of 218 cases, Can. J. Surg. **11**:369, 1968.
205. Shamma'a, M.H., and Benedict, E.B.: Esophageal webs, N. Engl. J. Med. **259**:378, 1958.
206. Sieracki, J.C., and Fine, G.: Whipple's disease—observations on systemic involvement. II. Gross and histologic observations, Arch. Pathol. **67**:81, 1959.
207. Sizer, J.S., Frederick, P.L., and Osborne, M.P.: Primary linitis plastica of the colon: report of a case and review of the literature, Dis. Colon Rectum **10**:339, 1967.
208. Skandalakis, J.E., Gray, S.W., and Shepard, D.: Smooth muscle tumor of the stomach, Int. Abst. Surg. **110**:209, 1960.
209. Smith, B.H., and Welter, E.H.: Pneumatosis intestinalis, Am. J. Clin. Pathol. **48**:455, 1967.
210. Smith, C.R., Jr., Bartholomew, L.G., and Cain, J.C.: Hereditary hemorrhagic telangiectasia and gastrointestinal hemorrhage, Gastroenterology **44**:1, 1963.
211. Sobel, H.J., et al.: Granulomas and peritonitis due to starch glove powder, Arch. Pathol. **91**:559, 1971.
212. Sohar, E., et al.: Familial Mediterranean fever: a survey of 470 cases and review of the literature, Am. J. Med. **43**:227, 1967.
213. Southwick, H.W., Harridge, W.H., and Cole, W.H.: Recurrence at the suture line following resection for carcinoma of the colon: incidence following preventive measure, Am. J. Surg. **103**:86, 1962.
214. Spira, I.A., Ghazi, A., and Wolff, W.I.: Primary adenocarcinoma of the duodenum, Cancer **39**:1721, 1977.
215. Starr, G.F., and Dockerty, M.B.: Leiomyomas and leiomyosarcomas of the small intestine, Cancer **8**:101, 1955.
216. Stempien, S.J., et al.: Hypertrophic hypersecretory gastropathy: analysis of 15 cases and a review of the pertinent literature, Am. J. Dis. **9**:471, 1964.
217. Stout, A.P.: Pathology of carcinoma of the stomach, Arch. Surg. **46**:807, 1943.
218. Stout, A.P.: Mesotheliomas of pleura and peritoneum, J. Tenn. Med. Assoc. **44**:409, 1951.
219. Stout, A.P., Hendry, J., and Purdie, F.J.: Primary solid tumors of the great omentum, Cancer **16**:231, 1963.
220. Strickland, R.J., and Mackay, I.R.: A reappraisal of the nature and significance of chronic atrophic gastritis, Am. J. Dig. Dis. **18**:426, 1973.
221. Tagart, R.E.B.: Endometriosis of the large intestine, Br. J. Surg. **47**:27, 1959.
222. Tallquist, A., Salmela, H., and Lindstrom, B.L.: Leiomyoblastoma of the stomach, Acta Pathol. Microbiol. Scand. **71**:194, 1967.
223. Tedeschi, C.G., and Botta, G.C.: Retractile mesenteritis, N. Engl. J. Med. **266**:1035, 1962.
224. Therkelsen, F.: On histological diagnosis of appendicitis, Acta Chir. Scand. **94**(suppl. 108):1, 1946.
225. Thompson, H.: Vascular pathology of the splanchnic circulation, Clin. Gastroenterol. **1**:597, 1972.
226. Thompson, H.L., and McGuffin, D.W.: Melena: study of underlying causes, J.A.M.A. **141**:1208, 1949.
227. Tonkin, R.D., Field, T.E., and Wykes, P.R.: Pancreatic heterotopia as a cause of dyspepsia, Gut **3**:135, 1962.
228. Torma, M.J., et al.: Necrotizing enterocolitis in infants: analysis of forty-five consecutive cases, Am. J. Surg. **126**:758, 1973.
229. Trier, J.S., et al.: Whipple's disease: light and electron microscope correlation of jejunal mucosal histology with antibiotic treatment and clinical status, Gastroenterology **48**:684, 1965.
230. Trier, J.S., et al.: Celiac sprue and refractory sprue, Gastroenterology **75**:307, 1978.
231. Tumen, H.J.: Intestinal obstruction. In Bockus, H.L.: Gastroenterology, ed. 2, Philadelphia, 1964, W.B. Saunders Co.
232. Turcot, J., Despres, M.P., and St. Pierre, F.: Malignant tumors of the central nervous system associated with familial polyposis of the colon, Dis. Colon Rectum **2**:465, 1959.
233. Valdes-Dapena, A., et al.: Adenocarcinoma of the small bowel in association with regional enteritis: four new cases, Cancer **37**:2938, 1976.
234. Waldmann, T.A., et al.: The role of the gastrointestinal system in "idiopathic hypoproteinemia," Gastroenterology **41**:197, 1961.
235. Wangensteen, O.H., and Dennis, C.: Experimental proof of the obstructive origin of appendicitis in man, Ann. Surg. **110**:629, 1939.
236. Wayte, D.M., and Helwig, E.B.: Colitis cystica profunda, Am. J. Clin. Pathol. **48**:159, 1967.
237. Wayte, D.M., and Helwig, E.B.: Small-bowel ulceration—iatrogenic or multifactorial origin? Am. J. Clin. Pathol. **49**:26, 1968.
238. Weedon, D.D., et al.: Crohn's disease and cancer, N. Engl. J. Med. **289**:1099, 1973.
239. Weinstein, E.C., Cain, J.C., and ReMine, W.H.: Meckel's diverticulum: 55 years of clinical and surgical experience, J.A.M.A. **182**:251, 1962.
240. Weinstein, W.M., et. al.: Collagenous sprue—an unrecognized type of malabsorption, N. Engl. J. Med. **283**:1297, 1970.
241. Wells, C.L, Moran, T.J., and Cooper, W.M.: Villous tumors of the rectosigmoid colon, with severe electrolyte imbalance: a cause of unexplained morbidity and sudden mortality, Am. J. Clin. Pathol. **37**:507, 1962.
242. Whitehead, R.: The pathology of ischemia of the intestines, Pathol. Annu. **11**:1, 1976.
243. Whitehead, R., Truelove, S.C., and Gear, W.L.: The histological diagnosis of chronic gastritis in fibre optic gastroscope biopsy specimens, J. Clin. Pathol. **25**:1, 1972.
244. Williams, E.D., and Sandler, M.: The classification of carcinoid tumors, Lancet **1**:238, 1963.
245. Windsor, C.W.O.: Ischemic strictures of the small bowel, Clin. Gastroenterol. **1**:707, 1972.
246. Winslow, D.J., and Taylor, H.B.: Malignant peritoneal mesotheliomas: a clinicopathological analysis of 12 fatal cases, Cancer **12**:127, 1960.
247. Wolf, S.: Summary of evidence relating life situation and emotional response to peptic ulcer, Ann. Intern. Med. **31**:637, 1949.
248. Yannopoulos, K., and Stout, A.P.: Primary solid tumors of the mesentery, Cancer **16**:914, 1963.
249. Yardley, J.H., Bayless, T.M., and Diamond, M.P.: Cancer in ulcerative colitis, Gastroenterology **76**:221, 1979.

CHAPTER 27 Liver

HUGH A. EDMONDSON
ROBERT L. PETERS

The subspecialty of liver disease is now known as hepatology, and clinicians with a major interest in this field are called hepatologists. Liver disease has steadily gained recognition as a major health problem, principally because of the worldwide distribution of viral hepatitis, the ubiquity of cirrhosis of the liver, and the relationship of both to the increasing incidence of one of the world's most common malignant tumors, hepatocellular carcinoma. The symptoms of liver disease, such as jaundice, fever, abdominal enlargement, and encephalopathy, are striking phenomena that may bring the patient to the physician. The need for interpretation of the increasing number of laboratory, ultrasonographic, and radiologic tests plus needle biopsy of the liver makes it imperative that the physician have a sound knowledge of the pathology of this most interesting organ and its multitudinous functions. In this chapter an attempt is made to present not only the pathology of liver disease but also many of the clinical and laboratory features as they apply to specific diseases of the liver.

GENERAL CONSIDERATIONS

Embryology and structure

The liver arises from the hepatic diverticulum in the 20- to 25-somite embryo. The primitive hepatic cells grow into the septum transversum, where the endodermal cells proliferate rapidly. At the same time, rapid growth of the mesoderm produces angioblasts and sinusoids.[40] The formation of hepatocytes is determined by an interaction between the endodermal cells and the precardiac mesoderm.[25] Glycogen granules are noted at 8 weeks. The development of intrahepatic bile ducts is complete at 3 months,[4,23] at which time bile secretion is said to begin. In the third month the liver begins to store iron and concurrently becomes the chief blood-forming organ of the embryo. The site of hematopoiesis is in the extravascular component of the lobule.[18,47] This hematopoietic function is gradually transferred to the bone marrow as it develops so that by the time of birth only an occasional focus of hematopoiesis remains. In premature infants areas of hematopoiesis are abundant. In the full-term baby the liver weighs about 135 g, ranging from 75 to 180 g, and projects well below the costal margin.[32] The left lobe is relatively large in the neonate. During fetal life this lobe receives well-oxygenated blood from the umbilical vein. The latter structure atrophies after parturition and becomes the round ligament. The omphalomesenteric veins drain predominantly into the large right lobe of the liver, and from these veins evolves the portal vein.

The liver grows at a relatively slower rate than the rest of the body, reaching approximately 1350 g in an adult. At maturity the liver is located most commonly at or above the costal margin. However, it is not unusual for the lower edge to be 1 to 3 cm below the costal margin. The right lobe becomes much larger than the left, and the organ is held firmly in the right hypochondrium and epigastrium by the falciform and triangular ligaments. Anatomically the dividing line between the right and left lobes is 1 to 1.5 cm to the right of the falciform ligament, approximating the gallbladder-caval line. The division of the liver into various segments, each with its separate blood supply, makes a study of surgical anatomy worthy of emphasis.[27,31]

A firm, smooth layer of connective tissue (Glisson's capsule) encloses the liver and is continuous with similar tissue in the porta hepatis, the latter forming a sheath around the portal vein, hepatic artery, and bile ducts that enter the hilum of the liver. This connective tissue surrounds all subdivisions of the blood vessels and ducts to the finest radicles, where it joins the inner aspect of Glisson's capsule. The portal vein, hepatic artery, and common hepatic duct divide in the porta hepatis into right and left branches that supply the two lobes of the liver. In their subsequent ramification through the liver, the branches of the artery, vein, and hepatic duct are always together in the portal tracts. Injection and corrosion methods have shown that among the structures of the portal triad, the portal vein is the largest. The hepatic artery, being much smaller, tends to twine about it like a vine over the trunk of a tree. The branches of the hepatic duct are about the same size as those of the hepatic artery. The latter are subject to many gross anatomic variations.[28]

The hepatic parenchyma, as one may see with the unassisted eye or more clearly with the microscope, is composed of innumerable small lobules, each with a diameter of 0.5 to 2 mm and the shape of an irregular and somewhat pyramidal hexahedron. At the center of each lobule is the intralobular or central efferent vein, and around the periphery are four or five portal spaces arranged at regular intervals. This is the classic lobule of the liver.[15]

Rappaport[35] has described the functioning lobule or liver acinus that has a portal triad at its center and portions of several classic lobules around its periphery. The liver acinus probably represents the true functioning unit of the liver, but because it is difficult to recognize grossly and microscopically, pathologists in their descriptions of gross and microscopic specimens most often use the term *lobule* in its classic sense. Rappaport has identified the periportal area as zone 1, the portion surrounding the terminal hepatic venule as zone 3, and the intermediate tissue as zone 2.

The acini (lobules) are composed of hepatocytes so arranged between sinusoids that at least two cells at their poles opposite the sinusoids may form bile canaliculi.[15] Depending on the angle at which the cells are sectioned for histologic preparation, one may see cell groups of variable thickness. It is important from the functional standpoint that a hepatocyte-sinusoidal system does exist so that every hepatic cell abuts on a sinusoid through which blood passes from the portal vessels to the terminal hepatic venules and that the cell has access to the bile canalicular system. Liver cell membranes form the lining of the canaliculi and are arranged as microvilli when viewed with the electron microscope.[42] The canaliculi form an interlacing network that impinges on at least one side of every hepatic cell. These lead into larger channels that finally join the bile ductules at the margin of the lobule. At the junction, biliary duct epithelium and liver cells join in an uneven manner over a short distance.[42] The passage is surrounded by a rosette of biliary epithelium, termed cholangiole, duct of Hering, or bile preductule.[42] The sinusoids form a radial network that allows the blood to come into contact with every parenchymal cell as it flows to the terminal hepatic venules.

The sinusoidal system is lined with two types of cells: Kupffer cells and endothelial cells. Kupffer cells are especially prominent at the angular junctions of the sinusoids. They are members of a family of cells scattered throughout the body that are known as the mononuclear phagocyte system, or the reticuloendothelial system (RES).[37,45] The cells of this system arise from a common precursor cell of the bone marrow, the monoblast. They divide into promonocytes and monocytes and finally, after circulation, come to reside in the tissue as tissue macrophages. It has been estimated that 50% of circulating monocytes ultimately become Kupffer cells.[8] The Kupffer cells perform most efficiently in clearing the circulation of bacteria, microorganisms, neoplastic cells, and senescent or dead cells that may be harmful to the body.[37] They also secrete active biologic substances. In addition to the Kupffer cells, endothelial lining cells and parenchymal cells are also able to take up many substances that in the past were believed to be cleared only by the RES.[34] These substances are taken into the endothelial and parenchymal cells by adsorptive endocytosis.

The lining cells are held in place by interdigitations of their microvilli with the microvilli of the parenchymal cells. The cytoplasm of lining cells contains perforations so that blood plasma may circulate freely into the space between the lining cells and the parenchymal cells (Fig. 27-1). This space is known as Disse's space. It is not large enough normally to accommodate erythrocytes or leukocytes but averages about 0.33 μm or 300 to 400 nm in width.

The hepatocytes have a polyhedral shape, a round nucleus, and a fairly prominent nucleolus. Their fine structure has been extensively investigated.[26] The surface of the liver cell is in contact with (1) its neighbors, from which it is separated by narrow intercellular spaces, (2) Disse's space, and (3) the bile canaliculus (Fig. 27-1). Desmosomes are present along the lateral intercellular surface. Near the canaliculus, tight junctions are formed by the fusion of the external leaflets of the neighboring plasma membranes. The bile canaliculi are lined by rather short microvilli of adjoining liver cells. A large portion of the surface of the parenchymal cell is exposed to Disse's space. Combined cytochemical and electron microscopic studies have shown that the plasma membrane along the sinusoidal surface has strong alkaline phosphatase and nucleoside monophosphatase activities; nucleoside triphosphatase is most active on the bile canaliculus side. The hepatocytes contain many mitochondria, more in the periportal (zone 1) than in the perivenular (zone 3) areas. The endoplasmic cisternae are part of the distribution system that transports nutrients to all parts of the cell.[26] The Golgi apparatus has a convex and concave surface and is located between the nucleus and the bile canaliculus. It is the "packaging plant" of the liver cell. The bilirubin-conjugating enzyme is present in the smooth endoplasmic reticulum, but the transport mechanism for bilirubin glucuronide is not known. Normally, glycogen is abundant throughout the cytoplasm. Lysosomes are numerous, and in the functioning liver vesicles and vacuoles of variable size are present near

Disse's space. Vesicular invaginations of the plasma membrane occur between the bases of microvilli that project into Disse's space. Much knowledge has accumulated regarding the relation of liver function to structure through the use of newer techniques such as morphometry, freeze-fracture, and scanning electron microscopy.[20] Study of the structure by these newer techniques has greatly clarified the relationship of organelles to hepatocyte function. This applies particularly to the endoplasmic reticulum and the Golgi apparatus. Bile canaliculi form a polygonal network throughout the lobule so that a small portion of every liver cell contributes to the canalicular system.[3] The terminal hepatic venules and veins course through zone 3 of the lobules in a longitudinal fashion and empty into sublobular veins. The sublobular veins have specialized connective tissue walls, and since they are not associated with arteries and bile ducts, they are distinguished from branches of the portal vein. The sublobular veins unite to form the hepatic veins. The latter combine to form two large trunks and several smaller ones that open into the inferior vena cava. The vena cava passes through a groove on the posterior surface of the liver. The veins from the caudate lobe drain directly into the vena cava at this point. Large trunks of the hepatic vein form a single branching system that is not nearly as angulated and tortuous as the large branches of the portal vein.

Circulation

The liver receives about 1500 ml of blood per minute into its sinusoidal system. It is estimated that about 600 ml comes from the hepatic artery and 900 ml from the portal vein. Some 50% to 60% of the oxygen is supplied by the portal vein.[43] The latter system differs from the systemic venous system in that the blood is under a pressure of 8 to 10 mm Hg and has a relatively high oxygen content, usually about 80% saturated. The mixture of blood from a high-pressure arterial system (90 mm Hg) and a low-pressure venous system (8 to 10 mm Hg) is accomplished by a drop in arterial pressure consequent to the fine subdivisions of the hepatic arterioles that form a periductular plexus before the blood enters the peripheral sinusoids. Some small branches from the hepatic artery empty directly into the peripheral sinusoids, where the arterial flow has a siphoning effect on the sinusoidal system as blood with a faster velocity flows to the

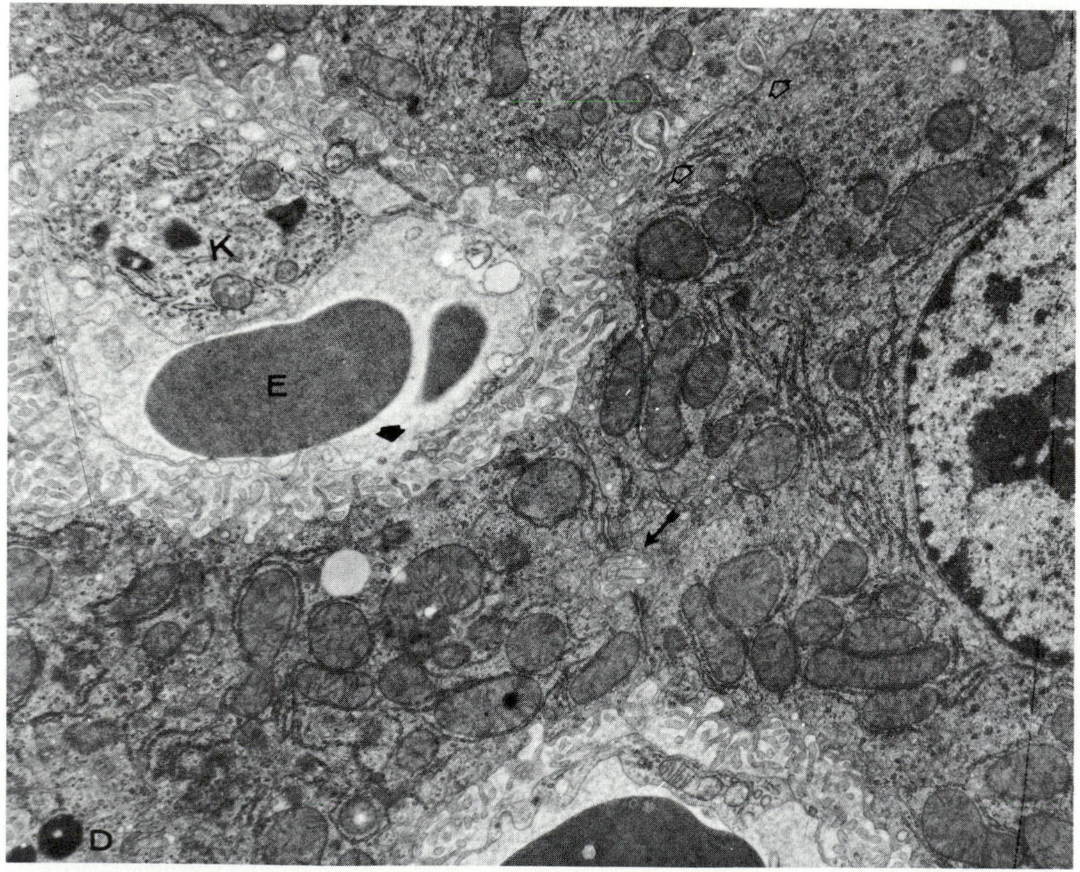

Fig. 27-1. Interlocking of liver cells is furnished by studlike projections of intercellular membrane *(open arrowheads). E,* Erythrocyte in sinusoid; *K,* Kupffer cell; *D,* dense body; *arrow,* bile canaliculus; *black arrowhead,* pore in endothelium lining.

terminal hepatic venules.[35] An intermittent type of flow has been observed that is no doubt regulated by the tonus of the hepatic arteriolar system and precapillary sphincters.[24]

Function and laboratory diagnosis

Healthy hepatocytes perform a multitude of functions that are concerned with the following[36]:

1. Secretion of bile and other substances
2. Intermediate metabolism of proteins, lipids, and carbohydrates
3. Storage of certain foodstuffs and minerals
4. Detoxification of various compounds and metabolism of hormones and drugs

In disease, one or more of these vital functions may be disturbed and can be measured by laboratory tests (Table 27-1), or the cause can be diagnosed by tissue examination. Among the laboratory tests used in the evaluation of liver disease are those related to the liver functions as just outlined. Other procedures measure either soluble enzymes that enter the blood when the liver cells are injured by disease or abnormal substances (proteins or otherwise) that are elaborated by diseased liver cells. Tests that measure specific antibodies produced by the reticuloendothelial system in certain diseases are widely used.

Tests of hepatocyte uptake and excretion

Bilirubin. Bilirubin is a product of hemoglobin degradation, and its accumulation is a measure of binding, conjugating, and excretory capacity of the hepatocyte relative to the erythrocyte degradation rate. Although not a sensitive indicator, bilirubin levels may rise in diseases of hepatocytes (necrosis), of excretion (duct obstruction) defects in conjugating enzymes (Gilbert's disease), and in hemolysis.

Bromosulfophthalein (BSP). This dye is removed from circulation by the same binding, conjugating, and excretory mechanisms as bilirubin. However, since a measured amount of BSP is introduced and measurement of residua made after a specific time lapse, greater sensitivity results from BSP than from bilirubin determination. Measurement of BSP removal has been useful in detecting liver disease when other tests have been normal, but the test has been largely supplanted by other techniques.

Tests of hepatocyte synthesis

Bile acids. The primary bile acids, cholic and chenodeoxycholic acids, are formed entirely in the hepatocyte from cholesterol and from recirculating bile acids. The bile acids are conjugated with the amino acids glycine or taurine in the hepatocyte and sequestered during the night in the normal gallbladder where a 10-fold concentration of the liver bile occurs. Feeding causes gallbladder contraction by stimulating the intestinal production of cholecystokinin. This in turn results in extrusion of a bolus of the conjugated bile acids into the gut, where these acids are deconjugated and absorbed or partially dehydrated into secondary bile acids and largely absorbed. Only 10% of the total bile acids is excreted in the feces as unabsorbable toxic lithocholic acid. Most of the reabsorbed bile acids enter the splanchnic bed and are removed in a single pass through a normal liver, reconjugated, and excreted. However, diseases involving function of the parenchymal cells are associated with failure of the hepatocytes to take up the bile acids from portal blood or to conjugate and excrete them. Diseases of cholestasis have restricted transport of bile acids through the duct system to the gut. Such diseases are associated with increased serum levels of bile acids. Cirrhosis or portal hypertension is associated with shunts of portal blood around the liver vascular bed, resulting in particularly high levels of postprandial bile acids.[33]

Serum proteins. Most serum proteins are produced by the hepatocytes and are synthesized in decreased amounts in hepatocellular disease. The serum levels of individual proteins in hepatocellular diseases are a function of biologic half-life and biologic "order of importance" in terms of diminished production.

Albumin. Albumin has a long biologic half-life; serum levels are diminished in chronic liver diseases but not in acute hepatocellular disease, unless it is protracted for 3 or 4 weeks.

Prothrombin. Prothrombin, as well as most other coagulation factors, is produced by the hepatocytes, and levels are reduced in severe chronic hepatocellular disease. Prothrombin and factor VII levels, because of their short half-lives, are also reduced in severe acute hepatocyte damage. Because of easier analysis, prothrombin activity is the preferred determination. Since vitamin K is required in the conversion of immunologically assayable prothrombin precursor (preprothrombin) to the active form, prothrombin activity is also reduced in vitamin K deficiency. Vitamin K assimilation is reduced either as a result of diminution of bile acid flow that normally emulsifies and permits absorption of fat-soluble vitamin K or because warfarin-like vitamin K antagonists have been administered. If vitamin K deficiency is the cause of low prothrombin levels, amounts of the precursor preprothrombin will be nearly normal in blood at a time the prothrombin activity is significantly reduced, and a correction of prothrombin activity occurs after parenteral administration of vitamin K. Both prothrombin and preprothrombin are decreased in hepatocellular disease, and vitamin K administration does not result in increased levels of either.[7,12]

Alpha-1-antitrypsin. Alpha-1-antitrypsin, an inhibitor of multiple proteases, is synthesized by the hepatocyte and is diminished in serum only in severe, acute hepatocellular necrosis, in severe chronic liver disease, or in genetically controlled production of aberrant types of the

Table 27-1. Laboratory findings in acute and chronic liver disease*

Normal values	Transferases (AST, 5-46 units; ALT, 8-40 units)	Bilirubin (1.2 mg/dl or less)	Urine urobilinogen (positive in 1:4 dilution)	Alkaline phosphatase†	Prothrombin: Percentage of normal level (normal = 100%)	Prothrombin: Response to vitamin K	Serum proteins (albumin, 3.5-4.5 g; globulin, 3-4 g)
ACUTE LIVER DISEASE							
Necrosis							
Viral hepatitis	High elevation (500-4000) early; ALT usually >AST	Mild to sharp increase (2-40)	Increased early and late but may be absent during phase of deepest jaundice	Normal or mild increase	Moderate to sharp decrease (10%-80%)	Poor	Normal except in a prolonged course or in elderly patients
Infectious mononucleosis	Moderate elevation (100-500)	Normal or mild increase (2-5)	Mild or moderate increase	Normal or mild increase	Normal or mild decrease	Poor	Normal
Chemical (CCl_4, methyldopa, halothane, isoniazid, paracetomol)	High elevation (500-5000), ALT usually >AST	Mild to sharp increase (2-40)	Usually increased but may be decreased during period of deepest jaundice	Normal or mild increase	Moderate to sharp decrease (5%-80%)	Poor	Normal
Acute alcoholic liver disease	AST, 75-300; ALT, 50	Usually moderately elevated	Mild to moderate increase	Slight elevation	Normal to sharp decrease	Poor	Albumin acutely decreased; globulin normal in early stage
Cholestasis (drug-induced)	Mild to moderate elevation (usually <300); AST and ALT approximately equal	Mild to moderate increase (3-15)	Variable—mild decrease to mild increase	Moderate to sharp increase	Normal or mild decrease (50%-100%)	Good	Normal
Extrahepatic obstruction Stone	Mild to moderate increase (100-300), AST and ALT equal	Mild to moderate increase; fluctuations (2-15)	Variable—may be absent but occasionally increased	Moderate to sharp increase	Normal or moderate decrease (40%-100%)	Good	Normal
Cancer	Same as for stone	Moderate elevation without fluctuation (10-20)	Absent	Moderate to sharp increase	Variable decrease, mild to sharp (20%-80%)	Good	Normal except for possible decrease in albumin because of malnutrition

*Many tests are necessarily omitted; for example, the BSP retention test is valuable but is used only for anicteric patients.
†May be measured in King-Armstrong units, Bodansky units, Bessey-Lowry units, or International units.

Table 27-1. Laboratory findings in acute and chronic liver disease—cont'd

Normal values	Transferases (AST, 5-46 units; ALT, 8-40 units)	Bilirubin (1.2 mg/dl or less)	Urine urobilinogen (positive in 1:4 dilution)	Alkaline phosphatase†	Prothrombin		Serum proteins (albumin, 3.5-4.5 g; globulin, 3-4 g)
					Percentage of normal level (normal = 100%)	Response to vitamin K	
CHRONIC LIVER DISEASE							
Biliary cirrhosis							
Secondary	Mild to moderate increase (100-300); AST often >ALT	Mild to moderate increase (3-15)	Variable—decreased to increased	Moderate to sharp increase	Mild to moderate decrease	Variable, poor to good	Albumin decreased; globulin increased
Primary	Same as for secondary	Same as for secondary	Same as for secondary	Sharp increase	Mild to moderate decrease	Variable, poor to good	Albumin decrease; globulin increased
Alcoholic cirrhosis	Same as for biliary cirrhosis	Anicteric to episodes of jaundice (2-40)	Usually increased	Normal or mild increase	Moderate to sharp decrease	Poor	Albumin decreased; globulin increased
"Lupoid" cirrhosis or chronic active hepatitis	Sharp increase during jaundice episodes (500-1500); AST often >ALT	Mild to moderate increase (2-20)	Usually increased	Variable—normal to sharp increase	Moderate to sharp decrease	Poor	Albumin decreased; globulin increased (often sharply)
OTHER LESIONS							
Abscess	Mild increase (<200)	Normal or slightly elevated	Normal	Normal to moderate increase	Normal		Albumin may be decreased if chronic
Cancer, primary or metastatic	Mild increase (<200)	Normal unless major bile ducts involved	Normal	Usually a moderate to sharp increase	Normal		Usually normal, but albumin may be decreased
Granulomas	Mild increase (<200)	Normal	Normal	Same as for cancer	Normal		Normal

protease inhibitor. Phenotyping of alpha-1-antitrypsin is used to identify the genetic variants that may occur; specifically, the homozygosity of the abnormal Z gene is associated with very low alpha-1-antitrypsin levels and often with juvenile cirrhosis.

Ceruloplasmin. Ceruloplasmin, another protein synthesized in the hepatocyte, has a function in copper transport. In hepatolenticular degeneration, a genetic disease, depressed serum ceruloplasmin levels are related to storage of huge amounts of copper in tissues and to the development of cirrhosis. Ceruloplasmin synthesis is stimulated by progestational oral contraceptives; conversely, nongenetically reduced levels occasionally may be found in patients with far advanced chronic liver disease, usually as a finding in a patient close to death.

Alpha-fetoprotein (AFP). Alpha-fetoprotein, the principal serum protein of the early fetus, is synthesized by the adult hepatocyte during reversion to a more primitive cell, as occurs during some types of active cell replication. As such, the AFP level is a measure of extent of regenerative activity in hepatitis B. Its principal use in study of liver disease has been for detection of hepatocellular carcinoma (HCC). Seventy-five percent of patients with HCC arising in B viral cirrhosis have AFP in excess of 500 ng/ml. HCC arising in a previously normal liver is associated with such levels of AFP in only 33% of cases. Other less common embryonal tumors (testicular embryonal carcinoma, choriocarcinomas, yolk sac tumor) also produce AFP, and during pregnancy the AFP of the fetus enters maternal circulation sufficiently to raise the AFP level in maternal serum.

Globulin. Globulin, in the broad sense, refers to the nonalbumin serum protein. The gamma globulins, which constitute the major fraction of the total globulins, are produced by the reticuloendothelial system as a response to inflammation. Total and gamma globulin levels are raised in many chronic liver diseases, as they are in many nonhepatic inflammatory diseases.

Cell products stimulated by disease. Some cellular enzymes are released in increased amounts in disease as a result of increased production.

Alkaline phosphatase activity. Alkaline phosphatase, or more precisely the phosphomonoesterases with optimal activity in the alkaline pH range, are grouped together and called serum alkaline phosphatase.[21] Alkaline phosphatases are present in endothelium, surface epithelia of many mucosal surfaces, neutrophils, placenta, bone, renal tubules, and, to some extent, liver canaliculi.[6] Despite the uncertain source and largely undetermined function, serum alkaline phosphatase activity is a valuable and sensitive liver test. For practical purposes, only liver diseases, bone abnormalities, bone growth, and late pregnancy are associated with elevations in activity. Although the serum alkaline phosphatase activity may rise in the presence of any liver disease, the greatest elevations occur in biliary tract obstruction. Increase in alkaline phosphatase activity found in a patient with a space-occupying mass in the liver may be the only abnormality in the usual screening panel of laboratory tests.

Electrophoretic studies of elevated alkaline phosphatase in the serum suggest that one band, L, is the isoenzyme derived from the liver. The isoenzymes from the intestine and bone are indicated as band I and band B. Increase in "liver" alkaline phosphatase may be associated with liver disease, but the same fraction is elevated in some patients with bone disorders and in others with no hepatic disease.[5] Thus it appears that alkaline phosphatase isoenzyme levels still lack good clinical correlation.

Leucine aminopeptidase (LAP, leucine arylamidase) and 5′-nucleotidase (5′-nase). Leucine aminopeptidase and 5′-nucleotidase are enzymes that have widespread distribution in body tissues, but serum activity levels are rarely elevated except in obstructive diseases of the biliary tract. Either test is helpful in patients who have elevated alkaline phosphatase activity without evidence of liver disease. Because bone disease is not associated with elevated serum activities of LAP or 5′-nase, an increase in LAP and 5′-nase levels indicates that the elevation of alkaline phosphatase activity is related to hepatobiliary disease.[39]

Alpha-glutamyl-transpeptidase (GGTP). Alpha-glutamyl-transpeptidase is an enzyme abundant in the kidney and somewhat less so in the pancreas, but the liver is apparently the source of the enzyme found in serum. The normal function of the enzyme is to catalyze a reaction between glutathione and an amino acid. Serum levels of GGTP activity are erratic and quantitatively unrelated to the extent of hepatocellular necrosis. However, the test is useful in detecting some additional abnormality in patients with quiescent liver disease. In alcoholic patients who have regained a stable pattern of laboratory test values, elevated GGTP levels develop if they start drinking again. The GGTP may be the only test that shows abnormal results in sera of patients who have resumed alcoholism.

Tests of hepatocyte disruption

Aminotransferases (transaminases). Serum aspartate aminotransferase (AST) and alanine aminotransferase (ALT) are the two hepatic parenchymal cell enzymes that are most frequently quantitatively assessed in the evaluation of liver cell necrosis. Hepatocellular damage brings about the release of many cytoplasmic components. Some are unstable and others, which may also originate in extrahepatic tissues, are unsuitable for diagnosis. ALT is fairly restricted to liver tissue. It is unbound to ultrastructures, is quite soluble,[38] and apparently leaks through damaged but viable cell membranes. AST is present in other tissues but in smaller quantities than in the liver.[29] Earlier and still commonly used terms for AST and ALT are glutamic oxaloacetic transaminase (GOT) and glutamic pyruvic transaminase (GPT), respectively.

Lactic acid dehydrogenase fraction 1, isocitric dehydrogenase, sorbital dehydrogenase, glutamate dehydrogenase, ornithine carbamyl transferase, alcohol dehydrogenase, and guanase. These enzymes, present in liver in much higher quantities than in other tissues, are released as a result of hepatocellular damage. The determination of levels in sera seems to have no diagnostic advantage over assessing the AST and ALT levels, since the latter two enzymes have well-established use. Serum guanase activity, however, does appear to be a simple, precise, and reproducible indicator of liver cell death.

Tests for specific etiologic agents or antibodies to agents

Hepatitis B surface antigen (HBsAg). The hepatitis B surface antigen, a 20 nm particulate material, is a noninfective product of hepatitis B virus. The hepatitis virus, which proliferates in the hepatocytes, produces its surface coating in great excess, to be released into the serum as HBsAg. HBsAg can be demonstrated histologically in the liver tissue in some patients with chronic varieties of hepatitis B.[9,13,14] Demonstration in tissues is by immunofluorescent or immunoperoxidase reaction specifically toward HBsAg[1,19] or by the orcein stain.[41] The latter apparently demonstrates the disulfide bonding of HBsAg. HBsAg has been demonstrated in tissue of some patients with chronic liver disease when serum levels of the antigen were undetectable.[1] A confirmed positive test for HBsAg is definitive proof of infection (either acute or chronic) by hepatitis B.

Anti–hepatitis B core (anti-HBc). Anti–hepatitis B core is an antibody to the protected core of the hepatitis B virus. It develops in essentially all patients with hepatitis B, becoming detectable at about the time of maximum elevation of serum aminotransferase activities. Anti-HBc remains elevated but at lower titers for a long period of time, apparently years. Patients who retain the hepatitis B virus in the liver maintain a high titer of anti-HBc. Testing for anti-HBc is by radioimmunoassay or quantitative enzyme-linked immunosorbant assay (ELISA).[17]

Another antigen-antibody system associated with hepatitis B is the e system (HBeAg and anti-HBe): HBe antigenemia is closely associated with a hepatitis viral DNA polymerase and the presence of infective viral particles. Anti-HBe is a marker indicating low or no infectivity. HBeAg is present early in sera of all patients with acute hepatitis B, and either HBeAg or anti-HBe can be detected in the sera of patients with chronic varieties of hepatitis B.[17]

Ameba antibodies. Antibodies to *Entamoeba histolytica* commonly develop in patients with extracolonic tissue invasion by the organism. Usually this means the development of a hepatic amebic abscess. The antibody levels are often elevated at the time the patient enters the hospital with symptoms of a liver abscess, but the height of antibody titer is not related to severity of illness or to the size of the abscess(es). The antigen used in testing is the extract of a mutant strain of *E. histolytica* that can be grown on artificial cell-free culture media.

Nonspecific reactions to specific diseases

Smooth muscle antibody. In many diseases associated with hepatic necrosis, an antibody develops to components of muscle, apparently actin.[11] Seemingly the hepatocyte has a protein that is immunologically similar to actomyosin.[10] In many disorders, hepatic or otherwise, an antibody of IgM type is detectable, and detection of IgM-type smooth muscle antibody has little diagnostic value. However, an IgG class of antibodies to smooth muscle is detectable in high titer in sera of patients with chronic active lupoid hepatitis and in some with cryptogenic cirrhosis. The test is useful in detecting "autoimmune" liver disease, but attempts to improve specificity of the reaction by alternative methods of antibody detection have not indicated high levels of specificity.[16]

Mitochondrial antibody. For inexplicable reasons, an antibody against mitochondrial membranes develops in patients with primary biliary cirrhosis. The antibody is IgG type and is demonstrated in a fashion similar to that for smooth muscle antibody. About 84% of patients with primary biliary cirrhosis have mitochondrial antibodies. In a properly controlled laboratory, there are few false-positive results.[22]

Liver-kidney microsomal antibodies (LKM antibodies). A rare antibody to microsomal membranes distinct from, but easily confused with, mitochondrial antibodies has been demonstrated by immunofluorescence in a manner similar to that for smooth muscle and mitochondrial antibodies. Localization is in hepatocytes and renal proximal convoluted tubules in a very fine particulate distribution. The antibody has been detected in a very small percentage of patients with liver disease, but about 75% of those with LKM antibody have chronic liver disease.

Radiologic diagnosis of liver disease

During the past decade, great advances have been made in the radiologic diagnosis of liver disease. These advances are the result of new techniques and new instrumentation. A constant flow of new reports appears in the medical literature. The various approaches used have been classified as either noninvasive or invasive. Among the noninvasive methods, radiocolloid scintigraphy has been in use for some 20 years.[2] In this procedure technetium 99m sulfur colloid is given intravenously and is phagocytized by the Kupffer cells. The technique outlines focal lesions, and the size, location, and shape of the liver and spleen can be determined. Gallium 67 and technetium 99m HIDA are also being used.

Ultrasonography has proved to be of great value in the diagnosis of a wide variety of liver and bile duct diseases because it is a fairly inexpensive, easily performed, noninvasive approach. Computed tomography is also a suitable approach[30] but is more costly and exposes the patient to radiation.[46] In selected cases, after one or more of these tests have been used, further studies by invasive methods are indicated. These include percutaneous transhepatic cholangiography and endoscopic retrograde cholangiopancreatography (ERCP) for outlining most clearly the bile duct system. Hepatic angiograms via the injection of dye into the celiac or hepatic artery give useful information concerning the size, location, and nature of certain tumors and tumorlike lesions. Angiograms using the portal vein and hepatic veins are helpful in the diagnosis of selected disorders.[44]

BASIC HEPATIC HISTOPATHOLOGY

Hydropic change

The descriptive term *hydropic change* is given to hepatocytes because the cells are pale, watery, and usually swollen. A wide variety of conditions may produce the relative or absolute decrease of eosinophilia of the hepatocytes. Mitochondria and ribosomes of the rough endoplasmic reticulum are the principal subcellular components responsible for eosinophilic staining characteristics. Physiologic causes for reduction of eosinophilia include an increased storage of glycogen after high-carbohydrate feeding and proliferation of smooth endoplasmic reticulum (SER), occurring at the expense of the eosinophilic rough endoplasmic reticulum (RER) and seen when there is induction of a specific enzymatic system, such as that produced by protracted phenobarbital administration. Active regeneration of hepatocytes may result in swollen hydropic cells. Hydropic swelling is also a common early sign of cellular damage. Often the change seems related to increased cellular water content, perhaps reflecting cell membrane alteration. This effect frequently follows exposure of the hepatocyte to a toxin. In the latter instance hydropic swelling may be localized to only part of the cell, usually the part adjacent to the sinusoidal surface of the hepatocyte, with displacement of the eosinophilic portion of the cytoplasm to a pericanalicular position. This change is often striking in viral hepatitis and in drug-induced damage. In the hydropic hepatocytes of the acute alcoholic patient, frequently a cell that appears hydropic under ordinary microscopy actually will have fine, foamy vacuoles that can be recognized as lipid by use of fat stains or electron microscopy.

Atrophy

Generalized atrophy may occur in old age and in starvation states, such as anorexia nervosa. The atrophy may or may not be accompanied by an increase of lipochrome that gives the liver a deep brown appearance. In the atrophic state the liver often weighs less than 1000 g, and the hepatocytes appear shrunken and deeply eosinophilic.

Fatty change

The accumulation of neutral triglycerides in hepatocytes is one of the most common pathologic changes in the hepatocyte. The liver is a focal point in the assimilation of dietary and depot lipids. Accumulation of hepatocellular fat may occur when there is (1) a sudden increased mobilization of depot fat to the liver, (2) relative unavailability of protein or protein precursors necessary for cellular release of hepatic lipid, (3) intracellular shunting of metabolic pathways in the liver resulting in increased hepatic lipid formation, or (4) decreased fatty acid utilization. Probably all mechanisms are important in some instances of lipid accumulation in the hepatocyte. The pathogenic importance of lipoperoxide formation in causing cytoplasmic damage is still debated. In automobile accident victims at autopsy, a considerable percentage of the "normal" population has shown fatty change on examination of the liver.[67]

Normally about 5% of the wet weight of the liver is fat. In some conditions, particularly alcoholic liver disease, greater than 50% of the wet weight of the liver may be fat; in such a case the liver is grossly lardaceous. On ordinary histologic sections, fat in the liver appears as a globular intracytoplasmic clear space, since the fat is removed by routine tissue processing and only the sharp interface that the lipid body forms with remaining aqueous cytoplasm remains. Fat droplets may be multiple and only a micrometer or less in diameter, requiring electron microscopy for identification, or more commonly they may be so large that the hepatocyte membrane is stretched several fold to surround a single fat globule. Only an occasional fat droplet may be found within a single lobule, or in extreme cases every hepatocyte may be bloated with fat. Deposition of large fat globules alone has not been shown to impair cellular function; the usual fatty hepatocyte has its nucleus displaced, but the thin rim of cytoplasm that surrounds the fat globule is rich in enzyme activity and mitochondria are abundant.

The most common cause of large amounts of hepatic fat in patients in the United States is chronic alcoholism, but small amounts of fat are common in acute illnesses or acute alcoholism, probably as a result of increased mobilization of depot fat.

Kwashiorkor, a common disease of infants in Africa and other tropical regions, results from a protein-energy malnutrition. Because of a variety of circumstances that led to a similar protein deficiency, sporadic cases have been noted in the United States. Hypoglycemia is a common finding.[57] On entry to the hospital the patients may be lethargic or comatose. Edema and hypoalbuminemia are present and differentiate kwashiorkor from marasmus. In kwashiorkor, fatty change in the liver may be extreme.[102] The fat accumulates in large vacuoles, sometimes forming fatty cysts.[105]

Cytoplasmic condensation, hyaline bodies, and inclusions

Cytoplasmic condensation and droplets occur in several types of cell injury. Cytoplasmic condensation is a clumping or aggregation of eosinophilic or polychromatophilic material, which results in the displacement of RER material to pericanalicular and perinuclear positions by hydropic change beneath the cell membrane. Such condensation occurs in acute viral hepatitis or in toxic damage to the hepatocyte and is apparently a reversible change. In some types of cell damage the ribosomes are displaced from the RER and aggregate in one part of the hepatocyte. A special type of condensation results in the Mallory body (MB)[78] or alcoholic hyalin, a change not always reversible. The MB initially develops in a hydropic bloated hepatocyte as ropy eosinophilic strands that appear to condense to become an irregular but discrete intracytoplasmic mass of homogeneous-appearing material. It may have staining characteristics ranging from only slightly more eosinophilic than the surrounding cytoplasm to a nearly purple discrete coagulum. MBs are seen with an electron microscope as microfilaments that are randomly oriented, interposed among endoplasmic reticulum from which the ribosomes have been displaced.[89,107] The ribosomes often form a loose cuff around the clustered microfilaments. The composition of MBs is similar to that of prekeratin filament protein[59] and may, by immunologic studies, be altered cytoskeletal filaments.[61,82]

MBs develop in widely varied conditions; by far the most common is alcoholic liver disease. MBs are found occasionally in livers of patients with Wilson's disease,[101] primary biliary cirrhosis,[77,81] hepatocellular carcinoma (within the tumor cells),[72] jejunoileal bypass,[49,87] and Indian childhood cirrhosis[49] and after extensive small bowel resection.[90] Occasionally it has been described in alpha-1-antitrypsin disease[88] and after treatment with perhexiline maleate,[76] diethylaminoethoxyhexestrol,[71] and protracted glucocorticoid therapy.[70] MBs may occur in abetalipoproteinemia,[86] Weber-Christian disease,[74] or obesity or from unknown causes.[48] Very rarely, MBs may be seen associated in small numbers with almost any disease. It is debatable whether the MB plays any part in the genesis of alcoholic liver disease or if it is merely a frequently found signpost along the road to cell destruction in certain diseases.

Markedly enlarged mitochondria (megamitochondria), occasionally up to 5 μm, are fairly common in acute alcoholic liver disease as discrete, round, eosinophilic structures.[108] They have also been described in other conditions.[55] Megamitochondria can be produced in ethionine-treated animals[92]; at one time these bodies were mistaken for alcoholic hyalin in experimental animals.

Mitochondria of near-normal size, visible as pinpoint dots in microscopic thin sections but not large enough to appear as eosinophilic globules, are more obvious in livers with certain kinds of acute cell damage, including those related to alcoholism, aflatoxins, and Reye's syndrome, to name a few.

Lysosomes in the form of 0.5 to 1 μm, round phagocytic vacuoles may resemble megamitochondria but are less discrete and contain stainable glycoproteins, allowing recognition.[52,68,85] Hepatocytic lysosomes become particularly abundant in certain types of acute cell damage, as in severe acute alcoholic liver disease. Kupffer cell lysosomal activity is prominent whenever phagocytic activity occurs.

Many other types of hepatocytic cytoplasmic bodies may be found. Large cytoplasmic inclusions without a membrane but with a finely granular appearance are found in patients who have chronic forms of hepatitis B, called ground-glass cells or Hadziyannis cells.[65] These bodies consist of proliferated endoplasmic reticulum and hepatitis B surface antigen, a product of hepatitis B virus. Similar bodies may be seen rarely in livers of patients taking certain drugs. Disulfiram (Antabuse)[104] has been reported to be associated with cytoplasmic bodies, and we have observed cytoplasmic bodies in association with azathioprine (Imuran). Occasionally, endocytosis by the hepatocyte results in membrane-bound cytoplasmic pale bodies that contain plasma proteins. Such endocytosis occurs in severe anoxia, occasionally in liver tumors, and for reasons unknown. Cytoplasmic bodies that appear similar to these are found in hepatocytes (and in neurons) of patients with a familial myotonic epilepsy and Lafora's disease.[83] On occasion, usually in cirrhotic livers, hepatocytes are bloated with mitochondria, imparting an eosinophilic oncocytic appearance.[63] Striking cytoplasmic bodies in the periportal hepatocytes appear in patients with anomalous Z phenotype of alpha-1-antitrypsin. These bodies, which are intracisternal accumulations of alpha-1-antitrypsin,[109] are discrete, round, and eosinophilic. They resemble megamitochondria, except for (1) their periportal, rather than perivenular, location and (2) their glycoprotein content, which gives a strong diastase-resistant periodic acid–Schiff reaction.

Necrosis

Death of hepatocytes may assume several patterns, with respect both to lobular distribution and to the morphologic appearance of the involved hepatocytes.

Liver cell necrosis, depending on its distribution within the lobule, is divided into focal, zonal, and diffuse patterns. The various etiologic agents tend to produce the same pattern of injury from one patient to another. Detailed descriptions of focal and diffuse necrosis are included in the following sections concerned with specific diseases.

Zonal necrosis. Zonal necrosis is the usual reaction to many of the hepatotoxins. Apparently, liver cells in corresponding lobular areas have a similar sensitivity. Depending on the noxious agent, necrosis may be perivenular (zone 3), midzonal (zone 2), or periportal (zone 1). Perivenular necrosis is the most common. It is most often caused by ischemia, particularly in patients with congestive heart failure or shock from any cause. Most necrotizing hepatotoxins have a perivenular effect; these are discussed in the section on drug-induced disease. Midzonal necrosis of yellow fever is discussed in Chapter 10.

Periportal necrosis has been described in phosphorus poisoning and in eclampsia. Yellow phosphorus in sufficient doses leads to peripheral fatty change and necrosis of liver cells.[60] Perivenular necrosis has also been described after phosphorus poisoning.[97]

Hepatocyte death and dissolution (hepatocytolysis). Hepatocytolysis may occur in such rapid sequence that dead cells are not seen, such as in viral hepatitis and with certain toxins. A type of lytic necrosis of perivenular hepatocytes occurs in alcoholic patients, perhaps representing the final stage of hydropic and foamy degeneration. In coagulative necrosis, a common type of necrosis in other parts of the body, the parenchymal cells retain their cytoplasm, which assumes an eosinophilic, granular, or waxy appearance. After 2 or 3 days the nucleus loses its basophilia and becomes indiscernible. The cell shrinks, rounds up slightly, and disappears slowly after infiltration by inflammatory cells. Coagulative necrosis is a characteristic of anoxia; other causes of coagulative necrosis may be based on damage to fundamental cellular respiratory systems, whereby lysosomes fail to be activated.

Acidophilic necrosis. Acidophilic necrosis is a peculiar patchy change of single hepatocytes in which the cell configuration changes from polyhedral to globose and the cytoplasm becomes more eosinophilic. The shrunken, rounded hepatocyte sloughs from its place in the liver cord, loses its pyknotic nucleus, and is ultimately phagocytosed by Kupffer cells. The acidophilic bodies, or Councilman bodies as they were formerly known (in recognition of the medical officer who described them in livers of patients dying of yellow fever),[100] are found scattered throughout the liver, particularly in the liver infected by the hepatitis virus but also with certain other diseases. On ultrastructural examination it appears that cytoplasmic dehydration has occurred: the mitochondria

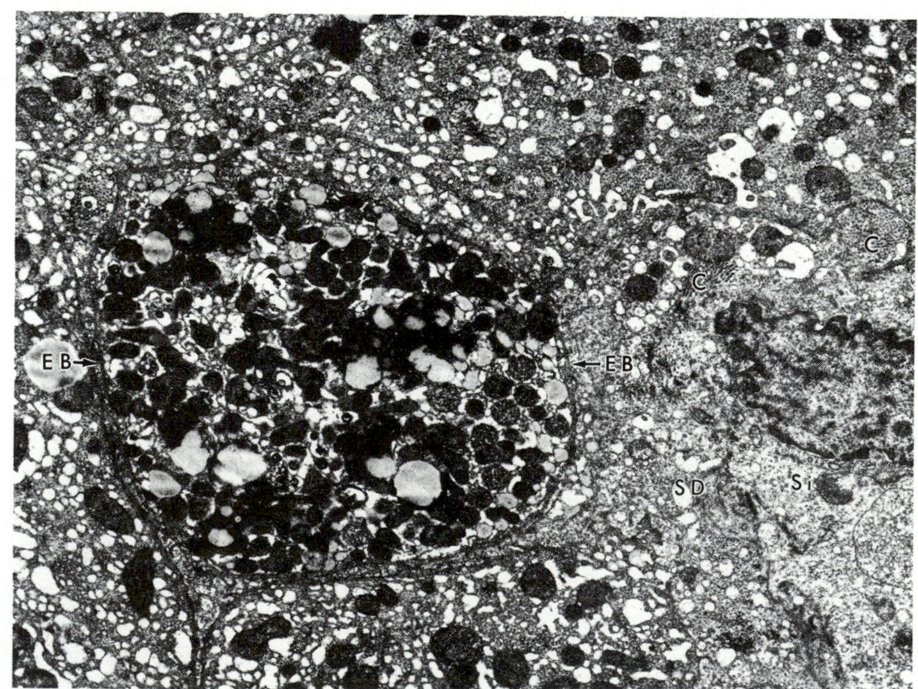

Fig. 27-2. Electron photomicrograph of acidophilic body just before extrusion into sinusoid. Note collagen in Disse's space, which is not generally detectable on light microscopy. *C,* Collagen; *EB,* eosinophilic (acidophilic) body; *SD,* Disse's space; *Si,* sinusoid. (Courtesy Dr. Hisando Kobayashi, Nagoya, Japan.)

remain visible as shrunken, osmophilic structures (Fig. 27-2).[73,115]

Immune cytopathic cell lysis

Although there has been conjecture that hepatocellular necrosis may in certain instances be immunologic in origin, proof of this mechanism is incomplete. In most cell systems immune lysis may be based on humoral events following activation of complement. Activation is initiated by a combination of antibody with cell surface antigen. A second mechanism involves the binding of a T lymphocyte to the target cell surface by the antibody. The Fab portion of the antibody, the portion that imparts specificity, attaches to cell surface antigen, and the remaining portion of the antibody (the Fc portion) is recognized by the Fc receptor on the lymphocyte. Either type of cascading events results in cell lysis, apparently initiating breakdown of the permeability barrier to small molecules, cell swelling, and, ultimately, osmotic lysis.[80,91]

Emperipolesis, the act of lymphocytes invaginating the hepatocyte membrane and ultimately entering the cell, can be seen in certain hepatic conditions. Although emperipolesis has been demonstrated to be a step in cell death involving other target cells, its importance in liver cell necrosis is unclear.

Inflammatory reaction

In addition to its role as a parenchymal organ, the liver includes a significant part of the lymphoid and reticuloendothelial systems of the body. The portal areas, which even in the 12- to 17-week embryo contain T cell precursors,[94] normally include lymphoid tissue in the adult. In common with lymphoid tissue elsewhere, the portal lymphoid component reacts to many nonhepatic inflammatory conditions by hyperplasia. Such hyperplasia, by itself, should not be considered a hepatic disorder, although portal lymphoid tissue also becomes hyperplastic in response to hepatic inflammatory conditions. Usually, portal lymphoid hyperplasia is confined within the limiting plate. The hyperplasia is rarely follicular; the cellular component includes lymphocytes, immunoblasts, plasma cells, and background histiocytes. Over a period of years, protracted or recurrent lymphoid hyperplasia often results in collagenous deposition and arteriolar sclerosis. Portal lymphoid hyperplasia is frequently accompanied by Kupffer cell hyperplasia. Confusion of the reactive changes of the reticuloendothelial component of the liver with an inflammatory condition in the liver must be carefully avoided.

Calcification

The differential diagnosis of calcifications within the right upper quadrant of the abdomen is clinically important. First, the intrahepatic calcifications must be differentiated from those in other tissues.[58] Worldwide, the most common causes of calcifications are tuberculosis, histoplasmosis, and hydatid cysts. Calcified granulomas vary in size from miliary to moderate. Punctate calcifications of 1 to 3 mm, when present in the spleen and lungs as well as the liver, are characteristic of histoplasmosis. Large solitary or multiple calcifications may result from pyogenic or amebic liver abscesses. A large percentage of patients with hydatid disease have calcifications that are arranged in a shell-like pattern.[106] In a few reported cases, primary tumors of the liver have shown areas of calcification. Among these are hepatocellular carcinoma, cholangiocarcinoma, and mixed hepatoblastoma in infancy and childhood.[66] Among the benign tumors, calcification is seen most often in cavernous hemangioma. Calcification in metastatic lesions, especially those from the colon, may occur.[64] The latter characteristically have a fine granular appearance and tend to coalesce into large aggregates without distinct margins.[79]

Cholestasis

The physiologist recognizes cholestasis as the reduction in bile flow that can be recognized when fasting serum bile acid levels become elevated.[51] It becomes evident to the morphologist only when bilirubin plugs in the canaliculi are seen. Microscopy is an insensitive measure of reduction of bile flow, but slight dilatation of canaliculi, as well as an increasingly discrete canalicular membrane, can be recognized before pigmented casts of bilirubin appear in the canalicular lumina. Since much of the bilirubin pigment is removed in routine tissue processing, correlation between serum bilirubin levels and the amount of bile pigment demonstrable histologically is poor; however, only rarely can canalicular bile plugs be seen when serum bilirubin levels are normal. The plugs are usually more prominent in the perivenular canaliculi, although in some conditions periportal plugs are found (see following sections on primary biliary cirrhosis and impaired regeneration). Bile plugs, most commonly associated with mechanical obstruction of the biliary tract, may be found in many instances of "medical jaundice," such as viral hepatitis and drug-induced cholestasis.

Bile droplets in hepatocytes are not readily appreciated after tissue processing. In some conditions, bile staining of hepatocytic cytoplasm is recognizable (see following sections on acute lytic necrosis in alcoholic liver disease). After cholestatic bile plugs have been present for a protracted period, they assume the appearance of microcalculi. Breakdown of hepatocytes allows the miniature casts to be released and phagocytosed by Kupffer cells as fragmented bile casts.

Pigmentation

Anthracotic pigment may be carried to the liver by the bloodstream after rupture into the pulmonary veins of a thoracic lymph node containing carbon pigment. The carbon particles are phagocytosed by the Kupffer cells and tend to be carried to portal spaces, where they accumulate.

Silver pigment may be found under the sinusoidal endothelial cells of the liver in argyria. After the injection of Thorotrast, macrophages in the periportal areas and Kupffer cells may store thorium for decades.

Hemosiderin accumulation in the liver is common. In hemolytic anemias the hemosiderin tends to be distributed diffusely. The pigment is found in both the hepatic cells and the phagocytic Kupffer cells of the sinusoids. In hemochromatosis the pigment is largely hemosiderin, but hemofuscin is present as well.

In malaria, hematin pigment may accumulate in large amounts, mainly in the Kupffer cells of the sinusoids. It may be sufficient to give the liver a dark gray-brown color. A similar pigment may be found in the liver in schistosomiasis.

Bile pigmentation of the liver is seen in any variety of jaundice. When seen fresh, the liver is yellowish but soon changes to green as a result of oxidation of the bilirubin to biliverdin. Masses of pigment may be seen distending the bile capillaries and small ducts and within the hepatic cells.

Patients with sufficient quantity of melanoma to produce melaninuria frequently have granules of melanin pigment in Kupffer cells.

The differential diagnosis of increased lipochrome in the liver as seen on biopsy is discussed in a later section.

Regeneration

The liver has a striking capacity for regeneration. In the normal adult rat the hepatocyte has an annual turnover rate of about one mitosis per year[62]; under maximum stimulus the rate is greatly accelerated. Following 70% hepatectomy, liver weight doubles in 48 hours, is almost normal size in 3 days, and reaches normal size in 6 days, although regeneration continues for 15 to 16 days. A burst of DNA synthesis begins 15 to 18 hours after partial hepatectomy, reaches a peak in about 24 hours, and then declines.[95] A second but lower maximum is reached at about 56 hours. Studies with tritiated thymidine have shown that the maximal labeling index is found in the periportal areas but not immediately adjacent to the triads; however, only about 30% of the hepatocytes are in DNA synthesis. Later, at 34 hours, the zone of maximal proliferation has shifted toward the perivenous zones of the liver lobule where about 20% of the hepatocytes are labeled. This potential has clinical and pathologic relevance, since some 70% of the liver may be resected for removal of neoplasms; usually lesser amounts are removed after trauma. The regenerative capacity diminishes with advancing age and is profoundly affected by many other factors, which are not yet defined. Cirrhotic livers have such poor regenerative power that large resections for neoplasms are not attempted.

Regenerating hepatocytes may divide more rapidly than their capacity to reestablish a sinusoidal pattern and thus maintain the liver plate-sinusoid-plate relationship. As a result, clusters of hepatocytes develop in areas of rapid replication, particularly in periportal areas where regeneration seems most active. Rapidly regenerating hepatocytes are swollen and hydropic compared with normal hepatocytes; their nuclei are enlarged with more crisply defined chromatin, and nucleoli are prominent. The functional capacity of actively regenerating hepatocytes is diminished compared with that of the normal hepatocyte. The regenerative response is rapid following partial hepatic resection or extensive necrosis.

The factors that initiate, potentiate, and, finally inhibit hepatocyte proliferation are termed hepatotrophic factors. Many of these have been identified, and their mode of action has been actively investigated. Other factors are unknown at present. It has long been shown that a flow of nonhepatic portal blood from the splanchnic area is a major factor in hepatic regeneration. The substances in this blood are called portal hepatotrophic factors; the best known of these is insulin. Glucagon and epidermal growth factor–urogastrone (EGF) from the gut are also considered to be essential.[75] Known nonportal factors include parathyroid hormone, calcitonin, and an insulin-like substance produced by the liver, somatomedin c. The insulin molecule attaches to the hepatic cell membranes, and the blood levels of insulin fall. The exact role of glucagon and EGF is not well understood. In tissue culture of rat hepatocytes under chemically defined conditions, insulin, glucagon, and EGF initiate DNA synthesis and mitoses. The earliest step is promotion of a membrane sodium ion flux activity by peptides similar or identical to EGF; subsequently these are potentiated by the combined action of insulin plus glucagon.[54] There is evidence that initiation of proliferation is caused by some substance within the liver.[98] An inhibitory factor or factors stop proliferation when the liver reaches normal size. In the process of regeneration, no new lobules are formed. The pathologic process is one of hyperplasia. In addition to the increase in hepatocytes, there is a concomitant lengthening of blood vessels and bile ducts. Angiographic studies show that during regeneration the arteries probably hypertrophy and appear stretched, but no new vessels are observed.[50] The entire subject of liver regeneration concerned with the various hepatotrophic factors has been the topic of an international symposium.[56]

Blood flow and vascular changes

The normal liver, with its double vascular supply, is less at risk to develop hypoxic conditions than most active parenchymal organs. Therefore thrombosis or arteriosclerosis of the hepatic artery is not a significant cause of liver disease. However, venous stasis related to problems of pulmonary vascular flow is a common occurrence. When venous stasis is prolonged, it may result in perivenular liver cell atrophy and, ultimately, hepatocyte dropout. Coagulative necrosis of perivenular hepatocytes may occur if there is reduced blood supply to the liver in addition to venous stasis, a combination seen in shock, myocardial infarction, or arrhythmia. The production of necrosis of both parenchymal cells and stroma is indeed rare in the liver with normal architecture. However, such coagulative necrosis is common in cirrhotic nodules following shock from variceal hemorrhage. The latter circumstance combines reduced arterial flow (shock), diminished portal vein flow from the pressure drop of variceal hemorrhage, impaired hepatic vein drainage related to cirrhosis, and the precarious blood supply that many cirrhotic nodules have.

A change in hepatocytes that may be associated with hypoxia is the formation of intracytoplasmic pale bodies by endocytosis. This change was originally described under electron microscopy,[53,84] but it can be seen with the light microscope in about 25% of the livers of people dying of heart failure.[103]

Postmortem changes

Postmortem autolytic changes develop rapidly in the liver, producing a soft, even mushy, organ. Such changes occur more rapidly in patients with an acute necrotizing hepatic process, such as fulminant hepatitis or acute alcoholic liver disease. Microscopically, all cell detail may be lost. Portions of the liver adjacent to the transverse colon often show a bluish black discoloration. The most striking postmortem change is the "foamy" liver, which is caused by postmortem growth in the liver of anaerobic gas-producing organisms from the intestinal tract. The liver becomes soft and spongy, with the bubbles of gas producing a honeycombed effect in the hepatic tissue. Numerous bacilli may be evident, particularly in blood vessels.

Fibrosis

The deposition of collagen is the most important feature of chronic liver disease. Normally approximately 4% of the liver protein is collagen, an amount that undergoes a twofold to sixfold increase in cirrhosis.[96] Humans have a far more exuberant collagen response to injury than do other animals, and an equivalent extent of collagenosis in the liver of humans is not duplicated in lower animals, even other primates.[99] Collagen is now recognized as a family of similar but chemically and immunologically distinct entities, of which type III is apparently laid down in the liver in response to injury. Type I collagen, the type found as the principal structural protein in normal organs, including liver, gradually replaces the type III collagen as the fibrous tissue ages. However, the basic cellular interactions—the role of circulating factors on local collagenosis—is unclear. Normal collagen in the liver becomes denser and more compact with advancing age, just as it does in other parts of the body. In very advanced years it may become hyalinized. After repeated bouts of reactive inflammatory hyperplasia, often reflected in the lymphoid tissue of the portal areas, there is some increase in portal collagen. No demonstrable ill effects of the portal collagen change occur with advancing age. Collagen is deposited in areas of chronic inflammation in the liver but in quantitatively and perhaps qualitatively different patterns in different disorders. In bile duct obstruction the collagen is circumferentially arranged about the ducts initially in a loose, edematous fashion and later as a dense, compact sheath. At the same time an increase in portal collagen, accompanied by cellular inflammatory response, causes destruction of the limiting plate and widening of the entire portal area.

Simple hepatocyte necrosis results in the formation of little new collagen; thus the collapsed stroma of severe viral hepatitis or drug necrosis provides a convenient framework for repair. Broad areas of collapse may remain as compressed stroma. Repeated or continuous necrosis is associated with fibrosis; however, some inflammatory diseases are more often associated with fibrosis than others. Among the most striking depositions of collagen is that found in alcoholic liver disease in which little of the collagen represents condensation of collapsed stroma. The fibrosis in alcoholic liver disease occurs pericellularly in the spaces of Disse and in sinusoids, particularly in the perivenular region. Portal fibrosis also develops. Fibrosis in the liver of the alcoholic patient apparently need not be antedated by necrosis, and requirement for prior inflammatory reaction has not been proved.

Aside from the sequelae of chronic inflammation, neoplasia may be accompanied by fibrosis. An ineffective fibrous barrier may form between metastatic carcinoma and adjacent liver, a pattern often seen with metastatic squamous cell carcinoma. In other tumors a fibrous reaction around each tumor duct or gland develops (metastatic carcinoma from pancreas or breast), to the extent that far more liver destruction and replacement may result from the fibrosis than from the direct growth of tumor cells. Whereas most hepatocellular carcinomas do not excite fibrosis, some do, and adenocarcinoma of the intrahepatic bile ducts usually is very fibrogenic. In contrast, metastatic malignant melanomas and bronchogenic oat cell carcinomas usually stimulate no fibrosis in the liver. The nature of stimulus to fibrosis, or its absence, relative to metastatic tumor is still a mystery, and the protective or invasive implications remain unknown.

Collagens are formed by fibroblasts and perhaps by other cells. The exact role of the latter is unknown. In experimental animals the formation of new collagen is accompanied by an increase in prolyl hydroxylase. This enzyme has been found to be increased in needle biopsy specimens as well as in the blood.[93] The degree of fibrosis in any one liver depends on the interplay of the fibroblast-stimulating factors that produce new collagen versus collagen degradation by collagenase.[96] The difference in the degree of fibrosis and cirrhosis indicates that the interplay of these factors must vary greatly. Early in fibrosis the connective tissue is often loosely arranged and fibers are separated by considerable matrix. Later in the cirrhotic process the connective tissue is much more dense and poorly cellular.

Cirrhosis

Cirrhosis is a term defined by agreement among hepatologists as "altered reconstruction of the lobular parenchyma with both extensive fibrosis and regenerative nodules."[69] The regenerative nodule, by definition, is not only an area of hepatocytes surrounded by fibrosis but a spherical structure, formed by replication of the hepatocytes, that compresses the surrounding stroma or collagen and thus distorts the lobular architecture of the liver. Nodules may range from microscopic to well over 1 cm in diameter. The cirrhotic liver, because of the distortion of architecture and the obliteration of terminal vessels and sinusoids, has an irregularly distributed blood supply. This results in severe impediment to portal blood flow through the liver and consequent elevation of portal hydrostatic pressure. The elevated pressure leads to the establishment of portal-systemic venous collaterals that permit, and even force, much of the splanchnic blood flow to bypass the liver.

The formation of a cirrhotic liver is a dynamic process. The changing morphology of cirrhosis causes difficulty in formulating a relevant classification. Most cirrhotogenic conditions are characterized by episodic destruction and inflammatory activity, followed by relative quiescence during which nodular regeneration occurs at an accelerated rate. The size and structure of the nodules are related to the duration of the cirrhotic process and also to the etiology and the individual reaction to the specific disease. For example, in the liver of the alcoholic patient, collagen is deposited pericellularly within the nodule, as well as in fibrous septa around nodules. Consequently the encased nodules do not bulge greatly on the cut surface. Most persons with alcoholic cirrhosis continue drinking after cirrhosis develops, and continuing destruction of nodules and invasive collagenosis prevent large nodule formation. About 2 weeks after the patient stops drinking, regeneration is histologically demonstrable. But the dense and infiltrative nature of the collagen in the alcoholic person inhibits the development of large nodules unless alcohol is discontinued for months or years. Protracted alcohol abstinence after cirrhosis develops provides the opportunity for vascularization and some reabsorption of the dense, hard collagen.

Table 27-2. More common types of cirrhosis in adults

Preferred name	Etiology or associations	Liver size (g)	Nodular size (cm)	Collagen density
Alcoholic cirrhosis	Chronic alcoholism	Early >1800 Late <1200	Usually <0.3; occasionally >0.5	Hard, rarely loose
B-viral cirrhosis	Chronic active hepatitis B	<1500	Early—granular; late—usually >0.3	Usually loose
NAB viral cirrhosis	Chronic active hepatitis non-A, non-B	<1500	Granular to 0.3	Usually loose
Autoimmune cirrhosis	Laboratory evidence of autoimmune features (LE, ANA)	<1500	Late—0.3 to 1	Usually loose
(Drug name) cirrhosis (as distinct from submassive necrosis)	Follows drug-induced chronic active hepatitis with some drugs (oxyphenisatin, selacryn, methotrexate, dantrolene)	Variable	Variable	Variable
Primary biliary cirrhosis	Unknown	>1500	0.3 to 0.5	Variable
Secondary biliary cirrhosis	Chronic obstruction to biliary flow	>1500	0.3 to 0.5	Firm
Hemochromatosis	Abnormal iron absorption	<1500	0.1 to 0.3	Usually loose
Wilson's disease (W-D) cirrhosis	Genetic abnormality in handling copper		≥0.3	Loose to hard
Pi ZZ juvenile cirrhosis	Associated with alpha-1-antitrypsin type ZZ		0.1 to 0.3	
Pi ZZ adult cirrhosis	Associated with alpha-1-antitrypsin, develops late in life		0.5 to 1	
Pi MZ, SZ, MS cirrhosis	Questionable relationship			
Cryptogenic cirrhosis	Unknown	Variable	Variable	Variable
Miscellaneous	Jejunoileal bypass, syphilis, parasitic disease, tyrosinemia, galactosemia, cardiac disease	Variable	Variable	Variable

It may be difficult to recognize such a cirrhotic liver as alcoholic in type when the alcoholic cirrhotic person has stopped drinking for 3 or 4 years. Alternatively, the patient whose drinking pattern is steady and substantial, day by day, throughout many years but who maintains a good diet may never show signs of acute alcoholic liver disease, but cirrhosis may develop insidiously. Such a patient may seldom or never have been intoxicated.

Cirrhosis following chronic active hepatitis has a different pathogenesis from alcoholic cirrhosis. Although initially characterized grossly by a uniform finely granular pattern that represents the widened portal areas, chronic active hepatitis becomes quiescent, with respect to continuing necrosis, several years before clinical signs of cirrhosis appear. Because the collagen deposition within nodules in the liver is far less in chronic active hepatitis than in alcoholism, hepatic nodules in the former grow to a much larger size by the time of death. Thus nodular size and discreteness are the result of both density of collagen and freedom of continued regeneration, without disrupting necrotizing activity. Functionally more important than nodular size in cirrhosis is the size of the entire hepatic mass, which can be estimated with radioisotope scans. The more common types of cirrhosis are listed in Table 27-2.

INFECTIOUS DISORDERS

Viral hepatitis

Viral hepatitis is a necrotizing inflammatory lesion of the liver produced by any one of at least four infective agents. Two of these agents have been isolated and characterized as viruses; two others have distinctive electron microscopic features and have been shown to produce immunologically separate infections in chimpanzees (Table 27-3).[155] Acute viral hepatitis (AcVH), predominantly type A, is the most common acute liver disease of children and adolescents, occasionally assuming epidemic proportions when hygienic conditions are poor. The severity of viral hepatitis ranges from subclinical disease in a majority of patients to rapidly fatal illness in a few. Hepatitis results in chronic liver disease in a relatively small number of patients, but a chronic form of one of the hepatitis virus infections underlies one of the most common malignant tumors worldwide. Most chronic hepatitis infections follow an initial subclinical disease.

In usage the term *viral hepatitis* has not included certain other uncommon and geographically localized but admittedly viral infections of the liver, such as yellow fever,[234] Lassa fever,[138,232] Bolivian and Argentinean hemorrhagic fever,[124] Rift Valley fever,[238] Marburg virus infection,[112] Ebola virus,[119,160,189] or the many other viruses that usually affect other organs predominantly (only rarely is the liver affected in a clinically significant fashion) such as herpes simplex, variola, varicella, measles, cytomegalovirus, and Epstein-Barr virus.

The hepatitis viruses are hepatitis A virus (HAV), an orally acquired, fecally excreted agent representing 39% of adult infections by hepatitis agents in Los Angeles during 1981; hepatitis B virus (HBV), a percutaneously acquired and transmitted agent, representing 36% of adult hepatitis infections; and the hepatitis non-A, non-B viruses (H-NAB-V), a designation for the composite remaining agents that include both orally and percutaneously transmitted agents and represent 24% of acute hepatitis infections.[199a] A temporary designation of NAB-1 and NAB-2 has been suggested to more precisely designate two of the NAB agents.[236]

At our current state of knowledge, the pathologic changes of acute viral hepatitis (AcVH), whether resulting from A, B, or NAB agents, are similar with all agents. They are discussed on p. 1117.

Hepatitis A

Etiologic agent. Viral hepatitis A (also known as VH-A, epidemic hepatitis, infectious hepatitis, infective hepatitis, Botkin's disease, and, in older usage, catarrhal jaundice) is caused by an orally acquired, fecally excreted RNA virus that is 27 nm in diameter[122] (Fig. 27-3) and has been demonstrated in cytoplasm of hepatocytes of infected humans, marmosets, and chimpanzees.[178,179,195,211] No other organ has been shown to be a source of HAV proliferation. The agent can be inoculated into and passed in tissue culture of green monkey kidney cells,[130] in which it produces no cytopathic effect.

HAV infectivity is totally destroyed by heating to 100° C for 5 minutes, reduced in infectivity by heating to 60° C for 1 hour, almost completely inactivated by ultraviolet irradiation, and destroyed after 3 days of incubation at 37° C in 1:4000 formalin.[195] Infectivity is neutralized by addition of convalescent serum. HAV infection in the subhuman primate produces mild histologic hepatic changes, but rarely significant illness.[134,140,156]

Hepatitis A particles have not been demonstrated in sera of infected persons, but their brief presence in serum is inferred because, experimentally, serum taken from a patient in the prodrome of VH-A is infective for a second susceptible human. Although HAV theoretically can be transmitted by percutaneous routes, it is not, for practical purposes, an agent that produces posttransfusion hepatitis (PTH).[193,219] Hepatitis A particles are demonstrable for a brief period in the stool of infected patients[145]; the viral particles in ultracentrifugal fractions of the stool are agglutinated by convalescent sera, allowing the electron microscopic visualization of not only the clusters of the 27 nm round structures but also the halo of antibodies attached to the viral bodies. The particles appear in the stool about 2 weeks before symptoms and 5 days before development of abnormal transaminase levels and remain until nearly peak serum transaminase levels are reached.[134,170]

Table 27-3. Viral hepatitis

Clinical disease	Abbreviation	Older names	Agent
Acute viral hepatitis type A	AcVH-A	Infectious hepatitis Catarrhal jaundice Epidemic hepatitis MS-1	HAV
Acute viral hepatitis type B	AcVH-B	Serum hepatitis Homologous serum jaundice MS-2	HBV
Fulminant viral hepatitis type B	FVH-B	Acute red atrophy Acute yellow atrophy Subacute yellow atrophy	HBV
Viral hepatitis type B, impaired regeneration syndrome	VH-B-IRS	Subacute yellow atrophy Subacute hepatic necrosis Chronic aggressive hepatitis (?) Protracted hepatitis	HBV
Persistent viral hepatitis type B	PVH-B	Transaminitis Chronic hepatitis Unresolved viral hepatitis B Chronic persistent hepatitis	HBV
Chronic active viral hepatitis	CAVH-B	Chronic hepatitis Subacute hepatitis Chronic aggressive hepatitis	HBV
Active (or) inactive viral cirrhosis type B		Postnecrotic cirrhosis Posthepatitis cirrhosis Macronodular cirrhosis	HBV
Acute viral hepatitis non-A, non-B*	AcVH-NAB*	Infectious hepatitis Serum hepatitis	Not identified

*Apparently all of the patterns of disease that occur with hepatitis B virus may also be found with hepatitis non-A, non-B; the percentages are unknown. They

Clinical and immunologic aspects. HAV is highly infective, and infection confers lifetime immunity with no chronic carrier or chronic disease state. Thus it occurs in epidemics, in densely populated areas, and predominantly in children. The disease is usually overlooked because it may be symptomless or appear as a mild influenza-like illness. When a clinical illness does develop after a 15- to 45-day incubation period, it is ushered in with fatigue, nausea, vomiting, and anorexia. A distaste for cigarettes often develops. Patients with symptomatic acute viral hepatitis type A (AcVH-A) also usually have fever, lymphadenopathy, and tender hepatomegaly. Biliuria is followed by icterus; the highest serum bilirubin level is usually reached 1 to 2 weeks after onset of jaundice, at which time the patient usually becomes subjectively improved. All of the signs and symptoms usually disappear by 6 weeks after onset of jaundice. Fatalities are uncommon; between 1% and 13% of deaths from viral hepatitis can be attributed to HAV.[180,196] Chronic liver disease caused by HAV has not been demonstrated.

Patients with AcVH-A rapidly produce specific IgM-type antibody that appears about 2 weeks after infection and usually persists for 2 months but may last for several months.[161] Its presence is considered diagnostic of acute or recent VH-A. A specific IgG-type antibody follows about 5 weeks after infection, rising in titer as the titer of IgM falls. The IgG antibody persists throughout the patient's life, conferring immunity.[121,146]

Passive transfer of small amounts of convalescent serum to a patient at risk protects the patient from clinically evident infection for about 6 months. Commercially available "hyperimmune" gamma globulin contains antibody to HAV of titers between 1:2000 and 1:8000.

Epidemiology. VH-A has a worldwide distribution and apparently is primarily a disease of humans; other primates are only occasional secondary hosts, deriving the disease from humans.[140] In 1960 it was found that certain

Infective material	Transmission methods	Incubation (days)	Antigen and antibody	Course
Stool 4^+ Urine 3^+ Blood 1^+	Fecal-oral	15-45	Blood anti-HA Stool HAV	Recovery
Blood 4^+ Body fluid 1 to 3^+ Stool 0	Percutaneous, unknown	45-180	Early: HBsAg Recovery: anti-HBs anti-HBc	Recovery 85% Fulminant 1% Subacute (impaired regeneration) fatal $<$ 0.2% Persistent viral hepatitis 10%-12% Chronic active viral hepatitis type B $<$ 3%
(As above)	Percutaneous, unknown	45-180	Early: HBsAg Late: not applicable	Death in days 75% Complete recovery 25% (age related)
(As above)	Percutaneous, unknown	45-180	Early: HBsAg Recovery: anti-HBs anti-HBc	Slow recovery in elderly Fatal in 50%
(As above)	Transplacental, percutaneous, unknown	45-180	Anti-HBc HBsAg	Continued antigenemia nonprogressive 90% Recovery 10%
(As above)	Transplacental, percutaneous, unknown	45-180	Anti-HBc HBsAg	Progression to cirrhosis probably 100%
(As above)	Transplacental, percutaneous, unknown	45-180	Anti-HBc HBsAg	Death from complication of cirrhosis
Body fluid?	Percutaneous, unknown	Peaks at 45	Unknown	Recovery 50%-85%; persistent hepatitis, 25%-45%; CAH, 5%-25%

apparently do not develop or rarely develop with hepatitis A viruses.

mollusks harvested from polluted seawater concentrated the virus, and ingestion of raw or partially cooked mollusks was associated with an occasional epidemic.[137] Because of its high infectivity, its mode of transmission, the apparent rarity of either animal vectors or a chronic carrier state, and the immunity conferred by HAV infection, VH-A tends to occur in epidemics only as a susceptible population reaches an age at which there is intimate contact with older children. The continual entry of new susceptible persons is necessary for the maintenance of the virus. For unknown reasons, incidence figures for VH-A also show seasonal variation. In most countries of the world the incidence of AcVH-A is decreasing, but in certain countries, including Yugoslavia, Taiwan, and Israel, nearly 100% infection rate has been acquired by midadult life.[220] In New York City, 72% to 80% of adults in lower socioeconomic groups have acquired an immune status, compared with 18% to 30% of persons in upper-middle socioeconomic groups.[218] The disease is common

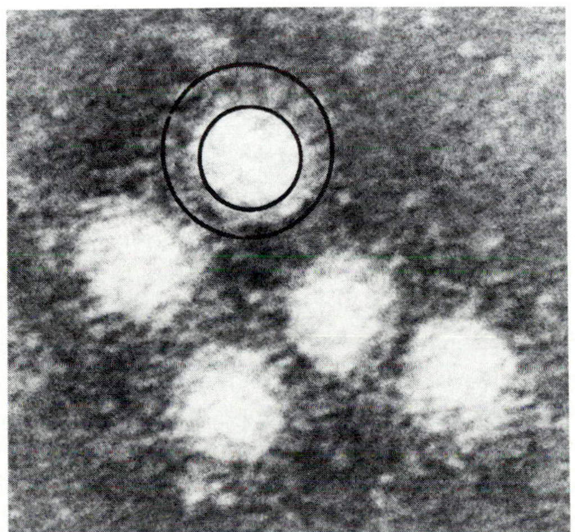

Fig. 27-3. Hepatitis A particles from stool of infected patient, agglutinated by anti-HA. Note fuzzy halo around particles representing antibodies. (One particle and halo are encircled.) (Courtesy Dr. Jorge Rakela, Rochester, Minn.)

in homosexual men, particularly those participating in oral-anal sexual activities.[136]

Hepatitis B

Etiologic agent. Viral hepatitis B (VH-B, serum hepatitis, syringe jaundice, homologous serum hepatitis) is caused by a percutaneously transmitted virus that has a complicated morphology and life cycle.[224] HBV is a member of a new, unnamed class of viruses. The B virus resembles, but is antigenetically separate from, other members of the group, which include the following: woodchuck hepatitis virus (WHV), ground squirrel hepatitis virus (GSHV), and Peking duck hepatitis B virus (DHBV).[116,147] A similar agent is also said to be present in prairie dogs. The complete virion of HBV is a 40 nm double-shelled structure called the Dane particle in humans, after one of the investigators who first described the form. It is sparsely distributed in serum of infected persons.[131] The outer shell of the Dane particle is a lipoprotein with the antigenic specificity identified as hepatitis B surface antigen (HBsAg). Beneath the HBsAg of the Dane particle is a 28 nm hexagonal core that is antigenically dissimilar to HBsAg; the antigen characteristic of the core is called hepatitis B core antigen (HBcAg).[129] DNA is apparently associated with the core. It has been claimed that DNA polymerase is sandwiched between the outer HBsAg shell and the inner HBcAg of the Dane particle. Dane particles are very sparse in serum; however, large amounts of material are antigenically identical to the outer surface of the Dane particle but without core DNA or DNA polymerase. This "excess" surface material is in the form of 20 nm spheres or 20 nm diameter tubular structures of variable lengths. The abundant HBsAg is detectable in the patients' sera and is the basis of the most common tests for HBV infection. The excess material is apparently an aberrant noninfective byproduct of viral replication. There are antigenic subtypes of HBsAg: a universal type (a) and sets of alleles (d and y, w and r, as well as others less well characterized), which have different geographic distributions.[173] The subtypes are characteristics of the virus, not the host. The manner in which the virus infects the hepatocyte is unclear. After infection, however, the core apparently replicates in the nucleus of the infected hepatocyte, whereas the HBsAg originates in cytoplasm, probably in the endoplasmic reticulum as a thin filamentous material that undergoes additional morphologic rearrangement before release from the hepatocyte, either as the protective coating of the Dane particle, as 20 nm spheres, or as the tubular structures (Fig. 27-4). Apparently WHV, GSHV, and DHBV have similar developmental stages.

Recently, there has been some evidence to suggest that HBV may replicate in the pancreas[154,213,214] and in the salivary gland.

An additional antigenic substance in sera of patients with acute viral hepatitis B (AcVH-B), e antigen (HBeAg), is related to infectiveness and is a feature of the virion rather than of HBsAg. The presence of HBeAg in sera correlates closely with presence of DNA polymerase, Dane particles, or HBcAg.[206] Serum of HBsAg-positive patients seems relatively less infective if it contains anti-HBe, which develops after HBeAg disappears.

In vitro digestion of HBcAg has produced substances with some of the antigenic specificity of HBeAg[125]; thus it would appear that HBeAg may consist of certain polypeptide components of HBcAg, and its appearance in serum is a reflection of the quantity or the turnover of HBcAg (that is, infective material). HBeAg persists longer in serum than DNA polymerase or the virus particle (Dane particle), probably reflecting only a longer degradation time.

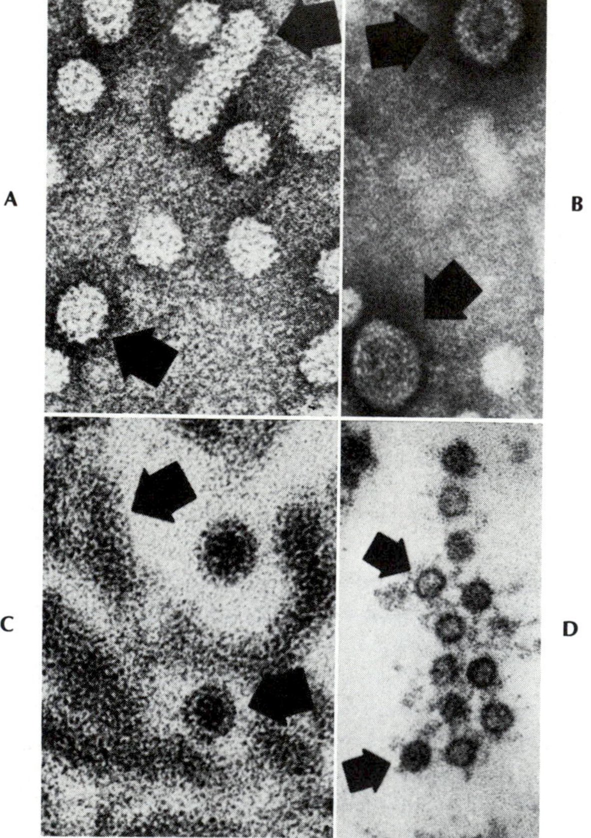

Fig. 27-4. Electron microscopic appearance of components of hepatitis B virus. HBsAg is found in serum, **A,** as 20 nm spheres *(left arrow)* or tubular structures *(right arrow)* but is also found sparsely in serum, **B,** as the Dane particle *(arrow),* apparently the complete virion. In hepatocyte cytoplasm, **C,** HBsAg is form of long filamentous structures; rarely a spherical shell surrounds a hexagonal core, apparently the complete virus *(arrow).* Liver cell nuclei contain core, which is inner part of Dane particle without HBsAg envelope, **D.** (Courtesy Alfred E.G. Dunn, Los Angeles.)

Recently an additional antigen-antibody system, the delta system, has been described in association with VH-B, usually in the chronic form of the B viral infection.[203] Delta antigen, a 68,000 dalton molecular weight protein originally isolated from the liver of a patient with B viral cirrhosis, is apparently found transiently in the liver of a small proportion of patients with AcVH-B, but in greater amounts in hepatocyte nuclei of some patients with chronic forms of VH-B. The relative numbers of chronically HBV-infected patients who also have delta antigen depend on the geographic locale of the patients.[203] Usually delta-infected patients have a history of intravenous drug use. Delta antigen can be transmitted to chimpanzees only if the animals are carriers of HBV.[204,205] Delta antigen may be an incomplete virus that requires HBV components for replication. What effect delta antigen has on HBV infection is unclear, but reports have suggested that progressive forms of chronic VH-B occur more often in patients who have superinfection with the delta agent.[118] The antibody to delta agent has been found in a larger number of patients with chronic VH-B in the Mediterranean area.[204]

Clinical and immunologic aspects. HBV infection involves adults more frequently than does VH-A and is more often associated with serious liver disease. Whether the diseases differ in severity in age-matched individuals is unclear, but many clinicians believe that even in age-matched patients, VH-B is still a more severe illness than VH-A.

Although it is unlikely that chronic liver disease ever follows VH-A, chronic liver infection in some form follows VH-B in 12% or more of patients. Prodromal influenza-like symptoms, joint swelling, and effusion, all apparently manifestations of acute immune-complex disease, are more common in the prodrome of AcVH-B than in VH-A or viral hepatitis non-A, non-B (VH-NAB).[183] Prodromal skin rashes and pruritus occur in about equal frequency in AcVH-B and in acute viral hepatitis non-A, non-B (AcVH-NAB). Some patients develop no prodrome with AcVH-B. Patients with VH-B may have fewer gastrointestinal symptoms than do patients with VH-A, but nausea, vomiting, and fatigue are the principal symptoms of VH-B.

The serologic manifestations of HBV infection are indicated in Fig. 27-5. HBsAg may be detectable 1½ months after percutaneous inoculation with HBV, but it takes 2 to 6 months for clinical symptoms to develop. The rise of bilirubin levels lags behind the rise in ALT and AST activities.

After active HBV infection, anti-HBc in particular remains in the serum, probably indefinitely. One study has shown that 98% of drug addicts in the United States have serologic evidence of previous HBV infection; of those with evidence of prior infection, 11% have chronic HBs antigenemia, 67% have both anti-HBs and anti-HBc, 20% have anti-HBc alone, and only 2% have anti-HBs alone.[187] However, in a population survey a relatively larger number of persons who have never had clinically evident HBV infection may be shown to have anti-HBs without anti-HBc. It is possible that subclinical infection with HBV may result in a serologic pattern that differs from that found in patients who have had clinically evident disease. Since successful vaccination against HBV results in the appearance of anti-HBs only,[181,222]

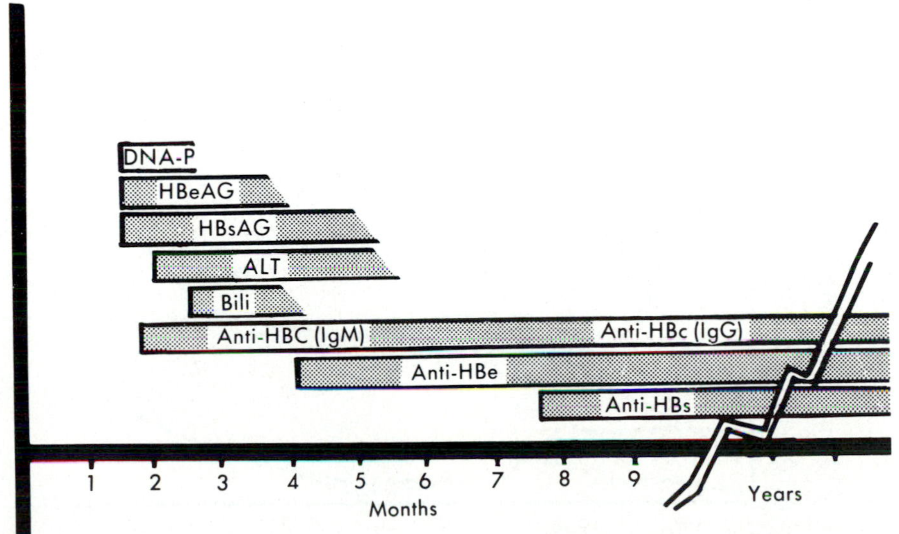

Fig. 27-5. Laboratory changes associated with acute hepatitis B infection. *DNA-P*, DNA polymerase; *HBeAg*, hepatitis B e antigen; *HBsAg*, hepatitis B surface antigen; *ALT*, alanine transferase; *Bili*, bilirubin; *anti-HBc*, antibody to hepatitis B core antigen; *IgM*, immunoglobulin M; *IgG*, immunoglobulin G; *anti-HBs*, antibody to hepatitis B surface antigen.

the question has been raised that perhaps persons with anti-HBs but without anti-HBc may have been naturally immunized but not actually infected by the HBV agent.

Epidemiology. VH-B has a worldwide distribution but, in contrast to VH-A, a large reservoir of asymptomatic carriers exists. Although transmission of HBV in the United States is often by inoculation of human blood products, HBV is not dependent on such artificial techniques for its propagation. Since HBsAg has been encountered in saliva,[208,227] tears, ascitic fluid, sneeze droplets,[227] blood-sucking insects,[191,192] menstrual fluid,[132] semen,[208] gingival and anorectal mucosa,[201] and, rarely, urine,[227] many mechanisms of person-to-person transmission have been suggested. These have included kissing,[227] biting,[176] sharing of razors and toothbrushes,[185] homosexual and heterosexual activities,[151,152] and transmission transplacentally or perinatally.[194,207]

The incidence of VH-B increased in large cities at alarming rates until 1970, mostly because of the practice of needle sharing by parenteral drug users. It is uncertain whether a recent decrease has resulted from diminished percutaneous drug abuse or the creation of immunity among drug users.

In the late 1970s the number of patients with VH-B related to illicit drug use declined (Fig. 27-6), and the high incidence of VH-B in male homosexuals became apparent. The high transmission rate of HBV among homosexuals led to the use of the homosexual community in controlled vaccine studies.[222] Approximately 8.2% of homosexuals in the Los Angeles area are chronic carriers of HBV, between 20- and 40-fold more than the remaining population.[146a] Transmission of the infection among homosexual men is correlated with punctate anal and gingival mucosal lesions.[201]

An important discovery of worldwide significance was the demonstration that HBV could be transmitted in the perinatal period and, occasionally, transplacentally from infected mother to offspring. The transmissibility in the perinatal period is strongly associated with the positive HBeAg status. Infants who acquire HBV in this fashion seldom develop a clinical illness; only 17% become icteric; 25% develop aminotransferase levels rising above 500 units, without icterus; whereas 58% develop a low-level persistent elevation of aminotransferase activities. Most infants infected in the first month of extrauterine life who develop icteric disease lose the virus on recovery from the acute illness. Conversely, those whose hepatitis is asymptomatic retain the virus and often the HBeAg into adult life; consequently, the females may transmit HBV to their subsequent offspring. Thus perinatal infection is the leading cause for a high incidence of chronic HBV infections, including cirrhosis and resulting hepatocellular carcinoma in the Orient and, probably, in Africa.

Offspring of women with AcVH-A do not develop an infection during the neonatal period. It is unclear whether they would do so if born while the mother was in the prodrome of hepatitis A, that is, when fecal viral content is high and before transplacentally acquired or breast-secreted HAV antibody is available.

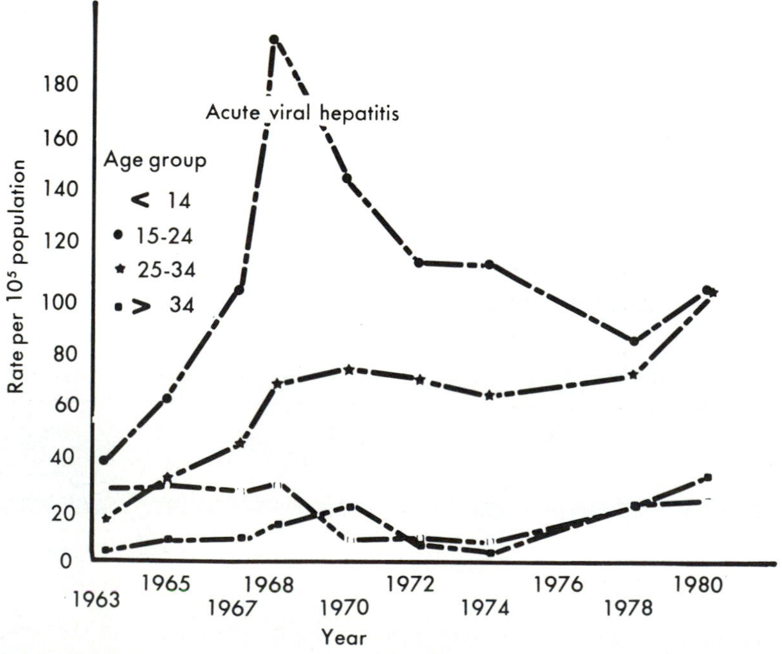

Fig. 27-6. Changing annual incidence of acute viral hepatitis in different age groups in California, 1963-1980. Despite increased incidence in 15- to 24-year-olds, age group with hepatitis most often related to transfusion has no change of incidence over 10-year period.

Screening candidate blood donors for HBsAg reduced the total incidence of posttransfusion hepatitis by about 25%. Despite sensitive screening of donor blood, a few cases of posttransfusion hepatitis are still type B. Pooling of blood products may increase the risk of transmitting the agent; however, pooling also adds anti-HBs, which is protective. Were it not for the addition of anti-HBs, every large pool of human blood products used in the past would have been infective. Blood fibrinogen carries a particularly high risk of transmitting HBV,[117] a risk reduced, but not eliminated, by HBsAg screening of donors. However, heat-treated serum albumin and Cohn-fractionated gamma globulin are free of infectivity.[186] Reports of removal of the risk of posttransfusion hepatitis by reconstituting washed, frozen erythrocytes[126] have been largely discounted.[150] Passive protection against HBV has been achieved by inoculation of high-titer anti-HBs.[171,217] Inoculation of heated HBsAg, as in some lots of human albumin, confers active immunization against HBV.[153,169,222] Protection is conferred apparently because of the immune response that develops to HBsAg, even though HBsAg itself is not infective.

Finally, a vaccine made up of treated HBsAg has been shown to be effective in producing protection against infection.[172,209,221] Although the vaccine use could theoretically bring about the disappearance of VH-B and reduction in incidence of hepatocellular carcinoma, the amount available precludes epidemiologic control in the immediate future.

Hepatitis non-A, non-B

There is ample clinical, epidemiologic, and experimental evidence for at least two hepatitis agents that are neither type A nor type B.[155,164,236] By 1982, at our liver unit, 24% of patients with clinically apparent acute viral hepatitis had H-NAB-V infections.[199a] A study in West London indicated 13% of the patients with acute viral hepatitis to be H-NAB-V type.[142] All but a few patients who develop posttransfusion hepatitis after receiving blood screened for HBsAg have H-NAB-V types. H-NAB-V has been transmitted percutaneously to produce at least two different infections that elicit no cross-immunity.[155,236] One candidate agent has been described in hepatocyte nuclei of chimpanzees and another in cytoplasm.[135,226,236] It is not known whether the agent that has produced at least one fecal-oral epidemic in New Delhi is yet another virus[233]; the clinical characteristics of the New Delhi illness were relatively more severe than most cases of acute viral hepatitis seen elsewhere. Similar epidemics of viral hepatitis that are non-A and non-B but which may differ from H-NAB-V types seen in the United States have been reported from the Kashmir Valley in India.[164,165]

Fifty percent of infants born of mothers with AcVH-NAB are reported to have minor elevations in serum levels of aminotransferase activities, but no sequelae in the infants have been recognized.[225]

Although greater concern has usually centered around VH-B with respect to severity, 42% of cases of fatal viral hepatitis at the USC Liver Unit have been from H-NAB-V type, and of patients with fulminant hepatitis, the mortality is higher in those with H-NAB-V type (see discussion of fulminant hepatitis). Chronicity occurs with greater frequency after VH-NAB than after VH-B, but the prognosis of the chronic disease that develops needs further clarification and may differ with the type of H-NAB-V involved (see discussion of chronic active hepatitis).

Pathology of viral hepatitis

AcVH is associated with histologic changes that vary considerably, depending on the temporal stage of the disease, severity of the process, and individual cellular and reparative response. Any differences in morphology produced by the various hepatitis agents are less than the variation in severity, response, or regeneration seen with any one of the virus infections.

In a liver biopsy specimen taken before the onset of symptoms and before there is biochemical evidence of cell necrosis, there is only nonspecific change. The hepatic cords are straight and regular; the hepatocytes have slightly enlarged nuclei and sharp nuclear membranes. The size and number of Kupffer cells, as well as the number of lymphocytes in the sinusoids, are increased, but portal lymphoid hyperplasia is lacking. Sparse foci of cell dropout or hepatocytolysis may be seen, but generalized liver cell hydropic swelling develops just before the onset of symptoms and simultaneously with serum biochemical abnormalities.

Three nearly concurrent, independently variable, morphologic changes characterize viral hepatitis at the height of clinical disease: (1) hepatocyte damage, (2) lymphoid and reticuloendothelial reaction, and (3) hepatocyte regeneration.

The hepatocyte damage is generalized. All the cells become swollen with a watery-appearing cytoplasm; this change is most severe in the perivenular regions, where the hydropic change at the sinusoidal margin of the hepatocyte contrasts sharply with the perinuclear and pericanalicular condensation of cytoplasm. In the early stage the hepatocyte cord arrangement becomes disrupted because of the cytoplasmic swelling and onset of heptocyte regeneration (Fig. 27-7). The nuclei are slightly, but uniformly, enlarged with finely divided, granular nuclear chromatin, a prominent nucleolus, and a sharp nuclear membrane. Hepatocytolysis is not randomly distributed throughout but is most prominent in the perivenular regions, where the intercellular membranes often become indistinct and structures that resemble syncytial giant cells are often seen. Rarely, severe confluent cell destruction may leave only a spongy stromal network in

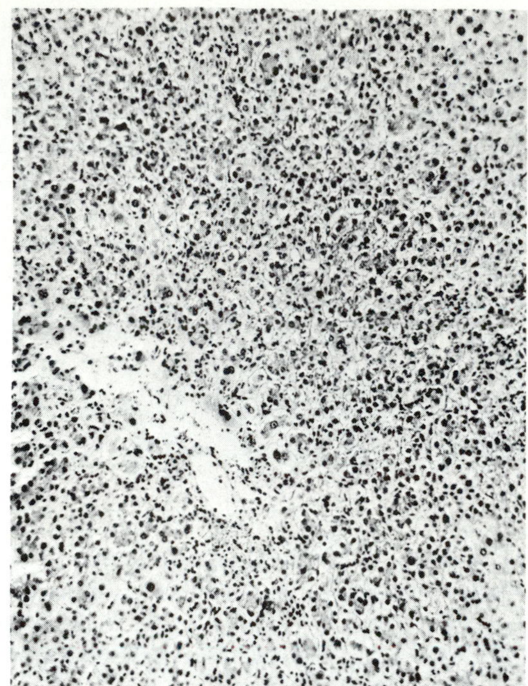

Fig. 27-7. Acute viral hepatitis. Appearance is that generally seen on needle biopsy. Note swollen liver cells, lack of cord pattern, and focal necrosis.

the perivenular areas. The lysis of dying cells is rapid, and dead liver cells are not identifiable on biopsy. An exception is the type of cell death that results in the acidophilic body, examples of which are often scattered throughout the lobule (see discussion of necrosis, Fig. 27-2, and Plate 3, *A*).

The hepatic lymphoid and reticuloendothelial response usually produces the most prominent histologic change in acute viral hepatitis. Kupffer cell activity is greatly increased, and unicellular foci of hepatocytolysis usually are identified by the histiocytes, which along with Kupffer cells phagocytose cell debris. The histiocytes usually are filled with glycoprotein, apparently representing activated lysosomes, and also contain lipochrome pigment. The foci of hepatocytolysis are further marked by numerous lymphocytes and a few plasma cells, which also are in sinusoids and spaces of Disse, often forming a cuff around hepatocytes. In the portal areas proliferative cholangiolar epithelium and poorly formed duct structures are found; lymphocytes, plasma cells, and mononuclear cells often transverse the limiting plates of portal zones, producing a saw-toothed effect, often referred to as piecemeal necrosis. Although piecemeal necrosis has often been described as a feature of chronic liver disease, it is usually present in acute viral hepatitis.

Concurrently with acute damage and necrosis, regeneration without nodularity occurs. Regeneration is manifest by zones of clustered hepatocytes without the regular contiguous relationship of hepatocytes to sinusoids. The periportal cells, particularly, have a solid pavement appearance early in the disease and consist of closely packed clusters of pale, swollen cells.

Perivenular canalicular cholestasis is variable, but even when extensive, there is poor correlation with clinical features that usually characterize cholestatic disease. Conversely, patients who have unusually high elevations of alkaline phosphatase activity in association with acute viral hepatitis do not have unusual cholestasis on biopsy. If jaundice is prolonged, the Kupffer cells also contain bile pigment, but there is usually little bile staining of the cytoplasm of the swollen hepatocytes.

Late histologic changes. After a patient's clinical recovery, although the serum transaminase levels approach normalcy, histologic changes persist. Pigment-laden and glycoprotein-rich histiocytes remain in scattered foci of previous cell necrosis, and hepatic parenchymal cells develop a cobblestone configuration, whereas the perivenular accentuation of cell damage disappears. A slow establishment of the sinusoidal and cord pattern often requires a year, and the portal lymphoid hyperplasia often remains prominent for months.

Electron microscopic studies. HAV, which is associated with cytoplasmic antigenic material in the liver even after the virus becomes undetectable in stool,[178] has been associated with cytoplasmic, viruslike, round bodies packaged in a saclike structure.[194,211] Although HAV antigenic material is found in Kupffer cells by immunofluorescent microscopy, there are no reports that these cells contain hepatitis A viral particles when studied under the electron microscope.

Electron microscopic studies disclose that viral particles are extremely sparse during AcVH-B, but the opposite is true of the liver of the patient who is a chronic carrier or who has HBsAg-positive chronic liver disease.

At least two electron microscopically different virallike structures have been described in AcVH-NAB. Except for one report, however, these particles have been described only in studies of VH-NAB in chimpanzees. One type of particle has a tubular ultrastructure with double-membrane walls enclosing electron-dense material found in hepatocyte cytoplasm during acute viral hepatitis[148,212,226,235,236] and is said to have an incubation period of 2 to 4 weeks in chimpanzees.[236] An agent with an incubation time of 5 weeks in a chimpanzee produces a disease without cytoplasmic tubular structures[236] but with poorly defined spherical structures that apparently develop in hepatocyte nuclei. Equivocal cytoplasmic tubules and nuclear particles have been described in humans, occurring simultaneously in both acute and chronic VH-NAB,[135] but the development of well-formed cytoplasmic and nuclear forms in humans has not been demonstrated. One study in chimpanzees showed that the same inoculum produced nuclear particles in one chimpanzee and cytoplasmic particles in another.[226] Thus the electron microscopic features of viruses responsible for VH-NAB remain controversial and unsettled.

Other ultrastructural changes observed in liver cells and Kupffer cells are nonspecific[223] and are apparently similar for hepatitis A, B, and NAB. Early in the disease the endoplasmic reticulum becomes irregularly dilated and vesicular and often is separated or destroyed by ballooning of the cytosol. The nuclei enlarge, and nucleoli are prominent. Free ribosomes increase in the cytoplasm, and glycogen deposition is irregular. The intercellular membranes, instead of disappearing as one would anticipate from light microscopy, actually develop microvilli. The space between adjacent cells is widened. Fine strands of collagen are occasionally found in Disse's space and in the intercellular space (Fig. 27-2).

The acidophilic, or Councilman-like, body is observed often in viral hepatitis, although it may be seen in many other diseases in humans and animals. Councilman described the bodies in yellow fever.[216] Although some doubt has been expressed as to whether the bodies are the same as those seen in viral hepatitis, most hepatopathologists use the terms *acidophilic body* and *Councilman's body* interchangeably. The acidophilic body is composed of condensed cytoplasm from which ribosomes have largely disappeared but in which the shadowy, electron-dense remains of many cell organelles are still visible.[115,128]

Several histologic variants of AcVH may occur, apparently based on host response and not on differences of viral strains or expressions of antigenic subgroups. The immunologic reaction and parenchymal reparative properties of the host may be affected by external environmental factors.

The pathogenesis of viral hepatitis (A, B, or NAB) is unsettled. The older concept that hepatocyte death results from a viral cytopathic effect has not been disproved but seems inadequate to explain the variations in course. It has been proposed that viral components incorporated in hepatocyte cell membranes act as the target for a cellular immune response.[139] However, no direct proof exists that cell death in viral hepatitis is immunocytopathic.

Viral hepatitis in homosexuals

A leading reservoir for HAV and HBV in large American cities is the male homosexual. Of the hepatitis agents, HBV has been studied most thoroughly. In Los Angeles 8.2% of homosexual men have a chronic HBV infection, whereas many more have serologic evidence of previous HBV infection. In Boston 70% of acute hepatitis infections in homosexuals in 1981 were type A. Of the remainder of homosexual men tested, 70% had serologic evidence of previous HAV infection.[144]

In New York over a 2-year period, 34.5% of the homosexual men studied developed serologic evidence of new HBV infection.[221] The high rate of infectivity is apparently related in part to promiscuity. Heterosexual contact between an acutely infected and a susceptible person results in as high as a 40% transmission rate[199]; heterosexual transmission rarely becomes epidemic, however. Experimental transmission studies have shown semen of HBV-infected persons to transmit HBV and have demonstrated that HBV can be acquired transvaginally. When there are breaks in oral mucosa, as can occur after brushing of teeth, HBV may be transmitted orally. There is evidence that the infection can be transmitted rectally, apparently through asymptomatic rectal mucosal abrasions[201]; whether the agent traverses intact mucosa is unclear.

Viral hepatitis in intravenous drug users

Although it appears that AcVH-B is on the decrease, as perhaps is the illicit use of intravenous drugs, an increased frequency of viral hepatitis among drug addicts has been recognized for many years, reaching a peak during the late 1960s.[174] In one study in 1981, 97% of the intravenous drug users had serologic evidence of chronic or healed VH-B.[187]

In some studies, up to 82% of intravenous drug users have heavy alcoholic consumption; thus assessment of the liver disease in this group is often difficult. Chronic HBs antigenemia has been reported to occur in over 10% of chronic intravenous drug users.[187]

Some intravenous drug users develop icteric hepatitis on more than one occasion; some have had four or five episodes; many have had three. The multiple attacks led to the recognition that there were indeed several types of virus involved, even before discovery of the B virus or demonstration of HAV. Occurrence of multiple bouts of icteric viral hepatitis is rare in non–drug users, including individuals who receive hundreds of units of blood or blood products. Immunoglobulin levels in addicts who have multiple attacks of hepatitis are not depressed.

On biopsy the liver of the percutaneous drug user with hepatitis often has more lymphoid proliferation in the portal areas than seen in typical AcVH; occasionally, formation of lymph follicles occurs. The lymphoid hyperplasia may be related to the repeated inoculations of foreign material. After the patient has had multiple bouts of hepatitis, the portal areas may become widened, but nodular regeneration does not develop. At one time in many cities, heroin and other opiates were often adulterated or "cut" with substances that included talclike particles; the repeated intravenous injection of these drugs resulted in accumulation of polarizable crystals in the portal areas and in Kupffer cells. The crystals rarely cause true granulomas but are often associated with mild nonprogressive increase of connective tissue. In addition, the high incidence of alcoholism in drug users is reflected by the large proportion of liver biopsies that show increased collagen and confuse the diagnosis.

Fatal viral hepatitis

Fulminant viral hepatitis. Fulminant hepatic failure is the clinical designation for the abrupt onset of liver failure with coma that always results from acute massive hepatic necrosis and usually occurs after severe submassive hepatic necrosis. The most common cause of severe, coma-producing hepatic necrosis in the United States is viral hepatitis. About 1% of patients hospitalized with viral hepatitis during the 1960s and 1970s developed abrupt and severe liver cell necrosis, producing hepatic insufficiency. During the early 1980s the percentage of patients with overt hepatitis who developed fulminant disease was about 3%, with about 66% mortality (Fig. 27-8, *bars 1-3*). In patients designated as having fulminant viral hepatitis, coma usually develops after less than 4 weeks of symptoms. Death usually follows coma within 24 hours to a few days. The liver morphology is determined by the extent of necrosis, amount of regeneration, and duration of survival of the patient after onset of fulminant disease.

Recovery of patients with AcVH is based on a balance of four semi-independent factors: (1) extent of hepatocellular loss, (2) extent and rapidity of regeneration of residual hepatocytes, (3) adequacy of functional activity of residual hepatocytes, and (4) adequacy of mechanisms of defense against continued viral replication and activity. The relationship of the clinical course to the sum of the effects of necrosis, adequacy of regeneration, and function of residual liver is charted in Table 27-3.

Patients with fatal fulminant hepatitis are divided into two major groups based on morphology: those who have less than a single layer of hepatocytes around the portal areas and no islands of viable parenchyma are classified as having acute massive necrosis; those with larger numbers of hepatocytes, either as islands of regenerating tissue or as evenly distributed periportal cells, are classified as having acute submassive necrosis (Plate 4, A).

In acute massive necrosis the liver weighs from 1 to 1.2 kg, only slightly less than normal. The liver capsule is smooth, but the liver is limp. When the liver is sectioned, the portal connective is accentuated; the remaining tissue is deep red and retracted. The liver in acute massive necrosis simulates the appearance of spleen, a pattern once referred to as acute red atrophy (Fig. 27-9). With complete necrosis there has usually not been sufficient time for bile pigment to accumulate, and there are no hepatocytes to extract it from blood; thus neither the patient nor the liver is deeply icteric.

Microscopic study reveals the destruction of hepatocytes. The Kupffer cells are large and numerous, and

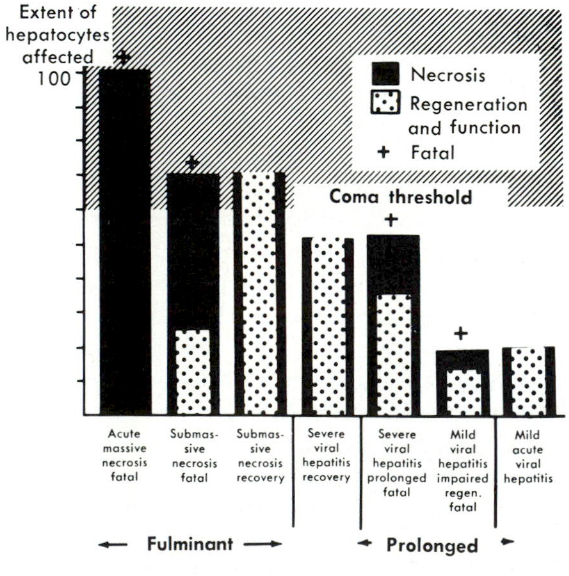

Extent of hepatocytes affected
100
Necrosis
Regeneration and function
+ Fatal
Coma threshold
Acute massive necrosis fatal
Submassive necrosis fatal
Submassive necrosis recovery
Severe viral hepatitis recovery
Severe viral hepatitis prolonged fatal
Mild viral hepatitis impaired regen. fatal
Mild acute viral hepatitis
← Fulminant →
← Prolonged →

Fig. 27-8. Schematic relationship between extent of necrosis, regeneration and function, and survival. First three bars reflect extensive necrosis to extent that coma develops (fulminant). First bar depicts total destruction (thus no regeneration or function). Second bar has regeneration and function inadequate to regain original mass. Third bar reflects recovery because of greater regeneration, despite amount of necrosis similar to that of second bar. Remaining bars indicate that, with less necrosis, death may still occur if regeneration and function are impaired.

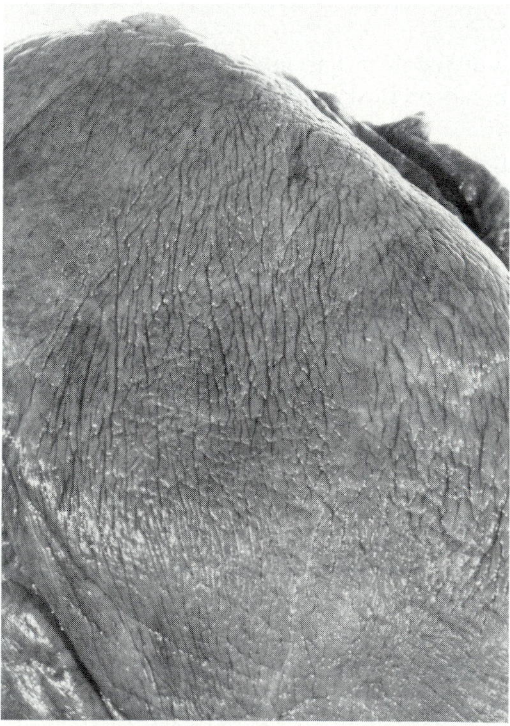

Fig. 27-9. Fulminant viral hepatitis occurring after blood transfusions given 140 days before onset of jaundice. Note typical wrinkling of capsule of liver when flexed.

there is a minimum amount of lymphocytic infiltrate and hyperplasia. The liver stroma is intact, and little collapse is noted. The bile ducts show little hyperplasia unless the fulminant episode occurred late in the course of ordinary hepatitis. Since all hepatocytes are destroyed, the factors of regeneration, function, and continued viral activity are not a consideration (Fig. 27-8, *bar 1*).

A patient with submassive necrosis (Fig. 27-8, *bars 2 and 3*) of the liver may die in less than 1 week but may live for 2 or 3 weeks when there is enough surviving liver parenchyma or greater regenerative and functional capacity.

The livers of patients who survive less than a week (stage I) are slightly shrunken, limp, and finely mottled. The deeply icteric swollen parenchymal cells remaining in periportal areas impart a golden yellow color that caused Rokitansky in 1842 to use the term *acute yellow atrophy* to describe such a liver. If the patient survives more than a week after developing hepatic coma from submassive necrosis, all of the parenchymal cells may disappear in some large zones, whereas in other areas yellow periportal parenchyma remains and replicates (Fig. 27-10).

The pattern of collapse and regeneration may become irregular. There may be some areas of considerable residual periportal liver parenchyma fading into zones of sharply defined perivenular collapse. These areas gradually merge into those where the periportal rims of residual hepatocytes are narrower or nonexistent and the corresponding stromal collapse of the remaining lobules more extensive (stage II). The liver is shrunken to a weight of about 800 to 900 g. It is wrinkled and deeply icteric (Fig. 27-9), particularly in the areas of less collapse.

In patients who survive 3 weeks or more (stage III), the liver is characterized grossly by islands of yellow liver parenchyma bulging above the surrounding dark collapsed stroma. In the past, this stage was called subacute yellow atrophy. However, the necrosis is acute, even though the patient may have survived longer because there was enough functionally active residual liver. If the patient lives for several weeks after the episode of submassive hepatic necrosis, the blood channels in the collapsed stroma of the liver may sclerose, and areas of collapse may become pale and lose the congested "splenic" appearance. The residual and regenerating liver is nearly devoid of inflammatory exudate (Fig. 27-10, *B*).

These patterns, often misinterpreted as cirrhosis or precursors to cirrhosis, are called early (I), middle (II), and late (III) stages of submassive necrosis. Microscopically in late submassive necrosis there are striking numbers of bile plugs and microconcretions of bile in periportal canaliculi.

In both massive and submassive necrosis, changes such as minimal ascites, pleural effusion, and peripheral edema are often present. The regional lymph nodes and spleen are generally enlarged at autopsy. Hemorrhagic areas often are found in various tissues because of deficiency of coagulation factors normally produced by the liver. Hemorrhages are often present in the intestine,

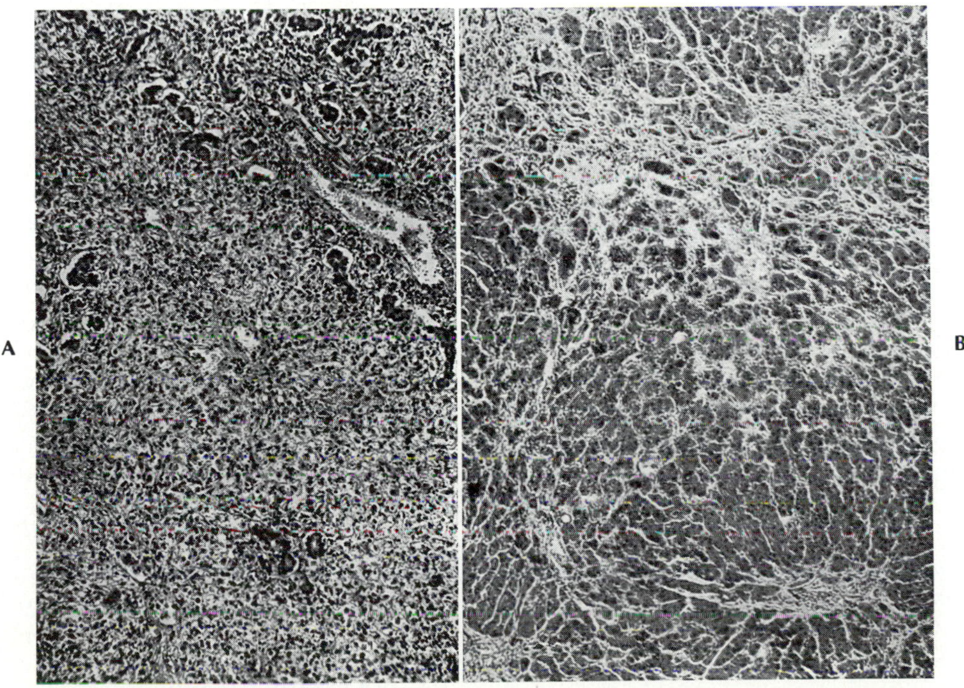

Fig. 27-10. Fatal viral hepatitis. **A,** Appearance of liver on ninety-third day, showing collapsed areas. **B,** Residual liver. (From Lucké, B.: Am. J. Pathol. **20:**595, 1944.)

lungs, and mesentery, and gastrointestinal bleeding occasionally contributes to death.

Mortality. The survival rate in patients with fulminant viral hepatitis has varied in different studies. One important factor in outcome has been the age of the patient. Chance of survival is greater in younger individuals; of 81 patients with fulminant hepatitis admitted to our liver unit from 1965 to 1972, there was a 47.3% survival of the 11- to 20-year age group; 25% survival in the 21- to 40-year age group; and none in those over 40 years.[200] Since 1965, all but one of 22 survivors of fulminant hepatitis at our liver unit have been under 30 years of age. None of 22 survivors of the 81 cases of clinically fulminant hepatitis has developed cirrhosis or any other hepatic sequela.[162]

However, a report from the National Acute Hepatic Failure Study Group indicated a difference in prognosis for patients with fulminant hepatitis B, in contrast to those with fulminant hepatitis non-A, non-B (NAB). Patients with fulminant hepatitis NAB had only a 13% overall survival, in contrast to a 33% survival in the patients with fulminant hepatitis B. In addition, patients under 24 years of age with fulminant hepatitis NAB had a 21% survival; those 25 to 44 years, a 5% survival; those over 45 years, a 16% survival.[196] Since 60% of the patients with fulminant hepatitis at the USC Liver Unit had type B hepatitis, compared with 31% in the national study group,[113] survival expectations might be expected to differ not only with respect to patient age but also with respect to the infective agent.

Infectivity of patients with fulminant hepatitis. Patients with fulminant hepatitis B are HBeAg positive but DNA polymerase negative at the time of development of coma[196a]; thus they have much lower infectivity than patients with ordinary AcVH or, for that matter, many patients with chronic active hepatitis or B viral cirrhosis. There is neither documentation of needle-stick transmission of hepatitis B from a patient with fulminant hepatitis nor evidence of an autopsy prosector contracting hepatitis B after being cut during the course of autopsy of such a patient. Although data are less complete regarding infectivity of fulminant hepatitis NAB, there is no evidence of greater risk to medical personnel by patients with more serious illness. Since HAV is demonstrable in the liver of patients dying of fulminant hepatitis A, one might suspect a greater hazard at autopsy from fulminant hepatitis A than B, but there are no data to clarify that point and only about 1% or less of the fulminant hepatitis in the United States is caused by HAV.

Viral hepatitis with impaired regeneration syndrome (VH-IRS), protracted viral hepatitis, and subacute hepatic necrosis. A small but significant segment of the patients who die following AcVH undergo a protracted nonfulminant form of the disease. Twenty-two percent of the patients who have died of viral hepatitis at the USC Liver Unit have had such a protracted, rather than fulminant, pattern. Because the basic difficulty appears to be related more to the failure to regenerate than to the amount of necrosis, we have called this pattern the impaired regeneration syndrome (VH-IRS).[190] Patients who fit into the category average 60 years of age, in contrast to the 20- to 30-year-old patients dying of fulminant disease; the average duration of illness of patients with VH-IRS is 75 days rather than 14 and 20 days for acute massive and submassive necrosis, respectively. The percentage of patients who survive after developing the IRS is unclear because there is a degree of impaired regeneration in the clinical pattern of most elderly patients with viral hepatitis; viral hepatitis in older patients is regularly protracted and the cholestasis more prominent even after transaminase activities have dropped to nearly normal range.

Liver biopsies from patients with IRS who ultimately recover show regular, straight liver cords that are frequently somewhat shrunken, apparently a reflection of the failure of those cells to proliferate at an accelerated rate. Otherwise, in initial aspects of the disease the histologic appearance is similar to AcVH. However, when the necrosis is more severe, areas of confluent hepatocellular destruction are not replaced by rapidly regenerating hepatocytes, as they are in younger individuals with hepatitis, but are marked by collapsed stroma. When this stroma produces "bridging" bands that connect adjacent portal areas or perivenular regions throughout the biopsy specimen, the pattern has been referred to as subacute hepatic necrosis (SHN).[120] Bridging, however, can be seen as a result of severe acute necrosis if biopsies are performed as early as it is safe to do so; it also may be seen in chronic active hepatitis and after there has been only an ordinary degree of necrosis with impaired regeneration. Thus the prognosis of patients with the bridging lesion depends on the underlying hepatic disorder in which the bridging is recognized.[229]

The liver of the patient who dies with the bridging lesion of VH-IRS is shrunken and slightly toughened but limp. Its surface is bumpy or irregular with few regenerative areas. Microscopic examination shows shrunken hepatocytes and little exudate in the parenchyma; hyperplasia of the lymphoid and reticuloendothelial system within widened portal areas is somewhat less than in ordinary viral hepatitis. There is also considerable collapse within each lobule. Thin fingers of collapsed stroma and collagen extend from both the portal and the perivenular areas. Regeneration is minimal; thus the hepatic cords are straight and obvious. Cholestasis is striking in the liver of many patients with VH-IRS, producing periportal biliary concretions that may result in acute cholangitis around the plugged interlobular duct radicals.

Relapse of viral hepatitis

About 2% of patients with AcVH have a relapse of their disease within 3 months after recovery. The symptoms are indistinguishable from the initial episode, although the disease is usually somewhat milder. Occasionally the relapse may be more severe, but it is rarely fatal. The biopsy changes in the liver are similar to those of the initial attack. Recovery occurs after the relapse.

Chronic varieties of hepatitis

The foregoing discussion has dealt with the relationship between the extent of necrosis, regenerative capacity, and adequacy of hepatocellular functional activity. A fourth variable in the recovery or nonrecovery from viral hepatitis deals with the ability or inability of patients to rid themselves of the virus. The definition of chronic forms of viral hepatitis involves the failure to terminate the viral infection.

There are considerable differences in chronicity that follow infection by different viral agents. HAV infection has not been shown to progress to chronicity. A great deal is known about chronic forms of HBV infection, and although the non-A, non-B viruses are less well studied, there is good evidence that chronic viral infection following VH-NAB occurs more often than does chronicity after HBV infection. It is not clear whether chronic forms of VH-NAB have a course identical to or widely divergent from that of VH-B. Since NAB viruses constitute a group of possibly unrelated agents, the final answer will not be forthcoming until specific agents can be identified.

Chronic forms of VH-B

In approximately 10% to 12% of adults with overt AcVH-B, a chronic form of the disease develops.[195,198] In a much higher percentage, up to 50% in the pediatric age group, chronic disease develops when the acute illness is subclinical.[135,169] There are two classes of chronic hepatitis B: a nonprogressive, benign form termed persistent viral hepatitis type B (PVH-B) and a progressive form, termed chronic active viral hepatitis B (AVH-B) (Fig. 27-11). During the acute stage there is no way to predict in which patients a chronic form of VH-B will develop or to assess, in those in whom VH-B becomes chronic, the features that cause one patient to have a progressive form and another a nonprogressive disorder. In our experience at the USC Liver Unit, we have not found that PVH-B, *as we define it,* progresses to a more serious form of chronic liver disease, but many investigators have speculated that patients may vacillate between the two forms of chronic hepatitis.

In a large population, between 0.1% (United States) and 15% (Taiwan) of the population asymptomatically have HBsAg in their sera. Most have had no signs or symptoms of AcVH. The initial infection was therefore subclinical by definition. A small percentage of these "asymptomatic" carriers have AVH-B, but most have the clinical and histologic features of PVH-B. Many investigators have demonstrated HBsAg in hepatocyte cyto-

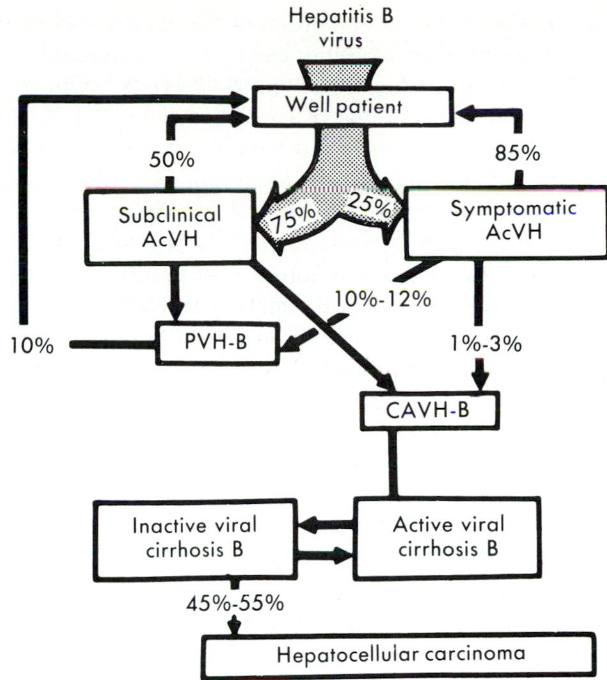

Fig. 27-11. Relationship of acute viral hepatitis B to chronic forms of disorder.

plasm and HBcAg in hepatocytic nuclei of such carriers. Worldwide, it is estimated that 200 million persons are chronically infected with HBV, providing the major source of virus for continued infection of susceptible individuals. Most patients chronically infected with HBV are HBeAg positive early in the course but, over the years, lose HBeAg and acquire anti-HBe.[157] From a practical standpoint, HBeAg-positive persons represent the important transmitters of HBV, doing so by sexual contact, perhaps by kissing, by percutaneous inoculation of various sorts, or during the birth process. Chronically HBV-infected persons who are HBeAg negative have distinctly lower infectivity, requiring a substantial percutaneous inoculation of blood or fluid into a susceptible person to bring about infection. In the Orient and probably in Africa and the Pacific Islands, the major source of chronic hepatitis B is perinatal infection. Individuals who have acquired their hepatitis at birth apparently retain not only their infection but also their infectivity (HBeAg) longer, even into the childbearing age. In the United States most of the 0.1% to 0.4% of chronically HBsAg-positive women have acquired the virus in adolescence or young adulthood, and many more become HBeAg negative at an earlier age. Thus a low incidence of HBeAg positivity in the women of childbearing age is critical in a population, since the HBsAg-positive childbearers who are also HBeAg positive are responsible for perpetuating the infection from generation to generation. The advent of immunoglobulin and vaccine and the apparent effectiveness in aborting the perinatal transmission may bring about resolution of this worldwide problem, although the economic barriers are formidable.

Persistent viral hepatitis type B. PVH-B is the most common form of chronic disease caused by VH-B. Ten percent of the patients who have overt VH-B develop this benign, "normal carrier" state. The patient is asymptomatic, although during the first 5 years or so serum transaminase activities remain elevated in the 50- to 200-unit range. Recurrence of jaundice or progression of the condition does not occur. Ultimately, transaminase activities return to normal, and about 10% of the patients lose HBsAg and acquire anti-HBs over the years.[175] While HBsAg is present, however, the titer is always high.

The morphologic pattern of the liver in PVH-B changes somewhat with time. The changes are minimal, initially resembling healed hepatitis. Uniformity is maintained within the lobule and from one lobule to another. For the first few years the hydropic appearance of hepatocytes and lack of distinct cord pattern is present throughout the lobule. There are usually unicellular foci of hepatocytolysis, only one to four per lobule, replaced by an accumulation of lymphocytes and macrophages condensed into the site of a lysed hepatocyte (Fig. 27-12). About one third of the patients with PVH-B have portal lymphoid hyperplasia, one third have patchy lymphoid hyperplasia in portal areas, and one third have normal portal areas. Clearly the reticuloendothelial component of the liver is not reacting similarly in all patients. In time, usually years, the hydropic change diminishes, and a regular cord pattern may be recognized. The HBsAg accumulates in some hepatocytes and produces a characteristic body that occupies part or nearly all of the cytoplasm of scattered hepatocytes. These faintly granular cells are called ground-glass (GG) cells or Hadziyannis cells, after the individual who described them and recognized their relationship to VH-B (Fig. 27-13).[149] GG cells are found in any type of chronic hepatitis B and never in AcVH-B. In PVH-B, GG cells, when present, are regularly distributed throughout the liver, unlike the distribution in AVH-B, in which they are frequently in clusters and quite irregular in distribution. The GG cells actually consist of closely packed smooth endoplasmic reticulum with tubular structures composed of HBsAg. Specific immunoperoxidase stains[110] or orcein stains for disulfide bonds[210] establish the presence of large amounts of HBsAg (Fig. 27-14).

Chronic active hepatitis (CAH). Originally the term *chronic active hepatitis* was a clinical designation for patients who had repeated, usually mild, bouts of a hepatitis-like illness, interrupted by remissions that progressed to cirrhosis. It is now known that most CAH is subclinical, just as the initial hepatitis infection is usually subclinical. Only 15% of patients with B-viral cirrhosis have a history of symptoms of liver disease before onset of symptoms of advanced cirrhosis or hepatocellular carcinoma. The causes of CAH are multiple, and the ultimate prognosis depends on the causative agent and its propensity to persist.

Morphology of chronic active hepatitis type B (CAVH-B) and B-viral cirrhosis. The initial lesion of CAVH-B is usually seen fortuitously because the onset is usually mild or subclinical and only occasionally follows ordinary AcVH. Usually a biopsy is performed because the patient is found to have either asymptomatic abnormal serum transaminase activities or recurrent clinical episodes of a hepatitis-like illness. Histologically, CAVH-B is usually described as active or quiescent. Activity, as most hepatologists use the term, refers to the amount of inflammatory and necrotizing processes, not to the regenerative activity. The active and quiescent phases differ microscopically; however, as the disease progresses to cirrhosis, there may be a greater difference in the inflammatory and the necrotizing activity from one nodule or zone to another. In the early stage (active phase) the disease resembles AcVH. Hepatocytes are swollen, some having cuffs of lymphocytes, and there is poorly defined hepatocytolysis and portal exudative reaction. The dissimilarity from AcVH lies in the localization of the changes. In ordinary AcVH the changes are uniform from one lobule to the next, and the greatest inflammatory and necrotizing changes are perivenular (zone 3 of Rappaport), whereas regenerative changes are periportal. In CAVH-B there is no perivenular accentuation of necrosis and exudate; instead, those changes may be greater in the periportal area or uniform throughout a lobule, and there may be considerable variation from one lobule to the next (Fig. 27-15). Regeneration is also irregularly distributed and is not necessarily periportal. Regenerating areas are often poorly defined but are made up of larger, more hydropic hepatocytes among which there is little if any necrosis or exudate. The portal areas are usually wider in CAVH-B than in AcVH. Portal widening in CAVH-B usually includes a deposition of collagen that, although not heavy, distorts the relationship of the portal components. Destruction of the portal limiting plate by necrosis and exudate (so-called piecemeal necrosis) occurs in both AcVH and CAVH-B, and widening of the portal areas by intense lymphoid hyperplasia is particularly prominent in livers of some illicit percutaneous drug users at the time of hepatitis. It is now apparent that an exuberant inflammatory response is not related to chronicity.[143] GG cells or cells staining positively for HBsAg are sparse in the active phases of CAVH-B, but when present, they are irregularly distributed, unlike persistent hepatitis in which the distribution of GG cells is regular (Fig. 27-16).

During the quiescent phases of CAVH-B, when the patient is asymptomatic and the serum aminotransferase levels are normal or nearly so, necrosis and exudate are reduced or absent. Morphologic abnormalities may be

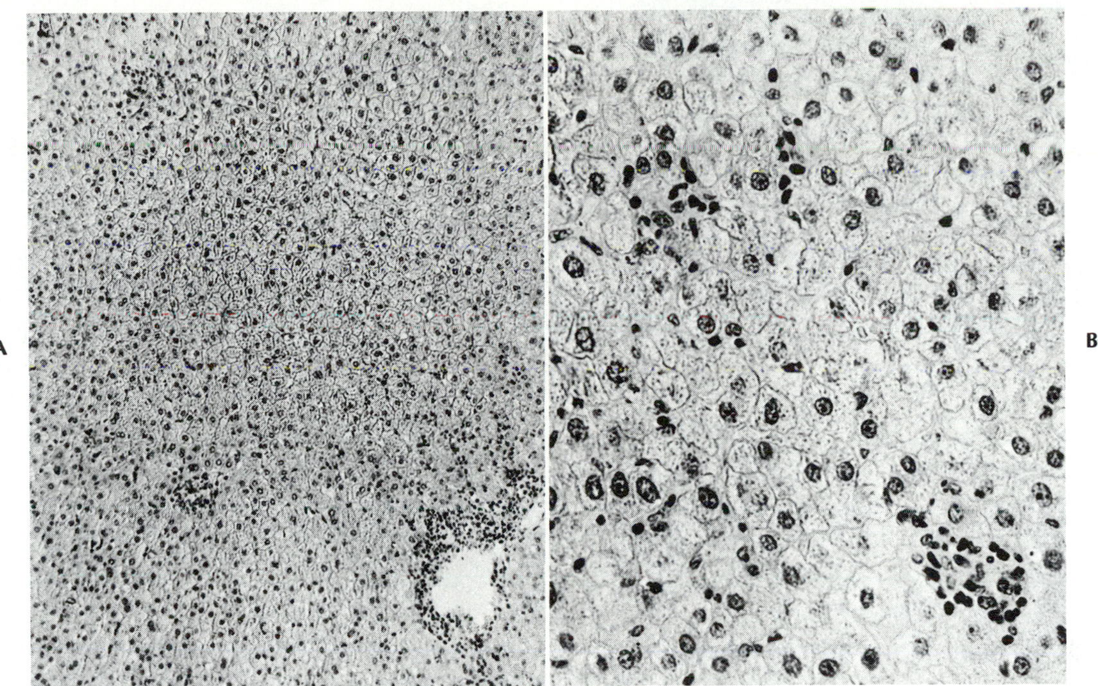

Fig. 27-12. A, Persistent viral hepatitis. Note cobblestone pattern of liver cells and scattered areas of focal necrosis. **B,** Higher magnification, emphasizing focal necrosis.

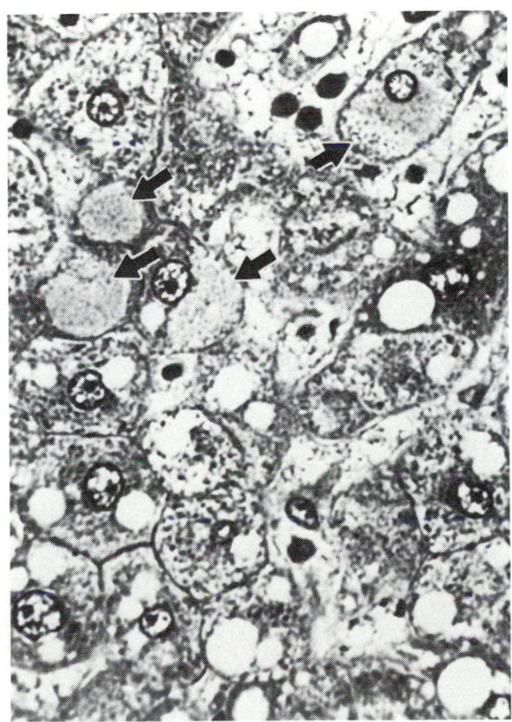

Fig. 27-13. "Ground-glass" hepatocytes of Hadziyannis *(arrows)* may be found either in persistent viral hepatitis B or in chronic active viral hepatitis B.

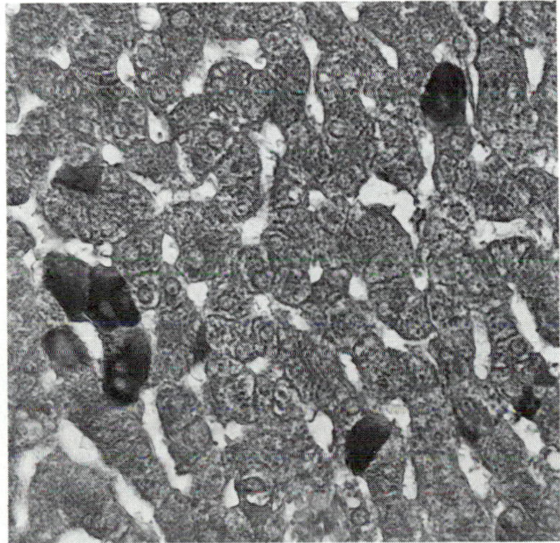

Fig. 27-14. Immunoperoxidase stains reveal HBsAg in "ground-glass" cells of Hadziyannis. (Courtesy Dr. Angelos Afroudakis, Athens, Greece.)

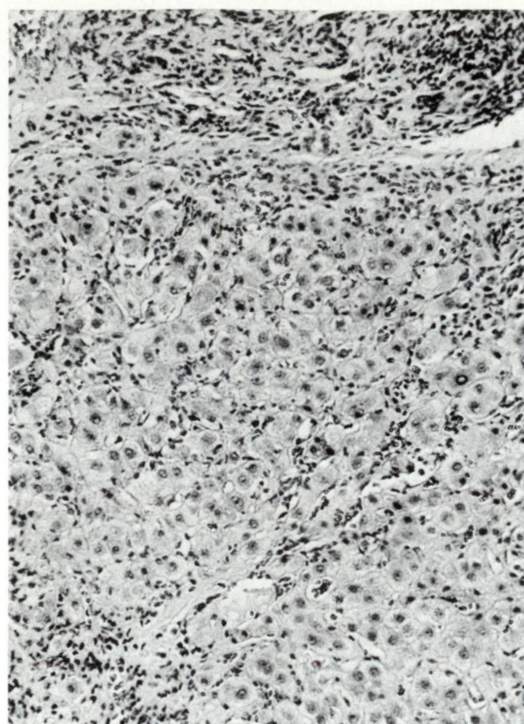

Fig. 27-15. Diffuse inflammation and liver cell necrosis in regenerative nodule from liver in chronic active hepatitis.

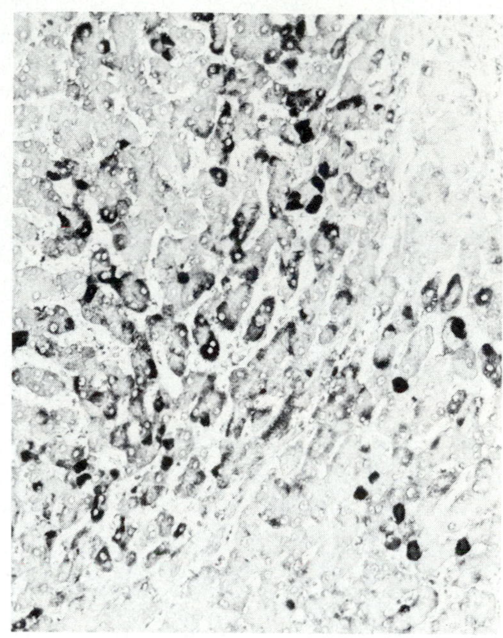

Fig. 27-16. Immunoperoxidase demonstration of HBsAg in chronic active viral hepatitis B. (Courtesy Dr. Angelos Afroudakis, Athens, Greece.)

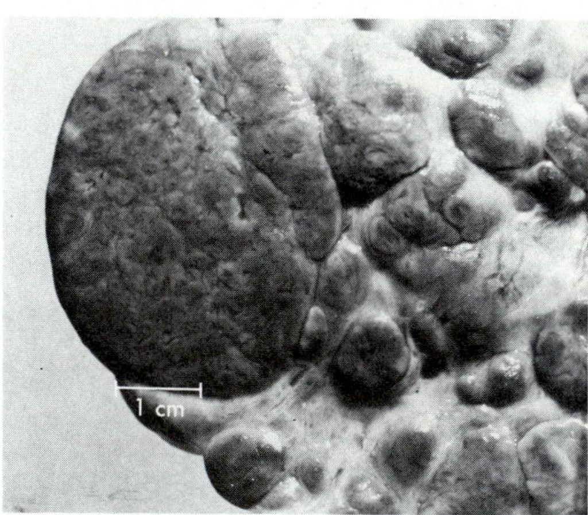

Fig. 27-17. Cut surface of atrophic, firm, megalonodular B-viral cirrhosis.

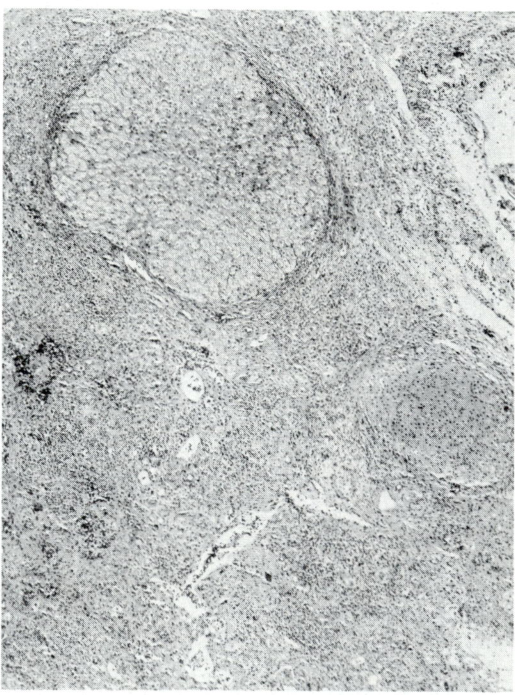

Fig. 27-18. Well-defined regenerative nodule amid collapsed inflamed stroma in coarsely nodular cryptogenic cirrhosis.

restricted to irregularly distributed, poorly defined zones of regenerating hepatocytes that subtly compress adjacent hepatocytes. Some areas have hepatocytes with dyplastic or polyploid nuclei, and others are interspersed with increased Kupffer cells. Portal areas are usually larger than normal with increased amounts of collagen or lymphoid tissue. HBsAg-containing hepatocytes or GG cells are irregularly distributed, usually sparing zones of the more actively regenerating hepatocytes. GG cells may be extremely abundant or nonexistent. The hepatic morphologic changes during the early, inactive phase of CAVH-B are so vague and nonspecific that the diagnosis often cannot be made during quiescent phases on morphologic changes alone unless the HBsAg-containing GG cells are recognized, identifying the disease as a form of CAVH-B. The distinction from PVH-B is based on the uniformity of cell arrangement of the latter. Changes similar to those of the quiescent phase of an early CAVH-B may, except for the GG cells, be seen in nonprogressive hepatic disorders.

In spite of the paucity of necrosis and inflammation that may be a feature of CAVH-B, progression to cirrhosis proceeds relentlessly in both the subclinical (quiescent) and the clinically apparent (active) forms of the disease, with cirrhosis developing between 1 and 3 years after acquisition of the infection. After the development of frank cirrhosis, even the disease of those patients with earlier episodes of jaundice and elevated aminotransferase activities tends to become quiescent, and a latent period of 5 to as much as 50 years may elapse before either hepatocellular carcinoma or the consequences of portal hypertension supervene. From 40% to 45% of patients dying of B-viral cirrhosis have hepatocellular carcinoma; in the United States, where B-viral cirrhosis is relatively uncommon, this results in relatively low incidence of hepatocellular carcinoma. However, in the Orient and in Africa, where B-viral cirrhosis is the leading form of cirrhosis, the resultant neoplastic development makes hepatocellular carcinoma one of the most common neoplasms in the world.

The cirrhosis that develops from CAVH-B is called B-viral cirrhosis. Although the nodules in B-viral cirrhosis have their origin in small, poorly defined areas of regeneration, the nodules are usually large by the time symptoms of portal hypertension or hepatic failure develop (Fig. 27-17). However, hepatocellular carcinoma may develop while the nodules are still small or poorly defined. The average weight of the liver involved at the end stage of B-viral cirrhosis at autopsy is 860 g, ranging from 400 to 1600 g. Nodules are from 0.3 to 1 cm in diameter, septa are usually thin, and the collagen is loose (Fig. 27-18) rather than hard and leathery as it is in the alcoholic person. On cut surface the nodules bulge, reflecting the paucity of collagen within them.

Chronic forms of hepatitis non-A, non-B

Although by 1982 there were no reliable serologic or tissue markers to identify chronic forms of VH-NAB, there is substantial evidence that chronicity exists.[159,168,197] Since the number of H-NAB-V agents that may be responsible for chronicity is unknown and the differing characteristics (if they do differ) of the chronic disorders associated with each H-NAB-V agent are similarly unclear, prediction of events in individual instances is not based on well-defined criteria. Between 20% and 50% of patients who develop VH-NAB continue to have elevated levels of aminotransferase activity and histologic alterations beyond the 6-month period usually allotted to the course of AcVH.

Persistent viral hepatitis non-A, non-B (PVH-NAB)

The persistent form of non-A, non-B hepatitis is more common but more elusive than PVH-B. More than 50% of the patients who develop AcVH-NAB related to percutaneous injections of illicit drugs continue to have elevated serum levels of aminotransferases for longer than 6 months. Very few, less than 1%, develop progressive liver disease. A similar percentage of patients who develop VH-NAB following transfusion have protracted elevation of aminotransferase activities, but about 40% of the patients who develop chronically elevated serum aminotransferase levels after transfusion-transmitted VH-NAB progress to cirrhosis. Of patients who have no obvious source for the acquisition of hepatitis, only 20% have continued elevation of serum aminotransferase levels, and few (less than 1%) of these patients develop progressive hepatic lesions.[197] It is unclear whether the differences in course are a result of different viral infection(s) or are related to the means of acquisition. As with PVH-B, patients with PVH-NAB have a slow diminution of serum aminotransferase levels and of histologic alterations. There is no way, at present, to know whether or not PVH-NAB has healed.

The pathologic changes of PVH-NAB are difficult to separate from the changes associated with continued intravenous drug use, which in itself results in reactive inflammatory hyperplasia. However, the changes in PVH-NAB include portal lymphoid hyperplasia and Kupffer cell hyperplasia, with scattered focal hepatocytolysis. The cobblestone pattern often associated with PVH-B may be lacking. There is no regenerative activity or nodularity, but the portal areas are often somewhat widened. This histologic appearance is not as bland as it is with PVH-B. Because of the lack of a serologic marker for PVH-NAB, we cannot tell if the lesion heals, if it progresses to cirrhosis, or, as with PVH-B, if the patient has no progressive disease but is part of an infective pool. It has been suggested that transmission of the H-NAB-V agents from mother to newborn occurs,[225] but conclusive evidence of continued H-NAB-V infection of the children is lacking.

Chronic active hepatitis, non-A, non-B, and NAB viral cirrhosis

Chronic active hepatitis non-A, non-B (CAVH-NAB) is a lesion whose etiology is difficult to establish. The lack of serologic or tissue markers restricts the use of the term *chronic active viral hepatitis non-A, non-B* to patients whose chronic disease follows an episode of acute hepatitis. If, as with hepatitis B, most chronic illness is derived from initially mild or subclinical acute disease, a substantial number of cases would be anticipated. Instead, HBsAg-negative chronic active hepatitis is uncommon in both drug users and male homosexuals, although both groups of individuals have a high incidence of acute viral hepatitis A, B, and NAB. But CAVH-NAB is common as a sequela to posttransfusion hepatitis NAB. In brief, it seems that either a large inoculum is necessary for the induction of CAVH-NAB or a different agent is inoculated in blood transfusion than is transmitted by illicit drug use.

Pathology. Although livers of many patients with CAVH-NAB have changes indistinguishable from those of CAVH-B, often the converse is true. CAVH-NAB often features less regenerative activity, a tendency toward more intrasinusoidal and pericellular fibrosis, and scattered fat droplets. Other features of CAVH-B such as randomly distributed focal hepatocytolysis, irregular distribution of regeneration, and portal widening are present. The rate of progression of CAVH-NAB is unclear. In at least some instances the progression is more rapid than in CAVH-B and results in a cirrhotic liver that, at time of death from hepatic failure, has small, poorly defined nodules. The nodules are invaded by fine collagen fibers, but the connective tissue is loose, thus differing from the dense, hard liver in cirrhosis of the alcoholic individual. However, since there are no markers to identify H-NAB-V agents, it is uncertain whether progression of CAVH-NAB is, at times, self-limiting; it is possible that the H-NAB-V agent(s) may not persist as tenaciously as the HBV agent does in CAVH-B. On the contrary, it is not clear how many of the patients with cryptogenic cirrhosis or with cryptogenic chronic active hepatitis derive their diseases from the H-NAB-V agent(s).

The prognosis of the patient with cirrhosis following VH-NAB is similar to that of patients with other types of cirrhosis. Hepatocellular carcinoma may develop less frequently than it does in patients with B viral cirrhosis, but even that relationship is not certain.

Chronic active autoimmune (lupoid) hepatitis (CALH)

Autoimmune (lupoid) hepatitis is a variety of chronic active hepatitis in which the patient has one or more immunologic abnormalities. Although the disease has no known viral relationship, the possibility of a viral-host interaction to produce a "foreign" antigen has been proposed by some investigators.

Some 85% to 90% of patients with autoimmune hepatitis are women, principally those of childbearing age. Early symptoms include the development of amenorrhea or systemic complaints long before liver disease is manifest. The name "lupoid" was based on the finding of positive lupus erythematosus preparations (LE "preps") in peripheral blood. In addition to positive LE preps, biologic false-positive tests for syphilis occur in 25% of patients with lupoid hepatitis[177,202]; 50% have positive latex fixation reaction for rheumatoid arthritis; 75% have antinuclear antibodies[177]; and 90% or more have a positive reaction for IgG type of smooth muscle antibodies.[231]

Autoimmune hepatitis responds to immunosuppressant therapy in a fashion not paralleled by other forms of CAH.[199a] Without such therapy, fatal submassive hepatic necrosis often develops, a complication rarely found in other forms of CAH. At the USC Liver Unit, 50% of patients with autoimmune hepatitis died in fulminant failure after submassive necrosis, whereas only one of 63 patients dying of CAVH-B had a terminal fulminant course. Although immunosuppressants are effective in aborting such episodes in autoimmune hepatitis, the effect on the ultimate course is unclear, and the oncogenic potential of protracted immunosuppression is still an unsettled question. Recently, two patients with autoimmune hepatitis who had taken steroids for years developed hepatocellular carcinoma. The infrequency of HCC in patients with CALH may be related to the preponderance of females with autoimmune hepatitis, whereas hepatocellular carcinoma is far more common in men.

Chronic active hepatitis may result from certain idiosyncratic drug reactions and must be considered in the differential diagnosis. Some patients develop abnormal serologic findings, usually associated with chronic active autoimmune hepatitis, when administered certain drugs to which they are sensitive. Very few drugs truly initiate chronic active hepatitis, although many cases of submassive necrosis have been considered incorrectly to be chronic active hepatitis (see discussion of drug necrosis).

Cryptogenic chronic active hepatitis (CCAH)

The cryptogenic form of CAH includes those cases of CAH and even cirrhosis in which all other etiologies have been excluded. As this group is reviewed and new etiologies are elucidated, the category designated *cryptogenic* should shrink. In some livers previously classified as showing CCAH, HBV infection may be present in hepatocytes without HBsAg in serum.[111,163,167,188] In our series of previously diagnosed cryptogenic cirrhosis patients, one third had demonstrable HBcAg in hepatocyte nuclei. In addition, some individuals with CCAH undoubtedly have CAVH-NAB infection. Certain other

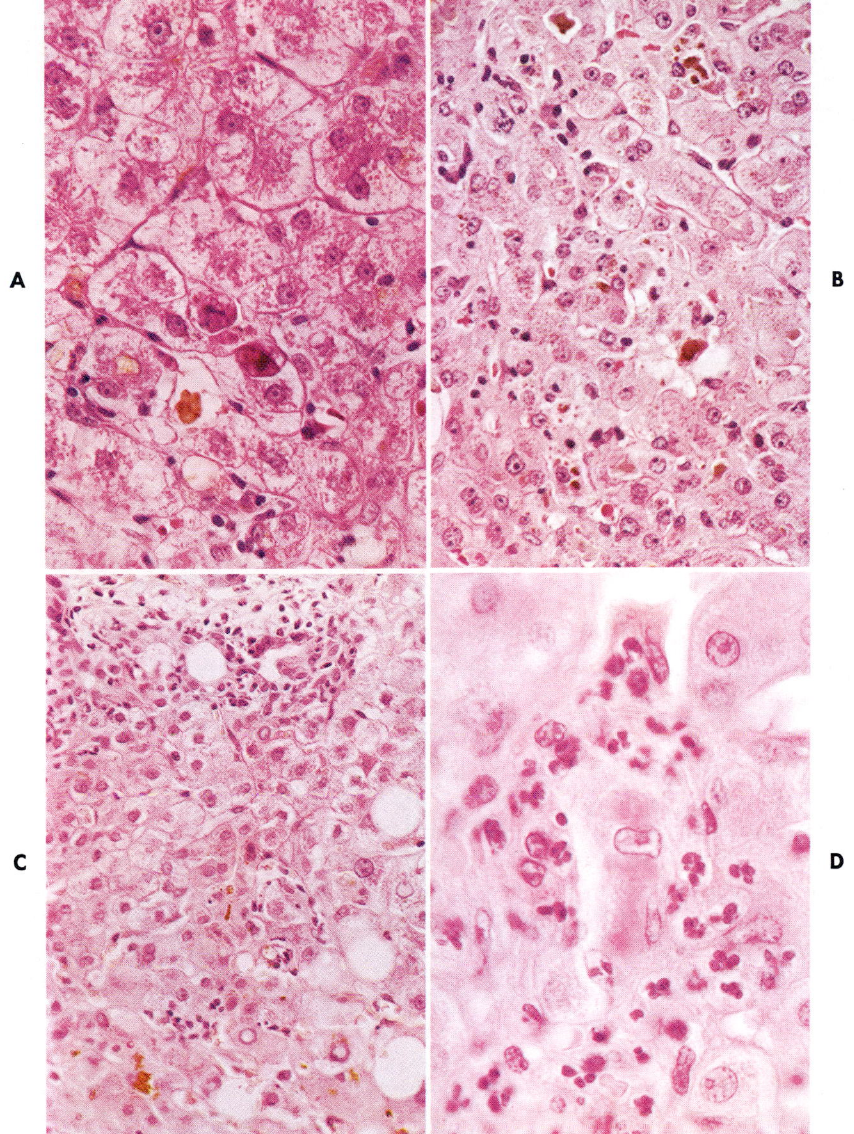

Plate 3

A, Needle biopsy in acute hepatitis A. Two acidophilic bodies are present near bottom. Cytoplasm is swollen and granular and cell membranes are indistinct.

B, Centrilobular bile stasis in patient taking oral contraceptive.

C, Acute pericholangitis and cholestasis in needle biopsy. Later at surgery, stone was removed from common bile duct.

D, Hyaline necrosis in alcoholic patient. Many neutrophils are in sinusoids.

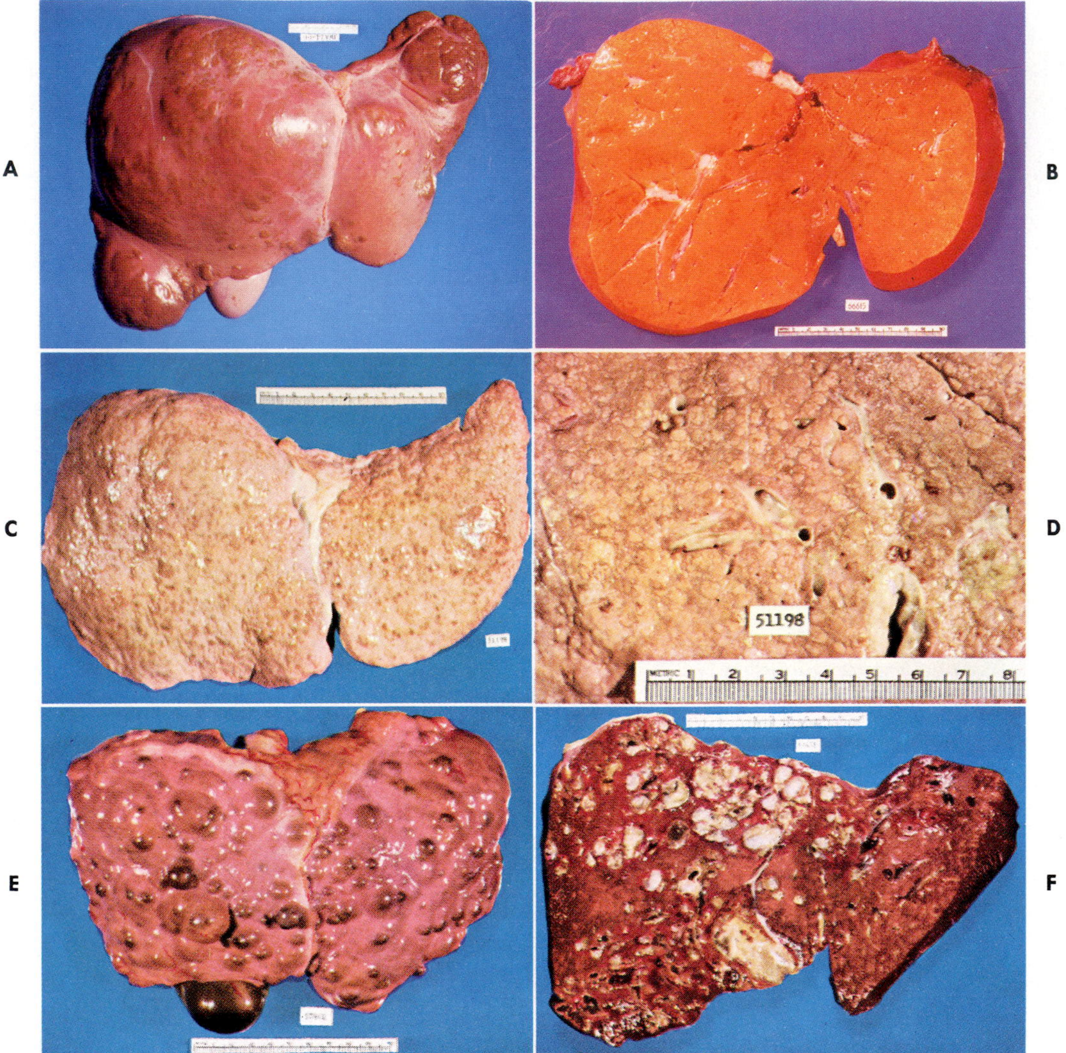

Plate 4

A, Submassive hepatic necrosis from viral hepatitis, with bulging areas of residual liver and much shrinkage and collapse of left lobe. Patient lived 24 days after onset of clinical symptoms.

B, Hypertrophic, firm, smooth alcoholic fatty liver.

C, Eutrophic, hard, finely pseudolobular alcoholic cirrhosis in 65-year-old man.

D, Cut surface of alcoholic cirrhosis showing pseudolobular pattern.

E, Atrophic, firm, megalonodular lupoid cirrhosis, quiescent in 20-year-old woman.

F, Suppurative cholangitis with multiple abscesses resulting from carcinomatous obstruction of common duct.

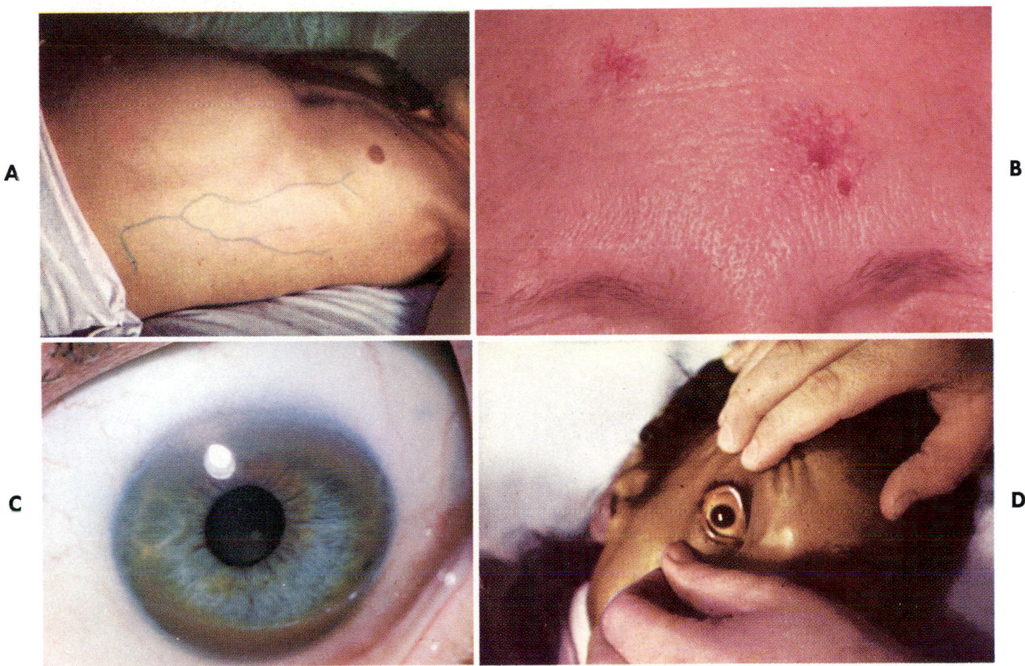

Plate 5

A, Hepatic cirrhosis. Ascites, congested veins, pigmented male nipple, axillary alopecia, and absence of striae.

B, Arteriovenous fistulas (vascular spiders) in diabetic cirrhosis. Arterial blood supply in center of lesion.

C, Kayser-Fleischer ring in Wilson's disease.

D, Jaundice and biliary cirrhosis after ligation of common bile duct.

(**A** and **D,** From Wiener, K.: Skin manifestations of internal disorders, St. Louis, 1947, The C.V. Mosby Co.)

diseases of specific causes must also be excluded, such as Wilson's disease (p. 1164) and alpha-1-antitrypsin aberrant types (p. 1159). The gross and microscopic changes of CCAH and cirrhosis are similar to those of B viral cirrhosis (Fig. 27-29).

Other acute infections

There are other acute infectious diseases of the liver that occur much less frequently than viral hepatitis. In this group are certain viral, bacterial, rickettsial, and other diseases that involve the liver primarily or in some secondary fashion.

Other viral infections may involve the liver, some producing extensive hepatic necrosis with high incidence of fatality.[238] Most of these diseases are uncommon (Lassa fever,[138,184,232] yellow fever, Ebola virus,[119,166,219] and Marburg viral hepatitis).[112,215] Other viral infections may involve the liver of patients who have systemic infection, but rarely do such viruses produce hepatic symptoms.[228] An exception is herpes simplex, which in the immunosuppressed patient may produce extensive fatal hepatic necrosis. Varicella, rubeola, and hemorrhagic fevers[141,228] may produce incidental hepatic lesions that are usually asymptomatic.

The involvement of the liver by Epstein-Barr virus (EBV) in patients with the clinical features of infectious mononucleosis has long been recognized. The hepatic involvement is usually clinically mild but may be associated with hyperbilirubinemia. The liver has marked atypical mononuclear cell hyperplasia in the portal areas, with striking atypical lymphocytosis and Kupffer cell hyperplasia in the lobules. The hepatocytes are not ordinarily swollen or in disarray, as they are in viral hepatitis, but there may be punched-out foci of nonepithelioid granulomatous necrosis. Patients with symptomatic infectious mononucleosis almost always have histologic hepatic involvement whether or not hepatic symptoms are found. Abnormal findings in hepatic tests are usually present in such patients. The liver does not progress to cirrhosis; fatal fulminant disease, although reported, is a rarity.[127]

Cytomegalovirus (CMV) infections in the liver have grown in incidence with increased blood usage, homosexuality,[158] and treatment modalities that reduce immune response but may be contracted by normal individuals who have no obvious source and no apparent immune defect. CMV disease may be associated with fatigue or only with chronic fever; rarely are aminotransferase activities above 300 units, and jaundice is not a feature. Microscopically there may be only Kupffer cell hyperplasia or a pattern indistinguishable from infectious mononucleosis. There is no evidence of progression of CMV liver disease to cirrhosis.

Herpes simplex viruses, both type 1 and type 2, have become important etiologic agents of severe hepatic necrosis. Hepatic herpes simplex infection is usually restricted to neonates, malnourished infants, pregnant women, and patients undergoing immunosuppressive therapy or with diseases associated with depressed immune response.[114] Systemic symptoms are nonspecific, but the disease is generalized, with death occurring in 90% of patients 1 to 2 weeks after onset. The involved liver is enlarged and mottled with sharply defined yellow areas or multiple 0.1 to 0.2 cm yellowish foci. Microscopically the yellow areas represent coagulative necrosis of hepatocytes. The margins of the areas of necrosis are made up of deeply eosinophilic degenerated hepatocytes. Many viable hepatocytes at the margins of the areas of necrosis have nuclei with large eosinophilic inclusion bodies. The inclusions can be identified as herpes simplex type 1 or 2 by immunoperoxidase or immunofluorescence techniques.

Bacterial infections arising in nonhepatic locations may cause jaundice, the exact mechanism of which is unknown. Infections caused by gram-negative organisms may affect both the neonate (see p. 1160) and the adult.[237] In both age groups cholestasis is the chief microscopic finding, usually with some degree of Kupffer cell hyperplasia. There is little or no necrosis. Experimental evidence indicates that the effect of endotoxin on cell membranes may be the causative factor.[237] Typhoid fever is accompanied by hyperbilirubinemia in a sizable percentage of cases. Focal necrosis (typhoid nodules) of the liver is common in typhoid fever, but microscopically the diffuse cholestasis bears no relationship to the foci of necrosis. The cause of jaundice is unclear.[133] In adults, septicemia caused by both gram-negative and gram-positive organisms may cause jaundice within a few days after onset of sepsis. A large number of organisms and sources of infections have been reported.[237] It has been suggested that jaundice accompanying severe bacterial infection is caused by a selective defect in the excretion of conjugated bilirubin because there is a disproportionate increase in serum bilirubin as compared to serum alkaline phosphatase and AST.[182] Jaundice is also known to occur in patients with lobar pneumonia, probably caused by hepatocellular injury. This type of jaundice is more common in Africa and the southwest Pacific area.[237] More recently, bacterial hepatitis, proved by culture of a biopsy specimen, has been reported.[231]

The principal rickettsial disease that may cause hepatic symptoms is Q fever, discussed on p. 341. Although rare, Weil's disease (p. 219), caused by a spirochete, should be suspected when there are jaundice, high fever, and sore muscles.

CHEMICAL AND DRUG INJURY

Hundreds of compounds, both inorganic and organic, are capable of causing liver injury when they gain access to the body. This may be by inhalation, by injection, or, most commonly, via the intestinal tract. Among the inorganic compounds are arsenic, phosphorus, copper, and iron salts. The organic agents include certain naturally occurring plant toxins, such as the pyrrolizidine alkaloids; mycotoxins, of which aflatoxin is an example; and bacterial toxins. The synthetic group of organic compounds is by far the most important, especially the medicinal agents used for the diagnosis and treatment of disease. In addition, exposure to hepatotoxic compounds[299] may be occupational, environmental, or domestic, including accidental, homicidal, or suicidal ingestion.

The incidence of hepatotoxic injury is low compared with other forms of acute liver disease, being far less than viral hepatitis or alcoholic liver disease. However, among patients with fatal hepatocellular disease, the percentage who have drug-related injury is much higher. All patients with acute liver disease should be questioned regarding drug usage and exposure to known hepatotoxins. Furthermore, in patients receiving the drugs that are most commonly hepatotoxic, it is worthwhile to check liver enzyme and serum bilirubin levels routinely for the first few months. This is especially true of drugs such as isoniazid that are capable of causing fatal liver cell necrosis.

The role of the liver in drug metabolism and the mechanism of drug-related injury have been the subject of intensive research. Most of the synthetic drugs are lipid soluble and easily absorbed from the intestines, but their elimination from the body requires the addition of polar groups to make them water soluble. This conjugation occurs in the liver. The enzyme systems responsible for the metabolism of the lipid-soluble drugs are located in the smooth endoplasmic reticulum (SER). These enzymes, present in the SER fragments (microsomal fraction), may be isolated by centrifugation at high speeds and are known as microsomal enzymes. Because of the diversity of the reactions attributed to microsomal enzymes, the term *mixed-function oxidase system* (MFO system) has been used to describe them. The MFO system includes cytochrome P450, NADPH-cytochrome c reductase, and phosphatidylcholine, a lipid. Apparently the key component is cytochrome P450, and there is strong evidence of its important role in the metabolism of drugs in humans.[250] Two reactions are necessary for the biotransformation of the lipid-soluble drugs. In phase 1 a polar group, either oxygen or a hydroxyl, is added. This is known as a nonsynthetic reaction. In phase 2 conjugation with a glucuronide, a sulfate group, or other anions makes the compound soluble in water and thus excretable in the urine or the bile. The metabolite formed by the addition of a polar group may make the activity of the metabolite less than, the same as, or greater than that of the parent compound.

Some drugs, such as barbiturates and phenytoin, when taken over a long period are enzyme inducers, increasing the amount of SER and of cytochrome P450. The metabolic pathway is nonspecific, however, and any one of many drugs or chemicals can be detoxified at an increased rate. These increase the rate of drug oxidation and may result in toxic metabolites. The marked increase in SER is prominent on electron microscopic examination. A biopsy discloses enlarged hepatocytes with abundant, finely reticular cytoplasm and a thickened cell membrane. These changes are most noticeable in the perivenular (zone 3) areas.[291] The lobules and even the liver may become enlarged.[240]

Many classifications of hepatotoxic injury have been proposed.[299] One of the more recent and all inclusive has first a group of intrinsic agents that act directly on the liver cells, such as carbon tetrachloride, or indirectly, such as acetaminophen. In the second group are the idiosyncratic reactions, either by hypersensitivity or through a secondary metabolite. The greatest advances have been made in the study of the latter group.

A condensed clinicopathologic approach is used in this chapter, with emphasis on the pathologic changes (Table 27-4). Occasionally some overlap from one group to another occurs. The changes produced by hepatotoxins vary from mild disease that is diagnosed only by a rise in serum enzymes to instances of massive necrosis and death. Some reactions are relatively innocuous, even though the patient is jaundiced. Two clinical groups are recognized: drugs that are administered for diagnosis or therapy and those that are not. In the latter the injurious agent may be taken accidentally or for suicidal or homicidal purposes. Also in the latter group are compounds that have a direct toxic reaction on the liver of humans and experimental animals that is dose related and fairly prompt. The morphologic expression commonly known as toxic hepatitis is usually uniform and predictable. Among these organic and inorganic hepatotoxins are carbon tetrachloride, chloroform,[292] chlorinated naphthalenes, phosphorus, and the toxins of mushrooms, all of which usually produce a zonal type of hepatic necrosis accompanied by fatty change. Other body organs may also be affected. If death from the acute exposure does not occur, hepatic recovery is complete. The best-known hepatotoxin in this group, often used in experimental pathology, is carbon tetrachloride. It is postulated that this compound is split by microsomal enzymes into the free radicals —CCl_3 and —Cl. These attack methylene bonds of the unsaturated fatty acids of microsome membranes, producing lipoperoxidases that cause severe membrane alterations.[282,283] The free radicals also damage microsomal proteins and cytochrome P450. Cysteine protects the liver cell from necrosis, possibly by reducing the binding of the free radical to the microsomal proteins.[257] The ultrastructural changes in carbon tetrachloride injury include the dislocation of ribosomes and dilatation of cisternae.[244] An early morphologic change in the plasma membrane of isolated rat hepatocytes has also been demonstrated.[275]

Mushrooms of the *Amanita phalloides* group produce several cyclopeptides or amanitins that are among the most lethal poisons known.[267] The structural formula and mode of action of these toxins have been extensively studied.[298] The cyclopeptides act by inhibiting nuclear RNA polymerase B, and thus they interfere with RNA and DNA transcription. This results in necrosis of liver cells. Damage occurs to both nuclei and cytoplasm at the ultrastructural level, particularly in the periportal zone.[273] Fatty change has been observed in fatal cases.[273] Nonfatal cases are characterized by perivenular (zone 3) necrosis and collapse.[297] Many cases of nonlethal mushroom poisoning have been reported.[265]

Poisoning by inorganic compounds is rare, but the accidental ingestion of a large quantity of ferrous sulfate by children is a cause of periportal necrosis and jaundice[286] and may be fatal. Many hepatic features of copper poisoning are similar to results of iron toxicity, except that the perivenular zone (zone 3) is damaged.[251]

The largest and most important group of toxic reactions are those that occasionally follow the use of pharmaceutical compounds usually given for treatment but that may also be ingested in large quantities accidentally or for suicidal purposes. Some drugs taken in excessive amounts are intrinsic hepatotoxins; others act in an idiosyncratic fashion. The deleterious action of this group of compounds has been termed drug-induced jaundice or drug-induced liver disease. An important advance in knowledge occurred when it was shown that with many drugs the mechanism of injury was indirect and caused by the metabolites that, following oxidation, form covalent linkages to macromolecules that are vital to cell function. It was first shown in experimental animals that the drug metabolites would often bind to glutathione rather than structural macromolecules as long as glutathione was available, thus preventing hepatocellular necrosis. Cysteamine and other agents have been used successfully in therapy for patients with overdose of acetaminophen. The mode of action results either from the binding capacity of cysteamine[270,274,280,281] or because the toxic metabolite is reconverted to acetaminophen. Pretreatment of experimental animals with enzyme inducers causes an increased severity of the hepatic necrosis, presumably because of the increased production of toxic metabolite along the proliferated smooth endoplasmic reticulum.[252] Experimental studies have shown that various drugs form covalent linkage to macromolecules.[268]

Liver disease resulting from hypersensitivity is usually assumed when a drug causes injury in only a small percentage of patients, is not dose related, and is accompanied by allergic manifestations such as skin rash, fever, and eosinophilia.[268] The microscopic findings often include eosinophilic infiltrate or a granulomatous reaction.[299]

Genetic factors may also influence drug hepatotoxicity. For example, some patients are rapid acetylators, and others are slow acetylators. Acetylation rate has a genetic basis, and since many drugs are acetylated, genetic factors may play a part in toxic reactions noted when patients who are rapid acetylators are given isoniazid for the treatment of tuberculosis.

The pathologic changes include two large categories. In one there is acute liver disease characterized by one or more of the following: cholestasis, hepatocellular necrosis with or without inflammatory reaction, fatty change, and granulomatous formation. In the second category there is a chronic reaction with variable degrees of fibrosis and, rarely, cirrhosis or neoplasia.

Acute liver disease

The first group (Table 27-4) is usually characterized by simple cholestasis without cell necrosis or inflammation. It is likely that in simple cholestasis more than one defect exists in the normal steps of the physiologic flow of bile. Normally, the flow of bile depends on (1) transport of the basic constituents from sinusoidal blood into the hepatocytes, (2) the metabolic alteration of some of these constituents by the hepatocytes, (3) transport into the canaliculi, (4) passage along the bile ductules and ducts during which a varying degree of modification occurs, and (5) exit from the liver.[300] Cholestasis results from physiologic defects distal to the conjugation within the hepatocyte. The formation of canalicular bile follows its active transport across the cell membrane. First, a bile salt–dependent flow results from the osmotic pull of the bile salts after active transport into the canaliculi. Second, a bile salt–independent flow results from the osmotic pull of Na^+ (sodium pump). This occurs after the active transport of sodium into the canaliculus under the influence of canalicular Na^+, K^+-adenosine triphosphatase (ATPase).[256]

As a group, the cholestatic drugs produce reversible injury to the secretory mechanism that prevents bilirubin glucuronide from normally entering the canaliculi. The bilirubin that does enter the canaliculi tends to accumulate and form bile plugs that are obvious on microscopic examination, especially in the perivenular zones (Plate 3, *B*). Mild swelling or hydropic change of the hepatocytes is a usual finding. An occasional focus of liver cell necrosis may occur, and on rare occasions severe necrosis has been reported. The electron microscope discloses a distortion and disappearance of the canalicular microvilli and widening of the canalicular ectoplasm.[278] Damage to the pericanalicular microfilaments has been shown in experimental cholestasis. This may be important in the etiology of simple cholestasis.[277]

Women who have had a condition known as benign jaundice of pregnancy, presumably because of excess production of sex hormones, often have a recurrence of jaundice when they take one of the oral contraceptives

Table 27-4. Action of drugs

Common examples of drug action	Incidence	Pathologic condition	Symptoms	Bilirubin	Transaminases	Alkaline phosphatase	Prothrombin activity
CHOLESTATIC ACTION							
Anabolic steroids with a 17-alkyl group, methyltestosterone	High	Perivenular cholestasis	Uncomplicated jaundice	Elevated, usually 15 mg	Normal	Elevated often above 20 BL units	Normal
Oral contraceptives	1:10,000	Perivenular cholestasis	Itching and jaundice	Mild elevation	Mild increase	Elevation mild to moderate	Normal
CHOLESTASIS WITH NECROSIS							
Phenothiazine drugs	1%	Perivenular bile stasis and focal necrosis; lymphoid hyperplasia of portal areas in many instances	In addition to jaundice, may be fever, rash, and eosinophilia	Elevated, usually 15 mg	Mild rise, 500 units; occasionally 1000 units or more	Elevated	Normal
Sulfonamides	0.6%						
Thiouracil	Rare						
Mercaptopurine	5%						
Sulfonylureas	<1%						
NECROSIS							
Isoniazid	Very rare	Necrosis, inflammation	Jaundice	Increased	Increased	Variable	Decreased
Acetaminophen	Suicide, variable	Coagulative necrosis	Jaundice	Moderate elevation	Rise, 1000 to 2000	Normal	Often decreased
Phenytoin	Rare	Varies—necrosis to granulomas	Jaundice usually	Usually high	High		
Alpha-methyldopa	F:M::9:1	Necrosis, inflammation	Jaundice	Increased	High	Usually increased	Decreased
Halothane	1:10,000	Liver cell injury—massive necrosis or zonal necrosis	Severe usually; may proceed to hepatic coma and death	Moderate to high	Rise, 500 to 2000	Normal to mild elevation	Decreased
Phenylbutazone	Rare	Necrosis or mild reaction with granulomas	Jaundice	Increased	High	Slight to moderate increase	Decreased
CHRONIC ACTIVE HEPATITIS							
Alpha-methyldopa	Rare	Usually submassive necrosis at autopsy, cirrhosis rare	Jaundice	High	High	Variable	Decreased
Isoniazid	Rare	Same as above	Insidious, weakness	Normal or high	High	Variable	Decreased
Nitrofurantoin	Rare	Fibrosis and chronic inflammation	None	Normal	Increased	Normal	Decreased
OTHER							
Tetracycline, especially in pregnancy	Unknown	Fine, foamy fatty change	Jaundice, coma	Elevated	Rise, 500	Elevated	Moderate decrease
Novobiocin	Unknown	Cholestasis	Newborn infants more susceptible	Elevated unconjugated bilirubin	Normal	Normal	Normal
Methotrexate	High	Fibrosis, inflammation	Insidious	Normally not elevated	Often a mild increase	Variable	Decreased late

(Plate 2, *B*).[253] The estrogens appear to be responsible for the rare instances of jaundice that follow the use of oral contraceptives.[289] The 17-alpha-alkyl-19-norsteroids cause the most difficulty with bile secretion.[266]

In the second and largest group of acute drug-related reactions (Table 27-4), there is liver cell injury as well as cholestasis so that the laboratory findings often include a rise in the serum transaminase levels. This type of injury has been referred to as hepatocanalicular injury.[299] Among the drugs that cause it are the phenothiazines, sulfonamides, mercaptopurines, and organic arsenical drugs. On microscopic examination the findings are variable, but cell ballooning, focal necrosis of hepatocytes, cholestasis, and inflammation along the portal tracts are usually present. The reaction in the portal areas varies greatly. In some biopsies there is an increase of connective tissue and inflammatory exudate in which round cells, neutrophils, or eosinophils may predominate. Ductular proliferation may also be seen. Granulomas with eosinophilic infiltrate may result from sensitivity to one of the sulfonamide drugs. Most patients in the second group recover when the offending drug is discontinued.

In the third pattern of acute drug reaction (Table 27-4) liver cell necrosis occurs with a minimal to moderate inflammatory response accompanied by hyperbilirubinemia and high serum transaminase activity. Many commonly used drugs are included in this group. One of these is isoniazid, the most widely used drug in the treatment of tuberculosis. Mild subclinical liver injury, characterized by mild elevations of serum transferase activities, may occur within the first 3 months of treatment in 12% to 20% of patients, but the damage never progresses in most of the patients throughout the period of treatment. Most patients spontaneously improve, even while treatment continues. However, in about 0.5% of patients treated, a more serious reaction occurs in which there is hepatocellular necrosis. The occurrence of necrosis is distinctly age related; it is extremely rare in those under 20 years of age and occurs in about 0.3% of patients 30 to 40 years of age, 1.2% of patients 35 to 45 years of age, and 2.3% of patients over 50 years.[269] The extent of necrosis varies from a moderately severe disease that resembles viral hepatitis, both clinically and pathologically, to submassive or massive hepatocellular necrosis, also resembling hepatitis. In patients with the latter the mortality is high. Isoniazid-related hepatic necrosis, when it occurs, almost always develops within the first year of therapy; half of the time it is within the first 8 weeks of therapy.[269] It has been suggested that isoniazid liver injury is related to the rapid acetylation of the drug. Patients who are of the rapid acetylator phenotype hydrolyze a larger percentage of isoniazid to isonicotinic acid and the free hydrazine compound.[269] However, this theory has been questioned.[255]

Acetaminophen is another widely used drug that is assumed to be safe when used in recommended doses. When used to excess, as for suicidal purposes, there is a dose-related type of perivenular liver cell necrosis. Prognosis has been linked to the total quantity taken, rate of disposition, activity of the MFO system, and glutathione stores.[263,285,299] Moderately severe injury may occur with therapeutic doses when the MFO system has been stimulated by other drugs or alcohol.[287] Unlike isoniazid-indirect hepatic necrosis, acetaminophen toxicity is associated with little inflammatory reaction and is characterized by coagulative necrosis of perivenular hepatocytes. Dead hepatocytes are slowly removed by histiocytes over approximately a 1-week period.[279] Toxic hepatitis has also been claimed to result from long-term, moderate to excessive self-therapeutic use of acetaminophen.[243,247] Treatment with alternative binding agents, such as *N*-acetylcysteine, is very effective if these agents are administered within 12 hours after ingestion, before hepatic necrosis develops.[270,281]

Although phenytoin is widely used in the treatment of seizure disorders, hepatotoxic reactions are rare. Adverse reactions usually occur within 1 to 6 weeks after the beginning of therapy. The microscopic findings vary widely and include hepatocellular necrosis, granulomatous reaction, bile duct injury,[290] and ground-glass transformation of the hepatocytes.[271] The reaction appears to be caused by hepatic hypersensitivity, since most of the patients have fever, skin rash, chills, pruritus, and hepatomegaly associated with jaundice. Most hepatic reactions resemble hepatic involvement in infectious mononucleosis.

Alpha-methyldopa, an antihypertensive drug, occasionally causes acute necrosis of the liver as a short-term effect, especially in women. The clinical features are similar to those of acute viral hepatitis. In about 10% of the patients the disease is fatal, submassive necrosis being noted at autopsy. Long-term effects have also been reported.[241,242] These include fatty change and fibrous septa formation.

One drug, allopurinol, is unique in that the toxic reactions are of the hypersensitivity type, but the microscopic change varies greatly from patient to patient. Most patients have a centrilobular type of zonal necrosis, whereas others may have a granulomatous change along the portal tracts.[239] Halothane and similar compounds, such as methoxyflurane (Penthrane), occasionally are associated with liver necrosis.[262,276,288] It has been reported that the serum of patients with fulminant hepatic failure after halothane-induced anesthesia contains a circulating antibody that reacts specifically with the cell membrane of hepatocytes isolated from halothane-anesthetized rabbits.[294] The nature of the antigenic substance on the membrane of the hepatocytes is yet to be determined. The biotransformation of halothane has

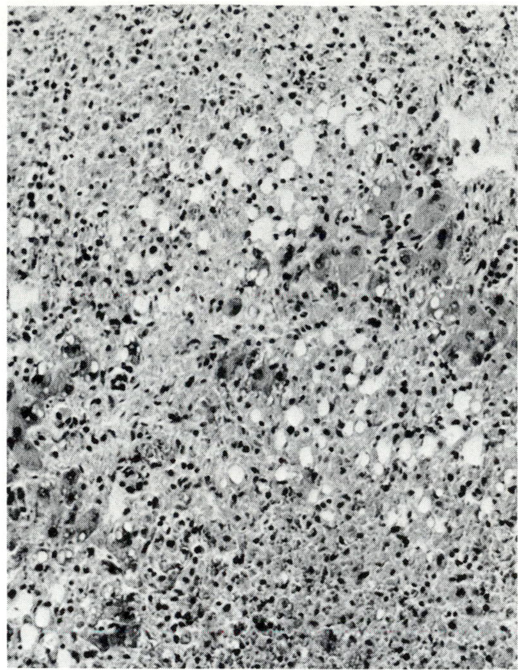

Fig. 27-19. Massive hepatocellular necrosis after halothane anesthesia. (From Peters, R.L., et al.: Am. J. Med. **47**:748, 1969.)

been extensively studied in rats, and it seems possible that liver cell necrosis may result from some reactive intermediary, particularly by means of a reductive or oxygen-deficient pathway.[249] A possible genetic factor in halothane-producing injury has also been proposed.[258] In most instances halothane-associated liver damage occurs after more than one exposure, usually in a patient who has had an unexplained fever after the first halothane-induced anesthesia.

In fatal massive necrosis after halothane anesthesia, three stages can be recognized: necrotic, absorptive, and regenerative. In the necrotic stage, dead liver cells are still recognizable and occur in the first 5 days after onset of jaundice (Fig. 27-19). In the absorptive stage the liver cells have disappeared, leaving areas of collapse. This is the period in which most of the patients die, usually 1 to 2 weeks after the onset of jaundice. In the regenerative stage submassive necrosis has occurred, and the patients live from 2 weeks to a month. These patients are older and have insufficient regenerative capacity to restore the liver parenchyma. Patients under 30 years of age who survive 3 weeks after the onset of jaundice may be expected to recover.

Phenylbutazone may cause a severe reaction with hepatocellular necrosis or a milder illness characterized by granulomas.[245] The toxic manifestations usually occur within 6 weeks after drug use begins. Clinical evidence indicates that drug sensitivity is a major factor.

A mild nonfatal hepatotoxic injury may follow the use of aspirin, sometimes with a marked hypertransaminasemia.[299] Hepatic injury is most likely to follow when the blood levels of salicylate are higher than 25 mg/dl.[301]

Effect of chronic drug use

After the chronic use of certain drugs, the histologic, clinical, and laboratory findings may closely resemble those of chronic active hepatitis of the immune or lupoid type (fourth group in Table 27-4). Relatively few drugs produce chronic active hepatitis, since most agents that produce hepatocellular necrosis will bring about massive necrosis and death if not discontinued when signs of liver disease develop. Production of drug-induced chronic active hepatitis requires either that the drug cause only a low level of necrosis with continued use, so that much of the disease is subclinical, or that repeated small doses of the hepatotoxin are administered with sufficient time between exposures to allow partial recovery. An example of the latter may occur in sensitive anesthesiologists who sniff halothane to assure themselves of adequate flow of the agent when administering anesthesia.[260] Chronic active hepatitis following self-medication with minimal toxic doses of acetaminophen[247] has been reported in a few patients.

The histologic findings of drug-related chronic active hepatitis may be essentially the same as those described on p. 1124. The drug oxyphenisatin, not now in use in the United States but still available in some countries, was a frequent cause of this disorder.[284] Alpha-methyldopa,[264] sulfonamides,[293] and isoniazid[246] have also been implicated, but the reported cases actually seem to represent examples of submassive necrosis. Nitrofurantoin, a drug used to treat urinary tract infections, may cause an acute cholestatic reaction with fever, skin rash, and eosinophilia in some patients and a more subtle chronic active hepatitis in others.[261] On withdrawal of the offending drug, patients with chronic active hepatitis–like disease almost invariably recover.

In addition to the chronic changes mentioned, a primary biliary cirrhosis–like disease may rarely occur in patients taking chlorpromazine, tolbutamide, or organic arsenical drugs. This disorder slowly resolves after cessation of drug therapy in nearly every case.[295]

In a small miscellaneous group (fifth group in Table 27-4), the abnormalities produced are distinctive for each drug.[254] There are no common findings in the liver. A characteristic foamy type of fatty change occurs in the liver after intravenous administration of large amounts of tetracycline (Fig. 27-20).[248] In this disorder the nucleus is not displaced as it is in the macrovesicular type of fatty change. The tetracycline interferes with the production of protein by RNA. Thus formation of lipoprotein, necessary for the transfer of fat from the liver, is blocked. Novobiocin inhibits the action of glucuronyl transferase, producing an unconjugated hyperbilirubinemia.

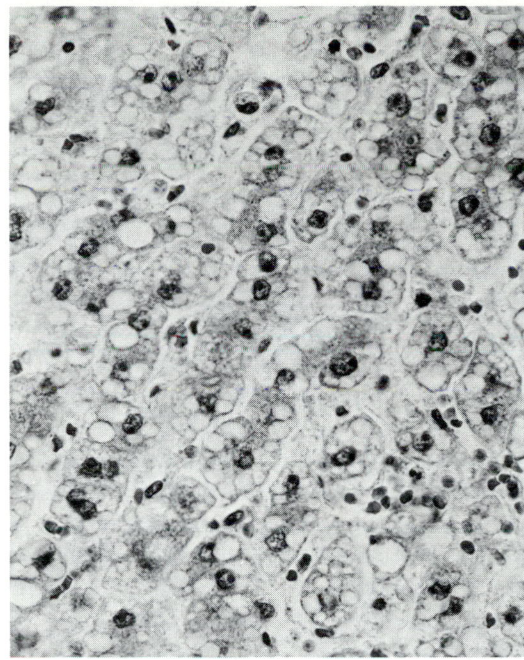

Fig. 27-20. Fine foamy vacuolization of liver after large amounts of intravenously administered tetracycline. (From Peters, R.L., et al.: Am. J. Surg. **113**:622, 1967.)

A true toxic cirrhosis caused by drugs has rarely been reported except in patients taking methotrexate.[259,272,296] A difference of opinion exists as to whether methotrexate is solely responsible for cirrhosis that may be seen in psoriatic individuals taking the drug. In our patients we have observed diffuse fibrosis along the sinusoidal walls, and the presence of megalohepatocytes is a characteristic change in patients taking methotrexate for a protracted period.

Several other adverse reactions to drugs and chemicals are more appropriately discussed elsewhere in this chapter. Among these are peliosis hepatis, thrombosis of the hepatic veins or Budd-Chiari syndrome, neoplasms, and granulomas.

ALCOHOLIC LIVER DISEASE

Since prehistoric times, alcohol has been the most widely used euphoriant. Probably the first alcoholic drink was mead made from fermented honey.[313] The long history of alcohol use and alcoholism has recently been reviewed.[318] The rise in the use of distilled liquor began in the eighteenth century and led to the early recognition of chronic liver disease, first by Matthew Baillie[302] in 1793 and by René Laënnec[322] in 1819. Since Laënnec introduced the term *cirrhosis* (from Gr. *kirrhos*, "tawny"), a multitude of diagnostic terms have been used for this most common type of cirrhosis. They include Laënnec's cirrhosis, alcoholic cirrhosis, portal cirrhosis, septal cirrhosis, diffuse cirrhosis, and hobnail cirrhosis.

Of the approximately 100 million of the U.S. population who use alcoholic beverages, about 10% become alcoholics. The definition of alcoholism is still controversial, but certain major and minor criteria have been established for its diagnosis by the National Council on Alcoholism.[307]

The frequency of cirrhosis at autopsy from all causes is alleged to vary between 1% and 10% throughout the world. In various centers in the United States the range is from 1.6% to 11%. Although alcoholic liver disease (ALD) may occur anytime from the third decade to senility, the peak incidence is in middle life (50 to 55 years), with most patients between 40 and 65 years of age. Men are affected more frequently than women; in the latter the peak age incidence is about a decade earlier than in men. In the Los Angeles County–University of Southern California Medical Center in 1970, at a time when 25% of deaths were caused by alcohol-associated diseases, the frequency of cirrhosis at autopsy was 11%, principally of the alcoholic type. Furthermore, ALD was the leading cause of death in those under 50 years of age.

Alcoholic cirrhosis follows the long-continued consumption of alcohol. The epidemiologic evidence indicates that the mortality from cirrhosis is directly related to the per capita consumption of alcohol from wine and spirits.[336] In India, Africa, and certain other parts of the world in which B viral cirrhosis is common, alcoholism is not etiologically important. However, in some countries an increase in alcohol consumption has been followed by an increase in alcoholic cirrhosis,[316] although there are differences in male-to-female ratio and the frequency of acute alcoholic hepatitis as compared with the United States. A relationship between alcoholism and cirrhosis is unquestionable, but the exact mechanism of the injurious effect of alcohol is unknown. Among patients with cirrhosis, a history of excessive use of alcohol has been found in 30% to 92% in various series in the United States. About 90% of patients have a history of 5 to 15 years of heavy consumption of alcohol. Many consume as much as a quart of whiskey or a gallon of wine per day. In addition to steady drinking, most patients periodically drink excessively for 1 or 2 weeks, during which time they eat little or no food. These bouts often terminate in an attack of jaundice, pneumonia, pancreatitis, or delirium tremens. The drinking patterns of alcoholics differ from one country to another and even within one country.

Ethanol metabolism

After ingestion and absorption from the stomach and small bowel, ethanol is distributed in the water space of the body. As ethanol circulates through the liver, it is removed by the hepatocytes where, by a two-step enzymatic process, some 90% of it is oxidized to acetate. Studies in humans indicate that 50% to 100% of ethanol entering the liver appears in the hepatic venous outflow as acetate.[327] Only a small percentage is oxidized elsewhere so that within 24 hours, 90% of the ingested ethanol is oxidized finally to carbon dioxide and water and a small amount (2% to 10%) is excreted unchanged by the lungs and kidneys.

The major pathway for hepatic ethanol oxidation is shown in Fig. 27-21. The enzyme alcohol dehydrogenase (ADH) present in the cytosol is sufficient to account for the maximal rate of ethanol metabolism. Because ADH has a wide range of substrates, the physiologic role of the enzyme has been debated. The finding of measurable levels of ethanol in the portal blood of nondrinking rats supports the concept that the primary function of ADH is ethanol oxidation.[320] As ethanol is oxidized to acetaldehyde by ADH, the cofactor nicotinamide-adenine dinucleotide (NAD) is reduced to NADH. The second enzymatic step occurs in the mitochondria where acetaldehyde is oxidized to acetate by acetaldehyde dehydrogenase (AcDH) and the same cofactor NAD is reduced to NADH. The acetate leaves the liver to be oxidized further to carbon dioxide and water in other tissues. Reduction in the NAD/NADH redox ratio is the fundamental biochemical alteration that occurs during ethanol metabolism. The free NAD/NADH ratio cannot be measured because of the binding of the pyridine nucleotides; therefore the ratio of oxidized and reduced metabolites is measured by showing that the lactate/pyruvate ratio and the beta-hydroxybutyrate/acetoacetate ratios are both increased, the former in the cytoplasm and the latter in mitochondria. In persons who drink excessively, the amount of NADH that is reoxidized becomes the rate-limiting factor for the oxidation of ethanol. Because the mitochondrial membranes are impenetrable to NADH, the reoxidation of this substance is accomplished by a shuttle system, whereby reducing equivalents enter the mitochondria. These shuttles are (1) the alpha-glycerophosphate shuttle, (2) the malate-asparate shuttle, and (3) the fatty acid elongation shuttle.[305] The mitochondrial respiratory chain is therefore ultimately responsible for the oxidation of NADH. As long as ethanol is available to the hepatocytes, it may replace up to 90% of all the substrates that are normally used by the liver, taking over almost the entire intermediary metabolism. Many of these substrates therefore cannot be metabolized by the liver. Furthermore, the continuous presence of alcohol causes a marked depression in the Krebs cycle. This particularly affects the metabolism of fat and leads to fatty liver, the most common microscopic observation in alcoholism. The disturbed lactate/pyruvate ratio probably decreases gluconeogenesis and could be partially responsible for the hypoglycemia that is sometimes seen in persons with alcoholism.

The total activity of ADH varies considerably in normal humans because of the presence of isoenzymes and enzyme polymorphisms.[324,337,342] A genetic model has been proposed that includes three autosomal gene loci that code for three subunits: alpha, beta, and gamma. Atypical subunits give rise to isoenzymes that show a higher specific activity. Among whites, only 5% to 20% are atypical phenotypes, whereas Orientals are predominantly atypical. Thus Orientals may oxidize alcohol at a faster rate on ingestion, leading to higher blood aldehyde levels; this may in turn be responsible for the well-known

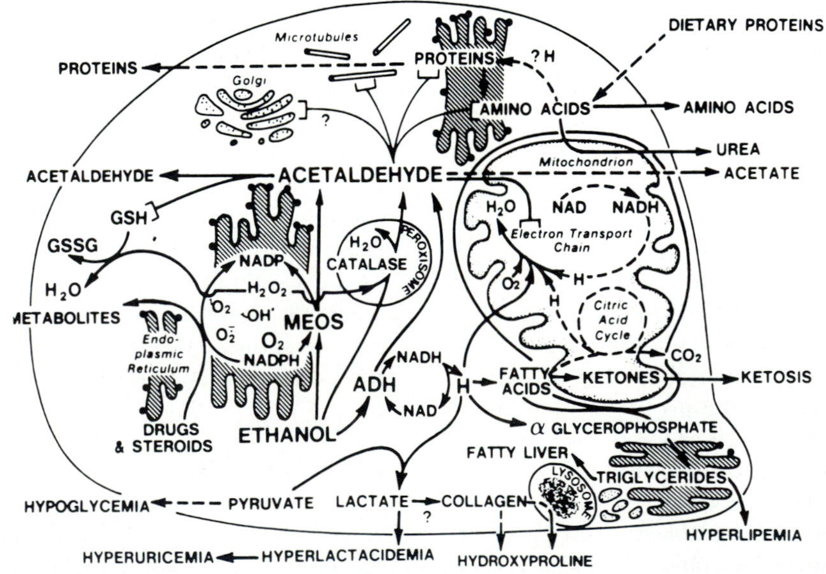

Fig. 27-21. Effects of oxidation of ethanol on intermediary metabolism in liver. *Broken lines*, Pathways inhibited by ethanol. Coupling of oxidation of ethanol with reduction of oxaloacetate is hypothetical. (From Lieber, C.S.: Clin. Gastroenterol. **10**:315, 1981.)

flushing syndrome that is so frequently recognized in some Orientals when they consume alcoholic beverages.

The oxidation of acetaldehyde to acetate occurs for the most part in the mitochondria. In the chronic alcoholic this second step in the metabolism of alcohol may be overburdened by the production of NADH. Under these circumstances it is thought that aldehyde may enter the bloodstream. The quantity, however, is unclear, primarily because of difficulty in its chemical determination. Furthermore, the pathologic significance of acetaldehyde that is not immediately oxidized to acetate but remains in the liver is unknown.

In chronic alcoholism there is an increase in SER, and alcohol is metabolized at an increased rate. This has led to the study of other pathways for the oxidation of alcohol. One of these is the microsomal ethanol-oxidizing system (MEOS), which is associated with the degradation of ethanol by microsomes.[305,326] Another alternative pathway is by means of catalase present in the peroxisomes.[326] The MEOS system may be of considerable importance in the chronic alcoholic. An additional metabolic pathway has been recently described in which acetaldehyde is converted to acetoin by the brain.[341] This substance undergoes reduction to 2,3-butanediol by the liver.

In advanced cirrhosis, poor nutrition and poor blood supply to the hepatocytes may alter the rate of oxidation of alcohol.[340]

Pathology

The chronic use of ethanol may produce one or more morphologic changes in the liver that are characteristic and allow a presumptive diagnosis of ALD to be made on these grounds alone. The spectrum of alterations includes hydropic change, fatty change, necrosis, regeneration, inflammation, and fibrosis. Some of these may occur singly, but often more than one microscopic change is seen. A major advance in the study of ethanol hepatoxicity was the production of the morphologic lesion of acute and chronic ALD in baboons given an alcoholic diet supplemented with adequate nutritional factors.[332] Therefore ethanol and its metabolites may produce both acute and chronic damage, but deficient diet is not required for liver injury in the person with chronic alcoholism. Among the millions of persons with chronic alcoholism, it has been estimated that only 5% to 15% will develop cirrhosis.[319] The exact percentage who develop some form of symptomatic or asymptomatic disease is unknown. Other factors that have been given consideration include genetic and constitutional status of the patient. It has been shown that children born of a biologic alcoholic parent have a significant increase in alcoholic-related problems.[308] Furthermore, it has been reported that patients with alcoholic cirrhosis have a higher frequency of HLA-B40 than (1) those patients with ALD but without cirrhosis, (2) those with miscellaneous liver disease, or (3) alcoholic persons without liver disease.[303] It is possible that severe dietary deficiency has an additive effect in ALD.[328] The observation that severe liver disease, indistinguishable from ALD, often occurs after a jejunoileal bypass for morbid obesity is an example of the role that other factors, possibly nutrition, play in another indistinguishable form of liver disease.[321]

The term *alcoholic liver disease* may be used for all lesions of the liver associated with excessive use of ethanol that cannot be ascribed to any other etiologic factor. Persons with chronic alcoholism may have liver disease, sometimes severe, that has a nonalcoholic etiology, or even a combination of alcoholic and nonalcoholic disease.[323] A clinicopathologic classification of ALD that we have found useful includes the following:

A. Early asymptomatic liver disease
B. Acute liver disease
  1. Fatty liver with or without cholestasis
  2. Acute foamy degeneration
  3. Fatty liver with lytic necrosis
  4. Sclerosing hyaline necrosis (SHN)
  5. Acute portal fibrosis
C. Chronic liver disease
  1. Chronic sclerosing hyaline disease (CSHD)
  2. Precirrhosis and cirrhosis
    a. Precirrhosis
    b. Early cirrhosis
    c. Moderate cirrhosis
    d. Advanced cirrhosis

Three clinicopathologic variations of ALD are recognizable: asymptomatic (any morphologic stage), acute liver disease ("alcoholic hepatitis"), and chronic liver disease (usually cirrhosis or precirrhosis). These may or may not progress from one to another. A patient may have several acute episodes that do not advance to cirrhosis. Often acute alcoholic liver disease is superimposed on chronic liver disease. Biopsies and autopsies disclose that, although the disease does often progress through the acute stages before cirrhosis occurs, many alcoholic persons are symptomless until the advanced stage of cirrhosis is reached. In this latter group the various steps leading to cirrhosis are unknown but are presumed to be similar to but less severe than those described below, allowing the patient to live to a more advanced stage without occurrence of the clinical features of acute alcoholic liver disease.

Early asymptomatic alcoholic liver disease

Before clinical disease is manifest, usually after a few years of heavy drinking, hepatomegaly may occur. This is caused by fatty or hydropic change. Although usually considered a benign disorder, a fatty liver may be associated with sudden death, the exact cause of which is uncertain. Hypoglycemia, hypomagnesemia, and the withdrawal syndrome have been considered.[333] Many patients with fatty liver are seen by the physician or hospitalized for any one of several nonhepatic complications of alcoholism. These include delirium tremens, nausea and vomiting, trauma, acute infection, and alcoholic pancreatitis. More severe changes, including alcoholic hepatitis and cirrhosis, have been noted in a small percentage of persons with asymptomatic alcoholism.[304] Hepatomegaly in asymptomatic alcoholism has been ascribed to hydropic change and excess protein in the hepatocytes.[325]

The time between the onset of heavy drinking and microscopic abnormalities in the liver is unknown. Alcohol given to young nonalcoholic volunteers produced fatty vacuolation in 2 days.[335] However, the fat was uniformly distributed throughout the lobule, and droplets were relatively small (usually from 5 to 15 μm) and different from the fat deposition of symptomatic stages of alcoholic liver disease.

A biopsy performed in the asymptomatic stage usually reveals fatty change or hydropic vacuolization or both. Sometimes the hydropic change noted in the perivenular hepatocytes may be extreme. The nucleus is still apparent, but the cytoplasm is so watery that it is difficult to find any granular material (Fig. 27-22).

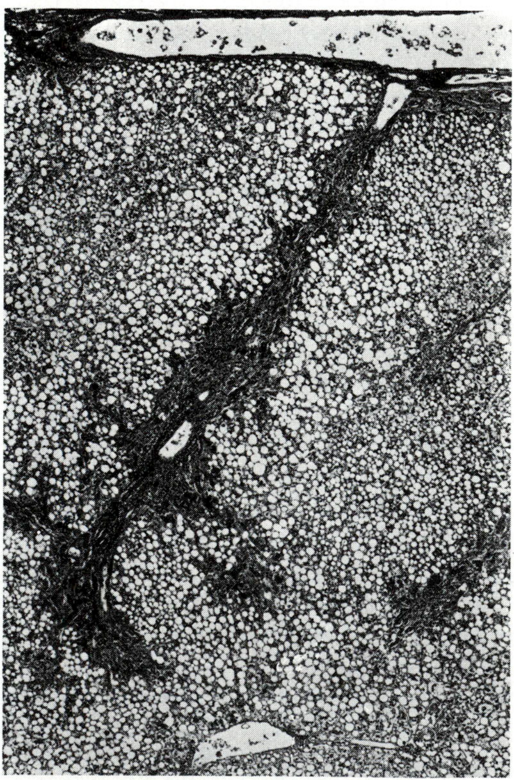

Fig. 27-22. Early stage of cirrhosis in fatty liver of alcoholic patient. Fibrosis and bile duct proliferation can be seen along terminal branch of portal tree. Irregular manner in which connective tissue invades periphery of lobules is clearly shown. There is little change around sublobular and central vein at bottom.

Another helpful finding in some biopsies performed in the early stages of ALD is the presence of giant mitochondria. These are easily seen with a light microscope because they are in the cytoplasm and are often approximately the size of an erythrocyte (Fig. 27-23).[306,343]

Acute liver disease

The onset of acute liver disease in alcoholism is difficult to predict but is usually associated with an increased intake of ethanol and poor eating habits. The symptoms differ somewhat, depending on the morphologic abnormalities in the liver, but most commonly the patient has a more or less sudden onset of jaundice that often is accompanied by fever. In the literature these patients have been described as having alcoholic hepatitis. A liver biopsy usually discloses one of four structural changes, each of which has certain identifiable features: (1) fatty liver with cholestasis; (2) fatty liver with foamy change, which in more severe cases undergoes a lytic type of necrosis; (3) sclerosing hyaline necrosis; and (4) acute portal sclerosis. There may be some overlap between the first of these and the other three.

The simplest microscopic change is a fatty liver with cholestasis. A mild thickening of sinusoidal and central vein walls is common, but little or no increase of portal connective tissue is seen. On hospitalization, the patients usually recover in a period of a few weeks. It is remarkable how rapidly a large fatty liver shrinks when

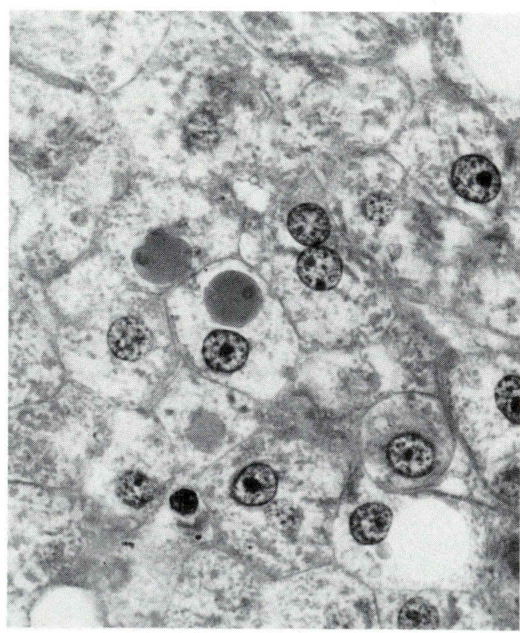

Fig. 27-23. Megamitochondria in hepatocytes of chronically alcoholic patient.

the patient partakes of an adequate diet and abstains from alcohol. In addition to hyperbilirubinemia, the hepatic tests usually show a moderate rise in alkaline phosphatase levels. Rarely a patient with severe fatty change and cholestasis may die of liver failure.[329] The cause or causes of fatty liver in the person with alcoholism are still under discussion.[338] It seems likely that the major factor is concerned with beta oxidation of fatty acids.[341]

A second acute clinicopathologic syndrome in the precirrhotic alcoholic patient is alcoholic foamy degeneration (AFD). Patients with AFD may have very transient elevations of both the ALT and AST activities to over 300 units; the elevated ALT level is often missed because it may be in an elevated range for only 24 hours.[315] The perivenular hepatocytes are bloated with fine, fatty vacuoles, separated by a delicate cytoplasmic interface (Fig. 27-24). The hepatocytes are deficient in mitochondrial enzyme activity and by electron microscopic study are virtually lacking in mitochondria.[339] The nuclei of these foamy cells are often pyknotic. The foamy cell change may be the early change, still reversible, that when severe leads to lytic necrosis.

On rare occasions, a fatty liver may undergo a lytic type of necrosis.[309] Most patients who die in hepatic failure with only fatty livers or fatty livers with fibrosis have severe perivenular lytic necrosis of the hepatocytes. The lytic foci are devoid of inflammatory exudate. Cholestasis, bile staining of cytoplasm, and bile in Kupffer cells are uniformly present. Some of the patients become critically ill and die in hepatic coma. At autopsy the liver is hypertrophic, weighing as much as 5000 g; the capsule is smooth and usually tautly stretched around bulging, fatty icteric parenchyma. However, if lytic necrosis is sufficiently severe and the patient has survived for more than a week or so in coma, the parenchyma is limp and soft. In such instances of severe necrosis there is perivenular depression and deep bile staining. Microscopically the bloated, hydropic perivenular hepatocytes appear foamy and partially autolyzed; the periportal cells usually contain a large single fat globule. The laboratory findings are similar to those in patients with fatty liver and cholestasis alone, except that the AST level may reach 300 units, and the ALT remains normal. The prothrombin activity may be decreased to the range of 20%. Since prothrombin activity precludes early biopsy, it has not been proved that lytic necrosis is a more severe stage of acute foamy degeneration, but clinically it would appear to be so.

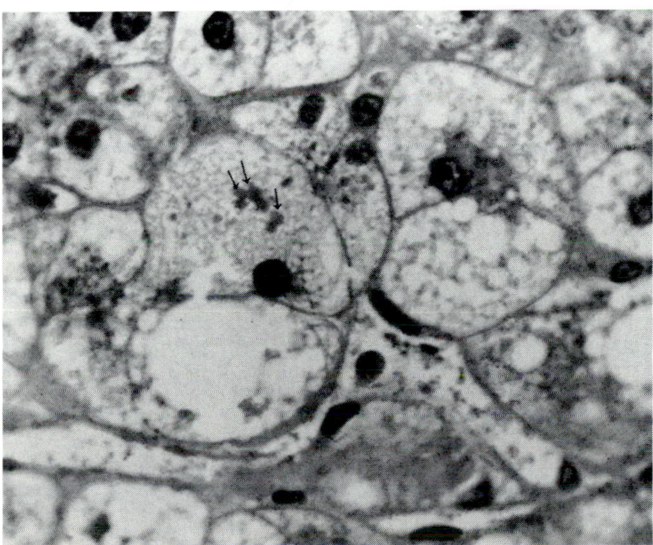

Fig. 27-24. Acute foamy degeneration in alcoholic patient. Note foamy vesicles and pale cytoplasm. This pattern may be found in liver of patient with acute alcoholism. Note megamitochondria *(arrows)*, somewhat smaller than those in Fig. 27-23.

A third type of microscopic change is now known as alcoholic hepatitis, although we continue to use the term *sclerosing hyaline necrosis*.[310] In this disorder the perivenular hepatocytes undergo hydropic and hyaline change that precedes necrosis. This change is most striking in a liver with few fat vacuoles, although fatty livers are not spared. The hyalin first appears as clumps in the cytoplasm and then as large masses that often have an eccentric location in the cell (Plate 3, *D*). Usually there are many neutrophils in the sinusoids around the necrotic cells that may even penetrate the cytoplasm of the cell and possibly assist in its death or liquefaction. The latter appears to be a slow process. Various stages in the progression of hyaline necrosis are seen in the liver at any one time. A remarkable increase in collagen occurs in the perivenular areas (Fig. 27-25). This is associated with increased numbers of cells that appear to be derived from endothelial lining cells and function as fibroblasts. Recent reports indicate that the fibrosis is associated with many myofibroblasts.[325] Much of the new formation of collagen has been shown to occur in the space of Disse. A highly significant correlation has been noted between the amount of collagen and the intrahepatic portal venous pressure.[330] The increased connective tissue leads to obliteration of many of the perivenular sinusoids and terminal hepatic veins. The changes in sclerosing hyaline necrosis may be so severe that death ensues, but many patients recover. The necrotic cells finally disappear; the connective tissue condenses, and although the regenerative response is poor, the remaining cells in the altered lobules resume their functions. In the acute phase the patients often have jaundice, ascites, abdominal pain, and an exceptional neutrophilic leukocytosis.[310] Ultrastructural studies have shown that hyaline bodies are composed of light and dark conglomerate filaments. These are surrounded by proliferated rough endoplasmic reticulum (RER) from which ribosomes have been shed, hypertrophied Golgi complex, and enlarged mitochondria that often contain matrical granules.[331] Almost always there is a cuff of the detached ribosomes around the hyaline bodies. Similar changes may be seen in hepatocytes without alcoholic hyaline but which probably represent an early stage in the development of the disease. Branching and tubular microfilaments have been recognized. Electrophoretic and immunologic studies of the isolated and homogenized hyaline bodies show several bands identical to protein bands in normal liver. Mallory bodies are antigenic and contain similar antigenic determinants in common with the axial filaments of the hepatocyte.[311] The exact role of any antigen-antibody reaction in the pathogenesis of acute alcoholic hepatitis remains to be proved. It has been proposed that a continuous pattern of deposition of IgA in the hepatic sinusoids is specific for ALD.[317]

It has been shown that when Mallory bodies are present, T lymphocytes in the liver are increased as compared with their numbers in the peripheral blood, indicating that a cell-mediated immune response has occurred.[312]

Acute portal fibrosis is a rare complication of alcoholism we have recognized in recent years. The portal tracts are moderately enlarged by a profuse increase of connective tissue that obliterates many of the portal vein and hepatic artery branches. Fatty change is usually present. The patients are jaundiced and have an elevated alkaline phosphatase.

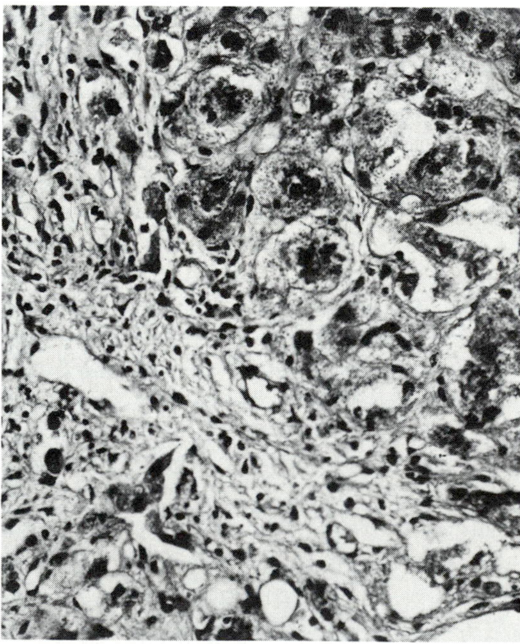

Fig. 27-25. Cytoplasm of hepatic cells contains eosinophilic granular material, so-called alcoholic hyalin. Cells appear swollen, and cell borders are indistinguishable. Sclerosis of vascular walls has begun. Needle biopsy of liver of 42-year-old Native American, chronic alcoholic who had been on long drinking spree before entering hospital.

Chronic alcoholic liver disease

As the early changes of ALD evolve toward cirrhosis, several different patterns are recognizable. In one of these, perivenular fibrosis is a major pathologic component, whereas portal fibrosis is minor. This lesion, termed chronic sclerosing hyaline disease, may follow acute sclerosing hyaline necrosis, but more often symptoms of acute disease have been subclinical. The intense sclerosis that obstructs the venous outflow tract at the level of the terminal venules and sublobular veins becomes condensed (Fig. 27-26, *A*). Patients with chronic sclerosing disease have an indolent clinical

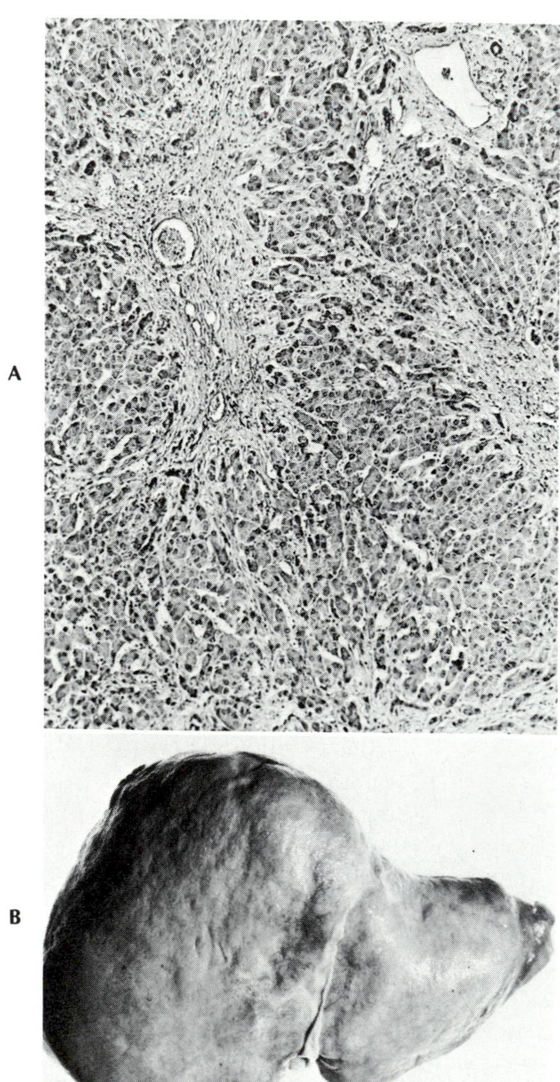

Fig. 27-26. Chronic sclerosing hyaline disease with eutrophic, hard, granular, precirrhotic pattern. **A,** Fibrous destruction of centrilobular areas and slight widening of portal areas. **B,** Surface has sandstone appearance.

course characterized by muscle wasting, resistant ascites, and frequently, functional renal failure. Jaundice is not usually present. Wedged hepatic vein pressure is nearly always elevated.[334] At autopsy the liver may be eutrophic or atrophic but has a smooth or fine sandstone-like thickened capsule that encloses a tough hard parenchyma (Fig. 27-26, *B*). The presence of dense perivenular fibrosis at biopsy in patients with acute alcoholic hepatitis may be the forerunner of chronic sclerosing hyaline disease.

Precirrhosis and cirrhosis

In some patients precirrhotic changes occur in a fatty liver in which the portal tracts have an increase in amount and density of connective tissue, along with bile duct proliferation. There is little or no perivenular change. The widened portal area assumes an arachnoid configuration as the limiting plate disappears. Irregular prolongation of the portal connective tissue encroaches on the periphery of the lobules and may extend directly along the sinusoids (Fig. 27-22). In this type of portal fibrosis there is little or no necrosis and not necessarily any regenerative nodules. The liver is always hypertrophic, sometimes weighing as much as 2000 to 5000 g. The capsule has finely granular regular areas of retraction and is unthickened but taut. The liver is yellow with fat or is yellow-green with bile and fat. There is slight to moderate increased resistance on cutting, to a degree that would be characterized as firm. The bulging parenchyma is greasy, and thin sections of the liver may float in water. The lobules are enlarged, and the terminal hepatic venules may be indistinct.

In the most common precirrhotic pattern there is both a perivenular and a portal component, and both fatty change and perivenular sclerosis are observed. The lobular pattern is altered, small regenerative nodules are seen, and communicating septa often connect perivenular and portal areas. This stage is called alcoholic fatty liver with perivenular and portal fibrosis. Should the patient discontinue alcohol consumption, the fat will disappear in about 3 months; however, the fibrosis will remain, displaced somewhat by the concomitant hepatocellular regeneration that begins about a week after alcohol consumption is discontinued.

Although there are all degrees of severity in the cirrhotic process, the next step in progression may be called cirrhosis. The morphologic pattern that develops in the alcoholic patient is a result of the continual encroachment of collagen fibers into regenerating nodules that proliferate most exuberantly during periods of improved nutrition and cessation of alcoholic intake. The outcome is a cirrhotic liver, usually made up of poorly defined, irregularly sized nodules with thin collagen fibers insinuated between the hepatocytes. In this early stage the liver is hypertrophic, weighs 2000 to 4000 g, and has a firm rubbery quality. It is more resistant to cutting, and the fibrous septa delineate fairly uniform-sized nodules 1 to 2 mm in diameter. As the cirrhosis progresses to the moderate stage, one or more areas of dense scarring may develop. The scars are irregular in configuration and are up to about 1.5 cm in greatest dimension. At the margin of the scars the pseudolobules are smaller than those in liver remote from the scar. Near the center of the scar the pseudolobules are absent. The pathogenesis of these scars is unknown; the area most frequently involved is in a line between the gallbladder bed and the hepatic vein orifices, a less vascular area in that the line drawn between these structures represents the boundary separating the true median portion of left lobe from the true right lobe. Often the scarring results in a U-shaped area of retraction of the capsule over the dome of the liver. In alcoholic cirrhosis, severe obliterative change along the hepatic venous outlow tract is noted in nearly all cases. The terminal hepatic veins disappear or are in the process of obliteration (Fig. 27-27). The small hepatic veins (sublobular veins) are severely damaged, and even larger veins are sclerosed in some areas, particularly where there is gross scarring. The vascular sclerosis probably occurs after earlier subclinical attacks of sclerosing hyaline necrosis, although a milder degree of connective tissue proliferation about hepatic venous tributaries does occur in fatty livers in which there has been no demonstrable sclerosing hyaline necrosis. There are no lobules

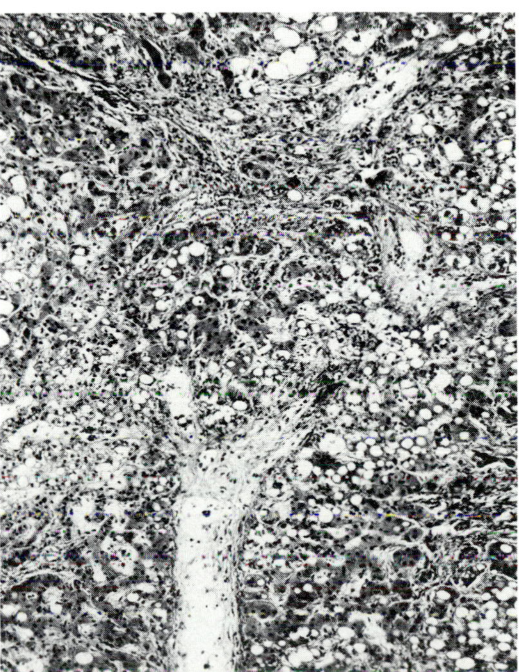

Fig. 27-27. Moderate cirrhosis. There are fatty change and early obliteration of central and subhepatic veins. This is granular fatty liver of 25-year-old Mexican man with history of chronic alcoholism.

with a normal pattern. Instead, arachnoid connective tissue septa surround and invade pseudolobules of various sizes. Regeneration occurs in some portions of the liver, and this further distorts the normal architecture so that the hepatic and portal veins may come to occupy positions near one another in the fibrous septa. Infiltration with round cells and occasionally neutrophils may occur in the septa. Fatty change is usually found in the early stages of alcoholic cirrhosis; however, if alcoholism is discontinued at any stage, the fat is diminished and parenchymal regeneration becomes prominent, resulting in the formation of larger, more discrete regenerative nodules.

In the histogenesis of moderately advanced stages of cirrhosis, there is both portal and centrilobular sclerosis. Attacks of necrosis may result in subdivision of preexisting nodules. The necrosis in turn acts as a stimulus to further regeneration, and larger nodules form, particularly if there is cessation of alcoholic intake for a while. The patients who die in this stage of cirrhosis are most often in hepatic coma but may also die of bleeding or intercurrent infection, especially pneumonia.

In the advanced stage of alcoholic cirrhosis the liver is atrophic, weighing between 800 and 1200 g. The nodules are usually well defined and are described as nodular if they bulge hemispherically and as insular if the cut surface is flat (Fig. 27-28). Nodules are usually between 1 and 4 mm in diameter (referred to as finely nodular or insular), but occasionally individual nodules may be as large as 1 cm (referred to as coarsely nodular between 0.4 and 1 cm). The capsular surface is deformed by the projecting nodules (Plate 4, *C*). The liver is resistant to cutting, and after sectioning, the characteristic yellow–mahogany brown nodules are sharply outlined and appear to have been embedded in the pale gray bands of connective tissue (Plate 4, *D*). In some irregular areas parenchymal tissue may be completely absent. On microscopic examination the liver is composed entirely of pseudolobules and wide bands of connective tissue (Fig. 27-29). Much of the outflow tract is obliterated, especially its smaller radicles. The larger and thick-walled hepatic veins that remain may be near some of the larger portal triads, the two being separated only by the connective tissue bands.

There is usually diminution or absence of fat in the atrophic stage. The collagenous connective tissue is dense, but there may be small foci of hyaline necrosis, usually without inflammatory exudate or sclerosis of sinusoids. Focal areas of cholestasis resulting from loss of communication between the regenerative nodules and functioning bile ducts may be observed. Often the liver

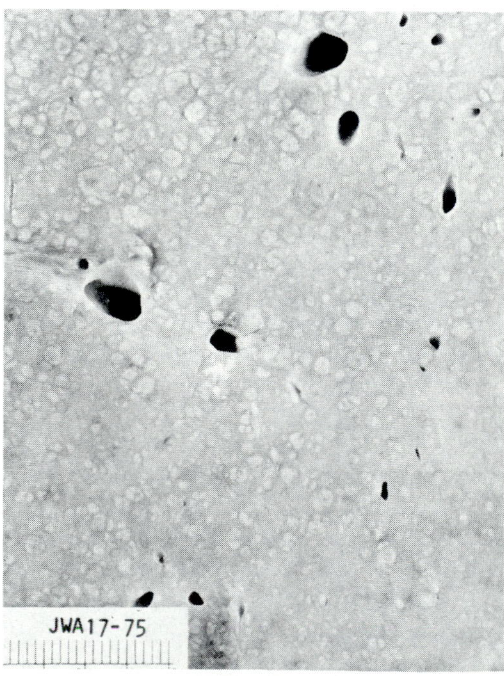

Fig. 27-28. Cut surface of liver of alcoholic cirrhotic patient with atrophic, sclerotic, finely insular alcoholic cirrhosis. Note denser scarring on right of photograph.

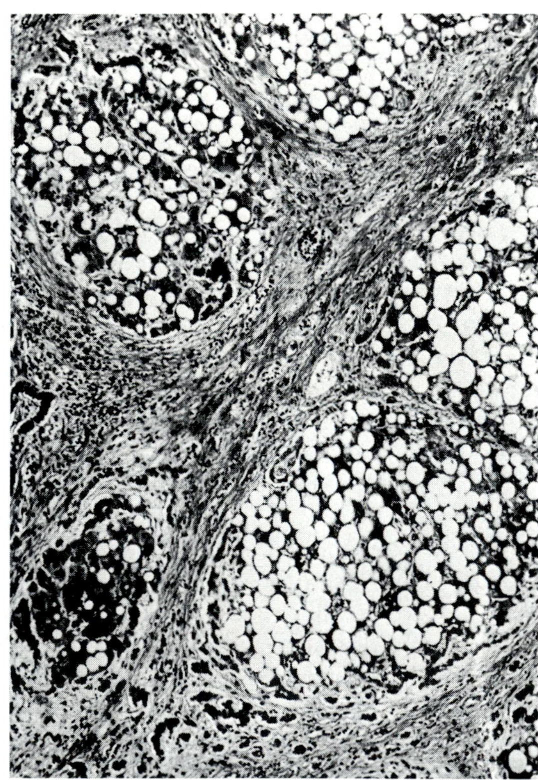

Fig. 27-29. Advanced stage of cirrhosis in 49-year-old white woman, known alcoholic for many years. Increase of connective tissue forms septa that subdivide liver into many small pseudolobules. Patient died in hepatic coma. Portacaval shunt was done 1 year before death, but patient continued to drink excessively.

cells in the hyperplastic nodules have abnormally large hyperchromic nuclei or even two nuclei. The cells in areas of recent regeneration lack any lipochromic pigment. In the atrophic stage the cord pattern usually becomes reestablished and regular within the nodules; apparently the stimulus for or the response to regeneration was abated. Adenomatous hyperplasia occasionally occurs in quiescent alcoholic cirrhosis, and the scattered nodules are two or three times larger than their neighbors and are dark brown. Since such nodules are more common in patients who have a hepatocellular carcinoma elsewhere, it is possible that the adenomatous nodules are preneoplastic.

Some cirrhotic patients after portacaval anastomosis will abstain from further use of alcohol, and the biopsy specimens taken at surgery may be compared with autopsy material many years later. There is usually considerable improvement or at least an increase in regenerated liver parenchyma at the expense of the connective tissue septa, which after revascularization have become thinner and less cellular. The portal lymphatics are less prominent, the liver cells in the pseudolobules often are normal in appearance, and the liver cord pattern is reestablished. The person with alcoholism with early or moderate cirrhosis who discontinues alcohol consumption will demonstrate similar improvement. The degree of reversibility after cessation of drinking is of clinical importance. The lack of further episodes of necrosis and jaundice as a result of excessive alcohol use plus the disappearance of fat and any acute change provides maximal opportunity for limited recovery. These patients, with or without portacaval shunt, may enter the phase of compensated cirrhosis. Even those who continue to drink much less may survive many years with few or no symptoms of cirrhosis.

In some patients with alcoholism the first symptoms of hepatic disease may not develop until the advanced stage of atrophic cirrhosis. There may be nothing in the history to indicate that a patient with an attack of jaundice ever had a large fatty liver that would cause necrosis of liver cells. It would seem that in some of these individuals the cirrhotic process may progress through various stages of severity to the atrophic and coarsely nodular liver with little or no fat demonstrable on biopsy. The quantitative aspects of alcohol consumption and malnutrition may well determine whether fibrosis and pseudolobules occur with or without fatty changes. Certainly in the presence of severe fatty change, the sequence of necrosis of hepatic cells, jaundice, and coma is more likely to develop. Also, alcoholic patients who develop fatal infections, pancreatitis, and delirium tremens seem to have such occurrences at the fatty liver stage more often than not.

It has been shown by injection-corrosion casts of normal and cirrhotic livers that in cirrhosis the hepatic arteries and arterial bed are enlarged, with an increased number of communications between the hepatic arteries and portal veins.[314] The portal and hepatic venous systems are reduced in size, the change being much more severe on the hepatic vein side. The reduction of venous systems often is associated with fibrosis. Anastomotic channels are occasionally seen between portal and hepatic veins, but no significant differences were observed in the vascular pattern of alcoholic liver disease when compared with that of coarsely nodular cryptogenic cirrhosis.

In the advanced stages of alcoholic cirrhosis, portal hypertension with variceal bleeding, hepatic failure with encephalopathy, and functional renal failure are the most common causes of death. An increased frequency of peptic ulcer also occurs in these patients, and bleeding from this source must always be considered. In some patients, ascites may become chronic and resistant to treatment, whereas in others the ascites is easily controlled or spontaneously disappears. Hepatic encephalopathy is easily precipitated by hemorrhage, infection, or further insults to the liver.

PATHOPHYSIOLOGY OF CHRONIC LIVER DISEASE

Many pathophysiologic phenomena are associated with chronic liver disease. Although some of these are the direct results of hepatic disease, others are unexplained. The concept that hepatic failure or insufficiency may occur to a variable degree is important. The most severe form of hepatic failure is coma. Only occasionally does the cirrhotic patient die in deep coma without some complication. The patient may from time to time have episodes of encephalopathy that are reversible. Some of these mild forms of encephalopathy are indicated by an inability to perform simple mental tests. More severe forms include flapping tremor, agitation, and disorientation.

In addition to encephalopathy, the more common complications of chronic liver disease in its progression to cirrhosis are portal hypertension, esophageal varices, and ascites.

Encephalopathy

The chief manifestation of hepatic failure is encephalopathy. This occurs in both acute and chronic liver disease. In fulminant hepatitis the onset is sudden and the mortality high.[347] In chronic liver disease the symptoms are more likely to be mild and the onset gradual. The manifestations are of a neuropsychiatric nature, varying from minor disturbances of consciousness and behavior to drowsiness, confusion, and coma. Often a flapping tremor of the extremities is evident. Despite the severe neurologic features that may develop, histopathologic changes at autopsy are minimal, apparently limited to enlargement and increased numbers of protoplasmic astrocytes.[350] One of the surprising aspects of hepatic coma is the rapid and complete recovery that may occur if hepatic failure is ameliorated.

The cause of hepatic encephalopathy is unknown, but four major hypotheses have been developed, each of which has devoted adherents.[386]

The first and foremost hypothesis is concerned with certain toxic metabolites formed in the gut or in the process of intestinal absorption that are usually removed by a normal liver but accumulate when there is hepatic malfunction. These substances interact, synergistically producing alteration of neural transmission and ultimately coma. The foremost of the toxic metabolites is ammonia, produced excessively in the breakdown of animal proteins and also by urea-splitting organisms in the gut. Reduction of meat in diet and sterilization of the gut have been the principal effective methods of reducing the development of encephalopathy.

Although ammonia is considered the most important toxic metabolite, methylmercaptan and short- and medium-chain fatty acids are believed to be contributory, and hypoxia, hypoglycemia, and electrolyte imbalances also offer synergistic effects. Methylmercaptan with its metabolites is believed to be the source of hepatic fetor, the peculiar breath odor of patients in hepatic coma or impending coma. Patients who have had surgical anastomoses of the portal vein to the vena cava to reduce the pressure in the splanchnic bed (portacaval shunt), particularly those patients who are over 60 years of age, are at high risk of encephalopathy. The encephalopathy develops because the blood is deviated from the gut into the systemic circulation without passing through the liver.

A second hypothesis is that efflux of aliphatic amino acids and glutamine from brain tissue is associated with an influx of aromatic amino acids, resulting in increased production of inhibitory transmitter (serotonin) and decreased synthesis of excitatory neurotransmitters such as dopamine and norepinephrine. However, efflux of glutamine may be the result of increased levels of blood ammonia that will increase brain glutamine severalfold.

A third hypothesis holds that gamma-aminobutyric acid (GABA), synthesized by gut bacteria, also becomes increased in serum when an intact liver is not available for adequate removal. At the same time, the permeability of the blood-brain barrier is increased, and larger numbers of central nervous system–binding sites for GABA form. GABA is a major component of the inhibitory neurotransmitter system of the mammalian brain. In excessive amounts it is alleged to induce coma.[378]

The fourth hypothesis proposes that encephalopathy is a result of impaired energy metabolism by the brain, based on the observation that oxygen consumption and glucose use by the brain are markedly reduced. However, the impaired metabolism is only measurably diminished after 24 hours or more of encephalopathy or coma.[386]

Meager but demonstrable morphologic changes occur in the brains of patients with encephalopathy. Alzheimer II astrocytes form in brains of these patients (Chapter 44).[350] Changes in astrocytes, indistinguishable from those found in the brain of a patient in hepatic coma, can be induced by ammonia,[386] by portacaval shunts in normal chimpanzees,[381] or by inducing ischemic hepatic necrosis in animals.[368]

Portal hypertension

Resistance to the flow of blood within the liver in chronic liver disease is the most common cause of portal hypertension. Such portal hypertension is intrahepatic, in contrast to the posthepatic type caused by lesions of the hepatic veins or the prehepatic type in which the obstruction is caused by disease of the portal vein or its radicles.

Intrahepatic portal hypertension. Any form of cirrhosis may be associated with intrahepatic portal hypertension. The mechanism of obstruction was once attributed to compression by regenerative nodules.[355] However, at least in the alcoholic patient, significant portal hypertension develops in response to perivenular intrasinusoidal collagen deposition before the development of regenerative nodules.[375] Whether or not small arterioportal shunts contribute to portal hypertension in cirrhotic livers is not established, but in the patient with hepatocellular carcinoma (HCC), arterial supply to the tumor associated with egress of blood from the tumor into the portal venous system is apparently the usual flow pattern.[367] How much the arterial portal shunt contributes to portal hypertension in the patient with HCC is unclear. The normal pressure in the portal vein is 6 to 10 mm Hg.[374] In cirrhosis it may rise to 20 to 30 mm Hg. The rise in pressure is directly related to the resistance to blood flow within the liver.

In about 15% of patients in whom portacaval shunt has been performed, the pressure on the hepatic side of a clamp placed on the vein is higher than it is on the splanchnic side, indicating that there is a reversal of portal vein blood flow in these patients. The pressure within the portal system may be measured indirectly with a fair degree of accuracy by introducing a catheter, through the inferior vena cava, into a small branch of the hepatic venous system. The catheter, when wedged into the vein, gives a pressure reading similar to the pressure within the portal vein system.[376] The so-called wedged hepatic vein pressure is helpful in determining whether the point of obstruction is within the liver or is extrahepatic. In the latter, normal wedged pressures are observed.

The portal pressure can also be measured directly, either by threading a firm catheter through the loose connective tissue of the closed umbilical vein into the left portal vein branch or by thin needle insertion into the liver percutaneously, directly into one of the major portal vein branches. The latter has become the more popular method of measurement of portal pressure.

The portal vein averages 7 cm in length and is formed by the confluence of the superior mesenteric and splenic veins. The inferior mesenteric vein joins the latter about 3 cm from its junction point. Thus the portal blood is received from the gastrointestinal tract, mesentery, spleen, gallbladder, and pancreas. Obstruction to the flow of blood through the portal trunk results in hypertension throughout the system. In cirrhosis this develops slowly but finally results in chronic passive hyperemia of the tissues drained by the portal vein. The intestines and peritoneum appear congested and edematous. The spleen is usually enlarged in portal hypertension, although how much of the cause is fibrocongestive, as once stated, is not clear. In the alcoholic cirrhotic patients who regularly have splenic lymphoid atrophy, only 23% have spleens weighing more than 400 g. Patients with cirrhosis of other types, however, may have spleens that weigh as much as 1000 g, and occasionally even more. There is poor correlation between spleen size and the severity of portal hypertension.

Posthepatic portal hypertension. Posthepatic portal hypertension is rare. It results from impeded egress of blood from the hepatic vein into the vena cava. Neoplastic obstruction, thrombosis of the hepatic veins or of the inferior vena cava, and prolonged congestive heart failure may transmit elevated pressure through the hepatic vascular bed to the portal vein.

Prehepatic portal hypertension. Prehepatic portal hypertension is an uncommon condition in which a block is hypothesized to occur before the portal blood reaches the sinusoidal bed. The liver is presumed not to be involved. Idiopathic portal hypertension is the principal example (see p. 1175). Classically, extrahepatic portal vein thrombosis has been considered a cause of prehepatic portal hypertension. However, neoplastic occlusion of the extrahepatic portal vein produces neither portal hypertension nor splenomegaly. When thrombosis of the portal vein associated with splanchnic portal hypertension occurs, quite possibly sludged blood already under increased pressure allowed the thrombus to form.[365] Congenital absence of the portal vein has been reported.[369]

Myelofibrosis rarely produces portal hypertension, probably because of the fibrous involvement of all the intrahepatic portal structures rather than increased blood flow through the enlarged spleen.

A condition known as nodular regenerative hyperplasia is often associated with portal hypertension believed to be prehepatic. Patients with Felty's syndrome (arthritis, leukopenia, and splenomegaly) often have nodular regenerative hyperplasia.

Esophageal varices. As a result of the increase in pressure within the portal system, the blood tends to bypass the liver and return to the heart by various collaterals (Fig. 27-30). These develop more prominently cephalad than caudad. Although hemorrhoids are common, they do not cause serious complications. More important are the large varices, susceptible to erosion and fatal bleeding, that arise in the mucosa at the lower end of the esophagus (Fig. 27-31). The blood entering these veins is short-circuited from the portal system through the coronary veins of the stomach and also the left gastroepiploic vein and vasa brevia. In the lower third of the esophagus the submucosal veins are poorly supported and are subjected to trauma by the passage of food. They may also be eroded by regurgitation of gastric juice. However, microscopic analyses of varices that have ruptured do not show overlying esophagitis or ulceration. It is unknown why the precipitating event that causes repeated variceal bleeding in some patients may seldom cause it in other patients who have even higher portal pressures. In patients with cirrhosis both esophagoscopy and roentgenograms are used to demonstrate the presence of varices. The exsanguination that follows rupture of the esophageal varices is a precipitating cause of death in 15% of cirrhotic patients. An additional 35% die of liver failure after esophageal hemorrhage.

Other anastomoses between the portal circulation and systemic veins may develop between the hilum of the liver and the umbilicus along the paraumbilical plexus of veins. These may cause enlargement of the umbilicus (caput medusae). When paraumbilical veins are greatly enlarged, the term *Cruveilhier-Baumgarten syndrome* sometimes is applied, especially when a murmur is heard. The cutaneous vessels over the upper abdomen may be enlarged (Plate 5, *A*). Other communications may be established through the veins of Retzius in the posterior mesentery and directly through the diaphragm via the veins of Sappey. It has been demonstrated that blood may even find its way through the periesophageal veins directly to the pulmonary veins and left atrium.[349]

In patients who have esophageal varices demonstrable by esophagoscopy or by roentgenograms and who may or may not have had an episode of hemorrhage, the construction of a portal-systemic shunt[363] is often performed to decompress the portal system. This is usually of the portacaval type. If an end-to-side anastomosis is used, it prevents any possible retrograde flow in the portal vein through anastomoses with branches of the hepatic artery within the liver. Patients with thrombosed hepatic veins profit by side-by-side anastomosis, which helps the

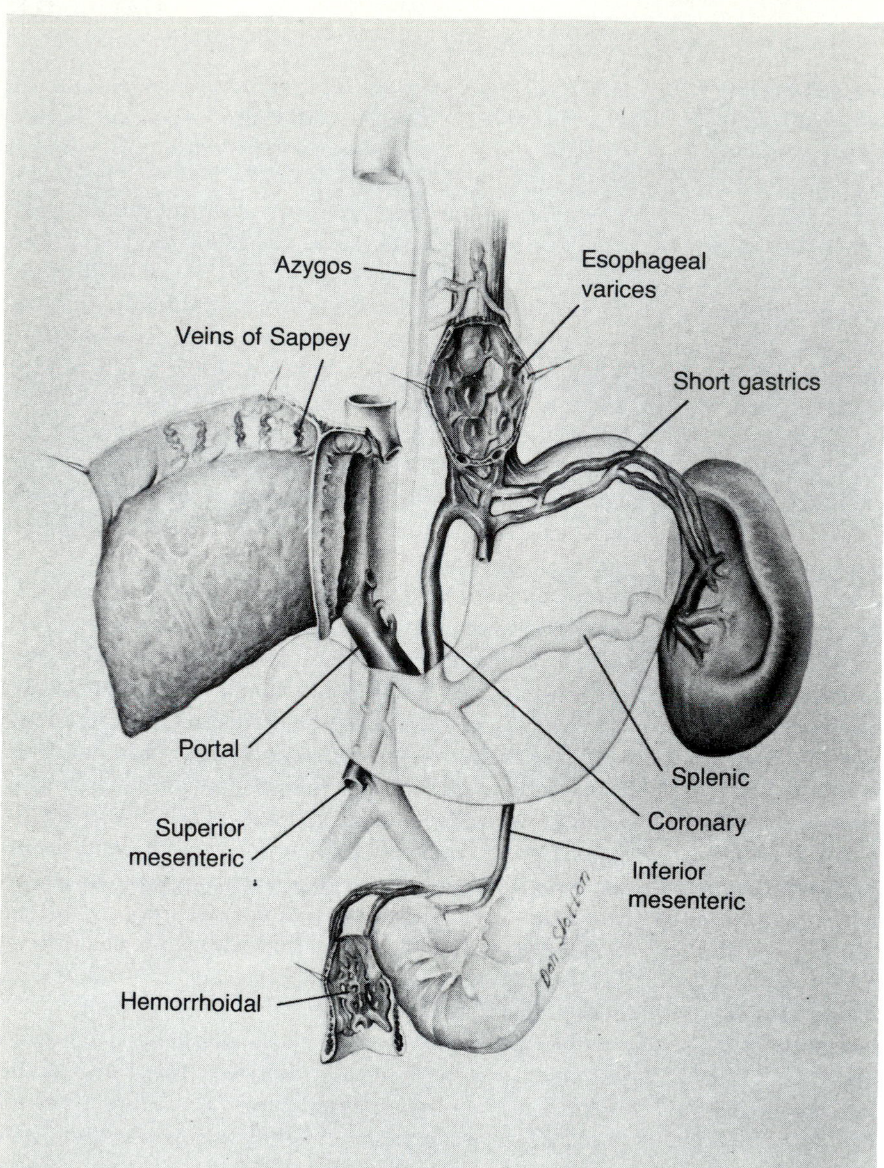

Fig. 27-30. Portal vein and its major tributaries showing most important routes of collateral circulation between portal and caval systems.

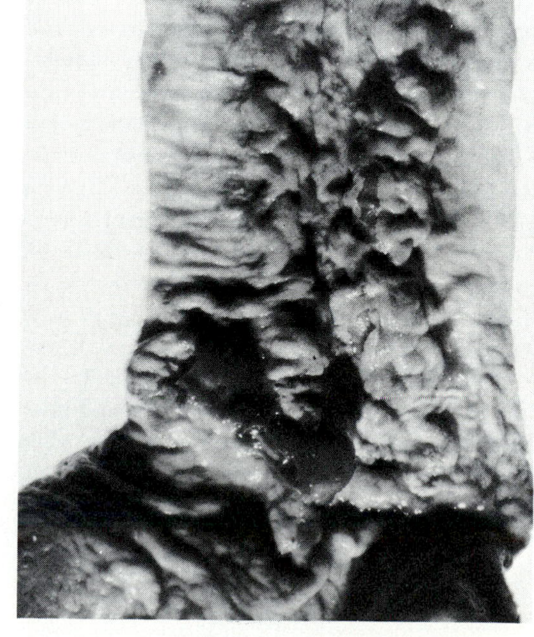

Fig. 27-31. Large esophageal varices on mucosal surface of opened esophagus.

nutrition of the liver by allowing more hepatic artery blood to circulate through the parenchyma and then out through the portal vein (reversed flow). In the past several years a selective portacaval shunt, reducing pressure in the esophagus and stomach without forcing blood from the small and large intestines to bypass the liver, has been popular. This procedure, a distal splenorenal shunt, achieves selective amelioration by dividing the splenic vein and swinging its splenic end to an end-to-side anastomosis into the renal vein. The hepatic side of the divided splenic vein is ligated, as is the coronary vein. Following shunting procedure, the varices tend to decrease in size, as does the spleen in about one half of the patients. Further variceal hemorrhage is rare. The status of the fibrotic process in the liver is unaffected by surgery. Proper diet and abstinence from ethanol are of most value in slowing the progress of the disease. In extrahepatic portal vein thrombosis a portacaval shunt is usually impossible, and a splenorenal shunt may be done. In recent years injection of sclerosing agents into varices through the esophagoscope has had a resurgence of popularity. Repeated injections, as needed, may prove to be as effective therapeutically and more cost effective than shunting. Whether patient survival time is actually increased by portal system shunt procedures remains undetermined. Clearly, however, such procedures markedly reduce the demands for scarce blood for transfusions.

Ascites. Ascites often accompanies portal hypertension, especially in the advanced stages of cirrhosis (Plate 5, *A*). The ascitic fluid, by definition, is a transudate, having a specific gravity of around 1.010. The mechanism of formation is complex, and many factors are involved: (1) portal hypertension and increased capillary filtration pressure, (2) postsinusoidal block, (3) hypoalbuminemia, (4) impaired renal function, (5) inferior vena cava hypertension, and (6) hyperaldosteronism.

The simple elevation of portal pressure and increased capillary filtration pressure may produce a soft tissue transudate from the entire splanchnic bed and liver surface. Postsinusoidal block is believed to be the fundamental mechanism of ascites formation. Not only does increased lymph form, but the liver surface tends to weep considerable amounts of fluid. Hypoalbuminemia may contribute to ascites by reduction of osmotic pressure in plasma, but its importance is believed to be minimal.

Impaired renal function. Impaired renal function in cirrhosis may be caused by pooling of splanchnic blood that results in a diminution of effective blood volume, reduced glomerular filtration rate, and sodium retention. There is also evidence that renal dysfunction is related to hepatic disease by changes other than blood flow. It has been suggested that in some unexplained fashion the liver may have a direct effect on the ability of the kidney to excrete sodium. The failure to excrete sodium would be responsible for increased blood volume and partially responsible for ascites.[357]

Other changes

Inferior vena cava hypertension. Inferior vena cava hypertension has been proposed as a contributing feature in the formation of ascites.[366] Frequently in cirrhosis an enlarged caudate lobe compresses the inferior vena cava into an elliptical shape that may lead to a pressure differential between the abdominal and the thoracic inferior vena cava. It has been suggested that such narrowing may impair both the hepatic venous and the renal venous returns, thus accentuating hepatic postsinusoidal portal hypertension and renal sodium clearance.

Aldosterone has strong sodium-retaining properties and is frequently increased in the plasma and urine of the cirrhotic patients, particularly those with ascites.[360,370] Whether the elevated levels are a primary or secondary feature in relation to ascites is unknown. Certainly hyperaldosteronism is not a prerequisite for ascites.

On occasion ascites may be associated with right-sided hydrothorax as a result of small defects that develop in the diaphragm.[358,359]

Arteriovenous fistulas of skin. Arteriovenous fistulas of skin, also called vascular spiders, are often observed in chronic liver disease (Plate 5, *B*). Similar lesions in the lung have been described and recognized as a possible cause of finger clubbing and cyanosis that are common in patients with alcoholic cirrhosis.[348] Other findings in the cirrhotic patient may include palmar erythema,[344] pallor of the fingernails, enlargement of the salivary glands, and Dupuytren's contractures of the palmar fascia. In women with alcoholic cirrhosis a decrease in menstruation or amenorrhea is frequent.

Testicular atrophy. Testicular atrophy almost invariably accompanies cirrhosis in the patient with alcoholism but not most other types of cirrhosis.[345] This is often accompanied by signs of feminization in those with alcoholic liver disease.[382] These include a decrease in beard, development of gynecomastia, and impotence. The plasma levels of testosterone are decreased, and those of estradiol are normal or slightly increased. Plasma gonadotropin levels are elevated. It appears that the testicular dysfunction and anatomic changes are the product of alcoholism, not of cirrhosis.[383]

Renal failure. Renal failure is a common cause of death in cirrhotic patients or patients with fulminant hepatic necrosis; 80% of patients with terminal cirrhosis or fulminant necrosis have elevated levels of blood urea.[345] Elevated creatinine levels, followed by a less striking rise of serum urea, often develop in patients with ascites. Although it is well established that functional renal failure occurs after reduced renal plasma flow and an even more pronounced decrease in glomerular filtration rate, the pathogenesis is unknown. The total plasma volume actually is increased, although it is possible that splanchnic pooling of blood, resulting from portal hypertension, may reduce effective plasma volume.[351,372] The liver disease is linked somehow with the impaired renal capacity to excrete sodium and with consequent fluid retention.

It is believed that there are two varieties of renal failure in patients with advanced liver disease. In the first type urinary sodium levels are low because of accentuated renal tubular absorption that results from reduced glomerular infiltration rate. This is called functional renal failure. A second type of renal failure is hypothesized to represent acute tubular necrosis because of the failure to conserve sodium.[361,377] The kidneys at autopsy in either type of renal failure have unusually well-preserved but slightly dilated tubules.

Proximal convoluted tubular epithelial proliferation. Proximal convoluted tubular epithelial proliferation occurs in patients who die of hepatic failure. The parietal layer of Bowman's capsule may be involved by a peculiar proliferation of the proximal convoluted tubules. Only scattered glomeruli may be involved. The cause of hepatic failure seems unimportant.

Spur cell hemolytic anemia and cirrhosis. Spur cell hemolytic anemia occurs in patients with either cirrhosis or other liver diseases. These patients may develop a hemolytic process with large numbers of circulating erythrocytes that have spurlike projections from their surface, producing distortion. The spurlike formation is accentuated by absence of the spleen. The syndrome is associated with anemia and hyperbilirubinemia, predominantly in the indirect fraction. Conflicting experimental results have been reported regarding whether the defect is in the erythrocytic cell membrane[379] or in a plasma fraction.[352] The prognosis is poor. Occasionally, hypersplenism is associated with portal hypertension.

Folate deficiency. Folate deficiency is relatively common in alcoholic liver disease, producing anemia but only rarely significant megaloblastosis. Usually folate deficiency is blamed on inadequate dietary intake,[354] but possibly the damaged liver may be incapable of adequate storage.

Hemorrhagic phenomena. Hemorrhagic phenomena are common in patients with hepatic disease. A number of defects in the clotting mechanism have been studied.[373] Fibrinogen, prothombin, and factors VII, IX, X, and V all are produced by the liver parenchymal cell, and the platelet count may be reduced by hypersplenism. In addition, an abnormal fibrinogen molecule may be produced,[380] and defects of fibrin polymerization have been reported.[353]

Immunologic defects. Immunologic defects are widely known in patients with cirrhosis, particularly those with the alcoholic type who often die of severe bacterial infection. A severe leukotactic defect attributable to the presence of abnormally high levels of chemotactic factor inactivator has been reported.[362] An increase in the number of T cells and a failure to develop delayed hypersensitivity have been noted.[346] Hyperglobulinemia is commonly observed. It has been suggested that this may be caused by the failure of the liver to sequester antigens absorbed from the intestine, since these circulate through the rest of the body because of the collateral circulation in cirrhosis.

• • •

Many other associations of extrahepatic diseases with hepatic disorders have been recognized: pulmonary hypertension and chronic active hepatitis have been reported to coexist,[356] although the relationship is unclear, and Graves' disease has a deleterious effect on the course of acute viral hepatitis. Muscle degradation in hepatic failure has been shown to be increased in cirrhotic patients; it has been hypothesized that the increased breakdown is a result of the increase in glucagon levels that is attained because the normal hepatic catabolism of glucagon is defective in hepatic failure. Glucagon accentuates muscle degradation. Cardiomyopathy and pancreatitis occur in alcoholic patients and are not necessarily related to liver disease, but cardiomyopathy is also apparently associated with the accentuated protein degradation of cirrhosis.[385] Vasculitis and glomerulonephritis have been associated with chronic active hepatitis B.[364]

CHOLESTATIC DISORDERS

Biliary tract disease and liver abscess

Many important diseases involve the intrahepatic biliary tract in adults: they may be primary or secondary. The latter are much more common, occurring when the extrahepatic flow of bile is obstructed, usually by stone, cancer, or stricture. Primary disease of the intrahepatic ducts, principally primary biliary cirrhosis (PBC), is now being diagnosed more frequently because of the use of laboratory screening that on occasion shows a high alkaline phosphatase activity or mitochondrial antibodies in an asymptomatic patient.

Biliary tract disease, either primary or secondary, is usually manifested by jaundice sometime in the course of the disease. The use of ultrasonography and cholangiograms, either transhepatic cholangiography or endoscopic retrograde cholangiopancreatography (ERCP), has resulted in a high degree of accuracy in the diagnosis of biliary tract disease in its various stages. Both PBC and secondary biliary tract disease may lead to cirrhosis.

Biliary obstruction

The extrahepatic biliary tract may be obstructed at any point from the hilus of the liver to the papilla of Vater by stone, carcinoma, or stricture. Taken as a group, these obstructive diseases produce many common features, although individual differences in clinical course, laboratory findings, and cholangiograms exist. Since jaundice is the outstanding symptom, mechanical obstruction of the biliary tree is also referred to as surgical jaundice.

Carcinoma of the bile ducts or the head of the pancreas usually produces complete obstruction with pronounced dilatation of the biliary tree, easily seen on cholangiograms (Fig. 27-32). There is jaundice accompanied by little or no pain. In obstruction caused by choledocholithiasis there is often a history of gallbladder disease, and jaundice is usually accompanied by pain. Although a calculus impacted in the papilla of Vater may produce complete obstruction, stones in the common duct are usually mobile and the jaundice tends to fluctuate or even disappear for varying periods of time. Cholangiograms are often diagnostic. Benign stricture of the extrahepatic bile ducts may follow surgical mishaps during cholecystectomy[442] or arise in the intrapancreatic portion of the common bile duct as a result of chronic alcoholic pancreatitis.[451] In the former the common hepatic duct is clamped or injured during surgery. Such surgical damage is followed by excessive drainage and usually jaundice within 1 week. Repair of the stricture is often difficult, and many of the patients have chronic jaundice and ultimately other complications, such as cholangitis and biliary cirrhosis. Obstruction of the common duct attributable to carcinoma causes a prompt rise in the serum alkaline phosphatase that precedes the rise in serum bilirubin, which, with complete obstruction, can reach levels of 20 to 25 mg/dl and even higher if there is renal failure (Table 27-1). The blood prothrombin activity decreases, the preprothrombin levels remain near normal, and the prothrombin activity rises after parenteral administration of vitamin K. Bile appears in the urine, and there is an absence of stercobilin in the stool. In choledocholithiasis the serum bilirubin level often fluctuates and usually does not go as high as it does when the duct is obstructed by carcinoma. Serum bilirubin levels are stable at a high level with neoplastic obstruction. The alkaline phosphatase level likewise does not show the constant elevated level in choledocholithiasis that is usually seen in cancerous obstruction. Since patients with postoperative strictures are usually subjected to multiple attempts at surgical repair, from time to time the laboratory and physical findings vary considerably. Chronic alcoholic pancreatitis may cause stricture of the common duct with jaundice and a bilirubin level that is usually less than 10 mg/dl.[445,451] Calcific alcoholic pancreatitis may produce partial obstruction only, marked by a very high alkaline phosphatase and little if any elevation of serum bilirubin.

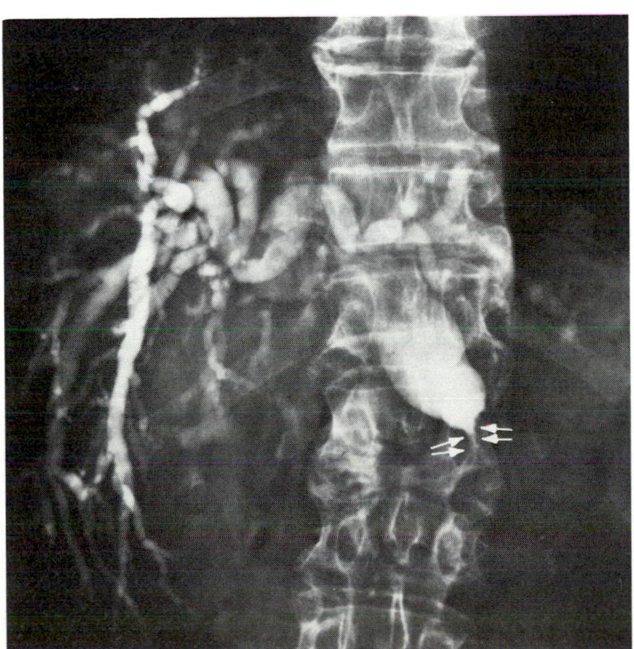

Fig. 27-32. Transhepatic cholangiogram showing extreme dilatation of extrahepatic and intrahepatic bile ducts caused by carcinoma of head of pancreas, narrowing intrapancreatic portion (*arrows*).

The bile acids in the serum have been studied extensively in patients with biliary obstruction and other forms of chronic liver disease. An increased level of serum bile acids is held responsible for the pruritus that is common in patients with chronic biliary obstruction.[439]

The sequence of events that follows obstruction of the bile duct depends to some extent on the severity of obstruction and infection that so often occurs in the stagnant column of bile in the dilated ducts behind the obstructing lesion. The early microscopic changes seen soon after obstruction include dilatation of the small ducts and, particularly, prominence of the ductules where they penetrate the limiting plate to join the canaliculi. The dilated ductules are usually outlined by neutrophils just beneath their basement membranes. Bile accumulates in the perivenular canaliculi, forming green-yellow to brown plugs (Plate 3, *C*). Later in unrelieved obstruction the ducts enlarge further and may proliferate. The bile canaliculi become more distended with bile plugs. In this state clinical symptoms of acute cholangitis may supervene, characterized by chills and fever in addition to the jaundice. The periductal neutrophils become more numerous and penetrate the lumen of the ducts. The cholangitis is of bacterial origin. Organisms often are found in stagnant bile when obstruction is attributable to stone or stricture, but only rarely are they present in surgical specimens when the obstruction is caused by tumor.[440] Electron microscopic studies of the livers of patients with duct obstruction show flattening of the canalicular microvilli and condensation of the pericanalicular ectoplasm.[392]

Studies of the intercellular junctions by the freeze-fracture method in biopsy material from patients with extrahepatic obstruction have shown discontinuities that might well allow the leakage of the bile directly from the canaliculi into the sinusoidal system.[434] The liver cells often contain intracytoplasmic bile, and Kupffer cells are enlarged by easily discernible masses of bile pigment. Foci of necrosis may appear within the lobules, with transformation to bile lakes and a rise in the serum transaminase levels. Often a feathery type of degeneration of liver cells is noted.[409] Increased connective tissue around the bile ducts may assume a lamellar arrangement, and small prolongations enter the periphery of the lobules. The patient with calculous obstruction, in particular, may have repeated attacks of chills, fever, and jaundice that last only a few days, a triad known as Charcot's intermittent hepatic fever.[398] In some patients with obstruction a more severe and life-threatening situation arises, characterized by fever, chills, a serum bilirubin level above 4 mg/dl, systemic sepsis, and a fall in blood pressure. These are caused by suppurative cholangitis, which is treated as a surgical emergency. Suppurative cholangitis is most often a complication of cancerous obstruction.[395] It is less often seen in calculous obstruction and is rarely seen in patients with a benign stricture. The actual presence of pus in the obstructed ducts is not always noted at surgery.

The borderline between suppurative cholangitis and multiple liver abscesses, particularly microabscesses, is indistinct because both may be present. In addition to surgical intervention and drainage of the common duct, percutaneous transhepatic cholangiography and drainage have been used successfully in diagnosis and treatment at this stage of the disease.[446] Thus the spectrum of changes that follow obstruction begins with a mild pericholangitis and includes the various stages of infectious cholangitis, multiple liver abscesses, and even biliary cirrhosis. The severity of infection and abscess formation may vary considerably from one part of the liver to another.

The prognosis in obstructive disease varies with the cause: cancerous obstruction has a poor prognosis, with the patients dying of their disease or of cholangitis. Choledocholithiasis is usually relieved by surgery, although occasionally death is caused by cholangitis or, rarely, biliary cirrhosis. Postoperative benign strictures are difficult to treat with bypass surgery and often lead to biliary fibrosis or cirrhosis. Bypass procedures for strictures caused by calcific pancreatitis may be successful.

Among the unusual types of cholangitis is massive hepatobiliary ascariasis in childhood. This disease is characterized by severe right upper quadrant pain accompanied by vomiting, fever, and often findings indicative of right upper quadrant (local) peritonitis. A diagnosis of massive intrahepatic involvement of the bile duct by the worms can be made by ultrasonography. In some cases conservative management fails and surgical drainage of the liver lesion is necessary. Cholangitis and multiple small abscesses are usually present.[419]

Because fatal cholangitis may occur quickly after obstruction by a stone in the duct of the diabetic patient, the screening of all diabetics past 40 years of age for cholelithiasis by ultrasonography should be a clinical consideration. In a small percentage of patients with choledocholithiasis, clinical features of acute cholangitis occur in the absence of jaundice.

Biliary cirrhosis

Obstruction of the biliary tract (either extrahepatic or intrahepatic) may, if prolonged, lead to cirrhosis of the liver. The causes of biliary obstruction have already been discussed (p. 1149). The appearance of the liver in extrahepatic obstruction depends on the degree of blockage and the time factor. Neoplastic obstruction is usually complete, and the patient dies before a true cirrhosis develops. The biliary tree proximal to the neoplasm is greatly dilated. The liver is green to greenish brown and finely granular. An increase of connective tissue along the large bile ducts near the hilum of the liver usually is noted. The organ is often increased in size and palpable before death, although there is little increase in weight. Occasionally a carcinoma obstructing the ducts grows very slowly; the increase in connective tissue is such that the diagnosis of early biliary cirrhosis is justified. Obstruction of the common duct caused by a calculus or a benign stricture is usually incomplete. Therefore the distension of the ducts and bile stasis in the liver are not as extreme as with cancerous obstruction. On occasion a stone or a stricture may obstruct the common duct for years and lead to true biliary cirrhosis. We have observed several such cases caused by inapparent choledocholithiasis.

The liver in biliary cirrhosis has a granular appearance or may even be nodular. Fibrosis is as pronounced as it is in alcoholic cirrhosis. In neglected patients, biliary cirrhosis of this type may on rare occasions cause portal hypertension, splenomegaly, and hemorrhage from esophageal varices. A portacaval shunt may become necessary.[388]

In the early stage of extrahepatic obstruction, microscopic examination reveals that dilatation of the large ducts near the hilum is constant, whereas the size of the smaller ducts is variable. Some increase of fibroblastic activity with the formation of spurs is seen within 30 to 50 days.[443] Bile stasis is predominantly perivenular. In the intermediate stage, between 60 and 100 days, connective tissue is more abundant and often has a concentric configuration around the bile ducts. Both at this stage and in the later cirrhotic phase, the arrangement of the connective tissue may give a "pipestem" effect (Fig. 27-33). Bile duct proliferation is present in only a small percentage of the total. The mononuclear type of exudate may be

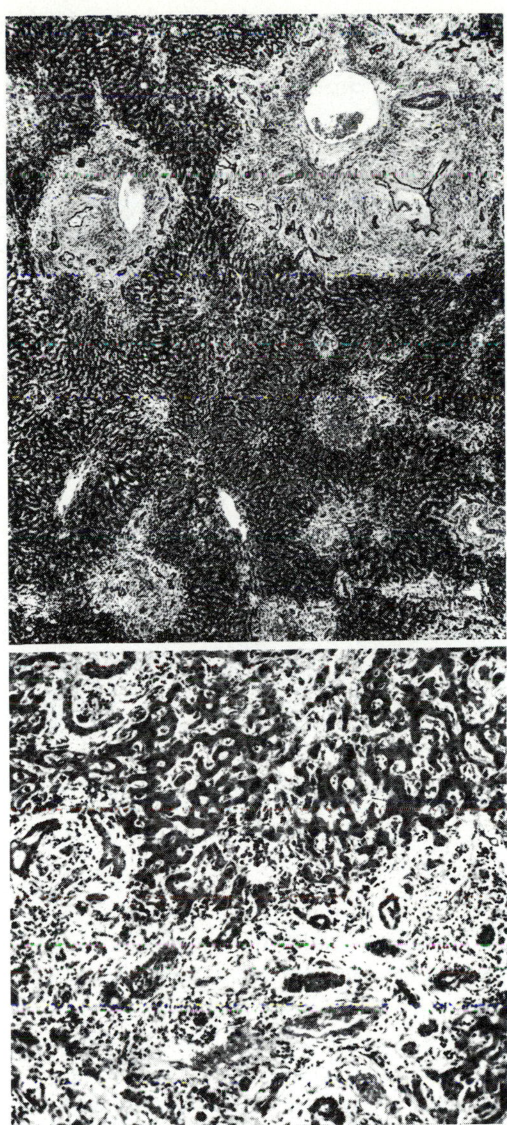

Fig. 27-33. Biliary cirrhosis.

increased. Focal necrosis of hepatic cells of either the lytic or the eosinophilic type is frequent. As the result of necrosis, particularly of cells in the peripheries of the lobules, bile lakes may form. The teminal hepatic veins are present, and a normal lobular architecture can be seen throughout most of the liver. A few abnormal hyperplastic nodules may make their appearance at this stage. Later, especially in patients with calculous obstruction or stricture, a well-developed cirrhosis is noted, with connective tissue septa outlining pseudolobules. Intralobular bile stasis is irregular but is now both perivenular and peripheral. There is usually no bile stasis within the interlobular ducts, probably because bile is absorbed within the lobule. Occasionally a liver may exhibit wide connective tissue septa with abundant bile duct proliferation. Fatty changes, extensive necrosis of parenchyma, and even abscesses may complicate the disease.

Primary biliary tract disease

There are three slowly progressive primary diseases of the intrahepatic biliary tract: primary biliary cirrhosis (PBC), primary sclerosing cholangitis (PSC), and Caroli's disease. The first two are of unknown etiology and are often associated with diseases of other organ systems, whereas Caroli's disease is a congenital disorder.

Primary biliary cirrhosis

Primary biliary cirrhosis (PBC), or chronic nonsuppurative destructive cholangitis, is a complex autoimmune disorder that is characterized by destruction of the interlobular bile ducts. The name *PBC* is somewhat misleading because the end stage of cirrhosis may not be reached until 5 to 10 years or more after diagnosis. Hanot first recognized the disorder in 1876, using the term *hypertropic cirrhosis with jaundice*.[435]

Little attention has been given to the geographic aspects of PBC, since most studies of the disease have been in the United States and Europe. In the United States about 94% of the PBC patients are women with a mean age of 52, 95% between 32 and 72 years of age.[431] PBC in patients under 30 years of age is rare. The frequency in the general population is unknown; however, the routine use of biochemical screening that includes determination of serum alkaline phosphatase levels has resulted in an increased number of cases being diagnosed in the asymptomatic stage.[405] In about 20% of all patients with PBC the disease is diagnosed at this stage. Liver biopsies in this subclinical stage have shown that any one of the various pathologic stages of PBC may be present, even cirrhosis.

The onset is generally insidious, beginning with pruritus that may be present for several months to years before the onset of dark urine or icterus.[400] A few patients have darkening of the skin well before the onset of pruritus and jaundice. After jaundice has been present for months, the patient may notice foul fatty stools, and slowly over the years the skin manifestations of hyperlipemia may become noticeable as xanthomas or fine yellowish deposits in the creases of the palms of the hands, antecubital spaces, and elsewhere (Fig. 27-34).

From the outset there is hepatomegaly, and about one half of the patients have splenomegaly. The impaired flow of bile into the intestine causes a deficiency of the absorption of vitamin D and calcium that results in osteomalacia, often with bone pain and even compression fractures of the vertebrae. Weight loss is noted as greater amounts of ingested fat are excreted in the stool, and a defect in glucose absorption occurs.[448] The course is one of slow deterioration, with the duration of life from 5 to 15 years after the diagnosis is established. In the end

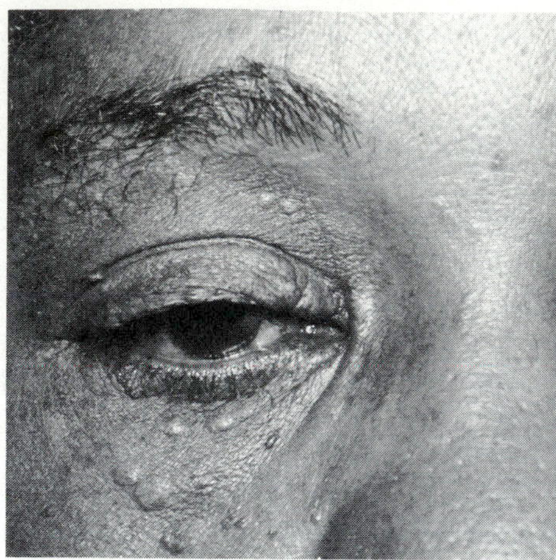

Fig. 27-34. Xanthomas of eyelid in primary biliary cirrhosis.

stage of cirrhosis, ascites, hepatic coma, and bleeding from esophageal varices are common features.

The laboratory findings consist of positive results of a properly performed mitochondrial antibody test, an increase in IgM, and an elevated alkaline phosphatase. In PBC there is often a familial type of hypergammaglobulinema.[414] The serum copper level is moderately elevated in symptomatic PBC. Abnormalities of serum complement levels have been noted; these are difficult to interpret, but they do demonstrate a marked hypercatabolism of C3.[406] Immune complexes are usually present in serum. The withered biliary tree seen on cholangiograms is characteristic of the disease.

More than any other liver disease, PBC is associated with a number of immune-type disorders. Among these are Sjögren's syndrome, scleroderma, arthritis, lupus erythematosus, interstitial pneumonitis, and thyroiditis.[401] Sjögren's syndrome (dry eyes and mouth) is the most common autoimmune type of disorder noted. Rheumatoid arthritis occurs in a relatively small percentage of patients.[394] An additional asymptomatic erosive type of arthritis involving the distal small joints of the hands has been described.[423] The arthritis is usually symptomless and is accompanied by osteopenia in a majority of patients. Association with thyroiditis has been noted in about one third of patients with PBC.[442] Scleroderma may occur alone or with Raynaud's phenomenon, calcinosis cutis, sclerodactyly, and telangiectasia; the latter is known as the CRST syndrome.[433] Immune complexes may usually be demonstrated in sera of patients with PBC.

Four pathologic stages, from the earliest changes seen on biopsy to the end stages of cirrhosis, have been described[420] in our patients, now consisting of over 140 cases in the last 5 years, and there is considerable overlap of staging features within the same biopsy specimen. Thus in the biopsy diagnosis we use only rough approximations and find staging, as described, inexact with respect to the clinical course of disease.

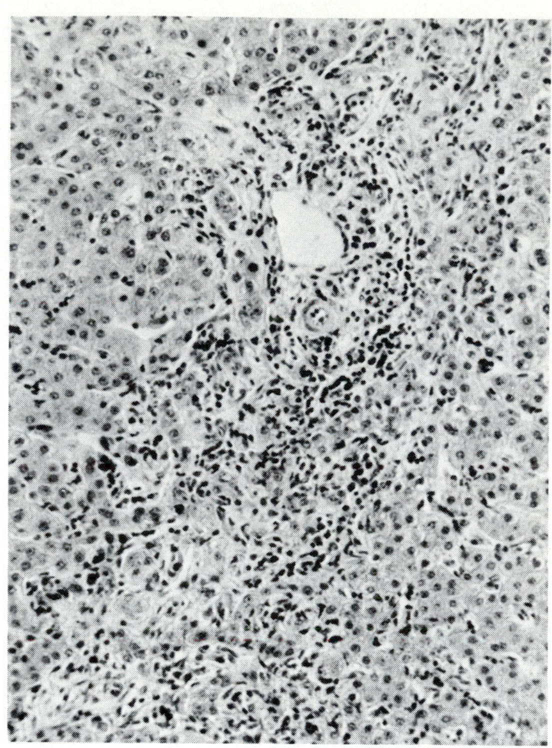

Fig. 27-35. Destruction of bile ducts and limiting plate in primary biliary cirrhosis.

In the early stages of the disease there is destruction of interlobular bile ducts as well as obliteration of the limiting plate (Fig. 27-35). The ducts show various stages of damage and are surrounded by a dense infiltrate of lymphocytes, plasma cells, and a few eosinophils. The lymphocytes often form follicles that impinge on or surround the affected ducts. In the destructive process the ductal epithelium shows cytoplasmic vacuolization, nuclear pyknosis, and karyorrhexis, along with some degree of atypical epithelial proliferation. The limiting plate is infiltrated with mononuclear cells and is difficult to define. The periportal hepatocytes may show degenerative hydropic change, and about 10% of the patients have scanty alcoholic hyalin in the hydropic periportal hepatocytes. Histiocytes may form granulomatous collections, more often in the portal areas than within the lobules. True epithelioid granulomas with giant cells are rare, occurring in about 10% to 20% of cases. With progression the portal areas become wider and fibrotic. The inflammatory reaction tends to regress, and the interlobular bile ducts disappear. More than 60% of the portal tracts ultimately become devoid of interlobular bile ducts, whereas the liver in other hepatic diseases shows less than 15% destruction.[390] Along with the reduction of the interlobular bile ducts, the proliferation of atypical "pseudoductules" is prominent. These little ducts have flat irregular epithelium and a tiny or absent lumen, are located at the peripheral zone of the portal tract, and probably represent transformed hepatic cords. The hepatic cords show little damage with the exception of those in the periportal areas, where necrosis, fibrosis (stage 3 or 4), and periportal cholestasis are often apparent. In the later stages of PBC, fibrous septa connect adjacent portal areas and also split the lobules. Finally, encircled nodules join to form biliary cirrhosis. In the final stages of the disease, perivenular cholestasis may occur. Marked copper accumulation may occur in livers of patients with chronic jaundice. Appropriate stains on either biopsy or autopsy material disclose large quantities of copper, fairly uniformly distributed in the periportal hepatocytes.

The piecemeal necrosis that occurs in the periportal areas has been reported to correlate with the presence of an antibody to human hepatocyte membrane lipoprotein.[448]

Primary sclerosing cholangitis

Primary sclerosing cholangitis (PSC) is predominantly a disease of men (80%) with an average age range of 25 to 45 years. It is characterized by jaundice, pruritus, and hepatomegaly.[417,450] In about one half to three fourths of patients the disease coexists with chronic ulcerative colitis but not or only rarely with Crohn's disease[397,450] It has occurred with an immunodeficiency syndrome.[432] PSC has a moderately progressive course, and many patients die of biliary cirrhosis within 5 years. Grossly the extrahepatic bile ducts are usually sclerosed and hard; the intrahepatic ducts are likewise affected, but increased numbers of patients with only intrahepatic PSC and "normal" extrahepatic ducts are now being recognized.[393] In the liver there is bile duct proliferation, fibrosis, and cholestasis that progresses to biliary fibrosis, often to cirrhosis. The ductal involvement has a very irregular distribution; thus the biopsy pattern is highly variable from one area to another. Some areas resemble the changes from mechanical obstruction; others simulate the changes of primary biliary cirrhosis. The regions of intrahepatic sclerosis have prominent thickening of ducts with intramural inflammation, and some areas have practically no changes. As with other types of biliary cirrhosis, a large amount of copper is present in hepatocytes of protracted cases but less than that found in patients with PBC. Cholangiograms in PSC are diagnostic (Fig. 27-36). Recently the disease has been reported in children.[449]

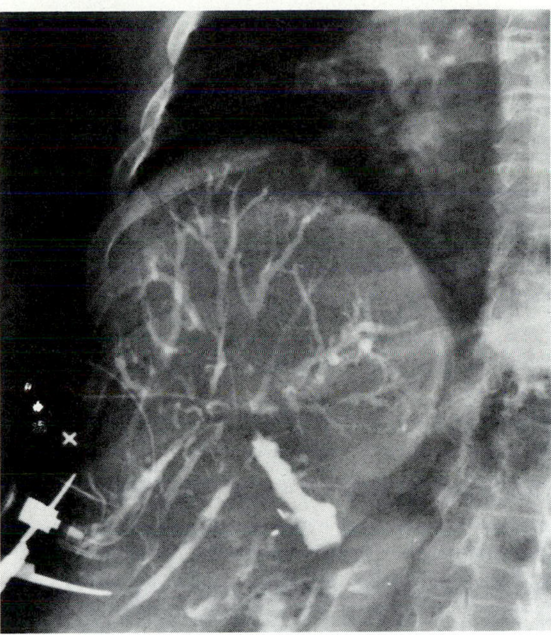

Fig. 27-36. Cholangiogram of patient with intrahepatic sclerosing cholangitis. Note irregular diameter of intrahepatic duct radicals, some of which appear amputated.

Caroli's disease

Congenital cystic dilatation of the intrahepatic bile duct (choledochal cyst or Caroli's disease) is a rare familial disorder. The cystic dilatations are easily seen on cholangiograms and may involve many of the intrahepatic bile ducts. The dilatations are filled with bile and have a characteristic gross and microscopic appearance.[447] Calculi may form within the cystic areas. Cholangitis and liver abscesses may be fatal. The disease may consist only of an isolated choledochal cyst or may be associated with renal tubular ectasia and other forms of cystic diseases of the kidneys. Carcinoma of the intrahepatic bile ducts has also been noted.[410] A form of the disease may be associated with congenital hepatic fibrosis.[408]

Other diseases

Other diseases of the intrahepatic bile ducts include hemobilia and pneumobilia. The clinical entity of hemobilia or hemorrhage into the biliary tract is characterized by biliary colic, gastrointestinal hemorrhage, and often bilirubinuria and clinical jaundice. Both melena and hematemesis may be present. Unrecognized hemobilia has a high mortality. Among the causes of hemobilia are trauma (p. 1170), needle biopsy of the liver,[391] transhepatic cholangiography,[403] neoplasms of the intrahepatic bile ducts or of the hepatic parenchyma, and aneurysms (hemocholecyst)[438] of the hepatic artery. Diseases of the gallbladder and extrahepatic ducts may also give rise to hemobilia. Superior mesenteric angiography is considered the best diagnostic procedure for the diagnosis of hemobilia. Air in the intrahepatic biliary tract, or pneumobilia, in the patient who has not had surgery may be associated with emphysematous cholecystitis, incompetence of the sphincter of Oddi, or biliary enteric fistula or may result from blunt abdominal trauma. Pneumobilia is a common finding in patients who have undergone biliary bypass surgery. In addition to ultrasonography, radionuclide scans, and plain abdominal roentgenograms, computed tomography is an excellent means of diagnosing air in the intrahepatic biliary tract.[441] Acquired bile duct cysts have been reported that result from liver infarcts caused by polyarteritis nodosa.[404]

Abscesses

Since the study by Ochsner, DeBakey, and Murray[426] on liver abscesses in 1938, there has been a considerable change in the etiologic background, diagnosis, and treatment of liver abscesses. Most abscesses are of bacterial pyogenic origin, a lesser number by *Entamoeba histolytica* and rarely by actinomycosis. They can be diagnosed by liver scans, computed tomography, and angiography. The occurrence of liver abscesses may constitute a severe clinical disorder, often with a delay in diagnosis and treatment and a high mortality. Conversely, the symptoms may be rather subtle and systemic manifestations mild.[387,429]

Pyogenic abscesses

Liver abscesses of pyogenic origin are far more common than those caused by amebas, although cases of the latter do occur in the southern United States and also in travelers to parts of the world where amebic dysentery is endemic. Pyogenic liver abscesses (Table 27-4) have been classified on the basis of the mode of entry, that is, (1) through ascension of the biliary tract (acute cholangitis), (2) by means of the hepatic artery (septicemia), (3) through the portal vein (pylephlebitis), (4) by direct extension (subphrenic abscess), (5) following trauma, and (6) from unknown sources. The pathologic changes vary from multiple microscopic lesions to single or multiple macroscopic abscesses.[436] The gross pattern of pyogenic abscess depends primarily on the source of infection and the accompanying pathologic changes in the liver and elsewhere.

Acute cholangitis. Multiple abscesses (Plate 4, *F*) most often follow acute cholangitis as the result of obstruction of the common duct. These abscesses are intimately associated with the biliary tree, often causing destruction of the walls of the dilated bile ducts.

Septicemias. Septicemias may produce multiple liver abscesses of variable size and abscesses of other organs in adults, infants, and children. In children they usually occur before the age of 5 years, particularly in patients with acute blastic leukemia.[402] In the neonate, liver abscesses may complicate umbilical infections or sepsis.[425] Chronic granulomatous disease (CGD) caused by an inherited defect in the bactericidal capacity of polymorphonuclear neutrophils may occur in both children and adults[428] and may result in hepatic abscesses.

Pylephlebitis. Pylephlebitis in the early part of the century was a well-known complication of acute appendicitis. This source of infection is now almost nonexistent in the United States but still occurs in some parts of the world. Pylephlebitis may complicate other types of intra-abdominal suppuration, such as diverticulitis. However, in recent decades suppurative pylephlebitis that extends from the source of the infection to involve the major portion of the extrahepatic portal system is rare indeed. In autopsy material, pylephlebitis that involves the hilar areas of the liver or portions of the intrahepatic portal branches still occurs, especially after attacks of acute cholangitis caused by obstructive biliary tract disease. Extensive involvement of the intrahepatic portal venous system is a common complication of recurrent pyogenic cholangitis, seen primarily in Asians.[452] Intrahepatic phylephlebitis may be present without liver abscesses; often, however, suppuration follows and microscopic or gross abscesses develop. Pylephlebitis with or without abscesses may occur in one lobe only. Thrombosis of intrahepatic branches of the portal vein may accompany carcinomas of the biliary tract or the head of the pancreas and produce multiple infarcts. If obstructive cholangitis is present, some of the infarcts may suppurate.

Suppurative abdominal disease. Suppurative abdominal disease with or without pylephlebitis may result in emboli or bacteria being carried to the liver by the portal vein, giving rise to liver abscesses. These most often occur in the right lobe when the suppurative disorder is drained by the superior mesenteric vein, whereas disease on the left side of the abdomen may cause suppuration in one or both lobes.[418]

Solitary abscesses. Solitary abscesses may complicate both penetrating and nonpenetrating injuries to the liver or arise from contiguous infections.[436] These abscesses are often anticipated and clinical diagnosis is easily made. A much more difficult problem is the patient with a solitary abscess or multiple large abscesses, in which case there is no recognizable source of infection. In the distant past, fever, chills, septicemia, and a large tender liver pointed the way toward the diagnosis of liver abscess. However, in recent years there appears to be milder reaction to pyogenic liver abscess.[427,444] Most abscesses are now seen in the elderly, are of bacterial origin, and can be diagnosed with liver scans.[436] The symptoms may be rather subtle and the systemic manifestations mild.[427] In many patients with solitary hepatic abscesses, no recognizable source can be found. Such abscesses have been reported in diabetic patients.[413]

Laboratory examination reveals a leukocytosis, elevated alkaline phosphatase level, hypoalbuminemia, and often a positive blood culture.[399] Chest roentgenograms may disclose basilar atelectasis or pneumonitis, an elevated right diaphragm, and a pleural effusion. A high degree of accuracy in diagnosis is achieved by the use of sonograms and scintiscans. Ultrasonography discloses a round to ovoid lesion with discrete, irregular, echo-poor margins. The walls are rather ragged. Liver scans are also used; however, lesions less than 2 cm in diameter are difficult to demonstrate.[416] In nonicteric patients with a solitary hepatic abscess, a filling defect is demonstrable on scintiscan far more often than in patients with multiple small hepatic abscesses. Some abscesses are characterized by gas formation, which is easily recognized on a plain film of the abdomen.[415] Computed tomography and angiograms are also useful in diagnosis.[407,412]

A wide variety of organisms have been cultured both from pyogenic abscesses and from the blood. Although *E. coli* seems to be the most common, many other organisms have been noted. Among these are streptococci, staphylococci, and *Klebsiella pneumoniae*.[437] Septicemia caused by melioidosis is another cause of liver abscesses.[430] Anaerobic cultures should always be performed on any aspirate. Although surgery is the generally accepted treatment for large abscesses, medical treatment has also proved successful.[421]

Amebic abscesses

Amebic abscesses of the liver are much less common than pyogenic abscesses but have many similar features. They are caused by the spread of *Entamoeba histolytica* from intestinal lesions by way of the portal vein. It is predominantly a disease of men, about 4:1, occurs before the age of 50 years, and is one of the serious diseases noted among travelers exposed to the organism. It is rare in persons who have not been outside the United States but does occur in some areas. Children are also susceptible to abscess formation.[429] A history of diarrhea weeks or months before onset of symptoms is obtained from approximately 50% of patients with hepatic amebic abscess. However, trophozoites are usually not demonstrable in the stools. Fever, leukocytosis, pain in the upper right quadrant, and a tender enlarged liver are common findings. In the diagnosis of amebic liver abscess the indirect hemagglutination test is highly sensitive, with a positive titer of at least 1:128 in 90% of patients. Effective demonstration of the organism in aspirated abscess contents is difficult but should be attempted on the last few drops of the aspirate.[429] Ultrasonography can also determine the size and number of the abscesses and is of great value in early diagnosis. Antiamebic therapy usually leads to rapid recovery. Scintiscans show that healing takes 2 to 4 months in most patients.[441]

The amebic abscesses recognized clinically may vary greatly in size but are usually solitary and often located in the superoposterior portion of the right lobe (Fig. 27-37). However, in autopsy series as many as 57% of the cases are reported to be multiple, attesting in part to a higher fatality rate in patients with multiple abscesses.[396] Left lobe abscesses have the highest incidence of rupture, especially into the pericardial and pleural cavities.[389] The contents of an abscess vary in appearance, probably depending on age and degree of parenchymal necrosis. Some observers have noted the contents to be more liquid early but becoming thick with age. This is not entirely in accord with our experience in autopsy material. The aspirate may vary in appearance from light tan to chocolate or "anchovy sauce." The lining of the abscess is usually gray-white and round, and small necrotic penetrations into the surrounding liver are seen. A striking "foam rubber" lining has been noted in much of our material. The abscess wall has an irregular lining composed of exudate and necrotic liver tissue. The contents usually stain deeply with hematoxylin, in contrast to pyo-

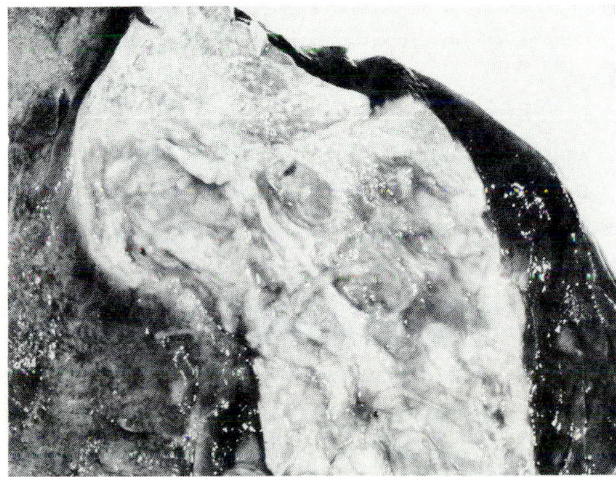

Fig. 27-37. Amebic liver abscess with rough, irregular lining of necrotic tissue.

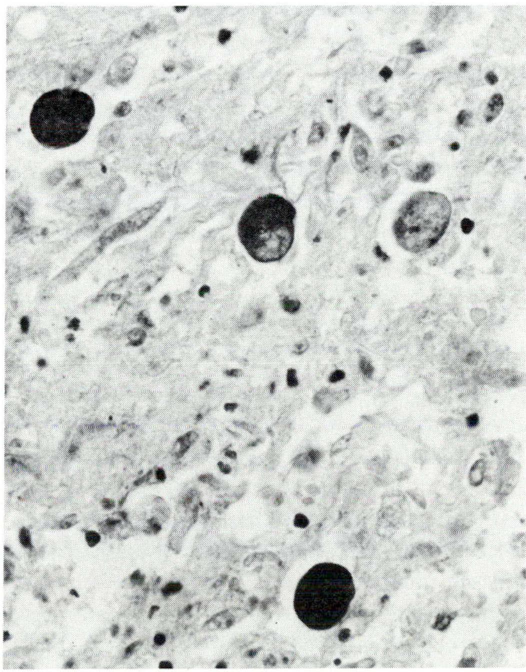

Fig. 27-38. Amebas in necrotic wall of liver abscess. (Periodic acid–Schiff stain.)

genic abscess. Amebas are most easily found in the marginal liver tissue, often in colonies with a clear zone about each ameba. A periodic acid–Schiff stain accentuates the contrast between ameba and body cells (Fig. 27-38). The amebic infection may involve the branches of the portal and hepatic veins, producing an amebic phlebitis and thrombosis, thus accentuating the necrotic process.

Actinomycotic abscesses of the liver usually have a pathogenesis similar to that of pyogenic pylephlebitic abscesses. Spread to the liver from intestinal lesions is by the portal venous channels. Multiple, small ragged abscess cavities are produced in which the actinomycotic colonies can be found.[424] A honeycomb type of calcification is sometimes seen on roentgenograms.

LIVER DISEASES IN INFANTS AND CHILDREN

The differential diagnosis of liver disease in a neonate, infant, or child includes a multitude of disorders. When age, symptoms, and etiology are considered, most of the disease entities may be discussed in a few broad categories, although there is a considerable overlap. One group is made up of neonates and those up to 3 months of age with jaundice. A second group includes older infants and children with acute or chronic liver disease. Finally, there is a small group of infants and children in whom the chief finding is hepatomegaly. In general the etiologic factors include infections, genetic or familial diseases, and congenital anatomic disorders, and there is a sizable group in which the cause is unknown.

Neonatal jaundice

Neonatal jaundice may arise from any one of many disturbances of bilirubin metabolism, varying from physiologic jaundice to fatal disease of the liver.[513,548] The various diseases are now included in one of two groups that consist of the indirect-acting (approximately unconjugated) and the direct-acting (approximately conjugated) hyperbilirubinemias. However, this separation does not become too evident until the fifth to seventh days of life when the liver has enough glucuronyl transferase to conjugate bilirubin.

Physiologic neonatal hyperbilirubinemia

Normally an acholuric indirect-acting type of hyperbilirubinemia is noted in most full-term infants on the second to fourth days of life, and in premature infants on the fifth or sixth days of life. A maximum level of approximately 6 mg/dl is present in the full-term neonate and 10 to 12 mg/dl in the premature neonate. Levels exceeding 12 mg/dl in the full-term neonate and 15 mg/dl in the premature neonate require further studies as to the cause of jaundice.[457] In the full-term baby the hyperbilirubinemia usually disappears by the seventh day and in the premature baby by the ninth or tenth day. Many factors may contribute to physiologic jaundice. One of these is an increased bilirubin load caused by the erythrocyte volume in the neonate and a shorter life span of the erythrocytes. Second is the decreased amount of glucuronyl transferase necessary for bilirubin conjugation. This is most noticeable in premature babies. A third factor is the lack of ligandins, the intracellular acceptors of bilirubin.[508] These proteins, also termed Y and Z, are the organic anion-binding proteins that facilitate the transfer of both bilirubin and sulfobromophthalein. A change in hepatic blood supply during transit from fetal to newborn life may also transiently impair hepatic function. It has been suggested that there is a correlation between elevated levels of alpha-fetoprotein and physiologic jaundice.[486]

In indirect-acting hyperbilirubinemia less than 15% of the total bilirubin is of the direct-reacting type. When the serum bilirubin rises above 20 mg/dl, irreversible damage to the central nervous system, called kernicterus, may be caused by unconjugated bilirubin entering nerve cells, particularly those in the basal ganglia. Despite extensive research, the exact mechanism of brain damage in kernicterus is still unknown.[501] Inasmuch as unconjugated bilirubin circulates bound to albumin, a low level of serum albumin or drug therapy that replaces the bilirubin bound to albumin will allow central nervous system damage at levels lower than 20 mg/dl. This is especially true in premature infants[509]; the presence of pulmonary hyaline membrane disease accentuates the risk. Ethnic differences in the frequency of neonatal jaundice have been observed.[495]

Because of the danger of kernicterus, severe hyperbilirubinemia often is treated by exchange transfusions with good results. The indications for exchange tranfusions include (1) bilirubin level approaching 20 mg/dl at any time during the first few days of life in a full-term infant without evidence of acidosis or respiratory distress; (2) bilirubin level of 10 to 15 mg/dl at any time in a premature infant with evidence of hypoxia, acidosis, or respiratory distress; (3) severe erythroblastosis fetalis and severe anemia (hemoglobin value of less than 10 g/dl), with or without evidence of fetal hydrops at birth; (4) clinical signs suggesting kernicterus at any time or at any bilirubin level; and (5) low unsaturated albumin binding level as determined by a reliable method, irrespective of serum bilirubin level at any age.[457] Phototherapy of the infant and phenobarbital treatment before delivery have also proved useful.[457,468]

Many disorders must be considered in the etiology of indirect-acting hyperbilirubinemia.[506] At one time the most important was hemolytic anemia of the newborn caused by an isoimmunization syndrome that occurred when Rh-positive infants produced anti-Rh factors in Rh-negative mothers. The disease condition occurs only after an earlier sensitization, either an earlier pregnancy or a transfusion of Rh-positive blood. In the past, this disease was known as erythroblastosis fetalis or icterus gravis neonatorum; it has been largely prevented by administering anti-Rh serum (anti-D) to Rh-negative mothers after they delivered their first Rh-positive infant and after the delivery of each subsequent Rh-positive infant.[559] Usually in erythroblastosis the liver is unable to secrete the large amount of unconjugated bilirubin that results from the hemolysis of erythrocytes, and jaundice appears in the first 24 hours. In fatal instances there is an even distribution of bile in canaliculi and also in the hepatic cells. Liver cell necrosis of variable degree may occur and could account for the increase in conjugated bilirubin that is sometimes seen in hemolytic disease of the newborn. However, additional factors may be involved.[490] Extramedullary erythropoiesis is common and may be extensive, not only in the liver but also in other organs. When hemolytic disease is caused by ABO incompatibility, the jaundice is usually mild, although kernicterus can occur if the serum bilirubin level rises excessively. ABO hemolytic disease is now the most common cause of neonatal jaundice, occurring almost exclusively in infants of group A or B having mothers of group O. The highest percentage of jaundiced babies are those who have a positive direct antiglobulin test. These infants also have the most severe jaundice.[476]

Maternal diabetes mellitus, newborn infection, glucose 6-phosphate dehydrogenase defect,[485] polycythemia, metabolic errors, conjugation defects, breast milk syndrome,[458,534] hypothyroidism, intestinal obstruction, and hematomas all are factors that may produce neonatal jaundice of the indirect-acting type.

In the children of diabetic mothers, the infants are usually large and hypotonic and have hypoglycemia. Infections that occur early, that is, during the first few days after birth or in the first 2 weeks of life, may be caused by any of many different organisms, although there has been a rise in the frequency of beta-hemolytic *Streptococcus* infections.[480,543] Rarely do the nonhemolytic indirect-acting hyperbilirubinemias require exchange transfusions.[519]

Direct-acting hyperbilirubinemia

Although any one of several diseases may cause an increase in direct-acting bilirubin,[467] such diseases may not become manifest until after the first week of life, for the liver is incapable of conjugating a large amount of bilirubin. Among the large number of diseases to be considered (Table 27-5),[459] three are most often responsible: biliary atresia, alpha-1-antitrypsin deficiency, and an idiopathic group collectively called neonatal hepatitis, although "hepatitis" may be a misnomer because evidence of infection is equivocal and inflammation is negligible. Other diseases, such as galactosemia, tyrosinemia, and fructosuria are far less common, although early diagnosis is imperative because of the irreversible

Table 27-5. Conjugated hyperbilirubinemia

Disease	Features	Diagnostic tests
Biliary atresia	40% to 50% of neonatal jaundice; surgically treated (Kasai procedure)	Diethyl IDA, biopsy of the liver
Neonatal "hepatitis"	Most familial cases progress; most nonfamilial heal	Biopsy of the liver
Choledochal cyst	2% of neonatal jaundice; surgically treated	Mass on ultrasound
Alpha-1-antitrypsin deficiency	Only in Pi ZZ (0.07% of population)	Alpha-1-antitrypsin level
Infections		
Sepsis	*E. coli;* beta-hemolytic streptococci groups A, B	Blood cultures
Syphilis	Rash, anemia	Cord blood/infant VDRL
Viral hepatitis A and B	Birth to 8 to 12 weeks; mother HBsAg positive	HBsAg, HAV-Ab
Toxoplasmosis	Progressive liver dysfunction	Sabin-Feldman dye test positive
Rubella	Congenital heart disease, hepatomegaly, occasionally jaundice (15%)	Fluorescent antibody test
Cytomegalovirus	Jaundice, hepatosplenomegaly, hemolytic anemia	Fetal viruria by culture, fluorescent antibody test for CMV-specific IgM antibody
Herpes simplex	Usually jaundice and hypoprothrombinemia; liver may not be palpable; skin vesicles	Viral culture
Metabolic diseases		
Galactosemia	Cataracts, ascites, cirrhosis	Clinistix/Galactostix
Fructosemia	Hypoglycemia, seizures	Enzyme assay, liver biopsy serum and urine levels
Tyrosinemia type 1	Aminoaciduria, aminoacidemia; autosomal recessive; liver cell carcinoma	Serum level of tyrosine
Parenteral nutrition	Cholestasis, fibrosis	Biopsy

changes that may occur in many organs if recognition and treatment are not prompt.

Biliary atresia

It is important to differentiate between neonatal hepatitis and biliary atresia because the latter is often amenable to surgical treatment. Hepatic portoenterostomy (the Kasai operation),[502] a surgical procedure whereby a limb of jejunum is anastomosed to the hilum of the liver at the site of amputated sclerotic duct, has been successful at least for a short term in many cases.[453,483] Long-term defects may still develop in many if not all of the successfully treated patients.

Many clinical, laboratory, and radiologic tests have been used to differentiate biliary atresia from other forms of intrahepatic cholestasis. Clinically in biliary atresia the earlier age at onset of acholic stools, a higher birth weight, and a large firm or hard liver are helpful clues in differentiating biliary atresia from neonatal "hepatitis" or alpha-1-antitrypsin deficiency.[453]

Among the abnormal laboratory test results, the presence of glutamyl transpeptidase (GGT) above the level of 780 IU/liter is a sensitive test for the differentiation of biliary atresia from neonatal hepatitis and cholestatic diseases.[493] Recently the use of *N*-substituted iminodiacetic acid (IDA) derivatives, especially diethyl IDA labeled with ^{99m}Tc, has proved helpful in the differential diagnosis of cholestatic disease.[530] In neonatal hepatitis after injection of diethyl IDA, the curve of hepatic-timed activities peaks early with a median of 1 minute and decays rapidly whereas in biliary atresia the curves peak in 10 minutes and decay more slowly.[493] Because irreversible cirrhosis may be present within 3 months, surgical exploration is very important before this age in infants with biliary atresia.[492]

Grossly biliary atresia may involve a short segment or nearly all of the extrahepatic duct system, including the gallbladder. The involved segments are reduced to cordlike structures. A Kasai operation is successful only when the right and left ducts are present and can be anastamosed to the bowel.

Both needle and excision biopsies are helpful in differentiating biliary atresia from neonatal hepatitis and other causes of intrahepatic cholestasis.[467] Portal fibrosis, ductular proliferation, and bile thrombi in the portal and periportal areas are the most constant findings in biliary atresia (Fig. 27-39). Giant cell transformation of a variable degree is common. Excision biopsies of the extrahepatic ducts at surgery may show (1) fibrosis with complete absence of any glands or ductal structures, (2) one or more clusters of lumina lined with cuboidal epithelium, seen peripherally, or (3) the presence of bile ducts at the center of concentrically arranged connective tissue.[453] Surgical treatment is more successful in the last group.[453] The Kasai operation, in which an anastomosis is made between the region of hepatic duct bifurcation and a loop of jejunum, relieves jaundice in some patients who have remained asymptomatic on follow-up studies.[453] Other studies of sequential biopsies indicate that fibrosis of the liver may continue and result in biliary cirrhosis with portal hypertension, even though bile flow is maintained.[455,487] Failure of establishment of a patent biliary tree produces severe perivenular cholestasis, bile duct proliferation, and periductal fibrosis that finally leads to biliary cirrhosis. At autopsy one third or more of the liver may be composed of fibrous tissue. However, there is considerable variation in severity not related to the duration of the obstruction. Children with unrelieved atresia who survive a few years may develop portal hypertension and die of bleeding esophageal varices.

Obstructive conditions other than extrahepatic biliary atresia, such as choledochal cysts and inspissated bile plugs,[482] may cause similar clinical findings. Hypoplasia of the extrahepatic bile ducts is a rare entity that has been diagnosed only with laparotomy and operative cholangiography.[511]

Neonatal "hepatitis" (NNH)

Neonatal hepatitis is a serious disorder of hepatocytes of unknown cause that may or may not be a true inflammatory disease. However, the term and its synonym, *giant cell hepatitis*, have been used for a long time in the pediatric literature.

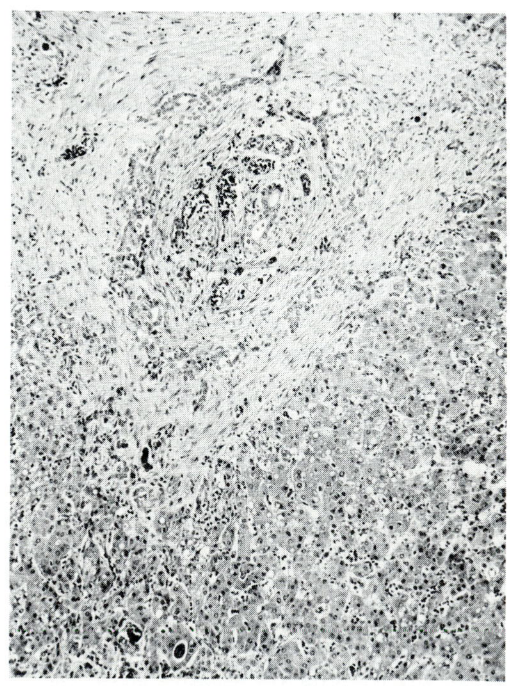

Fig. 27-39. Concentric bands of periportal connective tissue and bile stasis characteristic of biliary cirrhosis. Patient was 5-month-old infant with atresia of common bile duct.

NNH has about the same frequency as biliary atresia and much the same symptoms and laboratory findings. The disease is more prevalent in males with a birth weight less than those with biliary atresia.[453] If all known cholangitic factors and relationships are excluded, about 85% of the patients recover; the other 15% die of chronic liver disease. Of those developing chronic liver disease, 60% have family histories of similar hepatic illnesses.[524] Microscopically, NNH is characterized by transformation of hepatocytes to gigantic multinucleated syncytial cells (Fig. 27-40) that may have eight to 40 nuclei. The hepatocytes are usually hydropic and contain bile pigment. With progression of the disease, the giant multinucleated cells become more numerous, bile stasis is more prominent, and often there are intralobular tubules filled with bile. Rather characteristic is the diffuse formation of intralobular connective tissue that tends to sharply surround the circumscribed giant cells. Excess hepatic hematopoiesis is nearly always present. A majority of patients have an increased amount of iron in the liver cells and usually excess iron in the spleen.[531] There is ordinarily some increase in connective tissue in the periportal spaces, but the bile ducts are usually not as prominent as they are in biliary atresia.

Alpha-1-antitrypsin deficiency

Sixteen percent to 20% of jaundice in neonates previously included in the catchall term *neonatal hepatitis* is related in some way to aberrations in the genetically controlled protease inhibitor (Pi) system. The principal Pi of the body is produced by the liver and known as alpha-1-antitrypsin. There are 26 Pi types or alleles, with new ones added yearly. Each allele is given an alphabetic designation that relates to its relative rate of electrophoretic migration on acid starch gel. There is one additional allele, called null, that in the homozygous state is associated with complete absence of protease inhibitor. About 90% of the population is homozygous for type M. The allele of recognized pathologic importance is Pi, type Z, which occurs in heterozygous form in 3% to 4% of the population and is associated with low serum levels of the Pi. It is the homozygous state of Pi Z that is related to liver disease in neonates, juveniles, and, rarely, adults. Not all patients homozygous for Pi Z have liver disease; some estimates have placed the association as low as 10%.[460] Clinically alpha-1-antitrypsin liver disease may cause jaundice at about 1 month of age. At this stage the liver biopsy usually shows only cholestasis, liver cell swelling, and often diminutive portal tracts (Fig. 27-41). Usually eosinophilic droplets in periportal hepatocytes can be found. The droplets are alpha-1-antitrypsin and can be specifically identified by immunoperoxidase or immunofluorescence methods. Alpha-1-antitrypsin is a glycoprotein and thus is readily demonstrated by periodic acid–Schiff stain after diastase digestion. Occasionally the bile ducts are markedly hyperplastic, and in some patients, considerable portal fibrosis develops during the first few months of life.[488] In a few patients the disease progresses to cirrhosis within a year, but the

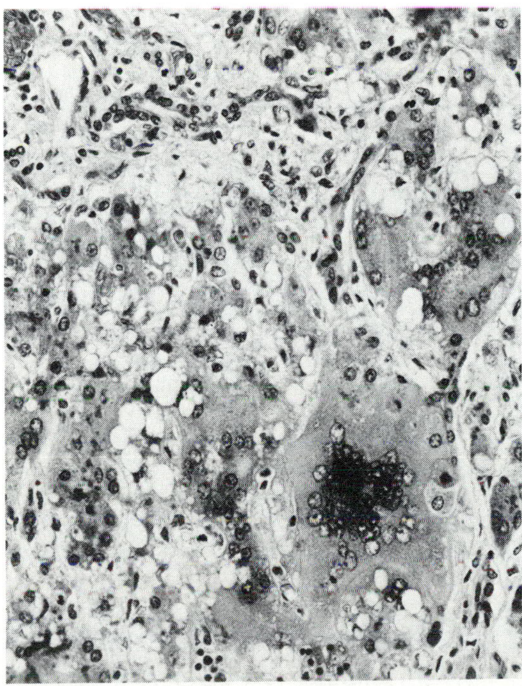

Fig. 27-40. Neonatal hepatitis (3-week-old male infant). Multinucleated giant cells compose most of parenchyma. Increased connective tissue can be seen along sinusoids and in periportal space. Intracanalicular bile stasis is at upper right and lower left.

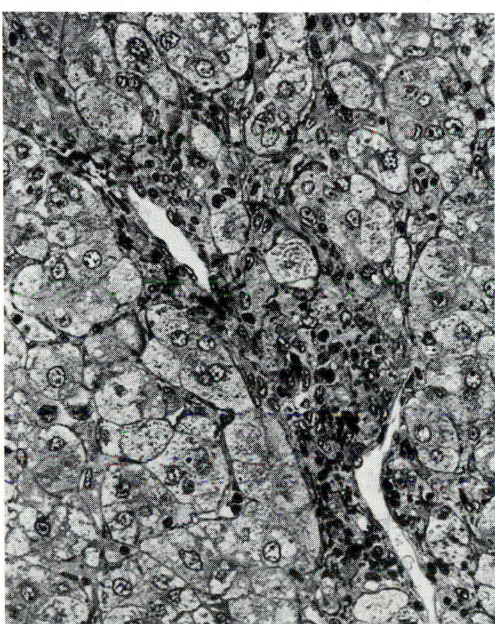

Fig. 27-41. Biliary dysgenesis associated with Pi ZZ. Note poorly defined portal area with deficient duct structures.

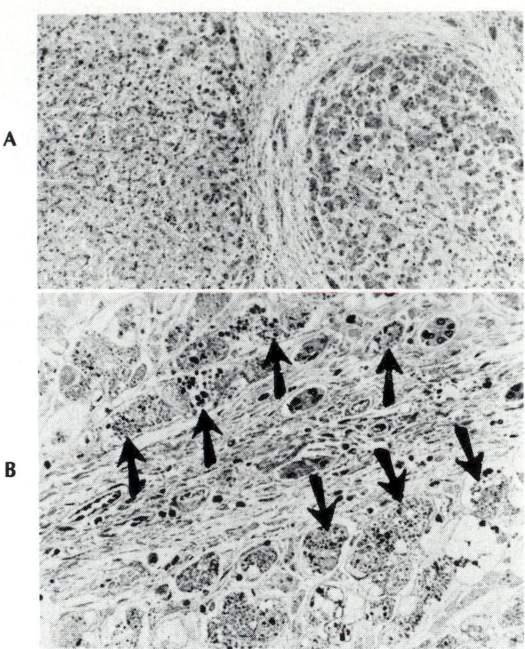

Fig. 27-42. Juvenile cirrhosis in alpha-1-antitrypsin deficiency (Pi ZZ). **A,** Lamellar fibrosis and duct deficiency. **B,** Marginal hepatocytes filled with glycoprotein droplets *(arrows)*.

majority of patients become asymptomatic before 6 months of age, only to develop signs of chronic liver disease, including varices and hepatic failure, during the late juvenile, adolescent, or young adult periods of life. The cirrhosis that develops is distinctly biliary in type. Parallel layers of collagen surround the cirrhotic nodules, interlobular bile ducts are absent (Fig. 27-42), and copper stains reveal copper binding protein and copper content that rivals the amount seen in Wilson's disease or primary biliary cirrhosis. The eosinophilic droplets of alpha-1-antitrypsin are in periportal hepatocytes and range in size from barely discernible to an occasional globule that fills the entire cytoplasm.

Ultimately, patients who develop cirrhosis die of hepatic failure or gastrointestinal bleeding from varices. Undoubtedly, in the past, many of the juvenile cirrhotic patients with Pi ZZ were considered to have Wilson's disease. Liver transplantation has been performed successfully in several patients.[494,529] Some patients who have Pi ZZ develop cirrhosis at ages 50 to 60 without having had an episode of neonatal jaundice,[551] and others are devoid of liver disease.

The importance of the heterozygous state in disease is unsettled. Many, probably most, patients with MZ do not develop liver disease, but there are numerous case reports of instances of cirrhosis with MZ phenotype and no other recognized basis for liver disease. There is disagreement about whether the coincidence of MZ and cirrhosis is greater than by chance. The number of reported cases of adult cirrhosis associated with heterozygosity of two abnormal Pi types, SZ, seems inordinately high.

Less common causes of jaundice

Among the less common causes of direct-acting hyperbilirubinemia in the first 3 months of life are infections, inborn errors of metabolism, and a number of other diseases.

In addition to bacterial infections that occur in the perinatal period,[544] gram-negative infections caused by *E. coli,* involving particularly the urinary tract, may cause jaundice.[561] The same is true in hepatic abscesses that complicate sepsis, vessel cannulation, or abdominal surgery.[519] Coxsackie viremia may cause extensive necrosis of the liver and jaundice.[504] Massive necrosis may also occur after echovirus infection.[496]

Another group of infections is now known as the TORCH group, that is, toxoplasmosis, rubella, cytomegalovirus, and herpes.[521] These diseases are discussed in detail in Chapters 7 and 10. Congenital toxoplasmosis in its generalized form may cause hepatomegaly and jaundice.[475] In fatal cases the microscopic findings in the liver are usually nonspecific. Severe extramedullary hematopoiesis is common, as in bile stasis. Small foci of necrosis may be present. The disease may be difficult to diagnose with laboratory tests.[544] Severe hepatitis with cholestasis and giant cell change has been observed in the rubella syndrome.[533] Coagulative necrosis also has been reported.[545] In cytomegalic inclusion disease bile stasis is prominent.[461,522,523] Multinucleated giant cells may be seen, but necrosis of liver cells is variable. When present, the giant intranuclear inclusions in the bile duct epithelium are diagnostic (Fig. 27-43). The hepatic lesions may persist into infancy. As a rule the inclusions are more easily found in the kidney. Cytomegalovirus hepatitis may produce jaundice in the adult.[557]

Herpes simplex infection in the neonate usually occurs on the fourth to seventh days of life and results in high mortality. The disease is acquired during passage through the genital tract in women who are infected. The liver and adrenal gland are most often involved. In the liver there are coagulative necrosis and nuclear inclusions without inflammation.[540,541] There are two types of nuclear inclusions. One is an amphophilic, glassy body that occupies most of the nucleus. The second is small, round, and surrounded by a halo. The first of these is the active infectious agent. Transplacental means of infection are rare.

Congenital syphilis still occurs, although in far lower incidence than 50 years ago. It may be manifested as hepatosplenomegaly and either a conjugated or an unconjugated hyperbilirubinemia. Fibrosis, cellular injury, and cholestasis are the usual microscopic findings.[558] The presence of the organism and increase in fibrous tissue have been shown by electron microscopy.[466] It has been noted that results of serologic tests on the neonate who has congenital syphilis of the liver may be negative, whereas results of tests on the mother are positive.[535]

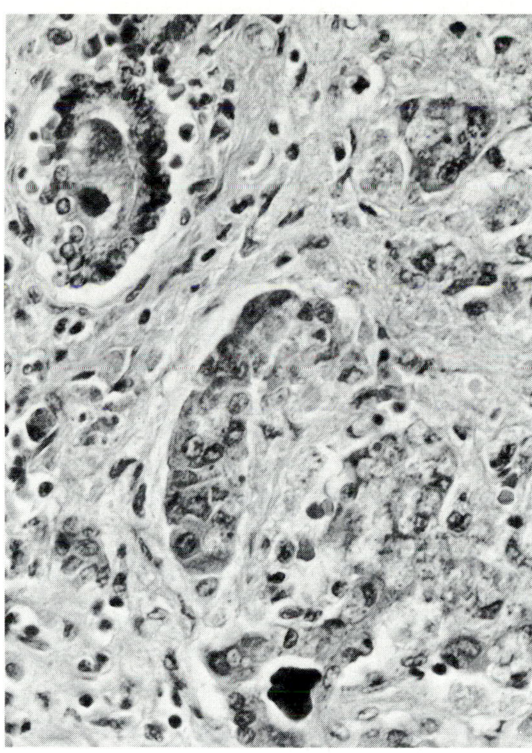

Fig. 27-43. Cytomegalic inclusion body in bile duct epithelial cell at upper left. Cholestasis and liver cell necrosis are evident. Patient had jaundice since birth and died at 2½ months of age.

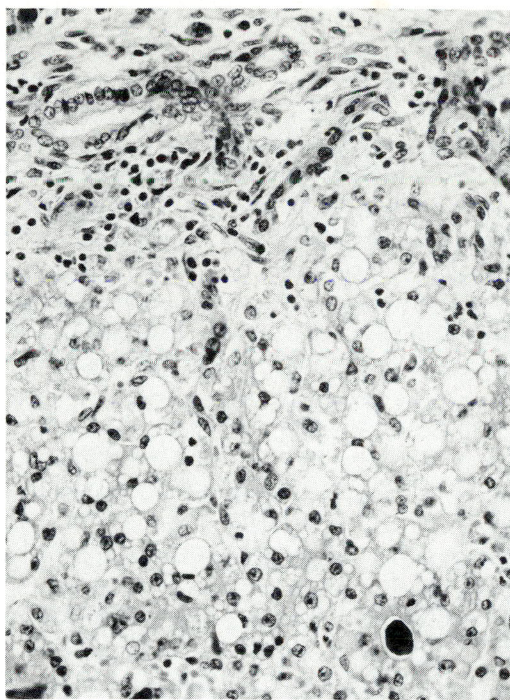

Fig. 27-44. Fatty change, intralobular bile stasis, and some increase of periportal connective tissue are characteristic of galactosemia. Patient was 3-week-old white male infant.

Acute viral hepatitis in the neonate as a cause of jaundice is uncommon, although there is a high incidence of transmission of the hepatitis B virus in the perinatal period. Usually the infant does not develop a clinical disorder.[536,537,550] However, there are examples of severe and even fatal cases of hepatitis in infants who have acquired the disease perinatally from infected mothers.[479]

Infants who do not acquire hepatitis from blood transfusions or an infected mother rarely develop hepatitis until they are in contact with many other children, as in nursery school. Hepatitis A acquired at this time results in a mild illness or is asymptomatic. Hepatitis B may follow contact with blood or blood products, saliva, or other infected blood fluids. Infants and children who acquire hepatitis B are more likely to develop chronic active hepatitis B than are adults.

Metabolic defects

Three inborn errors of metabolism cause severe liver disease when left untreated. The first symptom of each is often jaundice. These diseases are galactosemia, fructosemia, and tyrosinemia. All are autosomal recessive disorders in which an important metabolic enzyme is absent. In galactosemia, galactose-1-phosphate uridyltransferase is deficient. This enzyme in normal persons catalyzes formation of uridine diphosphate (UDP)-galactose and glucose-1-phosphate from galactose-1-phosphate and UDP-glucose. The deficiency causes galactose-1-phosphate to accumulate in the lens, liver, brain, and kidneys of infants who receive galactose in their diet. In addition to hepatic disease, the toxic effects of galactose accumulation are noted in the eye, where lenticular opacities may develop quickly, and in the brain, where degeneration and mental retardation may result.[549] The diagnosis of this condition is highly important because the removal of galactose from the diet relieves the symptoms.[473] Recognition of the disease may be delayed for a few months, depending on the symptoms. Various screening methods have been used for its detection.[510,514]

The liver in galactosemia is enlarged and fatty and may become cirrhotic. Microscopically the lobules are large; a moderate to severe degree of fatty change is present, and bile stasis is the rule. The bile plugs are contained within large acini. Often numerous bile ducts entering the periphery of the lobules are likewise filled with bile (Fig. 27-44). An irregular increase in connective tissue widens and lengthens the periportal spaces, sometimes connecting adjacent ones, so that cirrhosis can be diagnosed. The combination of large liver lobules, fatty changes, and bile stasis seems to be characteristic of galactosemia. More rarely in galactosemia, the liver contains an excess of glycogen, with the cytoplasm of the cells being almost water-clear; delicate septa connect the periportal spaces, resulting in a different type of cirrhosis. In both of the foregoing morphologic patterns the terminal hepatic veins are visible and regenerative change seems to be minimal. In children with proven cirrhosis and ascites, proper treatment results in an apparent cessation of the disease process.

In hereditary fructose intolerance, a deficiency of the enzyme fructose-1-phosphate aldolase, which is responsible for catalyzing the hydrolysis of fructose-1-phosphate into glyceraldehyde and dihydroxyacetone phosphate,[481,560] fructose-1-phosphate accumulates in the liver and other organs. The disease becomes manifest when the infant receives fruit or fruit juice. Vomiting, abdominal pain, excessive sweating, diarrhea, and even coma and convulsions may occur within 30 minutes after ingestion. Hypoglycemia, hypophosphatemia, hypermagnesemia, hyperuricemia, hyperfructosemia, and fructosuria are the most common laboratory findings. Aminoaciduria and other findings of the Fanconi syndrome may occur. All symptoms disappear on a fructose-free diet. Patients who continue to take fructose may develop fibrosis, fatty change, or even cirrhosis of the liver,[527] in addition to hyperbilirubinemia. Tyrosinemia type 1 is apparently caused by deficiency of the enzyme *p*-hydroxyphenylpyruvic acid oxidase, which converts *p*-hydroxyphenylpyruvic acid to homogentisic acid.[539] Symptoms may begin during the first month of life, with death resulting from liver failure within 6 to 8 months.[517] More often the course is chronic, with later onset of jaundice, ascites, hypoglycemia, hypoprothrombinemia, and finally, evidence of cirrhosis.[489,497] There are tyrosinemia, multiple renal tubular defects, and increased urinary excretion of phenolic acids.[484] On microscopic examination, regeneration, fatty change, and fibrosis are noted. Liver cell carcinoma may arise in the course of the disease.[555] The management of tyrosinemia type 1 is difficult. In addition to the restriction of tyrosine and phenylalanine, the restriction of methionine has now been added.[517]

With present-day laboratory methods tyrosinemia, galactosemia, and hereditary fructosemia can be differentiated from one another. Other enzyme defects do exist that affect the metabolism of galactose and tyrosine; however, these do not cause liver disease.

Several other diseases may produce jaundice in the first 3 months of life. Among these are hereditary cholestasis, parenteral nutrition–related cholestasis, and hereditary lymphedema.

A poorly understood but important anatomic disorder is known variously as hereditary cholestasis, Alagille's syndrome, intrahepatic atresia, and arteriohepatic dysplasia. Intrahepatic cholestasis, the retention of bile acids, impaired bile pigment excretion, elevated blood lipid levels, peripheral pulmonary stenosis, and vertebral anomalies have all been described.[454,459,491,553] The disease usually starts as a neonatal cholestasis but eventually becomes partial cholestasis with pruritus. The prognosis with respect to liver disease seems to be good, but death from cardiopulmonary disorder often occurs in early adult life. Clinical diagnosis is aided by the characteristic facies; the eyes are deeply set, the forehead is broad, and the chin is pointed.

Parenteral nutrition (PN) in sick infants is often associated with development of severe cholestasis, especially in premature babies. Jaundice is noted, usually within 3 weeks after PN is initiated. Biopsy material discloses severe cholestasis accompanied by inflammation along the portal tracts, consisting of round cells, neutrophils, portal fibrosis, and bile duct proliferation. After cessation of PN the jaundice clears, but biopsies months later often disclose some residual fibrosis and cholestasis.[474] In infants who received total parenteral nutrition (TPN) for more than 300 days, severe hepatic fibrosis and fatal liver failure have been reported.[528] The effect of prolonged fasting as an etiologic factor in the production of hepatobiliary dysfunction has been suggested.[462]

An unusual disease of the liver that produces hyperbilirubinemia in the first weeks of life is hereditary lymphedema. These cases have been particularly noted in Norway.[538]

Liver diseases of postneonatal infancy

The frequency of liver disease with onset in infants past 3 months of age, in children, and in juveniles is less than in the younger age group, although some of the diseases that start in the early months may continue as chronic liver disease and eventually develop into cirrhosis. These include the more common diseases already described. There are a number of acute or chronic diseases that begin or become manifest in the older pediatric group. Among these are certain metabolic disorders, anatomic abnormalities, intrahepatic cholestasis of childhood (familial cholestasis), and a miscellaneous group.

Among the metabolic disorders, many of which are familial, are those caused by excess glycogen storage, Niemann-Pick and Gaucher's diseases, Wilson's disease, hemochromatosis, and gangliosidosis. Glycogenosis has been defined as any condition in which the glycogen concentration of a tissue is increased.[516] Normally the glycogen concentration in the liver should not exceed 6% of the net weight. Glycogen-storage disease of the liver is now divided into types I to X, each with its specific enzyme defect. Hepatic fibrous septa only have been observed in types III, VI, IX, and X, whereas type IV may progress to cirrhosis that is fatal, usually in childhood. In type IV, intracellular hyaline deposits may be present in the periportal areas and are difficult to distinguish from alpha-1-antitrypsin deficiency.[516] In type I the liver is enlarged and fatty, but chronic changes do not occur. A similar change is noted in type III. Clinical, laboratory, and morphologic studies are helpful, but the final diagnosis rests on quantitative biochemical analysis of the tissue.[516] The absence of glycogen synthase leads to inadequate glycogen formation and severe fatty change in the liver.[472]

In Niemann-Pick disease there is an accumulation of sphingomyelin and other lipids in the body that particularly affects the liver and spleen and is accompanied by severe mental retardation. Five clinical categories have been recognized and are designated types A to E. Jaundice and severe liver changes, in both the hepatic reticuloendothelial system and the hepatocytes, have been noted.[465] A perivenular distribution of Kupffer cell storage has also been described.[477]

Gaucher's disease is an inherited disorder in which there is a deficiency of the lysosomal enzyme, glucocerebrosidase.[489] Gaucher's cells are commonly present in the liver, but symptoms of liver disease are rare, although fibrosis associated with Gaucher's cells may lead to scarring and eventually to a nodular liver. Liver changes may be observed in some of the mucopolysaccharidoses.[489] In the Hurler-Hunter syndrome, fibrosis and cirrhosis may occur, usually in older children and adults. In Hurler's syndrome (gargoylism) there is an excess of dermatan sulfate and heparan sulfate in the urine and tissues, along with a decrease of alpha-galactosidase in the tissues. GM_1 gangliosidosis is a genetically determined deficiency of alpha-galactosidase. Light and electron microscopy disclose many vacuoles in the hepatocytes and Kupffer cells. These have a characteristic ultrastructural appearance.[526] Wilson's disease and hemochromatosis are also inheritable disorders that may become manifest in childhood. These are discussed elsewhere in this chapter.

Two anatomic abnormalities, cystic fibrosis and congenital hepatic fibrosis, may become symptomatic or cause liver disease in infants and children. In cystic fibrosis the liver may contain focal areas of fibrosis associated with dilated bile ducts containing eosinophilic casts. Prolonged jaundice with cholestasis may be observed in neonates.[552] In more advanced states of liver disease a true cirrhosis may develop with formation of nodules of variable size. Portal venous hypertension may result.

Congenital hepatic fibrosis is a variant of polycystic disease[499]; microcysts are present in the dense fibrous tissue that surrounds the lobules. These are sometimes associated with tubular ectasia or polycystic disease of the kidney. The disease was first recognized in children[503] but may not become symptomatic until adulthood.[520] Although results of liver function tests are normal, portal hypertension is the predominating symptom. Portacaval shunts are usually successful, and hepatic encephalopathy does not develop.[456] Cholangitis may be a complication. The disease is characterized by an excessive amount of dense connective tissue that connects one portal tract with another and includes supernumerary small bile ducts.[479,548]

The term *juvenile cirrhosis* is sometimes used for patients in this particular age group. With careful study, most of these cases can be put in one of the various etiologic types of cirrhosis already described, particularly alpha-1-antitrypsin deficiency, Wilson's disease, or chronic active hepatitis of unknown etiology.

In addition to the intrahepatic cholestatic diseases, such as galactosemia and alpha-1-antitrypsin deficiency, there is a group of patients in whom the cause of liver disease is unknown. These include a broad spectrum of diseases that vary from benign recurrent jaundice to fatal familial cholestasis or Byler's disease. Fatal intrahepatic cholestasis may be familial or may occur sporadically. The familial form, known as Byler's disease, is named for the Byler family, whose seven children had the disease.[470] Usually the disease begins in the first few months of life and is characterized by jaundice, pruritus, and failure to thrive. The disease progresses rapidly or slowly over a period of months or years; ultimately, most of the patients die of a biliary type of cirrhosis. Biopsies performed early in the disease disclose intense cholestasis. Bile acid studies show high serum levels and a very low content in the duodenum, but these are also noted in other forms of cholestasis. In the sporadic form a number of unusual features have been observed. Kayser-Fleischer–like rings may develop in the eyes.[498] Studies of copper metabolism show high plasma copper concentration and increased urinary copper excretion, in contrast to the finding in patients with Wilson's disease. The early age of onset, the predominantly cholestatic clinical picture, and familial history all aid in diagnosis.[478]

A severe familial cholestasis has been noted in a group of North American Indian children, 90% of whom developed cirrhosis. Neonatal hepatitis was documented in the majority of the cases. Electron microscopic studies disclosed evidence of microfilament dysfunction of the hepatocytes.[554] In yet another group of patients, familial or sporadic cirrhosis may occur that is not characterized by jaundice. No specific etiologic agent has been identified.[505] The prognosis in some of these patients is yet to be determined; however, biopsy findings have disclosed advanced cirrhosis of the postnecrotic type. In other familial types of cirrhosis, Kayser-Fleischer rings have been noted.[500]

Miscellaneous diseases

In India a disease known as Indian childhood cirrhosis (ICC) may be seen in patients from 6 months to 14 years of age. Five different histologic types have been recognized. The largest number of patients were in group II, which is predominantly a degenerative disease characterized by ballooning of liver cells, hyaline necrosis, neutrophilic exudate, and giant cell transformation. Fibrosis and loss of lobular architecture are also present. It seems that only children in India are affected by the group II type of change. The other four types are not distinctive. In the limited material available for our study, we have had difficulty in distinguishing the changes in group II from sclerosing hyaline necrosis seen in alcoholic patients.

In the cerebrohepatorenal syndrome (Zellweger's syndrome) there are both a metabolic disorder and congenital anomalies. Jaundice with conjugated hyperbilirubinemia is often present in the first 2 weeks of life and is followed by progressive liver disease. Diffuse fibrosis of the lobules is characteristic of the early disease. With electron microscopy, mitochondrial defects have been noted that may be related to abnormal metabolism of the bile acids. Failure to oxidize the cholesterol side chain to form C-24 bile acids apparently leads to increased amounts of trihydroxycoprostanic acid, varanic acid, and dihydroxycoprostanic acid.[515]

In Reye's syndrome there is acute encephalopathy with fatty degeneration of the viscera, chiefly the liver.[532] The disease begins as an acute illness in a previously healthy infant or child and is characterized by vomiting that is usually followed within 24 hours by lethargy, stupor, convulsions, and coma. Death or recovery occurs within a few days. A wide range of laboratory findings may be present. Among these are hypoglycemia, hyperammonemia, hypertransaminasemia, and a prolonged prothrombin time. Liver biopsies performed within 48 hours usually disclose a fine foamy type of fatty change without nuclear displacement that is best seen in frozen sections stained for lipids. The hepatic lesion has been subdivided into three types, depending on the degree of glycogen deficiency: mild, type 1; moderate, type 2; and total, type 3.[464] The degree of depletion seems to correlate well with the occurrence of hypoglycemia, the severity of encephalopathy, and the mortality. The depletion of activity of several mitochondrial enzymes during the period of rapid lipid accumulation and low hepatic (manganese) content, coupled with the rarefied mitochondrial matrix and enlarged ameboid mitochondria seen on electron microscopy, suggest that a relationship exists between transient mitochondrial dysfunction and the fatty change, glycogen depletion, hypoglycemia, and hyperammonemia.[464,518] Reye's syndrome has now been associated with some 16 groups of viruses, particularly influenza A and B,[512] and a number of other possible etiologic agents.[463,469,542,546] The possibility that aspirin is involved in the etiology of Reye's syndrome is a recent proposal.[471] The patients are not jaundiced. At autopsy the liver is usually yellow and there is cerebral edema.

Lastly, consideration must be given to a physical finding, hepatomegaly, and to a serious physiologic disorder, hypoglycemia. In the pediatric group symptomless hepatomegaly may be noted at any age. Often this solitary finding is caused by a neoplasm or cyst.

Hypoglycemia in the neonate, as well as in infants and children, deserves special consideration because its recognition and treatment may be lifesaving.[472] Among the causes of hypoglycemia in the neonate are the hepatic enzyme deficiencies[525] such as glycogen-storage disease, fructose intolerance, galactosemia, glycogen synthase deficiency, and fructose 16-diphosphatase deficiency. Tyrosinemia and erythroblastosis may also be associated with hypoglycemia. In many of these diseases, jaundice is present. Neonatal cholestasis and hypoglycemia associated with endocrine disorders are possibly caused by cortisol deficiency.[507] Hypoglycemia must be defined relative to infant age. The following levels are considered to be hypoglycemic: (1) whole blood glucose concentrations less than 20 mg/dl (25 mg/dl serum or plasma) in the preterm, low–birth weight infant; (2) whole blood glucose values less than 30 mg/dl (35 mg/dl serum) from birth to 72 hours of age; and (3) whole blood levels less than 40 mg/dl (46 mg/dl serum) in the full-sized or full-term infant after 72 hours of age.[472] Prompt diagnosis and treatment are all important.

Hypoglycemia in infancy is comparatively rare but is caused by the same enzyme deficiencies just noted, and in addition, acquired liver diseases, such as hepatitis, cirrhosis, malnutrition with fatty liver,[556] and Reye's syndrome, must be considered.

LESS COMMON LIVER DISEASES

Wilson's disease (hepatolenticular degeneration)

Wilson's disease is a hereditary liver disease transmitted as an autosomal recessive trait. Cirrhosis and neurologic defects first become apparent between late juvenile and young adult ages. In 7.5% of the cases the disease does not become apparent until the third decade, and rare cases have been reported that are not symptomatic until the fourth decade.[643] It is a disease associated with abnormalities in copper metabolism.

The homeostatic role of the liver in copper metabolism has been well established. Both a deficiency and an excess of this element may result in clinical disease. As in the case of iron, the liver is the chief storage organ. In the normal neonate the copper concentration is six to eight times the level in the adult.[567] Within the first 6 months of life the hepatic copper level decreases to that seen in a normal adult, which is about 30 μg of copper per gram of dry tissue. Copper balance is achieved by an X-linked intestinal transport mechanism plus the regulation of copper stores by the liver. About 50% of the average daily intake, 2 to 5 mg, is absorbed into the blood and is loosely bound to albumin; this constitutes about 5% to 10% of the total copper circulating in the plasma. The absorbed copper is quickly cleared by the hepatocytes, in which two thiol-rich cytosol protein fractions are capable of storing the metal. One of these proteins has a higher molecular weight, 30,000 to 40,000 daltons, and has been termed superoxide dismutase. The lower–

molecular weight proteins of about 10,000 daltons probably consist of both metallothionein and nonmetallothionein. These two protein fractions contain about 80% of the copper in the normal adult liver.[639] The remainder is incorporated into cytochrome *c* oxidase and ceruloplasmin or is present in lysosomes before being excreted in bile. The latter is the principal means of achieving copper balance, since about 1.5 mg of copper is excreted each day in the bile, bound to a carrier that prevents its reabsorption from the gut. A small portion of hepatic copper, approximately 0.5 to 1 mg daily, is incorporated into ceruloplasmin, a blue copper glycoprotein, and released into the blood.[639] Radioactive studies have shown that this incorporation occurs in the first few hours after absorption. The turnover rate of this copper in ceruloplasmin is high.

In Wilson's disease the patient is in positive copper balance, and excess quantities of copper are stored, first in the liver and eventually in other tissues, especially the brain, cornea, and kidney. The disease occurs in homozygotes who have inherited a pair of autosomal recessive genes, one from each parent. It is estimated that the frequency in heterozygotes is 1 in 200 and in homozygotes, 5 in 1 million,[639] although in one family the frequency was unusually high.[614] In the homozygote several abnormal physiologic phenomena occur, the exact mechanism of which is unclear. Foremost is the failure of the liver to excrete copper in the bile. Other changes measurable in the laboratory consist of an increased storage of copper in the dry liver tissue, about 50 μg/g; serum ceruloplasmin less than 20 μg/dl; and increased urinary copper greater than 50 μg/day. A prominent finding is the presence of Kayser-Fleischer rings. These are areas of brown pigmentation of Descemet's membrane at the limbus of the cornea (Plate 5, *C*). Once considered pathognomonic of Wilson's disease, it is now known that Kayser-Fleischer rings may be found on rare occasions in chronic cholestatic disorders, characterized by an excessive copper storage such as primary biliary cirrhosis.[589]

The excess copper in the liver and later in the central nervous system, eyes, kidneys, and other organs leads to symptoms after 6 years of age; 50% of homozygotes have symptoms by 15 years of age.[639] These symptoms cover an extraordinarily wide range, most important being those caused by liver and basal ganglia involvement (Chapter 44). The liver disease may be manifested by symptoms of either acute or chronic liver disease and can be confused with acute viral hepatitis or chronic active hepatitis.[582,633] Occasionally cirrhosis may be diagnosed in an asymptomatic patient. Acute hemolytic anemia may occur during periods of acute accumulation of copper[581] and is an ominous sign. Various stages have been described in the progress of liver disease; however, the sequence probably varies from patient to patient. The earliest microscopic findings consist of fatty change, vacuolization of nuclei, and focal necrosis. In this stage the copper is present in the cytoplasm. In the next stage patients may have histologic changes indicative of chronic active hepatitis with peripheral necrosis. In these there may be stainable copper and atypical lipofuscin in the hepatocytes. Finally, cirrhosis of a nonspecific type, with either large nodules or both large and small nodules, is present, especially in patients dying of liver disease. In this latter stage, Mallory bodies may occur (Fig. 27-45). In the cirrhotic liver there may be sharp differences in the appearance of the hepatocytes from one pseudolobule to another or within the same lobule. This is noted particularly in regard to fatty change and the amount of lipochrome pigmentation. The septa in the cirrhosis of Wilson's disease vary greatly in thickness. Some are rather thin, whereas others are much thicker. These changes often give a nonuniform appearance to the cirrhosis of Wilson's disease. A copper stain is positive in about 90% of the cirrhotic livers, although in the early stage the regenerative nodules may not stain positive for copper. Electron microscopic studies have shown that early in the course of the disease the increase in hepatocytic copper is present in the cytoplasm,[595] where the copper ion is capable of causing episodes of necrosis. These may produce attacks of jaundice and a rise in the serum transaminase levels. Once cirrhosis has occurred, the copper is stored in lysosomes. Occasionally Wilson's disease may manifest biochemical and histologic characteristics that closely simulate those of active hepatitis. The diagnosis is even more difficult if Kayser-Fleischer

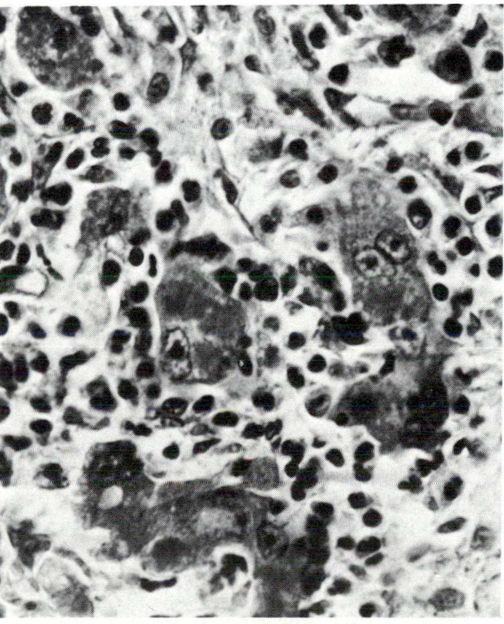

Fig. 27-45. Hyaline necrosis of hepatocytes in Wilson's disease. Abundant neutrophilic and round cell infiltrate in sinusoids.

rings are absent.[633] Prognosis of this pattern in Wilson's disease is frequently poor because it does not respond to D-penicillamine therapy. The use of radioactive copper may be helpful in differentiating the patient with Wilson's disease but who has low-normal ceruloplasmin levels and the histologic features of chronic active hepatitis from the non-Wilsonian patient with chronic active hepatitis. It is also useful in distinguishing the homozygote with low-normal ceruloplasmin from the heterozygote. In Wilson's disease there is no positive slope for the labeled copper within 4 to 48 hours after oral administration.[640] These distinctions are of major importance because the homozygotes should be treated with D-penicillamine for the remainder of their life.

Increased storage of hepatic copper also occurs in patients with chronic cholestasis, such as primary biliary cirrhosis,[617] extrahepatic biliary obstruction,[579] intrahepatic cholestasis of childhood (IHCC),[588] cirrhosis of alpha-1-antitrypsin, and biliary atresia.[637] In IHCC the hepatic copper levels are equal to those in Wilson's disease. The serum copper level is abnormally elevated, whereas the urinary copper level is normal or very slightly elevated. An increase of hepatic copper may also occur in patients who do not have chronic cholestasis: excess copper has been noted in 30% of patients with alcoholic liver disease.[566] Excess copper has also been reported in livers of patients with chronic active hepatitis[637] and Indian childhood cirrhosis.[619,645] The Bedlington terrier has a copper storage disease that closely simulates Wilson's disease in the humans.[610]

Iron metabolism and liver disease

The liver is a major participant in the metabolism of iron because it stores the metal and also synthesizes transferrin, an iron-binding protein necessary for the transport of iron. Transferrin is responsible for the movement of iron from its absorption in the small bowel to storage in the liver and other tissues and to the most active metabolic area—in the bone marrow. An easily mobilized form of iron is stored as ferritin in the hepatocyte. Ferritin is a large protein molecule composed of 24 subunits that form a shell capable of storing some 4000 atoms of iron. Some 20 or so isoferritins have been identified; these vary from one tissue to another. Subunit analyses indicate that these isoferritins are derived from two or perhaps three subunit types.[584] The origin of serum ferritin is unknown. It does not bind as much iron as does tissue ferritin. In excess iron storage, ferritin apparently is degraded to hemosiderin and stored in lysosomes, known as siderosomes. Hemosiderin is rich in iron and poor in protein. The iron in hemosiderin is difficult to mobilize for transfer to bone marrow. Details of iron metabolism and storage are given in Chapter 3. Normally the body contains 4 to 5 g of iron, most of which is present in hemoglobin. Storage iron, present mostly in the liver, spleen, and bone marrow, has been estimated at some 800 mg in adult men and 300 mg in women in the reproductive age.[621]

Idiopathic hemochromatosis

Iron overload may occur by any one of several mechanisms: (1) inappropriate mucosal absorption of iron; (2) absorption related to chronic anemia, decreased gut iron binding, or increased dietary intake; and (3) parenteral administration of iron, in the form of either blood transfusions or therapeutic injections. In the first category there is an appropriate increase in iron absorption with parenchymal deposition of iron, eventual tissue damage, and functional insufficiency of the organs involved, especially the liver, pancreas, and heart.[621] This disease, known as idiopathic hemochromatosis (IHC), is an inheritable disorder. Iron overload caused by parenteral administration or blood transfusions is deposited in the reticuloendothelial system and is known as hemosiderosis. However, in the latter, parenchymal cell deposition may eventually occur, and a secondary type of hemochromatosis is seen. It is still not clear whether the parenchymal iron deposition follows the parenteral administration of blood or results from the increased iron absorption from the gut, stimulated by the chronic anemia that was the purpose of the transfusion therapy. Excessive dietary intake, as seen in the Bantu of South Africa, usually leads to reticuloendothelial system overload but can also cause hemochromatosis and cirrhosis.

Idiopathic hemochromatosis has been the subject of intense research in recent years. Family studies on the genetic abnormality have shown that IHC is inherited as an autosomal recessive trait. The abnormal homozygote with clinical manifestations of the disease carries two hemochromatosis alleles on chromosome 6 close to the HLA locus. The pattern of transmission of the predisposing alleles in a family has been traced by typing for the A and B alleles of the HLA complex.[565,570,648] In addition to the homozygotes with full expression of the disease, heterozygotes and normal persons have been identified in the pedigree studies.

In the homozygote with IHC there is an increase in iron absorption from early in life that is steady until about 60, at which time approximately 18 g of iron may be present in the liver of men but less in women because of menstrual loss. The mechanism for the unusual absorption is unknown. There is also an increase in hepatic uptake of iron, even when the serum iron is normal in patients with treated hemochromatosis. This occurs whether or not cirrhosis is present.[563] Actually, free iron may be absorbed into the portal vein blood and removed by the liver. The serum ferritin is increased in hemochromatosis, its levels increasing with the increase in iron stores. In normal persons and those with a modest iron overload, each microgram of serum ferritin per liter is equivalent to 8 mg of iron in storage.

The symptomatic homozygous state is usually diagnosed around 50 years of age. The laboratory findings most helpful in diagnosis[570] include an increased serum iron, usually 200 μg/dl (normal is 100 μg/dl); transferrin saturation above 80% (normal is less than 50%, average about 30%); and serum ferritin mean 2099 ng/ml in men and 301 ng/ml in women (normal is 93 in men and 48 in women). The hepatic iron in men with hemochromatosis averages 877 μg/100 mg wet liver and 478 in women; in normal persons iron levels are less than 29 in men, 20 in women. A major iron load is defined as a transferrin saturation above 79% and hepatic iron concentration above 400 μg/100 mg of wet liver in men and above 250 μg/100 mg in women. A minor iron load is defined as a transferrin saturation greater than 50% or a hepatic iron concentration of 30 to 400 μg/100 mg wet liver in men and of 20 to 250 μg/100 mg in women.

Early in IHC, there may be little dysfunction of the organs with a heavy iron overload. Recognizing this stage of disease in patients is important because phlebotomy may arrest the course of the disease. In untreated patients the liver becomes cirrhotic, and pancreatic deposition may result in diabetes. Other tissues that frequently have striking iron deposits and associated dysfunction include myocardial fibers, gastric mucosa, endocrine epithelium, and the testes. The classic clinical triad (seen after years of iron accumulation) is hepatomegaly, diabetes, and skin pigmentation. However, the mode of presentation varies greatly. The patient may complain of impotence, easy fatigability, or arthopathy and may have signs of heart failure. The arthropathy involves the second and third metacarpophalangeal joints of each hand.[626,631] Signs or symptoms of hepatic failure or portal hypertension are not the usual initial features. In spite of the known diagnostic aids, a delay of several years often occurs before a correct diagnosis of IHC is made.[585] In one series of patients, the mean age at diagnosis of homozygous men was 52 years; for the homozygous woman the mean age was 44.8 years. In heterozygotes there are no clinical manifestations of iron overload, but biochemical abnormalities may occur. The mean transferrin percentage saturation may reach 51% in men but much less in women.[570] Iron loading in the liver in the heterozygous men may increase sevenfold or eightfold over the normal. Some of these patients, although asymptomatic, have been subjected to phlebotomy until the iron reserves were depleted.

Early in IHC, hemosiderin is present microscopically in all the hepatocytes, but there is some predilection for the periportal areas. The intracytoplasmic iron is usually most prominent around the canaliculi. Kupffer cell iron is insignificant, and fibrosis is absent. With advancement of disease, a variable degree of fibrosis occurs along the portal tracts and within the lobules, leading to well-defined cirrhosis (Fig. 27-46).

Although there is usually some correlation between the amount of iron present and the severity of cirrhosis, occasionally some livers with advanced cirrhosis have less stainable iron than those with poorly developed septa. As the iron increases, the aggregates become larger and cellular detail may be obscured. Masses of hemosiderin are also seen within Kupffer cells, although this does not usually parallel the amount of hemosiderin within the hepatic cells. Focal areas of necrosis may occur, and after healing, such areas are marked by closely packed macrophages whose cytoplasm contains dense accumulations of hemosiderin. After necrosis, regenerative nodules develop that have little or no stainable iron within their cells. Fibrous septa connecting the portal spaces are similar to those in alcoholic cirrhosis except for iron-filled macrophages and, occasionally, iron-encrusted connective tissue fibers. An iron-free pigment, hemofuscin, may accumulate within both the fibrous tracts and the hepatic cells. Fatty change is seen in a small proportion of patients but is most prevalent in those who have diabetes mellitus. The latter, when present, is usually mild. The presence of increased iron in sweat glands or melanin in the skin may give the patient a blue-gray or bronzed appearance, hence the name *bronze diabetes* for this complication of hemochromatosis. In many patients with pigmentary cirrhosis there is a long course (10 years or more) that exceeds the duration of most other types of cirrhosis. Portal hypertension and ascites are not common complications, but

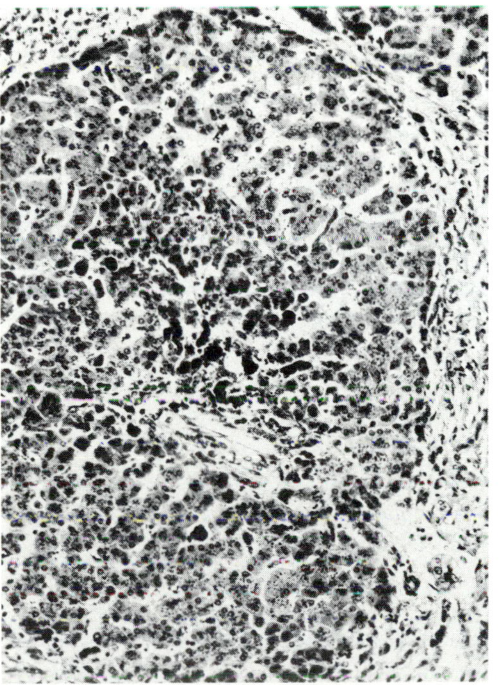

Fig. 27-46. Idiopathic hemochromatosis with pigmentary cirrhosis in 54-year-old white man who died of hepatocellular carcinoma of liver. Liver cells and Kupffer cells contain fine granules of hemosiderin. In area of recent necrosis near center, histiocytes are filled with hemosiderin.

primary carcinoma of the liver occurs more often than in most types of cirrhosis, to 25% of patients in some series.[622]

The question of whether iron produces fibrous scarring is unanswered. There is clinical evidence suggesting that iron is involved in the pathogenesis of hemochromatosis.[620] In our experience there does not seem to be an association between the density of iron deposition and the degree of fibrosis in both liver and pancreas. The Bantu who stores large amounts of iron absorbed from his diet, however, develops a meager degree of fibrosis. Iron-loading experiments have usually failed to produce significant fibrosis, with notable exceptions.[608]

The mechanism by which iron may damage the liver and pancreas, producing necrosis and fibrosis, is not known. Studies with the electron microscope show that iron is deposited within the lysosomes of the liver cell and, to lesser extent, in some of the mitochondria. The latter may then degenerate. It is likely that a point is reached at which some of the liver cells populating the lobules are unable to survive with so much of their cytoplasm occupied by iron.[646]

The presence of fibrosis preceding any evidence of cellular injury indicates that, by some mechanism, iron stimulates the synthesis of collagen.[599]

Few electron microscopic studies have been performed on liver biopsy material in idiopathic hemochromatosis.[600,627] In patients with thalassemia major, electron microscopic studies have shown that ferritin molecules are present in the cell sap and lysosomes.[599]

Secondary hemochromatosis and siderosis

Hepatic iron stores may become greatly increased in certain other disorders. Quantitative analysis generally reveals that this deposition is much less in secondary hemochromatosis; liver iron usually is calculated to be less than 2 g/100 g dry weight of liver when the iron loading is the result of another disorder. Iron overload alone, without cirrhosis of the liver dysfunction, is usually called hemosiderosis of the liver. In addition to idiopathic hemochromatosis, excess iron is found in the following:

1. Any chronically anemic patient, except one having iron deficiency
2. Patients with multiple transfusions, especially more than 100 units (such patients are usually chronically anemic)
3. A small percentage of patients with any type of cirrhosis, especially alcoholic liver disease
4. A small percentage of patients who have undergone a portacaval shunt for portal hypertension
5. Some patients with porphyria cutanea tarda
6. Patients who have excessive dietary intake of iron salts, particularly if protein intake is low

Patients in the last group are principally South African Bantus, who ingest the large quantities of iron in food or drink prepared in iron utensils. This condition has been known as Bantu siderosis. It may lead to increased iron absorption and storage within the reticuloendothelial system and liver.[568] When the iron content of the liver is more than 2% of the dry weight, classical signs of hemochromatosis may develop. The effect of vitamin C deficiency on the deposition of iron in the Bantu is of interest because the excess iron is found in the reticuloendothelial cells of the spleen, liver, and pancreas; the heart and other endocrine glands are usually spared. The nearly normal serum iron level in the Bantus rises when they are given vitamin C. This may possibly have a deleterious effect.[616] In refractory anemias, especially those characterized by accelerated erythropoiesis and defects in normoblast maturation, secondary hemochromatosis and cirrhosis may eventually develop.[603,604] Iron overload after multiple transfusions has now been studied in some detail.[628] Severe hemosiderosis and focal portal fibrosis are observed, along with a widespread subclinical organ dysfunction similar to that seen in idiopathic hemochromatosis. Total iron content in 100 transfusions is 20 g. In an autopsy series of patients who had thalassemia with and without transfusions, a definite relationship of fibrosis to quantity of iron and age of patient was observed.[625] After portacaval shunt for cirrhosis, increased hepatic iron stores may develop. Occasionally the classical picture of hemochromatosis develops.[618]

Liver diseases in pregnancy

The frequency of jaundice in pregnancy is about 1 in 1500 patients.[593] A few liver diseases occur almost exclusively in pregnancy, although other more common illnesses such as viral hepatitis, choledocholithiasis, and drug jaundice must also be considered.[574,641] Viral hepatitis occurring during pregnancy seems to be no different from that seen in nonpregnant women.[593] In our series of cases of fatal fulminant hepatitis from 1918 to 1981, two of the patients were pregnant, both in the first trimester, and another patient had recently given birth. This is in sharp contrast to a variety of non-A, non-B hepatitis with fecal-oral transmission, reported from Kashmir, in which both the incidence and the severity of disease were far greater in pregnant women.[605,649] Other reports of epidemics of hepatitis occurring in the Near East have similarly referred to the high fatality in pregnant women.[641] Unfortunately, there has been little morphologic comparison with fulminant hepatitis seen in the United States. During the nineteenth century, "acute yellow atrophy" of the liver seemed more common in pregnant women; although some would probably now be called fatty liver of pregnancy (see the following), there may have been a disorder akin to that now seen in the Near East. Choledocholithiasis is a rare complication of pregnancy.

Among the disorders peculiar to pregnancy is obstetric cholestasis or recurrent jaundice of the third trimester.

The condition is often familial and most often has its onset in the third trimester. It is accompanied by pruritus and tends to recur with succeeding pregnancies. Pruritus of pregnancy without jaundice is a variant. Recent investigations disclose a high perinatal mortality with low–birth weight babies and a higher frequency of postpartum hemorrhage.[601] Obstetric cholestasis is probably caused by an increased level of hormones in susceptible patients, especially since it has been shown that the same patients who develop recurrent jaundice of pregnancy may develop similar cholestasis and symptoms after the use of estrogens, progesterone, or both, as in oral contraceptives.[573,583] The possibility that intrahepatic cholestasis of pregnancy may represent an abnormal reaction to estrogen in predisposed persons is suggested.[623] A biopsy discloses perivenular cholestasis without necrosis. Laboratory findings include a serum bilirubin level of less than 10 mg/dl, a sharp elevation of serum alkaline phosphatase, and only a mild rise in AST levels. An associated rise in plasma bile acids is probably responsible for the pruritus.

Idiopathic fatty liver of pregnancy, initially described in 1940,[636] is a rare disorder that occurs in the third trimester. Although this is usually considered a highly fatal disease, a recent report indicates otherwise.[575] Many cases of fatty liver of pregnancy were reported during the early 1960s, but most of them occurred after the intravenous administration of tetracycline for the treatment of pyelonephritis.[576,607] It became apparent that tetracycline hepatotoxicity in pregnancy produced a fatty liver indistinguishable from the idiopathic type. Both are characterized by epigastric pain, vomiting, jaundice, and symptoms of hepatic and renal failure. The laboratory findings usually consist of hyperbilirubinemia, lactic acidosis, azotemia, hyperamylasemia, and depressed prothrombin activity. The transaminase levels are usually less than 500 units.[607] Those who survive an attack of idiopathic fatty liver of pregnancy may subsequently have an uncomplicated pregnancy.[575,611] At autopsy the liver is moderately decreased in size and is soft. Fatty change of a fine foamy type is present, the fat being most prominent on the sinusoidal border of the liver cell with the displacement of the granular portion of the cytoplasm to the pericanalicular area. Cholestasis is not prominent. Necrosis is slight, but syncytial change of hepatocytes is prominent in the perivenular zones. Pathologic changes also are seen in the renal tubules, pancreas, and brain. It is probable that tetracycline inhibits the synthesis of the proteins essential to the formation of lipoproteins, the principal form by which fat leaves the liver, thus leading to fatty liver.[607,615] The pathogenesis of the idiopathic fatty liver of pregnancy may be similar. Disseminated intravascular coagulation may complicate acute fatty liver of pregnancy.[569]

Eclampsia only rarely produces hepatic symptoms or clinical liver disease. Only one instance of fatal hepatic failure associated with the liver lesion of eclampsia was found at the Los Angeles County–University of Southern California medical complexes from 1918 to 1981. Jaundice in preeclampsia caused by disseminated intravascular coagulation has been reported.[609] However, hepatic fibrin deposition in preeclampsia that does not produce symptoms is common.[562] The overall problem of fibrin deposition is a subject of ongoing research.[638] Despite the absence of hepatic symptoms, patients who die of eclampsia generally have a mottled discoloration of the liver, with hemorrhagic areas alternating with zones of pale, ischemic necrosis and intact liver (Fig. 27-47). The periportal regions often have fibrin in the sinusoids and are necrotic. The small branches of the portal vein may be thrombosed. Zones of infarction may cover several lobules. Occasionally, such hepatic alterations develop without the convulsions of eclampsia.[564,572,594] Rarely, diffuse coagulative necrosis occurs as a terminal event. Spontaneous rupture of the liver is a rare complication, usually in the third trimester of a multiparous woman who has toxemia, with or without eclampsia. The rupture most often occurs in the right lobe as a complication of subcapsular hematoma.[564,594,597] Rupture of the liver may occur in women taking contraceptive drugs.[592]

Liver disease during pregnancy is often difficult to evaluate because of alterations of laboratory values that are associated with pregnancy. The serum albumin level is ordinarily depressed to a range of 2.8 to 3.7 g/dl (nor-

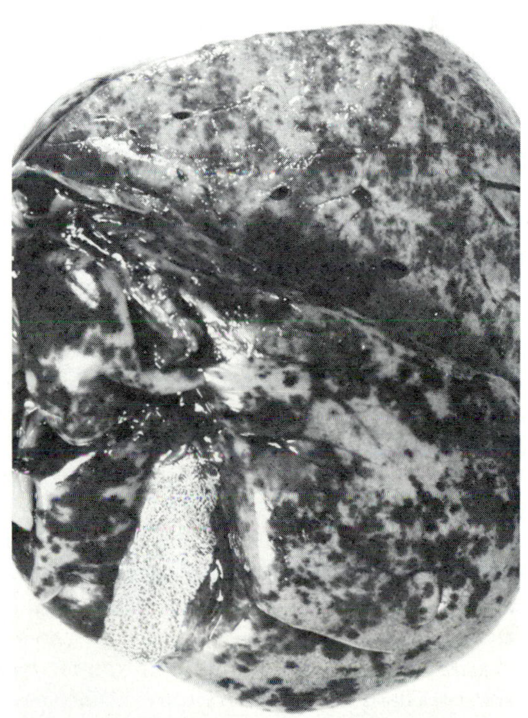

Fig. 27-47. Liver in eclampsia showing hemorrhagic appearance.

mal is 3.5 to 4.8 g/dl), and the alkaline phosphatase activity often is elevated to as much as twice the upper limits of normal. Most chronic diseases of liver preclude pregnancy, although patients with chronic active viral hepatitis B apparently have no impairment in ability to become pregnant.[632] In nonviral chronic active hepatitis, fertility is apparently reduced, but those pregnancies that do occur may proceed without detriment to the mother provided prednisone treatment is maintained. Babies may be born prematurely, and a higher than normal fetal loss can be expected.[642] The problem of acute liver disease with encephalopathy and renal failure in late pregnancy and early puerperium has been reviewed. The patients usually have recurrent pain and vomiting.[575]

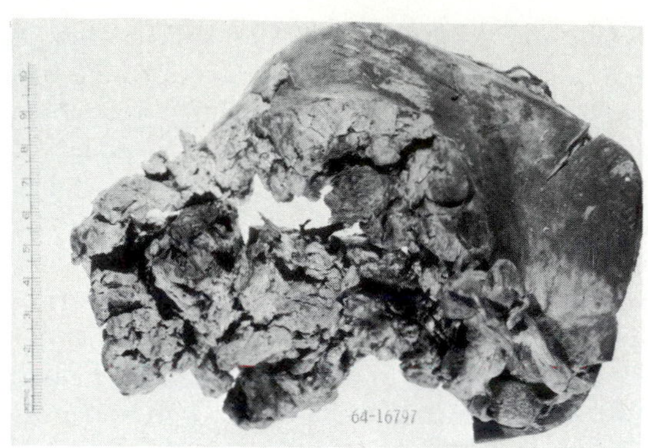

Fig. 27-48. Shattered right lobe of liver after bullet wound. Specimen was surgically resected.

Hepatic injuries

One of the various forms of hepatic injury constitutes the major indication for liver surgery in the United States. About 60% are caused by gunshot wounds, 20% by knife wounds, and 20% by blunt trauma. The mortality is high, between 10% and 20%, hemorrhage being the leading cause of death.[580,587] The liver, because of its size, weight, and soft consistency, is susceptible to blunt injury in high-speed vehicular accidents. The impact of the victim's body colliding with the steering wheel can be particularly harmful to the liver. Blunt injuries most often affect the right lobe, producing lacerations of variable configuration and severity that require surgery. Severe injury, without laceration of the capsule, may cause continued bleeding that results in a subcapsular hematoma and delayed rupture into the abdominal cavity 24 hours or more after the accident. A peritoneal tap may aid in the diagnosis of intrahepatic hemorrhage.[647] In some instances an intrahepatic hematoma ruptures into the biliary tract with resultant hemobilia,[624] in which the patient has gastrointestinal bleeding, often with hematemesis. Gunshot wounds may destroy much of the liver (Fig. 27-48).[613,647]

Liver injuries have been graded, based on the severity of the trauma, including whether bleeding is present.[580] Most traumatic lesions can be handled by simple surgical techniques; however, those with lobal destruction, central hematomas, and hepatic venous or retrohepatic vena caval injury require special techniques. Such severe injuries constitute only 10% of total cases of hepatic trauma. Extensive ligation of the hepatic artery and portal vein branches may be necessary to control hemorrhage. The highest mortality is from gunshot blasts and blunt trauma. Injury to other organs also increases the mortality. In traumatized liver removed at surgery there is a variable amount of hemorrhage and necrosis of the injured parenchyma, often with a neutrophilic exudate. On rare occasions an arteriovenous fistula has been known to occur after liver injury.[590] These are often present for many years before they are diagnosed. They are curable by surgery, but only if treated early. Left untreated, they lead to portal hypertension and ascites. Another rare complication of hepatic trauma is a biliary pleural fistula.[591]

Subcapsular hematomas of small or large size occur occasionally in newborn infants, especially those born prematurely, although they may require surgery or prove fatal. The frequency of unruptured hematomas as incidental findings in newborn premature infants makes it probable that many, or most, reabsorb without rupture. These hematomas may be caused by trauma during birth or may accompany blood dyscrasias, such as erythroblastosis fetalis.

Hereditary hyperbilirubinemia

Several syndromes that are caused by inborn errors in the metabolism of bilirubin have been described.[629,630] These may be divided into two groups. In Crigler-Najjar syndrome and Gilbert's syndrome, there are unconjugated hyperbilirubinemia and defects in the glucuronyl transferase system in the hepatocytes. In the second group, composed of Dubin-Johnson (Sprinz-Nelson) and Rotor's syndromes, conjugation of bilirubin occurs, but secretion is blocked. Some features of these disorders are given in Table 27-6. The Crigler-Najjar syndrome occurs in two forms: type 1 and type 2. In type 1 glucuronyl transferase is absent and hyperbilirubinemia is severe, usually greater than 20 mg/dl; the bile is almost completely colorless and contains only traces of unconjugated bilirubin (UCB). A similar disease occurs in the Gunn rat. In type 2 the patients have a partial deficiency of glucuronyl transferase, probably of the plasma membrane transglucuronidation enzyme. The hyperbilirubinemia is less severe, and the bile contains some bilirubin monoglucuronide. The conjugation defect in the first type is transmitted as an autosomal recessive trait and in the second type as an autosomal dominant characteristic. The jaundice appears in the neonate and persists with

Table 27-6. Hereditary hyperbilirubinemias

Syndrome	Age of onset of jaundice	Symptoms and course	Serum bilirubin			BSP excretion	Physiologic defect	Pathologic condition
			Range (mg/dl)	Conjugated	Unconjugated			
Crigler-Najjar								
Type 1	Neonate	Jaundice at birth with or without kernicterus; death in first year of life	>20	—	Increased	Normal	Absence of glucuronyl transferase	Few bile thrombi
Type 2	Neonate	May live past 50 years	<20 mg	—	Increased	Normal	Partial deficiency of glucuronyl transase	Few bile thrombi
Gilbert's	Birth to middle age (average 18 years)	Jaundice may be precipitated by fasting, fatigue, intermittent infections, alcohol, and stress	<5	Normal	Increased	Normal	Deficiency of transglucuronidation enzyme	Hypertrophy of smooth endoplasmic reticulum
Dubin-Johnson								
Classic	Most often 15 to 25 years	Pain over liver and hepatomegaly, especially during attacks of jaundice; dyspepsia; problem exists throughout life with fluctuations of jaundice	Normal to 6	Increased	Increased	Retention with late rise after 90 minutes		Pigment in liver, nature unknown
Variants in family members	Mild elevation of serum bilirubin after 10 years	None	>1 in 20% of family	Normal or increased	Normal or increased	Normal		Pigment in many but not related to increased bilirubin
Rotor's	Early life, usually before 20 years	Jaundice fluctuates	Normal to 6	Increased	Increased	Retention with no late rise		None

high concentrations of unconjugated bilirubin in the blood serum. Patients with type 1 often die in infancy, whereas those with type 2 have been known to survive past 50 years of age without neurologic disorders.[596] Administration of phenobarbital increases the hypertrophy of the smooth endoplasmic reticulum and lowers the serum UCB in type 2 patients only. As in Gilbert's disease, dietary restriction increases the UCB and a normal diet restores the former level. The intravenous administration of glucose after dietary restriction does not lower the UCB.[596]

Gilbert's syndrome (GS) is the most common of the hereditary hyperbilirubinemias.[629] Its frequency may total 2% to 6% of the population, as suggested by measurement of UCB. The frequency of jaundice, which usually begins after puberty, is much lower. The jaundice tends to be intermittent and may be precipitated by fasting. The most useful diagnostic test is the fasting test. Intravenous nicotinic acid is also used; either of these tests usually results in 100% rise in the serum bilirubin. However, fasting does not produce this result if the patient is not jaundiced at the time of the test.[598] All patients with GS have a defect in glucuronyl transferase, as shown on needle biopsy specimens. The defect has been postulated to be at the plasma membrane, since the bilirubin diglucuronide is decreased in the duodenal bile. However, two subpopulations of patients with GS have been recently reported. In one group endoplasmic reticulum is markedly increased, whereas the other group shows no increase. Patients with hypertrophy of the endoplasmic reticulum show a higher percentage of response to both caloric restriction and nicotinic acid injection.[577,578] No evidence of any defect is noted in the plasma membrane, either biochemically or by electron microscopy. In addition to the difficulty in the excretion of bilirubin that is attributable to the lack of glucuronyl transferase, there may also be a problem in bilirubin uptake in GS.[612]

Included in the second group of hereditary hyperbilirubinemia are the Dubin-Johnson (Sprinz-Nelson) and Rotor's syndromes. The Dubin-Johnson syndrome is characterized by a chronic or intermittent nonhemolytic type of jaundice in which there is an increase of both conjugated[602] and unconjugated bilirubin, although mostly of the conjugated type. Glucuronide formation is presumed to be normal, but the hepatocytes have difficulty secreting bilirubin. Similarly the secretion of sulfobromophthalein and iopanoic acid is affected so that there is BSP retention and the gallbladder cannot be viewed roentgenographically. Most helpful in diagnosis is the abnormal excretion of coproporphyrin isomers in the urine. Isomer I is increased and isomer III is decreased.[606] The parenchymal cells, especially in the perivenular zone 3, contain large granules of lipochrome pigment (Fig. 27-49), often in such amounts that the liver is black. The electron spin resonance study of this pigment indicates that it is not melanin.[644] It is excreted in the urine in large amounts in patients with Dubin-Johnson syndrome who have acute viral hepatitis. During this time it disappears from the liver but reappears after recovery. The pigment is located within lysosomes.[634] A similar disease is seen in a Corriedale sheep mutant.[571] The disease in the human is inherited as an autosomal recessive trait with a high frequency of consanguinity of parents.[586] Improvement in the handling of bilirubin and sulfobromophthalein is noted in some patients after the use of phenobarbital, an enzyme inducer.[635]

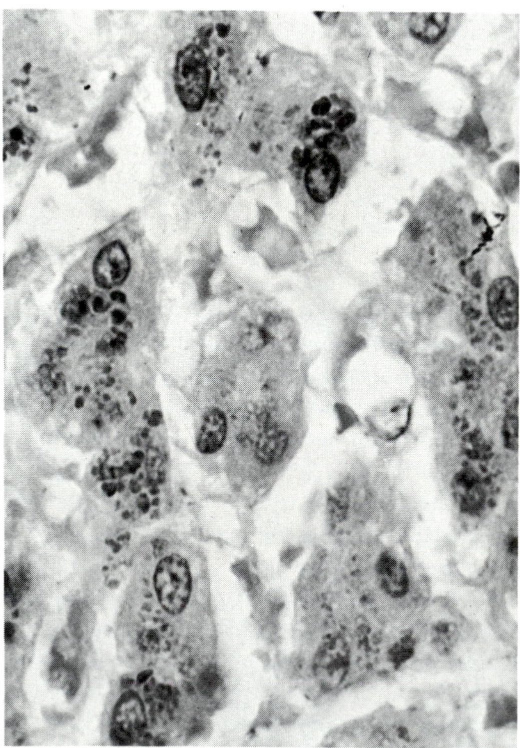

Fig. 27-49. Large masses of intracytoplasmic brown pigment in Dubin-Johnson syndrome.

In Rotor's syndrome there is likewise an increase in both conjugated and unconjugated serum bilirubin but no pigmentation of the liver cells. There is sulfobromophthalein retention but a normal view of the gallbladder. It has been suggested that Rotor's syndrome is a variant of the Dubin-Johnson syndrome.

CIRCULATORY DISTURBANCES

Hypoxic necrosis

Any circulatory disorder that results in prolonged hypoxia may cause recognizable pathologic changes in the liver. The damage may be acute or chronic in nature, depending on the underlying disease responsible for the lack of oxygen. For example, the hypotension of shock may produce perivenular necrosis, whereas chronic heart failure often results in perivenular atrophy and occasionally fibrosis. The acute changes may be observed in a liver that was previously normal, or the changes may be superimposed on chronic passive congestion or cirrhosis. Trauma, hemorrhage, heart failure, and endotoxic shock resulting from septicemia are the most common causes.[654] Normally, endotoxins in portal blood are removed in the liver.[673] Shock lasting longer than 24 hours usually is associated with liver cell necrosis.[654] In a study of 1000 patients with cardiac dysfunction, perivenular necrosis was associated with shock and with other sequelae of arterial hypotension, including acute tubular necrosis of the kidney and corticomedullary junction necrosis of the adrenal.[651] Left-sided congestive heart failure apparently was not a factor. In the same study chronic passive congestion of the liver without necrosis was associated with right-sided heart failure and other conditions associated with elevated systemic venous pressure.[651] Other studies indicate that perivenular necrosis may complicate severe heart disease and cardiogenic shock resulting from heart failure, whether it is right sided, left sided, or both. Occasionally, hypoxic necrosis in the absence of any demonstrable hypotension may be seen. Jaundice is rare but does occur in endotoxic shock and in cardiac conditions. When anoxic necrosis is associated with a marked increase of transaminase, it may be confused with acute viral hepatitis.[658]

In noncirrhotic individuals hypoxic perivenular necrosis usually has a uniform distribution involving about one half of the perivenular area. Grossly the areas of necrosis may or may not be recognized, but often the perivenular zones have a characteristic dull yellow to yellow-brown appearance. Microscopically coagulative necrosis is apparent with intensely acidophilic hepatocytes whose nuclei stain poorly or have disappeared. Neutrophils may be abundant, especially around the periphery of the necrotic zones. The degree of centrilobular hyperemia varies greatly; it may be so extreme that pools of blood fill the necrotic area. A distinctive perivenular hepatic lesion, characterized by hepatic cords filled with erythrocytes, has been described in patients with heart failure.[674] In some instances of hypoxic perivenular necrosis, a narrow rim of intact hepatocytes remains around the terminal venules. Although hypoxic necrosis is predominantly perivenular, the midzonal area is often affected. The necrotic cells slowly disappear, and in biopsy specimens taken in the healing stage, only dilated sinusoids and pigmented macrophages are seen, a histologic change difficult to distinguish from other types of healing centrilobular zonal necrosis.

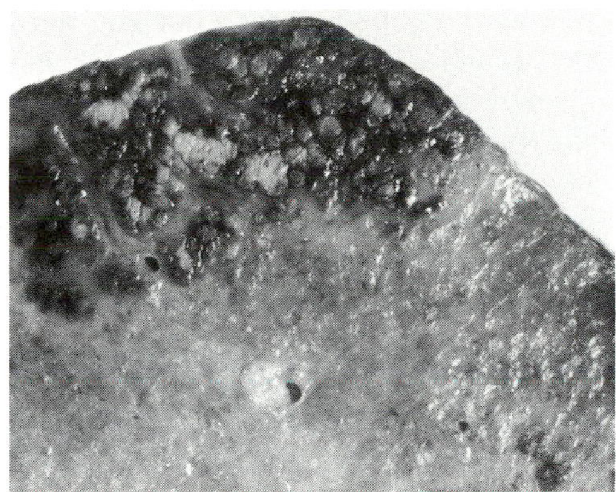

Fig. 27-50. Anoxic necrosis of liver. Alcoholic cirrhosis with fatal hemorrhage from duodenal ulcer.

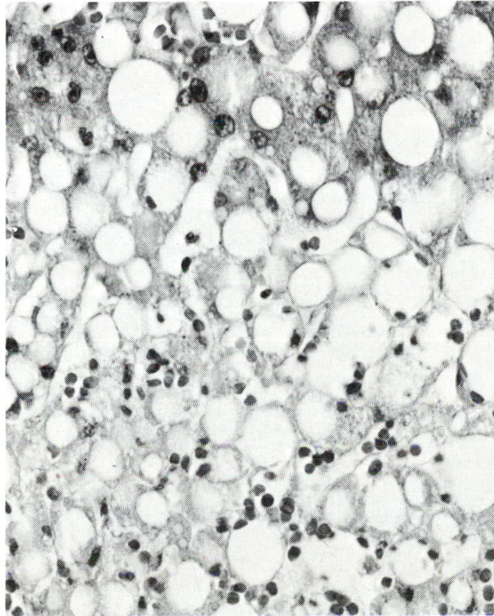

Fig. 27-51. Anoxic centrilobular necrosis in fatty liver of alcoholic patient who was in shock after variceal bleeding.

The cirrhotic liver is particularly prone to hypoxic pseudolobular necrosis when there is bleeding from varices. The large pseudolobules of cirrhosis are probably poorly oxygenated as a result of an abnormal inflow and outflow pattern. Furthermore, much of the portal vein blood may be shunted around the liver so that a fall in hepatic artery pressure during shock would lead rapidly to hypoxic necrosis. The areas of necrosis are often large and pale yellow-white and may be surrounded by a thin zone of hemorrhage (Fig. 27-50). Portions or entire pseudolobules may be involved by hypoxic necrosis (Fig. 27-51). It is likely that some of the depressed scars seen in the liver of cirrhotic patients who have bled from varices in the past may be of hypoxic origin.

Passive hyperemia and cardiac cirrhosis

Passive hyperemia of the liver is most often the result of cardiac disease with congestive failure, but also may result from compression and obstruction of the inferior vena cava or obstructions of the pulmonary circulation, leading to right-sided cardiac failure. Increased pressure in the venous system affects the liver severely because of the short distance between the point of entry of hepatic veins into the vena cava and the entry of the latter into the right auricle. Because the liver cells are particularly sensitive to hypoxia, the decreased oxygen content of the hepatic blood and the diminished flow in congestive failure are probably responsible for much of the histologic change that is observed.

In the early stages of passive congestion dilatation of only terminal hepatic veins and sinusoids is seen. Atrophy and disappearance of liver cells later lead to larger pools of blood in the dilated channels. Fragments of former sinusoidal walls remain, but the normal architectural arrangement around the central vein tends to disappear. Often a correlation is lacking between the clinical course and severity of atrophy. When the perivenular one third to one half of the lobule has undergone atrophy, fatty change of the remaining liver cells near the margin is often present and is responsible for the gross "nutmeg" appearance (Fig. 27-52). However, in many instances the pale peripheral lobular zones do not contain fat vacuoles. The reason for their pallor is not apparent. An increase of fibrous tissue may ensue coincidentally with the perivenular atrophy.[696] Occasionally, especially in patients with tricuspid valvular disease, fibrosis links the perivenular areas together, and a diagnosis of cardiac cirrhosis may be made (Fig. 27-53). It has been suggested that perivenular fibrosis and cardiac cirrhosis may follow repeated acute attacks of hypoxic necrosis.[710] This remains to be proved by the use of repeated needle biopsies.

Portal fibrosis with communicating septa to the central

fibrous areas is rare but does occur. Hyperplasia of the peripheral portions of the lobules is occasionally seen, sometimes in conjunction with cardiac cirrhosis.

Grossly the liver in cardiac cirrhosis is of normal or slightly reduced size, firm, and dark red-brown or purple-red. The surface is only slightly nodular, and the capsule is thickened. The cut surface shows a mottling of gray or yellow-gray areas separated by brown-red zones of variable size and shape. The hepatic veins are uniformly dilated, sometimes strikingly so, and their walls are thickened. Ill-defined nodules may be present in proximity to the portal tracts. Whether true cirrhosis of congestive origin exists is questionable. A small percentage of patients with long-standing congestive failure do have esophageal varices, but these rarely bleed.[678] In our experience the wedged hepatic vein pressure is not elevated in patients with congestive failure.

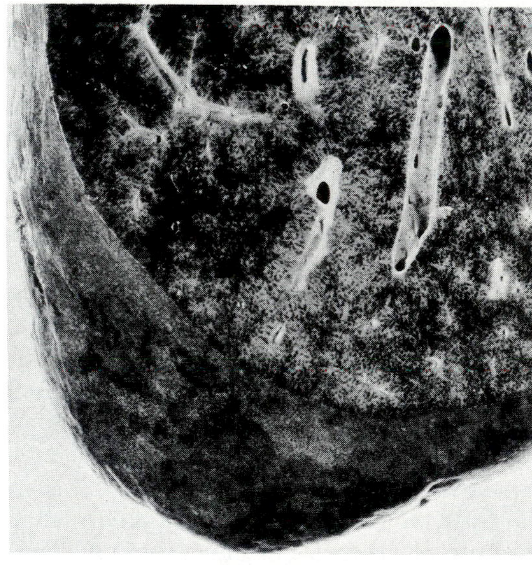

Fig. 27-52. "Nutmeg liver" in chronic passive congestion of liver.

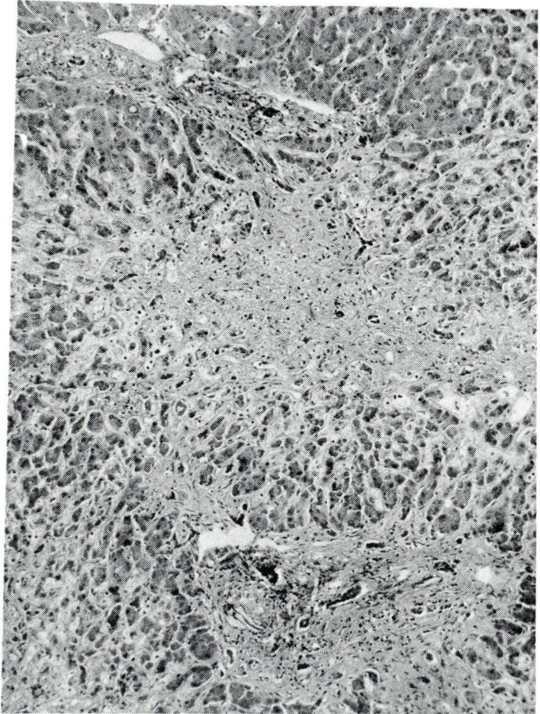

Fig. 27-53. Severe centrilobular fibrosis (cardiac cirrhosis) in patient with tricuspid stenosis and chronic heart failure.

Vascular diseases—infarction

Several pathologic entities may affect the blood vessels of the liver, often producing clinical symptoms. Most of these diseases can be diagnosed by angiography. The diseases of the hepatic artery include arteriosclerosis, embolism, aneurysm, polyarteritis nodosa, and hepatoportal arteriovenous fistula.

Infarction of the liver is rare; most cases result from obstruction of the hepatic artery or some of its branches by arteriosclerosis or aneurysms, as well as by bland or septic emboli from the heart.[698] Obstruction of the proper hepatic artery beyond the gastroduodenal and right gastric arteries is most likely to result in infarction. Ligature proximal to the latter arteries is well tolerated because of retrograde flow of blood through the right gastric artery from its anastomoses. Ligature of the hepatic artery is sometimes accidental but also may be necessary in treating severe trauma to the liver.[679] Polyarteritis nodosa is a rare cause of multiple infarcts (Fig. 27-54). Thickening of the walls of hepatic arteries has been observed in women taking oral contraceptives[712] and in orthotopic transplants.[702]

Hepatoportal arteriovenous fistulas may occur after trauma or biopsy.[690,708] Large fistulas necessitate obliter-

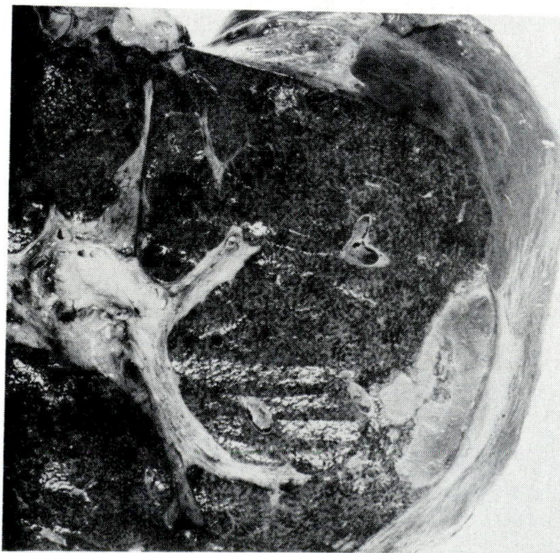

Fig. 27-54. Subcapsular infarct attributed to polyarteritis nodosa.

ation either by surgical means or by embolization to prevent portal hypertension. Smaller fistulas may close spontaneously or do not require treatment. There are anastomoses between the arteries supplying hepatocellular carcinoma (HCC) and the branches of the portal veins in a high percentage of cases. These shunts especially occur because of the tendency of HCC to grow into branches of the portal vein carrying along its arterial supply.[650,686,690] Most hepatic artery aneurysms occur in the extrahepatic portion; however, mycotic aneurysms resulting from bacterial endocarditis or sepsis have been reported.[693] Other causes include arteriosclerosis and trauma.[666]

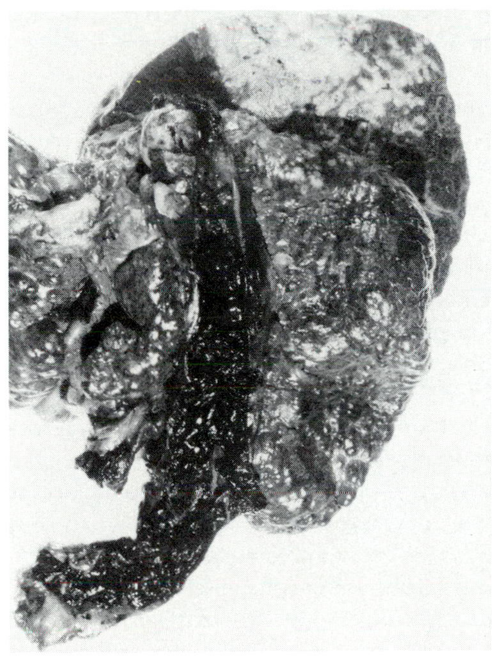

Fig. 27-55. Portal cirrhosis and thrombosis of portal vein. (Courtesy Dr. G. Lyman Duff.)

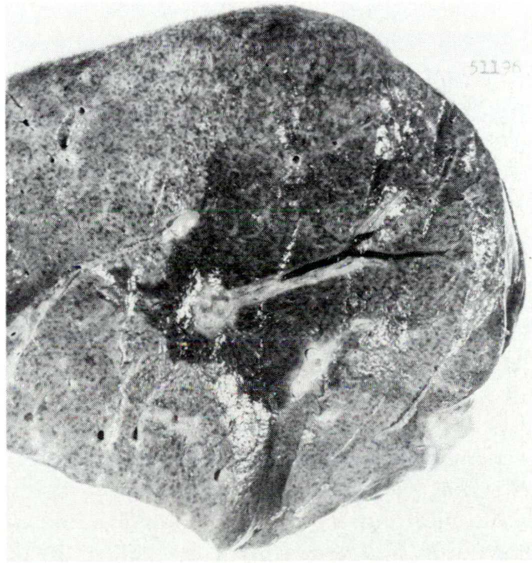

Fig. 27-56. Infarct of Zahn, area of dusky hyperemia attributed to thrombosis of branch of portal vein.

Occlusion of the portal vein or one or more of its branches usually results from another disease (Fig. 27-55), such as cirrhosis of the liver, idiopathic portal hypertension, pancreatitis, hepatocellular carcinoma, carcinoma of the pancreas that grows into the intrahepatic portal veins, or pylephlebitis that follows abdominal suppuration or umbilical infection of the newborn infant. Among cirrhotic patients undergoing decompressive procedures for variceal bleeding, approximately 20% have portal vein thrombosis.[697] In these patients the mortality is higher because of rebleeding. Intrahepatic obstruction of the portal vein or one of the major branches usually causes only the atrophic red infarct of Zahn (Fig. 27-56), a discolored zone that does not show necrosis on microscopic examination. Occasionally thrombosis or neoplastic invasion of the trunk of the portal vein causes areas of necrosis in the liver. True infarcts may also follow thrombosis of both hepatic and portal veins.[664]

In an adult, gas in branches of the portal veins noted on x-ray examination is a sign of serious abdominal disease and necessitates surgery, except in patients with chronic ulcerative colitis.[677]

Idiopathic portal hypertension

Idiopathic portal hypertension is a term used for a syndrome first described by Banti.[667] The syndrome is characterized by esophageal varices, hypersplenism, and portal hypertension but no cirrhosis. The disease is more common in India[656] and Japan[672] than in the United States. In the United States most patients first seek medical care for bleeding esophageal varices, at which time splenomegaly and mild pancytopenia are noted. Hepatic function is normal, at least initially.

Grossly the liver surface is smooth, the edges are blunted, and the parenchyma is slightly firmer than normal. Microscopically the relationship between terminal hepatic venules and portal areas is inconstant. Two or more outflow venules are often found in a lobule. The portal area is widened within an intact limiting plate, and there are increased numbers of dilated, thin-walled angiomatous structures. The major intrahepatic portal veins have sclerotic walls (Fig. 27-57). As the disease progresses, collagen becomes more dense in the portal areas and may extend beyond the confines of the limiting plates to adjacent portal areas. The terminal portal vein radicles may become thickened. The end stage of idiopathic portal hypertension is a fibrotic, shrunken liver without regenerative nodules.

Both the pathogenesis and the cause of idiopathic por-

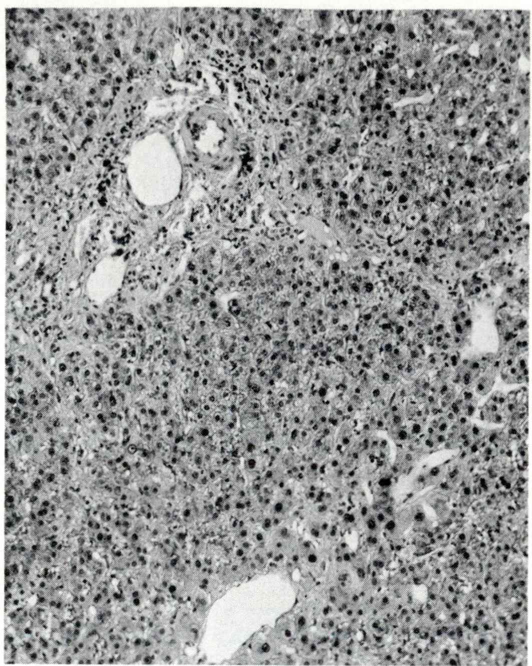

Fig. 27-57. Idiopathic portal hypertension with large vessels and increase of connective tissue in portal areas. Central veins are enlarged and prominent.

tal hypertension are unknown. There is general agreement that increased portal vein flow from an enlarged spleen could not produce portal pressure levels equivalent to those found in this disorder. Small segments of occlusion or narrowing have been demonstrated in the intrahepatic portal vein radicals,[655,684] but similar portal vein lesions were also found in incidental autopsy findings in significant numbers of patients who had no signs of portal hypertension.[709] Sclerosis and thickening of portal vein walls have also been described, but it is unclear whether thrombosis of diverse cause or phlebosclerosis is the pathogenic mechanism in such patients. The possibility of aberrant hepatic artery–portal vein communication has not been thoroughly explored. The histolic changes of idiopathic portal hypertension are similar to the changes in the livers of patients who have acquired an arterioportal fistula and consequent portal hypertension.[660] Abnormalities in hepatic veins that include unusual anastomoses by way of capsular veins to adjacent hepatic vein segments have been reported.[691]

Several etiologic factors and associations have been proposed, including induction of portal venular sclerosis by chronic inflammatory reaction or hepatitis, chronic arsenic exposure (a possible cause in India),[659] chronic exposure to vinyl chloride or polyvinylchloride,[692,707] and even cytomegalovirus infection.[661] The disease has also been reported after renal transplantation.[689]

A number of patients with the foregoing findings have thrombotic or sclerotic occlusion of the extrahepatic portal vein. This occlusion is considered by many investigators to be the cause of extrahepatic portal hypertension, whereas others[682] have suggested that the portal vein occlusion occurs after idiopathic portal hypertension, just as it occasionally occurs after portal hypertension associated with cirrhosis.

Hepatic veins

The blood from the liver drains into the inferior vena cava via three large venous trunks—the right, middle, and left—plus some direct branches, chiefly from the caudate lobe.[688] Although trauma is the most common disorder affecting the veins, often necessitating surgery, there are two rather rare, intrinsic diseases that may involve the hepatic veins. One of these is hepatic vein thrombosis (HVT), which affects the larger trunks and is known clinically as the Budd-Chiari syndrome (BCS). The other, veno-occlusive disease (VOD), is a specific entity that affects the terminal hepatic and sublobular veins. This disorder most often follows the ingestion of one of the pyrrolizidine alkaloids[680] present in a wide variety of plants in many parts of the world.

Budd-Chiari syndrome

In the Budd-Chiari syndrome obstruction to the flow of blood usually occurs slowly and, over a period of weeks or months, ascites and a large tender liver become manifest. However, a few patients may have an acute onset with abdominal pain and a rapid accumulation of ascites. Portal hypertension, esophageal varices, and hematemesis commonly occur late in the course of the disease. When the vena cava is occluded, collateral veins may be noted along the anterior and posterior thorax.

Among the etiologic factors that have been implicated are polycythemia vera,[671] paroxysmal nocturnal hemoglobinuria (PNH),[676] oral contraceptives,[675] pregnancy,[705] neoplasms, chemotherapy,[652] graft-versus-host reaction,[653,700] radiation,[663] familial immune deficiency,[681] and membranes across or sclerosis of inferior vena cava near the mouths of the hepatic veins.[687] However, in approximately half of the patients with BCS, there is no recognizable etiologic factor. Polycythemia vera and PNH are among the most common causes of BCS when a cause can be identified. PNH is particularly likely to have an acute onset.[676] Although there are many reports of HVT following use of oral contraceptives, whether there is a real increase of the disease in women of childbearing age might be questioned.

In BCS two diagnostic tests have been found useful[676]: the liver scan showing the hepatic and splenic enlargement, along with an increased uptake in the caudate lobe,[668] and percutaneous hepatography that often shows the site and nature of the outflow block. The pathology in BCS depends on the duration of the disease and to a lesser extent on the cause. An early biopsy discloses severe perivenular congestion, a variable degree of necrosis, and fibrin thrombi in terminal hepatic venules. Erythrocytes are often present in the space of Disse and between the hepatocytes. Atrophy and fibrosis of the liver, along with closure of vessels, is evident later. In autopsy material there are both thrombosis and sclerosis of the larger venous trunks. Many become fibrotic, but recanalization is not prominent. Atrophy of the liver parenchyma may be extensive, but cholestasis is not noted. Since the blood from the caudate lobe is drained by several small veins directly into the inferior vena cava, this lobe is often uninvolved or less involved than the main right and left lobe. Thus as the remainder of the liver undergoes atrophy in BCS, the caudate lobe becomes enlarged because of hyperplasia. This may be sufficient to impinge on the inferior vena cava, causing venous collaterals to form.[685,706] The prognosis is poor in patients with hepatic venous thrombosis. More than 50% die within a few months. Side-to-side portacaval shunt has been used in the treatment of BCS.[694]

Membranous obstruction of the inferior vena cava (MOVC) may produce a second and different type of BCS that is associated with signs and symptoms of inferior vena cava hypertension. These membranes affect both the inferior vena cava and the hepatic veins in some 72% of the cases. In the remainder the obstruction may be only of the inferior vena cava or only of the hepatic veins.[687] Although the membrane may be thin, usually it is a sclerotic segment of vena cava just above the diaphragm. Symptoms usually develop slowly over a period of years, and surgery is often successful.[662] Since hepatic vein thrombosis may occur late in the disease, early diagnosis and treatment are important. The disease has been reported mostly from Japan, but the occurrence is far greater in blacks in South Africa and is associated with hepatocellular carcinoma in 47.5% of cases.[701] The diagnosis is made with cavogram.

Veno-occlusive disease

Veno-occlusive disease (VOD) occurs in widespread locations throughout the world and is caused by one or more of the pyrrolizidine alkaloids. The disease also produces fatalities among livestock. In the West Indies, both children and adults who have ingested "bush tea" made from boiling the leaves of foliage that includes *Crotolaria fulva* and *Senecio* plants may develop occlusive disease of the terminal hepatic and sublobular veins with resultant hepatomegaly, ascites, and, often, jaundice (Fig. 27-58).[657,699,704] The disease has also been reported in South America[665] and, occasionally, in Native Americans in the western United States.[703] The venous lesion is first characterized by edema and, later, by collagenization. The large hepatic veins usually are unaffected. The sinusoids are remarkably congested, and the perivenular hepatic cells atrophy. Later, in chronic cases a nonportal type of cirrhosis may develop. A similar disease apparently occurs after the use of flour contaminatd with *Senecio* in Africa.[699] Egyptian children also suffer

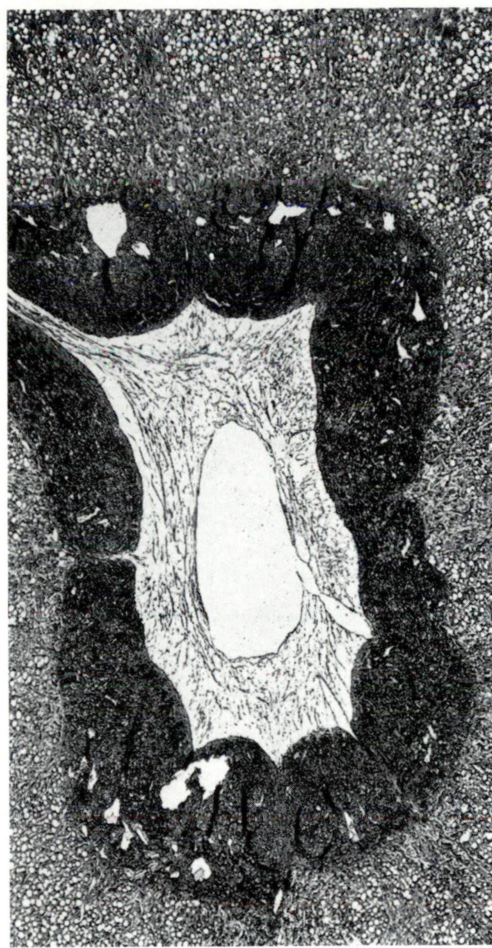

Fig. 27-58. Veno-occlusive disease of liver. (Courtesy Dr. G. Bras.)

from a disease involving the hepatic veins.[669] A severe outbreak of VOD, caused by *Heliotropium* plant seeds contaminating wheat used for human consumption, occurred in 1972 in Afghanistan. This involved several thousand patients and was usually fatal.[683] Another form of VOD with a high mortality has been noted after allogeneic bone marrow transplantation. Most of the patients who died had been treated for leukemia and had received chemoradiotherapy. In one report the VOD was most marked in patients who had received dimethyl busulfan.[700,711]

In symptomless disease of the hepatic veins sometimes seen at autopsy, small segments of the hepatic veins may be closed by thrombi or even by tumors that produce infarction. Primary carcinomas of the liver often grow into the hepatic veins but rarely fill the entire system.

Radiation injury

Heavy irradiation of the liver, 3000 to 5900 rad, produces perivenular necrosis, intense hyperemia, and damage to the small hepatic veins that taken together resemble VOD.[695] However, fibrin in the terminal hepatic veins and sinusoids has been observed in patients who had received fractionated radiation with total doses of 1850 to 4050 rad or single doses of 1000 rad.[663]

The microscopic changes in a needle biopsy specimen taken in the acute stage of irradiation damage are most difficult to distinguish from idiopathic BCS. In the chronic stage, after several months, there is a shrunken, atrophied liver with lobular collapse and portal tract fibrosis. Vascular damage is still present. The presence of both acute and chronic changes may represent an intermediate stage of damage. The disease may be fatal and may be considered a form of VOD. Experimentally irradiation produces a fine structural change in the rough endoplasmic reticulum, characterized by the formation of dense membranes.[670]

CHRONIC INFECTIONS AND OTHER CHRONIC DISORDERS

Granulomatous hepatitis—chronic infections

Hepatic granulomas have been reported in 10% or less of all needle biopsies of the liver. In our patients in Los Angeles, the percentage has dropped over the years to 2.5% in 1981. The indications for biopsy in patients with proven granulomas include a fever of unknown origin, hepatomegaly, and a high serum alkaline phosphatase level. A small percentage of patients may have jaundice or a tender liver. The presence of granulomas in needle biopsy specimens may be a confirmatory finding for the clinicians, but in some patients granulomatous disease is unexpected. Extensive bacteriologic, viral, and radiologic studies; skin testing; and even biopsies of other tissues may be necessary to establish a diagnosis. Etiologic classification of granulomatous hepatitis includes infectious diseases, drug sensitivity, granulomas associated with neoplasms, foreign body reaction, and a large and important group, including sarcoidosis, the etiology of which is not known.[723] Clinicopathologically, hepatic granulomas may be associated with (1) systemic granulomatosis, such as tuberculosis that involves one or more other organs; (2) another liver disease, such as primary biliary cirrhosis; and (3) a nonhepatic, nongranulomatous disease, such as abdominal cancer.[729] Most granulomas of the liver are nonnecrotizing and bear a certain similarity to one another, and in some instances very small aggregates of macrophages are difficult to categorize as granulomas. The definition of a granuloma as a "focal organized collection of mononuclear phagocytes"[713] seems applicable to the liver.

In our patients and probably in most large medical centers in the United States the major granulomatous diseases to be considered are sarcoidosis, tuberculosis, and granulomas associated with primary biliary cirrhosis and drug sensitivity. Other specific granulomas are rare, such as Q fever, but even after exhaustive studies, about 15% cannot be diagnosed. Tuberculous and sarcoid granulomas are the most frequently seen, and their differentiation is of practical importance. The lesion of sarcoidosis is composed of epithelioid cells with no particular arrangement. Caseation necrosis is not seen, and a few lymphocytes usually surround the granulomas (Fig. 27-59). Larger lesions are composed of multiple units, often with an occasional multinucleated giant cell. In some instances the noncaseating lesions of sarcoidosis are observed in the walls of the terminal hepatic and sublobular veins. In healing, sarcoid granulomas usually become surrounded by concentric layers of connective tissue. Tubercles often have a caseous center, the epithelioid cells are arranged in a radial fashion at the periphery, and the exudate contains both lymphocytes and other mononuclear cells. Langhans' giant cells are frequent. Fibrin is often present, which helps to distinguish tuberculosis from sarcoidosis. In the small early lesions of tuberculosis, there may be no caseation, and the differentiation from sarcoidosis and leprosy is most difficult. An acid-fast stain should always be done on any granulomatous lesion that resembles tuberculosis. Occasionally the tubercles are concentrated along the portal tracts, and the bile ducts may be destroyed. In a patient so affected, jaundice may occur. More rarely, solitary or multiple tuberculomas have been observed. Tubercle bacilli may reach the liver from either an active pulmonary or an abdominal focus.

In addition to tuberculosis, sarcoidosis must also be

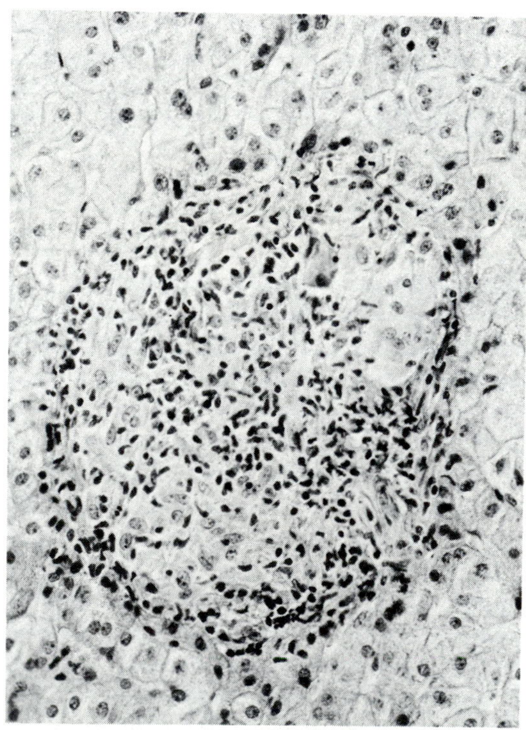

Fig. 27-59. Irregular arrangement of epithelioid cells and scanty lymphoid infiltrate in sarcoid granuloma of liver.

differentiated from PBC. Usually the clinical and laboratory findings suffice, but occasionally the presence of granulomas on biopsy is the first indication of early PBC. These granulomas are usually along the portal tracts and may be in close proximity to diseased bile ducts. They are also found within the lobules. These are usually solitary and do not have the complex structure of sarcoid. In the advanced stage of PBC, if extensive granulomas are present, the differentiation from sarcoidosis is difficult.[752] Also, on rare occasions sarcoidosis destroys branches of the intrahepatic bile ducts, producing chronic cholestasis and microscopic findings that are similar to PBC.[739]

Among the infectious granulomas, two are of major importance outside the United States. Schistosomiasis is a common cause of granulomas in which a specific diagnosis can be made by finding the larvae or the ova in the lesions. Liver involvement is also common in lepromatous leprosy and to a lesser extent in tuberculoid leprosy. The organisms are easily demonstrated with the Fite stain, especially in the foam cells. Leprosy involvement of the liver is usually symptomless; lesions are the result of bacteremia.[720]

Brucellosis infection causes a poorly defined granuloma or pseudogranuloma that consists of a jumblelike arrangement of epithelioid cells or round cells. They are located within the lobule and are associated with necrosis of hepatocytes.[738,750] Q fever produces rather characteristic lesions of variable size that often show a bright band of acidophilic material, apparently arising in the sinusoidal wall. These produce a doughnutlike lesion in the center of which is often a multinucleated giant cell.[716,721] The granulomas are present both in the triads and within the lobules and may at times form fairly large conglomerate lesions. Central vein involvement is noticed occasionally.

In visceral larva migrans the presence of the larvae of *Toxocara canis*, *T. cati*, or other parasites in the liver causes distinctive granulomas that may reach a diameter of several millimeters and are composed of a necrotic center surrounded by epithelioid cells having a radial arrangement, many eosinophils, and giant cells. The larvae may be identified on serial sectioning. The disease is seen in children, usually from 1½ to 6 years of age, who eat dirt (pica) and associate with dogs or cats. The syndrome is characterized by fever, hepatomegaly, eosinophilia, and hyperglobulinemia.[730] A reliable intradermal test using *Toxocara* antigen has been found useful.[754] *Toxoplasma gondii* occasionally causes a granuloma-like lesion of the liver.[717]

Where histoplasmosis is endemic, it is a fairly common cause of hepatic granulomas. In other parts of the United States, it is a rare cause.[737] In addition to granulomas, the organisms are commonly found in the Kupffer cells. Coccidioidal granulomas are of rare occurrence. Both histoplasmosis and coccidioidal organisms may be demonstrated with periodic acid–Schiff stains. Neonatal coccidioidomycosis with involvement of the liver has been observed.[749] Tularemia is discussed in Chapter 7.

The frequency of granulomas following drug use seems to be increasing. In one report nearly one third of patients with granulomatous hepatitis had acquired it following the use of drugs.[733] These granulomas are noncaseous and characterized by epithelioid cell reaction with giant cells and eosinophils. The presence of large numbers of the latter should make the pathologist suspect drug-induced or parasitic liver disease.[733] Among the more common drugs reported in association with granulomas are methyldopa,[735] hydralizine,[727] chlorpropamide,[744] quinidine,[718] allopurinol,[748,756] phenylbutazone,[715] and sulfonamides.

A rare disease characterized by granulomatous hepatitis, increased platelet aggregation, and hypercholesterolemia has been reported,[755] as has a single case of granulomatous disease of the small hepatic and portal veins.[740]

Numerous types of foreign material have been recognized as the cause of granulomas. Among these are copper, which has been noted in vineyard sprayers,[742] talcum crystals in narcotic addicts,[736] fluid silicone,[722] and silica in patients with advanced pulmonary silicosis.[719]

In the miscellaneous granuloma group associated with nonhepatic nongranulomatous disorders, there are abdominal neoplasms, Hodgkin's disease,[747] and Crohn's disease. Ileal bypass for obesity may also be complicated by nonnecrotizing granulomas in about one fourth of the patients. These granulomas do not seem to have clinical significance.[714]

Lastly, there are many cases (about 15% in our patients) in which no etiologic agent or association with another disease is ever demonstrated. The prognosis in these patients seems to be favorable.[743]

Syphilis of the liver

In congenital syphilis of the liver, now a rare entity, there is an overgrowth of mesenchymal tissue along the sinusoids that causes wide separation of the hepatic cells. Small gummas, or even large soft ones, occasionally are seen. Usually spirochetes are easily demonstrable. Syphilitic cirrhosis rarely occurs.

Secondary syphilis may rarely involve the liver, causing jaundice, a rise in the serum alkaline phosphatase, and mild rise in the AST.[731] The microscopic findings vary; usually there are portal tract inflammation, focal necrosis, disruption of the bile duct epithelium,[745] and occasional noncaseating granulomas. Spirochetes are difficult to demonstrate. Anal lesions are common.

Although common at one time, tertiary syphilis of the liver, complicating acquired syphilis, is now a rare disorder.[751] Gummas may be solitary or multiple and confluent, sometimes forming a large mass. On sectioning they have a dull gray-yellow area of central necrosis, an irregular outline, and a marginal zone of gray-white, glassy-appearing granulation tissue. They are often widespread, and, in healing, the scar tissue replacing them contracts to form deep scars that may incompletely divide the liver into masses of irregular size—hepar lobatum (Fig. 27-60). In other instances the crevices are not so deep, but stringy adhesions may bridge the indentations. More rarely, the liver is deformed by linear depressions. This occurs alone or in combination with the deeply scarred organ. Beneath these linear deformities are bands of connective tissue that do not have the appearance of healed gummas. In hepar lobatum syphiliticum, there may be little more than the normal amount of connective tissue or, on the contrary, the connective tissue may be diffusely increased.

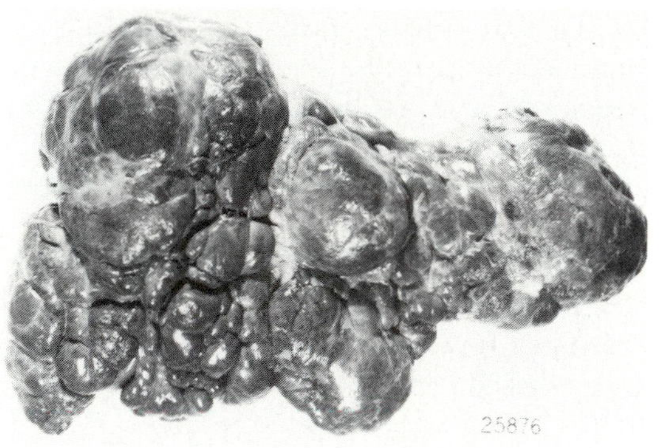

Fig. 27-60. Deeply scarred liver (hepar lobatum syphiliticum) that weighed only 710 g. Patient was 79-year-old white woman, known syphilitic, who had received some antisyphilitic therapy 3 years before death. Several large hyperplastic nodules are present. Stringy adhesions bridge some deep transverse fissures.

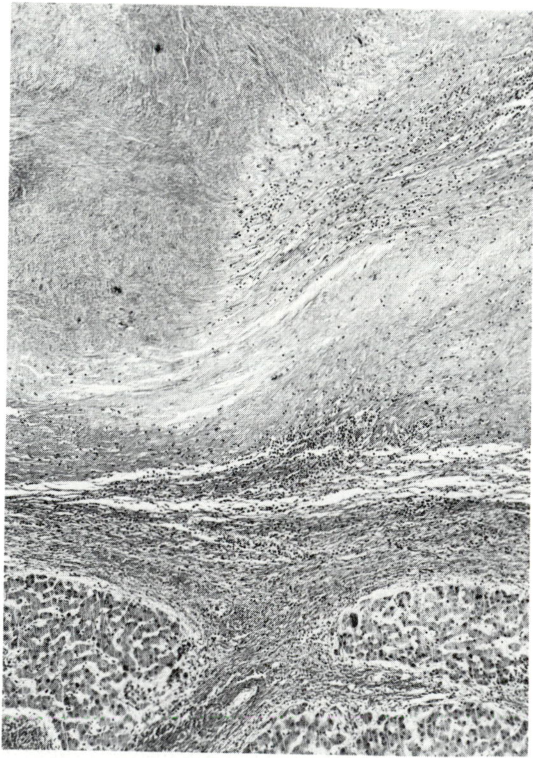

Fig. 27-61. Margin of gumma showing irregular outline, sparsity of epithelioid cells, and zone of granulation tissue. Patient was 41-year-old woman who died of massive gastrointestinal hemorrhage; syphilis was not diagnosed before death.

Microscopically in the gummatous stage there are isolated areas of necrosis surrounded by granulation tissue relatively poor in fibroblasts and usually sparse in epithelioid cells (Fig. 27-61). The granulation tissue impinges on the liver parenchyma, and necrosis of the latter appears to occur at this junction. Lymphocytes and plasma cells are common, both around the areas of gummatous necrosis and along the portal tracts. Later, wide bands of scar tissue are irregularly distributed throughout the liver, sometimes in combination with unhealed gummas.

Amyloidosis

In systemic amyloidosis the liver is commonly involved. Usually, however, there is only symptomless hepatomegaly that may be accompanied by bromosulfophthalein retention and increase in serum alkaline phosphatase.[734,746] Rarely jaundice and even ascites may occur, both of which are poor prognostic signs. Amyloidosis occurs in about equal frequency in primary (immunocyte dyscrasia with amyloidosis) and secondary (reactive systemic amyloidosis).[725] Grossly the liver is large, firm, much lighter in color than normal, and waxy in appearance. Microscopically amyloid may be predominantly intralobular (reticular), portal (collagenous), or globular in form. Amyloidosis that produces symptoms is usually of the intralobular variety. The amyloid is deposited in Disse's space, and the hepatocytes are severely compressed or may nearly disappear.[741] Cholestasis is noted in the few patients who are jaundiced.[746] Portal amyloidosis involves the blood vessels and is symptomless, but the distribution pattern is that seen in patients with plasma cell dyscrasias. The third type of amyloidosis of the liver is the recently reported globular form that may be associated with systemic amyloid involvement, including adrenal glands and kidneys.[724,728] Globular amyloid has not been associated with dysproteinemia or myeloma; similarly, intralobular (reticular) amyloid seems unassociated with myeloma. An immense amount of research has been done on the biochemistry, fine structure, and classification of amyloidosis (see p. 90).[726]

Parasitic cirrhosis

Although many different species of parasites may cause infestation of the liver, *Schistosoma mansoni* and *S. japonicum* are most likely to cause chronic liver disease, even cirrhosis. It has been estimated that 100 million people have schistosomiasis and that portal hypertension with esophageal varices is probably present in several million patients.[753] The pathology of all parasitic diseases is described in Chapter 12. The pathology of schistosomiasis was first described in Egypt in 1904. The pipestem fibrosis of schistosomiasis causes a presinusoidal bloc in the absence of any marked changes in liver function tests.[732,753]

CONGENITAL AND ACQUIRED ABNORMALITIES OF FORM AND POSITION

Congenital abnormalities of the liver are uncommon. Reidel's lobe is a downward projection of the right lobe, which may be mistaken for a tumor or believed to be a displaced kidney. The liver may be displaced in position in association with a congenital diaphragmatic hernia. Severe abnormalities that require surgery are seen rarely.[759] Supradiaphragmatic accessory liver lobes have been described.[761] Although rare, accessory lobes within the abdomen may occur.[760]

Aberrant adrenal tissue is sometimes seen beneath the capsule of the right lobe, and at least one functioning adrenocortical tumor of the liver has been reported.[757]

Acquired abnormalities of position are mainly downward or upward displacement by some extrahepatic cause, such as a subdiaphragmatic abscess or an abdominal tumor. Abnormalities of form may be the result of contraction of scar tissue (for example, hepar lobatum), nodularity from irregular regenerative hyperplasia, or neoplastic growth. Transverse, oblique, or sagittal grooves on the upper or anterior surface of the liver are common. They have been attributed to pressure of the ribs, folds of the diaphragm, and tight clothing. They are often associated with chronic cough, emphysema, and bronchitis caused by pressure from hypertrophied diaphragmatic muscle bundles. The capsule is thickened at the depths of the folds, and adjacent hepatic parenchyma may show slight atrophic changes. Such grooving does not appear to be of any functional significance.

Atrophy may affect only a liver segment or lobe. Certain diseases, especially alcoholic liver disease, chronic active hepatitis with cirrhosis, and hydatid disease, may bring about this change. Severe atrophy is chiefly caused by vascular or biliary obstruction, direct hepatic cell injury, or combinations of these factors. In some patients there are problems in diagnosis and treatment.[758] In our patients atrophy of the left lobe in alcoholic liver disease is the most common example. It is important to remedy any correctable cause when such changes are seen at surgery.

NEEDLE BIOPSIES

The indications for a needle biopsy of the liver are continually undergoing revision as more refined methods of diagnosing liver disease appear. However, in many patients indications for needle biopsy do exist, even after the most elaborate clinical and laboratory study. Included in these indications is hepatomegaly, especially when amyloidosis or cancer is suspected. Unexplained jaundice and abnormal liver tests constitute another category. The presence or absence of cirrhosis in chronic liver disease and the stage of cirrhosis if present are of importance to the clinicians. Repeated biopsies to monitor the course of certain diseases, such as chronic viral hepatitis, are indicated in some cases. Among the contraindications are prothrombin activity less than 40%, thrombocytopenia less than 60,000/mm^3, suspected vascular tumor, abscess or hepatic rupture, ascites, and extrahepatic bile duct obstruction. The most common complication of a needle biopsy is hemorrhage. Microscopic interpretation depends on an adequate biopsy specimen, sometimes defined as a specimen 2 cm long that contains at least five triads. Recently needle aspiration has become useful in diagnosis of hepatic tumors, particularly when guided by ultrasonography.[763]

Interpretation of needle biopsies

First each anatomic subunit is carefully scrutinized for normality. The structures in the triads must be recognized and studied. The size of the hepatic artery approaches that of the bile duct, whereas the portal vein branch is much larger. The connective tissue within the portal triad is scanty in infants, develops with maturity, and often increases moderately in old age. The borderline between a normal and an abnormal amount of portal lymphoid issue is difficult to establish. The triads may be considered somewhat analogous to the submucosa of the gut, where the lymphoid tissue has the capacity to become hyperplastic under conditions that cause lymphoid hyperplasia elsewhere. Such hyperplasia may widen the triads, but the limiting plate is intact. Although lymphoid and reticular elements may proliferate, follicles rarely appear. In the absence of intralobular disease, this hyperplasia should not be considered an infiltrate or exudate, and the term "triaditis" is misapplied to this nonspecific lymphoid response.

The lobules are examined for size, cord pattern, sinusoidal appearance, and the presence of central veins. Individual attention must be given to the hepatocytes, bile canaliculi, and Kupffer cells.

Normally, hepatocytes do not differ greatly from one biopsy to another. In old age, atrophy of the cells, as well as decrease in individual size, may decrease lobular diameter. Liver cells may lose glycogen and appear shrunken in starvation, in conditions causing negative nitrogen balance, and in biliary tract obstruction. Although hydropic change in any one of many acute liver diseases is discussed elsewhere, a similar abnormality occurs in patients with a high fever, in a liver undergoing regeneration, and in diabetic patients treated for hyperglycemia in whom there is a strong glycogen influx. There may be considerable variation in hepatocytic nuclear size, both in specific diseases such as viral hepatitis and in nonspecific reactions. Often perivenular liver cells have numerous polyploid nuclei that may be related to an abortive attempt at regeneration in those who are extremely ill, elderly, or undergoing chemotherapy. Vacuolated glycogen-filled nuclei are observed in a variety of metabolic disorders, especially in diabetic patients.

Kupffer cells, as part of the reticuloendothelial system, may increase in any chronic inflammatory reaction. Inflammatory conditions within the liver, extrahepatic infections, and fever of unknown origin may be responsible for Kupffer cell hyperplasia.

The differential diagnosis of cholestasis often arises in the various forms of acute liver disease. Rarely is viral hepatitis difficult to diagnose, but the differentiation between drug-induced jaundice, extrahepatic biliary obstruction, and simple cholestasis is often difficult or impossible. In extrahepatic bile duct obstruction, the prominence of the small interlobular bile ducts, infiltration of a few circumductal neutrophils, and perivenular cholestasis are most often seen.

In the incipient stages of primary biliary cirrhosis, cholestasis is usually absent, and the early destruction or even absence of interlobular bile ducts are the only findings. Since there is excess copper storage in chronic cholestastic disorders, a copper stain should be performed. In drug cholestasis the findings are variable, but usually the inflammatory changes in and around the small bile ducts are absent. Simple perivenular bile stasis is seen in some forms of drug jaundice, occasionally in heart failure, and in some instances of metastatic carcinoma of the liver.

A perivenular type of zonal necrosis may occur after exposure to halothane anesthesia, ingestion of carbon tetrachloride, or drug therapy and is occasionally seen in a needle biopsy. Peripheral lobular change attributable to phosphorus or to eclampsia is extremely rare. In a small percentage of biopsy specimens, occasional foci of cellular dropout marked by a few round cells are present, usually with mild Kupffer cell hyperplasia. An increase in round cells in the portal areas is often present. These specimens are taken, as a rule, from febrile patients who have minimal or no laboratory evidence of liver disease. No etiologic factors have been established.

Because of the small size of a needle biopsy, the diagnosis of cirrhosis should be made with care unless unequivocal septa and nodules are seen. The diagnosis of specific types of cirrhosis may or may not be possible. In alcoholic liver disease the fatty change and sclerosis of the perivenular area are the most helpful criteria. In chronic active hepatitis the diffuse round cell infiltrate, continuing focal necrosis, and areas of collapse are the chief indicators. Septa and nodules composed of fairly normal hepatocytes without infiltrate suggest cryptogenic cirrhosis. In primary biliary cirrhosis the lack of bile ducts and periportal cholestasis accompanied by penetration of the lobules by proliferating connective tissue should be kept in mind. Biopsy specimens from patients with cirrhosis often contain only fragments of pseudolobules, apparently because the needle fails to penetrate thick septa. These fragments are often larger than normal lobules and contain no bile ducts. A few islands of liver cell cancer present among cirrhotic nodules on a biopsy are easy to overlook.

Granulomas are discussed elsewhere in this chapter. Occasionally there is only a solitary lesion, best seen in only one fragment.

Increased quantities of intracytoplasmic pigment may pose a diagnostic problem. Since it is not always possible to distinguish parenchymal cell iron from lipochrome, an iron stain should be performed. Iron deposition is usually greatest in the periportal zones. Lipochrome predominates in the perivenular areas. A large quantity of fine brown pigment is usually lipochrome and of no diagnostic concern, but, occasionally, such pigment is seen in patients who have ingested large quantities of analgesic compounds containing phenacetin, salicylate, and caffeine. The chronic use of cascara compounds also may cause a pigmented liver. Large globules of pigment are seen in Dubin-Johnson syndrome (Fig. 27-49). Recently lipofuscinosis of the liver was reported in patients with a specific central nervous system disease.[762]

Mild degrees of passive congestion, indicated by dilatation of the terminal hepatic veins and sinusoids, should always be reported. Needle biopsies rarely are performed on patients with advanced passive congestion. Marked congestion with disappearance of liver cells and conversion of large portions of the lobules to blood channels is seen in Budd-Chiari syndrome and radiation damage of the liver. An unusually intense congestion with preservation of cord pattern occasionally is observed in sickle cell disease. The sickled cells form sludged lumps and are unable to move through the sinusoids in a normal manner.

When all structures appear normal, a diagnosis of "needle biopsy of liver, apparently normal" can be made. This does not mean, however, that a local lesion, such as a neoplasm or abscess, might not be present a few centimeters from the location where the specimen was taken.

Any abnormalities noted in the specimen should be carefully described and reported to the clinician, along with the pathologist's interpretation. Some lesions are specific and may involve only a single microscopic subunit, such as Gaucher's disease and polyarteritis nodosa. Others, such as neoplasms and amyloidosis, have identifiable features that allow a positive diagnosis. However, in most diseases seen on biopsy, there is more than one microscopic alteration, so that a discussion of the diagnostic probabilities is in order. Such suggestions are often helpful to the clinician.

DIFFERENTIAL DIAGNOSIS OF JAUNDICE

A rise in either the indirect- or direct-reacting bilirubin fraction in the blood results in yellow pigmentation of the skin or jaundice. More than 97.5% of normal persons have serum bilirubin levels between 0.1 and 1 mg/dl. Although a serum bilirubin above 1.2 mg/dl is abnormal, jaundice does not become manifest until a level of 2 mg/dl or more is reached. Since jaundice is dependent on bilirubin in tissue fluids, there may be a lag between the rise of the serum bilirubin level and evident jaundice. Minimal jaundice is best detected by examination of sclerae. Because bilirubin has an affinity for elastic connective tissue, these structures are more deeply pigmented (Plate 5, *D*). However, in severe jaundice the skin, interstitial fluids, and most of the body tissue (with the exception of the central nervous system) become bile stained. In chronic jaundice the skin may appear a deep green-yellow, and in a few instances an increase in melanin may result in dark brown to black skin.

Pigments other than bilirubin may cause a yellow skin. Patients who ingest large quantities of carrots or carrot juice may have carotenemia. This pigment is best seen in the palms of the hands but not in the sclerae. Quinacrine hydrochloride (Atabrine), an antimalarial drug, also is capable of causing a yellow skin, as is dinitrophenol.

When confronted with a jaundiced patient, the physician has the responsibility of making an etiologic diagnosis as quickly as possible. The use of the terms *medical jaundice* and *surgical jaundice* emphasizes the importance of etiology. Medical jaundice is caused by hepatocellular diseases, most commonly viral hepatitis and drug-induced changes in patients under 40 years of age. Surgical jaundice is related to obstruction of the extrahepatic biliary tract, seen most often after 40 years of age. Jaundice may occur in cirrhosis in all age groups.

A careful history and physical examination, followed by the performance of certain essential hepatic tests, usually lead to a correct diagnosis. The patient should be questioned about exposure to other jaundiced individuals and about transfusions and needle sharing, all high-risk factors for contracting viral hepatitis. Further questioning about ingestion of hepatotoxic drugs or exposure to hepatotoxic chemicals is necessary.

A family history of jaundice may suggest an inheritable disease or a common infective, toxic, or dietary disorder. Questions regarding alcohol intake are important but often are ignored in the private hospital. Travel outside the United States may point to hepatitis A. If pain is present, its location, type, severity, and areas of radiation are important. The patient should be questioned about pruritus and a change in stool color. The presence or absence of previous attacks of jaundice should be ascertained. Neoplasms usually cause an unremitting jaundice, whereas calculus obstruction, cirrhosis, and chronic active hepatitis are usually intermittent.

On physical examination the size and consistency of the liver and the presence or absence of tenderness, nodules, or masses should be determined. A normal liver may extend below the costal margin but is too soft to palpate. The cirrhotic liver has a firm, palpable edge. Even in advanced cirrhosis when the liver is contracted, the lower margin may be felt on deep inspiration. In early to moderate cirrhosis the liver is usually enlarged and the edge may be as low as the umbilicus. A small liver rarely is associated with biliary tract obstruction but often is the result of liver cell necrosis. Careful palpation for an enlarged gallbladder, splenomegaly, and minimal ascites is likewise helpful in diagnosis. Splenomegaly, ascites, and many vascular spiders suggest chronic liver disease in the jaundiced patient. Primary carcinoma of the gallbladder may produce a hard palpable organ that is associated with jaundice as the initial symptom. A tense distended gallbladder favors neoplastic obstruction rather than choledocholithiasis. In cholelithiasis the gallbladder usually becomes too fibrotic to undergo distension when the common bile duct is obstructed by a stone.

Usually no single laboratory test is relied on to diagnose the cause of jaundice, but certain combinations of abnormal tests (Table 27-1) help to delineate various subgroups that narrow the possibilities to be considered by the clinician. The total serum bilirubin, as well as the direct- and indirect-reacting fractions, always is determined. The test is usually performed at frequent intervals to provide valuable information as to the course of the disease.

Jaundice may be associated with an elevation of the indirect-reacting fraction of the serum bilirubin or, far more commonly, an elevation of both the direct- and indirect-reacting fractions. The Van de Bergh reactions show that only a few diseases cause an excess of indirect-reacting bilirubin alone in the adult. Among these is the excess production of bilirubin that follows severe hemolysis. Congenital hemolytic anemia, mismatched blood transfusions, and severe hemorrhage into tissues or body cavities are examples. A different etiology is noted in Gilbert's disease, in which there is a failure to remove a normal quantity of unconjugated bilirubin from the blood. Jaundice caused by a lack of UDP–glucuronyl transferase (Crigler-Najjar disease) may occur in both infants and adults.

The drug novobiocin may inhibit glucuronyl transferase and thus cause an unconjugated hyperbilirubinemia. Occasionally patients with alcoholic cirrhosis may have a predominance of indirect-reacting bilirubin that is often associated with spur cell anemia or hypersplenism. Since the unconjugated bilirubin does not filter through the glomerulus, there is no bilirubinuria as is seen in jaundice caused by conjugated hyperbilirubinemia.

In most cases of jaundice (that is, those caused by viral hepatitis, cirrhosis, biliary tract obstruction, and drugs), there is an increase in both direct- and indirect-reacting bilirubin. Indirect-reacting bilirubin is usually about 50% of the total bilirubin. The level of the total bilirubin may bear some relationship to the severity of disease in patients with liver cell necrosis and obstruction of bile ducts but is more useful in following the course of the disorder. Declining levels of the serum bilirubin reflect the healing phase of hepatitis, drug jaundice, and other disorders. The level of the serum bilirubin is regulated not only by degree of hepatic dysfunction and red cell destruction but also by rate of excretion of the water-soluble conjugated fraction in the urine. This fraction binds to albumin and is not freely excreted. For unknown reasons, the direct-reacting bilirubin may rise to higher levels in parenchymal cell disease than in obstructive disease. Although biliuria is prominent early in viral hepatitis, a decrease occurs as jaundice deepens, even though the direct-reacting bilirubin in serum rises.

Patients with hyperbilirubinemia who have greatly elevated serum transaminase levels and little or no rise in the alkaline phosphatase level are considered to have liver cell necrosis or hepatocellular jaundice. Viral hepatitis, chemicals, poisons, and certain drugs must be considered in a differential diagnosis. In some instances a rise in alkaline phosphatase occurs in viral hepatitis and may, in older patients, be difficult to differentiate from obstructive biliary tract disease, particularly if the patient's disease is at the stage in which serum aminotransferase levels have dropped to a range of 500 units or less. Patients in shock or severe heart failure may have hypoxic perivenular necrosis associated with high serum aminotransferase levels and jaundice, but usually the bilirubin levels are in the range of 5 mg/dl or less.

An increase in serum bilirubin levels accompanied by a high alkaline phosphatase level usually is associated with intrahepatic or extrahepatic biliary obstruction. Although extrahepatic biliary obstruction caused by stone, cancer, or stricture is a well-known cause of jaundice with a high alkaline phosphatase level, the possibility of drug-induced liver disease must always be ruled out. On occasion, obstructive disease may be accompanied by a moderate rise in serum aminotransferase levels (Table 27-1). The prothrombin activity may be reduced in either hepatocellular or prolonged obstructive disease. Administration of parenteral vitamin K corrects prothrombin deficiency induced by biliary tract obstruction but has little effect on the impairment caused by liver cell necrosis.

The diagnosis of obstructive biliary disease and its differentiation from cholestatic drug jaundice, primary biliary cirrhosis, and other forms of medical jaundice can now be made in nearly 100% of cases by clinical means plus certain noninvasive and invasive tests. Patients with choledocholithiasis tend to have a painful disorder often associated with cholangitis that produces bed-shaking chills, fever, and a high incidence of gram-negative bacteremia. Similar episodes of cholangitis may develop in the patient with a bile duct stricture but are uncommon in those with a malignant obstruction. The clinical background of patients with PBC and drug jaundice is described elsewhere in this chapter. A logical approach to the use of important diagnostic noninvasive and invasive aids has been published.[764,765] Aids include a plain roentgenogram of the abdomen, gray-scale ultrasonography, computed tomography, transhepatic cholangiography, and ERCP. Ultrasonography, a noninvasive technique, has been reported to show dilated bile ducts in obstructive disease in some 95% of cases, computed tomography is accurate in 90%, and transhepatic cholangiography, an invasive technique, is nearly 100% successful in diagnosing obstruction of the extrahepatic biliary tract.

Occasionally more than one etiologic factor is responsible for the presence of jaundice. Examples are post-traumatic jaundice and benign postoperative cholestasis. Many of these patients have a complicated postoperative course or soft tissue injuries. Sepsis may be present and blood transfusions may have been given. Patients with the benign type of postoperative jaundice may be deeply jaundiced, but their transaminase and alkaline phosphatase levels show little change. Usually the only diagnostic test necessary is ultrasonography for evaluation of the extrahepatic and intrahepatic bile duct system.[765] Among the rare causes of postoperative jaundice is fat embolism.[766]

Benign recurrent intrahepatic cholestasis is a rare disease characterized by attacks of jaundice that usually last from 2 to 3 months and seem to have a seasonal occurrence. Liver biopsies disclose severe cholestasis, predominantly centrilobular. Patients feel well between attacks, and there is no progression of the disease.[768]

Patients with sickle cell disease may have brief periods of jaundice known as a hepatic crisis. In this disorder bile stasis is only occasionally seen. A more serious disorder concerns the entity of sickle cell intrahepatic cholestasis, which has a high fatality rate. Sickled erythrocytes obstruct the hepatic sinusoids. The Kupffer cells undergo hypertrophy, and the canaliculi contain bile plugs. Treatment by exchange transfusion has been recommended.[767]

The presence of underlying chronic liver disease in the jaundiced patient usually is manifested by a low serum albumin and a high serum globulin. An enlarged firm liver, splenomegaly, vascular spiders, and ascites are nearly conclusive evidence of chronicity. The first symptom of chronic active hepatitis and alcoholic liver disease may be jaundice, even though chronic liver disease already is present. The jaundice that occurs in the patient with chronic liver disease is usually of limited duration, but more than one episode is not uncommon.

The diagnosis, care, and management of the jaundiced patient remain a challenge to the clinical acuity of the physician. This has been true for over 100 years, since the pioneers in the study of liver disease first published their observations.

LIVER DISEASE IN NONHEPATIC DISORDERS

Cirrhosis and other lesions may complicate the course of other serious diseases that are systemic or that primarily involve another organ or organ system in the body. Liver abnormalities are common in patients with inflammatory bowel disease.[772] Ulcerative colitis may be associated with fatty change, portal inflammation and fibrosis, chronic active hepatitis (which may follow transfusion), granulomas, amyloidosis, cirrhosis, bile duct carcinoma, pericholangitis (intrahepatic sclerosing cholangitis), and panductal sclerosing cholangitis.[778,779] The most common single laboratory finding is an elevated alkaline phosphatase level that is not associated with the cholestasis.[783] In patients with Crohn's disease the liver changes may be similar to those in ulcerative colitis but occur with much less frequency.[774] Pericholangitis and fibrosis may lead to protracted jaundice and, finally, a biliary type of cirrhosis. The liver in both ulcerative colitis and Crohn's disease may have an increased copper content.[781] The liver in both has occasionally been reported to improve after removal of the diseased bowel but in most instances seems unrelated to the course or the treatment of the colon disorder.

Fatty change, pericentric fibrosis, and even intracellular Mallory bodies may be observed in diabetes mellitus. Whether there is a progression from fatty change and a variable degree of fibrosis to cirrhosis is yet to be determined. An increased incidence of cirrhosis in diabetics has been suggested, but this is controversial.[775] It is well known that patients with alcoholic cirrhosis may secondarily become diabetic. Hepatic dysfunction in rheumatoid arthritis is common but usually asymptomatic. A rise in alkaline phosphatase, retention of sulfobromophthalein, and hepatomegaly are the more common findings.[776,777] In addition, infiltration of the portal tracts with round cells,[773] PBC, amyloidosis, and other findings have been recorded. Rarely the hepatic arteries are affected by rheumatoid arteritis.[777] The existence of liver disease in patients with systemic lupus erythematosus has been noted. A wide variety of changes occur, sometimes progressing to cirrhosis.[782] Regional enteritis, scleroderma,[770] rheumatic fever, hyperthyroidism,[769] and various bacterial infections occasionally may be complicated by cirrhosis. A mild degree of cirrhosis is not infrequently noted in the liver of elderly persons. This seems to be a slowly progressive disease that occurs in patients in whom there are no etiologically demonstrable factors, except possibly poor eating habits. In Boeck's sarcoidosis, the lesions in the liver may progress to cirrhosis.[780] Sickle cell anemia may be complicated by an unexplained type of micronodular cirrhosis. Presumably this follows vascular obstruction by the sickled cells, necrosis of hepatocytes, fibrosis, and regeneration.[771] A hemochromotatic type of cirrhosis may also occur. There is also the complication that non-A, non-B hepatitis followed by cirrhosis may develop in patients who receive many transfusions related to nonhepatic diseases. Thus one must be cautious not to ascribe cirrhosis or chronic active hepatitis too freely to some of the above mentioned diseases. As an example, most cases of chronic active hepatitis associated with inflammatory bowel diseases are probably a result of posttransfusion chronic active hepatitis.

TUMORS AND TUMORLIKE LESIONS

The liver provides a suitable milieu for the growth of neoplastic cells, especially for metastatic tumor. In addition, the lymphomas, leukemias, and primary carcinoma all grow readily within this organ. Its size, anatomic location, dual blood supply, and the ready availability of nutritional material are factors that influence the deposition and growth of neoplasms. Between 40% and 50% of all primary cancers in the body are noted at death to have metastases within the liver.[809] Primary neoplasms and tumorlike lesions of liver occur much less frequently in the United States but nevertheless are important inasmuch as they may enter into the differential diagnosis of an enlarged liver noted clinically or observed at laparotomy. In Asia and Africa the most common malignant tumor is cancer originating in the liver. Hepatomegaly, often symptomless, is a common finding in neoplastic liver disease. Malignant tumors usually are associated with weight loss. Fever and jaundice are less common. Esophageal varices may occur as a complication of both primary and secondary tumors.[839] Laboratory findings often include an elevation of the serum alkaline phosphatase level and sulfobromophthalein retention. Angiograms, scintiscans, echograms, and computed tomography are useful in determining the size, number, and anatomic location of hepatic neoplasms.

Percutaneous fine-needle aspiration biopsy of the liver, guided by radioisotope scintigrams and the fluoroscope, has proved to be highly successful in the diagnosis of malignant tumors of the liver.[822]

Primary growths may arise from hepatic cells, bile duct epithelium, or mesodermal structures; except for cavernous hemangioma, benign tumors are uncommon and include cavernous hemangiomas, hemangioendotheliomas, bile duct adenomas and cystadenomas, and liver cell adenomas.

Benign tumors and tumorlike lesions of duct epithelium

Cysts

Cysts in the liver are commonly of three types: congenital, solitary, and hydatid *(Echinococcus)* (Fig. 27-62).

Congenital cysts. Congenital cysts are not common[851] but may be associated with congenital cystic disease of the kidneys or other organs. They are usually small and cause no disturbance; however, cysts of large size do occur, and patients may have an abdominal mass, hepatomegaly, and occasionally abdominal pain or jaundice.[879] The cysts are lined by flattened or cylindrical epithelium, may be prominent just under the capsule, and contain clear fluid (Fig. 27-63). In some instances small gray-white areas are seen throughout the liver, and the cysts are barely visible or are of microsopic size. In this microcystic form of polycystic disease, the tubules are surrounded by dense connective tissue and may contain bile pigment. On rare occasions the amount of connective tissue and number of ducts are so great that entire lobules are surrounded, a condition known as congenital hepatic fibrosis (see pp. 1153 and 1163).[169]

Solitary or nonparasitic cysts. Solitary or nonparasitic cysts occur at any age but mostly in middle-aged women (male/female ratio is 4 or 5:1). Abdominal enlargement and a palpable mass are the usual findings. Jaundice is rare.[844] The cysts usually have a bluish appearance when seen beneath Glisson's capsule and may reach a diameter of 15 to 20 cm. They have a low columnar to cuboid epithelial lining and are filled with serous fluid. Occasionally a cyst is lined with squamous epithelium, or it is difficult to find any well-preserved epithelium. The wall is composed of compact fibrous tissue with an outer well-vascularized layer. Surgical treatment of symptomatic cysts has been successful.[821]

Hydatid (Echinococcus) cysts. Hydatid *(Echinococcus)* cysts are discussed in Chapter 12.

Bile duct cystadenomas. Bile duct cystadenomas are noted almost exclusively in women, usually in the middle-aged group. They may grow to 15 to 18 cm in diameter, producing abdominal enlargement and sometimes pain. Usually the tumor is composed of cysts of variable size; occasionally there is one large cyst and several smaller ones. These multilocular lesions are lined with a columnar mucin-secreting epithelium that is often arranged in folds. The connective tissue stroma, especially in the subepithelial area, is densely cellular and often contains areas of old hemorrhage. A few have undergone malignant change. The treatment is surgery.[848] Ductal cystadenomas have been reported.[886]

Bile duct adenomas. Bile duct adenomas are firm,

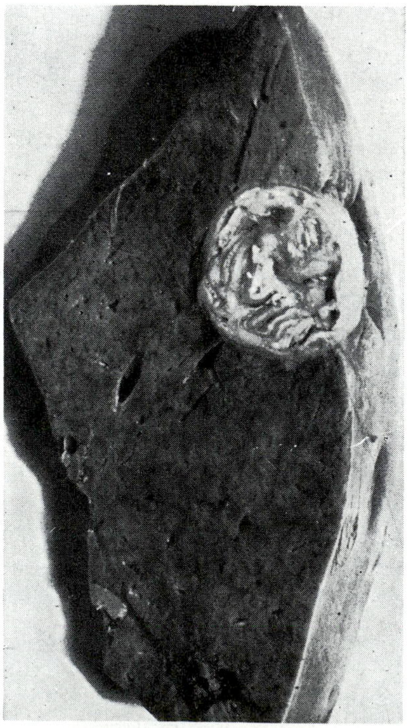

Fig. 27-62. *Echinococcus* cyst of liver. Note convoluted membranous content.

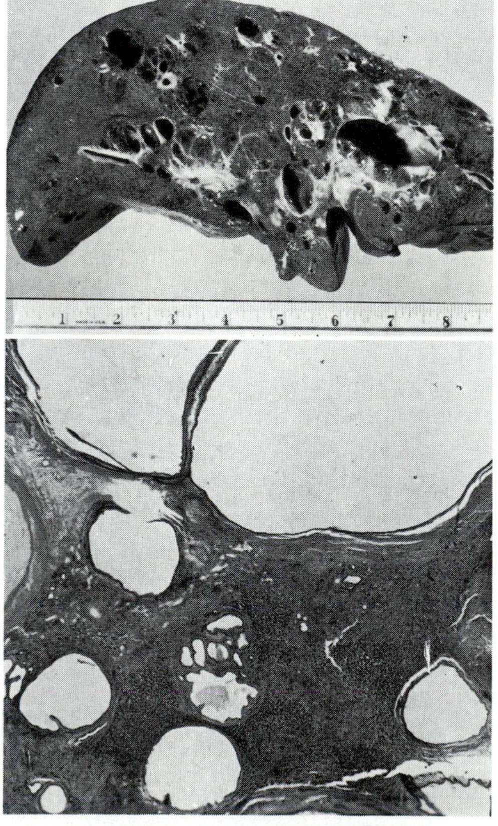

Fig. 27-63. Congenital cysts of liver.

gray-white areas, rarely over 1 cm in diameter, and usually located beneath Glisson's capsule. They are composed of a multitude of tiny acinar structures that are lined with a bile duct type of epithelium. The connective tissue stroma is sparse.

Benign tumors and tumorlike lesions of vascular origin

Cavernous hemangiomas. Cavernous hemangiomas usually are noted incidentally at necropsy, but a few become manifest clinically,[807,831] especially in multiparous women, possibly as a result of an increase of circulating estrogenic hormones during pregnancy. Angiomatous lesions of the gingiva and skin may likewise appear. Calcified hemangiomas of the liver have been reported in older women in association with hypertension.[871] Rarely a hemangioma may rupture into the peritoneal cavity, necessitating emergency surgery.[883] Surgery may also be necessary for large hemangiomas in adults[893] and for giant congenital hemangiomas.[849] Angiograms showing puddles of contrast material have proved most useful in the diagnosis of hemangiomas.[816]

Hemangiomas appear as circumscribed, dark red-purple areas that vary from a few millimeters to several centimeters in diameter. They may bulge beneath Glisson's capsule or may be located deep within the liver (Fig. 27-64, *A*). The presence of cavernous spaces gives them a spongy appearance. Microscopically the large, blood-filled spaces are lined by a single layer of endothelium and are separated by connective tissue that often has a myxomatous appearance (Fig. 27-64, *B*). Hemangiomas apparently grow for a limited length of time, and some eventually undergo fibrosis that obliterates the cavernous spaces. Rarely the liver may be diffusely involved by small hemangiomas. Steroid therapy has been used for cavernous hemangiomas in the newborn.[849]

Infantile hemangioendotheliomas. Infantile hemangioendotheliomas are congenital lesions that may be noted at birth or during the first 6 months of life or, rarely, up to 4½ years of age. Prematurity is common, and girls are affected more often than boys. The most common symptom is abdominal enlargement, but vascular arterial venous shunts within the lesions may cause congestive failure. The presence of a large liver, cutaneous hemangiomas, and congestive failure is considered diagnostic of the disease. Sequestration of platelets in the angiomas may cause thrombocytopenia. Scintigrams and angiograms may be used to establish the size and location of the tumors.[828,889,892] Radiotherapy,[878] prednisone,[863] or supportive treatment alone has been used successfully in the treatment of infantile hemangioendotheliomas.[797, 806]

Grossly, the liver most often contains multiple red nodules averaging 1.5 to 2 cm in diameter with uniform distribution. The tumors are rarely solitary. Microscopically hemangioendotheliomas are characterized by anastomosing vascular channels that are lined with one or more layers of hyperchromatic endothelial cells. The tumor grows along the sinusoids of the lobules, often replacing liver tissue. In a few cases malignant change has occurred.

Cystic lymphangiomatosis may involve the liver, spleen, and skeleton. The prognosis is poor, but some patients live to adult life. The liver contains innumerable endothelium-lined spaces filled with eosinophilic material.[788]

Peliosis hepatis is a rare, diffuse angiomatoid change of the liver.[908] Angiomatoid spaces filled with blood are distributed throughout the liver, varying in size from less than 1 mm to several centimeters. The pathogenesis is uncertain, but the disorder possibly stems from miliary necrosis. It may be innocuous, especially in patients who are not receiving any of the androgenic anabolic steroids; however, in the latter, patients may die of liver failure or rupture of one of the blood-filled spaces.[789] Peliosis hepatis may also be a fatal complication of Thorotrast-induced liver disease.[861] Peliosis hepatis has been known to regress with the discontinuation of androgenic steroid therapy.[856]

Peliosis hepatis must be distinguished from hereditary hemorrhagic telangiectasia (Osler-Rendu-Weber disease). In the latter there is ectasia of the blood vessels, in

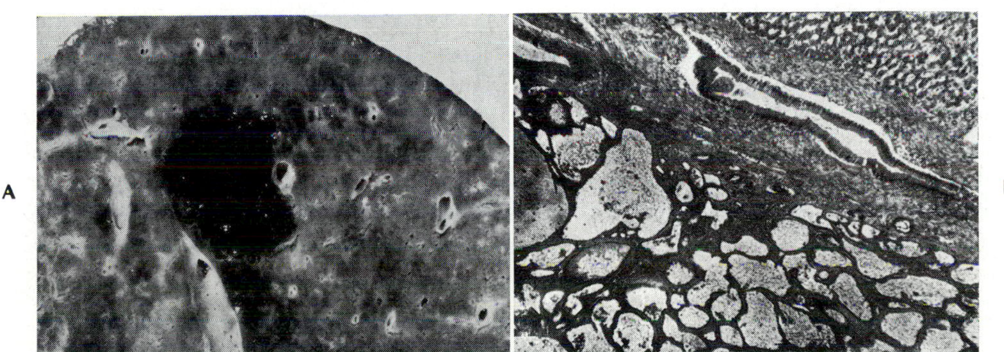

Fig. 27-64. A, Cavernous hemangioma of liver. **B,** Hepatic parenchyma at upper right.

both the portal and the intralobular areas. These vessels have a distinct endothelial lining and may be accompanied by fibrosis and occasionally by cirrhosis.[852] One patient with portal hypertension, a young woman taking oral contraceptives whose only histologic finding was peliosis hepatis, has been reported,[800] and peliosis hepatis has developed in some patients who have undergone renal transplantation.[804]

Benign hepatocellular tumors and tumorlike lesions

The benign hepatocellular tumors and tumorlike lesions include adenomas, focal nodular hyperplasia, adenomatous hyperplasia, and nodular regenerative hyperplasia.

Hepatocellular adenomas. Adenomas derived from hepatic cells were actually rare until the use of oral contraceptives. Since the first report of adenomas associated with the use of oral contraceptives in 1973, many similar cases have been published. Estrogen is believed to be responsible. In the United States the estimated risk in long-term users of low-potency oral contraceptives is 3.4 per 100,000.[877] The risk is greater in women over 30 years of age who have been taking oral contraceptives longer than 5 years. Liver cell adenomas following oral contraceptive use are usually solitary, but 10% are multiple. As a rule, they are encapsulated and somewhat lighter in color than the surrounding liver. About two thirds of the tumors have varying degrees of infarction and hemorrhage, particularly in their central portions (Fig. 27-65, *A*). Microscopically the neoplastic hepatocytes have a pronounced cordlike arrangement with tiny canaliculi (Fig. 27-65, *B*). Bile formation and fatty change are sometimes observed. There are no bile ducts or other evidence of portal structures.

A high percentage of adenomas that occur during pregnancy or the postpartum period may rupture.[833] Regression usually but not always occurs when oral contraceptives are discontinued.[811,846] A new tumor develops in 25% of women who resume oral contraceptive use after surgery for an adenoma.[877] A few adenomas in women not taking contraceptives have been reported. These rarely undergo infarction and hemorrhage. Hepatocellular carcinoma may occur in young women who are taking oral contraceptives.[857] Some of these may have areas of benign adenoma.[898] The etiologic relationship of oral contraceptives to liver cell carcinoma is not clear.

Androgen-induced primary tumors have followed the use of oxymetholone and methyltestosterone in the treatment of Fanconi's anemia, aplastic anemia, cryptorchidism, male impotence, and female-to-male transsexualism. Many of these have been reported as benign hepatomas but apparently are adenomas.[793,864] The majority of the patients have been young men. Many of these adenomas are characterized by large acinar formations, thus differing markedly from the estrogen-induced adenomas. Androgen-associated tumors tend to regress on cessation of therapy.

Multiple adenomas of the liver are common in patients with glycogen-storage disease type Ia; by the middle teenage years, nearly all such patients have evidence of tumors on scintigrams. These have been shown to regress when the patient's hypoglycemia is controlled by nocturnal feedings.[865] Multiple adenomas are also seen in infants with tyrosinemia. These often become malignant.[907]

Focal nodular hyperplasia. Focal nodular hyperplasia occurs predominantly in women between 20 and 50 years of age, the average age being about 32 years. In focal nodular hyperplasia, there is a firm, circumscribed, gray-brown tumor that usually measures 1 to 8 cm in diameter. It is always lighter in color than the surrounding liver. Although sharply circumscribed, the tumors do not have a true capsule. They may be single or multiple. Most often they are seen beneath the liver capsule, but they can arise deep within the liver.

Rarely are the tumors pedunculated. Ordinarily there is a stellate mass of connective tissue in the center of the lesion with radiation of the connective tissue toward the periphery. The nodules are composed of fairly normal-appearing liver cells arranged in small pseudolobules. Often the liver cells are arranged in individual units that surround small transformed ducts and vessels. The larger lesions have an abundant arterial supply.

Increase in the frequency of focal nodular hyperplasia in women taking oral contraceptives is yet to be proved. Liver scans and angiograms are helpful in distinguishing focal nodular hyperplasia from adenomas.[814,835] An occasional tumor has ruptured, and surgical removal has been performed on several occasions. The liver in these patients may also be extensively involved by nodular regenerative hyperplasia,[896] discussed in the following.

Adenomatous hyperplasia. In both cirrhosis and submassive necrosis, large nodules of adenomatous hyperplasia may occur. These may assume tumorlike proportions and become palpable. Sometimes this has led to unnecessary surgery. The large areas of hyperplasia that occur after submassive necrosis are usually lighter in color and sometimes bile stained. They stand out in sharp contrast to the surrounding dark-brown collapsed parenchyma. Areas of adenomatous hyperplasia in cirrhosis may reach a size of several centimeters. These are outlined by surrounding septa that contain blood vessels and bile ducts and thus do not form a true capsule. Adenomatous hyperplasia differs from a true adenoma in that small bile ducts and blood vessels ramify into its interior from the periphery. The same is true of adenomatous hyperplasia in submassive necrosis. Large areas of hyperplasia in regenerating liver have a characteristic angiographic pattern.[875]

Nodular regenerative hyperplasia. Nodular regenera-

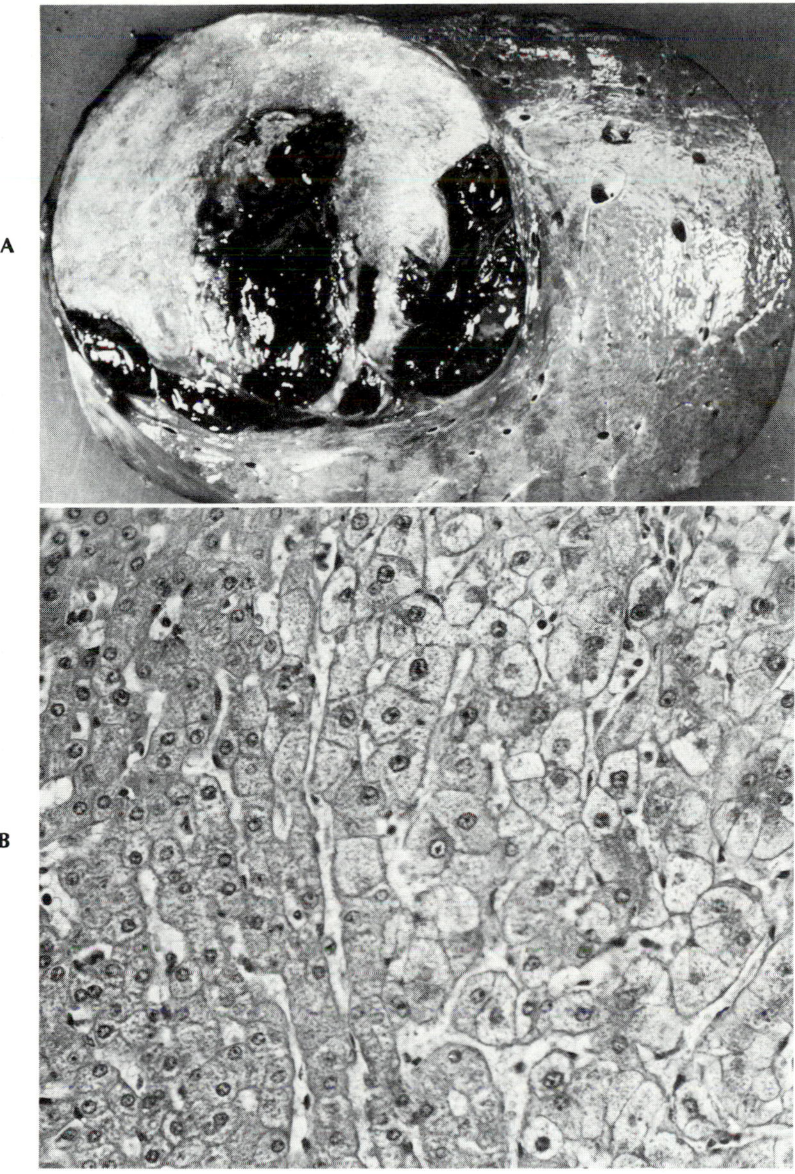

Fig. 27-65. Hepatic adenoma. **A,** Grossly mass is well defined with hemorrhage into tumor. **B,** Microscopically there is transition zone between adjacent liver and adenoma cells. Note larger size of adenoma cells and more distinct cord arrangement around canaliculi.

tive hyperplasia, also known as noncirrhotic nodulation and nodular transformation, is an uncommon condition in which nodules are formed in the liver without fibrous septa. It may occur as a complication of rheumatoid arthritis (especially Felty's syndrome), heart disease, drug therapy of many years' duration, immunologic dysfunction, diabetes mellitus,[900] and extrahepatic neoplasm.[894] In patients taking androgenic steroids the hyperplastic lesions may be present with or without liver cell adenomas. Grossly the liver is involved by a multitude of small hyperplastic lesions that vary from 1 mm to 4 or 5 mm in diameter and occasionally up to 1 cm or more (Fig. 27-66). The nodules are lighter colored than the normal liver. Grossly the liver may appear either cirrhotic or filled with neoplasms. Microscopically the lesion may be overlooked, since the nodules are composed of rounded masses of hepatocytes that compress surrounding parenchyma in a subtle fashion without collapse or fibrous septa. They are best demonstrated with a reticulum stain. The disease may be an incidental finding, or it may be associated with noncirrhotic portal hypertension, varices, splenomegaly, and ascites. It has been suggested that intrahepatic portal vein radicals are occluded in nodular regenerative hyperplasia,[906] making its pathogenesis similar to that suggested for idiopathic portal hypertension, which also has irregular arrange-

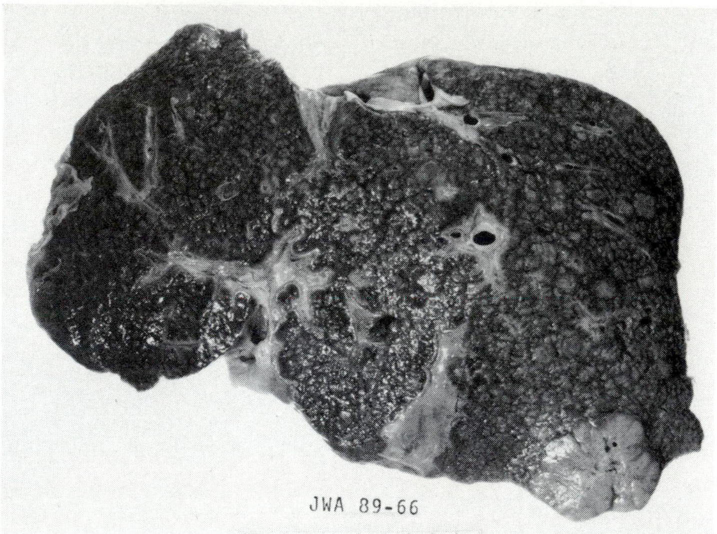

Fig. 27-66. Light yellow nodules of regenerative hyperplasia are present throughout liver.

ment of components of the liver lobules but does not have true nodularity.

Mesenchymal hamartoma. Mesenchymal hamartomas are gray-white to red-purple cystlike lesions that most often arise at the lower margin of the right lobe of the liver in the first 2 years of life. They tend to grow rapidly because of accumulation of fluid in the cystlike areas, often causing respiratory distress and occasionally edema of the lower extremities because of pressure on the inferior vena cava.[891] Surgical excision has proved successful.

Microscopically hamartomas are composed of remnants of triads with bile ducts, periportal hepatocytes, and fluid-filled spaces.[808] Electron microscopic studies disclose that the bile ducts and hepatocytes are typical of those in the normal liver, whereas the myxomatous foci consist of fibroblasts, mature collagen, and a few endothelium-lined spaces.[805] It is probable that these lesions represent an abnormal development of mesenchymal tissue in the infant.[808]

Primary carcinoma

Carcinoma primary in the liver occupies a unique position among neoplasms because of its propensity for arising in an organ that is already severely damaged by another disease—cirrhosis. Of the hepatocellular carcinomas studied in our liver unit, 77% arose in cirrhotic livers, 9% in what might be characterized as precirrhotic livers, and 14% in normal livers. Carcinomas most often are derived from hepatocytes, but a small percentage (less than 20%) are of bile duct origin. The preferred term for malignant tumors derived from hepatocytes is hepatocellular carcinoma (HCC), not "primary" hepatocellular carcinoma, a clearly redundant term, but one that with "hepatoma" and "liver cell carcinoma" continues to be used in the literature. There has been great interest in hepatic tumors over the past few decades but especially in recent years because of recognition of the part that hepatitis B virus plays in the etiology of HCC, particularly in the Orient and in Africa, where HCC is the leading malignant tumor. Hormones and environmental toxins may play additional roles. Incidence of HCC is reported to be between 0.2 per 100,000 population (about 0.1% of autopsies) in the British Isles[786] and about 173 per 100,000 in Taiwan.[790] Over a 60-year period in autopsies in Los Angeles, HCC has been found in 0.3% (0.15% in and before 1953, 0.88% by 1978); it comprises 1.8% of the malignant tumors studied at autopsy. In the Philippines, 4.5% of the deaths from malignancy are from HCC[843]; in Taiwan, 20% of all malignancies in both sexes combined are HCC.[907]

The second major type of carcinoma primary in the liver arises from or resembles bile duct epithelium and is called cholangiocarcinoma. Cholangiocarcinomas may arise at any point in the biliary tree: those arising at or near the level of interlobular ducts are called peripheral cholangiocarcinomas (PCC); the rare instances of primary tumor in the major intrahepatic ducts are called cholangiocarcinoma of right or left hepatic duct; those at the bifurcation of the common hepatic duct are called hilar cholangiocarcinomas. The carcinomas arising in the remaining extrahepatic duct system are collectively called extrahepatic cholangiocarcinomas. A rare intrahepatic tumor that resembles the epithelium of the cholangiole throughout the tumor is called cholangiolocellular carcinoma.

Many hepatic carcinomas have tumor cells resembling hepatocytes with ductal elements also present; occasionally the ductal elements comprise the major portion of the tumor. Many tumors with a continuum between hepatocyte and duct epithelium arise predominantly in the setting of hepatocellular carcinomas. Because the biologic activity of the tumor more closely resembles hepatocellular carcinoma, we have considered such tumors to be HCC, reserving the term *combined* for cases in which there are separate HCC and peripheral cholangiocarcinomas in the same liver.

PCC is much less common than HCC, representing only 10% of liver cancers at our hospital but 16% in Japan. There is no apparent relationship between cholangiocarcinomas and hepatitis B virus.

Clinically HCC or PCC complicating cirrhosis is difficult to distinguish from cirrhosis alone. An enlarged abdominal mass, pain in the right upper quadrant (often severe), weight loss, rapidly accumulating ascites, and blood-stained ascitic fluid on paracentesis point toward a diagnosis of carcinoma of the liver. Jaundice is usually not severe and occurs in a third or less of patients. The liver is enlarged and is hard and tender in nearly every symptomatic patient. The tumor has often been present in the liver for years before symptoms develop. Usually symptoms occur when enough liver is replaced to produce some degree of hepatic failure, and symptoms develop earlier in cirrhotic patients than in noncirrhotic patients. Occasionally the tumor invades the portal vein or hepatic duct or metastasizes before a large tumor or liver replacement has developed. Such anomalous types of spread produce a different set of symptoms, earlier diagnosis, and usually earlier death with respect to tumor size. Exceptionally rapid rates of tumor growth seem to occur in the HCC developing in patients in parts of Africa, particularly Mozambique.

Hepatocellular carcinoma

Etiology

The most important feature in the etiology of HCC is cirrhosis or precirrhotic changes. There are clear differences in the propensity of different kinds of cirrhosis to give rise to HCC. Some types of cirrhosis (such as tyrosinemia) have a high incidence of development of HCC[907] but are rare entities; others (such as biliary atresia and familial cholestatic disorders) have a progression of the cirrhosis that is too rapid to allow sufficient survival time for the development of HCC. In another example, patients with alcoholic cirrhosis have a far shorter life expectancy after development of cirrhosis than do patients with B-viral cirrhosis, a factor that should be considered in comparing the incidence of HCC in the two. A third factor to be considered is that many types of chronic liver disease are labeled "cirrhosis" long before the development of nodular regeneration. PBC is an example: the time from the development of nodules to death is relatively short in PBC, even though the span of disease is well over a decade. Correspondingly, the percentage of patients with PBC who develop HCC is low, although cases have been reported.[836]

In all patients with cirrhosis the frequency of HCC is related to etiology of the particular types of cirrhosis. There are patients with certain very protracted types of cirrhosis who have a lower incidence of HCC than do patients with other etiologic types of cirrhosis. An example of long-term cirrhosis with low incidence of HCC occurs in Wilson's disease. With D-penicillamine therapy, patients may live 20 years or more with established cirrhosis. Only two HCCs arising in livers of patients with acceptably proven Wilson's disease have been reported.[838] In all patients with cirrhosis the frequency of HCC is related to the etiology.

Hepatitis B appears to be the most important etiologically related factor in hepatic carcinogenesis worldwide. In Taiwan, where about 80% of patients with HCC have a chronic form of hepatitis B,[901] the incidence of HCC in persons who are HBsAg positive is 1158:100,000, compared with 5:100,000 in HBsAg-negative patients.[790] Data from Hong Kong, Japan, the Philippines, and the United States indicate that between 40% and 45% of patients dying of B-viral cirrhosis also have hepatocellular carcinoma,[809] whereas more precise data from Taiwan indicate that HCC develops in HBsAg carriers.[790] Thus it is unnecessary to hypothesize a cocarcinogen reacting with HBV infection in Asia or Africa to explain the high incidence of HCC in those countries. Differences in the incidence of HCC result from the difference in chronic HBsAg infection from one country to another. The high familial incidence of both HCC and chronic HBV infection in several countries[858,859,902] offers evidence for perinatal acquisition of HBV infection that is followed several decades later by development of HCC. Recent studies have detected hepatitis B-viral DNA incorporated into the DNA of hepatocellular carcinoma.[847,873] Some patients with HCC but with no serologic evidence of past or current hepatitis B infection have been reported to have such B-viral DNA incorporated into the tumor DNA.[798]

For purposes of comparison, since alcoholic cirrhosis is uncommon in Asia and Africa, if one excludes the patients with HCC arising in alcoholic cirrhosis in our series of patients with HCC from Los Angeles, more than 70% of the remaining patients with HCC arising in cirrhotic livers have chronic HBV infection.[869] Thus it appears that although chronic HBV infection is important in the etiology of HCC in the United States, it occurs about 1% as often in the United States as in parts of Asia.

HCC is much less likely to develop in alcoholic cirrhotic patients than in patients with many other types of cirrhosis, but since alcoholic cirrhosis is much more common than other types of cirrhosis in the United States and Europe, it forms the basis for the greatest number of cases of HCC. Overall in the United States only about 4% of patients with alcoholic cirrhosis studied at autopsy have HCC. However, when HCC arises in the alcoholic cirrhotic liver, it does so only in the advanced cirrhotic liver, a stage reached by only a small percentage of alcoholic cirrhotic patients in the United States. In France and Italy, where average alcohol consumption is higher but less intense per alcoholic than in the United States, HCC is more likely to develop in the cirrhotic livers.[808,868] If the alcoholic cirrhotic patient discontinues alcohol consumption and thus prolongs survival, the chances of developing HCC increase.[841] Thus the patient may live long enough to develop HCC.

Aflatoxin, a product of *Aspergillus flavus*, may be involved in the etiology of liver cell carcinoma. This fungus has widespread distribution, growing on peanuts, soybeans, and cereals in humid parts of the world. Aflatoxin B_1, the most toxic of the aflatoxins, is highly carcinogenic for some animal species, particularly rats. As little as 15 μg/kg body weight/day produces cancer. The relationship of aflatoxin intake to primary carcinoma of the liver has been studied in Kenya,[884] Thailand,[866] and Mozambique. The last has the highest frequency of HCC in the world and also has the highest per capita intake of aflatoxins. It has been estimated that in Mozambique one male in each 40 households will die of HCC. There may be a short induction time after exposure to aflatoxins.[785,905] In studies of both biopsy and autopsy specimens in Bantus of Lourenço Marques, toxic changes that differed from viral hepatitis seen in the same population were observed. It has been suggested that these changes may be precancerous.[903] Yet on a case by case basis the relationship of HCC to high dietary aflatoxin intake has not been established. Because of the carcinogenic effect of single large doses of aflatoxins, an effect of these agents cannot readily be excluded, and many investigators propose a cocarcinogenic effect between hepatitis B and aflatoxins. This is difficult to prove, since the increased incidence of HCC in most Asian and African countries can probably be explained on the basis of increased incidence of chronic forms of hepatitis B alone. Since aflatoxins are apparently not cirrhotogenic, the best areas for study of possible aflatoxin contribution include Mozambique and parts of South Africa where HCC frequently arises in younger individuals without predisposing cirrhosis.[791,792]

Hemochromatosis is relatively uncommon in the United States and Western Europe and therefore is not a major cause of HCC. However, HCC or cholangiocarcinoma develops in approximately 20% of patients with hemochromatosis. It is unclear whether treatment of hemochromatosis by iron removal reduces the incidence of development of HCC[872] or allows longer survival and higher incidence of HCC.[795,796] Many cirrhotic livers have secondary increases in iron stores, ranging from only slightly more than normal quantities to amounts comparable to those in livers of patients with idiopathic hemochromatosis. Whether these increased stores contribute to carcinogenesis is unclear.

Hormones. A relationship between benign hepatocellular tumors and oral contraceptives has been discussed (see p. 1188); a much less frequent association of oral contraceptives and HCC has also been reported.[803,874,899] Although cases of HCC associated with oral contraceptives have been collected by various investigators from a candidate population of approximately 12 to 15 million in the United States alone, there is little available information regarding the HCC incidence in the control population.

Anabolic steroids administered to young patients in treatment of aplastic anemia, particularly Fanconi's anemia, have been linked to occurrence of HCC. We are aware of no instances as yet of relationship between anabolic steroid use and HCC in athletes, many of whom use the agents to increase muscle mass.

Cryptogenic cirrhosis. HCC arises in livers of about 10% of patients who have cirrhosis of unknown etiology. Supposedly rare, there are reports of HCC rising in autoimmune cirrhosis.[799,830] Thirteen percent of the small series of lupoid cirrhotic patients studied at autopsy in our unit (8% of women with that disease and 50% of the men) have had HCC. However, nearly half of the patients with autoimmune liver disease died of submassive necrosis in a precirrhotic stage of chronic liver disease.

Non-A, non-B viral cirrhosis. The relationship between non-A, non-B viral hepatitis and cirrhosis is difficult to establish; undoubtedly many patients with so-called cryptogenic cirrhosis actually have chronic non-A, non-B viral infection. Although we have studied two patients who died of HCC arising in posttransfusion NAB cirrhosis, we have no solid information regarding the total number of cirrhotic patients in our hospital whose cirrhosis is NAB type.

Membranous obstruction of the vena cava. Membranous obstruction of the vena cava (MOVC) is a peculiar condition, rare in the United States[825,880] but frequently encountered in the Orient[834] and quite common in the black population in Pretoria, South Africa.[888] Of the African patients who died of MOVC, 47.5% also had HCC. The weblike obstruction apparently has its origin in utero or during early extrauterine life and is usually not recognized until adulthood. Because of the chronicity, MOVC is not quite comparable to hepatic vein occlusion, but HCC has been reported in patients with chronic Budd-Chiari disease.[868]

Several rare diseases that do not contribute significantly to the total HCC incidence but have a significant coincidence with HCC include alpha-1-antitrypsin, aberrant Pi Z,[813,817,820] chronic immunodeficiency,[787,887] postradiation venous occlusion,[801,854] biliary atresia,[837] and tyrosinemia.[907]

Carcinoma of the liver may occur in infancy and childhood, especially in male infants before 2 years of age. Among adults the disease in Europe and the United

States is most common in men between 40 and 50 years of age, whereas in Africa the average is nearer 30 years of age. When carcinoma arises in an otherwise completely normal liver, females are affected as often as males.

Pathologic anatomy

Hepatocellular carcinomas may be spreading, expanding, or multifocal. They usually arise as nodular or pseudolobular growths in a liver that is the seat of advanced cirrhosis.[810] A liver involved by HCC usually weighs between 2 and 3 kg but may be of normal size and weight. The right lobe is more frequently involved than the left in either the spreading or the expanding form. The cancer nodules often bulge beneath Glisson's capsule and are much softer to palpation than are areas of nodular regeneration. The nodules are rarely umbilicated.

In the expanding form of carcinoma the right lobe particularly may be largely replaced by well-circumscribed, soft, yellow-brown tumor (Fig. 27-67). Expanding type of tumor growth is more common in noncirrhotic livers. Small secondary nodules are sometimes present in other parts of the liver.

In the spreading type there is usually one mass that is larger, appears older, and is more circumscribed than any other lesion. Such a tumor may be regarded as the primary lesion (Fig. 27-63). Ordinarily nodules of smaller size are present throughout the remainder of the liver. Invasion of branches of the portal vein is usually demonstrable and is probably responsible for the rapid spread to all parts of the liver. Hemorrhage, necrosis, and bile staining may produce a wide variety of color changes within the nodules. It appears that the tumor nodules arise in multiple foci. This has been emphasized by the African investigators.[815]

The growth of carcinoma in the branches of the portal vein may lead to a tumor thrombus of the portal trunk and sudden increase of portal hypertension. Less often, the hepatic veins are invaded, and a tumor thrombus extends into the inferior vena cava. By this route the cancer may spread to the lungs and more distant structures.

Tumor cells of HCC simulate normal liver cells, being characterized by large, round, hyperchromatic nuclei, prominent nucleoli, abundant granular eosinophilic cytoplasm, and a tendency toward arrangement in trabeculae that are usually two to eight cells wide (Fig. 27-68). They retain another feature indicative of their origin: the trabeculae (and liver cords) are covered by a thin connective tissue envelope having, external to this envelope, endothelial cells. This arrangement is particularly noted when the cancer grows into blood vessels. In the expanding carcinomas arising in previously normal liver, the trabecular pattern may not be so obvious. Regardless of variations in pattern, however, most HCCs are composed only of malignant cells and a capillary stroma. The excess connective tissue that characterizes most adenocarcinomas is usually absent. Some carcinomas form acini that may or may not contain bile. Many of the functions of normal liver cells are retained in carcinomas, such as the ability to secrete bile and to store fat and glycogen. It has been suggested that the large amount of glycogen stored in a liver cell carcinoma is not available

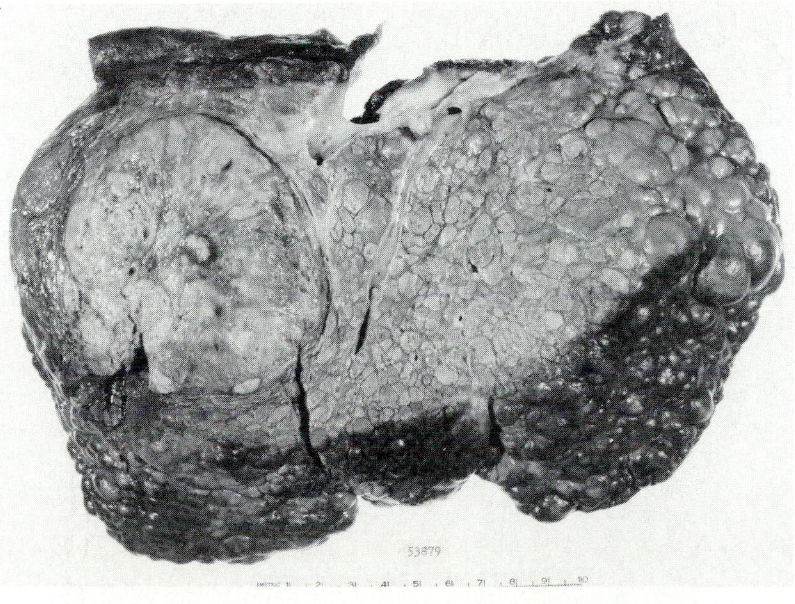

Fig. 27-67. Large, encapsulated, nodular liver cell carcinoma of right lobe arising in liver of 38-year-old Oriental man.

to form glucose, and this may result in hypoglycemia. Cytoplasmic hyaline inclusions, either globular or small Mallory bodies, are present in some neoplastic hepatocytes.[832] A few HCCs are highly undifferentiated, forming spindle and giant cell types. In some carcinomas complicating cirrhosis there is a combination of liver cell and bile duct carcinoma, with the former predominating as a rule. Rarely, calcification of the stroma in liver cell carcinoma has been observed.[853]

Hepatocellular carcinomas in infants and children are large, multinodular lesions that, with rare exception, arise in noncirrhotic livers. Congenital defects have been noted in an abnormally high percentage of these patients,[815] These tumors are classified as hepatoblastomas and hepatocarcinomas.[827] The cell type is smaller than that seen in adults, and bile plugs are frequent. Some of the tumors contain mesenchymal sarcoma and osteoid tissue. The name *mixed hepatoblastoma* has been suggested for this type.[826,827] The electron microscopic studies of the epithelial component of these hepatoblastomas disclose a variable degree of organelle development.[819] Biochemical studies have shown a lack of zinc in hepatoblastomas.[855] Surgical treatment of malignant tumors in infants affords the only chance of cure.[812] Rupture of hepatocellular carcinoma with abdominal bleeding may require emergency surgery.[862] Patients with inoperable disease may receive chemotherapy.[823]

Cholangiocarcinoma

Cholangiocarcinomas may arise from bile ducts within the liver (peripheral cholangiocarcinoma) but originates most often from the large hilar ducts (hilar cholangiocarcinoma) or from the extrahepatic ducts. These are usually mucin-producing, well-differentiated, sclerosing adenocarcinomas that on histologic examination are difficult to distinguish from mestastatic adenocarcinomas. In our patients in Los Angeles we have found that 25% of peripheral cholangiocarcinomas arise in cirrhotic livers.

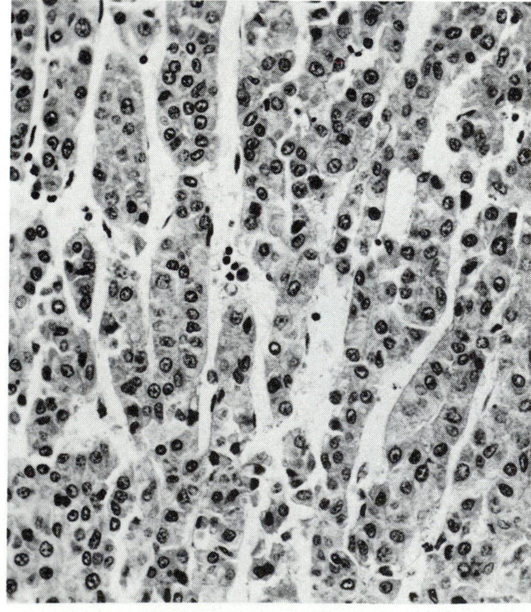

Fig. 27-68. Trabecular liver cell carcinoma with characteristic capillary pattern.

Etiology

Cholangiocarcinoma is known to follow Thorotrast injection,[867,890] *Clonorchis sinenis* infestation,[818] hemochromatosis, polycystic disease, and duct ectasia disease,[824] and occasionally the tumor arises in patients with chronic ulcerative colitis.[876] In patients with the last the risk of cholangiocarcinoma is said to be 10-fold higher than in normal individuals. Peripheral cholangiocarcinoma is not as likely as HCC to grow within branches of the portal and hepatic veins, although it metastasizes just as widely to other organs but in a different pattern from HCC, favoring abdominal nodes, bones, and serosal structure.

Hilar cholangiocarcinoma

Hilar cholangiocarcinoma represents 25% of the total cholangiocarcinomas arising within the liver in our patients in Los Angeles. Reports from Japan indicate that in that country about 30%[897] to 50%[860] of the carcinomas are hilar in location. These carcinomas are characterized by slow growth; only about 15% have metastases at autopsy.[842] The predisposing factors are similar to those for PCC and include many of the same conditions, such as congenital cystic diseases of the duct system,[870] inflammatory bowel disease,[885] and *Clonorchis sinensis*.[818] Hilar cholangiocarcinoma, unlike peripheral cholangiocarcinoma, is characterized by pruritus and icterus at the onset. The course may be protracted, lasting more than 3 years on occasion.

Mesodermal tumors

Malignant tumors of mesodermal origin are rare. Hemangioendothelial sarcomas form bulky hemorrhagic masses and may metastasize to the lungs, portal lymph nodes, and spleen. It has been possible to remove some of these vascular sarcomas surgically.[784] Microscopically they are vasoformative tumors characterized by malignant endothelial lining cells. They may occur after ionizing radiation from Thorotrast[882] and after exposure to arsenic, both in vineyard workers and after the ingestion for therapeutic purposes.[840] In recent years much publicity has been given to the occurrence of angiosarcoma in vinyl chloride workers.[794,802] Nonmalignant lesions in vinyl chloride workers consist of portal fibrosis, sinusoidal dilatation, and atypical sinusoidal lining cells. The toxicity of vinyl chloride and polyvinylchloride has been the subject of a conference.[881] Hemochromatosis associated with hemangioendothelial sarcoma has been reported.[895]

Embryonal rhabdomyosarcoma and malignant mesenchymal sarcomas occasionally are seen, especially in infancy and childhood.[807] Although Kupffer cell sarcomas have been reported, this term should be restricted to vasoformative tumors in which the malignant cells are actively phagocytic. Some highly vascular sarcomas of the liver contain large stromal cells in variable quantity that appear to be myosarcomatous. A few cases of fibrosarcoma[904] and leiomyosarcoma have been reported.

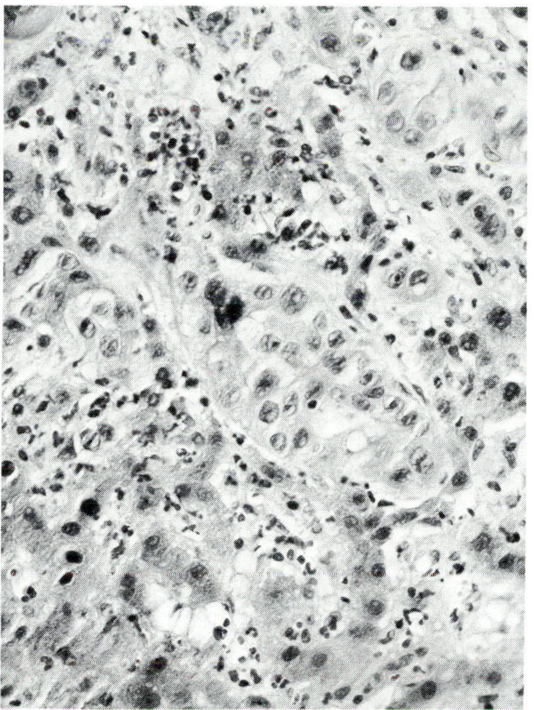

Fig. 27-69. Intrasinusoidal growth of metastatic carcinoma of liver.

Metastatic tumors

In metastatic cancer both lobes of the liver usually are involved, producing an enlarged nodular organ that is easily palpable in life. The cancer cells may reach the liver through the portal vein, hepatic artery, or hilar lymphatics or occasionally by direct extension. Once implanted, the cells may form small or large nodules or grow diffusely throughout the liver. Metastatic carcinoma often grows within sinusoids. The sinusoidal lining cells may be seen on biopsy around tiny metastatic growths (Fig. 27-69). In about 10% of the cases metastatic nodules are solitary. Characteristically, nodules of irregular size bulge beneath Glisson's capsule and are consistently depressed in their central portions (umbilicated) because of necrosis or fibrosis with contraction. Umbilication is practically never seen in HCC.

The pattern of growth of metastatic cancer appears to depend somewhat on the source; for example, carcinoma of the colon or stomach often produces large mucin-containing nodules that have a pebbled appearance on cut surface (Fig. 27-70). Breast cancer often forms smaller, discrete lesions, frequently oval in outline as seen beneath Glisson's capsule.

Metastatic carcinoma is usually gray to grayish white, but necrosis, hemorrhage, and mucus may add a variety of colors. Extensive hemorrhagic lesions are characteristic of choriocarcinoma and metastatic carcinoid. Malig-

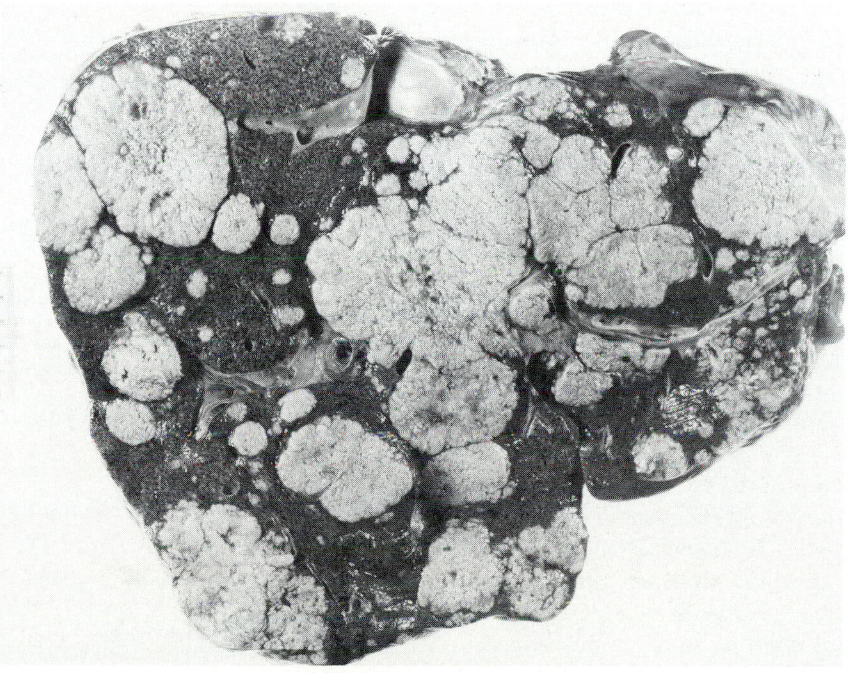

Fig. 27-70. Large metastatic nodules from primary carcinoma of stomach.

nant melanoma is black or brown but sometimes only faintly so.

Occasionally metastatic carcinoma may grow from the hilum outward along the portal tracts, causing them to be unusually prominent. Cancer from the gallbladder may grow directly into the liver, forming a solid mass along with smaller satellite deposits that decrease in size with increase in distance from their origin.

In 60% of the patients with metastatic carcinoma, the disease was demonstrated by a needle biopsy of the liver. If possible, a biopsy should be performed on a palpable nodule.

Metastatic carcinoma usually grows rapidly in the liver, with patients rarely living more than a year after the diagnosis is made.[829] There are two notable exceptions: metastatic malignant carcinoid is not incompatible with survival of 5 to 25 years, and metastatic neuroblastoma of the adrenal gland in infancy may apparently be cured with radiotherapy. Metastasis to the liver occurs in 38% of all cancers (41% of lung cancers; 56% of colon cancers; 70% of pancreatic cancers; 53% of breast cancers; and 44% of gastric cancers).[809]

Surgical treatment of metastatic cancer is limited to palliative procedures, although occasionally a solitary metastasis may be resected. Hepatic dearterialization[845] has been performed in some cases, since metastatic carcinoma, like HCC, derives its blood from the hepatic artery. These operations may prolong life somewhat and ameliorate symptoms in metastatic carcinoids.[850]

TRANSPLANTATION

Many orthotopic liver transplants have now been performed. Initially, many of the patients had primary carcinoma of the liver, but more recently patients with congenital biliary atresia, chronic aggressive hepatitis, primary liver malignancy, primary biliary cirrhosis, or alcoholic cirrhosis have been selected.[910,911,913,914] At present about 50% of the patients survive for 1 year or more. An occasional patient has survived as long as 12 years. Early graft failure results most often from mechanical and technical problems. These include difficulty in biliary drainage, intraoperative bleeding, hepatic artery kinking, and sepsis. Rejection of the graft may occur at any time, either immediately or within a matter of years. Immunosuppression involves the use of prednisone, azathioprine, and cyclosporine. In the past, infection resulting from the immunosuppression has been a major problem. Cyclosporine is promising because of the more specific T cell inhibition it induces. Graft rejection may be expected when there is a rise in alkaline phosphatase and aminotransferase levels, followed by jaundice. At autopsy the changes in the liver that are attributable to rejection alone are difficult to evaluate. These include a dense mononuclear cell infiltrate in the triads and sinusoids with prominent immunoblasts. Centrilobular necrosis and cholestasis are present. Immunoblastic and lymphocytic infiltration about portal and, later, central vein branches seems to be a characteristic feature. After recovery from apparent rejection occurs, collagen fibers may be seen in the space of Disse. The vascular changes consist of a thickened arterial intima, many lipophages, and disruption of the internal elastic lamina. The results of transplantation in 74 cases have been published.[912] Experience has shown that certain diseases, such as chronic active viral hepatitis and malignant tumors, cannot be successfully treated by a liver transplant. Some congenital disorders have lent themselves well to transplantation; among these is alpha-1-antitrypsin cirrhosis. After successful transplantation the new liver continues to produce its genetic type of alpha-1-antitrypsin, and there is no reversion to the ZZ type of the host.[910]

REFERENCES

General

1. Afroudakis, A., Liew, C.T., and Peters, R.L.: An immunoperoxidase technic for the demonstration of the hepatitis B surface antigen in human livers, Am. J. Clin. Pathol. **65**:533, 1976.
2. Ashare, A.B.: Radiocolloid liver scintigraphy: a choice and an echo, Radiol. Clin. North Am. **18**:315, 1980.
3. Bhathal, P.A., and Christie, G.W.: Fluorescence microscopy of terminal and subterminal portions of biliary tree, Lab. Invest. **20**:472, 1969.
4. Bloom, W.: The embryogenesis of human bile capillaries and ducts, Am. J. Anat. **36**:451, 1926.
5. Brensilver, H.L., and Kaplan, M.M.: Significance of elevated liver alkaline phosphatase in serum, Gastroenterology **68**:1556, 1975.
6. Colowick, S.P., and Kaplan, N.D.: Methods in enzymology, vol. 2, New York, 1955, Academic Press, Inc.
7. Corrigan, J.J., and Earnest, D.L.: Factor II antigen in liver disease and warfarin-induced vitamin K deficiency: correlation with coagulant activity using Echis venom, Am. J. Hematol. **8**:249, 1980.
8. Crofton, R.W., Diesselhoff-den Dulk, M.M.C., and Van Furth, R.: Origin, kinetics and characteristics of Kupffer cells in the normal steady state, J. Exp. Med. **148**:1, 1978.
9. Edgington, T.S., and Ritt, D.J.: Intrahepatic expression of serum hepatitis virus-associated antigen, J. Exp. Med. **134**:871, 1971.
10. French, S.W., and Davies, P.L.: Ultrastructural localization of actin-like filaments in rat hepatocytes, Gastroenterology **68**:765, 1975.
11. Gabbiani, G., et al.: Human smooth muscle autoantibody: its identification as antiactin antibody and a study of its binding to "non-muscular" cells, Am. J. Pathol. **72**:473, 1973.
12. Girolami, A., et al.: An immunological study of prothrombin in liver cirrhosis, Blut **41**:61, 1980.
13. Gudat, F., et al.: Pattern of core and surface expression in liver tissue reflects state of specific immune response in hepatitis B, Lab. Invest. **32**:1, 1975.
14. Hadziyannis, S.T., et al.: Cytoplasmic localization of Australia antigen in the liver, Lancet **1**:976, 1972.
15. Ham, A.W.: Histology, ed. 8, Philadelphia, 1979, J.B. Lippincott Co.
16. Hamlyn, A.N., and Berg, P.A.: Haemagglutinating anti-actin antibodies in acute and chronic liver disease, Gut **21**:311, 1980.
17. Hoofnagle, J.H.: Type B hepatitis: virology, serology and clinical course, Semin. Liver Dis. **1**:7, 1981.
18. Hoyes, A.D., Riches, D.J., and Martin, B.G.H.: The fine structure of haemopoiesis in human fetal liver. I. Haemopoietic precursor cells, J. Anat. **115**:99, 1973.

19. Huang, S.N.: Immunohistochemical demonstration of hepatitis B core and surface antigens in paraffin sections, Lab. Invest. **33**:88, 1975.
20. Jones, A.L., and Schmucker, D.L.: Current concepts of liver structure as related to function, Gastroenterology **73**:833, 1977.
21. Kaplan, M.A.: Akaline phosphatase, Gastroenterology **62**:452, 1972.
22. Klatskin, G., and Kantor, F.S.: Mitochondrial antibody in primary biliary cirrhosis and other diseases, Ann. Intern. Med. **77**:535, 1972.
23. Koga, A.: Morphogenesis of intrahepatic bile ducts of human fetus: light and electron microscopic study, Z. Anat. Entwicklungsgesch. **135**:156, 1971.
24. Lautt, W.W.: Hepatic vasculature: a conceptual review, Gastroenterology **73**:1163, 1977.
25. LeDouarin, N.M.: An experimental analysis of liver development, Med. Biol. **53**:427, 1975.
26. Ma, M.H., and Biempica, L.: Normal human liver cell: cytochemical and ultrastructural studies, Am. J. Pathol. **62**:353, 1971.
27. Madding, G.F., and Kennedy, P.A.: Trauma to the liver, ed. 2, Philadelphia, 1971, W.B. Saunders Co.
28. Michels, N.A.: Variant blood supply and collateral circulation of liver, Am. J. Surg. **112**:337, 1966.
29. Mueller, A.F., and Leuthardt, F.: Conversion of glutamic acid to aspartic acid in liver mitochondria, Helv. Chir. Acta **33**:268, 1950.
30. Munro, C.J.: Computed tomography of the liver, Radiology **47**:73, 1981.
31. Nakamura, S., and Tsuzuki, T.: Surgical anatomy of the hepatic veins and the inferior vena cava, Surg. Gynecol. Obstet. **156**:43, 1981.
32. Palmer, E.D.: Palpability of liver edge in healthy adults, U.S. Armed Forces Med. J. **9**:1685, 1958.
33. Pare, P., Hoefs, J.C., and Ashcavai, M.: Determinants of serum bile acids in chronic liver disease, Gastroenterology **81**:959, 1981.
34. Praaning-van Dalen, D.P., Brouwer, A., and Knook, D.L.: Clearance capacity of rat liver, Kupffer, endothelial, and parenchymal cells, Gastroenterology **81**:1036, 1981.
35. Rappaport, A.M.: Microcirculatory hepatic unit, Microvasc. Res. **6**:212, 1973.
36. Read, A.E.: Clinical physiology of the liver, Br. J. Anaesth. **44**:910, 1972.
37. Rogoff, T.M., and Lipsky, P.E.: Role of the Kupffer cells in local and systemic immune responses, Gastroenterology **80**:854, 1981.
38. Rowsell, E.V.: Transaminations with L-glutamate and L-oxoglutarate, Biochem. J. **64**:235, 1956.
39. Rutenburg, A.M., et al.: A comparison of serum aminopeptidase and alkaline phosphatase in the detection of hepatobiliary disease in anicteric patients, Ann. Intern. Med. **61**:50, 1964.
40. Severn, C.B.: Morphologic study of development of human liver. II. Establishment of liver parenchyma, extrahepatic ducts, and associated venous channels, Am. J. Anat. **133**:85, 1972.
41. Shikata, T., et al.: Staining methods for Australia antigen in paraffin sections, Jpn. J. Exp. Med. **44**:25, 1974.
42. Steiner, J.W., and Carruthers, J.A.: Structure of terminal branches of biliary tree: morphology of normal bile canaliculi, bile preductules, and bile ductules, Am. J. Pathol. **38**:639, 1961.
43. Tygstrup, N., et al.: Hepatic arterial blood flow and oxygen supply during surgery, J. Clin. Invest. **41**:447, 1962.
44. Widrich, W.C., and Sequeria, S.R.: Interventional radiology of the liver and related structures, Radiol. Clin. North Am. **18**:297, 1980.
45. Wisse, T.M., and Knook, D.L.: Kupffer cells and other liver sinusoidal cells, Amsterdam, 1977, Elsevier/ North Holland.
46. Yeh, H.C., and Rabinowitz, J.G.: Ultrasonography and computed tomography of the liver, Radiol. Clin. North Am. **18**:321, 1980.
47. Zamboni, L.: Hemopoietic activity of fetal liver, J. Ultrastruct. Res. **12**:525, 1965.

Basic hepatic histopathology

48. Adler, M., and Schaffner, F.: Fatty liver hepatitis and cirrhosis in obese patients, Am. J. Med. **67**:811, 1979.
49. Aikat, B.K., Bhattacharaya, T., and Walia, B.N.S.: Morphological features of Indian childhood cirrhosis: the spectrum of changes and their significance, Indian J. Med. Res. **62**:953, 1974.
50. Bengmark, S., Engevik, L., and Rosengren, K.: Angiography of regenerating human liver after extensive resection, Surgery **65**:590, 1969.
51. Berk, P., and Javitt, N.B.: Hyperbilirubinemia and cholestasis, Am. J. Med. **64**:311, 1978.
52. Biava, C.: Electron microscopic studies on periodic acid–Schiff–positive non-glycogenic structures in human liver cells, Am. J. Pathol. **46**:435, 1965.
53. Brewer, D.B., and Heath, D.: Electron microscopy of anoxic vacuolization in the liver cell and its comparison with sucroseravacuolization, Pathol. Bacteriol. **90**:437, 1965.
54. Bucher, N.L.: Regeneration of mammalian liver, Int. Rev. Cytol. **15**:245, 1963.
55. Chedid, A., Jao, W., and Port, J.: Megamitochondria in hepatic and renal disease, Am. J. Gastroenterol. **73**:319, 1980.
56. Ciba Foundation Symposium 55: Hepatotrophic factors, New York, 1978, Elsevier/ North Holland, Inc.,
57. Coward, W.A., and Lunn, P.G.: The biochemistry and physiology of kwashiorkor and marasmus, Br. Med. Bull. **37**:19, 1981.
58. Darlak, J.A., Moskowitz, M., and Kattan, K.R.: Calcifications in the liver, Radiol. Clin. North Am. **18**:209, 1980.
59. Denk, H., et al.: Formation and involution of Mallory bodies in murine and human liver revealed by immunofluorescence microscopy with antibodies to prekeratin, Proc. Natl. Acad. Sci. U.S.A. **76**:4112, 1979.
60. Fletcher, G.F., and Galambos, J.T.: Phosphorus poisoning, Arch. Intern. Med. **112**:846, 1963.
61. French, S.W.: The Mallory body: structure, composition, and pathogenesis, Hepatology **1**:76, 1981.
62. Gartner, U., et al.: Modulation of the transport of bilirubin and asialoorosomucoid during liver regeneration, Hepatology **1**:99, 1981.
63. Gerber, M.A., and Thung, S.N.: Hepatic oncocytes, Am. J. Clin. Pathol. **75**:498, 1981.
64. Green, P.A., and Stephens, D.H.: Hepatic calcification in cancer of the large bowel, Am. J. Gastroenterol. **55**:466, 1970.
65. Hadziyannis, S.T., et al.: Cytoplasmic hepatitis B antigen in "ground-glass" hepatocytes of carriers, Arch. Pathol. **96**:327, 1973.
66. Hall, P.M., et al.: Calcification in the liver: an unusual feature of ductal cell hepatic carcinoma, Cleve. Clin. Q. **37**:93, 1970.
67. Hilden, M., et al.: Liver histology in a "normal" population: examinations of 503 consecutive fatal traffic casualties, Scand. J. Gastroenterol. **12**:593, 1977.
68. Hruban, Z., et al.: Focal cytoplasmic degeneration, Am. J. Pathol. **42**:657, 1963.
69. International Association for Study of Diseases of the Liver and Biliary Tract: Standardization of nomenclature, diagnostic criteria and prognostic methodology: Fogarty International Proceedings No. 22, Pub. No. 76-725, Washington, D.C., 1976, Department of Health, Education, and Welfare.
70. Itoh, S., Igarash, M., and Tsukada, Y.: Nonalcoholic fatty liver with alcoholic hyalin after long-term glucocorticoid therapy, Acta Hepatogastroenterol. **24**:415, 1977.
71. Itoh, S., and Tsukada, Y.: Clinicopathological and electron microscopical studies on a coronary dilation agent 4-4' diethylaminoethoxyhexestrol-induced injuries, Acta Hepatogastroenterol. **20**:204, 1973.
72. Keeley, A.F., Iseri, O.A., and Gottlieb, L.S.: Ultrastructure of hyaline cytoplasmic inclusions in a human hepatoma: relationship to Mallory's alcoholic hyalin, Gastroenterology **62**:280, 1972.
73. Kerr, J.F.R.: Shrinkage necrosis: a distinct mode of cellular death, J. Pathol. **105**:13, 1971.
74. Kimura, H., et al.: Alcoholic hyalin (Mallory bodies) in a case of Weber-Christian disease: electron microscopic observations of liver involvement, Gastroenterology **78**:807, 1980.

75. Leffert, H.L., and Koch, K.S.: Ionic events at the membrane initiate rat liver regeneration, N.Y. Acad. Sci. **339**:201, 1980.
76. Lewis, C., et al.: Liver damage associated with perhexiline maleate, Gut **20**:186, 1979.
77. MacSween, R.N.M.: Mallory's (alcoholic) hyalin in primary biliary cirrhosis, J. Clin. Pathol. **26**:340, 1973.
78. Mallory, F.B.: Cirrhosis of liver, N. Engl. J. Med. **205**:1231, 1932.
79. Miele, A.J., and Edmonds, H.W.: Calcified liver metastasis: a specific roentgen diagnostic sign, Radiology **80**:779, 1963.
80. Miller, M.W., and Shamoo, E.A.: Membrane toxicity, New York, 1977, Plenum Publishing Corp.,
81. Monroe, S., French, S.W., and Zamboni, L.: Mallory bodies in a case of primary biliary cirrhosis: an ultrastructural and morphogenic study, Am. J. Clin. Pathol. **59**:254, 1973.
82. Morton, J.A., et al.: Mallory bodies in alcoholic liver disease, Gut **22**:1, 1981.
83. Nishimura, R.N., et al.: Lafora's disease: diagnosis by liver biopsy, Ann. Neurol. **8**:409, 1980.
84. Ouclea, P.R.: Anoxic changes of liver cells: electron microscopic study after injection of colloidal mercury, Lab. Invest. **12**:386, 1963.
85. Pariente, E.-A., et al.: Hepatocytic PAS-positive diastase-resistant inclusions in the absence of alpha-1-antitrypsin deficiency, Am. J. Clin. Pathol. **76**:299, 1981.
86. Partin, J.A., et al.: Liver ultrastructure in abetalipoproteinemia: evolution of micronodular cirrhosis, Gastroenterology **67**:852, 1974.
87. Peters, R.L.: Hepatic morphologic changes after jejunoileal bypass. In Popper, H., and Schaffner, F., editors: Progress in liver disease, vol. 6, New York, 1979, Grune & Stratton, Inc.
88. Peters, R.L., Gay, T., and Reynolds, T.B.: Postjejunal bypass hepatic disease: its similarity to alcoholic hepatic disease, Am. J. Clin. Pathol. **63**:318, 1975.
89. Petersen, P.: Alcoholic hyalin, microfilaments, and microtubules in alcoholic hepatitis, Acta Pathol. Microbiol. Scand. **85**:384, 1977.
90. Peura, D.A., Stromeyer, F.W., and Johnson, L.F.: Liver injury with alcoholic hyaline after intestinal resection, Gastroenterology **79**:128, 1980.
91. Podleski, W.K.: Cytodestructive mechanisms provoked by lymphocytes, Am. J. Med. **61**:1, 1976.
92. Porta, E.A., Koch, D.R., and Hartroft, W.S.: A new experimental approach in the study of chronic alcoholism, Lab. Invest. **20**:562, 1969.
93. Prockop, D.J., et al.: The biosynthesis of collagen and its disorders (in two parts), N. Engl. J. Med. **301**:13, **301**:77, 1979.
94. Pyke, K.W., and Gelfand, E.W.: Detection of T-precursor cells in human bone marrow and foetal liver, Differentiation **5**:189, 1976.
95. Rabes, H.M.: Kinetics of hepatocellular proliferation as a function of the microvascular structure and functional state of the liver. In Ciba Foundation Symposium 55: Hepatotrophic factors, New York, 1978, Elsevier/North Holland, Inc.
96. Rojkind, M., and Dunn, M.A.: Hepatic fibrosis, Gastroenterology **76**:849, 1979.
97. Salfeider, K., Seelkopf, C., and Inglessis, G.: Phosphorus poisoning, Zentralbl. Allg. Pathol. **108**:524, 1966.
98. Starzl, T.E., and Terblanche, J.: Hepatrophic substances. In Popper, H., and Schaffner, F., editors: Progress in liver disease, vol. 6, New York, 1979, Grune & Stratton, Inc.
99. Stern, R.: Experimental aspects of hepatic fibrosis. In Popper, H., and Schaffner, F., editors: Progress in liver disease, vol. 6, New York, 1979, Grune & Stratton, Inc.
100. Sternberg, G.M.: Report on the etiology and prevention of yellow fever, U.S. Marine Hosp. Pub. Health Bull. **2**:151, 1890.
101. Stromeyer, F.W., and Ishak, K.G.: Histology of the liver in Wilson's disease, Am. J. Clin. Pathol. **73**:12, 1980.
102. Theron, J.A., and Liebenberg, N.: Fine cytology of parenchymal liver cells in kwashiorkor patients, J. Pathol. Bacteriol. **86**:109, 1963.
103. Uchida, T., et al.: Personal communication.
104. Vasquez, J., and Pardo-Mindan, J.: Liver cell injury bodies similar to Lafora's in alcoholics treated with disulfiram (Antabuse), Histopathology **3**:377, 1979.
105. Webber, B.L., and Frieman, I.: Liver in kwashiorkor: a clinical and electron microscopic study, Arch. Pathol. **98**:400, 1974.
106. Whitcomb, F.F., Parikh, N.K., and Sedgwick, C.E.: Hydatid cyst disease, Am. J. Dig. Dis. **15**:711, 1970.
107. Wiggers, K.D., French, S.W., and Carr, B.N.: The ultrastructure of Mallory body filaments, Lab. Invest. **29**:652, 1973.
108. Yokoo, H., Singh, S.K., and Hawasli, A.H.: Giant mitochondria in alcoholic liver disease, Arch. Pathol. Lab. Med. **102**:213, 1978.
109. Yunis, E.J., Agostini, R.M., and Glew, R.H.: Fine structural observations of the liver in alpha-1-antitrypsin deficiency, Am. J. Pathol. **82**:265, 1976.

Infectious disorders

110. Afroudakis, A., Liew, C.T., and Peters, R.L.: An immunoperoxidase technic for the demonstration of the hepatitis B surface antigen in human livers, Am. J. Clin. Pathol. **65**:533, 1976.
111. Afroudakis, A., et al.: The immunohistochemical detection of HBsAg in liver tissue of serologically negative HBsAg patients (abstract), Am. J. Clin. Pathol. **66**(suppl.):461, 1976.
112. Bechtelsheimer, H., Korb, G., and Gedigk, P.: The morphology and pathogenesis of "Marburg virus" hepatitis, Hum. Pathol. **3**:255, 1972.
113. Berk, P.D., and Popper, H.: Fulminant hepatic failure: chairman's summary—a final evaluation, Am. J. Gastroenterol. **69**:349, 1978.
114. Bernuau, J., et al.: Non-inflammatory herpes simplex hepatitis in an adult with chronic neutropenia, Liver **1**:244, 1981.
115. Biava, C., and Mukhlova-Montiel, M.: Electron microscopic observation on Councilman-like acidophilic bodies, Am. J. Pathol. **46**:775, 1965.
116. Blumberg, B.S.: Viruses similar to hepatitis B virus (icrons), Hum. Pathol. **12**(12):1107, 1981.
117. Boeve, N.R., Winterscheid, L.C., and Merendino, K.A.: Fibrinogen-transmitted hepatitis in surgical patient, Ann. Surg. **170**:833, 1969.
118. Bonino, F., et al.: Outcome of chronic hepatitis in HBsAg carriers: delta hepatitis, a progressive disease with poor prognosis (abstract), Hepatology **1**:497, 1981.
119. Bowen, E.T.W., et al.: Viral haemorrhagic fever in southern Sudan and northern Zaire, Lancet **1**:571, 1977.
120. Boyer, J.L., and Klatskin, G.: Pattern of necrosis in acute viral hepatitis: prognostic value of bridging, N. Engl. J. Med. **283**:1063, 1970.
121. Bradley, D.W., and Maynard, J.E.: Serodiagnosis of viral hepatitis A by radioimmunoassay, Lab. Management **16**:29, 1978.
122. Bradley, D.W., et al.: CsCl banding of hepatitis A associated virus-like particles, J. Infect. Dis. **131**:304, 1975.
123. Brensilver, H.L., and Kaplan, M.M.: Significance of elevated liver alkaline phosphatase in serum, Gastroenterology **68**:1556, 1975.
124. Buchmeier, M.J., Monoclonal antibodies to lymphocytic choriomeningitis virus react with pathogenic arenaviruses, Nature **288**:486, 1980.
125. Budkowska, A., Kalinowska, B., and Nowoslawski, A.: Communications: identification of two HBeAg subspecificities revealed by chemical treatment and enzymatic digestion of liver-derived HBcAg, J. Immunol. **123**:1415, 1979.
126. Carr, J.B., de Guesada, A.M., and Shires, D.L.: Decreased incidence of transfusion with reconstituted frozen erythrocytes, Ann. Intern. Med. **78**:693, 1973.
127. Chang, M.Y., and Campbell, W.G.: Fatal infectious mononucleosis: association with liver necrosis and herpes-like virus particles, Arch. Pathol. **99**:186, 1975.
128. Child, P.L., and Ruiz, A.: Acidophilic bodies, Arch. Pathol. **85**:45, 1968.
129. Committee on Viral Hepatitis of the National Research Council–National Academy of Science: Nomenclature of antigens associated with viral hepatitis type B, J. Infect. Dis. **130**:92, 1974.

130. Daemer, R.J., et al: Propagation of human hepatitis A virus in African green monkey kidney cell culture: primary isolation and serial passage, Infect. Immun. **32**:388, 1981.
131. Dane, D.S., Cameron, C.H., and Briggs, M.: Virus-like particles in serum of patients with Australia-antigen–associated hepatitis, Lancet **1**:695, 1970.
132. Darani, M., and Gerber, M.: Hepatitis B antigen in vaginal secretions, Lancet **2**:1008, 1974.
133. DeBrito, T., Viera, W.T., and Dias, M.D.A.: Jaundice in typhoid hepatitis: light and electron microscopic study based on liver biopsies, Acta Hepatogastroenterol. **24**:426, 1977.
134. Deinhardt, F., et al.: Studies on the transmission of human viral hepatitis to marmoset monkeys. I. Transmission of disease, J. Exp. Med. **125**:673, 1967.
135. De Wolf-Peeters, C., et al.: Human non-A, non-B hepatitis: ultrastructural alterations in hepatocytes, Liver **1**:50, 1981.
136. Dienstag, J.L.: Hepatitis A virus: virologic, clinical, and epidemiologic studies, Hum. Pathol. **12**:1097, 1981.
137. Dougherty, W.J., and Altman, R.: Viral hepatitis in New Jersey: 1960-1961, Am. J. Med. **32**:704, 1962.
138. Drew, R., Edington, G.M., and White, H.A.: The pathology of Lassa fever, Trans. R. Soc. Trop. Med. Hyg. **66**:381, 1972.
139. Edgington, T.S., and Chisari, F.V.: Immunological aspects of hepatitis B virus infection, Am. J. Med. Sci. **270**:213, 1975.
140. Eichberg, J.W., and Kalter, S.S.: Hepatitis A and B: serologic survey of human and non-human primate sera, Lab. Anim. Sci. **39**:5411, 1980.
141. Elsner, B., et al.: Pathology of 12 fatal cases of Argentine hemorrhagic fever, Am. J. Trop. Med. Hyg. **22**:229, 1973.
142. Farrow, L.J., et al.: Non-A, non-B hepatitis in West London, Lancet **1**:982, 1981.
143. Fauerholdt, L., et al.: Significance of suspected chronic aggressive hepatitis and acute hepatitis, Gastroenterology **73**:543, 1977.
144. Fawaz, K.A., and Matloff, D.S.: Viral hepatitis in homosexual men, Gastroenterology **81**:537, 1981.
145. Feinstone, S.M., Kapikian, A.Z., and Purcell, R.H.: Detection by immune electron microscopy of virus-like antigen associated with acute illness, Science **182**:1026, 1973.
146. Flehmig, B., et al.: Solid-phase radioimmunoassay for detection of IgM antibodies to hepatitis A virus, J. Infect. Dis. **140**:169, 1979.
146a. Francis, D., and Hadler, S.: Personal communication.
147. Francis, D.P., Favero, M.S., and Maynard, J.E.: Transmission of hepatitis B virus, Semin. Liver Dis. **1**:27, 1981.
148. Gerety, T.E., et al.: Acute non-A, non-B hepatitis: specific ultrastructural alterations in endoplasmic reticulum of infected hepatocytes, Lancet **1**:1249, 1979.
149. Hadziyannis, S., et al.: Cytoplasmic hepatitis B antigen in "ground glass" hepatocytes of carriers, Arch. Pathol. **96**:327, 1973.
150. Haugen, R.K.: Hepatitis after the transfusion of frozen red cells and washed red cells, N. Engl. J. Med. **301**:393, 1979.
151. Henigst, W.: Sexual transmission of infections associated with hepatitis B antigen, Lancet **2**:1395, 1973.
152. Hersh, T., et al.: Non-parenteral transmission of viral hepatitis type B (Australia antigen-associated serum hepatitis), N. Engl. J. Med. **285**:1363, 1971.
153. Hilleman, M.R., et al.: Development and utilization of complement-fixation and immune adherence tests for hepatitis A virus and antibody, Am. J. Med. Sci. **270**:93, 1975.
154. Hoefs, J.A., et al.: Hepatitis B surface antigen in pancreatic and biliary secretions, Gastroenterology **79**:191, 1980.
155. Hollinger, F.B., et al.: Experimental medicine, J. Infect. Dis. **142**:400, 1980.
156. Holmes, A.W., et al.: Transmission of human hepatitis to marmosets: further coded studies, J. Infect. Dis. **124**:520, 1971.
157. Hoofnagle, J.H.: Type B hepatitis: virology, serology and clinical course, Semin. Liver Dis. **1**:7, 1981.
158. Immunocompromised homosexuals (editorial), Lancet **2**:1325, 1981.
159. Iwarson, S., Lindberg, J., and Lundin, P.: Progression of hepatitis non-A, non-B to chronic active hepatitis, J. Clin. Pathol. **32**:351, 1979.
160. Johnson, K.M., et al.: Isolation and partial characterization of a new virus causing acute haemorrhagic fever in Zaire, Lancet **1**:569, 1977.
161. Kao, A.H., Tumas, V., and Redeker, A.G.: The duration of hepatitis A IgM antibody after acute clinical hepatitis A (abstract), Clin. Res. **30**:92A, 1981.
162. Karvountzis, G., Redeker, A.G., and Peters, R.L.: Long term follow-up studies of patients surviving fulminant viral hepatitis, Gastroenterology **67**:870, 1974.
163. Katchaki, J.N., Siem, T.H., and Browser, R.: Serological evidence of presence of HBsAg undetectable by conventional radioimmunoassay, in anti-HBc positive donors, J. Clin. Pathol. **31**:837, 1978.
164. Khuroo, M.S.: Study of an epidemic of non-A, non-B hepatitis: possibility of another human hepatitis virus distinct from post-transfusion non-A, non-B type, Am. J. Med. **68**:818, 1980.
165. Khuroo, M.S., et al.: Incidence and severity of viral hepatitis in pregnancy, Am. J. Med. **70**:252, 1981.
166. Kiley, M.P., Regnery, R.L., and Johnson, K.M.: Ebola virus: identification of virion structural proteins, J. Gen. Virol. **49**:333, 1980.
167. Kojima, M., et al.: Correlation between titer of antibody to hepatitis B core antigen and presence of viral antigens in the liver, Gastroenterology **73**:664, 1977.
168. Koretz, R.L., Stone, O., and Gitnick, G.L.: The long-course of non-A, non-B post-transfusion hepatitis, Gastroenterology **79**:893, 1980.
169. Krugman, S., and Giles, J.P.: Viral hepatitis, type B (MS-2 strain): further observations on natural history and prevention, N. Engl. J. Med. **288**:755, 1973.
170. Krugman, S., Giles, J.P., and Hammond, J.: Infectious hepatitis: evidence for two distinctive clinical, epidemiological and immunological types of infection, J.A.M.A. **200**:365, 1967.
171. Krugman, S., Giles, J.P., and Hammond, J.: Viral hepatitis type B (MS-2 strain) prevention with specific hepatitis B immune serum globulin, JAMA **218**:1665, 1971.
172. Krugman, S., McAuliffe, V.J., and Purcell, R.H.: Hepatitis B vaccines: present status, Semin. Liver Dis. **1**:81, 1981.
173. Le Bouvier, G., and Williams, A.: Serotypes of hepatitis B antigen (HBsAg): the problem of new determinants, as exemplified by "+," Am. J. Med. Sci. **270**:165, 1975.
174. Levine, R.A., and Payne, M.A.: Homologous serum hepatitis in youthful heroin users, Ann. Intern. Med. **53**:164, 1960.
175. Lindsay, K.L., Redeker, A.G., and Ashcavai, M.: Delayed HBsAg clearance in chronic hepatitis B viral infection, Hepatology **1**:586, 1981.
176. MacGuarries, M.B., Forghani, B., and Wolochow, D.A.: Hepatitis B transmitted by a human bite, J.A.M.A. **230**:723, 1974.
177. MacLachlan, M.J., et al.: Chronic active "lupoid" hepatitis, Ann. Intern. Med. **62**:425, 1965.
178. Mathiesen, L.R., et al.: Localization of hepatitis A antigen in marmoset organs during acute infection with hepatitis A virus, J. Infect. Dis. **138**:369, 1978.
179. Mathiesen, L.R., et al.: Immunofluorescence studies of hepatitis A virus and hepatitis B surface and core antigen in liver biopsies from patients with acute viral hepatitis, Gastroenterology **77**:623, 1979.
180. Mathiesen, L.R., et al.: Hepatitis type A, B, and non-A, non-B in fulminant hepatitis, Gut **21**:72, 1980.
181. Matsaniotis, N., et al.: Immune responses to hepatitis B vaccine, Lancet **1**:210, 1981.
182. Miller, D.J., et al.: Jaundice in severe bacterial infection, Gastroenterology **71**:94, 1976.
183. Mirise, R.T., and Kitridou, R.C.: Arthritis and hepatitis, West. J. Med. **130**:12, 1979.
184. Monath, T.P., et al.: Lassa fever in the Eastern province of Sierra Leone: 1970–1972. II. Clinical observations and virological studies, Am. J. Trop. Med. Hyg. **23**:1140, 1974.
185. Mosley, J.W.: The epidemiology of viral hepatitis: an overview, Am. J. Med. Sci. **270**:253, 1975.
186. Mosley, J.W., et al.: Hepatitis B virus subtypes ad and ay among blood donors in the Greater Los Angeles area, Transfusion **14**:372, 1974.

187. Novick, D.M., et al.: Hepatitis B serologic studies in narcotic users with chronic liver disease, Am. J. Gastroenterol. **75**:111, 1981.
188. Omata, M., et al.: Comparison of serum hepatitis B surface antigen (HBsAg) and serum anti-core with tissue HBsAg and hepatitis B core antigen (HBcAg), Gastroenterology **75**:1003, 1978.
189. Pattyn, S., et al.: Isolation of Marburg-like virus from a case of haemorrhagic fever in Zaire, Lancet **1**:573, 1977.
190. Peters, R.L., et al.: Protracted viral hepatitis. In Vyas, G.N., Cohen, S.N., and Schmid, R., editors: Viral hepatitis, Philadelphia, 1978, The Franklin Institute Press.
191. Plainos, R.C., et al.: Dane particles in homogenates of mosquitoes fed with HBsAg-positive human blood, Lancet **1**:1334, 1975.
192. Prince, A.M., et al.: Hepatitis B antigen in wild-caught mosquitoes in Africa, Lancet **2**:247, 1972.
193. Prince, A.M., et al.: Long-incubation post-transfusion hepatitis without serological evidence of exposure to hepatitis B virus, Lancet **2**:241, 1974.
194. Proceedings of a symposium on viral hepatitis, Am. J. Med. Sci. vols. 270 and 271 (special issues), 1975.
195. Provost, P.J., et al.: Physical chemical and morphologic dimensions of human hepatitis: a virus strain CR326 (38578), Proc. Soc. Exp. Biol. Med. **148**:532, 1975.
196. Rakela, J.: Etiology and prognosis in fulminant hepatitis: Acute Hepatic Failure Study Group represented by J. Rakela (abstract), Gastroenterology **77**:A33, 1979.
196a. Rakela, J., and Hevia, F.: Personal communication.
197. Rakela, J., and Redeker, A.F.: Chronic liver disease after acute non-A, non-B hepatitis, Gastroenterology **77**:1200, 1979.
198. Redeker, A.G.: Viral hepatitis: clinical aspects, Am. J. Med. Sci. **270**:9, 1975.
199. Redeker, A.G., et al.: Hepatitis B immune globulin as a prophylactic measure for spouses exposed to acute type B hepatitis, N. Engl. J. Med. **293**:1055, 1975.
200. Redeker, A.G., and Yamahiro, H.S.: Controlled trial of exchange transfusion therapy in fulminant hepatitis, Lancet **1**:3, 1973.
201. Reiner, N.E., et al.: Asymptomatic rectal mucosal lesions and hepatitis B surface antigen at sites of sexual contact in homosexual men with persistent hepatitis B virus infection, Ann. Intern. Med. **96**:170, 1982.
202. Reynolds, T.B., et al.: Lupoid hepatitis, Ann. Intern. Med. **61**:650, 1964.
203. Rizzetto, M., et al.: Incidence and significance of antibodies to delta antigen in hepatitis B virus infection, Lancet **2**:986, 1979.
204. Rizzetto, M., et al.: Transmission of the hepatitis B virus-associated delta antigen to chimpanzees, J. Infect. Dis. **141**:590, 1980.
205. Rizzetto, M., et al.: Experimental HBV and delta infections of chimpanzees: occurrence and significance of intrahepatic complexes of HBcAg and delta antigen, Hepatology **1**:567, 1981.
206. Rizzetto, M., et al.: A radioimmunoassay for HBcAg in the sera of HBsAg carriers, Gastroenterology **80**:1420, 1981.
207. Schweitzer, I.L., et al.; Viral hepatitis B in neonates and infants, Am. J. Med. **55**:762, 1973.
208. Scott, R.M., et al.: Experimental transmission of hepatitis B virus by semen and saliva, J. Infect. Dis. **142**:67, 1980.
209. Seeff, L.B.: Immunoprophylaxis and treatment of viral hepatitis B, Semin. Liver Dis. **1**:69, 1981.
210. Shikata, T., et al.: Staining methods for Australia antigen in paraffin sections, Jpn. J. Exp. Med. **44**:25, 1974.
211. Shimizu, Y.K., et al.: Localization of hepatitis A antigen in liver tissue by peroxidase-conjugated antibody method: light and electron microscopic studies, J. Immunol. **121**:1671, 1978.
212. Shimizu, Y.K., et al.: Non-A, non-B hepatitis: ultrastructural evidence for two agents in experimentally infected chimpanzees, Science **205**:197, 1979.
213. Shimoda, T., et al.: Light microscopic localization of hepatitis B virus antigens in the human pancreas, Gastroenterology **81**:998, 1981.
214. Shorey, J.: Does hepatitis B virus grow outside the liver? Gastroenterology **79**:391, 1980.
215. Smith, D.H., et al.: Marburg-virus disease in Kenya, Lancet **1**:816, 1982.
216. Sternberg, G.M.: Report on the etiology and prevention of yellow fever, U.S. Marine Hosp. Pub. Health Bull. **2**:151, 1890.
217. Szmuness, W., et al.: Hepatitis B serum globulin in prevention of nonparenterally transmitted hepatitis B, N. Engl. J. Med. **290**:701, 1974.
218. Szmuness, W., et al.: Distrubution of antibody to hepatitis A antigen in urban adult population, N. Engl. J. Med. **295**:755, 1976.
219. Szmuness, W., et al.: Hepatitis type A and hemodialysis: a seroepidemiologic study in 15 U.S. centers, Ann. Intern. Med. **87**:8, 1977.
220. Szmuness, W., et al.: The prevalence of antibody to hepatitis A antigen in various parts of the world: a pilot study, Am. J. Epidemiol. **106**:392, 1977.
221. Szmuness, W., et al.: A controlled trial of the efficacy of the hepatitis B vaccine (Heptavax-B): a final report, Hepatology **1**:377, 1981.
222. Szmuness, W., et al.: Passive-active immunization against hepatitis B: immunogenicity studies in adult Americans, Lancet **1**:575, 1981.
223. Teodori, U., Gentilini, P., and Surrenti, C.: Electron microscope observation of forms of viral hepatitis, Gastroenterologia (Basel) **108**:105, 1967.
224. Tiollais, P., Charnay, P., and Vyas, G.N.: Biology of hepatitis B virus, Science **213**:406, 1981.
225. Tong, M.J., et al.: Studies on the maternal-infant transmission of the viruses which cause acute hepatitis, Gastroenterology **80**:999, 1981.
226. Tsiquaye, K.N., et al.: Ultrastructural changes in the liver in experimental non-A, non-b hepatitis, Br. J. Exp. Pathol. **62**:41, 1981.
227. Villarejos, V.M., et al.: Role of saliva, urine and feces in the transmission of type B hepatitis, N. Engl. J. Med. **291**:1375, 1974.
228. Viral haemorrhagic fevers (editorial), Lancet **2**:1325, 1981.
229. Ware, A.J., et al.: A prospective trial of steroid therapy in severe viral hepatitis, Gastroenterology **80**:219, 1981.
230. Weinstein, L.: Bacterial hepatitis, N. Engl. J. Med. **229**:1052, 1979.
231. Whittingham, S., et al.: Smooth muscle autoantibody in "autoimmune" hepatitis, Gastroenterology **51**:490, 1966.
232. Winn, W.C., Jr., et al.: Lassa virus hepatitis: observations on a fatal case from 1972 Sierra Leone epidemic, Arch. Pathol. **99**:599, 1975.
233. Wong, D.C., et al.: Epidemic and endemic hepatitis in India: evidence for a non-A, non-B hepatitis virus aetiology, Lancet **2**:876, 1980.
234. Yellow fever (editorial), Br. Med. J. **3**:121, 1975.
235. Yoshizawa, H., et al.: Virus-like particles in a plasma fraction in the circulation of apparently healthy blood donors capable of inducing non-A, non-B hepatitis, Gastroenterology **79**:512, 1980.
236. Yoshizawa, H., et al.: Demonstration of two different types of non-A, non-B hepatitis by reinjection and cross-challenge studies in chimpanzees, Gastroenterology **81**:107, 1981.
237. Zimmerman, H.J., et al.: Jaundice due to bacterial infection, Gastroenterology **77**:362, 1979.
238. Zuckerman, A.J., and Simpson, D.I.H.: Exotic virus infections of the liver. In Popper, H., and Schaffner, F., editors: Progress in liver disease, vol. 6, New York, 1979, Grune & Stratton, Inc.

Chemical and drug injury

239. Al-Kawas, F.H., et al.: Allopurinol hepatotoxicity: report of two cases and review of the literature, Ann. Intern. Med. **95**:588, 1981.
240. Altmann, H.W.: Drug-induced liver reactions: a morphological approach. In Grundmann, E., editor: Drug induced pathology, New York, 1980, Springer-Verlag, New York, Inc.

241. Arranto, A.J., and Sotaniemi, E.A.: Histologic follow-up of alpha-methyldopa-induced liver injury, Scand. J. Gastroenterol. **16**:864, 1981.
242. Arranto, A.J., and Sotaniemi, E.A.: Morphologic alterations in patients with alpha-methyldopa-induced liver damage after short- and long-term exposure, Scand. J. Gastroenterol. **16**:853, 1981.
243. Barker, J.D., deCarle, D.J., and Anuras, S.: Chronic excessive acetaminophen use and liver damage, Ann. Intern. Med. **87**:299, 1977.
244. Bassi, M.: Electron microscopy of rat liver after carbon tetrachloride, Exp. Cell Res. **20**:313, 1960.
245. Benjamin, S.B., et al.: Phenyl-butazone liver injury: a clinical pathologic survey of 23 cases and review of literature, Hepatology **1**:255, 1981.
246. Black, M., et al.: Isoniazid-associated hepatitis in 114 patients, Gastroenterology **69**:289, 1975.
247. Bonkowsky, H.L.: Chronic hepatic inflammation and fibrosis due to low doses of paracetamol, Lancet **1**:1016, 1978.
248. Breitenbucher, R., and Crowley, L.: Hepatorenal toxicity of tetracycline, Minn. Med. **53**:949, 1970.
249. Brown, B.R., and Sipes, I.G.: Biotransformation and hepatotoxicity of halothane, Biochem. Pharmacol. **26**:2091, 1977.
250. Burke, M.: Cytochrome P-450: a pharmacological necessity or a biochemical curosity? Biochem. Pharmacol. **30**:181, 1981.
251. Chutlani, H.R.: Acute copper sulfate poisoning, Am. J. Med. **39**:849, 1965.
252. Deo, M.G., Roy, H., and Ramalingaswami, V.: Protein deficiency in carbon tetrachloride-induced hepatic lesions, Arch. Pathol. **99**:147, 1975.
253. Drill, A.: Benign cholestatic jaundice of pregnancy and benign cholestatic jaundice from oral contraceptives, Am. J. Obstet. Gynecol. **119**:165, 1974.
254. Edmond, M., et al.: Effect of novobiocin on liver function, Can. Med. Assoc. J. **94**:900, 1966.
255. Ellard, G.A.: The hepatotoxicity of isoniazid among the three acetylator phenotypes, Am. Rev. Respir. Dis. **123**:568, 1981.
256. Erlinger, S.: Cholestasis: pump failure, microvilli defect or both, Lancet **1**:533, 1978.
257. Ferreyra, E.C., et al.: Prevention and treatment of carbon tetrachloride hepatotoxicity by cysteine: studies about its mechanism, Toxicol. Appl. Pharmacol. **27**:558, 1974.
258. Hoft, R.H., et al.: Halothane hepatitis in three pairs of closely related women, N. Engl. J. Med. **304**:1023, 1981.
259. Horvath, E., et al.: Fine structural changes in the liver of methotrexate-treated psoriatics, Digestion **17**:488, 1978.
260. Klatskin, G., and Kimberg, B.B.: Recurrent hepatitis attributable to halothane sensitization in an anesthetist, N. Engl. J. Med. **280**:515, 1969.
261. Klemola, H., et al.: Anicteric liver damage during nitrofurantoin medication, Scand. J. Gastroenterol. **10**:501, 1975.
262. Kline, M.A.: Enflurane-associated hepatitis, Gastroenterology **79**:126, 1980.
263. Lauterburg, B.H., and Mitchell, J.R.: Toxic doses of acetaminophen suppress hepatic glutathione synthesis in rats, Hepatology **2**:8, 1982.
264. Maddrey, W.C., and Boitnott, J.K.: Drug-induced chronic liver disease, Gastroenterology **72**:1348, 1977.
265. McCormick, D.J., Avbel, A.J., and Gibbons, R.B.: Nonlethal mushroom poisoning, Ann. Intern. Med. **90**:332, 1979.
266. Metreau, J.M., Dhumeaux, D., and Berthelot, P.: Oral contraceptives and the liver, Digestion **7**:313, 1972.
267. Mitchel, D.H.: Amanita mushroom poisoning, Ann. Rev. Med. **31**:51, 1980.
268. Mitchell, J.R., and Jollows, D.J.: Metabolic activation of drugs to toxic substances, Gastroenterology **68**:392, 1975.
269. Mitchell, J.R., et al.: Isoniazid liver injury: clinical spectrum, pathology and probable pathogenesis, Ann. Intern. Med. **84**:181, 1976.
270. Mitchell, M.C., et al.: Cimetidine protects against acetaminophen hepatotoxicity in rats, Gastroenterology **81**:1052, 1981.
271. Mullick, F.G., and Ishak, K.G.: Hepatic injury associated with diphenylhydantoin therapy: a clinicopathologic study of 20 cases, Am. J. Clin. Pathol. **74**:442, 1980.
272. Nyfors, A., and Hopwood, D.: Liver ultrastructure in psoriatics related to methotrexate therapy, Acta Pathol. Microbiol. Scand. **85**:787, 1977.
273. Panner, B.J., and Hanss, R.J.: Hepatic injury in mushroom poisoning, Arch. Pathol. **87**:35, 1969.
274. Paracetamol hepatoxicity (editorial), Lancet **2**:1189, 1975.
275. Perrissoud, D., et al.: The effect of carbon tetrachloride on isolated rat hepatocytes: early morphological alterations of the plasma membrane, Virchows Arch. (Cell Pathol.) **35**:83, 1981.
276. Peters, R.L., et al.: Hepatic necrosis associated with halothane anesthesia, Am. J. Med. **57**:748, 1969.
277. Phillips, M.J., Oda, M., and Kazuo, F.: Evidence for microfilament involvement in norethandrolone-induced intrahepatic cholestasis, Am. J. Pathol. **93**:729, 1978.
278. Popper, H., and Schaffner, F.: Cholestasis: concepts and mechanisms. In Bockus, H., editor: Gastroenterology, ed. 3, Philadelphia, 1976, W.B. Saunders Co.
279. Portmann, B., et al.: Histopathological changes in the liver following a paracetamol overdose: correlation with clinical and biochemical parameters, J. Pathol. **117**:169, 1975.
280. Prescott, L.F., Ballantyne, A., and Park, J.: Treatment of parecetomal (acetaminophen) poisoning with *N*-acetylcysteine, Lancet 2:432, 1977.
281. Prescott, L.F., et al.: Successful treatment of severe paracetamol (acetaminophen) overdose, Lancet **2**:829, 1976.
282. Recknagel, R.: Carbon tetrachloride hepatotoxicity, Pharmacol. Rev. **19**:145, 1967.
283. Recknagel, R.O., and Ghoshal, A.K.: Lipoperoxidation as vector in carbon tetrachloride hepatotoxicity, Lab. Invest. **15**:132, 1966.
284. Reynolds, T.B., Peters, R.L., and Yamada, S.: Chronic active and lupoid hepatitis caused by a laxative, oxyphenisatin, N. Engl. J. Med. **285**:813, 1971.
285. Robertson, W.O.: Changing perspectives on acetaminophen, Am. J. Dis. Child. **132**:459, 1978.
286. Rubotham, J.L., Troxler, R.F., and Lietman, P.S.: Iron poisoning: another energy crisis, Lancet **2**:664, 1974.
287. Sato, C., Matsuda, Y., and Lieber, C.S.: Increased hepatotoxicity of acetaminophen after chronic ethanol consumption in the rat, Gastroenterology **80**:140, 1981.
288. Sherlock, S.: Halothane hepatitis, Lancet **2**:364, 1978.
289. Smith, R.L.: Biliary excretion and hepatotoxicity of contraceptive steroids, Acta Endocrinol. **185**:149, 1973.
290. Spechler, S.J., Sperber, H., and Doos, W.G.: Cholestasis and toxic epidermal necrolysis associated with phenytoin sodium ingestion: the role of bile duct injury, Ann. Intern. Med. **95**:455, 1981.
291. Stenger, R.J.: Organelle pathology of the liver—the endoplasmic reticulum, Gastroenterology **58**:554, 1970.
292. Storms, W.W.: Chloroform parties, J.A.M.A. **225**:160, 1973.
293. Tonder, M., Nordoy, A., and Elgio, K.: Sulfonamide-induced chronic liver disease, Scand. J. Gastroenterol. **9**:93, 1974.
294. Vergani, D., et al.: Antibodies to the surface of halothane-altered rabbit hepatocytes in patients with severe halothane-associated hepatitis, N. Engl. J. Med. **303**:66, 1980.
295. Walker, C.O., and Combes, B.: Biliary cirrhosis induced by chlorpromazine, Gastroenterology **51**:631, 1966.
296. Weinstein, G., et al.: Psoriasis-liver methotrexate interactions, Arch. Dermatol. **108**:36, 1973.
297. Wepler, W., and Opitz, K.: Histologic changes in the liver biopsy in *Amanita phalloides* intoxication, Hum. Pathol. **3**:249, 1972.
298. Wieland, T., and Faulstich, H.: Aflatoxins, phallotoxins, phallolysin, and anatamanide: the biologically active components of poisonous *Amanita* mushrooms, C.R.C. Crit. Rev. Biochem. **5**:185, 1978.
299. Zimmerman, H.J.: Classification of hepatotoxins and mechanisms of toxicity. In Zimmerman, H.J., editor: Hepatotoxicity, New York, 1978, Appleton-Century-Crofts.
300. Zimmerman, H.J.: Intrahepatic cholestasis, Arch. Intern. Med. **139**:1038, 1979.

301. Zimmerman, H.J.: Effects of aspirin and acetaminophen on the liver, Arch. Intern. Med. **141**:333, 1981.

Alcoholic liver disease

302. Baillie, M.: The morbid anatomy of some of the most important parts of the human body, vol. 28. In Rodin, A.E.: The influence of Matthew Baille's morbid anatomy, Springfield, Ill., 1973, Charles C Thomas, Publisher.
303. Bell, H., and Nordhagen, R.: HLA antigens in alcoholics, with special reference to alcoholic cirrhosis, Scand. J. Gastroenterol. **15**:453, 1980.
304. Bruaguera, M., Bordas, J.M., and Rodes, J.: Asymptomatic liver disease in alcoholics, Arch. Pathol. Lab. Med. **101**:644, 1977.
305. Cederbaum, A.I.: Regulations of pathways of alcohol metabolism by the liver, Mt. Sinai J. Med. **47**:317, 1980.
306. Chedid, A., Jao, W., and Port, J.: Megamitochondria in hepatic and renal disease, Am. J. Gastroenterol. **73**:319, 1980.
307. Criteria Committee, National Council on Alcoholism: Criteria for the diagnosis of alcoholism, Ann. Intern. Med. **77**:249, 1972.
308. Deitrich, R.A., and McClearn, G.E.: Neurobiological and genetic aspects of the etiology of alcoholism, Fed. Proc. **40**:2051, 1981.
309. Edmondson, H.A.: Pathology of alcoholism, Am. J. Clin. Pathol. **74**:725, 1980.
310. Edmondson, H.A., et al.: Sclerosing hyaline necrosis of the liver in the chronic alcoholic: a recognizable clinical syndrome, Ann. Intern. Med. **59**:646, 1963.
311. Fleming, K.A., et al.: Mallory bodies in alcoholic and nonalcoholic liver disease contain a common antigenic determinant, Gut **22**:341, 1981.
312. French, S.W., et al.: Lymphocyte sequestration by the liver in alcoholic hepatitis, Arch. Pathol. Lab. Med. **103**:146, 1979.
313. Gayre, G.R.: Wassail! In Mazers of mead, London, 1948, Phillimore & Co., Ltd.
314. Hales, M.R., Allan, J.S., and Hall, E.M.: Injection corrosion studies of normal and cirrhotic livers, Am. J. Pathol. **35**:909, 1959.
315. Kao, H., Uchida, T., and Peters, R.L.: A clinical evaluation of acute hepatic decompensation in alcoholic liver disease (abstract), Hepatology **1**:522, 1981.
316. Karasawa, T., et al.: Morphologic spectrum of liver diseases among chronic alcoholics, Acta Pathol. Jpn. **39**:505, 1980.
317. Kater, L., et al.: Alcoholic hepatic disease: specificity of IgA deposits in liver, Am. J. Clin. Pathol. **71**:51, 1979.
318. Keller, M.: A historical overview of alcohol and alcoholism, Cancer Res. **39**:2822, 1979.
319. Klatsky, A.L., Friedman, G.D., and Siegelaub, A.B.: Alcohol and mortality: a ten-year Kaiser-Permanente experience, Ann. Intern. Med. **95**:141, 1981.
320. Krebs, H.A., and Perkins, J.R.: The physiologic role of liver alcohol dehydrogenase, Biochem. J. **118**:635, 1970.
321. Kroyer, J.M., and Talbert, W.M.: Morphologic liver changes in intestinal bypass patients, Am. J. Surg. **139**:855, 1980.
322. Laënnec, R.T.H.: Traite' de l'ausculatation mediate, Paris, 1826, Chaude.
323. Levin, D.M., et al.: Nonalcoholic liver disease: overlooked causes of liver injury in patients with heavy alcohol consumption, Am. J. Med. **66**:429, 1979.
324. Li, T.-K.: Human alcohol dehydrogenase isoenzyme (B), Alcoholism **5**:451, 1981.
325. Lieber, C.S.: Alcohol, protein metabolism, and liver injury, Gastroenterology **79**:373, 1980.
326. Lieber, C.S., and de Carli, L.M.: Hepatic microsomal ethanol-oxidizing system: in vitro characteristics and adaptive properties in vivo, J. Biol. Chem. **245**:2505, 1970.
327. Lundquist, F., et al.: Ethanol metabolism and production of free acetate in the human liver, J. Clin. Invest. **41**:955, 1962.
328. Mezey, E.: Alcoholic liver disease: roles of alcohol and malnutrition, Am. J. Clin. Nutr. **33**:2709, 1980.
329. Morgan, M.Y., Sherlock, S., and Scheuer, P.J.: Acute cholestasis, hepatic failure and fatty liver in the alcoholic, Scand. J. Gastroenterol. **13**:299, 1978.
330. Orrego, H., et al.: Correlation of intrahepatic pressure with collagen in the Disse space and hepatomegaly in humans and in the rat, Gastroenterology **80**:546, 1981.
331. Petersen, P.: Alcoholic hyalin, microfilaments, and microtubules in alcoholic hepatitis, Acta Pathol. Microbiol. Scand. **85**:384, 1977.
332. Popper, H., et al.: Histogenesis of alcoholic fibrosis and cirrhosis in the baboon, Am. J. Pathol. **98**:695, 1980.
333. Randall, B.: Fatty liver and sudden death: a review, Hum. Pathol. **11**:147, 1980.
334. Reynolds, R.B., et al.: Portal hypertension without cirrhosis in alcoholic liver disease, Ann. Intern. Med. **70**:497, 1969.
335. Rubin, E., and Lieber, C.S.: Alcohol-induced hepatic injury in nonalcoholic volunteers, N. Engl. J. Med. **278**:869, 1968.
336. Schmid, W., and Popham, R.E.: The role of drinking and smoking in mortality from cancer and other causes in male alcoholics, Cancer **47**:1031, 1981.
337. Smith, M., Hopkinson, D.A., and Harris, H.: Developmental changes and polymorphism in human alcohol dehydrogenase, Ann. Hum. Genet. **34**:251, 1971.
338. Stanko, R.T., et al.: Prevention of alcohol-induced fatty liver by natural metabolites and riboflavin, J. Lab. Clin. Med. **91**:228, 1978.
339. Uchida, T., et al.: Alcoholic foamy degeneration of the liver: a pattern in acute alcoholic patients (abstract), Gastroenterology **80**:1352, 1981.
340. Van Thiel, D.H., et al.: Gastrointestinal and hepatic manifestations of chronic alcoholism, Gastroenterology **81**:594, 1981.
341. Veech, R.L.: Metabolism of alcohol: enzymes, pathways, and metabolites (A), Alcoholism **5**:451, 1981.
342. Von Wartburg, J.P.: Alcohol metabolism and alcoholism: pharmacogenetic consideration, Acta Psychiatr. Scand. **62**(suppl. 286):179, 1980.
343. Yokoo, H., Singh, S.K., and Hawasli, A.H.: Giant mitochondria in alcoholic liver disease, Arch. Pathol. Lab. Med. **102**:213, 1978.

Pathophysiology of chronic liver disease

344. Bean, W.B.: Vascular "spiders" and palmar erythema, Am. Heart J. **25**:463, 1943.
345. Bennett, H.S., Baggenstoss, A.H., and Butt, H.R.: Testis, breast, and prostate of men who die of cirrhosis of liver, Am. J. Clin. Pathol. **20**:814, 1950.
346. Berenyi, M.R., Straus, B., and Avila, L.: T-rosettes in alcoholic cirrhosis of the liver, J.A.M.A. **232**:44, 1975.
347. Berk, P.D., and Popper, H.: Fulminant hepatic failure: chairman's summary—a final evaluation, Am. J. Gastroenterol. **69**:349, 1978.
348. Berthelot, P., et al.: Arterial changes in the lungs in cirrhosis of the liver, N. Engl. J. Med. **274**:291, 1966.
349. Calabresi, P., and Abelmann, W.H.: Portopulmonary anastomoses, J. Clin. Invest. **36**:1257, 1957.
350. Cavanagh, J.B., and Kye, M.H.: The astrocyte in liver disease, Lancet **2**:1189, 1971.
351. Eisenmenger, W.J.: Ascites in patients with cirrhosis, Ann. Intern. Med. **37**:261, 1952.
352. Grahn, E., et al.: Burr cells, hemolytic anemia and cirrhosis, Am. J. Med. **45**:78, 1968.
353. Green, G., et al.: Association of abnormal fibrin polymerisation with severe liver disease, Gut **18**:909, 1977.
354. Herbert, V.: Hematopoietic factors in liver diseases, Prog. Liver Dis. **2**:57, 1965.
355. Kelty, R.H., Baggenstoss, A.H., and Butt, H.R.: Portal hypertension, Gastroenterology **15**:285, 1950.
356. Kissane, J.M.: Chronic active hepatitis and pulmonary hypertension. In Cryer, P.E., editor: Clinicopathologic conference, Am. J. Med. **63**:604, 1977.
357. Lieberman, F.L., Ito, S., and Reynolds, T.B.: Effective plasma volume in sclerosis of ascites, J. Clin. Invest. **48**:975, 1969.
358. Lieberman, F.L., and Peters, R.L.: Cirrhotic hydrothorax, Arch. Intern. Med. **125**:114, 1970.

359. Lieberman, F.L., et al.: Pathogenesis and treatment of hydrothorax complicating cirrhosis with ascites, Ann. Intern. Med. **64**:341, 1965.
360. Liebowitz, H.R.: Pathogenesis of ascites in cirrhosis of liver, N.Y. J. Med. **69**:2012, 1969.
361. Liver disease and the renal prostaglandin system (editorial), Gastroenterology **77**:391, 1979.
362. Maderazo, E.G., Ward, P.A., and Quintiliani, R.: Defective regulation of chemotaxis in cirrhosis, J. Lab. Clin. Med. **85**:621, 1975.
363. McDermott, W.V., Jr.: Surgery of the liver and portal circulation, Philadelphia, 1974, Lea & Febiger.
364. Michalak, T.: Immune complexes of hepatitis B surface antigen in the pathologenesis of periarteritis nodosa: a study of seven necropsy cases, Am. J. Pathol. **90**:619, 1978.
365. Mikkelsen, W.P., et al.: Extra- and intrahepatic portal hypertension without cirrhosis (hepato-portal sclerosis), Ann. Surg. **162**:602, 1965.
366. Mullane, J.F., and Gliedman, M.L.: Elevation of pressure in inferior vena cava, Surgery **59**:1135, 1966.
367. Nakashima, T.: Vascular changes and hemodynamics in hepatocellular carcinoma. In Okuda, K., and Peters, R.L., editors: Hepatocellular carcinoma, New York, 1976, John Wiley & Sons, Inc.
368. Norenberg, M.D., et al.: Division of protoplasmic astrocytes in acute experimental hepatic encephalopathy, Am. J. Pathol. **67**:403, 1972.
369. Olling, S., and Olsson, R.: Congenital absence of portal venous system in a 50-year-old woman, Acta Med. Scand. **196**:343, 1974.
370. Orloff, M.J., et al.: Experimental ascites, Surgery **56**:83, 1964.
371. Palmer, E.D.: Management of esophageal varices, Prog. Liver Dis. **1**:329, 1961.
372. Papper, S.: Role of kidney in Laënnec's cirrhosis, Medicine **37**:299, 1958.
373. Ramoff, O.D.: Hemostatic mechanisms in liver disease, Med. Clin. North Am. **47**:721, 1968.
374. Reynolds, T.B.: Portal hypertension. In Schiff, L., editor: Diseases of the liver, ed. 4, Philadelphia, 1975, J.B. Lippincott Co.
375. Reynolds, T.B., et al.: Portal hypertension without cirrhosis in alcoholic liver disease, Ann. Intern. Med. **70**:497, 1969.
376. Reynolds, T.B., Redeker, A.G., and Geller, H.M.: Wedged hepatic pressure, Am. J. Med. **22**:341, 1959.
377. Ring-Larsen, H., and Palazzo, U.: Renal failure in fulminant hepatic failure and terminal cirrhosis: a comparison between incidence, types, and prognosis, Gut **22**:585, 1981.
378. Schafer, D.F., and Jones, E.A.: Hepatic encephalopathy and the γ-aminobutyric-acid neurotransmitter system, Lancet **1**:18, 1982.
379. Silber, R., et al.: Spur-shaped erythrocytes in Laënnec's cirrhosis, N. Engl. J. Med. **275**:639, 1966.
380. Soria, J., et al.: Study of acquired dysfibrinogenaemia in liver disease, Thromb. Res. **19**:29, 1980.
381. Taylor, P., et al.: Quantitative changes in astrocytes after portacaval shunting in chimpanzees and in man, Arch. Pathol. Lab. Med. **103**:82, 1979.
382. Van Thiel, D.H., Lester, R., and Sherins, R.J.: Hypogonadism in alcoholic liver disease: evidence for a double defect, Gastroenterology **67**:1188, 1974.
383. Van Thiel, D.H., et al.: Patterns of hypothalamic-pituitary-gonadal dysfunction in men with liver disease due to differing etiologies, Hepatology **1**:39, 1981.
384. Wilkinson, S.P., et al.: Kidney failure in liver disease, Br. Med. J. **1**:1375, 1978.
385. Wuhrmann, F.: Hepatogenic myocardosis, Scand. J. Gastroenterol. **7**(suppl.):97, 1970.
386. Zieve, L.: The mechanism of hepatic coma, Hepatology **1**:360, 1981.

Cholestatic disorders

387. Abul-Khair, M.H., et al.: Ultrasonography and amoebic liver abscesses, Ann. Surg. **193**:221, 1981.
388. Adson, M.A., and Wychulis, A.R.: Portal hypertension in secondary biliary cirrhosis, Arch. Surg. **96**:604, 1968.
389. Alkan, W.J., Kalmi, B., and Kauderon, M.: The clinical syndrome of amebic abscesses of the left lobe of the liver, Ann. Intern. Med. **55**:800, 1961.
390. Baggenstoss, A.H., et al.: The pathology of primary biliary cirrhosis with emphasis on histogenesis, Am. J. Clin. Pathol. **42**:259, 1964.
391. Ball, T.J., et al.: Hemobilia following percutaneous liver biopsy, Gastroenterology **68**:1297, 1975.
392. Biava, C.G.: Fine structure of normal bile canaliculi, Lab. Invest. **13**:840, 1964.
393. Blackstone, M.O., and Nemchausky, B.A.: Cholangiographic abnormalities in ulcerative cholitis associated pericholangitis which resembles sclerosing cholangitis, Dig. Dis. Sci. **23**:579, 1978.
394. Bodenheimer, H.C., and Schaffner, F.: Primary biliary cirrhosis and the immune system, Am. J. Gastroenterol. **72**:285, 1979.
395. Boey, J.H., and Way, L.W.: Acute cholangitis, Ann. Surg. **191**:264, 1980.
396. Brandt, H., and Tamayo, R.P.: Pathology of human amebiasis, Hum. Pathol. **1**:351, 1970.
397. Chapman, R.W.G., et al.: Primary sclerosing cholangitis: a review of its clinical features, cholangiography, and hepatic history, Gut **21**:870, 1980.
398. Charcot, J.M.: Leçcons sur les maladies du foie; des voies biliares et des reins: recueillies et publiées par Bourneville et Sèvestre, Paris, 1877, Progrès Médical.
399. Cheung, N.K., et al.: Pyogenic liver abscess, Am. Surg. **44**:272, 1978.
400. Christensen, E., Crowe, J., and Doniach, D.: Clinical pattern and course of disease in primary biliary cirrhosis based on an analysis of 236 patients, Gastroenterology **78**:236, 1980.
401. Crowe, J.P., et al.: Primary biliary cirrhosis: the prevalence of hypothyroidism and its relationship to thyroid autoantibodies and sicca syndrome, Gastroenterology **78**:1437, 1980.
402. Dehner, L.P., and Kissane, J.M.: Pyogenic hepatic abscesses in infancy and childhood, J. Pediatr. **74**:763, 1969.
403. Delamarre, J., et al.: Traumatic hemobilia: a complication of Chiba needle transhepatic cholangiography (letter), Gastroenterology **75**:771, 1978.
404. Doppman, J.L., et al.: Bile duct cysts secondary to liver infarcts: report of a case and experimental production by small vessel hepatic artery occlusion, Radiology **130**:1, 1979.
405. Fleming, C.R., Ludwig, J., and Dickson, E.R.: Asymptomatic primary biliary cirrhosis: presentation, histology, and results with *d*-penicillamine, Mayo Clin. Proc. **53**:587, 1978.
406. Frank, M.M.: Reticuloendothelial complement: specific clearance of circulating particles—primary biliary cirrhosis and the complement system, Ann. Intern. Med. **90**:72, 1979.
407. Freeny, P.C.: Acute pyogenic hepatitis: sonographic and angiographic findings, A.J.R. **135**:388, 1980.
408. Fujiwara, Y., et al.: Congenital dilatation of intrahepatic and common bile ducts with congenital hepatic fibrosis, J. Pediatr. Surg. **11**:273, 1976.
409. Gall, E.A., and Dobrogorski, O.: Obstructive jaundice, Am. J. Clin. Pathol. **70**:226, 1960.
410. Gallagher, P.J., Millis, P.R., and Mitchinson, M.J.: Congenital dilatation of the intrahepatic bile ducts with cholangiocarcinoma, J. Clin. Pathol. **25**:304, 1972.
411. Grant, E.G., et al.: Pneumobilia: a comparison of four imaging modalities, J. Comput. Assist. Tomogr. **4**:630, 1980.
412. Haaga, J.R., and Weinfield, A.J.: CT-guided percutaneous aspiration and drainage of abscesses, A.J.R. **135**:388, 1980.
413. Holt, J.M., and Spry, C.J.F.: Solitary pyogenic liver abscess in patients with diabetes mellitus, Lancet **2**:198, 1966.
414. Jaup, B.H., Lennart, S.W., and Zettergren, S.W.: Familial occurrence of primary biliary cirrhosis associated with hypergammaglobulinemia in descendants, Gastroenterology **78**:549, 1980.
415. Kanner, R., Weinfeld, A., and Tedesco, F.J.: Hepatic abscess—plain film findings as an early aid to diagnosis, Am. J. Gastroenterol. **71**:432, 1979.

416. Lawson, T.L.: Hepatic abscess: ultrasound as an aid to diagnosis, Dig. Dis. Sci. **22**:33, 1977.
417. Lefkowitch, J.H.: Primary sclerosing cholangitis, Arch. Intern. Med. **142**:1157, 1982.
418. Lin, C.S.: Suppurative pylephlebitis and liver abscess complicating colonic diverticulitis: report of two cases and review of literature, Mt. Sinai J. Med. N.Y. **40**:48, 1973.
419. Lloyd, D.A.: Massive hepatobiliary ascariasis in childhood, Br. J. Surg. **68**:468, 1981.
420. Ludwig, L., Dickson, E.R., and McDonald, G.S.A.: Staging of chronic non-suppurative destructive cholangitis (syndrome of primary biliary cirrhosis), Virchows Arch. (Pathol. Anat.) **379**:103, 1978.
421. Maher, J.A., Reynolds, T.B., and Yellin, A.E.: Successful medical treatment of pyogenic liver abscess, Gastroenterology **77**:618, 1979.
422. Maingot, R.: Postoperative strictures of the bile ducts: causes, prevention, repair procedures, Br. J. Clin. Pract. **31**:117, 1977.
423. Marx, W.J., and O'Connell, D.J.: Arthritis of primary biliary cirrhosis, Arch. Intern. Med. **139**:213, 1979.
424. Meade, R.H., III: Primary hepatic actinomycosis, Gastroenterology **78**:355, 1980.
425. Moss, T.J., and Pysher, T.J.: Hepatic abscess in neonates, Am. J. Dis. Child. **135**:726, 1981.
426. Ochsner, A., DeBakey, M., and Murray, S.: Pyogenic abscess of the liver. II. An analysis of forty-seven cases with review of the literature, Am. J. Surg. **40**:292, 1938.
427. Palmer, E.D.: The changing manifestations of pyogenic liver abscess, J.A.M.A. **231**:192, 1975.
428. Perry, H.B., Boulanger, M., and Pennoyer, D.: Chronic granulomatous disease in an adult with recurrent abscesses, Arch. Surg. **115**:200, 1980.
429. Peters, R.S., Gitlin, N., and Libdke, R.D.: Amebic liver abscesses, Annu. Rev. Med. **32**:161, 1981.
430. Piggott, J.A., and Hochholzer, L.: Humen melioidosis, Arch. Pathol. **90**:101, 1970.
431. Quispe-Sjogren, M., Uchida, T., and Peters, R.L.: Comparative clinico-histopathological study among PBC, PSC and liver disease (abstract), Gastroenterology **80**:1354, 1981.
432. Record, C.O., et al.: Intrahepatic sclerosing cholangitis associated with a familial immuno-deficiency syndrome, Lancet **2**:18, 1973.
433. Reynolds, T.B., et al.: Primary biliary cirrhosis with scleroderma, Raynaud's phenomenon and telangiectasia, Am. J. Med. **50**:302, 1971.
434. Robenek, H., Herwig, J., and Themann, H.: The morphologic characteristics of intercellular junctions between normal human liver cells and cells from patients with extrahepatic cholestasis, Am. J. Pathol. **100**:93, 1980.
435. Rolleston, H.D.: Diseases of the liver, gallbladder, and bile ducts, Philadelphia, 1905, W.B. Saunders Co.
436. Rubin, R.H., Swartz, M.N., and Malt, R.: Hepatic abscess: changes in clinical, bacteriologic, and therapeutic aspects—a review, Ann. Intern. Med. **57**:601, 1974.
437. Sabbaz, J., Sutter, V.L., and Finegold, S.M.: Anaerobic pyogenic liver abscess, Ann. Intern. Med. **77**:629, 1972.
438. Sandblom, P.: Hemobilia (biliary tract hemorrhage): history, pathology, diagnosis, treatment, Springfield, Ill., 1972, Charles C Thomas, Publisher.
439. Schoenfield, L.J., Sjovall, J., and Perman, E.: Bile acids on skin of patients with pruritic hepatobiliary disease, Nature **212**:93, 1967.
440. Scott, A.J., and Khan, G.A.: Origin of bacteria in bile-duct bile, Lancet **2**:790, 1967.
441. Sheehy, T.W., et al.: Resolution of an amebic liver abscess, Gastroenterology **55**:26, 1968.
442. Sherlock, S., and Scheurer, P.J.: The presentation and diagnosis of 100 patients with primary biliary cirrhosis, N. Engl. J. Med. **289**:674, 1973.
443. Shorter, R.G., and Baggenstoss, A.H.: Extrahepatic cholestasis. III. Chronology of histologic changes in the liver, Am. J. Clin. Pathol. **32**:10, 1959.
444. Silver, S., Weinstein, A., and Cooperman, A.: Changes in the pathogenesis of intrahepatic abscess, Am. J. Surg. **137**:608, 1979.
445. Snape, W.J., et al.: Marked alkaline phosphatase elevation with partial common bile duct obstruction due to calcific pancreatitis, Gastroenterology **70**:70, 1976.
446. Takada, T., et al.: Severe choledochocholangitis causing numerous cystlike hepatic abscesses, Int. Surg. **59**:180, 1974.
447. Thung, S.N., and Gerber, M.A.: Caroli's disease: a rarely recognized entity, Arch. Pathol. Lab. Med. **103**:650, 1979.
448. Tsantoulas, D., et al.: Antibodies to a human liver membrane lipoprotein (LSP) in primary biliary cirrhosis, Gut **21**:557, 1980.
449. Werlin, S.L., et al.: Sclerosing cholangitis in childhood, J. Pediatr. **96**:443, 1980.
450. Wiesner, R.H., and LaRusso, R.F.: Clinicopathologic features of the syndrome of primary sclerosing cholangitis, Gastroenterology **79**:200, 1980.
451. Yadegar, J., et al.: Common duct stricture from chronic pancreatitis, Arch. Surg. **115**:582, 1980.
452. Yellin, A.E., and Donovan, A.J.: Biliary lithiasis and helminthiasis, Am. J. Surg. **142**:128, 1981.

Liver disease in infants and children

453. Alagille, D.: Cholestasis in the first three months of life. In Popper, H., and Schaffner, F., editors: Progress in liver disease, vol. 6, New York, 1979, Grune & Stratton, Inc.
454. Alagille, D., et al.: Hepatic ductular hypoplasia associated with characteristic facies, vertebral malformations, J. Pediatr. **86**:63, 1975.
455. Altman, P.R., Chandra, R., and Lilly, J.R.: Ongoing cirrhosis after successful porticoenterostomy in infants with biliary atresia, J. Pediatr. Surg. **10**:684, 1975.
456. Alvarez, F., et al.: Congenital hepatic fibrosis in children, J. Pediatr. **99**:370, 1981.
457. Amanullah, A.: Neonatal jaundice, Am. J. Dis. Child. **130**:1274, 1976.
458. Arias, I.M., et al.: Prolonged neonatal unconjugated hyperbilirubinemia associated with breast feeding and a steroid, J. Clin. Invest. **43**:2037, 1964.
459. Balistreri, W.F., and Schubert, W.L.: Liver disease in infancy and childhood. In Schiff, L., and Schiff, E.R., editors: Diseases of the liver, ed. 5, New York, 1982, J.P. Lippincott Co.
460. Bearn, A.G.: Alpha-1-antitrypsin deficiency: a biological enigma, Gut **19**:470, 1978.
461. Becroft, D.M.O.: Prenatal cytomegalovirus infection. In Rosenberg, H.S., and Bernstein, J., editors: Perspectives in pediatric pathology, vol. 6, New York, 1981, Masson Publishing U.S.A., Inc.
462. Benjamin, D.R.: Hepatobiliary dysfunction in infants and children associated with long-term total parenteral nutrition: a clinico-pathologic study, Am. J. Clin. Pathol. **76**:276, 1981.
463. Bourgeois, C., et al.: Encephalopathy and fatty degeneration of the viscera: a clinicopathologic analysis of 40 cases, Am. J. Clin. Pathol. **56**:558, 1971.
464. Bove, K.E., et al.: The hepatic lesion in Reye's syndrome, Gastroenterology **69**:685, 1975.
465. Brady, R.O.: Sphingomyelin lipidosis: Niemann-Pick disease. In Stanbury, J.B., et al., editors: The metabolic basis of inherited disease, New York, 1978, McGraw-Hill Book Co.
466. Brooks, S., et al.: Hepatic ultrastructure in secondary syphilis, Arch. Pathol. Lab. Med. **103**:451, 1979.
467. Brough, A.J., and Bernstein, J.: Conjugated hyperbilirubinemia in early infancy: a reassessment of liver biopsy, Hum. Pathol. **5**:507, 1974.
468. Brown, A.K., and McDonagh, A.F.: Phototherapy for neonatal hyperbilirubinemia: efficacy, mechanism and toxicity, Adv. Pediatr. **27**:341, 1980.
469. Chalhub, E.G., et al.: Reye's syndrome complicated by a generalized herpes simplex virus type I infection, J. Pediatr. **98**:73, 1981.
470. Clayton, R.J., et al.: Byler disease—fatal familial intrahepatic cholestasis in an Amish kindred, Am. J. Dis. Child. **117**:112, 1969.

471. Committee on Infectious Disease: A special report: aspirin and Reye's syndrome, Pediatrics **69**:810, 1982.
472. Cornblath, M., and Schwartz, R.: Disorders of carbohydrate metabolism in infancy, Philadelphia, 1976, W.B. Saunders Co.
473. Craig, J.M., Geliis, S.S., and Hsia, D.Y.: Cirrhosis of the liver in infants and children, Am. J. Dis. Child. **90**:299, 1956.
474. Dahms, B.B., and Halpin, T.C., Jr.: Serial liver biopsies in parenteral nutrition-associated cholestasis of early infancy, Gastroenterology **81**:136, 1981.
475. Dische, M.R., and Gooch, W.M., III: Congenital toxoplasmosis. In Rosenberg, H.S., and Bernstein, J., editors: Perspectives in pediatric pathology, vol. 6, New York, 1981, Masson Publishing U.S.A., Inc.
476. Dufour, D.R., and Monoghan, W.P.: ABO hemolytic diseases of the newborn, Am. J. Clin. Pathol. **73**:369, 1980.
477. Elleder, M., et al.: Niemann-Pick disease: analysis of liver tissue in sphingomyelinase-deficient patients, Virchows Arch. (Pathol. Anat.) **385**:215, 1980.
478. Evans, J., Newman S., and Sherlock. S.: Liver copper levels in intrahepatic cholestasis of childhood, Gastroenterology **75**:875, 1978.
479. Fawaz, K.A., et al.: Repetitive maternal-fetal transmission of fatal hepatitis B, N. Engl. J. Med. **293**:1357, 1975.
480. Freedman, R.M., et al.: A half century of neonatal sepsis at Yale, Am. J. Dis. Child. **135**:140, 1981.
481. Froesch, E.R.: Essential fructosuria, hereditary fructose intolerance, and fructose-1, 6-diphosphatose deficiency. In Stanbury, J.B., et al., editors: Metabolic base of inherited disease, ed. 4, New York, 1978, McGraw-Hill Book Co.
482. Gates, G.F., Sinatra, F.R., and Thomas, D.: Cholestatic syndrome in infancy and childhood, Am. J. Pathol. **134**:1141, 1980.
483. Gautier, M., and Eliot, N.: Extrahepatic biliary atresia: morphological study of 98 biliary remnants, Arch. Pathol. Lab. Med. **105**:397, 1981.
484. Gentz, J., Jagenburg, R., and Zetterstrom, R.: Tyrosinemia, J. Pediatr. **66**:670, 1965.
485. Gibbs, W.N., Gray, R., and Lowry, M.: Glucose-6-phosphate dehydrogenase deficiency and neonatal jaundice in Jamaica, Br. J. Haematol. **43**:263, 1979.
486. Goldstein, A.I., and Farrell, R.C.: Physiologic jaundice of the newborn: relation to maternal serum and amniotic fluid alphafetoprotein, Obstet. Gynecol. **51**:315, 1978.
487. Haas, J.E.: Bile duct and liver pathology in biliary atresia, World J. Surg. **2**:561, 1978.
488. Hadchouel, M., and Gautier, M.: Histopathologic study of the liver in the cholestatic phase of alpha-1-antitrypsin deficiency, J. Pediatr. **89**:211, 1976.
489. Hardwick, D.F., and Dimmick, J.E.: Metabolic cirrhoses of infancy and childhood, Perspect. Pediatr. Pathol. **3**:103, 1976.
490. Hegyi, T., Polin, R.A., and Driscoll, J.M.: The pediatric corner: conjugated hyperbilirubinemia in infants with erythroblastosis fetalis, Am. J. Gastroenterol. **72**:297, 1979.
491. Henriksen, N.T., Drablos, P.-A., and Aagenaes, O.: Cholestatic jaundice in infancy: the importance of familial and genetic factors in aetiology and prognosis, Arch. Dis. Child. **56**:622, 1981.
492. Hirsig, J., and Rickham, P.P.: Early differential diagnosis between neonatal hepatitis and biliary atresia, J. Pediatr. Surg. **15**:13, 1980.
493. Hitch, D.C., et al.: Differentiation of cholestatic jaundice in infants: utility of diethyl-IDA, Am. J. Surg. **142**:671, 1981.
494. Hood, J.M., et al.: Liver transplantation for advanced liver disease with alpha-1-antitrypsin deficiency, N. Engl. J. Med. **302**:272, 1980.
495. Horiguchi, T., and Bauer, C.: Ethnic differences in neonatal jaundice: comparison of Japanese and Caucasian newborn infants, Am. J. Obstet. Gynecol. **121**:71, 1975.
496. Hughs, J.R., et al.: Echovirus 14 infection associated with fatal neonatal hepatic necrosis, Am. J. Dis. Child. **123**:61, 1972.
497. Jagenburg, R., et al.: Hereditary tyrosinemia: metabolic studies in a patient with partial *p*-hydroxyphenlpyruvate hydroxylase activity, J. Pediatr. **80**:994, 1972.
498. Jones, E.A., et al.: Progressive intrahepatic cholestasis of infancy and childhood: a clinicopathological study of a patient surviving to the age of 18 years, Gastroenterology **71**:675, 1976.
499. Jorgensen, M.: Stereological study of intrahepatic bile ducts: congenital hepatic fibrosis, Acta Pathol. Microbiol. Scand. **82**:21, 1974.
500. Kaplinsky, C., et al.: Familial cholestatic cirrhosis associated with Kayser-Fleischer rings, Pediatrics **65**:782, 1980.
501. Karp, W.B.: Biochemical alterations in neonatal hyperbilirubinemia and bilirubin encephalopathy: a review, Pediatrics **64**:361, 1979.
502. Kasai, M., et al.: Surgical treatment of biliary atresia, J. Pediatr. Surg. **3**:665, 1968.
503. Kerr, D.N.S., et al.: Congenital hepatic fibrosis, Q. J. Med. **30**:91, 1961.
504. Kibrick, S., and Benirschke, K.: Severe generalized disease in newborn infant due to infection with coxsackievirus, group B, Pediatrics **22**:857, 1958.
505. Kocak, N., and Ozsoylu, S.: Familial cirrhosis, Am. J. Dis. Child. **133**:1160, 1979.
506. Lanzkowsky, P.: The jaundiced newborn: causes and importance. 2. Hematological diseases in children, monograph series, Evansville, Ind., 1975, Mead Johnson Laboratory.
507. Leblanc, A., et al.: Neonatal cholestasis and hypoglycemia: possible role of cortisol deficiency, J. Pediatr. **99**:577, 1981.
508. Levi, A.J., Gatmaitan, Z., and Arias, I.M.: Deficiency of hepatic organic and anion-binding protein, impaired organic anion uptake and "physiologic" jaundice in newborn monkeys, N. Engl. J. Med. **283**:1136, 1970.
509. Levine, R.L.: Bilirubin, Pediatrics **64**:380, 1979.
510. Levy, H.L., and Hammersen, G.: Newborn screening for galactosemia and other galactose metabolic defects, J. Pediatr. **93**:871, 1978.
511. Longmire, W.P.: Congenital biliary hypoplasia, Ann. Surg. **159**:335, 1964.
512. Luscombe, F.A., Monto, A.S., and Baublis, J.V.: Mortality due to Reye's syndrome in Michigan: distribution and longitudinal trends, J. Infect. Dis. **142**:363, 1980.
513. Maisels, M.A.: Neonatal jaundice. In Avery, G.B., editor: Neonatology, Philadelphia, 1981, J.B. Lippincott Co.
514. Masters, P., et al.: Galactosaemia: case for neonatal screening illustrated by recent Australian experience, Med. J. Aust. **2**:348, 1978.
515. Mathis, R.K., et al.: Liver in the cerebro-hepato-renal syndrome: defective bile acid synthesis and abnormal mitochondria, Gastroenterology **29**:1311, 1980.
516. McAdams, A.J., Hug, G., and Bove, K.E.: Glycogen-storage disease, types I to X: criteria for morphologic diagnosis, Hum. Pathol. **5**:463, 1974.
517. Michals, K., Matalon, R., and Wong, P.W.K.: Dietary treatment of tyrosinemia type I, Research **73**:507, 1978.
518. Mitchell, R.A., et al.: Comparison of cytosolic and mitochondrial hepatic enzyme alterations in Reye's syndrome, Pediatr. Res. **14**:1216, 1980.
519. Moss, T.J., and Pysher, T.J.: Hepatic abscess in neonates, Am. J. Dis. Child. **135**:726, 1981.
520. Murray-Lyon, I.M., Ockenden, B.G., and Williams, R.: Congenital hepatic fibrosis: is it a single clinical entity? Gastroenterology **64**:653, 1973.
521. Nahmias, A.J.: The TORCH complex, Hosp. Pract. **9**:65, 1974.
522. Nankervis, G.A., Cox, F.C., and Kumar, M.L.: Diseases produced by cytomegalovirus and its effect on the fetus, Pediatr. Res. **7**:148, 1973.
523. Nankervis, G.A., and Kumar, M.L.: Diseases produced by cytomegaloviruses, Med. Clin. North Am. **62**:1021, 1978.
524. Odievre, M., et al.: Long-term prognosis for infants with intrahepatic cholestasis and patent extrahepatic biliary tract, Arch. Dis. Child. **56**:373, 1981.
525. Pagliara, A.S., et al.: Hypoglycemia in infancy and childhood, J. Pediatr. **82**:365, 1973.

526. Petrelli, M., and Blair, J.D.: Liver in GM, gangliosidosis types 1 and 2: light and electron microscopical study, Arch. Pathol. **99**:111, 1975.
527. Phillips, M.J., Little, J.A., and Ptak, T.W.: Subcellular pathology of hereditary fructose intolerance, Am. J. Med. **44**:910, 1968.
528. Postuma, R., and Trevenen, C.L.: Liver disease in infants receiving total parenteral nutrition, Pediatrics **63**:110, 1979.
529. Putman, C.W., et al.: Liver replacement for alpha-1-antitrypsin deficiency, Surgery **81**:258, 1977.
530. Ram, P., and Poe, N.: Hepatobiliary imaging by radionuclide scintigraphy, West. J. Med. **134**:434, 1981.
531. Reubner, B.H., and Miyai, K.: Neonatal hepatitis and biliary atresia: hemopoiesis and hemosiderin deposition, Ann. N.Y. Acad. Sci. **111**:375, 1963.
532. Reyes, R.D.K., Morgan, G., and Baral, J.: Encephalopathy and fatty degeneration of the viscera, Lancet **2**:749, 1963.
533. Rosenberg, H.S., Openheimer, E.H., and Esterly, J.R.: Congenital rubella syndrome. In Rosenberg, H.S., and Bernstein, J., editors: Perspectives in pediatric pathology, vol. 6, New York, 1981, Masson Publishing U.S.A., Inc.
534. Saland, J., McNamara, H., and Cohen, M.I.: Navajo jaundice: a variant of neonatal hyperbilirubinemia associated with breast feeding, J. Pediatr. **85**:271, 1974.
535. Saxoni, F., Lapatsanis, P., and Pontelakis, S.N.: Congenital syphilis, Clin. Pediatr. **6**:687, 1967.
536. Schweitzer, I.L., et al.: Hepatitis and hepatitis-associated antigen in 56 mother-infant pairs, J.A.M.A. **220**:1092, 1972.
537. Schweitzer, I.L., et al.: Factors influencing neonatal infection by hepatitis B virus, Gastroenterology **65**:277, 1973.
538. Sharp, H.L., and Krivit, W.: Hereditary lymphedema and obstructive jaundice, J. Pediatr. **78**:491, 1979.
540. Singer, D.B.: Pathology of neonatal herpes simplex virus infection. In Nahmias, A.J., et al., editors: The human herpes viruses, an interdisciplinary perspective, New York, 1980, Elsevier North-Holland, Inc.
541. Singer, D.B.: Pathology of neonatal herpes simplex virus infection. In Rosenberg, H.A., and Bernstein, J., editors: Perspectives in pediatric pathology, vol. 6, New York, 1981, Masson Publishing U.S.A., Inc.
542. Sinniah, D., and Baskaran, G.: Margosa oil poisoning as a cause of Reye's syndrome, Lancet **1**:487, 1981.
543. St. Geme, J.W., Jr.: Perinatal and neonatal infections, West. J. Med. **122**:359, 1975.
544. Stagno, S.: Congenital toxoplasmosis, Am. J. Dis. Child. **134**:1980.
545. Strauss, L., and Bernstein, J.: Neonatal hepatitis in congenital rubella, Arch. Pathol. **86**:317, 1968.
546. Tanaka, K.K., Kean, E.A., and Johnson, B.: Jamaican vomiting sickness, N. Engl. J. Med. **295**:461, 1976.
547. Thaler, M.M.: Jaundice in the newborn—algorithmic diagnosis of conjugated and unconjugated hyperbilirubinemia, J.A.M.A. **237**:56, 1977.
548. Thaler, M.M., et al.: Congenital fibrosis and polycystic disease of liver and kidneys, Am. J. Dis. Child. **126**:374, 1973.
549. Tolstrup, N.: Clinical and biochemical aspects of galactosemia, Scand. J. Clin. Lab. Invest. **18**(suppl. 92):148, 1966.
550. Tong, M.J., et al.: Studies on the maternal-infant transmission of the viruses which cause acute hepatitis, Gastroenterology **80**:999, 1981.
551. Triger, D.R., et al.: Alpha-1-antitrypsin deficiency and liver disease in adults, Q. J. Med. **45**:351, 1976.
552. Valman, H.B., France, N.E., and Wallis, P.G.: Prolonged neonatal jaundice in cystic fibrosis, Arch. Dis. Child. **46**:805, 1971.
553. Watson, G.H., and Miller, B.: Arteriohepatic dysplasia: familial pulmonary arterial stenosis with neonatal liver disease, Arch. Dis. Child. **48**:459, 1973.
554. Weber, A.M., et al.: Severe familial cholestasis in North American Indian children: a clinical model of microfilament dysfunction? Gastroenterology **81**:653, 1981.
555. Weinberg, A.G., Mize, C.E., and Worthen, H.G.: The occurrence of hepatoma in the chronic form of hereditary tyrosinemia, J. Pediatr. **88**:434, 1976.
556. Wharton, B.: Hypoglycemia in children with kwashiorkor, Lancet **1**:171, 1970.
557. Wills, E.J.: Electron microscopy of the liver in infectious mononucleosis/megalovirus hepatitis, Am. J. Dis. Child. **123**:301, 1972.
558. Wright, D.J.M., and Berry, C.L.: Liver involvement in congenital syphilis, Br. J. Vener. Dis. **50**:241, 1974.
559. Wysowski, D.K., et al.: RH hemolytic disease, J.A.M.A. **242**:1376, 1979.
560. Yudokoff, M., Cohn, R.M., and Segal, S.: Errors of carbohydrate metabolism in infants and children, Clin. Pediatr. **17**:820, 1978.
561. Zimmerman, H.J.: Jaundice due to bacterial infection, Gastroenterology **77**:362, 1979.

Less common liver diseases

562. Arias, F., and Jimenez, R.M.: Hepatic fibrinogen deposits in preclampsia, N. Engl. J. Med. **295**:578, 1976.
563. Batey, R.G., et al.: Liver physiology and disease: hepatic iron clearance from serum in treated hemochromatosis, Gastroenterology **75**:856, 1978.
564. Baumwol, M., and Park, W.: An acute abdomen: spontaneous rupture of liver during pregnancy, Br. J. Surg. **63**:718, 1976.
565. Beaumont, C., et al.: Serum ferritin as a possible marker of the hemochromatosis allele, N. Engl. J. Med. **301**:169, 1979.
566. Berresford, P.A., et al.: Histological demonstration and frequency of intrahepatocytic copper in patients suffering from alcoholic liver disease, Histopathology **4**:637, 1980.
567. Bloomer, L.D., and Lee, G.R.: Normal hepatic copper metabolism. In Powell, L.W., editor: Metals and the liver, New York, 1978, Marcell Dekker, Inc.
568. Bothwell, T.H., and Isaacson, C.: Siderosis in Bantu, Br. Med. J. **1**:522, 1962.
569. Cano, R.I., et al.: Acute fatty liver of pregnancy: complication by disseminated intravascular coagulation, J.A.M.A. **231**:159, 1975.
570. Cartwright, G.E., et al.: Hereditary hemochromatosis: phenotypic expression of the disease, N. Engl. J. Med. **304**:175, 1979.
571. Cornelius, C.E., Arias, I.M., and Osburn, B.: Syndrome in Corriedale sheep resembling Dubin-Johnson, J. Am. Vet. Med. Assoc. **146**:709, 1965.
572. Crawford, G., Cope, I., and Christie, A.: Liver failure in late pregnancy, Med. J. Aust. **2**:49, 1960.
573. Dalen, E., and Westerholm, B.: Occurrence of hepatic impairment in women jaundiced by oral contraceptives and in their mothers and sisters, Acta Med. Scand. **195**:459, 1974.
574. Davidson, C.S.: Hepatic disease and pregnancy, J. Reprod. Med. **10**:107, 1973.
575. Davies, M.H., et al.: Acute liver disease with encephalopathy and renal failure in late pregnancy and early puerperium, Br. J. Obstet. Gynaecol. **87**:1005, 1980.
576. Davis, J.S., and Kaufman, R.H.: Tetracycline toxicity: a clinicopathologic study with special reference to liver damage and its relationship to pregnancy, Am. J. Obstet. Gynecol. **95**:523, 1966.
577. Dawson, J., Seymour, C.A., and Peters, T.J.: Gilbert's syndrome: analytical subcellular fractionation of liver biopsy specimens, Clin. Sci. **57**:491, 1979.
578. Dawson, J., et al.: Gilbert's syndrome: evidence of morphological heterogeneity, Gut **20**:848, 1979.
579. Derring, T.B., et al.: Effects of D-penicillamine on copper retention in patients with primary biliary cirrhosis, Gastroenterology **72**:1208, 1977.
580. Dickerman, R.M., and Dunn, E.L.: Splenic, pancreatic, and hepatic injuries, Surg. Clin. North Am. **61**:3, 1981.
581. Diess, A., Lee, G.R., and Cartwright, G.E.: Hemolytic anemia in Wilson's disease, J. Intern. Med. **73**:413, 1970.
582. Don't forget Wilson's disease (editorial), Br. Med. J. **2**:1384, 1978.
583. Drill, A.: Benign cholestatic jaundice of pregnancy and benign cholestatic jaundice from oral contraceptives, Am. J. Obstet. Gynecol. **119**:165, 1974.

584. Drysdale, J.W., et al.: Human isoferritins in normal and disease states, Semin. Haematol. **14**:71, 1977.
585. Edwards, C.Q., et al.: Homozygosity for hemochromatosis: clinical manifestations, Ann. Intern. Med. **93**:519, 1980.
586. Edwards, R.H.: Inheritance of the Dubin-Johnson-Sprinz syndrome, Gastroenterology **68**:734, 1975.
587. Elerding, S.C., et al.: Fatal hepatic hemorrhage after trauma, Am. J. Surg. **138**:883, 1979.
588. Evans, J., Newman S., and Sherlock, S.: Liver copper levels in intrahepatic cholestasis of childhood, Gastroenterology **75**:875, 1978.
589. Fleming, D.R., et al.: Pigmented corneal rings in a patient with primary biliary cirrhosis, Gastroenterology **69**:220, 1975.
590. Foley, W.J., et al.: Intrahepatic arteriovenous fistulas between the hepatic artery and portal veins, Ann. Surg. **174**:849, 1971.
591. Franklin, D.C., and Mathai, J.: Biliary pleural fistula: a complication of hepatic trauma, J. Trauma **20**:256, 1980.
592. Frederick, W.C., Howard, R.G., and Spatola, S.: Spontaneous rupture of the liver in patient using contraceptive pills, Arch. Surg. **108**:93, 1974.
593. Geall, M.G., and Webb, M.J.: Liver disease in pregnancy: symposium on medical gynecology, Med. Clin. North Am. **58**:817, 1974.
594. Golan, A., and White, R.G.: Spontaneous rupture of the liver associated with pregnancy, S. Afr. Med. J. **56**:133, 1979.
595. Goldfischer, S., and Sternlieb, I.: Changes in distribution of hepatic copper in relation to progression of Wilson's disease, Am. J. Pathol. **52**:883, 1968.
596. Gollan, J.L., et al.: Prolonged survival in three brothers with severe type 2 Crigler-Najjar syndrome: ultrastructural and metabolic studies, Gastroenterology **68**:1543, 1975.
597. Hibbard, L.T.: Spontaneous rupture of the liver in pregnancy: a report of 8 cases, Am. J. Obstet. Gynecol. **126**:334, 1976.
598. Hollander, I.J.: Nonhemolytic hyperbilirubinemias, Ann. Clin. Lab. Sci. **10**:204, 1980.
599. Iancu, T.C., Neustein, H.B., and Landing, B.H.: The liver in thalassemia major: ultrastructural observations. In Porter, R., and Fitzsimons, D.W.: Iron metabolism (Ciba Foundation symposium new series 51), New York, 1977, Elsevier North-Holland, Inc.
600. Jacobs, A.: Iron overload: clinical and pathologic aspects, Semin. Hematol. **14**:89, 1977.
601. Johnston, W.G., and Baskett, T.F.: Obstetric cholestasis: a 14-year review, Am. J. Obstet. Gynecol. **133**:299, 1979.
602. Kawasaki, H., et al.: Unconjugated bilirubin kinetics in Dubin-Johnson syndrome, Clin. Chim. Acta **92**:87, 1979.
603. Kent, G., and Popper, H.: Secondary hemochromatosis and its association with anemia, Arch. Pathol. **70**:626, 1960.
604. Kent, G., and Popper, H.: Liver biopsy in diagnosis of hemochromatosis (editorial), Am. J. Med. **44**:837, 1968.
605. Khuroo, M.S., et al.: Incidence and severity of viral hepatitis in pregnancy, Am. J. Med. **70**:252, 1981.
606. Koskelo, P., and Mustajoki, P.: Altered coproporphyrin-isomer excretion in patients with the Dubin-Johnson syndrome, Int. J. Biochem. **12**:975, 1979.
607. Kunelis, C.T., Peters, R.L., and Edmondson, H.A.: Fatty liver of pregnancy and its relationship to tetracycline therapy, Am. J. Med. **38**:359, 1965.
608. Lisboa, P.E.: Experimental hepatic cirrhosis in dogs caused by chronic massive iron overload, Gut **12**:363, 1971.
609. Long, R.G., Scheuer, P.J., and Sherlock, S.: Pre-eclampsia presenting with deep jaundice, J. Clin. Pathol. **30**:212, 1977.
610. Ludwig, J., et al.: The liver in the inherited copper disease of Bedlington terriers, Lab. Invest. **43**:82, 1980.
611. MacKenna J., et al.: Acute fatty metamorphosis of the liver: a report of two patients who survived, Am. J. Obstet. Gynecol. **127**:400, 1977.
612. Macklon, A.F., Savage, R.L., and Rawlins, M.D.: Research review: Gilbert's syndrome and drug metabolism, Clin. Pharmacokinet. **4**:223, 1979.
613. Madding, G.F., and Kennedy, P.A.: Trauma to the liver, ed. 2, Philadelphia, 1971, W.B. Saunders Co.
614. Melendez, M.G., et al.: Clinical studies of a large family with Wilson's disease, South. Med. J. **73**:607, 1980.
615. Mistilis, A.P.: Liver disease in pregnancy, Aust. Ann. Med. **17**:248, 1968.
616. Nienhuis, A.W.: Vitamin C and iron, N. Engl. J. Med. **304**:170, 1981.
617. Owens, C.A., et al.: Hepatic sub-cellular distribution of copper in primary biliary cirrhosis: comparison with other hyperhepatocupric states, Mayo Clin. Proc. **52**:73, 1977.
618. Plumb, V., Ho., K.J., and Mihas, A.A.: Hemochromatosis associated with side-to-side portacaval shunt, South. Med. J. **70**:1369, 1977.
619. Popper, H., et al.: Cytoplasmic copper and its toxic effects: studies in India childhood cirrhosis, Lancet **1**:1205, 1979.
620. Powell, L.W., Bassett, M.L., and Halliday, J.W.: Hemochromatosis: 1980 update, Gastroenterology **78**:374, 1980.
621. Powell, L.W., Halliday, J.W., and Bassett, M.L.: Recent advances in iron metabolism, Aust. N.Z. J. Med. **9**:578, 1979.
622. Powell, L.W., Mortimer, R., and Harris, O.D.: Cirrhosis of the liver: a comparative study of the four major etiological groups, Med. J. Aust. **1**:941, 1971.
623. Reyes, H., et al.: Sulfobromophthalein clearance tests before and after ethinyl estradiol administration, Gastroenterology **81**:226, 1981.
624. Richardson, R.E., Gumbert, J.L., and Gale, S.Q.: Traumatic intrahepatic hematoma, Arch. Surg. **95**:940, 1967.
625. Risdon, R.A., Barry, M., and Flynn, D.M.: Transfusional overload: the relationship between tissue iron concentration and hepatic fibrosis in the thalassemia, J. Pathol. **116**:83, 1975.
626. Rosen, I.A., et al.: Arthropathy, hypouricemia and normal serum iron studies in hereditary hemochromatosis, Am. J. Med. **70**:870, 1981.
627. Ross, C.E., et al.: Hemochromatosis: pathophysiologic and genetic considerations, Am. J. Clin. Pathol. **63**:179, 1975.
628. Schafer, A.K., et al.: Clinical consequences of acquired transfusional iron overload in adults, N. Engl. J. Med. **304**:319, 1981.
629. Scharschmidt, B.F, and Gollan, J.L.: Current concepts of bilirubin metabolism and hereditary hyperbilirubinemia. In Popper, H., and Schaffner, F., editors: Progress in liver disease, vol. 6, New York, 1979, Grune & Stratton, Inc.
630. Schmid, R., and McDonagh, A.F.: Hyperbilirubinemia. In Stanbury, J.B., Wyngaarden, J.B., and Fredrickson, D.S., editors: The metabolic basis of inherited disease, New York, 1978, McGraw-Hill Book Co.
631. Schumacher, H.R.: Hemochromatosis and arthritis, Arthritis Rheum. **7**:41, 1964.
632. Schweitzer, I.L., and Peters, R.L.: Pregnancy in hepatitis B antigen positive cirrhosis, Obstet. Gynecol. **48**(suppl.):53s, 1976.
633. Scott, J., et al.: Wilson's disease presenting as chronic active hepatitis, Gastroenterology **74**:645, 1978.
634. Seymour, C.A., Neale, G., and Peters, T.J.: Lysosomal changes in liver tissue from patients with the Dubin-Johnson-Sprinz syndrome, Clin. Sci. Mol. Med. **52**:241, 1977.
635. Shani, M., et al.: Effect of phenobarbital on liver functions in patients with Dubin-Johnson syndrome, Gastroenterology **67**:303, 1974.
636. Sheehan, H.L.: Yellow atrophy: chloroform poisoning, J. Obstet. Gynecol. Br. Emp. **47**:49, 1940.
637. Smallwood, R.A.: Other liver diseases associated with increased liver copper concentration. In Powell, L.W., editor: Metals and the liver, New York, 1978, Marcel Dekker, Inc.
638. Stalker, A.L.: Fibrin deposition in pregnancy, J. Clin. Pathol. **29** (suppl. 10):70, 1976.
639. Sternlieb, I.: Copper and the liver, Gastroenterology **78**:1615, 1980.
640. Sternlieb, I., and Scheinberg, I.H.: The role of radiocopper in the diagnosis of Wilson's disease, Gastroenterology **77**:138, 1979.
641. Steven, M.M.: Pregnancy and liver disease, Gut **22**:592, 1981.
642. Steven, M.M., Buckley, J.D., and Mackay, I.R.: Pregnancy in chronic active hepatitis, Q. J. Med. (new series 48) 519, 1979.
643. Strickland, G.T., and Leu, M.-L.: Wilson's disease: clinical and laboratory manifestations in 40 patients, Medicine **54**:113, 1975.

644. Swartz, H.M., Sarna, T., and Varma, R.: On the nature and excretion of the hepatic pigment in the Dubin-Johnson syndrome, Gastroenterology **76**:958, 1979.
645. Tanner, M.S., and Portmann, B.: Indian childhood cirrhosis, Arch. Dis. Child. **56**:4, 1981.
646. Theron, J.J., et al.: Experimental dietary siderosis, Am. J. Pathol. **43**:73, 1963.
647. Trunkey, D.D., Shires, G.T., and McClelland, R.: Management of liver trauma in 811 consecutive patients, Ann. Surg. **179**:722, 1974.
648. Valbert, L.S., et al.: Clinical and biological expression of the genetic abnormality in idiopathic hemochromatosis, Gastroenterology **79**:884, 1980.
649. Viswanathan, R.: Certain epidemiological features of infectious hepatitis during the Delhi epidemic, 1955-1956. In Hartman, F.W., et al., editors: Hepatitis frontiers, Boston, 1957, Little, Brown & Co.

Circulatory disturbances

650. Adler, J., et al.: Arteriovenous shunts involving the liver, Radiology **129**:315, 1978.
651. Arcidi, M.M., Jr., Moore, G.W., and Hutchins, G.M.: Hepatic morphology in cardiac dysfunction: a clinicopathologic study of 1000 subjects at autopsy, Am. J. Pathol. **104**:159, 1981.
652. Asbury, R.F., et al.: Hepatic veno-occlusive disease due to DTIC, Cancer **45**:2670, 1980.
653. Berk, P.D., et al.: Veno-occlusive disease of the liver after allogenic bone marrow transplantation, Ann. Intern. Med. **90**:158, 1979.
654. Birgens, H.S., et al.: The shock liver: clinical and biochemical findings in patients with centrilobular liver necrosis following cardiogenic shock, Acta Med. Scand. **204**:417, 1978.
655. Boyer, J.L., Hales, M.R., and Klatskin, G.: "Idiopathic" portal hypertension due to occlusion of intrahepatic portal veins by organized thrombi, Medicine **53**:77, 1974.
656. Boyer, J.L., et al.: Idiopathic portal hypertension, Ann. Intern. Med. **66**:41, 1967.
657. Bras, G.: Veno-occlusive disease of liver with nonportal type of cirrhosis occurring in Jamaica, Arch. Pathol. **57**:285, 1954.
658. Cohen, J.A., et al.: Left-sided heart failure presenting as hepatitis, Gastroenterology **74**:583, 1978.
659. Datta, D.B., et al.: Chronic oral arsenic intoxication as a possible aetiological factor in idiopathic portal hypertension (non-cirrhotic portal fibrosis) in India, Gut **20**:358, 1979.
660. Donovan, A.J., et al.: Systemic-portal arteriovenous fistulas: pathological and hemodynamic observations in two patients, Surgery **66**:474, 1969.
661. Dresler, S., and Linder, D.: Noncirrhotic portal fibrosis following neonatal cytomegalic inclusion disease, J. Pediatr. **93**:887, 1978.
662. Espana, P., et al.: Membranous obstruction of the inferior vena cava and hepatic veins: Budd-Chiari syndrome? A treatable disease, Am. J. Gastroenterol. **73**:28, 1980.
663. Fajardo, L.F., and Colby, T.V.: Pathogenesis of veno-occlusive liver disease after radiation, Arch. Pathol. Lab. Med. **104**:584, 1980.
664. Ghandur-Mnaymneh, L.: Anemic infarction of the liver resulting from hepatic and portal vein thrombosis, Johns Hopkins Med. J. **139**:78, 1976.
665. Grases, P.J., and Beker, S.: Veno-occlusive disease of the liver: case from Venezuela, Am. J. Med. **53**:511, 1972.
666. Guida, P., and Moore, S.W.: Aneurysm of the hepatic artery, Surgery **60**:299, 1966.
667. Guido Banti: 1852-1925 (editorial), J.A.M.A. **201**:693, 1967.
668. Hartmann, R.C., et al.: Fulminant hepatic venous thrombosis (Budd-Chiari syndrome) in paroxysmal nocturnal hemoglobinuria, Johns Hopkins Med. J. **146**:247, 1980.
669. Hashem, M.: Etiology and pathology of types of liver cirrhosis in Egyptian children, J. Egypt Med. Assoc. **22**:319, 1939.
670. Hendee, W.R., Alders, M.A., and Garciga, C.E.: Development of ultrastructural radiation injury, Am. J. Roentgenol. **105**:147, 1969.
671. Hendrix, T.R., et al.: Clinical conferences at the Johns Hopkins Hospital, Johns Hopkins Med. J. **147**:41, 1980.
672. Imanga, H., Yamamoto, S., and Kuroyanagi, Y.: Surgical treatment of portal hypertension, Ann. Surg. **155**:42, 1962.
673. Jacob, A.I., et al.: Endotoxin and bacteria in portal blood, Gastroenterology **72**:1268, 1977.
674. Kanel, G.C., et al.: A distinctive perivenular hepatic lesion associated with heart failure, Am. J. Clin. Pathol. **73**:235, 1980.
675. Kent, D.R., Nissen, E., and Goldstein, A.I.: Oral contraceptives and hepatic vein thrombosis, J. Reprod. Med. **68**:113, 1981.
676. Leibowitz, A.I., and Hartmann, R.C.: Annotation: the Budd-Chiari syndrome and paroxysmal nocturnal haemoglobinuria, Br. J. Haematol. **48**:1, 1981.
677. Liebman, P.R., et al.: Hepatic-portal venous gas in adults: etiology, pathophysiology and clinical significance, Ann. Surg. **187**:281, 1978.
678. Luna, A., Meister, H.P., and Szanto, P.: Esophageal varices in absence in cirrhosis, Am. J. Clin. Pathol. **49**:710, 1968.
679. Madding, G.F., and Kennedy, P.A.: Trauma to the liver, ed. 2, Philadelphia, 1971, W.B. Saunders Co.
680. McLean, E.K.: The toxic actions of pyrrolizidine (Senecio) alkaloids, Pharmacol. Rev. **22**:429, 1970.
681. Mellis, C., and Bale, P.M.: Familial hepatic venoocclusive with probable immune deficiency, J. Pediatr. **88**:236, 1976.
682. Mikkelsen, W.P., et al.: Extra- and intrahepatic portal hypertension without cirrhosis (hepato-portal sclerosis), Ann. Surg. **162**:602, 1965.
683. Mohabbat, O., et al.: An outbreak of hepatic veno-occlusive disease in North-western Afghanistan, Lancet **2**:269, 1976.
684. Mukherjee, A.K., Ramaliangaswami, V., and Nayak, N.C.: Hepatoportal sclerosis: its relationship to intrahepatic portal venous thrombosis, Indian J. Med. Res. **69**:152, 1979.
685. Mullane, J.F., and Gliedman, M.L.: Elevation of pressure in inferior vena cava, Surgery **59**:1135, 1966.
686. Nagasue, N., et al.: Hepatoportal arteriovenous fistula in primary carcinoma of the liver, Surg. Gynecol. Obstet. **145**:504, 1977.
687. Nakamura, S., and Toshiharu, T.: Surgical anatomy of the hepatic veins and the inferior vena cava, Surg. Gynecol. Obstet. **152**:43, 1981.
688. Nakamura, T., et al.: Obstruction of the inferior vena cava in the hepatic portion and the hepatic veins, Angiology **19**:479, 1968.
689. Nataf, C., et al.: Idiopathic portal hypertension (perisinusoidal fibrosis) after renal transplantation, Gut **20**:531, 1979.
690. Okuda, K., et al.: Frequency of intrahepatic arteriovenous fistula as a sequela to percutaneous needle puncture of the liver, Gastroenterology **74**:1204, 1978.
691. Okuda, K., et al.: Anatomical basis for hepatic venographic alterations in idiopathic portal hypertension, Liver **1**:255, 1981.
692. Popper, H.: Alterations of liver and spleen among workers exposed to vinyl chloride, Ann. N.Y. Acad. Sci. **246**:172, 1975.
693. Porter, L.L., Houston, M.C., and Kadir, M.: Mycotic aneurysms of the hepatic artery: treatment with arterial embolization, Am. J. Med. **67**:697, 1979.
694. Prandi, D., Rueff, B., and Benhamou, J.P.: Side-to-side portacaval shunt in treatment of Budd-Chiari syndrome, Gastroenterology **68**:137, 1975.
695. Reed, G.B., Jr., and Cox, A.J., Jr.: Human liver after radiation injury, Am. J. Pathol. **48**:597, 1966.
696. Safran, A.P., and Schaffner, F.: Chronic passive congestion of liver in man, Am. J. Pathol. **50**:447, 1967.
697. Sarfeh, I.J.: Portal vein thrombosis associated with cirrhosis, Arch. Surg. **114**:902, 1979.
698. Seeley, T.T., et al.: Hepatic infarction, Hum. Pathol. **3**:265, 1972.
699. Selzer, G., and Parker, R.G.F.: Senecio poisoning exhibiting as Chiari's syndrome: report on 12 cases, Am. J. Pathol. **27**:885, 1951.
700. Shulman, H.M., et al.: An analysis of hepatic venoocclusive disease and centrilobular hepatic degeneration following bone marrow transplantation, Gastroenterology **79**:1178, 1980.

701. Simson, I.W.: Membranous obstruction of the inferior vena cava and hepatocellular carcinoma in South Africa, Gastroenterology **82**:171, 1982.
702. Starzl, T., et al.: Autopsy findings in a long-surviving liver recipient, N. Engl. Med. **289**:82, 1973.
703. Stillman, A.E., et al.: Hepatic veno-occlusive disease due to pyrrolizidine (Senecio) poisoning in Arizona, Gastroenterology **73**:349, 1977.
704. Stirling, G.A., Bras, G., and Urquhart, A.E.: Early lesion in veno-occlusive disease of liver, Arch. Dis. Child. **37**:535, 1962.
705. Sultan, K.M., and Datta, D.V.: Budd-Chiari syndrome following pregnancy: report of 16 cases with roentgenologic, hemodynamic and histologic studies of the hepatic outflow tract, Am. J. Med. **68**:113, 1980.
706. Tavill, A.S., et al.: Budd Chiari syndrome: correlation between hepatic scintigraphy and the clerical, radiological, and pathological findings in hepatic venous flow obstruction, Gastroenterology **68**:509, 1975.
707. Villeneuve, J.P., et al.: Idiopathic portal hypertension, Am. J. Med. **61**:459, 1976.
708. Vujic, I., Meredith, H.C., and Ameriks, J.A.: Embolization for hepatoportal arteriovenous fistula, Am. Surg. **46**:366, 1980.
709. Wanless, I.R., Bernier, V., and Seger, M.: Intrahepatic portal vein sclerosis in patients without a history of liver disease: an autopsy study, Am. J. Pathol. **106**:63, 1982.
710. Ware, A.J.: The liver when the heart fails, Gastroenterology **74**:62, 1978.
711. Woods, W.G., et al.: Fatal veno-occlusive disease of the liver following high dose chemotherapy, irradiation and bone marrow transplantation, Am. J. Med. **68**:285, 1980.
712. Zafrani, E.S., et al.: Focal necrosis of the liver—a clinicopathological entity possibly related to oral contraceptives, Gastroenterology **79**:1295, 1980.

Chronic infections and other chronic disorders

713. Adams, D.O.: The granulomatous, inflammatory response, Am. J. Pathol. **84**:164, 1976.
714. Banner, B.F., et al.: Hepatic granulomas following ileal bypass for obesity, Arch. Pathol. Lab. Med. **102**:655, 1978.
715. Benjamin, S.B., Ishak, K.G., and Zimmerman, H.J.: Phenylbutazone liver injury: a clinical pathologic survey of 23 cases and review of the literature, Hepatology **1**:255, 1981.
716. Bernstein, M., Edmondson, H.A., and Barbour, B.H.: The liver lesion in Q fever, Arch. Intern. Med. **74**:198, 1965.
717. Bohm, W., and Willnow, U.: Granulomartige hepatitis bei konnataler toxoplasmose, Z. Kinderheilk. **88**:215, 1963.
718. Bramlet, D.A., and Posalaky, Z.: Granulomatous hepatitis as a manifestation of quinidine hypersensitivity, Arch. Intern. Med. **140**:395, 1980.
719. Carmichael, G.P., et al.: Hepatic silicosis, Am. J. Clin. Pathol. **73**:720, 1980.
720. Chen, T.S.N., Drutz, D.J., and Whelan, G.E.: Hepatic granulomas in leprosy: their relation to bacteremia, Arch. Pathol. Lab. Med. **100**:182, 1976.
721. Dupont, H.L., et al.: Q fever hepatitis, Ann. Intern. Med. **74**:198, 1971.
722. Ellenbogen, R., et al.: Injectable fluid silicone therapy, J.A.M.A. **234**:308, 1975.
723. Fauci, A.S., and Wolff, S.M.: Granulomatous hepatitis. In Popper, H., and Schaffner, F., editors: Progress in liver disease, vol. 5, New York, 1976, Grune & Stratton, Inc.
724. French, S.W., Schloss, G.T., and Stillman, A.E.: Case reports: unusual amyloid bodies in human liver, Am. Soc. Clin. Pathol. **75**:400, 1981.
725. Glenner, G.G.: Amyloid deposits and amyloidosis: the betafibrilloses (in two parts), N. Engl. J. Med. **302**:1283, 1333, 1980.
726. Husby, G.: A chemical classification of amyloid, Scand. J. Rheumatol. **9**:60, 1980.
727. Jori, G.P., and Peschle, C.: Hydralizine disease associated with transient granulomas in the liver: a case report, Gastroenterology **64**:1163, 1973.
728. Kanel, G.C., and Peters, R.L.: Globular amyloid: an unusual morphologic presentation, Hepatology **1**:647, 1981.
729. Klatskin, G.: Hepatic granulomata: problems in interpretation, Mt. Sinai J. Med. **44**:798, 1977.
730. Kuzemko, J.A.: Toxocariasis, Arch. Dis. Child. **41**:221, 1966.
731. Lee, F.I., Murray, S., and Norfolk, D.R.: Cholestatis jaundice in secondary syphillis, Br. J. Clin. Pract. **33**:139, 1979.
732. Marcial-Rojas, R.A.: Parasitic diseases of the liver. In Gall, A., and Mostofi, F.K., editors: The liver, Baltimore, 1973, The Williams & Wilkins Co.
733. McMaster, K.R., and Hennigar, G.R.: Drug-induced granulomatous hepatitis, Lab. Invest. **44**:61, 1981.
734. Melkebeke, P., et al.: Huge hepatomegaly and portal hypertension due to amyloidosis of the liver, Digestion **20**:351, 1980.
735. Miller, A.C., and Reid, W.M.: Methyldopa-induced granulomatous hepatitis, J.A.M.A. **235**:2001, 1976.
736. Min, K.W., et al.: Talc granulomata in liver disease in narcotic addicts, Arch. Pathol. **98**:331, 1974.
737. Mir-Madjlessi, S.H., Farmer, R.G., and Hawk, W.A.: Granulomatous hepatitis: a review of 50 cases, Am. J. Gastroenterol. **60**:122, 1973.
738. Nagalotimath, S.J., Darbar, R.D., and Jogalekar, M.D.: Granulomatous hepatitis in brucellosis, J. Ind. Med. Assn. **72**:1, 1979.
739. Nakanuma, Y., et al.: Intrahepatic bile duct destruction in a patient with sarcoidosis and chronic intrahepatic cholestasis, Acta Pathol. Jpn. **20**:211, 1979.
740. Nakanuma, Y., et al.: Granulomatous liver disease in the small hepatic and portal veins, Arch. Pathol. Lab. Med. **104**:456, 1980.
741. Pfeifer, U., and Alterman, K.: Shedding of peripheral cytoplasm: a mechanism of liver cell atrophy in human amyloidosis, Virchows Arch. (Cell Pathol.) **29**:229, 1979.
742. Pimentel, J.C., and Meneges, A.P.: Liver granuloma containing copper in vineyard sprayer's lung, Am. Rev. Respir. Dis. **111**:189, 1975.
743. Reynolds, T.B., Campra, J.L., and Peters, R.L.: Hepatic granulomas. In Zakin, D., and Boyer, T., editors: Hepatology, a textbook of liver disease, Philadelphia, 1982, W.B. Saunders Co.
744. Rigberg, L.A., Robinson, M.J., and Espiritu, C.R.: Chlorpropamide-induced granulomas, J.A.M.A. **235**:409, 1976.
745. Romeu, J., et al.: Spirochetal vasculitis and bile ductular damage in early hepatic syphilis, Am. J. Gastroenterol. **74**:352, 1980.
746. Rubinow, A., Koff, R.S., and Cohen, A.S.: Severe intrahepatic cholestasis in primary amyloidosis: a report of four cases and a review of the literature, Am. J. Med. **64**:937, 1978.
747. Sacks, E.L., et al.: Epithelioid granulomas associated with Hodgkin's disease: clinical correlations in 55 previously untreated patients, Cancer **41**:562, 1978.
748. Simmons, F., et al.: Granulomatous hepatitis in a patient receiving allopurinol, Gastroenterology **62**:101, 1972.
749. Spark, R.P.: Does transplacental spread of coccidioidomycosis occur? Arch. Pathol. Lab. Med. **105**:347, 1981.
750. Spink, W.W., et al.: Histopathology of the liver in human brucellosis, J. Lab. Clin. Med. **34**:40, 1949.
751. Symmers, D., and Spain, D.M.: Hepar lobatum, Arch. Pathol. **42**:64, 1946.
752. Thomas, E., and Micci, D.: Chronic intrahepatic cholestasis with granulomas and biliary cirrhosis, J.A.M.A. **238**:337, 1977.
753. Warren, K.S.: Hepatosplenic schistosomiasis: a great neglected disease of the liver, Gut **19**:572, 1978.
754. Woodruff, A.W., and Thacker, C.K.: Infection with animal helminths, Br. Med. J. **1**:1001, 1964.
755. Yon, J.L., et al.: Granulomatous hepatitis, increased platelet aggregation, and hypercholesterolemia, Ann. Intern. Med. **84**:148, 1976.
756. Young, J.L., Boswell, R.B., and Nies, A.S.: Severe allopurinol hypersensitivity: association with thiazides and prior renal compromise, Arch. Intern. Med. **134**:553, 1974.

Congenital and acquired abnormalities of form and position

757. Dolan, M.F., and Janovski, N.A.: Adrenal dystopia, Arch. Pathol. **86**:22, 1968.

758. Ham, J.M.: Partial and complete atrophy affecting hepatic segments and lobes, Br. J. Surg. **66**:333, 1979.
759. Johnstone, G.: Accessory lobe of liver, Arch. Dis. Child. **40**:541, 1965.
760. Pujari, B.D., and Deodhare, S.G.: Symptomatic accessory lobe of liver with a review of the literature, Postgrad. Med. J. **52**:234, 1976.
761. Vercelli-Retta, J.: Fetal supradiaphragmatic accessory liver lobe: report of a case and review of the literature, Virchows Arch. (Pathol. Anat.) **378**:259, 1978.

Needle biopsies

762. Feldman, R.G., et al.: Familial intention tremor, ataxia and lipofuscinosis, Neurology **19**:503, 1969.
763. Ho, C.F., et al.: Guided percutaneous fine needle aspiration biopsy of the liver, Cancer **47**:1781, 1981.

Differential diagnosis of jaundice

764. Cello, J.P.: Diagnostic approaches to jaundice, Hosp. Pract. **17**:49, 1982.
765. Pitt, H.A.: The diagnosis of jaundice, West. J. Med. **133**:504, 1980.
766. Rasmussen, R.W., and McGill, D.B.: Fat embolism and postoperative jaundice: case report, J.A.M.A. **233**:271, 1975.
767. Sheehy, T.W., Law, D.E., and Wade, B.H.: Exchange transfusion for sickle cell intrahepatic cholestasis, Arch. Intern. Med. **140**:1364, 1980.
768. Summerfield, J.A., et al.: Benign recurrent intrahepatic cholestasis: studies of bilirubin kinetics, bile acids, and cholangiography, Gut **21**:154, 1980.

Liver disease in nonhepatic disorders

769. Ashkar, F.S., et al.: Liver disease in hyperthyroidism, South. Med. J. **64**:462, 1971.
770. Bartholomew, L.G., et al.: Liver disease in scleroderma, Am. J. Dig. Dis. **9**:43, 1964.
771. Bauer, T.B., Moore, G.W., and Hutchins, G.M.: The liver in sickle cell disease: a clinicopathologic study of 70 patients, Am. J. Med. **69**:833, 1980.
772. Dew, M.J., Thompson, H., and Allan, R.N.: The spectrum of hepatic dysfunction in inflammatory bowel disease, Q. J. Med. **48**:113, 1979.
773. Dietrichson, O., et al.: Morphological changes in liver biopsies from patients with rheumatoid arthritis, Scand. J. Rheumatol. **5**:65, 1976.
774. Eade, M.N., et al.: Liver disease in Crohn's colitis: a study of 21 consecutive patients having colectomy, Ann. Intern. Med. **74**:518, 1971.
775. Falchuk, K.R., et al.: Pericentral hepatic fibrosis and intracellular hyalin in diabetes mellitus, Gastroenterology **78**:535, 1980.
776. Fernandes, L., et al.: Studies on the frequency and pathogenesis of liver involvement in rheumatoid arthritis, Ann. Rheum. Dis. **38**:501, 1979.
777. Hocking, W.G., et al.: Spontaneous hepatic rupture in rheumatoid arthritis, Arch. Intern. Med. **141**:792, 1981.
778. Kolmannskos, F., et al.: Cholangiographic findings in ulcerative colitis, Acta Radiol. **22**:151, 1981.
779. Lupinetti, M., Mehigan, D., and Cameron, J.L.: Hepatobiliary complications of ulcerative colitis, Am. J. Surg. **139**:113, 1980.
780. Nelson, R.S., and Sears, M.E.: Massive sarcoidosis of liver, Am. J. Dig. Dis. **13**:95, 1968.
781. Ritland, S., et al.: Liver copper content in patients with inflammatory bowel disease and associated liver disorders, Scand. J. Gastroenterol. **14**:711, 1979.
782. Runyon, B.A., LaBrecque, D.R., and Anuras, S.: The spectrum of liver disease in systemic lupus erythamatosus: report of 33 histologically-proved cases and review of literature, Am. J. Med. **69**:187, 1980.
783. Samuelson, K., et al.: Evaluation of fasting serum bile acid concentration in patients with liver and gastrointestinal disorders, Scand. J. Gastroenterol. **16**:225, 1981.

Tumors and tumorlike lesions

784. Adam, Y.B., Huvos, A.G., and Hajdu, S.I.: Malignant vascular tumors of liver, Ann. Surg. **175**:373, 1972.
785. Aflatoxin and primary liver cancer (editorial), S. Afr. Med. J. **38**:2495, 1974.
786. Aoki, K.: Cancer of the liver: international mortality trends, World Health Stat. Rep. **31**:28, 1978.
787. Arbus, G.C., and Hung, R.H.: Hepatocarcinoma and myocardial fibrosis in an 8¾-year-old renal transplant recipient, Can. Med. Assoc. J. **107**:431, 1972.
788. Asch, M.J., Cohen, A.H., and Moore, T.C.: Hepatic and splenic lymphangiomatosis with skeletal involvement: report of case and review of literature, Surgery **76**:334, 1974.
789. Baghert, S.A., and Boyer, J.L.: Peliosis hepatis associated with androgenic-anabolic steroid therapy: severe form of hepatic injury, Ann. Intern. Med. **81**:610, 1974.
790. Beasley, R.P., et al.: Hepatocellular carcinoma and hepatitis B virus, Lancet **2**:1129, 1981.
791. Berman, C.: Primary carcinoma of the liver in the Bantu races of South Africa, S. Afr. J. Med. Sci. **5**:54, 1940.
792. German, C.: Primary carcinoma of the liver: a study of incidence, clinical manifestations, pathology and etiology, London, 1951, H.K. Lewis & Co.
793. Bird, D., Voweles, K., and Anthony, P.P.: Spontaneous rupture of a liver cell adenoma after long term methyltestosterone: report of a case successfully treated by right hepatic lobectomy, Br. J. Surg. **66**:212, 1979.
794. Block, J.B.: Angiosarcoma of liver following vinyl chloride exposure, J.A.M.A. **29**:53, 1974.
795. Bomford, A., Walter, R.J., and Williams, R.: Treatment of iron overload including results in a personal series of 85 patients. In Kief, H., editor: Iron metabolism and its disorders, New York, 1975, American Elsevier.
796. Bomford, A., and Williams, R.: Long-term results of venous section therapy in idiopathic hemochromatosis, Q. J. Med. **45**:611, 1976.
797. Braun, P., et al.: Hemangiomatosis of liver in infants, J. Pediatr. Surg. **10**:121, 1975.
798. Brechot, C., et al.: Evidence that hepatitis B virus has a role in liver-cell carcinoma in alcoholic liver disease, N. Engl. J. Med. **306**:1384, 1982.
799. Burroughs, A.K., et al.: Primary cancer in autoimmune chronic liver disease, Br. Med. J. **282**:273, 1981.
800. Chawla, S.K., et al.: Portal hypertension in peliosis hepatis: report of the first case, Am. J. Proctol. Gastroenterol. Colon Rectal Surg. **31**:11, 1980.
801. Chudecki, B.: Primary cancer of the liver following treatment of polycythemia vera with radioactive phosphorus, Br. J. Radiol. **45**:770, 1972.
802. Creech, J.L., Jr., and Johnson, M.N.: Angiosarcoma of liver in manufacture of polyvinyl chloride, J. Occup. Med. **16**:150, 1974.
803. Davis, M., et al.: Histological evidence of carcinoma in a hepatic tumour associated with oral contraceptives, Br. Med. J. **4**:496, 1975.
804. Degott, C., et al.: Peliosis hepatis in recipients of renal transplants, Gut **19**:748, 1978.
805. Dehner, L.P., Ewing, S.L., and Sumner, H.W.: Infantile mesenchymal hamartoma of liver: histologic and ultrastructural observations, Arch. Pathol. **99**:379, 1975.
806. Dehner, L.P., and Ishak, K.G.: Vascular tumors of the liver in infants and children, Arch. Pathol. **92**:101, 1971.
807. Edmondson, H.A.: Differential diagnosis of tumors and tumorlike lesions of the liver in infancy and childhood, Am. J. Dis. Child. **91**:168, 1956.
808. Edmondson, H.A.: Tumors of the liver and intrahepatic bile ducts. In Atlas of tumor pathology, section 7, fascicle 25, Washington, D.C., 1958, Armed Forces Institute of Pathology.
809. Edmondson, H.A., and Peters, R.L.: Tumors of the liver. In Schiff, L., and Eugene, R., editors: Diseases of the liver, ed. 5, Philadelphia, 1982, J.B. Lippincott Co.
810. Edmondson, H.A., and Steiner, P.E.: Primary carcinoma of the liver: a study of 100 cases among 48,900 necropsies, Cancer **7**:462, 1954.

811. Edmondson, H.A., et al.: Regression of liver cell adenomas associated with oral contraceptives, Ann. Intern. Med. **86**:180, 1977.
812. Ein, S.H.: Malignant liver tumors in children, J. Pediatr. Surg. **9**:491, 1974.
813. Eriksson, S., and Hagerstrand, I.: Cirrhosis and malignant hepatoma in alpha-1-antitrypsin deficiency, Acta Med. Scand. **195**:451, 1974.
814. Fechner, R.E., and Roehm, J.O.F., Jr.: Angiographic and pathologic correlations of hepatic focal nodular hyperplasia, Am. J. Surg. Pathol. **1**:217, 1977.
815. Fraumeni, J.F., Miller, R.W., and Hill, J.A.: Primary carcinoma of the liver in childhood: an epidemiologic study, J. Natl. Cancer Inst. **40**:1087, 1968.
816. Freeny, P.C., Vimont, T.R., and Barnett, D.C.: Cavernous hemangioma of the liver; ultrasonography, arteriography and computed tomography, Radiology **132**:143, 1979.
817. Ganrot, P.O., Laurell, C.B., and Eriksson, S.: Obstructive lung disease and trypsin inhibitors in alpha-1-antitrypsin deficiency, Scand. J. Clin. Lab. Invest. **19**:205, 1967.
818. Gibson, J.B., and Sun, T.: Clonorchiasis. In Marcial-Rojas, R.A., editor: Pathology of protozoal and helminthic disease, Baltimore, 1971, The Williams & Wilkins Co.
819. Gonzalez-Crussi, F., and Manz, H.J.: Structure of hepatoblastoma of pure epithelial type, Cancer **29**:1272, 1972.
820. Govindarajan, S., Ashcavai, M., and Peters, R.L.: Alpha-1-antitrypsin phenotypes in hepatocellular carcinoma (abstract), Hepatology **1**:628, 1981.
821. Hadad, A.R., et al.: Symptomatic nonparasitic liver cysts, Am. J. Surg. **134**:739, 1977.
822. Ho, C.F., et al.: Guided percutaneous fine needle aspiration biopsy of the liver, Cancer **47**:1781, 1981.
823. Holton, C.P., Burrington, J.D., and Hatch, E.I.: Multiple chemotherapeutic approach to management of hepatoblastoma: preliminary report, Cancer **35**:1083, 1975.
824. Homer, L.W., White, H.J., and Read, R.C.: Neoplastic transformation of Von Meyenburg complexes of the liver, J. Pathol. Bacteriol. **96**:499, 1968.
825. Horisawa, M., et al.: Incomplete membranous obstruction of the inferior vena cava, Arch. Surg. **111**:599, 1976.
826. Ishak, K.: Primary hepatic tumor in childhood. In Popper, H., and Schaffner, F., editors: Progress in liver disease, vol. 5, New York, 1981, Grune & Stratton, Inc.
827. Ishak, K.G., and Glunz, P.R.: Hepatoblastoma and hepatocarcinoma in infancy and childhood, Cancer **20**:396, 1967.
828. Jackson, C., et al.: Hepatic hemangioendothelioma: angiographic appearance and apparent prednisone responsiveness, Am. J. Dis. Child. **131**:74, 1977.
829. Jaffe, B.M., et al.: Factors influencing survival in patients with untreated hepatic metastases, Surg. Gynecol. Obstet. **127**:1, 1968.
830. Jenkins, P.J., et al.: Hepatocellular carcinoma in HBsAg-negative chronic active hepatitis, Gut **22**:332, 1981.
831. Kato, M., et al.: Hemangioma of the liver: a review of literature and presentation of illustrative case, Arch. Surg. **83**:105, 1975.
832. Keeley, A.F., Iseri, O.A., and Gottlieb, L.S.: Ultrastructure of hyaline cytoplasmic inclusions in a human hepatoma: relationship to Mallory's alcoholic hyalin, Gastroenterology **62**:280, 1972.
833. Kent, D.R., et al.: Effects of pregnancy on liver tumor associated with oral contraceptives, Obstet. Gynecol. **51**:148, 1978.
834. Kimura, C., et al.: Membranous obstruction of the hepatic portion of the inferior vena cava: clinical study of nine cases, Surgery **72**:551, 1972.
835. Knowles, D.M., II, et al.: The clinical radiologic, and pathologic characterization of benign hepatic neoplasms, Medicine **57**:223, 1978.
836. Krasner, N., et al.: Hepatocellular carcinoma in primary biliary cirrhosis: report of four cases, Gut **20**:255, 1979.
837. Kulkarni, P.B., and Beatty, E.C.: Cholangiocarcinoma associated with biliary cirrhosis due to congenital biliary atresia, Am. J. Dis. Child. **131**:442, 1977.
838. Kumakura, K., et al.: A case of Wilson's disease with hepatoma, Jpn. J. Intern. Med. **64**:22, 1975.
839. Kurtz, R.C., Sherlock, P., and Winawer, S.J.: Esophageal varices: development secondary to primary and metastatic liver tumors, Arch. Intern. Med. **41**:221, 1966.
840. Lander, J.J., et al.: Angiosarcoma of liver associated with Fowler's solution (potassium arsenite), Gastroenterology **68**:1583, 1975.
841. Lee, F.L.: Cirrhosis and hepatoma in alcoholics, Gut **7**:77, 1966.
842. Lees, C.D., et al.: Carcinoma of the bile ducts, Surg. Gynecol. Obstet. **151**:193, 1980.
843. Lingao, A.L., Domingo, E.O., and Nishioka, K.: Hepatitis B virus profile of hepatocellular carcinoma in the Philippines, Cancer **48**:1590, 1981.
844. Machell, R.J., and Calne, R.Y.: Solitary non-parasitic hepatic cysts presenting with jaundice, Br. J. Radiol. **51**:631, 1978.
845. Madding, G.F., and Kennedy, P.A.: Hepatic artery ligation, Surg. Clin. North Am. **52**:719, 1972.
846. Mariani, A.F., et al.: Progressive enlargement of an hepatic cell adenoma, Gastroenterology **77**:1319, 1979.
847. Marion, P.L., et al.: State of hepatitis B viral DNA in a human hepatoma cell line, J. Virol. **33**:795, 1980.
848. Marsh, J.L., Dahms, B., and Longmire, W.P., Jr.: Cystadenoma and cystadenocarcinoma of the biliary system, Arch. Surg. **109**:41, 1974.
849. Matolo, N.M., and Johnson, D.G.: Surgical treatment of hepatic hemangioma in newborn, Arch. Surg. **106**:725, 1973.
850. McDermott, W.V., Jr., and Hensle, T.W.: Metastatic carcinoid to the liver treated by hepatic dearterialization, Ann. Surg. **180**:305, 1974.
851. Melnick, P.J.: Polycystic liver: analysis of 70 cases, Arch. Pathol. **59**:162, 1955.
852. Michaeli, D., et al.: Hepatic telangiectases and portosystemic encephalopathy in Osler-Weber-Rendu disease, Gastroenterology **54**:929, 1968.
853. Moenandar, I.M.: Extensive calcification in stroma of a primary hepatic carcinoma, J. Pathol. **114**:53, 1974.
854. Moore, T.A., Ferrante, W.A., and Crowson, T.D.: Hepatoma occurring two decades after hepatic irradiation, Gastroenterology **71**:128, 1976.
855. Murphy, A.S.K., et al.: Biochemical studies on liver tumors of children, Arch. Pathol. **96**:48, 1972.
856. Nadell, J., and Kosek, J.: Peliosis hepatis: twelve cases associated with oral androgen therapy, Arch. Pathol. Lab. Med. **101**:405, 1977.
857. Neuberger, J., et al.: Oral-contraceptive associated liver tumors: occurrence of malignancy and difficulties in diagnosis, Lancet **1**:273, 1980.
858. Ohbayashi, A.: Genetic and familial aspects of liver cirrhosis and hepatocellular carcinoma. In Okuda, K., and Peters, R.L., editors: Hepatocellular carcinoma, New York, 1976, John Wiley & Sons, Inc.
859. Ohbayashi, A., Okochi, K., and Mayumi, M.: Familial clustering of asymptomatic carriers of Australia antigen and patients with chronic liver disease or primary liver cancer, Gastroenterology **42**:618, 1972.
860. Okuda, K., and the Liver Cancer Study Group of Japan: Primary liver cancers in Japan, Cancer **45**:2663, 1980.
861. Okuda, K., et al.: Peliosis hepatis as a late and fatal complication of Thorotrast liver disease: report of five cases, Liver **1**:110, 1981.
862. Ong, G.B., and Taw, J.L.: Spontaneous rupture of hepatocellular carcinoma, Br. Med. J. **4**:146, 1972.
863. Othersen, H.B., and Watanatittan, S.: Giant hemangiomatosis of the liver in infancy, Am. Surg. **20**:25, 1978.
864. Paradinas, F.J., et al.: Hyperplasia and prolapse of hepatocytes into hepatic veins during long term methyltestosterone therapy, Histopathology **1**:225, 1977.
865. Parker, P., et al.: Regression of hepatic adenomas in type Ia glycogen storage disease with dietary therapy, Gastroenterology **81**:534, 1981.
866. Peers, F.G., and Linsell, C.A.: Dietary aflatoxin and liver cancer: a population based study in Kenya, Br. J. Cancer **27**:473, 1973.

867. Person, D.A., Sargent, T., and Isaac, E.: Thorotrast-induced carcinoma of the liver, Arch. Surg. **88**:503, 1964.
868. Peters, R.L.: Pathology of hepatocellular carcinoma. In Okuda, K., and Peters, R.L., editors: Hepatocellular carcinoma, New York, 1976, John Wiley & Sons, Inc.
869. Peters, R.L., Afroudakis, A.P., and Tatter, D.: The changing incidence of association of hepatitis B with hepatocellular carcinoma in California, Am. J. Clin. Pathol. **68**:1, 1977.
870. Phinney, P.R., Austin, G.E., and Kadell, B.M.: Cholangiocarcinoma arising in Caroli's disease, Arch. Pathol. Lab. Med. **105**:194, 1981.
871. Plachta, A.: Triad syndrome inherent to calcified cavernous hemangioma of liver, Angiology **16**:594, 1965.
872. Powell, L.W.: Tissue damage in haemachromatosis: an analysis of the roles of iron and alcoholism, Gut **11**:980, 1970.
873. Prince, A.M.: Hepatitis B virus and hepatocellular carcinoma: molecular biology provides further evidence for an etiologic association, Hepatology **1**:73, 1981.
874. Pryor, A.C., Cohen, R.J., and Goldman, R.L.: Hepatocellular carcinoma in a woman on long term oral contraceptives, Cancer **40**:884, 1977.
875. Rabinowitz, J.F., Kinkabvalia, M., and Ulreich, S.: Macroregenerating nodules in the cirrhotic liver: radiologic features and differential diagnosis, Am. J. Roentgenol. Rad. Ther. Nucl. Med. **121**:401, 1974.
876. Rankin, J.G., Skyring, A.P., and Goulston, S.J.M.: Liver in ulcerative colitis: obstructive jaundice due to bile duct carcinoma, Gut **7**:433, 1966.
877. Rooks, J.B., et al.: Epidemiology of hepatocellular adenoma, J.A.M.A. **242**:644, 1979.
878. Rotman, M., et al.: Radiation treatment of pediatric hepatic hemangiomatosis and coexisting cardiac failure, N. Engl. J. Med. **302**:852, 1980.
879. Samelippo, P.M., Beahrs, O.H., and Weiland, L.H.: Cystic disease of liver, Ann. Surg. **179**:922, 1974.
880. Schaffner, F., et al.: Budd-Chiari syndrome caused by a web in the inferior vena cava, Am. J. Med. **42**:838, 1967.
881. Selikoff, I.J., and Hammond, E.C.: Toxicity of vinyl chloride–polyvinyl chloride, Ann. N.Y. Acad. Sci. **246**:5, 1975.
882. Selinger, M., and Koff, R.S.: Thorotrast and the liver: a reminder, Gastroenterology **68**:799, 1975.
883. Sewell, J.H., and Weiss, K.: Spontaneous ruptures of hemangioma of the liver, Arch. Surg. **83**:729, 1961.
884. Shank, R.C., et al.: Dietary aflatoxins and human liver cancer. III. Field survey of rural Thai families for ingested aflatoxins, Food Cosmet. Toxicol. **10**:61, 1972.
885. Sherlock, S., and Scheuer, P.J.: The presentation and diagnosis of 100 patients with primary biliary cirrhosis, N. Engl. J. Med. **289**:674, 1973.
886. Short, W.F., et al.: Biliary cystadenoma: report of case and review of the literature, Arch. Surg. **102**:78, 1971.
887. Simons, M.J., Yu, M., and Shanmugaratnam, K.: Immunodeficiency to hepatitis B virus infection and genetic susceptibility to development of hepatocellular carcinoma, Ann. N.Y. Acad. Sci. **259**:181, 1975.
888. Simson, I.W.: Membranous obstruction of the inferior vena cava and hepatocellular carcinoma in South Africa, Gastroenterology **82**:171, 1982.
889. Slovis, T.L., et al.: Hemangiomas of the liver in infants: review of diagnosis, treatment and course, A.J.R. **123**:791, 1975.
890. Smoron, G.L., and Battifora, H.A.: Thorotrast-induced hepatoma, Cancer **30**:1252, 1972.
891. Srouji, M.N., et al.: Mesenchymal hamartoma of the liver in infants, Cancer **42**:2483, 1978.
892. Stanley, P., et al.: Hepatic cavernous hemangiomas and hemangioendotheliomas in infancy, A.J.R. **129**:317, 1977.
893. Stern, Z., Gordon, R., and Gimmon, Z.: Surgical treatment of a solitary giant hemangioma of the liver presenting as an avascular mass, Int. Surg. **64**:27, 1979.
894. Stromeyer, F.W., and Ishak, K.G.: Nodular transformation (nodular "regenerative" hyperplasia) of the liver: a clinicopathologic study of 30 cases, Hum. Pathol. **12**:60, 1981.
895. Sussman, E.B., et al.: Hemangioendothelial sarcoma of the liver and hemochromatosis, Arch. Pathol. **97**:39, 1974.
896. Sweeney, E.C., and Evans, D.J.: Hepatic lesions in patients treated with synthetic anabolic steroids, J. Clin. Pathol. **29**:626, 1976.
897. Taksan, H., et al.: Clinicopathologic study of seventy patients with carcinoma of the biliary tract, Surg. Gynecol. Obstet. **150**:721, 1980.
898. Tesluk, H., and Lawrie, J.: Hepatocellular adenoma: its transformation to carcinoma in a user of oral contraceptives, Arch. Pathol. Lab. Med. **150**:296, 1981.
899. Thalassinos, N.C., and Lyberatos, C.: Liver cell carcinoma after long-term estrogen-like drug, Lancet **1**:270, 1974.
900. Thung, S.N., Gerber, M.A., and Bodenheimer, H.C., Jr.: Nodular regenerative hyperplasia of the liver in a patient with diabetes mellitus, Cancer **49**:543, 1982.
901. Tong, M.J., et al.: Hepatitis associated antigen and hepatocellular carcinoma in Taiwan, Ann. Intern. Med. **75**:687, 1971.
902. Tong, M.J., et al.: Evidence for clustering of hepatitis B virus infection in families of patients with primary hepatocellular carcinoma, Cancer **44**:2338, 1979.
903. Torres, F.O., Purchase, I.F.H., and Van der Watt, J.J.: Aetiology of primary liver cancer in the Bantu, J. Pathol. **102**:163, 1970.
904. Totzke, H.A., and Hutcheson, J.B.: Primary fibrosarcoma of the liver, South. Med. J. **58**:236, 1965.
905. Van Rensburg, S.J., et al.: Primary liver cancer rate and aflatoxin intake in a high cancer area, S. Afr. Med. J. **48**:2506, 1974.
906. Wanless, I.R., et al.: Nodular regenerative hyperplasia of the liver associated with macroglobulinemia, Am. J. Med. **70**:1203, 1981.
907. Weinberg, A.G., Mize, C.E., and Worthen, H.G.: The occurrence of hepatoma in the chronic form of hereditary tyrosinemia, J. Pediatr. **88**:434, 1976.
908. Yanoff, M., and Rawson, A.J.: Peliosis hepatis, Arch. Pathol. **77**:159, 1964.

Transplantation

909. Hood, J.M., et al.: Liver transplantation for advanced liver disease with alpha-1-antitrypsin deficiency, N. Engl. J. Med. **302**:272, 1980.
910. Porter, K.A.: Pathology of the orthotopic homograft and heterograft. In Starzl, T.E., editor: Experiments in hepatic transplantation, Philadelphia, 1969, W.B. Saunders Co.
911. Present state of liver transplantation (editorial), Br. Med. J. **1**:1441, 1979.
912. Roddy, H., Putnom, C.W., and Fennel, R.H.: Pathology of liver transplantation, Transplantation **22**:625, 1979.
913. Starzl, T.E., et al.: Fifteen years of clinical liver transplantation, Gastroenterology **77**:375, 1979.
914. Williams, R., et al.: Liver transplantation in man: the frequency of rejection, biliary tract complications, and recurrence of malignancy, Gastroenterology **64**:1024, 1973.

CHAPTER 28 Gallbladder and Biliary Ducts

KATHERINE DeSCHRYVER-KECSKEMETI

ANATOMY

The gallbladder is a pear-shaped bag, 9 cm long, with a capacity of about 50 ml. The fundus is the broad end and is directed forward; this is the part palpated when the abdomen is examined. The body extends into a narrow neck, which continues into the cystic duct. The valves of Heister are spiral folds of mucous membrane in the wall of the cystic ducts and neck of the gallbladder. Hartmann's pouch, a sacculation at the neck of the gallbladder, is a common site for a gallstone to lodge.

The hepatic ducts emerge from the right and left lobes of the liver and unite in the porta hepatis to form the common hepatic duct. This is soon joined by the cystic duct from the gallbladder to form the common bile duct.

The common bile duct, measured at operation, is about 0.5 to 15 mm in diameter and runs between the layers of the lesser omentum, lying anterior to the portal vein and to the right of the hepatic artery. Numerous anatomic variants of this relationship are known to occur. Passing behind the first part of the duodenum the common duct enters it, usually joining the main pancreatic duct to form the ampulla of Vater. In about 30% of subjects the biliary and pancreatic ducts open separately into the duodenum. The duodenal portion of the common bile duct is surrounded by a thickening of both longitudinal and circular muscle fibers derived from the intestine, called the sphincter of Oddi.

MORPHOLOGY

The biliary duct, as well as the gallbladder, are lined by tall columnar epithelium. The normal epithelium functions as an absorptive surface and has little mucin-secreting activity. Acinar glands producing a mucinous secretion are present only in the neck of the gallbladder and are absent in its body and fundus. Beneath the epithelium a delicate lamina propria contains capillaries. The mucosal surface of the gallbladder is immensely expanded by deep folds and ridges of varying heights. Microscopically the ridges are richly branching, and delicate connective tissue stalks are covered by tall columnar cells (Fig. 28-1). External to the lamina propria is a fairly dense, fibrous connective tissue making up the wall of the extrahepatic biliary ducts. In the gallbladder, external to the lamina propria, are smooth muscle bundles arranged longitudinally and external to that obliquely or circularly. The muscular coat is surrounded by the perimuscular layer composed of a narrow zone of loose connective tissue, sometimes interspersed with adipose cells. Serosa covers the perimuscular layer over the peritoneal surface of the gallbladder. In the gallbladder fossa the connective tissue of the wall is continuous with the periportal spaces of the liver. On the surface, aberrant bile ducts (Luschka ducts) frequently occur.

PHYSIOLOGY

The function of the gallbladder is to concentrate hepatic bile and deliver it at intervals into the intestine to aid in the digestion and absorption of fat. Despite its limited capacity the gallbladder concentrates and thus can accommodate up to half of the daily flow of hepatic bile and can sequester between meals the entire bile acid pool. The absorptive rate of the gallbladder, one of the highest among epithelia, is between 15% and 30% of intraluminal volume per hour, and the ionic profile of the residual concentrate is altered. Organic solutes comprise only 5% of human bile by weight and consist mainly of bile acid anions, phospholipids (mostly lecithin), and nonesterified cholesterol aggregated into mixed micelles.

Gallbladder motility, contraction, and choledochal relaxation are under the control of a peptide hormone, cholecystokinin (CCK), which is released from the proximal intestine by partly digested proteins and fatty acids.

The extent of neural control of gallbladder motor function is uncertain. Adrenergic innervation of gallbladder muscle is sparse; most of the adrenergic fibers in the

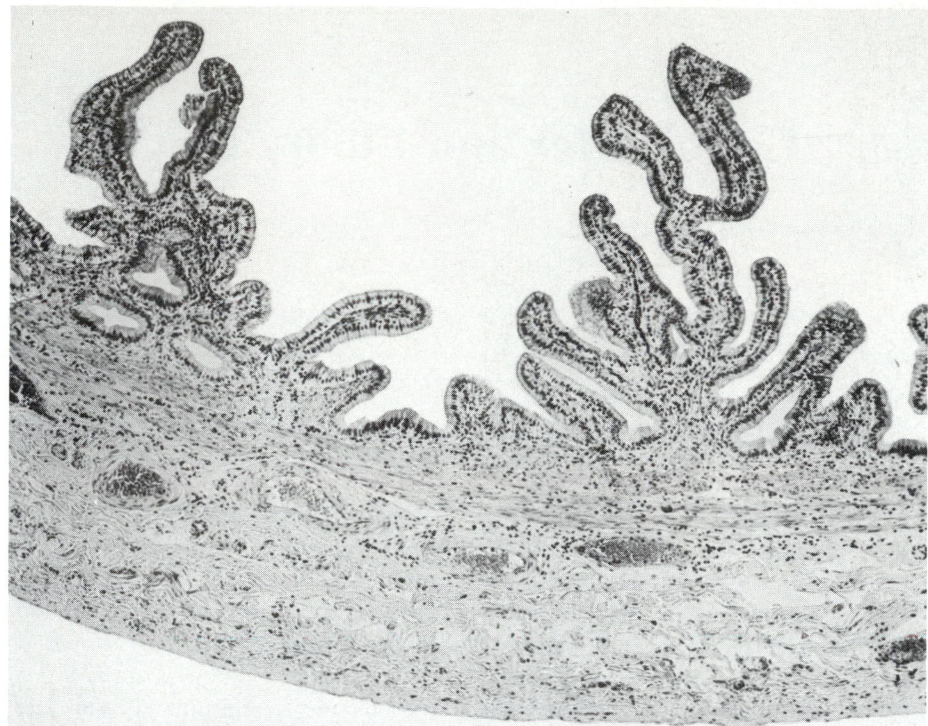

Fig. 28-1. Normal gallbladder in 33-year-old woman. In cross section of midportion, delicate connective tissue stalks are covered by tall columnar epithelium. Beneath tunica propria is muscular coat with smooth muscle bundles arranged longitudinally and then obliquely or circularly. External to muscular coat is perimuscular layer. (40×.)

human gallbladder are distributed to blood vessels. The extent of vagal cholinergic innervation of gallbladder smooth muscle has yet to be defined; vagotomy is said to decrease nerve fibers in the wall of the gallbladder by 10%. Cholinergic agonists contract, and beta-adrenergic agonists relax, gallbladder smooth muscle.

Vasoactive peptide (VIP), immunoreactive nerve fibers, and cell bodies have recently been demonstrated in muscle and submucosal layers of the gallbladder in humans and other mammals and appear to reach the gallbladder via the vagus nerve.[2] VIP relaxes gallbladder muscle and antagonizes the contractile effect of CCK.[1] It seems reasonable to speculate that VIP and CCK function as the neural and hormonal limbs of a peptide system for the control of gallbladder motor activity.

Certain substances, when injected intravenously or given by mouth, appear in the bile and reach the gallbladder. Some substances so administered accumulate in the gallbladder in concentrations not attained in the bile coming from the liver. Cholecystography, the visualization of the gallbladder roentgenographically, is based on this selective resorbing ability of the gallbladder. Radiopaque substances, after reaching the gallbladder, are resorbed more slowly than the bile, eventually attaining a concentration sufficient to cast a shadow on an x-ray film. Intraluminal lesions (stones or "polyps") appear as a radiolucent filling defect.

Congenital or developmental abnormalities

Many anomalous arrangements of the extrahepatic bile ducts and their arteries are usually asymptomatic and significant only for those involved in gallbladder surgery. Other abnormalities of the gallbladder include absence, duplication, and presence of heterotopic tissue. Agenesis may be associated with symptoms suggesting inflammatory disease of the gallbladder. Exploration and T-tube cholangiography establish the diagnosis. The remainder of the biliary tract is usually normally developed in these cases.[6] Duplication and lobulation show histologically normal features.

Heterotopic tissue is nearly always accompanied by inflammation and lithiasis.[7] Gastric tissue is the most frequent finding,[4] but adrenal,[3] pancreas,[9] and thyroid[5] tissues have all been reported.

A group of conditions with a probably related pathogenesis, which are designated infantile obstructive cholangiopathy, includes biliary atresia, choledochal cyst, and neonatal hepatitis.[8] They are now believed to be part of an acquired progressive process that occurs postnatally. They are discussed in detail on p. 1158.

Acquired disorders

Cholelithiasis

Cholelithiasis results from the interplay of numerous factors. It is more frequent in women than in men. The

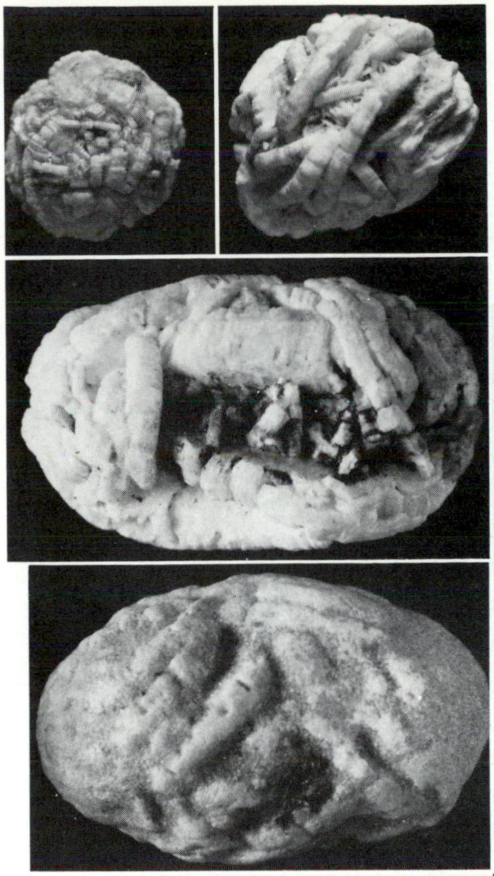

A

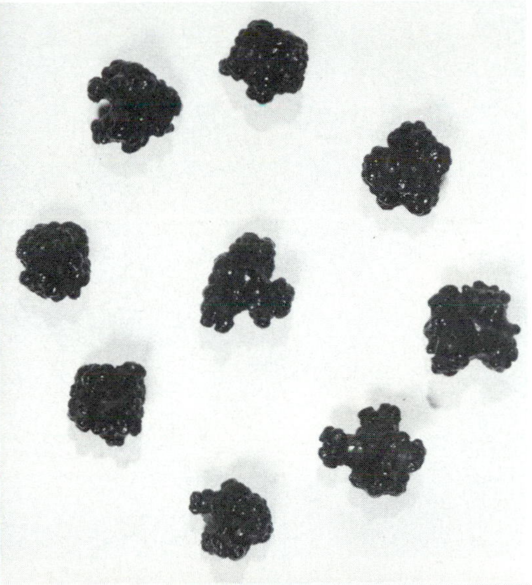

B

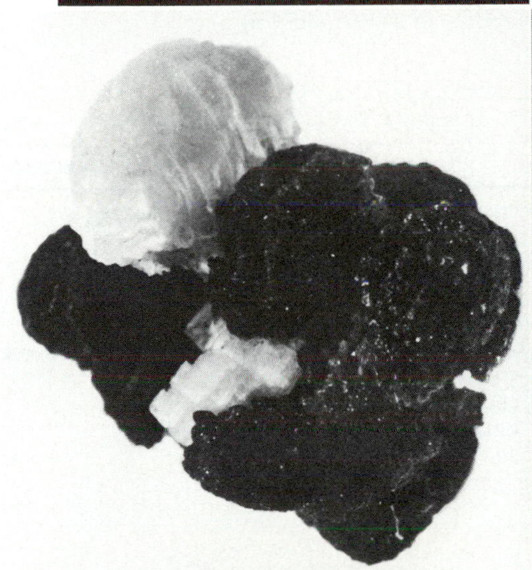

C

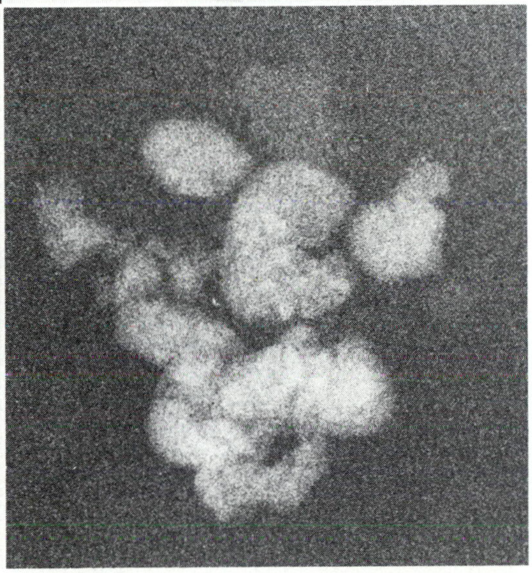

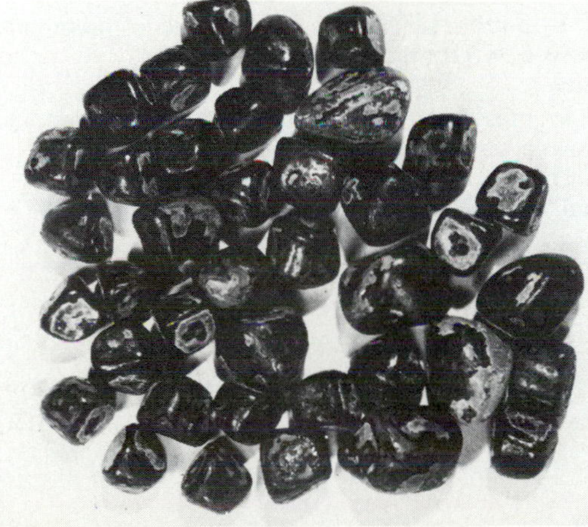

D

Fig. 28-2. A, Crystalline cholesterol stones of varying sizes, each from a different gallbladder. B, Calcium bilirubinate calculi from gallbladder in 78-year-old man. C, "Paired" pure gallstone from gallbladder in 41-year-old woman. Calculus is 0.9 cm in diameter. Attached to black calcium bilirubinate concretion are clusters of crystalline cholesterol. Calcium bilirubinate portion is radiopaque. D, Mixed gallstones from gallbladder in 68-year-old man. Calculi are of almost equal size with articulating faceted surfaces and are black with lighter black-brown centers. (A, 2×; A and C, courtesy Dr. Malcolm A. Hyman, New York.)

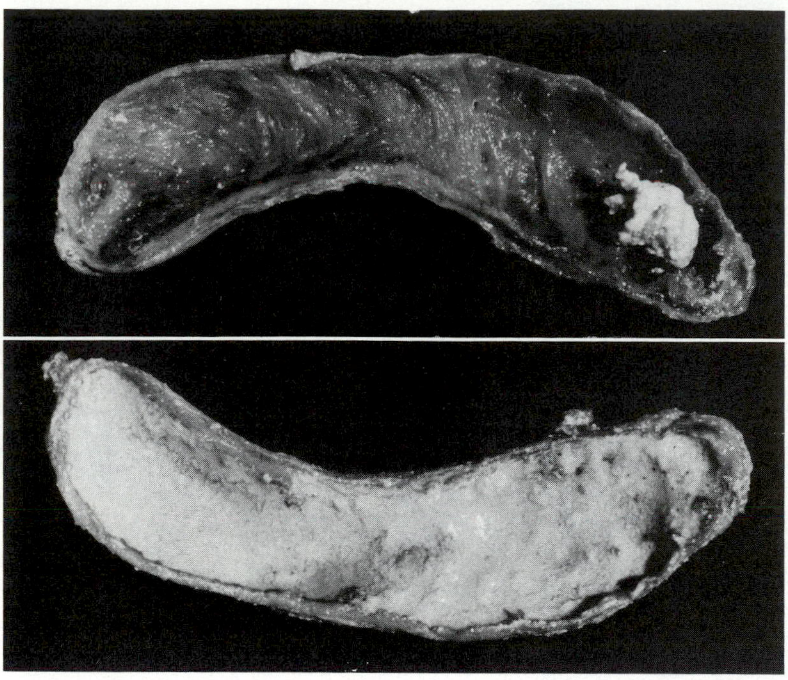

Fig. 28-3. Calcium carbonate stone and "lime paste" in gallbladder of 34-year-old man.

Table 28-1. Classification of gallstones

Type	Composition	Appearance	Factors in origin	Changes in gallbladder
Pure gallstones (10%)	Cholesterol (crystalline)	Solitary; crystalline surface	Increased cholesterol content in bile	Cholesterosis
	Calcium bilirubinate	Multiple; jet black; crystalline or amorphous	Increased pigment content in bile	No change
	Calcium carbonate	Grayish white; amorphous	Unknown	No change
Mixed gallstones (80%)	Cholesterol and calcium bilirubinate Cholesterol and calcium carbonate Calcium bilirubinate and calcium carbonate Cholesterol, calcium bilirubinate, and calcium carbonate	Multiple, faceted or lobulated, laminated, and crystalline on cut surfaces; hue depends on content: cholesterol, yellow; calcium bilirubinate, black; calcium carbonate, white	Chronic cholecystitis plus increased content in bile of cholesterol, calcium bilirubinate, or calcium carbonate	Chronic cholecystitis
Combined gallstones (10%)	Pure gallstone nucleus with mixed gallstone shell	Largest of gallstones when single; hue depends on composition of shell	As in pure gallstones, followed by chronic cholecystitis	Chronic cholecystitis
	Mixed gallstone nucleus with pure gallstone shell		As in mixed gallstones, followed by increased content in bile of cholesterol, calcium bilirubinate, or calcium carbonate	Chronic cholecystitis

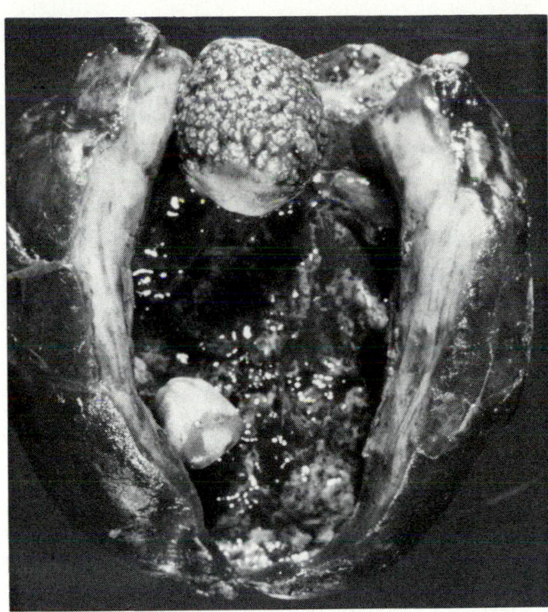

Fig. 28-4. Gross appearance of acute cholecystitis, superimposed on long-standing lithiasis. Hemorrhagic and fibrinopurulent deposits line gallbladder lumen, wall is markedly thickened, and stones are visible.

incidence in the general population of the United States is 11% according to the Framingham Study.[12] The incidence increases with age, so that at the age of 60 years, about 25% of women have stones. In the Native American population the incidence is considerably greater.[18]

Gallstones contain cholesterol, calcium bilirubinate, and calcium carbonate either in pure form or in various combinations (Figs. 28-2 and 28-3). About 20% contain sufficient calcium to be radiopaque. Others appear as a filling defect in an opacified gallbladder. About half of patients with lithiasis have a gallbladder that cannot be visualized. Ultrasonography and computed tomography are methods of choice for the investigation of symptoms referable to the gallbladder and common duct.[23] Ultrasonography has the advantage of being noninvasive, with no radiation exposure and modestly priced equipment, but it requires a high degree of interpretative skill.[21] Other procedures include percutaneous transhepatic cholangiography and endoscopic retrograde cholangiopancreatography (ERCP); these are invasive procedures and involve some radiation exposure but have high diagnostic accuracy.

Table 28-1 summarizes the appearance of various gallstones and the known factors in their formation. Intraluminal stones of different composition have different effects on the gallbladder mucosa. Gallbladders containing pure stones show little or no inflammatory reaction if the cystic duct is not obstructed. On the other hand, chronic cholecystitis is almost always present in gallbladders with mixed and combined gallstones, which represent the majority (90%) of cases of lithiasis (Fig. 28-4).

Numerous clinical and experimental studies have tried to elucidate the mechanism of stone formation in the gallbladder. It is increasingly evident that multiple factors are involved and that patients with cholecystolithiasis probably constitute a heterogeneous population. Some of the important factors identified in stone formation can be grouped according to three general categories[14]: (1) lithiasis resulting from abnormal composition of bile; (2) that resulting from abnormal contractility of the gallbladder; and (3) that resulting from abnormal epithelial secretion. However, in patients with lithiasis, the various factors exist synchronously, and their relative primary importance cannot be established independently. Supersaturation of bile in cholesterol is the major factor in gallstones associated with obesity and clofibrate therapy in coronary patients.[11] On the other hand, excessive bile salt loss is seen in lithiasis associated with intestinal bypass procedures and Crohn's disease.[17] Decreased bile acid secretion was identified in the lithogenic bile of the Native American women.

Cholelithiasis is rare in children.[20] A hemolytic disorder of one type or another is present in approximately 50% of afflicted children. These include congenital spherocytosis, sickle cell anemia, and thalassemia. In some of the other children there is a history of previous intra-abdominal sepsis.

Female sex hormones have long been suspected to have the side effect of gallstone formation by altering respective bile constituents. The female preponderance and the association of gallbladder stones and parity are well known. Gallbladder function in the last trimester of pregnancy has been examined by real-time ultrasonography; an abnormal contractility and a large residual volume resulting in stasis were observed, whereas in patients taking contraceptive steroids, gallbladder kinetics were normal.[10] Interestingly, progesterone has been shown experimentally to impair gallbladder response to exogenous cholecystokinin. There is a significant association between gallstones and oral contraceptives, replacement estrogen therapy, and estrogen given for coronary artery disease in men. The mechanism of this association is not determined but probably does not involve gallbladder motility per se. Vagotomy is said to predispose patients to lithiasis. Lastly, in an elegant series of in vitro studies,[15] excess mucin secretion by the gallbladder epithelium has recently been identified as the critical nucleation factor for stone formation.

Gallstones are formed in the gallbladder and may escape into the cystic duct or common duct. Approximately 15% of patients operated on for cholelithiasis also have concomitant choledocholithiasis.[23] In more than 1% of patients, symptoms of common duct lithiasis appear some time after cholecystectomy and are caused by stones overlooked at the time of operation.[13] The primary formation of stones in the extrahepatic ducts is so rare that common duct obstruction by stone is nearly always the result of gallbladder lithiasis. However, 20% of patients with agenesis of the gallbladder have had gallstones.[6] In rare cases, therefore, stones can and do form in the common duct. These so-called earthy stones are predominantly soft and dark in appearance. The common duct is invariably dilated.

Lithiasis, if untreated, has numerous complications.[16,22] Stones travel through the cystic duct to become impacted in the common duct or at the ampulla, causing intermittent jaundice and severe colicky pain. They are causes of obstruction with secondary acute cholecystitis. Gallstones may also lead to internal biliary fistulas, mostly between gallbladder and duodenum or gallbladder and colon. These result from inflammatory adhesions with subsequent perforation. Fistulas may be visualized on a plain film of the abdomen when an air column outlines the biliary tree. The rationale for removal of stones is thus the observed serious inflammatory and obstructive complications and not the possibility of associated cancer.[16,19,22]

ACUTE INFLAMMATION

Acute acalculous primary bacterial cholecystitis has been documented but is relatively rare in adults.[26] Strains of *Salmonella*, coliform bacteria, enterococci, and staphylococci have all been implicated in some cases. However, much more frequently, acute cholecystitis results from secondary bacterial infection caused by obstruction or impaction of a stone in the common duct. Thiazides have been incriminated in their ability to cause acute cholecystitis.[30] A temporary increase in bile salt content has also been shown experimentally to produce acute cholecystitis. Circulating bacterial toxins are also suspected to be able to damage gallbladder epithelium, as in the lesions of the toxic shock syndrome.[28]

In children, acute cholecystitis is more often the acalculous variety than in adults. Systemic infections such as scarlet fever, salmonellosis, and leptospirosis are considered significant factors in the etiology.[24] The exact mechanism by which acute inflammation of the gallbladder is initiated, however, is unknown.

In acute cholecystitis the clinical symptoms and signs are those of an acute inflammation in the right upper quadrant of the abdomen. Grossly the gallbladder is enlarged and firm, with a thickened wall oozing serous or serosanguineous fluid. There is marked edema, and the outer surface is a dusky reddish brown. The mucosa is congested and grayish red. The mucosa may be intact or may show focal or extensive areas of ulceration. Microscopic examination shows subserosal edema with all the layers spread apart, marked congestion, extravasation of red blood cells, and fresh thrombi within small veins. In distended capillaries, margination of white blood cells is conspicuous. A marked tissue reaction of polymorphonuclear cells is generally absent. Free perforation into the peritoneal cavity has become a rare complication. However, in an acutely distended gallbladder, bile may leak through the intact wall and cause bile peritonitis, which has a guarded prognosis. Hemorrhagic infarction of the gallbladder (gangrenous cholecystitis) may occur, often resulting from an impacted stone that interferes with the venous drainage of the gallbladder.

Occasionally a classic case of acute cholecystitis may show vasculitis with fibrinoid necrosis of the muscular arteries.[25,27,29] Some of these patients go on to full-blown multisystem disorders, whereas in others vasculitis-like changes are confined to the gallbladder.

CHRONIC INFLAMMATION

Chronic cholecystitis is rarely seen in the absence of lithiasis. The associated stones are of the mixed or combined type (Table 28-1). The gallbladder in chronic cholecystitis is characterized by prominent thickening and fibrosis of the wall, which may be grossly indistinguishable from sclerosing carcinoma (Fig. 28-5). Occasionally, diffuse calcification of the wall is also present (porcelain gallbladder, Fig. 28-6). The mucosal folds are coarse and may be completely obliterated. The surface may be trabeculated because of the muscular hyperplasia of the "fighting gallbladder" in the early phase of common duct obstruction (Fig. 28-7).

On microscopic examination the mucosa may be atrophic or show hyperplastic changes. The normal epithelium of the gallbladder does not secrete mucin, but in chronic inflammation, newly formed mucous glands arise from the epithelium in the depths of the folds and may become complex (Fig. 28-8). The recently redefined crucial role of epithelial mucin in the pathogenesis of lithiasis is relevant.[15] Endocrine cells may be increased.[7] The muscle usually becomes hyperplastic with mucosal diverticula (Rokitansky-Aschoff sinuses) between its fascicles (Fig. 28-9). These normally occur at a site of existing weakness of the wall, along the path of penetrating blood vessels. According to Halpert,[35] they result from inflammation and never occur in the normal gallbladder.[35] The perimuscular layer is fibrotic with coarse collagenous bundles. There is usually a moderate mixed inflammatory infiltrate involving all layers. Rarely, there is a prominence of lymphocytic infiltration with formation of lymph follicles and large germinal centers (chronic follicular cholecystitis).[33]

Numerous episodes of acute cholecystitis usually become superimposed on the chronic inflammatory process. Grossly the gallbladder appears acutely inflamed, red, and edematous with mucosal erosions and also contains stones (Fig. 28-4). Microscopically Rokitansky-Aschoff sinuses are numerous, and muscular hyperplasia and marked fibrosis of the wall are present. In addition, a

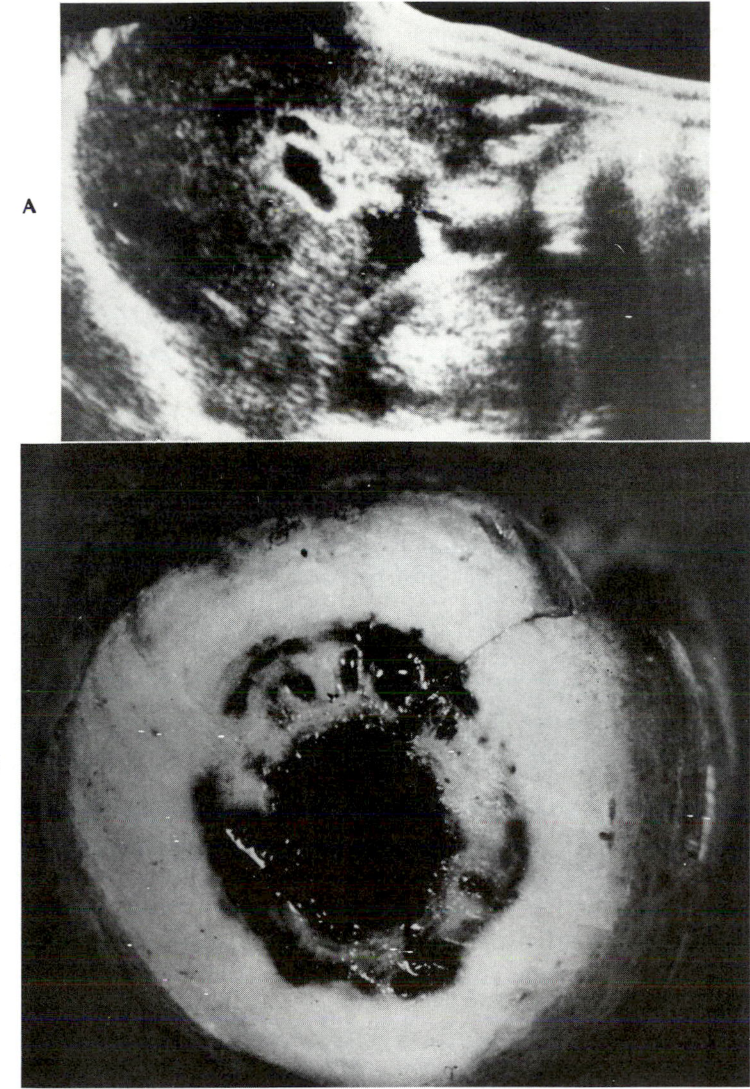

Fig. 28-5. Ultrasonogram, **A,** and transverse anatomic section of gallbladder, **B,** to show extent of thickening of wall in chronic cholecystitis. Appearance is grossly indistinguishable from that of sclerosing carcinoma.

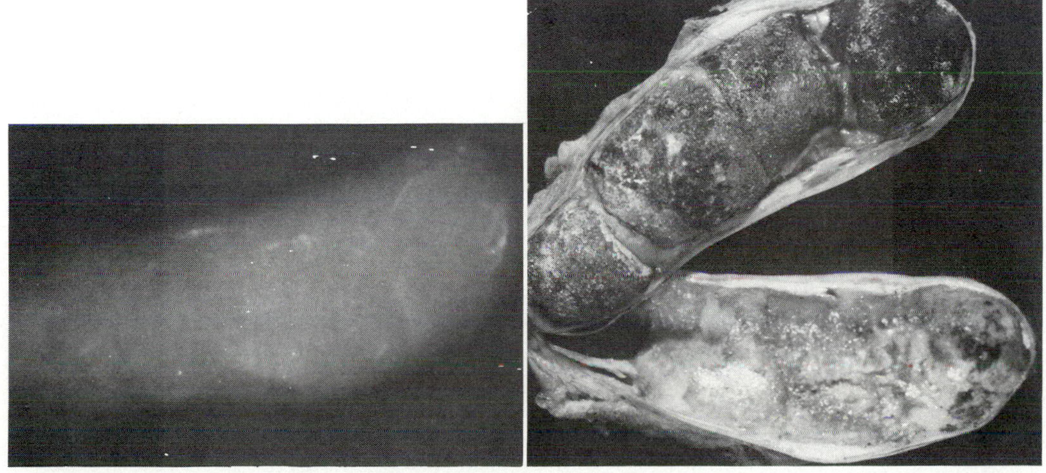

Fig. 28-6. Calcium impregnation of wall of gallbladder in 73-year-old man. Combined calculi with articulating faceted surfaces fill lumen. (Courtesy Dr. William R. Schmalhorst, Bakersfield, Calif.)

hemorrhagic fibrinopurulent exudate covers extended areas of the mucosa, and the inflammatory infiltrate contains sheets of polymorphonuclear cells in the interstitium. This is the condition that most frequently necessitates cholecystectomy. Localized tissue reactions with cholesterol crystals may be seen within the thickened fibrous wall underlying an ulcer (Fig. 28-10). Ceroid granulomas have recently been described in the gallbladder[31] and probably represent a form of chronic cholecystitis. Bile is postulated to serve as the substrate for the ceroid pigment formation within histiocytes (Fig. 28-11). What previously was called xanthogranulomatous cholecystitis probably represents the same entity.[4]

Strictures of the common duct usually result from operative trauma caused by inadvertent ligation. The numerous anatomic variants of the extrahepatic duct and their vessels mentioned earlier are contributing factors in causing the error. Rarely the common duct may participate and be encased in a process of idiopathic retroperitoneal fibrosis.[36] Surgical repair in all these cases is extremely difficult.

Sclerosing cholangitis, a rare disease of unknown etiology, is characterized by fibrosis and diffuse thickening of the wall, predominantly affecting the common duct.[34,32] However, more extensive involvement of the entire system can occur, sometimes including the intra-

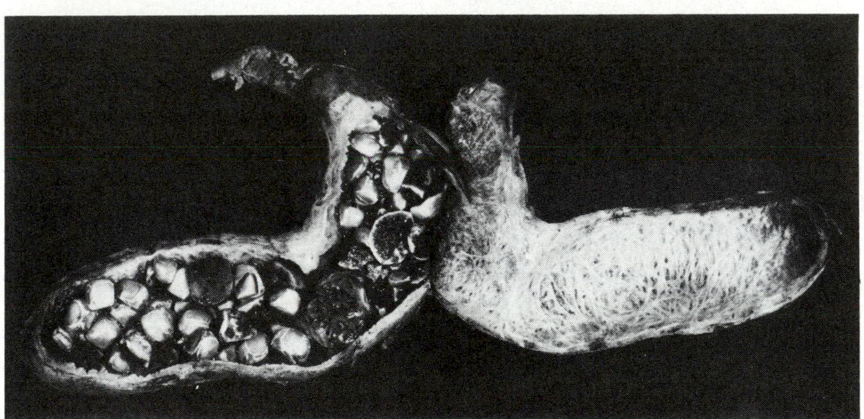

Fig. 28-7. Gallbladder with chronic cholecystitis containing mixed gallstones in 40-year-old man. There are noticeable trabeculations on mucosal surface. Calculi are faceted and yellow with brown centers.

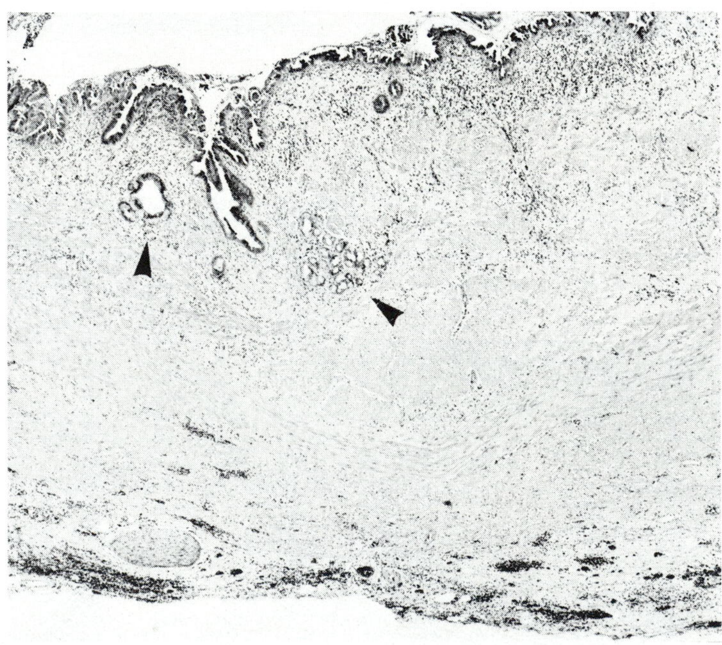

Fig. 28-8. Gallbladder in chronic cholecystitis. Compare thickness of wall to that in Fig. 28-1. Attenuation of mucosa and appearance of mucous cells (*arrows*) are characteristic. (Hematoxylin and eosin; 35×; WU 81-7968.)

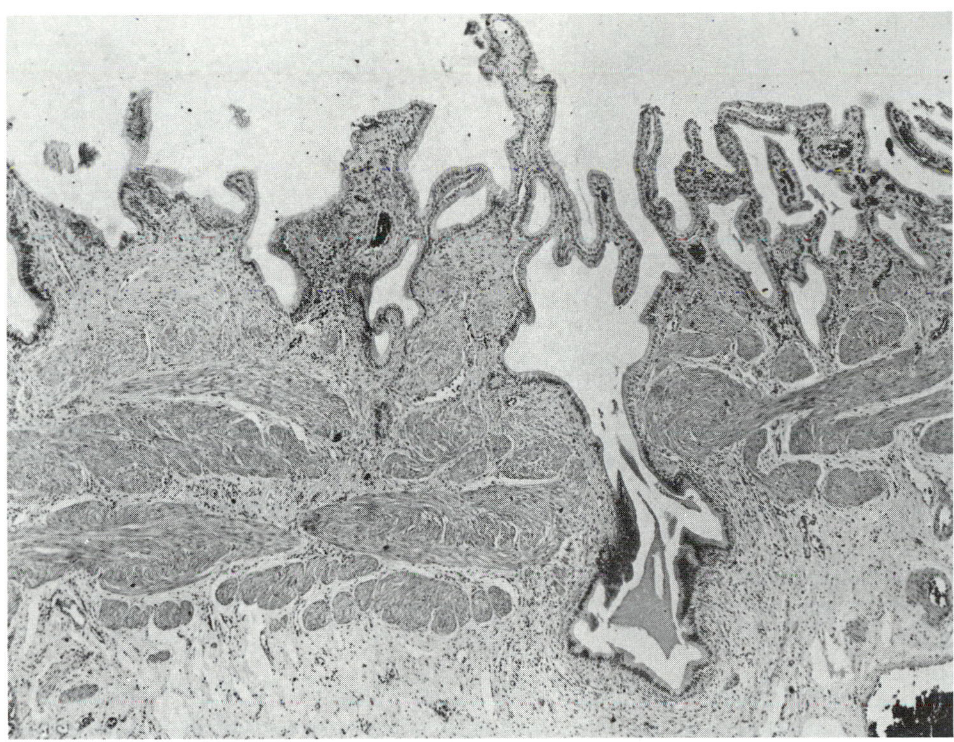

Fig. 28-9. Gallbladder with chronic cholecystitis that contained mixed gallstones in 57-year-old woman. In longitudinal section from body of viscus, folds of mucosa are coarse or delicate. Rokitansky-Aschoff sinus extends through entire thickness of greatly hypertrophied muscular coat. There is increase in connective tissue in tunica propria and between muscle bundles. Perimuscular layer is broad. In all layers there in slight infiltration with lymphocytes, plasma cells, large mononuclear cells, and some eosinophilic granulocytes. (Hematoxylin and eosin; 32×.)

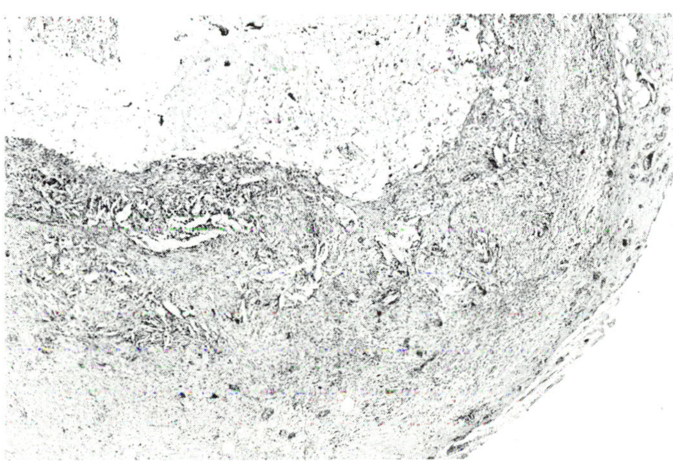

Fig. 28-10. Ulcerated gallbladder mucosa with underlying cholesterol granuloma that complicated long-standing lithiasis and chronic cholecystitis. (Hematoxylin and eosin; 35×; WU 81-7969.)

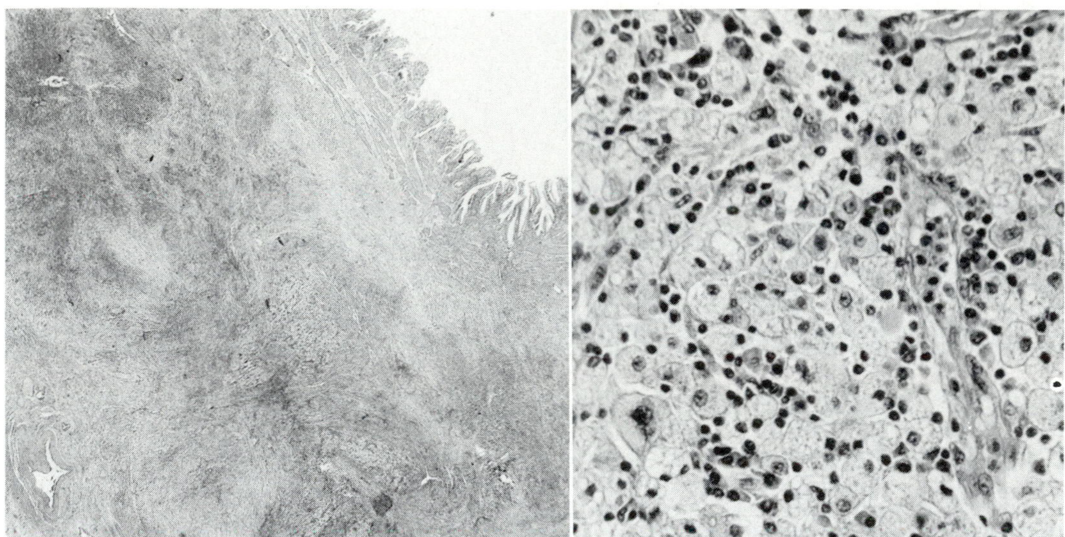

Fig. 28-11. Ceroid granuloma of gallbladder. Collections of pigmented histiocytes are seen deep in gallbladder wall, as is a chronic lymphoplasmacytic inflammatory infiltrate. (Hematoxylin and eosin; 10×; WU 81-10000; courtesy Dr. A.M. Wright, Penrose Hospital, Colorado Springs, Colo.)

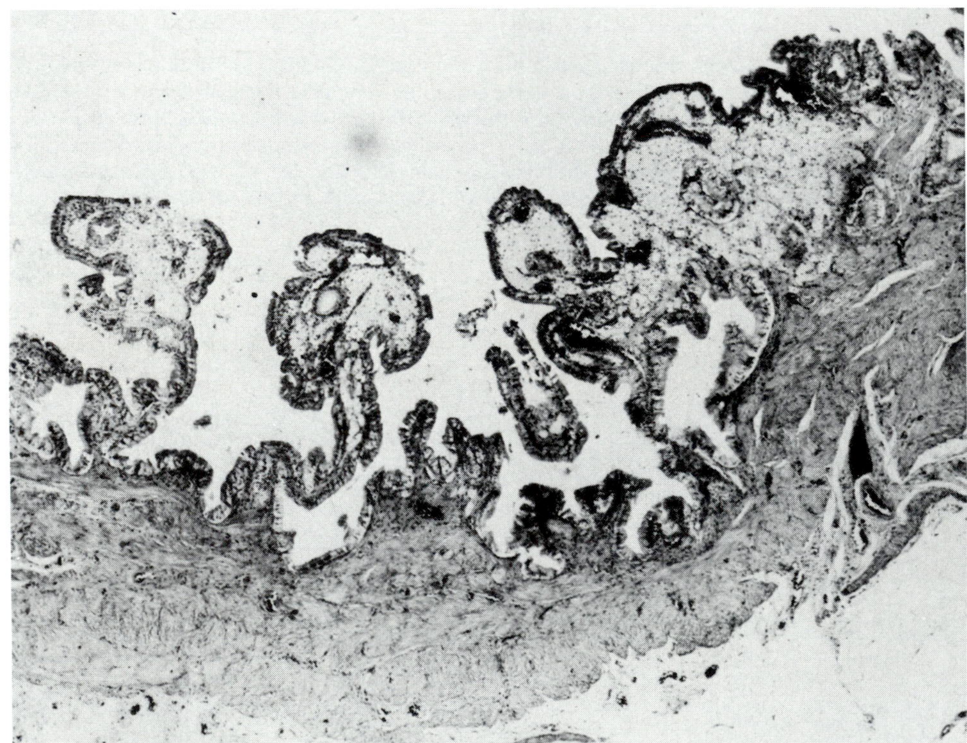

Fig.28-12. Gallbladder with cholesterosis of mucosa in 46-year-old woman. Viscus contained crystalline cholesterol stone. In cross section from near neck, folds are enlarged and rounded. Connective tissue stalks contain many large mononuclear cells with light-stained cytoplasm and eccentric nuclei. These cells contain anisotropic lipoid substances that can be demonstrated by fat stains. (Hematoxylin and eosin; 60×.)

hepatic ducts, in which case the characteristic changes may even be seen on liver biopsy. The diagnosis is best based on examination of a section of the common duct, which shows the chronic inflammatory and fibrosing changes involving submucosa and subserosa, whereas the mucosa is relatively intact. Well-differentiated sclerosing adenocarcinoma, the principal element of the differential diagnosis, must be ruled out. The diagnosis of sclerosing cholangitis should be made only in patients who do not have gallstones and who had no previous operations on the biliary tract. The disease may be found with ulcerative colitis.[37]

MISCELLANEOUS NONINFLAMMATORY CONDITIONS

Cholesterosis of the gallbladder has a characteristic morphologic pattern. Usually the lesion has no inflammatory component and the gallbladder mucosa is otherwise normal. Grossly the mucosa is congested and has yellow flecks of lipid in linear streaks. Cholesterol is increased in the bile but not in the blood. Microscopically collections of lipid-laden foamy cells are present in the lamina propria beneath a normal epithelium (Fig. 28-12).

Spontaneous perforation of the biliary tract occurs within the first year of life. It is usually solitary, and the most common site is the junction of the cystic duct and the common bile duct. The etiology is unclear, but a preexisting malformation of the wall has been postulated.[39] It is an acute abdominal emergency, and the treatment is surgical.

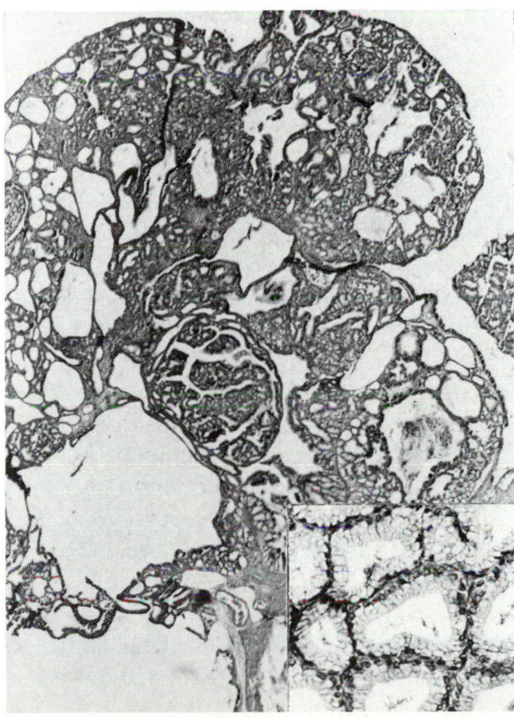

Fig. 28-13. Adenomatous polyp showing proliferated glands, some cystic, surrounded by scant connective tissue stroma. (Hematoxylin and eosin; 10×.)

Acute hydrops of the gallbladder is more often seen in children than in adults, and a precise cause had not been identified.[38] Right upper quadrant symptoms and often a mass are the clinical features. Grossly the gallbladder is distended without stones. The bile is pale, watery, or mucoid. The treatment is usually aspiration or cholecystotomy.

TUMORS

Benign tumors and pseudotumors

Benign true neoplasms of the gallbladder and common duct are extremely rare.[4] They include adenomatous polyps (Fig. 28-13), villous adenomas, and cystadenomas.[44] Granular cell myoblastomas have been reported in the biliary tract, and their morphology is similar to that at other sites seen by both light microscopy and electron microscopy.[42] Paragangliomas of the gallbladder have been reported,[45] as well as eosinophilic granuloma, which involved the common duct and occurred as a mass.[43]

More frequently, however, "masses" in the area of the gallbladder and extrahepatic system are "pseudotumors," including inflammatory polyps, cholesterol polyps, and reactive conditions. Cholesterol polyps are multilobular and yellow. Microscopically they consist of sheets of foamy histiocytes covered by an intact mucosa (Fig. 28-14). These may detach and become the nidus for stone formation.

Another condition, consisting of a complex system of tubular structures set within interlacing smooth muscle bundles, commonly involves the region of the fundus.[40] When sharply circumscribed, it appears grossly as a tumor (Fig. 28-15) and is called adenomyoma. The condition may involve the gallbladder in a more diffuse manner and is then labeled adenomyomatosis. It resembles cholecystitis glandularis and the various forms of gallbladder diverticuli. They probably all represent reactive conditions of the gallbladder mucosa.

Amputation neuromas have been described at the junction of the common and cystic ducts; some are isolated, and some are seen in conjunction with intriguing and complex syndromes, such as soft tissue tumors secreting nerve growth factor.[46] Ganglioneuromatosis of the gallbladder has been described in the multiple endocrine neoplasia 2b syndromes.[41]

Malignant tumors

Etiology and pathogenesis

Primary carcinoma of the gallbladder and biliary tract is not a rare disease, being the fifth most common of the digestive tract.[50] There has been an apparent increase in

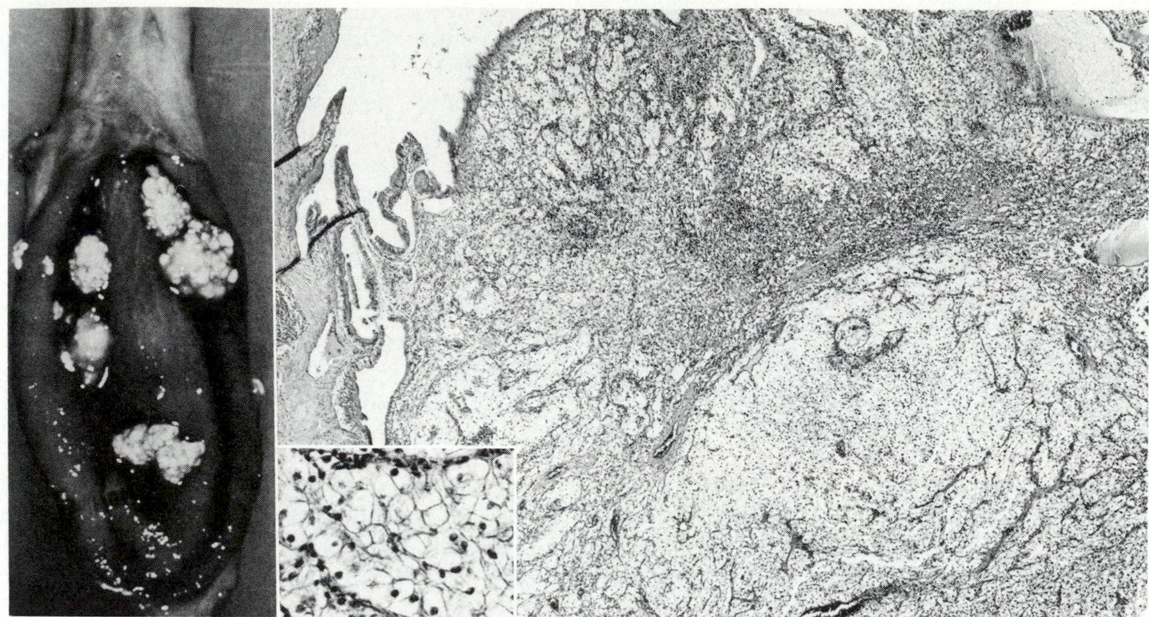

Fig. 28-14. Gross and microscopic appearances of pedunculated cholesterol polyps, consisting of sheets of foamy histiocytes lined by intact surface epithelium. (Hematoxylin and eosin; 35×; WU 81-7974.)

incidence during the last 15 years.[69] Whether this is real or only a reflection of more accurate reporting remains to be determined. Although the causes of this disease are unknown, several possible factors have been suggested.

Gallstones have long been thought to play a role in the genesis of gallbladder carcinoma. In one study the percentage of patients with gallbladder carcinoma who were definitely stated not to have stones accompanying the carcinoma varied only from 3.4% to 17%. Another series reported 29 cases of carcinoma among 1488 cholecystectomies, while stones were detected in 4459 patients by roentgenologic examination[72]; thus in the presence of cholelithiasis, the incidence of documented carcinoma in that study appears to be only 0.66%. In yet another cumulative series, only 0.4% of 1419 patients with known untreated gallstones developed gallbladder carcinoma when followed for 10 years.[69]

The role of chemical carcinogenesis in gallbladder cancer has also received considerable attention owing to the structural similarity of some known carcinogens to the naturally occurring bile acids. Animal studies have implicated methylcholantrene, *o*-amino-azotoluene, and various nitrosamines in the induction of gallbladder carcinoma.[53,69] Experimental animal studies, however, suffer from the problem of species differences in susceptibility and subsequent extrapolation to humans of data from animals. A higher incidence and earlier onset of cancer of the gallbladder have been reported in rubber industry workers.[65] Moreover, pesticides have been shown to be excreted in the bile. The therapeutic agent chenodeoxycholic acid, now available for the dissolution of cholesterol gallstones, may also have long-term effects that are not yet known.

There is a high prevalence of gallbladder carcinoma in certain population groups, such as Japanese immigrants[53] and Native Americans of the Southwest. In Native Americans the incidence of gallbladder carcinoma is six times that in whites.[55,58] The incidence of gallbladder cancer in the Hispanic population, which has a considerable Indian component in its gene pool, seems to be intermediate. Gallbladder cancer is extremely rare in the Bantu population. It has therefore been suggested that there is a strong genetic component in this disease, since many of these groups live under very different environmental conditions. However, gallbladder disease is also prevalent in these populations. The atypical epithelial lesions described in gallbladder of these populations, considered to be precursors to carcinoma, are invariably confined to the free surface epithelium and superficial epithelial invaginations. This observation suggests that the mucosal atypia in these cases may be related to exposure to substances in the gallbladder lumen, presumably contained in bile or stones.

A higher incidence of subsequent gallbladder carcinoma has also been reported in patients who had undergone previous operations on the biliary tract, usually a cholecystostomy. The association of chronic ulcerative colitis with carcinoma of the gallbladder had been reported, although the association with carcinoma of the bile

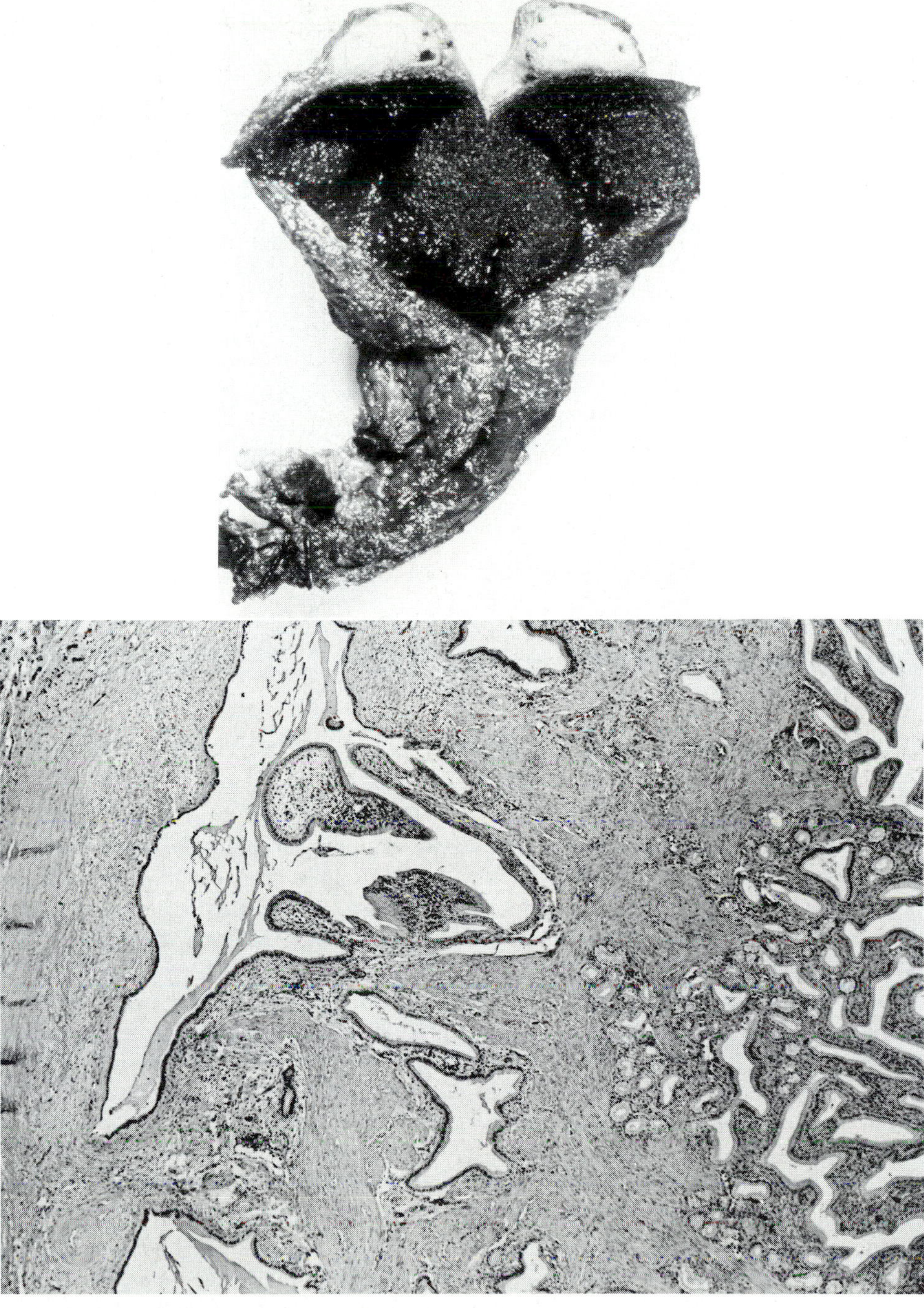

Fig. 28-15. Gross and microscopic appearances of adenomyoma of gallbladder that is localized to fundus. Sections show system of acinar tubular structures lined by cuboid or columnar cells in scanty connective tissue stroma. Interlacing smooth muscle bundles are also seen in stroma. (32×; courtesy Dr. Malcolm A. Hyman, New York.)

ducts is more frequent.[56,67] The tumors occur without preexisting hepatobiliary disease. Patients with ileal disease and those who have undergone bypass surgery are also at higher risk for gallbladder carcinoma. These same groups of patients, however, are also the ones with high incidence of gallbladder lithiasis.[60]

Liver fluke infections in the Orient are known promoters of bile duct carcinoma.[53] It is possible that the chronic inflammatory response they elicit potentiates the action of carcinogens in the bile. Similar conclusions have been drawn in experimental animals. There is an association of carcinoma with congenital cysts of the biliary tract, which may have a similar etiology.[62] In summary, chronic inflammation and fibrosis seem to be strongly associated with carcinoma of the biliary tract. It is interesting in this respect that patients with end-stage chronic cholecystitis, the calcified (porcelain) gallbladder, also have a very high incidence of malignancy.[70] The exact nature of the relationship, however, has been elusive both in clinical and in experimental studies. Nevertheless, in the United States the incidence of gallbladder cancer has recently stabilized, or possibly even declined, concurrent with a rise in the number of cholecystectomies.[58a]

Incidence and clinical presentation

The usual type of carcinoma of the gallbladder has a female preponderance (ratio of 4:1).[45] The mean age of 1728 patients was 65 years, with 0.1%, 1.5%, 8.9%, 19.6%, and 37% occurring in the third, fourth, fifth, sixth and seventh decades, respectively.[43] In patients over 70 years of age who underwent operations on the biliary tract, 10% to 17% were found to have carcinoma.

In a few instances, cancer arises from the hepatic duct in the region of the porta hepatis in relatively young persons (Fig. 28-16).[63] Some of these tumors are extremely well differentiated, with relatively slow growth. The presence and location of tumor are best demonstrated by percutaneous transhepatic cholangiography.

Bile duct carcinoma appears to be less frequent than gallbladder carcinoma,[76] and there is no sex difference in its incidence. Carcinoma of the terminal portion of the common bile duct and that of intrahepatic ducts are discussed elsewhere.

Clinically the lack of specific signs and symptoms prevents early detection of carcinoma of the gallbladder. The clinical presentation commonly mimics benign gallbladder disease, especially acute cholecystitis. As a result of the highly variable clinical presentation and the nonspecific physical, laboratory, and roentgenographic findings in gallbladder carcinoma, the mean correct preoperative rate of diagnosis is only 8.6%.[16] In diagnosed cases the tumor is advanced and usually inoperable. When the nature of the lesion becomes apparent to the surgeon at the time of exploration, the tumor is usually too advanced for cure. Results of a collective review of 993 patients revealed that 16% of patients underwent presumed complete resection of identified tumor and 72% underwent palliative procedures or biopsy alone. In a group of patients with a more favorable prognosis, however, "incidental" carcinoma was diagnosed only after microscopic examination of gallbladders that were removed for presumed benign disease.[52] In these cases the difficulty of diagnosis lies in the gross similarity with inflammatory fibrous tissue. Therefore microscopic examination of every excised gallbladder is mandatory.

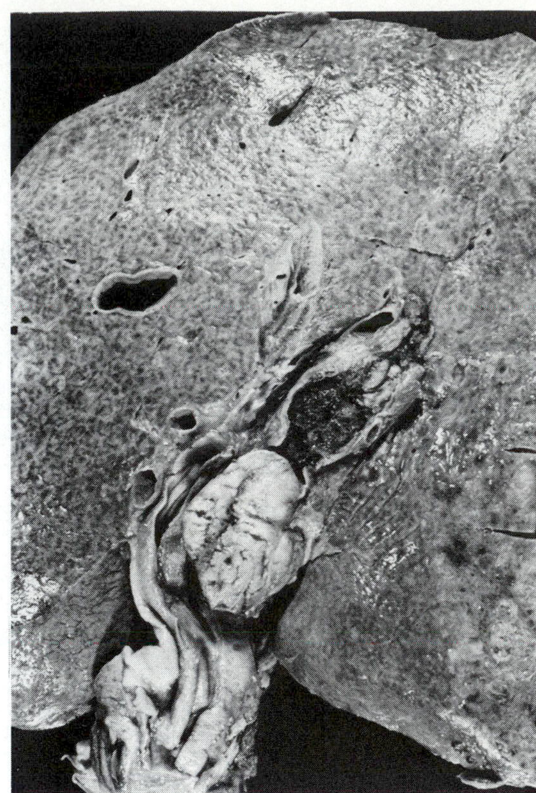

Fig. 28-16. Gross appearance of well-differentiated adenocarcinoma, "Klatskin tumor," arising in porta hepatis.

Pathology, clinicopathologic correlation, and rationale for treatment

Tumors may occur in all parts of the gallbladder but are most frequent in the fundus.[77] The gross pattern of growth assumes either a papillary or an infiltrative character, which may be superimposed on preexisting deformities because of chronic inflammation or lithiasis. Infiltrative carcinoma grows diffusely, imparting a firm, leatherlike quality to the wall, with considerable thickening. Papillary carcinoma is a less common variant. It may be localized or diffusely involve the entire mucosa. The papillary fronds are prone to necrosis and hemorrhage. Obstructive symptoms and development of

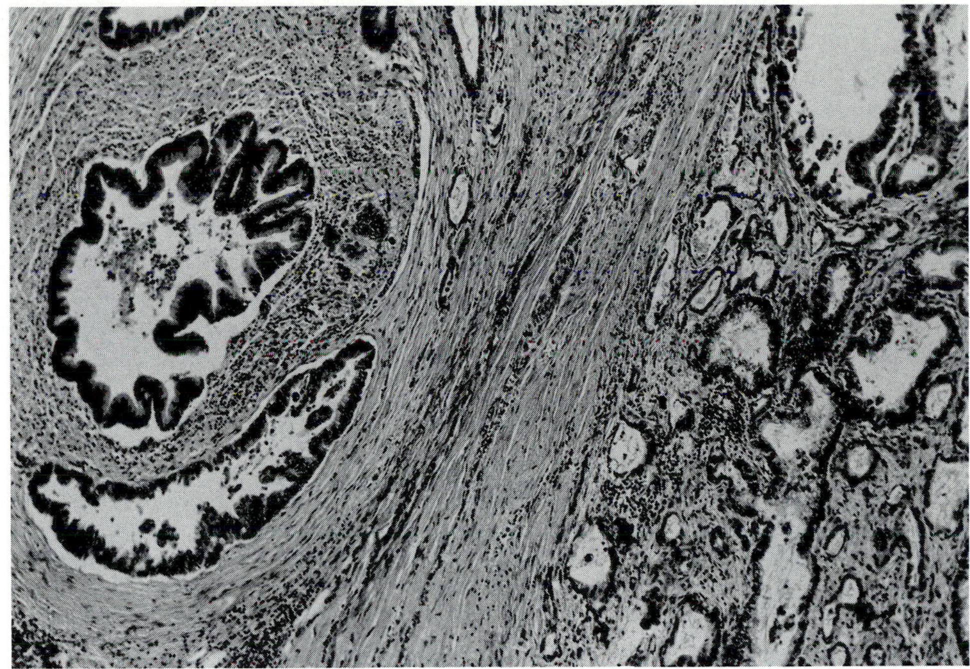

Fig. 28-17. Carcinoma of common bile duct in 83-year-old man. Neoplastic cuboid and columnar cells form acinar tubular structures or are mounted on delicate connective tissue stalks. Neoplastic cells are within sheath of nerve. There was complete obstruction of common bile duct but no involvement of regional lymph nodes and no distant metastasis. (Hematoxylin and eosin; 60×.)

hydrops are encountered in tumors in the neck. Tumors arising in the fundus usually remain asymptomatic. Gallstones are found in 80% to 90% of the cases.

Most gallbladder cancers are adenocarcinomas that are well differentiated and secrete variable amounts of mucin (Fig. 28-17). This is mainly sialomucin in character, in contrast to the sulfomucin type secreted by the normal or inflamed gallbladder. Adenocarcinomas may exhibit varying degrees of squamous metaplasia. In less differentiated tumors the glandular pattern may be partially or completely lost, and the tumor then grows in sheets (Fig. 28-18).

The precursor lesion of invasive gallbladder carcinoma has now been identified in a high-risk population for invasive carcinoma (Fig. 28-19).[48,54] It was concluded that a small number of hyperplasias of the gallbladder evolve toward atypical hyperplasia and that this in turn progresses to carcinoma in situ. The 10-year difference in the mean ages of patients with carcinoma in situ and those with invasive carcinoma gives additional support to the idea of progression of a precursor lesion.

Nevin and associates[68] classified gallbladder carcinoma on the basis of staging and histologic grading and found a good correlation with survival. Patients with stage I (carcinoma in situ and intramucosal lesions) and stage II (invasion of submucosa) were generally cured by cholecystectomy alone. Local recurrence has, however, been reported. In stages III (involvement of all three layers) and IV (involvement of all three layers and the cystic lymph node) the survival was 50%, whereas in stage V (involvement of the liver and other organs) the prognosis is hopeless. Well-differentiated papillary tumors also have a more favorable prognosis.

The biologic behavior of gallbladder carcinomas has been extensively studied by Fahim and co-workers.[59] The most common spread was shown to be lymphatic, vascular, neural, intraperitoneal, and intraductal, in decreasing order. Lymphatic drainage from the gallbladder is to lymph nodes along the cystic and common bile ducts and then via the pancreaticoduodenal nodes to the para-aortic chain. Venous drainage goes to the quadrate lobe of the liver. Vascular metastases to the liver are therefore localized near the gallbladder and are not in the whole liver as they are in other gastrointestinal carcinomas. Peritoneal seeding is rarely found.

Based on the knowledge that failure of treatment for gallbladder carcinoma results from local recurrence and not distant metastasis, radical cholecystectomy has been recommended as the treatment of choice.[69] More extensive resections have not yielded improvement in prognosis. Since a substantial number of carcinomas are known to be incidental, especially in women over 70 years of age who have lithiasis, and since these cases are known to have a more favorable prognosis,[52] all gallbladders in these cases should be carefully examined at the time of operation. Frozen section examination elucidates the

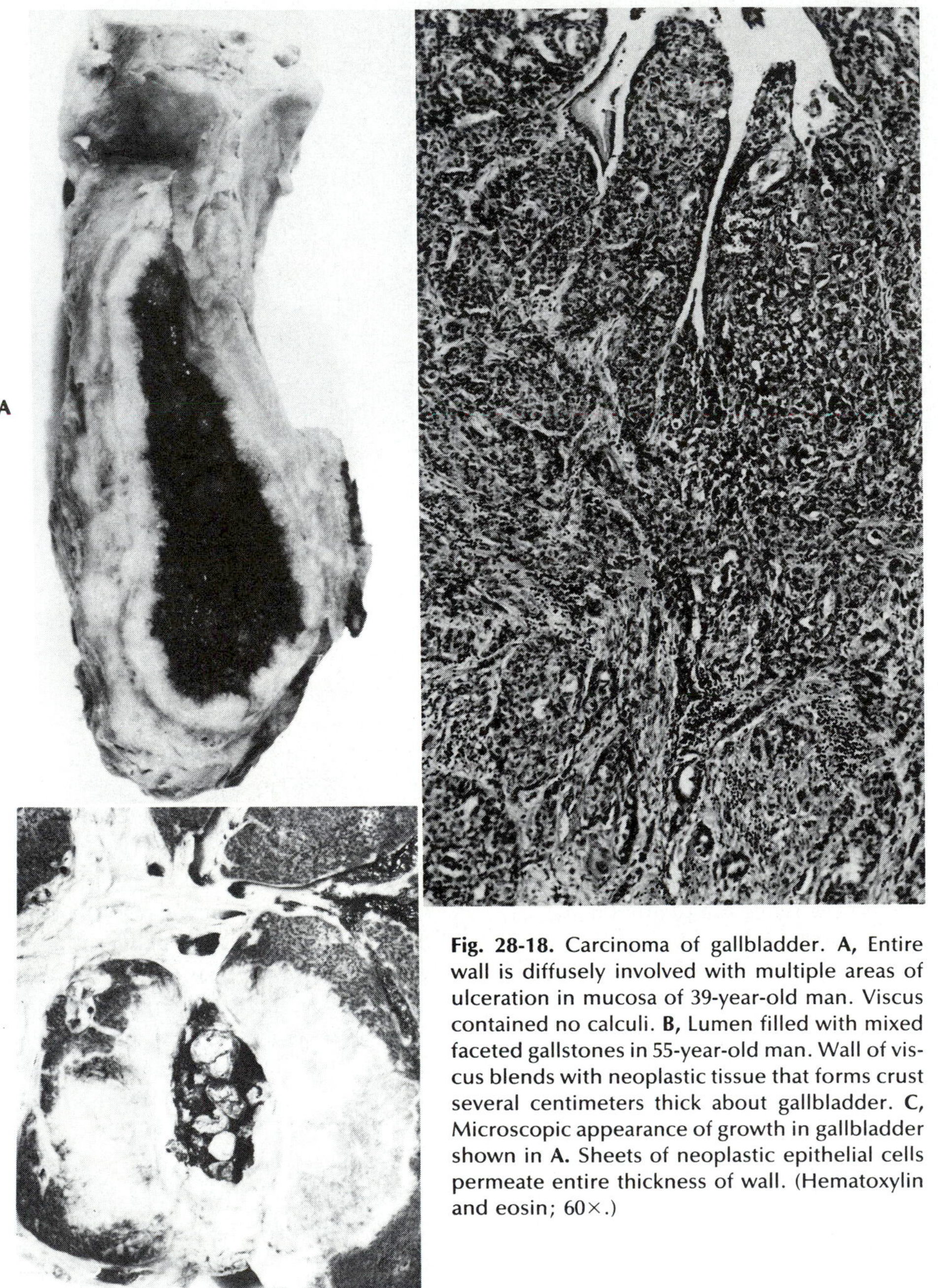

Fig. 28-18. Carcinoma of gallbladder. **A,** Entire wall is diffusely involved with multiple areas of ulceration in mucosa of 39-year-old man. Viscus contained no calculi. **B,** Lumen filled with mixed faceted gallstones in 55-year-old man. Wall of viscus blends with neoplastic tissue that forms crust several centimeters thick about gallbladder. **C,** Microscopic appearance of growth in gallbladder shown in **A.** Sheets of neoplastic epithelial cells permeate entire thickness of wall. (Hematoxylin and eosin; 60×.)

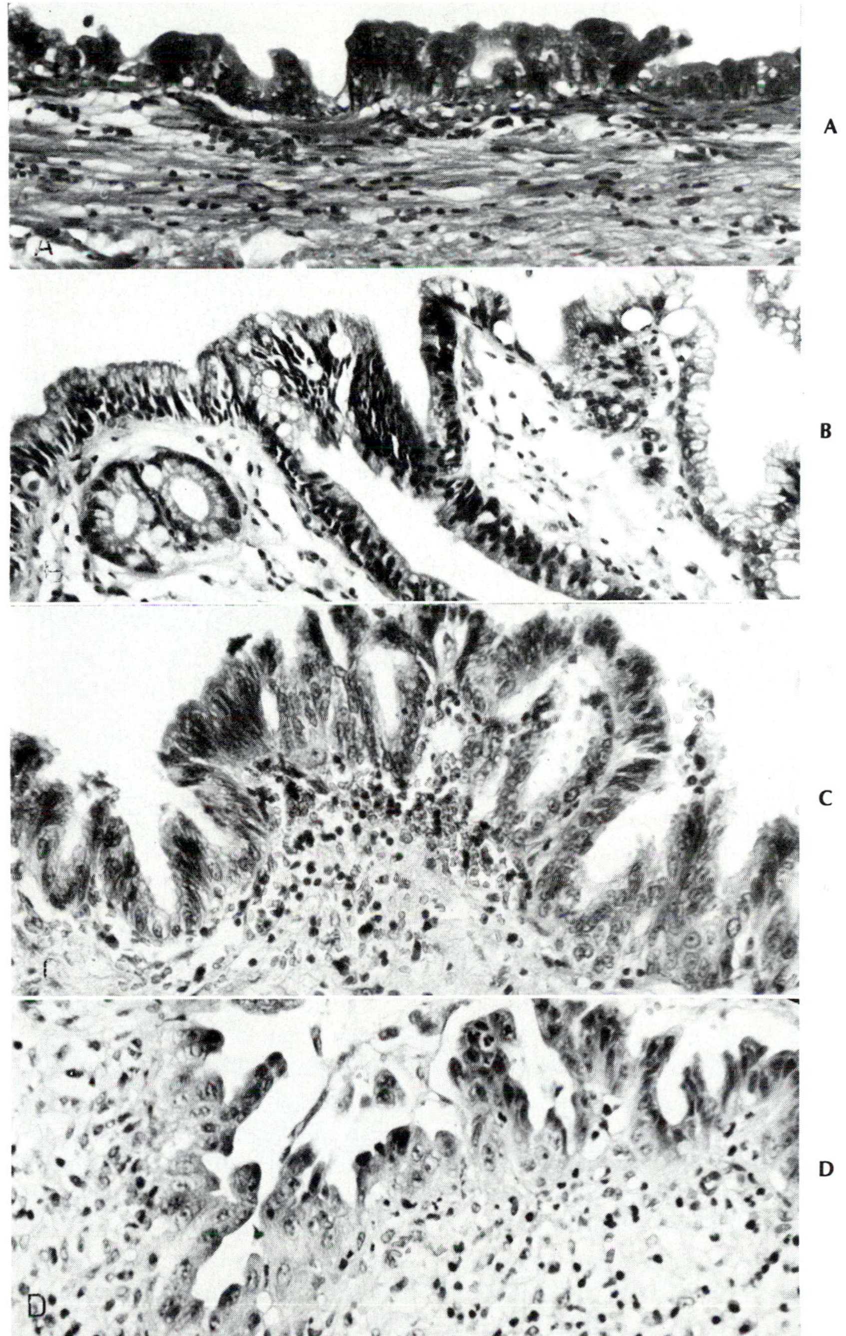

Fig. 28-19. A, Carcinoma in situ. Entire gallbladder wall was replaced by dense fibrous connective tissue, with no penetration of wall by cytologically malignant epithelium visible only on mucosal surface. Patient was free of disease at 4 years, one of the few survivors. **B,** Atypical hyperplasia indicated by variable enlargement of nuclei and crowding as seen especially in center of field. On right side is more normal epithelium for contrast. **C** and **D,** Similar microscopic changes in gallbladder mucosa at some distance from invasive adenocarcinomas. (Hematoxylin and eosin; 350×; courtesy Dr. William Black, University of New Mexico, Albuquerque; **C,** WU 81-10009; **D,** WU 81-10010.)

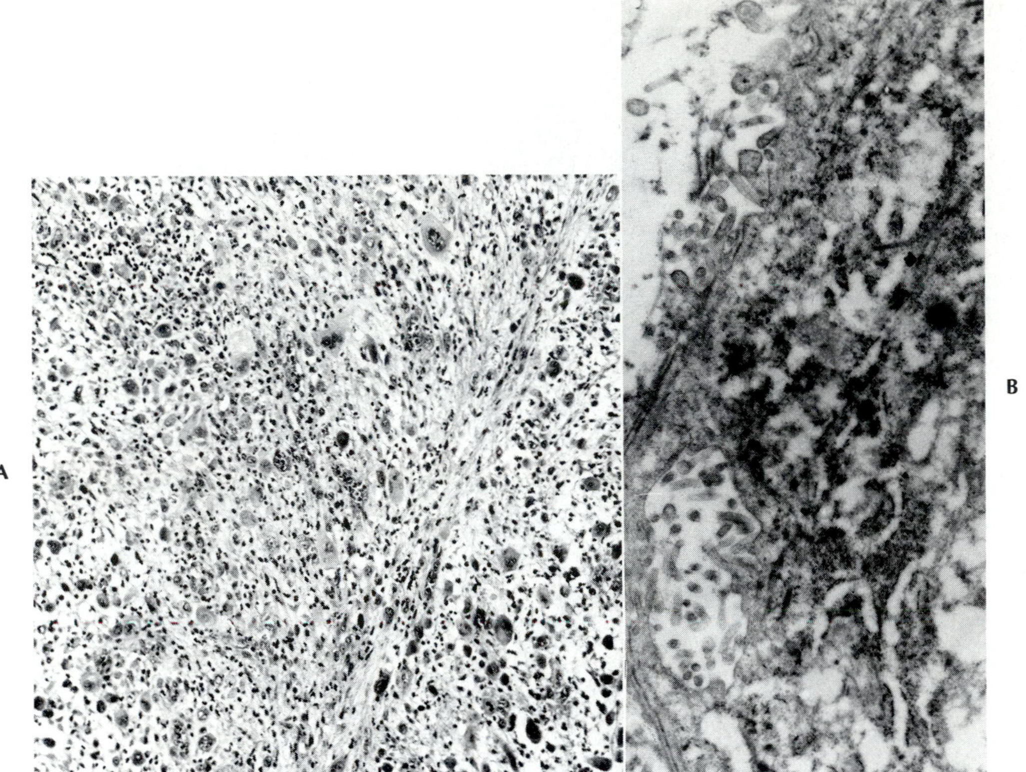

Fig. 28-20. A, Light micrograph of pseudosarcoma of gallbladder. Tumor cells grow without apparent cohesion, and multinucleated pleomorphic giant cells are numerous. **B,** By electron microscopy, however, intracellular lumina were present in tumor cells. Material was rescued from paraffin blocks. (**A,** Hematoxylin and eosin; 150×; WU 81-7976; **B,** uranyl acetate and lead citrate; 35,500×.)

nature of suspicious lesions. Radiotherapy has recently been used in addition to surgery, with better results in bile duct carcinoma than in gallbladder carcinoma.[74]

Since depth of tumor invasion is the determining factor in survival, efforts should be directed toward early detection in populations at risk. Cytologic examination of specimens obtained at ERCP may prove to be one such method in the future. A cell line from a human gallbladder carcinoma has now been established and characterized. In vitro approaches may prove useful in learning more about the biologic behavior of the tumor, with possible therapeutic implications.[64]

In the patient population in which gallbladder malignancy usually occurs, totally anaplastic carcinomas are rare and include giant cell and spindle cell variants, which simulate sarcomas.[47,49] By electron microscopy, a pleomorphic, spindle cell tumor of the gallbladder showed intracytoplasmic lumina with well-formed microvilli (Fig. 28-20). Pure sarcomas have been reported in the literature, without ultrastructural proof of their nonepithelial derivation.[71,78] Many probably also represent carcinomas with a pseudosarcomatous pattern.

Embryonal rhabdomyosarcoma of the biliary tract is rare,[57] but is the most common malignancy of extrahepatic ducts in children. There is a slight female preponderance, and the mean age at diagnosis is between 3 and 4 years. Fever, malaise, and obstructive jaundice are the major symptoms. There is marked dilatation of the common duct. Grossly the tumor is polypoid, and multiple mucoid glistening masses are attached to the mucosa. It has a deceptively benign soft polypoid appearance. Microscopically, loose myxoid tissue contains spindle-shaped tumor cells that are condensed beneath an intact ductal epithelium (Fig. 28-21). Some of these cases, when no ultrastructural studies are done, may well represent pleomorphic carcinomas as well (see preceding discussion). The prognosis is dismal because of local failure to control the disease.

Primary malignant melanomas have been documented, but metastatic melanomas are more common.[66] Metastatic involvement of the gallbladder in melanoma is rare but constitutes the most common metastatic lesion involving this organ.

Carcinoid tumors of the gallbladder have been reported.[51,73] About half were metastatic at the time of diagnosis. Some of these malignant endocrine tumors produce "ectopic" hormones,[75] whereas others are detected because of the obstructive picture they produce.[61]

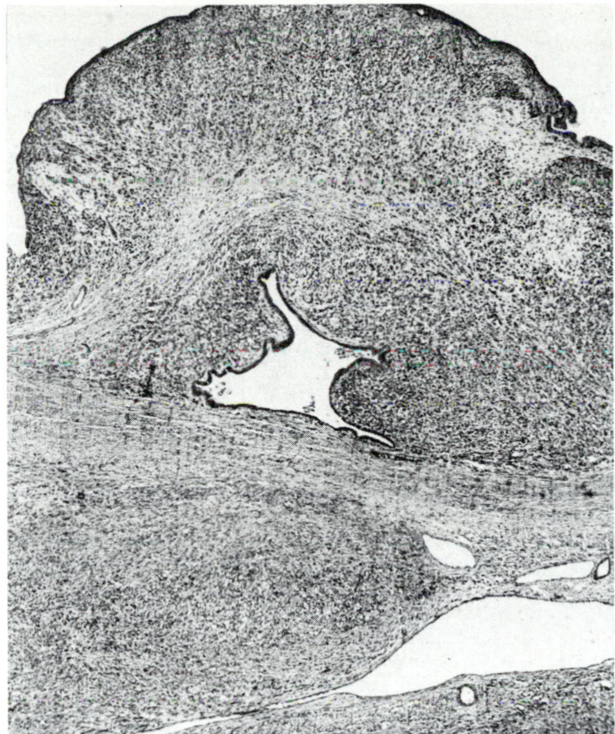

Fig. 28-21. Embryonal rhabdomyosarcoma of extrahepatic duct in child. There is condensation of spindle-shaped tumor cells under intact glandular and surface epithelium. (Hematoxylin and eosin; 33×; WU 81-10002; courtesy Dr. K.G. Ishak, Department of Hepatic Pathology, Armed Forces Institute of Pathology, Washington, D.C.)

REFERENCES

Normal morphology and brief overview of function

1. Ryan, J., and Cohen S.: Effect of vasoactive intestinal peptide on basal and cholecystokinin-induced gallbladder pressure, Gastroenterology **73**:870, 1977.
2. Sundler, F., et al.: VIP innervation of the gallbladder, Gastroenterology **72**:1375, 1977.

Abnormalities thought to be congenital or developmental

3. Busuttil, A.: Ectopic adrenal within the gallbladder wall, J. Pathol. **113**:231, 1974.
4. Christensen, A.H., and Ishak, K.G.: Benign tumors and pseudo tumors of the gallbladder: report of 180 cases, Arch. Pathol. **90**:423, 1970.
5. Curtis, L.E., and Sheahan, D.G.: Heterotopic tissues in the gallbladder, Arch. Pathol. **88**:677, 1969.
6. Gerwig, W.H., Jr., Countryman, L.K., and Gomez, A.C.: Congenital absence of the gallbladder and cystic duct: report of six cases, Ann. Surg. **153**:113, 1961.
7. Laitio, M.: Morphology and histochemistry of non-tumorous gallbladder epithelium: a series of 103 cases, Pathol. Res. Pract. **167**:335, 1980.
8. Landing, B.H.: Considerations of the pathogenesis of neonatal hepatitis, biliary atresia and choledochal cyst—the concept of infantile obstructive cholangiopathy, Prog. Pediatr. Surg. **6**:113, 1974.
9. Thorsness, E.T.: An aberrant pancreatic nodule arising on the neck of a human gallbladder from multiple outgrowths of the mucosa, Anat. Rec. **77**:319, 1940.

Acquired disorders

Lithiasis

10. Braverman, D.Z., Johnson, M.L., and Kern, F., Jr.: Effects of pregnancy and contraceptive steroids on gallbladder function, N. Engl. J. Med. **302**:362, 1980.
11. Coronary Drug Project Research Group: Gallbladder disease as a side effect of drugs influencing lipid metabolism, N. Engl. J. Med. **296**:1185, 1977.
12. Friedman, G.D., Kannel, W.B., and Dawber, T.R.: The epidemiology of gallbladder diseases: observations in the Framingham Study, J. Chron. Dis. **19**:273, 1966.
13. Glenn, F.: Retained calculi within the biliary ductal system, Ann. Surg. **179**:528, 1974.
14. LaMorte, W.W., et al.: The role of the gallbladder in the pathogenesis of cholesterol gallstones, Gastroenterology **77**:580, 1979.
15. Lee, S.P., Carey, M.C., and LaMont, J.T.: Aspirin prevention of cholesterol gallstone formation in prairie dogs, Science **211**:1429, 1981.
16. Lund, J.: Surgical indication in cholelithiasis: prophylactic cholecystectomy elucidated on the basis of long-term follow up on 526 nonoperated cases, Ann. Surg. **151**:153, 1960.
17. Marks, J.W., et al.: Gallstone prevalence and biliary lipid composition in inflammatory bowel disease, J. Dig. Dis. **22**:1097, 1977.
18. Morris, D.L., et al.: Gallbladder disease and gallbladder cancer among American Indians in tricultural New Mexico, Cancer **42**:2472, 1978.
19. Perpetuo, M.D.C.M.O., et al.: Natural history study of gallbladder cancer: a review of 36 years experience at M.D. Anderson Hospital and Tumor Institute, Cancer **42**:330, 1978.
20. Shrand, H., and Ackroyd, F.W.: Gallstones in children: case report, diagnostic clues and recent views on gallstone formation, Clin. Pediatr. **12**:191, 1973.
21. Simeone, J.F., and Ferrucci, J.T., Jr.: New trends in gallbladder imaging, J.A.M.A. **246**:380, 1981.
22. Wenckert, A., and Robertson, B.: The natural course of gallstone disease: eleven-year review of 781 nonoperated cases, Gastroenterology **50**:376, 1966.
23. Wilson, I.D., et al.: Choledocholithiasis, Gastroenterology **75**:120, 1978.

Inflammation—acute

24. Barton, L.L., et al.: Leptospirosis with acalculous cholecystitis, Am. J. Dis. Child. **126**:350, 1973.
25. Bohrod, M.G., and Bodon, G.R.: Isolated polyarteritis nodosa of the gallbladder, Am. Surg. **36**:681, 1970.
26. Campbell, C.W., and Eckman, M.R.: Acute acalculous cholecystitis caused by *Salmonella indiana*, J.A.M.A. **233**:815, 1975.
27. Dillard, B.M., and Black, W.C.: Polyarteritis nodosa of the gallbladder and bile ducts, Am. Surg. **36**:423, 1970.
28. Ishak, K.G., and Rogers, W.A.: Cryptogenic acute cholangitis—association with toxic shock syndrome, Am. J. Clin. Pathol. **76**:619, 1981.
29. LiVolsi, V.A., Perzin, K.H., and Porter, M.: Polyarteritis nodosa of the gallbladder, presenting as acute cholecystitis, Gastroenterology **65**:115, 1973.
30. Porter, J.B., Jick, H., and Dinan, B.J.: Acute cholecystitis and thiazides, N. Engl. J. Med. **304**:954, 1981.

Inflammation—chronic

31. Amazon, K., and Rywlin, A.M.: Ceroid granulomas of the gallbladder, Am. J. Clin. Pathol. 73:123, 1980.
32. Chapman, R.W.G., et al.: Primary sclerosing cholangitis: a review of its clinical features, cholangiography, and hepatic histology, Gut **21**:870, 1980.
33. Estrada, R.L., Brown, N.M., and James, C.E.: Chronic follicular cholecystitis: radiological, pathological and surgical aspects, Br. J. Surg. **48**:205, 1958.
34. Fee, H.J., et al.: Sclerosing cholangitis and primary biliary cirrhosis—a disease spectrum? Ann. Surg. **186**:589, 1977.
35. Halpert, B.: Morphologic studies on the gallbladder. II. The "true Luschka ducts" and "Rokitansky-Aschoff sinuses" of human gallbladder, Bull. Johns Hopkins Hosp. **41**:77, 1927.

36. Renner, I.G., et al.: Idiopathic retroperitoneal fibrosis producing common bile duct and pancreatic duct obstruction, Gastroenterology **79**:348, 1980.
37. Thorpe, M.E.C., Scheuer, E.P.J., and Sherlock, S.: Primary sclerosing cholangitis, the biliary tree, and ulcerative colitis, Gut **8**:435, 1967.

Miscellaneous noninflammatory conditions

38. Chamberlain, J.W., and Flight, D.W.: Acute hydrops of the gallbladder in childhood, Surgery **68**:899, 1970.
39. Prévot, J., and Babut, J.M.: Spontaneous perforations of the biliary tract in infancy, Prog. Pediatr. Surg. **1**:187, 1970.

Tumors

Benign neoplasms and pseudotumors

40. Beilby, J.O.: Diverticulosis of the gall bladder: the fundal adenoma, Br. J. Exp. Pathol. **48**:455, 1967.
41. Carney, J.A., et al.: Alimentary-tract ganglioneuromatosis: a major component of the syndrome of multiple endocrine neoplasia, type 2b, N. Engl. J. Med. **295**:1287, 1976.
42. Evagulis, J.E., et al.: Granular cell myoblastoma: a cause of biliary obstruction, Am. J. Dis. Child. **132**:68, 1978.
43. Jones, M.B., et al.: Multifocal eosinophilic granuloma involving the common bile duct: histologic and cholangiographic findings, Gastroenterology **80**:384, 1981.
44. Ishak, K.G., et al.: Biliary cystadenoma and cystadenocarcinoma: report of 14 cases and review of the literature, Cancer **38**:322, 1977.
45. Miller, T.A., Weber, T.R., and Appelman, H.D.: Paraganglioma of the gallbladder, Arch. Surg. **105**:637, 1972.
46. Waddell, W.R., et al.: Production of human nerve-growth factor in a patient with a liposarcoma, Lancet **1**:1365, 1972.

Malignant tumors

47. Albores-Saavedra, J., et al.: Unusual types of gallbladder carcinoma: a report of 16 cases, Arch. Pathol. Lab. Med. **105**:287, 1981.
48. Albores-Saavedra, J., et al.: The precursor lesions of invasive gallbladder carcinoma: hyperplasia, atypical hyperplasia and carcinoma in situ, Cancer **45**:919, 1980.
49. Appelman, H.D., and Coopersmith, N.: Pleomorphic spindle-cell carcinoma of the gallbladder, Cancer **23**:535, 1969.
50. Arminski, T.C.: Primary carcinoma of the gallbladder: a collective review with the addition of twenty-five cases from the Grace Hospital, Detroit, Michigan, Cancer **2**:379, 1949.
51. Bergdahl, L.: Carcinoid tumours of the biliary tract, Aust. N.Z. J. Surg. **46**:136, 1976.
52. Bergdahl, L.: Gallbladder carcinoma first diagnosed at microscopic examination of gallbladders removed for presumed benign disease, Ann. Surg. **191**:19, 1980.
53. Bismuth, H., and Malt, R.A.: Current concepts in cancer: carcinoma of the biliary tract, N. Engl. J. Med. **301**:704, 1979.
54. Black, W.C.: The morphogenesis of gall bladder carcinoma, Prog. Surg. Pathol. **2**:207, 1981.
55. Black, W.C., et al.: Carcinoma of the gallbladder in a population of Southwestern American Indians, Cancer **39**:1267, 1977.
56. Converse, C.F., Reagan, J.W., and DeCosse, J.J.: Ulcerative colitis and carcinoma of the bile ducts, Am. J. Surg. **121**:39, 1971.
57. Davis, G.L., Kissane, J.M., and Ishak, K.G.: Embryonal rhabdomyosarcoma (sarcoma botryoides) of the biliary tree: report of five cases and review of the literature, Cancer **24**:333, 1969.
58. Devor, E.J., and Buechley, R.W.: Gallbladder cancer in Hispanic New Mexicans. I. General population, 1957-1977, Cancer **45**:1705, 1980.
58a. Diehl, A.K., and Beral, V.: cholecystectomy and changing mortality from gallbladder cancer, Lancet **2**:187, 1981.
59. Fahim, R.B., et al.: Carcinoma of the gallbladder: a study of its modes of spread, Ann. Surg. **156**:114, 1962.
60. Hill, G.L., Mair, W.S.J., and Goligher, J.C.: Gallstones after ileostomy and ileal resection, Gut **16**:932, 1975.
61. Judge, D.M., Dickman, P.S., and Trapudki, B.S.: Nonfunctioning argyrophilic tumor (APUDOMA) of the hepatic duct: simplified methods of detecting biogenic amines arising in tissue, Am. J. Clin. Pathol. **66**:40, 1976.
62. Kagawa, Y., et al.: Carcinoma arising in a congenitally dilated biliary tract: report of a case and review of the literature, Gastroenterology **74**:1286, 1978.
63. Klatskin, G.: Adenocarcinoma of the hepatic duct at its bifurcation within the porta hepatis: an unusual tumor with distinctive clinical and pathological features, Am. J. Med. **38**:241, 1965.
64. Koyama, S., et al.: Establishment of a cell line (G-415) from a human gallbladder carcinoma, Gan **71**:574, 1980.
65. Mancuso, T.F., and Brennan, M.J.: Epidemiological considerations of cancer of the gallbladder, bile ducts and salivary glands in the rubber industry, J.Occupational Med. **12**:333, 1970.
66. McFadden, P.M., et al.: Metastatic melanoma of the gallbladder, Cancer **44**:1802, 1979.
67. Morowitz, D.A., et al.: Carcinoma of the biliary tract complicating chronic ulcerative colitis, Cancer **27**:356, 1971.
68. Nevin, J.E., et al.: Carcinoma of the gallbladder, Cancer **37**:141, 1976.
69. Piehler, J.M., and Greichlow, R.W.: Primary carcinoma of the gallbladder, Surg. Gynecol. Obstet. **147**:929, 1978.
70. Polk, H.C.: Carcinoma of the calcified gallbladder, Gastroenterology **50**:582, 1966.
71. Rose, A.G.: Primary sarcoma of the gallbladder: a case report, S. Afr. Med. J. **53**:909, 1978.
72. Russell, P.W., and Brown, C.H.: Primary carcinoma of the gallbladder, Ann. Surg. **132**:121, 1950.
73. Shiffman, M.A., and Juler, G.: Carcinoid of the biliary tract, Arch. Surg. **89**:113, 1964.
74. Smoron, G.L.: Radiation therapy of carcinoma of gallbladder and biliary tract, Cancer **40**:1422, 1977.
75. Spence, R.W., and Burns-Cox, C.J.: ACTH-secreting "apudoma" of gall-bladder, Gut **16**:473, 1975.
76. Stewart, H.L., Loeber, M.M., and Morgan, D.R.: Carcinoma of the extrahepatic bile ducts, Arch. Surg. **41**:662, 1940.
77. Thorbjarnarson, B., and Glenn, F.: Carcinoma of the gallbladder, Cancer **12**:1009, 1959.
78. Yasuma, T., and Yanaka, M.: Primary sarcoma of the gallbladder: report of three cases, Acta Pathol. Jpn. **21**:285, 1971.

CHAPTER 29 Pancreas and Diabetes Mellitus

JOHN M. KISSANE
PAUL E. LACY

NORMAL FORM AND DEVELOPMENT

The human pancreas is an elongated gland that extends from the concavity of the duodenal loop obliquely cephalad and to the left in the retroperitoneal space at the level of the junction between the first and second lumbar vertebrae, toward the hilum of the spleen. The adult gland is 12 to 15 cm long and weighs 60 to 100 g. The pancreas is subdivided into three topographic parts: (1) the head, dorsoventrally flattened, lying in the concavity of the duodenum with the uncinate (hooklike) process projecting ventromedially from the head of the pancreas to encompass the superior mesenteric artery and vein; (2) the body, the main portion of the gland; and (3) the thin, tapered tail extending toward the hilum of the spleen.

The pancreas is subdivided into rhomboid lobules by delicate connective tissue septa in which are found blood and lymphatic vessels, nerves, and ducts. The acini within the lobules are formed by pyramid-shaped acinar cells that contain numerous zymogen granules at their apices. Enzymes such as chymotrypsin, carboxypeptidase, and elastase have been demonstrated within individual zymogen granules by the fluorescent antibody technique. The basal portions of the acinar cells are basophilic and free of zymogen granules. Acini are intimately related to minute centroacinar ducts into which secretion products are discharged. Centroacinar ducts converge to form lobular ducts, which enter the major named pancreatic ducts. Islets possess no ductal system but release their secretory products—insulin, glucagon, gastrin, and perhaps others—directly into the circulation.

Ultrastructurally, zymogen granules appear as dense spherical structures encased within smooth membranous sacs. The basal portions of acinar cells are filled with a lamellar type of ergastoplasm with numerous ribonucleoprotein granules attached to the membranes. The ergastoplasm is responsible for the basophilic reaction of these cells. Electron microscopic and biochemical studies indicate that the zymogen granules are formed within the ergastoplasmic sacs, are subsequently transmitted to the Golgi zone where they apparently undergo further maturation, and finally move to the apical portion of the cell. After stimulation the zymogen granules with their encompassing sacs move to the apical surface of the cell; the membranous sacs fuse with the plasma membrane and rupture, and the zymogen granules are liberated into the lumina of the acini. The acinar and ductal cells are firmly attached by distinct desmosomes that prevent the enzymes within the zymogen granules from passing into the interstitial tissue. The precise intracellular metabolic changes that initiate the migration and liberation of the zymogen granules are unknown.

Development. Among the several segmental diverticula of the foregut that appear in 3 to 4 mm embryos, two persist and give rise to the definitive pancreas. The larger dorsal pancreatic diverticulum arises from the foregut just cephalad to the hepatic diverticulum and elongates to the left in the retroperitoneal space. The smaller ventral pancreatic diverticulum arises in the angle between the hepatic diverticulum and foregut and, after more rapid growth of the hepatic diverticulum, comes to arise from that structure. Differential growth rotates the developing duodenum to the right and shifts the ventral pancreatic anlage into the dorsal mesentery, where it fuses with the dorsal anlage and contributes the uncinate process and most of the head to the definitive organ.

Each pancreatic anlage possesses an axial duct. The distal end of the duct of the ventral pancreas ordinarily anastomoses with the duct of the dorsal pancreas and, as the duct of Wirsung, provides the major drainage for pancreatic secretions into the duodenum at the major duodenal papilla (of Vater). Distal to the point of anastomosis with the duct of Wirsung, the duct of the dorsal pancreas persists in about half of all individuals and, as the duct of Santorini, enters the duodenum at the minor duodenal papilla cephalad to the major papilla. In about 10% of individuals the duct of the ventral pancreas regresses, and the duct of Santorini provides the entire drainage into the duodenum. These relationships are important in the pathogenesis of acute pancreatitis (see p. 1237).

Pancreatic acini appear initially as buds from the ducts and subsequently differentiate into acinar cells containing zymogen granules. Lumina of the acini retain communication with the centroacinar ducts that converge and form a passageway for exocrine secretions of the pancreas into the duodenum. The islets of Langerhans also develop from the outer surfaces of the ultimate radicles of the pancreatic ducts. Solid masses of islet cells detach from the ducts and are vascularized by capillary sprouts. The first islets to be formed, primary islets, contain specific granules of beta cells as well as of delta cells. Insulin and several pancreatic enzymes have been identified very early in the primordial pancreas of rat embryos.[3] During the last 6 months of embryonic development, the primary islets undergo degeneration and a second generation of islet tissue originates from the ductal cells. Both primary and secondary islets arise from ductal tissue, not from acinar cells.

ABNORMALITIES OF FORM AND DEVELOPMENT

Annular pancreas

Annular pancreas results from failure of rotation of the ventral pancreas. When the ventral pancreas fuses with the dorsal, it forms a ring of pancreatic tissue that envelops the second portion of the duodenum. Usually the encirclement is complete, but occasionally a gap may be found anteriorly. In children an annular pancreas may be associated with atresia or stenosis of the duodenum that results in intestinal obstruction.[7] In adults an annular pancreas usually produces no symptoms, although in some instances duodenal obstruction, peptic ulceration, and pancreatitis may be present. The relationship of annular pancreas to these symptoms is not clearly understood.

Ectopic pancreas

Pancreatic tissue may be found in the gastrointestinal tract in loci other than its normal anatomic area. The most common locations of ectopic pancreas are the duodenum, stomach, jejunum, and Meckel's diverticulum. Usually, nodules of ectopic pancreatic tissue are small, less than 1 cm in diameter, and are located in the submucosa as circumscribed, mobile masses of firm yellow-white lobular tissue superficially suggesting a neoplasm. Microscopically the masses consist of normal-appearing pancreatic tissue, often including islets of Langerhans. Usually pancreatic heterotopias are asymptomatic. Rarely such masses may produce pyloric or duodenal obstruction, lead to an intussusception, ulcerate and bleed, or serve as the site for an ectopic islet cell neoplasm.

Cystic fibrosis

Cystic fibrosis (fibrocystic disease) of the pancreas is a hereditary disorder characterized by increased viscosity of mucous secretions, including those of the pancreas, intestinal glands, tracheal and bronchial glands, and mucous salivary glands, and by increased concentrations of electrolytes, especially sodium and chloride, in secretions of other glands, notably eccrine sweat glands and also parotid salivary glands. The disease is transmitted as a mendelian recessive trait with clinical consequences only in homozygotes. Other genetic mechanisms have been considered.[18]

The frequency of heterozygous carriers in most white populations must range between 2% and 5%. Factors that contribute to maintaining this very high gene frequency despite the virtually lethal aspect of the homozygous state may include an as yet uncharacterized reproductive advantage in heterozygotes. Cystic fibrosis has been referred to as the most common hereditary disease in white populations.[21] The disease is very rare in blacks and almost unknown in Orientals. It is responsible for approximately 5% of all deaths in infants and children who are born alive. Meticulous clinical management has conspicuously improved the prognosis of the disease so that approximately half of affected persons reach adulthood.

The nature of the basic biologic defect in cystic fibrosis is unknown.[19,22] The initially attractive hypothesis that the essential disorder consists of increased viscosity of mucous secretions gave rise to the early designation "mucoviscidosis" but could not be supported when more widespread disturbances, including those of eccrine sweat glands and serous glands such as parotid salivary glands, were discovered. In fact, the disease may represent the final pathophysiologic expression of several different basic abnormalities.

The traditional discussion of the disease among disorders of the pancreas is misleading on at least two counts; first, many organs other than the pancreas are involved, and second, the major clinical manifestations and chief threats to life result from pulmonary, not pancreatic, involvement. Lines of investigation of the basic defect in cystic fibrosis are currently directed in five, not necessarily exclusive, directions.

Biochemical composition of mucous secretions. Although results are not unanimous, the consensus is that mucous secretions of many origins from patients with cystic fibrosis are higher in the ratio of fucose to sialic acid than are secretions of normal individuals. The subject of glycoproteins in cystic fibrosis has been reviewed.[13]

Autonomic function. Many of the deviations from normal in the eccrine secretions of patients with cystic fibrosis resemble those that result from exhaustive parasympathetic stimulation of normal secretory mechanisms. Such nonsecretory autonomic mechanisms as the speed of pupillary mydriasis in the dark appear to be impaired in patients with cystic fibrosis.[35]

Electrolyte-concentrating mechanism. In the normal formation of sweat, a solution with composition essentially that of an ultrafiltrate of plasma accumulates in the coiled portions of eccrine sweat glands. Preferential absorption of sodium chloride in excess of water from the duct results in the excretion of the normally hypotonic sweat. Micropuncture studies[31] suggest that primary secretion in the coil is normal in those with cystic fibrosis and that defective absorption of solute from the duct results in hypertonicity of the sweat. Recently, diminished resorption of sodium and chloride has been demonstrated in rat parotid glands perfused with sweat from patients with cystic fibrosis.[31] Sweat from normal children had no effect on the absorptive mechanism.

Effect on ciliary motility. Asynchronous and uncoordinated ciliary motility has been observed in cultured explants of rat tracheal mucosa exposed to serum from patients with cystic fibrosis. The factor responsible for this disturbance in ciliary motility is heat labile and nondialyzable. Similar effects were produced by sera from some parents of patients with cystic fibrosis.[37]

Metachromasia in cultured fibroblasts. Studies have demonstrated that cultured fibroblasts from patients with cystic fibrosis elaborate metachromatic material either as discrete cytoplasmic granules or as diffuse cytoplasmic metachromasia. Cultured fibroblasts from parents and other relatives of patients showed the same type of metachromasia.[21]

Clinical features

Clinical features of cystic fibrosis are highly variable, even among affected siblings. From 10% to 15% of affected newborns have intestinal, usually distal ileal, obstruction by chalky masses of inspissated intestinal contents, meconium ileus. The frequency of associated ileal atresia supports an acquired mechanism for intestinal atresia. Intestinal perforation in utero with production of sterile meconium peritonitis may occur. Acute or episodic intestinal obstruction beyond infancy is increasingly reported as "meconium ileus equivalent."

Failure to gain weight despite adequate appetite, nonspecific feeding problems, steatorrhea, or other manifestations of intestinal malabsorption characterize one fourth to one third of all patients with cystic fibrosis. Rectal prolapse occurs in as many as one sixth of all patients. Heat prostration may be an early manifestation. In older children, ascites, bleeding from esophageal varices, or unexplained splenomegaly may be the first symptoms of cystic fibrosis.

Beyond infancy, respiratory complications are by far the most common manifestations of cystic fibrosis and comprise its chief threat to life. Recurrent bouts of pneumonia, bronchiolitis, or bronchitis are usual but not invariable manifestations of the disease. Signs and symptoms of chronic respiratory insufficiency or of right ventricular failure occasionally may precede any indication of infection of the lower respiratory tract. The finding of inflammatory nasal polyps in the upper respiratory tract of a prepubertal child compels consideration of the diagnosis of cystic fibrosis.

Pathologic changes

Most pathologic changes in fibrocystic disease are interpretable as resulting from obstruction by abnormally viscid mucus in a variety of viscera.

Pancreas. The pancreas is almost never normal in cystic fibrosis, although the degree of pancreatic involvement varies widely from case to case and correlates only crudely with age. Grossly, especially in infancy, the pancreas may appear deceptively normal (Fig. 29-1). Close examination even then, however, may disclose an almost too tidy demarcation of lobules and an increase in consistency. Later, pancreatic lobules come to assume an ovoid rather than a rhomboid or polyhedral contour and to bulge from the cut surface. Ultimately, the pancreas, still preserving relatively normal size and contour, represents gross fatty replacement of parenchyma. Fibrosis is rarely pronounced grossly, and macroscopic cysts are rarely discernible.

Microscopically, acinar atrophy and interlobular fibrosis are far out of proportion to the gross abnormality. Centroacinar ducts frequently contain laminated, eosinophilic concretions, and distal to these, acini are conspicuously atrophic, although stromal recapitulation of lobular architecture may be well preserved (Fig. 29-2). Islets persist until late in the evolution of the disease. Inflammation, fat necrosis, and pseudocyst formation are rarely prominent.

Intestine. In 12% to 15% of patients with cystic fibrosis, intestinal obstruction occurs in the newborn period. The obstructing lesion in meconium ileus is a plug of chalky, inspissated meconium in the distal ileum. Ileal atresia, volvulus, or perforation with the development of meconium peritonitis may occur secondarily, and total intestinal length usually is shortened. The occurrence of meconium ileus correlates more with dilatation of intestinal glands by inspissated mucous secretions than with the extent of pancreatic lesions.

Attention has been called to the occurrence of peptic ulcers in patients with cystic fibrosis.[16] Above-normal frequency of peptic ulcer in parents of patients with cystic fibrosis has been claimed.

Respiratory tract. In a typical case the lungs show gross compensatory overexpansion anteriorly, alternating posteriorly with areas of atelectasis and overt consolidation. Bronchi are dilated and contain inspissated mucopurulent exudate. Dilated small bronchi containing similar material usually can be appreciated in the centers of consolidated pulmonary lobules. Microscopically the pulmonary lesion is a purulent bronchitis and bronchiolitis with resulting bronchiectasis and bronchiolectasis accompanied by a limited peribronchiolar pneumonia. Parenchymatous purulent necrosis with abscess formation is distinctly unusual (see also p. 863).

Larynx, trachea, and major bronchi show chronic inflammation, often with foci of squamous metaplasia. Submucous glands are distended with inspissated secretions. In the upper respiratory tract, inflammatory nasal polyps may be found.

Liver. The liver is usually of normal size. Significant fatty metamorphosis is not common. Focal stellate areas of portal fibrosis and ductular proliferation may be seen, occasionally sufficiently extensive to justify the designation *focal biliary cirrhosis*. The lesion may produce por-

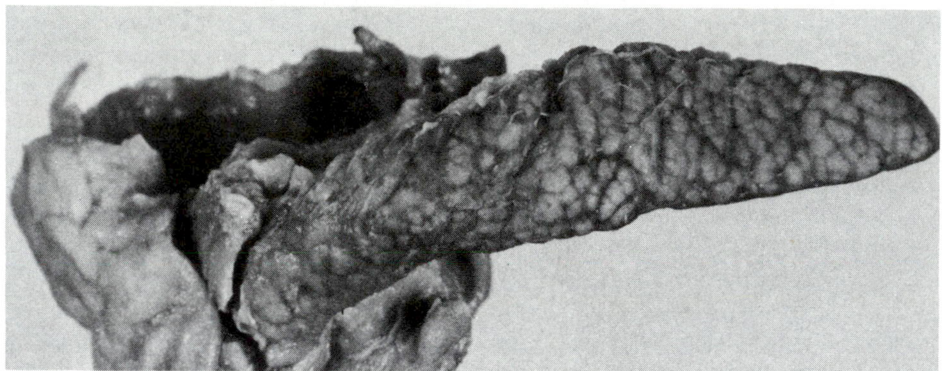

Fig. 29-1. Pancreas from child with cystic fibrosis showing accentuation of lobules but general preservation of size and contour of organ. (From Kissane, J.M., and Smith, M.G.: Pathology of infancy and childhood, ed. 2, St. Louis, 1975, The C.V. Mosby Co.)

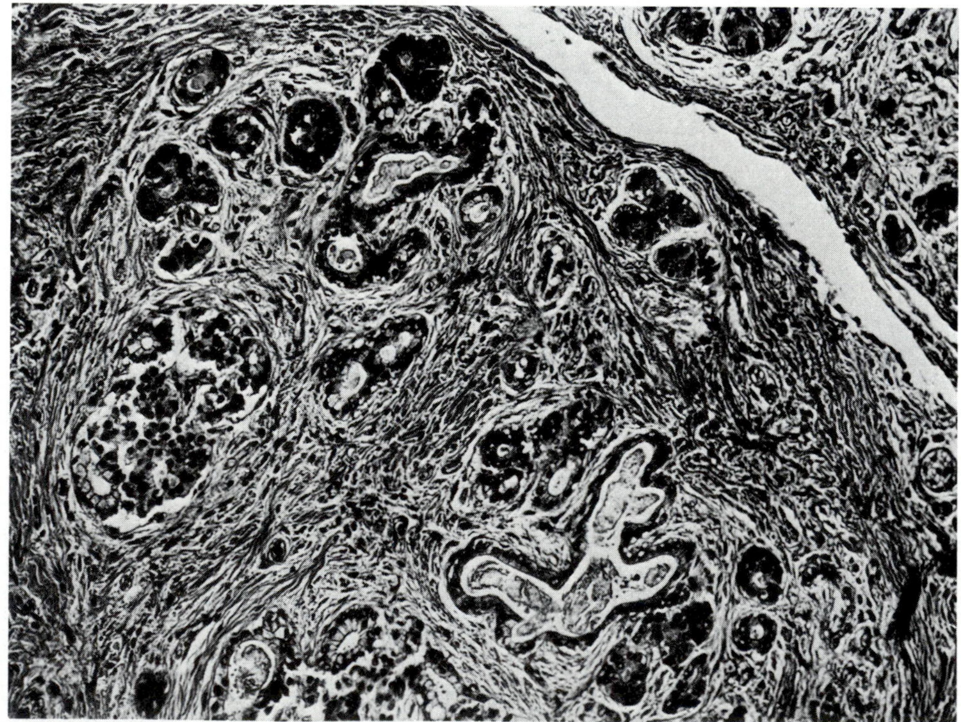

Fig. 29-2. Pancreas in cystic fibrosis showing dilated centrilobular ducts containing laminated concretions. Acini are almost totally replaced by fibrous tissue that still reflects lobular pattern of organ.

tal hypertension with its consequences—ascites, congestive splenomegaly, and gastroesophageal varices (see p. 1237).

Sweat glands. In view of the constancy and diagnostic importance of hypersecretion of sodium and chloride in the sweat, microscopic alterations in sweat glands are disappointingly scanty. Munger and associates[32] described diminished vacuolation of mucoid cells.

Reproductive system. The frequent finding of azoospermia in postpubertal males with cystic fibrosis is attributable to discontinuity of the male sex ducts. Only 1% to 2% of postpubertal males with cystic fibrosis are fertile. There is no anatomic correlate for the high maternal mortality among pregnant women with cystic fibrosis.

PANCREATITIS

Inflammation of the pancreas constitutes a spectrum of disorders that ranges from acute hemorrhagic pancreatitis, a prostrating, catastrophic disease with a high mortality, to chronic relapsing pancreatitis, a disorder characterized by recurring episodes of upper abdominal pain and eventual pancreatic insufficiency. Elaborate clinical systems of classification reflect the tendency of the disorder to recur.

Acute hemorrhagic pancreatitis

Acute hemorrhagic pancreatitis is almost entirely a disease of adults between 40 and 70 years of age, slightly more common in women than in men. The onset is abrupt and calamitous, often occurring after a heavy meal or an alcoholic debauch. Severe epigastric pain, especially radiating to the back; nausea; vomiting; and shock are prominent clinical features. Peculiar ecchymotic mottling of the skin of the flanks, Grey-Turner spots, may be seen in severe cases. Early in the disease, pancreatic enzymes are liberated into the bloodstream, and increased levels of amylase and lipase in the serum are important in establishing the diagnosis. The mortality, even with vigorous supportive measures, is between 15% and 25%.

Pathologic changes

In the first few days the pancreas is swollen and edematous. After 1 or 2 days, friable foci of necrosis appear, followed by interstitial hemorrhage that varies from reddish reticulation between pancreatic lobules to obliteration of grossly recognizable pancreatic tissue in a massive retroperitoneal hematoma. Foci of fat necrosis in the peripancreatic tissue, mesentery, and omentum appear rapidly as small, ovoid, yellow-white nodules of pasty, gritty material (Fig. 29-3). The peritoneal cavity usually contains a moderate effusion of turbid rusty fluid with high amylase activity. Rarely, remote adipose tissues such as subcutaneous fat and fatty marrow may contain foci of necrosis attributable to lipolysis by enzymes borne in the plasma.

Very early in the disease the pancreas microscopically shows only interstitial edema. Later the pancreas contains patches of coagulative necrosis rimmed by infiltrates of polymorphonuclear leukocytes (Fig. 29-4). Still later, necrosis of arteries and arterioles is responsible for gross hemorrhages. Veins often are thrombosed. Eventually, as bacteria lodge in the necrotic pancreas, via

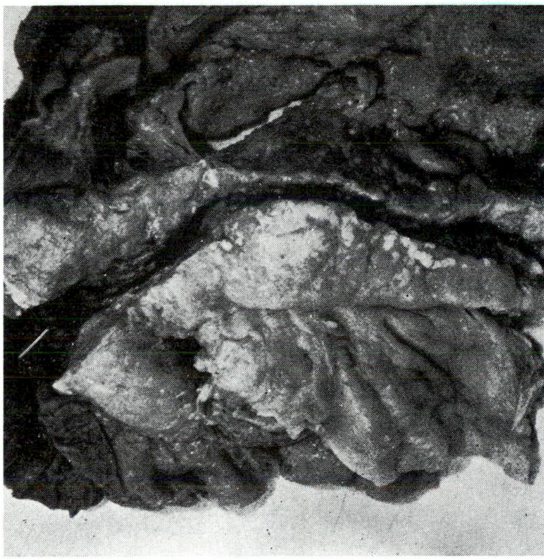

Fig. 29-3. Fat necrosis and acute pancreatitis. White opaque areas represent fat necrosis. Small white rod is in duct opening into duodenum.

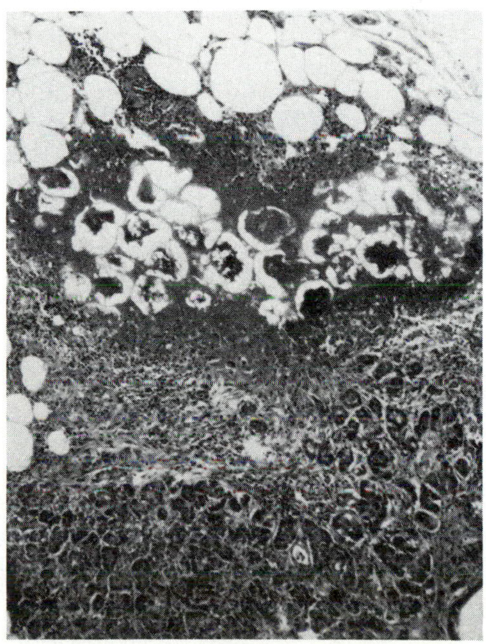

Fig. 29-4. Fat necrosis of pancreas.

either the ducts or the bloodstream, frank suppuration may occur.

A late complication of acute pancreatitis is the occasional development of a pseudocyst—an accumulation of enzyme-rich fluid, necrotic debris, and altered blood confined, not by an epithelial capsule, but by retroperitoneal connective tissue, adherent upper abdominal viscera, and the peritoneal components of the lesser omental sac. Pancreatic pseudocysts also may occur after blunt trauma to the abdomen.

Pathogenesis

The destructive changes that occur in the pancreas can be attributed to activation of proteolytic and lipolytic pancreatic enzymes and their liberation into the pancreatic interstitium. Normally the pancreas is protected from self-destruction by (1) synthesis and secretion of lytic enzymes as initially inactive proenzymes, which themselves require activation, often by trypsin; (2) elaborate compartmentalization of lytic systems within the cytoplasm of the acinar cell; and (3) the presence of trypsin inhibitors in acinar cells. Acinar cell injury by a variety of causes can disturb this relationship. When they gain access to the pancreatic interstitium,[50] active proteolytic enzymes such as trypsin and elastase produce necrosis of blood vessels, with resultant thrombosis and hemorrhage. Lipase liberated into the interstitial tissue causes necrosis of adipose tissue and the breakdown of triglycerides into fatty acids. Fatty acids combine with calcium in the interstitial tissue to form insoluble calcium soaps. This may produce a significant decrease in the level of serum calcium and lead to symptoms of hypocalcemia.

The pathogenesis of this sequence of events is not entirely clear. Experimentally, pancreatitis can be produced by injection of bile into the pancreatic duct at a pressure sufficient to rupture the ductal system. Opie's early report[52] of acute pancreatitis resulting from impaction of a gallstone in the ampulla of Vater directed perhaps undue attention toward the necessity for a "common channel" for biliary and pancreatic secretions to provide anatomically possible regurgitation of bile into the pancreatic duct. Detailed anatomic studies show that the configuration of the pancreatic ducts and common bile duct allows regurgitation of bile into the pancreatic duct in about 90% of specimens.[2]

Even in the presence of an anatomic common channel,

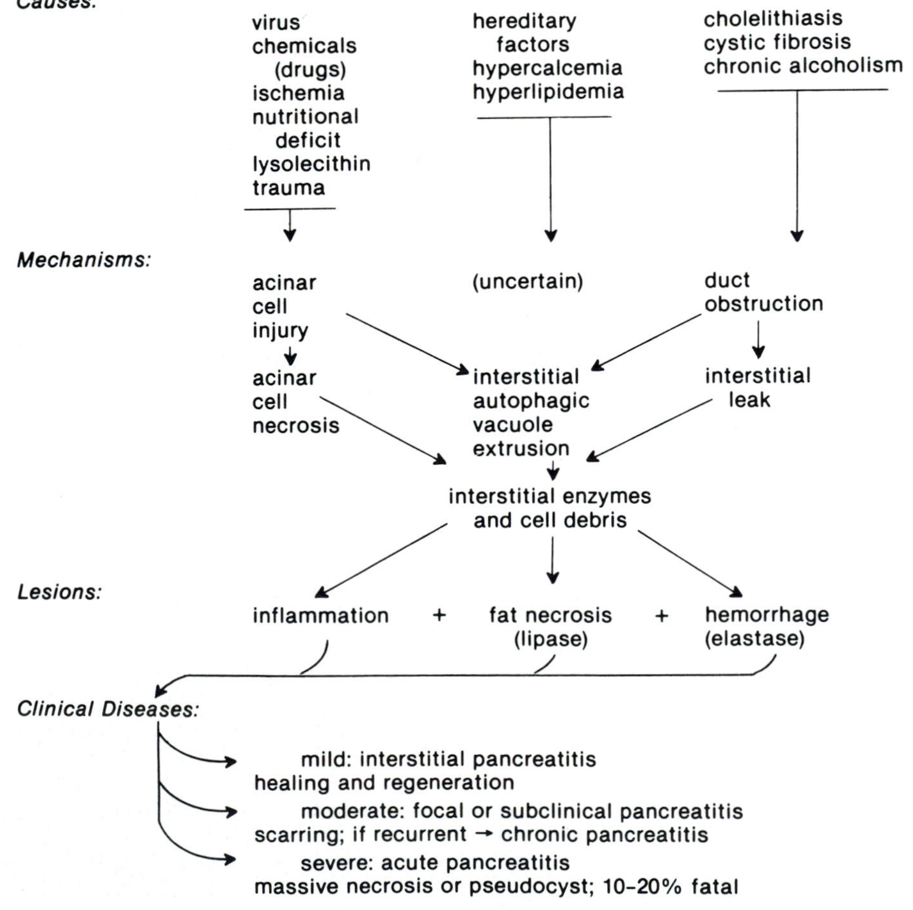

Fig. 29-5. Pathogenic mechanisms in pancreatitis. (From Longnecker, D.S.: Am. J. Pathol. **107**:103, 1982.)

measurements of pressures in the pancreatic duct and in the common bile duct indicate that the higher pressure in the pancreatic duct normally prevents the reflux of bile into the pancreatic duct. Increased intraductal pressure, whether from increased secretory pressure or as a result of duct obstruction, is, along with acinar cell injury, clearly a second general factor in the pathogenesis of pancreatitis. Fig. 29-5 diagrams these relationships.

The frequent association of chronic alcoholism suggests that alcohol functions not only by producing edema and partial obstruction of the sphincter of Oddi but also by stimulating pancreatic secretion. Pancreatic duct obstruction has been attributed to alcoholism.[56,57]

Ischemia has been implicated in the production of hemorrhagic pancreatitis, since it has been demonstrated experimentally that the pancreatic edema that occurs after ligation of the pancreatic duct in dogs can be transformed into acute hemorrhagic pancreatitis by the production of temporary ischemia in the pancreas. This factor alone is apparently not sufficient to produce the sequence of events, since vascular necroses in the pancreas in malignant hypertension are accompanied by only focal areas of necrosis, not a fulminating hemorrhagic pancreatitis.

Trauma also has been implicated as an etiologic factor. Acute pancreatitis is a recognized complication of closed abdominal trauma such as may result from "steering wheel" injuries to the abdomen. Acute pancreatitis also may complicate extensive surgery in the gastroduodenal area. On historical grounds, trauma can be excluded as a pathogenic mechanism in most cases.

Circulating antibodies to pancreatic tissue have been demonstrated in the bloodstream of patients with pancreatitis.[59] It is not clear whether these antibodies have an etiologic role in the production of pancreatitis or are simply immunologic by-products occurring after pancreatic necrosis in response to other factors. Fig. 29-5 summarizes current views as to pathogenic mechanisms.

Chronic pancreatitis

Chronic pancreatitis produces progressive destruction of the pancreas as the result of repeated episodes of necrosis of the parenchyma. Approximately one third of all patients who survive an episode of acute pancreatitis sustain subsequent acute episodes that ultimately progress to chronic pancreatitis. Some patients arrive at the stage of pancreatic insufficiency without sustaining a documented attack of acute pancreatitis. Chronic pancreatitis is a recognized manifestation of hyperparathyroidism and of a hereditary metabolic disorder usually, but not always, accompanied by aminoaciduria. The latter disorder accounts for only a small percentage of cases of chronic pancreatitis. Chronic relapsing pancreatitis occurs most frequently in the fourth or fifth decade. The disease is frequently associated with biliary tract disease or alcoholism.

Pathologic changes in the pancreas depend on the stage of development of the disease. In acute exacerbations, diffuse edema, local areas of necrosis, and peripancreatic inflammation may be present. After the acute attacks the pancreas will be firm and nodular, with areas of dense fibrosis, loss of acinar and islet tissue (Fig. 29-6), calcification in the interstitial tissue and pancreatic ducts, infiltration with plasma cells and lymphocytes, and formation of pseudocysts. The destruction of the pancreas eventually results in exocrine pancreatic insufficiency and, ultimately, diabetes mellitus.

Hereditary pancreatitis is a form of chronic pancreatitis that is transmitted as a mendelian dominant autosomal gene. In contrast to sporadic chronic pancreatitis, hereditary pancreatitis begins in childhood, and there is a relative infrequency of alcoholism and chronic biliary disease.[46]

PANCREATIC LESIONS IN SYSTEMIC DISEASE

Dilatation of acini and ducts of the pancreas occurs in approximately 40% to 50% of patients with uremia. The dilated structures contain eosinophilic inspissated material. In some instances the individual lobules are separated by edematous tissue with a mild infiltrate of neutrophils.

Histologic changes in the acinar cells of the pancreatic

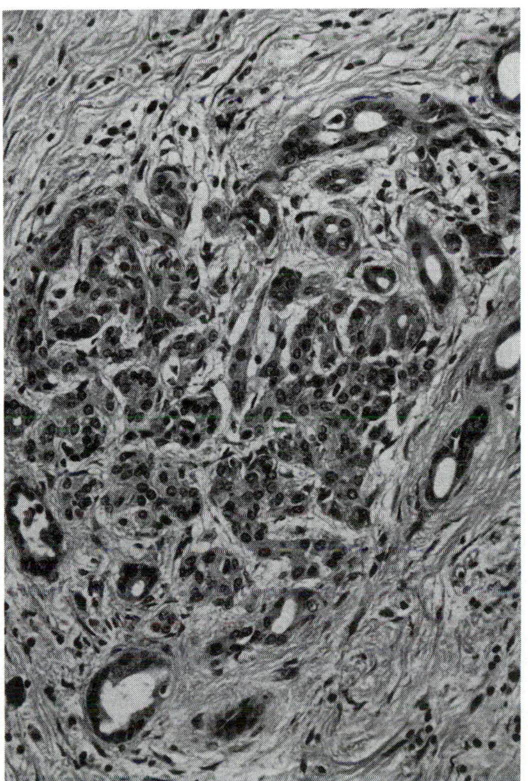

Fig. 29-6. Acinar atrophy occurring after pancreatic duct obstruction.

lobules may be present in chronic congestive heart failure. Peripheral acinar cells in the pancreatic lobules appear atrophic, with diminished zymogen granules and decreased basophils of their cytoplasm, whereas cells adjacent to islets retain their normal appearance. These histologic changes are apparently related to increased venous pressure and vascular stasis within the pancreatic venous circulation.

NEOPLASMS OF EXOCRINE PANCREAS

Cystadenoma

An uncommon but generally well-recognized pancreatic tumor is designated cystadenoma or mucinous cystadenoma. These lesions are more common in women than in men, are more common in the body or tail of the pancreas than in the head, and occur in middle-aged or elderly individuals in whom a detectable mass is usually the only clinical manifestation.

Grossly cystadenomas are bulky neoplasms partially or totally circumscribed by a dense capsule that radiates, centrally compartmentalizing the lesion into locules (Fig. 29-7).

Microscopically, two variants are distinguishable.[63] A microcystic or spongiform type features cuboidal, non-mucin-producing cells with clear cytoplasm lining small cystic spaces. The clear cytoplasm reflects accumulations of glycogen (hence "glycogen-neck cytoadenoma").[68] These lesions appear to be benign. The other variant (macrocystic) features tall, mucin-secreting cells that often fall into multilayered papillary folds about variable, mucin-filled cystic spaces. Distinction between benign and malignant variants may be impossible or even unjustified because metastases may occur many years after recognition of the lesion.[69]

Carcinoma

Carcinoma of the pancreas ranks fourth in frequency among fatal neoplastic diseases in the United States and is responsible for approximately 5% of all deaths caused by cancer. As a cause of death in the United States, carcinoma of the pancreas now exceeds such neoplastic diseases as carcinoma of the stomach, malignant lymphoma of all types, carcinoma of the prostate, and carcinoma of the cervix. Significantly increased risk of carcinoma of the pancreas has been attributed to and associated with disease of the gallbladder and extrahepatic biliary tree, cigarette smoking, consumption of alcoholic beverages, high levels of consumption of animal protein, and high daily average total caloric intake.[90] There is an increased risk of carcinoma of the pancreas among members of the American Chemical Society. Experimental models have been developed in animals.[71,75,85] Carcinoma of the pancreas is extremely rare before 40 years of age. Approximately two thirds of patients are over age 60. An uncommon, sluggishly malignant, histologically characteristic carcinoma of the pancreas has been described in children.[72] Its cell of origin appears to be the acinar cell.

Clinical symptoms of carcinoma of the pancreas depend on the site of the origin of the tumor. If it arises in the head of the pancreas, obstruction of the common bile duct occurs early, producing obstructive jaundice (Fig. 29-8, *A*). Clinical recognition of carcinoma of the body and tail is difficult because of the paucity of distinctive signs and symptoms. Pain is the most common initial symptom of carcinoma of the pancreas, regardless of its location. Symptoms that appear later in the disease include anorexia, weight loss, cachexia, and weakness. The majority of patients with carcinoma of the pancreas

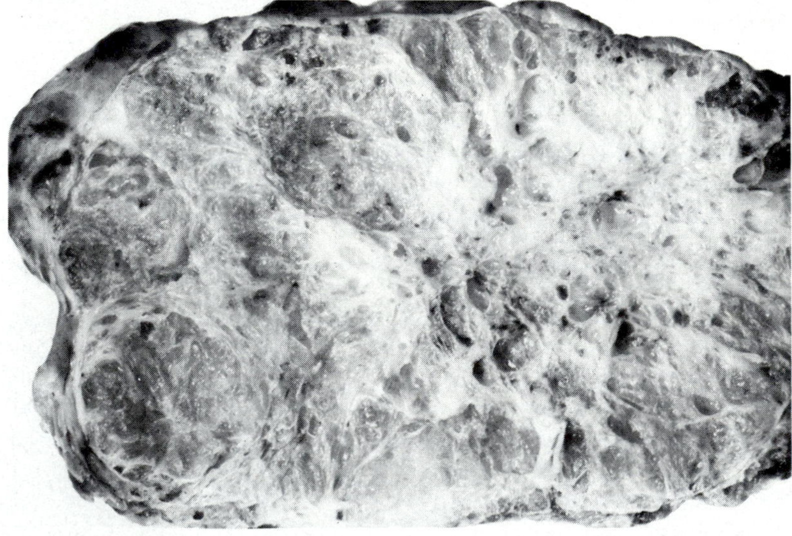

Fig. 29-7. Cystadenoma of pancreas. Coarse porous surface is typical. (From Rosai, J.: Ackerman's surgical pathology, ed. 6, St. Louis, 1981, The C.V. Mosby Co.)

are dead within a year after the onset of symptoms. The very high rate of failure of excisional surgery in the treatment of carcinoma of the pancreas has several possible explanations: initial symptoms are inconspicuous and nonspecific so that early diagnosis is difficult; the organ lies deep in the retroperitoneum intimately related to vital structures so that a conventional radical cancer operation is difficult; and multiple sites of origin within the pancreas have been described.[67]

Approximately one half of all deaths from carcinoma of the pancreas occur within 3 months of the onset of symptoms. Among selected patients with carcinoma of the pancreas who are subjected to radical pancreaticoduodenectomy, some 12% survive longer than 5 years.[88] This figure approaches 40% in cases of (usually well-differentiated) ampullary carcinoma, a lesion that should be distinguished from pancreatic carcinoma.

Approximately 70% of carcinomas of the pancreas occur in the head of the organ. The proximity of the neoplasm to the common bile duct results in neoplastic invasion of the wall of the duct, producing obstruction and dilatation. Obstruction of the common bile duct also occurs in cases of carcinoma of the body and tail of the pancreas. However, this is usually a late complication.

Carcinomas of the body and tail of the pancreas are, on the average, larger than those of the head. Metastases occur most frequently in the regional lymph nodes, liver, lungs, peritoneum, and adrenal glands. The incidence of metastases is higher in cases of carcinoma of the body and tail than that of the head of the pancreas.

A

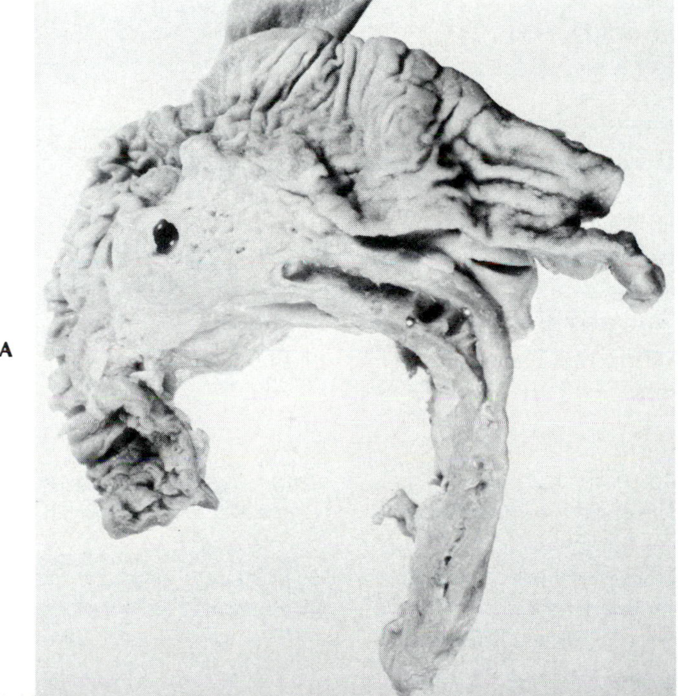

B

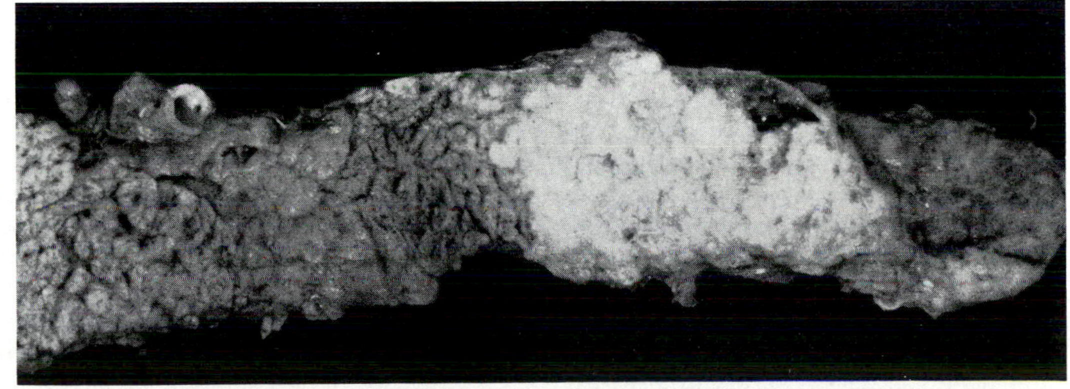

Fig. 29-8. Carcinoma of pancreas. **A,** Lesion of head of pancreas accompanied by atrophy of body and tail and dilatation of pancreatic duct. **B,** Lesion of body and tail of pancreas. (Courtesy Dr. Béla Halpert, Silver Spring, Md.)

Grossly the neoplasm is an ill-defined, firm expansion of a portion of the pancreas, with no sharp line of demarcation between the neoplasm and the surrounding parenchyma (Fig. 29-8).

The following is a classification of epithelial malignancies of the pancreas*:

A. Benign tumors
   1. Adenomas
      a. Clear cell adenoma
      b. Acinar cell adenoma
   2. Dermoid cyst
B. Malignant tumors
   1. Duct (ductular) cell origin
      a. Duct cell adenocarcinoma
      b. Giant cell carcinoma
      c. Giant cell carcinoma (epulis with osteoid)
      d. Adenosquamous carcinoma
      e. Microadenocarcinoma
      f. Mucinous ("colloid") carcinoma
      g. Cystadenocarcinoma
   2. Acinar cell origin
      a. Acinar cell adenocarcinoma
   3. Tumors of the immature pancreas, pancreatoblastomas
      a. Pleomorphic type, acinar differentiation
      b. Solid and papillary type, ductal or ductular differentiation
   4. Mixed type: acinar, duct, and islet-cell carcinoma
   5. Unclassified
      a. Large cell
      b. Small cell
      c. Clear cell

Most carcinomas of the pancreas are moderately well-differentiated adenocarcinomas believed to arise from ductal epithelium (Fig. 29-9). These tumors recapitulate tubular and ductlike structures lined by one or several layers of neoplastic cells supported by dense fibrous stroma (Fig. 29-10, *A*). Although histochemical demonstration of mucin secretion by neoplastic cells can often be demonstrated, conspicuous extracellular production of mucin is uncommon. Occasional carcinomas of the pancreas present a peculiar histologic dimorphism between tubular and ductular structures and a sarcomatous stroma (Fig. 29-10, *B*).[74] The pancreas is one of the more common sites for the occurrence of adenosquamous carcinoma, a carcinoma with both squamous and glandular elements.[66] Pure epidermoid carcinoma occurs. Undifferentiated small cell carcinoma of the pancreas may closely resemble the similar neoplasms of the lung (Fig. 29-10, *C*).[65] Acinar carcinoma is a rare neoplasm that recapitulates the pattern of acini in the normal pancreas. It may contain zymogen granules and manifest local features of lipolytic and proteolytic activity.[61,64] Peculiar giant cell tumors are rare.[87]

A
B

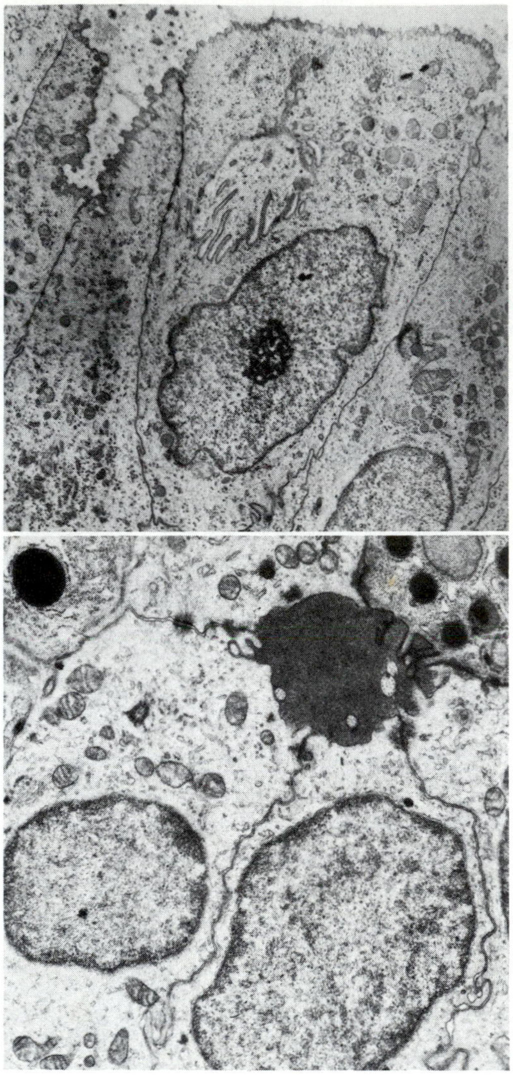

Fig. 29-9. Electron micrograph of pancreatic carcinoma compared with normal pancreatic ductule. **A,** Pancreatic adenocarcinoma. Cytoplasm of cell in center of field is traversed by canaliculus into which microvilli protrude. **B,** Normal pancreas shows a canaliculus with microvilli.

A mixed papillary and solid epithelial neoplasm with a definite predilection for girls and young women has been recognized.[84] Many have been detected incidentally, but these lesions are, at least sluggishly, malignant.

Adenocarcinoma of the pancreas frequently invades the perineural lymphatics (Fig. 29-10, *D*). This invasion of the nerves accounts for the frequency of abdominal pain in these patients. Multiple venous thromboses may be associated with carcinoma of the pancreas and occur more frequently when the neoplasm is in the body or tail of the pancreas. The veins most frequently involved are the iliac and femoral. The mechanism of thrombosis is not clearly defined.

*From Kissane, J.M.: Cancer Treat. Res. 8:99, 1982.

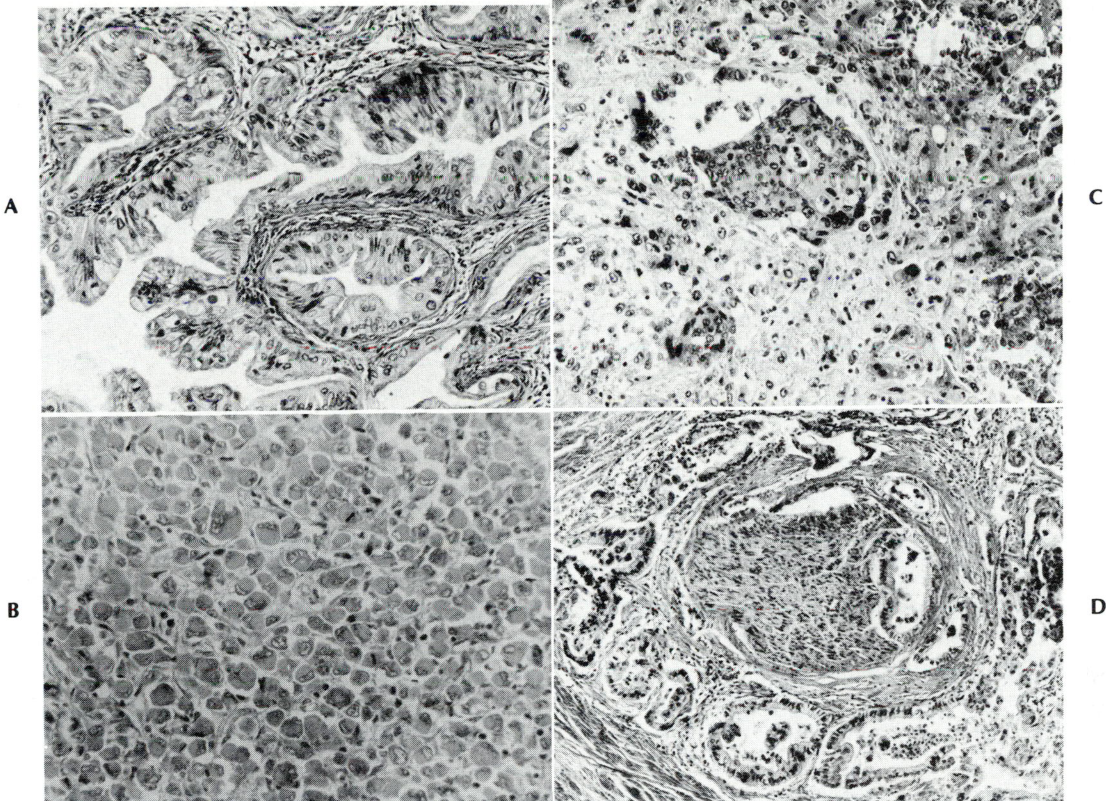

Fig. 29-10. Microscopic features of pancreatic carcinoma. **A,** Well-differentiated papillary adenocarcinoma. **B,** Adenosquamous carcinoma in which areas of epidermoid carcinoma occur in otherwise typical adenocarcinoma. **C,** Pleomorphic carcinoma, an anaplastic carcinoma consisting of large anaplastic cells in no particular architectural pattern. **D,** Invasion of nerve by pancreatic adenocarcinoma, a common microscopic feature.

ENDOCRINE PANCREAS

Diabetes mellitus

Diabetes mellitus is a hereditary disease that affects approximately 2% to 4% of the population of the United States. The discovery of insulin and the use of this hormone in treatment have saved and prolonged the lives of diabetic patients but have not cured the disease. Today the major problems associated with diabetes are the complications that may affect the eye with resultant blindness, the kidney with resultant renal failure, the cardiovascular system with accelerated arteriosclerosis, and the peripheral nervous system with the development of neuropathy.

Clinically the disease has been divided into three categories: juvenile-onset diabetes, maturity-onset diabetes, and maturity-onset diabetes of the young. In juvenile-onset diabetes the disease usually begins abruptly, early in life, with a gradual loss of insulin reserve in the pancreas; thus exogenous insulin is required for therapy. Maturity-onset diabetes occurs in older individuals and has an insidious onset; the insulin reserve in the pancreas may be normal or moderately decreased, and exogenous insulin therapy may not be required. This same type of diabetes with a slow, insidious onset may also occur in children and is called maturity-onset diabetes of the young.

Recently clinicians have recommended classifying diabetes into two types: insulin dependent as type 1 diabetes and noninsulin dependent as type 2 diabetes. Because this new clinical classification adds nothing to our understanding of diabetes, it is preferable to continue the use of the older clinical terms for describing diabetes until it can be reclassified based on specific etiologic factors.

Since diabetes mellitus affects so many different organ systems, it has been extremely difficult to determine the primary abnormality in these patients. Clinical studies indicate that the primary defect is in the B cells of the pancreas. In juvenile-onset diabetes the B cells are acutely and chronically destroyed, whereas in maturity-onset diabetes the B cells have a sluggish response to glucose stimulation.

An important question is whether genetic factors play a role in either the destruction or the alteration in function of B cells. This problem has been approached by long-term clinical studies of identical twins of whom one was diabetic. The surprising finding is that, if one twin had juvenile-onset diabetes, there was a 50% chance that the second twin would develop diabetes. In contrast, there was a 95% chance that the second twin would be diabetic if one of the identical twins had maturity-onset diabetes. These findings indicate that genetic factors play a role in the etiology of maturity-onset diabetes and suggest that environmental or endogenous factors may be responsible for diabetes in juvenile-onset diabetes. This raises the possibility that certain viruses may destroy B cells in the juvenile-onset diabetic.

Experimentally, infection with encephalomyocarditis virus produces destruction of B cells and diabetes in certain strains of mice. Epidemiologic studies in humans have provided suggestive evidence of a greater incidence of coxsackievirus B infection in juvenile diabetics than in controls. Recently a coxsackievirus B-4 was isolated from the pancreas of a diabetic child. The isolated virus caused destruction of B cells in tissue culture, and injection of this virus into a susceptible strain of mice produced diabetes. Since this particular case the infection with coxsackievirus B-4 was overwhelming, it is unknown whether the pancreas was secondarily involved or whether a coxsackievirus plays a primary role in causing destruction of B cells in juvenile-onset diabetics in general.

HLA typing of diabetics has shown that juvenile-onset diabetics have a higher incidence of HLA-B8, -BW15, -DW3, and -DW4 than the normal population. The strongest association occurred with HLA-DW3 and -DW4. Antibodies to islet cells have been demonstrated in approximately 50% of juvenile diabetics during the first 3 years of the disease. It has not been established whether these antibodies are cytotoxic for B cells. These intriguing findings have raised the possibility that the juvenile-onset diabetic may have a genetic susceptibility to an environmental viral or chemical agent that will damage the islet cells, and that autoimmunity may play a role in the continued destruction of B cells. At the present time this concept is purely hypothetical, and much more solid evidence will be needed to either establish or deny the validity of such a theory. In regard to maturity-onset diabetes, the clinical studies on identical twins provide evidence that genetic factors play a primary role in the development of diabetes; however, no genetic marker for diabetes has been identified in these patients.

The elucidation of the specific defect or defects in B cell secretion in diabetics and the possible role of the environment in the development of diabetes mellitus requires an understanding of the normal structure and function of the islet cells and the normal mechanism of insulin secretion. This information will permit a search for defects in the insulin-secretory process of diabetic subjects. While these investigations are in progress, attempts are also being made to replace the defective B cells with normal islet cells by transplantation.

Structure and function of B cells

The islets of Langerhans comprise about 1% to 3% of the weight of the pancreas, and the concentration of islets is greater in the tail than in the head or body of the pancreas. By use of immunohistochemical stains and electron microscopy, the islet cells of the human pancreas can be subclassified into A, B, D, F, and G cells (Fig. 29-11). Each cell type contains a specific hormone: A cell, glucagon; B cell, insulin; D cell, somatostatin; F cell, pancreatic polypeptide; and G cell, gastrin. Islets in the body and tail of the pancreas contain 60% to 70% B cells and 20% to 30% A cells; each of the remaining cell types comprises a small percentage of the islet population. In the head and uncinate process of the human pancreas are found islet cells that are composed of 95% F cells with a few A and D cells. Since somatostatin inhibits both insulin and glucagon secretion, the role of this hormone in the islet is not established. It has been suggested that secretion of somatostatin by the D cell may provide an intra-islet regulatory mechanism for insulin secretion and that this regulatory mechanism may be altered in diabetes. The normal hormonal action of pancreatic polypeptide is still unknown. When the normal role of this hormone is established, undoubtedly abnormalities of function of the F cells will be associated with a particular human disease state. Additional hormones have been demonstrated in islets and certain islet cell tumors; however, these hormones have not been localized to a specific type of islet cell. These include vasoactive intestinal polypeptide and serotonin.

Insulin synthesis. Insulin is stored in the B cell as secretory granules. Ultrastructurally the matrix of the mature B cell granules contain a crystalline structure with lines of repeating periodicity of 50 Å, which corresponds closely to the size of the hexameric, crystalline form of zinc insulin. Zinc is also present in B cell granules. Thus it would appear that the storage form of insulin is essentially a microcrystal of zinc insulin.

Stimulation of the B cell with glucose results in the immediate release of stored insulin and also initiates a series of events that leads to new formation of insulin. After glucose stimulation, proinsulin production is initiated in the endoplasmic reticulum. Human proinsulin is a single chain of 86 amino acids that consists of the A and B chains of insulin linked by a connecting peptide segment of 31 amino acids. This connecting segment is called the C peptide. Proinsulin is transferred by an energy-requiring mechanism to the Golgi complex where apparently the C peptide is split off by a specific proteolytic enzyme or enzymes. The newly formed insu-

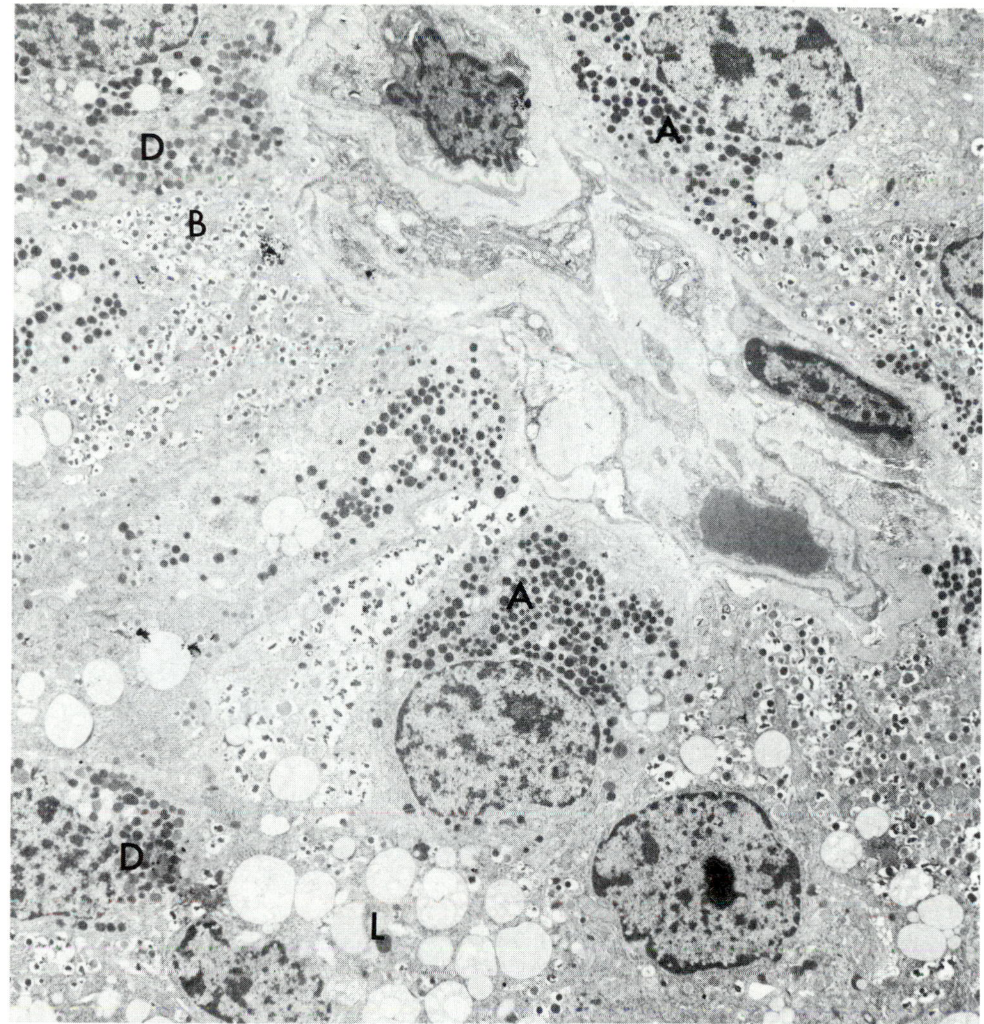

Fig. 29-11. Electron micrograph of islet cells of normal human pancreas. *A,* A cell; *B,* B cell; *D,* D cell. Lipochrome pigment, *L,* is present in cells. (Courtesy Dr. Marie Greider, St. Louis, Mo.)

lin and C peptide are packaged into secretory granules in the Golgi complex, then released into the cytoplasm after acquiring a membranous sac derived from the Golgi membranes. At some point in this process, zinc is transported into the B cell granule, resulting in the formation of zinc insulin crystals. Since C peptide is released with insulin and is also excreted in urine, it is possible to assess the endogenous secretion of insulin by measurement of C peptide in 24-hour urine specimens.

Insulin secretion. Understanding the biochemical and macromolecular events that link glucose stimulation with insulin release from the B cell is of vital importance in the search for defects in this mechanism in B cells of diabetic subjects. Glucose is the primary stimulus for insulin release, and the mechanism of induction of insulin release by this hexose is unknown. One theory is that glucose metabolism in the B cell initiates insulin release. Another is that glucose interacts with specific glucoreceptors in the B cell. It is probable that both theories are correct. The first phase of insulin release may result from an interaction of glucose with a glucoreceptor on the B cell membrane, resulting in membrane depolarization and the entrance of calcium into the cell, whereas the second phase of insulin secretion may be a result of the metabolism of glucose.

After initiation of insulin release by glucose the next step in the secretory process is to convey the packets of insulin to the B cell surface. This is accomplished by the microtubule-microfilament system in the B cell. In appropriate preparations examined with electron microscopy, linear bundles of microtubules separating columns of B cell granules can be demonstrated. It has been suggested that calcium interacts with the microtubule-microfilament system, an interaction that results in a contraction or a change in physical conformation of the system with the resultant displacement of B cell granules

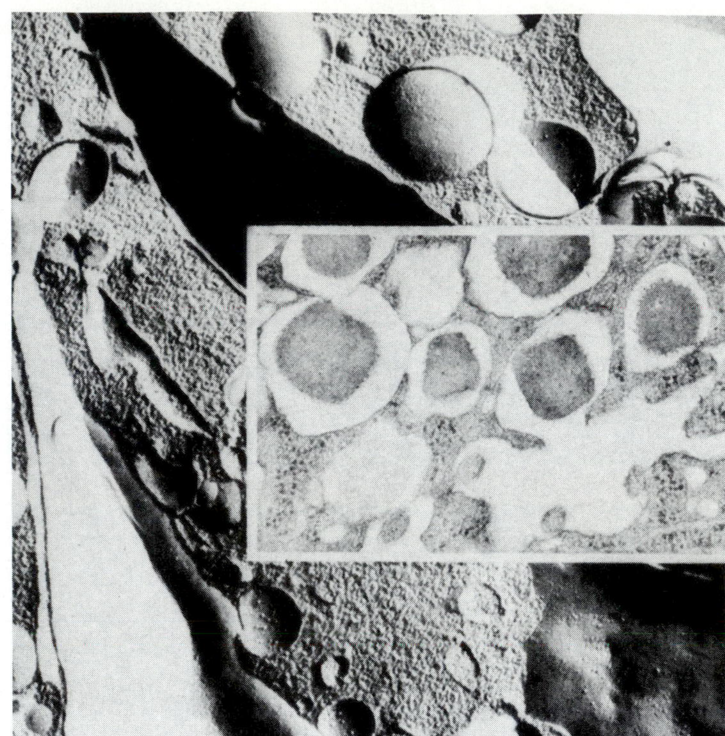

Fig. 29-12. Electron micrograph of freeze-fracture preparation of B cell demonstrating emiocytosis. *Inset,* Electron micrograph of section of stimulated B cell demonstrating release of B granule by emiocytosis. (Courtesy Dr. Lelio Orci, University of Geneva.)

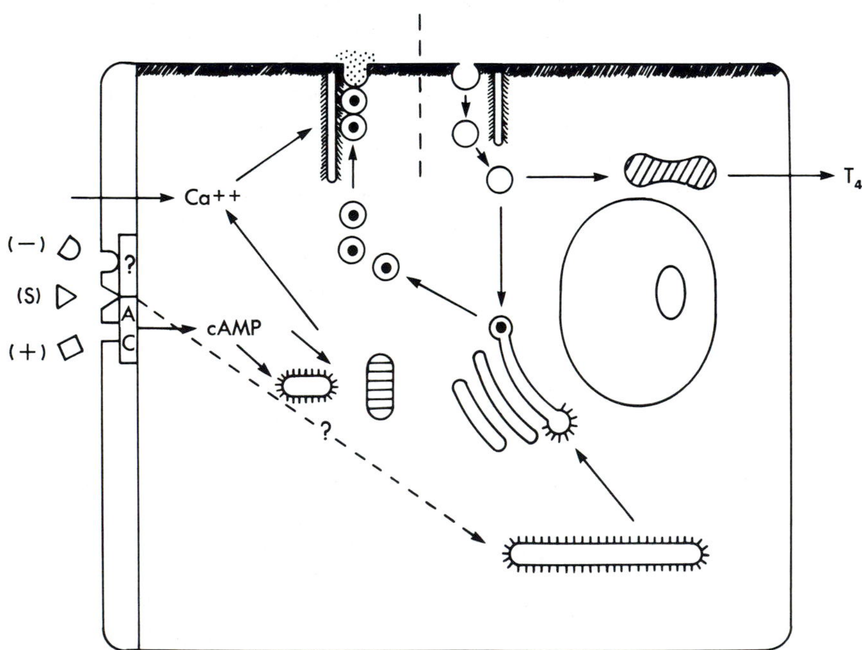

Fig. 29-13. Schematic representation of mechanism of B cell secretion. Glucose, *S,* interacts with presumed glucoreceptor on B cell membrane resulting in stimulation of adenylate cyclase system, *AC,* and influx of calcium into B cell, which results in displacement of B granules to cell surface by microtubular-microfilament system. Granules are released by emiocytosis, and membrane is recycled into cell. Thyroid secretion, T_4, would involve only recycling phase of secretory process. Proinsulin forms in endoplasmic reticulum, is transferred to Golgi complex, is converted to insulin, and is stored as B granules.

to the cell surface. Studies with transmission and freeze-fracture electron microscopy have demonstrated that the final step in the secretion of insulin is by emiocytosis (Fig. 29-12). This is accomplished by a fusion of the membranous sacs surrounding the B cell granules with the plasma membrane of the cell, resulting in the liberation of the granules and C peptide into the extracellular space where insulin and C peptide are then transported into the capillary system of the islets. The excess membrane incorporated into the plasma membrane as a result of emiocytosis is apparently recycled into the cytoplasm of the B cell. Recent studies indicate that this recycling involves a specific removal of the membranous sacs inserted into the plasma membrane, and this recycling mechanism may involve the microtubule-microfilament system. The involvement of the microtubule-microfilament system in the intracellular transport of the granules could also explain the biphasic pattern of insulin release. Those granules already associated with the system would be released immediately after glucose stimulation, whereas other stored granules and newly formed secretory granules would join the system at a later time, forming the second phase of insulin release.

This simple but elegant model for insulin secretion is shown in Fig. 29-13. It would appear that this model of endocrine secretion would be applicable to other endocrine glands, which may use either the entire system or only a portion of it. For example, in the thyroid gland only a portion of the mechanism would appear to be used. Stimulation with thyrotropic hormone results in increased pinocytosis of the apical portion of follicular cells with resultant accumulation of thyroglobulin droplets. The cytoplasm and the droplets are conveyed to lysosomes and degraded to thyroxine. Thus it would appear that only the recycling portion of the secretory process is used in the secretion of thyroxine in the thyroid gland.

A defect in any one of the steps in the secretory process could lead to an impairment or delay in the release of insulin by glucose. In maturity-onset diabetes the B cells do not respond immediately to glucose stimulation; thus a defect may exist in the putative glucoreceptor on the B cells, the calcium transport and metabolism may be altered, the microtubular-microfilament system may be defective, or the membranous fusion required for emiocytosis may be altered. An abnormality of the secretory mechanism for insulin release has been found in a hereditary form of diabetes in the spiny mouse. These animals respond sluggishly to glucose stimulation, as is the case in human maturity-onset diabetes. The B cells in the spiny mouse have been shown to be deficient in microtubular protein, and it has been suggested that this deficiency may impair the intracellular transport of B cell granules by the microtubular-microfilament system, with a resultant production of the diabetic state.

Pathologic changes in islets

The specific pathologic lesion(s) of the islet cells that would explain the etiology and pathogenesis of diabetes mellitus has not been elucidated. Despite this lack of specific knowledge, a number of pathologic changes have been demonstrated in the islets in association with diabetes. These include degranulation of B cells, amyloidosis, glycogenosis, and leukocytic infiltration. B cell degranulation is not a specific pathologic change, since it occurs as a result of hyperglycemia and simply represents a depletion of insulin reserve.

Distinct differences exist in the pathologic changes observed in the pancreases of individuals with classic juvenile- and maturity-onset diabetes. In juvenile-onset diabetes the B cell mass is reduced and fibrosis of the islets may be present, and, in occasional instances, lymphocytic infiltration is observed. In maturity-onset diabetes, the B cell mass and the degree of B cell degranulation may be normal or moderately reduced and amyloidosis may be present within the islets. In approximately 20% of patients with maturity-onset diabetes, no distinct light microscopic changes can be observed in the islets.

Amyloidosis of islets. By light microscopy, amyloid appears as an eosinophilic, amorphous material deposited around the capillaries of the islets, compressing and displacing the islet cells (Fig. 29-14). Previously, this change was called hyalinization of the islets of Langerhans and was one of the earlier morphologic findings observed in diabetic patients.

By electron microscopy the amyloid has a fibrillar appearance and is deposited between the two basement membranes, separating the islet cells from the capillaries. Amyloidosis does not involve all the islets within a single pancreas but has a patchy distribution. Amyloidosis of the islets is not limited to diabetic patients but has been found, to a minor degree, in about 2% of nondiabetic individuals over 40 years of age. It is unlikely that this pathologic change has a primary role in the etiology of the human diabetic state; however, it may play a role in the pathogenesis of the disease process once it is established.

Spontaneous diabetes has been described in many different species of animals. Amyloidosis of the islets has been described in spontaneous diabetes in monkeys and cats. In cats, occasional cases have been reported in which nearly all of the islets were replaced with amyloid and, in some instances, calcification of the amyloid was present. Amyloidosis of the islets has not been produced experimentally, and no information is available on the etiology and mechanism of development of this lesion.

Glycogenosis of B cells. Glycogen is deposited in B cells of the islets when there is a persistent hyperglycemia for a long period of time. Previously this lesion was called hydropic degeneration of B cells, since the cells

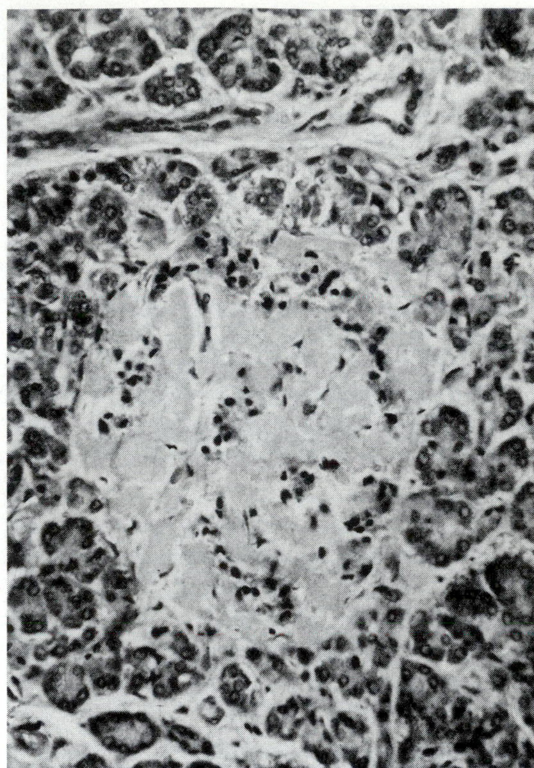

Fig. 29-14. Amyloidosis of islet of Langerhans in diabetic patient.

appeared greatly vacuolated and it was assumed that the vacuoles contained water. The use of special stains demonstrated that the vacuoles actually contained glycogen. Glycogenosis of B cells occurs in human diabetes as well as in experimental animals with diabetes (Fig. 29-15). Before the insulin era, glycogenosis of B cells was a common finding at autopsy in diabetic patients, but now it is rarely observed, since relatively few patients die in diabetic acidosis and severe hyperglycemia. Nevertheless, this lesion undoubtedly does occur during the life of diabetic subjects when there are periods of uncontrolled hyperglycemia.

Lymphocytic and eosinophilic infiltration of islets. Lymphocytic infiltration of the islets of Langerhans may be observed in juvenile diabetes. It is particularly evident when autopsy is performed within days or weeks after the onset of the disease process. Experimentally a similar type of lymphocytic infiltration occurs in virus-induced diabetes mellitus. Lymphocytic infiltration of the islets has also been observed in cattle and rabbits that were immunized with beef insulin. A permanent diabetic state was induced in some of the immunized rabbits. Both of these experimental findings relate to the question of a possible viral and autoimmune phenomenon in the pathogenesis of juvenile-onset human diabetes mellitus.

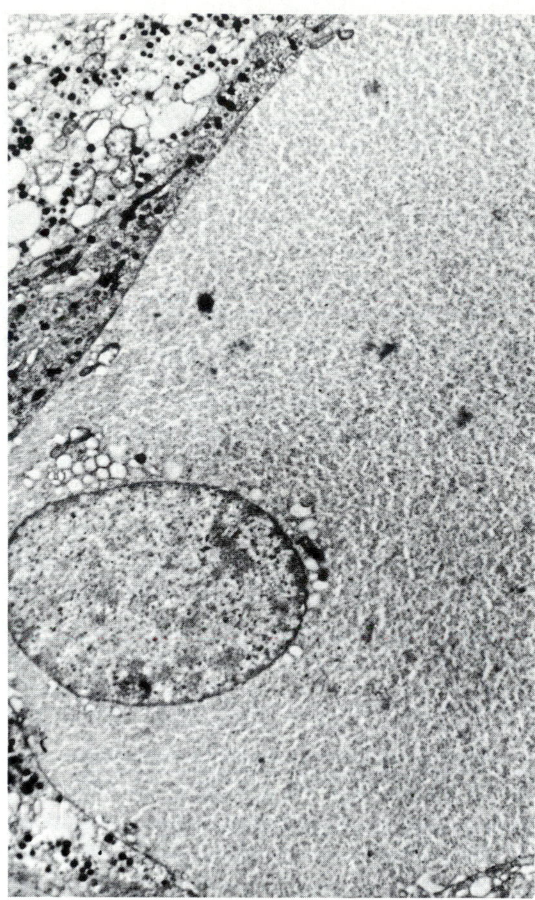

Fig. 29-15. Electron micrograph of B cell containing massive accumulation of glycogen in diabetic hamster. Glycogen accumulation presents appearance of hydropic degeneration in ordinary microscopic preparations.

Infiltration of eosinophils and lymphocytes within and around the islets and in the interstitial tissue of the pancreas is observed in approximately 25% of infants who are born to diabetic mothers and who die within 1 to 2 weeks after birth (Fig. 29-16). This infiltration is invariably associated with islet hypertrophy and hyperplasia and is diagnostic of diabetes mellitus in the mother. The appearance of an eosinophilic infiltration is not related to the severity of the diabetes or the form of therapy received by the mother. In some instances the mother has no clinical evidence of diabetes during pregnancy and may become diabetic within a period of months or years subsequently. Experimentally a morphologic counterpart of this lesion has been produced by acute injections of anti-insulin serum into rats. In these animals a severe diabetic state is produced and an infiltration of eosinophils and lymphocytes is present in the interstitial tissue and peri-insular areas of the pancreas. In monkeys with streptozotocin-induced diabetes, hyperplasia of the islets has been observed in the fetuses of the diabetic mothers; however, lymphocytic and eosinophilic infiltration was

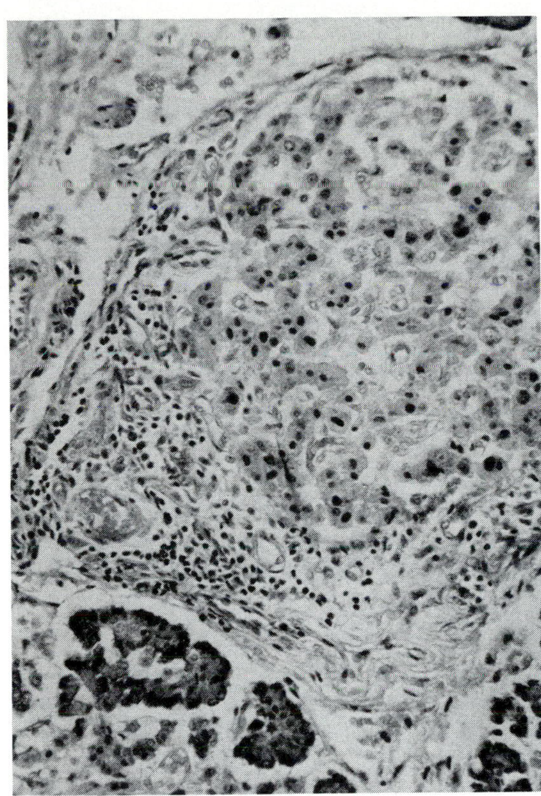

Fig. 29-16. Infiltration of eosinophils in peri-insular tissue of newborn infant of diabetic mother.

not present. It appears that the hyperplasia of the B cells is attributable to the hyperglycemia; however, the lymphocytic and eosinophilic infiltration may be caused by another factor involving an infectious agent or the transfer of specific antibodies to the fetus.

Hemochromatosis

Hemosiderin may be evident within acinar and B cells of the pancreas in hemochromatosis. The A cells are greatly reduced in number and do not contain hemosiderin. Atrophy of the acinar cells and interstitial fibrosis are usually present. The term "bronze diabetes" is sometimes used, since increased pigmentation of the skin, diabetes mellitus, and cirrhosis of the liver may be present in hemochromatosis (see also pp. 84 and 1166).

Diabetic microangiopathy

Pathologic changes in the small blood vessels and capillaries of the eye and kidney are responsible for the development of diabetic retinopathy and Kimmelstiel-Wilson syndrome in patients with diabetes mellitus. An important question is whether the changes in these small vessels in diabetics are limited to these two organs or whether they occur in small vessels throughout the body. The application of quantitative techniques to electron microscopic studies of capillaries in muscle biopsies from a large group of diabetic and nondiabetic patients has helped resolve this question as well as several others. Ultrastructural studies of the capillaries of the eye, kidney, muscle, and skin of diabetic patients have demonstrated a significant thickening of the basement membrane in each of these organs, which is specific for diabetes mellitus (Fig. 29-17). In nondiabetic persons, thickening of muscle capillary basement membranes occurs in a linear fashion in males with increasing age, whereas in females, the basement membrane thickness increases until about 40 to 50 years of age, reaches a plateau, and increases again between 60 and 70 years of age. In diabetics, the basement membrane is significantly thicker than in appropriate age- and sex-matched controls, and the thickening occurs segmentally and increases with the duration of the disease.

A significant question is whether the thickening of the basement membrane in diabetes is the result of a separate genetic defect or actually a complication of diabetes. Detailed and carefully controlled studies have now shown that the thickened basement membrane is a true complication of diabetes and is not the result of a separate genetic defect. These findings are of great importance, since they provide hope that, if the diabetic state could be reverted to normal by new therapeutic means, the early stages of the complications could be reversed and further progression of these lesions could be halted.

The structural components of a capillary are the endothelial cell, the basement membrane, and a supporting cell embedded in the basement membrane. This supporting cell is called a pericyte in skeletal muscle, a mural cell in the capillaries of the eye, and a mesangial cell in the glomerulus of the kidney. It is unknown whether the supporting cell or the endothelial cell is responsible for either the formation or the removal of the basement membrane. These fundamental questions must be resolved before one can attempt to understand why excess basement membrane is produced in patients with diabetes mellitus.

Kidney in diabetes

The nodular lesions of the glomeruli described by Kimmelstiel and Wilson are characteristic pathologic changes found in the kidney in diabetes mellitus. This lesion is the result of focal thickening of the basement membrane. Quantitative ultrastructural studies of the glomeruli in diabetic patients have demonstrated that the earliest change occurs in the mesangial area of the glomerulus. Initially there is thickening of the basement membrane in this area and an increase in the number of mesangial cells. Serial renal biopsies on these diabetic patients over a period of years have shown that the amount of basement membrane in the kidney gradually

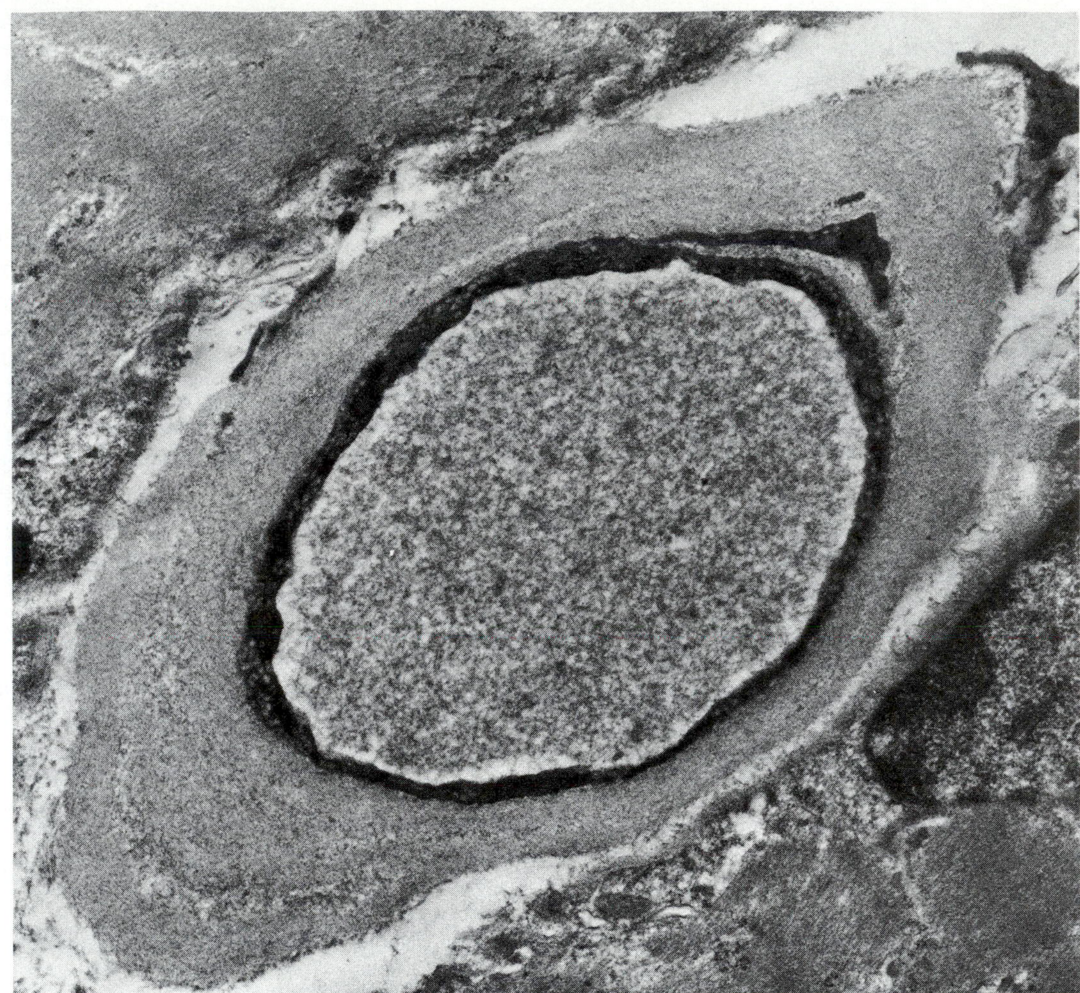

Fig. 29-17. Electron micrograph of capillary in skeletal muscle of diabetic patient. Basement membrane surrounding capillary tremendously thickened. (Courtesy Dr. Joseph R. Williamson, St. Louis, Mo.)

increases and results in the formation of the nodular lesions. These findings clearly indicate that the basement membrane changes result from the diabetic process. In experimentally induced diabetes in rats, an increase in the number of mesangial cells, a slight increase in basement membrane thickness, and the deposition of gamma globulin in the basement membrane have been observed. Islet transplants into these diabetic animals have returned the diabetic state to normal and have completely reversed the pathologic changes in the glomeruli (see also p. 754).

Vacuolization of the pars recta of the proximal convoluted tubules at the corticomedulary junction may be observed in patients dying of uncontrolled diabetes and severe hyperglycemia. These vacuoles represent areas of glycogen deposition within the tubules that disappear when the diabetic state is treated. This condition is called the Armanni-Ebstein lesion of the kidney.

Necrotizing renal papillitis is a rare but serious complication of diabetes mellitus. This condition is not limited to diabetic patients but also may occur in nondiabetic persons with obstructive lesions of the urinary tract. The condition is characterized clinically in the diabetic patient by the rapid onset of uremia and subsequent death caused by infarction and sloughing of the renal papillae.

Eye in diabetes

Diabetic retinopathy is now the second most and will soon become the most common cause of blindness in the United States. The sequence of events in the development of this lesion is changes in the pattern of blood flow through the retina with resultant areas of ischemia, occurrence of microaneurysms in the retinal capillaries, new formation of capillaries within the retina, subsequent hemorrhage into the vitreous, and formation of granulation tissue. The development of these lesions requires many years with a varying degree of severity in individual patients and long periods of remission with no further impairment of vision.

The earliest anatomic change observed in the retina of diabetic patients is a loss of mural cells in the capillaries. Ghostlike remnants of these cells persist for long periods of time. Presumably the loss of these cells affects the capillary tone and leads in some way to the change in the pattern of blood flow through the retina and the subsequent development of microaneurysms of the retina. The mechanism of destruction of the mural cells in the diabetic is unknown.

The earliest clinical change in the eyes of diabetic patients is an increase in permeability of retinal capillaries, which can be demonstrated by quantitative measurements of fluorescein leakage into the anterior chamber and vitreous of the eye. This same change has been demonstrated in rats with experimentally induced diabetes, and when the diabetic state reverts to normal after islet transplantation, the abnormal leakage from the retinal capillaries is also reversed.

Experimentally, microaneurysms and intraretinal hemorrhage have been observed in dogs with alloxan-induced diabetes. Tight control of these diabetic animals with insulin results in a sharp diminution in the number of microaneurysms, which adds further support to the concept that the vascular changes in the retina are associated with the diabetic state.

Peripheral nerves in diabetes

Peripheral neuropathy is particularly likely to occur in the older diabetic patient, with approximately 30% to 50% of the patients showing minor reflex changes and evanescent pains in the extremities. The basic pathologic change in the peripheral nerves is a segmental demyelination. The autonomic nervous system may also be involved in diabetic patients, with resultant development of severe diarrhea and abdominal pain. Greatly elevated levels of sorbitol and fructose have been demonstrated in peripheral nerves of animals with experimentally induced diabetes. The accumulation of sorbitol and fructose is apparently attributable to a partial shunting of the metabolism of glucose through the aldose reductase pathway. It is unknown whether this abnormal metabolism of glucose with the formation of sorbitol is responsible for the decreased nerve conduction and segmental demyelination in diabetic subjects. In experimental diabetes, degenerative changes have been found in autonomic nerve fibers of the intestinal tract of rats and were associated with the development of megacolon in these animals. Control of the diabetes by islet transplantation resulted in either prevention or disappearance of the degenerative lesions in the autonomic nerves.

Arteriosclerosis and diabetes

Diabetes mellitus accelerates the development of arteriosclerosis with a resultant earlier onset of coronary arteriosclerosis and atherosclerosis in general. The arteriosclerotic process also involves the vessels to the lower extremity with resultant production of gangrene of the toes and feet. Elucidation of the mechanism by which diabetes mellitus accelerates arteriosclerosis may provide insight into the etiology and pathogenesis of arteriosclerosis in general.

The precipitating causes of gangrene of the lower extremities are usually mechanical, thermal, or chemical trauma resulting in ulceration, infection, and subsequent gangrene. Comparison of the ultrastructure of dermal capillaries of the toes amputated from diabetic and nondiabetic individuals indicates that thickening of the basement membrane of the capillaries is limited to the diabetic group. The pronounced thickening in the basement membranes of the capillaries in diabetic patients may play some role in the inception and complication of the vascular insufficiency of the lower extremities, possibly by interference with nutrition and response of the tissues to injury.

Transplantation of pancreas and islets

Since the present therapeutic regimen for the treatment of diabetes mellitus does not prevent the complications of the disease process, studies are in progress to attempt to replace the defective B cells in the diabetic subject with normal-functioning B cells. The first approach to this problem was to transplant the whole pancreas into diabetic patients receiving kidney transplants for renal failure. Only a few of these pancreatic transplants have functioned normally beyond a few weeks or months, and no information is available as to whether the transplants affected the progression of the diabetic complications.

The ideal approach to transplantation would be to implant only the islets of Langerhans. The development of the collagenase technique for the isolation of intact islets has made this feasible in experimental animals. Using an inbred strain of rats, islets have been transplanted successfully into the liver via the portal vein, the spleen, and the peritoneal cavity of diabetic recipients. Fetal pancreatic tissue has also been successfully transplanted beneath the renal capsule and into the peritoneal cavity of diabetic animals. These transplants not only reversed the diabetic state to normal but also reversed early microvascular complications of diabetes occurring in the eyes and kidneys of these animals.

The major deterrent to the application of islet transplantation to human diabetics has been the immune rejection problem, since allografts of islets are rejected rapidly and immunosuppressive drugs would have to be administered continuously to diabetic patients to maintain the grafts. A remarkable series of recent findings has now shown that it is possible to transplant islets successfully across major histocompatibility barriers in rats and mice and across the species barrier of rat to mouse without the continuous use of immunosuppressive drugs. The concept behind these startling new findings is that passenger leukocytes contaminating the grafts are responsible for the initiation of immune rejection, whereas the islet cells alone are incapable of initiating the immune rejection. Removal or alteration of the passenger leukocytes was accomplished by in vitro incubation of the islets at a low temperature or in the presence of 95% oxygen before transplantation. These conditions did not affect the structure and function of the islets and permitted the successful transplantation of allografts and xenografts of islets into diabetic recipients. Recently it was shown that mouse islet cells lack IA antigens but express the other antigens of the H-2 complex. Since IA antigens are expressed on lymphoid cells and have been shown to be involved in the initiation of an immune reaction, a specific IA antisera was developed and used to treat the islets before transplantation. Allografts of mouse islets treated with specific IA antisera were not rejected and survived for more than 200 days. These recent findings not only provide hope for the eventual use of islet transplantation in human diabetics without the use of immunosuppressive therapy, but also raise the possibility of applying this technique to the transplantation of other tissues and organs.

NEOPLASMS OF PANCREATIC ISLETS

Several different types of islet cell tumors occur in the pancreas and produce specific hormones. These tumors cannot be differentiated on the basis of their morphologic appearance using hematoxylin and eosin preparations. To establish the specific identity of an islet cell tumor, immunohistochemical stains, electron microscopy, and immunoassay of the tumor for specific hormones are required. These procedures have revealed that islet tumors are composed of a predominant single type of islet cell and release a specific hormone but also contain minor elements of other types of islet cells and their hormones. It is mandatory that all of the specialized techniques be used in the diagnosis of islet cell tumors to permit accurate identification of the tumor and appropriate therapy for the patients.

B cell tumors (insulinomas)

Functioning B cell neoplasms retain the capacity to form, store, and release insulin into the bloodstream. The neoplastic B cells differ from normal in that they are no longer responsive to the normal control mechanisms affecting insulin release and thus release insulin at an uncontrolled rate, resulting in repeated attacks of hypoglycemia. Circulating levels of insulin are usually elevated in these patients during fasting and are increased during periods of hypoglycemia. Stimulation of insulin release from these neoplasms can usually be produced by the administration of either tolbutamide or arginine.

B cell tumors are most commonly found in the body and tail of the pancreas. Grossly the tumors are usually encapsulated and well circumscribed, varying from 5 mm to 10 cm in diameter. Their homogeneous color and increased consistency make them easy to delineate from the surrounding normal pancreas.

Microscopically the tumors usually have a gyroform pattern with ribbons or cords of cells passing between vascular sinusoids (Fig. 29-18). It is extremely difficult to assess the degree of malignancy of these neoplasms based on the presence of anaplasia and hyperchromatism of the nuclei, since these changes may be present in a circumscribed adenoma or in one that has metastasized. The degree of granulation within the neoplasms may vary from a few scattered granules to an intense granulation similar to the normal B cell. Measurements of insulin in microdissected neoplastic cells from freeze-dried sections confirm this striking variability in insulin content of the cells. On electron microscopic examination the neoplastic cells contain the typical, crystalline, rectangular granules that are present in normal B cells, and the number of crystalline granules varies noticeably within different neoplasms. Amyloid frequently is observed between the two basement membranes sepa-

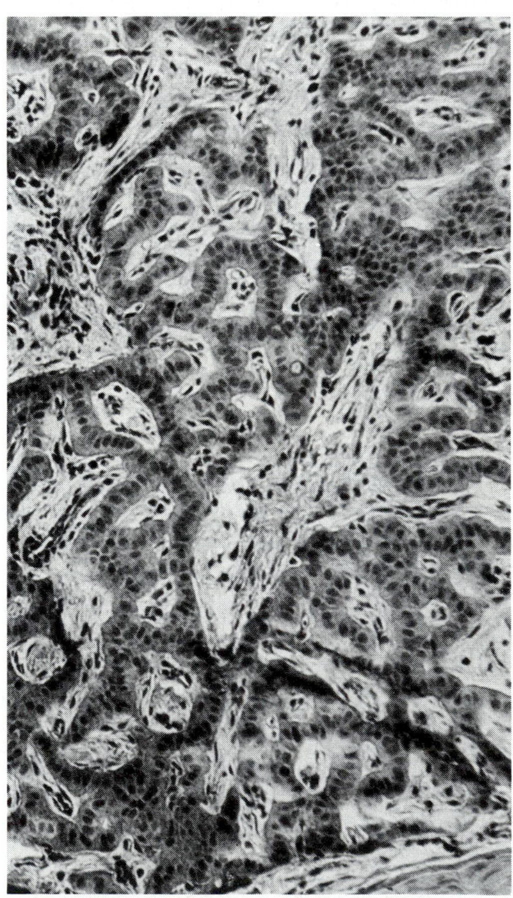

Fig. 29-18. B cell tumor. Gyroform pattern resulting from anastomosing cords of B cells. (Courtesy Dr. Marie Greider, St. Louis, Mo.)

rating the neoplastic cells from the capillaries, and in some instances calcification may be present in this area.

A cell tumors (glucagonomas)

A cell tumors are rare neoplasms of the islet cells. These tumors contain glucagon, and usually the level of circulating glucagon in the patient is greatly elevated. The clinical findings associated with high serum glucagon levels are a necrolytic migratory erythema, mild diabetes mellitus, and anemia. The skin rash is the main clinical diagnostic change that should arouse suspicion of hyperglucagonemia and the presence of an A cell tumor in the pancreas. By light microscopy the neoplasms have a gyroform pattern similar to that of the B cell tumors. Under electron microscopy the neoplastic cells have the ultrastructural appearance of normal A cells and contain numerous secretory granules. The secretory granules of the tumors are round with an extremely dense core and have a diameter of 225 to 425 nm.

G cell tumors (gastrinomas)

Zollinger and Ellison described a diagnostic triad that consists of a fulminating peptic ulcer diathesis persisting despite medical therapy or other radical procedures, gastric acid hypersecretion, and the presence of a non–B cell tumor in the pancreas. Approximately one third of the ulcers observed in these patients have been found in unusual locations, such as the esophageal, postbulbar, and jejunal areas. The tumors most frequently occur in the body and tail of the pancreas, and in a few instances the neoplasm has been found in the wall of the duodenum, apparently originating in heterotopic foci of pancreatic tissue. Multiple adenomas involving the pituitary, adrenal, and parathyroid glands and islets of Langerhans have been found in approximately one third of the patients.

Histologically the G cell tumors do not have a gyroform pattern as observed in A cell and B cell tumors. The neoplasms contain large, solid nests of cells with glandular structures (Fig. 29-19). Under electron microscopy the tumors are shown to contain small, round granules similar to the secretory granules of gastrin-producing cells of the pyloric antrum. Gastrin can be demonstrated in extracts of the tumor by immunoassay and in the tumor cells by immunohistochemical techniques.

D cell tumors (somatostatinomas)

Tumors of D cells have been described recently. Somatostatin has been isolated from the neoplasms and demonstrated in D cells of the tumors by immunohistochemical techniques. Elevated circulatory levels of somatostatin have been found in these patients. The number of cases is small; however, the clinical findings associated with this neoplasm appear to be diabetes, achlorhydria, steatorrhea, and cholelithiasis. These clinical changes are consistent with the inhibitory action of somatostatin on the secretion of gastrin, insulin, glucagon, and pancreatic enzymes as well as on gallbladder contraction.

Pancreatic polypeptide has been demonstrated as a minor component of several different islet cell tumors. Information is lacking on the precise site of action of pancreatic polypeptide in normal metabolism. Further investigations should establish the normal function of this hormone and delineate clinical features associated with an F cell tumor secreting predominantly pancreatic polypeptide.

Diarrheogenic tumors (vipomas)

Verner and Morrison described a clinical syndrome associated with non–B cell tumors of the pancreas that was characterized by profuse diarrhea with hypokalemia and achlorhydria. The tumors usually occurred in the head and tail of the pancreas and were solitary or occasionally multiple in the pancreas. Histologically the tumors had a pattern similar to that of G cell tumors, with glandular structures present in large solid nests of

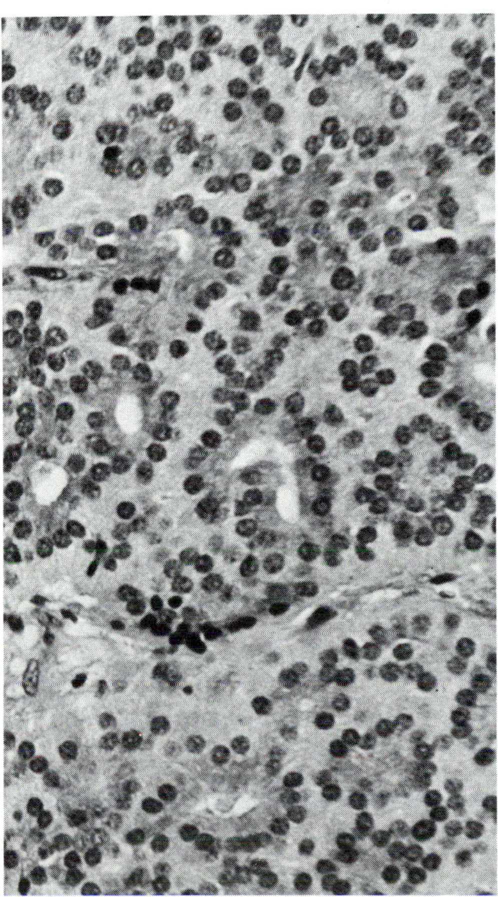

Fig. 29-19. Ulcerogenic tumor with glandular histologic pattern. (Courtesy Dr. Marie Greider, St. Louis, Mo.)

neoplastic cells. Vasoactive intestinal polypeptide (VIP) has been isolated from the tumors. Administration of VIP to experimental animals induces diarrhea and inhibits gastric acid secretion; thus VIP is apparently responsible for the clinical findings in patients with these neoplasms. VIP is present in autonomic nerve fibers, and it has been found that ganglioneuroblastomas may be associated with the clinical findings of diarrhea, hypokalemia, and achlorhydria. It is unknown at the present time whether VIP is produced by a specific type of islet cell.

Nesidioblastosis

Idiopathic hypoglycemia in infants is a sydrome encompassing several entities. The majority of these infants suffer from ketotic hypoglycemia, show leucine hypersensitivity, or are infants of diabetic mothers. The hypoglycemia may be transitory, as occurs following birth from a diabetic mother, or may undergo remission when the diet of the infant is altered to prevent ketogenesis or to lower the leucine intake. In approximately one third of the infants with this syndrome the hypoglycemia is persistent, with inappropriate insulin secretion and a high insulin/glucose ratio in the blood. A common finding in the pancreas is a continued formation of islet cells from pancreatic duct epithelium. This pathologic change is called nesidioblastosis. During normal embryologic development of the pancreas, islets form by budding from the ductular epithelium. In nesidioblastosis, new formation of islets continues after birth, and A, B, D, and F cells are present in these budding islets. Apparently abnormalities exist in the factors controlling the continued formation of islet cells after birth; however, it is unlikely that the hypoglycemia is simply the result of an increased mass of B cells. Undoubtedly the B cells are also defective, since the release of insulin is not controlled by the circulatory level of blood glucose, and leucine stimulates insulin release in many of these patients.

REFERENCES

Normal form and development

1. Liu, H.M., and Potter, E.L.: Development of human pancreas, Arch. Pathol. **74**:439, 1962.
2. Milbourn, E.: On the excretory ducts of the pancreas in man with special reference to their relationships to each other, to the common bile duct, and to the duodenum, Acta Anat. **9**:1, 1950.
3. Rutter, W.J., et al.: Epithelial-mesenchymal interactions, Baltimore, 1968, The Williams & Wilkins Co.
4. Wessells, N.K., and Cohen, J.H.: Early pancreas organogenesis: morphogenesis, tissue interactions, and mass effects, Dev. Biol. **15**:237, 1967.
5. Wessells, N.K., and Evans, J.: Ultrastructural studies of early morphogenesis and cytodifferentiation in the embryogenic mammalian pancreas, Dev. Biol. **17**:413, 1968.

Abnormalities of form and development

6. Barbosa, J.J. de C., Dockerty, M.B., and Waugh, J.M.: Pancreatic heterotopia: review of the literature and report of 41 authenticated surgical cases of which 25 were clinically significant, Surg. Gynecol. Obstet. **82**:527, 1946.
7. Elliott, G.B., Kliman, M.R., and Elliott, K.A.: Pancreatic annulus: a sign or cause of duodenal obstruction, Can. J. Surg. **11**:357, 1968.
8. Feldman, M., and Weinberg, T.: Aberrant pancreas: cause of duodenal syndrome, J.A.M.A. **148**:893, 1952.
9. Huebner, G.D., and Reed, P.A.: Annular pancreas, Am. J. Surg. **104**:869, 1962.
10. Lundquist, G.: Annular pancreas: pathogenesis, clinical features, and treatment with a report on two operation cases, Acta Chir. Scand. **117**:451, 1959.
11. Pearson, S.: Aberrant pancreas: review of literature and report of three cases, one of which produced common and pancreatic duct obstruction, Arch. Surg. **63**:168, 1951.
12. Van Der Horst, L.F.: Annular pancreas, Arch. Surg. **83**:249, 1961.

Cystic fibrosis

13. Alhadeff, J.A.: Glycoproteins and cystic fibrosis: a review, Clin. Genet. **14**:89, 1978.
14. Anderson, D.H.: Cystic fibrosis of pancreas and its relation to celiac disease: clinical and pathologic study, Am. J. Dis. Child. **56**:344, 1938.
15. Anderson, D.H.: Pancreatic enzymes in duodenal juice in celiac syndrome, Am. J. Dis. Child. **63**:643, 1942.
16. Aterman, K.: Duodenal ulceration and fibrocystic pancreas disease, Am. J. Dis. Child. **101**:210, 1942.
17. Bodian, M.: Fibrocystic disease of the pancreas, New York, 1953, Grune & Stratton, Inc.
18. Bowman, B.H., and Mangos, J.A.: Current concepts in genetics: cystic fibrosis, N. Engl. J. Med. **294**:937, 1976.
19. Changus, H.C., and Pitot, H.C.: Cystic fibrosis: a dilemma in metabolic pathogenesis of genetic disease, Arch. Pathol. Lab. Med. **100**:7, 1976.
20. Clarke, J.T., Elian, E., and Shwachman, H.: Components of sweat in cystic fibrosis of the pancreas compared with controls, Am. J. Dis. Child. **101**:490, 1961.
21. Danes, B.S., and Bearn, A.G.: Cystic fibrosis of the pancreas: a study in cell culture, J. Exp. Med. **129**:775, 1969.
22. di Sant'Agnese, P.A., and Davis, P.B.: Research in cystic fibrosis (in three parts), N. Engl. J. Med. **295**:481, 534, 597, 1976.
23. di Sant'Agnese, P.A., and Lepore, M.J.: Involvement of abdominal organs in cystic fibrosis of the pancreas, Gastroenterology **40**:64, 1961.
24. di Sant'Agnese, P.A., and Talamo, R.C.: Pathogenesis and physiopathology of cystic fibrosis of the pancreas: fibrocystic disease of the pancreas (mucoviscidosis) (in three parts), N. Engl. J. Med. **277**:1287, 1344, 1399, 1967.
25. Dische, Z., et al.: Composition of mucoprotein fractions from duodenal fluid of patients with cystic fibrosis of pancreas and from controls, Pediatrics **24**:74, 1959.
26. Farber, S.: Pancreatic function and disease in early life: pathologic changes associated with pancreatic insufficiency in early life, Arch. Pathol. **37**:238, 1944.
27. Farber, S.: Relation of pancreatic achylia to meconium ileus, J. Pediatr. **24**:387, 1944.
28. Frydman, M.I.: Epidemiology of cystic fibrosis: a review, J. Chronic. Dis. **32**:211, 1979.
29. Kaplan, E., et al.: Reproductive failure in males with cystic fibrosis, N. Engl. J. Med. **279**:65, 1968.
30. Macdonald, J.A., and Trusler, G.A.,: Meconium ileus: an eleven-year review at the Hospital for Sick Children, Toronto, Can. Med. Assoc. J. **83**:881, 1960.
31. Mangos, J.A., and McSherry, N.R.: Sodium transport inhibitory factor in sweat of patients with cystic fibrosis, Science **158**:135, 1967.
32. Munger, B.L., Brusilow, S.W., and Cooke, R.E.: An electron microscopic study of eccrine sweat glands in patients with cystic fibrosis of the pancreas, J. Pediatr. **59**:497, 1961.
33. Oppenheimer, E.H., and Esterly, J.R.: Pathology of cystic fibrosis: review of the literature and comparison with 146 autopsied cases, Perspect. Pediatr. Pathol. **2**:241, 1975.
34. Roberts, G.B.: Familial incidence of fibrocystic disease of the pancreas, Ann. Hum. Genet. **24**:127, 1960.

35. Rubin, L.S., et al.: Pupillary reactivity as a measure of autonomic balance in cystic fibrosis, J. Pediatr. **63**:1120, 1963.
36. Smoller, M., and Hsia, D.Y.: Studies on the genetic mechanism of cystic fibrosis of the pancreas, Am. J. Dis. Child. **98**:277, 1959.
37. Spock, A., et al.: In vitro study of ciliary motility to detect individuals with active cystic fibrosis and carriers of disease, Mod. Probl. Paediatr. **10**:200, 1967.
38. Taussig, L.M., et al.: Fertility in males with cystic fibrosis, N. Engl. J. Med. **287**:586, 1972.

Acquired diseases

39. Baggenstoss, A.H.: Pancreas in uremia, histopathologic study, Am. J. Pathol. **24**:1003, 1948.
40. Blumenthal, H.T., and Probstein, J.G.: Pancreatitis, Springfield, Ill., 1959, Charles C Thomas, Publisher.
41. Ciba Foundation Symposium: The exocrine pancreas, Boston, 1961, Little, Brown & Co.
42. Dreiling, D.A.: Pancreatic disease: a review, J. Mt. Sinai Hosp. N.Y. **36**:388, 1969.
43. Edmonson, H.A., and Berne, C.J.: Calcium changes in acute pancreatic necrosis, J. Surg. Gynecol. Obstet. **79**:240, 1944.
44. Elliott, D.W., Williams, R.D., and Zollinger, R.M.: Alterations in the pancreatic resistance to bile in the pathogenesis of acute pancreatitis, Ann. Surg. **146**:669, 1957.
45. Gambill, E.E.: Pancreatitis, St. Louis, 1973, The C.V. Mosby Co.
46. Gross, J.B., and Comfort, M.W.: Chronic pancreatitis, Am. J. Med. **33**:358, 1962.
47. Gross, J.B., Gambill, E.E., and Ulrich, J.A.: Hereditary pancreatitis: description of a 5th kindred and summary of clinical features, Am. J. Med. **33**:358, 1962.
48. Hanna, W.A.: Rupture of pancreatic cysts: report of a case and review of the literature, Br. J. Surg. **47**:495, 1960.
49. Hranilovich, G.T., and Gabbenstoss, A.H.: Lesions of the pancreas in malignant hypertension: review of 100 cases at necroscopy, Arch. Pathol. **55**:443, 1953.
50. Longnecker, D.S.: Pathology and pathogenesis of the diseases of the pancreas, Am. J. Pathol. **107**:103, 1982.
51. Murphy, R.F., and Hinkamp, J.F.: Pancreatic pseudocysts: report of 35 cases, Arch. Surg. **81**:564, 1960.
52. Opie, E.L.: The etiology of acute hemorrhagic pancreatitis, Bull. Johns Hopkins Hosp. **12**:182, 1901.
53. Ponka, J.L., Landrum, S.E., and Chaikof, L.: Acute pancreatitis in the postoperative patient, Arch. Surg. **83**:475, 1961.
54. Popper, H.L., Necheles, H., and Russell, K.C.: Transition of pancreatic edema into pancreatic necrosis, Surg. Gynecol. Obstet. **87**:79, 1948.
55. Rich, A.R., and Duff, G.L.: Experimental and pathologic studies on pathogenesis of acute hemorrhagic pancreatitis, Bull. Johns Hopkins Hosp. **58**:212, 1936.
56. Sarles, H.: Alcohol and the pancreas, Ann. N.Y. Acad. Sci. **252**:187, 1975.
57. Sarles, H., and Tiscornia, D.: Ethanol and chronic calcifying pancreatitis, Med. Clin. North Am. **58**:1333, 1974.
58. Szymanski, F.J., and Bluefarb, S.M.: Nodular fat necrosis and pancreatic disease, Arch. Dermatol. **83**:224, 1961.
59. Thal, A.P.: The occurrence of pancreatic antibodies and the nature of the pancreatic antigen, Surg. Forum **11**:367, 1960.
60. Tumen, H.J.: Pathogenesis and classification of pancreatic disease, Am. J. Dig. Dis. **6**:435, 1961.

Tumors

61. Auger, C.: Acinous cell carcinoma of pancreas with extensive fat necrosis, Arch. Pathol. **43**:400, 1947.
62. Bell, E.T.: Carcinoma of the pancreas, Am. J. Pathol. **33**:499, 1957.
63. Bogomoletz, W.V., et al.: Cystadenoma of the pancreas: a histologic, histochemical and ultrastructural study of seven cases, Histopathology **4**:309, 1980.
64. Burns, W.A., et al.: Lipase-secreting acinar cell carcinoma of the pancreas with polyarthropathy: a light and electron microscopic, histochemical and biochemical study, Cancer **33**:1002, 1974.
65. Carrin, B., et al.: Oat cell carcinoma of the pancreas with ectopic ACTH secretion, Cancer **31**:1523, 1973.
66. Cihak, R.W., Kawashima, T., and Steer, A.: Adenocanthoma (adenosquamous carcinoma) of the pancreas, Cancer **29**:1133, 1972.
67. Collins, J.J., Jr., Craighead, J.E., and Brooks, J.R.: Rationale for total pancreatectomy for carcinoma of the pancreatic head, N. Engl. J. Med. **274**:599, 1966.
68. Compagno, J., and Oertel, J.E.: Microcystic adenomas of the pancreas (glycogen-rich cystadenomas): a clinicopathologic study of 34 cases, Am. J. Clin. Pathol. **69**:289, 1978.
69. Compagno, J., and Oertel, J.E.: Mucinous cystic neoplasms of the pancreas with overt and latent malignancy (cystadenocarcinoma and cystadenoma): a clinicopathologic study of 41 cases, Am. J. Clin. Pathol. **69**:573, 1978.
70. Cubilla, A.L., and Fitzgerald, P.J.: Cancer of the pancreas (nonendocrine): a suggested morphologic classification, Semin. Oncol. **6**:285, 1979.
71. Druckrey, H., et al.: Erzeugung von Magen- und Pankreas-Krebs beim Meer-schweinchen durch Methylnitroso-harnstoff und-urethan, Z. Krebsforschung **72**:167, 1968.
72. Frable, W.J., Still, W.J.S., and Kay, S.: Carcinoma of the pancreas, infantile type: a light and electron microscopic study, Cancer **27**:667, 1971.
73. Frantz, V.K.: Tumors of the pancreas. In Atlas of tumor pathology, Section VII, Fascicles 27 and 28, Washington, D.C., 1959, Armed Forces Institute of Pathology.
74. Guillan, R.A., and McMahon, J.: Pleomorphic adenocarcinoma of the pancreas, Am. J. Gastroenterol. **60**:379, 1973.
75. Hayashi, Y., and Hasegawa, T.: Experimental pancreatic tumor in rats after intravenous injection of 4-hydroxyaminoquinoline 1-oxide, Gan **62**:329, 1971.
76. Hermreck, S., Thomas, C.Y., and Friesen, R.: Importance of pathologic staging in the surgical management of adenocarcinoma of the exocrine pancreas, Am. J. Surg. **127**:654, 1974.
77. Kaplan, N., and Angrist, A.: Mechanism of jaundice in cancer of the pancreas, Surg. Gynecol. Obstet. **77**:199, 1943.
78. Kenney, W.E.: Association of carcinoma in body and tail of pancreas with multiple venous thrombi, Surgery **14**:600, 1943.
79. Kissane, J.M.: Carcinoma of the exocrine pancreas: pathologic aspects, J. Surg. Oncol. **7**:167, 1975.
80. Kissane, J.M.: Tumors of the exocrine pancreas in childhood, Cancer Treat. Res. **8**:99, 1982.
81. Lafler, C.J., and Hinerman, D.L.: A morphologic study of pancreatic carcinoma with reference to multiple thrombi, Cancer **14**:944, 1961.
82. Mikal, S., and Campbell, A.J.A.: Carcinoma of the pancreas: diagnostic and operative criteria based on 100 consecutive autopsies, Surgery **28**:963, 1950.
83. Miller, J.R., Bagenstoss, A.H., and Comfort, M.W.: Carcinoma of the pancreas: effects of histological types and grade of malignancy on its behavior, Cancer **4**:233, 1951.
84. Oertel, J.E., Mendelsohn, G., and Compagno, J.: Solid and papillary epithelial neoplasms of the pancreas, Cancer Treat. Res. **8**:167, 1982.
85. Pour, P., et al.: Pancreatic neoplasms in an animal model: morphological, biological, and comparative studies, Cancer **36**:379, 1975.
86. Probstein, J.B., and Blumenthal, H.T.: Progressive malignant degeneration of a cystadenoma of the pancreas, Arch. Surg. **81**:683, 1960.
87. Rosai, J.: Carcinoma of pancreas simulating giant cell tumor of bone: electron microscopic evidence of its acinar cell origin, Cancer **22**:333, 1968.
88. Warren, K.W., Baasch, J.W., and Thum, C.W.: Carcinoma of the pancreas, Surg. Clin. North Am. **48**:601, 1968.
89. Weinstein, J.J.: Carcinoma of the head of the pancreas and periampullary area, Am. J. Gastroenterol. **37**:629, 1962.
90. Wynder, E.L., et al.: Epidemiology of cancer of the pancreas, J. Natl. Cancer Inst. **50**:645, 1973.

Diabetes mellitus

91. Allen, A.C.: So-called intercapillary glomerulosclerosis—a lesion associated with diabetes mellitus, Arch. Pathol. **32**:33, 1941.
92. Cerasi, E., and Luft, R.: The plasma insulin response to glucose infusion in healthy subjects and in diabetes mellitus, Acta Endocrinol. **55**:278, 1967.
93. Cogan, D.G., and Kuwabara, T.: Capillary shunts in the pathogenesis of diabetic retinopathy, Diabetes **12**:293, 1963.
94. Craighead, J.E., and Steinke, J.: Diabetes mellitus–like syndrome in mice infected with encephalomyocarditis virus, Am. J. Pathol. **63**:119, 1971.
95. Cudworth, A.G.: Type I diabetes mellitus, Diabetologia **14**:281, 1978.
96. Ehrlich, J.C., and Ratner, I.M.: Amyloidosis of the islets of Langerhans, Am. J. Pathol. **38**:49, 1961.
97. Ellenberg, M.: Current status of diabetes neuropathy, Metabolism **22**:657, 1973.
98. Faustman, D., et al.: Murine pancreatic B cells express H-2K and H-2D but not IA antigens, J. Exp. Med. **151**:1563, 1980.
99. Howell, S.L., Kostianovsky, M., and Lacy, P.E.: Beta granule formation in isolated islets of Langerhans: a study by electron microscopic radioautography, J. Cell Biol. **42**:695, 1969.
100. Irvine, W.J., et al.: Pancreatic islet-cell antibodies in diabetes mellitus correlated with the duration and type of diabetes, coexistent autoimmune disease, and HLA type, Diabetes **26**:138, 1977.
101. Kemp, C.B., et al.: Transplantation of isolated pancreatic islets into the portal vein of diabetic rats, Nature **244**:447,1973.
102. Kilo, C., Vogler, N., and Williamson, J.R.: Muscle capillary basement membrane changes related to aging and to diabetes mellitus, Diabetes **21**:881, 1972.
103. Kimmelstiel, P., and Wilson, C.: Intercapillary lesions in the glomeruli of the kidney, Am. J. Pathol. **12**:83, 1936.
104. Lacy, P.E.: Beta cell secretion—from the standpoint of a pathobiologist, Diabetes **19**:895, 1970.
105. Lacy, P.E.: Endocrine secretory mechanisms, Am. J. Pathol. **79**:170, 1975.
106. Lacy, P.E.: Transplantation of islet cells—isografts and allografts. In Fitzgerald, P.J., and Morrison, A.B., editors: Baltimore, 1980, The Williams & Wilkins Co.
107. Lacy, P.E., Davie, J.M., and Finke, E.H.: Prolongation of islet allograft survival following *in vitro* culture (24° C) and a single injection of ALS, Science **204**:312, 1979.
108. Lacy, P.E., Davie, J.M., and Finke, E.H.: Prolongation of islet xenograft survival without continuous immunosuppression, Science **209**:283, 1980.
109. Lacy, P.E., Davie, J.M., and Finke, E.H.: Transplantation of insulin producing tissue, Am. J. Med. **70**:589, 1981.
110. Lacy, P.E., and Wright, P.H.: Allergic interstitial pancreatitis in rats injected with guinea pig anti-insulin serum, Diabetes **14**:634, 1965.
111. Lazarus, S.S., and Volk, B.W.: The pancreas in human and experimental diabetes, New York, 1962, Grune & Stratton, Inc.
112. Malaisse, W.J.: Insulin secretion: multifactorial regulation for a single process of release, Diabetologia **9**:167, 1973.
113. McDaniel, M.L., et al.: Studies on the site of interaction for ninhydrin, alloxan, and D-glucose in insulin secretion by isolated islets *in vitro*, Endocrinology **105**:1446, 1979.
114. McGavran, M.H., and Hartroft, W.S.: The predilection of pancreatic beta cells for pigment deposition in hemochromatosis and hemosiderosis, Am. J. Pathol. **32**:631, 1956.
115. Nagler, W., and Taylor, H.: Diabetic coma with acute inflammation of islets of Langerhans, J.A.M.A. **184**:723, 1963.
116. Nerup, J., et al.: HLA, islet cell antibodies, and types of diabetes mellitus, Diabetes **27**:247, 1978.
117. Orci, L.: A portrait of the pancreatic B cell, Diabetologia **10**:163, 1974.
118. Oyer, P.E., et al.: Studies on human proinsulin, J. Biol. Chem. **246**:1375, 1971.
119. Schmidt, R.E., Nelson, J.S., and John, E.M., Jr.: Experimental diabetic autonomic neuropathy, Am. J. Pathol. **103**:210, 1981.
120. Silverman, J.L.: Eosinophile infiltration in the pancreas of infants of diabetic mothers, Diabetes **12**:528, 1963.
121. Steiner, D.F., et al.: Insulin biosynthesis: evidence for a precursor, Science **157**:697, 1967.
122. Tattersall, R.B., and Pyke, D.A.: Diabetes in identical twins, Lancet **2**:1120, 1972.
123. Toreson, W.E.: Glycogen infiltration (so-called hydropic degeneration) in the pancreas in human and experimental diabetes mellitus, Am. J. Pathol. **52**:1099, 1968.
124. Williamson, J.R., and Kilo, C.: Current status of capillary basement membrane disease in diabetes mellitus, Diabetes **26**:65, 1977.

Neoplasms of pancreatic islets
B cell tumors

125. Creutzfeldt, W.: Pancreatic endocrine tumors—the riddle of their origin and hormone secretion, Isr. J. Med. Sci. **11**:762, 1975.
126. Creutzfeld, W., et al.: Biochemical and morphological investigations of 30 human insulinomas, Diabetologia **9**:217, 1973.
127. Duff, G.L.: The pathology of islet cell tumors of the pancreas, Am. J. Med. Sci. **203**:437, 1942.
128. Frantz, V.K.: Tumors of islet cells with hyperinsulinism: benign, malignant, and questionable, Ann. Surg. **112**:161, 1940.
129. Howard, J.M., Moss, N.H., and Rhoads, J.E.: Hyperinsulinism and islet cell tumors of the pancreas, Int. Abstr. Surg. **90**:417, 1950.
130. Laidlaw, G.F.: Nesidioblastoma, the islet tumor of the pancreas, Am. J. Pathol. **14**:125, 1938.
131. Sieracki, J., Marshall, R.B., and Horn, R.C., Jr.: Tumors of the pancreatic islets, Cancer **13**:347, 1960.

Glucagonomas, gastrinomas, vipomas, somatostatinomas, and diarrheogenic tumors

132. Bloom, S.R., and Polak, J.M.: Glucagonomas, VIPomas and somatostatinomas, Clin. Endocrinol. Metabol. **9**:285, 1980.
133. Greider, M.H., and McGuigan, J.E.: Cellular localization of gastrin in the human pancreas, Diabetes **20**:389, 1971.
134. Greider, M.H., Rosai, J., and McGuigan, J.E.: The human pancreatic islet cells and their tumors. II. Ulcerogenic and diarrheogenic tumors, Cancer **33**:1423, 1974.
135. Greider, M.H., Steinberg, V., and McGuigan, J.E.: Electron microscopic identification of the gastrin cell of the human antral mucosa by means of immunocytochemistry, Gastroenterology **63**:572, 1972.
136. Heitz, P.U., et al.: Nesidioblastosis: the pathologic basis of persistent hyperinsulinemic hypoglycemia in infants, Diabetes **26**:632, 1977.
137. Krejs, G.J., et al.: Somatostatinoma syndrome, N. Engl. J. Med. **301**:285, 1979.
138. Mallison, C.V., et al.: A glucagonoma syndrome, Lancet **2**:1, 1974.
139. McGavran, M.H., et al.: A glucagon-secreting A cell carcinoma of the pancreas, N. Engl. J. Med. **274**:1408, 1966.
140. McGuigan, J.E., and Trudeau, W.L.: Immunochemical measurement of elevated levels of gastrin in the serum of patients with pancreatic tumors of the Zollinger-Ellison variety, N. Engl. J. Med. **278**:1308, 1968.
141. Zollinger, R.M., and Ellison, E.H.: Primary peptic ulcerations of the jejunum associated with islet cell tumors of the pancreas, Ann. Surg. **142**:709, 1955.

CHAPTER 30 Hemopoietic System: Reticuloendothelial System, Spleen, Lymph Nodes, Bone Marrow, and Blood

ARKADI M. RYWLIN

The cellular elements of the peripheral blood are red blood cells, granulocytes, lymphocytes, monocytes, and platelets. The hemopoietic system includes organs responsible for the formation of circulating blood cells: bone marrow, lymph nodes, and spleen. The thymus, tonsils, and lymphoid collections of the gastrointestinal tract, also responsible for lymphopoiesis, are discussed in other chapters. The reticuloendothelial system qualifies for the hemopoietic system because it is made up primarily of monocytes and their derivatives and interacts closely with lymphocytes in immune reactions.

RETICULOENDOTHELIAL SYSTEM (MONONUCLEAR PHAGOCYTE SYSTEM)[115]

Definition and terminology

The term *reticuloendothelial system* (RES) was coined by Aschoff and Kiyono[7] to cover, by an inclusive term, a system of cells found within and outside of organs and characterized functionally by phagocytosis and staining by vital dyes. Only cells that showed avidity for the vital dyes were included in the RES (see following outline).[197] Polymorphonuclear leukocytes were excluded because they did not take up carmine in solutions, even though they did phagocytose carmine granules. The endothelial cells of most of the blood and lymph vessels and the fibroblasts were not included because they took the dye only when vital staining had been carried to an advanced degree. Aschoff named phagocytic cells in direct contact with blood or lymph reticuloendothelia. Reticulum cells and reticuloendothelia share both the property of phagocytosis and that of forming argyrophilic fibers.[6] The following are cellular components of RES:

A. Intravascular cells
   1. Monocytes
   2. Endothelial cells
      a. Liver capillaries—Kupffer cells
      b. Lymph node sinuses
      c. Splenic sinuses
      d. Adrenal capillaries
      e. Hypophyseal capillaries

B. Extravascular cells
   1. Reticulum cells—fixed macrophages, related to reticulin fibers
   2. Histiocytes—wandering macrophages of connective tissue

Although there is general agreement that it is important to individualize a system of cells possessing the ability to phagocytose particulate material and colloidal solutions, there continues to be disagreement as to what cells should belong to this sytem and what the system should be named. Recently the term *mononuclear phagocyte system* has been introduced to include all avidly phagocytic mononuclear cells and their precursors. The microglia of the central nervous system, alveolar macrophages, serous membrane macrophages, and epidermal Langerhans cells are all included in this system.[115] There is also controversy about the origin and nomenclature of mononuclear phagocytic cells. Gall[73] found the term "reticulum cell" inexact and prefers to use "histiocyte" instead. "Histiocyte" was introduced by Aschoff and Kiyono[7] to denote the tissue origin of the mobile tissue macrophage, which was believed by Metchnikoff to be derived from the peripheral blood.[6] However, recent evidence shows that tissue macrophages are derived from blood monocytes originating in the bone marrow.[238] This consideration renders the term "histiocyte" somewhat inappropriate. For this reason many investigators prefer Metchnikoff's term "macrophage."

What seems reasonably well established is that there are fixed and mobile macrophages. The fixed macrophages are related to reticulin fibers and can be called reticulum cells. The reticulum cells and reticulin fibers form a fine, three-dimensional meshwork and constitute supporting elements of lymphoid tissue. The lymphoid tissue with its cellular and fibrous supporting meshwork is often called lymphoreticular tissue. The mobile tissue macrophages may be called histiocytes. Since in fixed, stained sections we cannot be sure whether a cell is mobile or fixed, the terms *reticulum cell* and *histiocyte* are often interchanged. These cells can be called macrophages, though some pathologists reserve this term for cells that have actually phagocytosed a substance, rather than for cells that are capable of phagocytosis.

Function

Phagocytosis is part of a broader concept—endocytosis, the common denominator of cells belonging to the RES. Endocytosis encompasses phagocytosis and pinocytosis. Phagocytosis is engulfment of particles visible by the light microscope. It is composed of two steps: (1) attachment of a particle to the cell membrane, and (2) ingestion or particle interiorization. Pinocytosis describes the ingestion of sub-light-microscopic particles, colloidal solutions, and fluid droplets. In both phagocytosis and pinocytosis there is invagination of the portions of the plasma membrane, resulting in phagocytic or pinocytic vesicles. Endocytosis requires energy, which is derived from anaerobic glycosis or oxidative phosphorylation or both.[157] Following endocytosis, the endocytic vesicles move away from the plasma membrane and fuse with lysosomes containing different enzymes. This fusion results in phagolysosomes (phagosomes) and pinolysosomes (pinosomes) in which the engulfed material is enzymatically degraded.

Even though endocytosis is the most fundamental property of the mononuclear phagocytic system, it has become clear in recent years that macrophages have an important secretory activity.[150] The secretory products of mononuclear phagocytes include enzymes, complement components, binding proteins (such as fibronectins), nucleosides and metabolites, pyrogens, reactive metabolites of oxygen, bioactive lipids (such as prostaglandin E_2 and thromboxane), chemotactic factor for neutrophils, factors promoting replication of erythroid, myeloid, and lymphoid cells, and factors inhibiting replication of tumor cells and viruses.

Pathophysiology

The physiology and pathophysiology of the RES are based on its functions of endocytosis and secretion. Because of these functions the RES is involved in the storage and clearance of a variety of metabolites, pigments, bacteria, fungi, and parasites. Pathogens that parasitize histiocytes and replicate within them include *Listeria*, *Salmonella*, *Brucella*, *Mycobacterium*, *Chlamydia*, *Rickettsia*, *Leishmania*, *Toxoplasma*, *Trypanosoma*, and *Legionella pneumophilia*. The RES is also involved in immune and inflammatory reactions.

Phagocytosis, storage, and clearance

Because of its phagocytic function the RES plays an important role in the removal of senescent or damaged cells and cell debris. When an erythrocyte is "worn out" at the end of its normal life span of about 120 days, it is disposed of by the phagocytic cells of the reticuloendothelial system. Since there are many phagocytes in the spleen and also in the liver, most of the phagocytic activity occurs in these organs. When disintegrating erythrocytes are removed from the blood by phagocytic cells in the spleen, the hemoglobin is broken down into the pigment moiety (bilirubin), the protein moiety (globin), and iron (Fig. 30-1).

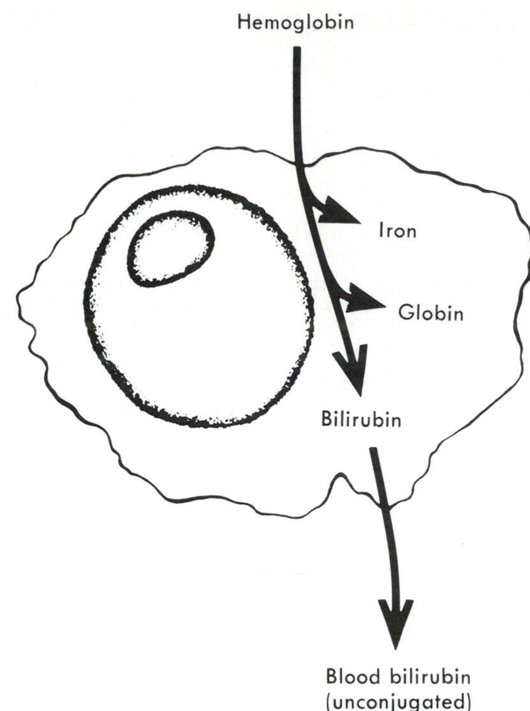

Fig. 30-1. Breakdown of hemoglobin within phagocytic reticuloendothelial cell (splenic macrophage, Kupffer cell in liver, alveolar macrophage of lung, and so on). Hemoglobin iron in form of hemosiderin is stored in phagocyte to various degrees, depending on body's need for iron, and is in equilibrium with plasma iron pool. Globin passes into plasma protein pool, whereas unconjugated bilirubin liberated into blood is cleared and conjugated in parenchymal cells of liver.

Macrophages are also involved in the debridement of wounds and possibly in the remodeling of tissues during embryogenesis.[38] When phagocytosed material accumulates in the histiocytes more rapidly than it can be catabolized or excreted morphologically, abnormal cells such as foam cells, Gaucher cells, and ceroid-containing histiocytes (sea-blue histiocytes) are produced. Such cells are often referred to as storage cells, and the diseases in which they occur are called storage diseases (see following discussion).

The RES also performs the phagocytic clearance of inert and metabolized foreign colloidal and particulate matter from the blood. In addition to its involvement in the metabolism of iron and bilirubin, the RES participates in lipid and protein metabolism.[208] It is also involved in the clearance of certain drugs, steroids, endotoxins, and microaggregates of fibrin.[208]

Role in immune reactions

The RES plays a major role in immune processes. It is the interaction between macrophages and lymphocytes that constitutes the cornerstone of immune responses. Although much knowledge in this field has been acquired in recent years, many unanswered questions remain.

Immune reactions can be divided into two types: (1) humoral immunity related to B lymphocytes (p. 453), associated with circulating immunoglobulins responsible for the immediate type of skin reactions and the Arthus phenomenon, and (2) cell-bound immunity depending on T lymphocytes (p. 453), associated with the delayed type of skin reaction and graft rejection.

In humoral immunity the macrophage plays a dual role: it protects the host against an overload of antigens by catabolizing them, and it presents the lymphocytes with antigenic material, which stimulates them to produce immunoglobulins. How the macrophage decides which antigen will be catabolized and which will be presented to lymphocytes is unknown.

In cell-bound immunity the macrophage becomes the effector cell. This is well illustrated by the Prausnitz-Küstner phenomenon in which a nonhypersensitive recipient is rendered hypersensitive by the injection of lymphocytes from a sensitized individual. These sensitized donor lymphocytes, when stimulated by the appropriate antigen, attract the recipient's macrophages with a resultant granulomatous inflammation characteristic of delayed hypersensitivity. The sensitized lymphocytes elaborate factors that attract monocytes (macrophages), inhibit their migration (migration inhibitory factor), and cause monocytic proliferation (blastogenic factor).[135]

Role in inflammation and infection

The RES responds to an inflammatory stimulus by a proliferation of histiocytes, resulting in the familiar granulomatous inflammation. Granulomatous inflammation is best defined as an inflammatory infiltrate with a predominance of histiocytes. The latter may proliferate diffusely in sheets (for example, lepromatous leprosy, leishmaniasis, histoplasmosis) or form fairly discrete nodules (sarcoidal or tuberculoid inflammation). Histiocytes are referred to as epithelioid cells when they resemble epithelial cells because they touch each other and possess abundant cytoplasm. The formation of giant cells (multinucleated cells) is one of the characteristics of histiocytes. Granulomatous inflammation is seen under many different circumstances, including acute bacterial infections such as typhoid fever (Mallory or Rindfleisch cells), listeriosis, and chronic mycobacterial and fungal diseases.

The mechanisms of histiocyte antimicrobial activity have been explored extensively in recent years. Human blood monocytes are similar to granulocytes in many aspects of their phagocytic behavior. Ingestion of bacteria induces increased oxygen consumption and production of hydrogen peroxide, superoxide, and chemiluminescent products, and stimulates hexose monophosphate shunt activity.[38] Among the oxygen-independent mechanisms of macrophage antimicrobial activity is rapid acidification of the phagocytic vacuoles to a pH of about 4.5 after lysosomal fusion.[150]

Proliferative disorders of the RES

Proliferation of histiocytes (macrophages, reticulum cells, monocytes) may be localized, multicentric, or systemic. It may be reactive (inflammatory) or neoplastic. The following is a classification of proliferative disorders of histiocytes*:

A. Localized
  1. Reactive or inflammatory: granulomatous inflammation
  2. Neoplastic
    a. Benign, such as fibrous histiocytoma, reticulohistiocytic granuloma
    b. Malignant, such as malignant fibrous histiocytoma, histiocytic sarcoma
  3. Uncertain whether reactive or neoplastic, such as juvenile xanthogranuloma, xanthomas

B. Multicentric or generalized
  1. Reactive or inflammatory, such as generalized miliary tuberculosis, sarcoidosis
  2. Neoplastic
    a. Eosinophilic granuloma, Hand-Schüller-Christian disease
    b. Reticulum cell sarcoma[121]
    c. Multicentric reticulohistiocytosis[13,232]
  3. Uncertain whether reactive or neoplastic: sinus histiocytosis with massive lymphadenopathy

C. Systemic (reticulosis, histiocytosis, reticuloendotheliosis)
  1. Reactive
    a. Storage diseases: Gaucher's disease, Nieman-Pick disease, ceroid histiocytosis
    b. Virus-associated hemophagocytic syndrome[188]
  2. Neoplastic
    a. Letterer-Siwe disease
    b. Malignant histiocytosis (histiocytic medullary reticulosis)
    c. Leukemic reticuloses
      (1) Monocytic leukemia
      (2) Leukemic reticuloendotheliosis (hairy cell leukemia)

The localized neoplastic proliferations of the RES are discussed under soft tissues and skin.

Multicentric or generalized proliferative disorders are characterized by several or many lesions without

*Modified from Rywlin, A.: Histopathology of the bone marrow, Boston, 1976, Little, Brown & Co., p. 114.

involvement of the entire RES. Sarcoidosis is a good example of a multicentric or generalized inflammatory reaction of the RES.

Neoplastic multicentric proliferative disorders are again characterized by multiple lesions without involvement of the entire RES. In a multicentric proliferative disorder such as reticulum cell sarcoma,[121] the patient has a dominant mass rather than the symmetric lymphadenopathy and hepatosplenomegaly characteristic of systemic proliferation. When a reticulum cell sarcoma generalizes, lesions appear away from the main mass. There is debate as to whether this generalization represents autochthonous multicentricity or metastatization. The secondary tumor nodules, whether autochthonous or metastatic, are usually sufficiently large to be visible with the naked eye. This contrasts with what is seen in the systemic proliferative disorders, where the proliferation of the RE cells is diffuse, causing enlargement of the liver and spleen without macroscopically visible nodules.

The hemopoietic system and RES are unique in exhibiting a systemic proliferation of reticuloendothelial cells. Systemic proliferation differs from multicentric proliferation in that all the cells of the system participate. This results in symmetric enlargement of lymph nodes, liver, and spleen. The proliferating cells are also found in the bone marrow. Systemic proliferation of the reticuloendothelial cells is often referred to as reticulosis, histiocytosis, or reticuloendotheliosis depending on the terminology.

A systemic proliferation may be reactive such as seen in the storage diseases or it may be neoplastic. A reactive systemic proliferation of histiocytes is seen in response to the accumulation of a catabolic product, which occurs because the patient is deficient in a specific enzyme necessary for the further degradation of the metabolite. Thus in Gaucher's disease the proliferated macrophages contain ceramide glucoside (glucocerebroside) because the patient is deficient in beta-glucosidase.

In neoplastic systemic proliferations the proliferating cells may spill over into the peripheral blood giving rise to a leukemia.

Storage diseases

In the storage diseases there is a systemic proliferation of histiocytes storing phagocytosed material. The accumulated material cannot be degraded and cleared because the histiocytes lack a specific enzyme. The proliferation of histiocytes causes an enlargement of organs housing the RES: spleen, liver, and lymph nodes. The "storage cells" proliferate also in the bone marrow, where they may displace hemopoietic cells, fat cells, and bone. We will discuss only storage diseases involving primarily the RES: Gaucher's disease, Niemann-Pick disease, and ceroid histiocytosis. The RES is involved to a lesser degree in other sphingolipidoses, mucopolysaccharidoses, and mucolipidoses.[224]

Gaucher's disease. Gaucher's disease is characterized by a benign systemic proliferation of histiocytes, whose cytoplasm is filled with a glucocerebroside (ceramide-glucose).[24] Clinically, there is a wide spectrum of severity, with some patients dying of the disease by their third decade and others leading relatively symptom-free lives for seven or eight decades.[168]

The dominant clinical features of Gaucher's disease are splenomegaly, hepatomegaly, erosion of cortices of the long bones, and generally mild anemia, leukopenia, and thrombocytopenia. Infantile, juvenile, and adult forms of Gaucher's disease are recognized.[23] Gaucher's disease is the result of a deficiency of beta-glucocerebrosidase, a catabolic enzyme required for the hydrolysis of the beta-glucosidic bond of glucocerebroside.

The accumulating glucocerebroside is a derivative of sphingosine to which a long-chain fatty acid is joined through an amide bond to the nitrogen atom on C-2. This *N*-acylsphingosine complex is called ceramide and is common to all the sphingolipids that accumulate in sphingolipidoses. In glucocerebroside a single molecule of glucose is joined by a beta-glycosidic bond to C-1 of ceramide. The major precursors of the glucocerebroside that accumulates in the histiocytes appear to be glycolipids from senescent red and white blood cells. Gaucher's disease is most prevalent in Ashkenazi Jews.

The spleen is greatly enlarged. The organ is firm, and the cut surface is red-gray and greasy. Microscopically the splenic cords and sinusoids show a diffuse and nodular infiltration with Gaucher's cells (Fig. 30-2). These are histiocytes whose cytoplasm is engorged with glucocerebroside (Fig. 30-3). These histiocytes are also present in the medullary portions of the lymph nodes, in sinusoids of the liver, and in the bone marrow. Gaucher's cells measure 20 to 80 μm, have a relatively small nucleus, and have a cytoplasm made up of a faintly eosinophilic, striated material often containing vacuoles. The cytoplasm is periodic acid–Schiff positive and shows autofluorescence. With the Prussian blue reaction for iron, the cytoplasm frequently exhibits a diffuse, pale blue hue caused by ferritin. Acid phosphatase is readily demonstrated in Gaucher cells using phenylphosphate substrates.[236] Acid phosphatase is found in all histiocytes but not to the extent that it is present in Gaucher's cells.

Gaucher's cells may be associated with an increased number of plasma cells, which may account for the increased occurrence of monoclonal gammopathies in Gaucher's disease.[174] Ultrastructural studies of Gaucher's cells reveal spindle- or rod-shaped membrane-bound cytoplasmic inclusions measuring 0.6 to 4 μm in diameter (Fig. 30-4). Gaucher-like cells have been described in chronic granulocytic leukemia, thalassemia, and hereditary dyserythropoietic anemia.[117] By light

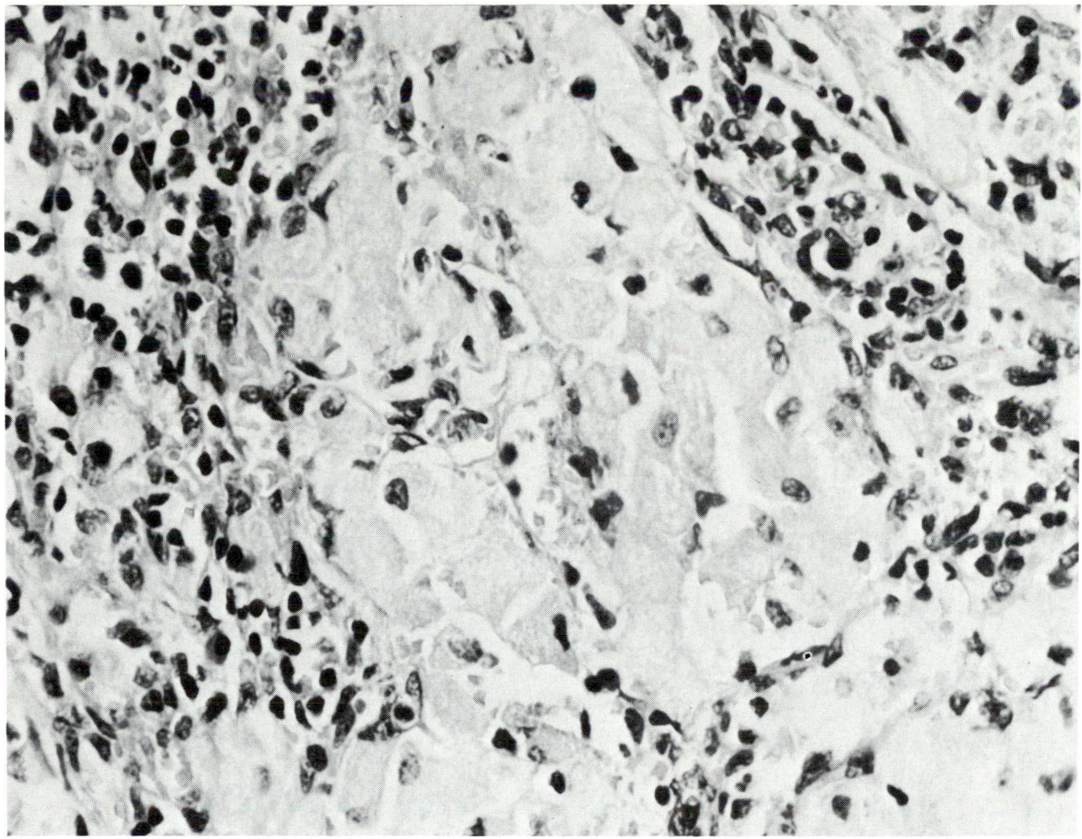

Fig. 30-2. Spleen in Gaucher's disease. Note nodule of Gaucher cells. (Hematoxylin and eosin; 250×.)

microscopy the Gaucher-like cells appear identical to true Gaucher's cells but are far less numerous. Ultrastructurally, significant differences have been reported between Gaucher-like and true Gaucher's cells.[117] It may be that the Gaucher-like cells result from the overtaxation of a normal enzyme system by an increased amount of globoside derived from an accelerated cellular destruction.

Niemann-Pick disease. Niemann-Pick disease classically affects infants and is characterized by hepatosplenomegaly, cachexia, and impaired mental development. Five types of the disease are distinguished depending on age of onset, degree of central nervous system involvement, and rapidity of progression.[69] The disease is characterized by the accumulation of sphingomyelin in histiocytes. Sphingomyelin is a ceramide derivative containing phosphorylcholine linked to C-1 of ceramide. The accumulating sphingomyelin may be derived from cell membranes, subcellular organelles of senescent cells, and myelin sheaths. In two of the types of Niemann-Pick disease the patients lack sphingomyelinase. In the other types the cause of the sphingomyelin accumulation is unknown.[69]

Histiocytes containing sphingomyelin appear as foam

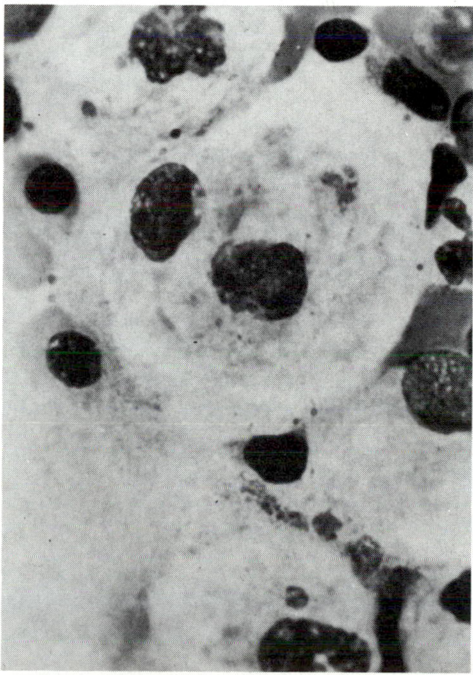

Fig. 30-3. Gaucher cell. (Spleen imprint; Wright's stain; 950×; from Miale, J.B.: Laboratory medicine—hematology, ed. 6, St. Louis, 1982, The C.V. Mosby Co.)

cells in paraffin-embedded, hematoxylin-and-eosin-stained sections. These cells are scattered throughout the spleen, bone marrow, liver, lymph nodes, and lungs. Hepatocytes and Kupffer cells are involved. The foam cells seen in Niemann-Pick disease may have a pale yellow to brown-yellow hue because of the presence of granules of ceroid. When stained with the Giemsa stain, these ceroid-containing histiocytes appear sea-blue and have been called sea-blue histiocytes.[202,211] The sphingomyelin that accumulates in the histiocytes is easily removed by fixation and embedding of tissues. Luxol fast blue, which stains phospholipids, should be applied to unfixed, frozen sections. Baker's acid hematin for phospholipids and the Schultz reaction for cholesterol are also positive. Ultrastructurally, concentrically laminated, myelin-like figures are seen in addition to granular lipid bodies.

Unlike the Gaucher's cell, the foam cell of Niemann-Pick disease is not diagnostic of this condition. A diagnosis of Niemann-Pick disease should not be based exclusively on morphologic and histochemical considerations. There is no stain that is pathognomonic for sphingomyelin. Chemical and enzymatic analyses should be performed to confirm the diagnosis.

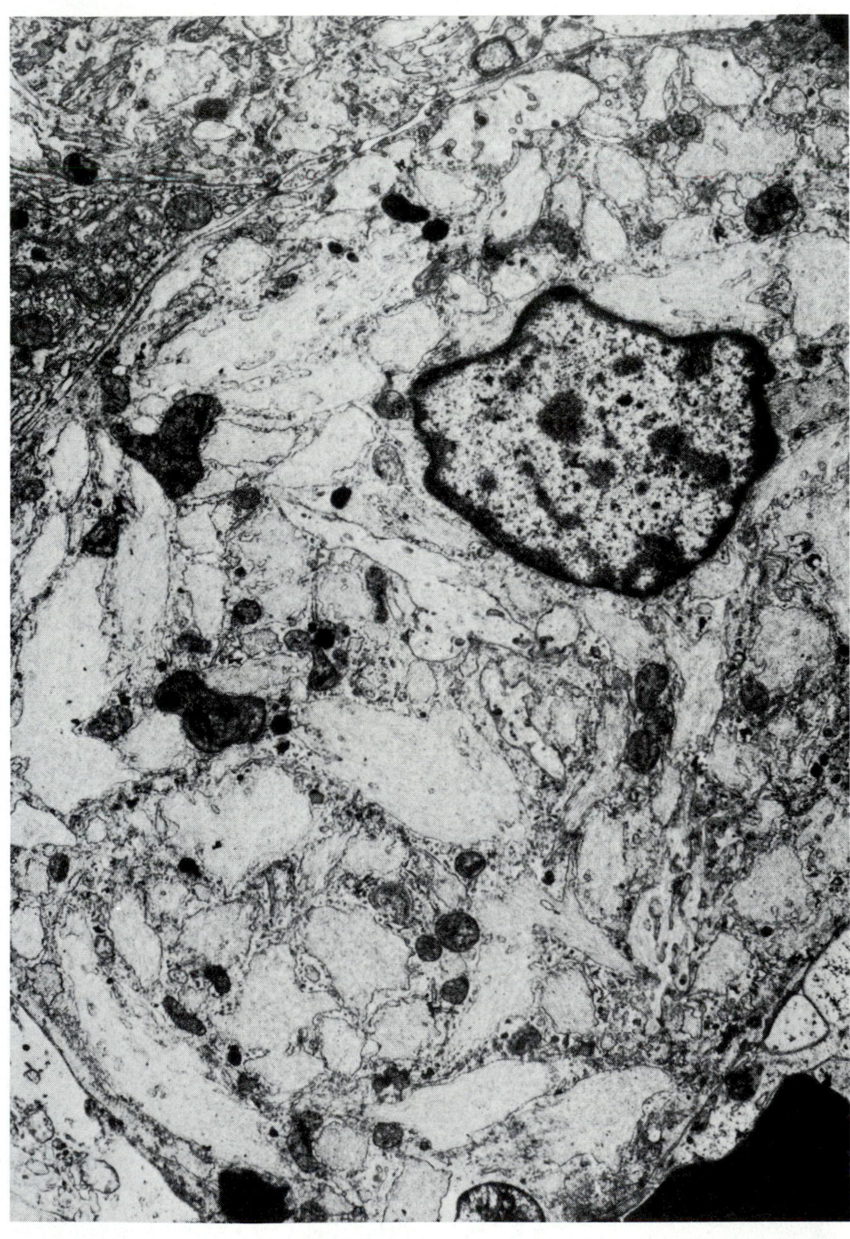

Fig. 30-4. Gaucher cell as seen by electron microscopy. Nucleus is irregular body in upper right area. Remainder is cytoplasm that contains lipid. (From Miale, J.B.: Laboratory medicine—hematology, ed. 6, St. Louis, 1982, The C.V. Mosby Co.)

Ceroid histiocytosis of spleen and bone marrow (syndrome of the sea-blue histiocyte). In 1970 Silverstein and associates[217] described the "syndrome of the sea-blue histiocyte," characterized by a relatively benign course, splenomegaly, thrombocytopenia, and the presence of sea-blue histiocytes in the bone marrow. Rywlin and coworkers[202,203] showed that the sea-blue granules observed in bone marrow smears with the Giemsa-Wright stains were made up of ceroid. Ceroid is a pale yellow to dark brown pigment that results from the peroxidation and polymerization of unsaturated lipids.[87] Ceroid is defined by its insolubility in hydrocarbon lipid solvents and its reactivity with fat stains such as Oil red O and Sudan black. The other histochemical reactions develop as the pigment ages: autofluorescence first, followed by diastase-resistant periodic acid–Schiff positivity and acid fastness.[87] Ceroid and lipofuscin share many physical and histochemical characteristics. Whether they are identical is still debated. At the present time lipofuscin seems the preferred term for naturally occurring, age-related pigment, whereas ceroid is used for a similar pigment seen in a variety of pathologic conditions. Ceroid-containing histiocytes (sea-blue histiocytes, blue-pigment macrophages) may be seen in the spleen and bone marrow in many different conditions (see list in the following and Fig. 30-5). The histiocytes may contain fat vacuoles only (foam cells), fat vacuoles and ceroid granules, or ceroid granules only. Before a diagnosis of idiopathic ceroid histiocytosis of the spleen and bone marrow can be made, all the known diseases that can give sea-blue histiocytes have to be eliminated by careful history and laboratory tests. Thus patients have to be tested for sphingomyelinase deficiency (to check for Niemann-Pick disease), for hyperlipoproteinemia, and for lecithin:cholesterol acyltransferase deficiency[95] before a diagnosis of idiopathic ceroid histiocytosis can be accepted. It is doubtful whether idiopathic ceroid histiocytosis exists. The following are conditions with ceroid-containing histiocytes in spleen or bone marrow*:

- Batten's disease
- Niemann-Pick disease
- Tay-Sachs disease
- Adult lipidosis resembling Niemann-Pick disease
- Wolman's disease
- Ceroid-storage disease
- Chronic granulomatous disease of childhood
- Familial lipochrome histiocytosis
- Ceroid histiocytosis of spleen with rupture in a vegetarian
- Vascular pseudohemophilia associated with ceroid pigmentophagia in albinos
- Hyperlipoproteinemia
- Ceroid histiocytosis of spleen and bone marrow in idiopathic thrombocytopenic purpura
- Syndrome of the sea-blue histiocyte (idiopathic ceroid histiocytosis of spleen and marrow)
- Familial lecithin:cholesterol acyltransferase deficiency
- Chronic granulocytic leukemia
- Sickle cell anemia
- Cirrhosis of the liver

Other proliferative disorders of the RES

Histiocytosis X (eosinophilic granuloma, Hand-Schüller-Christian disease, and Letterer-Siwe disease). Lichtenstein[123] views eosinophilic granuloma of bone, Hand-Schüller-Christian disease, and Letterer-Siwe disease as related manifestations of a single nosologic entity, which he named histiocytosis X. Other authors[124,159]

*Modified from Rywlin, A.M., and Ortega, R.S.: Am. J. Clin. Pathol. **57**:457, 1972.

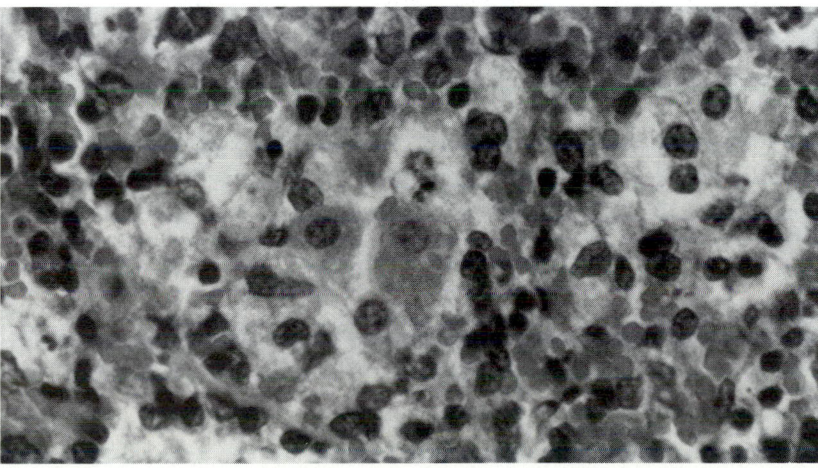

Fig. 30-5. Ceroid containing histiocytes in the spleen of patient with hyperlipoproteinemia. Note large cells with abundant granular cytoplasm. (Hematoxylin and eosin; high power.)

consider Hand-Schüller-Christian disease to be a multifocal or systemic variant of eosinophilic granuloma, unrelated to Letterer-Siwe disease. Eosinophilic xanthomatous granulomatosis has been proposed as a better term for these two entities.[159] The final word on the exact relationship of these disorders is not yet available.

The term *eosinophilic granuloma* is used for frequently solitary, bone-destroying lesions usually occurring in children. Histologically the lesion is characterized by sheets of well-differentiated histiocytes with interspersed eosinophils. The histiocytes contain an abundant eosinophilic cytoplasm.

Hand-Schüller-Christian disease consists of a multifocal or systemic proliferation of mature histiocytes with abundant cytoplasm and varying amounts of intracytoplasmic lipids consisting of cholesterol, cholesterol esters, and neutral fats (Fig. 30-6). The accumulation of intracellular lipid is not related to a primary derangement of lipid metabolism but appears to be attributable to phagocytosed lipids normally present in blood and tissues. A characteristic triad that prompts the suspicion of Hand-Schüller-Christian disease consists of punched-out bone lesions, exophthalmos, and diabetes insipidus. The spleen may be involved in a diffuse or nodular fashion. The infiltrates often have a yellow hue. Histologically there are sheets of mature histiocytes with varying numbers of foam cells, eosinophils, and fibroblasts.

The histiocytic cells have abundant cytoplasm with empty-appearing nuclei, which are often grooved. Nodules of histiocytes are separated by broad bands of fibrous tissue containing a few polymorphonuclear leukocytes and plasma cells.

We emphasize again that foam cells by themselves are not diagnostic of Hand-Schüller-Christian disease and can be seen with or without ceroid-containing histiocytes in many different conditions. Transitions between eosinophilic granuloma and Hand-Schüller-Christian disease have been observed, and some authors believe that there is no justification for using the term "Hand-Schüller-Christian disease" for multifocal eosinophilic granuloma.[124]

Letterer-Siwe disease is defined by Rappaport[178] as an acute or subacute progressive systemic proliferation of differentiated histiocytes. The disease affects infants and rarely develops in children more than 3 years of age. It is characterized by fever, prominent skin rash, and varying

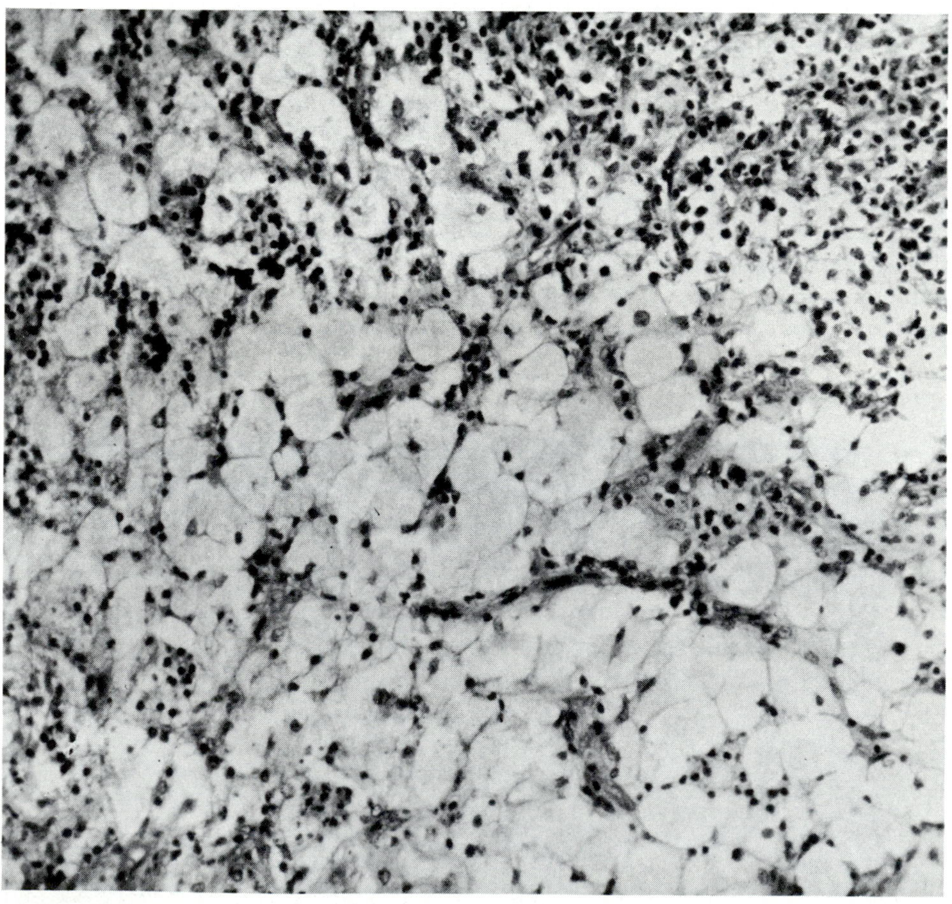

Fig. 30-6. Spleen in Hand-Schüller-Christian disease. (Hematoxylin and eosin; 250×.)

degrees of lymphadenopathy and hepatosplenomegaly. Authors who consider Letterer-Siwe disease to be distinct from Hand-Schüller-Christian disease point to the rapid course, the prominent involvement of the skin, and the lack of lipids in the diffusely proliferating histiocytes.[159] Those who view these diseases as part of a spectrum call attention to cases of Letterer-Siwe disease with a more chronic course and with partial lipidization of proliferating histiocytes.[178] The spleen in Letterer-Siwe disease may be greatly enlarged (Fig. 30-7, *A*). Foci of necrosis may be present. Microscopically there is a diffuse proliferation of differentiated histiocytes with a well-defined eosinophilic cytoplasm (Fig. 30-7, *B*). Mitoses are rare. Multinucleated cells are frequent. Phagocytosis by the proliferating histiocytes is not a prominent feature, at least in the early stages.

An additional argument in favor of a relationship among these three diseases is the presence of a distinctive ultrastructural, rod-shaped inclusion (Birbeck granule) in the cytoplasm of histiocytes in histiocytosis X. These inclusions are identical to those observed in the Langerhans cells of the epidermis.[233]

In a study of 51 children with histiocytosis X, Newton and Hamoudi[156] were able to distinguish two distinct groups. Seven children had a rapidly progressive fatal disease, with diffuse proliferation of large, pale histiocytes without lipidization of the cytoplasm. Eosinophils, giant cells, necrosis, and fibrosis were not evident. The remaining 44 children had a benign course with focal or multifocal involvement of the RES and histologic findings identical with those in Hand-Schüller-Christian disease. Langerhans cell granules were found only in patients who had a benign clinical course.

At the present time it is best to view eosinophilic granuloma and Hand-Schüller-Christian disease as parts of a spectrum of a single disease. Letterer-Siwe disease, although well defined clinically as a rapidly progressive, fatal disease of young children with diffuse involvement of the RES and the skin with proliferating, well-differentiated histiocytes, must be distinguished from monocytic leukemia, infectious diseases caused by intracellular mycobacteria, and malignant histiocytosis.

Histiocytosis X may also involve primarily the lymph nodes.[147,251] In such instances the differential diagnosis includes diseases involving the medullary areas of the lymph nodes, such as sinus histiocytosis with massive lymphadenopathy.

The introduction of the term "Langerhans cell granulomatosis"[234] as a substitute for histiocytosis X seems premature, since Langerhans cell granules cannot be found in all instances of this disease.

Virus-associated hemophagocytic syndrome. The symptoms of virus-associated hemophagocytic syndrome (VAHS)[140,188] are fever, pulmonary infiltrates, hepatosplenomegaly, generalized lymphadenopathy, varying cytopenias in the peripheral blood, abnormal liver function tests, and disseminated intravascular coagulation. VAHS is seen more frequently in renal transplant or immunosuppressed patients. There is often a history of a viral-like illness preceding VAHS by 2 to 6 weeks. VAHS is a nonneoplastic, potentially reversible process.[140]

Lymph nodes are enlarged and show small lymphoid follicles without germinal centers in the cortex. There is depletion of lymphocytes in the paracortical and medullary areas. At the periphery of the lymphoid follicles there is abundant nuclear debris, some lying free and some within the cytoplasm of proliferating histiocytes. Phagocytosis of red blood cells is variable. The spleen is enlarged and shows varying degrees of follicular destruction. The malpighian follicles are surrounded by a zone of nuclear debris and a concentric layer of eosinophilic material, probably representing fibrin (Fig. 30-8). Proliferating histiocytes exhibit extensive phagocytosis of nuclear debris. The histiocytic nuclei do not show significant atypia. The bone marrow shows varying degrees of histiocytic hyperplasia with prominent phagocytosis of red cells, platelets, and nucleated hemopoietic cells.

VAHS resembles familial hemophagocytic reticulosis,[61] familial erythrophagocytic lymphohistiocytosis,[167] and malignant histiocytosis. In malignant histiocytosis the histiocytic nuclei are markedly atypical.

Multicentric reticulohistiocytosis. Multicentric releculohistiocytosis (MRH) is a rare disease characterized clinically by polyarthritis, mucocutaneous nodules, fever, anemia, weight loss, and pleurisy.[13,232] An increased incidence of positive tuberculin skin tests and perhaps active tuberculosis may be seen.[13,78]

Histologically the lesions are composed of sheets of large mononucleated histiocytes, whose cytoplasm has a ground-glass appearance. Histochemically the cytoplasm contains a periodic acid–Schiff–positive, diastase-resistant material and exhibits acid phosphatase activity.

Malignant histiocytosis. Malignant histiocytosis (MH) is a usually rapidly fatal disease characterized by fever, weight loss, generalized lymphadenopathy, hepatosplenomegaly, jaundice, and pancytopenia. Occasionally the disease may be seen in asymptomatic patients who first show signs of splenomegaly.[239] The term was introduced by Rappaport, who described the disorder as a "systemic, progressive, invasive proliferation of morphologically atypical histiocytes and of their precursors."[178] This disease is also known as histiocytic medullary reticulosis, malignant reticulosis, and aleukemic reticulosis.[33] The disease may occur at all ages; men are affected more frequently than women. In one series of 24 patients the age range was from 3 to 62 years.[33] MH may occur in childhood and, in contrast to Letterer-Siwe disease, the patients are usually over 3 years of age.[257]

The spleen is greatly enlarged, and on cut section it shows vague, ill-defined bulging lesions. Discrete tumor

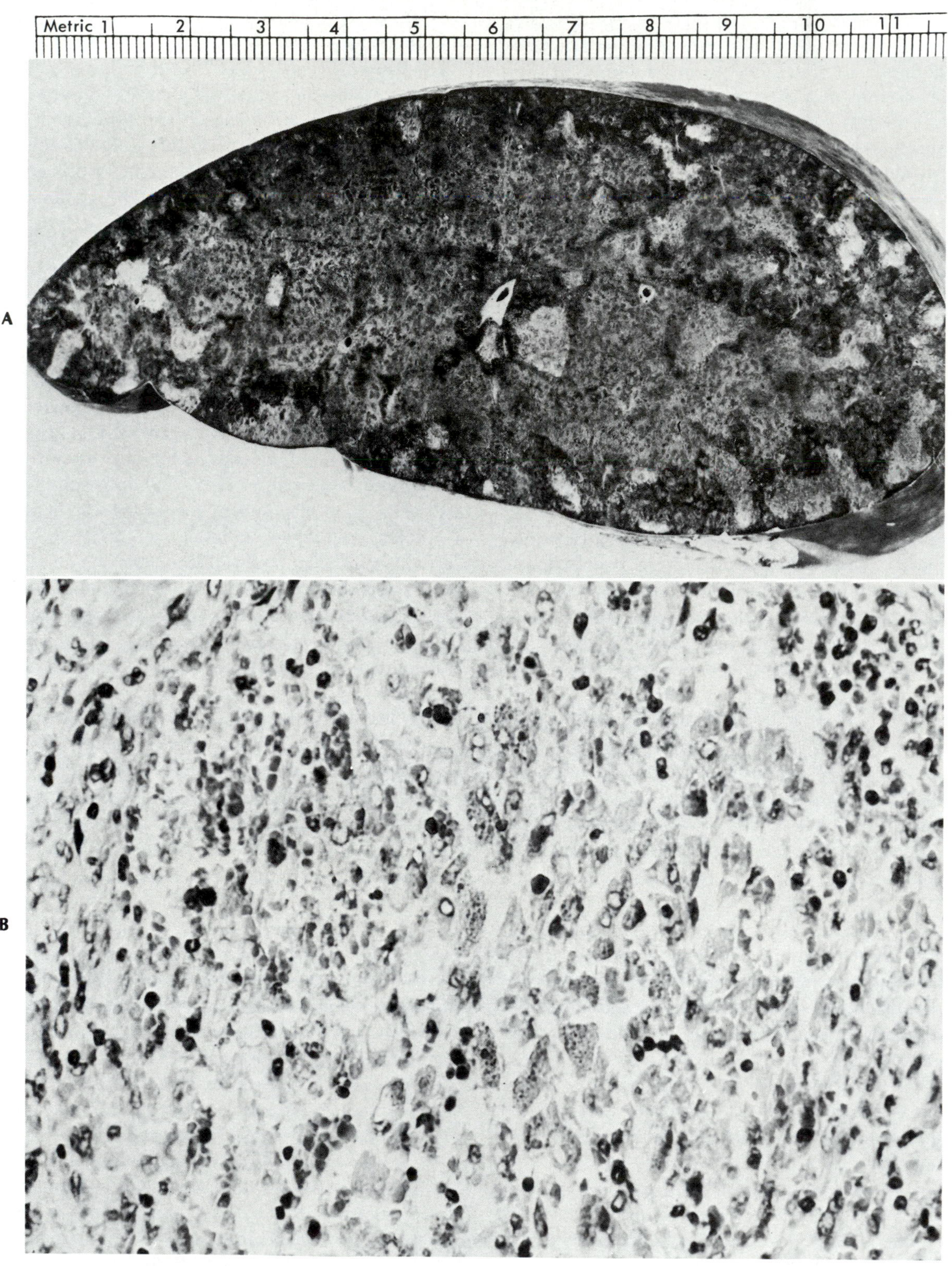

Fig. 30-7. Spleen in Letterer-Siwe disease. **A,** Gross appearance. **B,** Paraffin section. (**B,** Hematoxylin and eosin; 250×.)

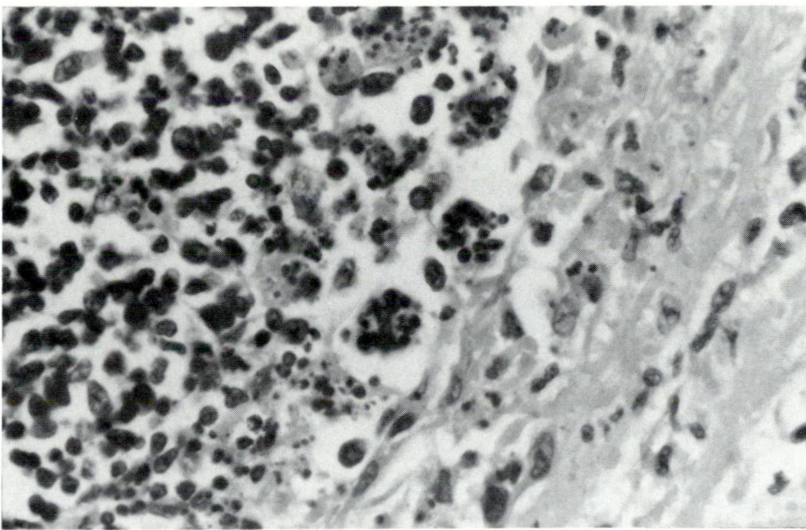

Fig. 30-8. Virus-associated hemophagocytic syndrome. Malpighian follicle with nuclear debris is at its periphery, some of it phagocytosed and a concentric layer of eosinophilic material probably representing fibrin. (Hematoxylin and eosin; high power.)

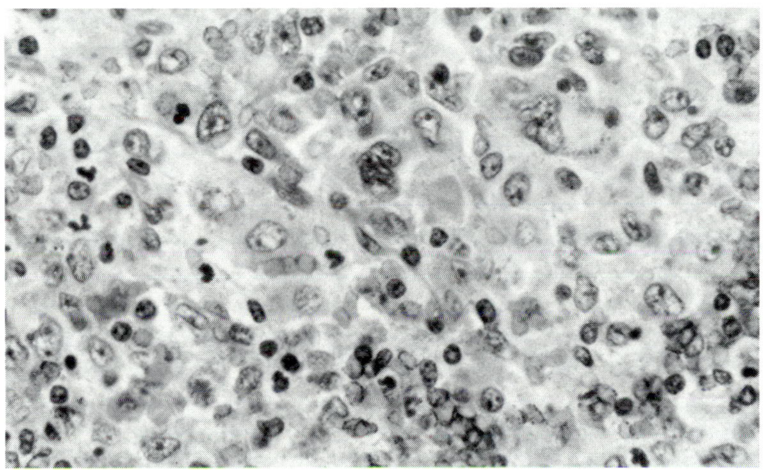

Fig. 30-9. Malignant histiocytosis. Spleen is infiltrated by large cells with atypical nuclei. Note some multinucleated cells and prominent nucleoli. (Hematoxylin and eosin; high power.)

nodules are not seen, so the pattern resembles leukemia rather than lymphoma.[246] Microscopically there is extensive infiltration of the red pulp and to a lesser extent of malpighian follicles, with histiocytes showing varying degrees of atypia (Fig. 30-9). Phagocytosis of red cells, white cells, platelets, and cellular debris can often be demonstrated but does not have to be prominent. Hemosiderin may be abundant. Multinucleated cells, some resembling Reed-Sternberg cells, may be seen. The lymph nodes are diffusely enlarged, and their normal architecture is attenuated or destroyed. In some areas the primary involvement of the sinusoids by the malignant histiocytes can be demonstrated. Plasma cells are almost always present and may be numerous. There may be a sprinkling of eosinophils. Phagocytosis may not be striking and is easier to demonstrate in imprints than in sections of lymph nodes.[189,246] The neoplastic cells may contain lipid inclusions mimicking signet-ring cells. The histiocytic nature of the neoplastic cells can be ascertained by diffuse cytoplasmic staining with the nonspecific esterase and acid phosphatase reactions as well as by ultrastructural studies.[189] Atypical histiocytes can usually be demonstrated in the bone marrow. Occasionally poorly circumscribed small nodules or sheets of malignant histiocytes are seen.[189] Soft tissue masses may develop in the course of the disease.[246] When the skin is involved, the infiltrate is perivascular and periadnexal, with more massive involvement of the lower portion of

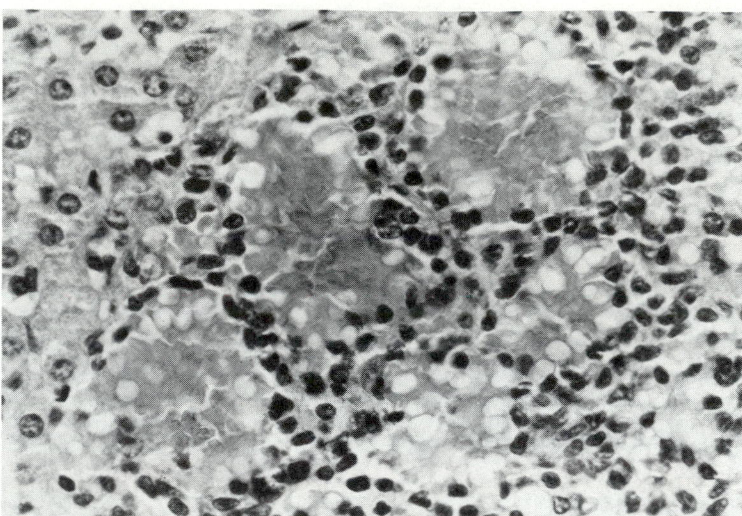

Fig. 30-10. Hairy cell leukemia. Liver with portal infiltrates. Pseudosinusoid contains red blood cells and is lined by neoplastic cells. (Hematoxylin and eosin; high power.)

the dermis and occasionally prominent infiltration of the subcutaneous fat. In contrast to histiocytosis X and mycosis fungoides, the infiltrate does not prominently involve the epidermis. Vascular invasion and destruction of adnexal structures by the infiltrate may be present. Leukemic forms of MH have also been described.[37]

Hairy cell leukemia. Hairy cell leukemia (HCL) has been described in the literature under terms such as lymphoid myelofibrosis,[51] histiolymphocytosis of the bone marrow and spleen,[64] and leukemic reticuloendotheliosis. There is no general agreement at present whether the proliferating cell belongs to the lymphoid or monocytic series or perhaps represents a hybrid.[30,36,43,96,211] The onset of the disease is insidious. Splenomegaly is frequently massive. Enlargement of lymph nodes is usually absent. Pancytopenia is frequent, and a "dry tap" or hypocellular specimen is obtained on bone marrow aspiration. In the peripheral blood, mononuclear cells with irregular, hairlike cytoplasmic projections are particularly well seen with phase microscopy. These cells contain a tartrate-resistant acid phosphatase isoenzyme.[254] They may also exhibit ultrastructurally a characteristic cytoplasmic inclusion referred to as ribosome-lamellar complex.[63,104] These can be recognized with the light microscope in Giemsa-stained smears as rod-shaped inclusions that are also pyroninophilic.[65,105]

The cut surface of the enlarged spleen does not reveal any tumor nodules. The trabecular and follicular pattern may be attenuated. Microscopically the red pulp is diffusely infiltrated with sheets of loosely arranged, monotonous-appearing cells with round to oval nuclei and inconspicuous nucleoli and cytoplasm. Mitotic figures are rare. Vascular channels are prominent, some representing dilated sinusoids and others pseudosinusoids.[149] The latter contain red blood cells, are lined by neoplastic cells rather than endothelial cells, and are not outlined by reticulin fibers (Fig. 30-10). Neoplastic cells may be seen in the subintimal lymphatics of trabecular veins, a finding usually limited to lymphoproliferative disorders. The reticulin stain reveals foci of well-preserved sinusoids, which are striking because the reticulin framework of the red pulp is attenuated. The pathologic findings in the spleen are specific and are considered by some to be pathognomonic of the disease.

The bone marrow involvment is focal or diffuse. When focal, it may be peritrabecular or removed from trabeculae. The bone marrow shows a characteristic loose infiltrate that contrasts with the tightly packed lymphocytes in lymphocytic leukemias and lymphomas (Fig. 30-11). Also, even when the infiltrate is focal, it is not in discrete nodules as seen in lymphoproliferative disorders. This loose "lymphoid" infiltrate is associated with marked reticulin myelofibrosis. The bone marrow findings have been described in detail by Burke[29] and by Vykoupil and associates.[243]

The prognosis of HCL is relatively good. The patients benefit from splenectomy and may be harmed by chemotherapy.

An increased incidence of mycobacterial infections and necrotizing vasculitis has been reported in HCL.[77,249] However, the significance of these findings is uncertain. Some authors think that HCL is a heterogeneous chronic lymphoproliferative disorder rather than a specific entity.[98,148]

Even though the exact definition of HCL remains uncertain, the diagnosis can be established on the basis

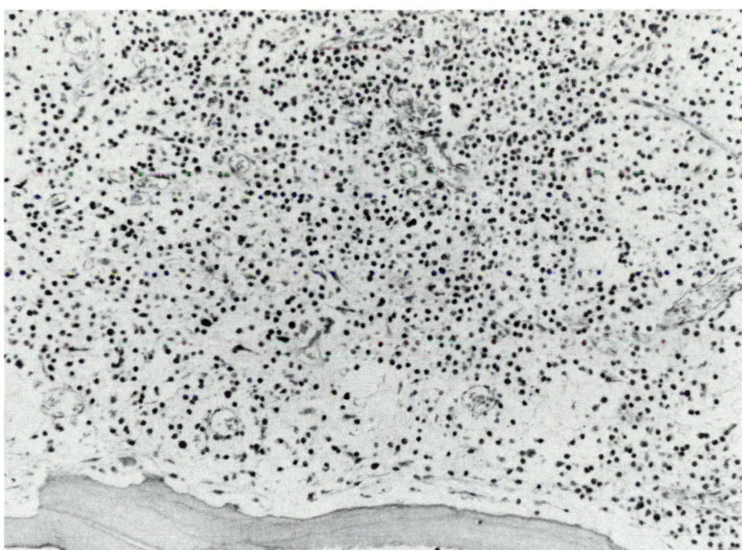

Fig. 30-11. Hairy cell leukemia. Bone marrow shows characteristic loose infiltrate with lymphoid cells. (Hematoxylin and eosin; medium power.)

of clinical findings, the tartrate-resistant acid phosphatase, and the characteristic pathologic findings in the spleen and marrow.

SPLEEN

Structure

The spleen comprises the largest single collection of lymphocytes and reticuloendothelial cells in the body. However, it is supplied by arterial blood by the splenic artery and is therefore in the vascular rather than the lymphatic system. It is roughly ovoid, with a convex upper surface and a concave surface below where the hilar vessels enter the organ. It lies beneath the ninth, tenth, and eleventh ribs, its long axis is parallel to them, and in the adult it weighs about 140 g (range 100 to 170 g). The capsule consists of a thin band of connective tissue with elastic fibers, covered by serous mesothelium. In humans, there is little if any smooth muscle in the capsule and thus, unlike in some animal species, there is no intrinsic contractile capability.

Grossly the surface is purple and the consistency friable. The cut surface shows tiny gray-white islands of white pulp scattered throughout the soft red-purple red pulp that makes up the bulk of splenic tissue. Scraping the normal surface with the edge of a knife yields a moderate amount of bloody cellular material.

The tiny nodules of white pulp are collections of small lymphocytes that form a sheath around arterioles of about 0.2 mm diameter and usually extend around even smaller arterioles. The lymphoid nodules are often called malpighian corpuscles. They may show germinal centers.

The red pulp as usually seen under the microscope does not seem particularly exciting, for the sinusoids are collapsed and one sees only many erythrocytes scattered, among which are a few neutrophils and phagocytic histiocytes. If the spleen is distended by injecting fixative through the splenic vein, however, the true structure is revealed. The framework of the organ consists of a mesh of argyrophilic reticulin fibers that are continuous with the collagen fibers of the capsule and trabeculae. Supported by this framework are many sinusoids lined with long narrow endothelial cells. The spaces between the sinusoids are referred to as the *cords of Billroth,* which contain red cells, reticulum cells, macrophages, some granulocytes, and plasma cells.

The vascular system of the spleen (Fig. 30-12) is not like that in any other organ. The splenic artery usually divides into several branches, which enter the organ at different points along the hilum. Each arterial branch enters the spleen within one of the large trabeculae of the capsule. When it leaves the trabecula, it becomes ensheathed with nodular collections of lymphocytes. The nodules of periarterial lymphocytes have been described previously as the white pulp of the spleen. The artery and arterioles within the white pulp are called follicular arteries. These leave the white pulp and enter the red pulp as straight arterioles called penicillary arteries.

There are several opinions as to the nature of the transition between the arterial and the venous vessels. It is agreed that between the two lie the sinusoids, but one opinion is that the penicillary arteries open directly into the sinusoids (the "closed" theory), whereas others believe that the artery opens into the pulp cords from which the blood enters the sinusoids through a discontinuous endothelial lining (the "open" theory). Knise-

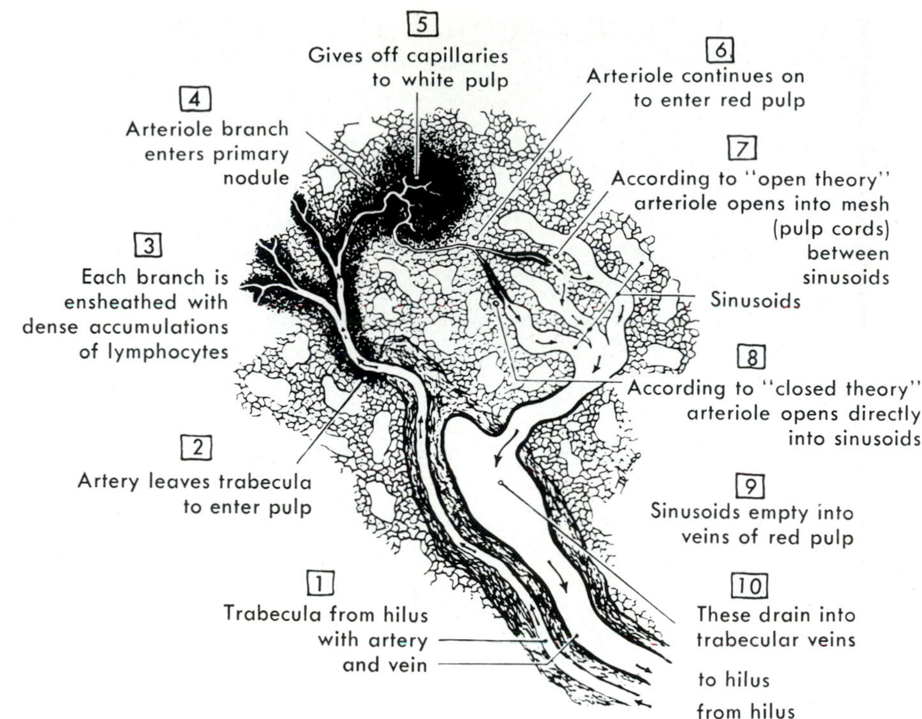

Fig. 30-12. Diagram of blood circulation through spleen. (From Blaustein, A.: The spleen, New York, 1963, copyrighted by McGraw-Hill Book Co.; used with permission.)

ly[112] described yet another system (in other species) made up of two portions: the arteriole empties directly into the sinusoid and a capillary shunt connects arterioles and venules.

It seems that both modes of microcirculation, the "open" and the "closed," occur in humans. The open circulation, in which cells from the peripheral blood percolate slowly through the cords of Billroth before entering the sinusoids seems to account better for the functions of the spleen. Indeed, during the slow circulation through the cords, the cellular elements of the peripheral blood are in close association with the macrophages, allowing for phagocytosis of abnormal cells, removal of abnormal inclusions, and fragmentation of abnormal erythrocytes. The veins leave the spleen at the hilum in association with the arteries that enter it.

The structure of the sinusoids deserves special mention. They do not have a basement membrane. They have been likened to a barrel, with the endothelial cells being arranged longitudinally, touching but not cemented together, with ring fibers running at right angles and binding them together. The ring fibers have cytochemical characteristics similar to those of the basement membrane of the renal glomerulus and have been shown by King and associates[109] not to have the properties of reticulum in the classic sense. It has been suggested that the absence of a basement membrane makes the sinusoidal wall discontinuous, allowing blood cells to pass through the spaces between the endothelial cells (Fig. 30-13).

The extent of the lymphatics in the spleen has been debated for many years. Goldberg,[79] on the basis of the location of tumor metastases, has presented evidence that lymphatic vessels do indeed extend deeply into the splenic parenchyma and that they are present in the adventitia of arteries and arterioles and in the subintima of trabecular veins.

Function

The function of the spleen can be classified under two general headings: (1) functions of the white pulp and (2) functions of the red pulp. The white pulp contains T lymphocytes in the periarteriolar sheaths and B lymphocytes in the malpighian corpuscles proper. The functions of the B and T lymphocytes are discussed on p 453. The functions of the red pulp are those of the RES.

After splenectomy, patients are susceptible to overwhelming infections[111,219,252] that begin with mild symptoms and rapidly lead to fulminant sepsis, which may be associated with disseminated intravascular coagulation and the Waterhouse-Friderichsen syndrome. The pneumococcus is responsible for one half to two thirds of the cases, and the meningococcus, streptococcus, and haemophilus account for an additional 25%.[252] The frequency of development of postsplenectomy sepsis depends on the age of the patient, the interval since splenectomy, and the reason for splenectomy. The younger the patient, the greater is the risk of postsplenectomy sepsis. The risk of sepsis is greatest in the first years after sple-

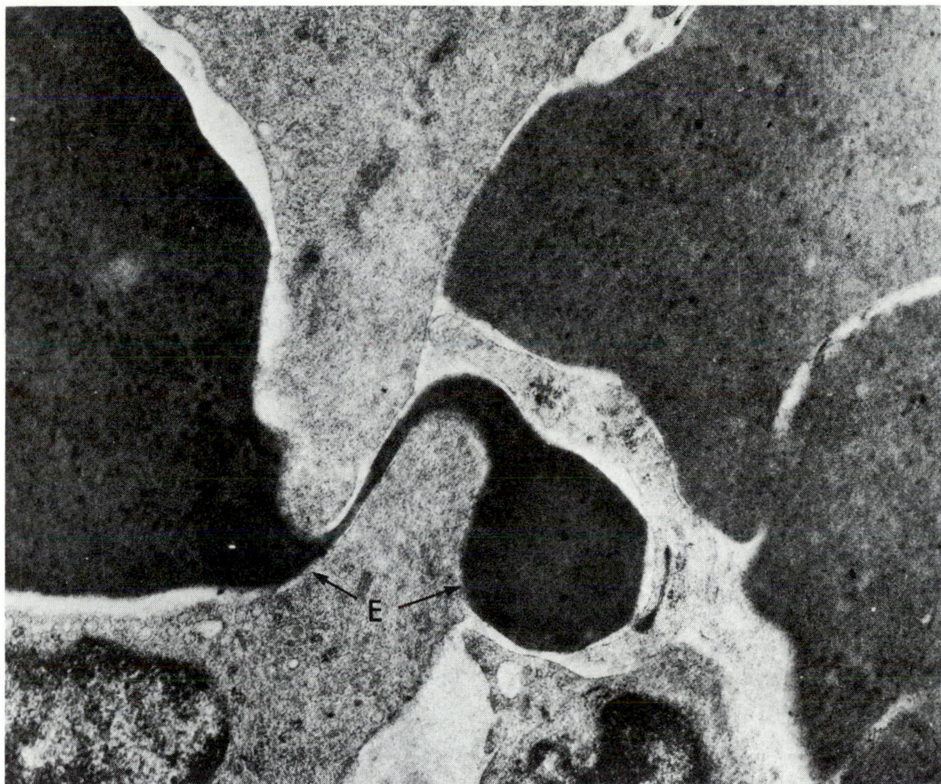

Fig. 30-13. Electron micrograph of spleen in hemoglobin H disease. Erythrocyte, *E,* lies partially within (smaller portion) and partially outside sinusoid. (From Wennberg, E., and Weiss, L.: Blood 31:778, 1968; by permission.)

nectomy. It is also greater if splenectomy if performed for a disease that is associated with decreased immunity (such as Hodgkin's disease) than if done because of trauma.

Splenic injury caused by therapeutic irradiation injures the lymphoid and RES components of the spleen and therefore may predispose patients to infections.[42]

Phagocytosis of erythrocytes and breakdown of the hemoglobin occur in the entire reticuloendothelial system, but roughly half of this catabolic activity is localized in the normal spleen. In splenomegaly the major portion of hemoglobin breakdown occurs in the spleen. The iron that is liberated is stored in the splenic phagocytes. These can be seen to be engorged with hemosiderin when erythrocyte destruction is accelerated, as in the hemolytic anemias. When there is an increase in stored iron, the spleen is said to be siderotic. Iron stored in the spleen can be used again for the synthesis of hemoglobin.

In addition to storing iron, the spleen participates in the storage diseases such as Gaucher's disease and Niemann-Pick disease. Abnormal lipid metabolites accumulate in all phagocytic reticuloendothelial cells but may so involve the many phagocytes in the spleen as to produce huge splenomegaly.

The functions of the spleen that are characteristic of this organ relate primarily to the circulation of erythrocytes through it. In a normal person the spleen contains only about 20 to 30 ml of erythrocytes, but in splenomegaly the reservoir function is increased greatly and the abnormally enlarged spleen contains many times this volume of red blood cells. The transit time through the cords of Billroth is lengthened, allowing for a longer exposure of red blood cells, granulocytes, and platelets to splenic macrophages. In part, stasis causes consumption of glucose, on which the erythrocyte is dependent for the maintenance of normal metabolism, and the erythrocyte is destroyed. Selective destruction of abnormal erythrocytes is also accelerated by the splenic pooling.

As erythrocytes pass through the spleen, the organ inspects them for imperfections and destroys those that it recognizes as abnormal or senescent. This is called the culling function. Even more remarkable is the pitting function, by which the spleen removes granular inclusions (Howell-Jolly bodies, siderotic granules, and so on) without destroying the erythrocyte. This normal function of the spleen keeps the number of circulating erythrocytes with inclusions to a minimum. By the same token, after splenectomy the peripheral blood reflects the loss of the pitting effect. Thus the postsplenectomy peripheral blood film shows Howell-Jolly bodies, siderotic granules, and flat target cells. The last is a consequence of the loss of normal surface membrane maturation, for the spleen is responsible for the rearrangement of lipid molecules at the surface of the erythrocyte to form the adult surface membrane.

The spleen also pools platelets in large numbers. The entry of platelets into the splenic pool and their return to the circulation are extensive. In splenomegaly the splenic pool may be so large as to produce thrombocytopenia. This lowering of the platelet count in splenomegaly has been erroneously interpreted as increased destruction of platelets in the spleen. The pooled platelets may be identified in the cords of Billroth as a granular eosinophilic material. Sequestration of leukocytes in the enlarged spleen in similar fashion may produce leukopenia.

The concept of hypersplenism, then, is that in some cases the sequestering effect on one or more of the three types of circulating blood cells (erythrocytes, granulocytes, and platelets) is so striking as to reduce the content of these cells in the peripheral blood. This sequestering effect can be demonstrated by the finding that isotope-labeled erythrocytes and platelets accumulate in the enlarged spleen, as evidenced by increased radioactivity of the organ.

The increased sequestration of circulating blood cells in the spleen may result in a compensatory hyperplasia of the precursors of these cells in the bone marrow.

Asplenia, polysplenia, and splenogonadal fusion

Asplenia refers to congenital absence of the spleen. In polysplenia, there are several, more or less equal splenic masses instead of a single spleen. Accessory spleens differ from polysplenia in that they are present in addition to the normal spleen. Asplenia and polysplenia are associated with extensive malformations. Moller and associates[146] state that polysplenia is a complex of bilateral left-sidedness (levoisomerism) in contrast to asplenia, which shows bilateral right-sidedness (dextroisomerism). Thus, in asplenia, the liver appears symmetric, as if made up of two right lobes, each lung has three lobes, and both bronchi are eparterial. In polysplenia, each lung may have two lobes, and the bronchi are hyparterial. Patients with asplenia and polysplenia may have a complete or partial situs inversus associated with complex cardiac malformations resulting in cyanotic heart disease.

Splenogonadal fusion is a rare malformation occurring much more frequently in males and involving primarily the left gonad.[176] In continuous splenogonadal fusion a cordlike structure connects the spleen to gonadal structures. The cord may be completely splenic, partly fibrous, or beaded with multiple masses of splenic tissue. In discontinuous splenogonadal fusion the splenogonadal mass has lost its continuity with the main spleen. This type is therefore a special variant of accessory spleen. The continuous type may be associated with peromelia and micrognathia. In both types the fused splenic tissue may swell and be painful in malarial attacks.

Regressive changes

Hyalinization

Hyaline degeneration of the arterial wall may be found in persons of any age, even the very young, and is nonspecific in nature. In young persons, hyaline thickening often accompanies hypertension. This degenerative change is most prominent in the sheathed arterioles of the lymphoid follicles. Central hyaline deposits in malpighian follicles of the spleen were studied by Stutte and Schulter,[229] who found them in 34% of autopsies and view them as being made up predominantly of fibrin.

Amyloidosis

Amyloid is deposited in the spleen under the same conditions as in other organs and is therefore found mainly when it occurs in other sites. In systemic diseases leading to amyloidosis, the spleen is the organ most frequently involved.

The spleen may be normal in size or considerably enlarged, depending on the amount and distribution of amyloid. Two types of involvement are seen: nodular and diffuse.

In the nodular or sago type, amyloid is found in the walls of the sheathed arteries and within the follicles but not in the red pulp. When so distributed, the nodules of amyloid are prominent on cut surface, and their waxy translucent appearance suggests the appearance of sago grains, hence the term *sago spleen*.

In the diffuse type the follicles are not involved, the red pulp is prominently involved, the spleen is usually greatly enlarged and firm, and the cut surface is characteristically waxy and translucent.

Atrophy

Atrophy of the spleen (50 to 70 g) is not uncommon in elderly persons. It also may occur in wasting diseases. In chronic hemolytic anemias, particularly in homozygous sickle cell anemia or hemoglobin S and C disease, there is progressive loss of pulp, increasing fibrosis, scarring from multiple infarcts, and incrustation with iron and calcium deposits (Fig. 30-14, *A*). In the final stage of atrophy the spleen may be so small as to be hardly recognizable (Fig. 30-14, *B*). Advanced atrophy sometimes is referred to as autosplenectomy.

Pigmentation

The pigments found in the spleen are (1) hemosiderin and hematoidin, derived from hemoglobin, (2) malarial pigment, (3) anthracotic pigment, and (4) ceroid.

Hemosiderin is the pigment form of excess iron, whether this is derived from endogenous or exogenous

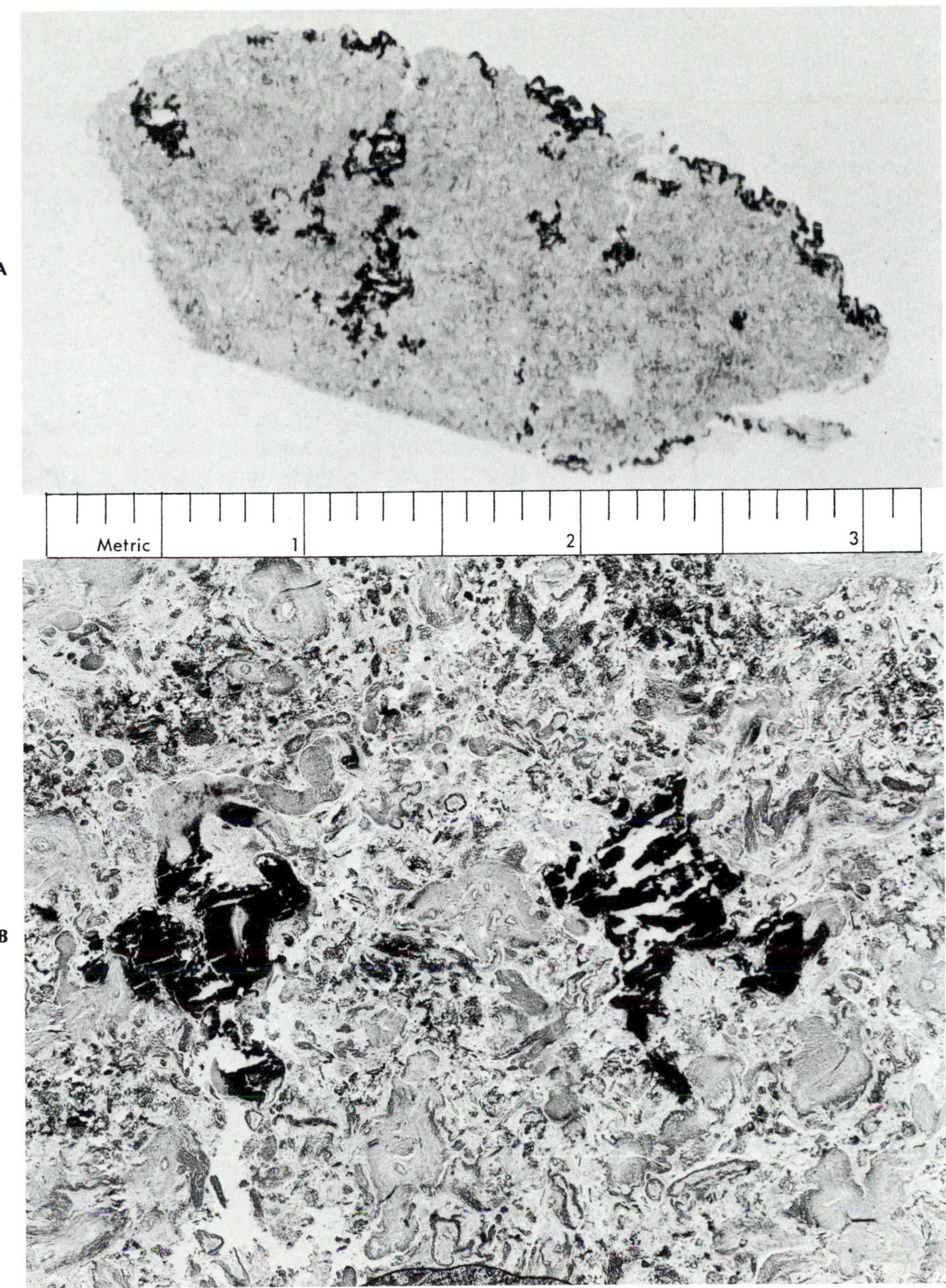

Fig. 30-14. Atrophy of spleen in long-standing sickle cell anemia. **A,** Gross appearance of bisected organ showing actual size of spleen bisected along its greatest dimension. **B,** Paraffin section. Note complete loss of normal architecture and replacement by fibrous tissue, pigment, and calcium deposits. (**B,** Hematoxylin and eosin; 25×.)

sources. It is seen readily in tissue sections as coarse brown granules within phagocytic cells. It gives a positive Prussian blue reaction and therefore contains ferric iron. Large amounts of hemosiderin are deposited in all phagocytic cells of the reticuloendothelial system when there is iron excess, as in chronic hemolytic anemia or after many blood transfusions. Deposition of hemosiderin iron in the spleen in abnormally large amounts is called siderosis or hemosiderosis of the spleen (Fig. 30-15).

Strictly speaking, hemosiderosis refers to iron deposits derived from heme, whereas siderosis should be used for iron derived from other sources, such as injections of medicinal iron or foreign bodies. The same descriptive terms are used for other organs. In moderate amounts, hemosiderin produces little reaction in the tissues. In large amounts, it stimulates proliferation of fibrous tissue. Hemosiderosis sometimes has been called secondary hemochromatosis to distinguish it from primary hemochromatosis, a primary metabolic defect in iron utilization and storage.

Hematoidin is formed in areas of hemorrhage or infarction, possibly in a hypoxic environment. It appears as golden brown burrlike or crystalline masses and does not give the Prussian blue reaction for ferric iron but gives a positive Gmelin reaction for bile pigments. From this one must infer that hematoidin is a non-iron-containing breakdown product of hemoglobin that is similar if not identical to bilirubin. Unlike hemosiderin, hematoidin is an extracellular pigment.

In malaria the black pigment imparts a dark brown color to the pulp of the spleen. The pigment is of the acid hematin type and is found within phagocytes.

Anthracotic pigmentation of the spleen is rare. Askanazy[8] describes finding anthracotic pigment in the bone marrow, liver, and spleen (his term *Kohlenmetastase*) in necropsy studies of anthracosis. The spread from the respiratory system is probably hematogenous.

Ceroid pigment is discussed in detail in the section on storage diseases.

Rupture

Rupture of a normal spleen may result from severe blunt trauma to the abdomen, or it may be associated with or caused by fractured ribs. An abscess of the spleen or an enlarged soft spleen, such as that seen in infectious mononucleosis, leukemia, malaria, or typhoid fever, ruptures easily with minimal trauma. The trauma may be so slight that the rupture is believed to be spontaneous. It is not unusual for such a spleen to be ruptured as the result of enthusiastic palpation maneuvers by the physician, straining at the stool, or even violent retching. In some cases rupture is delayed for some days after the trauma. The reason is that trauma causes an intrasplenic hemato-

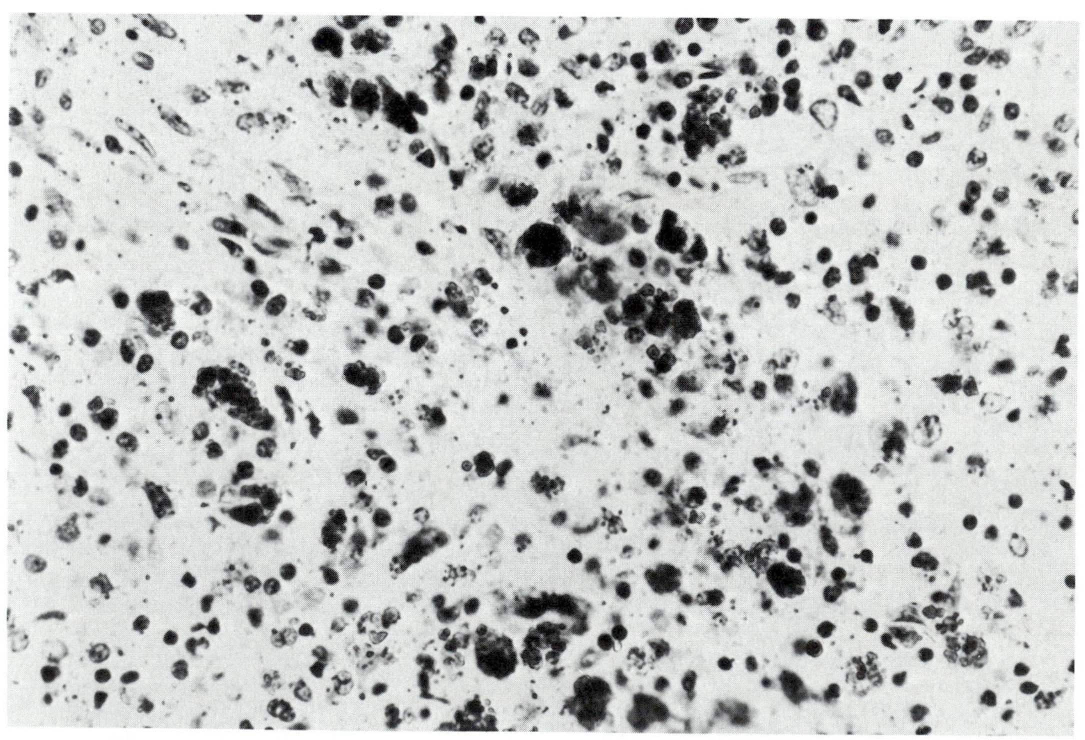

Fig. 30-15. Hemosiderosis of spleen. Most of hemosiderin lies within phagocytic histiocytes. (Hematoxylin and eosin; 125×.)

ma. As the hematoma enlarges, the capsule is put under tension and eventually ruptures.

One consequence of splenic rupture is autoimplantation of splenic tissue on the peritoneal surfaces, forming multiple implants (splenosis). Splenosis can be confused at the time of operative discovery with endometriosis, metastatic carcinoma, melanoma, or hemangioma and, if unrecognized, may lead to unnecessary surgical procedures.[25]

Circulatory disturbances

Active hyperemia

Active hyperemia accompanies the reaction in the spleen to acute systemic infections. This is called septic splenitis, acute splenic tumor, or acute reactive hyperplasia of the spleen (p. 1277). The spleen is moderately enlarged, the capsule is tense even though the organ is soft, and the cut surface is dark red and bulging, and its architecture is obscured by the bulging, cellular, bloody pulp.

Passive hyperemia and fibrocongestive splenomegaly

Passive hyperemia (chronic passive congestion) may be caused by increased pressure in the portal system or the venous systemic circulation. In passive hyperemia caused by cardiac disease, the spleen is only moderately enlarged and rubbery. The cut surface is dry, the cut edges are sharp, and the trabecular markings are increased. In long-standing cases there are thickening of the trabeculae, fibrosis of the red pulp (Fig. 30-16), and atrophy of lymphoid tissue.

Portal hypertension has many causes. The most frequent is cirrhosis of the liver, which is accompanied by splenomegaly in about 80% of the cases. Here, the obstruction to blood flow is intrahepatic. The obstruction may be extrahepatic, as in thrombosis of hepatic veins, thrombosis of the splenic vein with or without recanalization (cavernous transformation), or thrombosis of the portal vein. Portal hypertension may also be idiopathic, when neither intrahepatic nor extrahepatic obstruction is demonstrable.

In contrast to passive hyperemia from congestive heart failure, passive hyperemia from increased portal pressure causes considerable splenomegaly, often to 500 g or more. The spleen displays the full-blown picture of fibrocongestive splenomegaly. The malpighian follicles are atrophic and exhibit some periarterial fibrosis. Perifollicular hemorrhages may be present. As the latter become organized, siderotic nodules, also known as tobacco nodules or Gamna-Gandy bodies, are formed (Fig. 30-17). They consist of areas of fibrosis containing collagen fibers encrusted with iron and calcium. The cords of Billroth contain an increased number of macrophages, fibroblasts, and irregularly thickened reticulin fibers. The

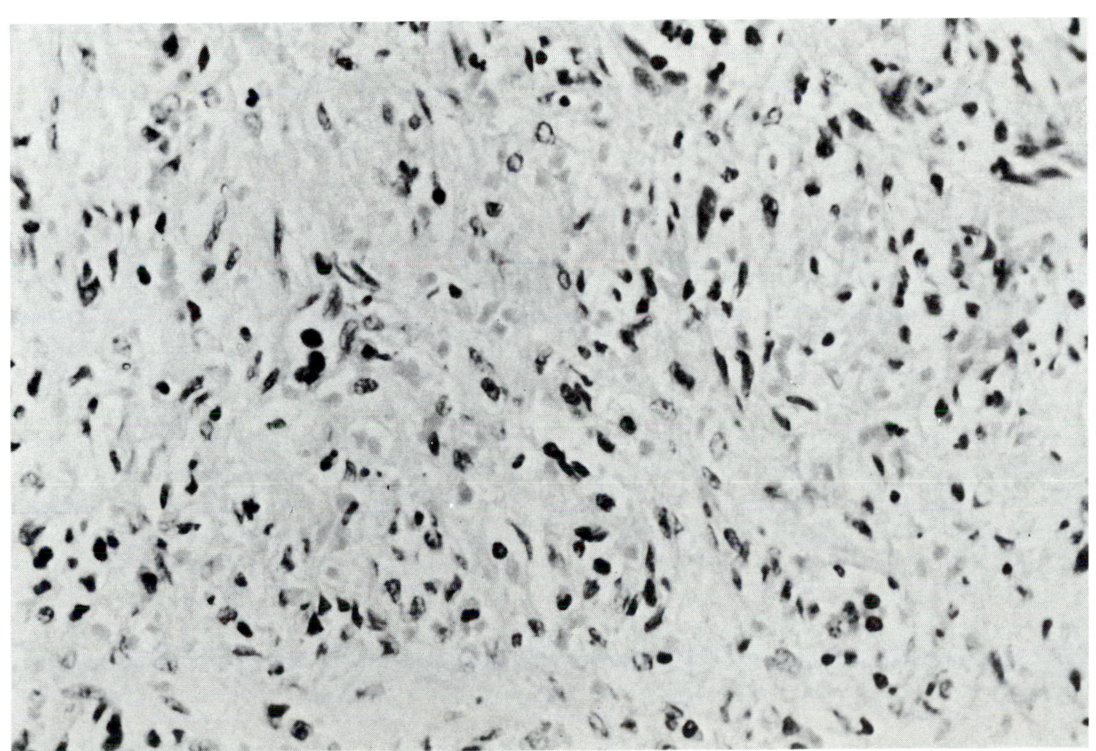

Fig. 30-16. Chronic passive congestion of spleen with fibrosis. Note pronounced fibrosis of red pulp. (Hematoxylin and eosin; 125×.)

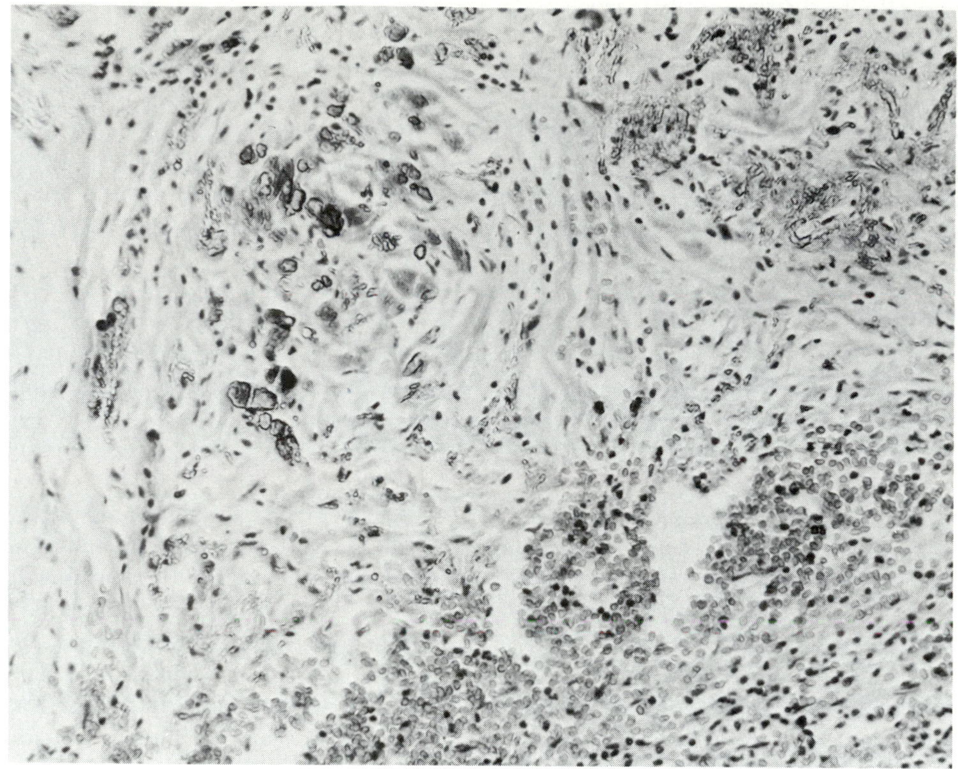

Fig. 30-17. Gamna-Gandy body consisting of fibrous tissue, hemosiderin, and hematoidin. (Hematoxylin and eosin; 125×.)

appearance of the sinuses may vary depending on the cause of the portal hypertension. They may be dilated and empty.[179] In portal hypertension from splenic vein thrombosis, the sinuses are narrower than normal but are greatly elongated.[228] The endothelial cells are prominent.

The term "Banti's syndrome" has been used for fibrocongestive splenomegaly associated with hypersplenism. Actually Banti described a disease characterized by enlargement of the spleen and anemia followed by digestive hemorrhages, cirrhosis of the liver, and ascites. The pathologic changes in the spleen, according to Banti, were characterized by "fibroadenie." Fibroadenie included fibrosis of malpighian corpuscles (lymphadenoid tissue) and glandlike appearance of the sinusoids because of prominent endothelial cells. The histologic appearance of the spleen is identical to that of fibrocongestive splenomegaly from splenic vein thrombosis.[228]

Whether Banti's disease exists is moot. Some observers apply the term to instances of splenomegaly with hypersplenism in which there are no demonstrable pathologic findings in the liver, portal, and splenic veins. The spleen in these instances shows varying degrees of fibrocongestive splenomegaly. Often there is only an increase in the red pulp. Some of these cases are associated with "idiopathic" portal hypertension; in others portal hypertension was not documented during surgery. We have followed a few such patients for several years. They remain cured of their hypersplenism and have not shown evidence of cirrhosis of the liver. Whether Banti's sequence with ascites and cirrhosis of the liver would have developed if the spleen had not been removed cannot be ascertained (see also p. 1175).

Infarction

Infarction results from occlusion of the splenic artery or branches. Occlusion may be caused by thrombosis, by emboli, by subendothelial infiltration with leukemic cells in chronic lymphocytic leukemia, or by obstruction of the microcirulation attributable to conglutination and sludging of red blood cells as is seen in sickle cell anemia, sickle cell trait, and sickle cell–hemoglobin C disease. Occlusion on the basis of emboli is most commonly seen in heart disease, either from mural thrombi in the left auricle or ventricle or from vegetations on the valves on the left side of the heart. Occasionally infarcts are found at necropsy without apparent cause for thrombosis and embolism.

Infarcts are sometimes conical, with the base at the capsular surface, and sometimes irregular in shape. Although they are classified as anemic or hemorrhagic on the basis of gross appearance (pale or red, respectively), most are hemorrhagic at first. Later, dehemoglobinization occurs and the infarcted area becomes pale and gray-

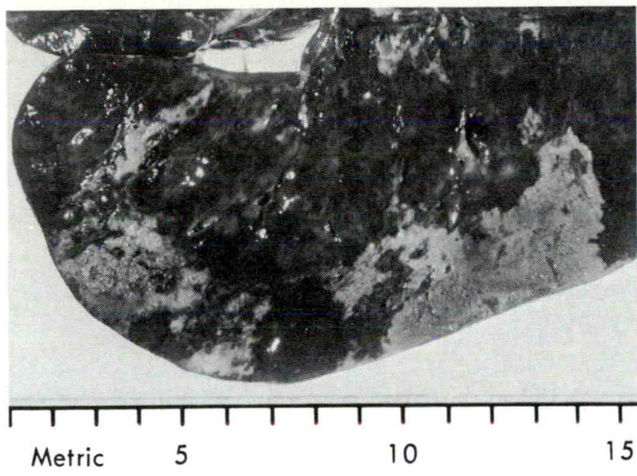

Fig. 30-18. Multiple infarcts of spleen. (From Rezek, P.R., and Millard, M.: Autopsy pathology, Springfield, Ill., 1963, Charles C Thomas, Publisher.)

white with a hyperemic border (Fig. 30-18). Later still, the necrotic tissue is replaced by fibrous tissue, which contracts and gives rise to a depressed scar.

If the embolus contains bacteria, as from vegetative endocarditis of the mitral or aortic valve, the infarct undergoes rapid softening and suppuration as the bacteria multiply. This is called a septic infarct.

A special type of ischemic necrosis may occur as a terminal event in uremia. The necrotic areas are white or yellowish and of varied sizes and irregular shapes, central as well as peripheral. The diffuseness of the necrosis gives the cut surface a spotted appearance—hence the term *Fleckmilz* (spotted spleen). Although not uncommon in uremia, this distribution of necrotic areas also is seen in systemic infections, with or without vascular occlusion. The areas of necrosis are probably the result of disseminated intravascular coagulation.

Occasionally patients with sickle cell trait who are deprived of an adequate supply of oxygen, as occurs when traveling at high altitudes, undergo infarction of the spleen. Such a spleen may present the picture of a pseudocyst filled with a brown, mushy, semifluid material.[198] The hypoxia reduces the hemoglobin S and leads to the formation of sickled cells. As a result the viscosity of the blood is increased, producing erythrostasis and further deoxygenation. In addition, a decrease in the tissue pH favors the production of sickled cells. The capillary circulation is blocked by the conglutinated sickled erythrocytes. The result is necrosis of tissue and formation of a pseudocyst. Electrophoretic studies of hemoglobin should be performed on all patients with pseudocysts of the spleen.

Spleen in systemic infections

General features

Enlargement of the spleen (250 to 350 g) is common in acute systemic infections. The enlarged, soft, even diffluent, cellular organ is then said to show acute reactive hyperplasia. Other terms used are acute inflammatory splenomegaly, septic splenitis, and acute splenic tumor.

The splenomegaly is caused in part by a true reactive hyperplasia of the myeloid and lymphoid cells of the pulp and in part by congestion with erythrocytes. The reaction may be to pathogenic organisms, but most often it is to the products of inflammation, substances responsible for the mobilization of neutrophils, lymphocytes, and eosinophils.[82] The spleen also can react to foreign substances not the product of inflammation, such as foreign protein or a distant focus of necrotic tissue. The spleen is not enlarged in bacterial peritonitis.

Acute reactive hyperplasia is characterized by an increase in the cells of the red pulp. Grossly the cut surface is red-gray and the follicles are prominent. Microscopically neutrophils are abundant, and some may be of intermediate maturity. The gray hue of the splenic surface is caused by the numerous polymorphonuclear leukocytes. There is also an increase in phagocytic cells, which contain ingested debris from dead leukocytes and erythrocytes and sometimes bacteria and other organisms. A number of plasma cells can also be found. The lymphoid follicles are usually hyperplastic, although the lymphoid hyperplasia may be obscured by the congestion of the red pulp. Sometimes the follicles have large reactive centers showing much phagocytic activity.

These general features are modified slightly in various infectious diseases but usually not sufficiently to enable one to make an etiologic diagnosis solely on the basis of morphologic changes.

Bacteremia and septicemia

In typhoid fever the spleen is greatly enlarged, soft, and cherry red. Infiltration with granulocytes is minimal, but mononuclear cells are numerous. There is much phagocytic activity. Focal necrosis, hemorrhage, and rupture are not uncommon.

In the septicemia caused by *Clostridium welchii*, hyperemia and congestion of the red pulp are intense, the sinusoids are collapsed, and there is evidence of extensive hemolysis of erythrocytes.

In streptococcal septicemia (whether acute or subacute), as in subacute bacterial endocarditis, the spleen is large and extremely soft and flabby. In subacute bacterial endocarditis, infarcts (both bland and septic) are not uncommon.

Infectious mononucleosis

The large soft spleen in infectious mononucleosis may rupture. This complication, necessitating splenectomy, has provided most of the material studied.[220] The spleen is enlarged to three or four times the normal size. Characteristic changes are as follows:

1. Large numbers of atypical lymphocytes like those found in the peripheral blood, bone marrow, and lymph nodes are seen in the red pulp.

2. The follicles are usually not hyperplastic.
3. The atypical lymphocytes usually infiltrate the capsule, trabeculae, adventitia of the arteries, subintima of the veins, and sinusoids.

Probably the cellular infiltration and edema of the capsule account for the high incidence of rupture.

Granulomatous inflammation

There are few features of granulomatous inflammation of the spleen that are not common to a given granulomatous inflammation in another organ or tissue. The spleen is normal in size or enlarged, depending on the extent of the inflammatory reaction. A few special features deserve mention.

In fibrocaseous tuberculosis of the lungs, the spleen is usually normal, but in tuberculous pneumonitis, it may be hyperplastic as part of the generalized reaction to severe acute infection. In miliary tuberculosis the spleen is almost always involved (Fig. 30-19). The tubercles may be few or very numerous, minute or readily visible. In any case, splenomegaly is slight. When numerous, the tubercles can be readily seen on cut surface or through the capsule. Occasionally, a large tumorlike tuberculoma, usually single and measuring several centimeters in diameter, is the only lesion found (see Chapter 22).

The lesions in syphilis depend on the stage of the disease. In congenital syphilis there is splenomegaly with hyperplastic changes in the red pulp, which contains an increased number of granulocytes, plasma cells, and phagocytic histiocytes. Spirochetes are very numerous and easily demonstrated by special staining techniques. In the acquired disease the spleen is normal during the primary stage. In the secondary stage it is enlarged and shows follicular hyperplasia and many plasma cells in the red pulp. In the tertiary stage it is generally normal except for the rare occurrence of the large spheroid lesions, call gummas, characteristic of tertiary syphilis. Occasionally splenomegaly in tertiary syphilis is the result of syphilitic cirrhosis of the liver with obstruction of the portal blood flow.

In sarcoidosis the spleen is involved quite often as part of the generalized disease, but occasionally the splenic involvement is so severe in proportion to lesions in other organs as to appear primary. The lesions vary from microscopic to grossly nodular. In the former they may be merely aggregates of epithelioid cells. In the latter they show the noncaseating type of granulomatous inflammation characteristic of sarcoidosis. It must be noted that sarcoidlike lesions (that is, noncaseating granulomas) may be found in a variety of conditions: leprosy,

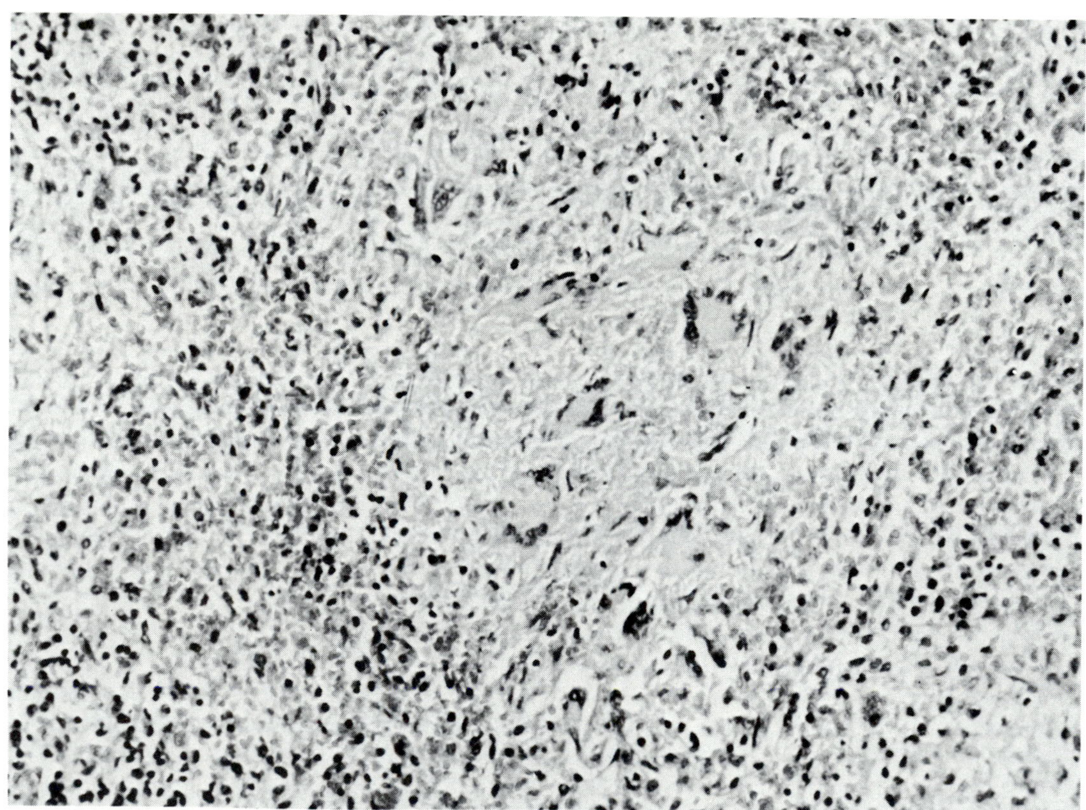

Fig. 30-19. Miliary tuberculosis of spleen. Tubercle is composed of epithelioid cells and Langhans' giant cells, and there is no caseous necrosis. (Hematoxylin and eosin; 125×.)

tularemia, histoplasmosis, brucellosis, berylliosis, splenic deposition of silica, lipid-storage diseases, Hodgkin's disease, and some reactions to parasites. To be distinguished from sarcoidosis are the rare cases of tuberculosis in which the tubercles fail to show central caseation. In granulomatous inflammation, calcification is common only in chronic brucellosis and in histoplasmosis.[209]

Spleen in parasitic infestation

Enlargement of the spleen is so common in malaria that this physical sign is used as presumptive evidence of infection when epidemiologists survey inhabitants of endemic areas. In the acute stages of malaria the febrile episodes are accompanied by reactive hyperplasia of the spleen. In chronic malaria the spleen is greatly enlarged. It is firm, the capsule usually is studded with pearly white thickenings ("ague cake spleen"), and the cut surface is slate gray because of large amounts of malarial pigment (hematin). Under the microscope, one sees malarial parasites and hematin in the sinus endothelium and the phagocytic cells of the red pulp. This pigment gives a negative reaction when stained for ferric iron. Fibrosis is prominent in infection of long duration. Rupture is not uncommon.

The spleen also enlarges in leishmaniasis (kala-azar). Except for the absence of pigmentation, the spleen is the same as described for malaria. Definitive diagnosis is based on identifying the many parasites *(Leishmania donovani)* in phagocytic cells.

Acute reactive hyperplasia of the spleen with varying degrees of infiltration with eosinophils may occur in schistosomiasis before the period of oviposition. In hepatosplenic schistosomiasis the splenomegaly is of the fibrocongestive type. Parasites or ova are found only exceptionally in the spleen. A few patients with hepatosplenic schistosomiasis and marked splenomegaly have retarded growth and sexual maturation. This schistosomal dwarfism is dramatically reversed by splenectomy.[138]

About 3% of *Echinococcus granulosus* cysts occur in the spleen.[223] These may cause pain and give rise to peritonitis on rupture. Some of the small hyalinized nodules in the spleen, usually interpreted as old granulomas, may result from pentastomiasis.[142]

Spleen in hemolytic anemia

Hemolytic anemia is the general term applied to anemia caused by decreased life span of the erythrocytes. When the rate of destruction is greater than can be compensated for by the bone marrow, anemia results. When destruction of erythrocytes is accelerated, the spleen's normal role in disposing of damaged erythrocytes is exaggerated and thus the spleen plays an important role in hemolytic disease.

Hemolytic anemia is a complex subject that cannot be covered here. For details, the reader is referred to standard texts in hematology. Some generalizations, however, can be made.

Decreased erythrocyte survival is the result of one of two abnormal situations: the erythrocyte is itself abnormal, an intrinsic defect, and therefore not able to survive normally, or there is an extrinsic influence that damages an otherwise normal erythrocyte and shortens its life span. The spleen seems to dispose of the defective erythrocytes in either case, but especially when the erythrocytes are intrinsically abnormal.

In congenital spherocytic hemolytic anemia (hereditary spherocytosis), an intrinsic abnormality of the erythrocytes gives rise to erythrocytes that are small and spheroid rather than the normal, flattened, biconcave discs. Although there is evidence that intracellular glycolysis and phosphorylation are abnormal, the nature of the intrinsic defect is unknown. The two components of the disease are the production of spherocytic erythrocytes by the bone marrow and increased destruction of these cells in the spleen. The spleen destroys spherocytes selectively, as shown by the following observations:

1. Normal erythrocytes transfused into a person having hereditary spherocytosis survive for a normal time.
2. Erythrocytes from a person with hereditary spherocytosis tranfused into a normal recipient are rapidly destroyed.
3. Erythrocytes from a person with hereditary spherocytosis transfused into a recipient previously subjected to splenectomy survive for a normal time.
4. In hereditary spherocytosis, splenectomy cures the hemolytic disease, even though the bone marrow continues to make spherocytes and the appearance of the peripheral blood smear is unchanged.

The spleen is always enlarged, and weights of 500 to 1000 g are not uncommon. The cut surface is deep red and hemorrhagic. The characteristic microscopic features (Fig. 30-20) are as follows:

1. Pronounced congestion of the cords of Billroth, possibly because the spheroid erythrocytes do not pass readily through the sinusoidal walls
2. Hyperplasia of the endothelial cells lining the sinusoids
3. Relatively empty sinusoids
4. Little or no hemosiderin, in contrast to many other hemolytic anemias

If accessory spleens are present, they not only show the same morphology but also, if not excised along with the principal spleen, take over the destructive function, and the original splenectomy is ineffective.

In sickle cell disease, as well as in some variants such as hemoglobin C and hemoglobin S thalassemia combinations, the spleen is severely involved. The changes are

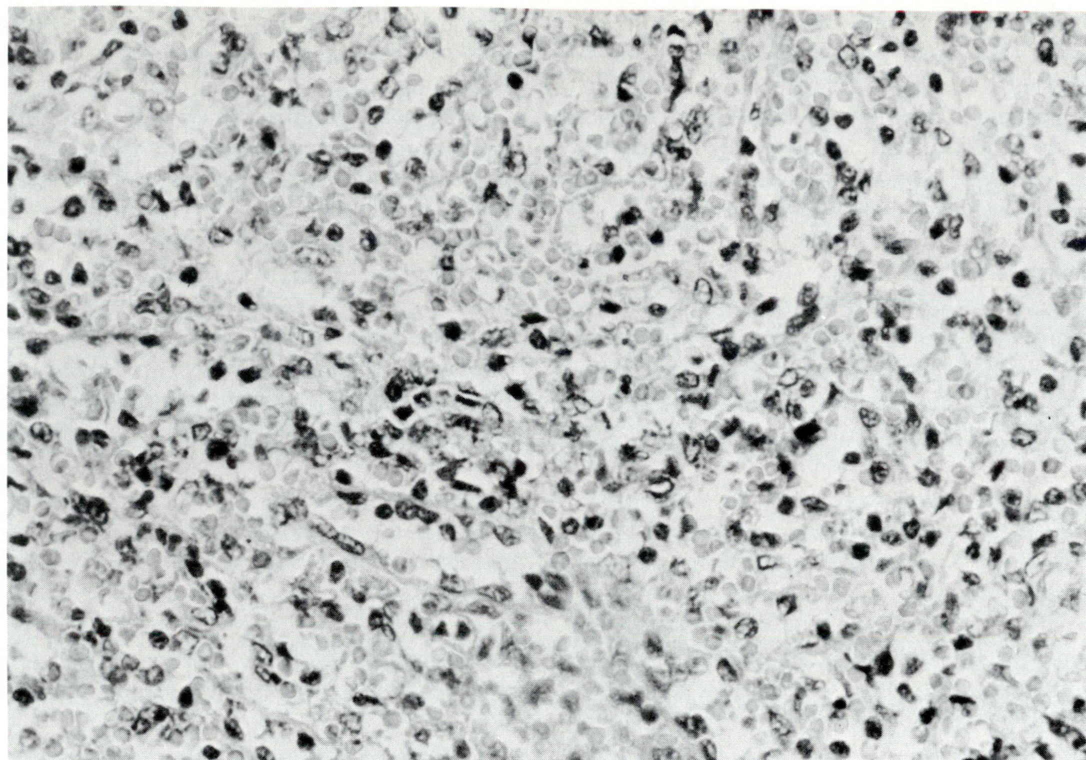

Fig. 30-20. Spleen in congenital spherocytosis. Note congestion of cords of Billroth and hyperplasia of endothelial cells lining sinusoids. (Hematoxylin and eosin; 125×.)

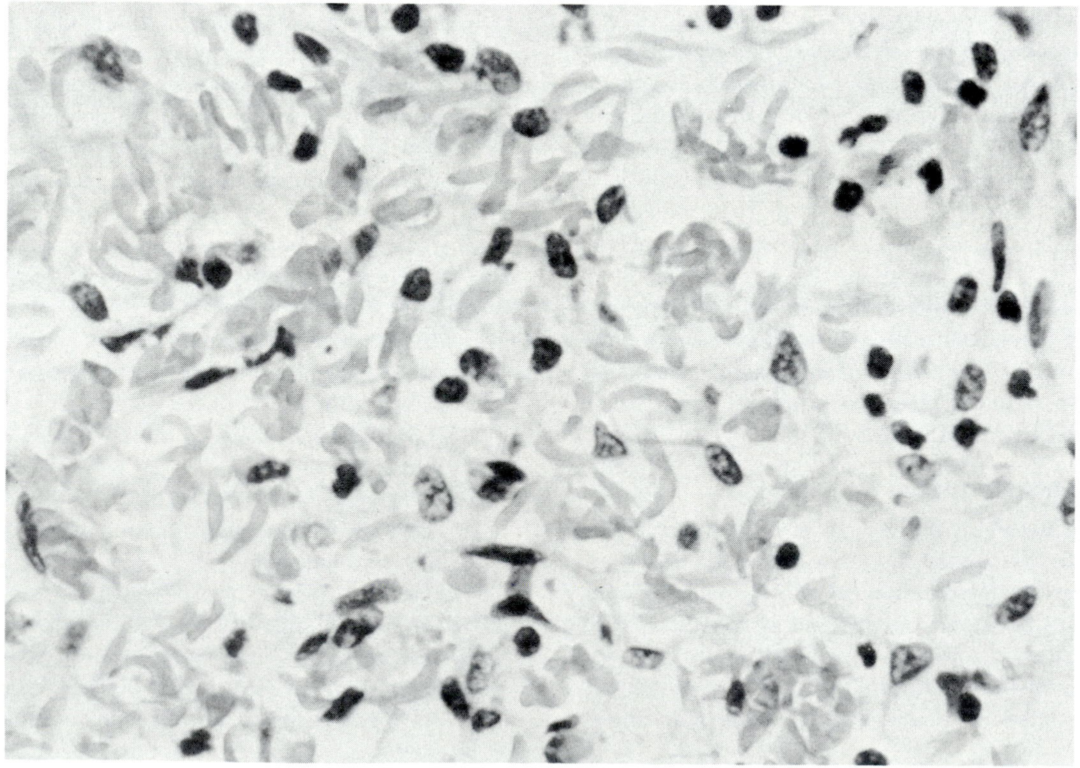

Fig. 30-21. Sickled erythocytes in spleen in sickle cell anemia. (Hematoxylin and eosin; 450×.)

progressive and are most severe in long-standing cases. As in hereditary spherocytosis, the defect in the erythrocytes is intrinsic, the content of hemoglobin S causing them to assume rigid, bizarre, sicklelike shapes under hypoxic conditions. The rigidity and peculiar shape of the erythrocytes cause them to plug up small blood vessels, and most of the clinical findings can be explained on the basis of obstruction of the microcirculation by conglutinated red cells. In the spleen they do not pass out of the splenic cords, which are congested and contain many sickled erythrocytes (Fig. 30-21). Later, the spleen shows the effect of repeated hemorrhages and infarcts; the hemorrhages lead to diffuse fibrosis with scattered siderotic nodules, whereas repeated infarction produces many large depressed scars. The most severe degree of fibrosis and atrophy has already been discussed and illustrated (Fig. 30-16).

The microscopic features that distinguish the spleen in sickle cell disease are as follows:

1. The sickled erythrocytes, always prominent in formalin-fixed tissue
2. The large amount of hemosiderin (unlike the spleen in congenital spherocytosis)
3. Progressive fibrosis
4. Numerous infarcts

It should be noted that some sickled erythrocytes are seen in any hemoglobinopathy in which hemoglobin S is one of the hemoglobins. Thus they may be seen in sickle cell trait (hemoglobin S plus hemoglobin A). Here, however, the spleen is relatively normal. Infarcts and pseudocysts of the spleen may occur in patients with sickle cell trait.

Patients with sickle cell anemia and its genetic variants are subject to periodic exacerbations or "crises" of their disease. In hemolytic crises there is an increase in the severity of the anemia because of a further shortening of the life span of the red cells. In aplastic crises the anemia becomes more severe because the bone marrow stops producing red blood cells. Nucleated red blood cells disappear from the marrow. In visceral or pain crises, deoxygenation causes sludging of red cells in the microcirculation in different organs simulating a variety of clinical conditions. Massive sickling involving large capillary territories may be responsible for sudden death.

In contrast to sickle cell disease, patients with hemoglobin C disorders (homozygous hemoglobin C and hemoglobin C and S disease) have large spleens exhibiting congestion of the cords of Billroth. Pregnancy is particularly dangerous for patients with hemoglobin C and S disease. In such patients severe visceral crises may develop in the third trimester of pregnancy, which may result in bone marrow necrosis with extensive fat and bone marrow emboli.[199]

In older patients with hemoglobin C and S disease the

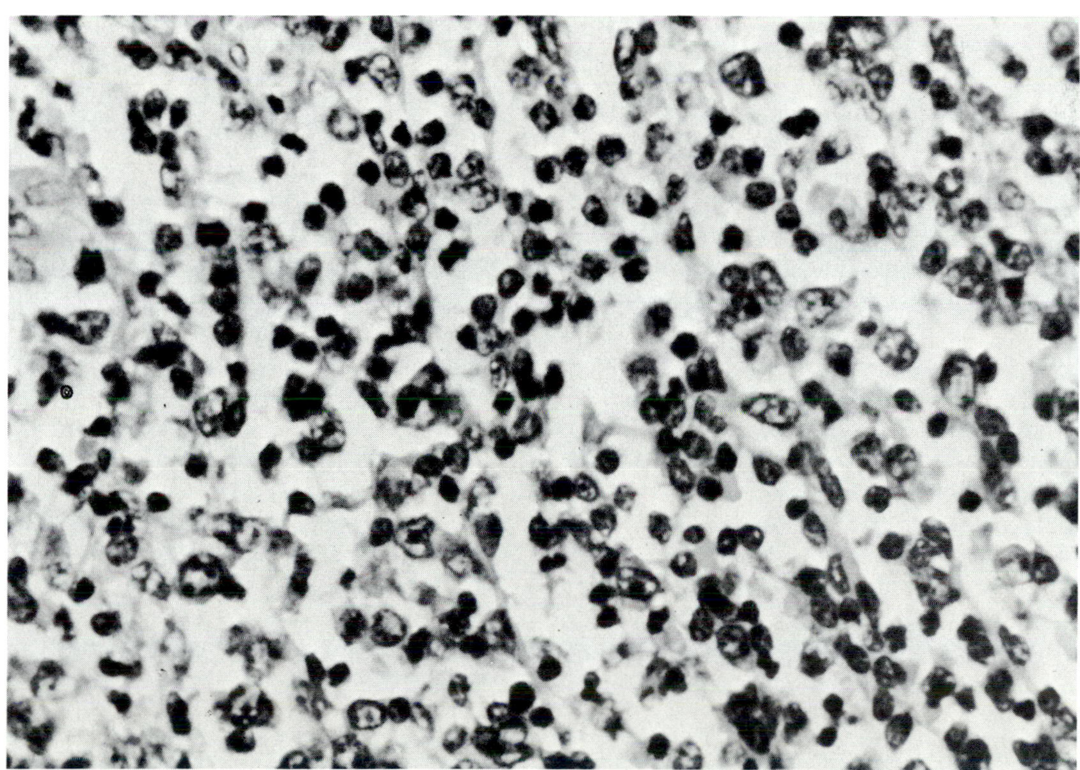

Fig. 30-22. Spleen in thalassemia. There are numerous large hyperplastic reticulum cells and some normoblasts. (Hematoxylin and eosin; 250×.)

spleen may be small and scarred. The spleen also is severely involved in thalassemia (Cooley's anemia, Mediterranean anemia). This hemoglobinopathy differs from the others in that an abnormal molecular form of hemoglobin is not present. Rather, there is a suppression of synthesis of beta-polypeptide chains (beta-thalassemia) or alpha-polypeptide chains (alpha-thalassemia) resulting in deficient synthesis of normal hemoglobin. Suppression of normal hemoglobin synthesis is accompanied by increased amounts of hemoglobin A_2 or hemoglobin F. The erythrocytes are not only deficient in normal hemoglobin (hypochromic) but also abnormal in shape, many being target cells, whereas the others vary greatly in size and shape. Their life span is short because they are destroyed in large numbers by the spleen.

The disease ranges in severity from mild to very severe. The changes in the spleen are greatest in the severe form called thalassemia major. The spleen is very large, often seeming to fill the abdominal cavity. The organ is firm and the capsule often thickened. The cut surface is dark red. Microscopically there are congestion, fibrosis, and hyperplasia of reticuloendothelial cells (Fig. 30-22). The one feature that is characteristic is the presence of foci of blood cell formation, extramedullary hemopoiesis. Also characteristic, but not as frequent, is the presence of foam cells in the red pulp. These are large and show a foamy cytoplasm that may contain ceroid. Siderotic nodules are sometimes found, but these are seen also in other anemias.

Spleen in other diseases of blood and blood-forming organs

In addition to the conditions already discussed, which may be considered to involve primarily some special splenic function, splenomegaly is found in hematologic disorders involving granulocytopoiesis, lymphopoiesis, and erythropoiesis. Enlargement of the spleen may occur in many other conditions, as follows:

A. Splenomegaly primarily caused by hemopoietic activity
   1. Granulocytopoiesis
      a. Reactive hyperplasia to acute and chronic infections
         (1) "Acute splenic tumor" of various acute infections
      b. Myeloproliferative syndromes
   2. Lymphopoiesis
      a. Generalized lymphocytic reactions
         (1) Infectious mononucleosis
         (2) Other viral infections
         (3) Hyperthyroidism
      b. Lymphocytic leukemia
      c. Malignant lymphomas
   3. Erythropoiesis
      a. Hemolytic anemias
      b. Myeloproliferative syndromes including polycythemia vera
      c. Erythroleukemia
      d. Extramedullary hemopoiesis
   4. Other cell types
      a. Reactive plasmacytosis
      b. Multiple myeloma
      c. Monocytic and histiocytic proliferative disorders

B. Splenomegally primarily caused by destructive activity
   1. Hemolytic anemias
   2. Thrombocytopenic purpura (rare)
   3. Splenic neutropenia

C. Splenomegaly caused by reticuloendothelial hyperactivity
   1. Reticuloendothelial hyperplasia in acute and chronic infections
   2. Disseminated lupus erythematosus
   3. Rheumatoid arthritis
   4. Felty's syndrome
   5. Hemochromatosis and hemosiderosis
   6. Gaucher's disease
   7. Niemann-Pick disease
   8. Amyloidosis
   9. Diabetes mellitus
   10. Gargoylism
   11. Sarcoidosis
   12. Infectious and parasitic diseases associated with diffuse proliferation of histiocytes or discrete granulomas
       a. Tuberculosis
       b. Syphilis
       c. Histoplasmosis
       d. Leishmaniasis
       e. Malaria
       f. Trypanosomiasis

D. Splenomegaly caused by vascular factors (congestive splenomegaly)
   1. Cirrhosis of liver
   2. Portal vein blockage
   3. Splenic vein thrombosis and other obstructions
   4. Cardiac failure
   5. Infarction

E. Splenomegaly caused by nonspecific afflictions
   1. Primary neoplasms and cysts
   2. Metastatic neoplasms
   3. Macrosomia

Primary tumors

The spleen is only rarely the site of primary tumor in the strict sense of the word. Thus most of the leukemias and lymphomas, which are multicentric in origin, are not considered to be primary splenic tumors.

Although usually affected as part of a generalized process, in some exceptional cases of malignant lymphoma the spleen may be the only detectable site of disease. The spleen harboring malignant lymphoma is enlarged and may show signs of hypersplenism. On gross examination the involved spleen contains a solitary large mass of malignant lymphoma, multiple smaller masses, or miliary nodules. The masses or nodules are firm and gray and may contain red and yellow areas corresponding to foci of hemorrhage and necrosis. Histologically the picture is similar to that seen in lymph nodes (see discussion of lymph nodes). The miliary nodules represent enlarged malpighian follicles. This pattern is particularly frequent in chronic lymphocytic leukemia and small cell malignant lymphoma. Often in lymphoproliferative disorders involving the spleen there is infiltration of the subintimal lymphatics in the trabecular veins. Patients with malignant lymphoma primarily involving the spleen may benefit from splenectomy.[218,226]

Other primary malignant tumors of the spleen are rare. They include fibrosarcomas, hemangiosarcomas, and spindle cell sarcomas, which may be difficult to classify. Primary benign tumors of the spleen include hemangiomas and lymphangiomas. Hemangiomas are sometimes only a few millimeters in diameter, more often measure 1 to 2 cm, and occasionally are so large as to cause splenomegaly (Fig. 30-23). Lymphangiomas may also be very large and may be present as multicystic lesions (Fig. 30-24). They are usually subcapsular or peritrabecular in location.[74] Other benign tumors (fibroma, chondroma, osteoma) are extremely rare.

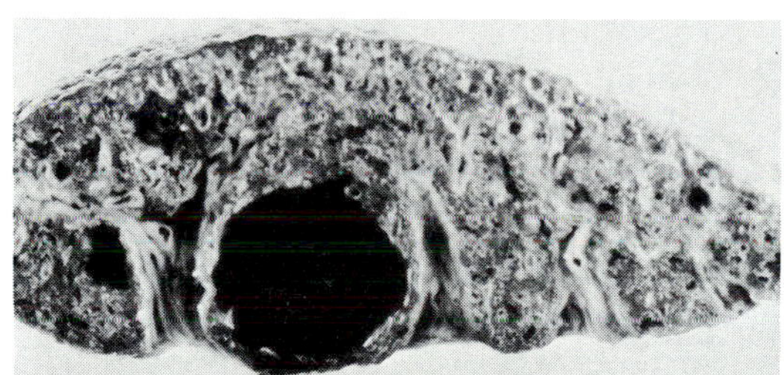

Fig. 30-23. Hemangioma of spleen with fibrosis.

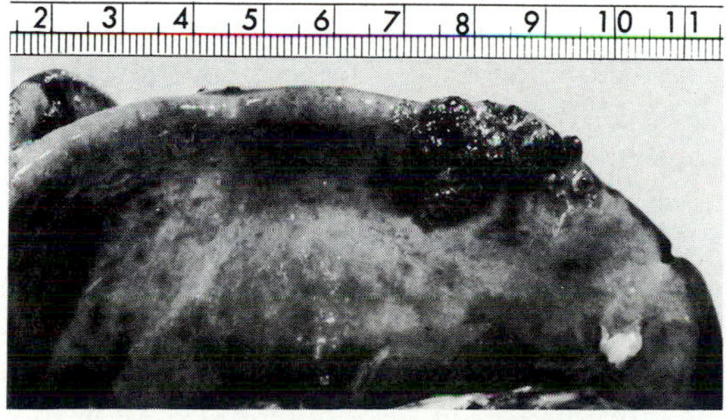

Fig. 30-24. Lymphangioma of spleen.

Occasionally well-circumscribed, but not encapsulated, nodules made up of splenic tissue resembling red pulp are seen within the splenic parenchyma. Well-formed malpighian follicles and trabeculae are rare. These nodules have been called hamartomas, splenomas, splenic adenomas, and intrasplenic accessory spleens.

Metastatic tumors

The frequency of involvement of the spleen by metastatic tumor ranges from rare to 50% in the various series reported. The higher values probably reflect the true incidence of metastases, for the more care taken to examine all of the spleen, both grossly and microscopically, the higher the incidence of metastatic tumor.

Metastases occur late in the course of the primary cancer and are not found in the absence of metastases to other organs. The primary tumors that metastasize to the spleen are many. The most common sites of origin, in order of decreasing frequency, are the lung, breast, prostate gland, colon, and stomach. Metastases may be either nodular or diffuse. Most represent hematogenous spread from the primary lesion, but some of the metastases are undoubtedly by lymphatic dissemination. In lymphatic dissemination, tumor cells are found subintimally in trabecular veins. Spleens showing only microscopic metastases range in weight from 60 to 400 g. Those showing large nodules of metastatic tumor range from 70 to 1100 g. Those showing diffuse gross involvement range from 100 to 3000 g.

Cysts

Cysts of the spleen are rare. They may be parasitic, of which those caused by *Echinococcus granulosus* are the most frequent, or nonparasitic. Nonparasitic cysts are more frequent in the United States,[74] whereas in other parts of the world parasitic cysts are more common. Nonparasitic cysts are divided into true cysts, exhibiting an epithelial lining, and secondary or false cysts or pseudocysts, which do not show an epithelial lining and are thought to result from trauma or hemorrhage. Pseudocysts are more frequent than epithelium-lined cysts. Their wall is made up of dense collagenous tissue that often contains deposits of calcium and hemosiderin. If remnants of an epithelial lining can be identified, the cysts should be classified as epidermoid cysts. Occasionally pseudocysts may result from massive necrosis of the spleen related to a hemoglobinopathy (p. 1277).

True cysts of the spleen are most frequently lined by squamous epithelium and are called epidermoid cysts (Fig. 30-25).[190,215] The epidermoid lining may contain mucous glands and an interrupted surface layer of mucus-containing cells.[215] The pathogenesis of epidermoid cysts is unclear; squamous metaplasia of mesothelial inclusions has been invoked.

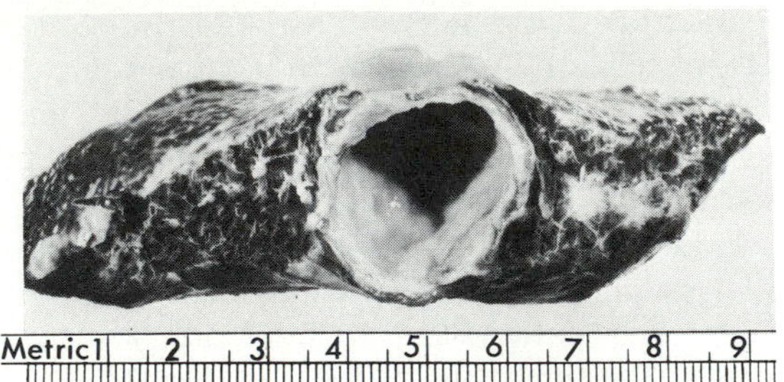

Fig. 30-25. Epidermoid cyst of spleen.

Dermoid cysts of the spleen contain, in addition to an epidermoid lining, sebaceous glands and hair follicles. They are exceedingly rare.

Spleen in autoimmune diseases

The concept of autoimmune disease, a direct and noxious attack by specific immunologic agents against cells and tissues, is based on firm experimental evidence. For example, allergic encephalomyelitis and thyroiditis can be produced by injecting organ extracts into animals, whereas graft-versus-host reactions may involve evidence of generalized disease such as Coombs-positive hemolytic anemia, polyarthritis, myocarditis, and nephritis. Although the experimental autoimmune diseases usually are characterized by the presence of tissue-specific antibodies in the blood, it does not necessarily follow that autoimmune antibodies in the blood in human diseases are in every instance directly toxic to cells and tissues. Nevertheless, it would seem that a common denominator in these diseases is the reaction of connective tissue. Since the spleen often is involved, the pathologic changes in this organ deserve brief mention.

Splenomegaly, with or without characteristic histologic alterations, is common to the entire group. In rheumatoid arthritis, for example, the spleen usually is enlarged but presents no diagnostic histologic changes. On the other hand, the spleen in systemic lupus erythematosus usually shows foci of degenerating collagen in the capsule and the characteristic periarterial "onion-skin" lesion (Fig. 30-26) that affects the central and penicillar arteries. By immunofluorescence, gamma globulin (Fig. 30-27), complement, and fibrinogen can be demonstrated in the laminae of the lesion.

There are two types of thrombocytopenic purpura in which the spleen shows recognizable involvement. In idiopathic thrombocytopenic purpura, an immunologic thrombocytopenia, the spleen is usually unremarkable. Occasionally the lymphoid follicles are hyperplastic (Fig. 30-28), megakaryocytes may be found in the red pulp, and there may also be occasional foamy histiocytes, with or without ceroid pigment. Thrombotic thrombocytopenic purpura, on the other hand, is believed not to be caused by an immunologic reaction. There is diffuse thrombosis of small blood vessels, once believed to be caused by platelet thrombi, but we have come to appreciate that the occlusion is caused by intravascular deposition of fibrin with secondary entrapment of platelets. The lesions can be found in the spleen as well as in most other organs.

LYMPH NODES

Structure

Lymph nodes are discrete nodules of lymphoid tissue located at anatomically constant points along the course of lymphatic vessels. Lymphoid tissue is not found exclusively in lymph nodes, for lymphoid aggregates are present in the submucosa of the intestinal tract and bronchi, in normal bone marrow, in the spleen, and diffusely in the thymus. However, as in the case of the spleen, lymph nodes are circumscribed and identifiable structures whose enlargement is easily discovered by palpation. As discrete structures, they can be excised and subjected to detailed bacteriologic, cytologic, and histologic study.

Lymph nodes have a fibrous capsule from which connective tissue trabeculae extend into the node in a roughly radial arrangement. The connective tissue framework between the trabeculae consists of a network of reticulin fibers, and this stroma supports primitive reticuloendothelial cells, scattered phagocytic histiocytes, and the predominant lymphocytes. In the central or medullary portion of the lymph node, the small lymphocytes are packed tightly in sheets and cords separated by medullary sinuses. In the peripheral or cortical portion, the lymphocytes are condensed into roughly spherical lymphoid nodules (primary follicles). These may consist entirely of small lymphocytes when the lymph node is in a completely resting or nonreactive state. When stimulated, the primary lymphoid nodules develop germinal or reactive centers (secondary follicles) that consist of small, intermediate, and large lymphoid cells. The germinal centers also contain dendritic, desmosome-containing reticulum cells, as well as macrophages with cytoplasmic inclusions known as tingible bodies (starry-sky macrophages).

The relationship between the small and large lymphoid cells has to be revised in the light of modern concepts (Fig. 30-29). When the small perifollicular lymphocytes are stimulated by antigens or mitogens, they enlarge and take on the appearance of blasts, that is, cells with round open nuclei, prominent nucleoli, large nuclear cytoplasmic ratios, and a rim of basophilic (Giemsa stain) and pyroninophilic cytoplasm. Such blast cells occur in normal germinal centers and have been called "large noncleaved cells" by Lukes and Collins[131] and "germinoblasts" and "centroblasts" by Lennert.[120]

Cells intermediate in development between the small lymphocyte and the centroblast are called centrocytes or

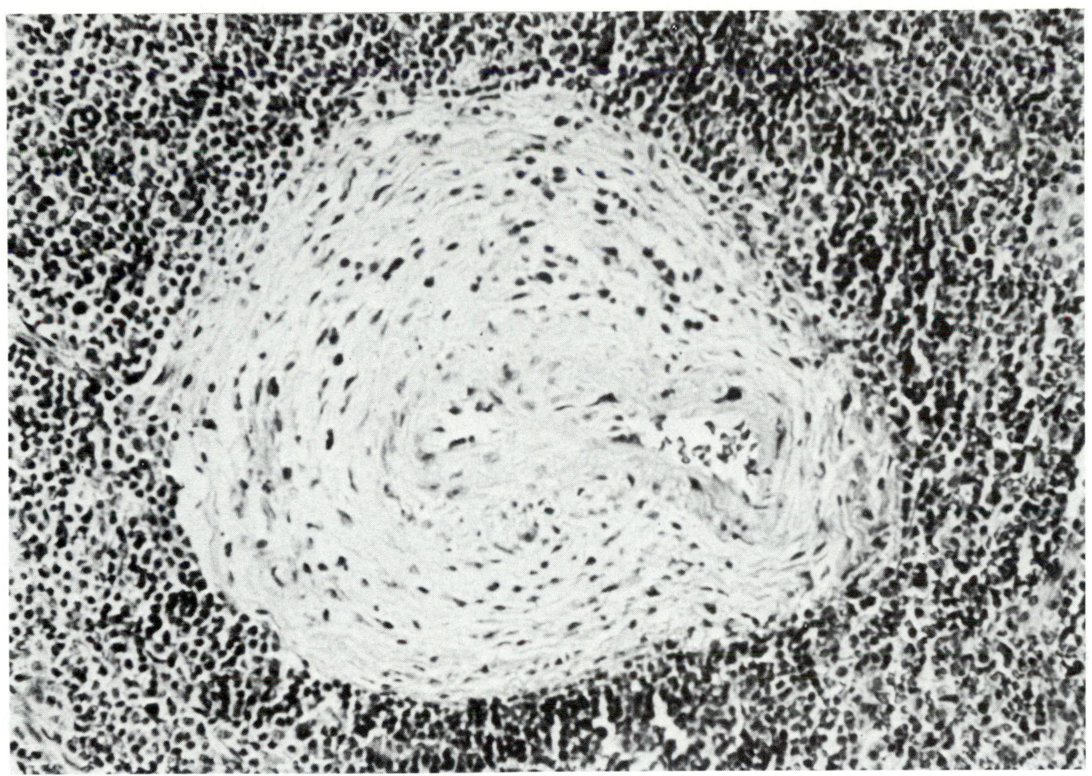

Fig. 30-26. Spleen in disseminated lupus erythematosus. Note onion-skin appearance of arteriolar wall. (Hematoxylin and eosin; 125×.)

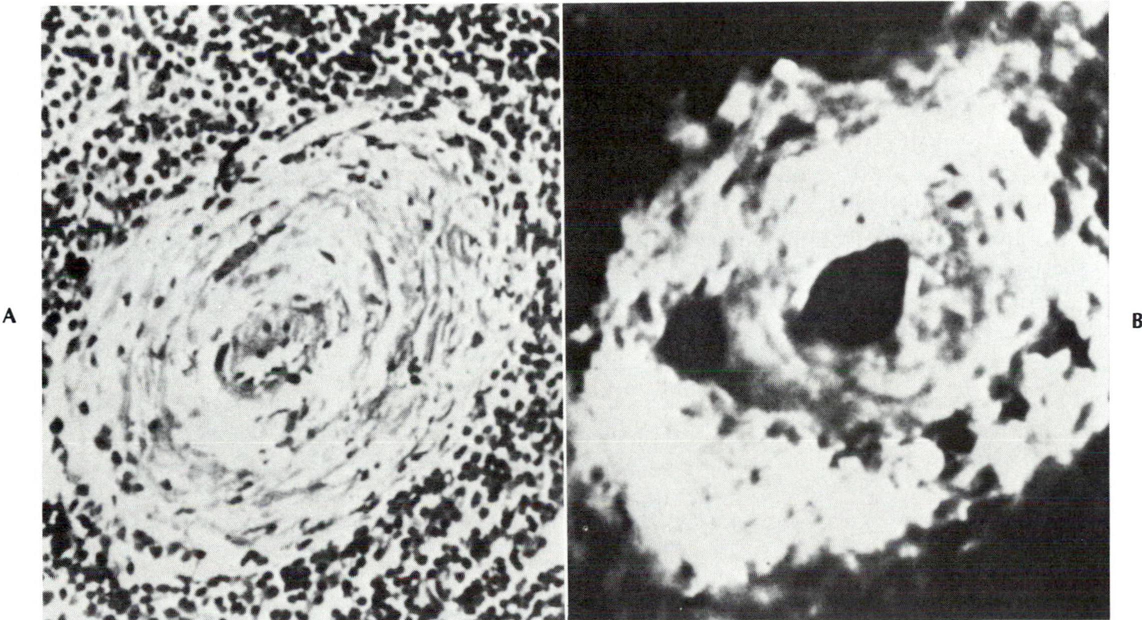

Fig. 30-27. Spleen in disseminated lupus erythematosus. **A,** Typical onion-skin appearance of arteriole. **B,** Immunofluorescence reaction with anti–gamma globulin serum showing deposition of gamma globulin. (From Miescher, P.A., and Muller-Eberhard, H.J.: Textbook of immunopathology, New York, 1968-1969, Grune & Stratton, Inc.; by permission.)

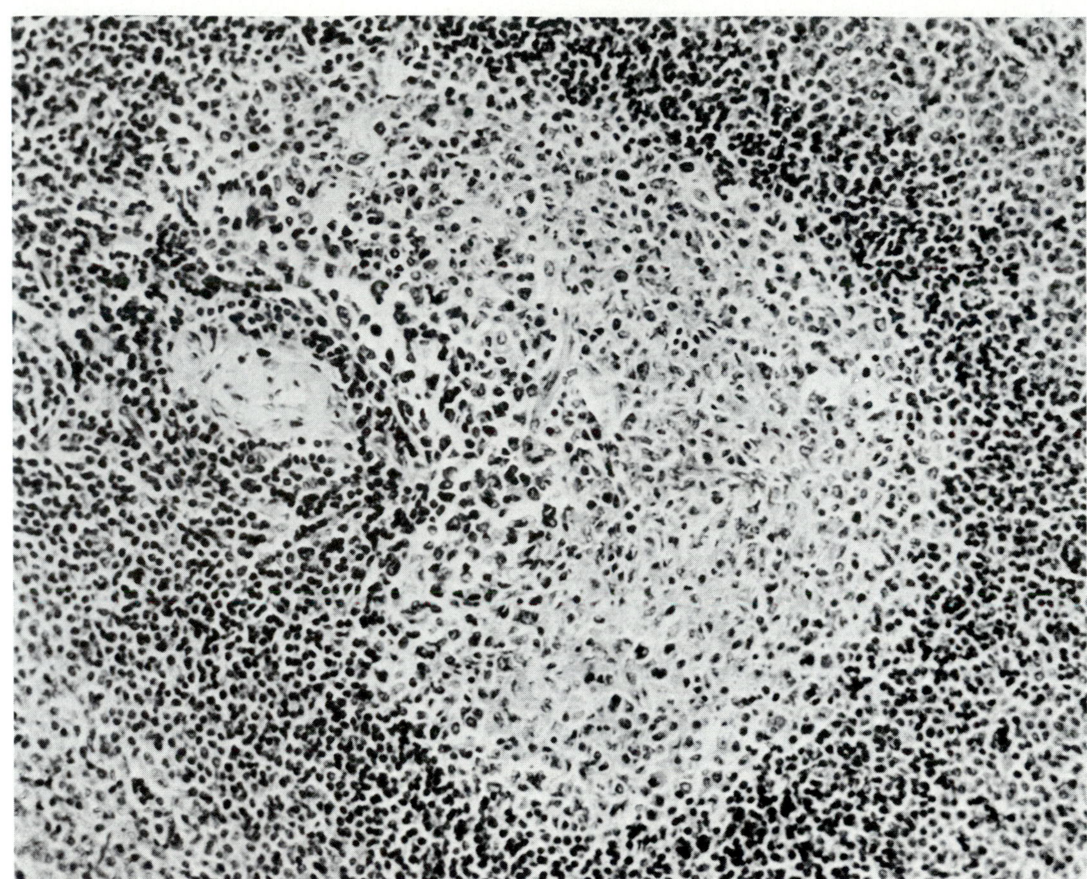

Fig. 30-28. Spleen in idiopathic thrombocytopenic purpura. There is striking hyperplasia of lymphoid follicle. (Hematoxylin and eosin; 125×.)

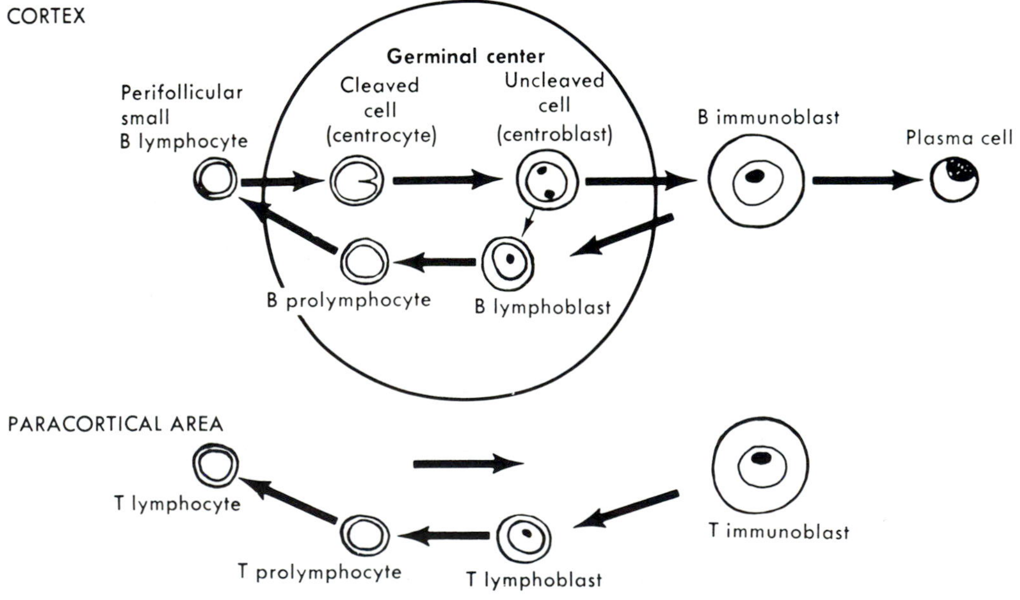

Fig. 30-29. Schematic representation of transformation of B and T lymphocytes.

cleaved cells because of the indentations of their nuclear membranes. According to Lennert, the centroblast is characterized by a round to oval nucleus with multiple nucleoli that are situated close to the nuclear membrane. The cytoplasm is narrow and basophilic and often contains vacuoles. The centroblast evolves into an immunoblast that is larger and contains a bigger, more centrally located nucleolus. The immunoblast possesses a wider rim of cytoplasm that ultrastructurally contains more rough endoplasmic reticulum and more polysomes than the centroblast. The B immunoblast gives rise to plasma cells. The centroblasts and immunoblasts also seem to participate in lymphopoiesis by becoming lymphoblasts, undergoing mitosis, and then developing into small, "mature" lymphocytes. This sequence is in line with the classical concept of lymphopoiesis: lymphoblast → prolymphocyte → lymphocyte. It is doubtful that a centrocyte can be distinguished from a prolymphocyte. T lymphocytes when stimulated are transformed into T immunoblasts, which probably also participate in T lymphopoiesis. T immunoblasts cannot be distinguished cytologically from B immunoblasts. They differ from B immunoblasts by their localization in the paracortical areas. Morphologically, in my opinion, lymphoblasts cannot be distinguished with certainty from centroblasts and immunoblasts.

The germinal center is pale staining and sharply circumscribed by the crowded dark-staining small lymphocytes that form a corona at its periphery. When studied in serial sections, the germinal centers can be shown to be spheroid with two poles. The superficial hemisphere, adjacent to the marginal sinus in a lymph node or epithelium in the intestine, is directed toward the nearest source of antigen and stains lightly because the cells are larger and have a more abundant cytoplasm. The deep hemisphere stains dark because the cells have scantier cytoplasm, and the corona of small lymphocytes is usually less distinct than at the upper pole. The polar structure corresponds to immunologic reactions, for it has been shown that bacterial antigens injected intravenously first localize in the perifollicular region and then migrate to the superficial or light area of the reactive center.[158]

The area of the lymph node between germinal centers and the subcapsular sinus is called the far cortical region. The deep cortex, or paracortex, is situated between the peripheral cortex with its germinal centers and the medulla of the lymph node. The deep cortex contains lymphocytes grouped around postcapillary venules (tertiary follicles). The postcapillary venules are also known as epithelioid venules because of the prominence of the endothelial cells. The bursa-dependent, or B, area of the lymph node includes the far cortical and germinal center regions, whereas the thymus-dependent, or T, area lies in the deep cortex (see p. 1355).

Lymph enters the node through afferent vessels and empties into a subcapsular sinus that is continuous with sinuses running along the trabeculae. The medullary sinuses ultimately form efferent lymphatics that leave the node at the hilum. The sinuses are lined by flat littoral or lining cells sometimes called endothelial, but littoral and endothelial cells are quite different when studied by electron microscopy.[21] The chief difference is that littoral cells are phagocytic, and, as such, they perform a housecleaning function on the lymph. Under pathologic conditions, these cells hypertrophy, multiply, and become detached as free phagocytes in the lymph sinus, the *Sinuskatarrh* of German authors, also known as sinus histiocytosis.

Study of the morphology of individual cells, as seen in imprints from the freshly cut surface of a lymph node or from smears of aspirated material, is a useful adjunct to the histopathologic appearance. Histologic sections are essential for determining the relationship of cells to each other and the architecture of the tissue, but cellular details are partially obscured by fixation and by the thickness of the section. On the other hand, imprints make possible a study of individual cells, as in a blood smear, and often reveal details of morphology that, in combination with the histologic appearance, are extremely useful in arriving at the correct diagnosis.

Imprints of a normal node show a predominance of small lymphocytes, as well as larger lymphoid cells, and scattered cells of other types. When the node is abnormal, quantitative and qualitative abnormalities will be found. Some of these will be illustrated in later discussions.

Function

The functions of the lymph nodes are three: (1) formation of lymphocytes, (2) production of antibodies, and (3) filtration of the lymph.

The lymph nodes are responsible for a portion of the total lymphocyte-producing capacity of lymphoid tissue. There is as yet no information on how many lymphocytes enter the total lymphocyte pool from lymph nodes and how many are produced elsewhere. On the basis of weight, lymph nodes contain about 100 g of lymphoid tissue as compared to 70 g in the bone marrow and 1300 g scattered throughout other tissues. Lymphocytes originating in lymph nodes enter the lymph channels on the efferent side. Some enter the bloodstream directly by passing through the walls of capillary vessels. According to modern concepts of lymphocytopoiesis and immunology, the lymphoid system is divided into a central portion, consisting of lymphoid tissue in Peyer's patches, appendix, and tonsils plus the lymphoid tissue in the thymus, and a peripheral portion consisting of spleen and lymph nodes. The spleen and lymph nodes not only generate new lymphocytes but also are populated by lym-

Table 30-1. Functional and anatomic characteristics of lymphoid and related cells

Cell type	Function	Location
T cells	Initiation of delayed hypersensitivity reactions Initiation of solid-tissue allograft rejection Initiation of graft versus host reactions Elaboration of lymphokines Defense against facultative intracellular bacterial and rickettsial pathogens, fungi, and many viruses Responsive to phytohemagglutinin or allogeneic cell stimulation in vitro Immunosurveillance against cancer (?)	Blood (65% to 80% of blood lymphocytes) Lymph node: deep cortical areas (paracortex) Spleen: perivascular areas of the white pulp (perivascular lymphocyte sheath)
B cells	Synthesis and secretion of immunoglobulins and specific antibodies (IgM, IgG, IgA, IgD, IgE) Progenitor of plasma cells Primary defense against high-grade encapsulated bacterial pathogens Detoxification of certain proteins, polypeptides, and other toxins Neutralization of viruses (especially secretory IgA in respiratory tract and gut) Interference with absorption of foreign proteins from respiratory tract and gut	Blood (15% to 25% of blood lymphocytes) Lymph node: germinal centers (lymphoid follicles, pyroninophilic cells) and medullary cords (secretory lymphocytes and plasma cells) Spleen: lymphoid follicles of white pulp and red pulp cords (chief site of splenic antibody production)
M cells (monocytes)	Phagocytosis of organisms and particles Major effector mechanism in defense against most bacterial, fungal, and probably viral pathogens Processing and presentation of antigen Removal of cellular debris	Blood: monocytes Tissue: macrophages, histiocytes, Kupffer cells of sinusoids of liver Lymph node: germinal center macrophages (tingible body macrophages) and medullary cord macrophages Spleen: present in both white pulp and red pulp
Dendritic reticulum cells	Apparently play crucial role in development of antibody response through adherence and presentation of antigen	Origin unknown; appear within germinal centers; extensive dendritic processes interdigitate with lymphocytes of the germinal center

From Hansen, J.A., and Good, R.A.: Hum. Pathol. **5**:567, 1974.

phocytes originating in the central tissues. The functional and anatomic characteristics of lymphoid cells and monocytes (M cells) are summarized in Table 30-1.

Lymph nodes play an obvious but relatively unimportant role as filters of particulate matter (anthracotic pigment, cellular debris, bacteria). Tumor cells carried by the lymph from the primary site to regional lymph nodes may implant and grow to form metastases.

Lymphadenitis

Lymph nodes may react to injury in unique patterns related to their structure and function. These patterns, collectively called reactive hyperplasia of lymph nodes, include follicular hyperplasia, paracortical hyperplasia, and sinus histiocytosis. In addition, lymph nodes may exhibit inflammatory reactions that are also seen in other tissues such as suppuration, necrosis, granulomatous inflammation, and infiltration with plasma cells. Combinations of reactive hyperplasia with other inflammatory reactions are seen in certain diseases. Some of these patterns are more or less specific, that is, suggest an etiologic agent; other patterns are nonspecific. Lymphadenitis may be caused by bacteria, fungi, viruses, protozoa, and helminths.

Reactive hyperplasia of lymph nodes

This group includes a number of histologic reaction patterns that are nonspecific, in the sense that they can be caused by a variety of stimuli.

Reactive hyperplasia of the follicular type (Fig. 30-30) is characterized by lymphoid follicles with large germinal centers exhibiting a high mitotic activity and numerous macrophages with tingible bodies. Plasma cells are numerous. The lymphoid follicles vary considerably in size but have well-defined margins surrounded by a mantle of small lymphocytes. This type of reaction pattern is caused by the stimulation of B lymphocytes. It may be seen in secondary syphilis, rheumatoid arthritis, and giant lymph node hyperplasia. It may simulate a malignant follicular lymphoma.

Reactive hyperplasia of the sinus histiocytosis type displays distension of the sinusoids by well-differentiated histiocyte-like cells. The significance of this reaction pattern is unknown. It is often observed in axillary lymph

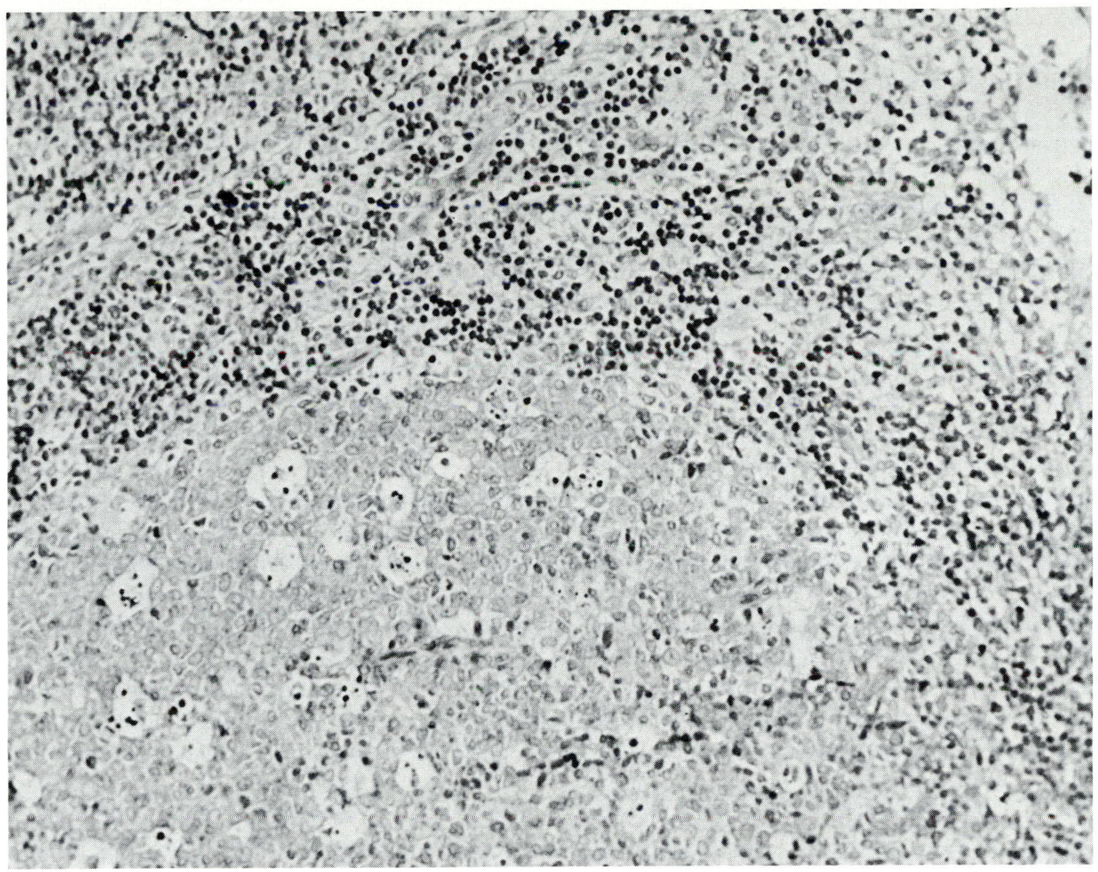

Fig. 30-30. Lymph node. Reactive hyperplasia, follicular type. (Hematoxylin and eosin; 125×.)

nodes from patients with carcinoma of the breast. In these cases the presence of a sinus histiocytosis pattern appears to indicate a more favorable prognosis.

This nonspecific sinus histiocytosis must be distinguished from histiocytic medullary reticulosis, histiocytosis X, and sinus histiocytosis with massive lymphadenopathy.

Paracortical lymphoid hyperplasia (T-area lymphoid hyperplasia) may be seen in antigenically stimulated lymph nodes. The paracortical areas show varying degrees of hyperplasia, which may attenuate the follicular and sinusoidal architecture of the lymph node. The paracortical areas display a considerable number of large lymphoid cells with prominent nucleoli and a basophilic cytoplasm with the Giemsa stain (immunoblasts). Under low-power magnification these cells impart a mottled appearance to the lymph node, since they are scattered among small lymphocytes.

Combination patterns between follicular, paracortical hyperplasia, and sinus histiocytosis types may be seen.

Suppurative lymphadenitis

An acute suppurative inflammatory reaction in a lymph node is caused by an inflammation in the area it drains. When the primary infection is caused by a pyogenic organism such as *Staphylococcus* or *Streptococcus*, the regional lymph node is enlarged and tender, and the pulp between follicles is hyperemic and infiltrated with neutrophilic leukocytes. Later, there is an exudation of monocytes and phagocytes, the latter containing ingested cellular debris. When bacteria have been carried to the node, they may multiply and produce hemorrhage and abscesses.

Necrotizing lymphadenitis

An extensive hemorrhagic and necrotizing lymphadenitis is characteristic of bubonic plague. Focal necrosis of lymph nodes is also seen in lupus erythematosus, in which it is associated with the deposition of hematoxylinophilic material. It has been observed in Dilantin hypersensitivity and infectious mononucleosis. Massive necrosis of lymph nodes has been attributed to thrombosis of hilar veins.[44]

Recently the terms *necrotizing lymphadenitis*,[237a] *histiocytic necrotizing lymphadenitis without granulocytic infiltration*,[171a] and *Kikuchi disease*[49a] have been applied to a fairly specific clinicopathologic entity of unknown etiology. The disease has a remarkable predilection for cervical lymph nodes of young women. Histologically the nodes show well-circumscribed paracortical foci of necrosis surrounded by aggregates of histiocytes. The necrotic foci contain karyorrhectic debris with some fibrin. There is a striking paucity of polymorphonuclear leukocytes. Spontaneous resolution of the lymphadenopathy seems to occur in most patients.

Idiopathic infarction of lymph nodes in patients with fever of unknown origin has been reported.[16,248] Infarction of lymph nodes may result in palisading necrotizing granulomas.[213] Varying degrees of necrosis are also seen in suppurative and granulomatous lymphadenitis.

Granulomatous lymphadenitis

Granulomatous lymphadenitis may be seen in bacterial, fungal, and viral diseases. Granulomas may also form as a response to various foreign bodies. Lipid granulomas are common in lymph nodes around bile ducts and the porta hepatis and in the mesentery.

Tuberculous involvement of lymph nodes presents the entire spectrum of the histopathology of tuberculosis, from the typical small tubercle to caseous necrosis, fibrosis, and calcification (Fig. 30-31). Lymph node involvement usually results from drainage from a primary site, as in involvement of hilar and peribronchial lymph nodes in the primary complex of pulmonary tuberculosis. In bronchogenic pulmonary tuberculosis or in organ tuberculosis, active lesions in satellite lymph nodes are relatively inconspicuous. Even when the lesion is typical, with caseous necrosis and giant cells, the diagnosis should be confirmed by bacteriologic culture of homogenized tissue. The demonstration of acid-fast bacilli in paraffin-embedded tissue is often disappointing. Furthermore, bacteriologic studies are necessary to identify the mycobacterium as being the typical *Mycobacterium tuberculosis* or one of the atypical varieties (see Chapter 22).

The lymph nodes are involved in sarcoidosis as part of the generalized disease. Characteristically the lesions are granulomatous and noncaseous and, in the later stages, fibrotic and hyalinizing. The early granuloma is composed of epithelioid cells and may contain giant cells of the Langhans type (Fig. 30-32). At this stage it may not be possible to determine the nature of the granuloma, for similar lesions are sometimes found in fungal infections, berylliosis, leprosy, toxoplasmosis, Hodgkin's disease, and early noncaseous tuberculosis and even in nodes draining a carcinomatous area (Fig. 30-33). Special mention should be made of the not uncommon occurrence of sarcoidosis-like lesions in scalene lymph nodes (lower deep jugular) draining a primary carcinoma of the lung.

Sarcoid lesions may contain foreign body formations (Schaumann's bodies, Fig. 30-34, and asteroids) that are not diagnostic of sarcoidosis, since they may be found in berylliosis and other conditions. In some cases small

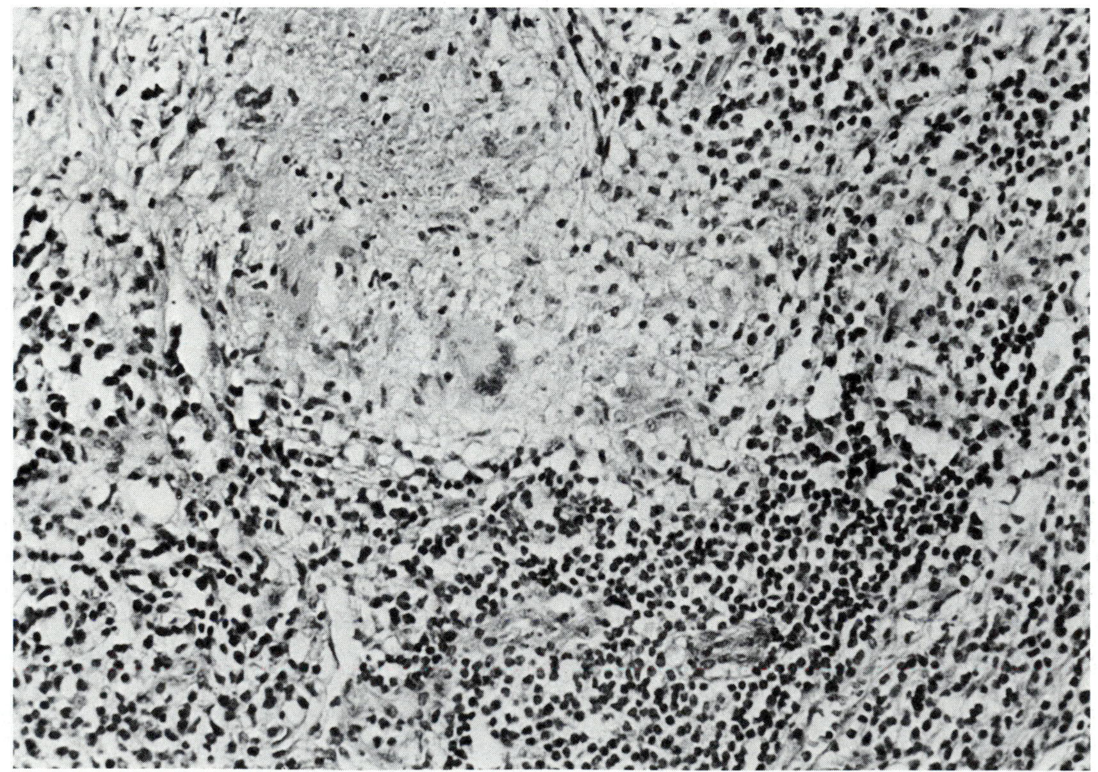

Fig. 30-31. Lymph node in tuberculosis. (Hematoxylin and eosin; 125×.)

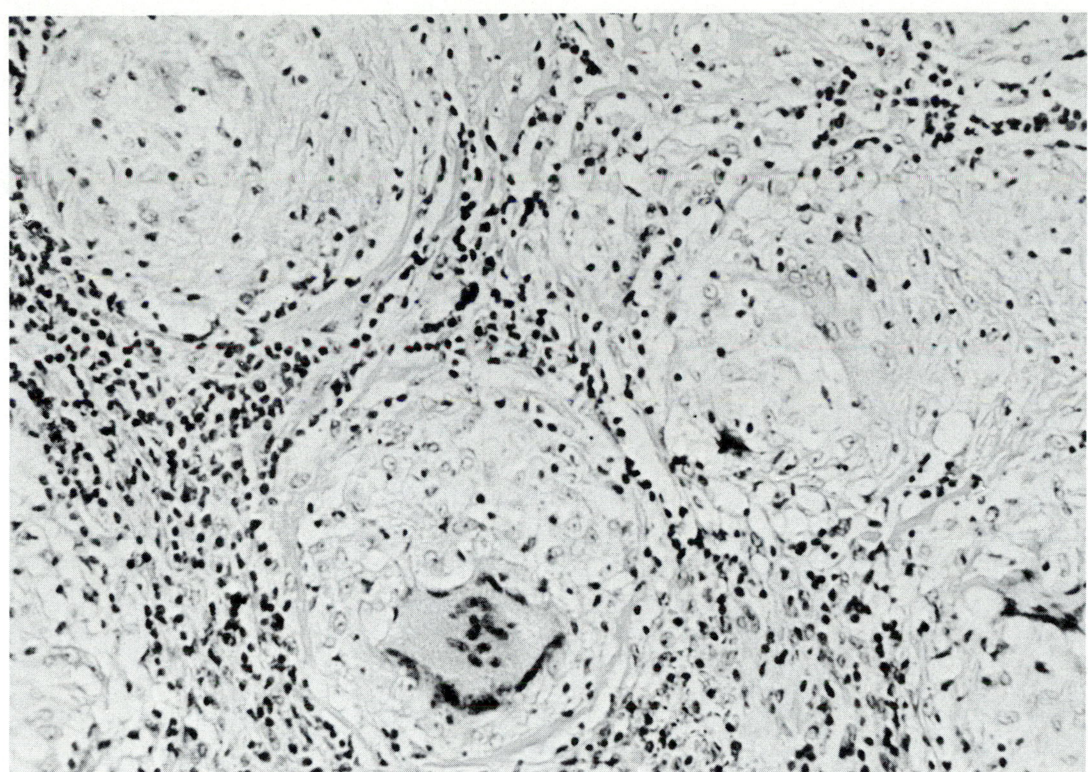

Fig. 30-32. Lymph node in sarcoidosis. (Hematoxylin and eosin; 125×.)

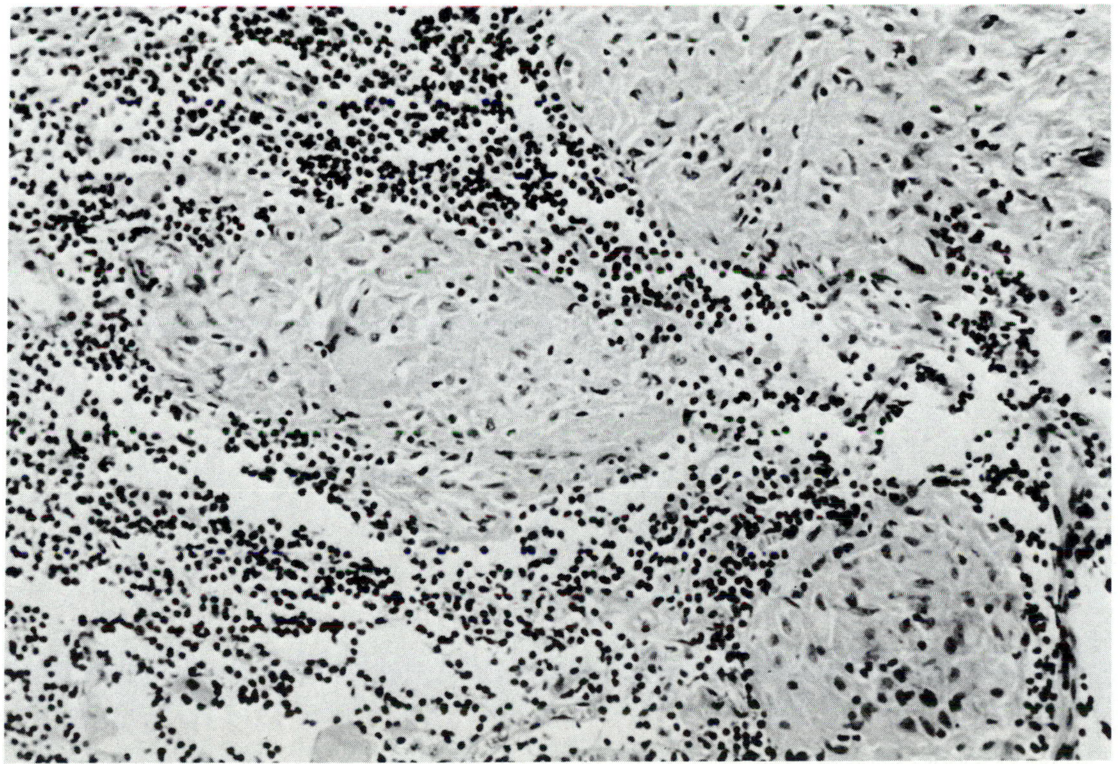

Fig. 30-33. Lymph node. Sarcoidosis-like lesions in cervical lymph node draining carcinomatous area. (Hematoxylin and eosin; 125×.)

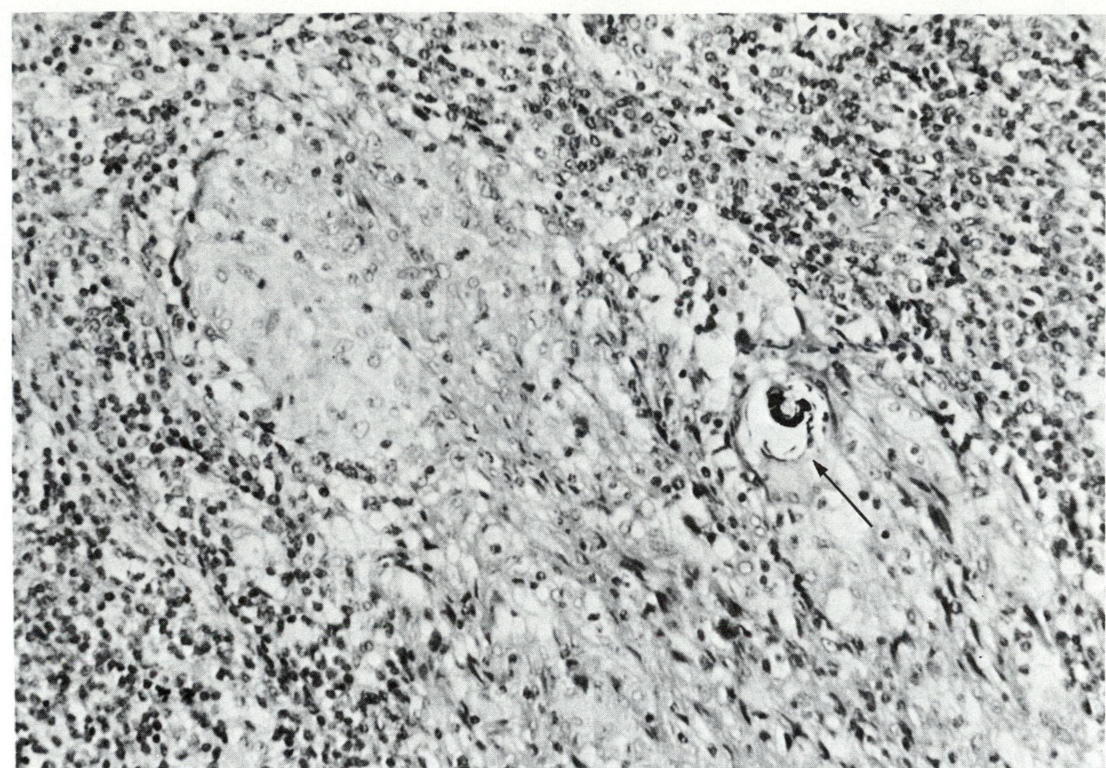

Fig. 30-34. Lymph node in sarcoidosis with Schaumann's body. (Hematoxylin and eosin; 125×.)

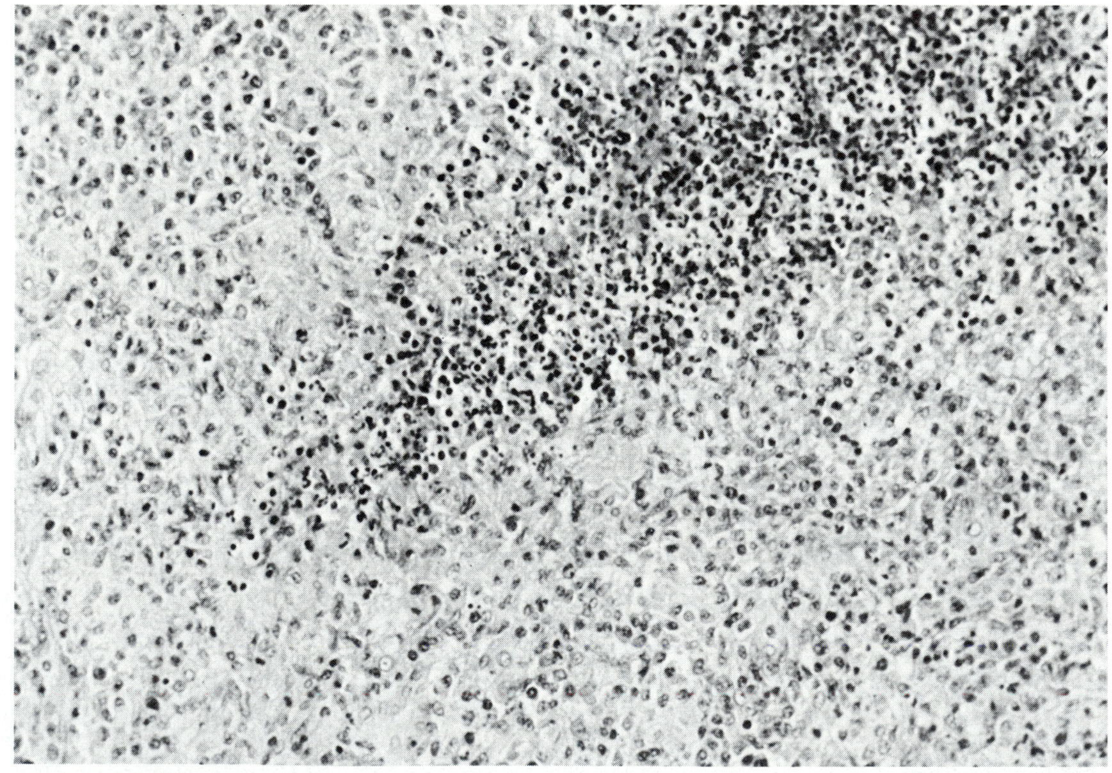

Fig. 30-35. Lymph node in cat-scratch disease; central abscess surrounded by epithelioid cells. (Hematoxylin and eosin; 125×.)

granular brown fusiform structures are seen that have been called Hamazaki-Wesenberg bodies. They exhibit the tinctorial characteristics of ceroid.[216] Sarcoid lesions do, at times, undergo central necrosis. The specific diagnosis of granulomatous inflammation is sometimes difficult and requires the correlation of clinical and laboratory data with the histologic appearance of the lesion.

Cat-scratch disease

Cat-scratch disease is one of the causes of enlargement of regional lymph nodes. There is tentative serologic evidence that the causative agent may be related to the chlamydiae of the psittacosis-lymphogranuloma group. However, recently delicate, pleomorphic, gram-negative bacilli were found in endothelial cells of capillaries and within microabscesses of the involved lymph nodes. These bacilli were best seen with the Warthin-Starry silver impregnation stain. They appear to be the causative agent of cat-scratch disease.[248a] The infectious agent is inoculated percutaneously by a cat scratch (60% of the cases), a cat bite (10%), or various injuries such as from splinters, thorns, pins, fishhooks, rabbit claws, and porcupine quills (5%). In about one fourth of the cases there is no known skin injury, although most of the patients are known to have had a cat in the household.

Since regional lymphadenopathy is the cardinal sign of cat-scratch disease, this disease must be considered in the differential diagnosis of lymphadenopathy. The histologic appearance of the lymph nodes is characterized by suppurative granulomas. These consist of a central necrotic area infiltrated with polymorphonuclear leukocytes surrounded by palisading epithelioid cells with occasional Langhans' giant cells (Fig. 30-35). This granulomatous inflammation is most noticeable in the cortical area of the lymph node. It usually extends to the perinodal tissue and to the medullary portion of the node. The remaining lymph nodal tissue shows follicular hyperplasia with prominent germinal centers, immunoblasts, plasma cells, and eosinophils. Suppurative granulomas are also characteristic of other diseases[119]: mesenteric adenitis attributable to *Yersinia enterocolitica*, tularemia, lymphopathia venereum, fungal infections, and melioidosis.

Toxoplasmic lymphadenitis

Toxoplasmic lymphadenitis involves primarily the cervical lymph nodes.[172] There is good correlation between toxoplasmic lymphadenitis and the Sabin-Feldman dye test and the IgM immunofluorescent antibody test.[49]

Histologically the involved lymph nodes show a striking degree of reactive follicular hyperplasia with large germinal centers containing many macrophages. The interfollicular zones contain small foci of epithelioid cells usually without giant cells. The epithelioid cells may be located within the germinal centers. An additional distinctive feature is the focal distension of sinuses by immature histiocytes. The medullary cords may contain increased numbers of plasma cells and immunoblasts. Toxoplasmic cysts are found very rarely in lymph nodes.

Postlymphangiography lymphadenitis

The angiographic contrast media used for studying the roentgenographic morphology of superficial and deep lymph nodes (lymphangiography) produce characteristic histologic changes.[183] They range from the early reaction consisting of exudation of neutrophils, eosinophils, and a few plasma cells to the chronic reaction characterized by foreign body giant cells surrounding droplets of contrast medium plus plasma cell infiltration.

Filarial lymphadenitis

Filarial lymphadenitis caused by *Brugia* species has been reported from New England, New Jersey, and New York.[41] The only naturally occurring *Brugia* species known in North America is *B. beaveri*, a lymphatic-dwelling parasite commonly found in raccoons. The infection is transmitted by mosquitoes. The patients are asymptomatic except for focal lymphadenopathy. The excised nodes show some degree of follicular hyperplasia with scattered eosinophils. The worm is small and may be found in only one of the sections made. It often lies in a lymphatic. A granulomatous reaction surrounding a degenerating worm may be seen. The worm must be distinguished from *Dirofilaria*, which has a much thicker, ridged cuticle. *Wuchereria bancrofti*, not indigenous to the continental United States, is considerably larger.

Infectious mononucleosis

Infectious mononucleosis, a disease of adolescents and young adults, is caused by Epstein-Barr virus.[90] Clinically it is demonstrated by cervical or generalized lymphadenopathy, splenomegaly in some cases, and a peripheral blood picture with an increased number of lymphocytes exhibiting considerable variability from small lymphocytes to blasts and intermediate forms. There is usually no anemia or thrombocytopenia.

The lymph nodes are enlarged, and the structure is partially effaced. Well-defined lymphoid follicles are present in most cases. There is also paracortical lymphoid hyperplasia with the appearance of blasts (immunoblasts), that is, large cells with nucleoli and a basophilic cytoplasmic rim with the Giemsa stain. These cells are also pyroninophilic. Small lymphocytes and intermediate lymphoid cells are present (Fig. 30-36). The sinusoids are distended with macrophages and blasts. Cells identical to Reed-Sternberg cells may be present.[142,245] Variable numbers of plasma cells are found within the sinuses and the medullary cords. At times focal necrosis is seen.

When Reed-Sternberg-like cells are present, Hodgkin's disease must be considered. The presence of follicles with reaction centers, detailed attention to the morphology of the Reed-Sternberg cells, and the partial preservation of the sinusoidal structure usually establish the diagnosis of infectious mononucleosis. These criteria may not be absolutely reliable, since occasionally follicles may be preserved in Hodgkin's disease and sinusoids may not be totally effaced. Close attention to clinical data and the peripheral blood smear may help to make the diagnosis.

The X-linked lymphoproliferative syndrome (XLP) is characterized by a combined variable immunodeficiency and vulnerability to Epstein-Barr virus infection with resulting fatal or chronic infectious mononucleosis, acquired agammaglobulinemia, aplastic anemia, or malignant B cell lymphoma.[175] Diagnosis of XLP requires documentation of two or more maternally related males with these phenotypes. The thymus-dependent regions in lymph nodes and spleen are depleted; numerous blasts with plasma cell differentiation are seen.

Postvaccinal lymphadenitis and viral lymphadenitis

Hartsock[88] (see also Lukes and Tindle[133]) has shown that the lymph nodes draining the site of smallpox vaccination undergo an intensive reaction that might, if not recognized, lead to an erroneous diagnosis of lymphoma. Similar reactions may occur after use of other vaccines such as those against tetanus, typhoid fever, diphtheria, pertussis, influenza, and poliomyelitis. Although there

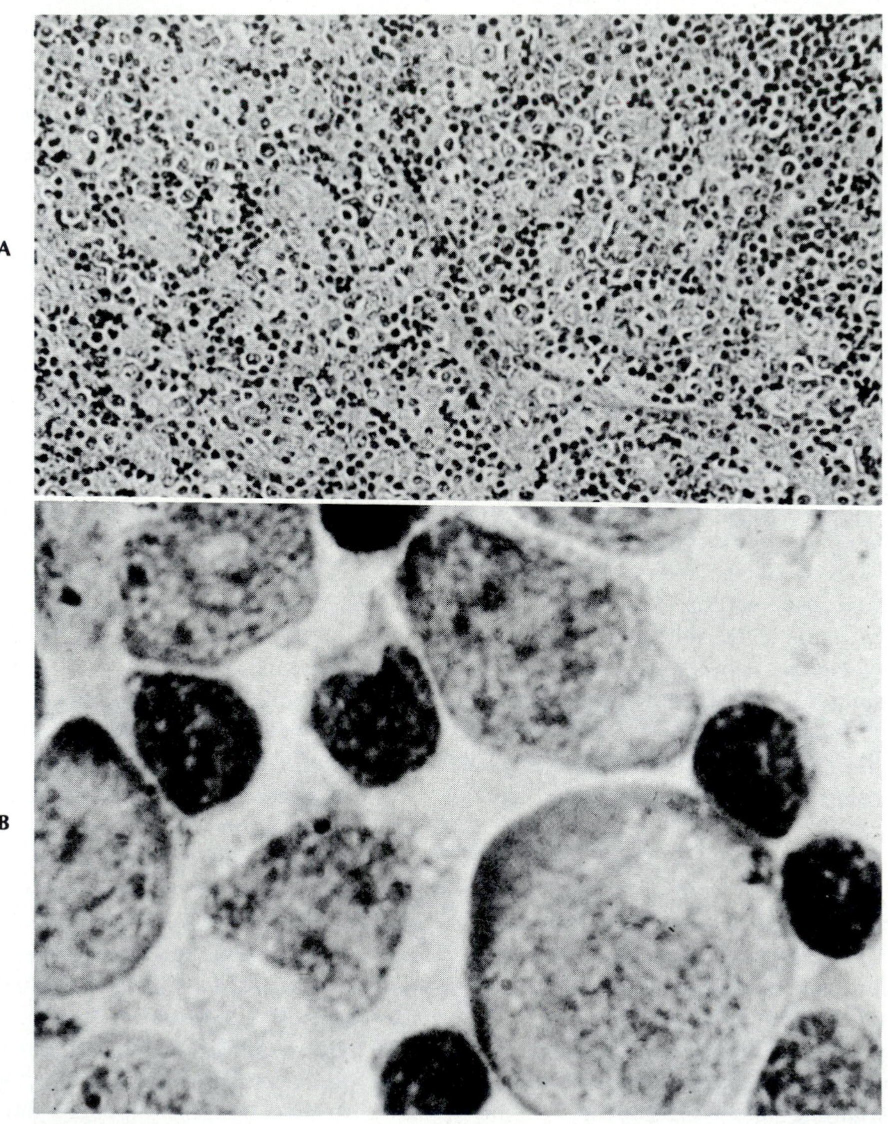

Fig. 30-36. Lymph node in infectious mononucleosis. **A,** Paraffin section. **B,** Imprint. (**A,** Hematoxylin and eosin; 100× **B,** Wright's stain; 1080×; **A** and **B,** courtesy Dr. Joseph C. Sieracki, Pittsburgh.)

should be no reason to excise a node draining a vaccination site, the history of vaccination may be overlooked. Of the 20 cases reviewed by Hartsock,[88] nine had been diagnosed as lymphoma, and in 14 the history of vaccination had been overlooked.

Histologically such a node shows (1) follicular or diffuse hyperplasia, (2) an increased number of immunoblasts (reticular lymphoblasts), (3) vascular and sinusoidal changes, and (4) a mixed cellular response. The hyperplasia involves primarily a proliferation of immunoblasts that, interspersed among other lymphocytes, produce a mottled appearance under low magnification. The immunoblasts have a single nucleus and one or more irregularly shaped nucleoli. The inconstant findings of focal dilatation of lymph sinuses, a mixed cellular response with scattered eosinophils, neutrophils, and plasma cells, and hypertrophy and hyperplasia of endothelial cells are not seen in non-Hodgkin's lymphoma.

Changes such as those described above may occur after the administration of live attenuated measles virus vaccine.[50] In such cases the lymph nodes contain Warthin-Finkeldey giant cells (mulberry cells), which are seen in the lymphoid tissue in the prodromal phase of measles.

Regional lymphadenopathy associated with or preceding herpes zoster skin lesions may mimic postvaccinal lymphadenitis.

Anticonvulsant drug lymphadenopathy (Dilantin lymphadenopathy)

Ingestion of anticonvulsant drugs (used in the treatment of epilepsy) sometimes produces an illness resembling malignant lymphoma both in the hematologic picture and in the histologic changes in lymph nodes and skin. One or more of the following may occur at any time after 1 week to many months of therapy: morbilliform skin rash, lymphadenopathy, fever, hepatosplenomegaly, and painful joints. Eosinophilia in the peripheral blood is not uncommon. The most common offending drugs are phenytoin (Dilantin) and mephenytoin (Mesantoin), but several other drugs of the same type also have been implicated.

The histologic appearance of the lymph nodes resembles postvaccinal lymphadenitis and may be mistaken for Hodgkin's disease. There is moderate to complete loss of normal architecture, focal or diffuse hyperplasia of immunoblasts, which may show pleomorphic nuclei, and diffuse infiltration with eosinophils, neutrophils, and plasma cells (Fig. 30-37). Mitotic figures are found, and infiltration of the capsule is common. One of the most common features is focal areas of necrosis accompanied by phagocytosis of nuclear debris.

In the differentiation of this lesion from the lymphomas, the clinical history is most important. It has been

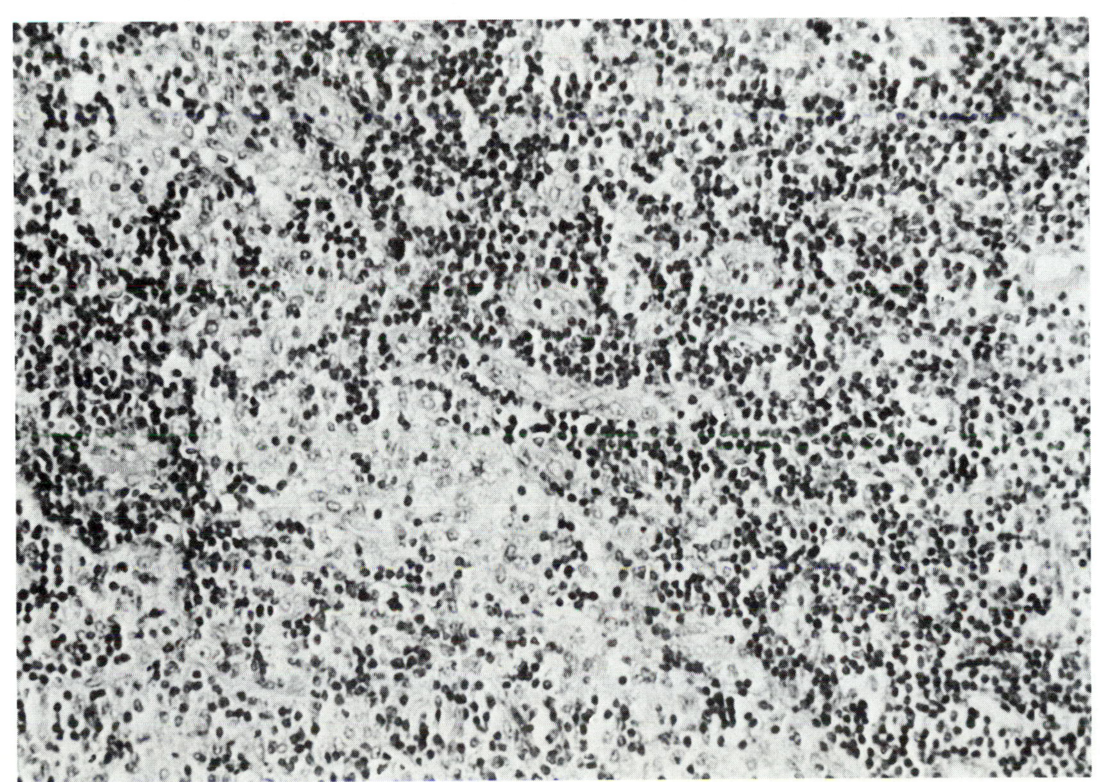

Fig. 30-37. Lymph node in pseudolymphomatous lymphadenitis resulting from ingestion of anticonvulsant drug. (Hematoxylin and eosin; 125×.)

estimated that there are 1 million epileptic patients in the United States. Most of these are receiving anticonvulsive therapy, so that pseudolymphomatous lymphadenitis may challenge the pathologist at any time. It also must be noted that in a patient with epilepsy under treatment a true lymphoma can develop, independent of other circumstances. It has been suggested, indeed, that the incidence of lymphoma is higher in epileptic patients under treatment than in the general population, but this is not based on good statistical evidence. Hyman and Sommers[91] have described the development of lymphoma in patients who had prolonged phenytoin therapy.

Dermatopathic lymphadenitis

Sometimes called lipomelanotic reticulosis, dermatopathic lymphadenitis is associated with chronic dermatoses particularly of the exfoliative type. When viewed with low magnification, it is characterized by a widened and pale-staining paracortical (T-zone) area (Fig. 30-38). Under higher power there is an increased number of epithelioid venules associated with lymphoid cells with cerebriform nuclei. In addition, there are foamy and vacuolated macrophages containing fat. Some macrophages contain melanin and varying amounts of hemosiderin (Fig. 30-39). Increased numbers of eosinophils, plasma cells, and immunoblasts may also be present.

The distinction between dermatopathic lymphadenitis and lymph node mycosis fungoides may be difficult. For the diagnosis of mycosis fungoides of the lymph node there must be at least focal infiltration of the node by atypical cells with cerebriform nuclei and effacement of normal lymph node architecture.[240]

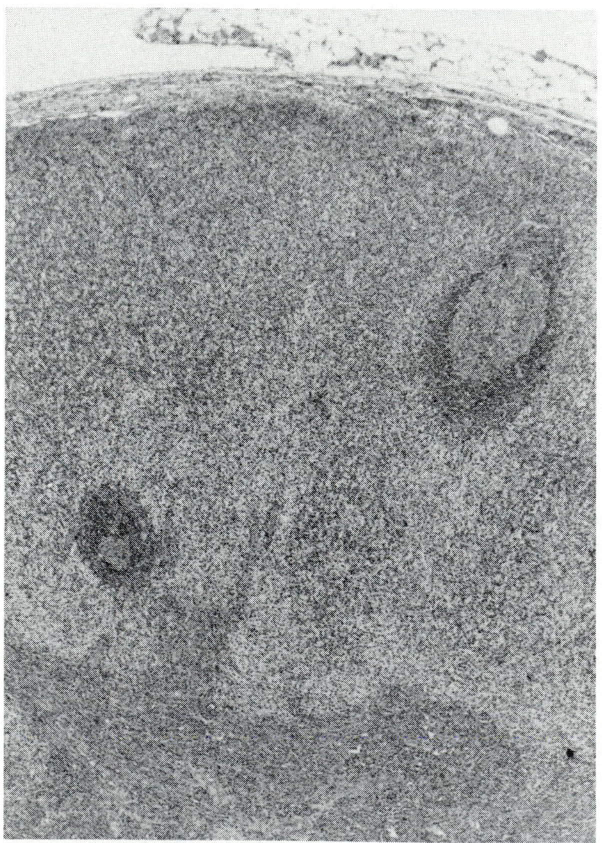

Fig. 30-38. Dermatopathic lymphadenitis. Note pale-staining, enlarged paracortical (T-zone) area and remaining small germinal centers. (Hematoxylin and eosin; low power.)

Miscellaneous lymphadenopathies

Miscellaneous lymphadenopathies include sinus histiocytosis with massive lymphadenopathy, immunoblastic lymphadenopathy, proteinaceous lymphadenopathy, and giant lymph node hyperplasia. It is unclear at present whether these entities represent an inflammatory or a neoplastic process.

Sinus histiocytosis with massive lymphadenopathy (Rosai-Dorfman disease)

This disease occurs most frequently in black children and is characterized by painless, often bilateral, cervical lymphadenopathy.[193] Other lymph node groups, Waldeyer's ring, and the orbit, skin, and bones may be involved.[245] Fever, leukocytosis, an elevated sedimentation rate, and polyclonal hypergammaglobulinemia are common features. The disease follows a protracted course with eventual complete recovery in most cases. The etiology and pathogenesis are unknown. An infectious process may be suspected because of the clinical course and the resemblance of the histologic features to those of rhinoscleroma.

The involved lymph nodes show a prominent sinusoidal infiltrate (Fig. 30-40) with compression of medullary cords, which contain large numbers of plasma cells. The sinusoids are filled with large histiocytes exhibiting large vesicular nuclei with prominent nucleoli. Moderate atypia and mitotic figures may be seen. The cytoplasm is abundant, granular, and vacuolated. At times it is conspicuously eosinophilic. Foamy histiocytes may be prominent. Well-preserved lymphocytes, as well as polymorphonuclear leukocytes, plasma cells, and red cells, may be found within the cytoplasm of the histiocytes (Fig. 30-41). Multinucleated histiocytes may also be seen. The differential diagnoses include histiocytosis X, malignant histiocytosis, nonspecific sinus histiocytosis, and metastatic malignancies, particularly melanoma and seminoma.

Proteinaceous lymphadenopathy

The term *proteinaceous lymphadenopathy* was coined by Osborne, Butler, and Mackay[162] to describe lymph nodes showing extensive replacement of their parenchyma with a hyaline material. The hyaline material is eosinophilic, is somewhat granular and fibrillary, and exhibits

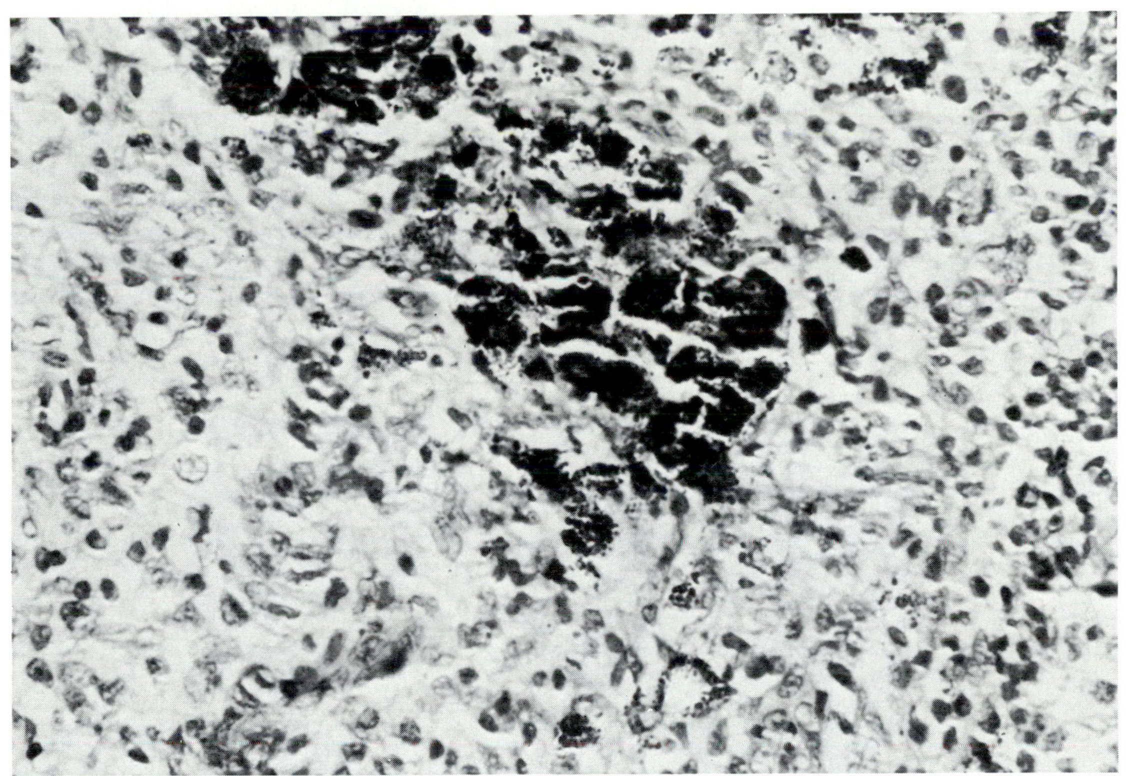

Fig. 30-39. Lymph node in dermatopathic lymphadenitis. Note macrophages containing melanin. (Hematoxylin and eosin; 250×.)

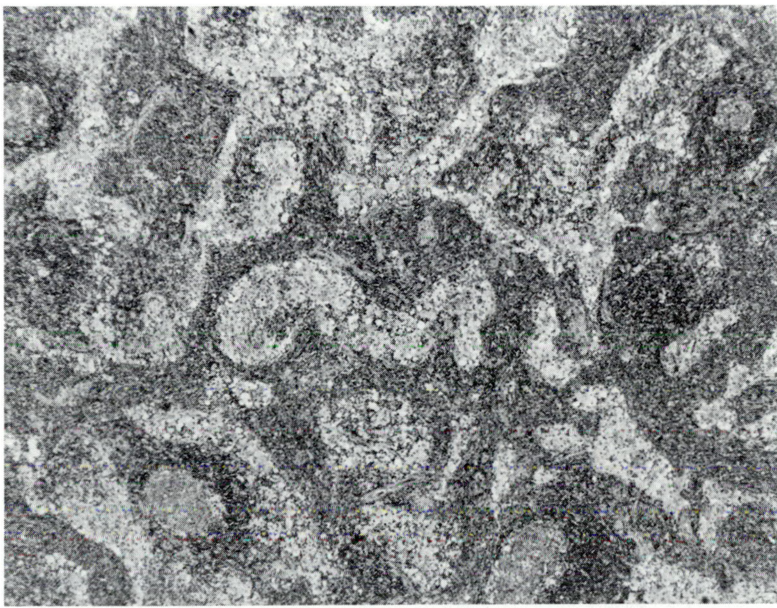

Fig. 30-40. Sinus histiocytosis with massive lymphadenopathy. Lymph node shows prominent sinusoidal pattern. (Hematoxylin and eosin; low power.)

a peculiar concentric arrangement (Fig. 30-42). It is strongly periodic acid–Schiff positive when still associated with lymphoid cells and stains more weakly in the areas where it has completely replaced the lymphoid tissue. This material probably represents an immunoglobulin elaborated by the lymphoid cells. I have observed such precipitates in patients with macroglobulinemia.

One of my patients with proteinaceous lymphadenopathy exhibited lymphoid nodules in the bone marrow, with hyaline material and extensive deposits of hyaline material in the lung associated with a lymphoid infiltrate, which appeared to be attenuated by the hyaline material.

Too few cases have been reported to establish a clinical presentation. Patients in the reported cases had lymphadenopathy and hypergammaglobulinemia.[162]

Immunoblastic lymphadenopathy[71,134]

Immunoblastic[134] or angioimmunoblastic lymphadenopathy with dysproteinemia[71] is an entity that may resemble Hodgkin's disease clinically and histologically. It is a disease of unknown etiology and pathogenesis. Clinically it is manifested by fever, sweats, weight loss, skin rash, generalized lymphadenopathy, and often hepatosplenomegaly. There is a polyclonal hyperglobulinemia and frequently hemolytic anemia. Histologically

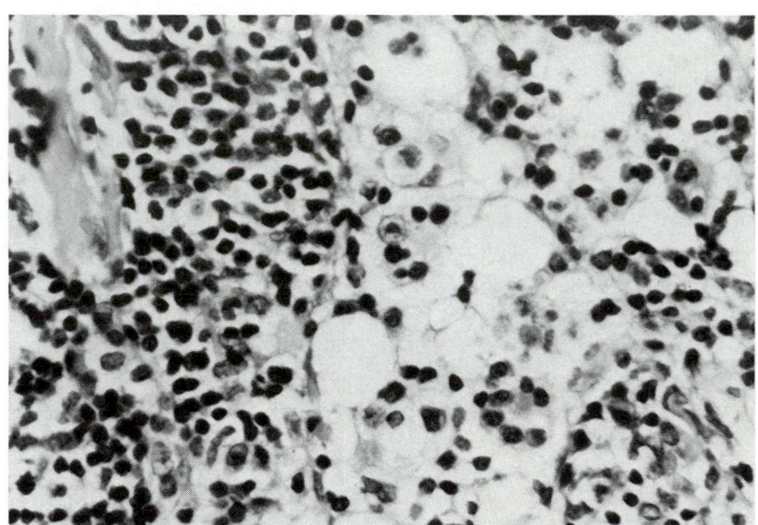

Fig. 30-41. Sinus histiocytosis with massive lymphadenopathy. Note foamy histiocytes with engulfed lymphocytes. (Hematoxylin and eosin; high power.)

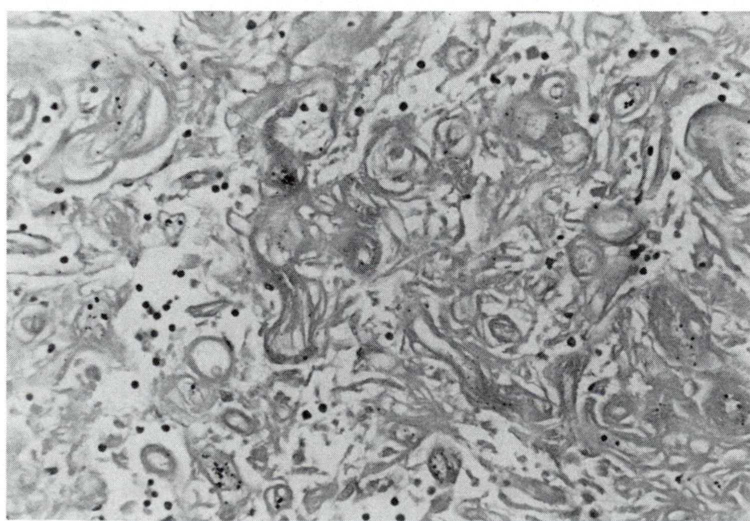

Fig. 30-42. Proteinaceous lymphadenopathy. Note concentric arrangement of hyaline deposits. (Hematoxylin and eosin; high power.)

the normal lymph node architecture is usually effaced, and lymphoid follicles and sinusoids are inconspicuous. There is abundant proliferation of arborizing small vessels associated with numerous immunoblasts and plasma cells, and the deposition of varying amounts of a homogeneous, eosinophilic, periodic acid Schiff positive material. Occasionally there may be abundant clusters of epithelioid cells.

Some investigators consider Lennert's lymphoma (lymphoepithelioid cell lymphoma) to be part of the spectrum of immunoblastic lymphadenopathy.[50]

Bone marrow lesions diagnostic of immunoblastic lymphadenopathy are found in 70% of patients.[164] Bone marrow involvement may be nodular or diffuse. The lesions may be paratrabecular. They replace fatty and hemopoietic marrow and are made up of lymphocytes, histiocytes, epithelioid cells, blasts, plasma cells, and eosinophils. Small blood vessels are increased, and fibroblasts are present. There is a moderate increase in the reticulin framework of the marrow. The course of the disease is usually progressive, with a median survival of 18 months reported in 18 fatal cases.[134] In three of the reported cases the disease evolved into a malignant lymphoma.[134]

In a few patients the disease remitted following lymph node biopsy or splenectomy.[50]

Giant lymph node hyperplasia (Castleman's disease)[106]

Giant lymph node hyperplasia has been described by a variety of names reflecting the different opinions concerning its histogenesis: angiomatous lymphoid hamartoma, angiofollicular lymph node hyperplasia, lymphoid hamartoma, benign giant lymphoma.[106] Clinically the patients most often have a mediastinal mass discovered on routine roentgenograms of the chest or because of pressure symptoms. Occasionally a palpable mass is present outside the thorax. Keller, Hochholzer, and Castleman[106] have studied 81 cases of this entity and have divided it into two histologic types, the hyaline-vascular type and the plasma cell type. The hyaline-vascular type is characterized by small lymphoid follicles that are rich in vessels, some of which enter the follicle in a radial fashion. The centers of the follicles contain varying amounts of hyaline material and superficially resemble Hassall's corpuscles of the thymus. The follicles show a tight concentric ("onion-skin") layering of small lymphocytes (Fig. 30-43). The interfollicular tissue is vascular and contains varying numbers of plasma cells, eosinophils, and immunoblasts.

The plasma cell type is much less frequent. It displays prominent germinal centers devoid of the rich vascularity of the hyaline-vascular type. The interfollicular tissue is vascular and contains sheets of plasma cells and some immunoblasts.

In my experience a clear separation of the two types is not always possible and transitions between the two types exist.

Systemic manifestations such as fever, anemia, and hyperglobulinemia have been observed in association with the plasma cell type of giant lymph node hyperplasia. These clinical signs disappeared after excision of the lesion.

A multicentric variant of giant lymph node hyperplasia has also been described.[71,72] In one of my patients the spleen weighed 900 g. The splenic malpighian follicles

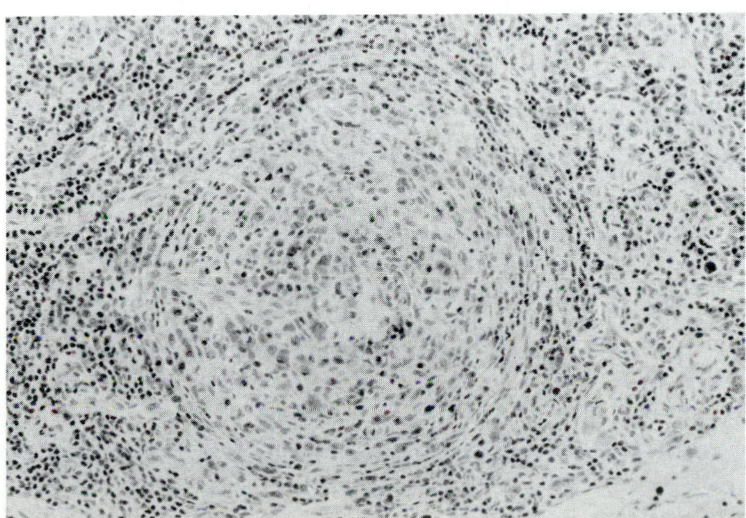

Fig. 30-43. Giant lymph node hyperplasia. Note vessels entering lymphoid follicle *(left)*, concentric layering of small lymphocytes, and hypervascularity of interfollicular tissue *(right)*. (Hematoxylin and eosin; medium power.)

were hypervascular and showed a hyaline material, which was periodic acid–Schiff positive, and an increased number of plasma cells. Histologically the differential diagnosis of giant lymph node hyperplasia includes thymoma if the biopsy specimen comes from the mediastinum, luetic lymphadenitis, Felty's syndrome, and Kaposi's sarcoma.[128,201] The possible relationship of multicentric lymph node hyperplasia to Kaposi's sarcoma is discussed in a later section.

Metastatic neoplasms

Since lymph drains from the site of a primary neoplasm to the regional lymph nodes, the latter are frequently the site of metastases. Carcinomas and malignant melanomas metastasize to lymph nodes much more frequently than do sarcomas. The tumor tissue in the lymph node usually, but not always, reproduces the cellular and architectural features of the primary tumor. Tumor cells or small nodules are first found in the subcapsular or paratrabecular lymph sinuses (Fig. 30-44). When there is extensive involvement, the normal architecture of the lymph node is completely destroyed.

When excising a primary neoplasm, the surgeon also is concerned with this potential involvement of the regional lymph nodes. In some circumstances, however, one may excise and examine a lymph node histologically to establish whether a primary neoplasm exists in the area or organ it drains. For example, intra-abdominal carcinoma, particularly carcinoma of the stomach, sometimes metastasizes to the left supraclavicular lymph nodes by way of the thoracic duct. An enlarged supraclavicular node containing tumor tissue sometimes is called Virchow's node. Another example is involvement of the scalene lymph nodes in intrathoracic tumors.

Lymph nodes may contain benign epithelial and nonepithelial inclusions. The benign epithelial inclusions include endometriosis, glandular inclusions associated with salpingitis isthmica nodosa,[108] thyroid follicles, and breast tissue.[237] Nonepithelial benign inclusions include nevus cells[187] and foci of angiomyolipoma.[126]

Kaposi's sarcoma

Lymphadenopathy related to Kaposi's sarcoma may be attributed to four distinct causes.[128] First, nonspecific inflammatory changes can be seen in a lymph node draining an area of ulcerated cutaneous Kaposi's sarcoma. Second, malignant lymphomas of various types occur significantly more frequently in patients with Kaposi's sarcoma.[184] Third, lymph nodes are frequently involved by Kaposi's sarcoma. This type of lymph node involvement may be seen in association with or without cutaneous Kaposi's sarcoma. It is particularly frequent in African children.[45] Grossly these lymph nodes show purple or brown nodules, which may be mistaken for melanoma.

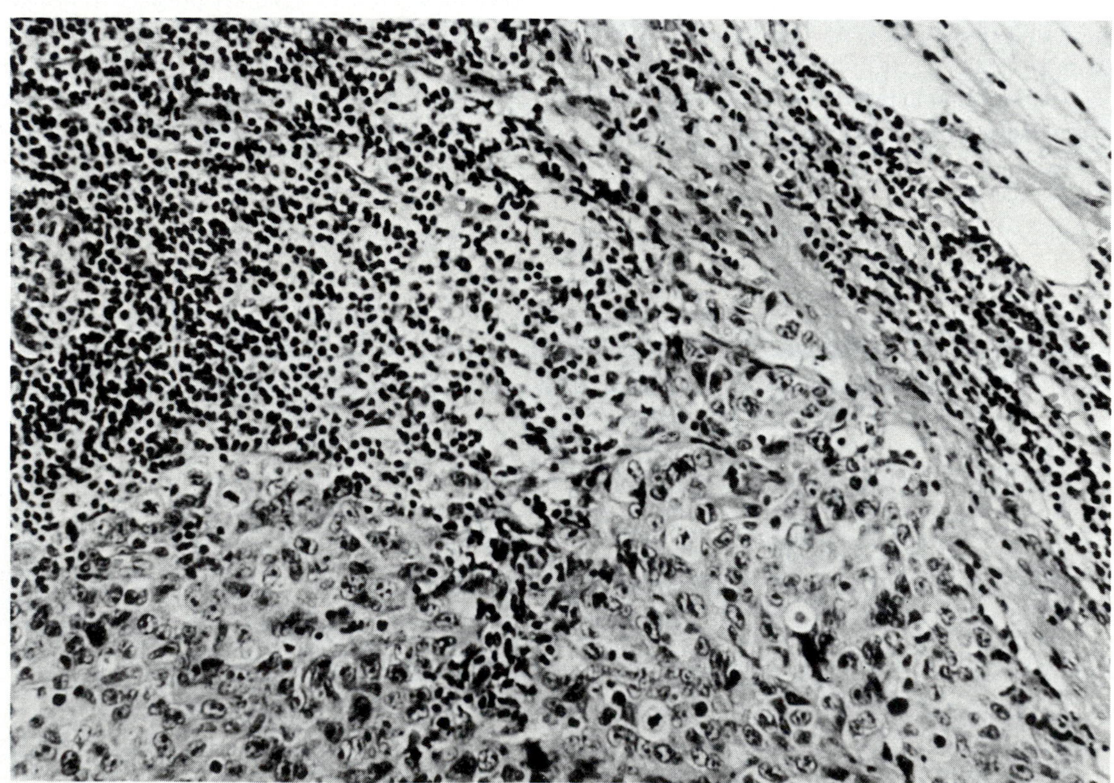

Fig. 30-44. Lymph node with metastatic carcinoma. (Hematoxylin and eosin; 125×.)

Microscopically the typical appearance of Kaposi's sarcoma with spindle cells, vascular slits, hemosiderin, and red cells is found (see p. 1627). Fourth, lymphadenopathy may be caused by an impressive, highly vascular follicular hyperplasia, associated with hypervascularity of the interfollicular tissue and a striking increase in plasma cells. Numerous sections may have to be examined before a diagnostic focus of Kaposi's sarcoma is found.

The highly vascular follicular hyperplasia associated with the plasmacytosis resembles angiofollicular lymphoid hyperplasia or giant lymph node hyperplasia. Because of the presence of foci of diagnostic, spindle-celled Kaposi's sarcoma, Rywlin, Marvan, and Robinson[201] interpreted these lesions as a manifestation of Kaposi's sarcoma. An alternate explanation would be that these lymph nodes contained two diseases, Kaposi's sarcoma and multicentric Castleman's disease. This view is supported by the fact that lymphoproliferative disorders are more frequent in Kaposi's sarcoma. It is also possible that at least the multicentric variant of giant lymph node hyperplasia is part of the histologic spectrum of Kaposi's sarcoma. The histologic constituents of the two diseases, proliferated blood vessels and plasma cells, are the same; foci of diagnostic Kaposi's sarcoma were found in some sections of the lymph nodes by Rywlin and associates.[201,204a] The clinical presentation of patients with Kaposi's sarcoma of lymph nodes associated with the highly vascular follicular hyperplasia was identical to multicentric giant lymph node hyperplasia. The patients had lymphadenopathy, fever, weight loss, anemia, and hypergammaglobulinemia. Additional studies are necessary to elucidate the precise relationship of these two diseases.

Vascular transformation of lymph node sinuses from venous obstruction[85] and nodal angiomatosis[62] should not be mistaken for Kaposi's sarcoma, although the former may be seen in association with this sarcoma. The characteristic proliferation of spindle cells with formation of vascular slits is not seen in these entities.

Malignant lymphomas

General considerations

Neoplastic proliferations of lymphocytes, monocytes (reticulum cells, histiocytes), and plasma cells are outlined in the following. By convention and somewhat arbitrarily the term "malignant lymphoma" is used collectively for some of the neoplastic proliferations listed: Hodgkin's disease, lymphocytic lymphomas, histiocytic lymphoma (reticulum cell sarcoma), Burkitt's tumor, and mycosis fungoides. Primarily it includes malignant lymphoreticular neoplasms that are localized at the time of diagnosis and arise preferentially in lymph nodes. The systemic and leukemic proliferations are not included under the lymphomas. One should also note that Burkitt's tumor usually occurs outside of lymph nodes and that mycosis fungoides is primarily, although not exclusively, a cutaneous neoplasm. Neoplastic proliferations of lymphocytes, monocytes (reticulum cells, histiocytes), and plasma cells are as follows:

1. Hodgkin's disease
2. Lymphocytic lymphomas, follicular and diffuse
3. Lymphocytic leukemias
4. Histiocytic lymphoma (reticulum cell sarcoma)
5. Malignant histiocytosis
6. Monocytic leukemias
7. Burkitt's tumor
8. Mycosis fungoides
9. Multiple myeloma
10. Waldenström's macroglobulinemia
11. Heavy-chain disease
    a. Alpha chain—Mediterranean lymphoma (Seligman's disease)
    b. Gamma chain—Franklin's disease
    c. Mu chain—mu chain disease

The term "lymphosarcoma" was coined by Virchow to describe primary malignant neoplasms originating in lymph nodes. Kundrat[114] believed that "lymphosarcomatosis" was more appropriate for these neoplasms, since they did not metastasize like other sarcomas. For the same reason other pathologists preferred the term "malignant lymphomas" for these neoplasms. Indeed hemopoietic and lymphoreticular malignancies exhibit a feature unique among malignant neoplasms: a tendency to multicentricity and systemic involvement with or without leukemic blood findings. Systemic involvement must be distinguished from widespread metastases. Metastases form grossly visible nodules that may involve many different tissues, whereas systemic involvement tends to be diffuse and is seen primarily in organs normally housing lymphoreticular tissues. Transition stages between a localized tumor mass, systemic involvement, and leukemia exist for neoplasias of lymphocytes, reticulum cells, plasma cells, and granulocytes. Transition stages between lymphoma and leukemia are sometimes called "leukosarcoma." Tumors formed by immature granulocytes are known as chloromas or granulocytic sarcomas.[178]

Virchow's lymphosarcomas were composed of small or large cells. Some pathologists believed that the large cell lymphosarcomas were derived from reticulum or reticuloendothelial cells rather than from lymphocytes and that they should be called "reticulum cell sarcomas." Others referred to them as "lymphosarcoma, reticulum cell type." Rappaport[178] views the large cell lymphomas as derived from histiocytes and calls them "histiocytic lymphomas." The term "histiocyte" was introduced by Aschoff and Kiyono[7] to denote that the wandering macrophages were of tissue rather than peripheral blood origin as believed by Metchnikoff. Modern investigators consider the wandering macrophages to be derived from

Table 30-2. Classification of lymphomas

Nodular	Diffuse
I. Lymphocytic lymphoma	**I.** Lymphocytic lymphoma
1. Poorly differentiated	1. Poorly differentiated
2. Moderately differentiated	2. Moderately differentiated
3. Well differentiated	3. Well differentiated
II. Lymphoma, mixed cell type	**II.** Lymphoma, mixed cell type
III. Reticulum cell sarcoma (histiocytic lymphoma, Gall)	**III.** Reticulum cell sarcoma (histiocytic lymphoma, Gall)

After Rappaport, H., Winter, W.J., and Hicks, E.B.: Cancer **9**:792, 1956.

monocytes arriving from the bone marrow in the peripheral blood.[238] The substitution of histiocytic lymphoma for reticulum cell sarcoma has not been universally accepted because it is impossible to determine by microscopic examination if a neoplasm has arisen from fixed macrophages (reticulum cells) or wandering macrophages (histiocytes). Also the term "histiocyte" appears to some investigators to be inappropriate for wandering macrophages arriving from the peripheral blood. Furthermore some "histiocytic" lymphomas either contain or secrete increased amounts of immunoglobulins indicating that they are of lymphoid rather than histiocytic origin. Malignant lymphomas made up of smaller cells were divided by Rappaport[178] into well-differentiated and poorly differentiated lymphocytic lymphomas (Table 30-2). These terms have also been criticized because from a functional point of view the larger cells are more differentiated than are the smaller lymphocytes. Indeed, when the small lymphocytes are stimulated by antigens or mitogens, they enlarge and take on the appearance of blasts (p. 1284).[120,131] Based on such considerations a a number of different terms have been proposed for malignant lymphomas believed to be derived from these cells: cleaved cell lymphoma (germinocytoma, centrocytic lymphoma), germinoblastoma (centroblastic lymphoma), immunoblastic sarcoma, and others (Table 30-5).

Another lymphoma that has given rise to considerable controversy was first described by Brill, Baehr, and Rosenthal[26] as "giant lymph follicle hyperplasia." It was later renamed "giant follicle lymphoblastoma."[10] The difficulty of distinguishing this entity from reactive follicular hyperplasia, the relatively good prognosis as compared with other lymphomas, and the tendency to develop a diffuse growth pattern and lose the nodular appearance were all recognized. Rappaport and co-workers[181] believed that follicular lymphoma is not a distinct lesion related to germinal centers but represents a nodular growth pattern of a lymphocytic or a histiocytic lymphoma. On the basis of cytologic and ultrastructural studies a number of investigators have contradicted this view.[120,122,131] They present evidence that follicular (nodular) lymphomas arise from or differentiate into germinal center lymphocytes, which according to Lukes and Collins[131] are derived from small B lymphocytes at the periphery of the germinal center. This small B lymphocyte is transformed into the noncleaved cell (centroblast of Lennert[120]) with intermediate cleaved cell (centrocyte) stages (see Fig. 30-29). Follicular (nodular) lymphomas are composed of these cells in relatively pure forms (centrocytic or centroblastic lymphoma) or varying mixtures of the two.[120]

In recent years markers have been developed to characterize B lymphocytes, T lymphocytes, and monocytes.[53,86] T cells can be identified by their ability to bind sheep erythrocytes, thus forming rosettes. Phytohemagglutinin causes transformation of T cells in vitro. They can also be identified by cytotoxicity or immunofluorescence by use of specific anti-T sera. Under the scanning electron microscope T cells appear relatively smooth surfaced.[173] B cells are characterized by surface-bound immunoglobulin, a receptor for the third component of complement and a receptor for the Fc portion of IgG. On scanning electron microscopy they exhibit a villous surface.[173] Monocytes also carry membrane receptors for the third component of complement and for the Fc fragment of IgG. However, in distinction to B lymphocytes, the Fc receptor in monocytes binds an antigen-antibody complex when presented as an IgG-coated erythrocyte. Monocytes have a ruffled surface on scanning electron microscopy.[173]

Applying these criteria to lymphoreticular neoplastic proliferative disorders, one can classify them as in the outline that follows. A word of caution is necessary. Neoplastic cells do not have to imitate normal cells in all their characteristics. It is likely that, as more studies become available, a clear-cut assignment to B lymphocytes, T lymphocytes, or monocytes will not always be possible. This is the case with hairy cell leukemia. The following is a classification of lymphoreticular malignancies by functional markers*:

1. B lymphocytes
   a. Chronic lymphocytic leukemia
   b. Malignant lymphoma, small cell type, follicular, and diffuse
   c. Malignant lymphoma, large cell type, follicular, and diffuse

*Modified from Hansen, J.A., and Good, R.A.: Hum. Pathol. **5**:567, 1974.

   d. Burkitt's tumor
   e. Multiple myeloma
   f. Heavy-chain diseases
2. T lymphocytes
   a. Mycosis fungoides
   b. Sézary's syndrome
   c. Mediastinal lymphoma of children
   d. Acute lymphoblastic leukemia (some cases)
3. Monocytes
   a. Hairy cell leukemia (?)
   b. Hodgkin's disease (?)
   c. Malignant histiocytosis

Clinical presentation and staging

The most common clinical presentation of malignant lymphoma is painless lymphadenopathy. The "lump" feels rubbery firm, and the diagnosis is established by biopsy and histologic examination. The lymph node(s) involved may be in any of the lymph node–bearing areas of the body. If internal lymph nodes are involved, the presenting symptoms may be the result of pressure by the nodes on important structures, such as pressure by hilar nodes on bronchi causing cough. If the disease is widespread, the patient may have systemic symptoms such as fever and weight loss. Mycosis fungoides is a special type of malignant lymphoma that is manifested by cutaneous plaques and tumors (p. 1631). Burkitt's tumor or lymphoma is predominantly a tumor of childhood that grows rapidly and is usually extranodal.

A detailed scheme for the clinical staging of Hodgkin's disease has been worked out.[35] It correlates well with prognosis and helps in deciding whether radiotherapy or chemotherapy should be used. The same clinical staging is also applicable to the non-Hodgkin's lymphomas, though less experience is available with staging in these entities. It must be emphasized that clinical and pathologic staging classifications apply only to the patient at the time of initial examination and before definitive therapy. The lymphatic structures are defined as the lymph nodes, spleen, thymus, Waldeyer's ring, appendix, and Peyer's patches. Stage I is involvement of a single lymph node region or of a single extralymphatic organ or site (I_E). Stage II is involvement of two or more lymph node regions on the same side of the diaphragm or localized involvement of an extralymphatic organ or site in addition to one or more lymph node regions on the same side of the diaphragm (II_E). Stage III is involvement of lymphatic structures on both sides of the diaphragm that may be associated with localized involvement of an extralymphatic organ or site (III_E), involvement of the spleen (III_S), or both (III_{SE}). Stage IV is diffuse or disseminated involvement of one or more extralymphatic organs or tissue with or without associated lymph node involvement. Each stage is further subdivided into A or B categories, B for those with defined general symptoms and A for those without. General symptoms include patients with (1) unexplained weight loss of more than 10% of the body weight in the 6 months before examination, (2) unexplained fever with temperatures above 38°C, and (3) night sweats.[35]

Gross appearance

Lymphomatous lymph nodes are enlarged and rubbery in contrast to lymph nodes containing metastatic carcinoma, which may be stony hard. Not uncommonly, several enlarged nodes are matted together into a large, firm nodular mass, which on cut surface shows the outline of the fused nodes. The cut surface is gray-cream in color, and the tissue has been likened to fish flesh. Foci of necrosis are common when the nodes are large. The different types of lymphoma cannot be distinguished grossly.

Histopathology

The first and most important decision the pathologist must make when examining a section of a lymph node is whether the histologic changes represent a reactive process or a lymphoma. Some general features can be outlined that, although not always present, help in making the distinction.

The most common feature of lymphoma is the effacement of the normal architecture of the node. The sinusoids, particularly the subcapsular, are no longer seen. There is no longer a distinction between the cortex of the node, with regularly spaced and clearly defined lymphoid nodules, and the medulla. Reticulin stains may be helpful in demonstrating loss of the normal pattern. In most of the lymphomas there is infiltration of the capsule and pericapsular fat by neoplastic cells. Infiltration of the capsule by normal lymphocytes sometimes is seen in reactive lymphadenitis, but the infiltration is seldom severe and the infiltrating cells are normal lymphocytes.

When sections are studied under high magnification, the population of cells in lymphoma varies, according to the disease, from well-differentiated small lymphocytes to highly pleomorphic and obviously malignant cells. The cell population in a reactive lymphadenitis is made up of small and large lymphocytes, histiocytes, neutrophil leukocytes, and some plasma cells. Of the lymphomas, only the mixed type of Hodgkin's disease shows eosinophils, neutrophils, and plasma cells. The final differential feature is the type of involvement of blood vessels. In lymphoma (and leukemia) the vessel wall is often infiltrated by neoplastic cells, whereas in benign hyperplasia there is no infiltration but frequently there is hyperplasia of endothelial cells.

Lymph nodes should be sectioned at a thickness no greater than 4 μm. Poor fixation of the tissue, too thick a section, and poor staining can make an already difficult

Table 30-3. Histologic types of Hodgkin's disease—comparison of old nomenclature, that proposed by Lukes and associates in 1966, and modified Lukes and associates classification recommended at the Conference on Hodgkin's Disease, Rye, N.Y., September 1965

Jackson and Parker*	Lukes et al., 1966†	Conference on Hodgkin's Disease, Rye classification, 1965‡
	I. Lymphocytic and histiocytic	**I.** Hodgkin's disease, lymphocytic predominance
Hodgkin's paragranuloma	**A.** Diffuse (lymphocytes predominant)	
	B. Nodular (lymphocytes predominant)	
	C. Nodular or diffuse (histiocytes predominant)	
	II. Nodular sclerosis	**II.** Hodgkin's disease, nodular sclerosis type
Hodgkin's granuloma	**III.** Mixed	**III.** Hodgkin's disease, mixed cellularity type
	IV. Diffuse fibrosis	**IV.** Hodgkin's disease, lymphocytic depletion type
	V. Reticular	
Hodgkin's sarcoma	**A.** With nonpleomorphic Reed-Sternberg cells	
	B. With pleomorphic Reed-Sternberg cells	

*From Jackson, H., and Parker, F.: Hodgkin's disease and allied disorders, New York, 1947, Oxford University Press.
†Slightly modified from Lukes, R.J., Butler, J.J., and Hicks, E.B.: Cancer **19:**317 1966.
‡From Lukes, R.J., et al.: Cancer Res. **26:**1311, 1966.

problem impossible to resolve. I also believe strongly that an excised lymph node should be sent to the surgical pathology laboratory promptly and nonfixed. The pathologist, in turn, should in each case make imprints from the freshly cut surface and, whenever possible, freeze a portion of the node for culture and immunoperoxidase study of T and B cells and their subsets should this be indicated.

Hodgkin's disease

Contrary to the non-Hodgkin's lymphomas, there is fairly good agreement as to the histologic classification of Hodgkin's disease. The current (Rye) classification is a simplification of the classification proposed by Lukes, Butler, and Hicks[130] (Table 30-3). It was established at a conference on Hodgkin's disease held in Rye, New York, in 1965. The older classification of Jackson and Parker[94] divided Hodgkin's disease into paragranuloma, granuloma, and sarcoma. It was not clinically useful because the majority of the cases were included in the granuloma group. A comparison of these three classifications is presented in Table 30-3.

According to the Rye classification, which has been almost universally adopted, Hodgkin's disease is subdivided into four types: (1) lymphocyte predominance, (2) nodular sclerosis, (3) mixed cellularity, and (4) lymphocyte depletion.[129] In general, the more mature lymphocytes there are, the better the prognosis. The various histologic types of Hodgkin's disease should not be considered as fixed and rigid categories.[129] Thus a patient who initially has the lymphocyte predominance type in time may change to the mixed and finally to the lymphocyte depletion type. However, the nodular sclerosis type of Hodgkin's disease remains the nodular sclerosis type, even though during its cellular phase it may present, in addition to the nodular structure, the bands of collagen, and the lacunar Reed-Sternberg cells, the diverse histologic appearance of the other types of Hodgkin's disease.

A histologic diagnosis of Hodgkin's disease requires the demonstration of Reed-Sternberg cells (Fig. 30-45). The classical or diagnostic type of Reed-Sternberg cell is a large cell with an abundant acidophilic to amphophilic cytoplasm, which is often pyroninophilic. It may contain two or more nuclei or a lobated nucleus with prominent, large, acidophilic, round, inclusion-like nucleoli that are surrounded with perinucleolar halos. In addition to this diagnostic type of Reed-Sternberg cell, there are three variants: (1) the lacunar type of Reed-Sternberg cell, characteristic of nodular sclerosis type of Hodgkin's disease; (2) a polyploid type of Reed Sternberg cells seen in the lymphocyte predominance type, and (3) the pleomorphic, sarcomatous variant seen in the lymphocyte depletion type.[129] In general the number of Reed-Sternberg cells found is inversely proportional to the number of lymphocytes present. One should remember that Reed-Sternberg cells by themselves are not sufficient for a diagnosis of Hodgkin's disease, since they can be seen

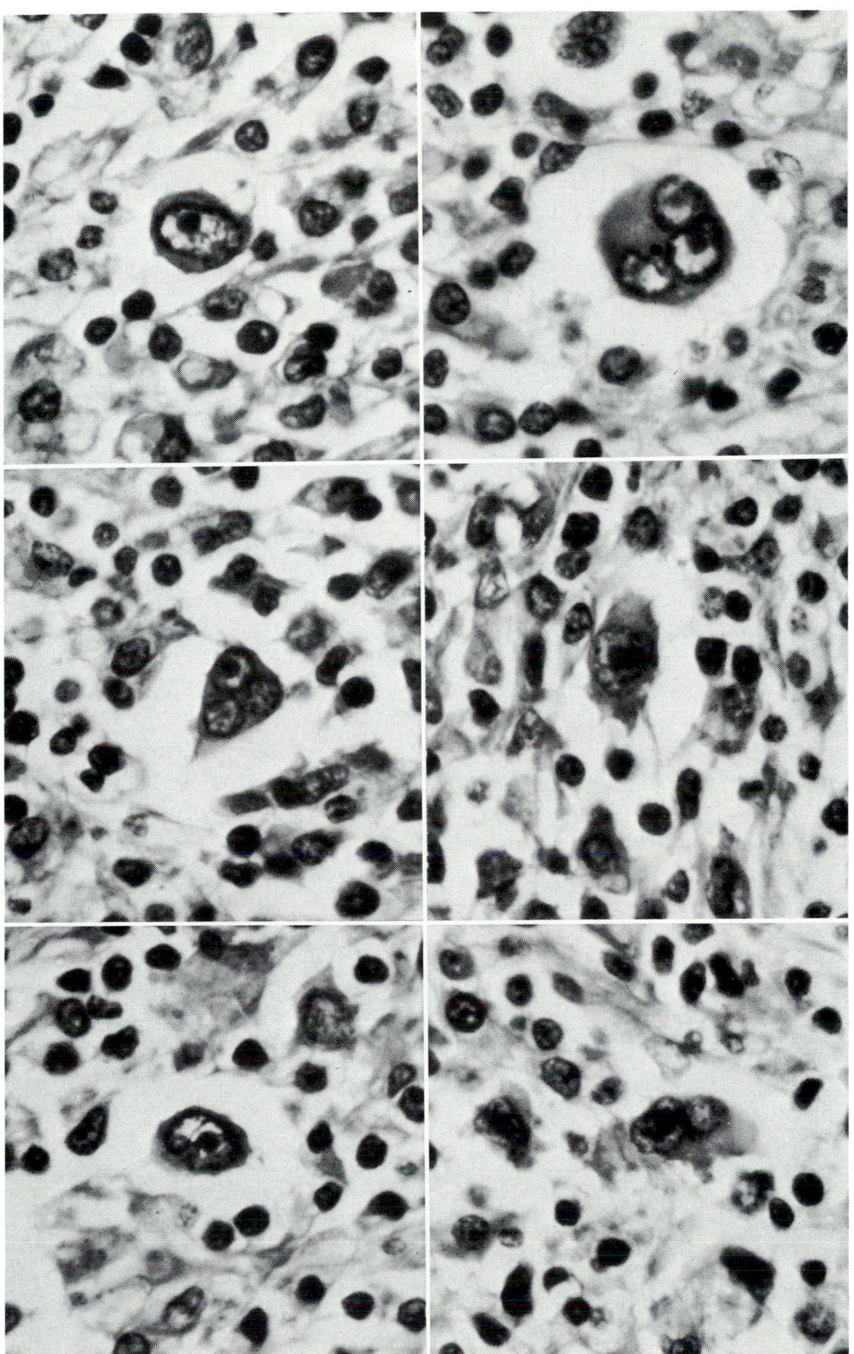

Fig. 30-45. Lymph node. Reed-Sternberg cells, Hodgkin's disease. (Hematoxylin and eosin; 450×.)

in other diseases, such as infectious mononucleosis. They have to be found in association with other characteristic histologic features before a diagnosis of Hodgkin's disease can be established.

Lymphocyte predominance type of Hodgkin's disease

The proliferation of small lymphocytes with a varying number of mature histiocytes may involve the lymph node diffusely or focally (Figs. 30-46 and 30-47). When the node is involved diffusely, it resembles a malignant lymphoma of the small (well-differentiated) lymphocytic type or chronic lymphocytic leukemia. The diagnosis of Hodgkin's disease is made when classical Reed-Sternberg cells are found. These are rare, and many sections may have to be examined before one is found. The scarcity of diagnostic Reed-Sternberg cells is as important for the diagnosis of the lymphocyte predominance type of Hodgkin's disease as is the abundance of lymphocytes. Besides the rare diagnostic Reed-Sternberg cell, a rather characteristic variant is more frequently found in the

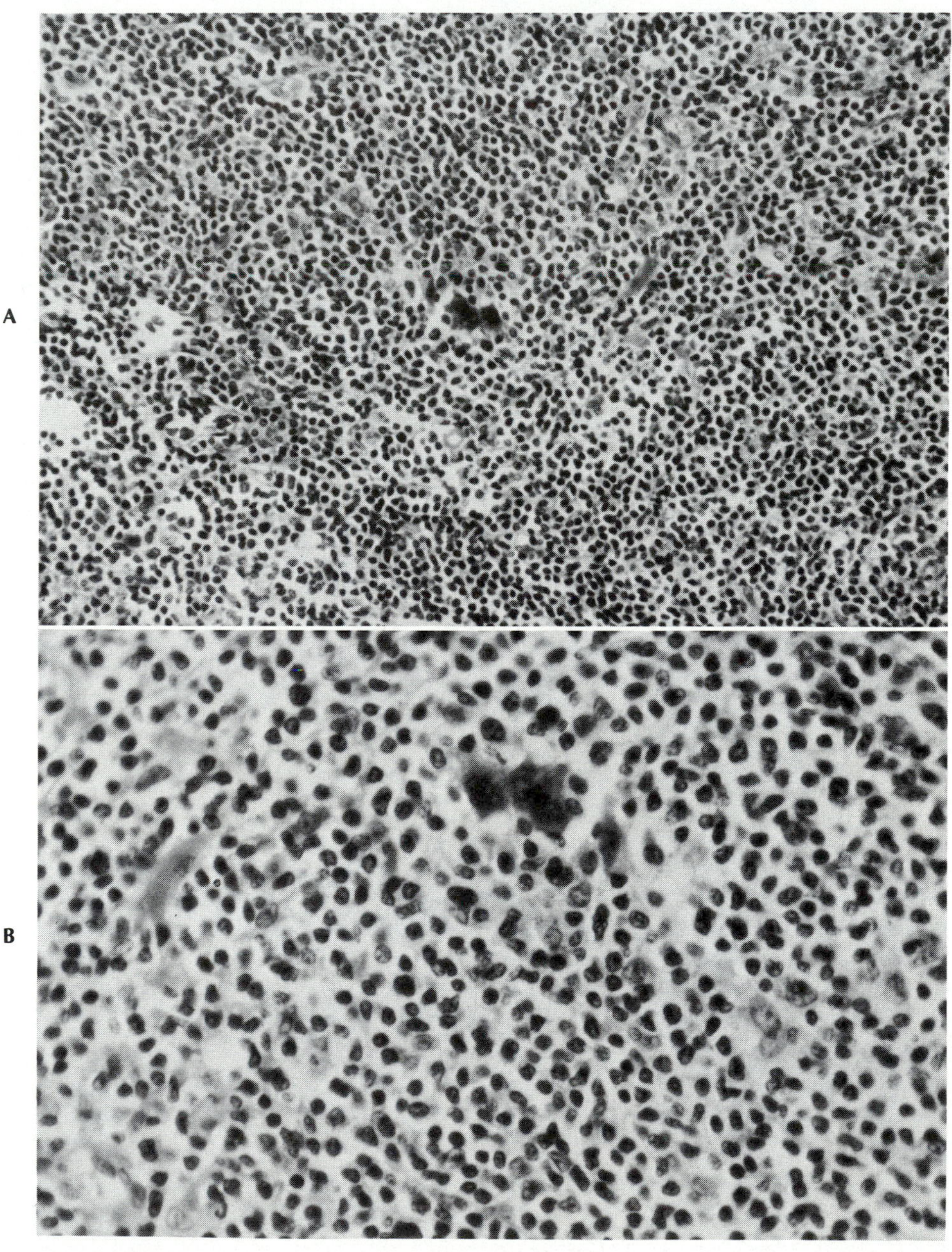

Fig. 30-46. Lymph node. **A,** Hodgkin's disease, lymphocytic predominance type. **B,** Note polyploid Reed-Sternberg cell, characteristic of Hodgkin's disease with lymphocytic predominance. (Hematoxylin and eosin; **A,** 125×; **B,** 250×.)

lymphocyte predominance type of Hodgkin's disease. It consists of a large, polypoid, twisted nucleus with fine nuclear chromatin and only small nucleoli.

Nodular sclerosis type of Hodgkin's disease (Figs. 30-48 and 30-49)

Two criteria are essential for the diagnosis of the nodular sclerosis type: bands of collagen and the lacunar type of Reed-Sternberg cell. The most distinctive feature of the lacunar Reed-Sternberg cell is a pericellular halo that is seen in formalin-fixed tissue and is caused by the retraction of the cytoplasm leaving only a small amount of perinuclear, acidophilic cytoplasm. The nuclei of the lacunar cells are hyperlobated and vary in size. Prominent nucleoli are always present. With Zenker's fixation the pericellular halo is not present and these cells may be overlooked.[129]

In addition to these two criteria, nodular sclerosis exhibits diverse histologic appearances resembling the other histologic types of Hodgkin's disease. Occasionally

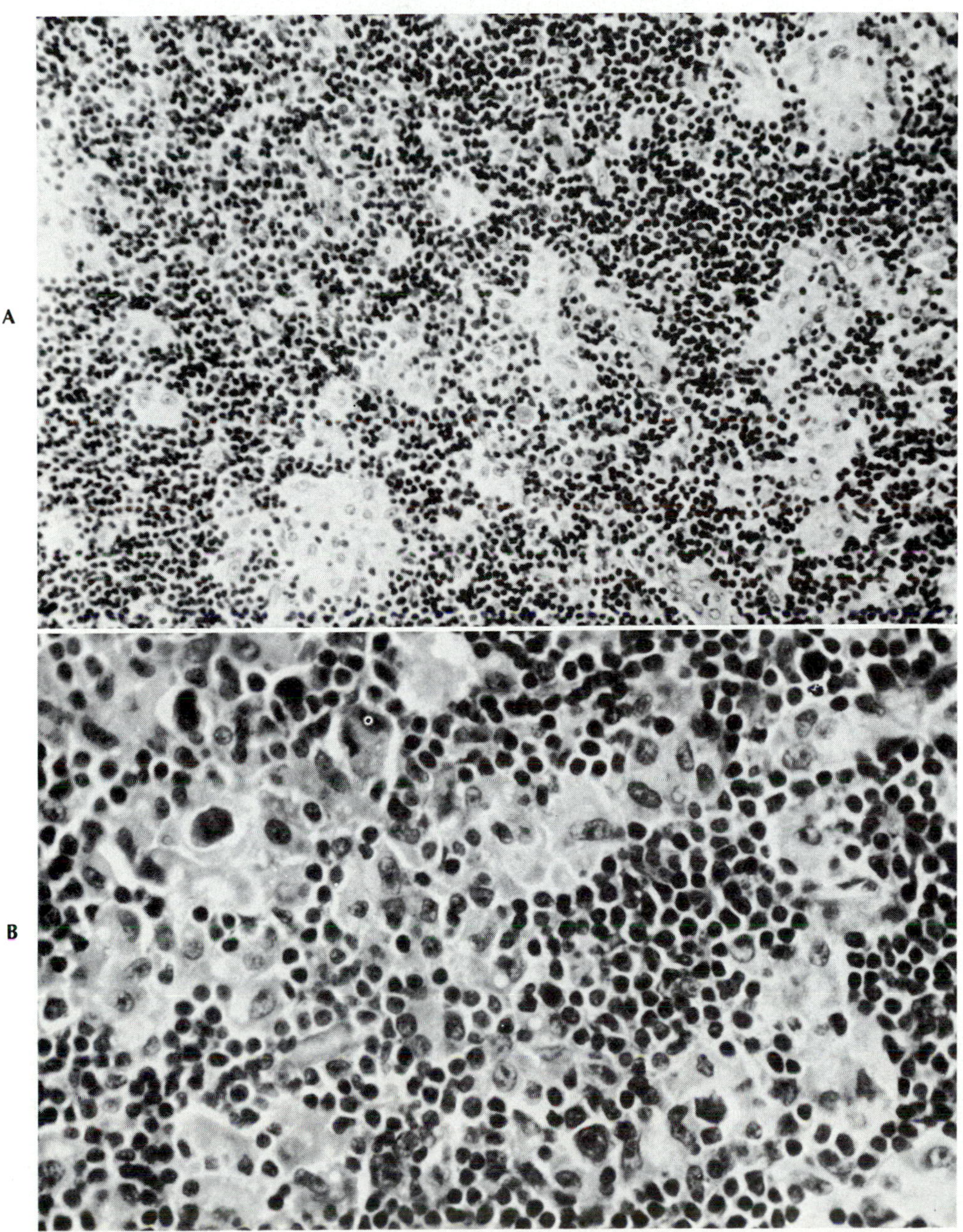

Fig. 30-47. Lymph node. Hodgkin's disease, lymphocytic predominance type. Note presence of numerous histiocytes. (Hematoxylin and eosin; **A,** 125×; **B,** 250×.)

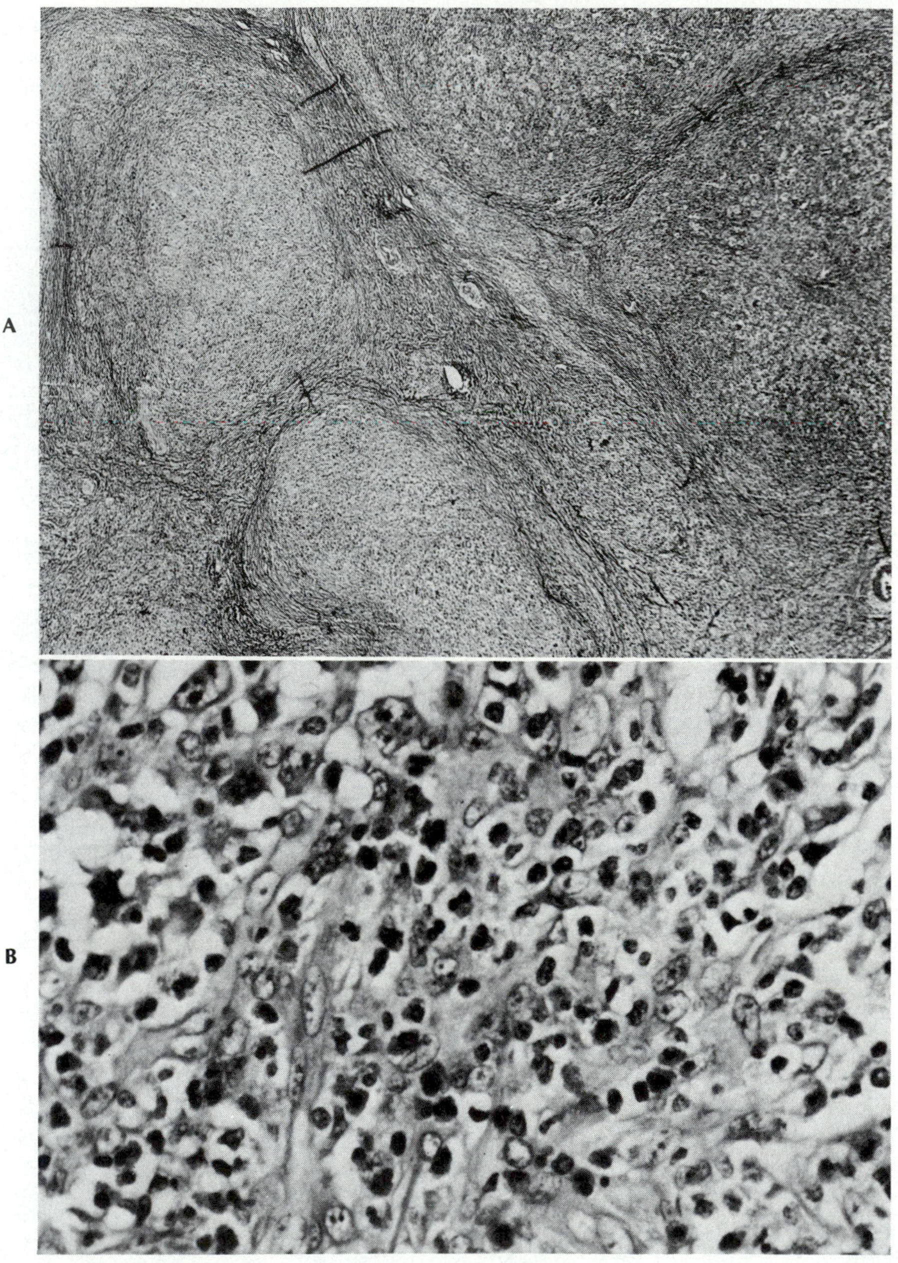

Fig. 30-48. Lymph node. Hodgkin's disease, nodular sclerosis. (Hematoxylin and eosin; **A,** 90×; **B,** 250×.)

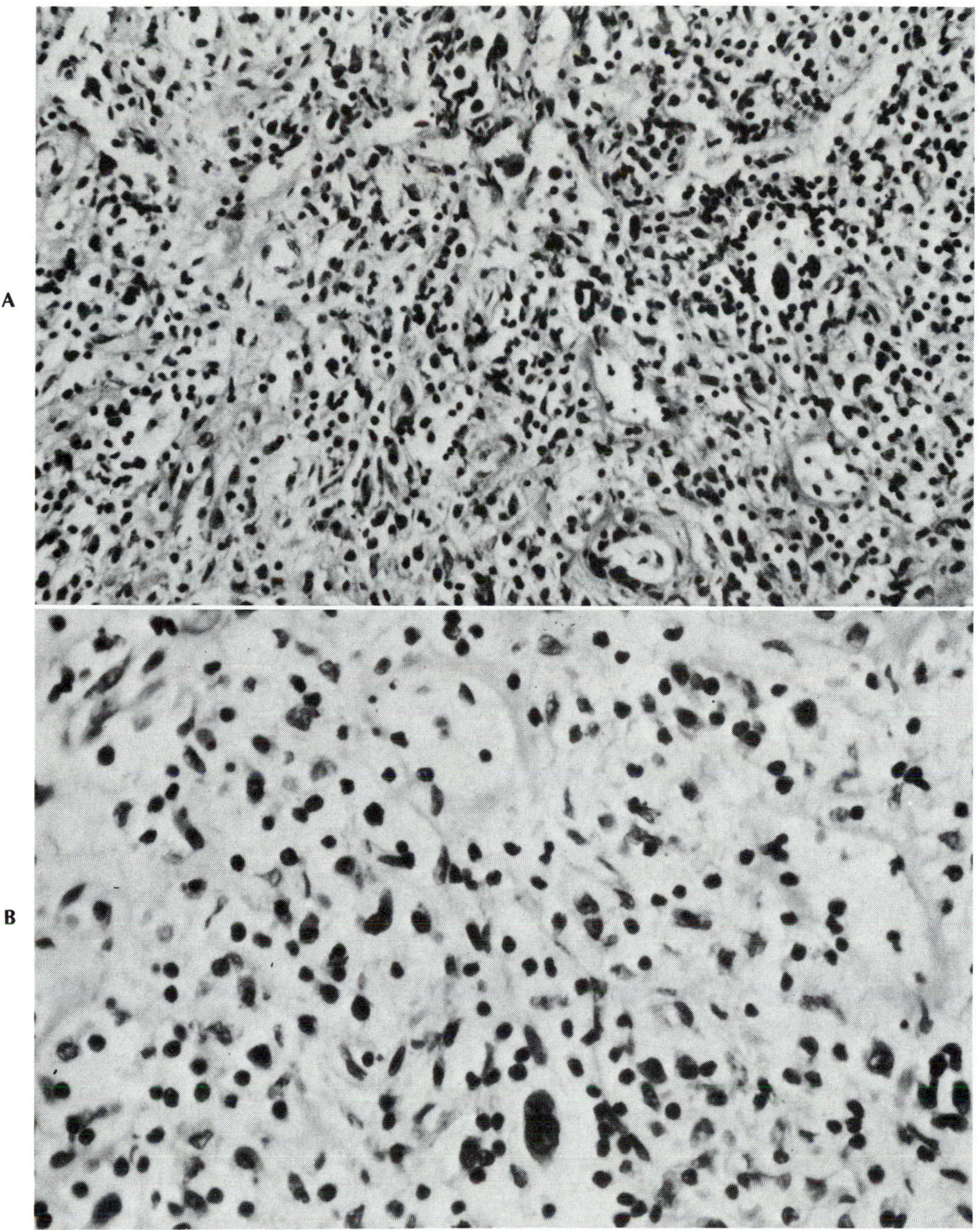

Fig. 30-49. Lymph node. Hodgkin's disease, nodular sclerosis type. Note halo around Reed-Sternberg cells. (Hematoxylin and eosin; **A,** 125×; **B,** 250×.)

the entire node may be replaced by dense, hyalinized collagen.

Nodular sclerosis is the most common histologic type of Hodgkin's disease. It is seen more frequently in women than in men and affects predominantly the mediastinal, supraclavicular, and cervical lymph nodes.

Mixed cellularity type of Hodgkin's disease

In the mixed cellularity type the architecture of the lymph node is obliterated by proliferating lymphocytes, histiocytes, eosinophils, polymorphonuclear leukocytes, and plasma cells (Fig. 30-50). Focal necrosis may be present. There is usually some fibrosis that varies in degree in different portions of the node. Diagnostic Reed-Sternberg cells are frequent. Mixed cellularity also serves as an unclassified type and includes all cases that lack the typical features of the remaining types.[129]

Lymphocyte depletion type of Hodgkin's disease

The lymphocyte depletion group contains the diffuse fibrosis and reticular types in the classification by Lukes and associates. Diffuse fibrosis is an inaccurate term for the histologic alteration observed. The lymph nodes are depleted of lymphocytes and exhibit a deposit of a homo-

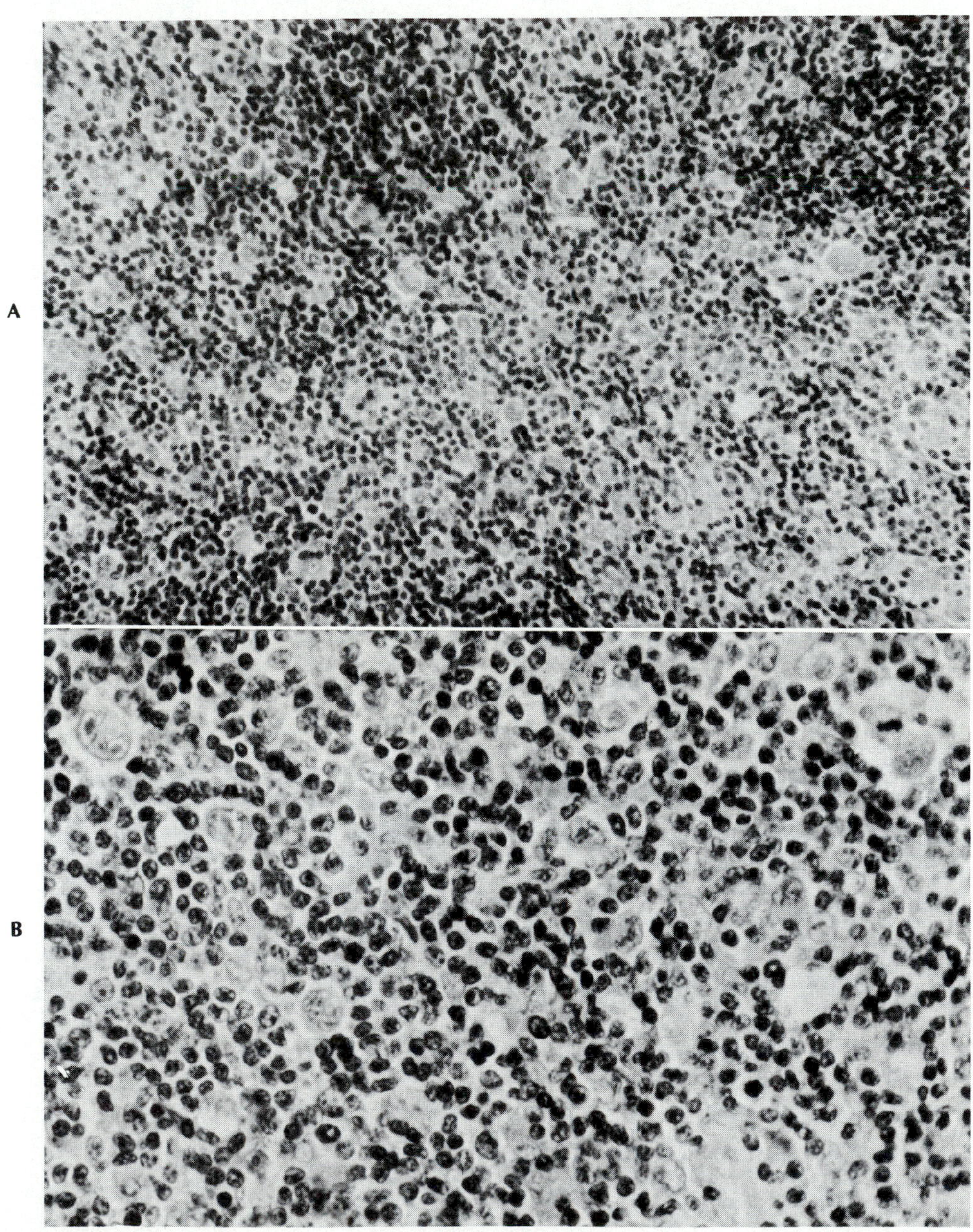

Fig. 30-50. Lymph node. Hodgkin's disease, mixed cell type. (Hematoxylin and eosin; **A,** 125×; **B,** 250×.)

geneous, nonfibrillary, nonbirefringent eosinophilic material, best described as hyalin. Stains for amyloid are negative. This hyalinosis is often associated with the reticular type of Hodgkin's disease, which slows proliferation, focal or diffuse, of highly atypical histiocyte-like cells, with varying numbers of diagnostic Reed-Sternberg cells (Fig. 30-51). In addition, there may be numerous pleomorphic Reed-Sternberg cells with bizarre nuclei and absent or giant eosinophilic nucleoli.

Lymphocyte depletion Hodgkin's disease is often a rapidly fatal disease with fever, pancytopenia, and lymphocytopenia, frequently without peripheral lymphadenopathy.[153] The distribution of the lesions is predominantly subdiaphragmatic with extensive involvement of the liver, spleen, retroperitoneal lymph nodes, and bone marrow.[153]

Staging laparotomy and criteria for the diagnosis of extranodal Hodgkin's disease

Staging laparotomy with splenectomy and biopsy of liver, retroperitoneal nodes, and bone marrow is performed to determine the extent of the disease, as well as the extent of radiotherapy or chemotherapy needed. This procedure is performed most often to confirm the

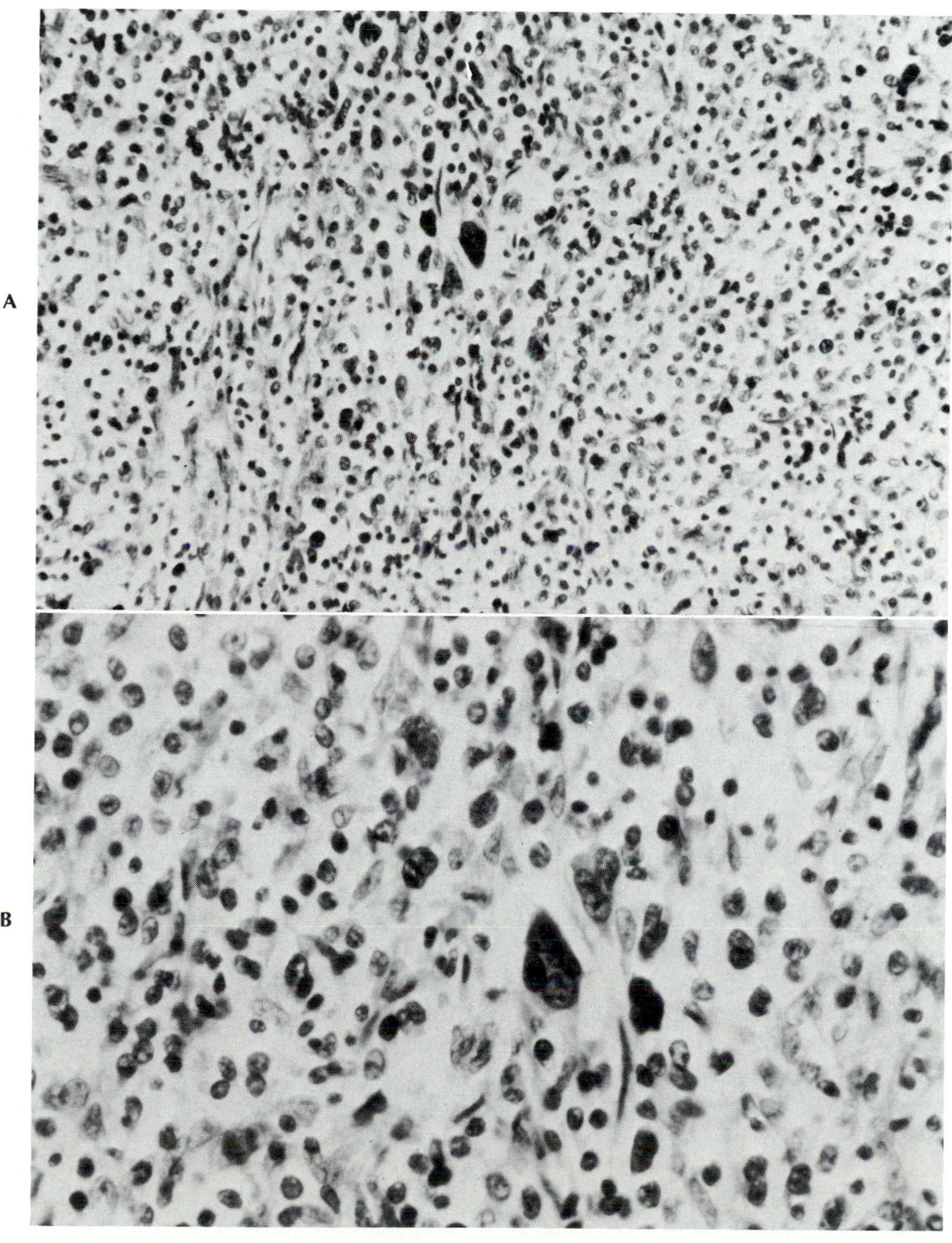

Fig. 30-51. Lymph node. Hodgkin's disease, lymphocyte depletion type with pleomorphic Reed-Sternberg cells. (Hematoxylin and eosin; **A,** 125×, **B,** 250×.)

extent of the disease in patients who clinically appear to have stage I or II disease. Approximately 25% of nonpalpable spleens removed at staging laparotomy contain clinically unsuspected Hodgkin's disease when studied by the pathologist.[195] Also, about 50% of spleens that are clinically enlarged do not exhibit Hodgkin's disease on detailed pathologic examination.[195]

In a study of 250 spleens from patients with Hodgkin's disease undergoing staging laparotomies, Diebold and Temmim[47] found Hodgkin's disease in 103. The weights of involved spleens varied from 100 to 2500 g. Of these spleens 36 weighed less than 200 g, 40 weighed between 200 and 300 g, and 27 exceeded 300 g. On gross examination the majority of the spleens showed multiple nodules of Hodgkin's disease. Single nodules were revealed in 9%, and 4% showed massive involvement of the spleen resulting from confluence of nodules. The gross appearance of individual nodules was similar to that in non-Hodgkin's lymphoma. Histologically the most frequent type of Hodgkin's disease was mixed cellularity, followed by nodular sclerosis, lymphocyte predominance, and lymphocyte depletion. The lesions of Hodgkin's disease seemed to start in the malpighian follicles. In uninvolved areas the malpighian follicles were normal, enlarged, or atrophic. In the lymphocyte depletion type the malpighian corpuscles were hyalinized and Reed-Sternberg cells were scarce. In the reticular variant of lymphocyte depletion, bizarre, pleomorphic Reed-Sternberg cells were frequent and associated with varying numbers of diagnostic Reed-Sternberg cells. The reticular variant must be distinguished from malignant histiocytosis.

When vascular invasion is observed in the spleen or in lymph nodes, there is a greater prevalence of disseminated and extranodal Hodgkin's disease.[227]

Of the 250 spleens studied by Diebold and Temmim,[47] 147 were uninvolved by Hodgkin's disease. In no case was Hodgkin's disease discovered microscopically when it was not seen grossly. Of the uninvolved spleens 10% were large enough to be clinically palpable. Lesions seen in the uninvolved spleens included hyperplasia and atrophy of the white pulp, sarcoid granulomas (10 cases), hemosiderosis, and infarcts.

It is unusual for the liver to be involved in the absence of splenic Hodgkin's disease. The overall demonstration of liver involvement by laparotomy is about 5%.[195]

The bone marrow must be examined histologically, not cytologically, to establish a diagnosis of Hodgkin's disease. Marrow for histologic examination may be obtained by aspiration[205] or by biopsy.

In Hodgkin's disease the marrow may be normal, show nonspecific changes, or be involved with Hodgkin's disease. The nonspecific reaction patterns include granulocytic, megakaryocytic, eosinophilic, and plasma cell hyperplasias. Nodular lymphoid hyperplasia and sarcoid granulomas may also be seen. The frequency of involvement of the bone marrow in Hodgkin's disease varies in different reports from 9%[194] to 29%.[52] The highest frequency occurs in stages III and IV and in the mixed cellularity and lymphocyte depletion types.

The involvement of the marrow in Hodgkin's disease is more often nodular than diffuse. The nodules are made up of atypical histiocytes admixed with lymphocytes, fibroblasts, plasma cells, and eosinophils. The reticulin framework is increased. The frequency of diagnostic Reed-Sternberg cells depends on the number of sections examined and the criteria considered essential for their diagnosis. At times when the bone marrow lesions are diffuse and associated with marked fibrosis, the pathologic findings may resemble agnogenic myeloid metaplasia. Megakaryocytes may be distinguished from Reed-Sternberg cells by their cytoplasmic periodic acid–Schiff positivity and by their close relationship to reticulin fibers. Also, immature myeloid cells, invariably present in agnogenic myeloid metaplasia, can be demonstrated by the naphthol AS-D chloroacetate (Leder) stain.

Staging laparotomies resulting in the submission to the pathologist of relatively small specimens of liver and bone marrow have raised the question as to minimal criteria necessary for the diagnosis of Hodgkin's disease.[182] The criteria are not as stringent as for the initial diagnosis of Hodgkin's disease, and diagnostic Reed-Sternberg cells with eosinophilic, inclusion-like nucleoli are not required. Mononuclear cells with nuclear features of Reed-Sternberg cells (Hodgkin cells) in one of the characteristic cellular environments of Hodgkin's disease should be regarded as indicative of liver or bone marrow involvement. The presence of atypical lymphoreticular cells that fall short of these criteria should be reported as "suggestive of Hodgkin's disease." The presence of nonspecific lymphoreticular infiltrates or sarcoidosis-like granulomas should not be considered evidence for Hodgkin's disease.[101] Focal fibrosis of the bone marrow associated with lymphoreticular cells, in the absence of mononuclear or multinuclear cells with nuclear features of Reed-Sternberg cells, should be regarded as strongly suggestive of Hodgkin's disease in an untreated person with histologically proved Hodgkin's disease.

Clinical correlations

Fig. 30-52 shows the correlation between the histologic type of Hodgkin's disease and survival as obtained from a study of 176 previously untreated cases of Hodgkin's disease.[107] After 6 years the highest number of survivors was in the lymphocyte predominance group. The largest histologic group, comprising half the cases, was the nodular sclerosis group. The second largest group was mixed cellularity. The lymphocyte predominance and lymphocyte depletion groups were about equal in frequency and constituted together approximately 10%

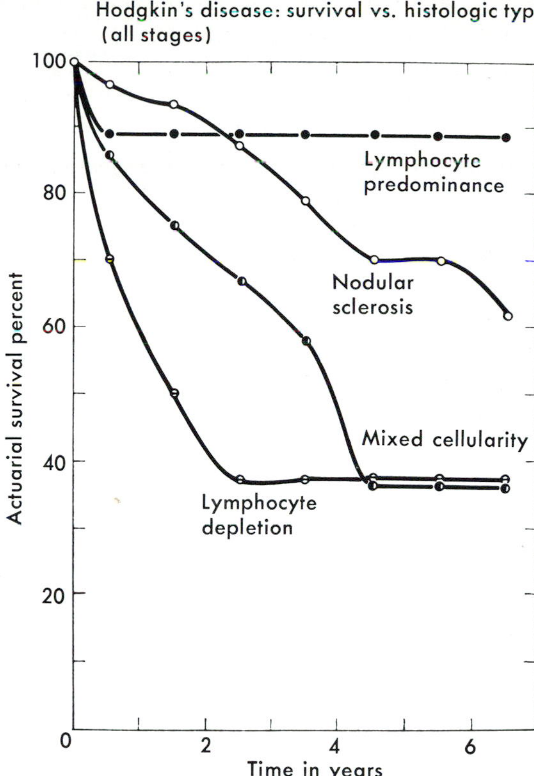

Fig. 30-52. Actuarial survival in 176 cases of Hodgkin's disease according to histologic types. Survival of nodular sclerosis and mixed cellularity groups at 5 years is significantly different ($p < .02$). (From Keller, A.R., et al.: Cancer **22:**487, 1968.)

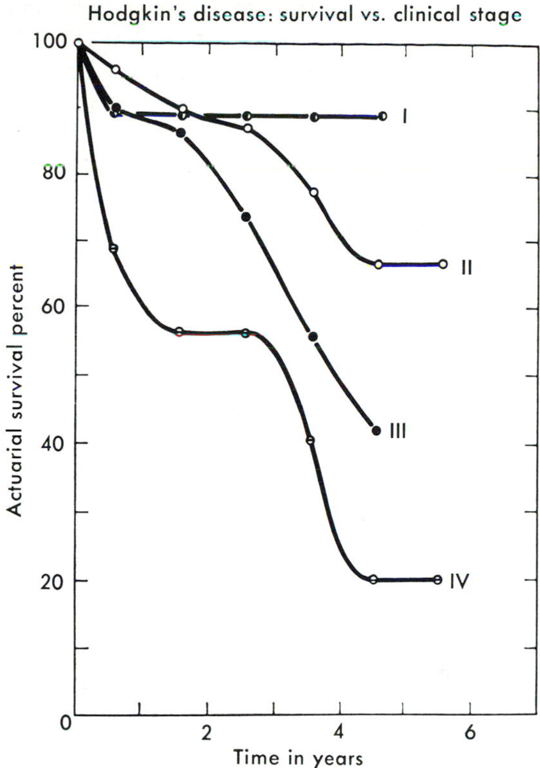

Fig. 30-53. Actuarial survival in Hodgkin's disease according to anatomic stages in 154 patients, all with lymphangiograms. Survival at 5 years of stages I and II, II and IV, and I and IV, are significantly different ($p < .02$). (From Keller, A.R., et al.: Cancer **22:**487, 1968.)

of the patients. Patients with lymphocyte predominance were almost entirely in clinical stages I and II, whereas lymphocyte depletion cases were largely in stages III and IV. Fig. 30-53 shows survival in relation to clinical stages.

There is a high degree of correlation between extensive disease and systemic symptoms. Thus nearly four fifths of stage IV cases had systemic symptoms, whereas three fourths of stage II cases had none.

The majority of patients with active Hodgkin's disease display a defect in cell-mediated immunity. This defect contributes to the variety of bacterial, viral, fungal, and protozoal infections to which these patients are prone.[1]

Non-Hodgkin's malignant lymphomas

At present there is no generally accepted classification of the so-called non-Hodgkin's lymphomas. The original classification included lymphosarcoma, reticulum cell sarcoma, and giant follicular lymphoblastoma (p. 1302). This was gradually replaced by Rappaport's classification[178] (Table 30-2). Rappaport's classification is simple and fairly well reproducible and has proved prognostically significant. There is, however, increasing evidence that it is histogenetically incorrect. Recent ultrastructural and immunofluorescence studies supplemented by techniques for membrane receptor sites (p. 1302) provide evidence for the origin of nodular lymphomas from follicular B lymphocytes.[75,118,120,122] The arguments against substitution of histiocytic lymphoma for reticulum cell sarcoma have been presented (p. 1302). There is also increasing evidence that most if not all lymphomas regarded as reticulum cell sarcomas (histiocytic lymphomas) are in fact derived from transformed B or T lymphocytes.

Many different classifications of the non-Hodgkin's lymphomas have been published in recent years (Table 30-4).[17,30,75] Despite the diversity of terminology used, there is general agreement that non-Hodgkin's lymphomas may exhibit a follicular or a diffuse growth pattern and that they may be composed of small and large cells. Based on these two accepted observations and the evidence of the relationship of follicular (nodular) lymphoma to germinal center cells, we propose the classification in Table 30-5. Some of the large cell lymphomas exhibit round nuclei with prominent nucleoli and a rim of fairly well-defined cytoplasm. The cytoplasm of these cells is pyroninophilic and deeply basophilic with the Giemsa stain. These lymphomas are called "blastic" lymphomas.

Table 30-4. Comparative classifications of non-Hodgkin's lymphomas

Lukes and Collins classification*	Kiel classification†	British classification‡	Dorfman's classification§
I. Undefined cell	Low-grade malignancy—(malignant) lymphoma	Grade 1 Follicular lymphomas Follicle cell, predominantly small Follicle cell, mixed (small and large Follicle cell, predominantly large	Follicular lymphomas (follicular or follicular and diffuse)
II. T-cell types (1) Convoluted lymphocyte (2) Immunoblastic sarcoma (T-cell)	Lymphocytic Lymphoplasmacytoid (immunocytic) Centrocytic Centroblastic-centrocytic follicular‖ Follicular‖ and diffuse Diffuse‖	Diffuse lymphomas Lymphocytic, well differentiated (small round lymphocyte) Lymphocytic, intermediately differentiated (small follicle cell)	Small lymphoid Mixed small and large lymphoid Large lymphoid
III. B-cell types (1) Small lymphocyte (CLL) (2) Plasmacytoid lymphocytic (3) Follicular center cell (follicular, diffuse follicular and diffuse, and sclerotic) (a) small cleaved (b) large cleaved (c) small noncleaved (d) large noncleaved (4) Immunoblastic sarcoma (B-cell)	High-grade malignancy Centroblastic Lymphoblastic Burkitt type Convoluted-cell type Others Immunoblastic	Grade 2 Lymphocytic, poorly differentiated (lymphoblast) Non-Burkitt's lymphoma Burkitt's tumor Convoluted-cell mediastinal lymphoma Lymphocytic cell, mixed (small and large) (mixed follicle cells) "Undifferentiated" large cell (large lymphoid cell) Histiocytic cell (mononuclear phagocytic cells) Plasma cell (extramedullary plasma cell) Unclassified Plasmacytoid differentiation in lymphocytic tumors and banded or fine sclerosis are recorded.	Diffuse¶ Small lymphocytic** Atypical small lymphoid Lymphoblastic Convoluted Nonconvoluted Large lymphoid** Mixed small and large lymphoid Histiocytic Burkitt's lymphoma Mycosis fungoides Undefined

From Rywlin, A.M.: Am. J. Dermatopathol. 2:17, 1980.
*From Lukes, R.J., and Collins, R.D.: Br. J. Cancer **31**:1, 1975.
†From Lennert, K.: Malignant lymphomas, Berlin, 1978, Springer-Verlag.
‡From Bennett, M.H., et al.: Lancet **2**:405, 1974.
§From Dorfman, R.F.: Lancet **1**:295, 1974.
‖With or without sclerosis.
¶Composite lymphomas comprise the following four types: two well-defined and apparently different types of lymphomas within the same tissue; lymphomas associated with sclerosis; lymphomas showing plasmacytoid differentiated**; those associated with epithelioid cells.

Other large cell lymphomas with more pleomorphic and bizarre nuclei but without a pyroninophilic or deeply basophilic cytoplasm with the Giemsa stain are called undifferentiated large cell lymphomas. It is important to distinguish the undifferentiated large cell lymphomas from anaplastic carcinomas and amelanotic melanomas. Pathologists with access to special techniques may extend this classification by marker studies that indicate whether the lymphoma is a B, a T, a subset of T, or a null cell type. Those who believe that they are able to subdivide the large cell lymphomas may do so by adding immunoblastic, centroblastic, or lymphoblastic subtype.

Normal germinal centers contain cells that are intermediate in size and nuclear structure between small lymphocytes and blasts (Fig. 30-29). These intermediate cells have been called cleaved cells, centrocytes, and prolymphocytes. I call malignant lymphomas resembling this intermediate cell, malignant lymphoma, intermediate cell type. Those who claim that they can tell a centrocyte from a prolymphocyte can add these terms to their diagnosis (Fig. 30-29). Other descriptive features, such as the presence of plasma cellular differentiation or of sclerosis, may also be added. Also, proliferating lymphoid cells may induce a stromal reaction that results in

Table 30-5. Proposed classification for non-Hodgkin's malignant lymphomas

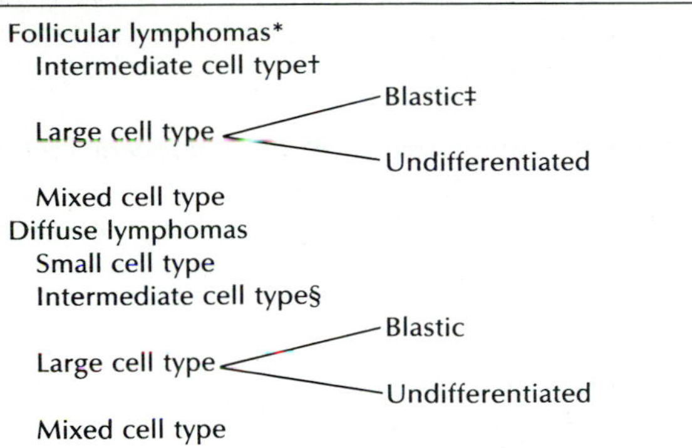

Follicular lymphomas*
Intermediate cell type†
Large cell type — Blastic‡ / Undifferentiated
Mixed cell type
Diffuse lymphomas
Small cell type
Intermediate cell type§
Large cell type — Blastic / Undifferentiated
Mixed cell type

From Rywlin, A.M.: Am. J. Dermatopathol. **2**:17, 1980.

*Follicular lymphomas exhibit a nodular growth pattern and originate from or differentiate into germinal center cells.

†This is the cleaved cell of Lukes and Collins or the germinocyte or centrocyte of Lennert; a follicular lymphoma made up of small, round, "mature" lymphocytes has not been described.

‡Identification of "blasts" is based on the presence of narrow blue rims of cytoplasm with the Giemsa stain in association with prominent nucleoli; the cytoplasm is also pyroninophilic. A large cell malignant lymphoma which does not exhibit a blue cytoplasmic rim with the Giemsa stain and/or pyroninophilia is called an undifferentiated type. It has to be distinguished from an anaplastic carcinoma or an amelanotic melanoma.

§This is the germinal center cell described in Footnote †; however, the growth pattern is diffuse.

an increased framework of reticulin. Any malignant lymphoma with many benign-appearing epithelioid histiocytes could be called Lennert's lymphoma.[197]

Burkitt's lymphoma is a blastic lymphoma with cytoplasmic vacuoles, numerous histiocytes containing tingible bodies, and certain clinical characteristics such as the occurrence in extranodal sites.[11] The blasts are somewhat smaller than in other large cell lymphomas. The "lymphoblastic lymphoma" seen in childhood and adolescents and often involving the mediastinum is composed of intermediate and blastic lymphocytes that may or may not have characteristic convoluted nuclei.[151]

This terminology can also be applied to the lymphocytic leukemias, which at present are classified according to the lymphoblast → prolymphocyte → lymphocyte arc (Fig. 30-29).

Recently the following "Working Formulation of Non-Hodgkin's Lymphomas for Clinical Usage" was proposed by a group of experts[20]:

- Low grade
  - Malignant lymphoma, small lymphocytic
  - Malignant lymphoma, follicular, predominantly small cleaved cell
  - Malignant lymphoma, follicular, mixed small cleaved and large cell
- Intermediate grade
  - Malignant lymphoma, follicular, predominantly large cell
  - Malignant lymphoma, diffuse, small cleaved cell
  - Malignant lymphoma, diffuse, mixed small and large cell
  - Malignant lymphoma, diffuse, large cell
- High grade
  - Malignant lymphoma, large cell, immunoblastic
  - Malignant lymphoma, lymphoblastic
  - Malignant lymphoma, small noncleaved cell
- Miscellaneous
  - Composite malignant lymphoma
  - Mycosis fungoides
  - Extramedullary plasmacytoma
  - Unclassifiable
  - Other

This formulation includes prognostic features (low, intermediate, and high grades), uses "follicular" instead of "nodular," relegates histiocytic lymphoma to a miscellaneous group, and substitutes large cell lymphoma for histiocytic lymphoma of Rappaport's classification. This formulation can easily be translated into the other classifications. Whether it will be universally accepted remains to be seen.

Follicular lymphomas

Follicular lymphomas are defined as malignant lymphomas arising from, or differentiating toward, germinal center cells. They exhibit a follicular or nodular growth pattern, which may be associated with a diffuse pattern. Occasionally a diffuse pattern only is seen, but a reticulin stain may still reveal remnants of a follicular pattern.

Lymphomas with a follicular pattern must be distinguished from reactive follicular hyperplasia. The criteria for separating these two entities are well summarized by Rappaport and co-workers.[152,180] They are based on architectural and cytologic features. In follicular lymphomas the architecture is partly or completely effaced. This is true of all malignant lymphomas and is best appreciated by a study of the subcapsular area normally occupied by the peripheral sinus. Obliteration of the subcapsular sinus is particularly well seen with reticulin stains. Neoplastic follicles vary moderately in size and shape and are evenly distributed throughout cortex and medulla. Reactive follicles are especially prominent in the cortical portion of the lymph node and vary considerably in size and shape. Reaction centers are more sharply demarcated than are neoplastic follicles. Reticulin fibers may be condensed at the periphery of neoplastic nodules, whereas they are slightly altered around reactive follicles. Cytologically, reactive follicles show debris-containing macrophages and frequent mitotic figures. In neoplastic follicles macrophages are inconspicuous and mitotic figures are scarce.

Follicular lymphomas have a better prognosis than do diffuse lymphomas. A follicular lymphoma made up of small, mature lymphocytes has not been identified.

Intermediate cell type. Synonyms for this type include nodular lymphoma, lymphocytic poorly differentiated; follicular lymphoma, small lymphoid type; prolymphocytic lymphoma, nodular; B cell lymphoma, cleaved cell type; germinocytoma; and centrocytic lymphoma.

This lymphoma consists of cells that are somewhat larger than the small, "mature" perifollicular lymphocyte, hence the term *intermediate cell*. The nuclear membranes may be distorted, partially collapsed, and cleaved. A few blasts are invariably present (Fig. 30-54).

Large cell type. Synonyms for this type include nodular lymphoma, histiocytic type; follicular lymphoma, large lymphoid type; B cell lymphoma, large noncleaved cell type; germinoblastoma; and centroblastic lymphoma.

These lymphomas exhibit a predominantly follicular or a follicular and diffuse growth pattern. When the large cells have a dark blue rim of cytoplasm with the Giemsa stain, they fall into the blast category. I believe that it is

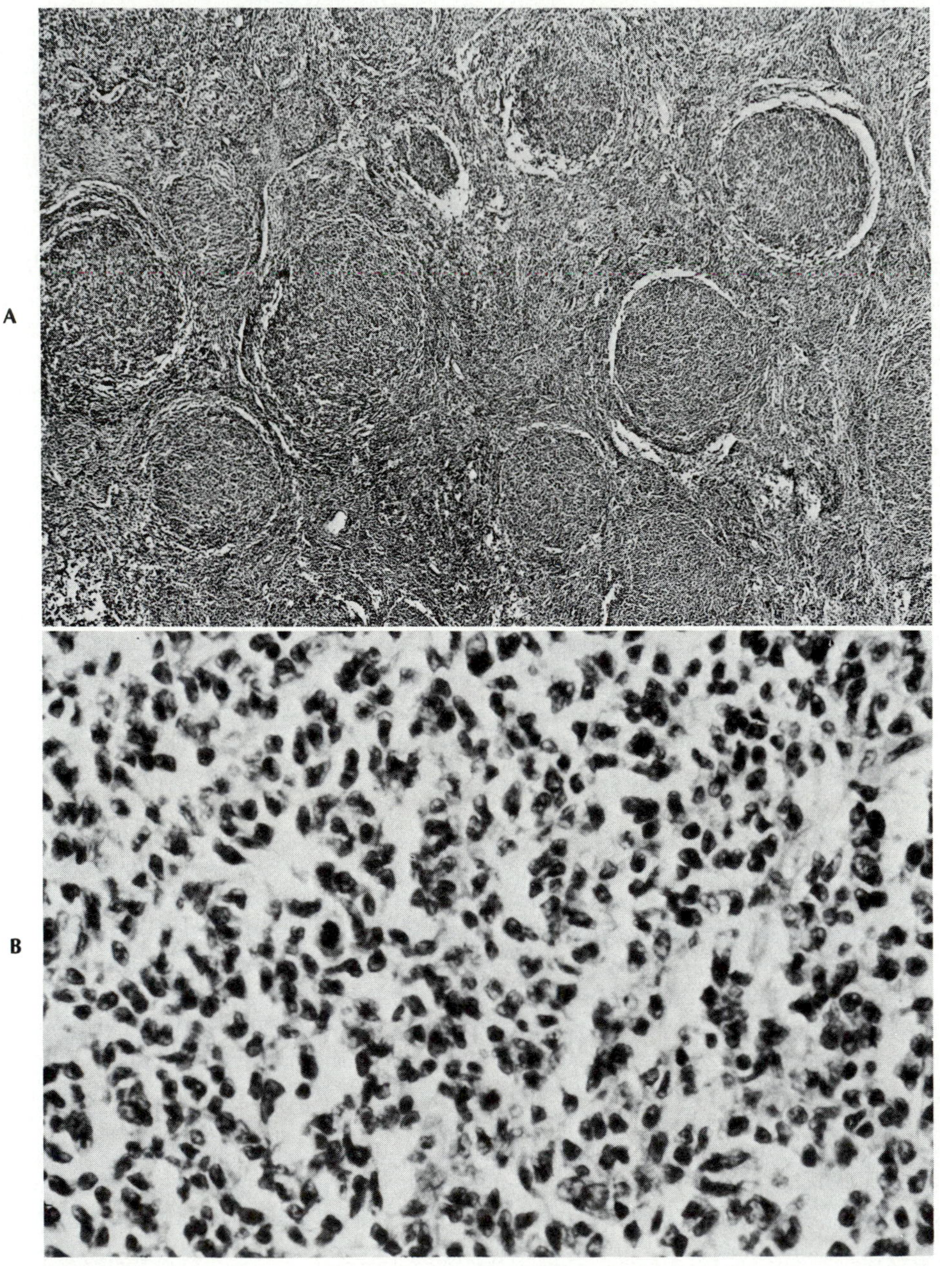

Fig. 30-54. Lymph node. Follicular lymphoma, intermediate cell type. Note follicular growth pattern, **A**, and distorted, irregular nuclear membranes, **B.** (Hematoxylin and eosin; **A**, 100×; **B**, 250×.)

impossible, at the present stage of knowledge, to clearly distinguish in neoplastic processes germinoblasts, immunoblasts, and lymphoblasts. The large cell lymphoma whose cells fail to exhibit pyroninophilia and basophilia of the cytoplasm is classified as an undifferentiated type. In large cell follicular lymphomas, mitotic figures may be abundant (Fig. 30-55).

Mixed cell type. Synonyms for this type include malignant lymphoma, nodular, mixed lymphocytic-histiocytic; follicular lymphoma, mixed small and large lymphoid; and centroblastic-centrocytic lymphoma.

This malignant lymphoma exhibits a follicular growth pattern and is composed cytologically of approximately equal numbers of the small and large cells described previously. Varying degrees of sclerosis may be present in this lymphoma (Figs. 30-56 and 30-57).

Diffuse lymphomas

Small cell type. Synonyms for this type include malignant lymphoma, well-differentiated lymphocytic diffuse; diffuse lymphoma, small lymphocytic type; B cell lymphoma, small lymphocytic type; lymphoplasmacytoid lymphoma; and immunocytic lymphoma.

This lymphoma exhibits a diffuse growth pattern only. The architecture of the lymph node is effaced. The lymph node is diffusely infiltrated with small, "mature" lymphocytes, exhibiting round to oval, hyperchromatic nuclei without any cleft formation (Fig. 30-58). The appearance of this lymph node is not distinguishable from chronic lymphocytic leukemia. A thorough search for Reed-Sternberg cells should be performed to exclude Hodgkin's disease with lymphocytic predominance. This type of malignant lymphoma is rare. In my experience most cases are examples of chronic lymphocytic leukemias.

This lymphoma may be associated with plasma cells, plasmacytoid lymphocytes, and cells with periodic acid–Schiff–positive cytoplasmic and intranuclear inclusions. A high percentage of such cases exhibit a monoclonal macroglobulinemia.

At times a malignant lymphoma of the small or intermediate cell type may exhibit plasmacytoid and plasma cells and giant Russell bodies that are strongly periodic acid–Schiff positive.[210] Benign-appearing histiocytes that have apparently phagocytosed the secreted immunoglobulin and have a granular periodic acid–Schiff–positive cytoplasm may also be seen.

Occasionally a malignant lymphoma with intracellular immunoglobulin mimics signet-ring cells of an adenocarcinoma.[242]

Intermediate cell type. Synonyms for this type are malignant lymphoma, diffuse, poorly differentiated lymphocytic; diffuse lymphoma, lymphocytic, intermediate differentiation (small follicle cell); malignant lymphoma, centrocytic, diffuse; malignant lymphoma, diffuse, cleaved cell or germinocytic type; and malignant lymphoma, diffuse, prolymphocytic.

This lymphoma exhibits a diffuse growth pattern and is identical cytologically to the follicular lymphoma of the intermediate cell type. It may have started with a follic-

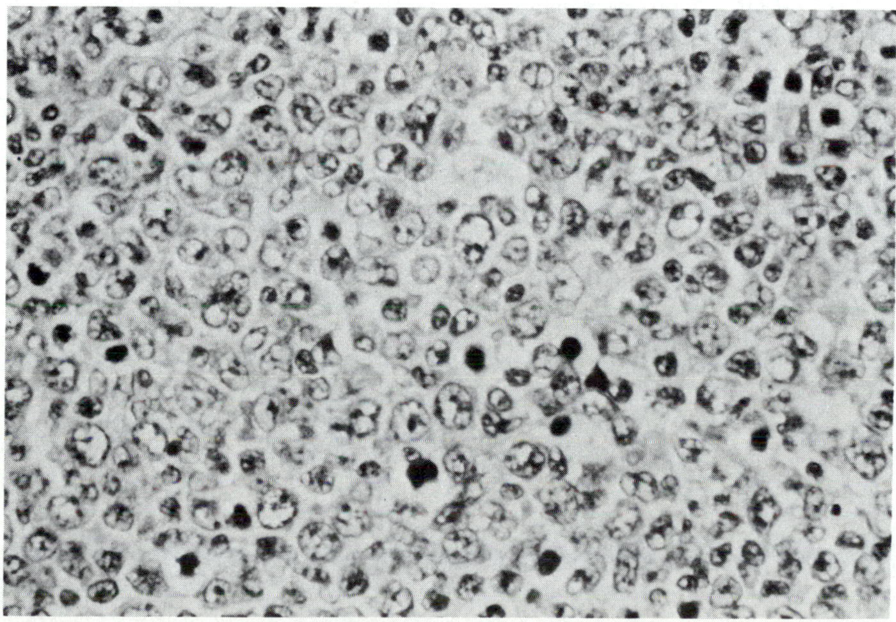

Fig. 30-55. Lymph node. Malignant lymphoma, follicular, large cell type. Follicular pattern cannot be appreciated with this magnification. (250×.)

ular growth pattern that became diffuse as the disease evolved. When this type of lymphoma becomes leukemic, the neoplastic cells in the peripheral blood correspond to "lymphosarcoma cells."

The "lymphoblastic lymphoma," also known as "malignant lymphoma, convoluted lymphocytic type,"[12] is primarily a tumor of children and adolescents. It arises in the thymus and progresses to acute leukemia in a high percentage of cases.[102,221] The cells are very similar to those of acute lymphocytic leukemia with T-markers. The nuclei may or may not have characteristic convolutions.[151] The term "lymphoblastic" for this tumor is unfortunate, since the cells do not display the features characteristic of blasts. They are smaller, nuclei may be convoluted, and nucleoli are small or inconspicuous. The nuclei exhibit a "dusty" chromatin pattern. The cytoplasm is scanty, and cytoplasmic pyroninophilia is difficult to demonstrate. A varying number of true blasts are present. This T cell lymphoma is a subcategory of the diffuse lymphoma, intermediate cell type.

Large cell type. Synonyms for this type are malignant lymphoma, diffuse, histiocytic type; reticulum cell sarco-

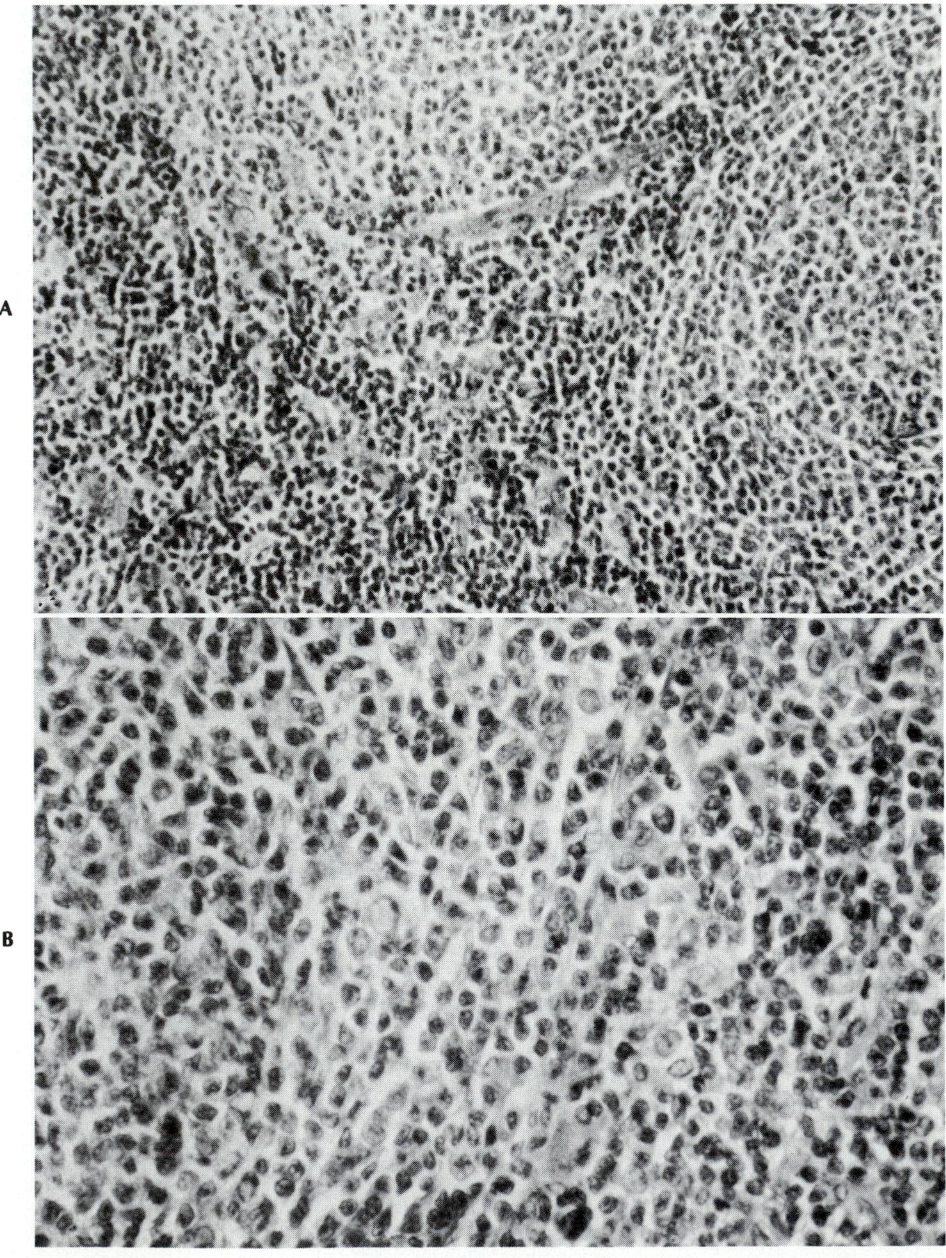

Fig. 30-56. Lymph node. Malignant lymphoma, follicular, mixed cell type. (Hematoxylin and eosin; **A,** 125×; **B,** 250×.)

ma; diffuse lymphoma, large lymphoid (pyroninophilic) type; B or T cell immunoblastic sarcoma; and lymphoblastic sarcoma.

This type of malignant lymphoma exhibits a diffuse growth pattern. On the basis of the Giemsa stain it can be divided into two types: "blastic" lymphoma and undifferentiated lymphoma. In the blastic lymphoma, the Giemsa stain reveals that the neoplastic cells possess a rim of dark blue cytoplasm (Figs. 30-59 and 30-60). The cytoplasm is also pyroninophilic. Pyroninophilia and basophilia with the Giemsa stain are indicative of high RNA content. Furthermore, the cells exhibit round to oval nuclei and prominent nucleoli. In the undifferentiated lymphoma, no dark blue rim of cytoplasm can be demonstrated. Also, the nuclei are more pleomorphic than those in the blastic type, and the cytoplasm is more irregular and eosinophilic (Fig. 30-61).

Burkitt's tumor or Burkitt's lymphoma is a diffuse, blastic lymphoma with characteristic clinical and histologic features. Burkitt's tumor was first reported as a jaw sarcoma of East African children.[32] It was identified as a malignant lymphoma by O'Connor and Davies.[160] In

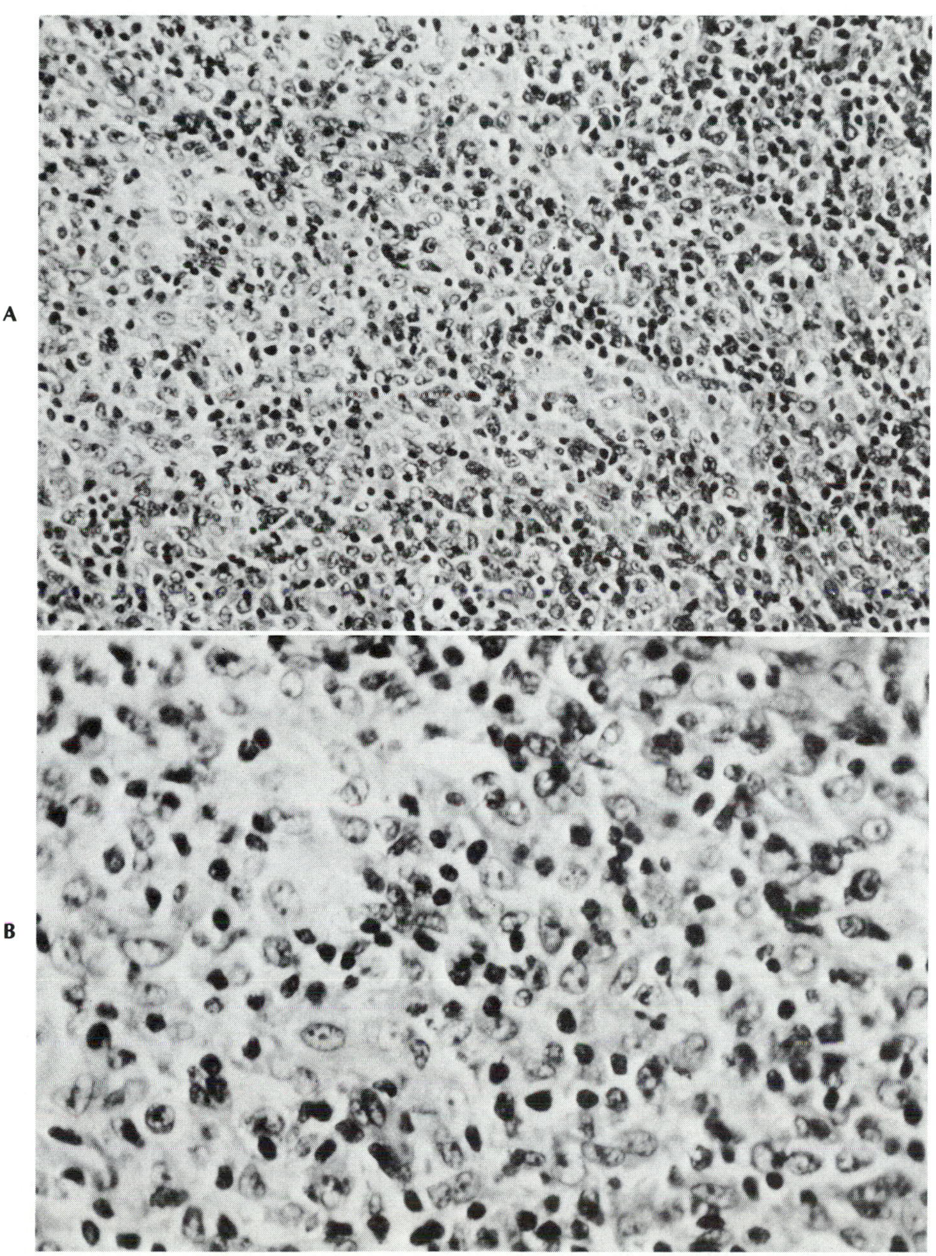

Fig. 30-57. Lymph node. Lymphoma, mixed cell type. (Hematoxylin and eosin; **A,** 100×; **B,** 250×.)

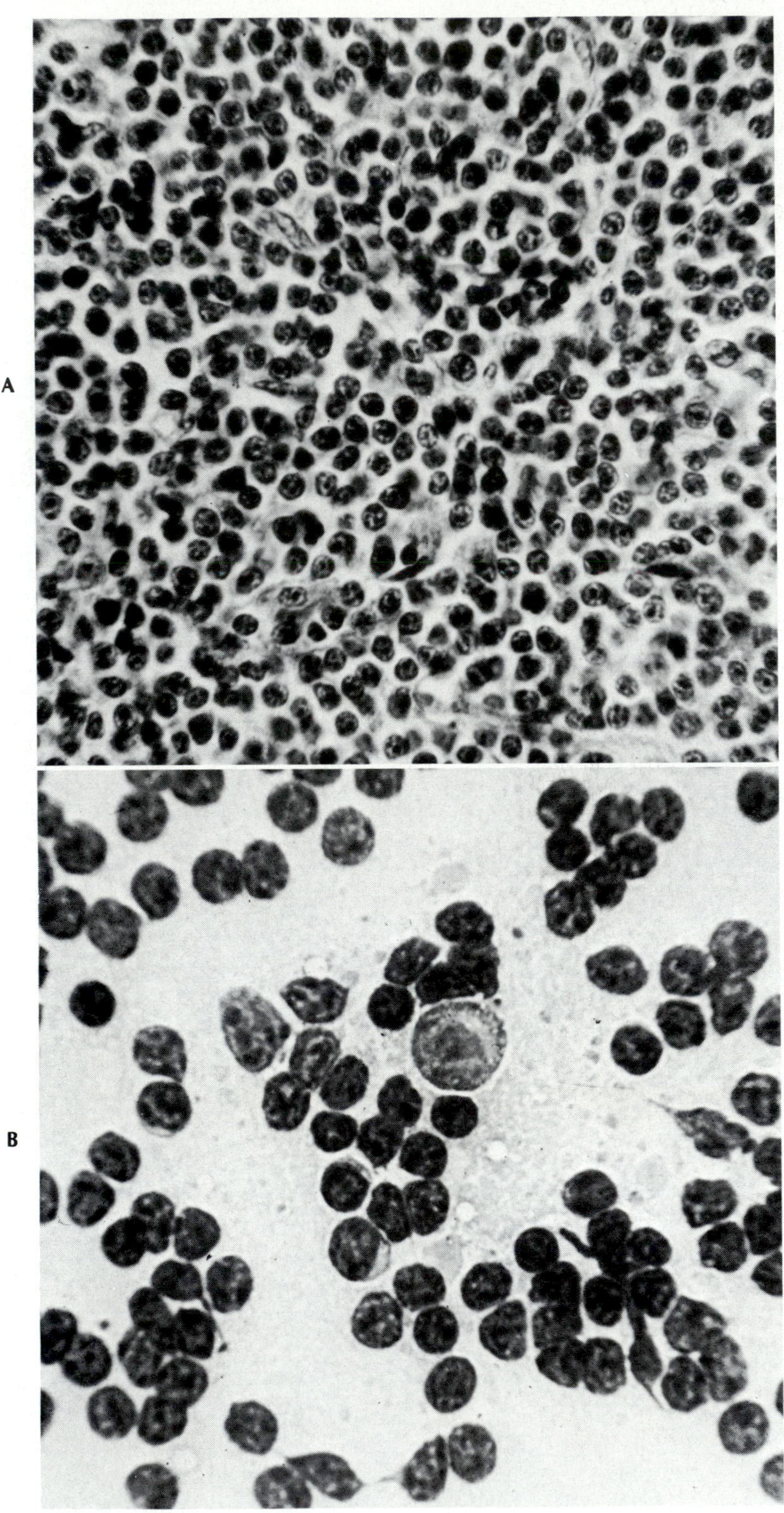

Fig. 30-58. Lymph node. Diffuse lymphoma, small cell type. Note small lymphocytes in imprint preparation, **B.** (**A,** Hematoxylin and eosin, 450×; **B,** Wright's stain; 1080×; **A** and **B,** courtesy Dr. Joseph C. Sieracki, Pittsburgh.)

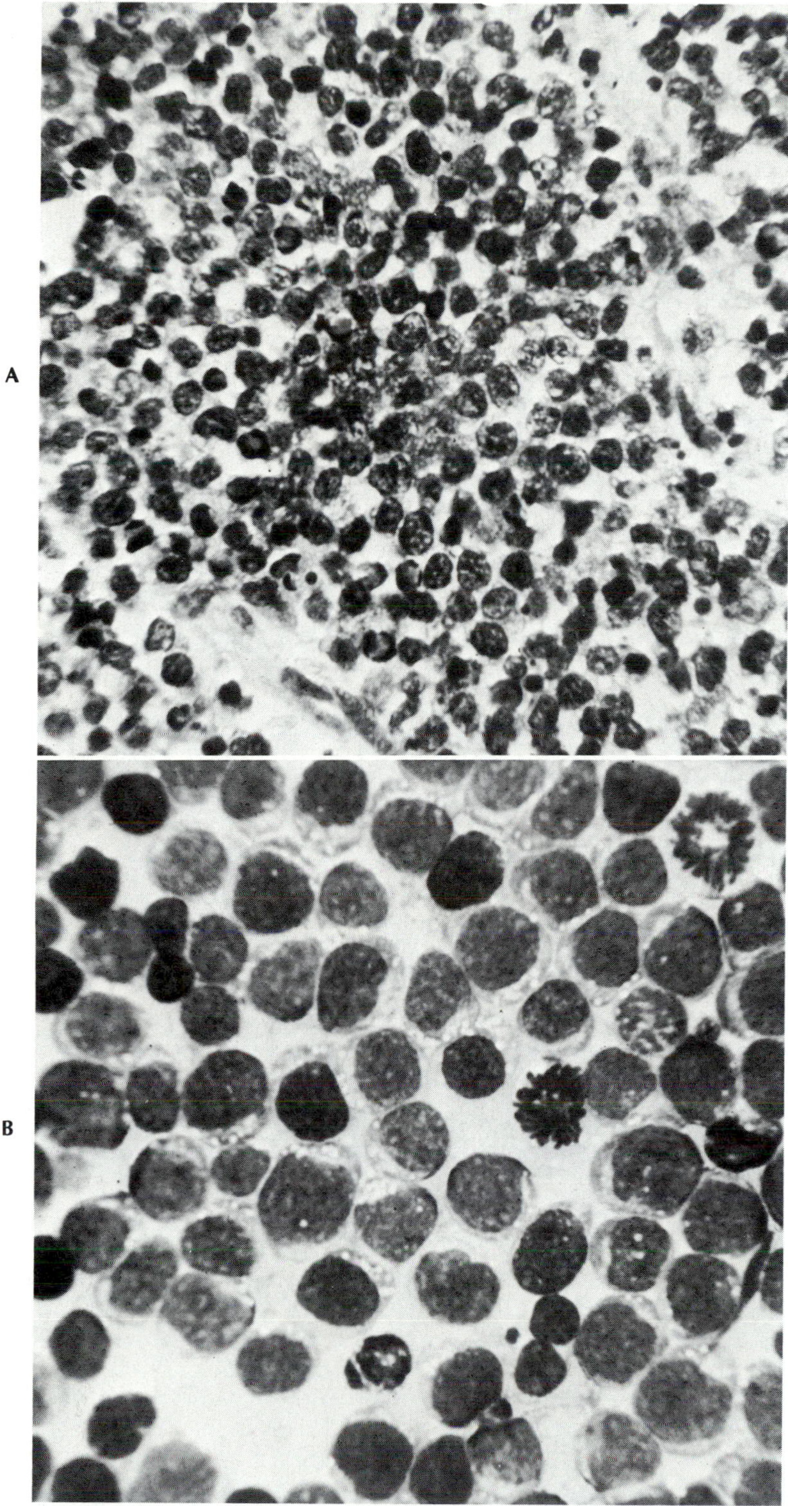

Fig. 30-59. Lymph node. Diffuse lymphoma, large cell type. Note blastic appearance of cell in imprint preparation, **B,** (**A,** Hematoxylin and eosin; 450×; **B,** Wright's stain; 950×; **A** and **B,** courtesy Dr. Joseph C. Sieracki, Pittsburgh.)

American patients, abdominal and pelvic involvement is far more frequent than jaw involvement. Bone marrow involvement is also more frequent in American patients. In a series of 30 American cases,[5,11] 23 had an abdominal tumor and four showed ovarian involvement. In only three was lymphadenopathy the sole presenting physical finding. Facial bones were involved in five cases. Involvement of the bone marrow was documented in five of the 26 patients whose bone marrows were available. Good correlation between lactic dehydrogenase values and stage of Burkitt's tumor has been reported.[5] Complete remissions were obtained in 13 of the 30 patients treated with chemotherapy.[5] Metabolic complications related to therapy included azotemia, hyperkalemia, hyperuricemia, hyperphosphatemia, and hypocalcemia. Of the 13 patients who had a complete remission, nine were free of disease for 37 to 80 months.[5]

Histologically Burkitt's tumor is composed of blasts with pyroninophilic and Giemsa-positive cytoplasmic rims. Nucleoli are prominent. Characteristic of this neoplasm is a "starry-sky" appearance because of benign-appearing phagocytic cells containing debris. Some periodic acid–Schiff–positive material can be identified in these macrophages. The histologic features of Burkitt's

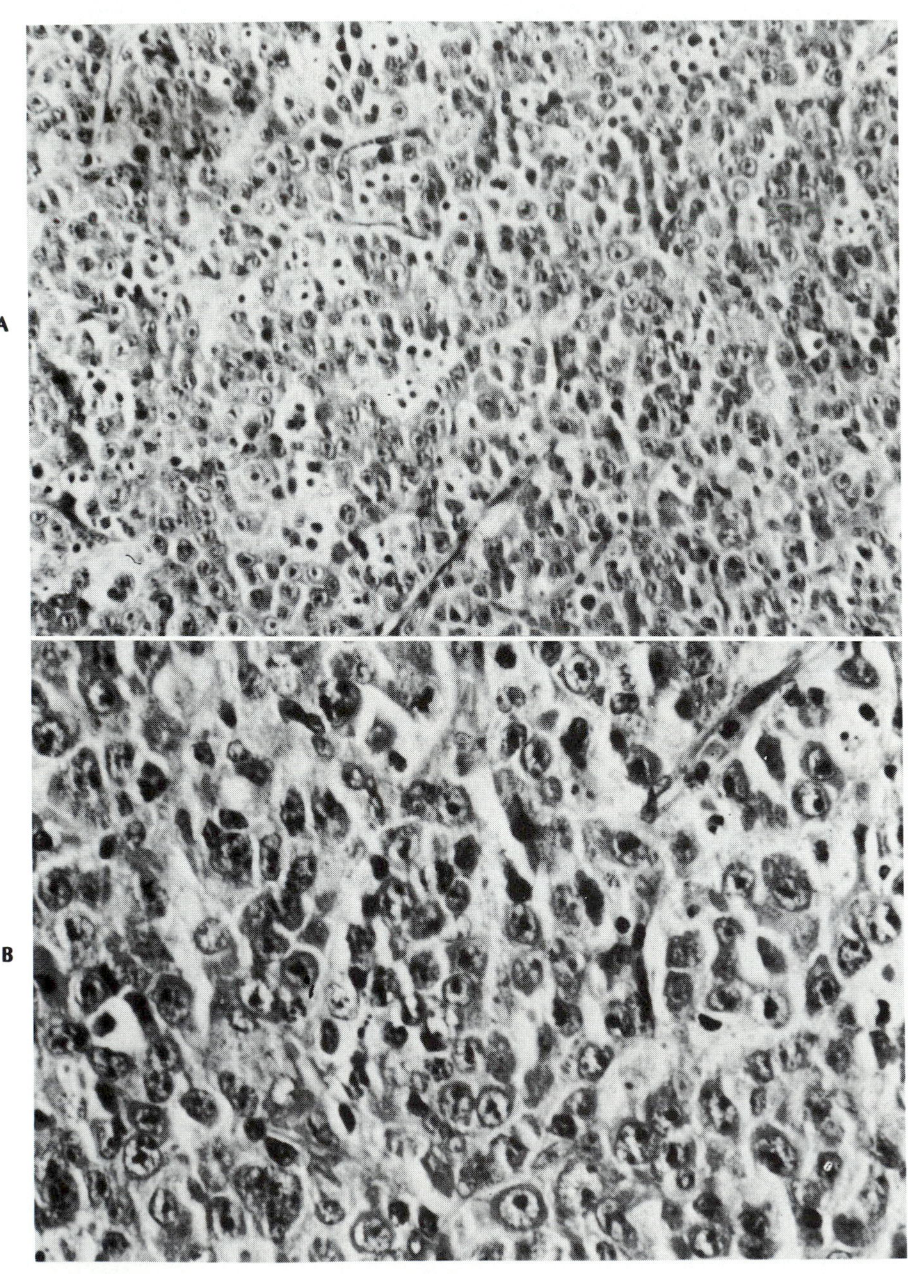

Fig. 30-60. Lymph node. Diffuse lymphoma, large cell type, "blastic." (Hematoxylin and eosin; **A**, 125×; **B**, 250×.)

tumor have been defined by the World Health Organization[19] and have been reviewed in detail by Wright.[253]

In 17 autopsied cases of Burkitt's tumor the most consistent feature was widespread organ involvement, predominantly in the extralymphatic sites.[11] All 17 patients had tumor in two or more gastrointestinal organs. Twelve patients had hepatic involvement, and 16 had tumor in the kidneys. Involvement of lungs was present in 11 cases, and of the central nervous system in nine. Cardiovascular organs and the musculoskeletal system were infiltrated with tumor in six patients. Diffuse peripheral lymph node involvement was seen in only one patient. The spleen was involved in 10 and the bone marrow in 12 of the 17 autopsied cases. Chemotherapeutic agents appeared to alter the cytologic appearance of the tumor. The cells exhibited pronounced pleomorphism resembling malignant histiocytes. Reed-Sternberg-like cells were seen occasionally.

Mixed cell type. Synonyms for this type include malignant lymphoma, diffuse, mixed lymphohistiocytic; malignant lymphoma, diffuse, mixed, small and large lymphoid; and diffuse lymphoma, mixed, small lymphoid and undifferentiated large cell.

This variety of lymphoma exhibits a diffuse growth pattern and is composed of approximately equal numbers of intermediate cells and large cells of the blast type. In every malignant lymphoma a few large cells can be found. Some of them are reticulum cells and perhaps are the result of an inductive effect of neoplastic lympho-

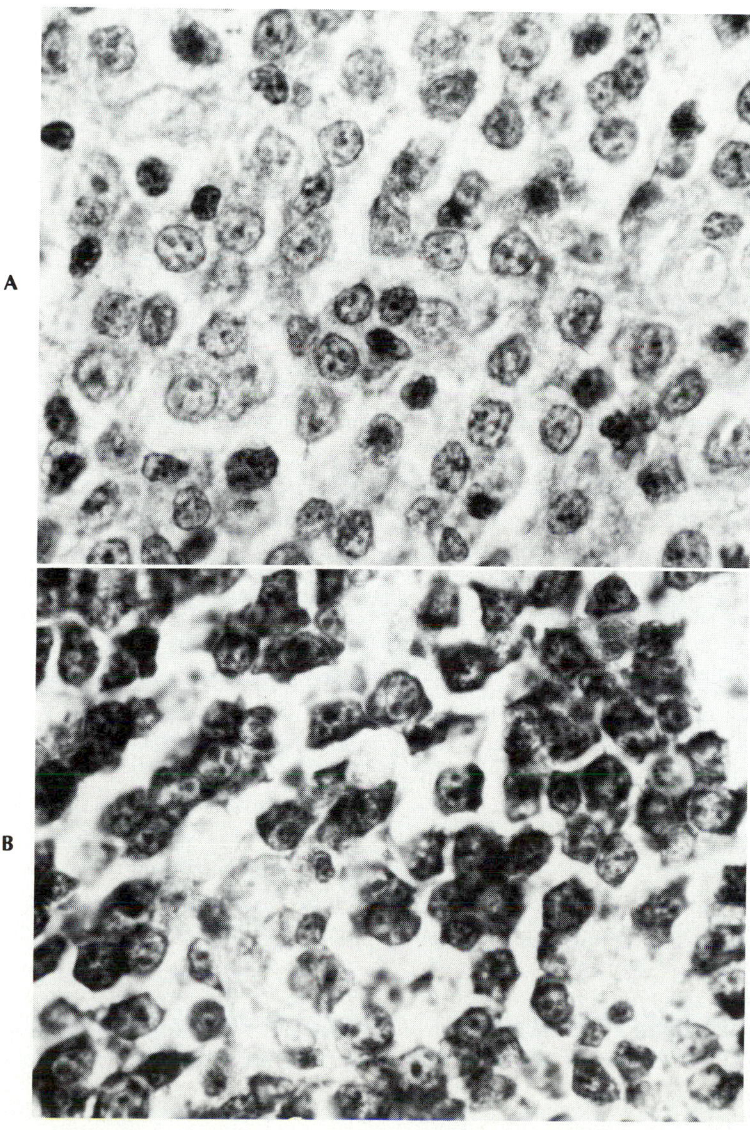

Fig. 30-61. A, Diffuse lymphoma, large cell type, undifferentiated. **B,** Diffuse lymphoma, diffuse blastic. Note dark blue rim of cytoplasm. (**A** and **B,** Giemsa stain, 882×.)

cytes on the stroma. Other large cells exhibit the characteristics of blasts. The presence of only a few large cells does not justify the diagnosis of a malignant lymphoma, mixed cell type.

When a malignant lymphoma shows pleomorphic cells with convoluted nuclei associated with epithelioid cells and numerous venules with prominent endothelial cells, one should suspect a malignant lymphoma of peripheral T lymphocytes.[244] This T cell lymphoma has to be distinguished from immunoblastic lymphadenopathy. In peripheral T cell lymphoma there are usually preserved lymphoid follicles that are not present in immunoblastic lymphadenopathy. However, hypergammaglobulinemia may occur in peripheral T cell lymphoma and may add to the difficulty in distinguishing it from immunoblastic lymphadenopathy.[247] At times T cell lymphomas may mimic B cell lymphomas of the large cell type.[163]

Bone marrow involvement in non-Hodgkin's lymphomas

The overall frequency of bone marrow involvement in non-Hodgkin's lymphoma is around 40%.[28,39] Follicular lymphomas affect the marrow as frequently as diffuse lymphomas. Bone marrow involvement is most frequent in small cell lymphomas and least frequent in large cell lymphomas.

The bone marrow lesions may be focal or diffuse, exhibiting complete replacement of hematopoietic and fatty marrow by lymphoma. In the small cell lymphoma the marrow picture may be identical to chronic lymphocytic leukemia. Patients with small cell malignant lymphomas of the bone marrow may exhibit chronic lymphocytic leukemia, monoclonal gammopathy, both chronic lymphocytic leukemia and monoclonal gammapathy, or neither.[59,165] In malignant lymphoma of the intermediate cell type (poorly differentiated lymphocytic) there is a tendency for the involvement of the peritrabecular marrow.

There is generally, although not always, good concurrence between the cell type of the original lymphoma and the lymphomatous cells in the marrow. At times lymphomatous nodules in the marrow may contain a large number of benign-appearing epithelioid cells simulating Lennert's lymphoma.[256]

Clinical correlations

There is less information available on clinicopathologic correlations for the non-Hodgkin's lymphomas than for Hodgkin's disease. In a large series of cases studied at Stanford University Medical Center,[100] follicular lymphomas were found in 44% of the group and diffuse lymphomas in 56%. Patients under 35 years of age and those over 60 tended to have diffuse lymphomas. Thirty-nine percent of the patients had stage IV disease at the time it was first diagnosed. Systemic symptoms did not adversely affect survival. They were present in 24% of patients with diffuse and 18% with follicular lymphomas. Patients with follicular lymphomas survived significantly longer than patients with diffuse lymphomas. Malignant lymphomas whether nodular or diffuse have a better prognosis if they exhibit a tendency to sclerosis.[145] The small cell lymphomas fare better than do the large cell lymphomas.

Left lower cervical or supraclavicular lymphadenopathy was significantly more often correlated with para-aortic lymphadenopathy than with involvement in the right lower neck region.

All patients with malignant lymphomas should have a serum protein electrophoresis and immunoelectrophoresis. Monoclonal gammopathies of various types may be encountered in the different forms of malignant lymphomas.

Heavy-chain diseases

Heavy-chain diseases are lymphocellular and plasmacellular proliferative disorders associated with an overproduction of Fc fragments of gamma (γ), alpha (α), or mu (μ) heavy chains.

Franklin's disease (gamma heavy-chain disease)[68]

The most frequent clinical presentation of Franklin's disease consists of painless cervical or axillary lymphadenopathy. Occasionally there is only thoracic or abdominal lymphadenopathy. Prominent involvement of Waldeyer's ring with erythema and swelling of the uvula was described in several cases. Hepatosplenomegaly was observed clinically or at autopsy in many of the cases. Fever was present in about half the reported cases. In the fatal cases the disease lasted from 6 months to a year. Anemia, leukopenia with lymphocytosis, atypical lymphocytes, peripheral blood plasmacytosis, and thrombocytopenia have all been reported. Most patients with Franklin's disease have hypoalbuminemia with a normal total serum protein level. An abnormal band of protein is usually present on electrophoresis. Immunoelectrophoresis of serum and urine reveals a precipitin arc with anti-IgG and anti-Fc serum. No light chains are found in the urine.

The infiltrate in the lymph nodes and other tissues consists of a varying mixture of lymphocytes, plasma cells, plasmacytoid cells, eosinophils, and histiocytes. Occasionally Reed-Sternberg-like cells have been reported.[57] The pathologist examining a lymph node may have considerable difficulty deciding whether an inflammatory or a neoplastic process is involved. It is essential that all the clinical and laboratory data be available before committing oneself to a definite diagnosis.

Mediterranean lymphoma (Seligman's disease, alpha heavy-chain disease)[212]

Mediterranean lymphoma is a term applied to a lymphoplasmacellular proliferative disorder occurring primarily in Mediterranean populations. It involves the small intestine with villous atrophy and malabsorption. In some patients with Mediterranean lymphoma, alpha-chain proteins are demonstrated in the serum on immunoelectrophoresis.[212] Whether all cases of Mediterranean lymphoma are associated with an alpha-chain peak remains unknown, since in many of the earlier cases alpha chains were not sought. Also, the amount present in the serum may be so small that it can be overlooked on routine electrophoresis.[68]

Morphologic findings in Mediterranean lymphoma are not uniform, and it is not settled whether we are dealing with different stages of one disease or with different lympho-proliferative disorders. Ramot[177] has divided 20 cases into three groups: (1) cases with massive plasma cell infiltration of the gut and lymph nodes without evidence of lymphoma (four cases); in two of these patients protein studies were performed and alpha heavy chains were found in the serum; (2) plasma cell infiltration of the intestine and malignant lymphoma in the mesenteric lymph nodes (two cases); and (3) malignant lymphoma of the small intestine with a heavy plasma cellular response (14 cases). No data on the presence of alpha chains were available for these patients. Reviewing this material, Rappaport and associates [182] concluded that the plasma cell infiltration, rather than the malignant lymphomas, was responsible for the malabsorption syndrome. There was no morphologic evidence that the malignant lymphomas were histogenetically related to the plasma cell infiltration. The possibility was suggested that the proliferation of plasma cells was a morphologic manifestation of an immune-deficiency state predisposing patients to the development of malignant lymphoreticular neoplasms.[180] Ramot[177] believes that the massive intestinal plasma cell infiltration should be considered neoplastic and classified as an extramedullary plasmacytoma.

Recently alpha heavy-chain disease has been reported with a diffuse lymphoplasmacellular infiltrate of the respiratory tract without intestinal involvement.[225]

Mu heavy-chain disease

Mu heavy-chain disease is the rarest of the heavy-chain diseases. The cases reported were in patients with long-standing chronic lymphocytic leukemia.[65,68] They had hepatosplenomegaly without peripheral lymphadenopathy. Routine electrophoresis revealed hypogammaglobulinemia; an abnormal component reacting with antisera to mu chains was discovered on immunoelectrophoresis. Mu chains have not been reported in the urine of these patients. Two of the reported patients had light chains in the urine.[68] There is evidence that the defect in mu-chain disease is a lack of normal coupling of light and heavy chains, rather than an overproduction of heavy chains, as is the case in alpha and gamma heavy-chain diseases.[118] Two of the reported patients had pathologic fractures and one had amyloidosis.[68] All the patients had vacuolated plasma cells in addition to lymphocytosis of the bone marrow.

BONE MARROW AND BLOOD

Structure and function

Two types of bone marrow can be clearly distinguished: yellow and red. Yellow marrow is made up of mature fat cells. Red marrow consists of fat cells and hemopoietic cells. The latter include cells of the megakaryocytic, erythrocytic, and granulocytic series with an admixture of lymphocytes, histiocytes, plasma cells, and mast cells. The red color of the hemopoietic bone marrow is determined by the number of cells in the erythrocyte series and by the amount of blood in the sinusoids.

At birth, all possible bone cavities contain active red marrow. By the age of 4 years, there is beginning replacement of red marrow by fatty marrow, and at the age of 20 years red marrow is found only in the skull, clavicles, scapulae, sternum, ribs, pelvis, and proximal ends of the long bones, whereas the distal portions of the long bones contain only fatty marrow. In the normal adult the ratio of red to fatty marrow is 1:1. Ellis[56] gives the total amount of active red marrow in a man weighing 70 kg as 1459 g, about equal to the weight of the liver, and gives data for distribution in various bones (Table 30-6). When marrow volume and cellularity are determined by means of radioisotopes of iron and gold, the values for the normal distribution are not changed appreciably, but these methods give interesting data concerning hematologic abnormalities.

The vascular bed of the bone marrow is unusual in several respects. For one thing, the rigid cortical bone that encases it makes an unyielding hydrostatic system in the marrow unlike that in any other organ. The arteries entering the marrow cavity have a normal structure, but soon after entering the marrow, the thick-walled arteries change abruptly into thin-walled arteries, the wall of which consists of a flattened thin tunica media and flat endothelium. The thin-walled arteries in turn open into

Table 30-6. Distribution of red marrow by weight in bones of normal 40-year-old man

	Weight of red marrow (g)	% total red marrow
Cranium and mandible	136.6	13.1
Humeri, scapulae, and clavicles	86.7	8.3
Sternum	23.4	2.3
Ribs	82.6	7.9
Vertebrae	297.8	28.4
Pelvis	418.6	40.0

Slightly modified from Ellis, R.E.: Phys. Med. Biol. 5:255, 1961; from Miale, J.B.: Laboratory medicine—hematology, ed. 6, St. Louis, 1982, The C.V. Mosby Co.

large sinuses. By electron microscopy the sinus walls can be seen to be made up of endothelium and adventitial or reticulum cells. Although there is an indistinct, flocculent, electron-dense material in the extravascular space beneath the endothelial cells, there is no distinct basal lamina. Scanning electron microscopy had shown a structural continuity of the walls of the myeloid sinuses.[46] It appears that the apertures described by earlier investigators were the result of artifactual mechanical injury. The delivery of cells from the marrow to the peripheral blood occurs via transcellular passage rather than migration through intercellular clefts.[46] In addition to the transmural passage of blood cells into the sinuses, there is also apparently transcellular penetration of platelet-forming megakaryocytic cytoplasm. Why the intravascular delivery of blood cells is limited to mature cells is not clear.

The bone marrow functions are formation of blood cells and endocytosis. The bone marrow is the chief site of the formation of erythrocytes, granulocytes, and platelets. It is involved also, although to a lesser extent, in the formation of monocytes, lymphocytes, and probably mast cells. As the cells in the different series mature, they go through stages of maturation. These can be recognized relatively easily in bone marrow smears stained with the Wright-Giemsa technique. These cells are well described in atlases of bone marrow cytology.[139] The maturation stages of the various cell series are more difficult to recognize in histologic sections. Certain general rules, with a few exceptions, should be kept in mind. The younger the cell, the larger its size and its nuclear cytoplasmic ratio. The blast stage, which is the youngest recognizable precursor of a cell series (myeloblast, lymphoblast, erythroblast or rubriblast, megakaryoblast), has a narrow rim of cytoplasm rich in RNA, which is therefore pyroninophilic and stains dark blue with the Giemsa stain. "Blasts" have large nuclei with a delicate chromatin pattern and a variable number of prominent nucleoli. As the cells mature they slowly acquire their cytoplasmic and nuclear characteristics. Thus for the myelocytic series, the promyelocyte is characterized by azurophilic granules and the myelocyte by specific neutrophilic, eosinophilic, or basophilic granules. In the metamyelocyte the nucleus begins to indent; when the indentation exceeds half the diameter of the nucleus, the cell is called a band-shaped polymorphonuclear leukocyte. Finally, when the lobes are connected by a very thin strand, the cell is a mature granulocyte or polymorphonuclear leukocyte. In the erythrocytic series, as it matures, the erythroblastic cytoplasm contains increasing amounts of hemoglobin and the nucleus undergoes progressive pyknosis until its final expulsion. This gives rise to the early, intermediate, and late normoblasts (still nucleated) and the mature erythrocyte (anuclear). In sections and in pathologic conditions special stains are helpful in identifying the various cell series (see the following discussion).

Because of its endocytic function, the bone marrow is an important part of the RES. The endothelial cells of the sinuses are the major cellular components responsible for the endocytic functions of the bone marrow.[46] In this respect they are similar to other endocytic endothelia such as those of the liver and lymphatic sinuses (see p. 1257). They are assisted by histiocytes and reticulum cells in the extravascular parenchyma.

Cytochemistry

Cytochemical studies are very useful in categorizing leukemic cells and in recognizing immature cells in smears and histologic sections.

The Leder or so-called specific esterase reaction using naphthol AS-D chloroacetate as a substrate is most useful in recognizing cells of the granulocytic series.[116] The esterase resides in azurophilic granules and therefore stains primarily promyelocytes and myelocytes. It also stains mature neutrophilic granulocytes, which contain a few azurophilic granules in addition to the neutrophilic granules. The Leder stain can be performed on paraffin-embedded histologic sections, provided EDTA is the decalcifying agent and a neutral fixative is used. Myeloblasts can be identified if there is some degree of maturation so that they are accompanied by promyelocytes. The Sudan black and peroxidase stains can also be used to identify the myelocytic series. They can be performed only on air-dried smears. Monocytic differentiation can be recognized by alpha-naphthyl acetate esterase positivity, which is inhibited by fluoride. An acid phosphatase stain can be used in smears. The immunoperoxidase technique allows staining of sections for muramidase and alpha-l-antichymotrypsin, which are useful markers for monocytes.[113] Leukemic red cells may exhibit granular or diffuse cytoplasmic staining with the periodic acid–Schiff stain. Glick and associates[76] have pointed out that granulocytic precursors reveal diffuse cytoplasmic periodic acid–Schiff positivity, whereas immature lymphoid cells show partial or block positivity.

Technical considerations

A complete evaluation of the bone marrow must include a study of smears and histologic sections. Satisfactory bone marrow sections can be obtained by aspiration[196] or by needle biopsy.[97] When using the aspiration technique, it is important to collect about 10 ml of marrow and eject it rapidly, before clotting, into a neutral buffered 10% formalin fixative. The formalin bone marrow mixture is then filtered to concentrate the particles. There is controversy as to whether the method of choice is aspiration or biopsy. Using standard techniques, that is, aspirating 10 ml of bone marrow and obtaining a 2 cm core with a regular adult Jamshidi needle, more marrow is obtained by aspiration than by biopsy.[93] Also, aspiration is superior to biopsy in the following ways:

1. Cytologic detail is sharper.
2. Giemsa and Leder stains are better.
3. Evaluation of hemosiderin is more accurate in aspirates because the leaching effect of an acid decalcifying solution is avoided. Also, decalcification with products containing hydrochloric acid may interfere with the demonstration of acid-fast organisms.[3]
4. Lymphoid nodules and granulomas are seen more frequently in aspirates than in biopsy specimens.
5. Obtaining marrow by aspiration yields material for sections and smears with a single procedure. If marrow is obtained by coring, the needle has to be replaced for aspiration so that a specimen can be secured for smears.
6. Aspiration can be performed in the sternum, which is not suitable for coring.
7. Aspiration can be done in the presence of thrombocytopenia.

On the other hand, a core biopsy must be obtained if aspiration results in a "dry tap." Furthermore, the core biopsy permits the recognition of paratrabecular location of lymphoid infiltrates, which may help to decide whether they are benign or malignant. Pathologic changes in bone can be evaluated only in core biopsy specimens.

Bone marrow examination is performed in the workup for anemia, leukopenia, and thrombocytopenia. It is also indicated in the workup for lymphoproliferative and myeloproliferative disorders, in the staging of malignant lymphoma and other malignant neoplasms, and in the follow-up of patients undergoing chemotherapy. Patients with hypercalcemia should have a core biopsy, since many of the conditions responsible for hypercalcemia can thus be diagnosed. These include Paget's disease, hyperparathyroidism, multiple myeloma, metastatic carcinoma, and sarcoidosis. The finding of granulomas and vascular lesions extends the indications for bone marrow biopsy to fever of unknown origin and the suspicion of vascular disease.

Necropsy

Bone marrow cells undergo degeneration soon after death. There is no relationship between rate of degeneration and age, sex, storage temperature, and mode of death, although some investigators believe that cellular damage is more rapid when death is the result of an infectious disease. Within the first 3 hours after death, the marrow cells are well preserved and can be identified easily in smears from aspirated material. After 3 hours there is progressive degeneration of the cells, the oldest cells such as mature granulocytes and mature normoblasts degenerating earlier than immature cells, lymphocytes, and plasma cells. After 15 or more hours from the time of death, cellular damage is so far advanced that aspirated material is practically worthless.

The degenerative change usually is called autolysis of the cells, but this may not be an accurate definition of what happens. For one thing, routine sections of paraffin-embedded marrow do not show much loss of cellular detail even when the tissue is obtained many hours after death. Also, it has been shown that if marrow is suspended in 5% bovine albumin and then smeared, the cells are well preserved and easily identifiable many hours after death. It would seem, then, that the postmortem change is not a true autolysis, which would be irreversible, but rather an increased fragility of the cytoplasm and possibly of the nucleus as well.

Relation to peripheral blood

The cellular population of the peripheral blood reflects the net of several effects: (1) rate of hemopoiesis in the bone marrow, (2) rate of release of cells from the bone marrow, and (3) rate of survival of cells in the peripheral blood. Hematologic diagnosis is based on making full use of all data that are pertinent to these basic mechanisms.

The hemopoietic activity of the bone marrow can be determined from the cellularity of the tissue sections and from the distribution of cells, according to type and degree of maturation. The rate of release of blood cells from the bone marrow into the peripheral blood is more difficult to establish. The presence of reticulocytes in normal number indicates normal release of erythrocytes. When the reticulocyte count is high, we can conclude that more young erythrocytes are being released than normal, and in this case the marrow shows hyperplasia of erythrocyte precursors. In special situations, such as the "aplastic crisis" of hemolytic anemia, the peripheral blood contains no reticulocytes, and we know that either the marrow maturation is arrested or no new cells are being released. It is not always possible to distinguish maturation arrest from lack of release. In pernicious anemia, for example, the marrow is hyperplastic, but the peripheral blood shows anemia and a low reticulocyte count. It can be shown that in this example the failure is partially in the release mechanism, for the marrow is full of reticulocytes that are not liberated into the blood. When vitamin B_{12} is given, one of the effects is to unblock the release mechanism and induce a shower of reticulocytes into the peripheral blood.

Finally, the rate of survival of erythrocytes can be established accurately by a variety of radioisotope methods; these also detect whether a decreased life span is attributable to an intrinsic defect in the erythrocytes or to extracorpuscular hemolytic mechanisms. Thus hemolytic disease is related to shortened life span of the erythrocytes and can be classified into two major categories, one related to intrinsic abnormality of the erythrocyte (hemoglobinopathy, enzyme deficiency, and so on) and the other to extracorpuscular factors (autoantibodies and so on). Life span of platelets is determined with only fair accuracy. Life span of leukocytes has so far defied an exact and direct definition.

Granulocytes are present in the peripheral blood in the circulation (circulating pool) and marginated to the blood vessel wall (marginated pool), where they are not included in the white blood cell count. Peripheral blood granulocyte counts do not necessarily correlate with the number of granulocytes in the bone marrow. Thus granulocytic hyperplasia of the bone marrow may be associated with normal, increased, or decreased numbers of granulocytes in the circulating pool. Peripheral blood leukocytosis may be present in the absence of granulocytic hyperplasia of the marrow. This "pseudoneutrophilia" is seen under stressful conditions when granulocytes are transferred from the marginated to the circulating pool.

Hypoplasia, aplasia, and hyperplasia

Bone marrow cellularity is evaluated by the relative amounts of hemopoietic and fat cells. The hemopoietic marrow is commonly referred to as cellular marrow. This term, although not quite correct because fatty marrow is also made up of cells, is generally accepted. Hartsock, Smith, and Petty[89] found a 79% cellularity during the first decade of life; it decreased to about 50% at 30 years of age and remained relatively constant until age 70, when the cellularity started to decline. It is important to evaluate overall cellularity of the bone marrow, since there may be considerable variation from area to area.

A marrow is hypoplastic (hypocellular) if the hematopoietic elements occupy less than 25% of the marrow. Almost complete disappearance of the marrow is termed aplasia of the marrow (Fig. 30-62). Only a few lymphocytes or reticulum cells are left. Hypoplasia or aplasia of the marrow may result from ionizing radiation, a variety of drugs and chemicals, and some infectious agents. Familial hypoplasia of the marrow with (Fanconi type) or without (Estren and Dameshek type) developmental anomalies may also be seen.

Hypoplasia can affect only one or two cell types, particularly when the offending agent is a myelotoxic drug. Such selective hypoplasia is reflected in the peripheral blood by a reduction of the corresponding circulating cells. Thus the peripheral blood may show leukopenia with neutropenia, thrombocytopenia, or anemia, or combinations of these. The term "aplastic anemia" refers specifically to the anemia resulting from bone marrow depression but is sometimes used loosely to refer to aplasia of the marrow and suppression of all cell types in the peripheral blood (pancytopenia). We know, however, that the pancytopenia in some cases is accompanied by

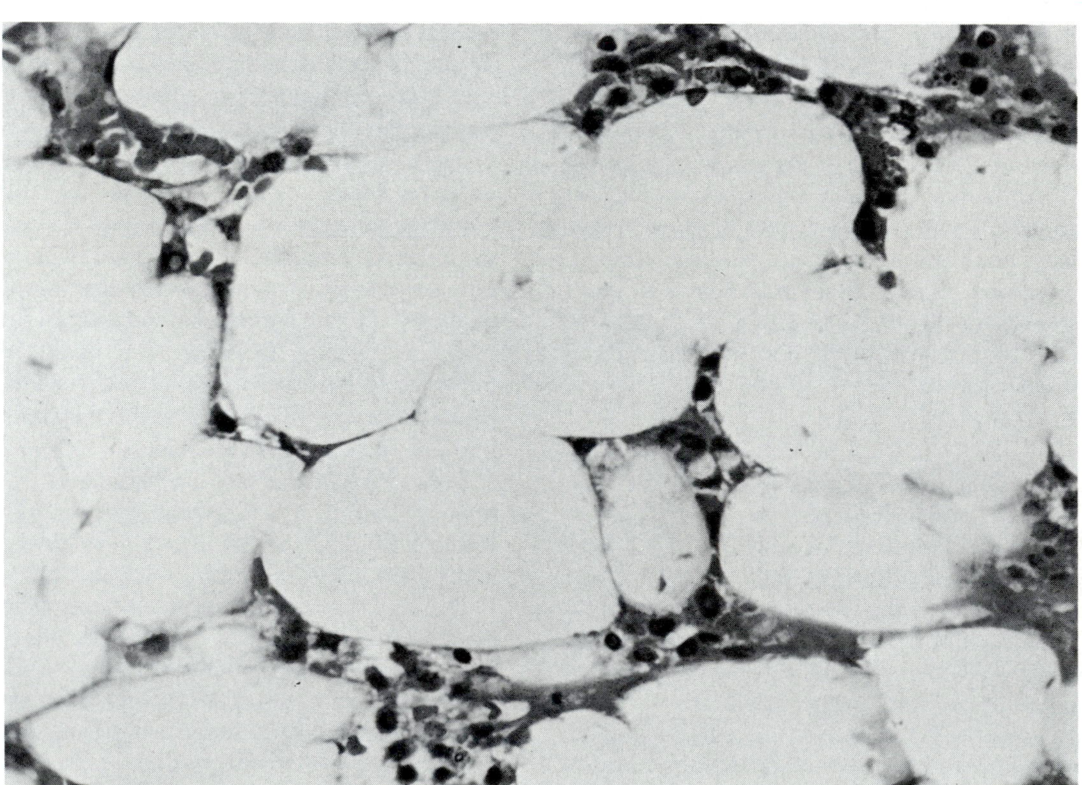

Fig. 30-62. Aplastic bone marrow caused by chloramphenicol. (Hematoxylin and eosin; 125×.)

hyperplasia of the bone marrow. This is why the term "aplastic anemia" has been replaced by "refractory anemia with hypocellular or hypercellular marrow." Refractory anemia may lead to leukemia or to progressive bone marrow failure.

Hyperplasia of the bone marrow may be selective or generalized. In most instances the hyperplasia is the result of a specific stimulation of one type of cell and is therefore selective. In most anemias, and particularly in hemolytic anemias, there is hyperplasia of erythroid cells to compensate for the anemia.

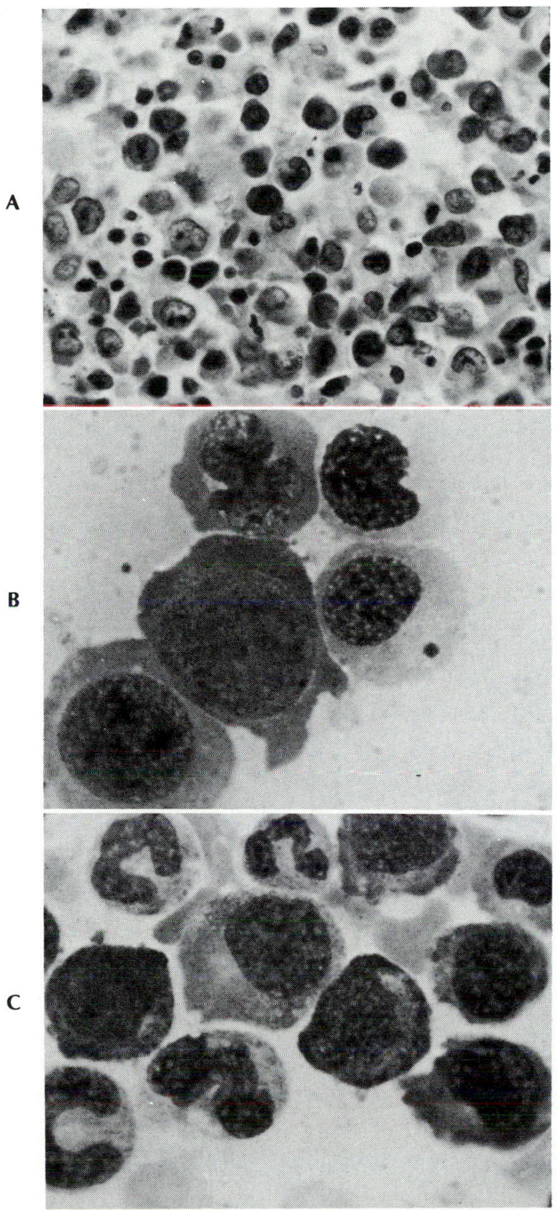

Fig. 30-63. Megaloblastic dyspoiesis in bone marrow. **A,** Paraffin section. **B,** Smear. All cells are megaloblasts. **C,** Smear. Note giant neutrophil metamyelocytes and stab cells. (**A,** Hematoxylin and eosin; 400×; **B** and **C,** Wright's stain; 950×.)

A special type of erythroid hyperplasia is seen in anemias caused by a deficiency of folic acid or vitamin B_{12}. Instead of the usual normoblastic maturation, there is a profound abnormality of maturation that affects all cell types, a dyspoiesis. The erythroid cells are large and atypical, resembling reticulum cells, and are called megaloblasts (Fig. 30-63, *A* and *B*). There is also abnormal maturation of granulocytes, and the metamyelocytes and bands are two or three times normal size (Fig. 30-63, *C*). Megakaryocytes are even more bizarre than usual. In infectious diseases characterized by leukocytosis, there is granulocytic hyperplasia. Hyperplasia of all cell types usually is seen in the myeloproliferative syndromes, although even in these, one series may be more hyperplastic than the others.

Leukemias

The leukemias are a malignant, neoplastic, systemic proliferation of hemopoietic cells, primarily in the bone marrow but with a tendency to involve the peripheral blood. They differ from other malignant neoplasms in that they are systemic; that is, they involve the bone marrow diffusely rather than in discrete tumors, and they often involve the peripheral blood. Tumor formation, medullary or extramedullary, may occur, either in the course of a leukemia or preceding it. These tumors are known as granulocytic sarcomas (myeloblastomas),[155] lymphoma (leukosarcomas), and monoblastic sarcomas.[169] Leukemias have been classified in different ways. Based on prognosis they may be divided into acute, subacute, and chronic. Based on the cell type involved they may be granulocytic, lymphocytic, or monocytic. Based on the maturity of the cell type, they may be blastic, made up of the pro- stages (promyelocytic, prolymphocytic), or of the mature cell types. Based on the number of leukemic cells released into the peripheral blood, leukemias may be subdivided into leukemic, aleukemic, and subleukemic types. In general, the acute leukemias are made up of immature cells, whereas in the chronic leukemias the cells are more mature.

Incidence

The incidence of leukemia has shown a steady increase during the past 40 years (Fig. 30-64). In the United States the mortality from leukemia rose from 3.9 per 100,000 in 1940 to 6.5 per 100,000 in 1954 and to 8 per 100,000 in 1964. In recent years a decline in the mortality of leukemia has been reported.[46a] Perhaps a portion of the increase in incidence can be ascribed to better diagnosis but, even when allowance is made for this and other factors, there remains what appears to be a true increase in incidence. There has been a proportionately greater increase in incidence in the older age groups. Only a small fraction of this can be attributed to greater longevity. The remarkable figures for improved longevi-

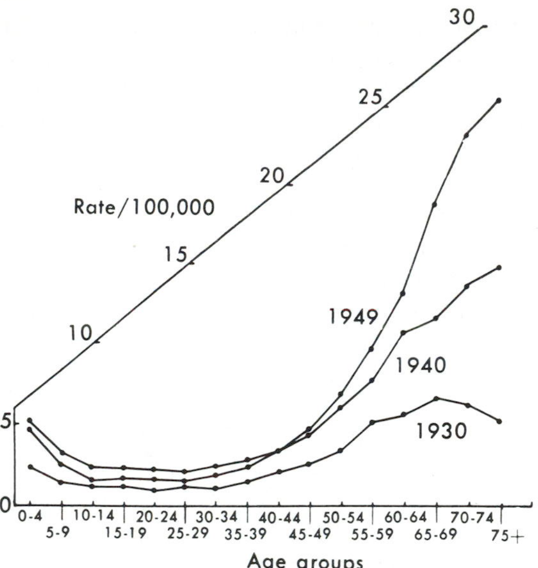

Fig. 30-64. Incidence of leukemia deaths by age in 1930, 1940, and 1949. (From Cooke, J.V.: Blood **9**:340, 1954; by permission.)

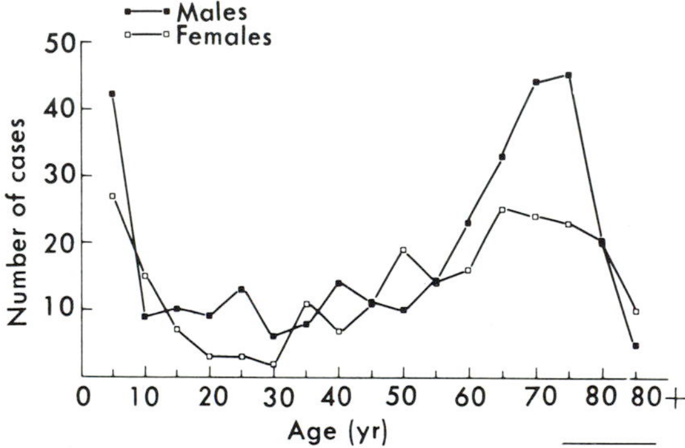

Fig. 30-65. Age and distribution of 553 cases of leukemia. (Data from Gunz, F.W., and Hough, R.F.: Blood **11**:882, 1956; from Miale, J.B.: Laboratory medicine—hematology, St. Louis, ed. 6, 1982, The C.V. Mosby Co.)

ty given by the biostatisticians reflect almost entirely improved neonatal and childhood survival, and the life expectancy for the middle-aged has improved only a little. In any case, if the incidence of all leukemias is plotted according to age (Fig. 30-65), two peaks are noted: one between the third and fourth year and one between the ages of 70 and 80 years. In the older age group the incidence in men is significantly higher than in women. In the younger age group, the incidence in white children is significantly greater than in black children (Fig. 30-66).

Although any type of leukemia can occur at any age, a consistent pattern is found in most large series. Acute leukemia is more common than chronic leukemia at all ages and is most frequent in children and in elderly per-

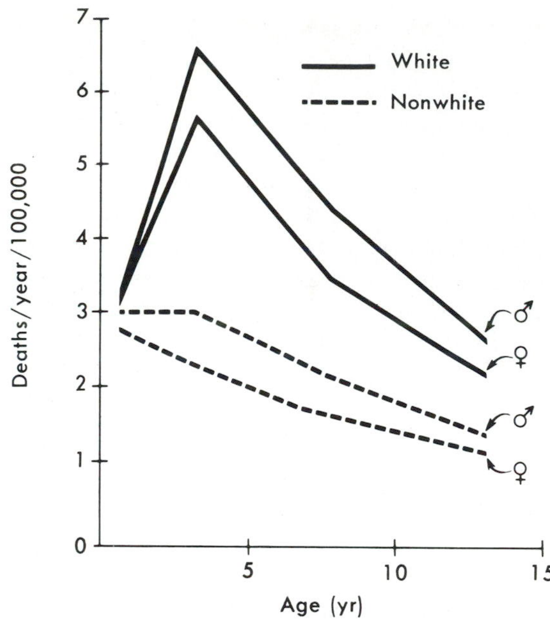

Fig. 30-66. Death rate from acute leukemia in white and black children, 1950-1959. (Data from Ederer, F., Miller, R.W., and Scotto, J.: J.A.M.A. **192**:593, 1965; from Miale, J.B.: Laboratory medicine—hematology, ed. 6, St. Louis, 1982, The C.V. Mosby Co.)

sons. Chronic myelocytic leukemia is rare in childhood, becoming increasingly more frequent in older age groups. Chronic lymphocytic leukemia is rare before the age of 35 years but is the most common type in elderly individuals. The overall distribution by type in the United States is as follows: chronic lymphocytic, 25%; chronic myelocytic, 22%; chronic myelomonocytic, 3%; acute lymphocytic, 20%; acute myelocytic, 20%; and acute myelomonocytic leukemia, 10%. Chronic lymphocytic leukemia is rare in China, Japan, and India. In children, almost all leukemias are acute lymphocytic (225 of 258 cases, with 13 acute myelocytic, 13 acute monocytic, four undifferentiated, and three chronic myelocytic leukemia).[141a]

Etiology and epidemiology

The etiology of leukemia is unknown. There are four partially overlapping approaches to the investigation of etiology: epidemiologic, the leukemogenic effect of ionizing radiation, the role of viruses, and the genetic (chromosomal) determinants.

Epidemiology. The epidemiology of leukemia shows some interesting but unexplained features. We know that there are some true differences in incidence among special groups:

1. The incidence in black children is lower than in whites and does not peak at 3 to 4 years of age.
2. The incidence of leukemia in Japan is about half of that in the United States, partly because of a lower

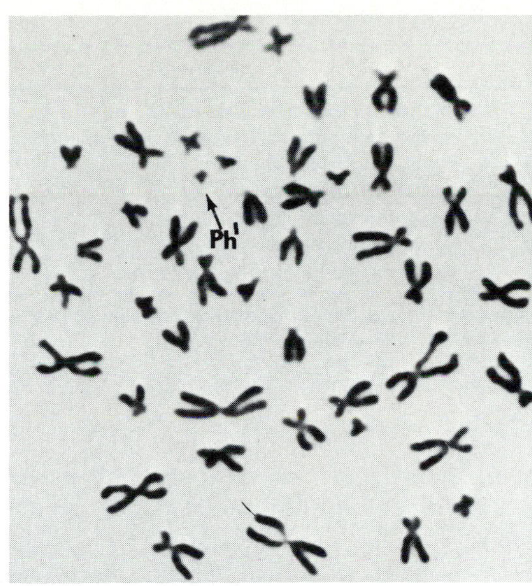

Fig. 30-67. Philadelphia chromosome *(Ph[1])*. Metaphase of diploid marrow cell in chronic myelocytic leukemia. (Courtesy Drs. Jacqueline Whang and J.H. Tjio, Bethesda, Md.)

incidence in middle-aged persons and partly because of the rarity of chronic lymphocytic leukemia in older Japanese.

3. African children have the lowest incidence of leukemia, even though the incidence of Burkitt's lymphoma is high.
4. There are occasional families with a high incidence of leukemia; it is noteworthy, however, that in these families the leukemia is sometimes of the same type (chronic lymphocytic) and sometimes of different types (the next most frequent association is chronic lymphocytic and chronic myelocytic leukemia).

Leukemogenic effect of ionizing radiation. There is no longer doubt that ionizing radiation is leukemogenic. Among survivors of the atomic explosion over Hiroshima, the first cases of leukemia appeared 18 months later and the peak incidence occurred 5 years later. The highest incidence was in those receiving the greatest dose of radiation. Of great interest is the finding that, in line with the low incidence of chronic lymphocytic leukemia in the Japanese, no case of chronic lymphocytic leukemia developed in the survivors. Therapeutic and diagnostic radiation also can be leukemogenic. The mechanism by which irradiation induces leukemia is not known.

Role of viruses. The induction by viruses of leukemia in fowls has been studied for over a half century. Gross[83] showed that mouse leukemia can be transmitted to newborn mice by cell-free filtrates. A viral etiology for human leukemia remains a likely possibility, but as yet no proof has been forthcoming. Direct transfusion of leukemic blood into normal recipients does not transmit leukemia. If a viral etiology is operative in human leukemia, one must suppose that there are other interacting factors such as genetic predisposition, ionizing radiation, and the latency of the virus until activated by intrinsic or extrinsic factors.

Chromosomal abnormalities. The association of chromosomal abnormalities with leukemia is well established. The most constant and characteristic change involves chromosome 21. In chronic myelocytic leukemia, a characteristic small chromosome, called the Philadelphia or Ph^1 chromosome (Fig. 30-67), is formed by deletion or translocation of portions of the normal 21 chromosome.

Some cases of chronic myelocytic leukemia without the Ph^1 chromosome also have been found. The high incidence of leukemia in children with Down's syndrome (17 times greater than in normal children) also suggests that abnormalities of chromosome 21 (children with Down's syndrome have trisomy 21) are related to the development of leukemia.

Acute myeloproliferative syndromes

The acute myeloproliferative syndromes encompass a spectrum of overlapping diseases, depending on the participation of the various cell series in the neoplastic process and on the presence of reticulin myelofibrosis (Table 30-7). The granulocytic, erythrocytic, megakaryocytic, and monocytic series share a common stem cell. A neoplastic proliferation may show no differentiation and may be made up of stem cells only. It may, however, show differentiation along granulocytic lines only or may also exhibit erythroid, megakarocytic, and monocytic features. It is perhaps best to view reticulin myelofibrosis as a reactive process that may or may not be present.

A group of French, American, and British hematologists has attempted to establish a classification of acute leukemias for use in the evaluation of different chemotherapeutic regimens.[18] Unfortunately, the authors used only smears and did not include such parameters as reticulin myelofibrosis or cellularity, which must be evaluated in histologic sections. Furthermore, no category for undifferentiated blastic leukemias is provided, even though it is well recognized that some leukemias do not show any differentiation even with cytochemical and ultrastructural studies. The French-American-British classification of acute leukemias categorizes the following myeloid forms.

M1: myeloblastic leukemia without maturation. Three percent or more of the blasts should be myeloperoxidase positive, and a varying proportion should contain at least a few azurophilic granules, Auer rods, or both.

M2: myeloblastic leukemia with maturation. The defining characteristic of this category is that maturation at or beyond the promyelocyte stage is present. The leukemic cells have varying amounts of cytoplasm, usually

Table 30-7. Spectrum of acute myeloproliferative disorders*

Granulocytes	Red cell series	Megakaryocytes	Reticulin myelofibrosis	Diagnosis
++++†	±	±	±	Acute myeloblastic leukemia or one of its variants
++++	±	±	+++	Acute myeloblastic leukemia with myelofibrosis
+++	+++	±	±	Acute erythroleukemia
+	++++	±	±	Acute erythemic myelosis
+	+	++++	±	Acute megakaryocytic myelosis
+++	+++	+++	±	Acute panmyelosis
+++	+++	+++	+++	Acute or malignant myelosclerosis

From Rywlin, A.M.: Bone marrow. In Silverberg, S.G., editor: Principles and practice of surgical pathology, New York, 1983, John Wiley & Sons, Inc.
*Other variants may occur. Thus, acute erythemic or megakaryocytic myelosis may be associated with reticulin myelofibrosis.
†Hyperplasia and/or atypia and/or shift to the left with presence of immature forms.

with many azurophilic granules. More than 50% of the bone marrow cells are myeloblasts and promyelocytes. Cells with Auer rods, almost always single, are common. In rare cases, almost all the myelocytes, metamyelocytes, and mature granulocytes are eosinophils. Erythroid hyperplasia may be present but does not show the atypia seen in erythemic myelosis or in erythroleukemia.

M3: hypergranular promyelocytic leukemia. The majority of the marrow cells are very heavily granulated atypical promyelocytes. The azurophilic granules are so dense that they obscure the cytoplasm. The nuclei vary in size and shape and may be reniform or bilobed. Cells containing bundles of Auer rods ("faggots") are almost invariably present in the bone marrow and sometimes in the peripheral blood.

M4: myelomonocytic leukemia. This form resembles M2 (myeloblastic leukemia with maturation), except that more than 20% of the nucleated marrow cells should belong to the monocytic series. Promonocytes and promyelocytes are not always readily distinguishable in Giemsa-Wright–stained smears. Special cytochemical reactions have to be used (p. 1326).

M5: monocytic leukemia. Two types are seen: poorly differentiated (monoblastic) and differentiated. In the poorly differentiated type the marrow exhibits large blasts with abundant basophilic cytoplasm and pseudopods. Rare azurophilic granules may be present. The nuclei have lacy chromatin and one to three prominent nucleoli. In the differentiated type the predominant cell in the bone marrow is the promonocyte, whereas monocytes predominate in the peripheral blood. The promonocyte has a less basophilic cytoplasm than the monoblast. The cytoplasm has a gray ground-glass appearance often with scattered azurophilic granules. Nucleoli may be present but are less frequent than in monoblasts. Less than 20% of the cells present should belong to the granulocytic series. Cytochemical methods are necessary to confirm the diagnosis.

M6: erythroleukemia. Fifty percent of the marrow cells should belong to the red cell series and should exhibit varying degrees of atypia. If the atypia is very severe, an erythropoietic component of 30% is adequate for the diagnosis of erythroleukemia. The granulocytic series must show an increased number of myeloblasts and promyelocytes. Abnormal megakaryocytes such as mononuclear forms or micromegakaryoblasts may be present.

• • •

Patients with an acute myeloproliferative syndrome have fever, pallor, and petechiae. The spleen may be enlarged, and bone pain may be elicited by pressure on the sternum. The peripheral blood shows anemia, thrombocytopenia, and varying elevations of the leukocyte count.

On histologic examination the bone marrow is usually markedly hypercellular, with almost complete disappearance of fat cells (Fig. 30-68). The megakaryocytic and red cell series are attenuated. The marrow is diffusely infiltrated with blasts. A naphthol AS-D chloroacetate esterase stain (p. 1326) reveals a sprinkling of promyelocytes and myelocytes. In erythroleukemia there is, in addition to the blasts, a hypercellular erythrocytic series, with varying degrees of atypia and megaloblastoid features and multinucleation. In acute panmyelosis (Table 30-7) the marrow exhibits the features of erythroleukemia, with an increased number of atypical megakaryocytes.

Acute or malignant myelosclerosis is a rapidly fatal disease with anemia, thrombocytopenia, and leukopenia.[15,127] The peripheral blood may show atypical nucleated red blood cells, immature granulocytes, abnormal platelets, and megakaryocytic nuclei. Bone marrow aspiration usually results in a dry tap. Core biopsy of the marrow shows panmyelosis with reticulin myelofibrosis. Some endosteal new bone formation may be present. As the disease progresses, the marrow may look more monotonous, resembling a blastic leukemia with reticulin myelofibrosis.

Chronic myeloproliferative syndromes

The chronic myeloproliferative syndromes include chronic granulocytic leukemia, polycythemia vera, and

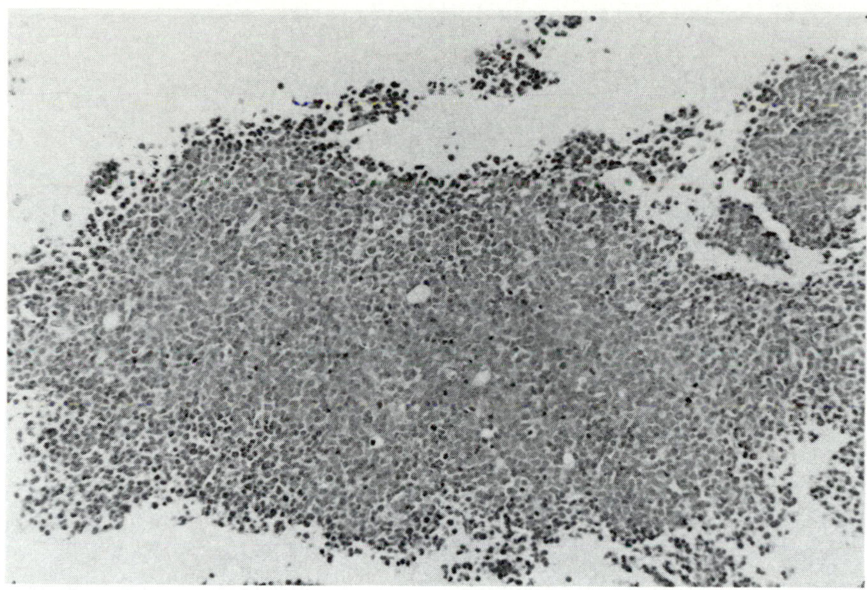

Fig. 30-68. Acute myelocytic leukemia. There is almost complete replacement of fat cells by leukemic cells. At periphery leukemic cells break away from particles. Note monotonous appearance of cells. (Hematoxylin and eosin; low power.)

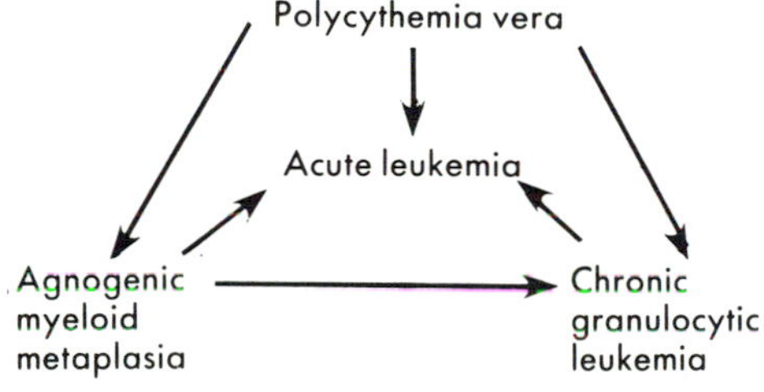

Fig. 30-69. Possible transitions between some myeloproliferative disorders.

agnogenic myeloid metaplasia. As in the acute myeloproliferative syndromes, there is a certain amount of overlap among these entities. Also, these conditions may develop a "blast crisis," which is essentially an acute blastic leukemia superimposed on the underlying disorder (Fig. 30-69).

Chronic granulocytic leukemia.

Chronic granulocytic leukemia (CGL) is found in all races and in both sexes and is primarily a disease of middle age. The onset of the disease is usually insidious; discomfort in the left upper quadrant seems to be the most frequent initial complaint. The peripheral blood shows varying degrees of a normochromic normocytic anemia, an increased number of platelets (which may reach 1 million/cu mm), and a leukocytosis commonly between 100,000 and 300,000/cu mm. There is an increased number of immature granulocytes, including a small percentage of myeloblasts and promyelocytes. Eosinophils and basophils are usually increased. The presence of a Philadelphia chromosome and a markedly decreased leukocyte alkaline phosphatase are helpful in confirming the diagnosis.

The bone marrow is markedly hypercellular. Megakaryocytes are increased in number and normal in appearance. The red cell series is attenuated. The granulocytic series is markedly hypercellular, with an increase in fully segmented polymorphonuclear leukocytes, myeloblasts, promyelocytes, and myelocytes (Fig. 30-70). Eosinophils and basophils are increased. The number of basophils can be evaluated only in smears.

The "blast crisis" complicating CGL may exhibit myeloid or, more rarely, lymphoid features.[170]

The spleen in CGL is enlarged and on cut section shows a uniform appearance. At times foci of necrosis (infarcts) are seen. The splenic parenchyma is pale red, the white pulp is inconspicuous, and the trabeculae are attenuated. On microscopic examination the red pulp is diffusely infiltrated with immature myeloid cells. Eosinophilic myelocytes are often prominent. A Leder stain (p. 1326) will confirm the myeloid nature of the infiltrating cells.

Polycythemia vera

Polycythemia vera (PV) occurs more often in men than in women and is more frequent in whites than in blacks. It is a disease of middle age and is rarely seen in children. The symptoms are insidious and are related to the increased red cell mass and the tendency to hemorrhage and thrombosis. The face often has a ruddy appearance and there may be a history of headaches and itching following a shower.

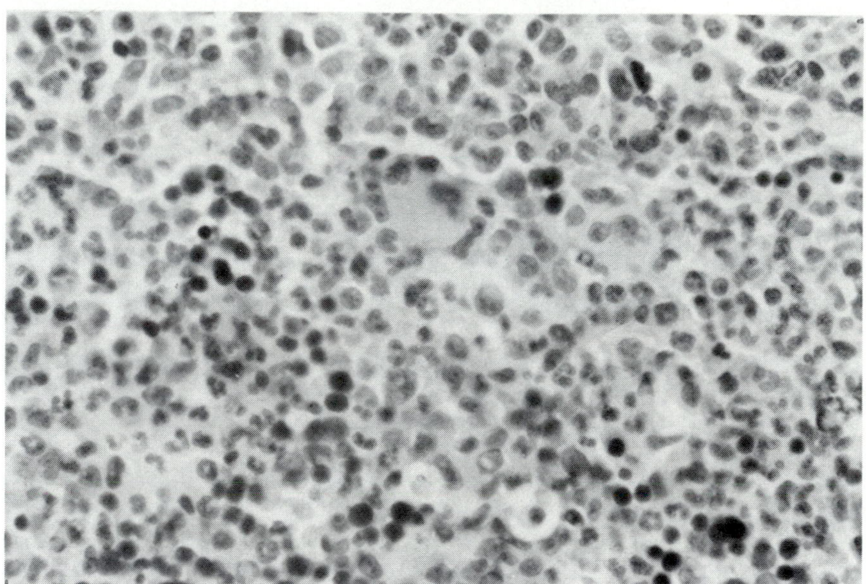

Fig. 30-70. Chronic granulocytic leukemia. Marrow is hypercellular, and no fat cells are seen. Megakaryocytes are increased and surrounded by many segmented polymorphonuclear leukocytes. (Hematoxylin and eosin; medium power.)

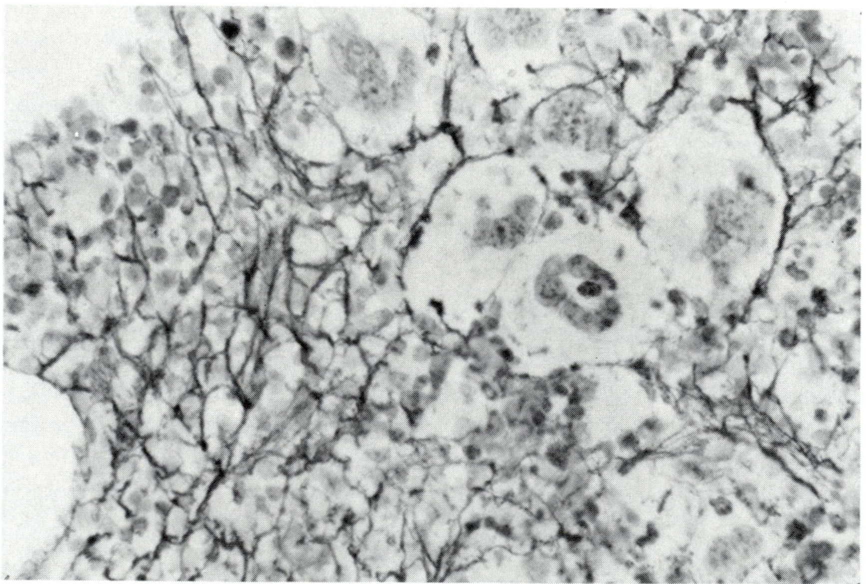

Fig. 30-71. Polycythemia vera. Note enlarged, atypical, and clustered megakaryocytes, some of which are surrounded by reticulin fibers. There is moderate reticulin myelofibrosis. (Gordon-Sweets reticulin stain; high power.)

The peripheral blood shows an elevated hemoglobin, hematocrit, and white cell and platelet count. The total red cell mass is increased, and the plasma volume may be normal or increased.

In the fully developed case the bone marrow is markedly hypercellular. Megakaryocytes are increased in number, clustered, and, in contrast to CGL, are enlarged and exhibit some atypia (Fig. 30-71). The red cell series is hypercellular. The hemosiderin stores are almost always depleted. The granulocytic series is also hypercellular and shows normal maturation. Eosinophils are often increased. Increased basophils can frequently be demonstrated in smears. In contrast to CGL, the reticulin framework of the marrow is increased, and, as in agnogenic myeloid metaplasia, the reticulin fibers ensheath individual megakaryocytes (Fig. 30-71). In secondary erythrocytosis the bone marrow contains considerably more fat, more hemosiderin, fewer megakaryocytes, and fewer eosinophils.

Few morphologic studies of the spleen in PV are available. It is enlarged, and sections show marked congestion of the red pulp. A few foci of extramedullary hematopoiesis may be seen. They are not diagnostic, since such foci may be seen in autopsies of patients without PV, particularly around infarcts. Foci of necrosis (infarcts) may be present.

Agnogenic myeloid metaplasia

Agnogenic myeloid metaplasia (AMM), also known as idiopathic or primary myelofibrosis, is a disease of middle age with an insidious onset. Weakness, fatigue, and upper abdominal discomfort caused by the enlargement of the spleen and liver are common initial symptoms. The spleen may be huge, extending into the pelvis.

The peripheral blood shows anemia with marked anisocytosis and poikilocytosis, tear-drop red cells, and nucleated red cells. The leukocyte count is usually elevated, and immature granulocytes are present. The platelet count may be normal, increased, or decreased. The platelets are often large.

Bone marrow aspiration is usually unsuccessful. Core biopsy of the marrow shows varying degrees of hypercellularity. The megakaryocytes are clustered, enlarged, and atypical. Their total number may be normal, increased, or decreased and varies from field to field. The red cell series shows normoblastic maturation and is attenuated. The hemosiderin stores may be normal, decreased, or increased, depending to some extent on the number of transfusions given to the patient. The granulocytic series shows normal maturation and may show hypocellularity or hypercellularity. There are extensive reticulin myelofibrosis and only mild collagen myelofibrosis. The reticulin fibers may ensheath megakaryocytes (Fig. 30-72). Dilated sinusoids may be prominent. Varying amounts of endosteal new bone formation are present. The variability of bone marrow histologic findings in AMM is related in part to the transition stages that exist between PV, CGL, AMM, and a "blast crisis" (Fig. 30-69). It has been recently postulated that the myelofibrosis is caused by a platelet-derived growth factor contained in the alpha granules of platelets.[166]

The spleen in agnogenic myeloid metaplasia is markedly enlarged and firm and often reveals areas of necrosis (infarcts). The cut surface is congested and of uniform appearance. The white pulp is attenuated. There is extensive extramedullary hemopoiesis with atypical megakaryocytes, nucleated red blood cells, and mature and immature granulocytic cells. The reticulin fibers are

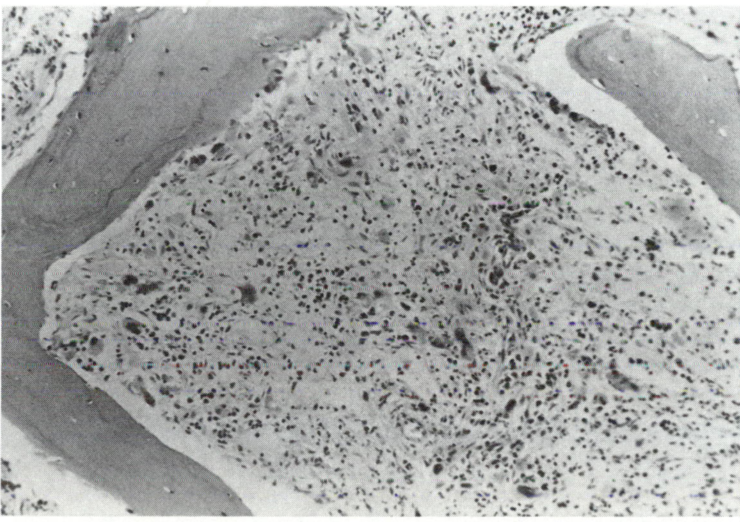

Fig. 30-72. Agnogenic myeloid metaplasia. There are increased atypical megakaryocytes and myelofibrosis. (Hematoxylin and eosin; high power.)

increased and thickened. The hemosiderin stores are increased. In addition, there may be fibrocongestive splenomegaly related to the hepatic fibrosis that may be seen in agnogenic myeloid metaplasia.

In this disease tumors made up of hemopoietic tissue may appear in the mediastinum and other extramedullary sites. Occasionally they may be very fibrotic, mimicking a fibrosarcoma or Hodgkin's disease. Megakaryocytes are strongly periodic acid–Schiff positive, whereas Reed-Sternberg cells are periodic acid–Schiff negative or weakly positive. With the Giemsa stain the nucleoli of Reed-Sternberg cells are very prominent and nucleoli of megakaryocytes are inconspicuous. Also, a Leder stain reveals some granulocytic precursors in these fibrous tumors, differentiating them from Hodgkin's disease, fibrous histiocytomas, and fibrosarcomas.

Lymphoproliferative disorders

Normal lymphoid nodules

Normal lymphoid nodules in the bone marrow have been reported in 1% to 62% of patients.[203] The incidence of lymphoid nodules increases with advancing age. Lymphoid nodules in the bone marrow can be divided into lymphoid follicles and lymphoid infiltrates.[203] Lymphoid follicles occur far more frequently than lymphoid infiltrates. They resemble the malpighian follicles of the spleen. Lymphoid infiltrates are irregular in shape, usually display preserved fat cells, and are composed of loosely arranged lymphocytes. Germinal centers are not seen in lymphoid infiltrates.

Nodular lymphoid hyperplasia

Nodular lymphoid hyperplasia (NLH) has been defined arbitrarily as the presence of four or more normal lymphoid nodules in any low-power field (eyepiece 10×, objective 4×). Another criterion for NLH is the presence of any lymphoid nodule exceeding 0.6 mm in greatest dimension.[203] NLH is more frequent in older patients and in women. Its clinical significance is unknown. It is important not to misdiagnose NLH as malignant lymphoma or the nodular type of bone marrow involvement seen in chronic lymphocytic leukemia.

Acute lymphocytic leukemia

Acute lymphocytic leukemia (ALL) is more common in children. Its clinical manifestations are similar to those of other acute leukemias. The bone marrow is hypercellular and the megakaryocytic, red cell, and granulocytic series are markedly attenuated. Mature granulocytes are rare. A Giemsa stain reveals the blastic appearance of the cells and the naphthol-ASD chloroacetate stain (Leder) shows sparse granulocytic precursors at the periphery of the infiltrates rather than intermingled with the blasts.

The French-American-British cooperative group has distinguished three types of ALL.[18] In LI the leukemic cells are relatively small, up to twice the diameter of the normal small lymphocyte. There is little cellular heterogeneity. The nuclear chromatin is finely dispersed and nucleoli are small. The cytoplasm is scanty. In LII the leukemic cells display considerable variation in size. Nuclear clefting and folding are characteristic. Nucleoli vary in size and number and are often large. The cytoplasm is abundant and often markedly basophilic. In LIII the leukemic cells are homogeneous and resemble those of Burkitt's lymphoma. The nucleus is oval to round, the chromatin is finely stippled, and one or more nucleoli are present. The cytoplasm is intensely basophilic and cytoplasmic vacuoles may be prominent.

B lymphocyte markers have been found in most cases of LIII, and T lymphocyte markers are present in about 25% of the non-LIII leukemias. LI is the common acute childhood leukemia.

Prolymphocytic leukemia

In prolymphocytic leukemia there is usually massive splenomegaly with absent or minimal peripheral lymphadenopathy and marked elevation of the peripheral blood lymphocyte count.[14] The leukemic cells are intermediate in size between small lymphocytes and blasts, and they exhibit a single prominent nucleolus. The bone marrow may show a nodular or diffuse infiltration.

Chronic lymphocytic leukemia

The onset of chronic lymphocytic leukemia (CLL) is insidious, and often the diagnosis is made in asymptomatic patients having a persistent peripheral blood lymphocytosis. At times the patient seeks medical advice because of enlarged peripheral lymph nodes. Physical examination usually reveals more or less symmetric enlargement of superficial lymph nodes and moderate splenomegaly. The peripheral blood shows an increased number of small lymphocytes and smudge cells and usually moderate anemia with normal or decreased platelets.

Four distinct patterns of bone marrow involvement can be seen in CLL: diffuse, interstitial, nodular, and mixed. In the diffuse type there is extensive replacement of hemopoietic and fat cells by sheets of small lymphocytes (Fig. 30-73). In the interstitial type of bone marrow involvement there is preservation of fat cells. The lymphocytes are located in the spaces among the fat cells, where they replace the normal hemopoietic elements. In the nodular type the lymphocytes are aggregated into nodular collections separated by normal marrow. In contrast to nodular lymphoid hyperplasia, the nodules vary considerably in size and shape. They are asymmetric, exhibit a tendency to confluence, and contain an increased number of intermediate lymphocytes and blasts. In the mixed type of marrow involvement there are combinations of diffuse, interstitial, and nodular pat-

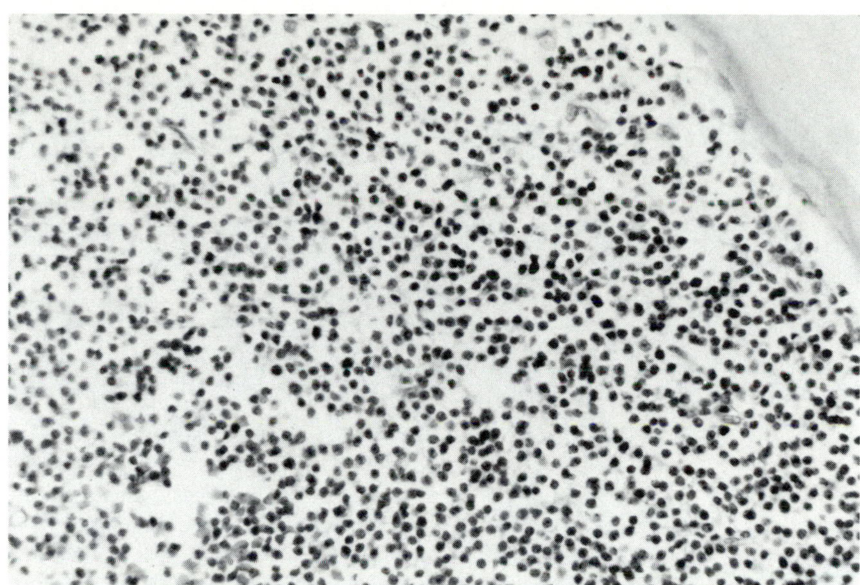

Fig. 30-73. Chronic lymphocytic leukemia, diffuse type of infiltrate. Note replacement of fat and hemopoietic cells by monotonous infiltrate of small lymphocytes. (Hematoxylin and eosin; medium power.)

terns. The diffuse and mixed types are seen most frequently. The diffuse pattern has the worst prognosis.[125]

At times the bone marrow shows the nodular pattern of CLL without any peripheral blood lymphocytosis. At autopsy the lymphoid infiltration may be limited to the bone marrow or may also involve lymph nodes, liver, and spleen. I have referred to such cases as aleukemic CLL.

The histologic appearance of the lymph nodes in CLL is similar to malignant lymphoma, diffuse, small cell type. In CLL, in contrast to small cell malignant lymphoma, the lymph node involvement is more symmetric and more generalized, usually without the presence of a dominant mass. Also, in CLL the liver involvement is microscopic without formation of grossly visible tumor nodules.

The spleen in CLL is enlarged and appears paler than normal on cut section. No grossly visible tumor nodules are seen. Microscopically the white pulp is enlarged. Small lymphocytes infiltrate both the white and red pulp, so that their normal sharp separation is obscured.

Richter's syndrome is the development of a large cell lymphoma in patients with CLL.[66,186] The clinical findings at the onset of Richter's syndrome include an abrupt deterioration of the clinical course with fever, asymmetric lymphadenopathy with the formation of tumor masses, and hepatosplenomegaly. The bone marrow shows, in addition to the CLL, nodules and sheets of malignant lymphoma composed of large lymphoid cells.

Proliferative disorders of plasma cells

In the normal bone marrow, plasma cells surround small blood vessels in a single layer. In reactive plasmacytosis the perivascular cuff may be several layers thick. Plasma cells are also seen at the edge of lymphoid nodules and at times mixed with other hemopoietic cells. In normal bone marrow it is unusual to find clumps containing more than four or five plasma cells. Between 2% to 3% is accepted as the upper normal limit of plasma cells in bone marrow smears. Plasma cells may contain round, cytoplasmic, eosinophilic inclusions called Russell bodies. Occasionally plasma cells contain eosinophilic, periodic acid–Schiff–positive, intranuclear inclusions referred to as Dutcher bodies. Angular, eosinophilic, periodic acid–Schiff–positive inclusions separated from each other by strands of compressed chromatin have also been described (Fig. 30-74).[204] These as well as the Dutcher bodies probably represent intranuclear cytoplasmic protrusions. Dutcher bodies and the angular inclusions are most frequently seen in monoclonal macroglobulinemia. They can also be found in polyclonal macroglobulinemia, in myelomas, and in malignant lymphomas associated with monoclonal gammopathies.

Bone marrow plasmacytosis is usually seen in diseases associated with hypergammaglobulinemia. Plasma cells are also increased in primary amyloidosis and in diseases characterized by the proliferation of histiocytes, such as Gaucher's disease or ceroid (sea-blue) histiocytosis. The increase in plasma cells in some histiocytic proliferations may be related to their tendency, even in normal bone marrow, to cluster around a histiocyte, a phenomenon

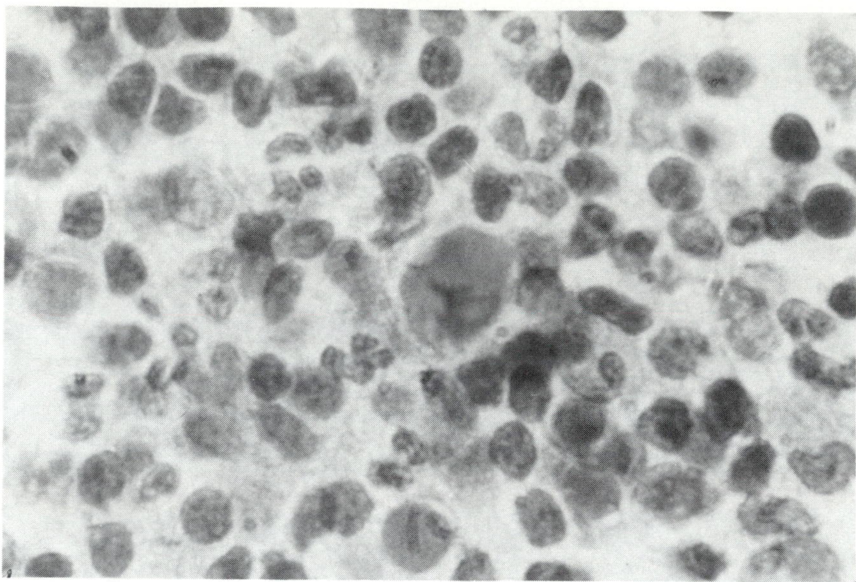

Fig. 30-74. Periodic acid–Schiff–positive intracytoplasmic inclusions compressing nuclear chromatin. (Periodic acid–Schiff, oil immersion.)

called plasmacytic satellitosis.[92] In hypogammaglobulinemia or agammaglobulinemia plasma cells may be absent from the bone marrow.

Multiple myeloma

Neoplastic proliferation of plasma cells initially appears as an extraskeletal plasmacytoma, as a solitary plasmacytoma of bone, or as multiple myeloma with a multifocal or diffuse replacement of normal hemopoietic and fatty marrow by neoplastic plasma cells. Transitions occur between solitary skeletal and extraosseous plasmacytomas and multiple myeloma. Multiple myeloma may show a terminal leukemic phase, plasma cell leukemia. Bone destruction is the usual manifestation of multiple myeloma. As a rule, it occurs in the form of osteolytic, punched-out lesions or diffuse osteopenia. Rarely, multiple myeloma may be associated with osteosclerosis.[192] In the uncommon, disseminated nonosteolytic myelomatosis, immature plasma cells infiltrate the marrow without causing any masses or osteolysis.[9]

Patients with multiple myeloma complain of bone pain and may have pathologic fractures. They are often anemic. Numerical abnormalities of the white cells and platelets are less common. Multiple myeloma is frequently diagnosed in asymptomatic patients who are found to have a monoclonal gammopathy in the serum (Fig. 30-75). Light chains (Bence Jones proteins) of the kappa or lambda type may be present in the urine. The monoclonal gammopathy is caused by the secretion by the neoplastic cells of an increased amount of one of the immunoglobulins, usually IgG or IgA. Rare IgD myelomas and even more unusual IgE myelomas have been described.[80,223] At times myeloma cells may produce an IgM monoclonal gammopathy or may secrete kappa or lambda chains only (light-chain myeloma). In the rare, nonsecretory myeloma there is no detectable monoclonal gammopathy.

The hyperglobulinemia is responsible for the rouleaux formation of red blood cells observed in the peripheral blood smear. The rouleaux formation causes a rapid sedimentation rate. The monoclonal immunoglobulin may exhibit properties of a cryoglobulin or pyroglobulin. The cryoglobulins, which are cold-precipitable proteins, may give rise to symptoms of cold sensitivity including Raynaud's phenomenon, circulatory impairment, and, at times, necrosis of fingers and toes. When the level of the immunoglobulin is very high, a hyperviscosity syndrome may result from impaired circulation in the brain and retina. This syndrome is more frequent in monoclonal macroglobulinemia because of the larger size of the immunoglobulin.

The diagnosis of multiple myeloma is established by the demonstration of a neoplastic proliferation of plasma cells in the bone marrow (Figs. 30-76 and 30-77). In early cases of myeloma or when the bone marrow aspiration or biopsy does not come from a fully developed lesion, the differential diagnosis between a neoplastic and an inflammatory proliferation of plasma cells may be difficult. The distinction can be made more accurately in histologic sections than in smears of bone marrow.[34] Criteria important in smears include a plasmacytosis exceeding 20% and cytologic features of malignancy such as large nucleoli (Fig. 30-77). Immunoperoxidase studies showing that the plasma cells are monoclonal, that is, that they secrete either kappa or lambda chains but not both, appear useful in difficult cases. Histologically the most helpful criterion in the diagnosis of neoplastic plasmacytosis is the presence of "solid" (absence of fat cells) collections of plasma cells (Fig. 30-76). At times a neoplastic plasma cell infiltrate may exhibit an interstitial pattern with preservation of fat cells but with replacement of hemopoietic cells. In some instances the plasma cells may be undifferentiated, resembling a large cell lymphoma. Careful attention to cytologic detail reveals evidence of plasmacellular differentiation. Rarely, solid collections of plasma cells may be associated with numerous lymphocytes, or irregular, fairly massive lymphoid infiltrates may be admixed with plasma cells. These cases are best diagnosed as malignant lymphoma with plasmacellular differentiation. The term *lymphoplasmacytic myeloma* has also been used for such entities.[230]

Since amyloidosis is a complication of multiple myeloma, amyloid deposits should be looked for in the bone marrow. They appear as homogeneous, eosinophilic deposits that, when stained with Congo red, exhibit dichroism, show metachromasia with crystal violet, and fluoresce when stained with thioflavine. At times the amyloid deposits may exhibit only some of the tinctorial characteristics of amyloid. Amyloid deposits may incite a foreign body granulomatous reaction. Amyloid deposits should not be confused with serous atrophy of fat or other hyaline deposits such as hyalinized collagen, immunoglobulin, or fibrin. Hyalinized collagen deposits may be seen in sarcoidosis or in Hodgkin's disease. In primary amyloidosis the bone marrow shows an increased number of plasma cells or, more rarely, lymphoid aggregates admixed with plasma cells. Occasionally it may be difficult to decide whether these cellular infiltrates represent a well-differentiated, nonosteolytic myeloma or lymphoma with plasmacellular differentiation, or a benign plasma cell or lymphoplasmacellular infiltrate.

At autopsy the gross appearance of the skeletal lesions in multiple myeloma varies considerably.[9] Most frequently the red marrow and to some extent the yellow marrow are replaced by confluent, poorly delineated, gelatinous, tan tumor nodules, seldom exceeding 1 cm in diameter. There is considerable bone destruction; collapsed vertebrae with compression of the spinal cord may be present. The appearance of discrete multiple plasmacytomas of the skeleton with normal-looking intervening bone marrow is uncommon. There is considerable overlapping between diffuse myelomatosis and the discrete plasmacytomas.[9]

Extramedullary plasmacellular infiltrates, seen frequently at autopsy, involve primarily the lymph nodes, spleen, and liver. Other organs, soft tissues, and skin may be involved. Visceral and cutaneous involvement seems to be relatively more frequent in light-chain and IgD myeloma.[80]

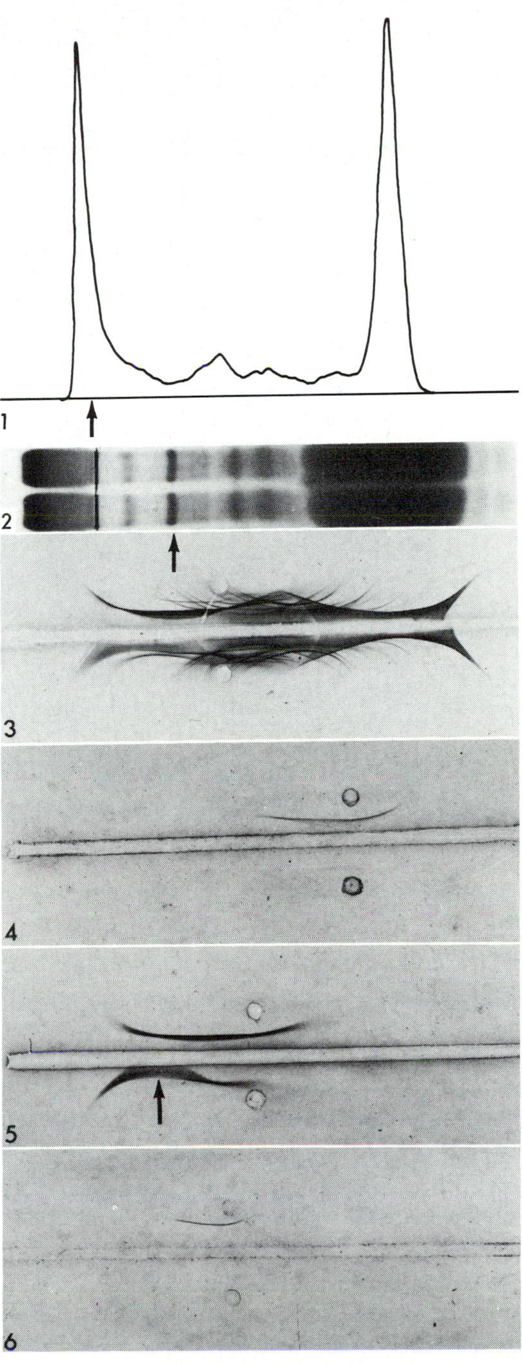

Fig. 30-75. Multiple myeloma. **1,** Electrophoretic pattern showing abnormal gamma peak *(arrow)*. **2,** Starch gel electrophoresis showing abnormal gamma band *(arrow)*. **3** to **6,** Immunoelectrophoresis: control subject *(top);* patient *(bottom)*. **3,** Polyvalent antiserum showing abnormal gamma components. **4,** Anti-IgA serum showing reduction of IgA. **5,** Anti-IgG serum showing abnormal and increased IgG component *(arrow)*. **6,** Anti-IgM serum showing decreased IgM. (From Miale, J.B.: Laboratory medicine—hematology, ed. 6, St. Louis 1982, The C.V. Mosby Co.)

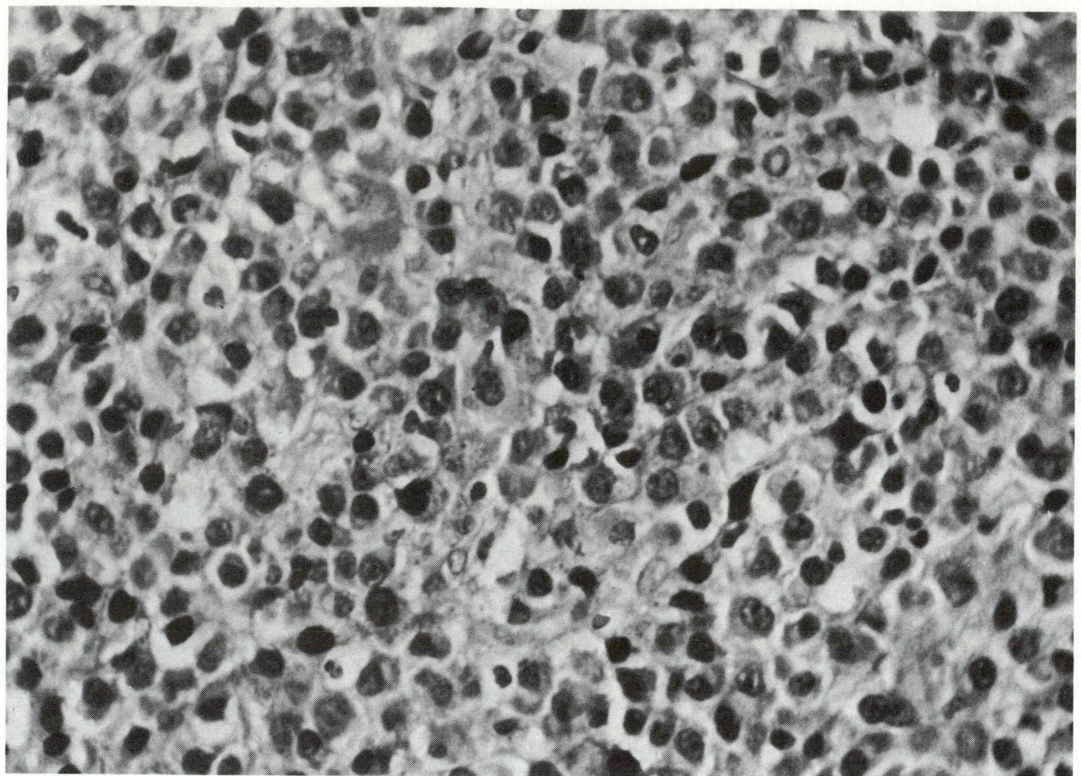

Fig. 30-76. Bone marrow in multiple myeloma. (Hematoxylin and eosin; 250×.)

Amyloid deposition may be extensive at autopsy and may involve the carpal tunnel, synovium, peripheral nerves, nerve roots, skeletal muscle, tongue, and heart. The distribution of amyloid is similar to that in primary amyloidosis. The deposits of amyloid may be associated with varying degrees of plasmacellular infiltration.

Renal dysfunction is frequently seen in patients with myeloma. Tubular casts surrounded by giant cells have been implicated in "myeloma kidney." At times extensive nephrocalcinosis is seen. Massive infiltration of the kidneys with plasma cells can also be seen, particularly in light-chain or IgD myeloma.

Benign monoclonal gammopathy

Benign monoclonal gammopathies are not associated with a demonstrable lymphoproliferative disorder or with myeloma. Laboratory data suggesting a benign monoclonal gammopathy include a mild elevation of the monoclonal immunoglobulin that does not increase significantly with the passage of time. In addition, there is no decrease in the levels of the other immunoglobulins, the serum albumin is normal, and in most cases there are no light chains in the urine. The bone marrow in such cases is normal or contains a moderately increased number of plasma cells. Solid collections of plasma cells are not present.

Monoclonal macroglobulinemia

Monoclonal macroglobulinemia may appear as a benign monoclonal gammopathy uncovered by immunoelectrophoresis. It is also seen in such entities as cold agglutinin disease, various lymphoproliferative disorders of the bone marrow including chronic lymphocytic leukemia, various types of nodal and extranodal malignant lymphomas, at times in association with carcinomas, and rarely with multiple myeloma.[207] As a rule, patients with lymphoproliferative disorders have higher levels of macroglobulins and may have symptoms of a hyperviscosity syndrome. The term *Waldenström's macroglobulinemia* has been applied to such instances.

The hyperviscosity syndrome includes circulatory impairment in the central nervous system with changing patterns of neurologic signs and symptoms such as transient paresis, deafness, and impairment of consciousness. The retina shows congested veins and hemorrhages, which may result in visual impairment. The bleeding diathesis in patients with macroglobulinemia may be the result of the formation of complexes between the macroglobulin and some coagulation factors. Interference with platelet function because of coating with IgM[136] and capillary damage resulting from increased viscosity are further contributing factors to the bleeding diathesis. Patients with macroglobulinemia may exhibit cryoglobu-

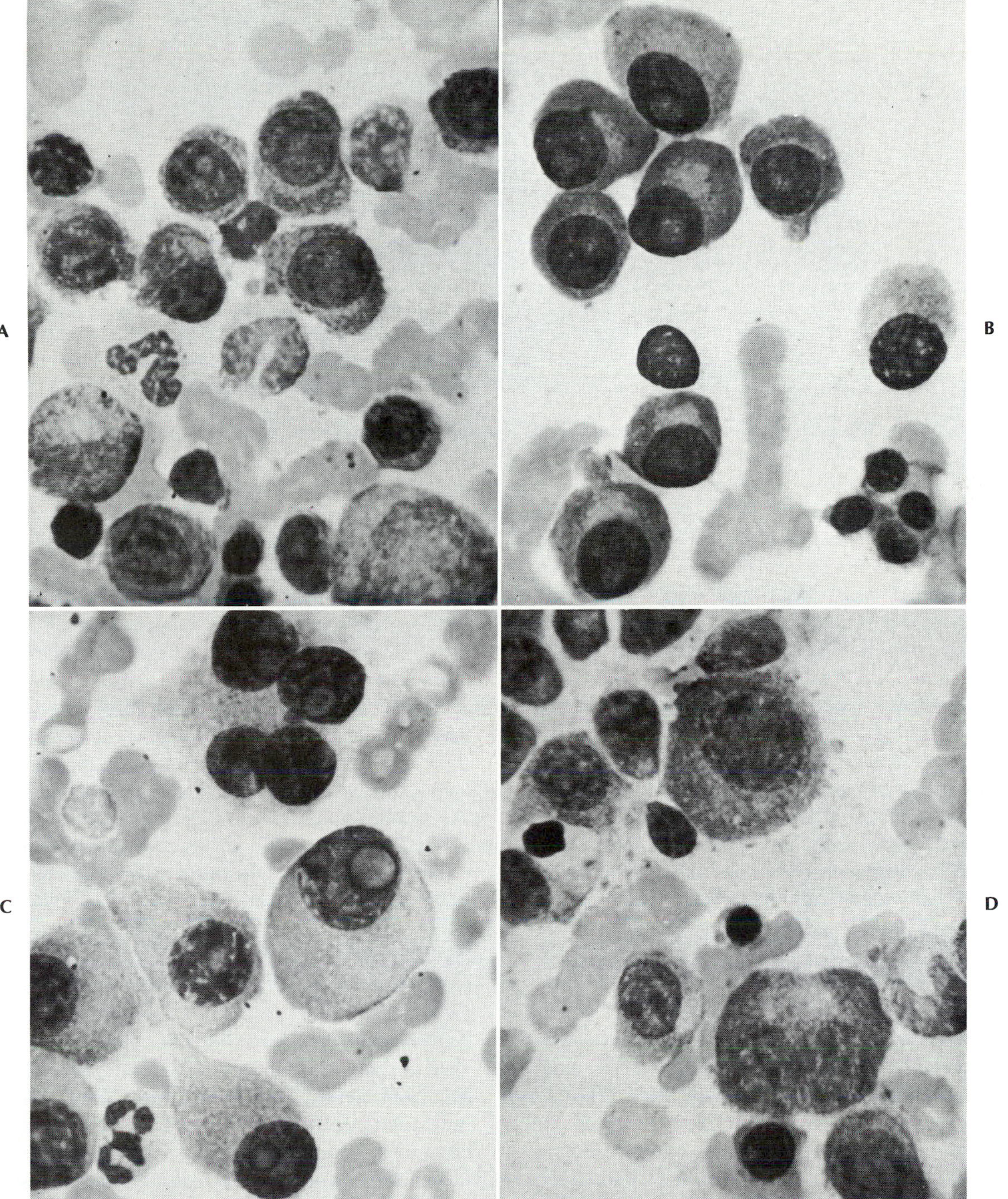

Fig. 30-77. Different degrees of maturity of plasma cells in multiple myeloma. Bone marrow smears from most mature **A,** to least mature, **D.** (Wright's stain; 950×; from Miale, J.B.: Laboratory medicine—hematology, ed. 6, St. Louis, 1982, The C.V. Mosby Co.)

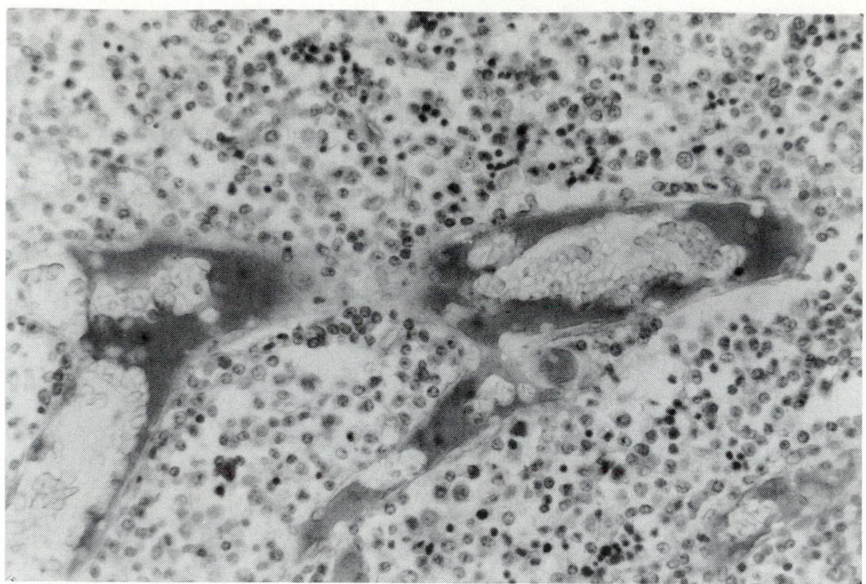

Fig. 30-78. Macroglobulinemia. Periodic acid–Schiff–positive intravascular plasma. (Periodic acid–Schiff; medium power.)

linema, amyloidosis, a susceptibility to infections, and neuropathy. Renal impairment appears less frequently than in myeloma.

The bone marrow findings in monoclonal macroglobulinemia are variable. Normal lymphoid nodules, nodular lymphoid hyperplasia, malignant lymphomas of different types, chronic lymphocytic leukemia, and rarely multiple myeloma may all be seen.[207] Morphologic features suggesting macroglobulinemia include plasmacytoid lymphocytes, Dutcher bodies and their variants (Fig. 30-74), periodic acid–Schiff–positive material in blood vessel walls and in lymphoid collections, as well as periodic acid–Schiff–positive intravascular plasma and extravascular lakelike and linear deposits (Fig. 30-78).

Proliferative disorders of mast cells

Mast cells may have different morphologic appearances. Most frequently, they have round to oval nuclei with an abundant, faintly granular cytoplasm. At times the nucleus is elongated and the cytoplasm is indistinct so that the cell resembles a fibroblast. Occasionally degranulated mast cells may be mistaken for histiocytes. The specific mast cell granules can be easily demonstrated with different special stains including Giemsa, chloroacetate esterase (Leder stain), toluidine blue, and Bismark brown. The distribution of mast cells varies from aspirated particle to particle. In general, mast cells are more abundant around blood vessels, sinusoids, and lymphoid nodules. In cored bone marrow biopsy specimens, mast cells are more numerous in the proximity of bone trabeculae. In bone marrow smears mast cells are most abundant in thick areas of crushed particles. The number of mast cells can be evaluated better in histologic sections than in smears of bone marrow.[99] Johnstone[99] found no mast cells in 30%, a few mast cells in 60%, and abundant mast cells in 10% of patients. Mast cells are increased in the marrow in the proliferative disorders of mast cells, some refractory anemias, lymphoproliferative disorders with macroglobulinemia, in some cases of osteoporosis,[67] and in uremic patients on dialysis,[163] Mast cell degranulation is associated with the release of the eosinophilic chemotactic factor of anaphylaxis,[105] which explains the frequent association of eosinophils with mast cell infiltrates.

Systemic mastocytosis

Mastocytoma and urticaria pigmentosa refer to unifocal and multifocal proliferations of dermal mast cells. The proliferation of mast cells may remain confined to the skin or may evolve into a systemic mastocytosis with involvement of liver, spleen, lymph nodes, and bone marrow. Systemic mastocytosis may rarely occur without cutaneous manifestations.[81] A leukemic picture may occur in systemic mastocytosis.[55] Systemic mastocytosis may be associated with flushing, urticaria, edema, pruritus, headache, tachycardia, and hypotension, presumably related to the release of histamine by the proliferating mast cells. The bone marrow in systemic mastocytosis shows sheets of mast cells replacing hemopoietic and fat cells. This replacement of hemopoietic elements may be responsible for the cytopenias observed in the peripheral blood. There may be an increased number of eosin-

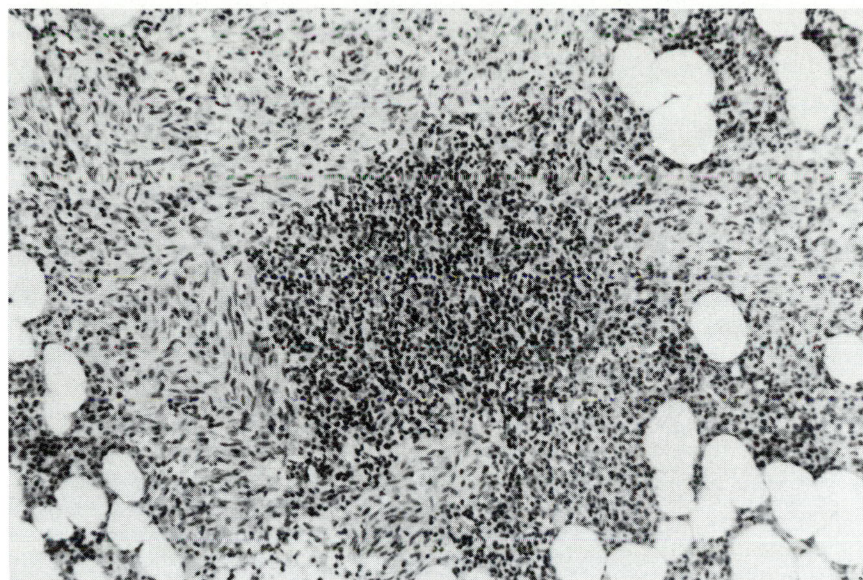

Fig. 30-79. Mastocytic eosinophilic fibrohistiocytic lesion. Lymphoid follicle is surrounded by mast cells characterized by regular, small, elongated nuclei. Eosinophils cannot be recognized at this magnification. (Hematoxylin and eosin; medium power.)

ophils in the bone marrow, sometimes associated with marked eosinophilia of the peripheral blood.[255] The bone marrow may also exhibit varying degrees of reticulin myelofibrosis. Osteosclerosis, resorption of bone, or a combination of both may be present. Mast cells may be partially or markedly degranulated and may be mistaken for histiocytes, myelocytes, or the cells of hairy cell leukemia.

Mastocytic eosinophilic fibrohistiocytic lesion[200]

In the mastocytic eosinophilic fibrohistiocytic lesion (MEFHL) the lesions consist of focal collections of cells characterized by regular, oval to spindle-shaped nuclei with an indistinct cytoplasm. Morphologically these cells have features of both fibroblasts and histiocytes.[200] Their mastocytic nature was recognized by de Velde and associates.[241] The lesions resemble granulomas and have been called mast cell granulomas.[60] These lesions are associated with an increased number of eosinophils, sometimes forming eosinophilic abscesses.[200] The lesions occur in four locations: (1) associated with lymphoid follicles (Fig. 30-79), (2) around blood vessels, (3) capping sinusoids, and (4) adjacent to bony trabeculae.

It appears that the MEFHL is distinct from systemic mastocytosis both clinically and histologically. Clinically, cutaneous manifestations and hepatosplenomegaly are less frequent. Signs and symptoms of hyperhistaminemia are absent or less striking than in the usual form of systemic mastocytosis. The most consistent clinical finding seems to be osteopenia.

Histologically the lesions are localized and do not replace the marrow extensively. The cells resemble fibrohistiocytes and are often degranulated. It may well be that the MEFHL represents the relatively benign end of the spectrum of mastocytic proliferations.

Stromal reactions

Serous (gelatinous) atrophy of fat

Serous or gelatinous atrophy of bone marrow is seen in cachectic patients. The fat cells become smaller, and the hemopoietic marrow between the fat cells is replaced by a faintly eosinophilic material made up of plasma, fibrin, and acid mucopolysaccharides.[2] With more advanced serous atrophy, the single fat vacuole seen in normal fat cells not only becomes smaller but breaks up into several smaller vacuoles.

Necrosis of bone marrow

Necrosis of the bone marrow may be seen in septicemia, in neoplastic diseases treated with chemotherapy or irradiation, and in sickle cell disease. Massive bone marrow necrosis may result in bone marrow and fat emboli, hypercalcemia, and peripheral blood cytopenias.[110] Small foci of bone marrow necrosis are seen in anergic miliary tuberculosis. Unless an acid-fast stain is employed, the diagnosis of tuberculosis may be missed.

In foci of bone marrow necrosis, the fatty and hemopoietic marrow is replaced by granular, eosinophilic debris. Marrow necrosis may be associated with hemorrhage. Fat necrosis of marrow is identical to that seen in other adipose tissues.

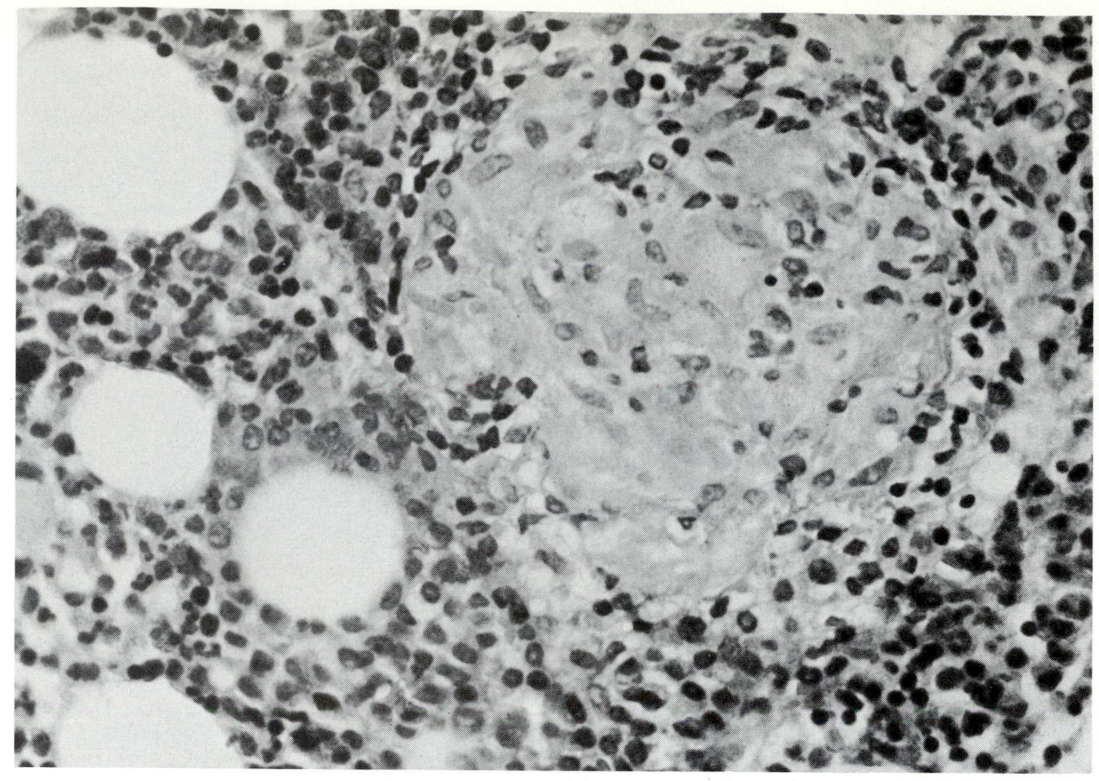

Fig. 30-80. Sarcoid granuloma in bone marrow. (Hematoxylin and eosin; 250×.)

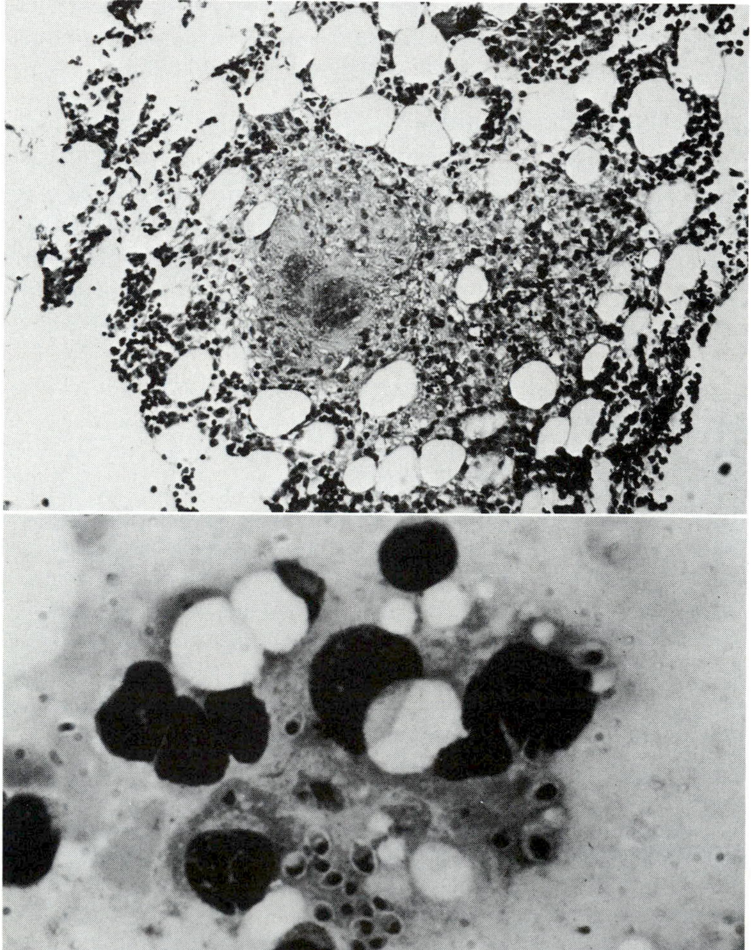

Fig. 30-81. Bone marrow in miliary tuberculosis. (Hematoxylin and eosin; 120x.)

Fig. 30-82. Bone marrow in histoplasmosis. Smear. (Wright's stain; 950x.)

Inflammation of bone marrow

Foci of acute myelitis are recognized by the exudation of fibrin associated with polymorphonuclear leukocytes. If the exudation of fibrin is not accompanied by polymorphonuclear leukocytes, the lesion is called fibrinous myelitis. It is seen in patients receiving chemotherapy or radiotherapy. Fibrinous myelitis is much richer in fibrin than serous atrophy of fat. In nonspecific chronic myelitis the normal marrow elements are replaced by a fibrinous exudate containing plasma cells and lymphocytes in addition to a few polymorphonuclear leukocytes.

Granulomas are frequently found in the bone marrow. The most commonly seen granuloma is the lipid granuloma.[200] It is identical to lipid granulomas found in the liver, spleen, and lymph nodes. Many lipid granulomas are rich in hemosiderin, and a few contain a finely granular, black pigment identical to anthracotic pigment. As the lipid granulomas age, they become sarcoidlike and may contain asteroid bodies. It is important to recognize this sarcoidlike appearance of some lipid granulomas to avoid making an unjustified diagnosis of sarcoidosis.

Sarcoidosis and miliary tuberculosis can be diagnosed from biopsies of bone marrow (Figs. 30-80 and 30-81). Burkhardt[31] claims that in sarcoidosis the marrow is involved more frequently than the liver. The bone marrow is often involved in lepromatous leprosy.[214] Even when histiocytes containing globi of *Mycobacterium leprae* are not seen, the Fite stain often reveals acid-fast organisms in histiocytes and endothelial cells and lying free in the tissue.

Nonspecific granulomas are found in typhoid fever, brucellosis, infectious mononucleosis, viral hepatitis, and Q fever, in which "doughnut-type" granulomas have been described.[161]

Specific granulomas are seen in the bone marrow in fungal diseases such as cryptococcosis and histoplasmosis (Fig. 30-82). The bone marrow may be prominently involved in leishmaniasis.

Granulomatous lesions may be seen in the bone marrow in drug reactions,[191] in Hodgkin's disease, and in the non-Hodgkin's lymphomas.[256]

Myelofibrosis

The term "myelofibrosis" is used by some hematologists as a synonym for agnogenic myeloid metaplasia. This is unfortunate because myelofibrosis means fibrosis of the marrow and can be seen in many different conditions. Fibrosis of the marrow can be seen in bone diseases such as osteitis fibrosa and Paget's disease. It can also be seen in a variety of hemopoietic disorders including myeloproliferative disorders, hairy cell leukemia, and systemic mastocytosis. Various inflammatory disorders of bone and marrow may also exhibit fibrosis of the marrow.

Myelofibrosis may be divided into reticulin and collagen types.[196] Reticulin myelofibrosis may precede but does not necessarily evolve into collagen myelofibrosis. The myelofibrosis associated with hemopoietic disorders is usually of the reticulin type, whereas the myelofibrosis seen with metastatic carcinoma is of the collagen type. Myelofibrosis may be associated with the formation of new endosteal or metaplastic bone. It may also be associated with resorption of bone.

Vascular lesions

Cholesterol emboli can be easily recognized in bone marrow specimens (Fig. 30-83). Widespread cholesterol

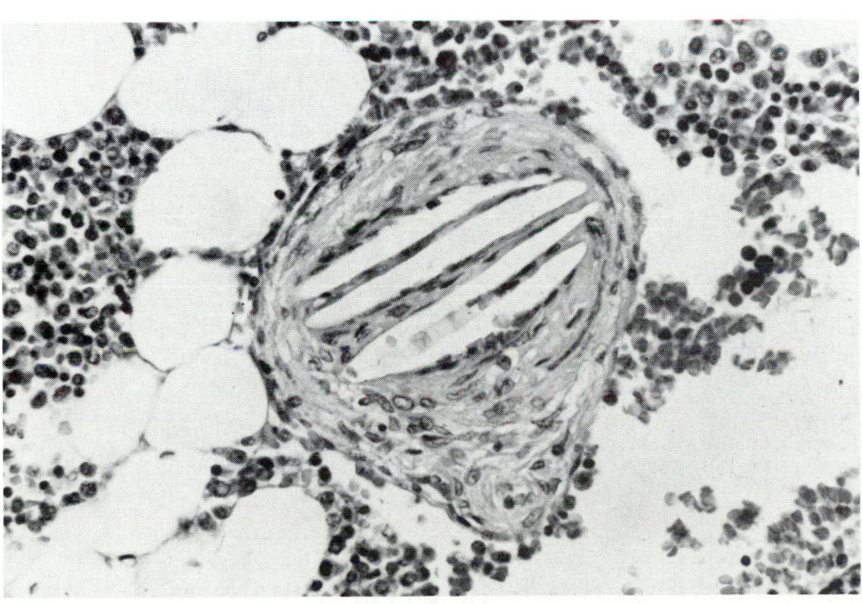

Fig. 30-83. Bone marrow. Arteriole contains cholesterol embolus. (Hematoxylin and eosin; medium power.)

emboli may appear clinically as a multisystem illness with neurologic and retinal changes, ischemic toes, renal failure, anemia, and eosinophilia.[171] Cholesterol emboli may be an incidental finding, indicating that the patient has ulcerating arteriosclerosis.

Characteristic vascular lesions in the marrow can be seen in the various types of polyarteritis, and hyaline thrombi are seen in thrombotic thrombocytopenic purpura.

Metastatic tumors

The incidence of metastases to the bone marrow in a study of autopsies of patients with carcinoma was found to be 34.5% by routine autopsy technique.[231] Examination of the marrow in patients with carcinoma by techniques used in living patients reveals metastatic tumor in nearly 10% of patients.[231] In one series, bone marrow metastases were most frequent in neuroblastoma (48.2%), followed by Ewing's sarcoma (35.5%), oat cell carcinoma of the lung (20.7%), prostate carcinoma (20.3%), breast carcinoma (19.6%), squamous cell carcinoma of the lung (15.7%), rhabdomyosarcoma (16.2%), and melanoma (6.8%).[4]

The marrow surrounding metastatic tumor deposits may be normocellular, hypercellular, or hypocellular. The hypercellularity may involve megakaryocytes, red cells, or granulocytes. At times only megakaryocytes will be increased; a marked increase in eosinophils or plasma cells may also be noted. In some instances there may be extensive collagen myelofibrosis with or without the formation of metaplastic bone. Endosteal new bone formation is frequently seen. Resorption of bony trabeculae may lead to osteopenia. The pathogenic factors determining formation or resorption of bone are not well understood.

In the presence of bone marrow metastases the peripheral blood may be normal or abnormal; when abnormal, hemoglobin may be decreased, and platelets and white cells may be increased or decreased. Occasionally there is marked eosinophilia. The presence of immature granulocytes and nucleated red blood cells—the classic leukoerythroblastic picture—is relatively rare.[196]

REFERENCES

1. Aisenberg, A.C.: Value of immunologic testing, J.A.M.A. **22**:1301, 1972.
2. Amrein, P.C., et al.: Hematologic changes in anorexia nervosa, J.A.M.A. **241**:2190, 1979.
3. Anderson, G., and Coup, A.J.: Effect of decalcifying agents on the staining of mycobacterium tuberculosis, J. Clin. Pathol. **28**:744, 1975.
4. Anner, R.M., and Drewinko, B.: Frequency and significance of bone marrow involvement by metastatic solid tumors, Cancer **39**:1337, 1977.
5. Arseneau, J.E., et al.: American Burkitt's lymphoma: a clinicopathologic study of 30 cases. I. Clinical factors relating to prolonged survival, Am. J. Med. **58**:314, 1975.
6. Aschoff, L.: Das Reticulo-endotheliale System, Ergeb. Inn. Med. Kinderheilkd. **26**:1, 1924.
7. Aschoff, L., and Kiyono: Zur Frage der Grossen Monouklearen, Folia Haematol. (Leipz.) **15**:385, 1913.
8. Askanazy, M.: Knochenmark. In Henke, F., and Lubarsch, O., editors: Handbuch der speziellen pathologischen Anatomie und Histologie, vol. I, Berlin, 1927, Julius Springer Verlag.
9. Azar, H.A., and Potter, M.: Multiple myeloma and related disorders, vol. I, New York, 1973, Harper & Row, Publishers, Inc.
10. Baehr, G., and Klemperer, P.: Giant follicle lymphoblastoma: benign variety of lymphosarcoma, N.Y. State J. Med. **40**:7, 1940.
11. Banks, P.M., et al.: American Burkitt's lymphoma: a clinicopathologic study of 30 cases. II. Pathologic correlations, Am. J. Med. **58**:322, 1975.
12. Barcos, M.P., and Lukes, R.J.: Malignant lymphoma of convoluted lymphocytes: a new entity of possible T-cell type. In Sinks, L.F., and Godden, J.O., editors: Conflicts in childhood cancer, New York, 1975, Alan R. Liss.
13. Barrow, M.V., and Holubat, K.: Multicentric reticulohistiocytosis: a review of 33 patients, Medicine **48**:287, 1969.
14. Bearman, R.M., Pangalis, G.A., and Rappaport, H.: Prolymphocytic leukemia, Cancer **42**:2360, 1978.
15. Bearman, R.M., Pangalis, G.A., and Rappaport, H.: Acute (malignant) myelosclerosis, Cancer **43**:279, 1979.
16. Benisch, B.M., and Howard, R.G.: Lymph node infarction in two young men, Am. J. Clin. Pathol. **64**:818, 1975.
17. Bennett, M.H., et al.: Classifications of non-Hodgkin's lymphomas, Lancet **2**:405, 1974.
18. Bennett, T.M., et al.: Proposals for the classification of acute leukemias, Br. J. Haematol. **33**:451, 1976.
19. Berard, C., et al.: Histopathological definition of Burkitt's tumour, Bull. WHO **40**:601, 1969.
20. Berard, C.W., et al.: A multidisciplinary approach to non-Hodgkin's lymphomas, Ann. Intern. Med. **94**:218, 1981.
21. Bernhard, W., and Leplus, R.: Fine structure of the normal and malignant human lymph nodes, New York, 1964, The Macmillan Co.
22. Blaustein, A.: The spleen, New York, 1963, McGraw-Hill Book Co.
23. Brady, R.O., and King, F.M.: Gaucher's disease. In Hers, H.G., and Van Hoof, F., editors: Lysosomes and storage diseases, New York, 1973, Academic Press, Inc.
24. Brady, R.O., et al.: Demonstration of a deficiency of glucocerebroside-cleaving enzyme in Gaucher's disease, J. Clin. Invest. **45**:1112, 1966.
25. Brewster, D.C.: Splenosis: report of two cases and review of the literature, Am. J. Surg. **126**:14, 1973.
26. Brill, N.E., Baehr, G., and Rosenthal, N.: Generalized giant lymph follicle hyperplasia of lymph nodes and spleen, J.A.M.A. **84**:668, 1925.
27. Brown, C.H.: Bone marrow necrosis: a study of seventy cases, Johns Hopkins Med. J. **131**:189, 1972.
28. Brunning, R.D., and McKenna, R.W.: Bone marrow manifestations of malignant lymphoma-like conditions, Pathol. Annu. **14**:1, 1979.
29. Burke, J.S.: The value of the bone marrow biopsy in the diagnosis of hairy cell leukemia, Am. J. Clin. Pathol. **70**:876, 1978.
30. Burke, J.S., Byrne, G.E., Jr., and Rappaport, H.: Hairy cell leukemia (leukemic reticuloendotheliosis). I. A clinical pathologic study of 21 patients, Cancer **33**:1399, 1974.
31. Burkhardt, R.: Farbatlas der Klinischen Histopathologie von Knochenmark und Knochen, Berlin, 1970, Springer-Verlag.
32. Burkitt, D.: A sarcoma involving the jaws of African children, Br. J. Surg. **46**:218, 1958.
33. Byrne, G.E., Jr., and Rappaport, H.: Malignant histiocytosis. In Akazaki, K., et al., editors: Malignant disease of the hematopoietic system, Gann Monogr. Cancer Res., no. 15, 1973, University of Tokyo Press.
34. Canale, D.D., and Collins, R.D.: Use of bone marrow particle sections in the diagnosis of multiple myeloma, Am. J. Clin. Pathol. **61**:382, 1974.

35. Carbone, P.P., et al.: Report of the Committee on Hodgkin's Disease Staging Classification, Cancer Res. **31**:1860, 1971.
36. Catovsky, D., et al.: The B-lymphocyte nature of the hairy cell leukaemic reticuloendotheliosis, Br. J. Haematol. **26**:29, 1974.
37. Clark, B.S., and Dawson, P.J.: Histiocytic medullary reticulosis presenting with a leukemic blood picture, Am. J. Med. **47**:314, 1969.
38. Cline, M.J.: Monocytes and macrophages: functions and diseases, Ann. Intern. Med. **88**:78, 1978.
39. Coller, B.S., Chabner, B.A., and Gralnick, H.R.: Frequencies and patterns of bone marrow involvement in non-Hodgkin's lymphomas: observations on the value of bilateral biopsies, Am. J. Hematol. **3**:105, 1977.
40. Cook, J.V.: The occurrence of leukemia, Blood **9**:340, 1954.
41. Coolidge, A., et al.: Zoonotic brugia filariasis in New England, Ann. Intern. Med. **90**:341, 1979.
42. Daily, M.O., Coleman, C.N., and Fajardo, L.F.: Splenic injury caused by therapeutic irradiation, Am. J. Surg. Pathol. **5**:325, 1981.
43. Davey, F.R., et al.: Immunological studies in hairy cell leukemia, Arch. Pathol. Lab. Med. **103**:433, 1979.
44. Davies, D.J., and Stansfeld, A.G.: Spontaneous infarction of superficial lymph nodes, J. Clin. Pathol. **25**:689, 1972.
45. Davies, J.N.P., and Lothe, F.: Kaposi's sarcoma in African children. In Ackerman, L.V., and Murray, J.F., editors: Symposium on Kaposi's sarcoma, Basel, 1963, S. Karger.
46. DeBruyn, P.P.H.: Structural substrates of bone marrow function, Semin. Hematol. **18**:179, 1981.
46a. Devessa, S.S., and Silverman, D.T.: Cancer incidence and mortality trends in the United States, J. Natl. Cancer Inst. **60**:545, 1978.
47. Diebold, J., and Temmim, L.: Etude anatomopathologique des prelevements effectures au cours de 250 laparotomies exploratrices pour maladie de Hodgkin, Ann. Anat. Pathol. **4**:341, 1980.
48. Dorfman, R.F.: Classification of non-Hodgkin's lymphomas, Lancet **1**:1295, 1974.
49. Dorfman, R.F., and Remington, J.S.: Value of lymph node biopsy in the diagnosis of acute acquired toxoplasmosis, N. Engl. J. Med. **289**:878, 1973.
49a. Dorfman, R.F., and Turner, R.R.: Letter, Am. J. Surg. Pathol. **8**:79, 1984.
50. Dorfman, R.F., and Warnke, R.: Lymphadenopathy simulating the malignant lymphoma, Hum. Pathol. **5**:519, 1974.
51. Duhamel, G.: Lymphoid myelofibrosis: about 10 further observations, Acta Haematol. **45**:89, 1971.
52. Duhamel, G., Najman, A., and Andre, R.: Les localisations a la moelle osseuse de la maladie de Hodgkin, La Presse Medicale **79**:2305, 1971.
53. Edelson, R.L., et al.: Identification of subpopulations of mononuclear cells in cutaneous infiltrates. I. Differentiation between B cells, T cells, and histiocytes, J. Invest. Dermatol. **61**:82, 1973.
54. Ederer, F., Miller, R.W., and Scotto, J.: U.S. childhood cancer mortality patterns, 1950-1959, J.A.M.A. **192**:593, 1965.
55. Efrati, P., Klajman, A., and Spitz, H.: Mast cell leukemia? Malignant mastocytosis with leukemia-like manifestations, Blood **2**:869, 1957.
56. Ellis, R.E.: The distribution of active bone marrow in the adult, Phys. Med. Biol. **5**:255, 1961.
57. Ellman, L.L., and Block, K.J.: Heavy-chain disease: report of a seventh case, N. Engl. J. Med. **278**:1195, 1968.
58. Estevez, J.M., Ureuta, E.E., and Moran, T.J.: Acute megakaryocytic myelofibrosis, Am. J. Clin. Pathol. **62**:52, 1974.
59. Evans, H.L., Butler, J.J., and Youness, E.L.: Malignant lymphoma, small lymphocytic type, Cancer **41**:1440, 1978.
60. Fallon, M.D., Whyte, M.P., and Teitelbaum, S.L.: Systemic mastocytosis associated with generalized osteopenia: histopathological characterization of the skeletal lesion using undecalcified bone from two patients, Hum. Pathol. **12**:813, 1981.
61. Farguhar, J.W., et al.: Familial haemophagocytic reticulosis, Br. Med. J. **2**:1561, 1958.
62. Fayemi, A.O., and Toker, C.: Nodal angiomatosis, Arch. Pathol. **99**:170, 1975.
64. Flandrin, G., et al.: Ilot erythroblastique anormal du au developement de jonctions intercellulaires (synartese erythroblastique) un noveau mecanisme d'anemia problemes posés par le diagnostique, Nouv. Rev. Fr. Hematol. **13**:609, 1973.
63. Flandrin, G., and Ripault, J.: Histio-lymphocytose medullaire et splenique de l'adulte: etude de 19 cases, actualités hematologiques, ser. 3, Paris, 1969, Masson & Cie.
65. Forte, F.A., et al.: Heavy chain disease of the μ (γ M) type: report of the first case, Blood **36**:137, 1970.
66. Foucar, K., and Rydell, R.E.: Richter's syndrome in chronic lymphocytic leukemia, Cancer **46**:118, 1980.
67. Frame, B., and Nixon, R.K.: Bone marrow mast cells in osteoporosis of aging, N. Engl. J. Med. **279**:626, 1968.
68. Frangione, B., and Franklin, E.C.: Heavy chain diseases: clinical features and molecular significance of the disordered immunoglobulin structure, Semin. Hematol. **10**:53, 1973.
69. Fredrickson, D.S., and Sloan, H.R.: Sphingomyelin lipidoses: Neimann-Pick disease. In Stanbury, J.B., Wyngaarden, J.B., and Fredrickson, D.S., editors: The metabolic basis of inherited disease, ed. 3, New York, 1972, McGraw-Hill Book Co.
70. Frizzera, G., Moran, E.M., and Rappaport, H.: Angio-immunoblastic lymphadenopathy with dysproteinaemia, Lancet **1**:1070, 1974.
71. Frizzera, G., et al.: Multicentric lymphoproliferative disorder with the morphologic features of Castleman's disease: a clinicopathologic study of ten patients, Lab. Invest. **42**:22, 1980.
72. Gaba, A.R., et al.: Multicentric giant lymph node hyperplasia, Am. J. Clin. Pathol. **69**:86, 1978.
73. Gall, E.A.: The cytological identity and interrelation of mesenchymal cells of lymphoid tissue, Ann. N.Y. Acad. Sci. **73**:120, 1958.
74. Garvin, D.F., and King, F.M.: Cysts and nonlymphomatous tumors of the spleen. In Sommers, S.C. and Rosen, P.P., editors: Pathology annual, New York, 1981, Appleton-Century-Crofts.
75. Gerard-Marchant, R., et al.: Classification of non-Hodgkin's lymphomas, Lancet **2**:406, 1974.
76. Glick, A.D., et al.: Acute leukemia of adults: ultrastructural, cytochemical and histologic observation in 100 cases, Am. J. Clin. Pathol. **73**:459, 1980.
77. Goedert, J.J., et al.: Polyarteritis nodosa, hairy cell leukemia and splenosos, Am. J. Med. **71**:323, 1981.
78. Gold, K.D., et al.: Relationship between multicentric reticulohistiocytosis and tuberculosis, J.A.M.A. **237**:2213, 1977.
79. Goldberg, G.M.: Metastatic carcinoma of the spleen resulting from lymphogenic spread: report of two cases, Lab. Invest. **6**:383, 1957.
80. Gomez, E.C., et al.: Cutaneous involvement by IgD myeloma, Arch. Dermatol. **114**:1700, 1978.
81. Conella, J.S., and Lipsey, A.I.: Mastocytosis manifested by hepatosplenomegaly, N. Engl. J. Med. **271**:533, 1964.
82. Gordon, A.S., et al.: Plasma factors influencing leukocyte release in rats, Ann. N.Y. Acad. Sci. **113**:766, 1964.
83. Gross, K.: "Spontaneous" leukemia developing in C3H mice following inoculation in infancy, with AK-leukemia extracts, or AK-embryos, Proc. Soc. Exp. Biol. Med. **76**:27, 1951.
84. Gunz, F.W., and Hough, R.F.: Acute leukemia over the age of fifty: a study of its incidence and natural history; etiologic implications, Blood **11**:882, 1956.
85. Haferkamp, O., Rosenau, W., and Lennert, K.: Vascular transformation of lymph node sinsuses due to venous obstruction, Arch. Pathol. **92**:81, 1971.
86. Hansen, J.A., and Good, R.A.: malignant disease of the lymphoid system in immunological perspective, Hum. Pathol. **5**:567, 1974.
87. Hartroft, W.S., and Porta, E.A.: Ceroid, Am. J. Med. Sci. **250**:324, 1965.
88. Hartsock, R.J.: Postvaccinal lymphadenitis: hyperplasia of lymphoid tissue that simulates malignant lymphomas, Cancer **21**:632, 1968.
89. Hartsock, R.J., Smith, E.B., and Petty, C.S.: Normal variations with aging of the amount of hematopoietic tissue in bone marrow

from the anterior iliac crest, Am. J. Clin. Pathol. **43**:326, 1965. Pathol. **5**:551, 1974.

91. Hyman, G.A., and Sommers, C.: The development of Hodgkin's disease and lymphoma during anticonvulsant therapy, Blood **28**:416, 1966.
92. Hyun, B.H., et al.: Reactive plasmacytic lesions of the bone marrow, Am. J. Clin. Pathol. **65**:921, 1976.
93. Ioannides, K., and Rywlin, A.M.: A comparative study of histologic sections of bone marrow obtained by aspiration and by needle biopsy, Am. J. Clin. Pathol. **65**:267, 1976.
94. Jackson, H., and Parker, F.: Hodgkin's disease and allied disorders, New York, 1947, Oxford University Press.
95. Jacoben, C.D., Gjone, E., and Hovig, T.: Sea-blue histiocytes in familial lecithin: cholesterol acyltransferase deficiency, Scand. J. Haematol. **9**:106, 1972.
96. Jaffe, E.S., et al.: Leukemic reticuloendotheliosis: presence of a receptor for cytophilic antibody, Am. J. Med. **57**:108, 1974.
97. Jamshidi, K., and Swaim, W.R.: Bone marrow biopsy with unaltered architecture: a new biopsy device, J. Lab. Clin. Med. **77**:335, 1971.
98. Jansen, J., et al.: Distinct subtype within the spectrum of hairy cell leukemia, Blood **54**:459, 1979.
99. Johnstone, J.M.: The appearance of significance of tissue mast cells in human bone marrow, J. Clin. Pathol. **7**:275, 1954.
100. Jones, S.E., et al.: Non-Hodgkin's lymphomas. IV. Clinicopathologic correlation in 405 cases, Cancer **31**:806, 1973.
101. Kadin, M.D., Donaldson, S.S., and Dorfman, R.F.: Isolated granulomas in Hodgkin's disease, N. Engl. J. Med. **283**:859, 1970.
102. Kaplan, J., Mastrangel, R., and Peterson, W.D.: Childhood lymphoblastic lymphoma, a cancer of thymus-derived lymphocytes, Cancer Res. **34**:521, 1974.
103. Katayama, I., and Finkel, H.E.: Leukemic reticuloendotheliosis: a clinicopathologic study with review of the literature, Am. J. Med. **57**:115, 1974.
104. Katayama, I., Nagy, G.K., and Balough, K. Jr.: Light microscopic identification of the ribosome-lamella complex in "hairy cells" of leukemic reticuloendotheliosis, Cancer **32**:843, 1973.
105. Kay, A.B., Stechschulte, D.J., and Austen, K.F.: An eosinophilic leukocyte chemotactic factor of anaphylaxis, J. Exp. Med. **133**:602, 1971.
106. Keller, A.R., Hochholzer, L., and Castleman, B.: Hyaline-vascular and plasma-cell types of giant lymph node hyperplasia of the mediastinum and other locations, Cancer **29**:670, 1972.
107. Keller, A.R., et al.: Correlation of histopathology with other prognostic indicators in Hodgkin's disease, Cancer **22**:487, 1968.
108. Kheir, S.M., Mann, W.J., and Wilkerson, J.A.: Glandular inclusions in lymph nodes: the problem of extensive involvement and relationship to salpingitis, Am. J. Surg. Pathol. **5**:353, 1981.
109. King, J.T., Puchtler, H., and Sweat, F.: Ring fibers in human spleens, Arch. Pathol. **85**:237, 1968.
110. Kiraly, J.F., and Wheby, M.S.: Bone marrow necrosis, Am. J. Med. **60**:361, 1976.
111. Kitchens, C.S.: Case report: the syndrome of post-splenectomy fulminant sepsis; case report and review of the literature, Am. J. Med. Sci. **274**:303, 1977.
112. Knisely, M.H.: Spleen studies: microscopic observations of circulatory system of living unstimulated mammalian spleens, Anat. Rec. **65**:23, 1936.
113. Koh, S.J., et al.: Malignant "histiocytic" lymphoma in childhood, Am. J. Clin. Pathol. **74**:417, 1980.
114. Kundrat, H.: Über Lymphosarkomatosis, Wien. Klin. Wochenschr. **6**:211, 1893.
115. Langevoort, H.L., et al.: The nomenclature of phagocytic cells. In van Furth, R., editor: Mononuclear phagocytes, Oxford, Eng., 1970, Blackwell Scientific Publications.
116. Leder, L.D.: The chloroacetate esterase reaction: a useful means of histological diagnosis of hematological disorders from paraffin sections of skin, Am. J. Dermatopathol. **1**:39, 1979.
117. Lee, R.E., and Ellis, L.D.: The storage cells of chronic myelogenous leukemia, Lab. Invest. **24**:261, 1971.
118. Lee, S.L., et al.: Mu-chain disease, Ann. Intern. Med. **75**:407, 1971.
119. Lennert, K.: Lymphknoten. In Uehlinger, E., editor: Handbuch der speziellen pathologischen Anatomie und Histologie, Heidelberg, 1961, Springer-Verlag.
120. Lennert, K.: Follicular lymphoma—a tumor of the germinal centers. In Akazaki, K., et al., editors: Malignant diseases of the hematopoietic system, Gann Monogr. Cancer Res., no. 15, 1973, University of Tokyo Press.
121. Lennert, K.: Malignant lymphomas, Berlin, 1978, Springer-Verlag.
122. Levine, G.D., and Dorfman, R.F.: Nodular lymphoma: an ultrastructural study of its relationship to germinal centers and a correlation of light and electron microscopic findings, Cancer **35**:148, 1975.
123. Lichtenstein, L.: Histiocytosis X: integration of eosinophilic granuloma of bone marrow, Letterer-Siwe disease and Schüller-Christian disease as related manifestations of a single nosologic entity, Arch. Pathol. **56**:84, 1953.
124. Lieberman, P.H., et al.: A reappraisal of eosinophilic granuloma of bone, Hand-Schüller-Christian syndrome and Letterer-Siwe syndrome, Medicine **48**:375, 1969.
125. Lipshutz, M.D., et al.: Bone marrow biopsy and clinical staging in chronic lymphocytic leukemia, Cancer **46**:1422, 1980.
126. Longo, S.: Benign lymph node inclusions, Hum. Pathol. **7**:349, 1976.
127. Lubin, J., Rozen, S., and Rywlin, A.M.: Malignant myelosclerosis, Arch. Intern. Med. **136**:141, 1976.
128. Lubin, J., and Rywlin, A.M.: Lymphoma-like lymph node changes in Kaposi's sarcoma: two additional cases, Arch. Pathol. **92**:338, 1971.
129. Lukes, R.J.: Criteria for involvement of lymph node, bone marrow, spleen and liver in Hodgkin's disease, Cancer Res. **31**:1755, 1971.
130. Lukes, R.J., Butler, J.J., and Hicks, E.B.: Natural history of Hodgkin's disease as related to its pathologic picture, Cancer **19**:317, 1966.
131. Lukes, R.J., and Collins, R.D.: New observations on malignant lymphomas. In Akazaki, K., et al., editors: Malignant diseases of the hematopoietic system, Gann Monogr. Cancer Res., no. 15, 1973, University of Tokyo Press.
132. Lukes, R.J., and Collins, R.D.: New approaches to the classification of the lymphomata, Br. J. Cancer **31**:1, 1975.
133. Lukes, R.J., and Tindle, B.H.: Immunoblastic lymphadenopathy: a hyperimmune entity resembling Hodgkin's disease, N. Engl. J. Med. **292**:1, 1975.
134. Lukes, R.J., et al.: Report of the Nomenclature Committee, Cancer Res. **26**:1311, 1966b.
135. Mackaness, G.B.: The monocyte in cellular immunity, Semin. Hematol. **7**:172, 1970.
136. MacKenzie, M.R., et al.: Waldenstrom's macroglobulinemia: correlation between expanded plasma volume and increased serum viscosity, Blood **35**:394, 1970.
137. Mark, T., and Levin, A.: Histologic examination of the bone marrow: aspiration or trephine? South. Med. J. **74**:1447, 1981.
138. McCully, R.M., Barron, C.N., and Cheever, A.W.: Schistosomiasis. In Binford, C.H., and Connor, D.H., editors: Pathology of tropical and extraordinary diseases, Washington, D.C., 1976, Armed Forces Institute of Pathology.
139. McDonald, G.A., Dodds, T.C., and Cruickshank, B., editors: Atlas of haematology, ed. 2, Baltimore, 1968, The Williams & Wilkins Co.
140. McKenna, R.W., Risdall, R.J., and Brunning, R.D.: Virus associated hemophagocytic syndrome, Hum. Pathol. **12**:395, 1981.
141. McMahon, N.J., Gordon, H.W., and Rosen, R.B.: Reed-Sternberg cells in infectious mononucleosis: report of a case, Dis. Child. **120**:148, 1970.

141a. Meighan, S.S.: Leukemia in children: incidence, clinical manifestations, and survival in an unselected series, J.A.M.A. **190**:578, 1964.

142. Meyers, W.M., Neafie, R.C., and Connor, D.H.: Pentastomiasis. In Binford, C.H., and Connor, D.H., editors: Pathology of

tropical and extraordinary diseases, Washington, D.C., 1976, Armed Forces Institute of Pathology.

143. Miale, J.B.: Laboratory medicine—hematology, ed. 6, St. Louis, 1982, The C.V. Mosby Co.
144. Miescher, P.A., and Muller-Eberhard, H.J.: Textbook of immunopathology, vol. 2, New York, 1963, Grune & Stratton, Inc.
145. Millett, Y.L., et al.: Nodular sclerotic lymphosarcoma: a further review, Br. J. Cancer **23**:683, 1969.
146. Moller, J.H., et al.: Congenital cardiac disease associated with polysplenia: a development complex of bilateral "left-sidedness," Circulation **36**:789, 1967.
147. Motoi, M., et al.: Eosinophilic granuloma of lymph nodes—a variant of histiocytosis X, Histopathology **4**:585, 1980.
148. Naeim, F.: "Hairy cell" leukemia: a heterogeneous chronic lymphoproliferative disorder, Am. J. Med. **65**:479, 1978.
149. Nanba, K., et al.: Hairy cell leukemia, Cancer **39**:2323, 1977.
150. Nathan, C.F., Murray, H.W., and Cohn, Z.A.: Current concepts: the macrophage as an effector cell, N. Engl. J. Med. **303**:622, 1980.
151. Nathwani, B.N., Kims, S., and Rappaport, H.: Malignant lymphoma, lymphoblastic, Cancer **38**:964, 1976.
152. Nathwani, B.N., et al.: Morphologic criteria for the differentiation of follicular lymphoma from florid reactive follicular hyperplasia: a study of 80 cases, Cancer **48**:1794, 1981.
153. Neiman, R.S., Bischel, M.D., and Lukes, R.J.: Uremia and mast cell proliferation, Lancet **1**:959, 1972.
154. Neiman, R.S., Rosen, P.T., and Lukes, R.J.: Lymphocytic-depletion Hodgkin's disease: a clinicopathological entity, N. Engl. J. Med. **288**:751, 1973.
155. Neiman, R.S., et al.: Granulocytic sarcoma: a clinicopathologic study of 61 biopsied cases, Cancer **48**:1426, 1981.
156. Newton, W.A., and Hamoudi, A.B.: Histiocytosis: a histologic classification with clinical correlation. In Rosenberg, H.S., and Bolande, R.P., editors: Perspectives in pediatric pathology, Chicago, 1973, Year Book Medical Publishers, Inc.
157. North, R.J.: Endocytosis, Semin. Hematol. **7**:161, 1970.
158. Nossal, G.J., et al.: Antigens in immunity. XII. Antigen trapping in the spleen, Int. Arch. Allergy Appl. Immunol. **29**:368, 1966.
159. Nyholm, K.: Eosinophilic xanthomatous granulomatosis and Letterer-Siwe's disease, Acta Pathol. Scand. **216**(suppl.):1, 1971.
160. O'Connor, G.T., and Davies, J.N.P.: Malignant tumors in African children with special reference to malignant lymphoma, J. Pediatr. **56**:526, 1960.
161. Okun, D.B., Sun, N.C.J., and Tanaka, K.R.: Bone marrow granuloma in Q fever, Am. J. Clin. Pathol. **71**:117, 1979.
162. Osborne, B.M., Butler, J.J., and Mackay, B.: Proteinaceous lymphadenopathy with hypergammaglobulinemia, Am. J. Surg. Pathol. **3**:137, 1979.
163. Palutke, M., et al.: T-cell lymphomas of large cell type: a variety of malignant lymphomas: "histiocytic" and mixed lymphocytic-"histiocytic," Cancer **46**:87, 1980.
164. Pangalis, G.A., Moran, E.M., and Rappaport, H.: Blood and bone marrow findings in angioimmunoblastic lymphadenopathy, Blood **51**:71, 1978.
165. Pangalis, G.A., Nathwani, B.N., and Rappaport, H.: Malignant lymphoma, well differentiated lymphocytic, Cancer **39**:999, 1977.
166. The pathogenesis of myelofibrosis in myeloproliferative syndromes (editorial), Ann. Intern. Med. **92**:877, 1980.
167. Perry, M.C., et al.: Familial erythrophagocytic lymphohistiocytosis: report of two cases and clinicopathologic review, Cancer **38**:209, 1976.
168. Peters, S.P., Lee, R.E., and Glew, R.H.: Gaucher's disease: a review, Medicine **56**:425, 1977.
169. Peterson, L.C., Bloomfield, C.D., and Brunning, R.D.: Blast crisis as an initial or terminal manifestation of chronic myeloid leukemia: a study of 28 patients, Am. J. Med. **60**:209, 1976.
170. Peterson, L., et al.: Extramedullary masses as presenting features of acute monoblastic leukemia, Am. J. Clin. Pathol. **75**:140, 1981.
171. Pierce, J.R., Wren, M.V., and Cousar, J.B.: Cholesterol embolism: diagnosis antemortem by bone marrow biopsy, Ann. Intern. Med. **89**:937, 1978.
171a. Pileri, S., et al.: Histiocytic necrotizing lymphadenitis without granulocytic infiltration, Virchows Arch. (Pathol. Anat.) **395**:257, 1982.
172. Piringer-Kuchinka, A., Martin, I., and Thalhammer, O.: Superior cervical-nuchal lymphadenitis with small groups of epitheliod cell proliferation, Virchows Arch. (Pathol. Anat.) **331**:552, 1958.
173. Polliack, A., et al.: Identification of human B and T lymphocytes by scanning electron microscopy, J. Exp. Med. **138**:607, 1973.
174. Pratt, P.W., Estren, S., and Kochwa, S.: Immunoglobulin abnormalities in Gaucher's disease: report of 16 cases, Blood **31**:633, 1968.
175. Purtilo, D.T.: X-linked lymphoproliferative syndrome: an immunodeficiency disorder with acquired agammaglobulinemia, fatal infectious mononucleosis, or malignant lymphoma, Arch. Pathol. Lab. Med. **105**:119, 1981.
176. Putschar, W.G.J., and Manion, W.C.: Splenic-gonadal fusion, Am. J. Pathol. **32**:15, 1956.
177. Ramot, B.: Intestinal lymphoma with malabsorption in Mediterranean populations, Isr. J. Med. Sci. **7**:1488, 1971.
178. Rappaport, H.: Tumors of the hematopoietic system. In Atlas of tumor pathology, Section III, Fascicle 8, Washington, D.C., 1966, Armed Forces Institute of Pathology.
179. Rappaport, H.: The pathologic anatomy of the splenic red pulp. In Lennert, K., and Harms, D., editors: The spleen, Berlin, 1970, Springer-Verlag.
180. Rappaport, H., Winter, W.J., and Hicks, E.B.: Follicular lymphoma: a re-evaluation of its position in the scheme of malignant lymphomas, based on a survey of 253 cases, Cancer **9**:792, 1956.
181. Rappaport, H., et al.: Report of the Committee on Histopathological Criteria Contributing to Staging of Hodgkin's Disease, Cancer Res. **31**:1864, 1971.
182. Rappaport, H., et al.: The pathology of so-called Mediterranean abdominal lymphoma with malabsorption, Cancer **29**:1502, 1972.
183. Ravel, R.: Histopathology of lymph nodes after lymphangiography, Am. J. Clin. Pathol. **46**:335, 1966.
184. Reynolds, W.A., Winkelman, R.K., and Soule, E.H.: Kaposi's sarcoma: a clinicopathologic study with particular reference to its relationship to the reticuloendothelial system, Medicine **44**:419, 1965.
185. Rezek, P.R., and Millard, M.M.: Autopsy pathology, Springfield, Ill., 1963, Charles C Thomas, Publisher.
186. Richter, M.N.: Generalized reticular sarcoma of lymph nodes associated with lymphatic leukemia, Am. J. Pathol. **4**:285, 1928.
187. Ridolfi, R.L., Rosen, P.P., and Thaler, H.: Nevus cell aggregates associated with lymph nodes: estimated frequency and clinical significance, Cancer **39**:164, 1977.
188. Risdall, R.J., et al.: Virus-associated hemophagocytic syndrome: a benign histiocytic proliferation distinct from malignant histiocytosis, Cancer **44**:993, 1979.
189. Risdall, R.J., et al.: Malignant histiocytosis: a light- and electron-microscopic and histochemical Study, Am. J. Surg. Pathol. **4**:439, 1980.
190. Robbins, F.G., et al.: Splenic epidermoid cysts, Ann. Surg. **187**:231, 1978.
191. Robinson, M.J., and Rywlin, A.M.: Granulomatous inflammation of bone marrow: a previously undescribed, probably drug-related lesion, Am. J. Clin. Pathol. **65**:268, 1976.
192. Rodriguez, A.R., Lutcher, C.L., and Coleman, F.W.: Osteosclerotic myeloma, J.A.M.A. **236**:1872, 1976.
193. Rosai, J., and Dorfman, R.F.: Sinus histiocytosis with massive lymphadenopathy: a pseudolymphomatous benign disorder; analysis of 34 cases, Cancer **30**:1174, 1972.
194. Rosenberg, S.A.: Hodgkin's disease of the bone marrow, Cancer Res. **31**:1733, 1971.
195. Rosenberg, S.A., et al.: Report of the Committee on Hodgkin's Disease Staging Procedures, Cancer Res. **31**:1862, 1971.
196. Rywlin, A.M.: Histopathology of the bone marrow, Boston, 1976, Little, Brown and Co.
197. Rywlin, A.M.: The reticuloendothelial system—distribution and function. In Gilson, A.J., Smoak, W.M., and Weinstein, M.B.,

editors: Hematopoietic and gastrointestinal investigations with radionuclides, Springfield, Ill., 1972, Charles C Thomas, Publisher.

197. Rywlin, A.M.: Non-Hodgkin's malignant lymphomas: brief historical review and simple unifying classification, Am. J. Dermatopathol. **2**:17, 1980.
198. Rywlin, A.M., and Benson, J.: Massive necrosis of the spleen with formation of pseudocyst, Am. J. Clin. Pathol. **36**:142, 1961.
199. Rywlin, A.M., Block, A.L., and Werner, C.S.: Hemoglobin C and S disease in pregnancy, Am. J. Obstet. Gynecol. **86**:1055, 1963.
200. Rywlin, A.M., Hoffman, E.P., and Ortega, R.S.: Eosinophilic fibrohistiocytic lesion of bone marrow: a definitive new morphologic finding, probably related to drug hypersensitivity, Blood **40**:464, 1972.
201. Rywlin, A.M., Marvan, P., and Robinson, M.J.: A simple technic for the preparation of bone marrow smears and sections, Am. J. Clin. Pathol. **53**:389, 1970.
202. Rywlin, A.M., and Ortega, R.S.: Lipid granulomas of the bone marrow, Am. J. Clin. Pathol. **57**:457, 1972.
203. Rywlin, A.M., Ortega, R.S., and Dominguez, C.J.: Lymphoid nodules of bone marrow: normal and abnormal, Blood **43**:389, 1974.
204. Rywlin, A.M., Recher, L., and Hoffman, E.P.: Lymphoma-like presentations in Kaposi's sarcoma, Arch. Dermatol. **93**:554, 1966.

204a. Rywlin, A.M., Rosen, L., and Cabello, B.: Coexistence of Castleman's disease and Kaposi's sarcoma, Am. J. Dermatopathol. **5**:277, 1983.

205. Rywlin, A.M., et al.: Ceroid histiocytosis of spleen and bone marrow in idiopathic thrombocytopenia purpura (ITP): a contribution to the understanding of the sea-blue histiocyte, Blood **37**:587, 1971.
206. Rywlin, A.M., et al.: Ceroid histiocytosis of spleen in hyperlipemia: relationship to the syndrome of the sea-blue histiocyte, Am. J. Clin. Pathol. **56**:572, 1971.
207. Rywlin, A.M., et al.: Bone marrow histology in monoclonal macroglobulinemia, Am. J. Clin. Pathol. **63**:769, 1975.
208. Saba, T.M.: Physiology and physiopathology of the reticuloendothelial system, Arch. Intern. Med. **126**:1031, 1970.
209. Salfelder, K., and Schwarz, J.: Histoplasmotische Kalkherde in der Milz, Dtsch. Med. Wochenschr. **92**:1468, 1967.
210. Schleicher, E.M.: Giant Russell bodies, Minnesota Med. 1125, 1965.
211. Schrek, R., and Donnelly, W.J.: "Hairy" cells in blood in lymphoreticular neoplastic disease and "flagellated" cells of normal lymph nodes, Blood **27**:199, 1966.
212. Seligmann, M., Mihaesco, E., and Frangione, B.: Alpha chain disease, Ann. N.Y. Acad. Sci. **190**:487, 1971.
213. Shah, K.H., and Kisilevsky, R.: Infarction of the lymph nodes: a cause of a palisading macrophage reaction mimicking necrotizing granulomas, Hum. Pathol. **9**:597, 1978.
214. Shepard, C.C., and Karat, A.B.A.: Infectivity of leprosy bacilli from bone marrow and liver of patients with lepromatous leprosy, Lep. Rev. **43**:21, 1972.
215. Shousha, S.: Splenic cysts: a report of six cases and a brief review, Postgrad. Med. J. **54**:265, 1978.
216. Sieracki, J.S., and Fisher, E.R.: The ceroid nature of the so-called "Hamazaki-Wesenberg bodies," Am. J. Clin. Pathol. **59**:248, 1973.
217. Silverstein, M.N., Ellefson, R.D., and Ahern, E.J.: The syndrome of the sea-blue histiocyte, N. Engl. J. Med. **282**:1, 1970.
218. Skarin, A.T., et al.: Lymphosarcoma of the spleen, Arch. Intern. Med. **127**:259, 1971.
219. Smith, C.H., et al.: Hazard of severe infections in splenectomized infants and children, Am. J. Med. **22**:390, 1957.
220. Smith, E.B., and Custer, R.P.: Rupture of the spleen in infectious mononucleosis: a clinicopathologic report of seven cases, Blood **1**:317, 1946.
221. Smith, J.L.: Characterization of malignant mediastinal lymphoid neoplasm (Sternberg sarcoma) as thymic in origin, Lancet **1**:74, 1973.
222. Sparks, A.K., Connor, D.H., and Neafie, R.C.: Echinococcosis. In Binford, C.H., and Connor, D.H., editors: Pathology of tropical and extraordinary diseases, Washington, D.C., 1976, Armed Forces Institute of Pathology.
223. Sparks, I., and Kahn, A.: Myelomatosis: fundamentals and clinical features, Basel, 1971, S. Karger.
224. Spranger, J.W., and Wiedemann, H.R.: The genetic mucolipidoses: diagnosis and differential diagnosis, Hum. Genet. **9**:113, 1970.
225. Stoop, J.W., et al.: Alpha-chain disease with involvement of respiratory tract in a Dutch child, Clin. Exp. Immunol. **9**:625, 1971.
226. Straus, D.J., et al.: Atypical lymphoma with prolonged systemic remission after splenectomy: description of three cases, Am. J. Med. **56**:386, 1974.
227. Strum, S.B., et al.: Further observations on the biologic significance of vascular invasion in Hodgkin's disease, Cancer **27**:1, 1971.
228. Stutte, H.J.: Round table discussion: splenopathic inhibition of bone marrow and Banti's disease. In Lennert, K., and Harms, D., editors: The spleen, Berlin, 1970. Springer-Verlag.
229. Stutte, H.J., and Schulter, E.: Zur Ätiologic von Fibrin pracipitaten in den Lymphofollikeln der menschlichen Milz, Virchows Arch. (Pathol. Anat.) **356**:32, 1972.
230. Sun, N.C.J., et al.: Lymphoplasmacytic myeloma: an immunological, immunohistochemical and electron microscopy study, Cancer **43**:2268, 1979.
231. Suprun, H., and Rywlin, A.M.: Metastatic carcinoma in histologic sections of aspirated bone marrow: a comparative autopsy study, South. Med. J. **69**:438, 1976.
232. Tani, M., et al.: Multicentric reticulohistiocytosis: electron microscopic and ultracytochemical studies, Arch. Dermatol. **117**:495, 1981.
233. Tarnowski, W.M., and Hashimoto, K.: Langerhans' cell granules in histiocytosis X: the epidermal Langerhans' cell as a macrophage, Arch. Dermatol. **96**:298, 1967.
234. Teplitz, C., and Goss, G.: Histiocytosis X—misnomer in systemic "Langerhans cell" proliferative disorders: ultrastructure of the distinctive infiltrative cell and the morphogenesis of its pathognomic granules (abstract), Lab. Invest. **32**:437, 1975.
235. Tindle, B.H., Parker, J.W., and Lukes, R.J.: "Reed-Sternberg cells" in infectious mononucleosis? Am. J. Clin. Pathol. **58**:607, 1972.
236. Tuchman, L.R., Goldstein, G., and Clyman, M.: Studies on the nature of the increased serum acid phosphatase in Gaucher's disease, Am. J. Med. **27**:959, 1959.
237. Turner, D.R., and Millis, R.R.: Breast tissue inclusions in axillary lymph nodes, Histopathology **4**:631, 1980.

237a. Turner, R.R., Martin, J., and Dorfman, R.F.: Necrotizing lymphadenitis, Am. J. Surg. Pathol. **7**:115, 1983.

238. van Furth, R.: Origin and kinetics of monocytes and macrophages, Semin. Hematol. **7**:125, 1970.
239. Vardiman, J.W., et al.: Malignant histiocytosis with massive splenomegaly in asymptomatic patients, Cancer **36**:419, 1975.
240. Variakojis, D., Rosas-Uribe, A., and Rappaport, H.: Mycosis fungoides: pathologic findings in staging laparotomies, Cancer **33**:1589, 1974.
241. Velde, J. de, et al.: The eosinophilic fibrohistiocytic lesion of the bone marrow, Virchows Arch. (Pathol. Anat.) **377**:277, 1978.
242. Vernon, S., et al.: Nodular lymphoma with intracellular immunoglobulin, Cancer **44**:1273, 1979.
243. Vykoupil, K.F., et al.: Hairy cell leukemia: bone marrow findings in 24 patients, Virchows Arch. (Pathol. Anat.) **370**:273, 1976.
244. Waldron, J.A., et al.: Malignant lymphoma of peripheral T-lymphocyte origin, Cancer **40**:1604, 1977.
245. Walker, P.D., et al.: The osseous manifestations of sinus histiocytosis with massive lymphadenopathy, Am. J. Clin. Pathol. **75**:131, 1981.

246. Warnke, R.A., Kim, H., and Dorfman, R.F.: Malignant histiocytosis (histiocytic meduallary reticulosis). I. Clinicopathologic study of 29 cases, Cancer **35**:215, 1975.
247. Watanabe, S., et al.: Adult T cell lymphoma with hypergammaglobulinemia, Cancer **46**:2472, 1980.
248. Watts, J.C., et al.: Idiopathic infarction of intraabdominal lymph nodes: a cause of fever of unknown origin, Am. J. Clin. Pathol. **74**:687, 1980.
248a. Wear, D.J., et al.: Cat scratch disease: a bacterial infection, Science **221**:1403, 1983.
249. Weinstein, R.A., et al.: Hairy cell leukemia: association with disseminated atypical mycobacterial infection, Cancer **48**:380, 1981.
250. Wennberg, E., and Weiss, L.: Splenic erythroclasia: an electron microscopic study of hemoglobin H disease, Blood **31**:778, 1968.
251. Williams, J.W., and Dorfman, R.F.: Lymphadenopathy as the initial manifestation of histiocytosis X, Am. J. Surg. Pathol. **3**:405, 1979.
252. Winkelstein, J.A.: Splenectomy and infection (editorial), Arch. Intern. Med. **137**:1516, 1977.
253. Wright, D.H.: Burkitt's lymphoma: a review of the pathology, immunology and possible etiology factors, Pathol. Annu. **6**:337, 1971.
254. Yam, L.T., Li, C.Y., and Finkel, H.E.: Leukemic reticuloendotheliosis: the role of tartrate-resistant acid phosphatase in diagnosis and splenectomy in treatment, Arch. Intern. Med. **130**:248, 1972.
255. Yam, L.T., Yam, C.F., and Yang Li, C.: Eosinophilia in systemic mastocytosis, Am. J. Clin. Pathol. **73**:48, 1980.
256. Yu, H.C., and Rywlin, A.M.: Granulomatous lesions of the bone marrow in non-Hodgkin's lymphomas, Lab. Invest. **42**:66, 1980.
257. Zucker, J.M., et al.: Malignant histiocytosis in childhood: clinical study and therapeutic results in 22 cases, Cancer **45**:2821, 1980.

CHAPTER 31 Thymus Gland

ROGERS C. GRIFFITH

The thymus gland is a complex, highly specialized lymphoreticular organ that has the central role in T lymphocyte ontogeny. This organ has become the focus of extensive research since Miller[84] conclusively proved in his classic thymectomy experiments in newborn mice that the thymus is essential for the development of cellular and most humoral immune responses. Information resulting from the ensuing two decades of research has redefined our concepts regarding the development of the thymus gland—its structure, its pathology, and its importance to the individual.

DEVELOPMENT

The morphogenesis of the human fetal thymus begins in the sixth gestational week. Paired cellular proliferations emerge from the endoderm of the ventral wing of the third pharyngeal pouch and from the ectoderm of the third pharyngeal cleft (Fig. 31-1). The inferior parathyroid glands arise similarly from the dorsal wing of the pharyngeal pouch. Both primordia separate from the pharyngeal wall and begin a caudal migration as the fetus grows. The thymic primordium leads and elongates, trailing the incipient upper lobes of the thymus gland behind. Small fragments may separate from the migratory primordium and persist postnatally along the migratory route. When the thymus gland ends its migration at the base of the heart, it lies anterior to the great vessels in the anterior, superior mediastinum, with the upper poles of its two lobes extending laterally along the trachea to the base of the thyroid gland.

The thymic primordial stroma is composed entirely of undifferentiated epithelial cells until the ninth gestational week, when hemopoietic precursor cells enter.[86] This influx of stem cells into the thymus occurs in successive waves[53,64] and is an active phenomenon[99] that depends on the maturational state of the thymic epithelium.[65] Lobulation occurs by the tenth week as the epithelial cells expand to surround mesenchymal septal ingrowths that communicate with the anlage through its surrounding basal lamina. Inductive tissue interactions between the epithelial and mesenchymal components are necessary for further normal development to occur.[3] The epithelial cells at the periphery develop a rounded contour, whereas those in the center appear more spindle shaped.[133] Adjacent epithelial cells are connected by well-developed desmosomes, but other large mesenchymal cells that are present in the septa and among the central epithelial cells lack intercellular junctions. These cells later differentiate into mononuclear cells that resemble the interdigitating reticulum cells of thymus-dependent regions of peripheral lymphoid tissue.[54] Rare cells containing myofilaments, described as myoid cells, are present in the central anlage as early as the eighth week. However, by the twelfth gestational week most of the nonepithelial cells present are lymphoid cells. Small cells are concentrated toward the center, and the larger lymphoblasts are present among the more peripheral epithelial cells, as are scattered macrophages. Normoblasts, residua from earlier hemopoiesis in the primordium, may also be present.

The presumptive precursors of the characteristic Hassall's corpuscles of the postnatal thymus are present in the central region of the thymus by the twelfth week. They appear as small, tubular structures composed of epithelial cells and often have microvilli projecting into the lumen. The histogenesis of these structures is still uncertain. Arguments for a direct, senescent derivation from central epithelial cells,[10,78] a specific differentiation of epithelial cells into stratified squamous epithelium,[134] or a separate postulated embryonic origin distinct from the principal primordium[23,116] have their proponents.

The development of the cortex and medulla is completed between the fourteenth and sixteenth gestational weeks, and any characteristic differences in the lymphocyte and epithelial cell populations of each region are apparent by this time. The mesenchymal septa extend to the corticomedullary junction and give rise to the perivascular spaces that enter the parenchyma of the gland.

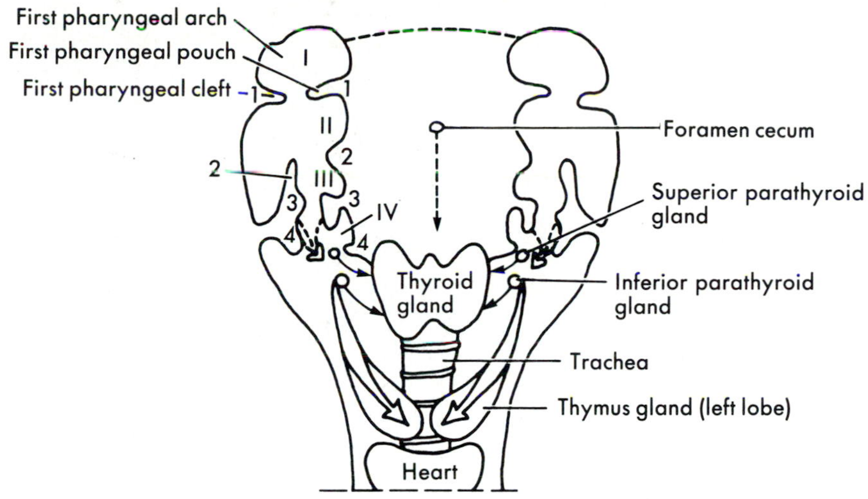

Fig. 31-1. Embryogenesis of thymus gland. In this schematic drawing of pharyngeal development, thymus gland originates from pouch and cleft of third pharyngeal structure.

Table 31-1. Weight of thymus

Age (yr)	Weight (g)		
	Minimum	Average	Maximum
Newborn	7.3	15.2	25.5
1-5	8.0	25.7	48.0
5-10	13.0	29.4	48.0
10-15	19.0	29.4	43.3
15-20	15.9	26.2	49.7
21-25	9.5	21.0	51.0
26-30	8.3	19.5	51.5
31-35	9.0	20.2	37.0
36-43	5.9	19.0	36.0
47-55	6.0	17.3	45.0
56-65	2.1	14.3	27.0
66-90	3.0	14.0	31.0

According to Hammar, J.A.: Die Menschenthymus in Gesundheit and Krankheit, Leipzig, 1926, Akademische Verlagsgesellschaft; from Fisher, E.R.: Pathology of the thymus and its relation to human disease. In Good, R.A., and Gabrielsen, A.E., editors: The thymus in immunobiology, New York, 1964, Paul B. Hoeber Medical Division, Harper & Row, Publishers, Inc.

The cortex is filled with immature and maturing thymocytes, whereas the medulla contains very few lymphocytes but many compact epithelial cells and interdigitating reticulum cells. This contrasting cellularity creates the distinct corticomedullary junction. The thymus at this stage of development resembles the postnatal thymus in all respects, except that it weighs only 0.2 g.

The thymus gland undergoes considerable growth before birth, when it attains its greatest weight in relation to body weight, weighing an average of 15 g. The thymus continues to increase in size until puberty, increasing in weight by another 50%. Afterward the process of natural involution occurs, with a gradual replacement of parenchyma by adipose tissue. This process is never complete.[33] Individuals display a considerable variation in thymic weight at all ages (Table 31-1).

STRUCTURE

The mature thymus gland maintains its fetal bilobed structure. Each lobe is separately encapsulated, and both lobes are invested in loose connective tissue that fuses into a continuous sheet anteriorly. Microscopically the basic structure of each lobe is the lobule, which is developed by the many invaginated mesenchymal septa (Figs. 31-2 and 31-3). Epithelial cells are stationary and provide the primary structure of the gland via their elongated interdigitating cytoplasmic projections. The histologic pattern of the lobule and its distinct corticomedullary junction are the result of the rich lymphocyte population of the cortex.

The epithelial cells appear strikingly similar throughout the thymus gland, although many observers have emphasized ultrastructural differences between the cells of the cortex and medulla.[46,133,134] Obvious differences are that the cortical cells are less densely arranged and have very elongated cytoplasmic branches that form interstices, where the mobile lymphoid cells are found. Similar attenuated cytoplasmic projections line the inner surface of the capsule. Basal lamina material is present over the surface of these cells and circumscribes all of the extrathymic areas, including the small blood vessels within the thymus.[9] The medullary cells are more densely associated and have blunted cytoplasmic projections. A consistent feature of these cells is the greater frequency of desmosomes and the dense tonofilaments in the cytoplasm that often insert into the desmosomes. These latter features are better developed in those attenuated cells that abut on Hassall's corpuscles. Otherwise, epithelial cells of either the cortex or the medulla lack spe-

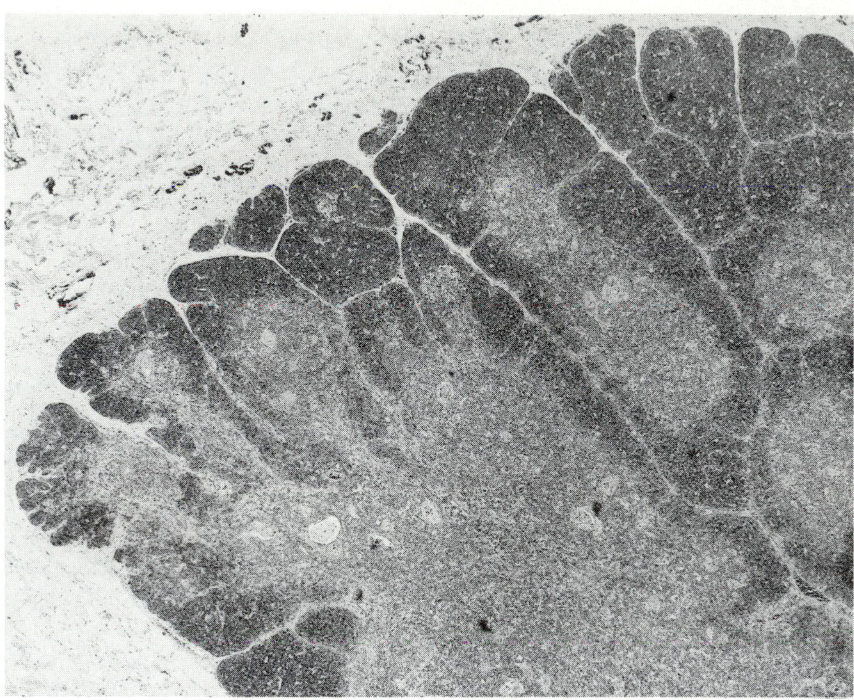

Fig. 31-2. Normal thymus gland from infant, showing lobulated structure, distinct corticomedullary junction, and prominent Hassall's corpuscles of medulla. (25×.)

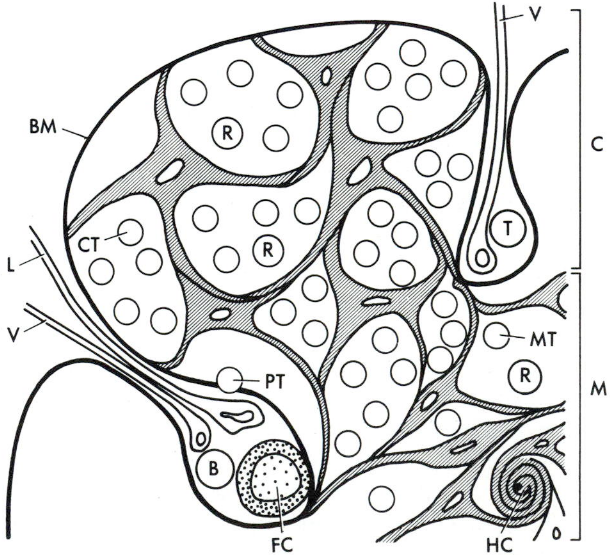

Fig. 31-3. Schematic representation of structural organization of mature thymus gland. Epithelial cells *(elongated shaded cells)* providing primary structure are more densely associated in medulla *(M)* than in cortex *(C)*. Basal lamina *(BM)* circumscribes thymic parenchyma proper in which freely moving thymocytes develop. *PT*, Prothymocyte; *CT*, cortical thymocytes; *MT*, medullary thymocytes; *HC*, Hassall's corpuscle; *R*, reticulum cells; *B*, B lymphocytes or plasma cells; *T*, T lymphocytes; *FC*, follicular center; *V*, blood vessels; *L*, lymphatic vessels.

cific cytoplasmic organelle specialization.

Hassall's corpuscles, the distinctive structures located within the medulla, are complex tubular arrays composed of the epithelial interdigitations of concentrically arranged epithelial cells. Basal lamina material, numerous desmosomes, and dense tonofilaments are prominent ultrastructural features. Keratinization occurs in Hassall's corpuscles, and related keratinic and cytoplasmic antigens have recently been demonstrated in the thymus and the epidermis.[131] Their central areas can be either cystic or solid, and degenerative changes with cellular debris may be observed centrally. Lymphocytes, macrophages, and eosinophils may also be found within these corpuscles.

The thymic cortex is replete with lymphocytes that en masse give the thymus gland its distinctive histologic appearance. Large, mitotically active lymphoblasts comprise about 15% of the lymphoid cells and are found predominantly in the subcapsular portion of the outer cortex.[22] A gradient of smaller, less mitotically active cells occurs from the outer cortex to the corticomedullary junction and to a much lesser degree into the medulla. In the subcapsular region of intense lymphopoiesis and to a lesser extent elsewhere in the cortex, lympholysis and active phagocytosis are indicative of the extensive amount of ineffective lymphopoiesis now considered a normal and constant finding in an active thymus gland.[113]

Other types of cells are found less frequently in the thymus gland. Macrophages are numerous in the cortex and in the medulla, and eosinophils, mast cells, plasma cells, and peripheral lymphocytes are frequently present in the extrathymic perivascular spaces. Lymphoid follicles with active germinal centers may also be found in an otherwise normal thymus, especially in children and adolescents.[83,130] These structures presumably arise within the perivascular spaces.[70] Myoid cells—cells with microscopic, ultrastructural, and immunohistochemical features of striated muscle—have been observed in the human thymic medulla of persons of all ages.[27,40,47] These cells, which are often found in the thymus of various lower vertebrates, have been extensively studied. Myoid cells are completely invested by epithelial cells, but evidence is lacking that these cells directly interact with epithelial cells or are derived from them. Their histogenesis or function in the human thymus is not known.

FUNCTION

The thymus provides the essential microenvironment for the differentiation and expansion of T lymphocyte subpopulations necessary to develop the complex network of immunoregulatory and cell-mediated effector functions attributable to mature T lymphocytes. Several distinct functional subpopulations have been identified primarily in rodents, and analogous subsets have also been found and are believed to function similarly in humans; these are outlined as follows:

1. Effector functions
   a. Cell-mediated cytotoxicity—killing of foreign antigen-bearing cells (allogeneic, virus-infected, or tumor cells)
   b. Lymphokine production—production of mediators of inflammation and nonspecific immunity (delayed-type hypersensitivity)
2. Regulatory functions
   a. Helper—enhancement of B lymphocyte responses to thymus-dependent antigens
   b. Suppressor—diminishing of thymus-dependent B lymphocyte responses and T lymphocyte helper, cytotoxic functions, or delayed-type hypersensitivity
   c. Amplifier—enhancement of T lymphocyte cytotoxic functions

These functional T lymphocytes and their precursors develop as a consequence of intrathymic and postthymic events.[126] This development begins after hemopoietic progenitor cells migrate from the bone marrow to the thymus. The process involves extensive cellular proliferation primarily in the outer cortex and intrathymic migration through the cortex to the medulla before exiting the thymus to the peripheral lymphoid compartment, where functional diversification is completed.[81,113] The intrathymic differentiation process requires direct interaction of the lymphoid precursor cells with the thymic epithelial cells, which also produce several hormonal factors that act to promote maturation of precursor cells that have undergone a primary event by direct contact with the epithelium.[5] The molecular events that are operative at this early stage of differentiation are not fully understood. However, the result of these interactions is the selection of a T lymphocyte repertoire that has the capacity to recognize gene products of the individual's own major histocompatibility complex (MHC) antigens but does not react with them.[142]

To fully understand the molecular basis of T cell repertoire development is to understand the basis of antigen recognition by the T lymphocyte, a persisting enigma of modern immunology. Current evidence indicates that effector T lymphocytes exhibit clonal recognition of specific antigens and that their activation results solely from the antigen being presented on the surface of another cell type. T cells recognize foreign antigens almost exclusively in the context of self-MHC antigens (antigens encoded by MHC genes) of the antigen-presenting cell, a phenomenon called MHC restriction. The particular restricting MHC products are different for different functional T cell subpopulations. Cytotoxic T cells recognize class I MHC products (HLA-A,B,C and H-2 K,D antigens in humans and mice, respectively), and T helper cells recognize class II MHC products (HLA-DR and H-2 Ia antigens). Recent evidence indicates that the development of MHC restriction in the individual is acquired during the process of intrathymic differentiation.[141]

The maturational effects of various thymic hormone preparations extracted from the thymus gland and presumably produced by the thymic epithelial cells are now well established. Although it was initially thought that these factors provided the sole stimulus for thymocyte development, it is now believed that these hormonal factors promote differentiation of the precursor cells and thymocytes during and after the cell-to-cell interactions that occur within the epithelial microenvironment. Thymic hormonal factors promote essentially two categories of effects in T lymphocyte differentiation: (1) they promote the expression of T cell differentiation antigens, and (2) they promote the development of the subspecialized T cell functions. The effects may be augmented and are probably completed through cell interactions outside thymic cortex and by lymphokines produced by mature T lymphocytes in the thymic medulla and peripheral lymphoid organs.[5] Several thymic hormone substances have been described since their existence was first discovered in 1966[4]: thynosine, thymopoietin, facteur thymic serique, and thymic humoral factor.

Many polypeptides have been isolated from these preparations, and their amino acid sequences have been

Table 31-2. Differentiation antigens of thymocytes defined by antibodies

Antigen or cell distribution	Designation	Reference
Heteroantisera		
Human T lymphocyte antigen	HuTLA	37
Human thymocyte antigen	HTA-1	37
Human Ia-like antigen	HLA-DR	48
Terminal deoxynucleotidyl transferase	TdT	15,16
Monoclonal antibodies		
HLA-A,B,C framework	HLA	21
HLA-DR framework	DR	21
Sheep erythrocyte receptor	OKT 11, Leu 5	45,59
Prethymocyte-cortical thymocyte	OKT 10	59
HTA-1 antigen	OKT 6, NA1/34, Leu 6	59,80
Peripheral T cells, medullary thymocytes	OKT 3, Leu 4	59,66
Helper inducer-associated antigen	OKT 4, Leu 3a	28,59
Suppressor cytotoxic-associated antigen	OKT 8, Leu 2a	28,59

determined. A pentapeptide has been isolated that reproduces some of the hormonal effects and whose sequence corresponds to positions 32 to 36 of thymopoietin.[34] As yet no amino acid sequence homology has been established between the sequenced polypeptides. This suggests that a family of hormones may exist, each of which is possibly produced by separate thymic epithelial cells and has qualitatively different effects on maturing T lymphocytes. Immunohistochemical techniques have been used to localize at least two of the isolates to the thymic epithelium.[85]

During the process of intrathymic differentiation to immunocompetent cells, thymocytes undergo a sequential modulation of cell surface antigens that reflects this differentiation process. Table 31-2 is a partial list of cell surface antigen markers that have been used to study this phenomenon by several investigators.[49,50,101,110] Such studies have provided insight into the cellular dynamics of intrathymic differentiation of thymocytes, as illustrated in the composite scheme of Fig. 31-4. Most of the medullary thymocytes express surface antigens and functional characteristics of peripheral T lymphocytes. In contrast, cortical thymocytes, which are in varying stages of immaturity, express surface antigens that are not usually detectable on mature, functional T lymphocytes.

Immunohistologic studies of the thymic epithelial cells

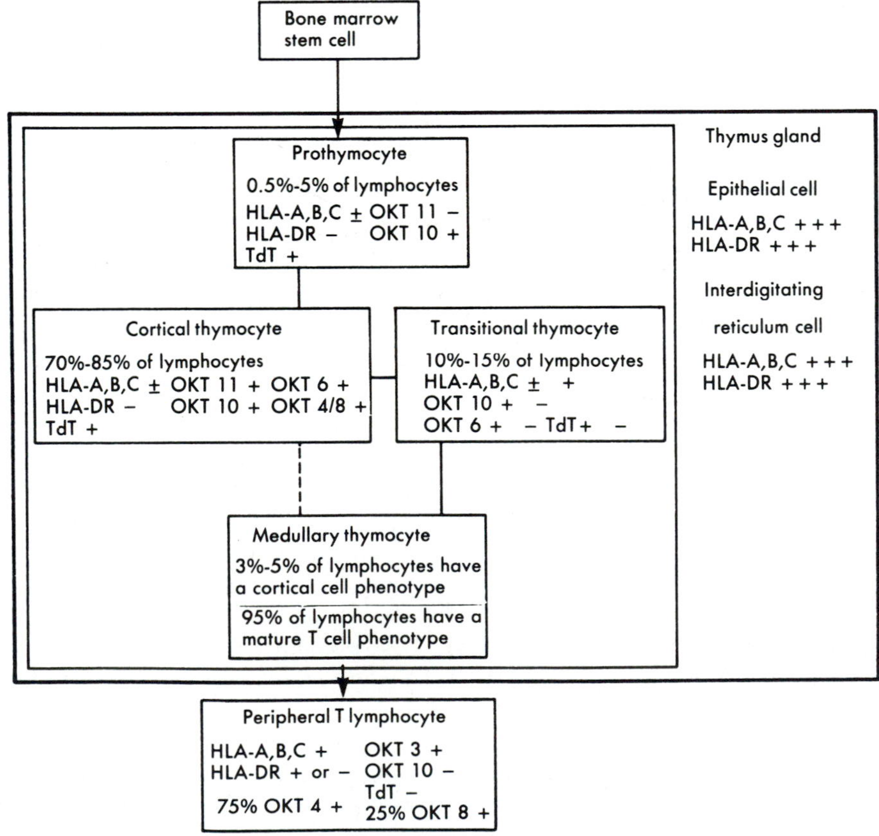

Fig. 31-4. Composite scheme of presumptive stages of intrathymic differentiation of thymocytes with correlation of cell-surface antigen expression.

indicate that cortical cells express large amounts of class II HLA antigens (HLA-DR) and moderate amounts of class I antigens (HLA-A,B,C). The more densely arranged medullary cells and the numerous interdigitating reticulum cells in the medulla express even larger amounts of both classes of antigen. In contrast, cortical thymocytes do not express detectable amounts of these antigens on their surfaces but do express large amounts of thymocyte-associated antigens and nuclear terminal deoxynucleotidyl transferase (TdT), a unique enzyme that may have the role of a somatic mutagen. The highly organized microenvironment of the thymic cortical epithelium permits an efficient interaction of cortical thymocytes that are deficient in MHC antigens with epithelial cells replete with these antigens in a milieu of very high concentrations of various hormonal factors. It is not yet known how these interactions influence the selection of precursor cells for survival, clonal expansion, and differentiation. It is known that the rate of differentiation from precursor to mature cell is very low, since about 95% of precursors die in situ.[81] This profound negative influence, possibly abetted by somatic mutation[51] in a strictly MHC antigen–controlled microenvironment, is believed to select for a T lymphocyte repertoire appropriate to the individual. Unlike cortical thymocytes, medullary thymocytes express MHC antigens and no nuclear TdT. Only rare medullary thymocytes express the phenotype of cortical thymocytes. These cells are thought to have just entered the medulla, where further maturation occurs before they exit to the peripheral lymphoid tissues.

INVOLUTION

The thymus gland normally decreases in size and weight with advancing age after puberty, resulting in the replacement of parenchyma by adipose tissue. This process of aging, called age or physiologic involution, is accompanied by gradual changes in thymocyte populations relative to different rates of involution of the cortical and medullary epithelium.[42,94,132] In the young adult the parenchymal loss is primarily that of decreasing numbers of cortical thymocytes, with relative sparing of the epithelial architecture. With advancing age the epithelial component becomes atrophied, and the gland consists of isles of spindle-shaped epithelial cells, with partially cystic, closely arranged Hassall's corpuscles and occasional small lymphocytes in abundant adipose tissue (Fig. 31-5). This gradual involution of the thymus after puberty is followed more gradually by a decrease in the volume of the peripheral T lymphocyte compartment.[77]

The thymus gland with active lymphopoiesis responds dramatically to episodes of severe stress by a loss in size

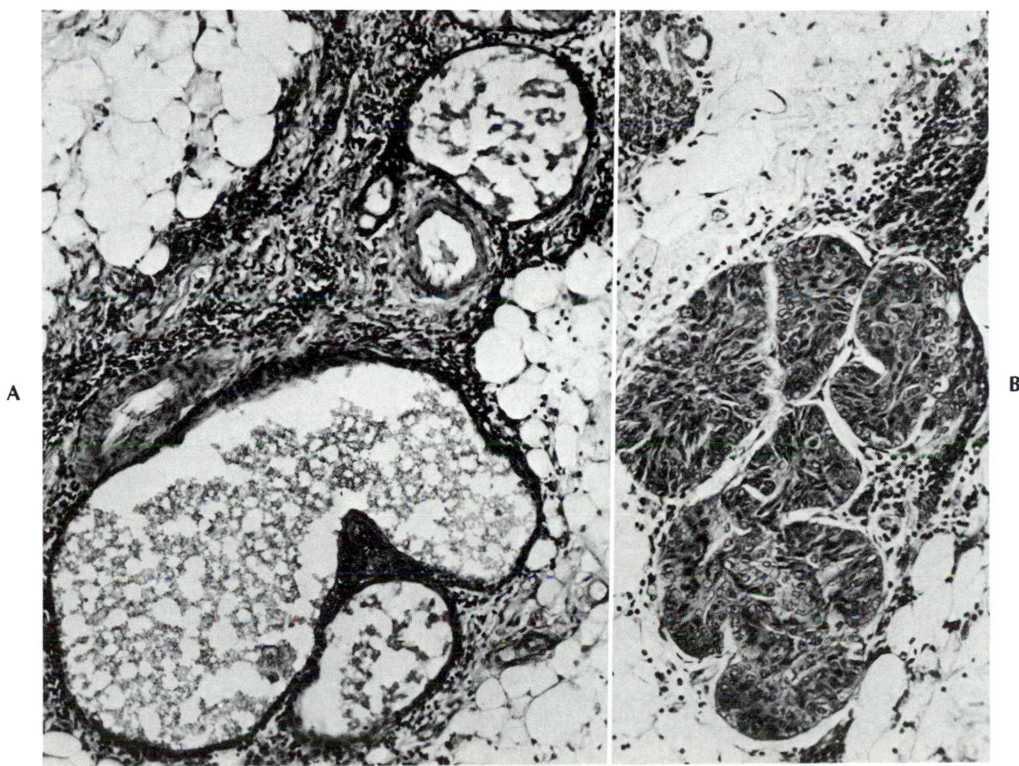

Fig. 31-5. Chronic involution of thymus. **A,** Cystic degeneration with epithelial cell atrophy and thymocyte depletion. **B,** Islets of spindle-shaped epithelial cells in abundant adipose tissue. (165×.)

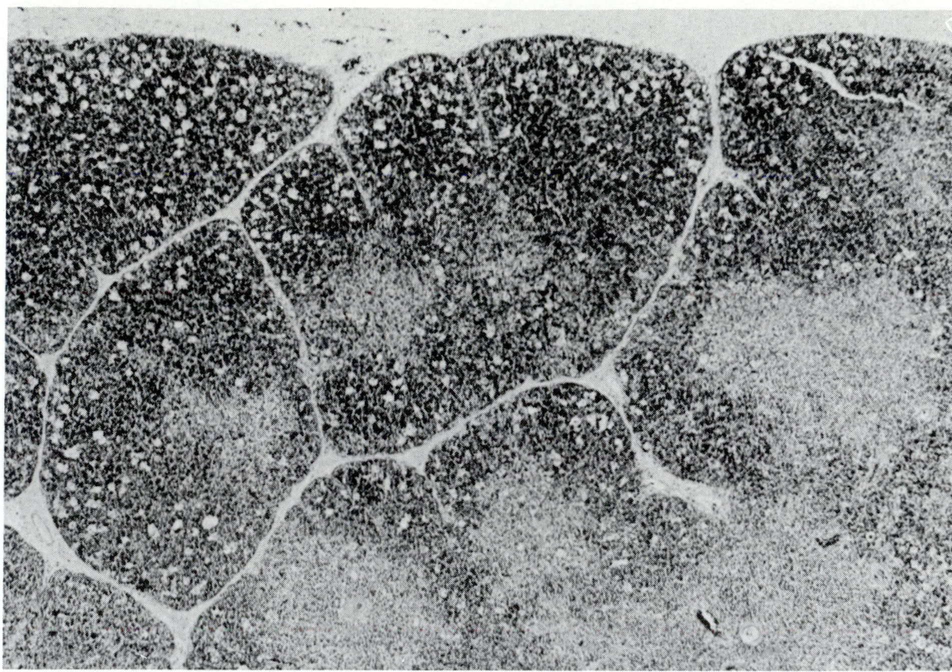

Fig. 31-6. Acute (stress or accidental) involution of thymus. Cortex exhibits prominent lympholysis and associated phagocytosis by macrophages—numerous "starry-sky" spaces. (55×.)

and weight, principally as a result of a loss of cortical thymocytes. A striking decrease in thymic size may be observed by roentgenogram within 24 hours of the onset of the illness. This process of accidental or stress involution is mediated in part by the release of corticosteroids from the adrenal cortex, which results in rapid lympholysis of the cortical lymphocytes. Microscopically a prominent karyorrhexis of lymphocytes and phagocytosis of debris by numerous macrophages are seen in the early period (Fig. 31-6). If the stimulus continues, the extensive lympholysis results in a loss of corticomedullary distinction and an accentuation of the epithelial cells, cystic Hassall's corpuscles, and elongated epithelial-lined cystic spaces. With further loss of thymocytes, the lobular architecture progressively collapses and fibrosis ensues. It is unlikely that this process ever results in a deficiency of the immune system after the patient recovers from the primary disease.

CONGENITAL ANOMALIES

Faulty embryogenesis of the thymus gland may result in a failure of migration, an aberrant localization of thymic tissue, or a failure of development associated with one of the varieties of primary immunodeficiency disorders (discussed in the next section). Failure of the thymic primordium to descend into the mediastinum may result in the development of one or both lobes in the neck, where it can produce symptoms of respiratory obstruction requiring its removal.[2] A more common occurrence is the appearance of thymic tissue nodules in the lateral neck or within or adjacent to the parathyroid or thyroid glands. Likewise parathyroid glands may be observed within the thymus gland, reflecting their close embryogenetic relationship. Cystic degenerative changes usually occur in the cervical thymic nodules, which leads to their clinical discovery. Such aberrant thymic nodules occur in perhaps 20% of the population[33] and may rarely be found outside the cervical migratory route.

PRIMARY IMMUNODEFICIENCY DISEASE

The primary immunodeficiency disorders are a heterogeneous group of genetic or acquired cellular defects that result in the faulty maturation, regulation, or function of antigen-specific lymphocytes. Concepts derived from the study of patients with these disorders as well as from experimental systems have rapidly expanded our understanding of developmental immunobiology. Only recently have these disorders been studied at the cellular and molecular levels in humans.[35,135] It may be hoped that the increasing understanding of the pathogenesis of these disorders will lead to the development of more specific approaches for the management of these patients.

The current classification of these disorders is based on criteria[32] that define an altered function of B or T lymphocytes or both. As a group, these disorders are rarely encountered in clinical medicine, since their frequency is less than 1 case per 50,000 to 100,000 individuals.[127] In patients with combined B and T lymphocyte immunode-

Table 31-3. Immunodeficiency disorders associated with an abnormal thymus gland

Syndrome	Inheritance	Associated findings
COMBINED IMMUNODEFICIENCIES		
Severe combined immunodeficiency		
Reticular dysgenesis	AR	Phagocytes absent
Swiss-type agammaglobulinemia	AR	
Thymic alymphoplasia	AR/ XL	
Adenosine deaminase	AR	Cartilage abnormalities
Ataxia telangiectasia	AR	Cerebellar ataxia Telangiectasia Chromosomal abnormalities Endocrine abnormalities Dyschrondroplasia
Wiskott-Aldrich syndrome	XL	Thrombocytopenia Eczema
Short-limbed dwarfism, type I	AR	Cartilage and hair hypoplasia Neutropenia
CELLULAR IMMUNODEFICIENCIES		
Thymic hypoplasia	S	HI variable Hypoparathyroidism Cardiovascular abnormalities Megaloblastic anemia
Nezelof syndrome	AR	HI variable
Purine nucleoside phosporylase deficiency	AR	HI variable Hypoplastic anemia
Short-limbed dwarfism, type II	AR	See type I

CMI, Cell-mediated immunity; *HI,* humoral immunity; *AR,* autosomal recessive; *XL,* X-linked recessive; *S,* sporadic.

ficiencies, dysplasia of the thymus is almost a constant feature. There are two exceptions: DiGeorge syndrome, or thymic hypoplasia, in which the thymus gland is hypoplastic or simply absent because of a variable failure in the embryogenesis of the pharyngeal pouches, and the two immunodeficiency disorders associated with defects in purine catabolism—adenosine deaminase deficiency and purine nucleoside phosphorylase deficiency—in which the thymus may appear normal, involuted, or dysplastic.[18,82] The thymus is generally normal in pure B lymphocyte deficiencies, except when accidental involution supervenes. Specific immunodeficiency diseases in which the thymus gland is abnormal are listed in Table 31-3.

The thymus gland that is fully dysplastic is often small, perhaps weighing as little as 1 g, and may not have completely descended into the mediastinum. It appears embryonal, with small lobules composed of spindle-shaped epithelial cells that are essentially devoid of lymphocytes (Fig. 31-7). Corticomedullary differentiation and Hassall's corpuscles are characteristically absent, although rudimentary development of these features may be present in some patients with cellular immunodeficiency. There is greater variation in the histology of thymic dysplasia in surgical biopsy specimens than in thymus glands examined at autopsy.[18,115] In some surgical biopsies the epithelial cells may be larger and less atrophic, and larger numbers of lymphocytes and phagocytic cells may be present. Often the degree of immune function abnormality does not correlate directly with the degree of dysplasia observed in the thymus. This range of morphologic expression of thymic dysplasia may reflect the heterogeneous nature of immunodeficiency, the stage of progression of the disorder, or the lack of involutional changes, which must compound the autopsy histologic findings. Thymic histopathologic characteristics similar to those of thymic dysplasia of primary immunodeficiency disease have been observed in infants as a consequence of graft-versus-host disease following blood transfusions.[114]

Recently it has been recognized that infants with combined immunodeficiencies have an increased incidence of malignant lymphoproliferative diseases.[122] These fatal lymphomas have occurred following immunoreconstitution with cultured thymic epithelium grafts and spontaneously in untreated persons.[17,58] Appreciable numbers of both non-Hodgkin's lymphomas and Hodgkin's disease have now been described.[31] The frequency distribution among the various subvarieties of both Hodgkin's and non-Hodgkin's lymphoma appears to be different from that of the general pediatric population, and among the non-Hodgkin's lymphomas of B lymphocyte origin, both clonal (expression of a single light chain by the tumor cells) and polyclonal tumors have been described.

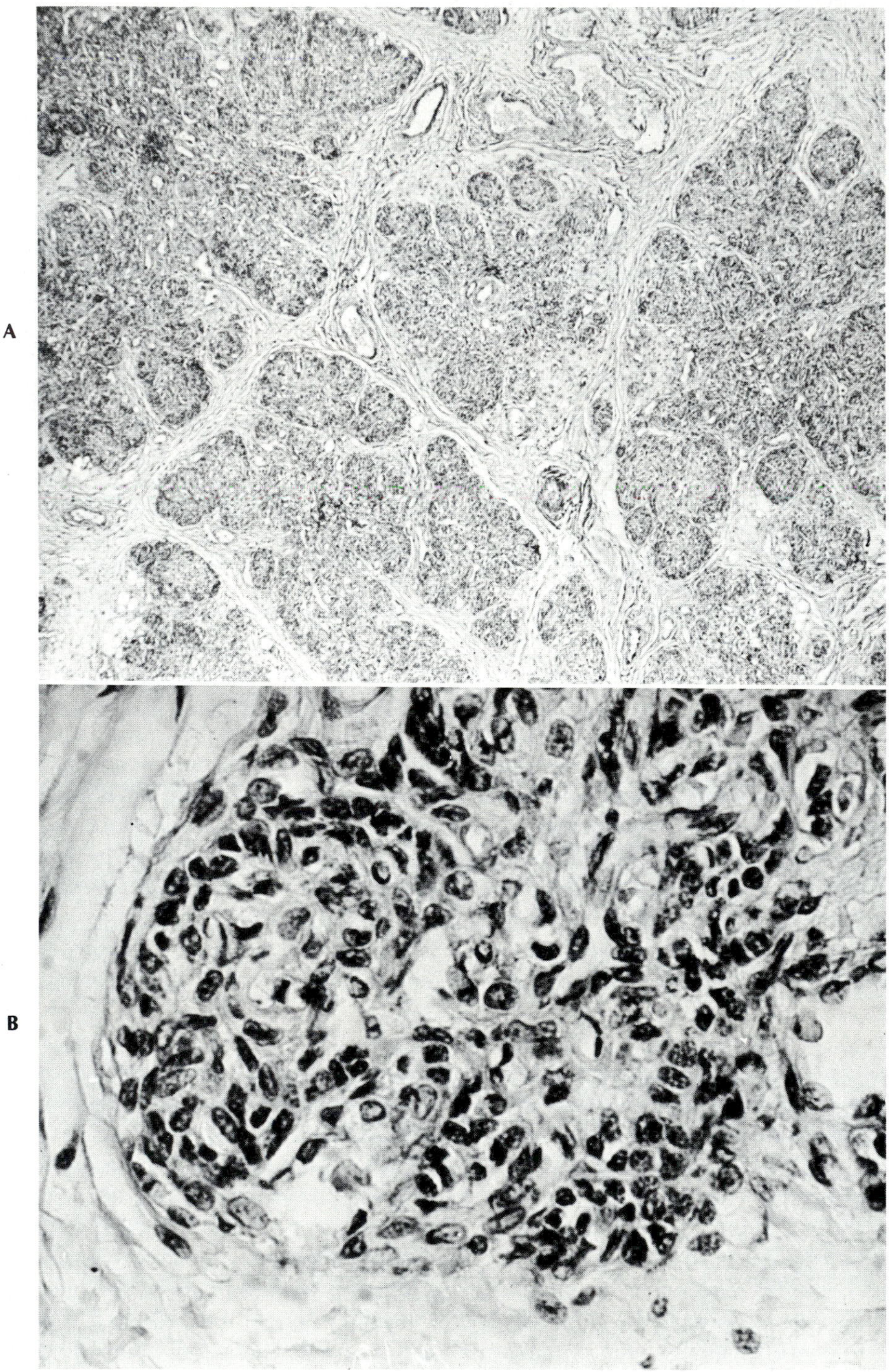

Fig. 31-7. Thymic dysplasia in severe combined immunodeficiency, thymic alymphoplasia. Poorly developed lobules are composed of spindle-shaped epithelial cells and are mostly devoid of thymocytes and Hassall's corpuscles. (**A,** 52×; **B,** 486×.)

The Epstein-Barr virus nuclear antigen has also been demonstrated within the neoplastic cell infiltrate of one polyclonal lymphoma following thymic epithelium engraftment.[100] This observation implicates one possible pathogenic mechanism for the increased incidence of fatal lymphomas in these patients, namely ineffective cellular immunity to ubiquitous agents that are trophic for B lymphocytes and vigorously stimulate their proliferation.[140]

THYMIC CYSTS

Cystic lesions of the thymus gland are acquired lesions of thymic tissue that may be found anywhere along the lines of thymic descent, from the angle of the mandible to the body of the sternum. Thymic cysts are distinguished from other cysts by the presence of thymic tissue in their walls. These simple cysts are lined by epithelium that may be flattened, columnar, squamous, or ciliated and are filled with accumulated fluid, cellular debris, and hemorrhagic extravasation. Leakage of these contents into the surrounding tissues may simulate infectious granulomatous inflammation. Although some may be developmental in origin and derived from the third bronchial pouch, the origin of most thymic cysts—whether mediastinal or cervical in location—appears to be degenerating Hassall's corpuscles or secondarily formed spaces in the thymus. An unusual intrathoracic thymic cyst that has been described in a 2-year-old girl contained not only thymic tissue in its walls but also parathyroid and salivary gland tissue, all tissue of pharyngeal origin.[20] Cystic lesions of other derivations arising in the thymus or in the same locations as thymic cysts include developmental cysts of the respiratory, gastrointestinal, pericardial, and lymphatic systems. Cystic degeneration of thymomas is common and may obscure the recognition of the neoplasm.

THYMIC HYPERPLASIA

The concept of thymic hyperplasia generically embrances two morphologic forms.[73] The first form, massive or giant thymic hyperplasia, is considered true hyperplasia and is a dramatic enlargement of the gland through an increase in the cellular elements, which remain normally organized. Because of the wide weight variation of normal thymus glands throughout the population, the establishment of borderline hyperplasia is frequently problematic. Before 1931 and the establishment of standard growth curves of the normal thymus,[139] a normally large thymus and proliferative lymphoid system were frequently misinterpreted as a contributing cause of sudden respiratory death in infancy and led to the now-archaic concept of "status thymolymphaticus." Nevertheless, thymus glands that are histologically unremarkable can weigh in excess of 200 g and are infrequently reported in infants[56,67,95] and children.[60] The pathogenesis and significance of enlargement to this degree are unknown. Lymphocytosis, presumably antigen-responsive T lymphocytes,[95] and an expansion of the thymus-dependent regions of lymph nodes often accompany thymic hyperplasia and resolve following thymectomy. Although patients have done well subsequently, selective hypogammaglobulinemia developed in one infant 2 years after operation.[67]

The second form of thymic hyperplasia is characterized by the presence of lymphoid follicles with active germinal centers in thymus glands that are infrequently increased in size or weight (Fig. 31-8). Lymphoid follicles are found in otherwise normal individuals, as judged by studies of thymus glands examined in victims of sudden accidental death[83] or removed incidentally during cardiac surgery.[130] The prevalence of lymphoid follicles in these studies ranged from 83% in patients under 20 years of age to 25% in young adults. General autopsy studies have reported incidences of from 0.01% to 11%. However, the populations in the latter studies suffer the bias of stress of chronic disease and various therapies that are capable of causing involution of lymphoid organs. A realistic overall incidence of follicular hyperplasia is somewhere between these extremes, perhaps 40%, with a greater prevalence in the young.

The presence of lymphoid follicles in the thymus gland is associated with a large number of diseases, most of which are believed to have an autoimmune basis or secondary immune complications: myasthenia gravis, primary hyperthyroidism, systemic lupus erythematosus, rheumatoid arthritis, scleroderma, allergic vasculitides, aplastic anemia, chronic liver disease, various endocrinopathies, and chronic glomerulonephritis. Myasthenia gravis is the disease most commonly associated with follicular hyperplasia, occurring in 85% of patients with this disease who have thymic abnormalities. It is the only disease among this large group in which follicular hyperplasia is most prevalent in and largely restricted to the thymus gland.[118] Thymic follicular hyperplasia associated with other disease processes appears to be a local manifestation of generalized follicular hyperplasia. The lymphoid follicles apparently arise at the corticomedullary junction or within the medulla and have been found to be no different morphologically, ultrastructurally, or immunologically from those of peripheral lymphoid organs.[70,123,128] Thymomas are often associated with many of these same disorders, implicating a role for the thymus gland in the pathogenesis of these diseases. The nature of this involvement is as yet unclear.

Equally unclear is the role that thymectomy should have in the therapy of nonthymomatous glands of patients with myasthenia gravis.[26,87] The principal advantage of thymectomy is the possibility of permanent improvement or remission that occurs in some cases after a 10-year interval.[1] Surgery is generally reserved for young patients who have moderately severe disease that is progressive despite medical treatment.

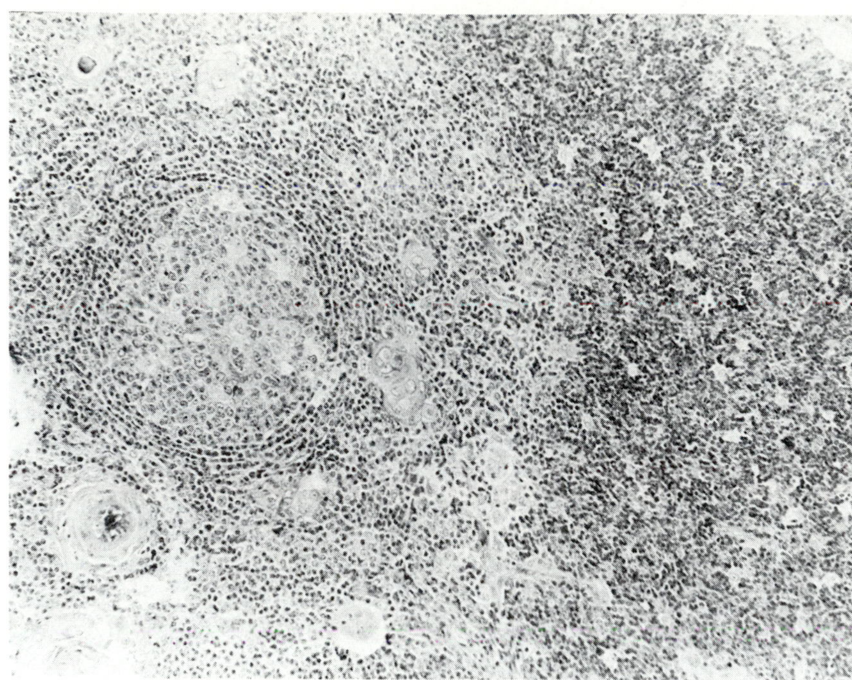

Fig. 31-8. Thymic hyperplasia. Active germinal centers in lymphoid constitute one form of hyperplasia. Although this form is often associated with myasthenia gravis, this patient was otherwise asymptomatic. (200×.)

NEOPLASMS

Thymoma

The generic term *thymoma* has been applied in the past to all neoplasms arising primarily in the thymus gland. More recently this designation has been restricted to neoplasms of the thymic epithelial cells based on pathobiologic considerations.[106] Other primary tumors of the thymus gland are now classified by their homologous identity to primary neoplasms in other locations—for example, malignant lymphomas, germ cell tumors, and neuroendocrine tumors.

The prevalence of thymomas in a population increases with increasing age of the individual until after the fifth decade, when it begins to decline. The expected incidence in a large metropolitan hospital is about 1 case per 10,000 to 20,000 admissions,[87] and the mean age of the patients at diagnosis is about 48 years. Thymomas are rarely seen before 20 years of age, and both sexes and different races are affected proportionally. In over 50% of patients, thymomas are asymptomatic and are discovered by routine roentgenographic examination, which shows lobated, anterior mediastinal masses. Linear calcification may be observed at the tumor's periphery in some cases. In the remaining patients, symptoms resulting from systemic diseases associated with thymoma, primarily myasthenia gravis, or symptoms resulting from the presence of the tumor itself, such as cough, dyspnea, dysphasia, chest pain, or superior vena cava compression, precede the tumor's discovery.[13,111] Superior vena cava syndrome or pain usually indicates tumor invasion. Evidence of associated systemic diseases is discovered in 65% to 70% of all patients with symptoms.[87]

Typically thymomas occur in the anterior mediastinum as well-encapsulated tumors that are easily removed surgically, although they can also arise in ectopic sites such as in the neck along the route of embryonic migration.[104] In about 20% to 25% of cases the tumor is adherent to surrounding tissues, and most often microscopic invasion of these tissues can be demonstrated.[79] Over half of the thymomas measure between 5 and 10 cm in greatest diameter and weigh an average of 150 g.[106] Tumors not associated with myasthenia gravis often weigh more. However, rare thymomas of microscopic size or of gigantic proportions weighing more than 5 kg do occur.[119] The cut surface of the neoplasm usually reveals a thick fibrous capsule surrounding tumor lobules of varying sizes that are separated by prominent, fibrous trabeculae. Cystic degeneration of thymomas is not uncommon and may be so extensive as to obscure the presence of the neoplasm (Fig. 31-9).

Thymomas display a wide variation in their microscopic appearances, a fact that has frustrated the development of an acceptable classification scheme. Most thymomas are composed of an admixture of epithelial cells and lymphocytes (Fig. 31-10), and they have been classified based on the ratio of these cell types—predomi-

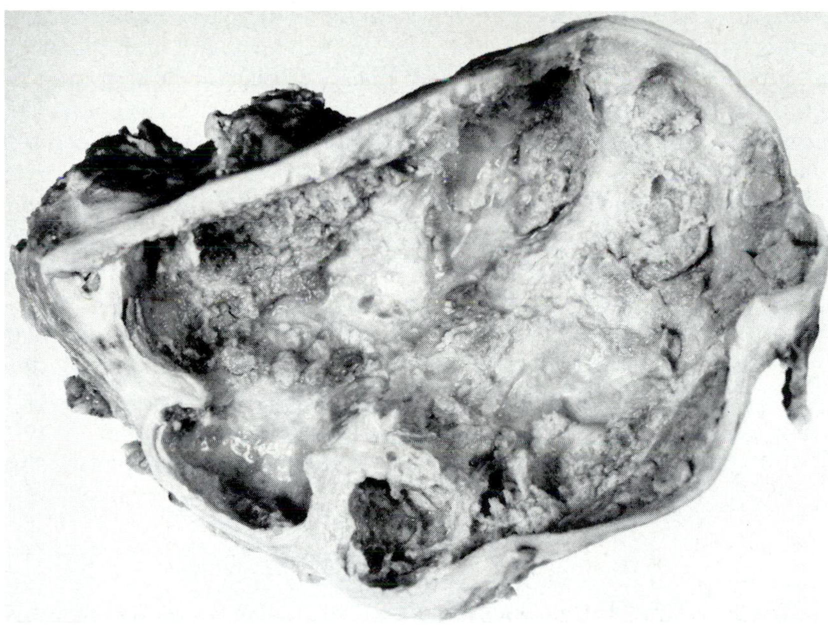

Fig. 31-9. Cystic degeneration of thymoma. Large central cyst was filled with necrotic, liquefied debris. Viable tumor was found microscopically in thick wall and in papillae that line cyst.

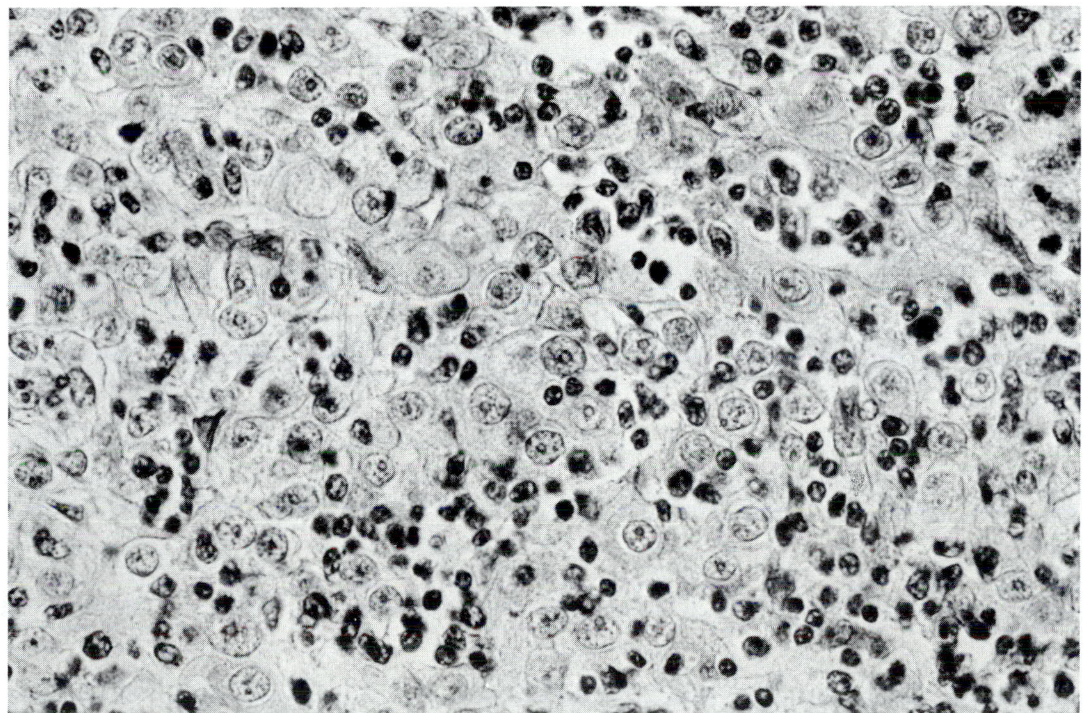

Fig. 31-10. Thymoma. Thymocytes are mixed with neoplastic epithelial cells. (585×.)

nantly lymphocytic, mixed, and predominantly epithelial. Only rarely are thymomas purely epithelial.[106] Thymomas have also been classified according to the cytologic structure of the neoplastic epithelial cells—round, polygonal, spindle, or mixed. These distinctions are arbitrary, since the ratio of lymphocytes to epithelial cells and the cytologic structure and growth patterns of the neoplastic epithelial component often show considerable variation even within the same tumor.

The neoplastic epithelial cells in thymomas are usually large, with a round or oval vesicular nucleus and indistinct, eosinophilic cytoplasm. The nucleolus is usually inconspicuous, although it may infrequently be prominent in some tumors. Mitoses are rare among the epithelial cells but may readily be present in the lymphocytic component, accompanied by prominent lympholysis and "starry-sky" phagocytosis of nuclear debris. Such cases can be misdiagnosed as malignant lymphoma if the arrangement and growth pattern of the epithelial component are not carefully observed. Electron microscopy can be especially useful in establishing or excluding the diagnosis of thymoma in such cases by demonstrating the epithelial qualities of the neoplastic cells.[74] Spindle-shaped cells are often present, and when they predominate, the tumor is described as a spindle cell thymoma. Transitional, polygon-shaped cells may be present in any tumor, or they may be the predominant cell type. Rare thymomas showing differentiation toward both epithelial cells and myoid cells have also been observed.[41] The growth patterns of the neoplastic epithelial cells may be strikingly variable (Fig. 31-11). Some tumors grow in prominent whorled, storiformed, or broad fasicular patterns. Others may show rosettelike or adenomatoid patterns or may resemble hemangiopericytomas.[106] Microcystic degeneration may be extensive in some tumors. Well-formed Hassall's corpuscles are rarely found in thy-

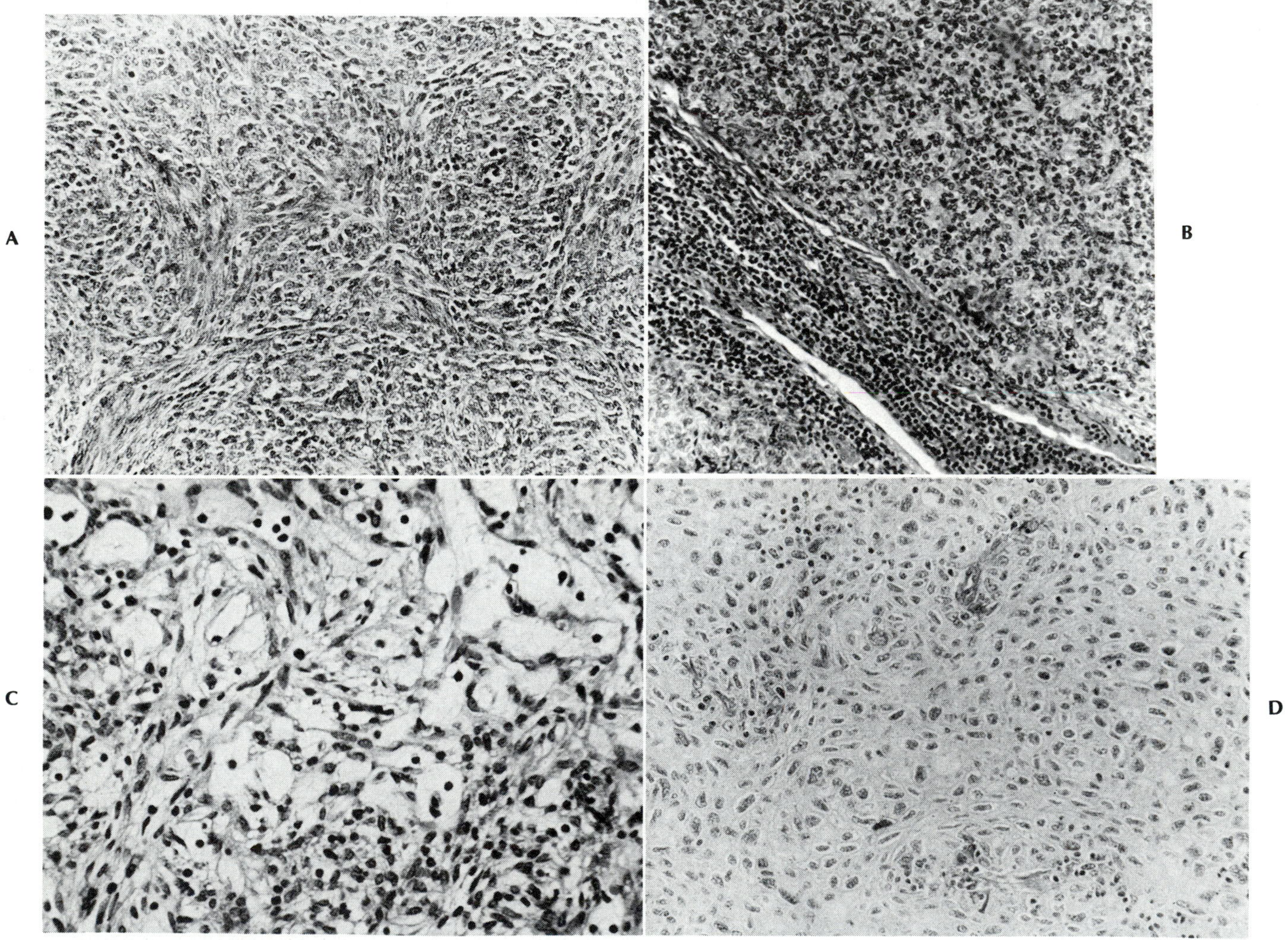

Fig. 31-11. Variable cytologic patterns exhibited by thymomas. **A,** Fascicular, spindled pattern. **B,** Rosettelike pattern. **C,** Microcystic pattern. **D,** Cytologically malignant pattern.

momas but may be entrapped by the growing tumor. Quite often normal thymic tissue is found adjacent to lobules of the thymoma. Thymic follicular hyperplasia may be observed in the adjacent tissue and, rarely, within the thymoma itself. This finding is common in cases associated with myasthenia gravis.[87]

The lymphocytic component of thymomas is not thought to be neoplastic, yet a close relationship appears to exist between lymphocytes and the tumor cells even in sites of metastases,[136] suggesting the persistence of the functional properties of the epithelial cell. Most lymphocytes in thymomas have cell surface antigens characteristic of normal thymocytes.[24,71] Interestingly, the maturational state of lymphocytes in predominantly lymphocytic thymomas is similar to that of the normal cortical thymocyte, whereas in predominantly epithelial tumors it resembles that of the more mature medullary thymocyte or peripheral T cell.[62,63] T cell lymphocytosis has also been observed in association with thymomas.[38,97]

Thymomas are extremely slow-growing neoplasms that usually remain localized even to one lobe of the thymus gland for many years before invading adjacent structures. Invasion of adjacent structures, such as lung or pericardium, occurs in about 20% to 25% of the patients, 66% of whom have symptoms.[13] Distant metastases occur very rarely and most frequently involve the lung, lymph nodes, liver, axial skeleton, and central nervous system.[36,39] Thymomas should be excised before invasion has occurred, since tumor recurrence and death as a direct result of noninvasive tumors are rare.[29,61,68] Even recurrences as localized mediastinal masses or pleural implants are amenable to secondary complete resection.[36] If primary or secondary complete resection is not accomplished, death from cardiorespiratory complications of tumor invasion will result. The histopathologic structure of the thymoma, other than the documentation of invasion (which may be difficult to ascertain macroscopically), provides little insight into a tumor's malignant biologic potential. However, some tumors do display marked cytologic atypia in the neoplastic epithelial component (Fig. 31-11, *D*) and should be considered cytologically malignant.[73] These true thymic carcinomas are more likely to be invasive and to metastasize. A diagnosis of thymic carcinoma implies the exclusion of secondary involvement of the thymus gland by metastatic carcinoma, especially from the lung. Pleomorphic sarcomatous thymomas of myoid cell derivation have also been reported.[30]

The long-term survival of patients with thymomas also depends on whether there is an associated systemic disease, primarily myasthenia gravis. Almost 90% of patients with fully excised, noninvasive tumors who do not develop myasthenia gravis are alive after 10 years, whereas there are no survivors with invasive thymomas plus myasthenia gravis. Considering all patients with thymoma, the survival rate at 1 year is 84%, at 3 years 77%, at 5 years 74%, and at 10 years 57%.[79] The 5-year survival rate for patients with localized or disseminated disease is 50%. Thymomas in children, although uncommon, are much more aggressive than those in adults and have a considerably poorer prognosis.[19,25] Adjuvant radiotherapy and chemotherapy are clearly indicated for patients after partial resection, but the role of postoperative irradiation after total resection of a noninvasive tumor is controversial.[1,8,12] Recent reports indicate that postoperative radiotherapy may be advantageous in reducing local tumor recurrences.[79,92]

Systemic disorders and thymomas

Thymomas have been described repeatedly in association with a large variety of systemic diseases.[121] These include myasthenia gravis (10% to 15% of cases),[87] acquired hypogammaglobulinemia (12% of cases),[98] erythroid hypoplasia (5% of cases),[43] and, less commonly (1% or less of cases), myositis, dermatomyositis, myocarditis, scleroderma, systemic lupus erythematosus, thyroiditis, Sjögren's syndrome, rheumatoid arthritis, pemphigus, and chronic mucocutaneous candidiasis. Cushing's syndrome, previously reported in association with thymomas, occurs in association with primary thymic neuroendocrine tumors (thymic carcinoid tumors).[105] A 20% incidence of nonthymic malignancy occurs in patients with thymomas.[120]

Various divergent mechanisms of autoimmunity are thought to function in each of these disease processes. What possible relationships exist in these infrequent associations with thymomas is unclear. As a group, myasthenia gravis patients with thymomas are older than myasthenia gravis patients without tumors but are younger than patients with thymomas that are not associated with myasthenia.[137] These patients generally have a more severe form of myasthenia and higher mortality than myasthenia patients without thymomas.[87] The correlation of the histologic appearance of thymomas and the presence or absence of an associated syndrome has not been successful, except perhaps in myasthenia gravis, in which spindle cell thymomas are rarely if ever observed. In patients with myasthenia gravis, thymectomy has been ineffectual or has resulted in clinical improvement and, less frequently, in remission of the disorder in some patients.[96] Parodoxically myasthenia gravis has also followed the complete excision of thymomas in other patients.[87] Resection of thymomas in patients with other associated diseases has resulted in improvement in only a minority of patients, principally those with erythroid hypoplasia. The clinical course of patients with an associated syndrome is determined less by the usually clinically benign thymic tumor than by the relentless progression of the systemic disease. This observation has been especially true for those patients with hemopoietic disorders and for patients with myasthenia gravis beyond the first 5 years, when survival differences become apparent.

Thymolipoma

Thymolipomas are rare, benign, encapsulated neoplasms of uncertain origin that arise within the thymus gland. They are usually seen initially as asymptomatic mediastinal masses that may attain a very large size, even more than 16 kg, although most tumors weigh from 500 to 2000 g.[106] These tumors generally assume the configuration of the normal gland and are composed histologically of normal thymic tissue, which in reality is excessive for age, and abundant mature adipose tissue.[14] One plausible explanation for this lesion is that it represents involution with compensatory fatty infiltration of previously unrecognized massive thymic hyperplasia. Although myasthenia gravis is not associated with thymolipomas, hyperthyroidism,[11] hypoplastic anemia,[7] and synchronous pharyngeal lipoma[129] have been observed in patients with thymolipomas.

Neuroendocrine (carcinoid) tumors

Until 1972, neoplasms arising from neuroendocrine cells of the thymus gland were confused with true thymomas of epithelial cell origin.[105] Rosai and Higa observed that these neoplasms have biologic and morphologic features that are distinctly different from those of thymomas; namely, they are malignant neoplasms that are often invasive and that metastasize in about 30% of the cases. These tumors, unlike thymomas, are associated with Cushing's syndrome in about one third of cases[73] but with no other endocrine aberrations. However, these neoplasms do occur in association with multiple endocrine adenomatosis[107] and with bronchial and gastrointestinal carcinoid tumors.[105]

Morphologically these neoplasms most often resemble carcinoid tumors by their pseudoacinar pattern of growth of well-defined, uniform tumor cells. Mitotic activity is often high, and necrosis with calcification may be present in areas of solid cell growth. Numerous neurosecretory granules are typically seen ultrastructurally. Several morphologic varieties of primary thymic neuroendocrine tumor occur: tumors resembling undifferentiated small cell carcinoma of the lung that are highly malignant[108]; tumors resembling spindle cell thymoma[72]; tumors that produce melanin[44]; and tumors resembling medullary thyroid carcinoma[69] with abundant amyloid deposition (Fig. 31-12). The treatment of these neoplasms is primarily surgical, since long-term survival has followed complete excision of these tumors.

Germ cell tumors

Primary germ cell tumors homologous to those in the gonads arise in the thymus and include adult teratoma, seminoma, embryonal carcinoma, teratocarcinoma, yolk sac tumor, and choriocarcinoma. It is generally accepted that these tumors have an origin similar to other midline extragonadal germ cell tumors—that is, an errant germ cell migration during embryogenesis[117]—but direct evidence of their cytogenesis is lacking. Mediastinal metastasis of primary gonadal tumors is rare but should always

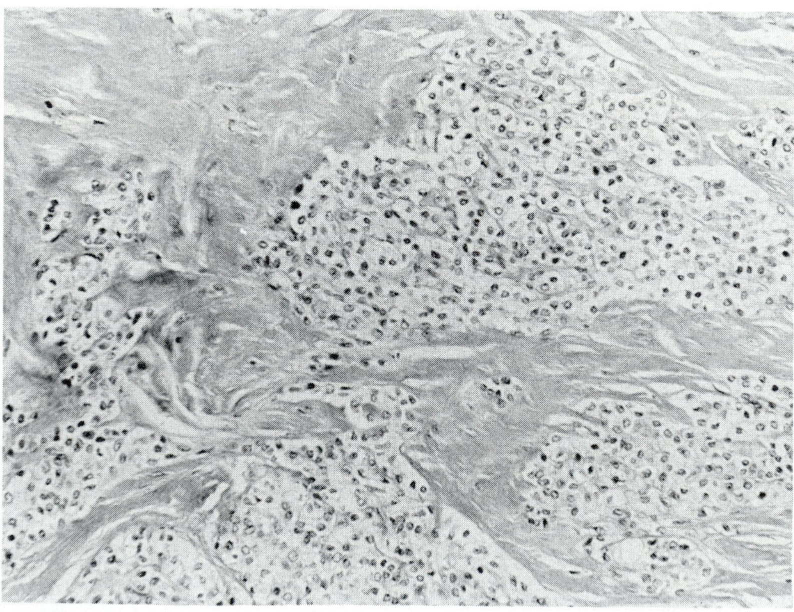

Fig. 31-12. Neuroendocrine (carcinoid) tumor. Tumor consists of solid areas of uniform cells with cleared cytoplasm arranged in abundant amyloid stroma. (900×.)

be considered as an alternative possibility. Most of the mediastinal germ cell tumors are benign adult teratomas. The malignant tumors have a predilection for men in the second and third decades of life, and as a group these tumors are highly malignant neoplasms that have poor prognoses. However, seminomas are highly radiosensitive, and postoperative radiotherapy affords an excellent prognosis in most cases.[112,124] Microscopically, thymic germ cell neoplasms resemble their gonadal counterparts (Fig. 31-13). Thymic tissue can usually be found within these neoplasms or in the walls of their capsules, and it is often possible to find teratoid elements in thymic seminomas. Thymic seminomas can be confused with thymomas and occasionally with granulomatous lesions, both benign and malignant. The excellent prognosis of such a tumor when properly treated, compared with thymomas and other malignant germ cell tumors, requires its separate recognition.[69]

Malignant lymphoma

Malignant lymphomas often involve the thymus gland primarily and by extension from parathymic lymph

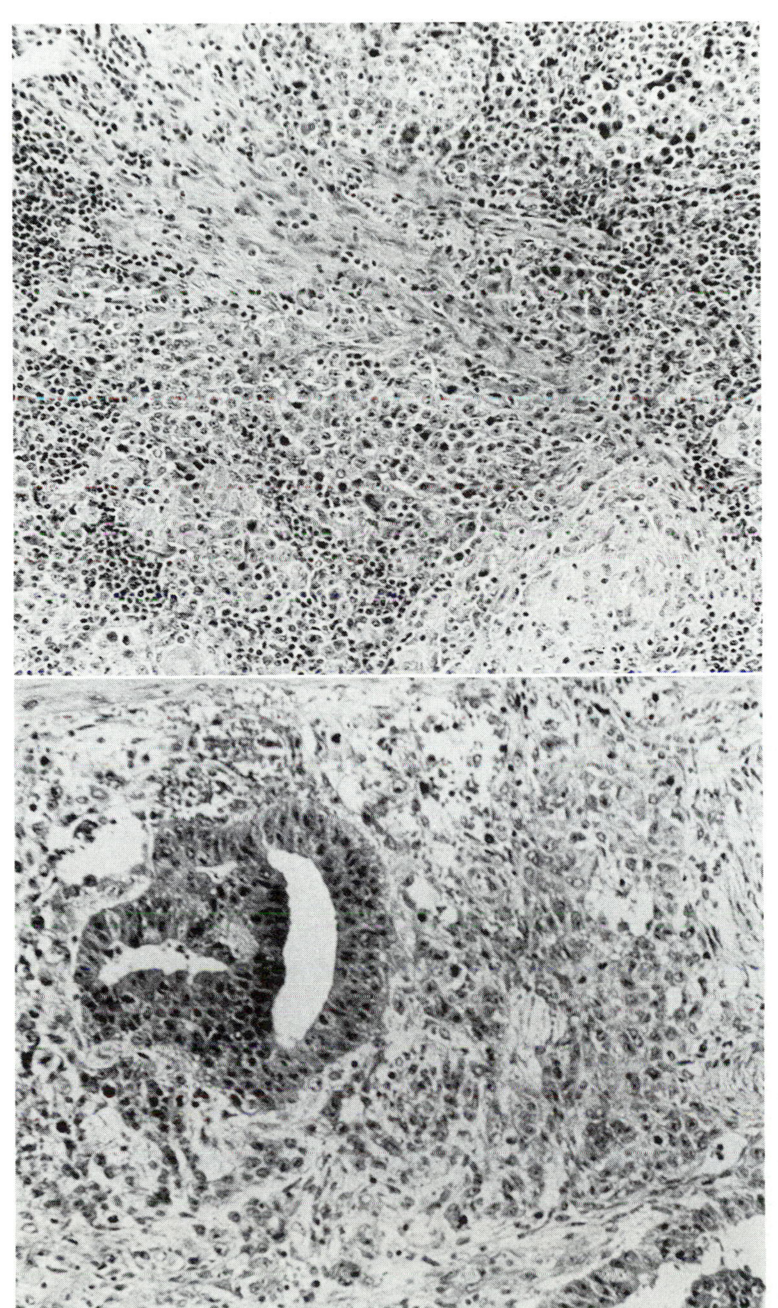

Fig. 31-13. Primary germ cell tumors of thymus gland. **A,** Seminoma. **B,** Teratocarcinoma. (900×.)

nodes; primarily, Hodgkin's disease, lymphoblastic lymphoma, and large cell lymphoma are encountered. Other varieties of lymphoma rarely involve the mediastinum initially. Although clearly distinct entities, these tumors may provide diagnostic difficulties with thymoma that ultrastructural and immunologic studies may not easily resolve. In contrast to thymomas, malignant lymphomas generally affect a younger population, demonstrate different patterns and more rapid rates of dissemination, and respond to nonsurgical therapeutic modalities (see Chapter 30).

Primary Hodgkin's disease of the thymus gland was once regarded as granulomatous thymoma, a variant of thymoma.[76] The nodular sclerosing variety is by far the most common subtype of Hodgkin's disease of the thymus gland (Fig. 31-14). Thymic involvement by Hodgkin's disease superficially resembles thymoma because of the nodular bands of fibrosis and the peculiar hyperplastic response of the thymic epithelial cells,[55] resulting in spindle cell areas and epithelium-lined cysts. However, in Hodgkin's disease the fibrous bands are rounded, not angulated, the epithelial hyperplasia is never pervasive throughout the tissue, and diagnostic Reed-Sternberg cells are identifiable, although occasionally with some difficulty.[91] Prognostic differences between thymic Hodgkin's disease and mediastinal lymph node disease have not been observed.[57] Only a single case of synchronously occurring thymoma and Hodgkin's disease of the thymus has been reported,[103] although one case each of thymic Hodgkin's disease,[93] myasthenia gravis,[93] and erythroid hypoplasia,[102] diseases of known association with thymoma, has been reported.

Lymphoblastic lymphoma was first recognized in 1905 as lymphocytic sarcoma involving the mediastinum that terminated in acute leukemia.[125] Characteristically the tumor is initially seen in adolescent males as a large mediastinal mass,[6,88] although this variety of lymphoma has been observed throughout the population and in many different primary sites.[89,109] Mediastinal enlargement develops in a significantly lower proportion of adult patients, and when this occurs the thymus gland may not be directly involved.[90] Conversely, early bone marrow involvement usually does occur and is followed rapidly by leukemia. There is also a relatively high frequency of central nervous system and gonadal involvement in the course of this disease. Intense leukemic therapy for these patients is advocated from the time of diagnosis.[138] The neoplastic cells of this lymphoma resemble the cortical thymocyte in size. They have a fine chromatin pattern and nuclear membrane convolutions, and they are mitotically active and express the cell markers of fetal thymocytes.[109] The rapidly proliferating cells expand the thymic lobules, surround persistent Hassal's corpuscles, infiltrate vessel walls, fibrous trabeculae, and the thymic capsule, and grow into the adjacent mediastinal adipose tissue. Observation of these features usually avoids a diagnostic confusion with lymphocyte-predominant thymoma.

Large cell lymphoma may be seen initially in the mediastinum in adults and less frequently in children as disease localized to the thymus gland with or without

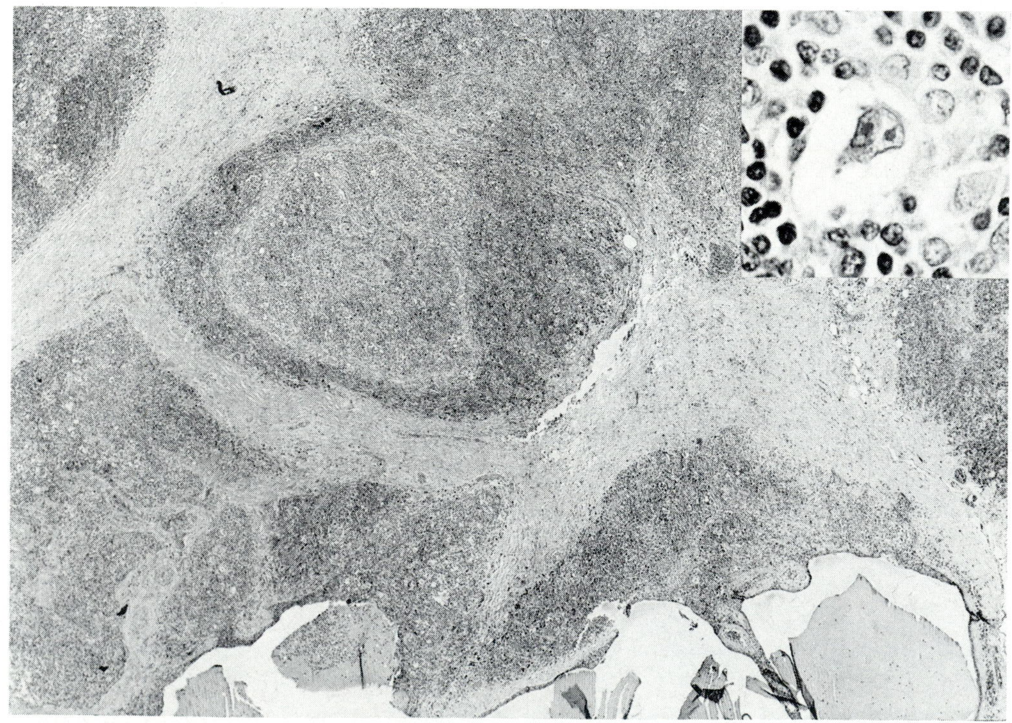

Fig. 31-14. Primary nodular sclerosing Hodgkin's disease of thymus gland. (80×.)

lymph node involvement.[52] Thymic lymphoma of the large cell type virtually always has a diffuse growth pattern and is often of the immunoblastic subtype.[75] Variable patterns of sclerosis may occur in over one third of cases. Large cell lymphoma in the thymus may occasionally be very difficult to distinguish from some thymomas, which have prominent nucleoli. Since the therapeutic approaches to these two neoplasms are vastly different, electron microscopy and immunologic cell surface antigen marker studies may be necessary to make this important distinction. Mediastinal large cell lymphomas have a rapid onset and are often accompanied by symptoms of cardiorespiratory failure including dyspnea, heart failure, and superior vena cava syndrome. Rapid systemic dissemination of these high-grade lymphomas is the rule, and they should be treated with an aggressive combined chemotherapy regimen.[75]

REFERENCES

1. Alpert, L.I., et al.: A histologic reappraisal of the thymus in myasthenia gravis: a correlative study of thymic pathology and response to thymectomy, Arch. Pathol. **91**:55, 1971.
2. Arnheim, E.E., and Gemson, B.L.: Persistent cervical thymus gland: thymectomy, Surgery **27**:603, 1950.
3. Auerback, R.: Morphogenetic interactions in the development of the mouse thymus gland, Dev. Biol. **2**:271, 1960.
4. Bach, J.F.: Thymic hormones, J. Immunopharmacol. **1**:277, 1979.
5. Bach, J.F., and Popiernik, M.: Cellular and molecular signals in T cell differentiation. In Porter, R., and Whelan, J., editors: Microenvironments in haemopoietic and lymphoid differentiation (Ciba Foundation Symposium 84), London, 1981, Pitman Medical Publishing Co., Ltd.
6. Barcos, M.P., and Lukes, R.J.: Malignant lymphoma of convoluted lymphocytes: a new entity of possible T-cell type. In Sinks, L.F., and Godden, J.O., editors: Conflicts in childhood cancer: an evaluation of current management, Progress in clinical and biological research, vol. 4, New York, 1975, Alan R. Liss.
7. Barnes, R.D.S., and O'Gorman, P.: Two cases of aplastic anemia associated with tumors of the thymus, J. Clin. Pathol. **15**:264, 1962.
8. Batata, M.A., et al.: Thymomas: clinicopathologic features, therapy, and prognosis, Cancer **34**:389, 1974.
9. Bearman, R.M., Bensch, K.G., and Levine, G.D.: The normal human thymic vasculature: an ultrastructural study, Anat. Rec. **183**:485, 1976.
10. Bearman, R.M., Levine, G D., and Bensch, K.G.: The ultrastructure of the normal human thymus: a study of 36 cases, Anat. Rec. **190**:755, 1978.
11. Benton, C., and Gerard, P.: Thymolipoma in a patient with Grave's disease: case report and review of the literature, J. Thorac. Cardiovasc. Surg. **51**:428, 1966.
12. Bergh, N.P., et al.: Tumors of the thymus and thymic region. I. Clinicopathological studies on thymomas, Ann. Thorac. Surg. **25**:91, 1978.
13. Bernatz, P.E., Harrison, E.G., and Clagett, O.T.: Thymoma: a clinicopathologic study, J. Thorac. Cardiovasc. Surg. **42**:424, 1961.
14. Boetsch, C.H., et al.: Lipothymoma: report of two cases, Dis. Chest **50**:539, 1968.
15. Bollum, F.J.: Antibody to terminal deoxynucleotidyl transferase, Proc. Natl. Acad. Sci. U.S.A. **72**:4119, 1975.
16. Bollum, F.J.: Terminal deoxynucleotidyl transferase as a hematopoietic cell marker, Blood **54**:1203, 1979.
17. Borzy, M.S., et al.: Fatal lymphoma after transplantion of cultured thymus in children with combined immunodeficiency disease, N. Engl. J. Med. **301**:565, 1979.
18. Borzy, M.S., et al.: Thymic morphology in immunodeficiency diseases: results of thymic biopsies, Clin. Immunol. Immunopathol. **12**:31, 1979.
19. Bowie, P.R., Teixeira, O.H.P., and Carpenter, B.: Malignant thymoma in a nine-year-old boy presenting with pleuropericardial effusion, J. Thorac. Cardiovas. Surg. **77**:777, 1979.
20. Breckler, I.A., and Johnston, D.G.: Choristoma of the thymus, Am. J. Dis. Child. **92**:175, 1956.
21. Brodsky, F.M., et al.: Monoclonal antibodies for analysis of the HLA system, Immunol. Rev. **47**:3, 1979.
22. Cantor, H., and Weissman, I.: Development and function of subpopulations of thymocytes and T lymphocytes, Prog. Allergy **20**:1, 1976.
23. Cordier, A.C., and Haumont, S.M.: Development of the thymus, parathyroids and ultimo-branchial bodies in NMRI and nude mice, Am. J. Anat. **157**:227, 1980.
24. Cossman, J., Deegan, M.J., and Schnitzer, B.: Thymoma: an immunologic and electron microscopic study, Cancer **41**:2183, 1978.
25. Dehner, L.P., Martin, S.A., and Sumner, H.W.: Thymus related tumors and tumor-like lesions in childhood with rapid clinical progression and death, Hum. Pathol. **8**:53, 1977.
26. Drachman, D.B.: Myasthenia gravis, N. Engl. J. Med. **298**:186, 1978.
27. Drenckhahn, D., et al.: Myosin and actin containing cells in the human postnatal thymus: ultrastructural and immunohistochemical findings in normal thymus and in myasthenia gravis, Virchows Archiv. **32**:33, 1979.
28. Engleman, E.G., et al.: Antibodies to membrane structures that distinguish suppressor/cytotoxic and helper T lymphocyte subpopulations block the mixed leukocyte reaction in man, J. Exp. Med. **154**:193, 1981.
29. Fechner, R.E.: Recurrence of noninvasive thymomas: report of four cases and review of literature, Cancer **23**:1423, 1969.
30. Friedman, N.B.: Tumors of the thymus, J. Thorac. Cardiovasc. Surg. **53**:163, 1967.
31. Frizzera, G., et al.: Lymphoreticular disorders in primary immunodeficiencies: new findings based on an up-to-date histologic classification of 35 cases, Cancer **46**:692, 1980.
32. Fudenberg, H., et al.: Primary immunodeficiencies: report of a World Health Organization committee, Pediatrics **47**:927, 1971.
33. Gilmour, J.R.: Some developmental abnormalities of the thymus and parathyroids, J. Pathol. Bacteriol. **52**:213, 1941.
34. Goldstein, G.: Isolation of bovine thymin: a polypeptide hormone of the thymus, Nature **247**:11, 1974.
35. Good, R.A., and Finstad, J.: Immunodeficiencies 1980: a summary and analysis of the International Conference on the Immunodeficiency Diseases. In Seligmann, M., and Hitzig, W.H., editors: Primary immunodeficiencies, New York, 1980, Elsevier/North Holland Biomedical Press.
36. Gravanis, M.B.: Metastasizing thymoma: report of a case and review of the literature, Am. J. Clin. Pathol. **49**:690, 1968.
37. Greaves, M.F., and Janossy, G.: Antisera to human T lymphocytes. In Bloom, B.R., and David, J.R., editors: In vitro methods in cell mediated and tumor immunity, New York, 1976, Academic Press, Inc.
38. Griffin, J.D., Aisenberg, A.C., and Long, J.C.: Lymphocytic thymoma associated with T-cell lymphocytosis, Am. J. Med. **64**:1075, 1978.
39. Guillan, R.A., et al.: Malignant thymoma associated with myasthenia gravis, and evidence of extrathoracic metastases: an analysis of published cases and report of a case, Cancer **27**:823, 1971.
40. Hayward, A.R.: Myoid cells in the human fetal thymus, J. Pathol. **106**:45, 1972.
41. Henry, K.: An unusual thymic tumour with a striated muscle (myoid) component (with a brief review of the literature on myoid cells), Br. J. Dis. Chest **66**:291, 1972.
42. Hirokawa, K.: Age-related changes of thymus: morphological and functional aspects, Acta Pathol. Jpn. **28**:843, 1978.
43. Hirst, E., and Robertson, T.I.: The syndrome of thymoma and erythroblastopenic anemia: a review of 56 cases including 3 case reports, Medicine **46**:225, 1967.

44. Ho, F.C.S., and Ho, J.C.I.: Pigmented carcinoid tumour of the thymus, Histopathology **1**:363, 1977.
45. Howard, F.D., et al.: A human T lymphocyte differentiation marker defined by monoclonal antibodies that block E-rosette formation, J. Immunol. **126**:2117, 1981.
46. Hwang, W.S., et al.: Ultrastructure of the rat thymus: a transmission, scanning electron microscope and morphometric study, Lab. Invest. **31**:473, 1974.
47. Ito, T., Hoskino, T., and Abe, K.: The fine structure of myoid cells in the human thymus, Arch. Histol. Jpn. **30**:207, 1969.
48. Janossy, G., et al.: Differentiation linked expression of p28,33 (Ia-like) structures on human leukaemic cells, Br. J. Haematol. **37**:391, 1977.
49. Janossy, G., et al.: The human thymic microenvironment: an immunohistologic study, J. Immunol. **125**:202, 1980.
50. Janossy, G., et al.: Distribution of T lymphocyte subsets in the human bone marrow and thymus: an analysis with monoclonal antibodies, J. Immunol. **126**:1608, 1981.
51. Jerne, N.K.: The somatic generation of immune recognition, Eur. J. Immunol. **1**:1, 1971.
52. Jones, S.E., et al.: Non-Hodgkin's lymphomas. IV. Clinicopathologic correlation in 405 cases, Cancer **31**:806, 1973.
53. Jotereau, F.V., Houssaint, E., and Le Douarin, N.M.: Lymphoid stem cell homing to the early thymic primordium of the avian embryo, Eur. J. Immunol. **10**:620, 1980.
54. Kaiserling, E., Stein, H., and Müller-Hermelink, H.K.: Interdigitating reticulum cells in the human thymus, Cell Tissue Res. **155**:47, 1974.
55. Katz, A., and Lattes, R.: Granulomatous thymoma or Hodgkin's disease of thymus: a clinical and histologic study and a re-evaluation, Cancer **23**:1, 1969.
56. Katz, S.M., et al.: Massive thymic enlargement: report of a case of gross thymic hyperplasia in a child, Am. J. Clin. Pathol. **68**:786, 1977.
57. Keller, A.R., and Castleman, B.: Hodgkin's disease of the thymus gland, Cancer **33**:1615, 1974.
58. Kersey, J.H., et al.: Lymphoma after thymus transplantation, N. Engl. J. Med. **302**:301, 1980.
59. Kung, P.C., et al.: Strategies for generating monoclonal antibodies defining human T-lymphocyte differentiation antigens, Transplant Proc. **12**(suppl. 1):141, 1980.
60. Lack, E.E.: Thymic hyperplasia with massive enlargement: report of two cases with review of diagnostic criteria, J. Thorac. Cardiovasc. Surg. **81**:741, 1981.
61. Lattes, R.: Thymoma and other tumors of the thymus: an analysis of 107 cases, Cancer **15**:1224, 1962.
62. Lauriola, L., et al.: Subpopulations of lymphocytes in human thymomas, Clin. Exp. Immunol. **37**:502, 1979.
63. Lauriola, L., et al.: Human thymoma: immunologic characteristics of the lymphocytic component, Cancer **48**:1992, 1981.
64. Le Douarin, N.M., and Jotereau, F.V.: Tracing of cells of the avian thymus through embryonic life in interspecific chimeras, J. Exp. Med. **142**:17, 1975.
65. Le Douarin, N.M., and Jotereau, F.V.: Homing of lymphoid stem cells to the thymus and the bursa of Fabricius studied in avian embryo chimeras. In Fouzereau, M., and Dausset, J., editors: Immunology 80, Prog. Immunol., vol. IV, London, 1980, Academic Press, Inc., Ltd.
66. Ledbetter, J.A., et al.: Evolutionary conservation of surface molecules that distinguish T lymphocyte helper/inducer and cytotoxic/suppressor subpopulations in mouse and man, J. Exp. Med. **153**:310, 1981.
67. Lee, Y., Moallem, S., and Lauss, R.H.: Massive hyperplastic thymus in a 22-month-old infant, Ann. Thorac. Surg. **27**:356, 1979.
68. Legg, M.A., and Brady, W.J.: Pathology and clinical behavior of thymomas: a review of 51 cases, Cancer **18**:1131, 1965.
69. Levine, G.D.: Primary thymic seminoma—a neoplasm ultrastructurally similar to testicular seminoma and distinct from epithelial thymoma, Cancer **31**:729, 1973.
70. Levine, G.D., and Bearman, R.: Electron microscopy of the thymus. In Johannessen, J.V., editor: Electron microscopy in human medicine, vol. 5, New York, 1980, McGraw-Hill Book Co.
71. Levine, G.D., and Polliack, A.: The T-cell nature of the lymphocytes in two human epithelial thymomas: a comparative immunologic, scanning and transmission electron microscopic study, Clin. Immunol. Immunopathol. **4**:199, 1975.
72. Levine, G.D., and Rosai, J.: A spindle cell variant of thymic carcinoid tumor: a clinical, histologic, and fine structural study with emphasis on its distinction from spindle cell thymoma, Arch. Pathol. Lab. Med. **100**:293, 1976.
73. Levine, G.D., and Rosai, J.: Thymic hyperplasia and neoplasia: a review of current concepts, Hum. Pathol. **9**:495, 1978.
74. Levine, G.D., et al.: The fine structure of thymoma, with emphasis on its differential diagnosis: a study of ten cases, Am. J. Pathol. **81**:49, 1975.
75. Lichtenstein, A.K., et al.: Primary mediastinal lymphoma in adults, Am. J. Med. **68**:509, 1980.
76. Lowenhaupt, E., and Brown, R.: Carcinoma of the thymus of granulomatous type, Cancer **4**:1193, 1951.
77. Makinodan, T.: The thymus in aging. In Greenblatt, R.B., editor: Geriatric endocrinology. Vol. 5. Aging, New York, 1978, Raven Press.
78. Mandel, T.: The development and structure of Hassall's corpuscles in the guinea pig: a light and electron microscopic study, Z. Zellforsch **89**:180, 1968.
79. Masaoka, A., et al.: Follow-up study of thymomas with special reference to their clinical stages, Cancer **48**:2485, 1981.
80. McMichael, A.J., et al.: A human thymocyte antigen defined by a hybrid myeloma monoclonal antibody, Eur. J. Immunol. **9**:205, 1979.
81. McPhee, D., Pye, J., and Shortman, K.: The differentiation of T lymphocytes. V. Evidence for intrathymic death of most thymocytes, Thymus **1**:151, 1979.
82. Meuwissen, H.J., Pollara, B., and Pickering, R.J.: Combined immunodeficiency disease associated with adenosine deaminase deficiency, J. Pediatr. **86**:169, 1975.
83. Middleton, G.: The incidence of follicular structures in the human thymus at autopsy, Aust. J. Exp. Biol. Med. Sci. **45**:189, 1967.
84. Miller, J.F.A.P.: Immunological function of the thymus, Lancet **2**:748, 1961.
85. Monier, J.C., et al.: Characterization of facteur thymique serique (FTS) in the thymus. I. Fixation of anti-FTS antibodies on thymic reticulo-epithelial cells, Clin. Exp. Immunol. **42**:470, 1980.
86. Moore, M.A.S., and Owen, J.J.T.: Chromosome marker studies on the development of the haematopoietic system in the chick embryo (in two parts), Nature **208**:956, 989, 1965.
87. Namba, T., Brunner, N.G., and Grob, D.: Myasthenia gravis in patients with thymoma, with particular reference to onset after thymectomy, Medicine **57**:411, 1978.
88. Nathwani, B.N., Kim, H., and Rappaport, H.: Malignant lymphoma, lymphoblastic, Cancer **38**:964, 1976.
89. Nathwani, B.N., et al.: Lymphoblastic lymphoma: a clinicopathologic study of 95 patients, Cancer **48**:2347, 1981.
90. Newcom, S.R., and Kadin, M.E.: T-cell leukemia with thymic involution, Cancer **43**:622, 1979.
91. Nickels, J., Franssila, K., and Hjelt, L.: Thymoma and Hodgkin's disease of the thymus, Acta Pathol. Microbiol. Scand. **81**:1, 1973.
92. Nordstrom, D.G., Tewfik, H.H., and Latourette, H.B.: Thymoma: therapy and prognosis as related to operative staging, Radiat. Oncol. Biol. Phys. **5**:2059, 1979.
93. Null, J.A., LiVolsi, V.A., and Glenn, W.W.L.: Hodgkin's disease of the thymus (granulomatous thymoma) and myasthenia gravis: a unique association, Am. J. Clin. Pathol. **67**:521, 1977.
94. Oosterom, R., and Kater, L.: The thymus in the aging individual. II. Thymic epithelial function in vitro in aging and in thymus pathology, Clin. Immunol. Immunopathol. **18**:195, 1981.
95. O'Shea, P.A., Pansatiankul, B., and Farnes, P.: Giant thymic hyperplasia in infancy: immunologic, histologic and ultrastructure observations (abstract), Lab. Invest. **38**:391, 1978.
96. Papastestas, A.E., et al.: Studies in myasthenia gravis: effects of thymectomy; results on 185 patients with nonthymomatous and thymomatous myasthenia gravis, Am. J. Med. **50**:465, 1971.

97. Pedraza, M.A.: Thymoma: immunological and ultrastructural characterization, Cancer **39**:1455, 1977.
98. Peterson, R.D.A., Cooper, M.D., and Good, R.A.: The pathogenesis of immunologic deficiency diseases, Am. J. Med. **38**:579, 1965.
99. Pyke, K.W., and Bach, J.F.: The in vitro migration of murine fetal liver cells to thymic rudiments, Eur. J. Immunol. **9**:317, 1979.
100. Reese, E.R., et al.: Lymphoma after thymus transplantation, N. Engl. J. Med. **302**:302, 1980.
101. Reinherz, E.L., et al.: Discrete stages of human intrathymic differentiation: analysis of normal thymocytes and leukemic lymphoblasts of T cell lineage, Proc. Natl. Acad. Sci. U.S.A. **77**:1588, 1980.
102. Remigio, P.A.: Granulomatous thymoma associated with erythroid hypoplasia, Am. J. Clin. Pathol. **55**:68, 1971.
103. Ridell, B., and Larsson, S.: Coexistence of a thymoma and Hodgkin's disease of the thymus, Acta Pathol. Microbiol. Scand. **88**:1, 1980.
104. Ridenhour, C.E., et al.: Thymoma arising from undescended cervical thymus, Surgery **67**:614, 1970.
105. Rosai, J., and Higa, E.: Mediastinal endocrine neoplasm, of probable thymic origin, related to carcinoid tumor: clinicopathologic study of 8 cases, Cancer **29**:1061, 1972.
106. Rosai, J., Hiza, E., and Davie, J.: Mediastinal endocrine neoplasm in patients with multiple endocrine adenomatosis: a previously unrecognized association, Cancer **29**:1075, 1972.
107. Rosai, J., and Levine, G.D.: Tumors of the thymus. In Firminger, H.I., editor: Atlas of tumor pathology, Series 2, Fascicle 13, Washington, D.C., 1976, Armed Forces Institute of Pathology.
108. Rosai, J., et al.: Carcinoid tumors and oat cell carcinomas of the thymus, Pathol. Annu. **11**:201, 1976.
109. Rosen, P.J., et al.: Convoluted lymphocytic lymphoma in adults: a clinicopathologic entity, Ann. Intern. Med. **89**:319, 1978.
110. Rouse, R.V., et al.: Expression of MHC antigens by mouse thymic dendritic cells, J. Immunol. **122**:2508, 1979.
111. Salyer, W.R., and Eggleston, J.C.: Thymoma: a clinical and pathological study of 65 cases, Cancer **37**:229, 1976.
112. Schantz, A., Sewall, W., and Castleman, B.: Mediastinal germinoma: a study of 21 cases with an excellent prognosis, Cancer **30**:1189, 1972.
113. Scollay, R.G., Butcher, E.C., and Weissman, I.L.: Thymus cell migration: quantitative aspects of cellular traffic from the thymus to the periphery in mice, Eur. J. Immunol. **10**:210, 1980.
114. Seemeyer, T.A., and Bolande, R.P.: Thymus involution mimicking thymic dysplasia: a consequence of transfusion-induced graft versus host disease in a premature infant, Arch. Pathol. Lab. Med. **104**:141, 1980.
115. Shearer, W.T., et al.: Successful transplantation of the thymus in Nezelof's syndrome, Pediatrics **61**:619, 1978.
116. Shier, K.J.: The thymus according to Schambacher: medullary ducts and reticular epithelium of thymus and thymomas, Cancer **48**:1183, 1981.
117. Simson, L.R., Lampe, I., and Abell, M.R.: Suprasellar germinomas, Cancer **22**:533, 1968.
118. Sloan, H.E., Jr.: The thymus in myasthenia gravis with observations on the normal anatomy and histology of the thymus, Surgery **13**:154, 1943.
119. Smith, W.F., DeWall, R.A., and Krumholz, R.A.: Giant thymoma, Chest **58**:383, 1970.
120. Souadjian, J.V., Silverstein, M.N., and Titus, J.L.: Thymoma and cancer, Cancer **22**:1221, 1968.
121. Souadjian, J.V., et al.: The spectrum of diseases associated with thymoma. Coincidence or syndrome? Arch. Intern. Med. **134**:374, 1974.
122. Spector, B.D., Perry, G.S., III, and Kersey, J.H.: Genetically determined immunodeficiency diseases (GDID) and malignancy: report from the Immunodeficiency-Cancer Registry, Clin. Immunol. Immunopathol. **11**:12, 1978.
123. Staber, F.G., Fink, U., and Sack, W.: B lymphocytes in the thymus of patients with myasthenia gravis, N. Engl. J. Med. **292**:1032, 1975.
124. Sterchi, M., and Cordell, A.R.: Seminoma of the anterior mediastinum, J. Thorac. Surg. **19**:371, 1975.
125. Sternberg, C.: Leukosarkomatose und myeloblastenleukaamie, Beitr. Pathol. **61**:75, 1916.
126. Stutman, O.: Intrathymic and extrathymic T cell maturation, Immunol. Rev. **42**:138, 1978.
127. Summary report of a Medical Research Council working-party: hypogammaglobulinemia in the United Kingdom, Lancet **1**:163, 1969
128. Tamaoki, N., Habu, S., and Kameyu, T.: Thymic lymphoid follicles in autoimmune diseases. II. Histological, histochemical and electron microscopic studies, Keio J. Med. **20**:57, 1971.
129. Trites, A.E.W.: Thyrolipoma, thymolipoma, and pharyngeal lipoma: a syndrome, Can. Med. Assoc. J. **95**:1254, 1966.
130. Vetters, J.M., and Barcley, R.S.: The incidence of germinal centers in thymus glands of patients with congenital heart disease, J. Clin. Pathol. **26**:583, 1973.
131. Viac, J., et al.: Epidermis-thymic antigenic relations with special reference to Hassall's corpuscles, Thymus **1**:319, 1980.
132. von Gaudecker, B.: Ultrastructure of the age-involuted adult human thymus, Cell Tissue Res. **186**:507, 1978.
133. von Gaudecker, B., and Müller-Hermelink, H.K.: Ontogeny and organization of the stationary non-lymphoid cells in the human thymus, Cell Tissue Res. **207**:287, 1980.
134. von Gaudecker, B., and Schmale, E.M.: Similarities between Hassall's corpuscles of the human thymus and the epidermis: an investigation by electron microscopy and histochemistry, Cell Tissue Res. **151**:347, 1974.
135. Waldmann, T.A., Strober, W., and Blaese, R.M.: T and B cell immunodeficiency diseases. In Parker, C.W., editor: Clinical immunology, Philadelphia, 1980, W.B. Saunders Co.
136. Wick, M.R., et al.: Malignant, predominantly lymphocytic thymoma with central and peripheral nervous system metastases, Cancer **47**:2036, 1981.
137. Wilkins, E.W., Jr., Edmunds, L.H., Jr., and Castleman, B.: Cases of thymoma at the Massachusetts General Hospital, J. Thorac. Cardiovasc. Surg. **52**:322, 1966.
138. Wollner, N., Exelby, P.R., and Lieberman, P.H.: Non-Hodgkin's lymphoma in children: a progress report on the original patients treated with LSA_2-L_2 protocol, Cancer **44**:1990, 1979.
139. Young, M., and Turnbull, H.M.: An analysis of the data collected by the Status Lymphaticus Investigation Committee, J. Pathol. Bacteriol. **34**:213, 1931.
140. Ziegler, J.L., et al.: Epstein-Barr virus and human malignancy, Ann. Intern. Med. **86**:323, 1977.
141. Zinkernagel, R.M.: Thymus and lymphohemopoietic cells: their role in T cell maturation in selection of T cells' H-2-restriction-specificity and H-2 linked Ir gene control, Immunol. Rev. **42**:224, 1978.
142. Zinkernagel, R.M., et al.: Restriction specificities, alloreactivity, and allotolerance expressed by T cells from nude mice reconstituted with H-2-compatible or -incompatible thymus grafts, J. Exp. Med. **151**:376, 1980.

CHAPTER 32 Pituitary Gland

NANCY E. WARNER

EMBRYOLOGY

The pituitary gland arises from two quite separate primordia that meet and join early in embryonic life to form the definitive organ. The adenohypophysis, or anterior lobe, is an ectodermal derivative that arises from Rathke's pouch, a midline diverticulum of the roof of the stomodeum, or primitive buccal cavity. The pouch grows upward through the transient craniopharyngeal canal to fuse with the infundibulum, the downgrowth from the floor of the diencephalon that forms the neurohypophysis. By rupture of its attachment, Rathke's pouch loses its connection with the roof of the pharynx and comes to lie within the developing sphenoid bone. Cells of Rathke's pouch proliferate to form the adenohypophysis; thus the lumen of the pouch is reduced to a narrow cleft, which is eventually obliterated, although remnants may persist as small cysts. The anterior part of the pouch becomes the definitive pars distalis. An upward extension of the developing adenohypophysis forms a cuff that surrounds the pituitary stalk, known as the pars tuberalis. The portion of the pouch that lies in contact with the neurohypophysis becomes the pars intermedia, which thus is delimited by the cleft from the developing pars distalis. In humans the pars intermedia remains rudimentary. The developing neurohypophysis differentiates into the infundibulum, the infundibular stem (or stalk), and the infundibular process, or neural lobe. Whereas the adenohypophysis loses its connection with the pharynx as the craniopharyngeal canal closes, the neurohypophysis permanently retains direct connections with the brain by the infundibular stalk (Fig. 32-1).

The adenohypophysis of the human fetus begins to produce growth hormone sometime between the twelfth and seventeenth weeks of pregnancy, as demonstrated by immunofluorescent staining. Hormones produced by the fetal hypophysis appear to have a crucial role in normal development of the thyroid and adrenal glands, since (1) congenital absence or hypoplasia of the human anterior lobe invariably leads to hypoplasia of thyroid and adrenals, and (2) experimental destruction of the fetal pituitary in the rat, mouse, and rabbit leads to reduction in size of the thyroid and adrenals, which can be avoided by injection of thyroid-stimulating hormone (TSH) or adrenocorticotropic hormone (ACTH) into the fetus.[5,13]

Remnants of Rathke's pouch regularly persist into postnatal life. The pharyngeal (caudal) end of the ruptured stalk of Rathke's pouch forms the pharyngeal pituitary.[3,6] The pharyngeal pituitary, which is present consistently in all age groups, is a small cylindrical body 5 to 6 mm in length, located in the midline in the roof of the nasopharynx, beneath the mucoperiosteum inferior to the vomerosphenoid junction (Fig. 32-2).[14] The extent of its function is uncertain. Other epithelial remnants

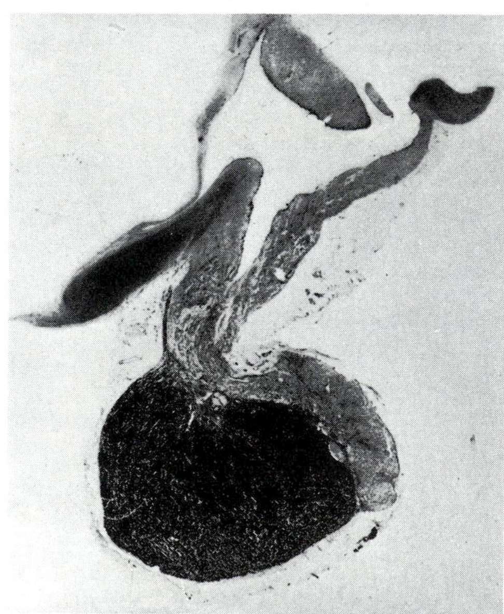

Fig. 32-1. Midsagittal section of pituitary gland to show neural attachments. (Hematoxylin and eosin; 4×; courtesy Drs. Dorothy S. Russell and A.R. Currie.)

include parapituitary epithelial residua, persistent Rathke's cleft within the gland, and remains of the craniopharyngeal stalk within the sphenoid bone[14]; these elements may be the source of cysts or tumors (see p. 1391).

ANATOMY

The pituitary gland in the adult is a small, bean-shaped, bilaterally symmetric organ that weighs 500 to 900 mg.[9] The gland is usually heavier in women, and its weight may reach 1100 mg or more during pregnancy[4] when hyperplasia normally occurs. The gland has two major anatomic divisions, the reddish brown adenohypophysis and the pale gray neurohypophysis. The adenohypophysis consists of the pars distalis (or pars anterior), the pars intermedia, and the pars tuberalis, which is an upward extension forming a cuff around the infundibular stem. The neurohypophysis consists of the pars nervosa (also known as the neural lobe, or infundibular process), the infundibular stem, and the infundibulum proper. The gland is attached to the brain by the stalk, which contains the nerve tracts and blood vessels, vital links to the hypothalamus. The stalk in turn merges with the infundibulum, a cone-shaped projection of the tuber cinereum of the hypothalamus; this region is referred to as the median eminence.

The pituitary gland is located in the hypophyseal fossa of the sella turcica, a midline cavity in the sphenoid bone. In this position deep inside the head, the gland is unusually well protected, but at the same time surgical approach is difficult. An extension of the dura mater lines the hypophyseal fossa and spreads out to form an incomplete covering for the sella, known as the diaphragma sellae. An extension of the leptomeninges blends with the surface of the pituitary, and a subarachnoid space of variable size may be present.

Knowledge of the anatomic relationships of the pituitary to its environs is essential in understanding the symptoms caused by pituitary tumors, which often compress the vital structures adjacent to the pituitary gland. The optic chiasm, hypothalamus, and third ventricle lie directly above the gland. Just lateral to the pituitary on each side are the cavernous sinuses, each containing the internal carotid artery and cranial nerves III, IV, V, and VI. Minor anatomic variations of these relationships are common, a matter of great concern to the neurosurgeon who is operating for tumor or palliative ablation of the hypophysis.[2,8]

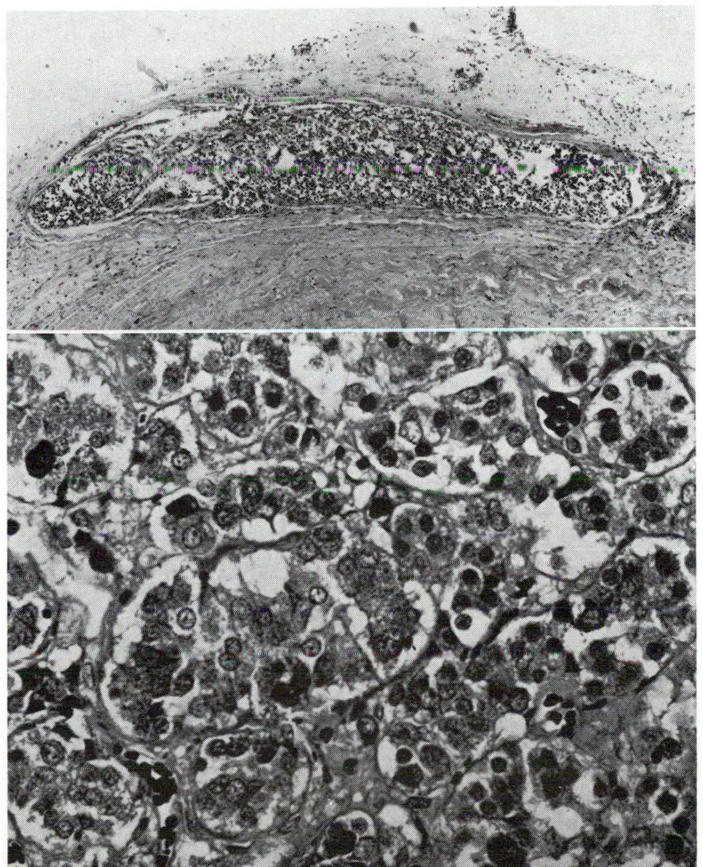

Fig. 32-2. A, Pharyngeal pituitary gland. **B,** Higher magnification showing typical configuration of adenohypohyseal cells in alveolar compartments. (**A,** Hematoxylin and eosin, 44×; **B,** acid fuchsin and aniline blue; 350×; courtesy Drs. Dorothy S. Russell and A.R. Currie.)

The arterial supply of the pituitary gland is derived from the internal carotid arteries by way of paired superior and inferior hypophyseal arteries. The neurohypophysis is supplied by direct branches of these arteries, which supply the superior and inferior regions of the neurohyphophysis, respectively.[15] In contrast, the arterial supply of the adenohypophysis is small[12] and probably insignificant.[1] Instead, the major blood supply of the adenohypophysis is derived from the hypophyseal portal system. The primary capillary bed of this portal system consists of capillaries in the infundibulum and infundibular stem; the secondary bed is the network of capillaries in the adenohypophysis.[16] The capillaries in the infundibulum and upper region of the stem are drained by the long portal veins, which course to the adenohypophysis through the stalk. The capillaries of the lower part of the stem are drained by the short portal veins, which are contained within the body of the gland. Therefore transection of the stalk will destroy the long portal veins, but the short veins may remain intact unless the stalk is divided at its junction with the gland.[10] The portal veins deliver blood to the secondary capillary bed of the adenohypophysis, each group of vessels supplying a specific territory in the pars distalis.[1] The capillaries of both the pars distalis and the pars nervosa drain into the dural venous sinuses surrounding the pituitary.

The neural and vascular pathways that link the hypothalamus to the pituitary warrant special consideration, since they are crucial in the regulation of the secretion of hormones by both neurohypophysis and adenohypophysis. The pathway between the hypothalamus and the neurohypophysis is a direct neural connection, the hypothalamohypophyseal tract, which originates from neurons in the supraoptic and paraventricular nuclei, traverses the pituitary stalk, and terminates in the pars nervosa. The supraoptic and paraventricular nuclei secrete vasopressin and oxytocin, octapeptide hormones with antidiuretic and oxytocic effects. These hormones become attached to carrier substances, the neurophysins, and are transported down the axons of the hypothalamohypophyseal tract to the pars nervosa, where they are stored before release into the capillaries of the neural lobe. Whereas the neurohypophysis is connected directly to the hypothalamus by a single link, the hypothalamohypophyseal nerve tract, the adenohypophysis is connected to the hypothalamus by a path consisting of two components, the tuberohypophyseal neural tract and the hypophyseal portal system. The tuberohypophyseal tract originates from neurons in the tuberal and other nuclei of the hypothalamus and terminates in the infundibulum, adjacent to the primary capillary beds of the hypophyseal portal system. Releasing and inhibiting factors synthesized in the cell bodies of tuberal nuclei pass down its axons and are deposited at the capillaries of the infundibulum, to be transported through the portal veins to the sinusoids of the adenohypophysis, where they control the release of hormones in the pars distalis.

HISTOLOGY AND FUNCTION

Adenohypophysis

The recognition of the hypothalamus as a higher center for integration of the pituitary has clarified the regulation of hypophyseal function.[7,11] That part of the hypothalamus concerned with hormonal regulation of pituitary function has been aptly termed the endocrine hypothalamus. The releasing and inhibiting substances produced by the endocrine hypothalamus are peptides. Those releasing hormones that have been identified are the thyrotropin-releasing hormone (TRH), follicle-stimulating hormone (FSH), and luteinizing hormone–releasing hormone (LHRH), or gonadotropin-releasing hormone (GnRH). Corticotropin-releasing factor (CRF) has been demonstrated, but its chemical structure is still unknown. The existence of a growth hormone–releasing factor (GHRF) and prolactin-releasing factor (PRF) is postulated. Hypothalamic release-inhibiting factors also have been established. Somatostatin, a tetradecapeptide, is the hormone that inhibits release of growth hormone; it also occurs outside the hypothalamus. Release of prolactin is inhibited by prolactin-inhibiting factor (PIF); the chemical structure is unknown as yet.

The pars distalis is composed of cords and clumps of epithelial cells separated by a network of capillaries, the secondary plexus of the hypophyseal portal bed. The capillaries are surrounded by perivascular spaces (best shown by electron microscopy) into which the secretory granules are released from the epithelial cells by exocytosis. Some of these cells are arranged in follicles, with a small central lumen containing colloid.

By light microscopy, the epithelial cells can be separated into chromophils, which have cytoplasmic secretory granules with a strong affinity for dyes, and chromophobes, smaller cells with cytoplasm having no visible granules by light microscopy and a lesser affinity for dyes. In hematoxylin and eosin–stained sections, three types of epithelial cells can be distinguished: chromophil cells with acidophilic granules (about 40%), chromophil cells with basophilic granules (about 10%), and chromophobe cells with no visible granules (about 50%). Efforts to subclassify the acidophils and basophils on the basis of special stains led to a succession of classifications[25,50] and resulted in chaos, principally for the reason that full understanding of functional cytology of the hypophysis was impossible without access to a broad range of techniques, some of which became available only recently. These techniques include histochemistry, enzyme immunohistochemistry (Fig. 32-3), electron microscopy of normal (Fig. 32-4) and abnormal hypophysis, ultrastructural analysis of cytoplasmic granules obtained by ultracentrifugation, autoradiography, and the histologic anal-

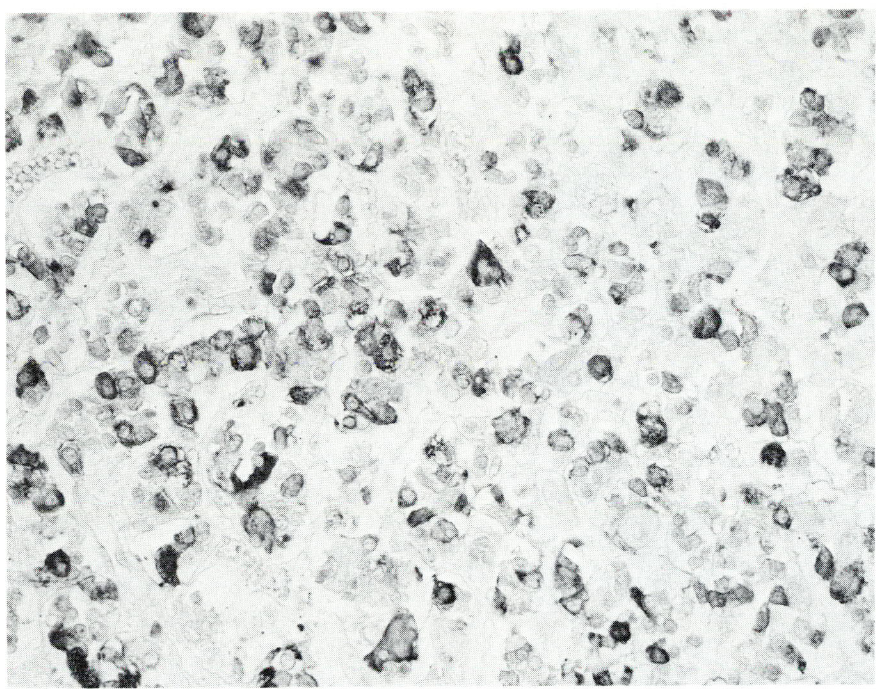

Fig. 32-3. Growth hormone–containing cells in adult human adenohypophysis. (Immunoperoxidase technique; 275×; courtesy Dr. Clive R. Taylor.)

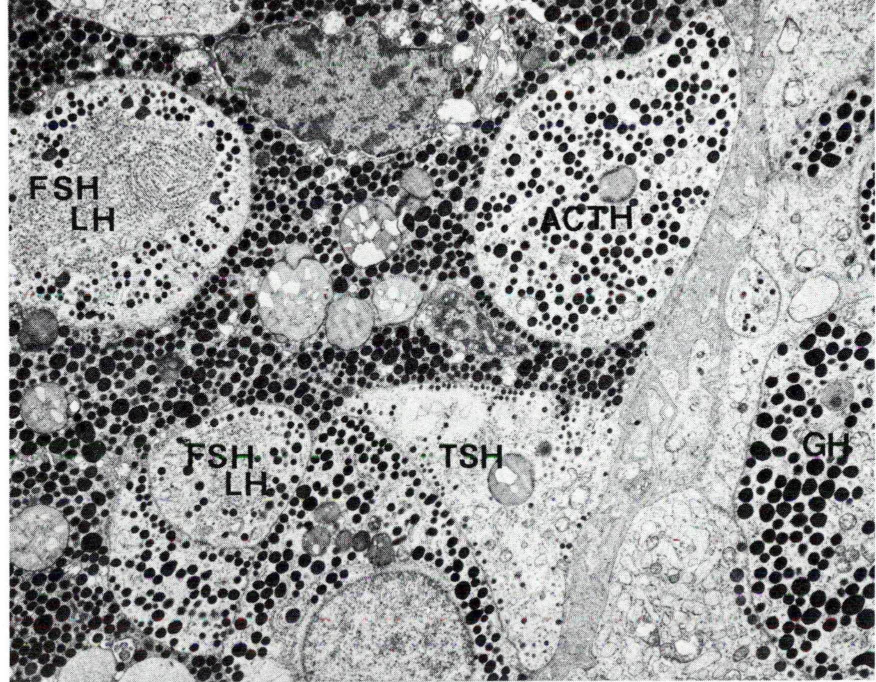

Fig. 32-4. Electron micrograph of normal pituitary removed transsphenoidally from 56-year-old woman with advanced mammary carcinoma. Smallest granules are in presumed thyrotroph (TSH) cell and largest granules are in presumed ACTH cell. Presumed FSH-LH cells have granules larger than TSH cell and smaller than ACTH cell. Mean granule sizes are TSH, 140 nm, FSH, 230 nm, ACTH, 330 nm, and GH, 470 nm. (4500×; courtesy Dr. I. Doniach.)

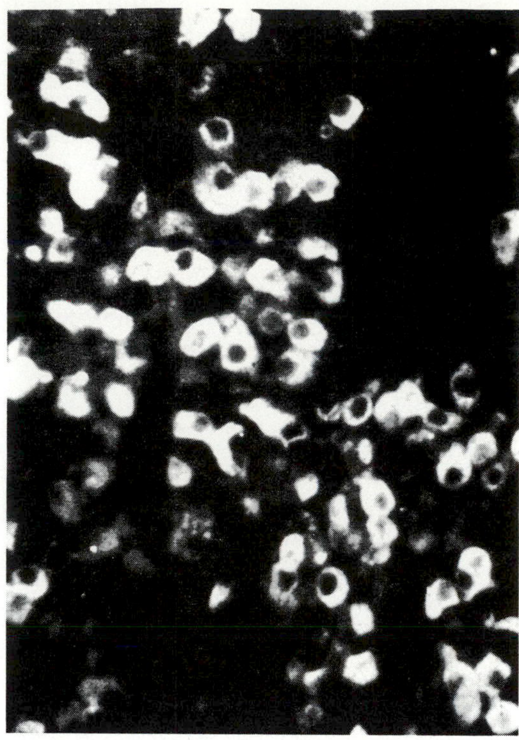

Fig. 32-5. Growth hormone–containing cells in adult human adenohypophysis. (Indirect immunofluorescence technique; 400×; from Porteous, I.B., Beck, J.S., and Currie, A.R.: J. Pathol. Bacteriol. **91**:539, 1966.)

ysis of antigen-antibody reactions by immunofluorescence (Fig. 32-5). The functional classification, in which each cell was named according to its secretory activity,[52] was proposed by the International Committee for Nomenclature of the Adenohypophysis. This functional classification has been widely accepted, and a tentative system of morphologic nomenclature has gradually emerged.[29] Previous classifications and recent developments are summarized in Table 32-1.

The designation alpha and beta granules instead of acidophil and basophil followed recognition that the staining reactions of chromophils were capricious and varied with fixation and pH of the medium. McManus[34] first reported periodic acid–Schiff–positive granules in hypophyseal cells, and Pearse[43] identified these cells as basophils (Fig. 32-6). These important discoveries marked the beginning of the histochemical studies that led ultimately to the demonstration of distinct classes of basophils.

The acidophils include somatotrophs and lactotrophs, which produce growth hormone (GH) and prolactin (PRL), respectively. Both hormones are simple proteins. In a horizontal section of the adenohypophysis, the acidophils are localized in the lateral wings.[29,41] Acidophils are readily identified by their affinity for eosin and other acidic dyes, such as orange G, erythrosin, and carmoisine.[19] Differentiation between the somatotrophs and lactotrophs is based on simultaneous use of orange G and

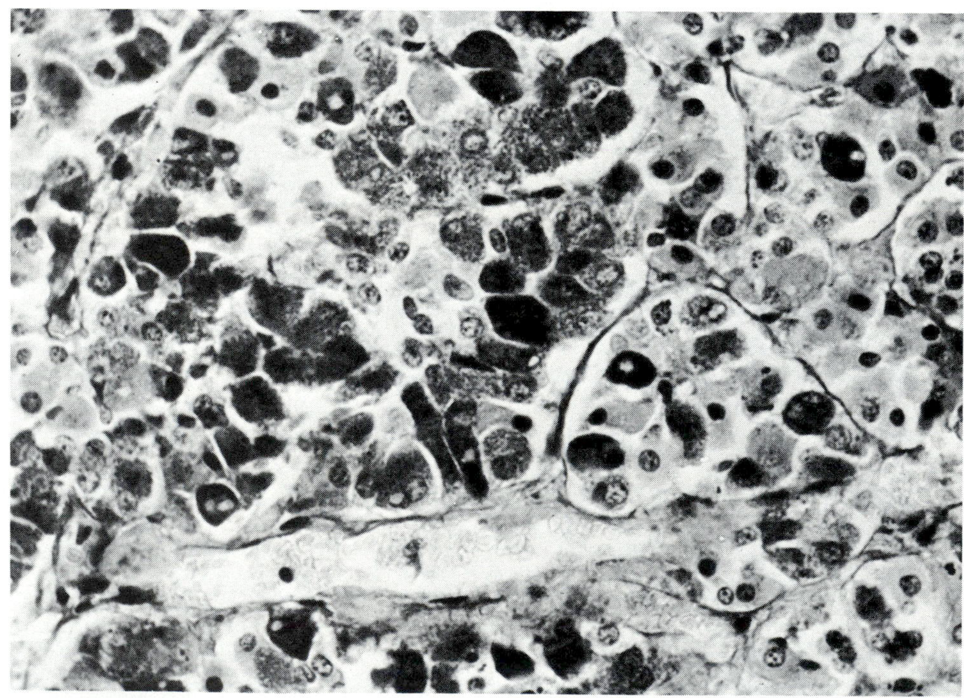

Fig. 32-6. Normal adult adenohypophysis showing groups of epithelial cells supported by connective tissue and sinusoids. Dark cells are basophils. (Periodic acid–Schiff–trichrome; 500×; courtesy Dr. A.R. Currie.)

Table 32-1. Cells of adenohypophysis and corresponding hormones

Hormone	Hematoxylin and eosin	Periodic acid–Schiff–orange G	Herlant's tetrachrome[31]	PM-AT-PAS-orange G*[25,40]	PFA-AB-PAS-orange G†[17,44]	Immunocytologic stains	Electron microscopy
Simple proteins **1.** GH	*Acidophils* (α cells)	*Acidophils* Orange G+	*Somatotrophs* Orange G+	*Acidophils* Orange G+	*Acidophils* Orange G+	*STH cell*	Granules 350-500 nm[45]; abundant; well-developed, rough endoplasmic reticulum
2. PRL			*Lactotrophs* Erythrosin+ (η cell)			*LTH cell*	Granules 275-350 nm[45]; distinctive rough endoplasmic reticulum
Mucoproteins **3.** FSH **4.** ICSH	*Basophils* (β cells)	*Mucoid cells* PAS+	*Basophils*	*Gonadotrophs* PAS+ (magenta granules); cell contour round (δ cells)	S^1 *cells*[44] Blue; granules PFA-susceptible	*FSH/LH cell*	Granules 275-375 nm[45]; density variable
5. TSH				*Thyrotroph*[23] Thionin+ (blue purple granules); cell contour angular (β_2 cell)	S^2 *cells*[44] Purple; granules PFA-susceptible	*TSH cell*	Granules 150-200 nm[45]; may be located peripherally
Polypeptides **6.** ACTH **7.** MSH **8.** LPH				*Corticomelanotrophs* PAS+ (red granules); cell contour oval (β_1 cell)	*R cells*[44] Red; granules PFA-resistant	*ACTH/MSH cell*	Granules 375-550 nm[45]; density variable; cytoplasmic filaments
(None)	*Chromophobes*	*Chromophobes* (No visible granules)	*Chromophobes* (No visible granules)	*Chromophobes* (No visible granules)	*Chromophobes* (No visible granules)		Sparse, fine granules[30]; 150 nm or less
						Chromophobes (No reaction)	No granules

*Permanganate–aldehyde thionine–periodic acid–Schiff–orange G.
†Performic acid–Alcian blue–periodic acid–Schiff–orange G.

erythrosin or carmoisine.[42] By electron microscopy, somatotrophs have abundant granules averaging 350 to 500 nm in diameter.[45] The lactotrophs have large, sparse granules measuring 275 to 350 nm and the most abundant rough endoplasmic reticulum of all the adenohypophyseal cells.[45] Concentric whorls of rough endoplasmic reticulum known as nebenkerns are a prominent feature. In pregnancy the distinction between the somatotrophs and lactotrophs can be made with hematoxylin and eosin stain alone, since the lactotrophs are considerably enlarged (pregnancy cells of Erdheim).[4]

The basophil cells include gonadotrophs, thyrotrophs, and corticotrophs. Differentiation of the basophils was accomplished by application of histochemistry, immunocytology, and electron microscopy, together with indirect evidence based on pathologic states, including deficiency, hyperactivity, and neoplasia. The histochemistry of the adenohypophysis is summarized in Girod's comprehensive monograph.[28] Basophils contain polysaccharides and protein, and they are known collectively as mucoid cells.[43] Oxidation of the polysaccharide with periodic acid results in formation of free aldehyde groups, which form visible purple complexes with Schiff's reagent, the basis for the periodic acid–Schiff–positive reaction of the basophil cells. Further differentiation of basophils was accomplished by Adams and Swettenham,[17] who found that the granules of corticotrophs are resistant (R) to performic acid and that they remain periodic acid–Schiff positive, whereas the granules of thyrotrophs and gonadotrophs are susceptible (S) but remain Alcian blue positive. Pearse and van Noorden[44] divided the susceptible cells into two types—blue S_1, associated with gonadotropins, and purple S_2, associated with thyrotropic hormone.

Gonadotrophs are the source of FSH, and LH or interstitial cell–stimulating hormone (ICSH) and thyrotrophs are the source of TSH. FSH, LH, and TSH are glycoproteins. They are composed of two polypeptides known as alpha and beta subunits, plus a polysaccharide portion. The alpha subunit of the polypeptide is identical in all three hormones. The beta subunit is unique to each one, conferring on the hormone its special properties. The corticotrophs produce ACTH, melanocyte-stimulating hormone (MSH, alpha and beta types), beta-lipotropin (LPH), and beta-endorphin.[20,33] ACTH, MSH, and LPH are simple peptides with a common heptapeptide core and overlapping properties.[37] Corticotrophs also are known as ACTH/MSH cells, corticolipotropic cells, or melanocorticotropic cells.

The important characteristics of the three types of basophils may be summarized as follows. The gonadotrophs have a round or oval contour and an eccentric nucleus; in horizontal section they are most numerous in the posterior portion of the median wedge[29] but are also found in the lateral wings.[27] Phifer and associates[46] showed that antisera to FSH and LH reacted with the same cell types, suggesting that FSH and LH are secreted by the same cell, hence the designation FSH-LH cell. With electron microscopy, the granules of gonadotrophs are 275 to 375 nm in diameter.[45] Some workers have described two ultrastructural types of gonadotrophs.[51] The thyrotrophs are angular cells that can be demonstrated selectively by Ezrin and Murray's permanganate-aldehyde thionine–periodic acid–Schiff–orange G stain.[28] In horizontal section, thyrotrophs are found in the median wedge, mainly in an anterior and subcapsular location.[29] The thyrotrophs stain with antibodies against TSH.[48] By electron microscopy, the cells have an irregular shape and contain small granules 125 to 200 nm in diameter, which may have a peripheral distribution.[45] The corticotrophs are oval cells, concentrated in the anterior part of the median wedge and adjacent lateral wings. A separate group of corticotrophs is found consistently in the pars nervosa, at the junction with the pars distalis; these cells may be remnants of pars intermedia,[36,49] and they may have a function as yet unidentified.[35] Immunostaining demonstrates ACTH, MSH, beta-lipotropin and beta-endorphin in the corticotrophs.[21,39] Phifer and associates[47] showed that the corticotroph contains alpha-MSH as well as beta-MSH, although the latter is the principal form in humans. With the electron microscope, the ACTH cell contains granules 375 to 550 nm in diameter,[45] and typical filaments may be found in the cytoplasm.[22] Large lysosomal structures known as enigmatic bodies are frequent.[24]

The classic chromophobes are small cells with scanty cytoplasm, no visible granules by light microscopy, and no secretory function. It was postulated that some might be primordial or resting cells. The finding of nongranulated cells with strongly basophilic cytoplasm suggested to earlier workers that some chromophobes might be actively secreting cells that failed to store granules. With the advent of electron microscopy, a large subpopulation of "chromophobes" has been shown to consist of poorly granulated cells with fine granules 150 nm or less in diameter that are invisible by light microscopy. These cells are associated with secretion of ACTH, TSH, or FSH-LH, and with immunostaining they may be classified as corticotrophs, thyrotrophs, or gonadotrophs. Another subgroup of chromophobes is follicular, or stellate, cells; they are best seen with electron microscopy. These elongated stellate elements are associated with follicles. Distinctive features include microvilli, cilia, junctional complexes at the apical pole, and elongated mitochondria.[18,38] Their function is uncertain.[32]

Neurohypophysis

The pars nervosa consists of interlacing nerve fibers and specialized glial elements known as pituicytes, with interspersed blood vessels. Granules of neurosecretory material, made up of the octapeptides vasopressin and oxytocin in association with carrier proteins termed neurophysins, are present throughout the neurohypophysis. The neurophysines are a useful marker of neurosecretion since they can be stained by the chrome alum–hematoxylin, the aldehyde fuchsin, or the performic acid–Alcian blue technique.[10] Vasopressin, or antidiuretic hormone (ADH), causes reabsorption of water from the renal tubules, and it is essential for maintaining osmolality of the plasma. Deficiency of ADH results in the condition known as diabetes insipidus, which is characterized by uncontrolled diuresis and polydipsia. Oxytocin is responsible for the ejection of milk from the lactating breast, by causing contraction of the mammary myoepithelium. It also stimulates contraction in the uterus at term.

The function of the pituicytes is unknown. Electron microscopy has revealed that pituicytes are closely apposed to neurosecretory fibers, and in lower animals a phagocytic function for disposal of neurophysins and membranes of granules has been suggested.[32]

PITUITARY IN PREGNANCY

The hypophysis undergoes a striking enlargement during pregnancy and lactation, when it may reach 1100 mg or more. Although involution occurs subsequently, the gland remains heavier in multiparous women.[4] The basis for enlargement is the pronounced hypertrophy and hyperplasia of the lactotrophs. In the pituitary of nonpregnant, nonlactating adults, the lactrotrophs are sparsely granulated and inconspicuous except with immunostains. However, during pregnancy and lactation the hypertrophic, hyperplastic lactotrophs can be recognized in hematoxylin and eosin–stained sections as enlarged acidophils, termed pregnancy cells.[4] The lactotrophs also are selectively stained with erythrosin in the tetrachrome method of Herlant and Pasteels[31] or Brookes' carmoisine technique.[19]

PITUITARY IN DISORDERS OF OTHER ENDOCRINE GLANDS

Hypofunction of the thyroid, adrenals, or gonads generally produces morphologic changes in the thyrotrophs, corticotrophs, or gonadotrophs, respectively, ascribed to lack of negative feedback. Hyperfunction of the adrenal glands has profound effects on the corticotrophs, and hyperthyroidism produces alterations in the thyrotrophs.[68] Experimental evidence suggests that the changes following hypofunction may be the result of stimulation of hypophyseal cells by hypothalamic-releasing hormones.[73]

Hypothyroidism

In untreated or inadequately treated myxedema caused by primary disease of the thyroid, hypertrophy and hyperplasia of the thyrotrophs lead to enlargement of the pituitary; weights up to 1.21 g have been recorded.[54] Historically such abnormal thyrotrophs have been designated thyroprival cells,[77] large chromophobes,[77] or hypertrophic amphophils.[55] With light microscopy the thyrotrophs can be recognized as large cells containing coarse vesicles, or droplets, in the cytoplasm; the typical basophil granules are lacking (Fig. 32-7). The droplets

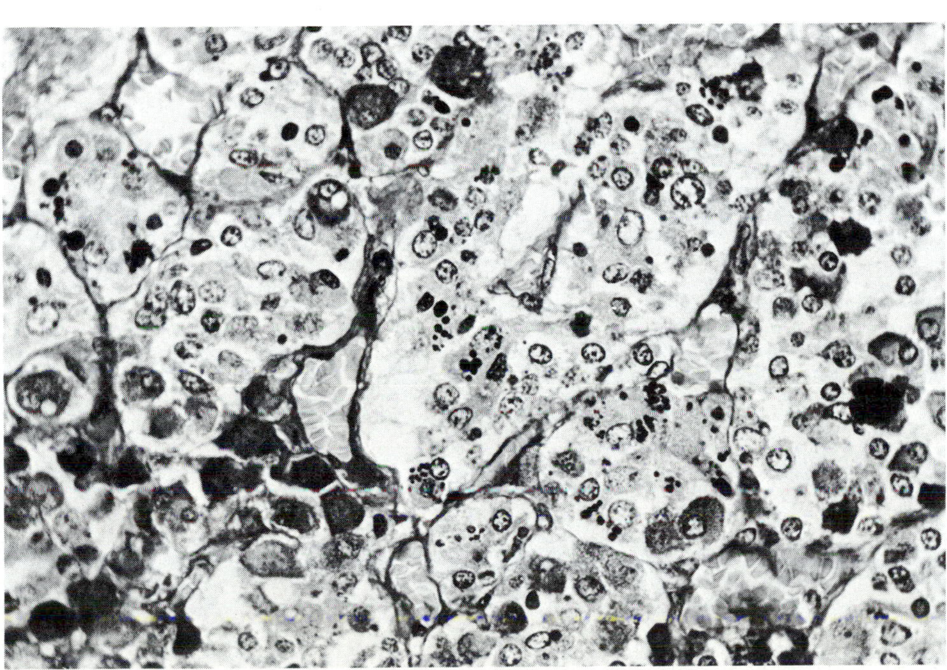

Fig. 32-7. Vesiculate cells in adenohypophysis of patient with myxedema. Note variation in size of periodic acid–Schiff–positive granules. (Periodic acid–Schiff–trichrome; 500×; courtesy Dr. A.R. Currie.)

are periodic acid–Schiff and aldehyde thionine positive. In rats, high-resolution autoradiography has demonstrated that thyroidectomy cells originate from division of preexisting TSH cells.[75] After administration of ^{131}I to mice with hypothyroidism, the thyroidectomy cells by electron microscopy show ballooning of the ergastoplasmic cisternae, and secretory granules are decreased or absent, resulting in a chromophobic appearance.[38] In such animals, hyperplasia of thyrotrophs is followed by the appearance of microadenomas and then gross tumors.[61] In humans with untreated primary hypothyroidism, thyrotroph cell adenomas are well documented.[76]

Hyperthyroidism

Ezrin has described regression of thyrotrophs in patients who died of hyperthyroidism.[23,68] The regressed TSH cells have small nuclei, a thin rim of cytoplasm, and a few aldehyde thionine–positive droplets. These alterations in the TSH cells are reversible. In contrast to the characteristic findings in the adenohypophysis in myxedema, the abnormalities in hyperthyroidism are not considered diagnostic.[29]

Addison's disease

In Addison's disease, gross enlargement of the hypophysis has been recorded, with a weight of 1.2 g.[69] The granulated basophils are reduced in number, the chromophobes are increased, and transitional forms of basophils are present.[58] Mitotic figures may be found.[69] Using special stains, Ezrin demonstrated that the apparent reduction in basophils is attributable to degranulation of those basophils associated with production of ACTH; these are transformed into actively secreting cells that resemble chromophobes by light microscopy. A similar sequence of events occurs in rats subjected to adrenalectomy; the ACTH cells enlarge and secretory granules are strikingly reduced.[74]

In patients with Addison's disease the number of thyrotrophs may be greatly increased.[25] This increase in thyrotrophs may be a reflection of the frequent association of idiopathic atrophy of the adrenal glands with atrophy of the thyroid, a condition known as Schmidt's syndrome, which apparently has an autoimmune basis.[53,56,64]

Hyperadrenocorticism

A typical cytoplasmic alteration known as Crooke's hyaline change was first observed in the basophils in cases of Cushing's syndrome.[57] Subsequently the abnormality was found in other conditions characterized by excess circulating adrenocortical hormones, including therapy with exogenous glucocorticoids[66] and hypercorticism resulting from ectopic production of ACTH in lung cancer.[65] The basophils that are affected are the ACTH cells.[63] In Crooke's change the granules disappear and the cytoplasm gradually becomes periodic acid–Schiff negative.[63,72] In hematoxylin and eosin–stained

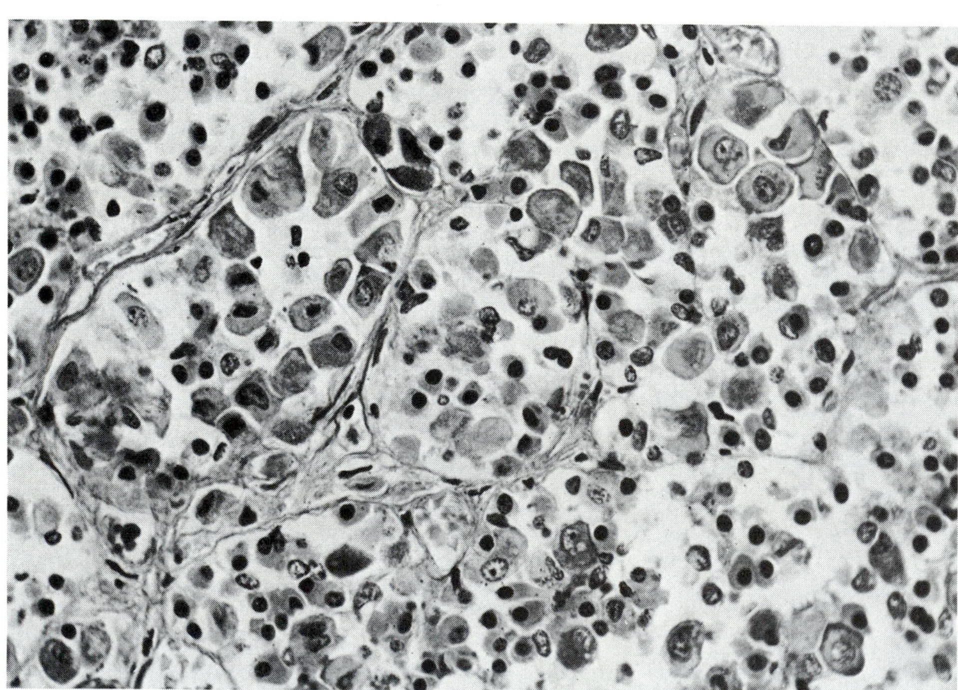

Fig. 32-8. Crooke's hyaline change in basophil cells in Cushing's syndrome. (Periodic acid–Schiff–trichrome; 500×; courtesy Dr. A.R. Currie.)

section, the cytoplasm assumes a ground-glass, pale gray appearance. The nucleus and the cell body enlarge, and a few cytoplasmic vacuoles may be present (Fig. 32-8). By electron microscopy, the hyaline substance is made up of a dense feltwork of fine filaments[22] of the same type that is found in the normal corticotroph.

Hyperadrenocorticism also affects the population of thyrotrophs, or TSH cells. Halmi and McCormick[62] found that the thyrotrophs were scanty or undetectable at autopsy in patients with elevated levels of glucocorticoids, whether exogenous or endogenous. They postulated that the paucity of thyrotrophs was the morphologic basis for the tonic depression of TSH secretion that is observed clinically in sustained hyperadrenocorticism.

Deficiency of gonadal hormones

In rodents, ovariectomy removes the negative feedback exerted by ovarian steroids on the pituitary gonadotrophs. In such animals the degranulated, hyperactive gonadotrophs acquire large vacuoles, assume a signet-ring appearance, and are known as castration cells. By electron microscopy the signet-ring morphology results from fusion of distended elements of the endoplasmic reticulum and enlargement of individual cisternae.[26,60]

Although the same feedback action exists in humans, distinctive signet-ring castration cells such as those found in rodents do not occur. Nonetheless, changes are found in the gonadotrophs of patients with deficiency of gonadal hormones. Russfield[70] observed cellular hypertrophy and enlargement of the Golgi complex in the gonadotrophs of patients with gonadal deficiency; the changes were reversible by hormone therapy. In a man who underwent castration for carcinoma of the prostate, Russfield and Byrnes[71] found hyperplasia of sparsely granulated, periodic acid–Schiff–positive cells, but the staining method did not differentiate between the types of basophils. Phifer and associates[46] observed an increase in the size and number of gonadotrophs in a woman castrated 5 years previously. By light microscopy Ezrin[59] noted enlarged, vacuolated gonadotrophic basophils resembling chromophobes in patients with hypogonadism and in postmenopausal women. With the electron microscope, extreme dilatation of cisternae of the endoplasmic reticulum of these hypertrophied cells has been observed.[67]

HYPOPHYSECTOMY

Hypophysectomy has been shown to produce temporary remission of symptoms in about one third of women with disseminated mammary cancer.[82] Relief from bone pain is especially gratifying. In treatment of metastatic carcinoma, total ablation of adenohypophyseal function is the goal. Thus hypophysectomy for palliation of breast cancer is an important cause of pituitary hypofunction.

The ability to predict the patient who will have a favorable response to endocrine ablation more accurately has been enhanced recently by the recognition of estrogen receptors in some mammary tumors. Evidence is incomplete, but it appears that women whose tumors contain such receptors are more likely to have a remission.[78,80,81]

Several lines of evidence suggest that the pharyngeal hypophysis is capable of active secretion of adenophypophyseal hormones in patients whose sellar hypophysis has been destroyed by tumor or hypophysectomy. In such patients Müller[86] reported "activation" of the cells of the pharyngeal pituitary, with typical acidophils and basophils, in contrast to the undifferentiated cells observed in the "inactive" state. McGrath[84] noted that acidophils predominated in the pharyngeal hypophysis after sellar hypophysectomy; basophils and chromophobes were also present. In extracts of pharyngeal hypophyses, McGrath[83] demonstrated PRL and GH. McPhie and Beck[85] found GH in acidophils of pharyngeal pituitary in patients without endocrine disease. These findings strongly suggest that the pharyngeal hypophysis is capable of active secretion. However, the extent to which this organ can compensate for absence of the sellar hypophysis is uncertain.[79]

HYPOPITUITARISM

Hypopituitarism, or pituitary insufficiency, may involve the neurohypophysis, the adenohypophysis, or both. The pathology of the major causes of insufficiency is discussed in detail in the later sections; some of the clinical features are described briefly here.

Deficiency of the neurohypophysis results in the syndrome known as diabetes insipidus because of the loss of vasopressin. The condition is characterized by diuresis, polyuria, and uncontrollable thirst.

Deficiency of the adenohypophysis may involve one, several, or all of the trophic hormones. Deficiency of all hormones (panhypopituitarism) follows destruction of 70% or more of the adenohypophysis. Infarction and tumor are the most common causes. Isolated hormonal deficiency may be associated with incomplete adenohypophyseal destruction, but it may also occur in the absence of a recognizable pathologic lesion. In such cases a functional disorder of the hypothalamus has been postulated.

The classic clinical syndrome of panhypopituitarism in adults is known as Simmonds' disease. The advanced cachexia that characterized the cases observed by Simmonds is rarely observed now, probably because of the advances in medical care since then.[87] From this heterogeneous group of cases described by Simmonds, Sheehan[89] separated the clinicopathologic entity of postpartum necrosis of the adenohypophysis, and this syndrome now bears his name.

The effects of isolated hormone deficiency depend on

the hormone involved and to some extent on the age of the patient. Deficiency of gonadotrophic hormones leads to hypogonadotrophic eunuchoidism in men and amenorrhea in women; before the age of puberty there are no clinical signs, but secondary sexual development fails to occur at adolescence.[88] Deficiency of corticotropin secretion leads to anorexia, weakness, weight loss, and hypoglycemia; in women axillary and pubic hair may be lost, and in girls it fails to appear. Isolated deficiency of thyrotropic hormone causes hypothyroidism in adults but has not been described in children. Isolated deficiency of growth hormone results in ateliotic dwarfism in children and microsplanchnia in adults.[59]

ANOMALIES

Agenesis

Agenesis of the pituitary is a rare anomaly that is almost always associated with cyclopia, a gross malformation involving the neural tube and axial skeleton. Even in this condition, agenesis is not universal, occurring in only about half the cases reported.[92] Agenesis of the anterior lobe has been described in a few normocephalic infants; in males the penis is unusually small, a finding that has been suggested as an external marker of this condition.[94] In such normocephalic infants, the sella turcica may appear normally formed but empty, or it may be smaller than normal with a persistent craniopharyngeal canal.[98] In all cases in which the anterior lobe of the pituitary is absent, the adrenal glands are hypoplastic and the thyroid gland is often similarly affected. The adrenal glands lack a fetal or "X" zone, and the layers of the cortex are irregular and disordered. That the function of these abnormal adrenal glands is defective is supported by the observation of stable, low maternal urinary estriol levels in the last weeks of pregnancy.[94] The hypoplastic thyroid is small and may lack an isthmus. The testes may also be hypoplastic, and absence of interstitial cells of Leydig has been reported.[91] Several of these infants have survived a decade or more, exhibiting mental deficiency, dwarfism, failure of development, myxedema, hypoglycemic convulsions, and undeveloped genitalia.[97]

Agenesis of the anterior pituitary may occur without any anomaly of the posterior pituitary.

Hypoplasia

Hypoplasia of the pituitary is a constant finding in anencephaly. In this condition the sella turcica is flattened and the exposed base of the skull is covered by a mat of spongy, vascular tissue. The hypophysis usually cannot be recognized grossly, but it can be found by en bloc removal of the entire sella, decalcification, and vertical sectioning of the central portion.[90] The size and shape of the gland are quite variable. Whereas the pars anterior is nearly always present, the pars nervosa is often absent.

The adrenals in anencephaly are invariably hypoplastic, and the X zone, or fetal cortex, is absent, so that the glands are miniature replicas of those of older infants,[95] with orderly cortical layers. The thyroid gland, gonads, and genitalia are unaffected.

Malposition

Malposition, or dystopia, of the hypophysis is a rare occurrence. Lennox and Russell[93] reviewed the literature and added two cases in which the pars nervosa lay between the infundibulum and the sella, being connected to the pars anterior by a stalk composed of pars tuberalis. No disorder of pituitary function was recognized. Another rare malposition occurs as a result of failure of contact between Rathke's pouch and the developing diencephalon, leading to displacement of pituitary tissue into a persistent craniopharyngeal duct.[86] In such cases, polypoid protrusion of pituitary anlage into the pharynx may occur. Adenomas may occur in ectopic pituitary tissue, and they have been reported in the nasal cavity, sphenoid sinus, sphenoidal wing, and temporal bone.[96]

EMPTY SELLA SYNDROME

Empty sella syndrome is characterized by an incomplete diaphragma sellae with extension of the subarachnoid space into the sella turcica. The sella may be enlarged and deformed, and the pituitary may be reduced to a flattened layer of tissue lining the floor of the sella.[103,104] Histologically the gland appears normal,[99,100] and endocrine function is not usually impaired. Hyperprolactinemia[102] and coexisting functional microadenoma have been reported in a few patients with empty sella syndrome.[101]

HEMORRHAGE

Severe skull trauma frequently injures the hypophysis, causing hemorrhage, laceration, and necrosis.[106] The patients who survive such injury may have diabetes insipidus as a result of damage to the neurohypophysis.[105,106] Hemorrhage in the posterior pituitary also occurs in patients who have cerebral hemorrhage, tumors of the brain, or "respirator brain" (deterioration of the brain that occurs as a complication of mechanical respirator therapy).[107]

PITUITARY APOPLEXY

Acute hemorrhage into a pituitary tumor is responsible for the condition known as pituitary apoplexy. It is characterized by sudden headache, ophthalmoplegia, meningismus, and signs of compression of the optic nerves or chiasm.[108] Sudden pituitary failure may result; impaction of the hypophysis by the expanding neoplasm has been cited as the mechanism. In some patients, pituitary apoplexy may be the first manifestation of hypophyseal tumor.

ISCHEMIA

Foci of ischemic necrosis are occasionally observed postmortem, with an incidence of 1% to 3% in unselected autopsies.[112] These almost always involve the adenohypophysis. The associated conditions are varied[113] and include such diverse entities as obstetric shock,[116] elevated intracranial pressure, diabetes mellitus,[111,114] craniocerebral trauma, cerebrovascular accident, shock, mechanical respirator therapy ("respirator brain"),[107,110,117] transection of the hypophyseal stalk,[10,109] overwhelming sepsis, and carcinomatous permeation of local blood vessels.[9] The common denominator in most of these conditions appears to be inadequate perfusion of the adenohypophysis, resulting in ischemia and coagulative necrosis. The "life support" of the adenohypophysis is the hypophyseal portal system, and the direct arterial supply to the anterior pituitary is not sufficient to sustain the cells.[1,10] This arrangement renders the adenohypophysis more vulnerable to episodes of stasis and ischemia. The pathogenesis of the ischemia has been ascribed to such mechanisms as embolism, thrombosis, Shwartzman phenomenon, vascular spasm, and vascular compression.[113] In many patients with infarcts, the lesions occur as a terminal complication of a severe systemic illness; hence they are of little importance clinically whether large or small. Survivors with microinfarcts do not have symptoms of hypopituitarism because insufficiency is not apparent until 70% of the adenohypophysis is destroyed.[70] However, survivors of large infarcts do suffer from hypopituitarism.

The most important cause of pituitary insufficiency from massive infarction is obstetric shock, usually related to hemorrhage at the time of delivery. Postpartum necrosis of the pituitary is known as Sheehan's syndrome. In severe cases the extent of necrosis of the adenohypophysis approaches 99% (Fig. 32-9).[11] A narrow

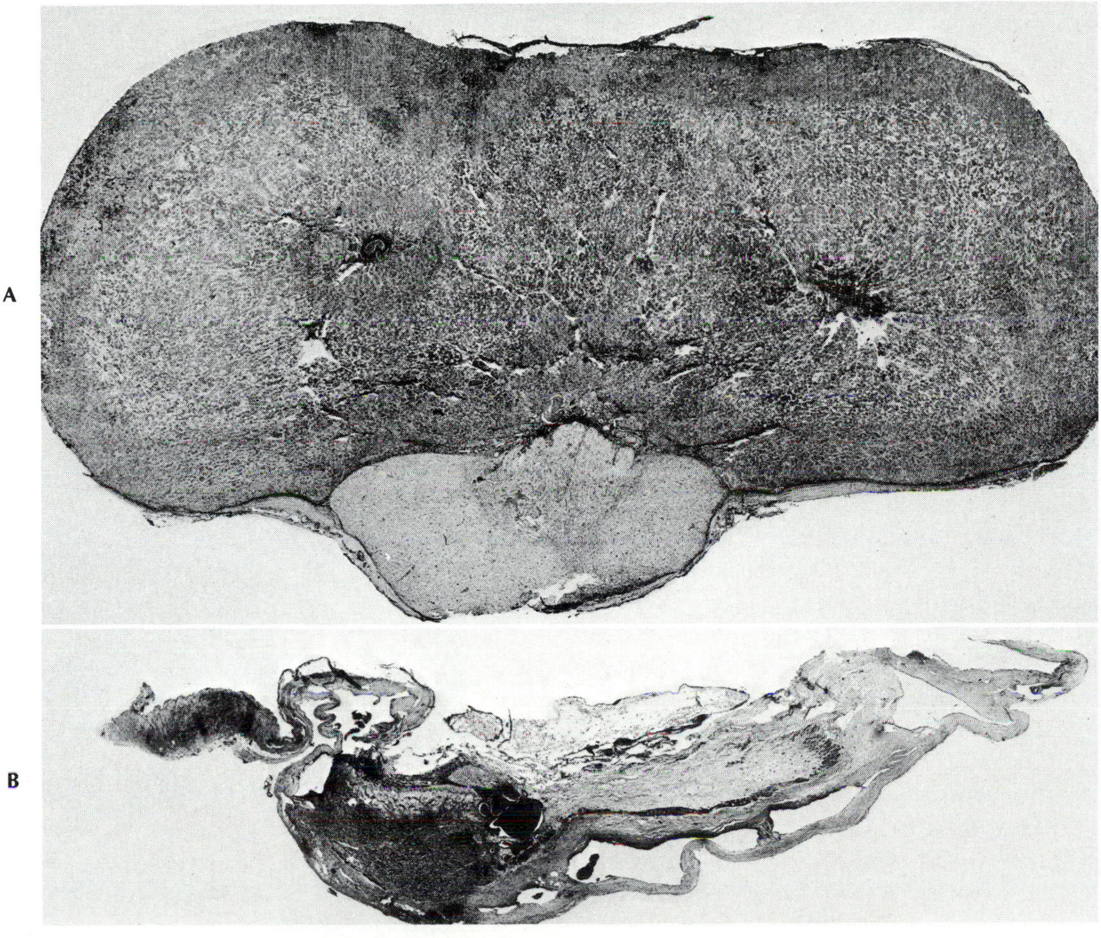

Fig. 32-9. Postpartum necrosis of pituitary gland. **A,** Most of anterior lobe affected. **B,** Gland shriveled and deformed. Patient survived for many years. (Hematoxylin and eosin; 10×; courtesy Prof. H.L. Sheehan and Dr. A.R. Currie.)

zone of tissue at the periphery may survive. The necrotic anterior lobe gradually shrivels and becomes replaced by a thin, semilunar collagenous scar (Fig. 32-9). The posterior lobe is unaffected. The degree of hypopituitarism depends on the extent of destruction. Failure of lactation may be the first sign, followed by amenorrhea and eventually by adrenocortical insufficiency and hypothyroidism.[115]

ACUTE INFLAMMATION

Acute purulent inflammation of the hypophysis may occur by direct extension of inflammation in an adjacent structure, by hematogenous dissemination during the course of overwhelming sepsis,[119] or as a complication of invasive pituitary adenoma.[120] Purulent meningitis causes acute hypophysitis by direct spread into the subarachnoid space surrounding the pituitary; inflammation in such a case may be limited to the surface of the gland. Rarely, the hypophysis is converted into a pus-filled sac.[118] Other causes include sinusitis, osteomyelitis of the sphenoid bone, thrombophlebitis of the cavernous sinus, and suppurative otitis media. In the case of hematogenous dissemination, microabscesses may form within the substance of adenohypophysis or neurohypophysis.[119]

CHRONIC INFLAMMATION

Granuloma

Granulomatous diseases may involve the pituitary and cause destruction of both adenohypophysis and neurohypophysis. Symptoms of hypopituitarism are proportional to the extent of destruction and localization of the involvement. Tuberculosis occurs by hematogenous dissemination or by direct extension from tuberculous meningitis; miliary tubercles or areas of caseous necrosis are found at autopsy. Syphilis of the pituitary may be congenital or acquired; in the acquired cases the lesion may be a diffuse fibrosis or gummatous necrosis.[122] Boeck's sarcoid can affect the central nervous system, with involvement of the base of the brain, hypothalamus, and pituitary including both neurohypophysis and adenohypophysis.[123] Noncaseating tubercles composed of epithelioid cells, lymphocytes, and giant cells of Langhans' type, which may contain asteroid bodies and Schaumann bodies, characterize the lesions. No etiologic agent can be demonstrated, and special stains for acid-fast organisms and fungi are negative.

The entity known as giant cell granuloma of the pituitary presents a histologic picture similar to Boeck's sarcoid, but unlike sarcoidosis, giant cell granuloma is not a disease of multiple systems. This rare disorder affects the anterior pituitary, and the involvement may progress to destruction of the adenohypophysis with consequent hypopituitarism and secondary atrophy of thyroid and adrenal glands. The hypophyseal lesions consist of noncaseating tubercles with Langhans' giant cells and associated chronic inflammatory cells. The condition occurs chiefly in middle-aged and elderly women.[124] The pathogenesis is obscure. In a few reported cases, similar granulomas were observed in the adrenals, and it has been suggested that giant cell granuloma may be an autoimmune or an infectious disorder.[121]

Lymphocytic hypophysitis

More recently, another variant of chronic inflammatory disease of the pituitary known as lymphocytic hypophysitis has been described in women, the majority of whom were postpartum.[124-126] In some patients the lesion appeared as a pituitary tumor.[124,126] Microscopically the adenohypophysis is involved by extensive nodular or diffuse infiltration of lymphocytes, sometimes with fibrosis. Concomitant thyroiditis and adrenalitis have been observed, with lymphoid infiltration in these organs. An autoimmune basis has been postulated for this disorder.

INFILTRATIONS AND METABOLIC DISORDERS

Amyloidosis

Generalized secondary amyloidosis may involve the pituitary.[129] In this condition, amyloid is deposited in the walls of the blood vessels of the adenohypophysis

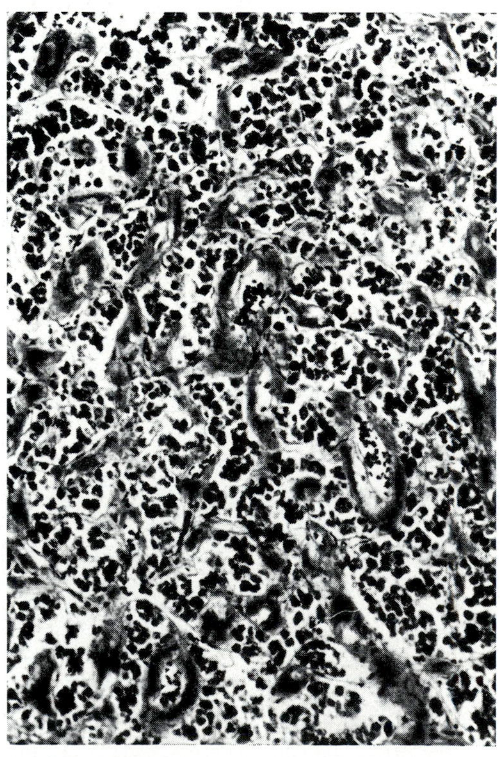

Fig. 32-10. Amyloid deposition in anterior lobe of pituitary gland. (Hematoxylin and eosin; 140×; courtesy Drs. Dorothy S. Russell and A.R. Currie.)

(Fig. 32-10). Amyloid may also be deposited in the pituitary in multiple myeloma.[127] Interstitial amyloid deposits may be found in pituitary adenomas,[133] and amyloid in the form of laminated concretions also has been described.[127,128,130,131]

Hand-Schüller-Christian disease

The posterior lobe, infundibular stem, and infundibulum are often involved by the xanthomatous deposits that characterize Hand-Schüller-Christian disease.[11] Usually the skull and dura mater adjacent to the hypophysis also are involved, with bony destruction. The infundibular lesions interfere with neurosecretion, and Hand-Schüller-Christian disease is an important cause of diabetes insipidus in children (see also p. 1263).

Hurler's syndrome (gargoylism)

The adenohypophyseal cells in Hurler's syndrome display a characteristic vacuolation with a foamy appearance, corresponding to the abnormal storage of mucopolysaccharides characteristic of this disorder. By electron microscopy the majority of the affected cells contain numerous membrane-bound vesicles. Lipid cytosomes with parallel-stacked or concentric osmiophilic lamellae known as "zebra bodies" also are present.[132]

TUMORS

Formerly cited at about 6%, the occurrence of symptomatic tumors of the pituitary has risen sharply in the past decade. This change is the result of the recognition of microadenomas (adenomas less than 10 mm) (Fig. 32-11) as a significant cause of the syndromes of pituitary hypersecretion. Although exact data are still lacking, it seems likely that their incidence may approach that of microadenomas at autopsy.[135] The early diagnosis of small intrasellar tumors has been greatly improved by advances in diagnostic radiology, clinical chemistry, and neurosurgery, the last enabling selective total adenomectomy without disturbing pituitary function. This turn of events has revolutionized the management of pituitary tumors.[136,137,139]

With improved clinical diagnosis of microadenomas and early surgical intervention, the role of frozen section for intraoperative diagnosis is changing. Although the neurosurgeon has little difficulty in identifying the tumor in a typical case, margins may present a problem.[140,142] Modified periodic acid–Schiff–orange G stain,[134,140] reticulin stain,[141] and fluorescent stains[138] using frozen sections have been suggested.

Tumors of the pituitary give rise to symptoms in two ways. Local effects result from expansion of the lesion, and distant effects are caused by hypersecretion or hyposecretion of trophic hormones or hypothalamic principles. Unchecked local growth and expansion will ultimately erode and enlarge the sella turcica, and extension upward into the suprasellar region impinges on optic chiasm, optic nerves, neurohypophysis, and adjacent cranial nerves (Fig. 32-12). At the same time, uninvolved portions of the pituitary may become compressed and attenuated, with insufficiency of trophic hormones or diabetes insipidus caused by pressure on the adenohypophysis or neurohypophysis, respectively. Displacement of the hypothalamus may impair production and transport of releasing hormones and inhibitory factors, causing further endocrine imbalance and abnormality. In fact, analysis of the effect of tumors has given considerable insight into the function of the hypophysis and hypothalamus.

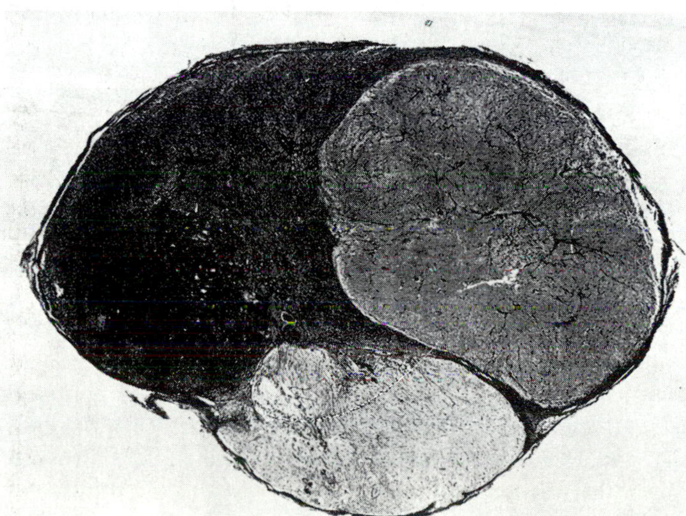

Fig. 32-11. Microadenoma of anterior lobe of pituitary gland. Clinically silent. (Acid fuchsin and aniline blue; 6×; courtesy Drs. Dorothy S. Russell and A.R. Currie.)

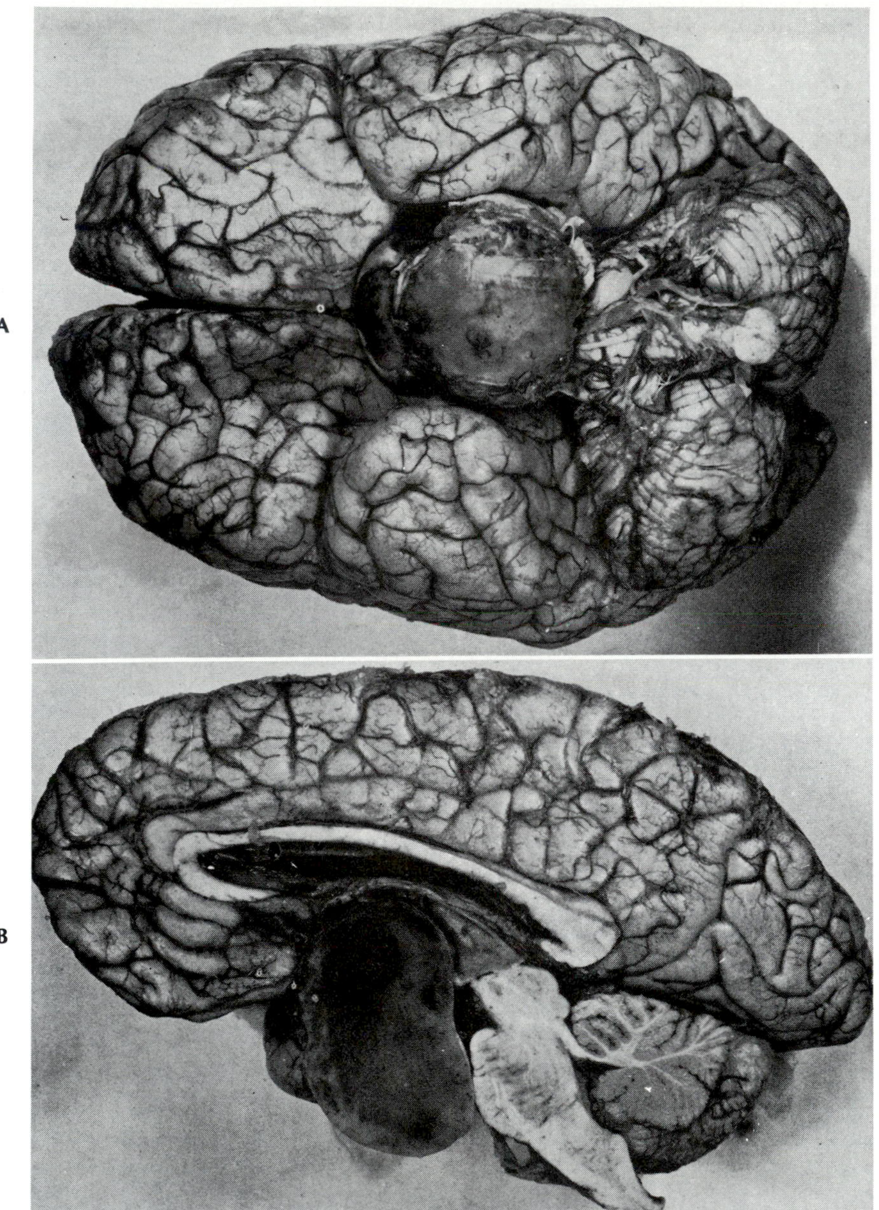

Fig. 32-12. A, Basal view of intrasellar part of large chromophobe adenoma. Note distortion of optic chiasm. **B,** Midsagittal view of same specimen shown in **A.** (Courtesy Drs. Dorothy S. Russell and A.R. Currie.)

Adenomas

Adenomas are the most common of the pituitary tumors, and their incidence in unselected autopsies is about 25%.[148,150,188] The simple but inadequate classification of adenomas as acidophil, basophil, or chromophobe that was proposed by early workers has been expanded and clarified by the remarkable advances of the past two decades, resulting in the functional classification of adenohypophyseal cells summarized in Table 32-1. Correlation of morphology with specific hormone production has given rise to the enlarged classification of pituitary adenomas that is now accepted by the World Health Organization[211]; a modified version is shown in Table 32-2. In the light of ultrastructural and immunocytochemical data, it is clear that many neoplasms formerly designated "chromophobe adenomas" are in reality tumors with granules too small or too sparse to be seen with the light microscope, explaining the paradoxical occurrence of "chromophobe" tumors in patients with clear-cut syndromes of hyperpituitarism such as acromegaly, Cushing's disease, or hyperthyroidism.

Some observers have suggested total rejection of the

Table 32-2. Classification of tumors of adenohypophysis

Hormone	Cell type		Syndrome
	Hematoxylin and eosin	Functional classification	
STH	Acidophil or chromophobe*	Somatotroph	Acromegaly
PRL		Lactotroph	Amenorrhea-galactorrhea
FSH-LH	Basophil or chromophobe*	Gonadotroph	—
TSH		Thyrotroph	Hyperthyroidism
ACTH-MSH		Corticomelanotroph	Cushing's syndrome, Nelson's syndrome
None	Chromophobe	No secretory function	Local compression: impaired vision, hypopituitarism

*Granules too small to be seen with light microscope.

classification of tumors as acidophil, basophil, or chromophobe. Instead, it seems more reasonable to retain the old terminology in screening hematoxylin and eosin–stained sections in analyzing a pituitary adenoma, recognizing that this procedure is a point of departure for application of the advanced techniques required for functional classification and final diagnosis.

Although the cause is usually unknown, failure of a target organ is a causative factor in some patients. Constant stimulation of pituitary cells by hypothalamic releasing hormones in the absence of feedback inhibition has been suggested as the mechanism.[213] Thus primary hypothyroidism, hypogonadism, or hypoadrenalism can lead to formation of a pituitary tumor. TSH cell adenomas and the sequence of events in their pathogenesis following thyroid ablation are well known in animals.[38,152,156] Basophil tumors also have been described in rats following gonadectomy.[159] The occurrence of thyrotroph cell adenoma associated with hypothyroidism in humans is well documented.[172] Pituitary tumors have also been reported in association with Addison's disease[153,162,169] and hypogonadism.[200]

Adenomas originate in the adenohypophysis and therefore arise in the hypophyseal fossa in the majority of cases. A few instances in which an adenoma originated outside the sella turcica, in an anomalous remnant of adenohypophysis, have been reported.[14,96]

Adenomas range from barely visible nodules (Fig. 32-11) to massive neoplasms with smooth or bosselated surfaces. Tumors less than 10 mm in diameter are termed microadenomas. Neurosurgeons have had the greatest experience in recognizing microadenomas; the consistency (soft, semisolid, or gelatinous) and color (creamy white, gray, or purple) of most microadenomas in contrast to the firm, yellow, "nonsuctionable" normal gland are regarded as diagnostic.[136,212] Externally, the adenohypophysis may appear normal, or symmetric and slightly enlarged. Microadenomas are typically discrete and well demarcated, but they lack a capsule. The larger tumors bulge upward from the sella turcica to encroach on the hypothalamus and third ventricle (Fig. 32-12). In such cases the tumor does not invade the brain, and it can be easily shelled from its bed in the compressed, invaginated cerebral tissue. Both large and small adenomas may be cystic, containing turbid or clear fluid. Also, infarction and hemorrhage may occur, producing the life-threatening syndrome of pituitary apoplexy in the case of larger tumors.[108]

With light microscopy, three patterns are observed: diffuse, sinusoidal, and papillary. The diffuse form is composed of polygonal cells arranged in sheets, with inconspicuous stroma (Fig. 32-13). The sinusoidal form more or less resembles the structure of the normal adenohypophysis. The cells tend to be columnar or fusiform, and the stroma has fibrovascular septa with sinusoidal blood vessels to which the cells are oriented, creating a perisinusoidal arrangement (Fig. 32-13). In the papillary form, which is a variant of the sinusoidal pattern, cuboidal or columnar neoplastic cells are arranged radially about papillae with a vascular core. In all three types the cells are quite orderly and mitoses are rare. Microscopic criteria for diagnosis of microadenoma include uniformity of cells, a well-defined margin, absence of the reticular pattern of the normal gland, and evidence of compression of the adjacent pituitary.[135,141,144,149,183] Reticulin stain is a useful adjunct in identifying the extent of the neoplasm, since the reticular pattern of the normal gland is lacking in the tumor (Fig. 32-14).

Acidophil adenoma

Acidophil tumors constitute well over half of the adenomas. In the past decade, the lactotroph, or prolactin cell adenoma, has become the most commonly diagnosed pituitary tumor.[155] Acidophil tumors that are sympto-

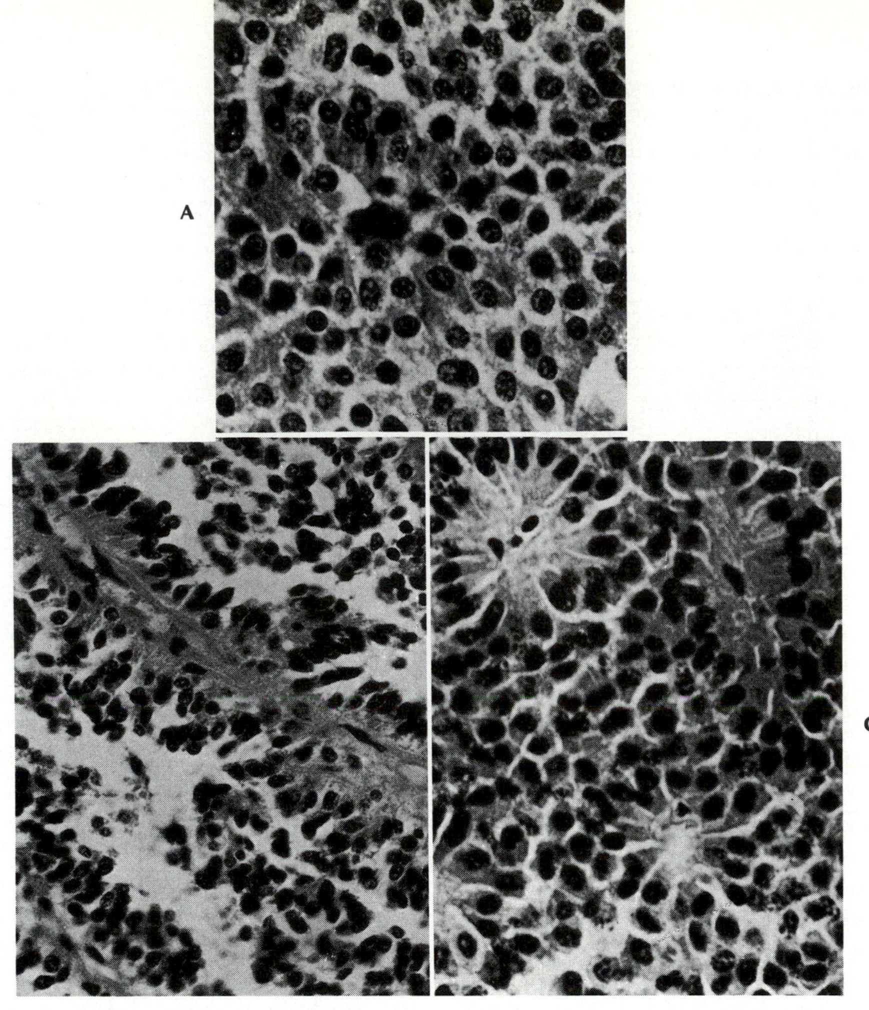

Fig. 32-13. Pituitary adenoma. **A,** Diffuse type. **B** and **C,** Perisinusoid type, with cells arranged about sinusoids. (**A** to **C,** Hematoxylin and eosin; **A,** 490×; **B,** 350×; **C,** 540×; courtesy Drs. Dorothy S. Russell and A.R. Currie.)

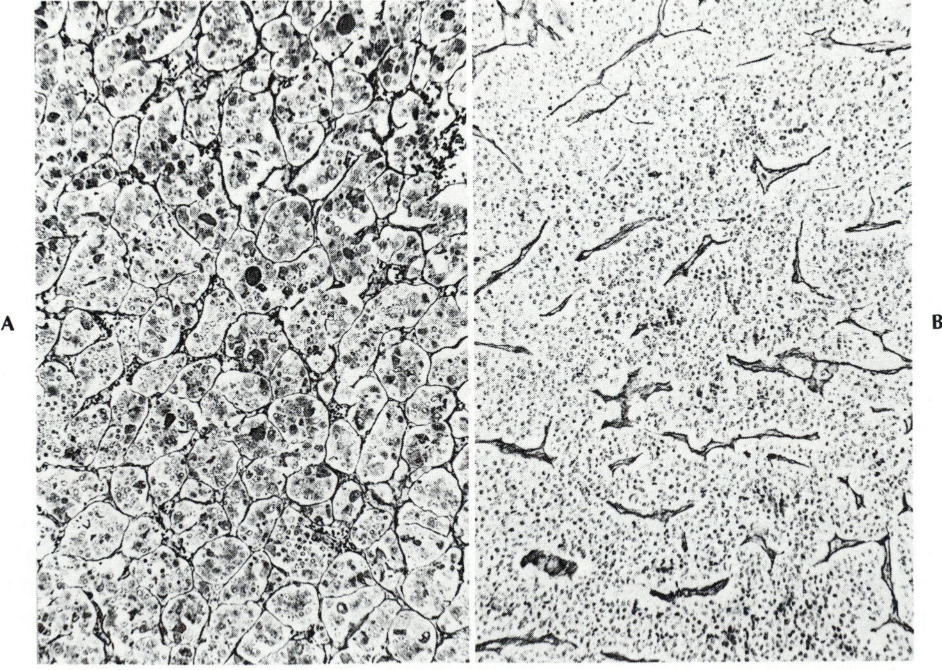

Fig. 32-14. Reticulin stain of, **A,** normal adenohypophysis and, **B,** pituitary adenoma. Normal alveolar pattern of reticulin is lost in tumor. (Gridley modification, silver impregnation method; 100×.)

matic usually do not reach massive proportions, although compression of adjacent hypophysis with hypophyseal insufficiency and suprasellar extension with compression of the optic chiasm and blindness may occur.

Acidophil adenomas are derived from the two types of acidophils normally present: somatotrophs (GH-secreting cells) and lactotrophs (PRL-secreting cells). They are best differentiated by immunocytochemical techniques. Neoplasms composed of a mixture of the two cell types are known as mammosomatotrophic tumors; they have been described in animals and humans.[146,160,175,187,190]

Acidophil microadenomas tend to localize in the lateral wings of the adenohypophysis, where acidophils are normally concentrated.[136] In all forms of acidophil adenomas, sparsely granulated or agranular hormone-secreting cells may be interspersed or may predominate; in hematoxylin and eosin–stained section, such a tumor may appear to be a chromophobe adenoma. In general, granules enlarge during storage,[183] and small, sparse granules correlate with rapid release of hormone and higher levels in the blood.[165,171,183] A subset of poorly granulated acidophil tumors associated with hyperprolactinemia or acromegaly, exhibiting immunostaining for GH and PRL, and having features of GH and PRL cells by electron microscopy has been designated acidophil stem cell adenoma.[166,168]

Somatotroph cell adenoma. Functioning GH-cell adenoma, may produce gigantism or acromegaly, depending on the patient's age. GH-cell adenoma that occurs in a prepubertal patient whose epiphyses have not closed leads to proportionate growth of the body with gigantism. In the adult, epiphyses are closed and abnormal growth is confined to the skull, jaw, hands, feet, and soft tissues, with enlargement of supraorbital ridges, the mandible, and phalanges, together with a characteristic coarsening of the features, thickening of heel pads, and enlargement of the viscera.

By light and electron microscopy, neoplastic acidophil cells may closely resemble their normal counterparts.[38,201] The GH cell has an abundant, well-developed, rough endoplasmic reticulum, a prominent Golgi apparatus, and round, oval, or pear-shaped granules from 100 to 500 nm.[182] Distinctive spherical filamentous aggregates may be found in the cytoplasm.[182,202]

Lactotroph (PRL) cell adenoma. The functioning PRL tumor produces prolactin (hence the designation prolactinoma). The excess prolactin may cause lactation. In women, increased prolactin blocks ovulation and amenorrhea results. The clinical picture of amenorrhea and galactorrhea produced by prolactinoma is known as the Forbes-Albright syndrome.[38,154,191] In men with prolactinoma, impotence, infertility, oligospermia, gynecomastia, and galactorrhea have been reported.[143,155,193,203]

PRL cells, which are erythrosin positive by light microscopy, exhibit a well-developed, rough endoplasmic reticulum, nebenkerns, a prominent Golgi apparatus, and granules of varying number, size, and shape. In general, the granules are large, averaging 600 nm; they may reach 1200 nm in heavily granulated tumors.[134] Misplaced exocytosis or release of secretory granules from cell surfaces not adjacent to perivascular spaces is characteristic.[164] Intra-adenomatous dystrophic calcification is a distinctive feature of PRL-secreting adenomas,[182] and formation of pituitary "stone" has been reported.[209]

Basophil adenoma

Basophil tumors are less common than acidophil adenomas, constituting less than 10% in most series. Basophil tumors are generally small, and the majority are microadenomas.[121,195] Three kinds of basophil adenomas are observed, corresponding to the three functional types of basophils in the normal hypophysis—gonadotrophs, thyrotrophs, and corticotrophs. Immunocytologic techniques are the best means for identification. Corticotroph tumors are the most common of these; TSH tumors are far less frequent, and FSH/LH tumors are rare.

Basophil microadenomas tend to localize in the median wedge or central core of the gland, where basophils are normally concentrated.[47,136] In hematoxylin and eosin–stained sections, the histologic patterns of basophil adenomas present no unusual features. Corticotroph adenomas are usually well granulated, but granules are sparse or absent in most reported thyrotroph and gonadotroph tumors, and thus they appear as chromophobe adenomas. Hormone-secreting oncocytic variants have also been documented.[158,170]

Basophil tumors secrete glycoprotein hormones, and elevation of alpha subunits has proved to be a useful marker in diagnosis of basophil adenomas.[167,173,194]

Corticotroph cell adenoma. Functioning corticotroph cell tumors are associated with two distinctive clinical disorders—Cushing's disease[151] and Nelson's syndrome.[189] In Cushing's disease the tumor causes hyperplasia of the adrenal cortex and overproduction of adrenal cortical hormones, thus producing the characteristic clinical findings that include truncal obesity, moon face, purple striae, muscular wasting, hypertension, and abnormal glucose tolerance. Cushing's belief that pituitary basophil adenomas were a significant cause of adrenal hypersecretion recently has been substantiated.[147,198,208]

The second disorder associated with corticotroph cell tumors is Nelson's syndrome—pituitary tumor and hyperpigmentation after bilaterial adrenalectomy.[189] When bilateral adrenalectomy is performed to control the clinical manifestations of hypercorticism, about 10% of patients develop cutaneous melanosis, signs and symptoms of a pituitary tumor, and elevated plasma ACTH. Whether the tumor was present at the outset and was the original cause of adrenal hyperplasia is not known at present.

Lamberts, deLange, and Stefanko[180] have found argyrophilic nerve fibers within some corticotroph adenomas and postulate that ACTH-secreting pituitary adenomas arise from basophils in two different locations, the adenohypophysis and cells of intermediate lobe incorporated within the neurohypophysis.

In addition to ACTH, corticotroph adenomas may also contain MSH, alpha endorphin,[204] beta-lipotropic hormone (β-LPH),[195] and beta endorphin.[39] The secretion of ACTH, LPH, and beta endorphin also has been confirmed in cultures of pituitary tumors.[157]

Pituitary adenomas containing immunoreactive 1-39 ACTH, α-17-39 ACTH or 19-39 ACTH, beta lipotropin, beta MSH, and alpha endorphin have been described in patients without hypercorticism.[167,206] Such tumors have been designated silent corticotroph adenomas.[167] Recently, Ridgway and associates[194] found isolated hypersecretion and serum elevation of the alpha subunit of glycoprotein hormones in two patients with no recognizable endocrine syndrome who had tumors staining as chromophobe adenomas.

With light microscopy, corticotroph cells more or less resemble their normal counterparts. Typically the cytoplasm contains abundant basophilic granules, is periodic acid–Schiff positive, and contains ACTH with immunoperoxidase technique. LPH[195] and endorphins[21] have also been demonstrated. The extent of granularity is variable, and cells resembling chromophobes may be interspersed or may predominate.

By electron microscopy, the secretory granules range from 250 to 700 nm, average 350 to 500 nm, and are spherical or irregular.[177,195] The perinuclear cytoplasm often contains microfilaments similar to those seen in Crooke's cells of patients with hypercorticism.[182,195]

Thyrotroph cell adenoma. Thyrotroph cell tumors are rare; only a few dozen cases have been reported. Clinically the tumor may be primary, arising autonomously in a previously euthyroid patient,[197,205] or it may be secondary to long-standing hypothyroidism.[172,199] Pituitary tumors that cause hyperthyroidism secrete TSH, which in turn stimulates the thyroid to produce excess hormones. Thus serum levels of T3, T4, and TSH are simultaneously elevated. The tumors that occur in association with hypothyroidism represent adenomatous transformation of thyrotroph cells in response to long-standing thyroid (end-organ) failure.

Most thyrotroph tumors have grown to the size of macroadenomas with suprasellar extension and visual disturbances before they are diagnosed. Usually hypothyroidism is recognized and treated first, and only after an asymptomatic interval of months or years do signs of intracranial tumor supervene.

Thyrotroph adenomas stain as chromophobe adenomas in hematoxylin and eosin–stained sections; the cells are typically small, angular, and polyhedral, resembling normal thyrotrophs. Granules positive for periodic acid–Schiff and aldehyde thionine may be present. TSH is demonstrated by immunocytochemical staining or by chemical extraction of the tumor tissue. A significant proportion of TSH-cell adenomas contain an admixture of cells producing a second hormone, usually PRL or GH.

By electron microscopy, the granules are small and sparse, measuring less than 200 nm. They are often in the periphery of the cell, localized along the cell membrane.

Gonadotroph cell adenoma. A number of cases of gonadotrophin-producing tumors verified by clinical, immunocytochemical, and ultrastructural data have now been reported.[207] Adenomas that secrete only FSH[177] and those that secrete a combination of FSH and LH have been described. Some patients have had long-standing hypogonadism[178,200]; in others, onset of disturbed gonadal function was recent. Most tumors have been macroadenomas, with disturbed vision or headache as an initial symptom.

Gonadotroph cell adenomas are chromophobe tumors in hematoxylin and eosin–stained sections. Scattered oncocytes (verified by electron microscopy) have been described.[207] Periodic acid–Schiff stains may reveal a few small positive granules. The tumor cells are small and polyhedral or angular. FSH and LH are demonstrated by immunohistochemical staining or extraction. Beta endorphin or TSH also has been found in some tumors.

Electron microscopy reveals small secretory granules averaging 150 to 200 nm, distributed throughout the cell or along the cell membrane.[178,207] Microtubules are generally abundant,[178] and nebenkern pattern has been observed.[207]

Chromophobe adenoma

Chromophobe tumors constitute about 20% of surgically treated adenomas.[182] These neoplasms also have been termed endocrine inactive adenomas[182] or null cell adenomas.[179] They are clinically silent until relatively far advanced. The first symptoms are headache and disturbed vision; ultimately, hypopituitarism caused by compression of uninvolved pituitary gland supervenes. Chromophobe adenoma is to be differentiated from the clinically silent adenoma composed of cells that are immunoreactive for pituitary hormones, that is, ACTH, beta endorphin or beta lipotropin,[161,167] the adenoma that produces biologically inactive substances immunologically related to pituitary hormones,[206] and the adenoma associated with isolated production of alpha subunits of glycoprotein hormone.[194]

Chromophobe tumors consist of small cells with scanty

cytoplasm and small, oval nuclei, exhibiting the usual diffuse, sinusoidal, or papillary patterns. The cytoplasm fails to stain with periodic acid–Schiff or lead hematoxylin, and the cells show no evidence of granules or production of hormones by electron microscopy or immunocytochemistry.[211] With electron microscopy, abundant microtubules have been described.[179]

Multiple endocrine adenomatosis

Adenomas of the pituitary occur as an integral part of Wermer's syndrome, or multiple endocrine adenomatosis (MEA) type I.[145] This genetic disorder is inherited as an autosomal dominant, and familial involvement is the rule.[210] The disease is characterized by multiple adenomas involving pancreatic islets, parathyroids, and the pituitary. The endocrine involvement may be sequential rather than simultaneous. Clinically the patient usually has a combination of Zollinger-Ellison syndrome, hyperparathyroidism, and signs of pituitary tumor, which is often a PRL-secreting neoplasm, chromophobic by light microscopy.[185,192] At least one case of a malignant pituitary tumor has been recorded in multiple endocrine adenomatosis.[186]

Oncocytic adenoma

Oncocytic adenomas are composed of cells with characteristic finely granular, eosinophilic cytoplasm, resembling acidophils except for their fine rather than coarse granularity.[174,184] The cytoplasm is densely packed with abnormal mitochondria, which is the basis for the acidophilia observed with the light microscope.[163] Thus positive identification of this tumor depends on electron microscopy. Some oncocytomas are nonfunctional, whereas others are responsible for hypersecretion, including Cushing's syndrome[158] or amenorrhea-galactorrhea syndrome.[170]

Carcinoma

Primary carcinoma

To identify a primary tumor of the adenohypophysis with distant metastases as a carcinoma presents no problem.[214,218] However, the characteristic tendency of tumors of the adenohypophysis to erode bone and displace or compress soft tissues as the tumors expand, which already has been emphasized, has led to considerable debate on the criteria for malignancy of tumors without distant spread. Evans[215] takes the sensible approach that all tumors that burst their capsules and directly invade the adjacent structures, especially the cavernous sinuses, the base of the cranium, and the sphenoidal sinuses, should be labeled malignant. It is clear that cytologic criteria are not absolute, since pleomorphism, hyperchromatism, and mitotic activity have been observed in tumors that are not infiltrative and tumors with none of these qualities have exhibited invasiveness.[215]

Carcinomas may originate from chromophobe or chromophil cells; chromophobe neoplasms are the rule. However, functioning tumors usually producing adrenocortical hyperplasia and Cushing's syndrome have been reported.[218]

Metastatic carcinoma

Metastases to the pituitary gland occur in patients having widespread metastatic carcinoma. The usual primary site is the breast, and carcinoma of the lung is the second most common.[217,219] Most observers have found the pars nervosa to be involved more frequently than the pars distalis. Destruction of the posterior pituitary by metastatic carcinoma is a significant cause of diabetes insipidus in patients with carcinomatosis.[216]

Craniopharyngioma

Craniopharyngioma is a benign tumor believed to originate in remnants of Rathke's pouch that persist into postnatal life. An alternative explanation that the neoplasm arises by metaplasia of adenohypophyseal cells has been proposed. The onset of these tumors in childhood favors the origin from embryologic rests.[215] Whichever theory is correct, it is a fact that most craniopharyngiomas originate outside the sella turcica and are usually suprasellar in location. Occurrence within the sphenoid bone has also been reported.

Craniopharyngiomas make up 1% to 3% of intracranial tumors.[227,234,235] They are most common in children and young adults but may occur in older persons as well.

Grossly the tumor is encapsulated and firmly adherent to surrounding tissues, which suffer compression as the neoplasm slowly enlarges. Thus the structures comprised are the brain above, the pituitary below, the optic chiasm anteriorly, and the circle of Willis at the periphery. The typical tumor is cystic, with intervening solid areas (Fig. 32-15). The content is fluid or semisolid, dark brown, greasy material containing cholesterol crystals, altered blood, and calcified debris.

Microscopically, the patterns are distinctive. The solid areas contain anastomosing cords of well-differentiated stratified squamous epithelium with a palisaded peripheral layer, set in a stroma of connective tissue (Fig. 32-16). Within the epithelium, areas composed of loosely arranged stellate cells may be found. Mitoses and cellular pleomorphism are uncommon. The cystic regions may be lined by similar epithelial cords, with lipid histiocytes in the stroma and desquamated keratin in the cysts. The ultrastructure of craniopharyngioma has been described by Ghatak and associates.[223]

The histologic patterns may strikingly resemble those of ameloblastoma, an epithelial odontogenic tumor of the jaw.[230] Consequently, craniopharyngioma also is known as ameloblastoma. That a craniopharyngioma should resemble an ameloblastoma is not surprising, since the adenohypophysis itself arises in primitive buccal epithe-

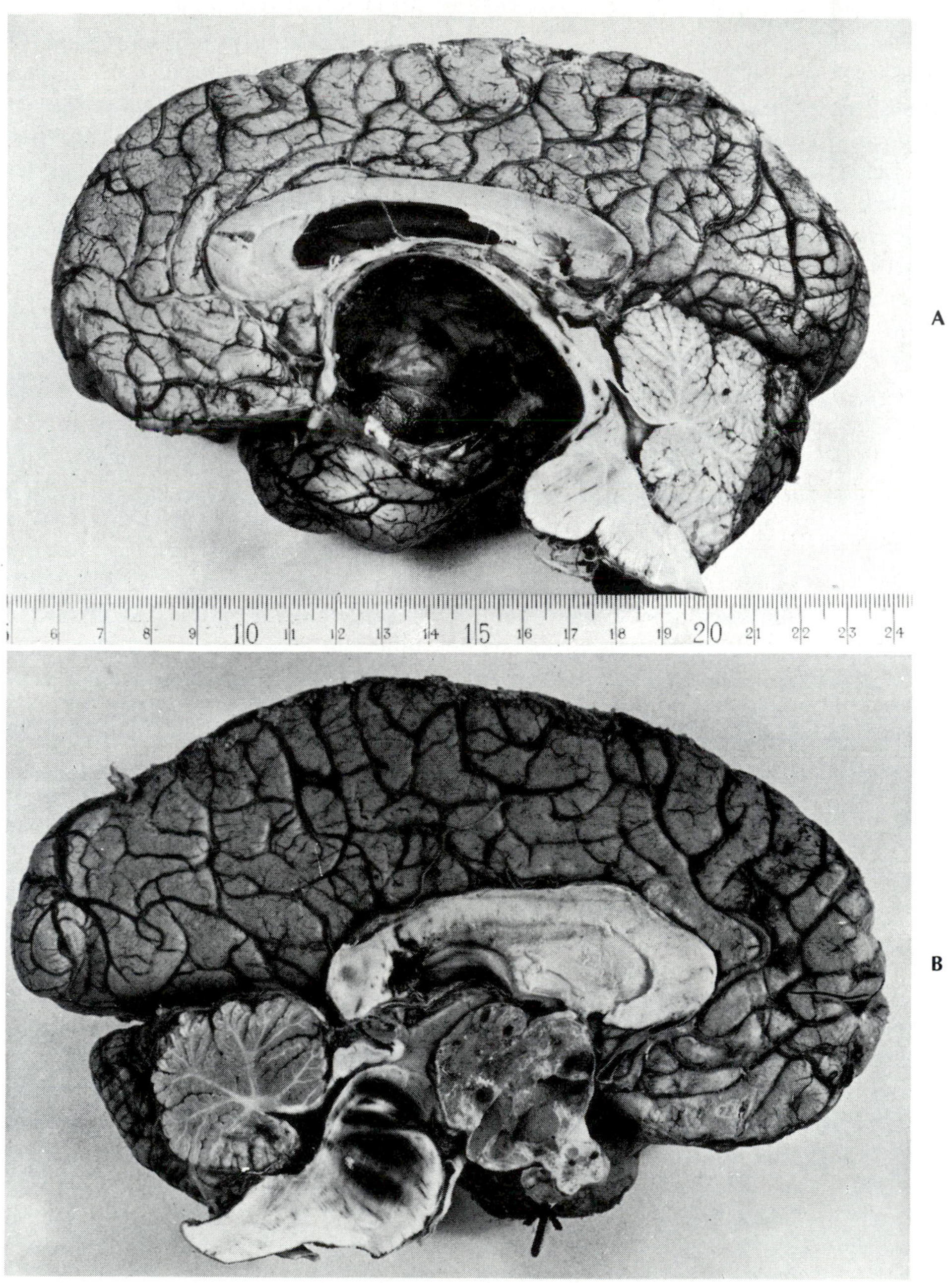

Fig. 32-15. A, Cystic suprasellar craniopharyngioma. **B,** Solid and cystic suprasellar craniopharyngioma. *Arrow,* Pituitary gland. (Courtesy Drs. Dorothy S. Russell and A.R. Currie.)

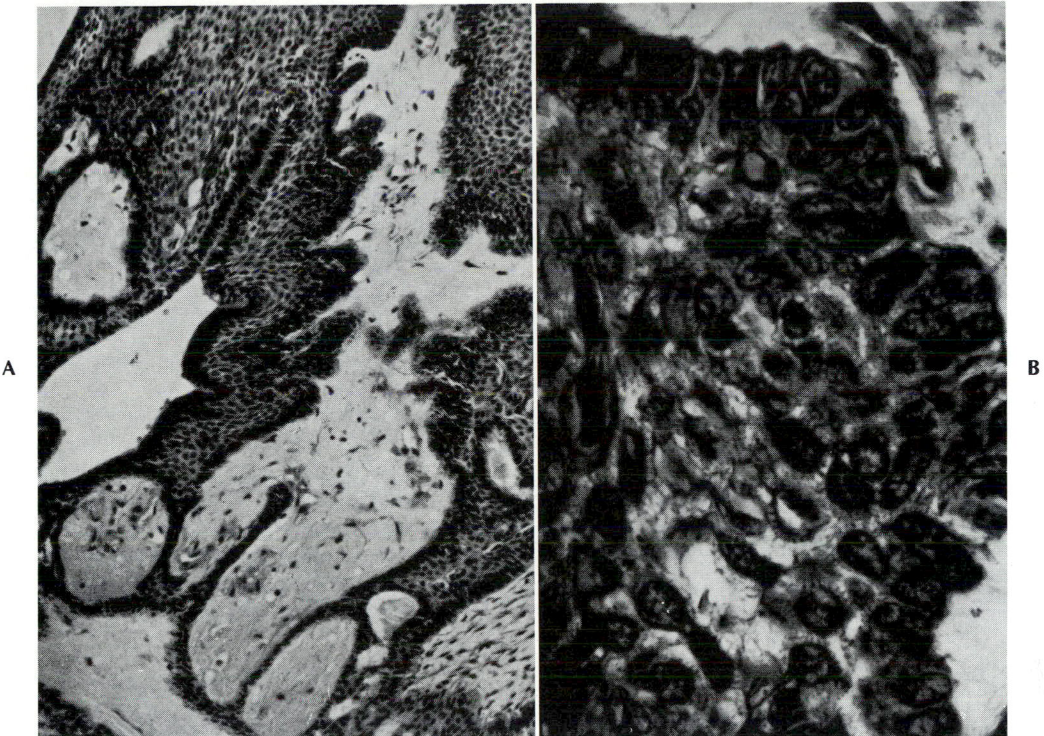

Fig. 32-16. Craniopharyngioma. **A,** Solid anastomosing trabeculae of cells. **B,** Surface cells of basal type and squamous cells. (**A,** Hematoxylin and eosin, 140×; **B,** phosphotungstic acid and hematoxylin, 850×; courtesy Drs. Dorothy S. Russell and A.R. Currie.)

lium. It follows that neoplasms of its developmental remnants might be expected to reflect kinship with other buccal derivatives.

Although craniopharyngioma is histologically benign and grows slowly, ablation is difficult because of its location, and progressive enlargement is the rule.

Intrasellar cyst

Colloid-filled, epithelium-lined, asymptomatic benign cysts of microscopic size are commonly found at the junction of the pars distalis and the pars nervosa.[231] Such cysts are interpreted as remnants of Rathke's pouch. Rarely, larger benign cysts producing symptoms occur. They may be located entirely within the sella, or they may protrude above it, producing a dumbbell shape. The intrasellar cysts are usually lined by simple cuboidal epithelium, which may be ciliated.[130,231] The suprasellar portion of a dumbbell cyst may be lined by stratified squamous epithelium.[9] Kepes[224] has described a unique transitional epithelial tumor arising in the wall of a Rathke's cleft cyst.

Granular cell tumor (choristoma)

The granular cell tumor arises in the neurohypophysis, and it is the most common primary tumor of the posterior lobe. Nearly always asymptomatic, granular cell tumor is usually identified as an incidental finding at autopsy in persons past 30 years of age.[225] The incidence in Luse and Kernohan's series of autopsies was 6.4%.[225] Originally the name "choristoma" was proposed in the belief that the condition was a developmental anomaly. More recently, origin from Schwann cells[220] or pituicytes[226] has been suggested.

Grossly the lesion is generally too small to be seen. Microscopically it is composed of orderly, large polygonal cells with abundant granular pale pink cytoplasm and small, oval, eccentrically placed nuclei. The resemblance to the tumor known as granular myoblastoma found in extracranial locations is striking.

Rarely, granular cell tumor of the neurohypophysis may be large enough to produce symptoms. Such patients have signs and symptoms of a space-occupying intracranial lesion[232] or loss of vision as a result of compression of the optic chiasm.[229,233]

Germinal tumors

Tumors histologically identical to germinoma (seminoma) and teratoma of the gonads may occur within and adjacent to the sella turcica.[222,228] Because these tumors are more common in the pineal region, formerly they were designated ectopic pinealoma when they occurred in the hypothalamic region or the sella. However, the identity of the pinealoma with the germinoma (seminoma) of the testis was recognized by Friedman,[221] who

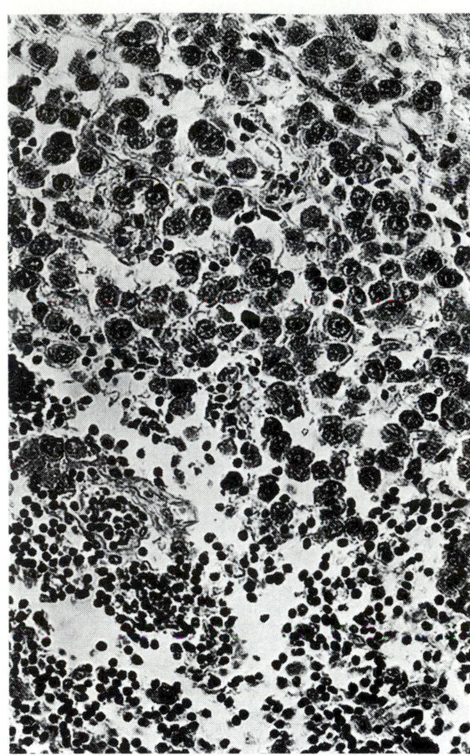

Fig. 32-17. Germinoma of pituitary stalk and posterior lobe of pituitary gland. (Hematoxylin and eosin; 260×; courtesy Drs. Dorothy S. Russell and A.R. Currie.)

emphasized their unmistakable morphologic congruity, and the term *germinoma* has become accepted.[228]

Grossly the germinoma is a fleshy, soft gray, diffusely infiltrating mass, frequently associated with hemorrhage. Microscopically the tumor is composed of large polygonal cells with abundant cytoplasm, a large vesicular nucleus, and one or more prominent nucleoli (Fig. 32-17). Mitoses are numerous. The cells are arranged in sheets or clusters separated by fibrovascular septa. Numerous small lymphocytes are usually present in the stroma. The resemblance to germinoma (seminoma) of the testis and dysgerminoma of the ovary is remarkable.

Teratomas also may occur in a suprasellar location. These neoplasms typically are cystic and are lined by ectodermal derivatives; bone and cartilage may be found in the wall.[228]

REFERENCES

Structure

1. Adams, J.H., Daniel, P.M., and Prichard, M.M.L.: Observations on the portal circulation of pituitary gland, Neuroendocrinology **1**:193, 1965-1966.
2. Bergland, R.M., Ray, B.S., and Torack, R.M.: Anatomical variations in the pituitary gland and adjacent structures in 225 human autopsy cases, J. Neurosurg. **28**:93, 1968.
3. Boyd, J.D.: Observations on the human pharyngeal hypophysis, J. Endocrinol. **14**:66, 1956.
4. Erdheim, J., and Stumme, F.: Über die Schwangerschaftsveränderungen bie der Hypophyse, Beitr. Pathol. Anat. **46**:1, 1909.
5. Jost, A.: Anterior pituitary function in foetal life. In Harris, G.W., and Donovan, B.T., editors: The pituitary gland, Berkeley, 1966, University of California Press.
6. Melchionna, R.H., and Moore, R.A.: The pharyngeal pituitary gland, Am. J. Pathol. **14**:763, 1938.
7. Pantić, V.R.: The specificity of pituitary cells and regulation of their activities, Int. Rev. Cytol. **40**:153, 1975.
8. Renn, W.H., and Rhoton, A.L., Jr.: Microsurgical anatomy of the sellar region, Neurosurgery **43**:288, 1975.
9. Russell, D.S.: Pituitary gland (hypophysis). In Anderson, W.A.D., editor: Pathology, ed. 4, St. Louis, 1961, The C.V. Mosby Co.
10. Russell, D.S.: Effects of dividing the pituitary stalk in man, Lancet **1**:466, 1956.
11. Sheehan, H.L., and Kovacs, K.: Neurohypophysis and hypothalamus. In Bloodworth, J.M.B., Jr., editor: Endocrine pathology, ed. 2, Baltimore, 1982, The Williams & Wilkins Co.
12. Stanfield, J.P.: The blood supply of the human pituitary gland, J. Anat. **94**:257, 1960.
13. Wells, L.J., and Highby, D.N.: Experimental evidence of production of adrenotrophin by the fetal hypophysis, Proc. Soc. Exp. Biol. Med. **68**:487, 1948.
14. Willis, R.A.: The borderland of embryology and pathology, London, 1958, Butterworth & Co.
15. Xuereb, G.P., Prichard, M.M.L., and Daniel, P.M.: Arterial supply and venous drainage of human hypophysis cerebri, Q. J. Exp. Physiol. **39**:199, 1954.
16. Xuereb, G.P., Prichard, M.M.L., and Daniel, P.M.: The hypophysial portal system of vessels in man, Q. J. Exp. Physiol. **39**:219, 1954.

Histology and function

17. Adams, C.W.M., and Swettenham, K.V.: Histochemical identification of two types of basophil cells in the normal human adenohypophysis, J. Pathol. Bacteriol. **75**:95, 1958.
18. Bergland, R.M., and Torack, R.M.: An ultrastructural study of follicular cells in the human anterior pituitary, Am. J. Pathol. **57**:293, 1969.
19. Brookes, L.D.: A stain for differentiating two types of acidophil cells in the rat pituitary, Stain Technol. **43**:41, 1968.
20. Celio, M.R.: Distribution of β-endorphin immunoreactive cells in human fetal and adult pituitaries and in pituitary adenomas, J. Histochem. Cytochem. **27**:1215, 1979.
21. Celio, M.R., et al.: "Proopiocortin fragments" in normal human adult pituitary, Acta Endocrinol. **95**:27, 1980.
22. deCicco, F.A., Dekker, A., and Yunis, E.J.: Fine structure of Crooke's hyaline change in the human pituitary gland, Arch. Pathol. **94**:65, 1972.
23. Ezrin, C.: Embryology and anatomy of thyrotrophin-secreting cell, the thyrotroph. In Werner, S.C., and Ingbar, S.H., editors: The thyroid, ed. 3, Hagerstown, Md., 1971, Harper & Row, Publishers, Inc.
24. Ezrin, C., Horvath, E., and Kovacs, K.: Anatomy and cytology of the normal and abnormal pituitary gland. In DeGroot, L.J., et al., editors: Endocrinology, New York, 1979, Grune & Stratton Inc.
25. Ezrin, C., and Murray, S.: The cells of the human adenohypophysis in pregnancy, thyroid disease and adrenal cortical disorders. In Benoit, J., and DeLage, C., editors: Cytologie de l'adénohypophyse, Paris, 1963, Centre National de la Recherche Scientifique.
26. Farquhar, M.G., Skutelsky, E.H., and Hopkins, C.R.: Structure and function of dispersed anterior pituitary cells: in vitro studies. In Tixier-Vidal, A., and Farquhar, M.G., editors: The anterior pituitary, New York, 1975, Academic Press, Inc.
27. Fowler, M.R., and McKeel, Jr., D.W.: Human adenohypophyseal quantitative histochemical cell classification, Arch. Pathol. Lab. Med. **103**:613, 1979.
28. Girod, C.: Histochemistry of the adenohypophysis. Handbuch der Histochemie, vol. 8, part 4, Stuttgart, 1976, Gustav Fischer Verlag.

29. Halmi, N.S.: Current status of human pituitary cytophysiology, N.Z. Med. J. **80**:551, 1974.
30. Herlant, M.: Introduction. In Tixier-Vidal, A., and Farquhar, M.G., editors: The anterior pituitary, New York, 1975, Academic Press, Inc.
31. Herlant, M., and Pasteels, J.L.: Histophysiology of human anterior pituitary, Methods Achiev. Exp. Pathol. **3**:250, 1967.
32. Holmes, R.L., and Ball, J.N.: The pituitary gland, Cambridge, Eng., 1974, Cambridge University Press.
33. Kovacs, K., Horvath, R., and Ryan, N.: Immunocytology of the human pituitary. In DeLellis, R., editor: Diagnostic immunohistochemistry, vol. 2, Monographs in diagnostic pathology, New York, 1981, Masson Publishing USA, Inc.
34. McManus, J.F.A.: Histological demonstration of mucin after periodic acid, Nature **158**:202, 1946.
35. McNicol, A.M.: Patterns of corticotropic cells in the adult human pituitary in Cushing's disease, Diagn. Histopathol. **4**:335, 1981.
36. Nieuwenhuijzen Kruseman, A.C., and Schröeder-van der Elst, J.P.: The immunolocalization of ACTH and a MSH in human and rat pituitaries, Virchows Arch (Cell Pathol.) **22**:263, 1976.
37. Norris, D.O.: Vertebrate endocrinology, Philadelphia, 1980, Lea & Febiger.
38. Olivier, L., et al.: Ultrastructure of pituitary tumor cells: a critical study. In Tixier-Vidal, A., and Farquhar, M.G., editors: The anterior pituitary, New York, 1975, Academic Press, Inc.
39. Osamura, R.Y., et al.: Adrenocorticotropic hormone cells and immunoreactive β-endorphin cells in the human pituitary gland, Am. J. Pathol. 99:105, 1980.
40. Paget, G.E., and Eccleston, E.: Simultaneous specific demonstrations of thyrotroph, gonadotroph, and acidophil cells in the anterior hypophysis, Stain Technol. **35**:119, 1960.
41. Paiz, C., and Hennigar, G.R.: Electron microscopy and histochemical correlation of human anterior pituitary cells, Am. J. Pathol. **59**:43, 1970.
42. Pasteels, J.L., et al.: Morphology of lactotropes and somatotropes of man and rhesus monkeys, J. Clin. Endocrinol. **34**:959, 1972.
43. Pearse, A.G.E.: Cytochemistry and cytology of the normal anterior hypophysis investigated by the trichrome-periodic acid-Schiff method, J. Pathol. Bacteriol. **64**:811, 1952.
44. Pearse, A.G.E., and van Noorden, S.: The functional cytology of the human adenohypophysis, Can. Med. Assoc. J. **88**:462, 1963.
45. Pelletier, G., Robert, F., and Hardy, J.: Identification of human anterior pituitary cells by immunoelectron microscopy, J. Clin. Endocrinol. **46**:534, 1978.
46. Phifer, R.F., Midgley, A.R., and Spicer, S.S.: Immunohistologic and histologic evidence that follicle-stimulating hormone and luteinizing hormone are present in the same cell type in the human pars distalis, J. Clin. Endocrinol. **36**:125, 1973.
47. Phifer, R.F., Orth, D.N., and Spicer, S.S.: Specific demonstration of human hypophyseal adrenocortico-melanotropic (ACTH/MSH) cell, J. Clin. Endocrinol. **39**:684, 1974.
48. Phifer, R.F., and Spicer, S.S.: Immunohistochemical and histologic demonstration of thyrotrophic cells of the human adenohypophysis, J. Clin. Endocrinol. **36**:1210, 1973.
49. Rasmussen, A.T.: Origin of the basophilic cells in the posterior lobe of the human hypophysis, Am. J. Anat. **46**:461, 1930.
50. Romeis, B.: Die mikroskopische Anatomie der Hypophyse. In von Möllendorff, W., editor: Handbuch der mikroskopischen Anatomie des Menschen, vol. 6, part 3, Berlin, 1940, Julius Springer Verlag.
51. von Lawzewitsch, I., et al.: Cytological and ultrastructural characterizaion of the human pituitary, Acta Anat. **81**:286, 1972.
52. van Oordt, P.G.W.J.: Nomenclature of the hormone-producing cells in the adenohypophysis: a report of the International Committee for Nomenclature of the Adenohypophysis, Gen. Comp. Endocrinol. **5**:131, 1965.

Pituitary in endocrine disorders

53. Bloodworth, J.M.B., Jr., Kirkendall, W.M., and Carr, T.L.: Addison's disease associated with thyroid insufficiency and atrophy (Schmidt syndrome), J. Clin. Endocrinol. **14**:540, 1954.
54. Boyce, R., and Beadles, C.F.: Enlargement of the hypophysis cerebri in myxoedema; with remarks upon hypertrophy of the hypophysis, associated with changes in the thyroid body, J. Pathol. Bacteriol. **1**:224, 1893.
55. Burt, A.S., Landing, B.H., and Sommers, S.C.: Amphophil tumors of the hypophysis induced in mice by I^{131}, Cancer Res. **14**:497, 1954.
56. Carpenter, G.C.J., et al.: Schmidt's syndrome (thyroid and adrenal insufficiency): a review of the literature and a report of fifteen new cases including ten instances of coexistent diabetes mellitus, Medicine **43**:153, 1964.
57. Crooke, A.D.: A change in the basophil cells of the pituitary gland common to conditions that exhibit the syndrome attributed to basophil adenoma, J. Pathol. Bacteriol. **41**:339, 1935.
58. Crooke, A.D., and Russell, D.S.: The pituitary gland in Addison's disease, J. Pathol. Bacteriol. **40**:255, 1935.
59. Ezrin, C.: The adenohypophysis. In Ezrin, C., et al., editors: Systematic endocrinology, Hagerstown, Md., 1973, Harper & Row, Publishers, Inc.
60. Farquhar, M.G., and Rinehart, J.F.: Electron microscopic studies of the anterior pituitary gland of castrate rats, Endocrinology **54**:516, 1954.
61. Furth, J., and Clifton, K.H.: Experimental pituitary tumors. In Harris, G.W., and Donovan, B.T., editors: The pituitary gland, vol. 2, Berkeley, 1966, University of California Press.
62. Halmi, N.S., and McCormick, W.F.: Effects of hyperadrenocorticism on pituitary thyrotrophic cells in man, Arch. Pathol. **94**:471, 1972.
63. Halmi, N.S., McCormick, W.F., and Decker, D.A., Jr.: The natural history of hyalinization of ACTH/MSH cells in man, Arch. Pathol. **91**:318, 1971.
64. Irvine, W.J.: Autoimmunity in endocrine disease, Proc. R. Soc. Med. **67**:548, 1974.
65. Ketelbant-Balasse, P., Herlant, M., and Pasteels, J.L.: Modifications hypophysaires dans un cas d'hypercorticisme para-néoplastique, Ann. Endocrinol. **34**:743, 1973.
66. Kilby, R.A., Bennett, W.A., and Sprague, R.G.: Anterior pituitary gland in patients treated with cortisone and corticotropin, Am. J. Pathol. **33**:155, 1955.
67. Kovacs, K., and Horvath, E.: Gonadotrophs following removal of ovaries: a fine structural study of human pituitary glands, Endokrinologie **66**:1, 1975.
68. Murray, S., and Ezrin, C.: Effect of Graves' disease on the "thyrotroph" cell of the adenohypophysis, J. Clin. Endocrinol. **26**:287, 1966.
69. Russfield, A.B.: The endocrine glands after bilateral adrenalectomy compared with those in spontaneous adrenal insufficiency, Cancer **8**:523, 1955.
70. Russfield, A.B.: Adenohyophysis. In Bloodworth, J.M.B., Jr., editor: Endocrine pathology, Baltimore, 1968, The Williams & Wilkins Co.
71. Russfield, A.B., and Byrnes, R.L.: Some effects of hormone therapy and castration on the hypophysis in men with carcinoma of the prostate, Cancer **11**:817, 1958.
72. Schochet, S.S., Jr., Halmi, N.S., and McCormick, W.F.: PAS-positive hyalin change in ACTH/MSH cells of man, Arch. Pathol. **93**:457, 1972.
73. Shiino, M.: Morphological changes of pituitary gonadotrophs and thyrotrophs following treatment with LH-RH or TRH in vitro, Cell Tissue Res. **202**:399, 1979.
74. Siperstein, E.R., and Miller, K.J.: Hypertrophy of ACTH-producing cell following adrenalectomy: a quantitative electron microscopic study, Endocrinology **93**:1257, 1973.
75. Stratmann, I.E., et al.: The origin of thyroidectomy cells as revealed by high resolution radioautography, Endocrinology **90**:728, 1972.
76. Takano, K., et al.: A TSH secreting tumor accompanied by high stature: presentation of a case and review of the literature, Endocrinol. Jpn. **28**:215, 1981.
77. Thornton, K.R.: The cytology of the pituitary gland in myxoedema, J. Pathol. Bacteriol. **77**:249, 1959.

Hypophysectomy

78. Block, G.E., Jensen, E.V., and Polley, T.Z., Jr.: The prediction of hormonal dependency of mammary cancer, Ann. Surg. **182**:342, 1975.

79. Crome, L.: Underdevelopment of the pituitary, Dev. Med. Child. Neurol. **16**:222, 1974.
80. Horwitz, K.B., et al.: Predicting response to endocrine therapy in human breast cancer: a hypothesis, Science **189**:726, 1975.
81. Landau, R.L.: Endocrine management of malignancies of the prostate, breast, endometrium, kidney, and ovary. In DeGroot, L.J., et al., editors: Endocrinology, vol. 3, New York, 1979, Grune & Stratton, Inc.
82. Manni, A., et al.: Transsphenoidal hypophysectomy in breast cancer, Cancer **44**:2330, 1979.
83. McGrath, P.: Prolactin activity and human growth hormone in pharyngeal hypophyses from embalmed cadavers, J. Endocrinol. **42**:205, 1968.
84. McGrath, P.: Extra-sellar post-hypophysectomy remnant, Br. J. Surg. **56**:64, 1969.
85. McPhie, J.L., and Beck, J.S.: Growth hormone in the normal human pharyngeal pituitary gland, Nature **219**:625, 1968.
86. Müller, W.: On the pharyngeal hypophysis. In Currie, A.R., and Illingworth, C.F.W., editors: Endocrine aspects of breast cancer, Edinburgh, 1958, E. & S. Livingstone, Ltd.

Hypopituitarism

87. Daughaday, W.H.: The adenohypophysis. In Williams, R.H., editor: Textbook of endocrinology, ed. 5, Philadelphia, 1975, W.B. Saunders Co.
88. Laron, Z.: The hypothalamus and the pituitary gland (hypophysis). In Hubble, D., editor: Paediatric endocrinology, Philadelphia, 1969, F.A. Davis Co.
89. Sheehan, H.L.: Post-partum necrosis of the anterior pituitary, J. Pathol. Bacteriol. **45**:189, 1937.

Anomalies

90. Angevine, D.M.: Pathologic anatomy of hypophysis and adrenals in anencephaly, Arch. Pathol. **26**:507, 1938.
91. Blizzard, R.M., and Alberts, M.: Hypopituitarism, hypoadrenalism, and hypogonadism in newborn infant, J. Pediatr. **48**:782, 1956.
92. Edmonds, H.W.: Pituitary, adrenal and thyroid in cyclopia, Arch. Pathol. **50**:727, 1950.
93. Lennox, B., and Russell, D.S.: Dystopia of the neurohypophysis: two cases, J. Pathol. Bacteriol. **63**:485, 1951.
94. Moncrieff, M.W., et al.: Congenital absence of pituitary gland and adrenal hypoplasia, Arch. Dis. Child. **47**:136, 1972.
95. Potter, E.L., and Craig, J.M.: Pathology of the fetus and infant, ed. 3, Chicago, 1975, Year Book Medical Publishers, Inc.
96. Rasmussen, P., and Lindholm, J.: Ectopic pituitary adenomas, Clin. Endocrinol. **11**:69, 1979.
97. Steiner, M.W., and Boggs, J.D.: Absence of pituitary gland, hypothyroidism, hypoadrenalism and hypogonadism in a 17-year-old dwarf, J. Clin. Endocrinol. **25**:1591, 1965.
98. Willard, D., et al.: La dysgénésie antéhypophysaire primitive, Nouv. Presse Med. **1**:2237, 1972.

Empty sella syndrome

99. Bergeron, C., Kovacs, K., and Bilbao, J.M.: Primary empty sella: a histologic and immunocytologic study, Arch. Intern. Med. **139**:248, 1979.
100. Doniach, I.: Histopathology of the anterior pituitary, Clin. Endocrinol. Metab. **6**:21, 1977.
101. Ganguly, A., et al.: Cushing's syndrome in a patient with an empty sella turcica and a microadenoma of the adenohypophysis, Am. J. Med. **60**:306, 1976.
102. Jones, J.R., et al.: Galactorrhea and amenorrhea in a patient with an empty sella, Obstet. Gynecol. **49**:(suppl. 1):9, 1977.
103. Kaufman, B.: The "empty" sella turcica—a manifestation of the intrasellar subarachnoid space, Radiology **90**:931, 1968.
104. Neelon, F.A., Goree, J.A., and Lebovitz, H.E.: The primary empty sella: clinical and radiographic characteristics and endocrine function, Medicine **52**:73, 1973.

Hemorrhage

105. Goldman, K.P., and Jacobs, A.: Anterior and posterior pituitary failure after head injury, Br. Med. J. **5217**:1924, 1960.
106. Kornblum, R.N., and Fisher, R.S.: Pituitary lesions in craniocerebral injuries, Arch. Pathol. **88**:242, 1969.
107. McCormick, W.F., and Halmi, N.S.: Hypophysis in patients with coma dépassé ("respirator brain"), Am. J. Clin. Pathol. **54**:374, 1970.

Pituitary apoplexy

108. Wakai, S., et al.: Pituitary apoplexy: its incidence and clinical significance, J. Neurosurg. **55**:187, 1981.

Infarction and necrosis

109. Adams, J.H., et al.: The volume of the infarct in pars distalis of a human pituitary gland, 30 hr after transection of the pituitary stalk, J. Physiol. **166**:39P, 1963.
110. Daniel, P.M., Spicer, E.J.F., and Treip, C.S.: Pituitary necrosis in patients maintained on mechanical respirators, J. Pathol. **111**:135, 1973.
111. Frey, H.M.: Spontaneous pituitary destruction in diabetes mellitus, J. Clin. Endocrinol. **19**:1642, 1959.
112. Kovacs, K.: Adenohypophysial necrosis in routine autopsies, Endokrinologie **60**:309, 1972.
113. Kovacs, K.: Necrosis of anterior pituitary in humans, Neuroendocrinology **4**:170, 1969.
114. Kovacs, K.: Pituitary necrosis in diabetes mellitus, Acta Diabetol. Lat. **9**:958, 1972.
115. Purnell, D.C., Randall, R.V., and Rynearson, E.H.: Postpartum pituitary insufficiency (Sheehan's syndrome): review of 18 cases, Mayo Clin. Proc. **39**:321, 1964.
116. Sheehan, H.L., and Davis, J.C.: Pituitary necrosis, Br. Med. Bull. **24**:59, 1968.
117. Towbin, A.: The respirator brain death syndrome, Hum. Pathol. **4**:583, 1973.

Acute inflammation

118. Dominguez, J.N., and Wilson, C.B.: Pituitary abscesses: report of seven cases and review of the literature. J. Neurosurg. **46**:601, 1977.
119. Simmonds, M.: Über embolische Prozesse in der Hypophyse, Virchows Arch. Pathol Anat. Physiol. **217**:226, 1914.
120. Zorub, D.S., et al.: Invasive pituitary adenoma with abscess formation: case report, Neurosurgery **5**:718, 1979.

Granuloma

121. Doniach, I.: Histopathology of the anterior pituitary, Clin. Endocrinol. Metab. **6**:21, 1977.
122. Oelbaum, M.H.: Hypopituitarism in male subjects due to syphilis, Q. J. Med. **21**:249, 1952.
123. Plair, C.M., and Perry, S.: Hypothalamic-pituitary sarcoidosis, Arch. Pathol. **74**:527, 1962.

Lymphocytic hypophysitis

124. Asa, S.L., et al.: Lymphocytic hypophysitis of pregnancy resulting in hypopituitarism: a distinct clinicopathologic entity, Ann. Intern. Med. **95**:166, 1981.
125. Cebelin, M.S., et al.: Galactorrhea associated with lymphocytic adenohypophysitis, Br. J. Obstet. Gynaecol. **88**:675, 1981.
126. Mayfield, R.K., et al.: Lymphoid adenohypophysitis presenting as a pituitary tumor, Am. J. Med. **69**:619, 1980.

Infiltrations and metabolic disorders

127. Barr, R., and Lampert, P.: Intrasellar amyloid tumor, Acta Neuropathol. **21**:83, 1972.
128. Bilbao, M.M., et al.: Pituitary adenoma producing amyloid-like substance, Arch. Pathol. **99**:411, 1975.
129. Kraus, E.J.: Die Hypophyse. In Henke, F., and Lubarsch, O., editors: Handbuch der speziellen Anatomie und Histologie, vol. 8, Berlin, 1926, Julius Springer Verlag.
130. Russell, D.S., and Rubinstein, L.J.: Pathology of tumours of the nervous system, ed. 4, Baltimore, 1977, The Williams & Wilkins Co.
131. Schober, R., and Nelson, D.: Fine structure and origin of amyloid deposits in pituitary adenoma, Arch. Pathol. **99**:403, 1975.
132. Schochet, S.S., Jr., McCormick, W.F., and Halmi, N.S.: Pituitary gland in patients with Hurler syndrome, Arch. Pathol. **97**:96, 1974.

133. Westermark, P., et al.: Amyloid in polypeptide hormone-producing tumors, Lab. Invest. **37**:212, 1977.

Tumors

134. Adelman, L.S. and Post, K.D.: Intra-operative technique for pituitary adenomas, Am. J. Surg. Pathol. **3**:173, 1979.
135. Burrow, G.N., et al.: Microadenomas of the pituitary and abnormal sellar tomograms in an unselected autopsy series, N. Engl. J. Med. **304**:156, 1981.
136. Hardy, J.: Transsphenoidal surgery of hypersecreting pituitary tumors. In Kohler, P.O., and Ross, G.T., editors: Diagnosis and treatment of pituitary tumors, New York, 1973, American Elsevier Publishing Co.
137. Horvath, E., and Kovacs, K.: Pathology of the pituitary gland. In Ezrin, C., et al., editors: Pituitary diseases, Boca Raton, Fla., 1980, CRC Press, Inc.
138. McKeever, P.E.: Personal communication, 1981.
139. Post, K.D.: General considerations in the surgical treatment of pituitary tumors. In Post, K.D., Jackson, I.M.D., and Reichlin, S., editors: The pituitary adenoma, New York, 1980, Plenum Publishing Corp.
140. Post, K.D., et al.: Selective transsphenoidal adenomectomy in women with galactorrhea-amenorrhea, J.A.M.A. **242**:158, 1979.
141. Velasco, M.E., Sindley, S.D. and Roessmann, U.: Reticulum stain for frozen-section diagnosis of pituitary adenomas, J. Neurosurg. **46**:548, 1978.
142. Wrightson, P.: The limitations of surgical treatment of pituitary microadenomas. In Faglia, G., Giovanelli, M.A., and MacLeod, R.M., editors: Pituitary microadenomas, Proceedings of the Serono Symposia, vol. 29, New York, 1980, Academic Press, Inc.

Adenomas

143. Abbassy, A.A., and Sakali, W.A.: Hyperprolactinemia and male infertility, Br. J. Urol. **54**:305, 1982.
144. Adelman, L.S.: The pathology of pituitary adenomas. In Post, K.D., Jackson, I.M.D., and Reichlin, S., editors: The pituitary adenoma, New York, 1980, Plenum Publishing Corp.
145. Ballard, H.S., Frame, B., and Hartsock, R.J.: Familial multiple endocrine adenoma–peptic ulcer complex, Medicine **43**:481, 1964.
146. Baskin, D.G., Erlandsen, S.L., and Parsons, J.A.: Functional classification of cell types in the growth hormone- and prolactin-secreting rat MtTW15 mammosomatotropic tumor with ultrastructural immunocytochemistry, Am. J. Anat. **158**:455, 1980.
147. Bigos, S.T., et al.: Cushing's disease: management by transphenoidal pituitary microsurgery, J. Clin. Endocrinol. Metab. **50**:348, 1980.
148. Burrow, G.N., et al.: Microadenomas of the pituitary and abnormal sellar tomograms in an unselected autopsy series, N. Engl. J. Med. **304**:156, 1981.
149. Carmalt, M.H.B., et al.: Treatment of Cushing's disease by transsphenoidal hypophysectomy, Q. J. Med. **46**:119, 1977.
150. Costello, R.T.: Subclinical adenoma of the pituitary gland, Am. J. Pathol. **12**:205, 1936.
151. Cushing, H.: The basophil adenomas of the pituitary body and their clinical manifestations (pituitary basophilism), Bull. Johns Hopkins Hosp. **50**:137, 1932.
152. Dingemans, K.P.: Development of TSH-producing pituitary tumors in mouse, Virchows Arch. (Cell. Pathol.) **12**:338, 1973.
153. Dluhy, R.G., Moore, T.J., and Williams, G.H.: Sella turcica enlargement and primary adrenal insufficiency, Ann. Intern. Med. **89**:513, 1978.
154. Forbes, A.P., et al.: Syndrome characterized by galactorrhea, amenorrhea and low urinary FSH: comparison with acromegaly and normal lactation, J. Clin. Endocrinol. **14**:265, 1954.
155. Frantz, A.G.: Prolactin, N. Engl. J. Med. **298**:201, 1978.
156. Furth, J., et al.: Thyrotrophic tumor syndrome: a multiglandular disease induced by sustained deficiency of thyroid hormones, Arch. Pathol. **96**:217, 1973.
157. Gillies, G., et al.: Secretion of ACTH, LPH, and β-endorphin from human pituitary tumours in vitro, Endocrinology **13**:197, 1980.
158. Gjerris, A., Lindholm, J., and Riishede, J.: Pituitary oncocytic tumor with Cushing's disease, Cancer **42**:1818, 1978.
159. Griesbach, W.E., and Purves, H.D.: Basophil adenomata in the rat hypophysis after gonadectomy, Br. J. Cancer **14**:49, 1960.
160. Guyda, H., et al.: Histologic, ultrastructural, and hormonal characterization of pituitary tumor secreting HGH and prolactin, J. Clin. Endocrinol. **36**:531, 1973.
161. Hassoun, J., et al.: Corticolipotropin immunoreactivity in silent chromophobe adenomas, Arch. Pathol. Lab. Med. **106**:25, 1982.
162. Himsworth, R.L., Lewis, J.G., and Rees, L.H.: A possible ACTH secreting tumour of the pituitary developing in a conventionally treated case of Addison's disease, Clin. Endocrinol. **9**:131, 1978.
163. Horvath, E., and Kovacs, K.: Pituitary chromophobe adenoma composed of oncocytes: a light and electron microscopic study, Arch. Pathol. **95**:235, 1973.
164. Horvath, E., and Kovacs, K.: Misplaced exocytosis: distinct ultrastructural feature in some pituitary adenomas, Arch. Pathol. **97**:221, 1974.
165. Horvath, E., and Kovacs, K.: Ultrastructural classification of pituitary adenomas, Can. J. Neurol. Sci. **3**:9, 1976.
166. Horvath, E., et al.: Acidophil stem cell adenoma of the human pituitary, Arch Pathol. Lab. Med. **101**:594, 1977.
167. Horvath, E., et al.: Silent corticotrophic adenoma of the human pituitary gland: a histologic, immunocytologic, and ultrastructural study, Am. J. Pathol. **98**:617, 1980.
168. Horvath, E., et al.: Acidophil stem cell adenoma of the human pituitary: clinicopathologic analysis of 15 cases, Cancer **47**:761, 1981.
169. Jara-Albaran, A., et al.: Probable pituitary adenoma with hypersecretion secondary to Addison's disease, J. Clin. Endocrinol. **49**:236, 1979.
170. Kalyanaraman, U.P., et al.: Prolactin-secreting pituitary oncocytoma with galactorrhea-amenorrhea syndrome, Cancer **46**:1584, 1980.
171. Kameya, T., et al.: Untrastructure, immunochemistry and hormone release of pituitary adenomas in relation to prolactin production, Virchows Arch. (Pathol. Anat.) **387**:31, 1980.
172. Katz, M.S., et al.: Thyrotroph cell adenoma of the human pituitary gland associated with primary hypothyroidism: clinical and morphological features, Acta Endocrinol. **95**:41, 1980.
173. Kourides, I.A., et al.: Thyrotropin-induced hyperthyroidism: use of alpha and beta subunit levels to identify patients with pituitary tumors, J. Clin. Endocrinol. Metab. **45**:534, 1977.
174. Kovacs, K., and Horvath, E.: Pituitary chromophobe adenoma composed of oncocytes: a light and electron microscopic study, Arch. Pathol. **95**:235, 1973.
175. Kovacs, K., Horvath, E., and Ezrin, C.: Pituitary adenomas. In Sommers, S.C., and Rosen, P.P., editors: Pathology annual, vol. 12, part 2, New York, 1977, Appleton-Century-Crofts.
176. Kovacs, K., et al.: Pituitary adenomas associated with elevated blood follicle-stimulating hormone levels: a histologic, immunocytologic and electron microscopic study of two cases, Fertil Steril. **29**:622, 1978.
177. Kovacs, K., et al.: Silent corticotroph cell adenoma with lysosomal accumulation and crinophagy, Am. J. Med. **64**:492, 1978.
178. Kovacs, K., et al.: Gonadotroph cell adenoma of the pituitary in a woman with long-standing hypogonadism, Arch. Gynecol. **229**:57, 1980.
179. Kovacs, K., et al.: Null cell adenoma of the human pituitary, Virchows Arch. (Pathol. Anat.) **387**:165, 1980.
180. Lamberts, S.W.J., de Lange, S.A., and Stefanko, S.Z.: ACTH secreting pituitary adenomas in Cushing's disease originate from the anterior or intermediate lobe—consequences for surgical therapy, Eur. J. Clin. Invest. **11**:18, 1981.
181. Lamberts, W.J.L., et al.: The dynamics of growth hormone and prolactin secretion in acromegalic patients with "mixed" pituitary tumours, Acta Endocrinol. **90**:198, 1979.
182. Landolt, A.M.: Progress in pituitary adenoma biology, Adv. Technol. Standards Neurosurg. **5**:4, 1978.
183. Landolt, A.M.: Biology of pituitary microadenomas. In Faglia, G., Giovanelli, M.A., and MacLeod, R.M., editors: Pituitary

microadenomas, Proceedings of the Serono Symposia, vol. 29, New York, 1980, Academic Press, Inc.
184. Landolt, A.M., and Oswald, U.W.: Histology and ultrastructure of an oncocytic adenoma of human pituitary, Cancer **31**:1099, 1973.
185. Levine, J.H., et al.: Prolactin-secreting adenoma as part of the multiple endocrine neoplasia-type I (MEN-I) syndrome, Cancer **43**:2492, 1979.
186. Marshall, A.H.E., and Sloper, J.C.: Pluriglandular adenomatosis of pituitary, parathyroid and pancreatic islet cells associated with lipomatosis, J. Pathol. Bacteriol. **68**:225, 1954.
187. Martinez, A.J., et al.: Pituitary adenomas: clinicopathological and immunohistochemical study, Ann. Neurol. **7**:24, 1980.
188. Mosca, L., et al.: Pituitary adenomas: surgical versus post mortem findings today. In Faglia, G., Giovanelli, M.A. and MacLeod, R.M., editors: Pituitary microadenomas, vol. 29, New York, 1980, Academic Press, Inc.
189. Nelson, D.H., Meakin, J., and Thorn, G.W.: ACTH-producing pituitary tumors following adrenalectomy for Cushing's syndrome, Ann. Intern. Med. **52**:560, 1960.
190. Parsons, J.A., et al.: Heterogeneity of the MtTW15 mammosomatotropic tumor, Anat. Rec. **190**:719, 1978.
191. Peake, G.T., et al.: Ultrastructural, histologic and hormonal characterization of a prolactin-rich human pituitary tumor, J. Clin. Endocrinol. **29**:1383, 1969.
192. Prosser, R.R., et al.: Prolactin-secreting pituitary adenomas in multiple endocrine adenomatosis, type I, Ann. Intern. Med. **91**:41, 1979.
193. Racadot, J., et al.: Adenomes hypophysaires à cellules à prolactine: étude structural et ultrastructurale, correlations anatomocliniques, Ann. Endocrinol. **32**:298, 1971.
194. Ridgway, E.C., et al.: Pure alpha secreting pituitary adenomas, N. Engl. J. Med. **304**:1254, 1981.
195. Robert, F., Pelletier, G., and Hardy, J.: Pituitary adenomas in Cushing's disease, Arch. Pathol. Lab. Med. **102**:448, 1978.
196. Saeger, W.: Licht- und elektronenmikroskopische Untersuchungen zur Klassification von Hypophysenadenomen, Z. Krebsforsch. **84**:105, 1975.
197. Saeger, W., and Lüdecke, D.K.: Pituitary adenomas with hyperfunction of TSH, Virchows Arch. (Pathol. Anat.) **394**:255, 1982.
198. Salassa, R.M., et al.: Transsphenoidal removal of a pituitary microadenoma in Cushing's disease, Mayo Clin. Proc. **53**:24, 1978.
199. Samaan, N.A., et al.: Endocrine and morphologic studies of pituitary adenomas secondary to primary hypothyroidism, J. Clin. Endocrinol. Metab. **45**:903, 1977.
200. Samaan, N.A., et al.: Reactive pituitary abnormalities in patients with Klinefelter's and Turner's syndromes, Arch. Intern. Med. **139**:198, 1979.
201. Schecter, J.: Electron microscopic studies of human pituitary tumors. II. Acidophilic adenomas, Am. J. Anat. **138**:387, 1973.
202. Schochet, S.S., McCormick, W.F., and Halmi, N.S.: Acidophil adenomas with intracytoplasmic filamentous aggregates: a light and EM study, Arch. Pathol. **94**:6, 1972.
203. Segal, S., Polishuk, W.Z., and Ben-David, M.: Hyperprolactinemic male infertility, Fertil. Steril. **27**:1425, 1976.
204. Singer, R., et al.: Demonstration of immunoreactive alpha-endorphin in corticotroph cell adenomas of the human pituitary, ICRS Med. Sci. **6**:250, 1978.
205. Tolis, G., et al.: Pituitary hyperthyroidism, Am. J. Med. **64**:177, 1978.
206. Tramu, G., et al.: Hypophysaire à cellules à a, 17-39 ACTH et b,MSH sans hypercorticisme, Ann. Endocrinol. **39**:51, 1978.
207. Trouillas, J., et al.: Human pituitary gonadotropic adenoma: histological, immunocytochemical, and ultrastructural and hormonal studies in eight cases, J. Pathol. **135**:315, 1981.
208. Tyrell, J.B., et al.: Selective trans-sphenoidal resection of pituitary microadenomas, N. Engl. J. Med. **298**:753, 1978.
209. Von Westarp, C., Weir, B.K.A. and Shnitka, T.K.: Characterization of a pituitary stone, Am. J. Med. **68**:949, 1980.
210. Wermer, P.: Endocrine adenomatosis and peptic ulcer in a large kindred, Am. J. Med. **35**:205, 1963.
211. Williams, E.D.: Histological classification of tumours of the anterior pituitary (adenohypophysis). In Williams, E.D., Siebenmann, R.E., and Sobin, L.H., editors: Histological typing of endocrine tumours, Geneva, 1980, World Health Organization.
212. Wilson, C.B., and Dempsey, L.C.: Transsphenoidal microsurgical removal of 250 pituitary adenomas, J. Neurosurg. **48**:13, 1978.
213. Woolf, P.D. and Schenk, E.A.: An FSH-producing tumor in a patient with hypogonadism, J. Clin. Endocrinol. Metab. **38**:561, 1974.

Carcinoma

214. D'Abrera, V.S.E., et al.: Carcinoma of pituitary gland, J. Pathol. **109**:335, 1973.
215. Evans, R.W.: Histological appearances of tumours, ed. 2, Edinburgh, 1966, E. & S. Livingstone, Ltd.
216. Houck, W.A., Olson, K.B., and Horton, J.: Clinical features of tumor metastasis to pituitary, Cancer **26**:656, 1970.
217. Kovacs, K.: Metastatic cancer of pituitary gland, Oncology **27**:533, 1973.
218. Queiroz, L. de S., et al.: Pituitary carcinoma with liver metastases and Cushing syndrome, Arch. Pathol. **99**:32, 1975.
219. Roessman, U., Kaufman, B., and Friede, R.L.: Metastatic lesions in the sella turcica and pituitary gland, Cancer **25**:478, 1970.

Other tumors

220. Fischer, E.R., and Wechsler, J.: Granular cell myoblastoma—a misnomer, Cancer **15**:936, 1962.
221. Friedman, N.B.: Germinoma of pineal—its identity with germinoma ("seminoma") of the testis, Cancer Res. **7**:363, 1947.
222. Ghatak, N.R., Hirano, A., and Zimmerman, H.M.: Intrasellar germinomas: a form of ectopic pinealoma, J. Neurosurg. **31**:670, 1969.
223. Ghatak, N.R., Hirano, A., and Zimmerman, H.M.: Ultrastructure of a craniopharyngioma, Cancer **27**:1465, 1971.
224. Kepes, J.J.: Transitional cell tumor of the pituitary gland developing from a Rathke's cleft cyst, Cancer **41**:337, 1978.
225. Luse, S.A., and Kernohan, J.W.: Granular-cell tumors of the stalk and posterior lobe of the pituitary gland, Cancer **8**:616, 1955.
226. Massie, A.P.: A granular-cell pituicytoma of the neurohypophysis, J. Pathol. **129**:53, 1979.
227. Petito, C.K., DeGirolami, U., and Earle, K.M.: Craniopharygiomas: a clinical and pathological review, Cancer **37**:1944, 1976.
228. Rubinstein, L.J.: Tumors of the central nervous system, Series 2, Fascicle 6, Atlas of tumor pathology, Washington, D.C., 1972, Armed Forces Institute of Pathology.
229. Satyamurti, S., and Huntington, H.W.: Granular cell myoblastoma of the pituitary: case report, J. Neurosurg. **37**:483, 1972.
230. Seemayer, T.A., Blundell, J.S., and Wiglesworth, F.W.: Pituitary craniopharyngioma with tooth formation, Cancer **29**:423, 1972.
231. Shuangshoti, S., Netsky, M.G., and Nashold, B.S., Jr.: Epithelial cysts related to sella turcica—proposed origin from neuroepithelium, Arch. Pathol. **90**:444, 1970.
232. Symon, L., Ganz, J.C., and Burston, J.: Granular cell myoblastoma of neurohypophysis: report of 2 cases, J. Neurosurg. **35**:82, 1971.
233. Waller, R.R., Riley, F.C., and Sundt, T.M., Jr.: A rare cause of the chiasmal syndrome, Arch. Ophthalmol. **88**:269, 1972.
234. Zimmerman, H.M.: Ten most common types of brain tumor, Semin. Roentgenol. **6**:48, 1971.
235. Zülch, K.J.: Brain tumors, their biology and pathology, ed. 2, New York, 1965, Springer Verlag.

CHAPTER 33 **Thyroid Gland**

KAARLE O. FRANSSILA

DEVELOPMENT, STRUCTURE, AND FUNCTION

The thyroid gland arises from a midline invagination at the base of the tongue. The invagination grows downward to the normal position of the thyroid, and its lowest part proliferates to form the gland. The thyroglossal duct that initially connects the gland to the pharyngeal floor disappears by the sixth week of embryonic life. Its proximal end is represented in adults by the foramen cecum at the base of the tongue and its lowest part by the pyramidal lobe of the thyroid, which occurs in about 40% of individuals. The other epithelial component of the thyroid, the C cells, are believed to have their origin in the neural crest.[3]

The thyroid in an adult weighs between 15 and 30 g, but this varies considerably in different areas of the world. The gland is composed of two lateral lobes connected by an isthmus that may have a pyramidal lobe that extends cranially. The cut surface is yellow-red and translucent.

The functional unit of the thyroid is a follicle, a spherical sac filled with acidophilic colloid and lined by cuboidal epithelium with a thin basement membrane. The follicles are separated from each other by delicate fibrous tissue containing the blood vessels, nerves, and lymphatics. Between 20 and 40 follicles are surrounded by a thicker connective tissue sheath, forming a lobule. The apical surface of the epithelial cells shows numerous microvilli extending to the colloid,[2] which is composed of the glycoprotein thyroglobulin.

Briefly, the synthesis of thyroid hormones is as follows. The epithelial cells absorb iodide from the blood, concentrate it more than 20 times, and oxidate it to iodine. Iodine attaches to tyrosine residues of thyroglobulin to form monoiodotyrosine (MIT) and diiodotyrosine (DIT), which couple to form triiodothyronine (T_3) and tetraiodothyronine (T_4, or thyroxine). Both the oxidation of iodide and the coupling of tyrosines require the presence of peroxidases. The release of thyroid hormones occurs through endocytosis of colloid and proteolysis of thyroglobulin by lysosomal enzymes. T_3 and T_4 are freed and discharged into blood, where they are bound to plasma proteins, mainly thyroxine-binding globulin. The synthesis and release of thyroid hormones are regulated by hypophyseal thyroid-stimulating hormone (TSH).

C cells, or parafollicular cells, are dispersed within the follicles, especially in the posterolateral parts of the lateral lobes. They make up about 0.1% of the epithelial mass.[5] These cells secrete a polypeptide hormone called calcitonin, which has a hypocalcemic effect. C cells are almost impossible to identify by light microscopy without the use of special techniques such as argyrophil silver stains[4] or immunohistochemical methods.[5] Ultrastructurally C cells contain secretory granules and occupy an intrafollicular position. They are separated from the interstitium by the follicular basement membrane and from the colloid by extensions of the follicular cell cytoplasm.[1]

FUNCTIONAL DISORDERS

Hypothyroidism

Hypothyroidism is defined as a clinical state that results from inadequate production of thyroid hormones or, very rarely, from resistance of the peripheral tissues to the influence of thyroid hormones. Hypothyroidism may be congenital or may appear in children or adults. Adulthood hypothyroidism shows about a 10-fold predominance among females and begins most often between the ages of 30 and 60 years.

The clinical features depend on the age at onset. Symptoms of overt adult hypothyroidism include lack of energy, cold intolerance, dryness of skin and hair, hoarseness of voice, and subcutaneous swelling that is most prominent around the eyes. This kind of advanced hypothyroidism with subcutaneous swelling is called myxedema. In mild hypothyroidism the symptoms are frequently minor or nonspecific. Serum T_4 concentrations are low in severe hypothyroidism, but within the normal range in mild cases. Because of a negative feedback control, serum TSH values are raised even before the patient has any symptoms (if the disease is not of hypophyseal origin). The causes of hypothyroidism are presented in the outline that follows.

A. Causes of congenital hypothyroidism
   1. Developmental anomalies
      a. Thyroid agenesis
      b. Ectopic thyroid
   2. Genetic defects in thyroid hormone synthesis (dyshormonogenesis)
      a. Iodide transport defect (inability to concentrate iodide in the thyroid)
      b. Organification defect (inability to bind iodide to thyroglobulin caused by deficiency in peroxidases)
      c. Coupling defect (inability to couple MIT and DIT to form T_3 and T_4)
      d. Dehalogenase defect (inability to deiodinate MIT and DIT caused by deficiency in dehalogenase)
      e. Defects in thyroglobulin synthesis
   3. Endemic goiter and cretinism
   4. Fetal exposure to iodides, antithyroid agents, or radioactive iodine
B. Causes of noncongenital hypothyroidism
   1. Autoimmune thyroiditis
      a. Hashimoto's thyroiditis
      b. Atrophic thyroiditis (spontaneous hypothyroidism)
   2. Ablation of thyroid by surgery or radiation
   3. Endemic and sporadic goiter
   4. Hypopituitarism
   5. Thyroid cancer destroying the gland
   6. Antithyroid drug administration
   7. Developmental anomalies and defects in thyroid hormone synthesis (mild cases, less than complete lack of thyroid hormone)

The most common cause of noncongenital hypothyroidism is autoimmune thyroiditis, especially its atrophic variant, and the next most common is ablation of the thyroid by radioactive iodine or surgery.

Cretinism is the term given to congenital hypothyroidism if the lack of thyroid hormone is complete or nearly complete and prolonged. Endemic cretinism occurs in the same areas as endemic goiter and is mainly caused by the lack of iodine. Sporadic cretinism, on the other hand, has many etiologies, the most common of which are developmental anomalies and genetic defects in thyroid hormone synthesis.[9] In cretinism there is, in addition to hypothyroidism, an associated intellectual defect and growth retardation, which are caused by thyroid hormone deficiency during fetal life. The early symptoms of cretinism, including decreased activity, feeding problems, enlarged tongue, and hoarse cry, appear during the neonatal period. However, the full picture, including physical and mental retardation, develops slowly over months.

Most endemic cretins also have neurologic defects such as deafmutism or spastic diplegia, but they do not always have postnatal hypothyroidism, and sometimes they have no intellectual defect.[7] Although endemic cretins have lack of iodine and thyroid hormones during fetal life, their thyroids are usually capable of producing hormones postnatally if iodine is available.

Hypothyroidism that develops in children after the first year results in growth retardation but usually no intellectual defect.

Hyperthyroidism

Hyperthyroidism, also called thyrotoxicosis, is defined as a hypermetabolic clinical state that results from increased production of thyroid hormones. It is characterized by emotional lability, nervousness, rapid pulse, weight loss, perspiration, heat intolerance, and fine tremor in the hands.

Hyperthyroidism may be caused by several diseases.[6] The most common in areas where there is no endemic goiter is Graves' disease, while in many endemic areas, toxic nodular goiter is the predominant cause.

Rarely, hyperthyroidism may be caused by hypersecretion of pituitary TSH owing to a pituitary tumor, or by hypersecretion of thyrotropin-releasing hormone (TRH). Exessive secretion of chorionic gonadotropin by trophoblastic tumors, such as hydatidiform mole and choriocarcinoma, or by testicular tumors containing trophoblastic elements is another rare cause of hyperthyroidism. (Chorionic gonadotropin has a weak thyrotropic effect on the thyroid.) Hyperthyroidism may also be caused by excessive doses of thyroid hormones or iodine (jodbasedow). Congenital hyperthyroidism may develop when the mother has Graves' disease, because the thyroid-stimulating immunoglobulins can cross the placental barrier. In the initial phase of granulomatous thyroiditis there may be a transitional hyperthyroid phase. Rarely, hyperthyroidism may be caused by metastatic tumors in the thyroid[8] or by thyroid hormones secreted by thyroid carcinoma or struma ovarii (teratoma with thyroid components).

DEVELOPMENTAL ANOMALIES

Developmental anomalies of the thyroid result from disturbances in the descent of the thyroid anlage. Although rare, they are the most common cause of sporadic cretinism.

Thyroid agenesis

A complete failure of the thyroid anlage to develop may occur. It results in total absence of thyroid tissue.

Children with thyroid agenesis are born as cretins. In hemiagenesis one of the thyroid lobes does not develop.

Ectopic thyroid

Ectopic thyroid can be seen anywhere along the route of the descent, usually between the normal position and the base of the tongue but sometimes caudally in the mediastinum.[11] The base of the tongue is the most common location. This lingual thyroid sometimes causes laryngeal or pharyngeal obstruction. Total absence of thyroid tissue from its normal location occurs in about two thirds of cases of ectopic thyroid.[11]

In patients with ectopic thyroid the presence and severity of hypothyroidism depend on the quantity of residual thyroid tissue. Hypothyroidism may not develop until late in childhood or in adulthood.

Lateral aberrant thyroid

Lateral aberrant thyroid, the term given to thyroid tissue occurring laterally in the neck, does not represent—at least in the great majority of cases—a developmental anomaly but may be a result of different disorders. It may represent a thyroid nodule connected to the gland by a very thin strand of tissue[15] or nonneoplastic thyroid tissue implanted to the operative area during thyroid operation. Thyroid follicles occurring in the lymph nodes appear practically always to represent metastasis from a papillary thyroid carcinoma that is often occult.[14] However, there remains a small possibility that some small clusters of normal-appearing thyroid follicles in lymph node sinuses represent nonneoplastic inclusions.[13] In metastatic papillary carcinoma at least some of the follicular cell nuclei usually, but not always,[14] have the ground-glass appearance typical of this tumor (see p. 1411).

Thyroglossal cyst

Remnants of the thyroglossal duct may give origin to cysts or sinuses. Thyroglossal cysts occur in the midline, most commonly in the region of the hyoid bone. They are lined by columnar or squamous epithelium, although this may be lacking because of inflammation.[10] Follicles are sometimes present in the wall of the cyst. Cysts may communicate with the pharynx at the foramen cecum and form fistulas. If they are inflamed, they may also rupture to the skin. Rarely, carcinoma may arise from a thyroglossal cyst.[12] It is usually of the papillary type.[12]

GRAVES' DISEASE (DIFFUSE TOXIC GOITER)

Graves' disease, also called Basedow's disease and primary hyperplasia, is characterized by hyperthyroidism, ophthalmopathy, and diffuse enlargement of the thyroid. In most countries it is the second most common thyroid disease, preceded only by nontoxic goiter. The disease occurs at all ages, most often in the third and fourth decades, and shows about a fivefold preponderance among females.

Low levels of circulating antibodies against various thyroid constituents are present in most cases of Graves' disease. In addition, almost all patients have circulating thyroid stimulators that have been shown to be immunoglobulins. There is strong evidence that they stimulate thyroid function on combination with the antigen, the TSH receptor of the follicular cell surface.[17,19] According to a recent hypothesis, thyroid enlargement in Graves' disease might be caused by another stimulator, the thyroid growth immunoglobulin.[21]

An aggregation of Graves' disease and Hashimoto's thyroiditis in the same families has been found, and it is expected that these two diseases are immunologically closely related autoimmune disorders.[19] The reason for the autoimmune reactions is unknown, but both diseases have been proposed to be caused by inherited defects in immunoregulation, possibly in suppressor T lymphocyte function.[19] Immunologic mechanisms also appear to be important in the development of the ophthalmopathy.[16]

Clinically patients with Graves' disease have the typical features of hyperthyroidism (see p. 1400) and diffuse goiter. In addition, eye symptoms occur in about one half of the patients; the mildest and most common form is exophthalmos, and the most severe form is limitation of eye movement and optic nerve damage. Rarely, patients also have pretibial myxedema or acropathy (peripheral soft tissue swelling and periosteal changes).

The thyroid is usually moderately and symmetrically enlarged; the weight in most cases is less than 70 g. The cut surface is homogeneous and hyperemic, and the normal colloidal appearance is lacking. Histologically, marked epithelial hyperplasia is seen; the follicles are small, and sometimes the epithelial cells occur in solid groups without any visible lumen. The follicular cells are tall and columnar and often form papillary infoldings that project into the colloid (Fig. 33-1). The enlarged nuclei, which may show some variation in size, lie at the base of the cell. Occasional mitoses may be seen. The colloid is light staining and often finely vacuolated. Some follicles may appear quite empty. The stroma is vascular. In addition to epithelial hyperplasia, foci of lymphatic tissue, often with germinal centers, are seen in many cases. It has been proposed that the amount of lymphatic tissue correlates positively to high microsomal antibody titers and to frequent occurrence of postoperative hypothyroidism.[17]

Histologic differential diagnosis from papillary carcinoma (p. 1412) and from chronic diffuse thyroiditis (p. 1405) may occasionally be difficult.

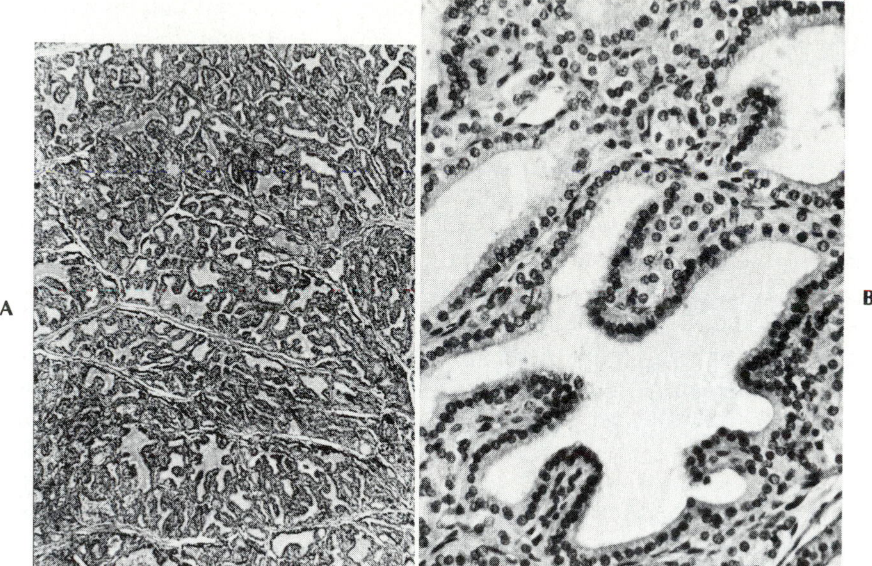

Fig. 33-1. Epithelial hyperplasia in Graves' disease. **A,** Note preserved lobular structure. **B,** Papillary infoldings projecting into the follicle, high columnar epithelium, solid cell groups, and pale staining colloid. (**A,** Low power; **B,** 300×.)

Operative specimens rarely show the typical hyperplastic features of Graves' disease because nearly all patients receive preoperative medication. Iodine inhibits hormone synthesis and release, resulting in thyroid involution with accumulation of colloid in the follicles and decrease in vascularity and follicular cell height. The histologic picture may appear quite normal, although usually some hyperplastic foci persist.

Antithyroid drugs inhibit thyroid hormone synthesis, resulting in an increase in the level of TSH. As a result the thyroid may become even more hyperplastic, although the patient is often clinically euthyroid.

Exophthalmos is caused by the increase in the volume of extraocular muscles and other orbital tissues. Histologically, deposits of material rich in mucopolysaccharides (glycosaminoglycans) are seen, as are edema and mononuclear inflammatory cells, followed later by fibrosis.[20] In pretibial myxedema, metachromatic material is seen in deeper parts of the dermis.[18]

Lymphatic hyperplasia may occur in Graves' disease in the thymus, spleen, and lymph nodes, in addition to the thyroid.

GOITER (NODULAR GOITER AND DIFFUSE NONTOXIC GOITER)

The term *goiter* refers to thyroid enlargement that is caused by compensatory hyperplasia in response to thyroid hormone deficiency. Diffuse thyroid enlargement is called diffuse nontoxic goiter; nodular enlargement is called nodular or adenomatous goiter. Although the term *goiter* is sometimes used for all kinds of thyroid enlargement, here it does not include thyroid enlargement caused by other thyroid diseases such as neoplastic growth or inflammation.

Etiology

Goiter occurs in two epidemiologic forms: (1) endemic, and (2) sporadic or nonendemic. A goiter prevalence higher than 10% indicates that the area is endemic.[24] Endemic goiter is prevalent in several high mountainous areas or areas far from the sea, such as the Alps, the Himalayas, and the Andes, where the content of iodine in drinking water and food is low. Endemic goiter is a common disease; in 1960 it was estimated that 200 million people in the world had endemic goiter.[25] Most endemic goiter is caused by lack of iodine,[24] although in some cases goitrogens and genetic features may be factors.

Sporadic goiter is also a common disease. A small proportion is caused by inborn errors in the synthesis of thyroid hormones. It has been suggested that this dyshormonogenetic goiter is inherited according to simple mendelian rules.[9,22] The different types of this disorder are presented on p. 1400.

Goitrogens, substances that interfere with the production of thyroid hormones, are a rare cause of goiter. The most common goitrogens are drugs used for treatment of hyperthyroidism. Goitrogens are able to cross the placental barrier and may cause congenital goiter.

In most cases of sporadic goiter the cause is unknown. On some occasions suboptimal iodine intake may predispose to goiter, especially during increased metabolic demands. Also, genetic factors and undefinable dyshormonogenetic defects may have influence on goiter development that is possibly multifactorial in origin.

Pathogenesis

The development of goiter is believed to be caused by long-lasting stimulation of TSH during a period of suboptimal production of thyroid hormones.[23] This stimulation leads to epithelial hyperplasia, which is often followed by involution. Both of these changes result in diffuse goiter. Nodular goiter is usually regarded as an end stage of diffuse goiter, resulting from cyclic changes of hyperplasia and involution. This is supported by the finding that in endemic areas the goiter is hyperplastic in childhood, diffusely enlarged with colloid accumulation in adolescence, and nodular in adulthood.

Some patients with nodular goiter develop hyperthyroidism, a condition often called toxic nodular goiter or Plummer's disease. It has been suggested that this is caused by long-standing hyperplastic nodules becoming autonomous.

Clinical features

Goiter is more common in females than in males. Diffuse goiter often appears at puberty or adolescence. It may regress, but if not, it often later turns nodular. Nodular goiter may produce compression symptoms, which may be severe if the goiter extends substernally.

Dyshormonogenetic goiters are detected in early childhood or not until adulthood. The thyroid may be diffuse or nodular.[26] In sporadic goiter compensatory mechanisms usually keep the patient euthyroid, but patients with dyshormonogenic goiter are usually hypothyroid, with the most severe cases involving cretinism. In endemic goiter hypothyroidism is rather common, varying in severity from clinical euthyroidism to cretinism. In toxic nodular goiter the symptoms of hyperthyroidism usually develop more slowly than in Graves' disease.[27] Ophthalmopathy does not occur, but cardiac symptoms are common.

Morphology

Diffuse goiter is symmetrically and diffusely enlarged and may weigh several hundred grams. Histologically, the hyperplastic stage is characterized by epithelial hyperplasia with small follicles, high epithelium showing papillary infoldings, and scanty colloid. The involution stage, the stage usually seen in histologic specimens, is characterized by large follicles distended by colloid and lined by flattened follicular cells. At this stage the cut surface is gelatinous and colloidal (colloid goiter).

Nodular goiter weighs 50 to 100 g in most cases but sometimes more than 500 g. The gland is usually asymmetric with nodules varying considerably in size (Fig. 33-2). Both grossly and histologically, it is characterized by marked heterogeneity in structure. The nodules may be colloidal or show degenerative features such as hemorrhages with hemosiderin deposits and cholesterol crystals, as well as calcifications, fibrous scarring, or cystic degeneration. The nodules are completely or partially encapsulated. The follicles may be small or large, and the epithelium varies from flat to high (Fig. 33-3). Some nodules may be composed of oxyphilic cells, often arranged in cords, and some of so-called macropapillary structures (Fig. 33-4) that may be erroneously diagnosed as papillary carcinoma.

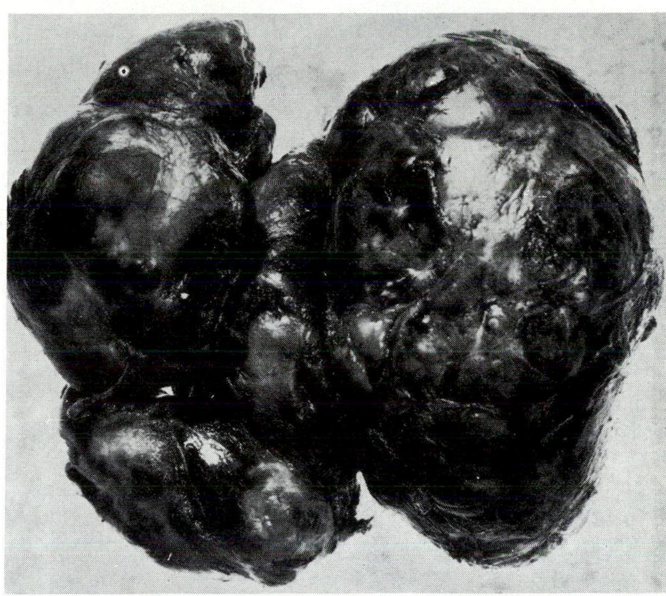

Fig. 33-2. Nodular goiter with areas of degeneration and hemorrhage. (From Anderson, W.A.D., and Scotti, T.M.: Synopsis of pathology, ed. 10, St. Louis, 1980. The C.V. Mosby Co.)

Dyshormonogenetic goiters often show an intense epithelial hyperplasia (Fig. 33-5), which may sometimes be difficult to differentiate from follicular carcinoma.

In toxic nodular goiter, focal areas of hyperplasia are seen. However, it is not possible to evaluate thyroid function on the basis of histologic features, since such hyperplastic areas also occur in thyroids of euthyroid patients.

THYROIDITIS

Infectious thyroiditis

Acute thyroiditis is an uncommon disease that usually develops as a complication of bacterial infection elsewhere, often in the oropharynx or tonsils.[38] Inflammation is usually suppurative, and the abscess may rupture to the skin, trachea, or esophagus. The thyroid is swollen and painful, and the patient usually has marked general symptoms such as fever and malaise.

Tuberculosis, syphilis, actinomycosis, and echinococcosis also occur in the thyroid but are very rare.[38]

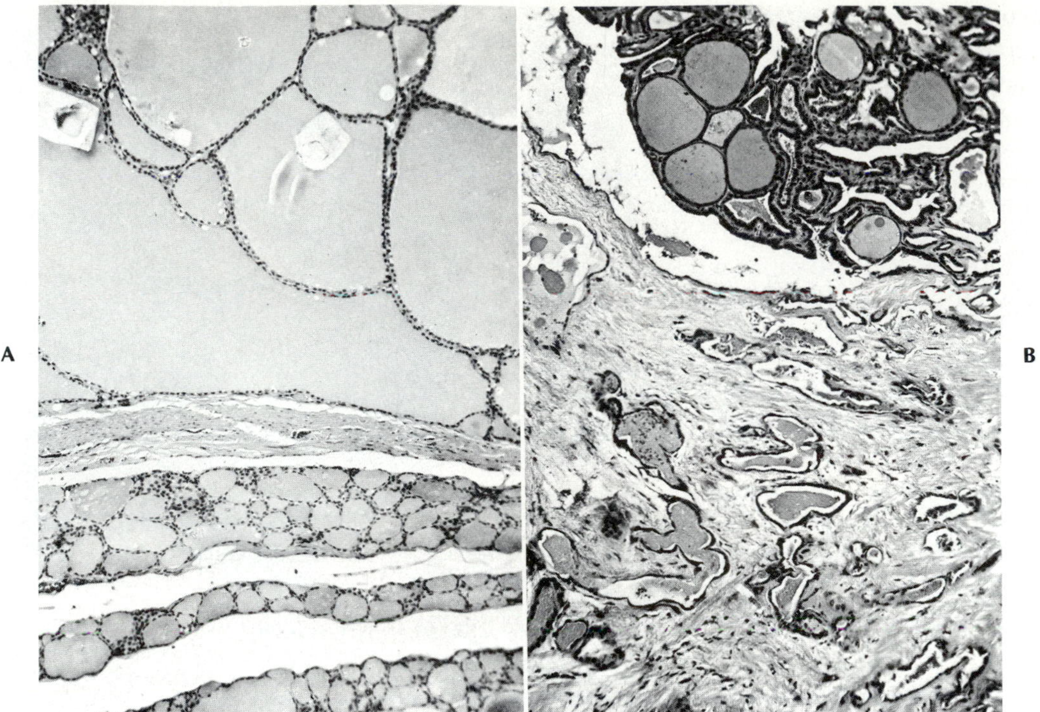

Fig. 33-3. Nodular goiter. **A,** Abundant colloid, flat epithelium, and fibrosis around upper nodule. **B,** Fibrosis and nodule with hyperplasia. (85×.)

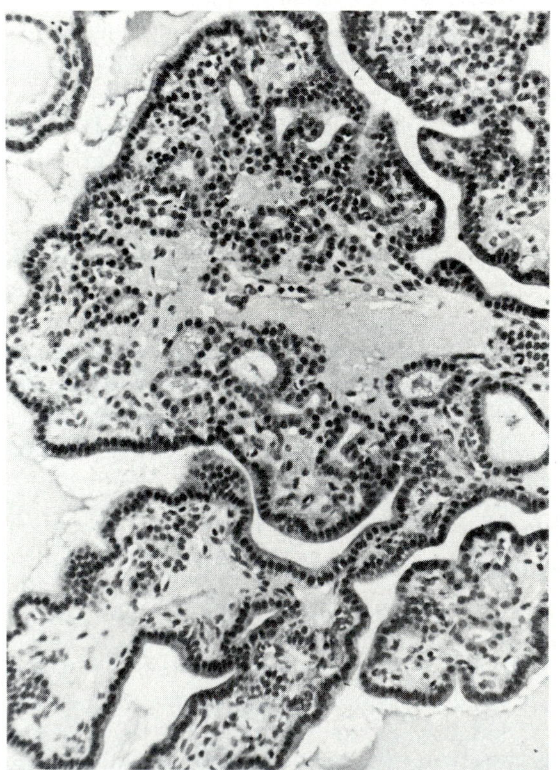

Fig. 33-4. Macropapillary structures in nodular goiter. Note tall epithelium, dark nuclei against basement membrane, and follicles within papillae. (150×.)

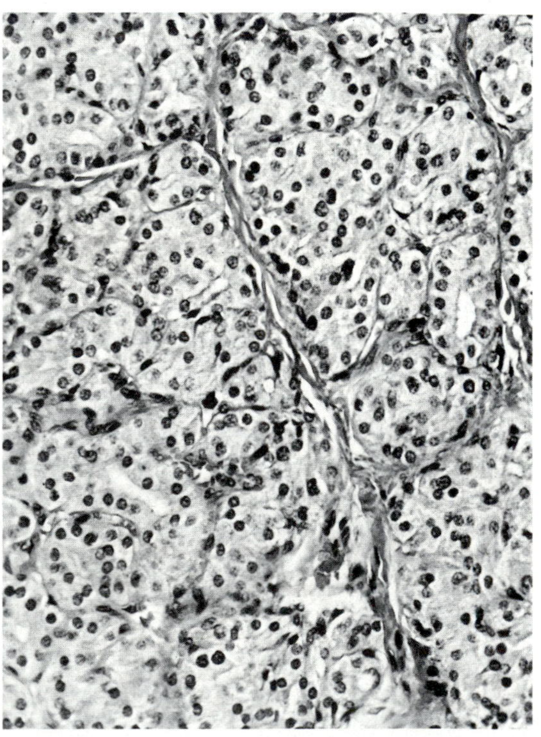

Fig. 33-5. Goiter from cretin with pale and notably hyperplastic epithelium. (240×.)

Granulomatous (de Quervain's) thyroiditis

Granulomatous thyroiditis is the same as subacute thyroiditis and giant cell thyroiditis. Its etiology is unknown, but a viral etiology is supported by clinical features such as a prodromal phase, often a preceding respiratory infection, and usually a complete recovery. The disease is fairly common and occurs mainly in middle-aged and young women.[38] The patient typically has a fever and a painful and moderately enlarged thyroid. Manifestations of hyperthyroidism are common in the early phases of the disease and are probably caused by the destruction of the follicles and the leakage of colloid.

Grossly the thyroid is slightly or moderately enlarged and often asymmetric. The involvement is irregular but usually bilateral. The involved areas are whitish and firm. Some slight adhesions may occur in the capsule, but the gland is easily separated from the surrounding structures.

The histologic findings vary according to the stage of the disease. The process appears to begin with destruction of follicular epithelium and infiltration of the disrupted follicles by neutrophils.[38,41] Neutrophils are replaced by histiocytes and multinucleated giant cells, which are situated inside the follicle and characteristically surround residual colloid (Fig. 33-6), producing the typical granulomatous appearance. The surrounding interstitium shows edema and an inflammatory infiltrate composed of lymphocytes and histiocytes. Later, fibroblastic proliferation and fibrosis are seen. The intensity of the process and its extent vary considerably, and there are often lesions at different stages of development in the same gland. The disease can be diagnosed with aspiration cytology; the diagnosis is based on the occurrence of giant cells, histiocytes, and lymphocytes.[34]

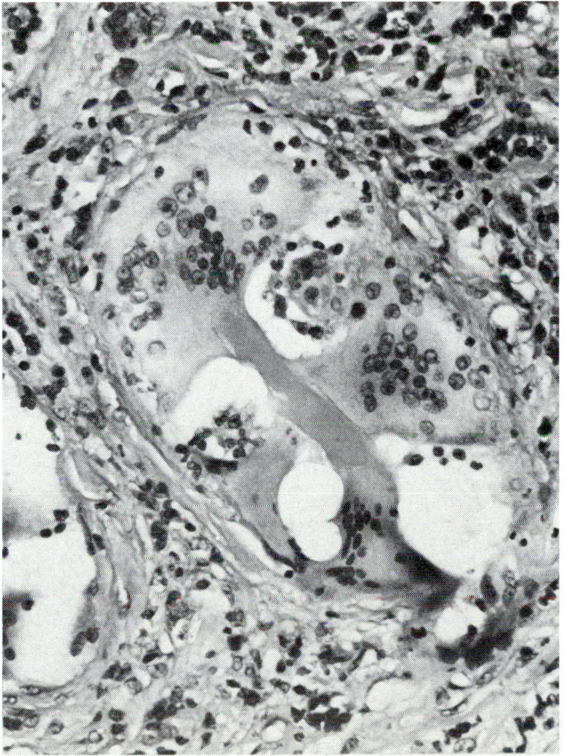

Fig. 33-6. Granulomatous (de Quervain's) thyroiditis. Multinucleated giant cells surround residual colloid in a follicle. Outside follicle are mononuclear inflammatory cells and fibrosis. (300×.)

Granulomatous thyroiditis should be differentiated from so-called palpation thyroiditis, which has been described to occur in most patients with thyroid disease and is believed to be caused by traumatic injury from palpation of the thyroid.[28] In this disorder there are scattered follicles containing foamy histiocytes, lymphocytes, desquamated epithelial cells, and occasional multinucleated giant cells, but there is no continuous spectrum from granuloma to scar like that seen in granulomatous thyroiditis.

Lymphocytic (autoimmune) thyroiditis

Lymphocytic thyroiditis includes Hashimoto's thyroiditis, atrophic thyroiditis, and focal lymphocytic thyroiditis. These diseases have in common lymphocytic infiltrates in the gland and the occurrence of thyroid antibodies, but in many other respects they differ from each other both morphologically and clinically.

Hashimoto's thyroiditis

Hashimoto's thyroiditis (diffuse lymphocytic thyroiditis, goitrous autoimmune thyroiditis) is characterized by thyroid enlargement, lymphocytic infiltration of the gland, and occurrence of thyroid antibodies. The disease is fairly common, especially in women around menopause (sex ratio about 10:1). Certain variants of the disease are seen in childhood and adolescence and make up about 40% of all nontoxic thyroid enlargement occurring in childhood.[29,35]

Hashimoto's thyroiditis is an autoimmune disease closely related immunologically to Graves' disease, and it often occurs in the same families as Graves' disease.[32] Antibodies against different thyroid antigens, such as the microsomal component and thyroglobulin, are present in the sera of almost 100% of patients,[29] but thyroid-stimulating immunoglobulins do not generally occur. The tissue destruction is believed to be caused both by cytotoxic antibodies and by cell-mediated immunity.[37] Immunocomplexes and natural killer cells are probably also important in inducing the changes.[32] The reasons for the autoimmune reactions are presented on p. 1401. According to a recent report,[40] the disease is associated with an excess of HLA-DR5.

Classically, the patient with Hashimoto's thyroiditis is clearly hypothyroid and has a large, rubbery hard goiter. Most patients are either euthyroid or only mildly hypothyroid and have only a slightly or moderately enlarged thyroid.[29]

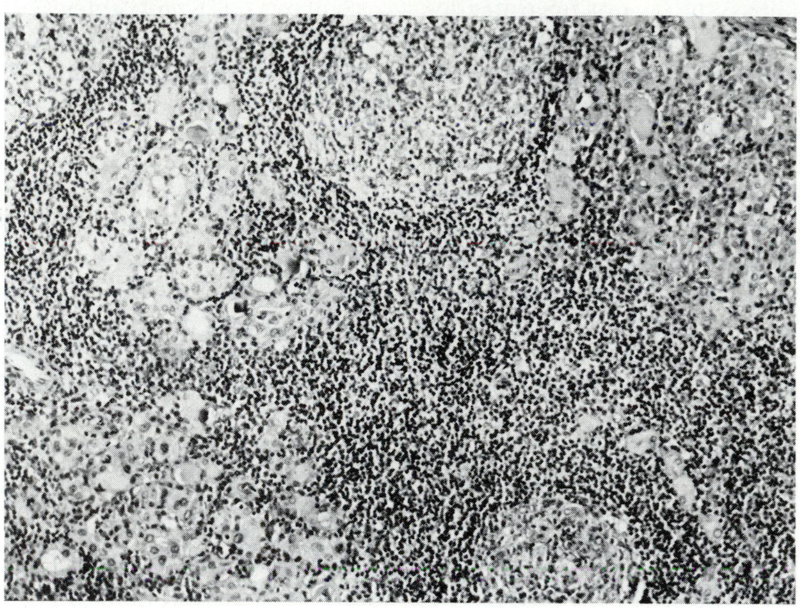

Fig. 33-7. Hashimoto's thyroiditis. Marked lymphocytic infiltration with germinal centers, and destruction of follicles. (150×.)

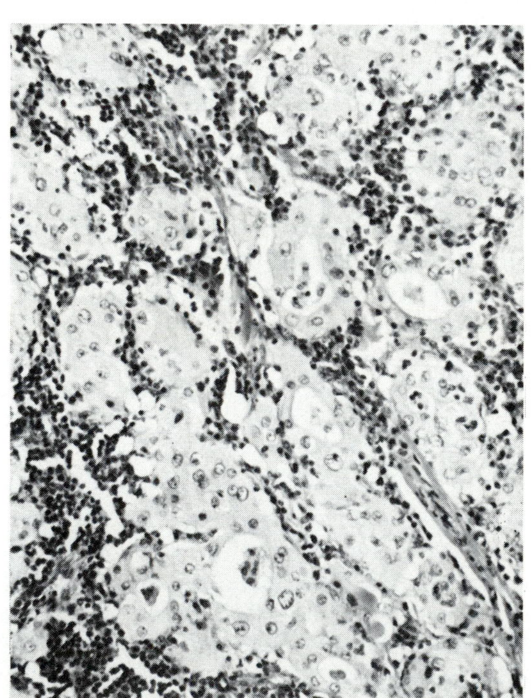

Fig. 33-8. Hashimoto's thyroiditis. Lymphocytic infiltration and oxyphilic cells with enlarged nuclei varying in size, and prominent nucleoli. (250×.)

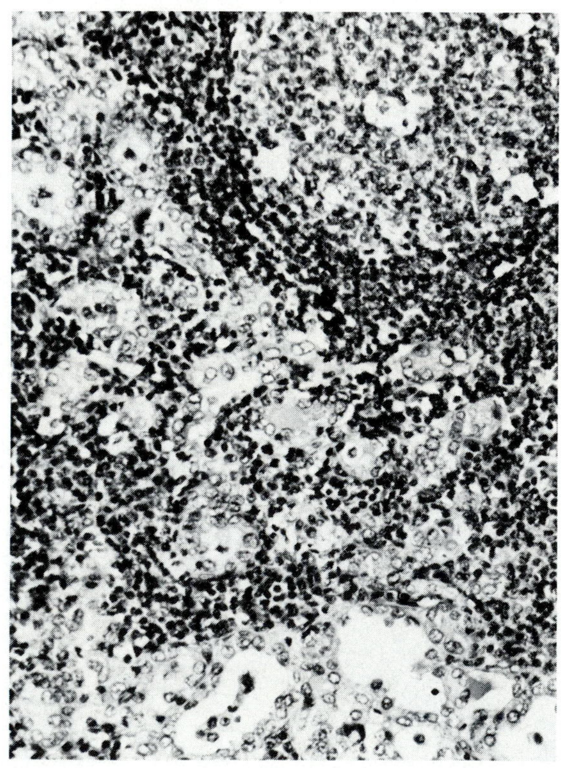

Fig. 33-9. Hashimoto's thyroiditis, juvenile variant. There is marked lymphatic hyperplasia with germinal center. Cuboidal epithelium, no oxyphilic change. Some macrophages in follicular lumina. (250×.)

The thyroid usually weighs around 40 to 60 g but sometimes as much as 350 g.[29] The consistency varies but is often firm or rubbery. The surface is smooth or slightly bosselated, and the capsule is thin and unaltered. The cut surface is uniform, faintly lobulated, and opaque.

Histologically, the most prominent feature is marked diffuse lymphocytic infiltration, which usually contains lymphatic follicles with germinal centers (Fig. 33-7).[38,41] Plasma cells are present in most cases. There is a decreased number of thyroid follicles, and the remaining follicles are generally small and often devoid of colloid. The epithelial cells usually have an abundant oxyphilic and faintly granular cytoplasm, an enlarged hyperchromatic nucleus, often varying in size, and a prominent nucleolus (Fig. 33-8). These oxyphilic cells, also called Askanazy or Hürthle cells, contain large numbers of mitochondria.[36] Slight fibrous thickening of the interlobular septa is common and gives the gland the typical lobulated appearance, but in most cases only slight fibrosis occurs outside the septa. The disease can be diagnosed by aspiration cytology, which reveals oxyphilic cells and lymphocytes.[34]

It is possible to separate from Hashimoto's thyroiditis some histologic variants that differ in their clinical features from the rest. In *juvenile thyroiditis* no oxyphil cells or only occasional ones are seen, but the epithelium is cuboidal or sometimes columnar (Fig. 33-9), and often has papillary infoldings that give it a hyperplastic appearance. The follicular lumina often contain clumps of macrophages. Germinal centers are abundant, and fibrosis is slight or absent. This type of thyroiditis occurs mainly in children and young women. The patients are usually euthyroid and symptomless, show only low titers of thyroid antibodies, and their thyroids are only slightly enlarged.[35,36]

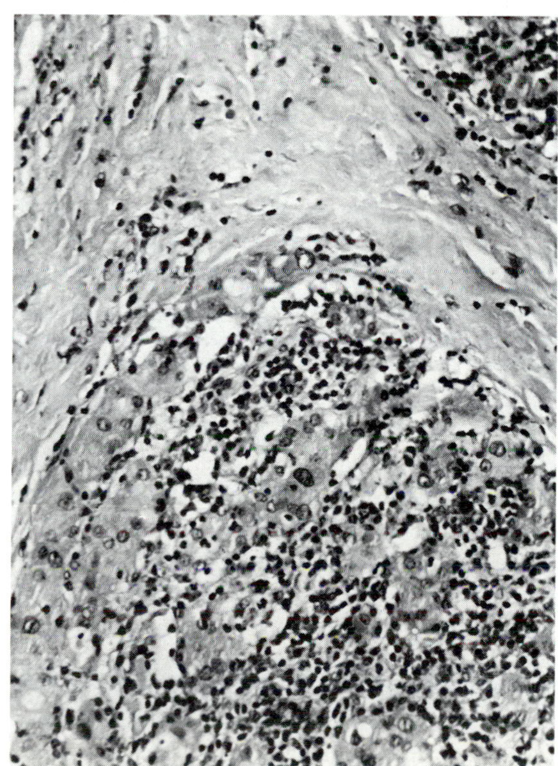

Fig. 33-10. Hashimoto's thyroiditis, fibrous variant. There are marked fibrous replacement of thyroid parenchyma, lymphocytic infiltration, follicle destruction with oxyphilic cytoplasmic chance. (250×.)

In about 10% of cases there is marked fibrous replacement of thyroid parenchyma (Fig. 33-10) often accompanied by squamous metaplasia,[31] which may simulate neoplastic growth. Patients with this *fibrous variant of Hashimoto's thyroiditis* have a firm and enlarged thyroid, often with compression symptoms and high thyroid antibody titers, and frequently clinical hypothyroidism.[31]

Histologic differential diagnosis of Hashimoto's thyroiditis from malignant lymphoma, follicular carcinoma, and Graves' disease may sometimes cause problems. In Graves' disease the lymphocytic infiltration is usually focal and milder, and there is no oxphilic change in the epithelium. However, epithelial hyperplasia occurs in addition to Graves' disease sometimes also in Hashimoto's thyroiditis, especially in the juvenile variant. For the relation of Hashimoto's thyroiditis to malignant lymphoma, see p. 1417.

Atrophic thyroiditis

Atrophic thyroiditis corresponds to the clinical condition called spontaneous hypothyroidism. In atrophic thyroiditis the thyroid is not enlarged but is often decreased in size. Thyroid antibodies are present. Histologically, lymphocytic infiltration, atrophy of the follicles, and fibrosis are seen. It is believed that this condition is closely related to Hashimoto's thyroiditis but that the thyroid has failed to regenerate; in Hashimoto's thyroiditis the thyroid enlargement is probably caused by regeneration of follicular epithelium induced by TSH.[37] It has been suggested that the lack of regeneration in atrophic thyroiditis might be caused by thyroid growth–blocking antibodies reported to occur in atrophic thyroiditis but not in Hashimoto's thyroiditis.[30]

Focal lymphocytic thyroiditis

In focal lymphocytic thyroiditis, focal aggregates of lymphocytes, often with germinal centers, are seen in the thyroid (Fig. 33-11). Especially in more severe forms, the areas involved may show oxyphilic changes in the follicular epithelium, but most of the epithelium appears unaltered. This lesion has been reported to occur in up to 36% of women and 18% of men in autopsy series and to be twice as common in glands that have some other abnormality (nodular goiter, adenoma, papillary carcinoma) than in otherwise normal glands.[39] The

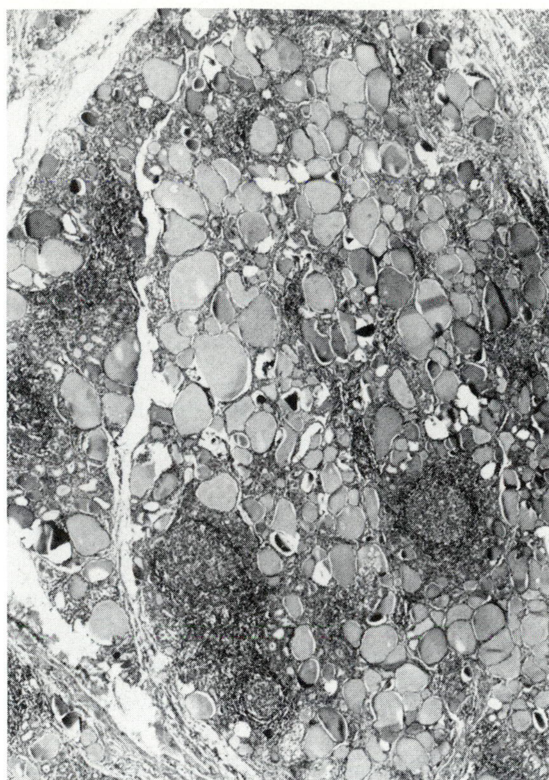

Fig. 33-11. Focal lymphocytic thyroiditis. Lymphocytic infiltrates have germinal centers. Follicles appear unaltered. (Low power.)

patients usually have low titers of thyroid antibodies, and the disease is usually included in autoimmune thyroiditis. The disorder does not usually appear to be progressive or to have clinical importance.[29]

Riedel's thyroiditis (invasive fibrous thyroiditis)

Riedel's thyroiditis is a rare disease; only 20 cases were found among 42,000 thyroidectomies.[41] The initial complaint of the patients is a stony hard goiter that is densely adherent to adjacent structures in the neck. Compression symptoms, such as dysphagia, may occur. Thus the clinical picture resembles that of cancer.

The cause is unknown, but it has been suggested that Riedel's thyroiditis belongs to the disease group of so-called multifocal idiopathic fibrosclerosis,[33] which also includes idiopathic retroperitoneal, mediastinal, or retro-orbital fibrosis and sclerosing cholangitis. These disorders may occur simultaneously.[33]

The process involves the whole gland or a part of one lobe. In addition, contiguous structures, most often muscle, are involved, which contrasts to the findings in de Quervain's thyroiditis and Hashimoto's thyroiditis. The involved areas are stony hard and whitish and show no lobulation on cross section. The thyroid capsule is not usually discernible. Histologically, fibrous tissue, accompanied by different inflammatory cells, replaces normal thyroid structures and invades the adjacent muscle tissue.[41] The fibrous tissue may be extensively hyalinized. Usually neither germinal centers nor oxyphilic cells are seen.

RADIATION CHANGES

After ionizing radiation, whether external or from radioactive iodine, interstitial fibrosis, thickening of blood vessel walls, cytoplasmic oxyphilia, and nuclear atypia are seen in the thyroid.[44] The nuclei are hyperchromatic and often bizarre and show considerable variation in size, with many giant forms. Marked morphologic variation is seen between different follicles as well as within the same follicle; some of the nuclei appear morphologically normal and some are hyperchromatic. The nuclear abnormalities appear some weeks after the radiation and persist for many years.[44] Late changes after low-dose irradiation have been described as including nodule formation, oxyphilic cell change, and focal lymphocytic thyroiditis.[43] For the relation of radiation to carcinogenesis, see p. 1411.

AMYLOIDOSIS

The thyroid may be involved in systemic amyloidosis. Occasionally the infiltrates may be so massive that they replace most of the thyroid tissue. This kind of lesion has been called amyloid goiter.[42]

TUMORS

Benign tumors

Follicular adenoma

Follicular adenoma is an encapsulated noninvasive tumor arising from follicular cells and showing a follicular or trabecular growth pattern.

Follicular adenoma is a common tumor that can occur at any age but mainly in young adults. It is about five times more common in females than males.[47] Clinically it is usually a solitary thyroid nodule that occasionally causes compression. A hemorrhage into an adenoma may cause pain and an acute increase in the size of the tumor.

Grossly adenomas are circumscribed and encapsulated spherical tumors that vary in size up to 10 cm in diameter. On section, the tumor is often less colloidal than the surrounding tissue, its color varies from white to red-brown, and its consistency varies from soft to firm. Degenerative features such as a central scar or calcifications and hemorrhages are often seen.

Histologically the tumor is surrounded by a fibrous capsule that often contains wide vascular spaces. The tumor cells form follicles, usually of small size (Fig. 33-12), or occur in cords (trabeculae) or solid groups with little follicle formation (Fig. 33-13). They are separated by a hyalinized or edematous stroma (Fig. 33-14) or by thin fibrous septa, often containing abundant thin-walled vascular spaces, which give a sinusoidal appearance (Fig. 33-15). The nuclei of the tumor cells are often enlarged,

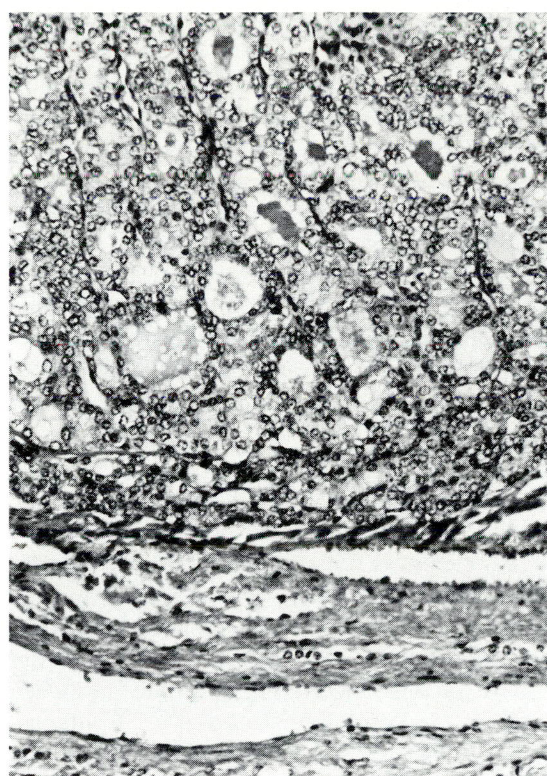

Fig. 33-12. Follicular adenoma. Encapsulated tumor is composed of follicles. Capsule contains wide vascular lumina. (250×.)

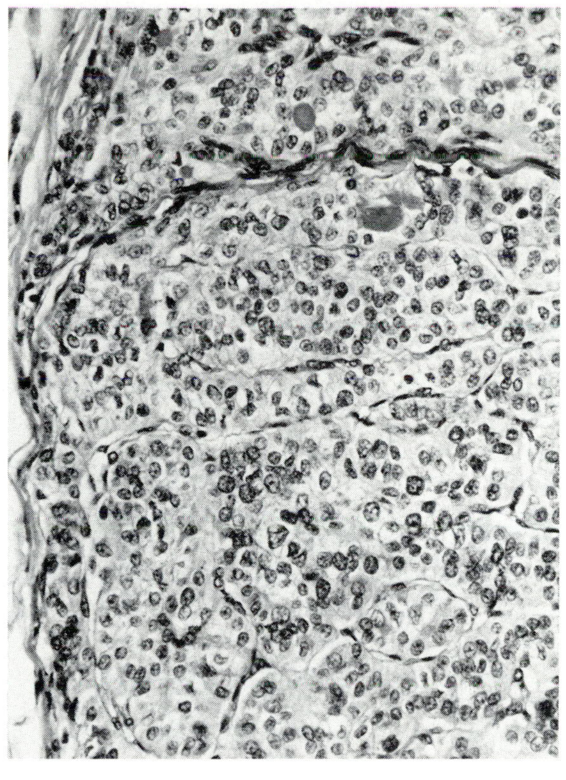

Fig. 33-13. Follicular adenoma. Trabecular growth pattern. Occasional colloid droplets are seen. (300×.)

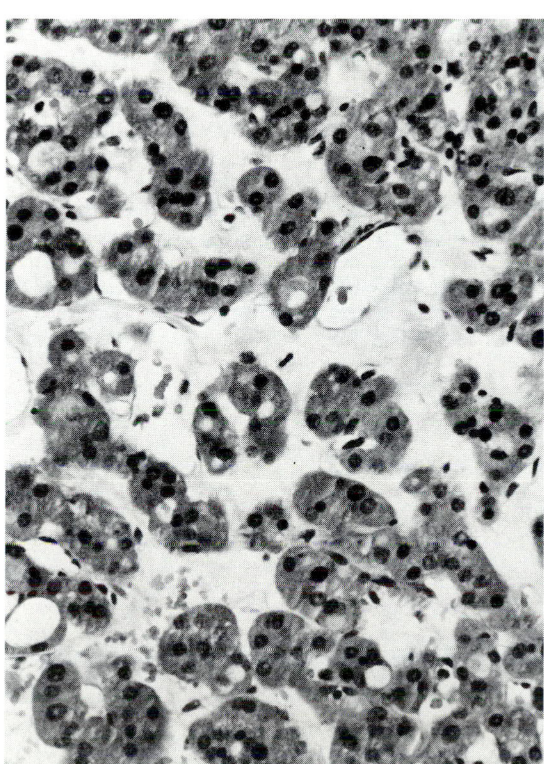

Fig. 33-14. Follicular adenoma. There are oxyphilic cells with trabecular growth pattern and occasional follicles. Note edematous stroma. (300×.)

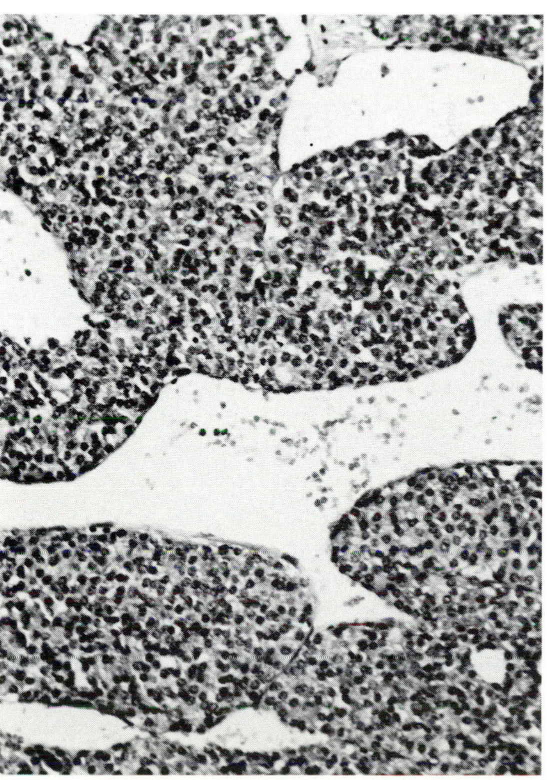

Fig. 33-15. Follicular adenoma. Cell cords are separated by wide vascular spaces giving a sinusoidal appearance. (100×.)

and there may be some variation in the size and shape, but mitoses are infrequent.

Follicular adenomas are often divided according to their pattern into several subgroups such as trabecular (old term "embryonal"), microfollicular ("fetal"), normofollicular ("simple"), and macrofollicular ("colloid") adenoma. Because adenomas are often composed of more than one type of structure and the subdivision does not show any clinical correlations, it can be regarded as unnecessary for practical purposes.

It may sometimes be difficult to differentiate follicular adenoma from follicular carcinoma (see p. 1413) and from nodular goiter. Follicular adenoma has been said to differ from a nodule of nodular goiter by having a continuous capsule, a clear distinction in the architecture inside and outside the capsule, a rather uniform histologic architecture inside the capsule, and compression of the surrounding thyroid tissue. Increased vascularity and small follicle size also support the diagnosis of adenoma. However, there are nodules in nodular goiter that fulfill these criteria. In practice, such nodules are usually called adenomas if they are single and nonneoplastic if they are multiple.

Hürthle cell adenoma (oxyphilic adenoma) is usually regarded as a subtype of follicular adenoma. It is composed of cells that have abundant oxyphilic cytoplasm and usually a trabecular growth pattern (Fig. 33-14) but may also occur in solid groups or form follicles. The nuclei are clearly enlarged and often vary considerably in size. The nucleolus is prominent. Ultrastructurally the cytoplasm is studded with mitochondria.[45,46] The tumor does not seem to differ in its clinical behavior from other follicular adenomas.

Clear cell adenoma is a term sometimes used for follicular adenomas composed of cells with clear cytoplasm.[45]

Atypical adenoma is a term that has been given to adenomas showing features that can be regarded as indicative of malignancy, such as high cellularity, nuclear atypia, and increased number of mitoses.[47]

Teratoma

Teratoma is a very rare tumor that occurs mainly in newborn infants.[48] Some teratomas may arise from the thyroid capsule, but others may originate from the adjoining structures. Teratomas are usually, but not always, histologically and clinically benign.[79] They may grow large and cause compression of adjacent structures.

Malignant tumors

Thyroid cancer is not a common disease; it makes up less than 1% of all human cancer. Carcinoma is clearly the most common type, but sarcomas and primary lymphomas also occur. Usually thyroid carcinoma is divided into four histologic types: papillary, follicular, medullary, and anaplastic (undifferentiated).[71,72] Epidermoid,[93] mucoepidermoid,[88a] and mucinous[61a] carcinomas have also been reported to occur in the thyroid, but they are rare. Most tumors with epidermoid differentiation represent epidermoid metaplasia in papillary carcinoma.

There is a good correlation between histologic findings and prognosis in thyroid cancer.[50,62,101] In addition to prognosis, the histologic picture of the tumor correlates to other features in the natural history of the disease better than in malignant tumors of most other organs (Table 33-1).[62,101] For these reasons an accurate histologic classification of thyroid cancer is important.

Table 33-1. Natural history in different types of thyroid carcinoma

	Papillary carcinoma	Follicular carcinoma	Medullary carcinoma	Anaplastic carcinoma
Age	All ages	Middle and old age	Middle and old age (familial cases also in children)	Old age
Female-to-male ratio	About 3:1	About 2.5:1	About 1:1	About 1.5:1
Primary tumor	Usually small	Usually small	Usually small	Usually large and invades contiguous structures
Regional metastases	Common	Very rare	Common	Common
Distant organ metastases	Rare	Common	Rare	Common
10-year survival	80% to 95%	50% to 70%	60% to 70%	5% to 10%, median survival about 2 months
Principal cause of death	Local invasion and distant metastases	Distant metastases	Distant metastases	Local invasion

Aspiration cytology is useful in the diagnosis of thyroid cancer.[84] However, follicular carcinoma and follicular adenoma cannot usually be cytologically differentiated.

Carcinoma

Papillary carcinoma. Papillary carcinoma is the most common type of thyroid carcinoma, comprising 45% to 70% of all.[50,62,102] It occurs at all ages, including children, but the incidence rises with advancing age. The tumor is about three times more common in females than males.[72]

It has been shown that people who have been exposed to irradiation in childhood have an increased risk of papillary carcinoma.[73,90,91] Radiation has been suggested to act as an initiating factor in thyroid carcinogenesis.[90] There appears to be a negative association between papillary carcinoma and endemic goiter; the incidence of the tumor is exceptionally high in Iceland, an iodine-rich area,[65,99] and the relative frequency of papillary carcinoma rose in Switzerland after administration of iodine in the diet.[74]

Papillary carcinoma is a slowly growing tumor that usually appears clinically as a solitary thyroid nodule. The primary tumor is in most cases limited to the gland, but especially in older people it may invade the surrounding structures, such as muscles, esophagus, or larynx. Regional lymph nodes in the neck are involved in almost one half of cases at the time of diagnosis,[62,86,101] and this may be the only symptom of the disease. Lymph node involvement is most common at young age.[62] Dis-

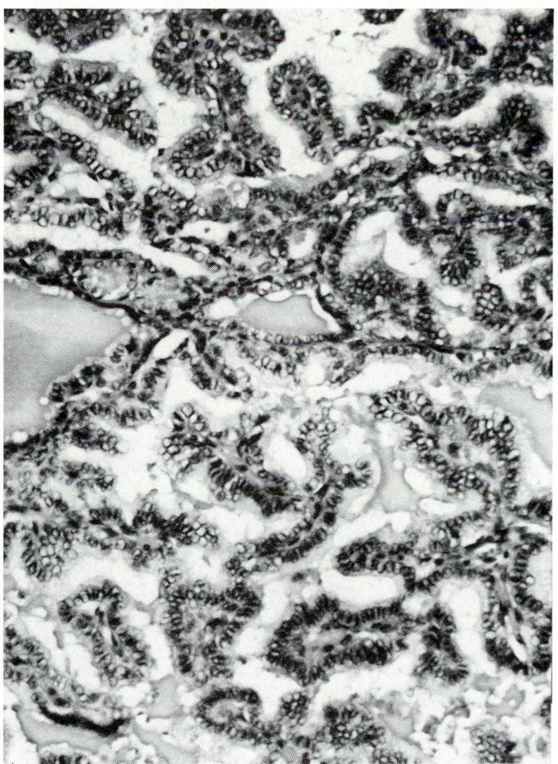

Fig. 33-16. Papillary carcinoma. Papillae have one layer of tumor cells, ground-glass nuclei. (150×.)

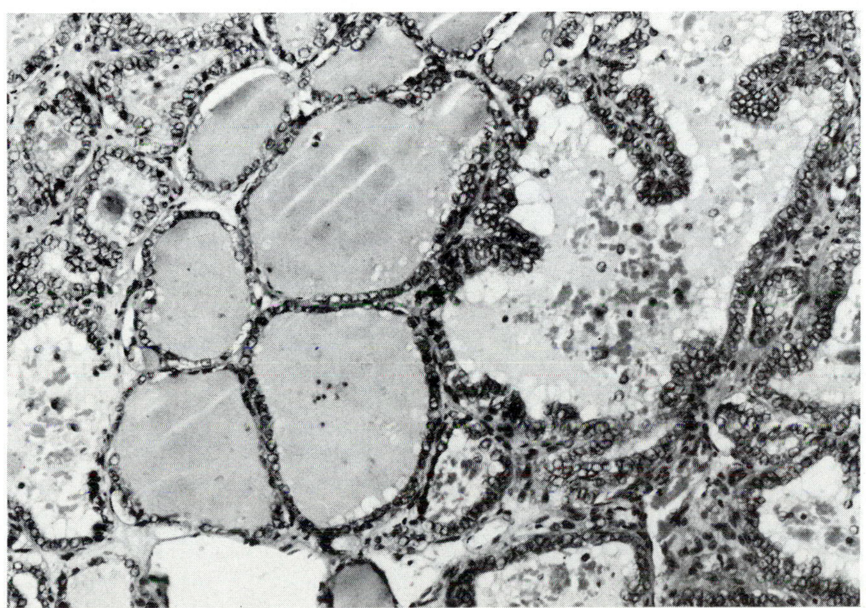

Fig. 33-17. Papillary carcinoma. Papillae are on right; follicles with colloid are on left. Note ground-glass nuclei. (150×.)

tant (organ) metastases occur mainly in the lungs but are rare; their frequency at diagnosis is less than 5%.[50,62,86,101]

The prognosis for papillary carcinoma is good, with a 10-year survival rate on the order of 80% to 95%.[64,86,101] Survival rate correlates to the extent of the primary tumor and the presence of distant metastases but unexpectedly not to the presence of regional metastases.[64,101] Young age is associated with good prognosis.[54,64]

Grossly the tumor is usually a whitish, hard, scarlike, poorly limited area, but it may also be cystic. The primary tumor may be extremely small, only a few millimeters in diameter, although it may have bulky regional metastases.

Histologically papillary carcinoma is composed of papillae, usually accompanied by follicles and sometimes by solid sheets of cells as well. The papillae are often long and slender and have a fibrovascular core that is usually thin but may be thick and hyalinized. The core is covered by one layer of tumor cells (Figs. 33-16 and 33-17). The follicles are usually well differentiated and often contain colloid (Figs. 33-17 and 33-20). The solid sheets of cells often occur at the periphery of the tumor (Fig. 33-18). These structures are most common in tumors of young people. The nuclei of the tumor cells are often overlapping and typically have the ground-glass appearance, that is, large and pale with an inconspicuous nucleolus. Ultrastructurally the nuclei often have deep infoldings containing cytoplasmic pseudoinclusions[77] that appear in light microscopy as intranuclear vacuoles. The ground-glass appearance, generally regarded as an important diagnostic criterion of papillary carcinoma,[59,63] is not always seen in all nuclei but is usually seen in at least some. In frozen material the nuclei usually lose this appearance.

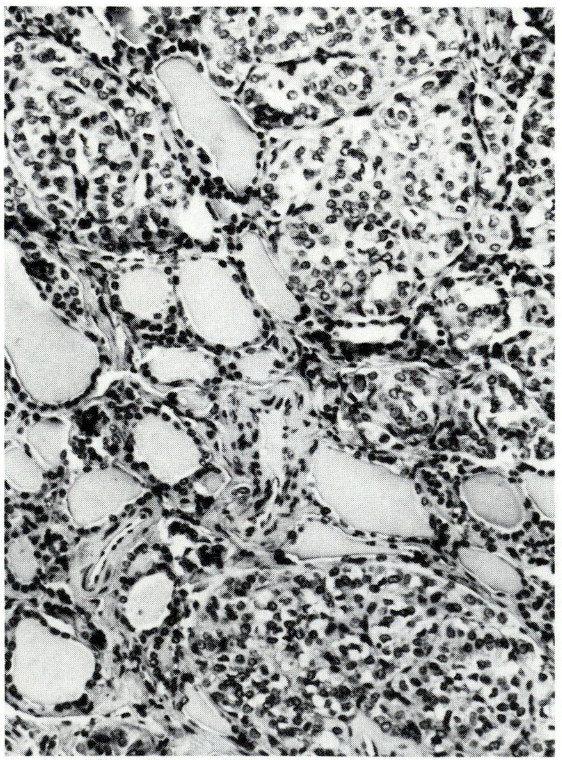

Fig. 33-18. Papillary carcinoma. Solid sheets of cells invade between normal follicles. Other parts of tumor showed papillae and follicles. (100×.)

Many authors include as papillary carcinomas those carcinomas composed solely of follicles and having ground-glass nuclei. These tumors usually have the typical growth pattern of papillary carcinoma. Their course of disease is like that of other papillary carcinomas and different from that of follicular carcinoma.[63] The smallest papillary carcinomas are often composed solely of follicles.

Papillary carcinoma is typically strongly invasive, and encapsulation is rare. Fibrosis and lymphocytic infiltration are often seen around the invading islands. Small foci of tumor tissue, possibly representing intrathyroid lymphatic metastases, often occur far from the tumor proper, even in the other thyroid lobe. Blood vessel invasion is rare. Psammoma bodies, which are small, concentric, calcified spherules, are seen in almost half of papillary carcinomas,[63] sometimes far from the tumor, and they have been regarded as diagnostic for it. They must, however, be differentiated from calcified colloid, which may occur in a variety of conditions. Calcified colloid is located inside the follicles, whereas psammoma bodies are usually seen in the stroma. Epidermoid metaplasia,[82] which morphologically appears benign, may occur in papillary carcinoma and apparently does not have any prognostic importance.[62]

All papillary neoplasias are usually considered malig-

Table 33-2. Histological differential diagnosis of papillary and follicular carcinomas

	Papillary carcinoma	Follicular carcinoma
Encapsulation	Rare	Common
Invasion	Strongly invasive, invades in small islands	Less invasive, invades in large islands with pushing border
Multiple tumor foci	Common	Rare
Blood vessel invasion	Rare	Common
Cellular pattern	Papillae, follicles, solid cell groups	Follicles, trabeculae, no papillae (pseudopapillary infoldings may occur)
Psammoma bodies	In about 50%	None (calcified colloid may occur)
Nuclei	"Ground glass," overlapping	Normochromatic or hyperchromatic, not overlapping

nant, regardless of the presence of encapsulation.

Sometimes it may be difficult to differentiate papillary carcinoma from follicular (Table 33-2) and medullary carcinomas (p. 1416) and from epithelial hyperplasia and macropapillary structures in nodular goiter. In epithelial hyperplasia the nuclei may resemble ground-glass nuclei, but there is no abrupt change in the nuclear type as is seen in the border of papillary carcinoma. The papillary infoldings projecting to the follicles are short in epithelial hyperplasia, and the normal lobular structure is preserved (Fig. 33-1), whereas it is distorted by fibrosis in papillary carcinoma. In macropapillary structures the nuclei are not of the ground-glass type and the papillae are short and broad and often contain follicles (Fig. 33-4), which does not commonly occur in papillary carcinoma.

Occult papillary carcinoma (occult sclerosing carcinoma) is a term given to small papillary carcinoma (usually defined as less than 1.5 cm in diameter) that often has a central fibrous scar. Its prevalence has been high, varying between 6% and 28%[66] in autopsy studies in which the thyroids were semiserially sectioned. The tumors may have regional lymph node metastases, although most tumors are detected as incidental findings in thyroids resected for another thyroid disease. Distant metastases or deaths from carcinoma are extremely rare in this tumor.[75] It has been suggested that occult carcinoma represents the initiation phase of papillary carcinoma.[90] Irradiation seems to increase its prevalence.[90]

Follicular carcinoma. Follicular carcinoma comprises about one fourth of all thyroid carcinomas. It is more common in females than in males[63,72] and is a disease of middle and old age. It has been claimed that there is a positive correlation between the risk of follicular carcinoma and endemic goiter,[99] but this is controversial.[65] The association between irradiation and follicular carcinoma is not clear.

The primary tumor in follicular carcinoma is in most cases confined within the thyroid capsule, but it may invade the surrounding structures. In contrast to papillary carcinoma, regional lymph node metastases are almost nonexistent, but distant metastases are common, occurring in as much as 25% at diagnosis.[63] Their most common sites are the bones and lungs. Symptoms caused by distant metastases, such as a pathologic fracture, are often the first symptom of the disease. The prognosis for follicular carcinoma is between that for papillary and anaplastic carcinomas.

Grossly, follicular carcinoma is usually circumscribed, resembling follicular adenoma in that respect. Histologically the tumor is often encapsulated. The capsule usually contains large, thin-walled blood vessels. Vascular invasion—often to these vessels—is common, which fits well with the frequent occurrence of distant blood-borne metastases in follicular carcinoma (Figs. 33-19 and 33-21). When tissue invasion occurs, the invading islands are usually large and have a pushing border. Only tumors that show vascular or capsular invasion are considered malignant.

Like follicular adenoma, follicular carcinoma is composed of follicular or trabecular structures or both. The degree of follicular differentiation varies, but usually the

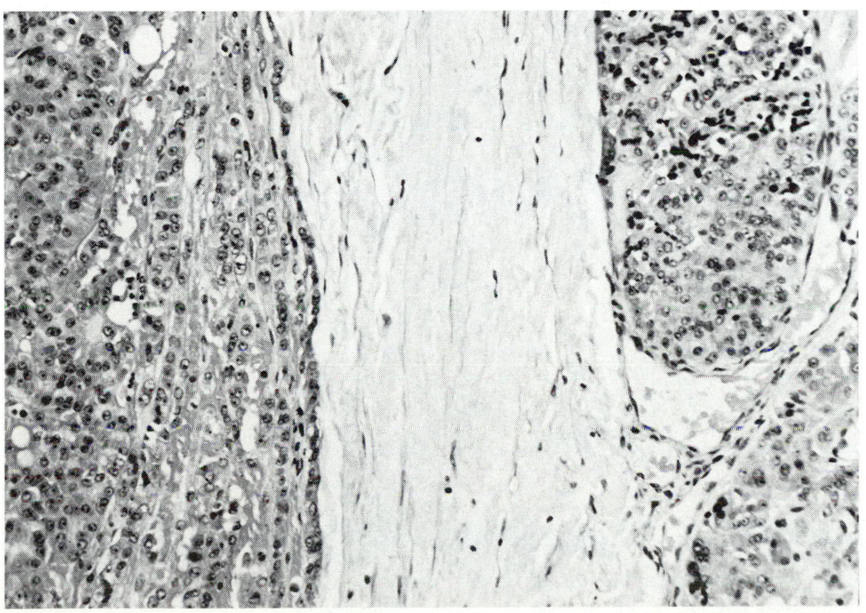

Fig. 33-19. Follicular carcinoma. Encapsulated tumor is composed of Hürthle cells with trabecular growth pattern. Tumor invades capsular vessel on right. Note compact tumor thrombus surrounded by endothelium. (150×.)

follicles are less well differentiated than the follicles in papillary carcinoma. Between the trabeculae and groups of follicles are often abundant thin-walled blood vessels, which may form a sinusoidal pattern. Neither papillary structures nor psammoma bodies occur, and the nuclei are not of the ground-glass type but are normochromatic or hyperchromatic (Fig. 33-20). The nuclear atypia varies but is usually not marked.

Follicular carcinoma is divided into two subtypes: *encapsulated* and *invasive*. In the first subtype the tumor is encapsulated and only minimal (difficult to find) vascular or capsular invasion is seen. In the second subtype the tumor is either nonencapsulated or encapsulated with marked invasion. These two subtypes should always be differentiated when evaluating the prognosis because the 10-year survival rate for the first type is 80% to 95% and for the second type 30% to 45%.[64,101]

Follicular carcinoma should be histologically differentiated from atypical follicular adenoma, atypical nodules of nodular goiter, papillary carcinoma (Table 33-2), and thyroiditis. Follicular carcinoma differs from adenoma and atypical nodules by showing capsular or vascular invasion.[47] Capsular invasion can be regarded as having occurred if tumor tissue is seen outside the capsule; tumor tissue within the capsular wall may be caused by capsular infoldings. Vascular invasion is considered real if there is a compact tumor thrombus surrounded by vascular endothelium in a vessel within or outside the capsular wall (Figs. 33-19 and 33-21).[69] Loose tumor cells in vascular lumina should not be accepted as vascular invasion because in most cases they appear to be caused by manipulation of the tumor.[69] It is usually impossible to evaluate blood vessel invasion inside the tumor tissue, because in most cases there is an intimate contact with

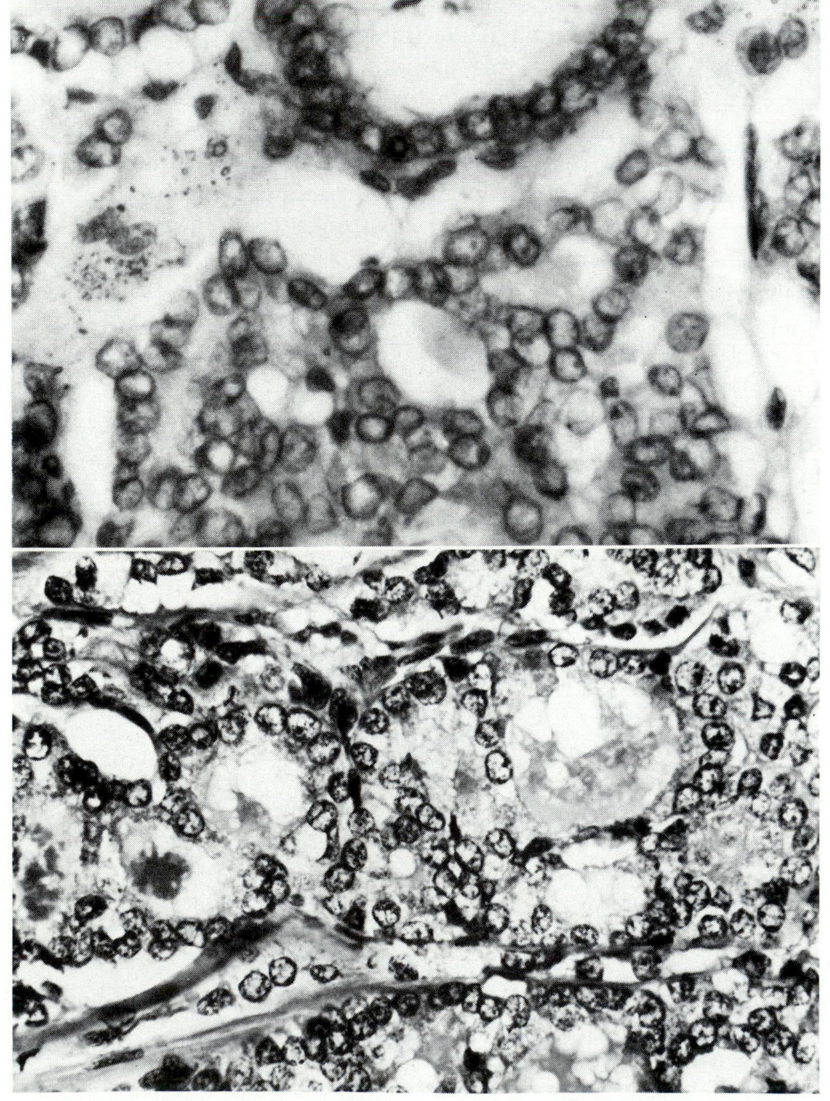

Fig. 33-20. A, Papillary carcinoma, follicular area. **B,** Follicular carcinoma. Note difference in nuclear type. In papillary carcinoma the nuclei are overlapping and of the ground-glass type. (400×.)

the tumor cells and the vascular endothelium. In Hashimoto's thyroiditis epithelial atypia may lead to erroneous diagnosis of follicular carcinoma.

Hürthle cell carcinoma. Carcinomas composed of Hürthle (oxyphilic) cells usually have a follicular or trabecular growth pattern and are classified as follicular carcinomas (Fig. 33-19). The criteria of malignancy are the same as for other follicular carcinomas. The course of disease also appears to be the same.[62]

Clear cell carcinoma. Cells with clear cytoplasm are fairly often seen in thyroid carcinomas. The clear appearance is caused by accumulation of glycogen.[97] Carcinomas composed solely of cells with clear cytoplasm are rare. They usually form follicles and are then classified as follicular carcinomas. It may be difficult to differentiate them from metastatic renal cell carcinoma, although renal cell carcinoma does not show periodic acid–Schiff–positive colloid droplets like those usually seen in clear cell thyroid carcinoma. Also, immunohistochemical methods based on the thyroglobulin content of most differentiated thyroid carcinomas may help in differentiation.[53]

Anaplastic (undifferentiated) carcinoma. Anaplastic carcinoma comprises 10% to 25% of all thyroid carcinomas.[62,101] The tumor is only slightly more common in women than in men and is a disease of old age. A differentiated component, either papillary or follicular carcinoma, is usually found if anaplastic carcinoma is studied with subserial sections,[89] and it has been assumed that the tumor derives from differentiated carcinoma.[49,67,76]

In contrast to differentiated carcinomas, the course of disease in anaplastic carcinoma is characterized by heavy invasion of the tumor into adjacent soft tissues and the trachea and esophagus. That is why the first symptom is often dyspnea, hoarseness, dysphagia, or a rapidly growing tumor in the neck. Prognosis is poor; the 5-year survival rate is only on the order of 10%, and the median survival about 2 months.[49,64] Death is usually caused by local invasion of the tumor, although the tumor also metastasizes into both regional nodes and distant organs, most often the lungs.

Grossly, anaplastic carcinoma is usually large and firm and shows necrotic areas. According to the histologic picture, the tumor is often divided into *spindle and giant cell carcinoma* and *small cell carcinoma*. The first type is composed mainly of spindle cells and therefore closely resembles sarcoma (Fig. 33-22). However, areas that appear epithelial are usually also found. Also, cells with

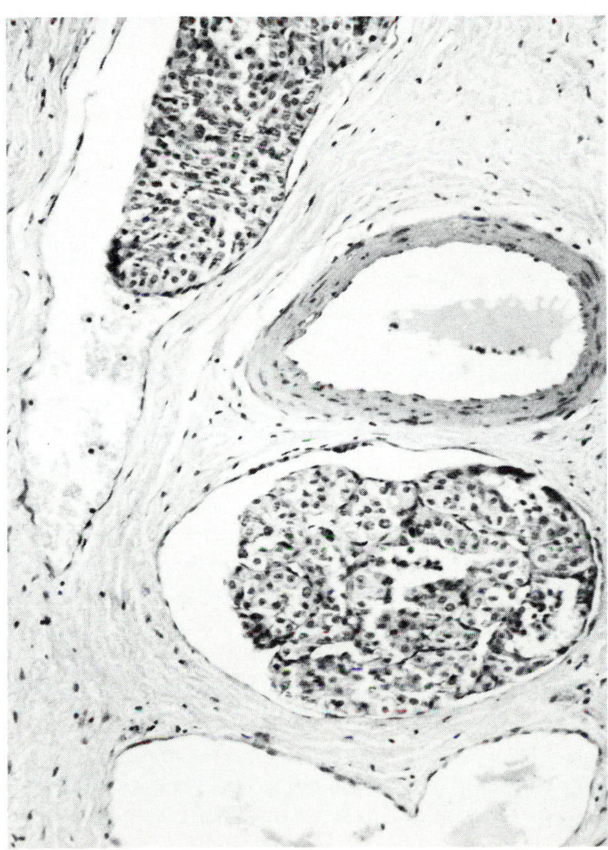

Fig. 33-21. Follicular carcinoma with blood vessel invasion. Tumor thrombi are compact and are surrounded by vascular endothelium. (80×.)

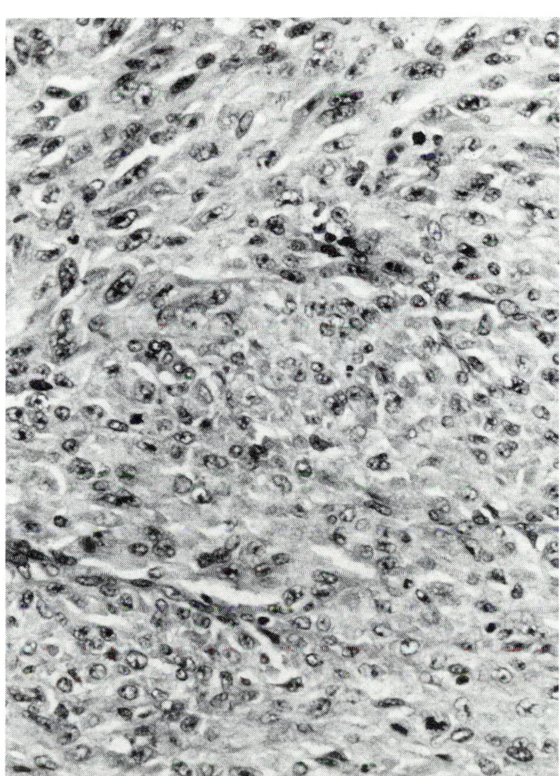

Fig. 33-22. Anaplastic carcinoma of spindle and giant cell type. Note spindle cells with mitoses. (200×.)

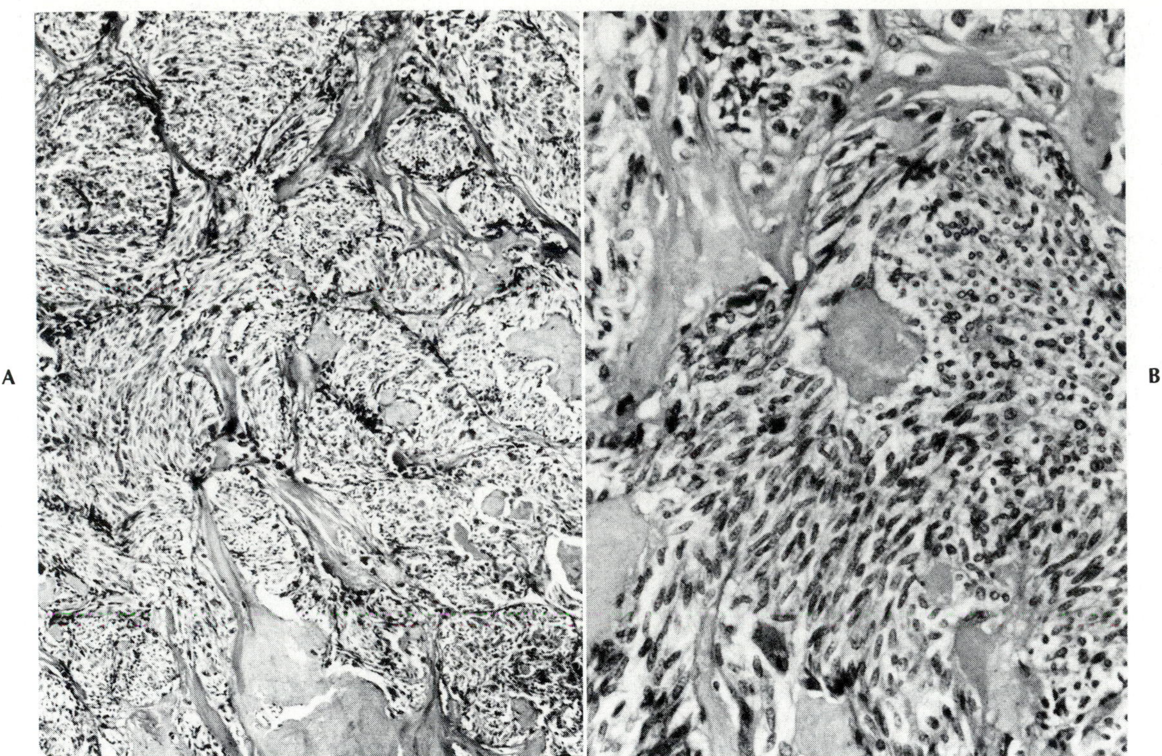

Fig. 33-23. Medullary carcinoma. **A,** Fibrous septa divide tumor cells into islands. **B,** Regular spindle-shaped tumor cells surround mass of amyloid. (**A,** 50×; **B,** 200×.)

giant nuclei are often seen, and multinucleated giant cells, resembling osteoclasts, occur occasionally. At present many authors are of the opinion that if a small cell anaplastic carcinoma occurs in the thyroid at all, it is very rare. Probably most undifferentiated small cell tumors with a diffuse growth pattern represent malignant lymphomas, and those with a solid growth pattern represent medullary carcinoma.

Anaplastic carcinoma is sometimes difficult to differentiate from spindle cell sarcoma and from medullary carcinoma.

Medullary carcinoma. Medullary carcinoma differs basically from the other thyroid carcinomas by arising from C cells (parafollicular cells), whereas all the other carcinomas originate from follicular cells. Like normal C cells, the tumor cells produce and secrete calcitonin. The tumor may also secrete prostaglandins,[68] histaminase,[68] and carcinoembryonic antigen (CEA),[61] and occasionally 5-hydroxytryptamine (5HT) or adrenocorticotropic hormone (ACTH).[68,78] Medullary carcinoma is regarded as one of the APUD tumors.[3]

Although most medullary carcinomas occur sporadically, about 10% have a genetic background.[69] The familial form has an autosomal dominant mode of inheritance and is often associated with pheochromocytoma and parathyroid hyperplasia or adenoma (multiple endocrine adenomatosis, MEN IIA)[51,83,95,98] or with pheochromocytoma and multiple mucosal neuromas (MEN IIB).[95] Although the sporadic carcinoma is generally unilateral, the familial tumor is usually bilateral and multicentric and often accompanied by C cell hyperplasia, which, it has been suggested, may precede the development of medullary carcinoma.[1,100] Also, the associated pheochromocytoma is usually bilateral and multicentric and is probably preceded by medullary hyperplasia.[60]

Medullary carcinoma is rather rare, comprising about 5% to 10% of all thyroid carcinomas. It is as common in men as in women and is usually detected at middle age. The most frequent finding is a solitary thyroid nodule, but sometimes enlarged cervical lymph nodes may be the first symptom. Regional lymph node metastases are common; they have been detected in about half of the patients at the time of surgery.[56] Distant metastases also occur but are less common. About one third of patients, mostly those with the most extensive disease, have diarrhea thought to be caused by calcitonin secretion.[58] Occasional patients have carcinoid syndrome, probably caused by serotonin secretion, and some have Cushing's syndrome, apparently caused by ACTH secretion.[68] The prognosis is moderate; the observed 10-year survival rate is on the order of 60% to 70%.[56,101] The presence of regional metastases correlates with poorer prognosis.[56] The familial form seems to have a better prognosis than the nonfamilial form.[56]

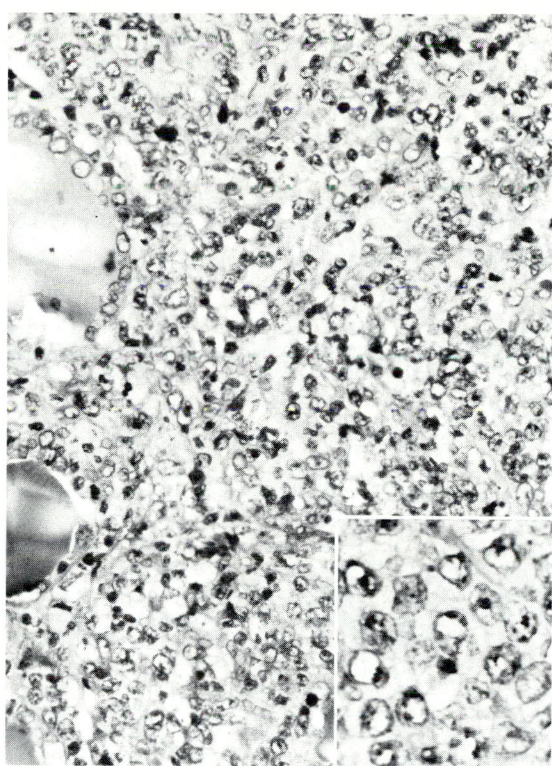

Fig. 33-24. Malignant lymphoma. Growth pattern is diffuse. Tumor cells invade between residual follicles on left. (200×.) *Inset,* Large vesicular nuclei and prominent nucleoli corresponding to large noncleaved cell lymphoma. (650×.)

Grossly the tumor is usually of hard consistency and rather well limited but not encapsulated. Histologically it is composed of sheets of tumor cells that are divided into groups by fibrous septa. The cells may be polygonal, spindle shaped, or round (Fig. 33-23). Sometimes they are arranged in ribbonlike structures or rosettes. In poorly fixed specimens, shrinkage may cause a pseudopapillary pattern. The cytoplasm is eosinophilic and finely granular, and the nuclei are usually uniform in shape, although binucleate cells and occasional giant nuclei occur. Mitoses are infrequent. There are often irregular calcifications in the stroma that may resemble psammoma bodies but do not show the regularity of lamination. Irregular masses of amyloid are seen between the tumor cells, sometimes in their cytoplasm. The amyloid stains with the usual staining methods, such as Congo red, and is believed to be stored calcitonin in the form of prohormone. It is not always possible to find amyloid in medullary carcinoma. In such cases the diagnosis can be confirmed by argyrophil silver stains[4] or immunohistochemical methods based on the calcitonin content of the cells.[61,87] The cells have also been reported to contain CEA,[61,80] histaminase,[87] and somatostatin[96] and sometimes 5HT[55] and ACTH.[55]

Differentiation of medullary carcinoma from papillary carcinoma may cause problems if pseudopapillary structures are present. Medullary carcinoma with rosettes may resemble poorly differentiated follicular carcinoma. It is important to differentiate medullary carcinoma with spindle cells from anaplastic carcinoma. Problems may arise especially in the rare cases in which medullary carcinoma contains clusters of bizarre giant cells.[88]

Malignant lymphoma

The thyroid is involved in about 20% of patients who die of generalized lymphoma. Also, primary lymphomas occur and comprise about 5% of all thyroid cancer. The tumor has a diffuse growth pattern; residual follicles are often seen within the tumor at the border (Fig. 33-24). Tumor cells may be seen in these follicles. Lymphomas are almost always of B lymphocyte origin,[52] and the most common types are large noncleaved cell[92] and immunoblastic[85] lymphomas. Hodgkin's disease probably does not involve the thyroid primarily. The prognosis is better than in anaplastic carcinoma; the 5-year survival rate is about 50%[52] and is higher in tumors confined within the thyroid capsule.[52,57,101] In most cases malignant lymphoma occurs together with lymphocytic thyroiditis,[57,85] which suggests evolution of the lymphoma from thyroiditis.

Sarcoma

Fibrosarcomas[70] and malignant hemangioendotheliomas may occur in the thyroid, but they are extremely rare. The existence of the latter tumor has been questioned.[81] In the past, sarcomas were rather common in studies from Central Europe, but most of these cases probably represented spindle cell and giant cell anaplastic carcinomas.[70]

Metastatic tumor

Although clinically demonstrable metastases are uncommon in the thyroid, thyroid metastases have been detected in autopsies in one fourth of patients dying of metastasizing neoplasm.[94] The most common primary tumors are malignant melanoma and carcinomas of the kidney and bronchus.

REFERENCES

Development, structure, and function

1. DeLellis, R.A., Nunnemacher, G., and Wolfe, H.J.: C-cell hyperplasia: an ultrastructural analysis, Lab. Invest. **36**:237, 1977.
2. Klinck, G.H., Oertel, J.E., and Winship, T.: Ultrastructure of normal human thyroid, Lab. Invest. **22**:2, 1970.
3. Pearse, A.G.E.: The APUD cell concept and its implications in pathology, Pathol. Annu. **9**:27, 1974.
4. Wilander, E., et al.: Staining of rat thyroid parafollicular (C-) cells with the Sevier-Munger silver technique, Acta Pathol. Microbiol. Scand. **88**:339, 1980.
5. Wolfe, H.J., Voekel, E.F., and Tashijian, A.H., Jr.: Distribution of calcitonin-containing cells in the normal adult thyroid gland: a correlation of morphology with peptide content, J. Clin. Endocrinol. Metab. **38**:688, 1974.

Functional disorders

6. Dorfman, S.G.: Hyperthyroidism: usual and unusual causes, Arch. Intern. Med. **137**:995, 1977.
7. Ibbertson, H.K.: Endemic goitre and cretinism, Clin. Endocrinol. Metab. **8**:97, 1979.
8. Shimaoka, K.: Thyrotoxicosis due to metastatic involvement of the thyroid, Arch. Intern. Med. **140**:284, 1980.
9. Stanbury, J.B.: Inborn errors of the thyroid, Prog. Med. Genet. **10**:55, 1974.

Developmental anomalies

10. Dalgaard, J.B., and Wetteland, P.: Thyroglossal anomalies: a follow-up study of 58 cases, Acta Chir. Scand. **111**:444, 1956.
11. Larochelle, D., et al.: Ectopic thyroid tissue: a review of the literature, J. Otolaryngol. **8**:523, 1979.
12. LiVolsi, V.A., Perzin, K.H., and Savetsky, L.: Carcinoma arising in median ectopic thyroid (including thyroglossal duct tissue), Cancer **34**:1303, 1974.
13. Meyer, J.S., and Steinberg, L.S.: Microscopically benign thyroid follicles in cervical lymph nodes: serial section study of lymph node inclusions and entire thyroid gland in 5 cases, Cancer **24**:302, 1969.
14. Sampson, R.J., et al.: Metastases from occult thyroid carcinoma: an autopsy study from Hiroshima and Nagasaki, Japan, Cancer **25**:803, 1970.
15. Sisson, J.C., Schmidt, R.W., and Beierwaltes, W.H.: Sequestered nodular goiter, N. Engl. J. Med. **270**:927, 1964.

Graves' disease

16. Doniach, D.: The pathogenesis of endocrine exophthalmos: a short review, Proc. R. Soc. Med. **70**:695, 1977.
17. Doniach, D., and Roitt, I.M.: Autoimmune thyroid disease. In Miescher, P.E., and Müller-Eberhard, H., editors: Textbook of immunopathology, ed. 2, New York, 1976, Grune & Stratton, Inc.
18. Johnson, W.C., and Hellwig, E.B.: Cutaneous focal mucinosis: a clinopathological and histochemical study, Arch. Dermatol. **93**:13, 1966.
19. Kidd, A., et al.: Immunologic aspects of Graves' and Hashimoto's diseases, Metabolism **29**:80, 1980.
20. Riley, F.C.: Orbital pathology in Graves' disease, Mayo Clin. Proc. **47**:975, 1972.
21. Thyroid autoimmune disease: a broad spectrum (editorial), Lancet **1**:874, 1981.

Goiter

22. Barsano, C.P., and DeGroot, L.J.: Dyshormonogenetic goitre, Clin. Endocrinol. Metab. **8**:145, 1979.
23. Hennemann, G.: Non-toxic goitre, Clin. Endocrinol. Metab. **8**:167, 1979.
24. Ibbertson, H.K.: Endemic goitre and cretinism, Clin. Endocrinol. Metab. **8**:97, 1979.
25. Kelly, F.C., and Snedden, W.W.: Prevalence and geographical distribution of endemic goitre. In Endemic goitre, World Health Organization Monograph no. 44, Geneva, 1960.
26. Kennedy, J.S.: The pathology of dyshormogenetic goiter, J. Pathol. **99**:251, 1969.
27. Miller, J.M.: Plummer's disease, Med. Clin. North Am. **59**:1203, 1975.

Thyroiditis

28. Carney, J.A., et al.: Palpation thyroiditis (multifocal granulomatous folliculitis), Am. J. Clin. Pathol. **64**:639, 1975.
29. Doniach, D., Bottazzo, G.F., and Russell, R.C.G.: Goitrous autoimmune thyroiditis (Hashimoto's disease), Clin. Endocrinol. Metab. **8**:63, 1979.
30. Drexhage, H.A., et al.: Thyroid growth-blocking antibodies in primary myxoedema, Nature **289**:594, 1981.
31. Katz, S.M., and Vickery, A.L.: The fibrous variant of Hashimoto's thyroiditis, Hum. Pathol. **5**:161, 1974.
32. Kidd, A., et al.: Immunologic aspects of Graves' and Hashimoto's diseases, Metabolism **29**:80, 1980.
33. Kraemmer Nielsen, H.: Multifocal idiopathic fibrosclerosis: two cases with simultaneous occurrence of retroperitoneal fibrosis and Riedel's thyroiditis, Acta Med. Scand. **208**:119, 1980.
34. Löwhagen, T: Thyroid. In Zajicek, J., editor: Aspiration biopsy cytology. Part I, Munich, Germany, 1974, S. Karger.
35. Rallison, M.L. et al.: Occurrence and natural history of chronic lymphocytic thyroiditis in childhood, J. Pediatr. **86**:675, 1975.
36. Shamsuddin, A.K.M., and Lane, R.A.: Ultrastructural pathology in Hashimoto's thyroiditis, Hum. Pathol. **12**:561, 1981.
37. Thyroid autoimmune disease: a broad spectrum (editorial), Lancet **1**:874, 1981.
38. Volpé, R.: The pathology of thyroiditis, Hum. Pathol. **9**:429, 1978.
39. Weaver, D.R., Deodhar, S.D., and Hazard, J.B.: A characterization of focal lymphocytic thyroiditis, Cleve. Clin. Q. **33**:59, 1966.
40. Weissel, M., et al.: HLA-DR and Hashimoto's thyroiditis, Tissue Antigens **16**:256, 1980.
41. Woolner, L.B.: Thyroiditis: classification and clinicopathologic correlation. In Hazard, J.B., and Smith, D.E., editors: The thyroid, International Academy of Pathology Monograph No. 5, Baltimore, 1964, The Williams & Wilkins Co.

Radiation changes, amyloidosis

42. James, P.D.: Amyloid goitre, J. Clin. Pathol. **25**:683, 1973.
43. Spitalnik, P.F., and Straus, F.H.: Patterns of human thyroid parenchymal reaction following low-dose childhood irradiation, Cancer **41**:1098, 1978.
44. Vickery, A.L., Jr.: Thyroid alterations due to irradiation. In Hazard, J.B., and Smith, D.E., editors: The thyroid, International Academy of Pathology Monograph No. 5, Baltimore, 1964, The Williams & Wilkins Co.

Benign tumors

45. Böcker, W., et al.: Immunohistochemical and electron-microscope analysis of adenomas of the thyroid gland. II. Adenomas with specific cytological differentiation, Virchows Arch. (Pathol. Anat.) **380**:205, 1978.
46. Heimann, P., et al.: Oxyphilic adenoma of the human thyroid: a morphological and biochemical study, Cancer **31**:246, 1973.
47. Lang, W., et al.: The differentiation of atypical adenomas and encapsulated follicular carcinomas in the thyroid gland, Virchows Arch. (Pathol. Anat.) **385**:125, 1980.
48. Silberman, R., and Mendelson, I.R.: Teratoma of the neck: report of two cases and review of literature, Arch. Dis. Child. **35**:159, 1960.

Malignant tumors

49. Aldinger, K.A., et al.: Anaplastic carcinoma of the thyroid: a review of 84 cases of spindle and giant cell carcinoma of the thyroid, Cancer **41**:2267, 1978.
50. Beaugié, J.M., et al.: Primary malignant tumors of the thyroid: the relationship between histological classification and clinical behaviour, Br. J. Surg. **63**:173, 1976.
51. Bigner, S.H.: Medullary carcinoma of the thyroid in the multiple endocrine neoplasia IIA syndrome, Am. J. Surg. Pathol. **5**:459, 1981.
52. Burke, J.S., Butler, J.J., and Fuller, L.M.: Malignant lymphomas of the thyroid: a clinical pathologic study of 35 patients including ultrastructural observations, Cancer **39**:1587, 1977.
53. Burt, A., and Goudie, R.B.: Diagnosis of primary thyroid carcinoma by immunohistological demonstration of thyroglobulin, Histopathology **3**:279, 1979.
54. Cady, B. et al.: Changing clinical, pathologic, therapeutic and survival patterns in differentiated thyroid carcinoma, Ann. Surg. **184**:541, 1976.
55. Capella, C., et al.: Multiple endocrine cell types in thyroid medullary carcinoma: evidence for calcitonin, somatostatin, ACTH, 5HT and small granule cells, Virchows Arch. (Pathol. Anat.) **377**:111, 1978.
56. Chong, G.C., et al.: Medullary carcinoma of the thyroid gland, Cancer **35**:695, 1975.

57. Compagno, J., and Oertel, J.E.: Malignant lymphoma and other lymphoproliferative disorders of the thyroid gland: a clinicopathologic study of 245 cases, Am. J. Pathol. **74**:1, 1980.
58. Cox, T.M., et al.: Role of calcitonin in diarrhoea associated with medullary carcinoma of the thyroid, Gut **20**:629, 1979.
59. Cuello, C., Correa, P., and Eisenberg, H.: Geographic pathology of thyroid carcinoma, Cancer **23**:230, 1969.
60. DeLellis, R.A., et al.: Adrenal medullary hyperplasia: a morphometeric analysis of patients with familial medullary thyroid carcinoma, Am. J. Pathol. **83**:177, 1976.
61. DeLellis, R.A., et al.: Calcitonin and carcinoembryonic antigen as tumor markers in medullary thyroid carcinoma, Am. J. Clin. Pathol. **70**:587, 1978.
61a. Deligdisch, L., Subhani, Z., and Gordon, R.E.: Primary mucinous carcinoma of the thyroid gland, Cancer **45**:2564, 1980.
62. Franssila, K.: Value of histologic classification of thyroid cancer, Acta Pathol. Microbiol. Scand. [A] **225**(suppl.):1, 1971.
63. Franssila, K.O.: Is the differentiation between papillary and follicular thyroid carcinoma valid? Cancer **32**:853, 1973.
64. Franssila, K.O.: Prognosis in thyroid carcinoma, Cancer **36**:1138, 1975.
65. Franssila, K., et al.: Incidence of different morphological types of thyroid cancer in the Nordic countries, Acta Pathol. Microbiol. Scand. [A] **89**:49, 1981.
66. Fukunaga, F.H., and Yatani, R.: Geographic pathology of occult thyroid carcinomas, Cancer **36**:1095, 1975.
67. Harada, T., et al.: Fatal thyroid carcinoma: anaplastic transformation of adenocarcinoma, Cancer **39**:2588, 1977.
68. Hazard, J.B.: The C cells (parafollicular cells) of the thyroid gland and medullary thyroid carcinoma: a review, Am. J. Pathol. **88**:214, 1977.
69. Hazard, J.B., and Kenyon, R.: Encapsulated angioinvasive carcinoma (angioinvasive adenoma) of thyroid gland, Am. J. Clin. Pathol. **24**:755, 1954.
70. Hedinger, C.E.: Sarcomas of the thyroid gland. In Hedinger, C.E., editor: Thyroid cancer, UICC Monograph Series No. 12, Berlin, 1969, Springer-Verlag.
71. Hedinger, C.E., and Sobin, L.H.: Histological typing of thyroid tumors. In International histological classification of tumours, vol. 11, Geneva, 1974, World Health Organization.
72. Heitz, P., Moser, H., and Staub, J.J.: Thyroid cancer: a study of 573 thyroid tumors and 161 autopsy cases observed over a thirty-year period, Cancer **37**:2329, 1976.
73. Hempelmann, L.H., et al.: Neoplasms in persons treated with x-rays in infancy: fourth survey in 20 years, J. Natl. Cancer Inst. **55**:519, 1975.
74. Hofstädter, F.: Frequency and morphology of malignant tumours of the thyroid before and after the introduction of iodine-prophylaxis, Virchows Arch. (Pathol. Anat.) **385**:263, 1980.
75. Hubert, J.P., Jr., et al.: Occult papillary carcinoma of the thyroid, Arch. Surg. **115**:394, 1980.
76. Jao, W., and Gould, V.E.: Ultrastructure of anaplastic (spindle and giant cell) carcinoma of the thyroid, Cancer **35**:1280, 1975.
77. Johannessen, J.V., Gould, V.E., and Jao, W.: The fine structure of human thyroid cancer, Hum. Pathol. **9**:385, 1978.
78. Jolivet, J., et al.: ACTH-secreting medullary carcinoma of the thyroid: monitoring of clinical course with calcintonin and cortisol assays and immunohistochemical studies, Cancer **46**:2667, 1980.
79. Kimler, S.C., and Muth, W.E.: Primary malignant teratoma of the thyroid: case report and literature review of cervical teratomas in adults, Cancer **42**:311, 1978.
80. Kodama, T., et al.: Identification of carcinoembryonic antigen in the C-cell of the normal thyroid, Cancer **45**:98, 1980.
81. Kriesch, K., et al.: Hemangioendothelioma of the thyroid gland—true endothelioma or anaplastic carcinoma, Pathol. Res. Pract. **170**:230, 1980.
82. LiVolsi, L.A., and Merino, M.J.: Squamous cells in the human thyroid gland, Am. J. Surg. Pathol. **2**:133, 1978.
83. Ljungberg, O.: On medullary carcinoma of the thyroid, Acta Pathol. Microbiol. Scand. [A] **231**(suppl.):1, 1972.
84. Löwhagen, T., et al.: Aspiration biopsy cytology (ABC) in nodules of thyroid gland suspected to be malignant, Surg. Clin. North Am. **59**:3, 1979.
85. Maurer, R., et al.: Non-Hodgkin lymphomas of the thyroid: a clinico-pathological review of 29 cases applying the Lukes-Collins classification and an immunoperoxidase method, Virchows Arch. (Pathol. Anat.) **383**:293, 1979.
86. Mazzaferri, E.L., et al.: Papillary thyroid carcinoma: the impact of therapy in 576 patients, Medicine **56**:171, 1977.
87. Mendelsohn, G., et al.: Calcitonin and histaminase in C-cell hyperplasia and medullary thyroid carcinoma: a light microscopic and immunohistochemical study, Am. J. Pathol. **92**:35, 1978.
88. Mendelsohn, G., et al.: Anaplastic variants of medullary thyroid carcinoma: a light microscopic and immunohistochemical study, Am. J. Surg. Pathol. **4**:333, 1980.
88a. Rhatigan, R.M., Roque, J.L., and Bucher, R.L.: Mucoepidermoid carcinoma of the thyroid gland, Cancer **39**:210, 1977.
89. Russel, W.O., et al.: Thyroid carcinoma: classification, intraglandular dissemination, and clinicopathological study based upon whole organ sections of 80 glands, Cancer **16**:1425, 1963.
90. Sampson, R.J.: Prevalence and significance of occult thyroid cancer. In DeGroot, L.J., et al., editors: Radiation-associated thyroid carcinoma, New York, 1977, Grune & Stratton, Inc.
91. Schneider, A.B., et al.: Characteristics of 108 thyroid cancers detected by screening in a population with a history of head and neck irradiation, Cancer **46**:1218, 1980.
92. Schwarze, E.W., and Papadimitriou, C.S.: Non-Hodgkin lymphoma of the thyroid, Pathol. Res. Pract. **167**:346, 1980.
93. Shimaoka, K., and Tsukada, Y.: Squamous cell carcinomas and adenosquamous carcinomas originating from the thyroid gland, Cancer **46**:1833, 1980.
94. Silverberg, S.G., and Vidone, R.A.: Metastatic tumors in the thyroid, Pacif. Med. Surg. **74**:175, 1966.
95. Sizemore, G.W., Heath, H., III, and Carney, J.A.: Multiple endocrine neoplasia type 2, Clin. Endocrinol. Metab. **9**:299, 1980.
96. Sundler, F., et al.: Somatostatin-immunoreactive cells in medullary carcinoma of the thyroid, Am. J. Pathol. **88**:381, 1977.
97. Valenta, L.J., and Michel-Béchet, M.: Electron microscopy of clear cell thyroid carcinoma, Arch. Pathol. Lab. Med. **101**:140, 1977.
98. Williams, E.D., Brown, C.L., and Doniach, I.: Pathological and clinical findings in a series of 67 cases of medullary carcinoma of the thyroid, J. Clin. Pathol. **19**:103, 1966.
99. Williams, E.D., et al.: Thyroid cancer in an iodide-rich area, Cancer **39**:215, 1977.
100. Wolfe, H.J., et al.: C-cell hyperplasia preceding medullary thyroid carcinoma, N. Engl. J. Med. **289**:437, 1973.
101. Woolner, L.B.: Thyroid carcinoma: pathologic classification with data on prognosis, Semin. Nucl. Med. **1**:481, 1971.
102. Woolner, L.B., et al.: Primary malignant lymphoma of the thyroid: reveiw of forty-six cases, Am. J. Surg. **111**:502, 1966.

CHAPTER 34 **Parathyroid Glands**

JAMES E. OERTEL

The parathyroid glands are important regulators of the metabolism of calcium and phosphorus and act to maintain normal levels of these elements in the blood.

DEVELOPMENT AND STRUCTURE

The parathyroid glands, usually four in number, are developed from endoderm of the third and fourth branchial pouches, in intimate relation to portions of the thymus but quite independent of the thyroid gland.[1-4] The superior pair of glands is derived from the fourth pharyngeal pouches, whereas the inferior pair, derived from the third pouches, outdistances the superior pair and the thyroid gland in caudal migration and takes the lower position. Their close connection with the development of the thymus explains the occasional occurrence of one or more parathyroid glands near or even embedded in thymic tissue. This possibility should be borne in mind during a search for parathyroid tissue or a parathyroid adenoma by surgical procedures or at autopsy.

Although four parathyroid glands are usually present, variations in number from two to 10 have been reported. The superior pair is nearly always situated on the medial part of the dorsal surface of each lobe of the thyroid gland, at about the junction of the middle and upper thirds, and lies close to ascending branches of the inferior thyroid artery. They often are embedded in thyroid substance but separated from it by a connective tissue capsule. The inferior parathyroid glands, more inconstant in position, are found usually on the dorsal surface of the lateral lobes of the thyroid gland, near the lower pole.

The parathyroid glands are brownish yellow, oval, somewhat flattened bodies, each measuring, in adults, about 1.5 by 3.5 by 6.5 mm and having a combined weight of about 120 to 130 mg (four glands). The amount of interstitial tissue is variable, but the mean weight of parenchymal tissue has been estimated to be about 80 to 90 mg (four glands).[5]

Each parathyroid gland possesses a capsule of connective tissue, from which bands pass through the gland. The parenchymal cells may be arranged in solid masses but frequently appear in cords or columns. Acinar or follicular structures may be found, tending to increase in frequency with age. These may contain colloid. Interstitial adipose tissue is present after puberty and tends to increase in proportionate amount with age until the middle of the fifth decade. This interstitial fat is replaced and decreases or disappears when there is hyperplasia or adenomatous growth of the parenchyma.

The parenchymal cells appear in three main forms: chief cells, water-clear cells, and oxyphil cells. Transitional forms occur.

The chief cell (6 to 8 μm in diameter) is the most numerous. Its cytoplasm is weakly acidophilic and may appear vacuolated by light microscopy. Electron microscopy indicates that the chief cell has cycles in which it changes from an inactive form to an actively synthesizing phase and again to an inactive form.[7] In the inactive phase the cell contains abundant glycogen, dispersed sacs of rough endoplasmic reticulum, a small Golgi apparatus, and rare secretory granules. The actively synthesizing cell has the expected increase in granular endoplasmic reticulum. This form is followed by a phase in which the cellular structures suggest transfer and packaging of the hormone into secretory granules. After releasing the hormone, the cell returns to the inactive phase. Individual cells do not appear to synchronize their cycles with their neighbors, which may account for the subtle differences in the appearance of adjacent cells that are visible with the light microscope.

The water-clear cell is larger (10 to 15 μm), has abundant clear cytoplasm and a relatively small pyknotic nucleus, and has well-defined cell borders, a feature often evident in all varieties of parathyroid cells. This cell is rare in normal glands. Large membrane-limited cyto-

The opinions or assertions contained herein are the private views of the author and are not to be construed as official or as reflecting the views of the Department of the Army or the Department of Defense.

plasmic vacuoles are the most conspicuous aspect of its fine structure. Dense secretory granules are sparse.

The oxyphil cell is 8 to 14 μm in diameter. Its eosinophilic granular cytoplasm is packed with mitochondria, secretory granules are rare, and glycogen is present in moderate amounts. Before puberty, oxyphil cells are uncommon. They increase in number with age and in certain diseases, such as chronic renal failure.

PARATHYROID HORMONE

Parathyroid hormone is a polypeptide that acts to elevate serum calcium and reduce serum phosphate. Reduction of serum ionized calcium promptly causes increased secretion of the hormone, whereas elevation of serum calcium results in decreased secretion. Elevation of magnesium ions in serum also causes decreased secre tion of the hormone; magnesium depletion impairs the secretion of parathyroid hormone.

Parathyroid hormone acts on the tubular cells of the nephrons to inhibit reabsorption of phosphate and to promote absorption of calcium and magnesium, causes resorption of bone matrix and bone mineral, and increases renal production of 1,25-dihydroxycholecalciferol (which in turn promotes the absorption of calcium from the small intestine).

REGULATION OF CALCIUM METABOLISM

The regulation of calcium metabolism is a complex mechanism involving the effects of hormones and ions on bone, the absorption of calcium and phosphate from the small intestine, and the loss of calcium and phosphate in the urine and feces. Parathyroid hormone maintains the level of calcium in the blood and other extracellular fluids by the actions mentioned in the previous section. Calcitonin opposes parathyroid hormone partly by preventing resorption of bone and partly by enhancing renal excretion of sodium, calcium, and phosphate. It is released in response to elevations of serum calcium and probably also by certain hormones of the alimentary tract.

Vitamin D is required for absorption of calcium ions from the intestine and for adequate growth and mineralization of the skeleton. Its most active metabolite, 1,25-dihydroxycholecalciferol, is formed in the kidney; synthesis is enhanced by parathyroid hormone and by hypophosphatemia.

Calcium metabolism is also affected by the corticosteroids, by some of the hormones of the alimentary tract, and by thyroid hormone. Estrogens, androgens, and growth hormone also have long-term effects on the skeleton, but their short-term influence on divalent cation metabolism is unknown.

PATHOLOGIC CALCIFICATION

Pathologic calcification is the deposition of mineral salts, including calcium, in tissues not normally calcified as well as in excretory or secretory ducts. Mineral deposits are found quite regularly in some soft tissues (for instance, the pineal gland after puberty). Calcium phosphate (present most often as hydroxyapatite) mixed with small amounts of calcium carbonate is the most common form. Calcium oxalate deposits may also be present, especially in the urinary tract.

Pathologic calcification has been described under the categories of dystrophic calcification, metastatic calcification, calcification in tumors, calcinosis, and calciphylaxis.

Dystrophic calcification is the deposition of calcium salts in injured or dead tissue. The systemic chemical balance is normal, but the local environment is altered to favor precipitation of the salts. Metastatic calcification is the deposition of calcium salts in soft tissue as a result of a systemic disturbance in calcium and phosphate metabolism. Calcification in tumors is a form of dystrophic calcification in which a tumor contains calcium salts either as irregular masses in the tissue, often associated with regions of necrosis, or as psammoma bodies (concentrically laminated bodies formed of calcium apatite). Calcinosis is local or generalized calcification in or under the skin, sometimes including muscles, fasciae, nerves, and tendons, and occasionally is associated with a collagen vascular disease. Tumoral calcinosis refers to a localized, often cystic, calcific mass in the soft tissue, usually next to a large joint and usually solitary. In some individuals there are disturbances in mineral metabolism; some cases are familial. Calciphylaxis is an experimental process in animals in which induced hypercalcemia is followed by injury to tissues by chemical or physical agents, and calcification of the damaged tissues results.

These categories of calcification of soft tissues are artificial because, regardless of whether there is an alteration in the levels of calcium and phosphate in the extracellular fluids or local injury to tissues, the mechanisms of calcification are similar. Current belief is that the avidity of mitochondria for calcium and their ability to store it lead to its accumulation within them. Elevated extracellular calcium and phosphate cannot be excluded by the cells (overloading the mitochondria), or an insult to the cells results in their inability to exclude extracellular calcium present in normal amounts (also overloading the mitochondria). Eventually the calcium salts interfere with mitochondrial metabolism, and the cell dies. Likewise, calcification of membrane-limited vesicles occurs within and outside cells in both metastatic calcification and dystrophic calcification, analogous to the matrix vesicles of cartilage and bone, which are instrumental in initiating mineralization.

Once the initial foci of calcium salts have been deposited, the growth of mineral crystals depends on the systemic chemical environment, local mechanisms for concentrating the ions, quantity and character of available matrix, and levels of inhibitors of calcification, such as pyrophosphate and proteoglycans. Major factors promoting calcification include elevation of the calcium-phosphate product (Ca × P in mg/100 ml) resulting from higher levels of calcium or phosphate or both, elevation of pH locally or systemically, and availability of a suitable matrix. The local elevation of pH in the eye and kidney (because the cells establish a hydrogen-ion gradient across their membranes) may enhance calcification.

HYPOPARATHYROIDISM

Diminution or absence of circulating parathyroid hormone causes a reduction of serum calcium (to as little as half the normal level) and an elevation of serum phosphate (to as much as three or four times normal levels). Little or no calcium appears in the urine. Tetany and other evidence of neuromuscular irritability are the most important clinical manifestations of hypoparathyroidism. If the disease is of long duration, the persons affected may have (in addition to tetany) skin disorders, abnormal nail growth, loss of hair, cataracts, a variety of disorders of the central nervous system, and roentgenographic evidence of increased bone density and calcification in the vessels of the basal ganglia of the brain. Convulsions, papilledema, and gastrointestinal disturbances may be present.

The most common cause of hypoparathyroidism is the removal of all or part of the parathyroid tissue during surgery on the neck, especially during thyroidectomy. If only part of the gland tissue is removed, or if the glands are partially injured by impairment of their blood supply or by postoperative edema, the hormonal deficiency will be temporary. Complete removal or more severe damage results in permanent impairment of function.

Temporary neonatal hypocalcemia may be a manifestation of the hypoparathyroidism that occurs normally in many infants for a brief period after birth. This state may persist in sick or injured infants and may become manifest as symptomatic hypocalcemia.[25,29]

So-called idiopathic hypoparathyroidism is a rare disease that is sporadic or familial and in some instances may be an autoimmune disorder. The glands either are replaced by fat or cannot be found.[26,28] Permanent idiopathic hypoparathyroidism developing during the first year of life may be associated with congenital hypoplasia or absence of the parathyroid glands and thymus, and the children usually die.[31] Another type of hypoparathyroidism that also occurs in childhood may be familial or sporadic and is associated with a variety of disorders, some of which are accompanied by autoimmune phenomena. These include idiopathic adrenocortical atrophy, lymphocytic thyroiditis, oophoritis, diabetes mellitus, gastric mucosal atrophy, hepatitis, alopecia totalis, and severe *Candida* infections.

PSEUDOHYPOPARATHYROIDISM

Pseudohypoparathyroidism and pseudo-pseudohypoparathyroidism are related disorders and may be called Albright's hereditary osteodystrophy. Pseudohypoparathyroidism is familial, with a female preponderance, and is characterized by clinical and chemical features suggestive of idiopathic hypoparathyroidism. Brachydactyly, short stature, and multiple foci of soft tissue calcification and ossification are additional distinctive features. Renal glomerular function is normal. Pseudo-pseudohypoparathyroidism is similar, but the serum calcium and phosphate levels are normal.

In these disorders the parathyroid glands are normal or hyperplastic. Parathyroid function is intact. Levels of circulating parathyroid hormone are increased. The disease results from the inability of the renal tubules to respond to parathyroid hormone.[24,27]

HYPERPARATHYROIDISM

Excessive production of parathyroid hormone results from several different disorders: from a disturbance of calcium and phosphorus metabolism originating elsewhere in the body (renal failure, vitamin D deficiency) and leading to secondary hyperplasia of parathyroid tissue, from primary hyperplasia of the parathyroid tissue, from benign and malignant tumors of the parathyroid glands, and from neoplasms not of parathyroid origin, such as carcinoma of the lung or of the kidney.

Hyperparathyroidism may occur at any age but is more likely after 30 years of age. It is more common in women, and there is evidence that primary hyperparathyroidism is especially likely to occur in women about the time of the menopause.

In some patients incidental laboratory tests reveal the disorder. The most common symptoms in symptomatic patients are weakness and fatigability, followed in frequency by signs and symptoms of urinary calculi. Renal manifestations also include nephrocalcinosis and uremia. Less common are signs and symptoms of skeletal disease, such as pathologic fractures, bone pain, and generalized demineralization of the skeleton. Gastrointestinal disorders occur, including epigastric discomfort, constipation, and vague abdominal complaints. More important, peptic ulcers occur in 10% to 15% of hyperparathyroid patients, especially men. Central nervous system disturbances may constitute an important part of the clinical picture. These include depressive reactions, confusion, stupor, and personality changes. Additional manifestations of hypercalcemia include polydipsia and polyuria. The ophthalmologist may find band keratopathy, a corneal opacity extending across the cornea from within the limbus, and also may note crystals in the conjunctivae. Some patients have hypertension, often the result of renal damage, although in certain instances the relationship to kidney disease is unclear because impairment of renal function cannot be demonstrated.[41]

Elevated levels of circulating parathyroid hormone cause increased urinary excretion of inorganic phosphate, decreased serum phosphate, and increased serum calcium. Intestinal absorption of calcium rises. If skeletal lesions are present, serum alkaline phosphatase is elevated, and the urinary excretion of hydroxyproline rises (see also p. 1425).

Hyperparathyroidism must be differentiated from other causes of hypercalcemia, such as hypervitaminosis A and D, hyperthyroidism, adrenocortical insufficiency, the milk-alkali syndrome (excessive ingestion of milk and absorbable alkalis, leading to hypercalcemia, alkalosis, and azotemia without hypophosphatemia), use of certain diuretics, sarcoidosis, tuberculosis, multiple myeloma, leukemia, lymphoma, and some other malignant neoplasms with and without metastatic foci in bone. Idiopathic hypercalciuria with normal serum calcium and repeated formation of renal stones and the hypercalciuria present in renal tubular acidosis are conditions that also must be distinguished from hyperparathyroidism.

Secondary hyperplasia

Disturbances in calcium and phosphorus metabolism not primarily involving the parathyroid glands may in time cause changes in the glands as they respond to the metabolic abnormalities. Chronic renal glomerular insufficiency resulting in retention of phosphate and depression of intestinal absorption of calcium is the most common cause of compensatory parathyroid hyperfunction and hyperplasia. Very high levels of circulating parathyroid hormone may be present, but the glands are still responsive to changes in serum calcium. Hyperplasia may occur in rickets and osteomalacia caused by vitamin D deficiency, with intestinal malabsorption syndromes causing deficiencies of calcium and vitamin D, and in pseudohypoparathyroidism.

Hyperplastic glands range from normal size to striking enlargement. Variations in the size of the individual glands in any one patient may be evident. As a rule the glands are not adherent to the surrounding tissue. The cut surfaces may be smooth or nodular. There is a decrease in or absence of stromal fat, and the glands are cellular, composed usually of pale and vacuolated chief cells (Fig. 34-1). Transitional oxyphil cells or transitional water-clear cells may predominate occasionally. The cells often are arranged in solid masses, but nests, cords, or acinar patterns may occur. Nuclei are normal sized or somewhat enlarged.

Primary hyperplasia

Hyperplasia of the glands in the absence of any known underlying metabolic disease is called primary hyperplasia. The cause of this disorder is unknown. It may be a familial disorder and may be associated with proliferative disorders of other endocrine glands, as in the syndromes of multiple endocrine adenopathy.

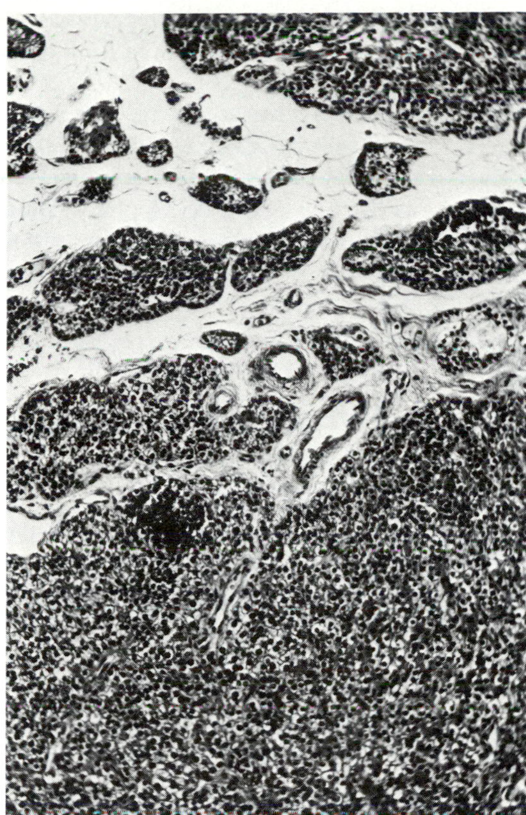

Fig. 34-1. Primary chief cell hyperplasia. Irregular involvement of gland can occur. Several small groups of cells appear to be normal.

The glands may be uniformly enlarged and have decreased or absent stromal fat and an approximately uniform proliferation of abnormal chief cells. However, a considerable number of these patients have uneven involvement of the glands, both within the individual glands and among the glands as a group. There may be nodular hyperplasia with parathyroid tissue that appears normal separating the foci of hyperplastic cells, or only one or two glands may be hyperplastic and the others appear normal. The cells may vary in appearance within a gland from slightly abnormal chief cells to transitional water-clear cells and transitional oxyphil cells. Mitotic figures, occasional degenerative changes, and fibrosis may be found in hyperplastic glands, making differentiation from parathyroid neoplasms difficult in some patients.

A small number of patients undergoing surgery because of elevated serum ionized calcium levels or other abnormalities suggestive of hyperparathyroidism have normal parathyroid glands by biopsy or have subtle abnormalities only suggestive of hyperplasia. Such instances may represent an early or mild form of hyperparathyroidism.

Primary water-clear cell hyperplasia is very rare and is probably a variant of long-standing primary chief cell hyperplasia. The glands are enlarged, irregular, chocolate brown, nonadherent, and soft. They are composed entirely of large water-clear cells that are 10 to 40 μm in diameter and have small dark-staining nuclei 4 to 8 μm in diameter.

Neoplasms

Parathyroid adenoma

Parathyroid adenoma (Fig. 34-2) is the cause of primary hyperparathyroidism in three fourths of patients with the disorder. Two or more adenomas are rare. They are more common in the lower pair of glands. Adenomas range in weight from less than 100 mg to several hundred grams (rarely), but most weigh only a few grams. Some are palpable on physical examination. There is a rough correlation between the size of the tumor and the degree of hyperfunction. The tumors are spherical to ovoid, soft, tan to reddish brown, or occasionally gray, have a delicate capsule, and are usually not adherent to the surrounding tissues. The cut surface may be focally hemorrhagic or cystic, and zones of fibrosis and calcification may be present. Deposits of brown pigment mark the sites of old hemorrhage.

The majority of adenomas are composed of chief cells, either normal or abnormal in appearance, but any cell type can predominate and any single tumor can contain a variety of cell types. Oxyphil cell tumors are often nonfunctional, but except for these, there is no correlation between the degree of function and the cell type. Giant nuclei, bizarre nuclei, and multinucleated cells are fairly common. Mitoses are rare.

The cells may be arranged as simply a solid mass, or they may form cords, nests, acini, or follicles resembling thyroid follicles. Nodules of single or mixed patterns may be evident. Commonly one histologic pattern predominates, but in some tumors a variety of patterns is visible.

The tissue of a gland containing an adenoma often forms a rim of normal tissue outside the capsule of the adenoma. Such a glandular remnant typically contains considerable adipose tissue and is composed of small chief cells and sometimes oxyphil cells. Considerable neutral lipid is usually present within these glandular cells, in contrast to its absence or the lesser amounts found in the cells of adenomas and hyperplastic tissue.

Adenoma (and also carcinoma) is occasionally accompanied by evidence of hyperplasia in the rest of the parathyroid glandular tissue, suggesting that the tumor is only part of a spectrum of parathyroid proliferative disorders. Adenoma may occasionally be difficult or impossible to differentiate from irregular or nodular hyperplasia. Despite these problems, if the surgeon removes the single largest gland from a patient who has primary hyperparathyroidism, the odds greatly favor cure of the disorder.

Carcinoma

Since nonfunctional parathyroid carcinomas are difficult to differentiate from thyroid carcinomas, most

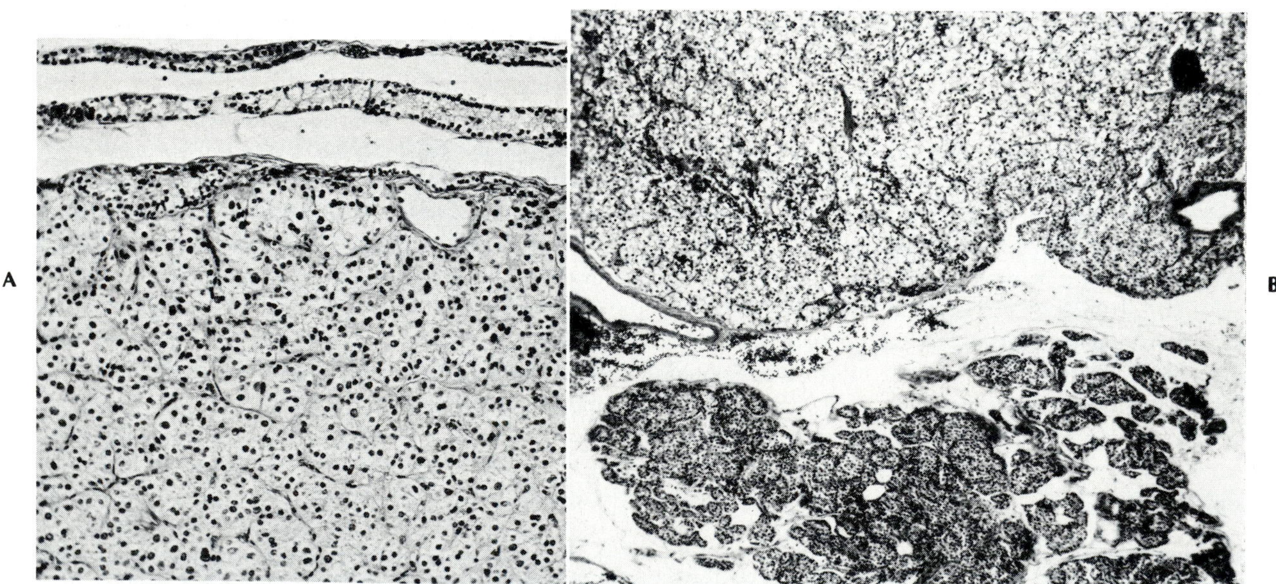

Fig. 34-2, A. Adenoma. Two delicate strands of remaining glandular tissue are above tumor. **B,** Remnant of normal tissue accompanies adenoma.

pathologists require the presence of hyperparathyroidism to make the diagnosis. Parathyroid hyperfunction is often pronounced. A moderate number of carcinomas are palpable on physical examination.

At surgery carcinoma is nearly always tightly adherent to surrounding tissue and is irregular in shape, but some resemble typical adenomas. The cut surface is gray, light tan, or brown and is firm, largely as a result of fibrous septa running through the tumor.

Typically carcinoma is surrounded by a thick capsule and is composed of solid masses of cells divided by irregular fibrous septa. The cells may be polygonal or elongated with clear, amphophilic, or eosinophilic cytoplasm. Nuclei are relatively large. The tumors may closely resemble adenomas, even on careful microscopic examination. Perivascular palisading and trabecular patterns are common. Mitotic figures are usually present.

The only certain criteria of malignancy are local invasion of adjacent tissues and distant metastatic lesions. Recurrence is common, and death may occur. Management of the patient is difficult because of the persistent or recurring hyperparathyroidism.

Lesions associated with hyperparathyroidism

The hypercalcemia of hyperparathyroidism may lead to the deposition of calcium salts (known as metastatic calcification) in a variety of soft tissues. Renal calculi occur in at least half the patients with symptomatic hyperparathyroidism and often are the reason the patient seeks medical aid. A considerably smaller number of patients have osteoporotic lesions of the skeletal system, a condition that when fully developed is known as generalized osteitis fibrosa cystica.

Metastatic calcification

The kidneys and blood vessels are the most frequent sites of metastatic calcification, but some deposits, especially in acute hyperparathyroidism, may be found in the lungs, stomach, heart, eyes, and other tissues. Calcific deposits are particularly abundant when there is renal failure with phosphate retention.

In blood vessels the calcification is mainly in the media and particularly involves elastic tissue, so the internal elastic lamella is often prominently calcified. The adjacent intima may be thickened by hyperplasia but is usually without calcification. Vascular calcification may be particularly severe in secondary renal hyperparathyroidism in which there is an increased level of blood phosphate. In some patients, ischemic muscle pains in the extremities and even gangrene have resulted.

Generalized osteitis fibrosa cystica

Osteitis fibrosa cystica (von Recklinghausen's disease) (Fig. 34-3) is essentially an osteoclastic resorption of bone and its replacement by connective tissue in which there are abortive attempts at new bone formation. The

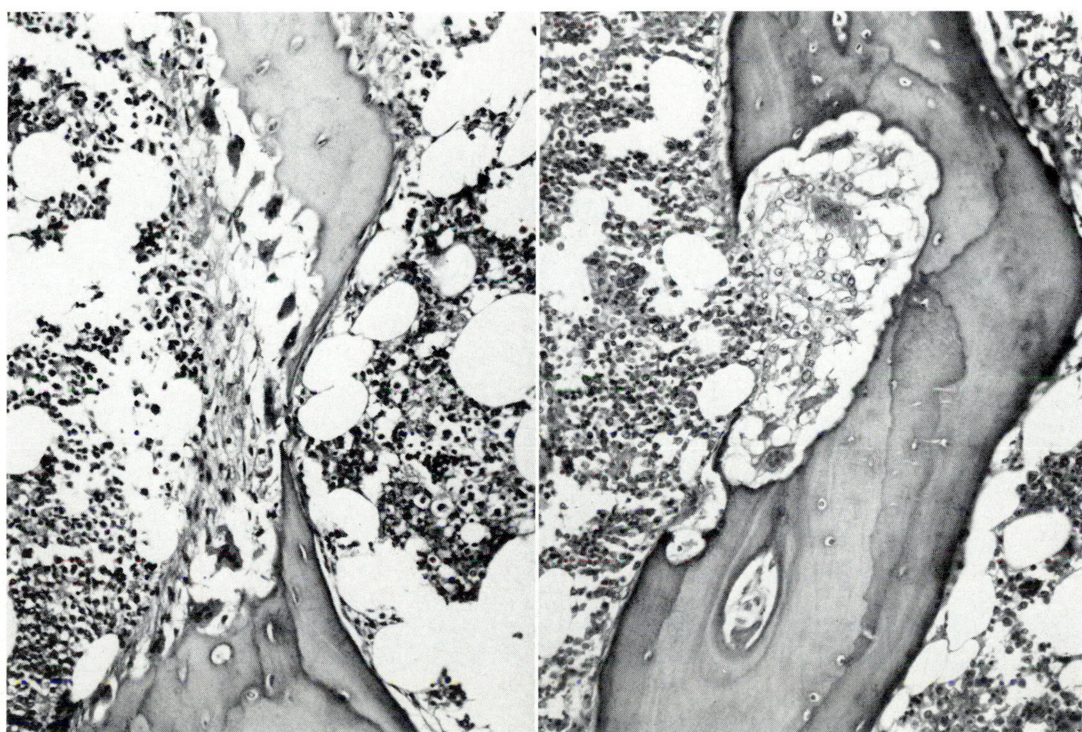

Fig. 34-3. Bone in hyperparathyroidism. Portions of trabeculae have been removed by osteoclasts, and small part of marrow has been replaced by fibroblasts.

changes range from a slightly increased porosity of the bones, because of an increase in osteoclasts removing trabecular and cortical bone with minimal replacement of the marrow by fibrous stroma, to a marked dissecting osteitis of the trabeculae and large cutting cores in the bony cortex in advanced cases. Immature and poorly calcified bone develops in the connective tissue. The newly formed bone may undergo resorption. While endosteal resorption occurs, periosteal deposition of bone is taking place. Osteoclasts are abundant. Large fibrous scars develop in place of the original spongy bone. Brown tumors, usually in the jaws or long bones, are colored by blood pigment and consist of multinucleated giant cells, cellular fibrous stroma, macrophages filled with hemosiderin, and newly formed vessels. Cysts lined by connective tissue may result from degeneration or hemorrhage but are not always present. Characteristic early roentgenographic changes include subperiosteal resorption of bone, most frequently seen along the margins of the middle phalanges of the fingers. Plasma alkaline phosphatase is increased. Because skeletal collagen is resorbed, urinary hydroxyproline excretion is increased.

Renal lesions

The kidneys may be severely damaged in hyperparathyroidism as a result of the deposition of calcium salts (nephrocalcinosis) and the formation of renal stones. Excess parathyroid hormone apparently interferes with the ability of the tubules to concentrate urine. In acute hyperparathyroidism, some of the nephrons show calcification of tubular epithelial cells and tubular basement membranes. Calcific casts are formed.

In the milder chronic cases, patchy calcification usually involves cells of the ascending limb of the loop of Henle, the distal convoluted tubule, and the collecting tubule.[40] Casts, usually calcific, are formed partly from desquamated cells and cellular debris and may cause obstruction of the nephron. Some interstitial calcification may occur. Foci of fibrosis with tubular and glomerular atrophy and infiltration by chronic inflammatory cells are common.

In advanced cases fibrosis, inflammation, and nephron destruction are extensive, and calcification of interstitial tissue may be striking. Both atrophy and cystic dilatation of the tubules proximal to obstructing calcific masses may be evident (Fig. 34-4).

Although hyperparathyroidism is an uncommon cause of renal calculi, its presence should be sought in every patient with renal stones. In some clinics, 4% of individuals with renal stones have hyperparathyroidism. The calculi are predominantly calcium oxalate or calcium phosphate. Kidneys containing stones may have only minor tubular damage, or they may be extensively involved by calcific deposits and the associated parenchymal damage. Hydronephrosis may occur. Pyelonephritis is common in kidneys damaged by stones and by calcinosis.

Renal osteodystrophy and secondary hyperparathyroidism

The osteodystrophy occurring in chronic renal failure is characterized by varying degrees of osteitis fibrosa, osteomalacia, osteoporosis, and osteosclerosis.[59] The clinical and pathologic features in a single patient depend

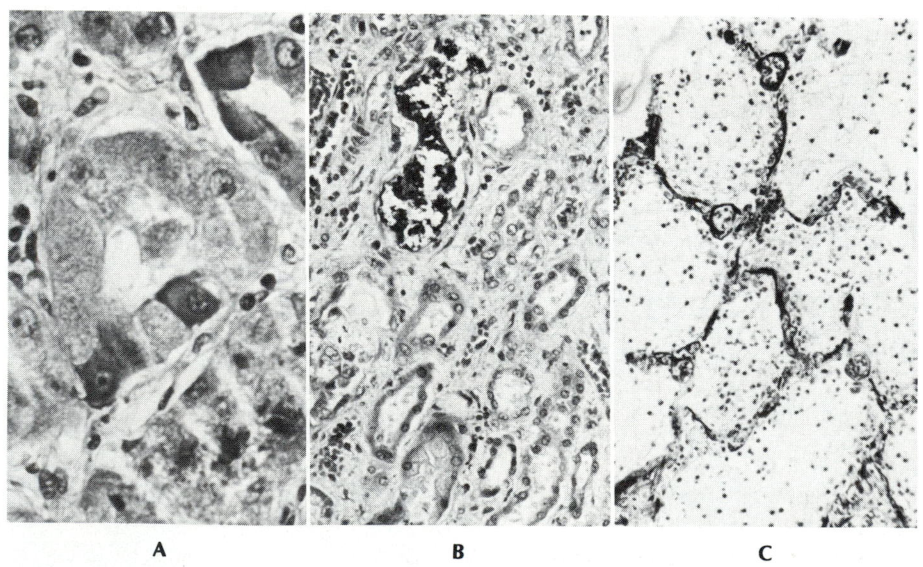

Fig. 34-4. Kidney and lung from 35-year-old man with large parathyroid adenoma. **A,** Several renal tubular cells have undergone calcification. **B,** Calcific material fills a renal tubule. **C,** Walls of alveoli and of blood vessels are calcified.

on the pathologic process that predominates during a particular time period. The pathologic processes, in turn, depend on which of the complex metabolic disturbances of uremia are most important in the person affected and how these disturbances are altered by therapeutic measures. Renal lesions of a type in which large amounts of renal parenchyma are lacking or destroyed and those that are stationary or very slowly progressive (renal insufficiency over a prolonged period) may result in these skeletal changes. Hemodialysis and renal transplantation prolong life and thereby have substantially increased the possibility that skeletal disease may develop.

One of the most important complications of the secondary hyperparathyroidism usually present in chronic renal disease is soft tissue calcification. Sites commonly involved are the arteries, heart, kidneys, lungs, stomach, soft tissues around joints, eyes, and skin and subcutaneous tissues. Arterial, myocardial, and renal calcification may have grave clinical effects.

In children, remarkable skeletal deformities and growth disturbances (dwarfism) may result because bone growth is incomplete and the epiphyses are not united. The underlying renal lesion is most commonly a developmental malformation in the kidneys or urinary tract, such as congenital hypoplasia, congenital polycystic disease, strictures of the ureters, or congenital valves of the urethra. Infection (pyelonephritis) may be added to hydronephrotic atrophy in cases of obstruction in the lower urinary tract and may further decrease the functioning renal parenchyma.

The characteristic changes in the epiphyseal cartilages are probably the result of abnormal metabolism of vitamin D as well as of hyperparathyroidism. The epiphyseal cartilages are greatly increased in bulk but show degenerative changes, defects of calcium deposition, and distortion. The cartilage may be bent and twisted and displaced from its normal position at the end of the shaft. Extreme deformity often results. The skull may be greatly thickened, and the appearance of the calvaria closely resembles that in Paget's disease of bone.

The kidneys show less calcium deposition than in primary hyperparathyroidism, and renal calculi are less frequent.

OTHER ABNORMALITIES

Parathyroid cysts large enough to be clinically apparent are rare. They may occur within the thyroid gland and the mediastinum as well as in the lower neck near the thyroid gland.

Inflammatory processes in parathyroid tissue are unusual. Sometimes inflammation in the thyroid gland extends into one or several glands. Rarely part of the gland tissue is replaced by amyloidosis or by secondary carcinoma, such as carcinomas of the lung and the thyroid gland.

REFERENCES

General; development and structure

1. Castleman, B., and Roth, S.I.: Tumors of the parathyroid glands. In Atlas of tumor pathology, Series 2, Fascicle 14, Washington, D.C., 1978, Armed Forces Institute of Pathology.
2. Gilmour, J.R.: The embryology of the parathyroid glands, the thymus, and certain associated rudiments, J. Pathol. Bacteriol. **45**:507, 1937.
3. Gilmour, J.R.: The gross anatomy of the parathyroid glands, J. Pathol. Bacteriol. **46**:133, 1938.
4. Gilmour, J.R.: The normal histology of the parathyroid glands, J. Pathol. Bacteriol. **48**:187, 1939.
5. Gilmour, J.R., and Martin, W.J.: The weight of the parathyroid glands, J. Pathol. Bacteriol. **44**:431, 1937.
6. Nilsson, O.: Studies on the ultrastructure of the human parathyroid glands in various pathological conditions, Acta Pathol. Microbiol. Scand. **263**(suppl.):1, 1977.
7. Roth, S.I., and Capen, C.C.: Ultrastructural and functional correlations of the parathyroid gland, Int. Rev. Exp. Pathol. **13**:161, 1974.

Hormones; regulation of calcium metabolism

8. Chase, L.R., and Aurbach, G.D.: Renal adenyl cyclase: anatomically separate sites for parathyroid hormone and vasopressin, Science **159**:545, 1968.
9. Fisken, R.A., et al.: Hypercalcaemia in hospital patients: clinical and diagnostic aspects, Lancet **1**:202, 1981.
10. Kyle, L.H.: Differentiation of hyperparathyroidism and the milk-alkalai (Burnett) syndrome, N. Engl. J. Med. **251**:1035, 1954.
11. MacIntyre, I.: Parathyroid hormone, calcitonin, and vitamin D, Curr. Top. Exp. Endocrinol. **2**:179, 1974.
12. Wang, C.-A.: The anatomic basis of parathyroid surgery, Ann. Surg. **183**:271, 1976.

Pathologic calcification

13. Anderson, H.C.: Calcification processes, Pathol. Annu. **15**(2):45, 1980.
14. Barr, D.P.: Pathological calcification, Physiol. Rev. **12**:593, 1932.
15. Dalinka, M.K., and Melchior, E.L.: Soft tissue calcifications in systemic disease, Bull. N.Y. Acad. Med. **56**:539, 1980.
16. Lutz, J.F.: Calcinosis universalis, Ann. Intern. Med. **14**:1270, 1941.
17. Mortensen, J.D., and Baggenstoss, A.H.: Nephrocalcinosis: review, Am. J. Clin. Pathol. **24**:45, 1954.
18. Mulligan, R.M.: Metastatic calcification, Arch. Pathol. **43**:177, 1947.
19. Parfitt, A.M.: Soft-tissue calcification in uremia, Arch. Intern. Med. **124**:544, 1969.
20. Selye, H.: Calciphylaxis, Chicago, 1962, University of Chicago Press.
21. Skrabanek, P., McPartlin, J., and Powell, D.: Tumor hypercalcemia and "ectopic hyperparathyroidism," Medicine **59**:262, 1980.
22. Stewart, A.F., et al.: Biochemical evaluation of patients with cancer-associated hypercalcemia: evidence for humoral and nonhumoral groups, N. Engl. J. Med. **303**:1377, 1980.
23. Veress, B., Malik, M.O.A., and El Hassan, A.M.: Tumoural lipocalcinosis: a clinicopathological study of 20 cases, J. Pathol. **119**:113, 1976.

Hypoparathyroidism; pseudohypoparathyroidism

24. Chase, L.R., Melson, G.L., and Aurbach, G.D.: Pseudohypoparathyroidism: defective excretion of 3′, 5′-AMP in response to parathyroid hormone, J. Clin. Invest. **48**:1832, 1969.
25. David, L., and Anast, C.S.: Calcium metabolism in newborn infants: the interrelationship of parathyroid function and calcium, magnesium, and phosphorus metabolism in normal, "sick," and hypocalcemic newborns, J. Clin. Invest. **54**:287, 1974.
26. Drake, T.G., et al.: Chronic idiopathic hypoparathyroidism: report of six cases with autopsy findings in one, Ann. Intern. Med. **12**:1751, 1939.
27. Drezner, M.K., et al.: 1,25-Dihydroxycholecalciferol deficiency: the probable cause of hypocalcemia and metabolic bone disease in

pseudohypoparathyroidism, J. Clin. Endocrinol. Metab. **42**:621, 1976.

28. Mann, J.B., and Alterman, S., and Hills, A.G.: Albright's hereditary osteodystrophy comprising pseudohypoparathyroidism and pseudo-pseudohypoparathyroidism, Ann. Intern. Med. **56**:315, 1962.
29. Roberton, N.R.C., and Smith, M.A.: Early neonatal hypocalcaemia, Arch. Dis. Child. **50**:604, 1975.
30. Spinner, M.W., Blizzard, R.M., and Childs, B.: Clinical and genetic heterogeneity in idiopathic Addison's disease and hypoparathyroidism, J. Clin. Endocrinol. Metab. **28**:795, 1968.
31. Taitz, L.S., Zarate-Salvador, C., and Schwartz, E.: Congenital absence of the parathyroid and thymus glands in an infant (3 and 4 pharyngeal pouch syndrome), Pediatrics **38**:412, 1966.

Hyperparathyroidism

32. Castleman, B., and Mallory, T.B.: The pathology of the parathyroid gland in hyperparathyroidism: a study of 25 cases, Am. J. Pathol. **11**:1, 1935.
33. Dekker, A., Watson, C.G., and Barnes, E.L., Jr.: The pathologic assessment of primary hyperparathyroidism and its impact on therapy: a prospective evaluation of 50 cases with oil-red-O stain, Ann. Surg. **190**:671, 1979.
34. Heath, H., 3rd, Hodgson, S.F., and Kennedy, M.A.: Primary hyperparathyrodism: incidence, morbidity, and potential economic impact in a community, N. Engl. J. Med. **302**:189, 1980.
35. Hellström, J., and Ivemark, B.I.: Primary hyperparathyroidism: clinical and structural findings in 138 cases, Acta Chir. Scand. **294** (suppl.):1, 1962.
36. Kelly, T.R.: Primary hyperparathyroidism: a personal experience with 242 cases, Am. J. Surg. **140**:632, 1980.
37. Larsson, L., Eneström, S., and Gillquist, J.: Biochemical and morphological findings in patients with increased serum ionized calcium, Acta Chir. Scand. **145**:435, 1979.
38. Lloyd, H.M.: Primary hyperparathyroidism: an analysis of the role of the parathyroid tumor, Medicine **47**:53, 1968.
39. Pugh, D.G.: Subperiosteal resorption of bone: a roentgenologic manifestation of primary hyperparathyroidism and renal osteodystrophy, Am. J. Roentgenol. **66**:577, 1951.
40. Pyrah, L.N., Hodgkinson, A., and Anderson, C.K.: Primary hyperparathyroidism, Br. J. Surg. **53**:245, 1966.
41. Rienhoff, W.F., Jr., et al.: The surgical treatment of hyperparathyroidism, Ann. Surg. **168**:1061, 1968.
42. Rogers, H.M., et al.: Primary hypertrophy and hyperplasia of the parathyroid glands associated with duodenal ulcer: report of an additional case, with special reference to metabolic, gastrointestinal and vascular manifestations, Arch. Intern. Med. **79**:307, 1947.

Hyperplasia

Secondary hyperplasia

43. Castleman, B., and Mallory, T.B.: Parathyroid hyperplasia in chronic renal insufficiency, Am. J. Pathol. **13**:553, 1937.
44. Pappenheimer, A.M., and Wilens, S.L.: Enlargement of the parathyroid glands in renal disease, Am. J. Pathol. **11**:73, 1935.

Primary hyperplasia

45. Albright, F., et al.: Hyperparathyroidism due to diffuse hyperplasia of all parathyroid glands rather than adenoma of one: clinical studies on three such cases, Arch. Intern. Med. **54**:315, 1934.
46. Black, W.C., III, and Utley, J.R.: The differential diagnosis of parathyroid adenoma and chief cell hyperplasia, Am. J. Clin. Pathol. **49**:761, 1968.
47. Castleman, B., Schantz, A., and Roth, S.I.: Parathyroid hyperplasia in primary hyperparathyroidism: a review of 85 cases, Cancer **38**:1668, 1976.
48. Cope, O., et al.: Primary chief-cell hyperplasia of the parathyroid glands: a new entity in the surgery of hyperparathyroidism, Ann. Surg. **148**:375, 1958.
49. Golden, A., Canary, J.J., and Kerwin, D.M.: Concurrence of hyperplasia and neoplasia of the parathyroid glands, Am. J. Med. **38**:562, 1965.

Neoplasms

50. Arnold, B.M., et al.: Functioning oxyphil cell adenoma of the parathyroid gland: evidence for parathyroid secretory activity of oxyphil cells, J. Clin. Endocrinol. Metab. **38**:458, 1974.
51. Harness, J.K., et al.: Multiple adenomas of the parathyroids: do they exist? Arch. Surg. **114**:468, 1979.
52. Schantz, A., and Castleman, B.: Parathyroid carcinoma: a study of 70 cases, Cancer **31**:600, 1973.
53. van Heerden, J.A., et al.: Cancer of the parathyroid glands, Arch. Surg. **114**:475, 1979.
54. Woolner, L.B., Keating, F.R., Jr., and Black, B.M.: Tumors and hyperplasia of the parathyroid glands: a review of pathological findings in 140 cases of primary hyperparathyroidism, Cancer **5**:1069, 1952.

Lesions associated with hyperparathyroidism

55. Andersen, D.H., and Schlesinger, E.R.: Renal hyperparathyroidism with calcification of the arteries in infancy, Am. J. Dis. Child. **63**:102, 1942.
56. Anderson, W.A.D.: Hyperparathyroidism and renal disease, Arch. Pathol. **27**:753, 1939.
57. Follis, R.H., Jr., and Jackson, D.A.: Renal osteomalacia and osteitis fibrosa in adults, Bull. Johns Hopkins Hosp. **72**:232, 1943.
58. Herbert, F.K., Miller, H.G., and Richardson, G.O.: Chronic renal disease, secondary parathyroid hyperplasia, decalcification of bone and metastatic calcification, J. Pathol. Bacteriol. **53**:161, 1941.
59. Kleeman, C.R., et al.: The problem and unanswered questions: renal osteodystrophy, soft tissue calcification, and disturbed divalent ion metabolism in chronic renal failure, Arch. Intern. Med. **124**:262, 1969.
60. Mehls, O., et al.: Renal osteodystrophy in uraemic children, Clin. Endocrinol. Metab. **9**:151, 1980.

Other abnormalities

61. Wood, J.W., Johnson, K.G., and Hinds, M.J.A.: Parathyroid cysts, Arch. Surg. **92**:785, 1966.

CHAPTER 35 Adrenal Glands

SHELDON C. SOMMERS

STRUCTURE AND FUNCTION

Ultrastructural, histochemical, biochemical, tissue culture, and immunopathologic analyses have recently greatly increased our understanding of the adrenal glands.

Embryologically the adrenal medulla is of neural crest ectodermal origin. The cortex originates from urogenital ridge mesoderm. Accessory cortical nodules are commonly present in the adrenal capsule. They are also scattered throughout the retroperitoneal space, in the testicular region in 7.5% and beneath the renal capsule in 1.2% of autopsies, and less often in the parametrium or elsewhere. Celiac accessory adrenal glands were found in 32% of autopsies. Tissue foci resembling the adrenal medulla and termed *paraganglia* are peppered throughout the retroperitoneum, forming the prominent infant organ of Zuckerkandl, which is more difficult to find after puberty.

The human adrenal gland passes through three major developmental phases—fetal, childhood, and adult. The prenatal cortex has an inner fetal zone, which disappears within months after birth, is responsive to ACTH, and produces dehydroepiandrosterone. Relative to body weight, the adrenal glands are large at birth, weighing 2 to 4 g each, or 8.2 ± 3.4 g together. In anencephalics the fetal cortical zone atrophies prematurely before the twentieth week of pregnancy, and at birth each adrenal gland weighs only about 8% of normal, with closely packed cortical cells that lack ultrastructural indications of steroidogenesis.

In late childhood, the adrenarche occurs, with increased prepubertal secretion of androgens and related compounds. By then the adult cortical zonation of glomerulosa, fasciculata, and reticularis has become established. At 11 to 15 years of age, the normal aggregate weight is 8.5 g in boys and 7.5 g in girls. Apparently normal adult adrenal glands removed surgically weigh 4.8 ± 0.8 g in men and 4.1 ± 0.8 g in women. After sudden death, the aggregate adrenal weight is 9.2 ± 1.8 g in the United States. In autopsies in other situations the normal range is 12 to 16 mg, or 0.21 to 0.26 g/kg body weight. The increase is ascribed to cortical hypertrophy in response to the stress of illness. Crowding of experimental animals leads to adrenocortical hypertrophy and gonadal shrinkage. Comparable effects may occur in humans. Most autopsies do not include careful stripping of the periadrenal fat or accurate weighing of the glands, and except for a few series, satisfactory baseline weights are difficult to find.

The flattened right and pyramidal left human adrenal glands each have a head, body, and tail region, with the medulla in the more medial aspect of the head and body. The zona fasciculata accounts for 69.3% of the total cortical volume. Medulla, capsule, connective tissue, and vessels make up about 21.5% of the whole gland volume. The normal cortex measures 1 to 2 mm in width. The total cortical width and zona fasciculata width are statistically significantly correlated with their volumes. The human zona glomerulosa is normally discontinuous.

On section the adrenal cortex is golden yellow with a brown pigmented inner zona reticularis and a gray medulla. In women of menopausal age the zona reticularis is often prominent. Abundant sudanophilic lipid and cholesterol are present in all three adrenocortical zones. The cells normally appear finely vacuolated in paraffin sections. Zonation may not be obvious histologically, but with experience aided by reticulin stains, the outer glomerulosa pattern, the linearly arranged fasciculata, and the diagonal network of slightly pigmented reticularis cells can be recognized. The irregularly arranged medullary cells have prominent nuclei and abundant amphophilic cytoplasm. Chromaffinity is a mahogany brown medullary tissue color produced by the oxidant effect of chromate salts or Helly's solution on epinephrine in unfixed tissues.

Electron microscopy demonstrates characteristic platelike mitochondrial cristae in the zona glomerulosa cells, in contrast to tubular mitochondria of zona fasciculata cells. Cortical cells have abundant smooth endoplasmic reticulum, like other steroid-secreting cells, and a less prominent rough endoplasmic reticulum. Although it contains isolated adrenocortical cells, the adrenal medulla is separated completely from the cortex by a basement membrane. The endothelium is fenestrated. Osmiophilic cytoplasmic catecholamine-storage granules in medullary cells are of pure epinephrine and norepinephrine types, each surrounded by limiting membranes. The latter have a clear peripheral halo.

Adrenocortical function involves the synthesis and secretion of steroids formed from cholesterol (Fig. 35-1). In the human adult these include aldosterone, chiefly from the zona glomerulosa, hydrocortisone (cortisol) from the zona fasciculata, and androgens and estrogens predominantly from the zona reticularis. The human fetal cortex responds to both ACTH and chorionic gonadotropin but has relatively little 3-beta-hydroxysteroid dehydrogenase activity, which prevents the formation of progesterone and hence of aldosterone and cortisol. Instead, dehydroepiandrosterone and its derivatives are the major steroids secreted, contributing to the placental synthesis of estrogens, particularly estriol.

At birth the fetal cortical zone degenerates, shrinks, and completely involutes within 3 to 12 months. Failure of the fetal cortex to involute or to develop 17-hydroxylase, 21-hydroxylase, and 11-beta-hydroxylase, which normally occurs after the first 10 weeks of pregnancy, may result in some instances of congenital adrenal hyperplasia.

CONGENITAL ANOMALIES

Absence of both adrenal glands is compatible with life if accessory cortical tissue is present in the retroperitoneum or testes or if sufficient corticosteroids are produced by the brown fat. Aberrant adrenal tissue also may occur in the pancreas or liver. Only one adrenal gland may develop, the two glands may be fused, or there may

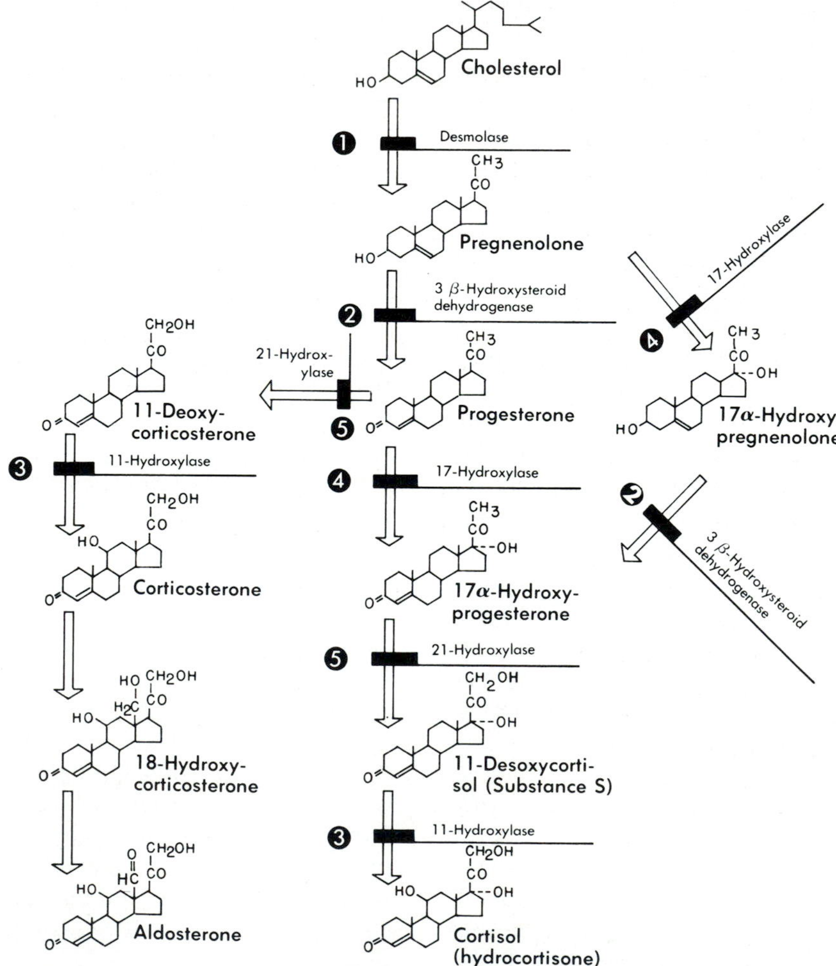

Fig. 35-1. Scheme of adrenocorticosteroid synthetic pathways. Enzymes underlined and numbered correspond to congenital enzymatic deficiencies that block reactions, as discussed in text.

be bilaterally double adrenal glands. Minor anomalies include adrenohepatic or adrenorenal fusion, usually unilateral and without functional importance.

Hypoplasia

Hypoplasia of the fetal cortical zone associated with anencephaly has been mentioned, and similar effects occur in pregnancies with subnormal maternal urinary estriol, preeclampsia, or both, as well as with prenatal pituitary or nervous system degeneration. Neonates with the respiratory distress syndrome had adrenal weights 19% less than normal, and their plasma cortisol was one third the expected levels. Cystic degeneration of the outer cortex is common in premature infants of less than 35 weeks' gestation.

Three types of adrenal hypoplasia are recognized in liveborn infants:

1. Precocious involution of the fetal cortex, which is found in postmaturity or various newborn illnesses. Destructive necrosis and hemorrhage of the fetal cortex are extensive, with infiltrates of neutrophils, and may destroy parts of the definitive cortex.
2. Idiopathic hypoplasia, in which the glands weigh only 0.3 to 1.8 g each, with miniature adult type of cortices some eight cells thick. Fetal cortex is decreased or absent. An ACTH-resistant familial variety is fairly typical in females. The affected infants typically suffer weight loss, dehydration, hyponatremia, hypoglycemia, and convulsions and die of adrenocortical insufficiency within 10 days.
3. Cytomegalic adrenocortical hypoplasia, which is rare, usually occurs in males, and evidently involves failure of the fetal cortical zone to involute and a related hypoplasia of the permanent outer cortex. Some instances are familial.

Anaplastic fetal adrenocortical cells are found in about 5% of infants at autopsy. Ordinarily, this focal cytomegaly and irregular nuclear polyploidy may only represent an atypical involutional change. Fetal adrenocortical cytomegaly is a characteristic of Beckwith's syndrome, which also includes macroglossia, abnormal umbilicus, somatic gigantism, and severe hypoglycemia. Adrenocortical carcinoma developed in three children with this syndrome. If bilateral adrenocortical cytomegaly is extensive, death from adrenal insufficiency may follow in about 1 month. The cytomegalic cells may be functional; ultrastructural features of steroidogenesis also are found.

Hyperplasia

Congenital adrenal hyperplasia with the adrenogenital syndrome is an uncommon condition believed to be attributable to autosomal recessive genes. Its importance lies in the associated anomalies of the external genitalia, the enzyme blocks responsible for the syndrome, and the interrelations of embryonic adrenal and genital tract differentiation thus revealed. The following classification of Bongiovanni and associates is useful, since it permits correlation of the individual enzyme deficiencies indicated in Fig. 35-1 with clinicopathologic alterations.

Patients with all types have a relative cortisol deficiency and consequent increase in pituitary ACTH secretion owing to decreased feedback control.

1. Desmolase deficiency is a rarity associated with lipid adrenal hyperplasia. The cortical cells contain excessive cholesterol and neutral lipid. Since practically all types of corticosteroid synthesis are blocked, there is no virilization, the blood pressure is low, salt and water loss are common, and death in infancy is frequent. Males usually are hypospadic and may be regarded as pseudohermaphrodites. Urinary ketosteroid levels are low.
2. 3-Beta-hydroxysteroid dehydrogenase deficiency is also rare and usually fatal. Affected males are hypospadic or may possess a vagina. Normal development of the male external genitalia is inhibited because the testis also lacks the enzyme, so testosterone and related steroids are not produced. Females may be moderately virilized at birth by the weakly androgenic effects of dehydroepiandrosterone and related delta$_5$-3-beta-hydroxysteroid compounds, which comprise almost all the urinary steroids. Ordinarily, low blood pressure, salt loss, hypoadrenal crises, failure to respond to treatment, and death ensue.
3. 11-Hydroxylase deficiency is the chief virilizing and hypertensive type of congenital adrenal hyperplasia. The dominant steroid is compound S, urinary 17-ketosteroids are increased, and salt wastage is uncommon. Urinary pregnanetriol is slightly elevated. Similar clinical and laboratory findings occur in some children with hypertension, adrenal adenoma, malnutrition, or diarrhea. A few postpubertal female patients with polycystic ovaries, virilism, or hypertension may have incomplete 11-hydroxylase deficiency. Adrenal hyperplasia is not always demonstrated.
4. 17-Hydroxylase deficiency is rare. No androgens or estrogens are produced. The urinary 17-ketosteroid levels are low. Aldosterone and cortisol are deficient. Hypertension is present without salt wastage, since the major steroids produced are deoxycorticosterone and corticosterone. Amenorrhea, incompletely developed secondary sex characteristics, and polycystic ovaries have been found. It is uncertain whether the enzyme deficiency is congenital or is associated with adrenal hyperplasia.

5. 21-Hydroxylase deficiency accounts for about 90% of all congenital adrenal hyperplasias. It produces the most familiar type of adrenogenital syndrome in infants and children. Virilization in both sexes is moderate and notable. Affected females have clitoral hypertrophy, and labial fusion may simulate a scrotum (Fig. 35-2). In males there may be precocious penile enlargement (macrogenitosomia). Both sexes have accelerated somatic growth. The dominant steroid is 17-hydroxyprogesterone, and more than 20 urinary steroids that lack C-21 hydroxyl groups are present, with androsterone and etiocholanolone predominant among the increased 17-ketosteroids. Pregnanetriol is one urinary 17-hydroxyprogesterone metabolite. The virilizing androgen is testosterone. Adult onset also occurs (Fig. 35-3).
6. The last types of enzyme deficiency involve 18-hydroxylase and 18-dehydrogenase without cortical hyperplasia.

In embryos, androgens inhibit differentiation of the genital tract along female lines, except in testicular feminization. One consequence is external genitalia of female pseudohermaphroditic appearance. The internal genitalia of embryos and children are less affected by androgens, whereas after puberty luteinized ovarian cysts or testicular Leydig cell hyperplasia may occur. In some cases there is testicular proliferation of accessory adrenocortical cells, but usually the testicular masses are hyperplastic Leydig cells. Female pseudohermaphroditism occasionally follows maternal therapy with progesterone, androgens, or estrogens. Since masculinization is progressive, early diagnosis and continuous cortisone type of steroid therapy are desirable.

In about 30% of patients with 21-hydroxylase deficiency, there are salt loss, a tendency to low blood pressure,

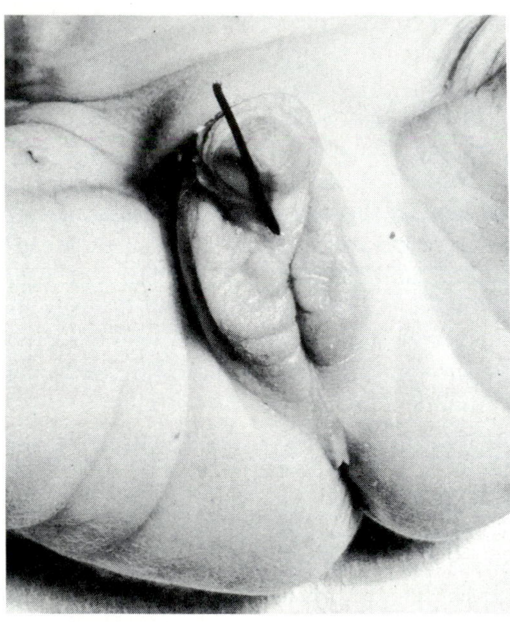

Fig. 35-2. External genitalia of female infant with 21-hydroxylase deficiency and adrenocortical hyperplasia. Appearance is typical of female pseudohermaphroditism with adrenogenital syndrome.

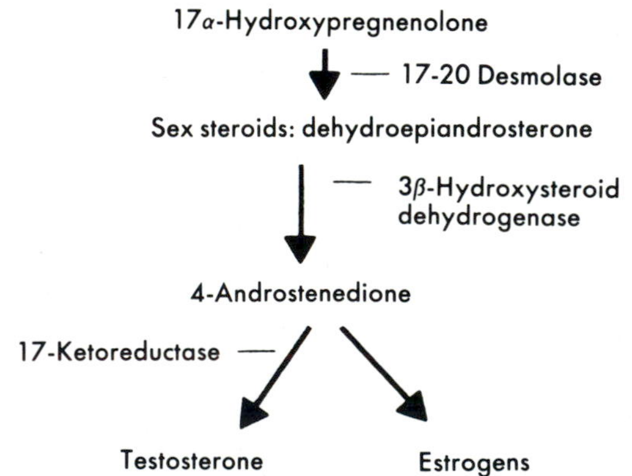

Fig. 35-3. Androgens and estrogens are synthesized from 17-alpha-hydroxypregnenolone, which is also included in Fig. 35-1.

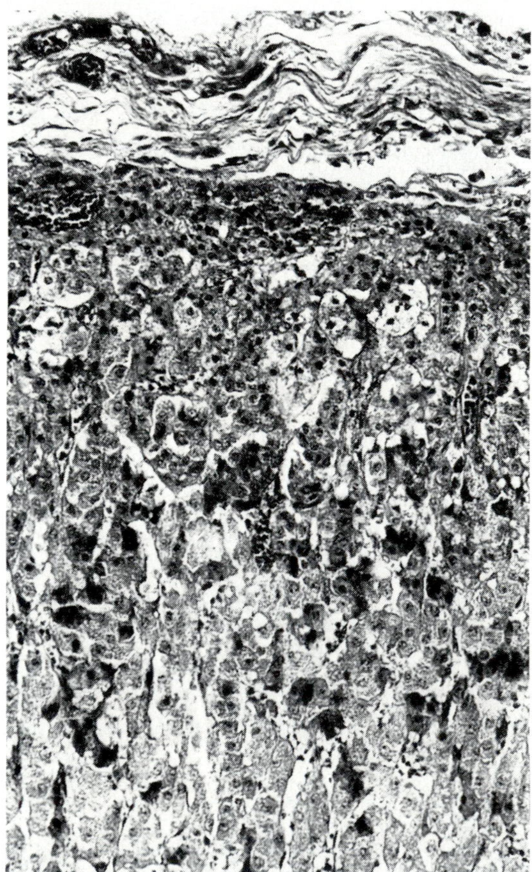

Fig. 35-4. Congenital adrenal hyperplasia associated with female pseudohermaphroditism. Cortical cells are irregularly enlarged, with acidophilic granular cytoplasm. (120×.)

sudden collapse with water restriction, and low serum sodium and high potassium levels, as well as hypoglycemia, susceptibility to infections, and brown skin pigmentation. Episodic fever may be attributable to etiocholanolone secretion. Supported by cortisone therapy, the individuals may survive to middle age or beyond.

Except for desmolase deficiency, the adrenal glands appear similar in all the congenital hyperplasias. The glands are up to five times normal size and may weigh 40 to 50 g each. The cortex is thickened and convoluted, with cells resembling the zona reticularis comprising two thirds of its total volume (Fig. 35-4). Apparently the hyperplasia does not represent persistent fetal adrenocortical tissue. In children the cells generally are not pigmented or stained by fuchsin. The zona fasciculata usually is identifiable microscopically. In adult female pseudohermaphrodites the hyperplastic zona reticularis is both pigmented and fuchsinophilic. Ultrastructurally the mitochondria in congenital hyperplasia resemble those of the zona reticularis (Fig. 35-5).

At least three other conditions with adrenal hyperplasia in the newborn infant have been reported. Infants of diabetic mothers may have increased urinary corticoids as part of an edematous, pseudoerythroblastosis syndrome, sometimes with an apparent increase of fetal cortical width. In infants dying of erythroblastosis fetalis or alpha-thalassemia, the fetal cortex is both thick and excessively vacuolated; the accompanying thymic atrophy suggests adrenal hyperfunction, possibly because of chronic intrauterine hypoxia. Antenatal infection also is reported associated with adrenocortical hyperplasia in the newborn.

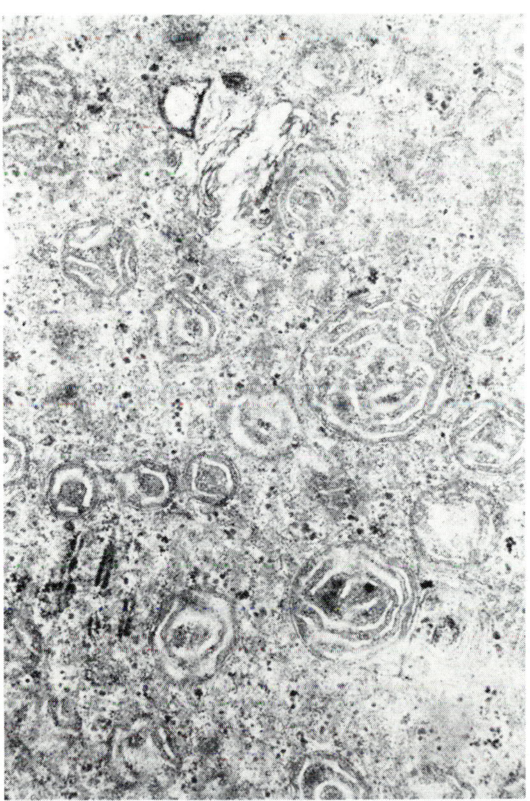

Fig. 35-5. Electron microscopy of predominant adrenocortical cells in congenital hyperplasia shows them to contain mitochondria with heavy internal structure found in the zona reticularis. (19,000×; from Tannenbaum, M.: Ultrastructural pathology of the adrenal cortex. In Sommers, S.C., editor: Pathology decennial 1966-1975, New York, 1975, Appleton-Century-Crofts.)

CHILDHOOD ABNORMALITIES

Hemorrhage

Certain adrenal lesions are more common before puberty, without necessarily being limited to children. Adrenal hemorrhage that destroys both the cortex and the medulla may reflect birth trauma, particularly after breech delivery. Waterhouse-Friderichsen syndrome involves bilateral, ordinarily fatal, destructive adrenal hemorrhages, classically associated with meningococcemia. Other gram-negative organisms such as colon bacilli may be responsible, and, less often, diphtheria, varicella, or measles. Gram-negative endotoxin shock, endothelial necrosis, sinusoidal thrombi, and intravascular consumption coagulopathy are implicated in the pathogenesis.

Necrosis

Hepatoadrenal necrosis is another usually fatal lesion, especially in premature infants with systemic herpes simplex infection acquired at birth, probably from maternal vaginitis. Both the adrenocortical and the hepatic cells are extensively destroyed. Some contain intranuclear Cowdry type A inclusion bodies. Cytomegalic inclusion disease is accompanied by typical, large, acidophilic intranuclear viral inclusions and cortical necrosis in about one third of generalized cytomegalovirus infections. A comparable adrenal involvement may occur in adults as a complication of lymphoma, leukemia, or peptic ulcer. Systemic *Pneumocystis* or *Cryptococcus* infections may localize in the adrenal glands. Varicella and herpes zoster of the adrenal glands produce medullary intranuclear inclusions.

Granulomas

In about half the autopsied cases of infantile toxoplasmosis, adrenal granulomas with or without recognizable organisms are found. In generalized histoplasmosis, coccidioidomycosis, and brucellosis, there occur epithelioid, caseous, or partly calcified adrenal granulomas, sometimes extensive enough to cause death from adrenocortical insufficiency. Congenital syphilis may show subcapsular adrenal fibrosis and abundant treponemes. Tuberculous Addison's disease of children is like the adult condition described in the following section.

Hypoplasia and degeneration

Adrenocortical cytotoxic hypoplasia, occasionally with persistent cytomegalic cortical cells, characterizes idiopathic Addison's disease of infancy. Histologically the adrenocortical cells are degenerated, with intermingled lymphocytes and macrophages. Several familial syndromes include childhood Addison's disease, most frequently combined with hypoparathyroidism and candidiasis or pernicious anemia. Adrenoleukodystrophy is characterized by ballooning degeneration and cytoplasmic striations affecting the cells of the zona fasciculata and zona reticularis accompanying cerebral demyelinization (Fig. 35-6). Another rare, sex-linked recessive condition is adrenocortical atrophy and cerebral sclerosis in males. Adrenocortical insufficiency and death from malnutrition at the age of 4 months or less occur in primary familial xanthomatosis (Wolman's disease). Among various xanthomatous lesions ascribed to inborn lysosomal acid lipase deficiency, the adrenal glands are notably enlarged by cortical foam cells. Adrenal cholesterol, over 90% esterified, is increased 20 fold. There are also adrenocortical necrosis, foreign body reaction to crystallized lipid, and diffuse punctate calcifications that may be radiologically diagnostic. In children, adrenal calcification also follows hemorrhage from birth trauma.

Cortical insufficiency

Partial adrenocortical insufficiency with selective familial cortisol deficiency in a child was correlated with absence of the zonae fasciculata and reticularis. Adrenal cortisol unresponsiveness to ACTH, mental retardation, typical facies, dwarfism, and obesity comprise the Prader-Willi syndrome. Familial hypoaldosteronism in infants with 18-hydroxylase deficiency occurs with hyponatremia and hyperkalemia. Urinary corticosterone and related dehydro and tetrahydro compounds are increased. At autopsy the adrenal glands are not enlarged. Small cells form tubular cords in the peripheral cortex. Functional, sometimes transient, hypoaldosteronism is reported in a few children and young adults but lacks a distinctive lesion.

Cortical hyperfunction

Adrenocortical hyperfunction in children is more often attributable to adrenal neoplasms than to hyperplasia. Boys may show the "infant Hercules" syndrome of pro-

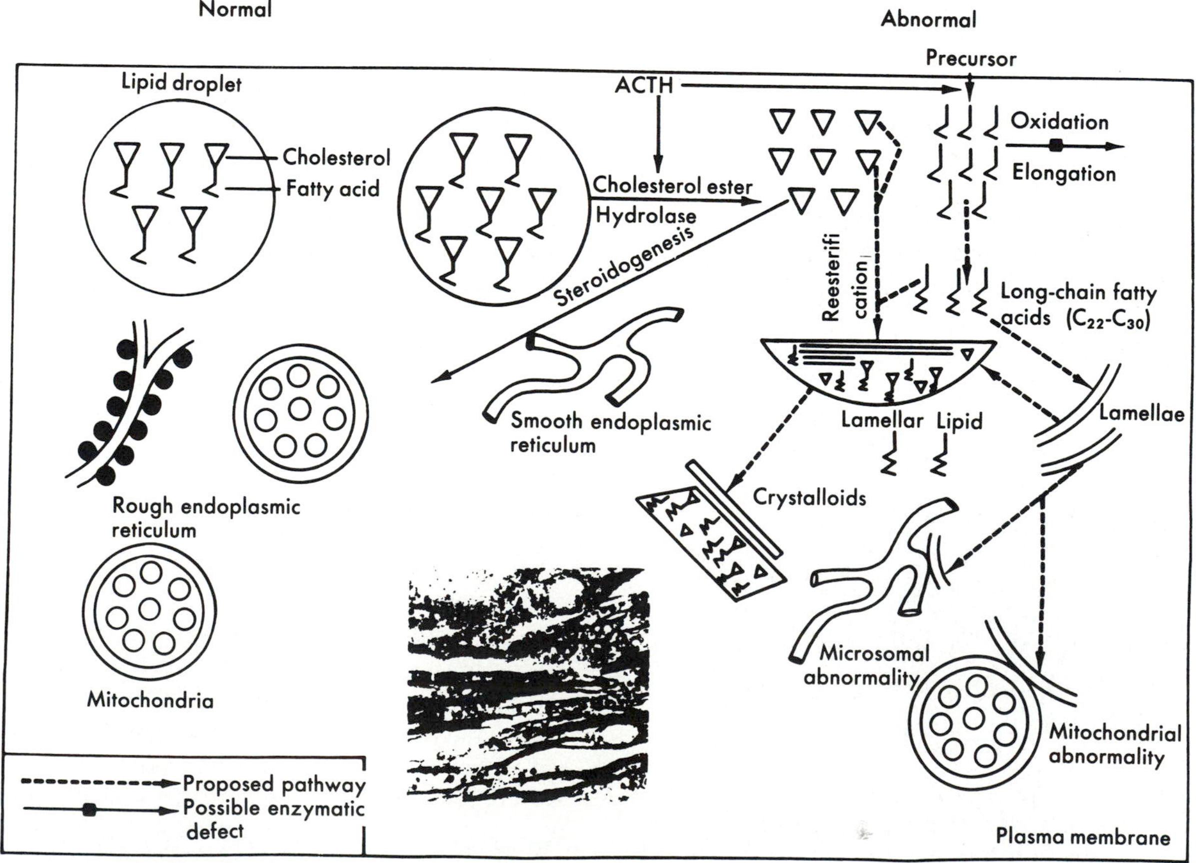

Fig. 35-6. Intracellular lesion in adrenoleukodystrophy involves formation of abnormal long-chain fatty acids that interfere with steroidogenesis and produce cytoplasmic lamellar lipid striations shown in inset. (22,000×; modified from Powers, J.M., et al.: Invest. Cell. Pathol. **3**:353, 1980.)

nounced muscular and somatic development with precocious pseudopuberty, comprised of macrogenitosomia and hirsutism but without testicular tubular or Leydig cell maturation. Girls with either neoplasms or adrenal hyperplasia are more often virilized, with some attributes comparable to those of Cushing's syndrome in adults. Adrenomedullary hyperplasia has been correlated with hypertension in two children and reported in pancreatic cystic fibrosis and in the sudden infant death syndrome.

Neuroblastoma

Neuroblastoma of the medulla is the chief infantile adrenal neoplasm, varying from incidentally found seedlings to massive retroperitoneal tumors. Next to retinoblastoma, this is the most common congenital cancer. The age at diagnosis is less than 1 year in 30% and below 5 years in 80%. Less than 5% of the patients are over 15 years of age. Extra-adrenal neuroblastomas arise elsewhere, particularly in the retroperitoneum and posterior mediastinum. When the primary tumor is small, metastases may first attract attention. Typical profuse osseous metastases, which include the skull and orbit, with resulting exophthalmos, are called the Hutchison type of neuroblastoma. Large hepatic neuroblastomatous metastases constitute the Pepper syndrome. Bilateral primary tumors exist.

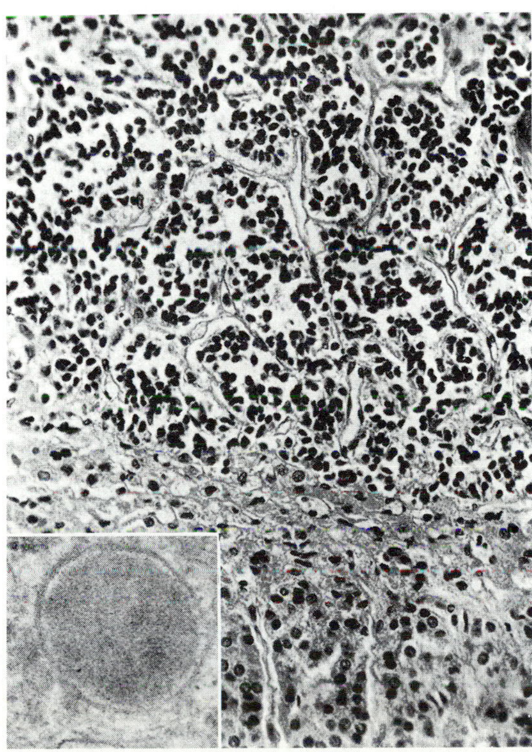

Fig. 35-7. Adrenomedullary neuroblastoma in newborn infant. (200×.) *Inset,* Membrane-enclosed catecholamine granule. (50,000×.)

Adrenal neuroblastomas are grossly or finely nodular, soft, gray-red, and vascular with a peripheral rim of persistent yellow adrenal cortex. Necrosis, hemorrhage, cystic degeneration, and calcification are seen. Microscopically the viable tumor is composed of small, dark-stained, rounded or unipolar cells, practically without cytoplasm or architecture, arranged among thin-walled sinusoidal vessels (Fig. 35-7). Rosettes with distinctive neuroblastic palisading around spaces resembling primitive neural canals or pseudorosettes similar to those in embryonic sympathetic ganglia distinguish about half of neuroblastomas. Neurites and rosettes are formed in neuroblastoma tissue cultures. Ultrastructurally, most neuroblastomas contain cytoplasmic catecholamine granules, and they occasionally secrete excessive epinephrine (Fig. 35-7, *inset*).

In related better-differentiated and less lethal neoplasms classified as ganglioneuroblastomas, foci of immature or mature neurons and nerve fibers are present. Fully differentiated ganglioneuromas are benign. In 11 cases, maturation has been observed from malignant neuroblastoma to benign ganglioneuroma. Sometimes neuroblastoma and the histologically indistinguishable retinoblastoma regress spontaneously. Nerve growth factor promotes the formation of neurite processes and maturation of neuroblastoma cells in tissue culture.

HEMORRHAGE AND NECROSIS

Adult adrenal apoplexy involves massive (usually bilateral) adrenal hemorrhage, complicating trauma, infections, malignant hypertension, myocardial infarction, toxemia of pregnancy, septic abortion, burns, or anticoagulant therapy. Vascular injury, parenchymal degeneration, venous thrombi, and generalized hemorrhage or intravascular coagulation are considered responsible.

Adrenocortical shrinkage or coagulative necrosis occurs focally in malaria, tetanus, typhus, Rocky Mountain spotted fever, epidemic hemorrhagic fever, and gram-negative bacterial or herpes infections, and may accompany acute peptic ulcers. It also occurs after abdominal operations. Diffuse bilateral adrenal necrosis and cortical insufficiency are more common in children than in adults but may complicate infected abortion, obstetric shock, and fatal pemphigus vulgaris. Focal necrosis more often occurs after thromboses of afferent capsular vessels and outer zonal sinusoids, whereas diffuse bilateral adrenocortical necrosis results from long-lasting sinusoidal obstruction and medullary venous thromboses. Combined arterial and venous damage exaggerates both parenchymal necrosis and the subsequent hemorrhage.

INFLAMMATION, ATROPHY, AND ADDISON'S DISEASE

Exudative inflammation is uncommon in the adrenal cortex because of the antiphlogistic effects of corticosteroids. Necrosis exceeds leukocytic infiltration in various viral, mycotic, and bacterial infections that involve the adrenal glands. Granuloma formation is retarded in adrenal tuberculosis, leprosy, coccidioidomycosis, and histoplasmosis, with relatively more organisms and parenchymal destruction and less epithelioid or giant cell reaction and fibrosis than in other tissues. In lesions of extra-adrenal infections, corticoid therapy also reduces granulomas and promotes increased organisms and necrosis.

Foci of lymphocytes and plasma cells localized around adrenal medullary veins usually are associated with comparable infiltrations in the splenic red pulp and surrounding the renal and retroperitoneal veins. These commonly indicate chronic pyelonephritis with retroperitoneal chronic phlebitis rather than intrinsic adrenal disease. Malakoplakia rarely does occur in the adrenal.

Bilateral destructive adrenocortical tuberculosis is the classic cause of Addison's disease. Weakness, pigmentation of the skin and mucous membranes, hypotension, hypoglycemia, hyponatremia and hyperkalemia, a tendency to dehydration, and adrenal crises with shock after trauma or infections are its salient characteristics. Both adrenal glands are enlarged and largely replaced by caseous granulomas (Fig. 35-8). Fifty years ago, 70% of Addison's disease was tuberculous, but idiopathic adrenocortical atrophy now predominates. Amyloidosis accounts for 1%, and adrenal replacement by metastatic carcinoma for less than 0.5%, of Addison's disease. Lymphoid tissues and pancreatic islets tend toward hyperplasia because of their release from adrenocortical control.

In idiopathic adrenal atrophy the gland weights are reduced to a range of 1.2 to 2.5 g each and the cortices are narrowed and largely replaced by fibrous tissue (Fig. 35-9). Sometimes nonspecific granulomas, giant cells, or infiltrates of lymphocytes are present in the cortices and medullae. These lesions comprise so-called cytotoxic atrophy. Lymphocytic adrenalitis is associated with familial immune disorders, with antibodies to adrenal, thyroid, gastric parietal, and gonadal cells, and sometimes with other endocrine deficiencies. Periadrenal brown fat may be conspicuous.

Combined nontuberculous Addison's disease, hypothyroidism resulting from chronic thyroiditis, and occasionally hypopituitarism associated with pituitary lymphoid infiltrates constitute Schmidt's syndrome. Circulating antiadrenal mitochondrial and microsomal antibodies are found in the sera of half the patients with nontuberculous Addison's disease. Diabetes mellitus, chronic hepatitis, gonadal failure, or pernicious anemia may accompany Addison's disease, a relationship that also

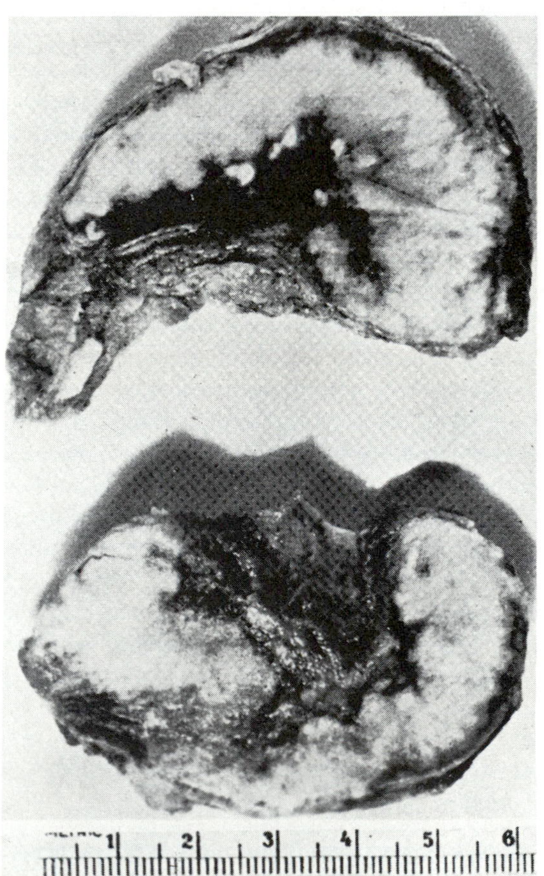

Fig. 35-8. Tuberculosis of adrenal glands in Addison's disease.

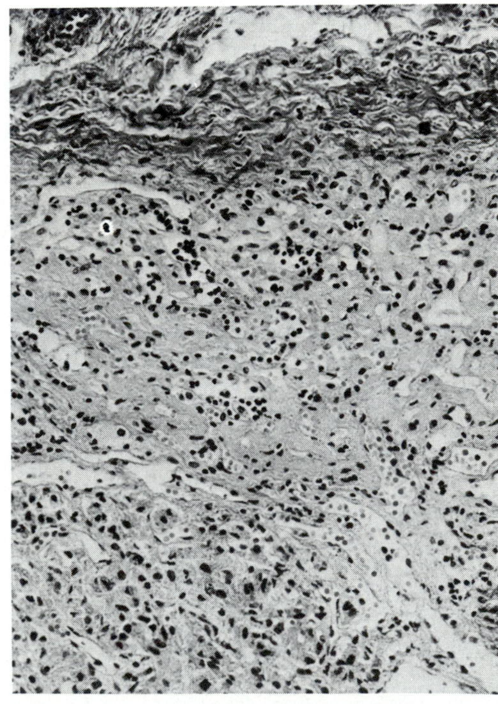

Fig. 35-9. Idiopathic adrenocortical atrophy with Addison's disease. Cortical cells have practically disappeared and stroma is collapsed. Adrenal medulla and central veins can be seen below. (120×.)

suggests autoimmune reactions. Experimental allergic adrenalitis can be transferred passively by lymphoid cells.

Adenocortical atrophy resulting from hypophysectomy or pituitary destruction by disease may be extreme. In one adult with panhypopituitarism the combined weight of the adrenal glands was only 0.8 g, with cortices 10 to 12 cells thick. Giant mitochondria occur after hypophysectomy in the zona fasciculata, reflecting a high progesterone/corticosterone ratio. Long-term cortisone type of therapy for connective tissue diseases, arthritis, or asthma reduces the gland weights by about half, with notable shrinkage of the zona glomerulosa (Fig. 35-10). In iatrogenic adrenocortical atrophy the collapsed, condensed cortical stroma may simulate fibrosis. Patients treated with both ACTH and cortisone demonstrate zona fasciculata cytolysis. Isolated pituitary ACTH deficiency rarely causes adrenocortical insufficiency.

DEGENERATION AND INFILTRATION

As corticosteroids are secreted in acute diseases, the adrenal cortex becomes rapidly depleted of both birefringent and sudanophilic lipid. After 6 days the cortical lipid is restored, but in the interval lipid depletion reflects recent hypersecretion. In chronically ill individuals, adrenal lipid also is frequently depleted. The outer zona fasciculata cells may be reduced in size, producing a lipid-depletion reversion pattern. In severe acute trauma, burns, toxemias, and infections such as diphtheria, besides the loss of lipid, hyaline protein droplets are found in cortical cells with necrobiosis. The outer zona fasciculata regenerates around the cytolysis, resulting in a hollow cylindrical appearance of the fasciculata cell cords termed Rich's tubular degeneration (Fig. 35-11). Excessive ACTH stimulation is considered responsible for tubular degeneration, but hyaline droplet change has been produced experimentally by methyl androstenediol. Similar hyaline droplets in adrenomedullary cells occur in various chronic diseases. Spironolactone, an aldosterone antagonist, produces laminated, sudanophilic, whorled, membranous, myelin-like bodies of altered smooth endoplasmic reticulum in active zona glomerulosa cells and aldosterone-secreting adenomas (Fig. 35-12).

Less specific degenerative changes include adrenal lymphocytic infiltrates near the corticomedullary junction associated with fragmented basement membranes. Hyaline fibrotic areas beneath the capsule or in the medulla are commonly the result of arteriolosclerosis. Heavy radiotherapy results in fibrosis of the juxtamedullary zona reticularis. In old age relatively little identifiable adrenal medulla may remain. Rarely there are also medullary calcification and functional insufficiency.

Amyloid is deposited in the zona fasciculata in about

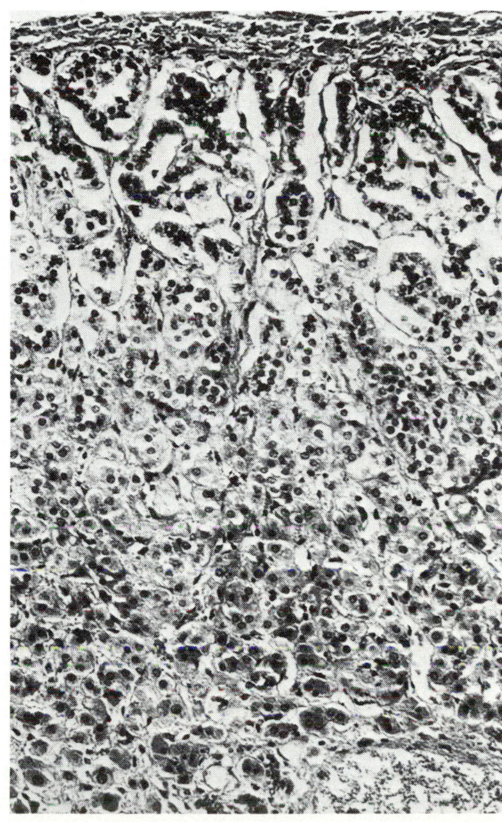

Fig. 35-10. After prolonged cortisone therapy, zona fasciculata cells become shrunken and cortical thickness is reduced to 0.5 mm, half the normal width. Zona glomerulosa and zona reticularis are unaffected and appear prominent. (120×.)

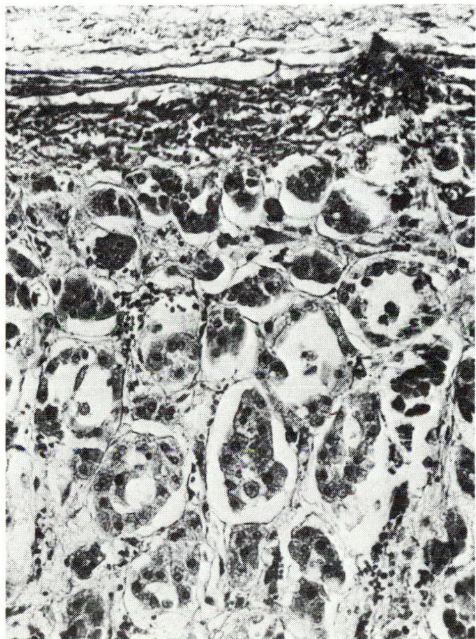

Fig. 35-11. Tubular degeneration resulting from cytolytic degeneration of zona fasciculata with regeneration to form hollow cylinders of cortical cells. (120×.)

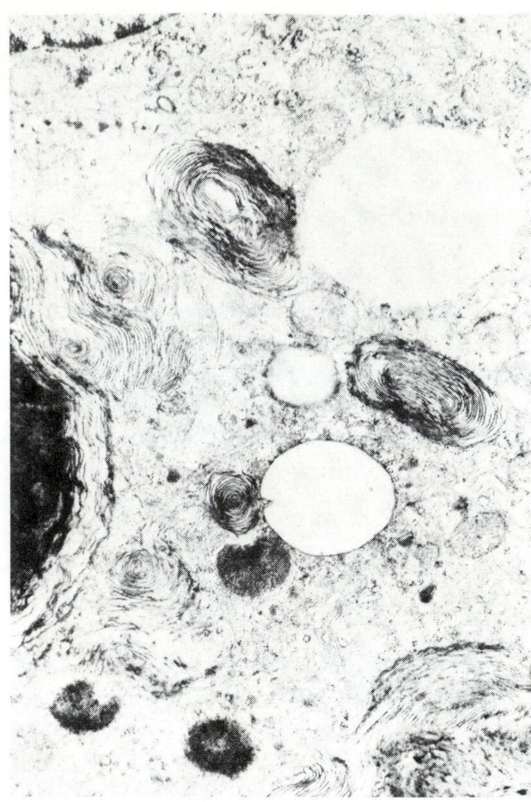

Fig. 35-12. Spironolactone bodies are complex whorled membranous structures in adrenal zona glomerulosa. (12,000×; from Bloodworth, J.M.B., Jr., Horvath, E., and Kovacs, K.: Fine structural pathology of the endocrine system. In Trump, B.F., and Jones, R.T., editors: Diagnostic electron microscopy, vol. 3, New York, 1980, John Wiley & Sons, Inc.)

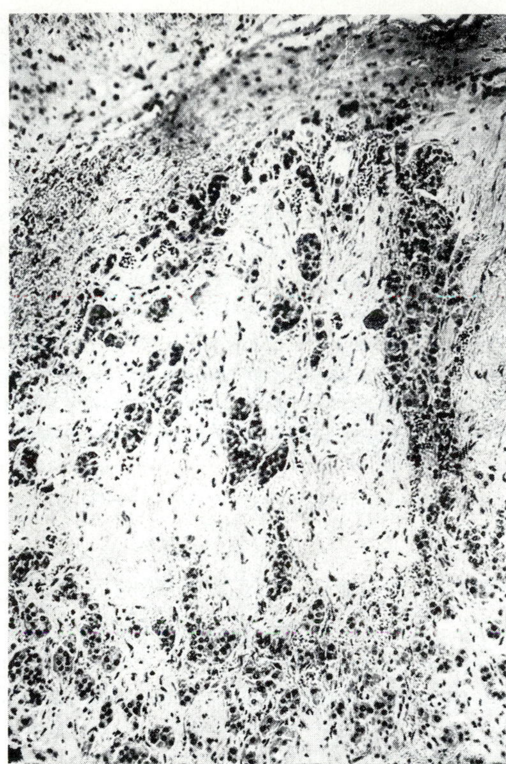

Fig. 35-13. Amyloidosis of adrenal cortex. Capsule at top and adrenocortical cells are largely replaced by deposits. (100×.)

80% of patients with generalized amyloidosis, with such deposition augmenting the adrenal weights. The zona glomerulosa is infiltrated last, and adrenocortical insufficiency is uncommon (Fig. 35-13). Purely localized adrenal deposits of amyloid have been found in 6% of autopsies. In primary amyloidosis, only the adrenal arteries may be involved.

The zona glomerulosa becomes pigmented in hemosiderosis, and additional hemosiderin is deposited there in hemochromatosis.

Fat replaces parts of the adrenal zonae fasciculata and reticularis occasionally without affecting adrenal weight. A few lymphocytes or hemopoietic foci may be associated with fatty infiltration. The adrenal cortex also is a site of myeloid metaplasia; hemopoiesis is evident in sinusoids of the deep zona fasciculata, compressing the cell cords without significant gland enlargement.

CORTICAL NODULARITY

Approximately half of all persons over 50 years of age have nonuniform adrenal cortices with multiple small rounded nodules of zona fasciculata. Regeneration after segmental ischemic adrenocortical atrophy attributable to local vascular disease accounts for many cortical nodules in older persons. The nodular foci may possess more or less lipid than the uninvolved cortex and also differ in histochemical succinic dehydrogenase, esterase, and acid phosphatase reactions. Nodularity is more common with cirrhosis, hypertension, and cancer than with other chronic conditions. Its functional importance is unknown.

HYPERPLASIA, CUSHING'S SYNDROME, AND ADRENAL VIRILISM

Adrenocortical hyperplasia may be either diffuse or nodular (finely or grossly), and it is usually bilateral. Criteria for the diagnosis include gland weights exceeding the top 5% of normal weights or above twice the standard deviation from the mean and cortices thicker than 2 mm. Usually hyperplasia involves the zona fasciculata. Exceptions in aldosteronism and adrenal virilism are noted in the following paragraphs. Additional less conclusive indications of hyperplasia are irregular extracapsular proliferations of cortical cells, nodules that bulge into the medulla, and prominent cortical cell cuffs around the central veins.

Nonspecific adrenocortical hyperplasia is most common with acromegaly, thyrotoxicosis, hypertension associated with arteriolosclerosis and arteriosclerosis, cancer, and diabetes mellitus. Some cases are unexplained. The adrenal glands of acromegalic patients usually are enlarged and nodular, with exaggerated androgen secretion after ACTH stimulation. Hyperplasia accompanies hyperthyroidism in about 40% of the patients, essential hypertension and arteriosclerosis in 16%, and diabetes mellitus in 3.4%. In both hyperthyroidism and hypertension, increased adrenal weights may be ascribed partly to the frequent terminal complication of congestive heart failure.

The best-understood specific adrenocortical hyperplasia accompanies Cushing's syndrome. As originally described, Cushing's *disease is* caused by an ACTH-secreting basophil pituitary adenoma, but in the much more common *syndrome*, no pituitary tumor is found. Typically the patient has a rounded moon-shaped face, obesity with a "buffalo hump" around the shoulders or a girdle distribution, a plethoric complexion associated with polycythemia, thin skin with easy bruising and abdominal striae, muscle weakness, hypertension, osteoporosis, and glucose tolerance test results indicating a diabetic type. Hirsutism in women, amenorrhea, and mental disturbances are frequent, and acne may be present. Since practically all these changes occur after sufficient cortisone or cortisol administration, Cushing's syndrome is attributable to hypercortisolism. Women are affected more frequently than men, in a ratio of about 3:1 (see also p. 1434).

In children, Cushing's syndrome is about equally commonly associated with adrenocortical hyperplasia and tumors, but after the age of 10 years, zona fasciculata hyperplasia accounts for approximately 70% of cases. The zona reticularis also may be increased. Cortical adenoma is responsible for about 20% of the cases of adult Cushing's syndrome and adrenocortical carcinoma for 10%. The uninvolved and contralateral cortices are atrophic. Surgically removed glands with diffuse hyperplasia together weigh 14 to 26 g or more in three fourths of the patients with Cushing's syndrome and 10 to 12 g in one fourth. The cortices are usually thicker than 2 mm. In equivocal cases, volumetric studies demonstrate zona fasciculata hyperplasia. A distinctive cytologic enlargement and increased cytoplasmic lipid are observed, producing clublike thickenings of the outer zona fasciculata cell cords, with occasional very large cells (Fig. 35-14). Ultrastructurally the mitochondria are increased in size and complexity, smooth endoplasmic reticulum is increased and dilated, and pericellular basal laminae are reduplicated. The hyperplastic zona fasciculata may compress, infiltrate, or replace the zona glomerulosa and zona reticularis and penetrate into the medulla. Hyperplasia also includes the zona reticularis in women with virilization; thus in clinical Cushing's syndrome the endocrine hyperfunction is not necessarily restricted to the zona fasciculata and hypercortisolism.

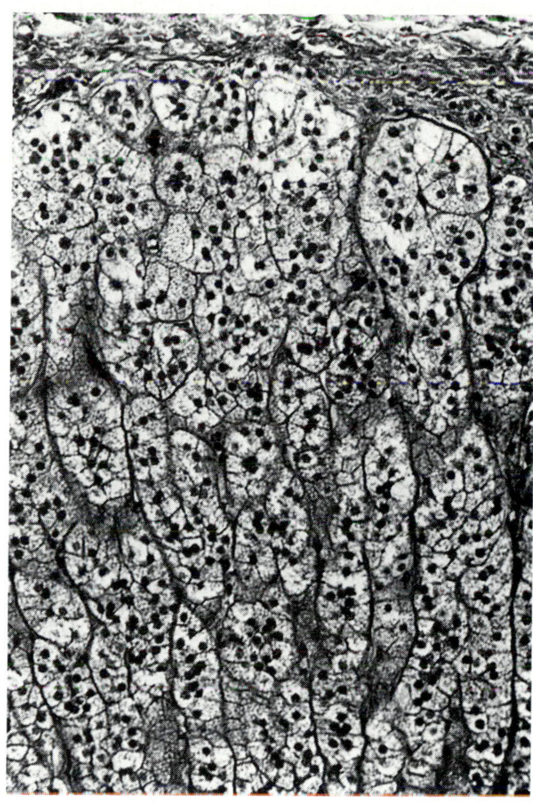

Fig. 35-14. Cushing's syndrome with diffuse adrenocortical hyperplasia. Outer zona fasciculata cells are typically enlarged to form club-shaped cords. (120×.)

Nodular hyperplasia involves increased adrenal weights and cortices thickened by rounded zona fasciculata nodules, usually 1 to 6 mm and occasionally up to 2 cm in diameter. Some individuals are apparently normal endocrinologically. Others have hypertension, edema, and hyperaldosteronism. Grossly, nodular hyperplasia with Cushing's syndrome involves bilateral adrenal hypertrophy (up to triple the normal weight) and multiple adenomatous nodules that are 1 to 5 cm in diameter and yellow, brown, black, or red according to their lipid content and lipochrome or heme pigmentation from hemorrhages. The nodules have variable lipid content and decreased glucose-6-phosphate dehydrogenase activity (Fig. 35-15). On electron microscopy the hyperplastic adrenocortical cells possess an abundant smooth endoplasmic reticulum and tubulovesicular mitochondria characteristic of the zona fasciculata.

Nodular adrenocortical dysplasia is an unusual lesion in infants or children with Cushing's syndrome. The glands are not enlarged, and the cortex contains multiple minute nodules up to 2 mm in diameter, notably pigmented by lipochrome and apparently arising from the zona reticularis. The intervening cortical tissue is atrophic. The cortical hyperfunction is unresponsive to ACTH or dexamethasone, unlike the more common

ACTH-dependent hyperplasia with Cushing's syndrome (Fig. 35-16).

Ectopic ACTH production by nonendocrine tumors is considered responsible for approximately 20% of the cases of Cushing's syndrome. Often the clinical findings are incomplete or absent, perhaps because the condition has developed rapidly, but hypokalemic alkalosis is a usual finding. Edema, skin pigmentation, and severe diabetes mellitus are more common than in idiopathic Cushing's syndrome. Oat cell carcinoma of the lung is the most frequently associated tumor. Pituitary hyaline basophils are increased, indicating increased circulating cortisone. Other recognized ACTH-secreting tumors include thymic oat cell carcinomas, pancreatic islet cell tumors, thyroid medullary carcinomas, and carcinoids of the lung or stomach, among diverse foregut endodermal neoplasms. Neuroblastomas and ovarian, testicular, and other neoplasms also have been implicated.

The adrenal glands in the ectopic ACTH syndrome usually are notably enlarged, two to five times the normal weight. Microscopically the zona fasciculata cells, particularly near the capsule, are distinctively enlarged, depleted of lipid, and acidophilic (Fig. 35-17). These are effects of maximal ACTH stimulation. Besides ACTH, some neoplasms also produce excessive melanocyte-stimulating hormone, parathyroid hormone, gastrin, glucagon, antidiuretic hormone, norepinephrine, calcitonin, or serotonin. Pancreatic tumors appear to be the most versatile. Patients with lung carcinomas that do not produce ACTH may secrete excessive 17-hydroxycorticosteroids and cortisone after ACTH administration, as occurs nonspecifically in other severe illnesses.

Iatrogenic adrenocortical hyperplasia has followed prolonged ACTH therapy in leukemic children and in adults with various chronic diseases. Gland weights are nearly doubled. Both the zona fasciculata and the zona reticularis are thicker, individual cells are enlarged, and cholesterol and lipid are reduced. The clinical and laboratory findings resemble those in Cushing's syndrome.

Cushingoid states have some attributes of Cushing's syndrome such as obesity, diabetes mellitus, hirsutism, or hypertension, without a clear-cut correlated hypercortisolism, pituitary and adrenocortical hyperplasia, or neoplasia.

Hyperplasia of the inner zona fasciculata and zona reticularis together characterize adrenal virilism, sometimes called the acquired or adult adrenogenital syn-

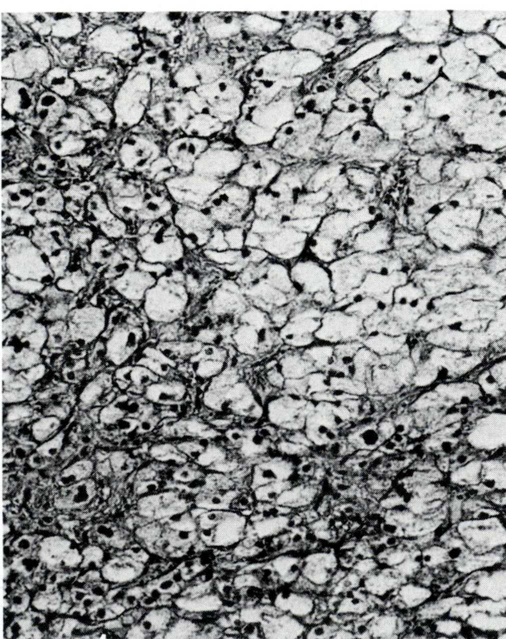

Fig. 35-15. Nodular hyperplasia of zona fasciculata with Cushing's syndrome associated with irregular cellular enlargement and locally increased lipid in adrenocortical cells. (120×.)

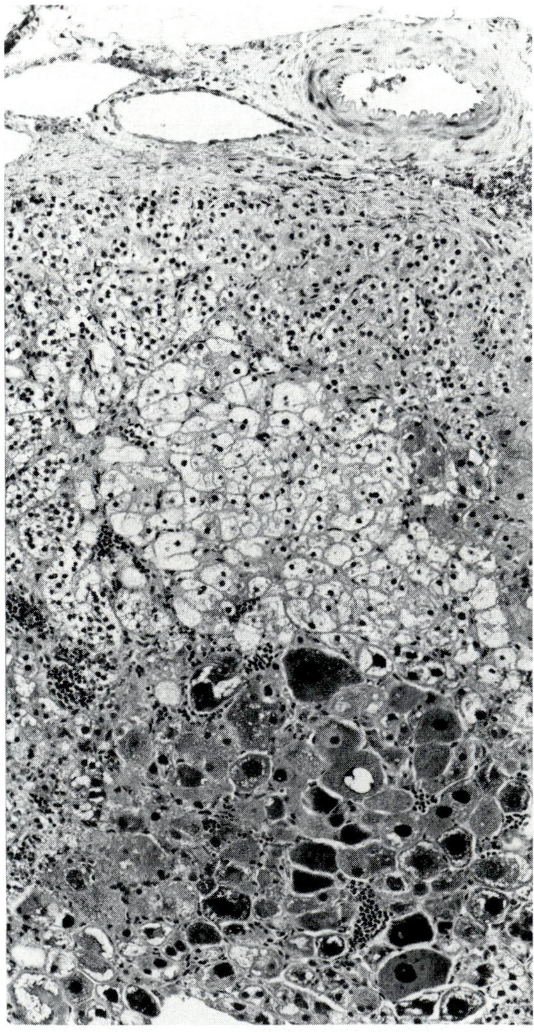

Fig. 35-16. Adrenalectomy specimen of normal-sized gland in adolescent with Cushing's syndrome showing notable nodularity and cytologic atypia of cells in deeper nodules. (100×.)

drome. In women, hirsutism, acne, temporal alopecia, squared body contours, deep voice, and clitoral enlargement to some degree frequently accompany Cushing's syndrome. Secretion of androgens, particularly dehydroepiandrosterone and 11-beta-hydroxyandrostenedione, is responsible. Cortisol and corticosterone also are increased. Pure adrenal zona reticularis hyperplasia is unusual. When mild, it may produce only hirsutism. Adrenal hirsutism is estimated to explain about 1% of excessive hair growth in women. Two distinctive characteristics of hyperplastic zona reticularis cells are lipochrome pigment and fuchsinophilia. Rarely, Leydig cells are present. Feminizing nodular hyperplasia also exists.

Zona glomerulosa hyperplasia, with enlarged lipid-containing cells forming a continuous subcapsular layer at least 100 μm wide, is associated with secondary aldosteronism fully developed as a complication of malignant or renovascular hypertension, nephrotic syndrome, cirrhosis with ascites, and other conditions. Nodular hyperplasia of both zona glomerulosa and zona fasciculata accompanies cases variously classified as idiopathic or pseudoprimary aldosteronism. Serotonin-mediated stimulation may be responsible. Unilateral nodular hyperplasia is a rare genuine cause of primary aldosteronism (Fig. 35-18). In sodium restriction the zona glomerulosa ordinarily is increased in thickness with depletion of the cytoplasmic lipid and cholesterol.

Medullary hyperplasia is considered later in the chapter.

NEOPLASMS

Adenoma, primary aldosteronism, and carcinoma

Adrenocortical adenoma is usually a relatively large, single, rounded mass of yellow-orange adrenocortical tissue, measuring 1 to 5 cm in diameter (Fig. 35-19). Larger adenomas up to 12 cm in diameter may show hemorrhages, cystic degeneration, and calcification. The tissue bulges from the cut surface, an indication of compression. Most adenomas are surrounded by a rim of stretched, uninvolved adrenal cortex and have an incomplete fibrous capsule or none. Histologically, adenomas are composed of relatively regular large cells with uniformly abundant lipid, arranged in nodules and cords with a vaguely fasciculate pattern. The margins of contact with uninvolved adrenal cortex are evident, since cells of the latter are zonated and smaller and contain less lipid.

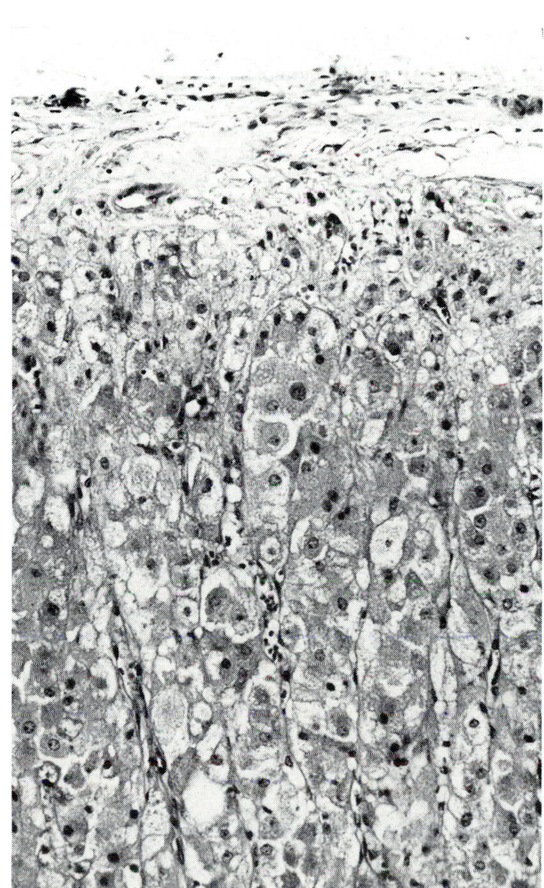

Fig. 35-17. Enlargement and lipid depletion of maximally stimulated outer zona fasciculata cells produced by ectopic ACTH. (120×.)

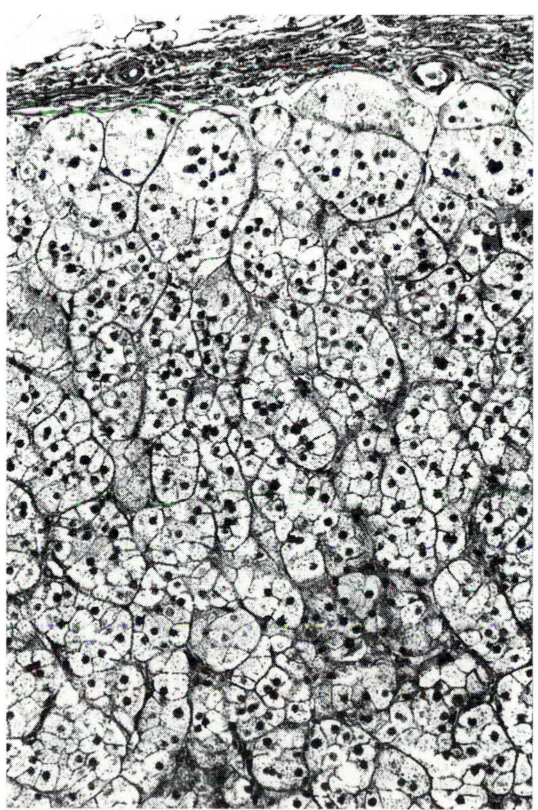

Fig. 35-18. Primary aldosteronism associated with unilateral adrenocortical hyperplasia. Zona glomerulosa cells are enlarged and finely granular. (120×.)

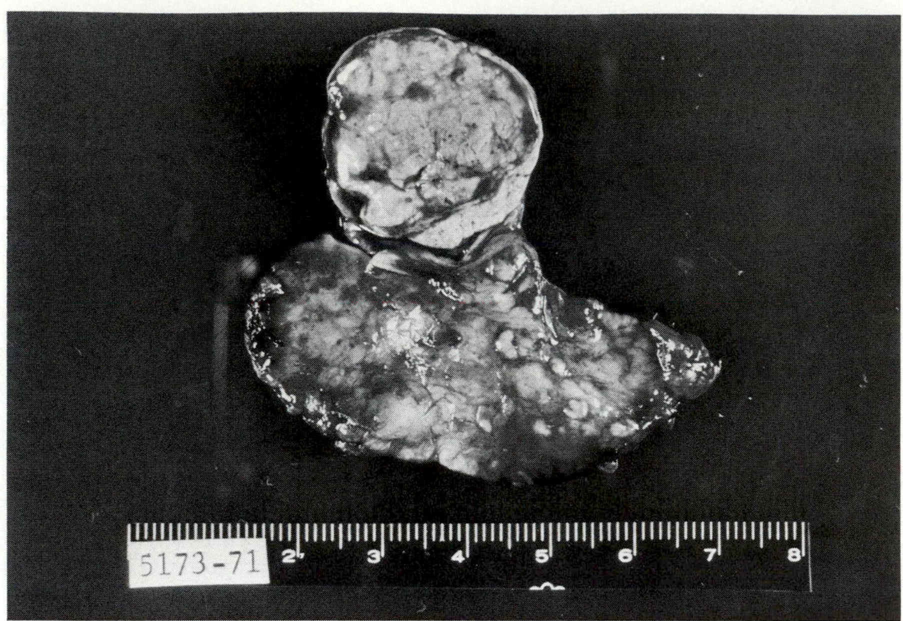

Fig. 35-19. Sectioned rounded mass above adrenal gland is cortical adenoma responsible for primary aldosteronism.

Giant cells with prominent nuclei and cellular polymorphism often present in adrenocortical adenomas are not considered evidence of cancer.

Nodules smaller than 9 mm in diameter sometimes are considered adenomas, but if they are multiple, bilateral, or zonated and lie in the capsule or outside, it is doubtful that they are true adenomas. A genuine adrenocortical adenoma usually is associated with either a normal or an atrophic homolateral and contralateral uninvolved gland. When the adrenal cortices are multinodular or hyperplastic, the largest masses represent dominant nodules rather than adenomas.

Adenomas located centrally in the adrenal gland may be difficult to distinguish from pheochromocytomas, and in extra-adrenal sites such as the retroperitoneum or ovary they may be confused with nonchromaffin paragangliomas, Leydig cell tumors, and hypernephroid or other neoplasms. Some differential diagnostic features are given in Table 35-1.

An adrenal adenoma is found in 2% to 8% of autopsies on adults. In the absence of overt endocrine effects and hormonal analyses, these are called nonfunctional adenomas. Adenomas have been found most commonly in autopsies of elderly, obese, diabetic patients (30%); women averaging 81 years of age (29%); hypertensive individuals (20%); and patients with the familial multiple endocrine neoplasia syndrome (MEN I) that also involves the pancreatic islets and the parathyroid, pituitary, and thyroid glands besides peptic ulcerations, gastric mucosal hyperplasia, and colonic villous adenomas.

About 75% of functioning adrenal tumors in children are benign adenomas, 10% of which are bilateral. The remaining one fourth are carcinomas. Practically all the carcinomas metastasize and prove fatal. Dehydroepiandrosterone is the chief steroid secreted by virilizing adenomas, and the urinary 17-ketosteroids are increased. Sometimes chiefly testosterone is produced. Androgens also promote somatic growth and maturation. The testicular tubules and Leydig cells remain undeveloped, or there is no menstrual activity, unlike the situation in precocious puberty. Cortisol hypersecretion typifies Cushing's syndrome. Combined virilization and estrogenization are associated with adrenocortical partial conversion of dehydroepiandrosterone to estradiol.

Table 35-1. Differential diagnostic features

Features	Adrenocortical tumor	Pheochromocytoma
Gross appearance	Yellow or orange	Gray, red, or brown
Histology	Cordlike arrangement	Sheets, nests, mosaic or twisted cord pattern
Cytology	Uniform size, squared shapes	Variable size, polyhedral shapes
	Cytoplasmic lipid vacuoles, Sudan- and cholesterol-positive	No lipid vacuoles
	Occasional mitoses	No mitoses
Chromaffinity	Negative	Positive
Ultrastructure	No catecholamine granules	Catecholamine granules

In adults with Cushing's syndrome, functioning adrenal adenomas characteristically reduce the plasma ACTH, unlike adrenocortical hyperplasia. Hirsutism and acne accompany adenoma less commonly than they do adrenal carcinoma. Virilizing and feminizing adrenal tumors are more often carcinomas than adenomas. Adenomas may produce mineralocorticoids as well as cortisone and may respond functionally to ACTH, dexamethasone, or chorionic gonadotropin. Receptors for diverse hormones are present.

Primary aldosteronism is associated with an adrenocortical adenoma in about 90% of cases and with carcinoma, multiple adenomas, and unilateral cortical hyperplasia in the remainder. Few authentic cases with adenomas have been reported in children. Before the age of 20 years, most instances of aldosterone hypersecretion are associated with either bilateral diffuse or nodular cortical hyperplasia. Conn's syndrome (Conn, Knopf, and Nesbit[118]) describes the combination of hypokalemic alkalosis, renal potassium loss, and hypertension, which may be cured by removing an aldosterone-secreting adrenal adenoma. Renin is characteristically suppressed, and the renal juxtaglomerular cells are atrophic. Aldosteronomas often are flattened tumors 0.9 to 1.5 cm in diameter. They may be impalpable and unidentified until multiple sections of the gland are made. A few are larger, and some have weighed more than 30 g. Characteristically they are more orange than yellow, are rich in lipid, and histologically resemble other adrenal adenomas, with either a fasciculate or a glomerulosal architecture (Fig. 35-20). Biosynthesis of cortisol, corticosterone, and aldosterone is demonstrable. Electron microscopy has shown the tumor mitochondria to possess the platelike cristae of zona glomerulosa cells, or tubulovesicular cristae like the zona fasciculata, or a combined "hybrid cell" type. Histochemically, 3-beta-hydroxysteroid dehydrogenase activity is reportedly intense. Some aldosteronomas are ACTH dependent.

Hypertension also occurs in association with adenomas that produce corticosterone, deoxycorticosterone, or, more rarely, tetrahydrodeoxycorticosterone. Unlike adenomas, adrenal carcinomas with aldosteronism usually show increased 17-ketosteroids and 17-hydroxycorticosteroids, and biosynthesis in vitro of hydrocortisone, cortisone, and corticosterone also is found.

Primary aldosteronism without hypokalemia or an aldosteronoma exists but is uncommon enough that the diagnosis should be questioned. The nature of cases with hyperaldosteronism and one or multiple cortical nodules 0.3 to 0.8 cm in diameter or bilateral hyperplasia is disputed. Conceivably, they represent transitions from adrenocortical hyperplasia to genuine adenomas. In contrast to other functioning adrenocortical neoplasms, the uninvolved homolateral and contralateral zona glomerulosa and zona fasciculata in primary aldosteronism have been reported as atrophic, normal, or hyperplastic.

Hypoaldosteronism as an isolated adult abnormality is also a puzzling condition. Instances have been observed in which an adenoma contained compound S, or with postoperatively recurrent hypercortisolism, prolonged heparin therapy, or excessive licorice ingestion, or as a functional deficiency with orthostatic hypotension. Some cases have accompanied hypopituitarism. Deficient renin secretion, a failure of angiotensin to stimulate aldosterone secretion, and renal tubular unresponsiveness to this hormone have been reported.

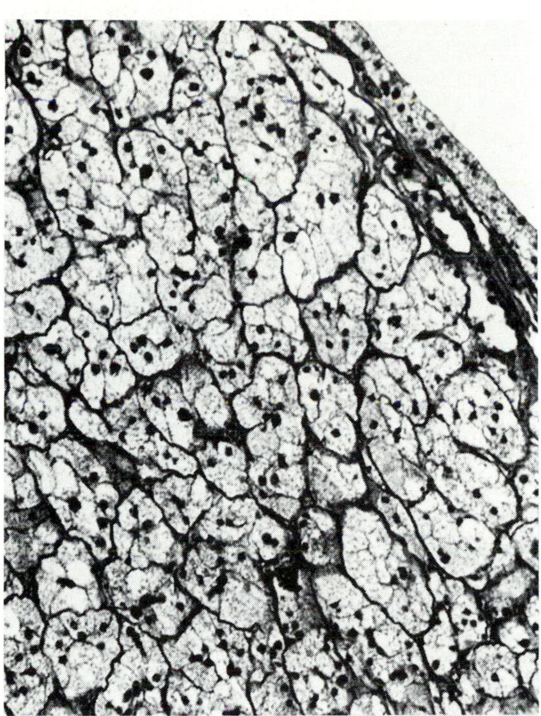

Fig. 35-20. Enlarged lipid-rich cells surrounded by fibrous capsule characterize adrenocortical adenomas, in this instance aldosteronoma. (120×.)

Pigmented adrenocortical adenoma, or so-called black adenoma, is usually without functional significance. Grossly and microscopically the cells contain so much brown pigment that they resemble a melanoma, but special stains demonstrate a periodic acid–Schiff–positive lipochrome like that of the zona reticularis. Rarely, Cushing's syndrome or hyperaldosteronism is associated with a black adenoma (Fig.35-21).

Adrenal carcinomas are distinguished from adenomas by capsular or blood vessel invasion and metastasis. Carcinomas are usually large when first discovered, 7 to 20 cm in diameter, and weigh 100 to 4500 g. Hemorrhage, necrosis, and calcification are more common in adrenal carcinomas than in adenomas (Fig. 35-22). Nuclear atypia, large nucleoli, multinucleated cells, mitoses, and compact acidophilic cells are typical of adrenocortical carcinomas, but demonstrable invasion or metastasis, or both, are necessary for definite diagnosis (Fig. 35-23). Most adrenal carcinomas metastasize widely and cause

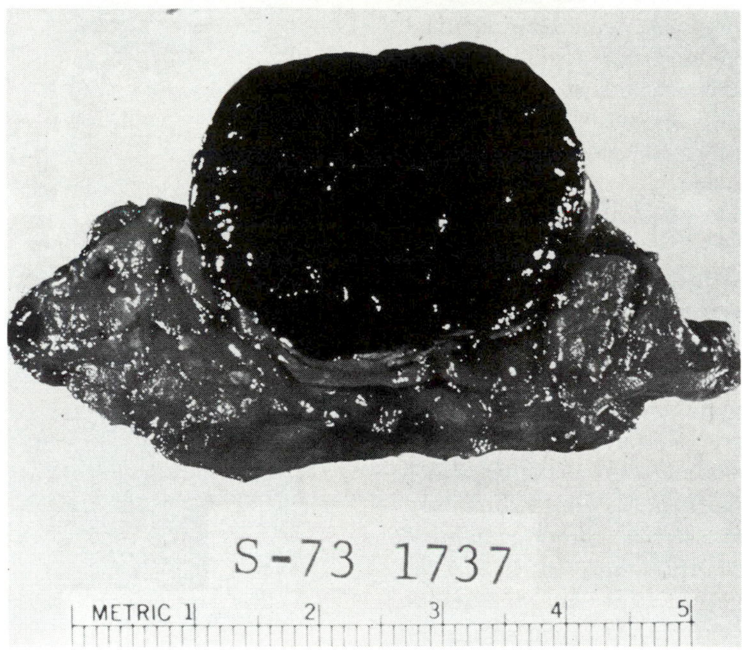

Fig. 35-21. Intense pigmentation of black adrenal adenoma is due to lipochromes. (Courtesy Dr. Mary B. King.)

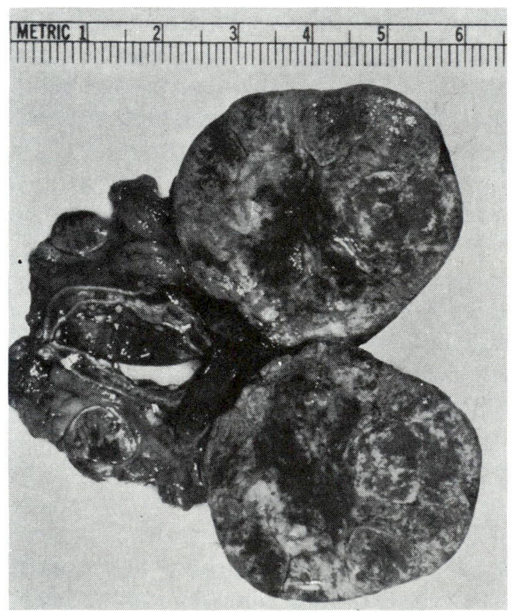

Fig. 35-22. Adrenal carcinoma associated with Cushing's syndrome.

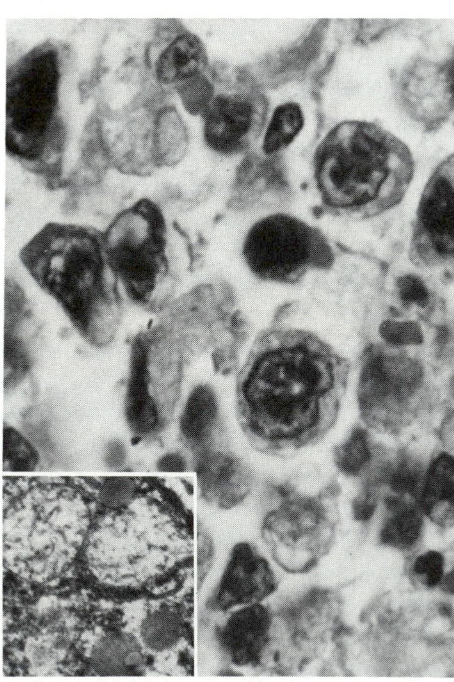

Fig. 35-23. Carcinoma of adrenal cortex. Tumor cells show considerable variation in size, shape, and intensity of staining. (900×.) *Inset,* Cytoplasmic lipid droplets and mitochondria of adrenocortical type. (5080×.)

death. Large anaplastic adrenocortical carcinomas may be difficult to recognize histologically, and the ultrastructural features may aid in their diagnosis (Fig. 35-23, *inset*). Judged from reported cases, about half of adrenal carcinomas are functional. Of these, 50% are associated with combined Cushing's syndrome and virilization, 30% with virilization, 12% with feminization, and 4% with aldosteronism and related conditions. Fever may attract attention to the nonfunctioning type. Some 12 large carcinomas have been observed in association with severe hypoglycemia.

About three fourths of feminizing adrenal neoplasms are carcinomas, and one fourth are adenomas. Most develop in men between 20 and 60 years of age, with bilateral gynecomastia, loss of libido, and atrophy of the testes and penis. Obesity, attributes of Cushing's syndrome, and feminine distribution of body hair may be present. The tumors are not distinguishable histopathologically from other adrenal neoplasms. Estrogen biosynthesis is demonstrable from pregnenolone, progesterone, androstenedione, and testosterone. In women, estrogen-producing adrenal tumors are associated with amenorrhea, hirsutism, and clitoral enlargement. No feminizing adrenocortical hyperplasia is known in adults.

Feminizing and virilizing adrenal neoplasms that arise in extra-adrenal rests are difficult or impossible to distinguish morphologically from Leydig cell tumors, ovarian lipid cell tumors, Sertoli cell type of androblastomas, or luteomas of pregnancy. These primary gonadal tumors are ordinarily virilizing and benign, whereas adrenocortical neoplasms that produce sex hormones are predominantly malignant.

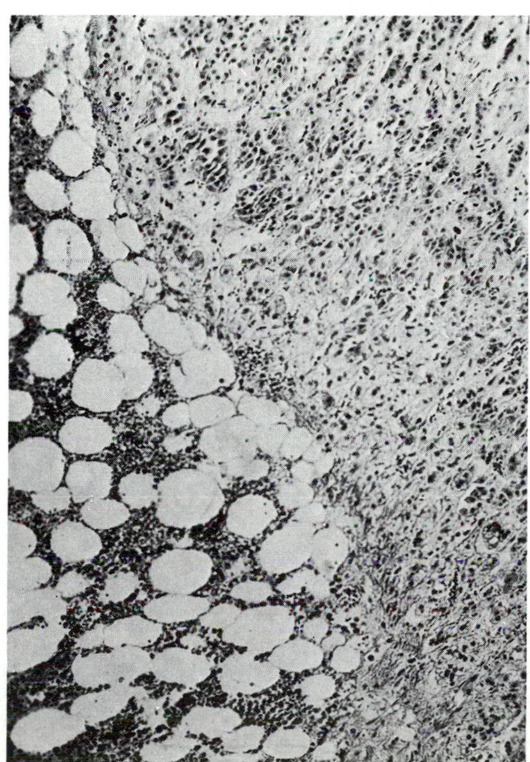

Fig. 35-24. Myelolipoma of adrenal gland. Tissue resembling bone marrow surrounded by adrenal cortex. (100×.)

One adrenal theca-granulosa cell tumor has been described; possibly it arose from ectopic ovarian stroma with thecal metaplasia.

Metastatic cancer in the adrenal glands is often bilateral, with tumors commonly less than 2.5 cm in diameter. Initially the medulla usually is involved. Carcinomas of the lung, particularly of the squamous cell type, form adrenal metastases in one third of cases. Carcinomas of the breast show metastases in 25% of adrenalectomy specimens and 30% at autopsy. Carcinomas of the stomach, large intestine, and pancreas frequently metastasize to the adrenal glands. Also melanomas, renal cell carcinomas, and thyroid carcinomas often spread to the adrenal glands.

Cysts

Aside from rare echinococcal cysts, found in less than 0.5% of patients with echinococcosis, most adrenal cysts are noninflammatory. Pseudocysts lined by fibrous tissue represent residues of remote hematomas or degenerated adenomas. Genuine cysts may be lined by glandular epithelium or by endothelium indicating a cavernous lymphangioma or hemangioma. Angiomas are the largest adrenal cysts, sometimes exceeding 20 cm in diameter. They may have partly calcified walls.

Myelolipoma

Myelolipoma of the adrenal gland is a fatty, gray or red spheroid mass apparently originating in the inner zona fasciculata, usually measuring 0.5 to 6 cm in diameter. One such tumor measuring 25 cm in diameter produced pressure symptoms. Histologically the structure simulates adult hemopoietic bone marrow, with comparable amounts of adipose and myeloid cells (Fig. 35-24). Myelolipomas are not clearly neoplasms and may represent enlarged mesenchymal rests. Sometimes they accompany obesity or bone marrow failure and may occur also in the intercostal spaces and retroperitoneal or pelvic connective tissue. A few have accompanied Cushing's syndrome and contained adrenocortical cells. One woman has been reported with bilateral adrenal tumors composed of brown fat or hibernomas.

Pheochromocytoma and chromaffin paraganglioma

A pheochromocytoma is a medullary adrenal neoplasm that typically secretes epinephrine or norepinephrine or both. Similar extra-adrenal tumors, conventionally termed chromaffin paragangliomas, may be retroperito-

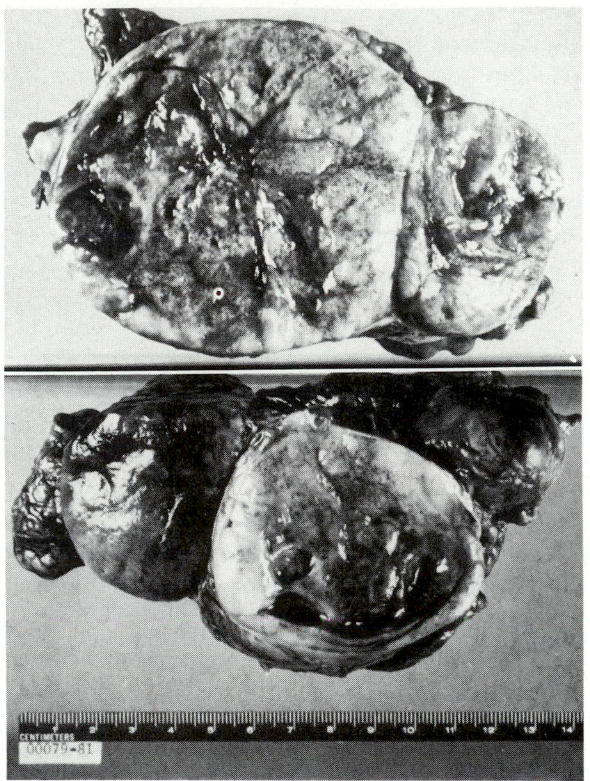

Fig. 35-25. Bilateral pheochromocytomas weighing 428 g on right *(above)* and 260 g on left *(below)*, removed surgically from young woman with MEN type IIA.

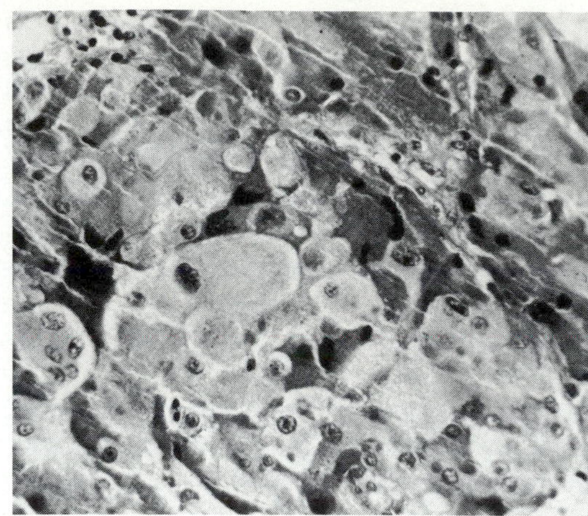

Fig. 35-26. Irregular size and shape of pheochromocytoma cells and nuclei, as well as variable staining of their cytoplasm, are characteristic. Darker-colored cells are brown because of chromaffin reaction. (350×.)

neal, above the aortic bifurcation or celiac in location, attached to the urinary bladder, in the ovary, or within mediastinal, intrathoracic, or intracranial areas. Sporadic pheochromocytomas may be unsuspected and often are found after an elective operation in a patient who develops acute hypertension and subsequent lethal shock under anesthesia. Patients with preoperatively recognized pheochromocytomas have paroxysmal or persistent hypertension, with increased urinary vanillylmandelic acid and other catecholamine metabolites. About two thirds have hyperglycemia ascribable to decreased insulin release, and three fourths are hypermetabolic. Occasionally, diabetes mellitus is cured by removal of a pheochromocytoma.

The tumors vary from incidental microscopic findings to masses over 2 kg in weight, but the average weight is 90 g and the size 5 to 6 cm in diameter. Grossly, pheochromocytomas are rounded, gray or red, and circumscribed and are surrounded by stretched adrenal cortex. Hemorrhages, cystic areas, calcification, or a central dense fibrous scar is common (Fig. 35-25). Chromaffin tests on fresh tissue characteristically color pheochromocytomas dark brown. Occasional tumors containing pure norepinephrine are chromaffin negative; these pheochromocytomas are more common in childhood. Tissue fixed in Helly's or Zenker's fluid demonstrates chromaffinity both grossly and microscopically.

Histologically, pheochromocytomas show notable variability of cell and nuclear size and arrangement. Basic twisted cell cord patterns, basophilic or acidophilic staining, and the presence of fine or coarse intracytoplasmic pigment granules and periodic acid–Schiff–stained secretory droplets aid in making the diagnosis (Fig. 35-26). Ultrastructurally identified epinephrine-containing cytoplasmic granules in pheochromocytomas are larger than in the normal medulla. Similar organelles in neuroblastomas and ganglioneuroblastomas explain their occasionally excessive secretion of catecholamines. Homolateral and contralateral hyperplasia of the predominant pheochromocytoma cell type has been reported. Catecholamines are stored and secreted from osmiophilic cytoplasmic granules. Differentiation from adrenocortical neoplasms may be difficult microscopically (Table 35-1). Adrenocortical adenoma and pheochromocytoma may occur in the same gland. The periadrenal adipose tissue in cases of pheochromocytoma typically has an excess of brown or hibernating fat.

Pheochromocytomas arise from nodular or diffuse adrenal medullary hyperplasia in familial cases. Malignant pheochromocytomas constitute about 6% of all cases. Some are microscopically atypical, more closely resembling neuroblastomas. Others are typical except for gross or microscopic invasion of the periadrenal fat or blood vessels. However, neither gross invasion nor microscopic pleomorphism is a reliable indication of likely recurrence of pheochromocytomas or metastasis, and the metastatic tumor histologically may still appear benign. Multiple benign chromaffin paragangliomas are to be distinguished from malignant pheochromocytoma.

Carney's triad comprises a functioning extra-adrenal paraganglioma, gastric leiomyosarcoma, and pulmonary chondroma (usually in women).

Several syndromes are associated with pheochromocytoma—including von Recklinghausen's neurofibromatosis, von Hippel-Lindau disease and cerebellar hemangioblastoma, Albright's syndrome, multiple mucocutaneous neuromas, and familial multiple endocrine neoplasms such as medullary thyroid carcinoma and hyperparathyroidism caused by parathyroid hyperplasia or adenomas. This last combination is also called Sipple's syndrome, or multiple endocrine neoplasia type II, to distinguish it from multiple adenomas of the pituitary gland, parathyroid glands, and pancreatic islets (type I) and combined papillary thyroid carcinoma and parathyroid adenoma (type III). MEN type IIB has mucosal neuromas, which are absent in type IIA. Pheochromocytomas are bilateral in about half the cases of familial pheochromocytoma, compared with 5% of sporadic cases. Autosomal dominant inheritance appears responsible for familial multiple endocrine neoplasia.

Cushing's syndrome caused by a cortisol-secreting pheochromocytoma has been recognized in about 12 cases, including one intrapancreatic chromaffin paraganglioma. Calcitonin, catecholamines, and cortisol were produced by a single tumor. Ectopic ACTH-producing pheochromocytomas have been reported in seven women.

Malignant melanoma and other adrenal neoplasms

Primary malignant melanoma in the adrenal gland has been recognized in 14 cases. Usually, multiple metastases are present elsewhere. The pigment is identified as melanin, and other possible primary sites are excluded. Neural crest melanoblasts are probably the cells of origin.

Other adrenal neoplasms are usually small benign connective tissue tumors, including neurilemoma, neurofibroma, lipoma, leiomyoma, osteoma, and angioma, as well as mixed mesenchymoma.

REFERENCES

Structure and function

1. Bech, K., Tygstrup, I., and Nerup, J.: The involution of the fetal adrenal cortex, Acta Pathol. Microbiol. Scand. **76**:391, 1969.
2. Black, V.H., et al.: A correlated thin-section and freeze-fracture analysis of guinea pig adrenocortical cells, Am. J. Anat. **156**:453, 1979.
3. Bloodworth, J.M.B., Jr.: The adrenal. In Sommers, S.C., editor: Endocrine pathology decennial 1966-1975, New York, 1975, Appleton-Century-Crofts.
4. Bloodworth, J.M.B., Jr., Horvath, E., and Kovacs, K.: Fine structural pathology of the endocrine system. In Trump, B.F., and Jones, R.T., editors: Diagnostic electron microscopy, vol. 3, New York, 1980, John Wiley & Sons, Inc.,
5. Branchaud, C.T., et al.: Steroidogenic activity of hACTH and related peptides on the human neocortex and fetal adrenal cortex in organ culture, Steroids **31**:557, 1978.
6. Cox, J.N., and Chavrier, F.: Heterotopic adrenocortical tissue within a placenta, Placenta **1**:131, 1980.
7. Gould, V.E., and Sommers, S.C.: Adrenal medulla and paraganglia. In Bloodworth, J.M.B., Jr., editor: Endocrine pathology, ed. 2, Baltimore, 1982, The Williams & Wilkins Co.
8. Gray, E.S., and Abramovich, D.R.: Morphologic features of the anencephalic adrenal gland in early pregnancy, Am. J. Obstet. Gynecol. **137**:491, 1980.
9. Kadair, R.G., et al.: "Masked" 21-hydroxylase deficiency of the adrenal presenting with gynecomastia and bilateral testicular masses, Am. J. Med. **62**:278, 1977.
10. Korth-Schutz, S., et al.: Evidence for the adrenal source of androgen in precocious adrenarche, Acta Endocrinol. **82**:342, 1976.
11. Magalhães, M.C., et al.: Ultrastructural changes in rat adrenal cortical cells after chronic stimulation with β^{1-24}-corticotropin, Cell Tissue Res. **204**:267, 1979.
12. Ryan, U.S., et al.: Fenestrated endothelium of the adrenal gland: freeze-fracture studies, Tissue Cell **7**:181, 1975.
13. Schulz, D.M., Giordano, D.A., and Schulz, D.H.: Weights of organs of fetuses and infants, Arch. Pathol. **74**:244, 1962.
14. Sizonenko, P.C., Paunier, L., and Carmignac, D.: Hormonal changes during puberty, Hormone Res. **7**:288, 1976.
15. Stirling, G.A., and Keating, V.J.: Size of the adrenals in Jamaicans, Br. Med. J. **2**:1016, 1958.
16. Symington, T.: Functional pathology of the adrenal gland, Baltimore, 1969, The Williams & Wilkins Co.
17. Symington, T.: The adrenal cortex. In Bloodworth, J.M.B., Jr., editor: Endocrine pathology, Baltimore, 1981, The Williams & Wilkins Co.
18. Wallace, E.Z., et al.: Endocrine studies in a patient with functioning adrenal rest tumor of the liver, Am. J. Med. **70**:1122, 1981.
19. Wasada, T., et al.: Adrenal contribution to circulating estrogens in woman, Endocrinol. Jpn. **25**:123, 1978.
20. Zoller, L.C., and Malamed, S.: Acute effects of ACTH on dissociated adrenal cells, Anat. Rec. **182**:473, 1975.

Congenital anomalies

21. Bell, J.E.: Fused suprarenal glands in association with central nervous system defects in the first half of foetal life, J. Pathol. **127**:191, 1979.
22. Birnbaum, M.D., and Rose, L.I.: The partial adrenocortical hydroxylase deficiency syndrome in infertile women, Fertil. Steril. **32**:536, 1979.
23. Blankstein, J., et al.: Adult-onset familial adrenal 21-hydroxylase deficiency, Am. J. Med. **68**:441, 1980.
24. Bongiovanni, A.M., et al.: Disorders of adrenal steroid biogenesis, Rec. Prog. Horm. Res. **23**:375, 1967.
25. Bricaire, H., et al.: Hyperandrogénies surrénaliennes par trouble enzymatique à révélation tardive chez la femme, Nouv. Presse Med. **8**:2663, 1979.
26. Favara, B.E., Franciosi, R.A., and Miles, V.: Idiopathic adrenal hypoplasia in children, Am. J. Clin. Pathol. **57**:287, 1972.
27. Feldman, A.E., Rosenthal, R.S., and Shaw, J.L.: Aberrant adrenal tissue, J. Urol. **113**:706, 1975.
28. Filippi, G., and McKusick, V.A.: The Beckwith-Wiedemann syndrome, Medicine **49**:279, 1970.
29. Holmes, L.B.: Inborn errors of morphogenesis, N. Engl. J. Med. **291**:763, 1974.
30. Honoré, L.H., and O'Hara, K.E.: Combined adrenorenal fusion and adrenohepatic adhesion, J. Urol. **115**:323, 1976.
31. Marsden, H.B., and Zakhour, H.D.: Cytomegalic adrenal hypoplasia with pituitary cytomegaly, Virchows Arch. (Pathol. Anat.) **378(2)**:105, 1978.
32. Mininberg, D.T., Levine, L.S., and New, M.I.: Current concepts in congenital adrenal hyperplasia, Invest. Urol. **17**:169, 1979.
33. Mininberg, D.T., Levine, L.S., and New, M.I.: Current concepts in congenital adrenal hyperplasia. Part 2, Pathol. Annu. **17**:179, 1982.
34. Nakamura, Y., Yano, H., and Nakashima, T.: False intranuclear inclusions in adrenal cytomegaly, Arch. Pathol. Lab. Med. **105**:358, 1981.
35. Oppenheimer, E.H.: Cyst formation in the outer adrenal cortex, Arch. Pathol. **87**:653, 1969.

36. Penny, R., Olambiwonnu, N.O., and Frasier, S.D.: Precocious puberty following treatment in a six-year-old male with congenital adrenal hyperplasia, J. Clin. Endocrinol. Metab. **36**:920, 1973.
37. Petersen, K.E., Tygstrup, I., and Thamdrup, E.: Familial adrenocortical hypoplasia with early clinical and biochemical signs of mineralocorticoid deficiency (hypoaldosteronism), Acta Endocrinol. **84**:605, 1977.
38. Rosenwaks, Z., et al.: An attenuated form of congenital virilizing adrenal hyperplasia, J. Clin. Endocrinol. Metab. **49**:335, 1979.
39. Russell, M.A., et al.: Sudden infant death due to congenital adrenal hypoplasia, Arch. Pathol. Lab. Med. **101**:168, 1977.
40. Spark, R.F., and Etzkorn, J.R.: Absent aldosterone response to ACTH in familial glucocorticoid deficiency, N. Engl. J. Med. **297**:917, 1977.
41. Tsutsui, Y., Hirabayashi, N., and Ito, G.: An autopsy case of congenital lipoid hyperplasia of the adrenal cortex, Acta Pathol. Jpn. **20**:227, 1970.
42. Wiener, M.F., and Dallgaard, S.A.: Intracranial adrenal gland, Arch. Pathol. **67**:228, 1959.

Childhood abnormalities

43. Azzarelli, B., et al.: Central neuroblastoma, J. Neuropathol. Exp. Neurol. **36**:384, 1977.
44. Bove, K.E., and McAdams, A.J.: Composite ganglioneuroblastoma. Arch. Pathol. Lab. Med. **105**:325, 1981.
45. Cheatham, W.J., et al.: Varicella, Am. J. Pathol. **32**:1015, 1956.
46. Coates, P.M., et al.: Prenatal diagnosis of Wolman's disease, Am. J. Med. Genet. **2**:397, 1978.
47. Davis, L.E., et al.: Adrenoleukodystrophy and adrenomyeloneuropathy with partial adrenal insufficiency, Am. J. Med. **66**:342, 1979.
48. deBaecque, C.M., Pollack, M.A., and Suzuki, K.: Late infantile neuronal storage disease with curvilinear bodies, Arch. Pathol. Lab. Med. **100**:139, 1976.
49. Forsyth, C.C., Forber, M., and Cummings, J.N.: Adrenocortical atrophy and diffuse cerebral sclerosis, Arch. Dis. Child. **46**:273, 1971.
50. Hawkins, E., and Singer, D.B.: The adrenal cortex in cystic fibrosis of the pancreas, Am. J. Clin. Pathol. **66**:710, 1976.
51. Kramer, S.A., Bradford, W.D., and Anderson, E.E.: Bilateral adrenal neuroblastoma, Cancer **45**:2208, 1980.
52. Meador, C.K., et al.: Primary adrenocortical nodular dysplasia: a rare cause of Cushing's syndrome, J. Clin. Endocrinol. Metab. **27**:1255, 1967.
53. Naeye, R.L.: Brain-stem and adrenal abnormalities in the sudden-infant-death syndrome, Am. J. Clin. Pathol. **66**:526, 1976.
54. Neville, A.M., and Symington, T.: Bilateral adrenocortical hyperplasia in children with Cushing's syndrome, J. Pathol. **107**:95, 1972.
55. Pegelow, C.H., et al.: Familial neuroblastoma, J. Pediatr. **87**:763, 1975.
56. Powers, J.M., and Schaumburg, H.H.: The testis in adreno-leukodystrophy, Am. J. Pathol. **102**:90, 1981.
57. Powers, J.M., et al.: A correlative study of the adrenal cortex in adrenoleukodystrophy, Invest. Cell. Pathol. **3**:353, 1980.
58. Reynolds, C.P., et al.: Catecholamine fluorescence and tissue culture morphology, Am. J. Clin. Pathol. **75**:275, 1981.
59. Rosen, P.P.: Cytomegalovirus infection in cancer patients, Pathol. Annu. **13(2)**:175, 1978.
60. Rudd, B.T., Chance, G.W., and Theodoridis, C.G.: Adrenal response to ACTH in patients with Prader-Willi syndrome, simple obesity, and constitutional dwarfism, Arch. Dis. Child. **44**:244, 1969.
61. Templeton, A.C.: Generalized herpes simplex in malnourished children, J. Clin. Pathol. **23**:24, 1970.
62. Van Hale, H.M., and Turkel, S.B.: Neuroblastoma and adrenal morphologic features in anencephalic infants, Arch. Pathol. Lab. Med. **103**:119, 1979.
63. Wilkerson, J.A., Van De Water, J.M., and Goepfert, H.: Role of embryonic induction in benign transformation of neuroblastomas, Cancer **20**:1335, 1967.

Hemorrhage and necrosis

64. Fox, B. Venous infarction of the adrenal glands, J. Pathol. **119**:65, 1976.
65. Greendyke, R.M.: Adrenal hemorrhage. Am. J. Clin. Pathol. **43**:210, 1965.
66. Joseph, T.J., and Vogt, P.J.: Disseminated herpes with hepatoadrenal necrosis in an adult, Am. J. Med. **56**:735, 1974.
67. Kaufman, G.: Adrenal cortical necrosis, Arch. Pathol. **97**:395, 1974.
68. Kerr, J.F.R.: Shrinkage necrosis, J. Pathol. **107**:217, 1972.
69. McGovern, V.J., and Tiller, D.J.: Adrenal necrosis and hemorrhage. In Shock, New York, 1980, Masson Publishing, Inc.
70. Smith, J.A., Jr., and Middleton, R.G.: Neonatal adrenal hemorrhage, J. Urol. **122**:674, 1979.
71. Xarli, V.P., et al.:: Adrenal hemorrhage in the adult, Medicine **57**:211, 1978.

Inflammation, atrophy, and Addison's disease

72. Arvanitakis, C., and Knouss, R.F.: Selective hypopituitarism, impaired cell-mediated immunity, and chronic mucocutaneous candidiasis, J.A.M.A. **225**:1492, 1973.
73. DeLellis, R.A., et al.: Adrenal medullary hyperplasia, Am. J. Pathol. **83**:177, 1976.
74. Dixon, R.B., and Christy, N.P.: On the various forms of corticosteroid withdrawal syndrome, Am. J. Med. **68**:224, 1980.
75. Griffel, B.: Focal adrenalitis, Virchows Arch. (Pathol. Anat.) **364**:191, 1974.
76. Irvine, W.J., and Barnes, E.W.: Addison's disease, ovarian failure, and hypoparathyroidism, Clin. Endocrine Metab. **4**:379, 1975.
77. Modhi, G., Bauman, W., and Nicolis, G.: Adrenal failure associated with hypothalamic and adrenal metastases, Cancer **47**:2098, 1981.
78. Nathan, C., et al.: Insuffisance surrénale et histoplasmose, Ann. Endocrinol. **32**:588, 1971.
79. Nerup, J.: Addison's disease, Dan. Med. Bull. **21**:201, 1974.
80. Neufeld, M., et al.: Islet cell and other organ-specific autoantibodies in U.S. caucasians and blacks with insulin-dependent diabetes mellitus, Diabetes **29**:589, 1980.
81. Sinclair-Smith, C., Kahn, L.B., and Cywes S: Malacoplakia in childhood, Arch. Pathol. **99**:198, 1975.
82. Slavin, R.E.: Late generalized tuberculosis, Pathol. Annu. **16(1)**:81, 1981.
83. Uei, Y., and Takahashi, Y.: An autopsy case of Schmidt's syndrome, Acta Pathol. Jpn. **20**:215, 1970.

Degenerations and infiltrations, cortical nodularity

84. Dekker, A., and Oehrle, J.S.: Hyaline globules of the adrenal medulla of man, Arch. Pathol. **91**:353, 1971.
85. Dobbie, J.W.: Adrenocortical nodular hyperplasia: the ageing adrenal, J. Pathol. **99**:1, 1969.
86. Hiraoka, K., et al.: A clinicopathological study on relationship of the focal hyperplasia of adrenal cortex to hypertension and arteriosclerosis in the aged, Jpn. Heart J. **12**:450, 1971.
87. Kovacs, K., Korvath, E., and Singer, W.: Fine structure and morphogenesis of spironolactone bodies in the zona glomerulosa of the human adrenal, J. Clin. Pathol. **26**:949, 1973.
88. Rodin, A.L., Hsu, F.L., and Whorton, E.B.: Microcysts of the permanent adrenal cortex in perinates and infants, Arch. Pathol. Lab. Med. **100**:499, 1976.
89. Sommers, S.C., and Carter, M.: Adrenocortical postirradiation fibrosis, Arch. Pathol. **99**:421, 1975.
90. Sugihara, H., Kawai, K., and Tsuchiyama, H.: Pathology of intracortical nodules in rat adrenal glands, especially on their finestructure, Acta Pathol. Jpn. **23**:253, 1973.
91. Tchertkoff, V., Salomon, M.I., and Garret, R.: Adrenal tumours and hypertension, Br. Med. J.**2**:444, 1975.
92. Wilbur, O.M., Jr., and Rich, A.R.: Study of role of adrenocorticotropic hormone (ACTH) in pathogenesis of tubular degeneration of adrenals, Bull. Johns Hopkins Hosp. **93**:321, 1953.

Hyperplasia, Cushing's syndrome, and adrenal virilism

93. Baer, L., Sommers, S.C., and Krakoff, L.R.: Pseudoprimary aldosteronism, Circ. Res. **27**(suppl. 1):203, 1970.

94. Boyar, R.M., and Hellman, L.: Syndrome of benign nodular adrenal hyperplasia with feminization and hyperprolactinemia, Ann. Intern. Med. **80**:389, 1974.
95. Hidai, H., et al.: Cushing's syndrome caused by multiple nodular hyperplasia of the adrenal cortex, Endocrinol. Jpn. **22**:555, 1975.
96. Horvath, E., et al.: Leydig-like cells in the adrenals of a woman with ectopic ACTH syndrome, Hum. Pathol. **11**:284, 1980.
97. Marek, J., and Motlik, K.: Ultrastructural changes of the adrenal cortex in Cushing's syndrome treated with aminoglutethimide (Elipten Ciba), Virchows Arch. (Cell Pathol.) **18**:145, 1975.
98. McArthur, R.G., et al.: Cushing's disease in children, Mayo Clin. Proc. **47**:318, 1972.
99. Migeon, C.E.: Adrenal androgens in man, Am. J. Med. **53**:606, 1972.
100. Raux, M.C., et al.: Studies of ACTH control in 116 cases of Cushing's syndrome, J. Clin. Endocrinol. Metab. **40**:186, 1975.
101. Schäfer, A., and Schnabel, K.H.: Zur Ultrastruktur der Nebennierenrinde bei Cushing-Syndrom ohne und mit Hyperaldosteronismus, Endokrinologie **65**:22, 1975.
102. Sober, A.J., et al.: Visceromegaly in acromegaly, Arch. Intern. Med. **134**:415, 1974.
103. Sommers, S.C.: Endocrine activities of tumors. In Bloodworth, J.M.B., Jr., editor: Endocrine pathology, ed. 2, Baltimore, 1982, The Williams & Wilkins Co.
104. Tască, C., and Stefăneanu, L.: Ultrastructural pathology of the adrenal gland in Cushing's syndrome, Endocrinologie **17**:157, 1979.
105. Tazaki, H., Murai, M., and Baba, S.: Human adrenal tumors and hyperplasias in vitro, Invest. Urol. **11**:288, 1974.
106. Thorn, G.W., and Lauler, D.P.: Clinical therapeutics of adrenal disorders, Am. J. Med. **53**:673, 1972.
107. Visser, J.W., and Axt, R.: Bilateral adrenal medullary hyperplasia, J. Clin. Pathol. **28**:298, 1975.

Neoplasms

Adenomas, primary aldosteronism, and carcinoma

108. Aiba, M., et al.: Enzyme histochemical and electron microscopic study of a virilizing adrenocortical adenoma, Acta Pathol. Jpn. **28**:615, 1978.
109. Aiba, M. et al.: Spironolactone bodies in aldosteronomas and in the attached adrenals, Am. J. Pathol. **103**:404, 1981.
110. Bahn, R.M., Battifora, H., and Shambaugh, G., III: Functional black adenoma of the adrenal gland, Arch. Pathol. **98**:139, 1974.
111. Blau, N., et al.: Spontaneous remission of Cushing's syndrome in a patient with an adrenal adenoma, J. Clin. Endocrinol. Metab. **40**:659, 1975.
112. Brown, J.J., et al.: Hypertension with aldosterone excess, Br. Med. J. **2**:391, 1972.
113. Caplan, R.H., and Virata, R.L.: Functional black adenoma of the adrenal cortex, Am. J. Clin. Pathol. **62**:97, 1974.
114. Cedermark, B.J., et al.: The significance of metastases to the adrenal glands in adenocarcinoma of the colon and rectum, Surg. Gynecol. Obstet. **144**:537, 1977.
115. Cedermark, B.J., et al.: The significance of metastases to the adrenal glands from carcinoma of the stomach and esophagus, Surg. Gynecol. Obstet. **145**:41, 1977.
116. Check, J.H., Rakoff, A.E., and Roy, B.K.: A testosterone-secreting adrenal adenoma, Obstet. Gynecol. **51**(suppl. 1):46s, 1978.
117. Clinicopathologic Conference: Hirsutism progressing to virilization in an older woman, Am. J. Med. **70**:1255, 1981.
118. Conn, J.W., Knopf, R.F., and Nesbit, R.M.: Clinical characteristics of primary aldosteronism from an analysis of 145 cases, Am. J. Surg **107**:159, 1964.
119. Didolkar, M.S., et al.: Natural history of adrenal cortical carcinoma, Cancer **47**:2153, 1981.
120. Fang, V.S., Furuhashi, N., and Gomez, O.: Human prolactin stimulates estrogen production by feminizing adrenal neoplastic cells, Proc. Soc. Exp. Biol. Med. **157**:159, 1978.
121. Fidler, W.J.: Ovarian thecal metaplasia in adrenal glands, Am. J. Clin. Pathol. **67**:318, 1977.
122. Gorgas, K., Böck, P., and Wuketich, S.: Fine structure of a virilizing adrenocortical adenoma, Beitr. Pathol. **159**:371, 1976.
123. Gross, M.D., et al.: Suppression of aldosterone by cyproheptadine in idiopathic aldosteronism, N. Engl. J. Med. **305**:181, 1981.
124. Guthrie, G.P., and Kotchen, T.A.: Hypertension and aldosterone overproduction without renin suppression in Cushing's syndrome from an adrenal adenoma, Am. J. Med. **67**:524, 1979.
125. Harrison, J.H., Mahoney, E.M., and Bennett, A.H.: Tumors of the adrenal cortex, Cancer **32**:1227, 1973.
126. Hogan, M.J., Schambelan, M., and Biglieri, E.G.: Concurrent hypercortisolism and hypermineralocorticoidism, Am. J. Med. **62**:777, 1977.
127. Hogan, T.F., et al.: A clinical and pathological study of adrenocortical carcinoma, Cancer **45**:2880, 1980.
128. Hough, A.J., et al.: Prognostic factors in adrenal cortical tumors, Am. J. Clin. Pathol. **72**:390, 1979.
129. Howard, C.P., Takahashi, H., and Hayles, A.B.: Feminizing adrenal adenoma in a boy, Mayo Clin. Proc. **52**:354, 1977.
130. Hsu, S.M., Raine, L., and Martin, H.F.: Spironolactone bodies, Am. J. Clin. Pathol. **75**:92, 1981.
131. Kano, K.I., and Sato, S.: Fine structure of adrenal adenomata causing Cushing's syndrome, Virchows Arch. (Pathol. Anat.) **374**:157, 1977.
132. King, D.R., and Lack, E.E.: Adrenal cortical carcinoma, Cancer **44**:239, 1979.
133. Komiya, I., et al.: Concurrent hypersecretion of aldosterone and cortisol from the adrenal cortical adenoma, Am. J. Med. **67**:516, 1979.
134. Kovacs, K., et al.: Ultrastructural features of an aldosterone-secreting adrenocortical adenoma, Horm. Res. **5**:47, 1974.
135. Krolner, B., Larsen, S., and Damkjaer Nielsen, M.: Corticosterone-secreting adrenal carcinoma and empty sella turcica, Acta Endocrinol. **91**:650, 1979.
136. Lewinsky, B.S., et al.: The clinical and pathologic features of "non-hormonal" adrenocortical tumors, Cancer **33**:778, 1974.
137. Longo, D.L., et al.: Pathology of the adrenal gland in refractory low-renin hypertension, Arch. Pathol. Lab. Med. **102**:322, 1978.
138. Matsukura, S., et al.: Multiple hormone receptors in the adenylate cyclase of human adrenocortical tumors, Cancer Res. **40**:3768, 1980.
139. McKenna, J., Miller, A.B., and Liddle, G.H.: Plasma pregnenolone and 17-hydroxy-pregnenolone in patients with adrenal tumors, ACTH excess, or idiopathic hirsutism, J. Clin. Endocrinol. Metab. **44**:231, 1977.
140. Mitschke, H., and Saeger, W.: Zur Ultrastruktur der atrophischen Nebennierenrinde bei dissoziierter, sekundärer Nebennierenrindeninsuffizienz, Virchows Arch. (Pathol. Anat.) **361**:217, 1973.
141. Mitschke, H., Saeger, W., and Breustedt, H.J.: Zur Ultrastruktur der Nebennierenrindentumoren beim Cushing-Syndrom, Virchows Arch (Pathol. Anat.) **360**:253, 1973.
142. O'Hare, M.J., Monaghan, P., and Neville, A.M.: The pathology of adrenocortical neoplasia, Hum. Pathol. **10**:137, 1979.
143. Onuigbo, W.B.: Human model for studying seed-soil factors in blood-borne metastasis, Arch. Pathol. **99**:342, 1975.
144. Orselli, R.C., and Bassler, T.J.: Theca granulosa cell tumor arising in adrenal, Cancer **31**:474, 1973.
145. Rizza, R.A., et al.: Visualization of nonfunctioning adrenal adenomas with iodocholesterol, J. Nucl. Med. **19**:458, 1978.
146. Saeger, W., and Mitschke, H.: Morphology of adrenal and ovarian tumors with androgen excess, Acta Endocrinol. **87**(suppl. 215): 47, 1978.
147. Sasano, N., Ojima, M., and Masuda, T.: Endocrinologic pathology of functional adrenocortical tumors, Pathol. Annu. **15**:105, 1980.
148. Schteingart, D.E., et al.: Virilizing syndrome associated with an adrenal cortical adenoma secreting predominantly testosterone, Am. J. Med. **67**:140, 1979.
149. Sommers, S.C., and Terzakis, J.A.: Ultrastructural study of aldosterone-secreting cells of the adrenal cortex, Am. J. Clin. Pathol. **54**:303, 1970.
150. Sultan, C., et al.: Pubertal gynecomastia due to an estrogen-producing adrenal adenoma, J. Pediatr. **95**:744, 1979.

151. Takahashi, H., et al.: A gonadotrophin-responsive virilizing adrenal tumor identified as a mixed ganglioneuroma and adrenocortical adenoma, Acta Endocrinol. **89**:701, 1978.
152. Tan, S.-Y., et al.: Steroid profile in a case of adrenal carcinoma with severe hypertension, Am. J. Clin. Pathol. **67**:591, 1977.
153. Tang, C.-K., Harriman, B.B., and Toker, C.: Myxoid adrenal cortical carcinoma, Arch. Pathol. Lab. Med. **103**:635, 1979.
154. Tannenbaum, M.: Ultrastructural pathology of the adrenal cortex. In Sommers, S.C., Pathology decennial 1966-1975, New York, 1975, Appleton-Century-Crofts.
155. Valente, M., et al.: Androgen producing adrenocortical carcinoma, Virchows Arch. (Pathol. Anat.) **378**:91, 1978.
156. Vetter, H., et al.: Aldosteron im Nebennierenvenenblut beim primären Aldosteronismus, Schweiz. Med. Wochenschr. **109**:1890, 1979.
157. Visser, J.W., Boeijinga, K.D., and Meer, C.V.: A functioning black adenoma of the adrenal cortex, J. Clin. Pathol. **27**:955, 1974.
158. Wenting, G.J., et al.: ACTH-dependent aldosterone excess due to adrenocortical adenoma, J. Clin. Endocrinol. Metab. **46**:326, 1978.
159. Wirth, T., et al.: Feminisierendes Nebennierenrindenkarzinom bei einem 66 jährigen Manne, Schweiz. Med. Wochenschr. **107**:411, 1977.
160. Wong. T.-W., and Warner, N.E.: Ovarian thecal metaplasia in the adrenal gland, Arch. Pathol. **92**:319, 1971.

Cysts, myelolipoma

161. Babin, J.-P., et al.: Les kystes de la surrénale chez le nouveau-né, Arch. Fr. Pediatr. **4**:130, 1977.
162. Bennett, B.D., et al.: Adrenal myelolipoma associated with Cushing's disease, Am. J. Clin. Pathol. **73**:443, 1980.
163. Boudreaux, D., et al.: Giant adrenal myelolipoma and testicular interstitial cell tumor in a man with congenital 21-hydroxylase deficiency, Am. J. Surg. Pathol. **3**:109, 1979.
164. Damjanov, I., et al.: Myelolipoma in a heterotopic adrenal gland, Cancer **44**:1350, 1979.
165. Ghandur-Mnaymneh, L., et al.: Adrenal cysts, J. Urol. **122**:87, 1979.
166. Incze, J.S., et al.: Morphology and pathogenesis of adrenal cysts, Am. J. Pathol. **95**:423, 1979.
167. Rubin, H.B., Hirose, F., and Benfield, J.R.: Myelolipoma of the adrenal gland, Am. J. Surg. **130**:354, 1975.

Pheochromocytoma, other neoplasms

168. Carney, J.A., Sizemore, G.W., and Sheps, S.G.: Adrenal medullary disease in multiple endocrine neoplasia, Type 2, Am. J. Clin. Pathol. **66**:279, 1976.
169. Chander, S., et al.: Triad of neoplasms (paraganglioma, gastric sarcoma, chondroma), N.Y. State J. Med. **81**:392, 1981.
170. Forman, B.H., et al.: Ectopic ACTH syndrome due to pheochromocytoma, Yale J. Biol. Med. **52**:181, 1979.
171. Kameya, T., et al.: Morphologic and functional aspects of hormone-producing tumors, Pathol. Annu. **15**:350, 1980.
172. Kamiyama, R., et al.: Malignant pheochromocytoma arising in the organ of Zuckerkandl, Acta Pathol. Jpn. **28**:731, 1978.
173. Kissel, P., et al.: Tumeur surrénalienne complexe bilatérale au cours d'un syndrome d'Albright, J. Genet. Hum. **23**(suppl.):223, 1975.
174. Lips, C.J.M., et al.: Evidence of multicentric origin of the multiple endocrine neoplasia syndrome type 2A (Sipple's syndrome) in a large family in the Netherlands, Am. J. Med. **64**:569, 1978.
175. Lips, C.J.M., et al.: Bilateral occurrence of pheochromocytoma in patients with the multiple endocrine neoplasia syndrome type 2A (Sipple's syndrome), Am. J. Med. **70**:1051, 1981.
176. Mackay, B., and Silva, E.G.: Diagnostic electron microscopy in oncology, Pathol. Annu. **15**:241, 1980.
177. Rothberg, M., et al.: Adrenal hemangiomas, Radiology **126**:341, 1978.
178. Sasidharan, K., et al.: Primary melanoma of the adrenal gland, J. Urol. **117**:663, 1977.
179. Shamsuddin, A.M., et al.: Multifocal malignant pheochromocytoma presenting as a lung tumor, Hum. Pathol. **12**:475, 1981.
180. Sutton, M.G., Sheps, S.G., and Lie, J.T.: Prevalence of clinically unsuspected pheochromocytoma, Mayo Clin. Proc. **56**:354, 1981.

CHAPTER 36 Female Genitalia

FREDERICK T. KRAUS

Abnormalities and diseases of the female genitalia have been the object of fascination for centuries and the basis for one of the oldest medical specialties. An abnormal external physical appearance may provide clues to significant underlying malformations, some of which are life threatening. The genital tract is the portal of entry for infectious diseases of remarkable variety with far-reaching effects on the patient and sometimes on her progeny. Neoplasms of the female genitalia are unsurpassed for bizarre appearance and variety of systemic effects and size; they also represent the second most common source of fatal cancer in women. Many insights into the biology of infections and neoplasms are afforded by a study of these conditions; the correct application of principles of prevention and treatment of these diseases may offer a greater prospect for relief of suffering and extension of life than is possible in any other area of the body.

EMBRYOLOGY OF FEMALE GENITAL TRACT

Knowledge of the anatomic changes in the early development of the female genitalia is helpful in understanding various pathologic conditions. Some malformations become recognizable as a failure in the completion of a developmental sequence. There is a close relationship between primitive urinary and genital structures, so that malformations often affect both systems, sometimes in predictable ways. For instance, recognition of ambiguous sexual differentiation of the vulva may be the first evidence of the potentially fatal, but curable, adrenogenital syndrome. Finally, the histologic similarities in neoplasms are understandable in terms of the embryologic relationships that form the basis of their classification. A brief summary of female genital tract embryology is supplied as a basis for such an understanding; for more detailed descriptions see standard texts.[10]

Genital ridges and müllerian ducts

With the exception of the germ cells, the internal genitalia arise from the mesoderm (celomic epithelium and adjacent mesenchyme) of the posterior body wall. Bilateral urogenital ridges are formed parallel to the body axis. In a 6 mm embryo (about 5 weeks old) each of these has become segregated longitudinally into a lateral mesonephric ridge and a medial genital ridge (Fig. 36-1).

By the end of the sixth week the primitive gonad is represented by proliferating surface epithelial cells and an inner blastema of loose mesenchymal cells. A lateral groove forms in the surface epithelium of each urogenital ridge, rolls inward, and closes to form the müllerian (paramesonephric) duct on each side. The cranial ends remain open and eventually become the fimbriated open ends of the uterine tubes. The caudal ends burrow medially in front of the mesonephric ducts and farther caudad toward the urogenital sinus. The point at which they end in the dorsomedial aspect of the urogenital sinus is transiently marked by a swelling, Müller's tubercle. The distal ends of the müllerian ducts fuse to become the uterus, cervix, and upper vagina. The myometrium and endometrial stroma differentiate from the surrounding mesenchyme (Fig. 36-2).

In a 60 mm embryo the ovary is suspended by its mesovarium from the ventral surface of the mesonephros, which is still prominent (Fig. 36-3). The mesonephric ducts are functional at this time and pass into the urogenital sinus through the lateral walls of the developing myometrium.

Differentiation of ovary

Each ovarian blastema is covered by a surface layer of celomic epithelium, closely related but not identical to the cells that form the müllerian ducts. Perhaps because of this close relationship in early development, the adenocarcinomas that arise from ovarian surface epithelium closely resemble typical adenocarcinomas of the tube, endometrium, cervix, and vagina. As a result of this similarity of patterns, it has become customary to regard the common ovarian epithelial neoplasms as müllerian, even though the ovary does not actually form from the müllerian duct. The advantage of conceptual understanding overshadows the sacrifice of conformity to rigid embryologic fact. Pelvic mesothelium and underlying mesenchyme also maintain the capacity to generate, rarely, primary epithelial and stromal neoplasms identical to those of the uterus, tubes, and ovaries.[31]

The germ cells originate in the yolk sac endoderm near the hindgut, move through the primitive hindgut mesentery, and finally settle in the blastemas of the primitive ovaries.[21] The segregation of an occasional straggler along the way may explain some retroperitoneal germ cell tumors and the development of heterotopic ovarian tissue along the trail of this migration. This migration is completed by the tenth week. The germ cells begin to proliferate by mitosis on arrival, notably after the eighth week; by the twelfth week some begin the first meiotic division. At birth, germ cell mitosis has ceased, and most ova, at this time called oogonia, are in the dictyotene stage of meiosis. The adjacent stromal cells differentiate into a single layer of flattened granulosa cells, forming a primary follicle. The granulosa cells proliferate; a cavity, the antrum, appears, forming a graafian follicle; follicles may be numerous and some are large at birth. The ovaries descend into the pelvis attached to connective tissue strands, the gubernacula, which will become the medial ovarian ligaments and the round ligaments, extending from the uterine horns to the labia majora.

Differentiation of müllerian ducts

The separate proximal portions of the müllerian ducts develop into the uterine (fallopian) tubes. The fused middle and distal portions complete their merger by the twelfth week, forming the uterus and upper part of the vagina, respectively. The myometrium differentiates from the surrounding mesenchyme, enveloping the adjacent segments of the withering mesonephric ducts.

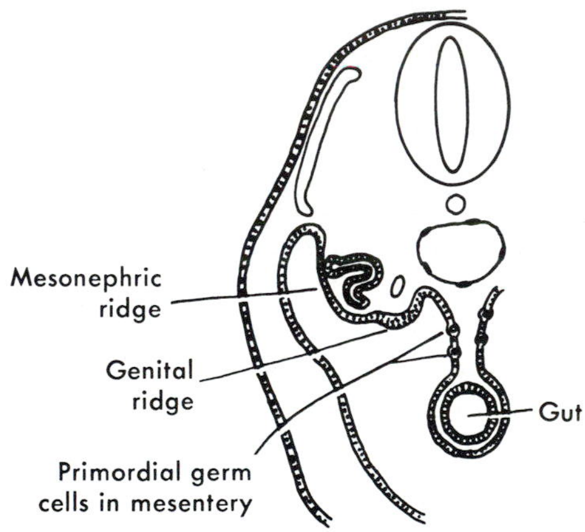

Fig. 36-1. Diagrammatic cross section of 6 mm embryo showing migrating germ cells, genital ridge, and mesonephros. (From Kraus, F.T.: Gynecologic pathology, St. Louis, 1967, The C.V. Mosby Co.)

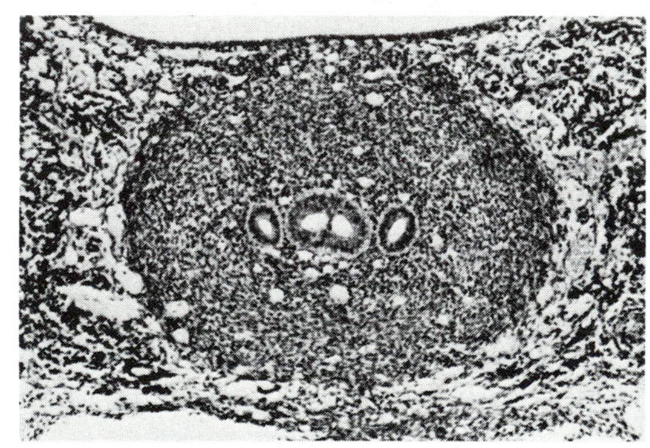

Fig. 36-2. Cross section of uterine anlage of 60 mm embryo. Müllerian ducts have nearly fused at center. Mesonephric ducts are situated on each side. Peritoneum of cul-de-sac is at top. (150×; from Kraus, F.T.: Gynecologic pathology, St. Louis, 1967, The C.V. Mosby Co.)

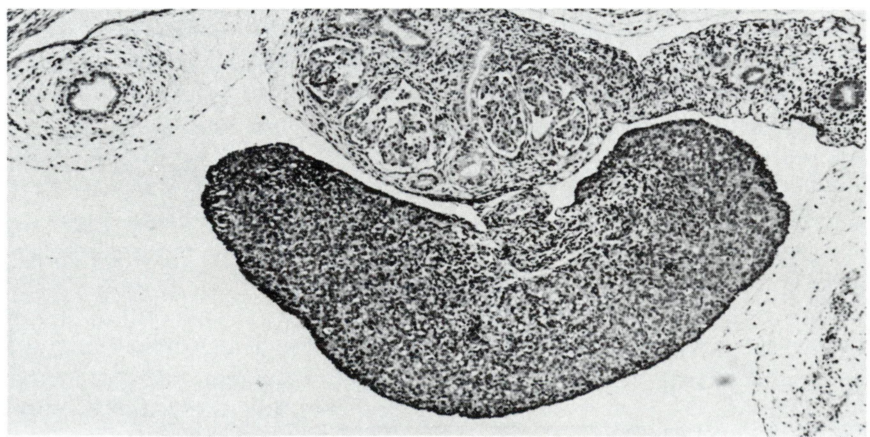

Fig. 36-3. Transverse section of ovary and adjacent mesonephros. Mesonephric glomeruli persist at this 60 mm stage. (90×; from Kraus, F.T.: Gynecologic pathology, St. Louis, 1967, The C.V. Mosby Co.)

Between the eighth and eleventh weeks the primitive vagina is a solid cord of epithelial cells ending distally in the urogenital sinus at Müller's tubercle. Evaginations of the urogenital sinus on either side of Müller's tubercle enlarge, fuse, and merge to form the hymen and distal vaginal wall. The lining of the vagina is formed by proliferation of epithelial cells from the dorsum of the urogenital sinus, extending craniad toward the cervix, which is lined by simple columnar epithelium. This process occurs between the twelfth and eighteenth weeks, which is a crucial period for female infants exposed in utero to the drug diethylstilbestrol and its derivatives.

Differentiation of vulva

The primitive hindgut, urinary ducts, and genital ducts all empty into a common chamber, the cloaca. By the sixth week the urorectal septum has formed as a transverse ridge separating the urogenital sinus and rectum. Müller's tubercle moves progressively caudad. The urinary bladder forms from the allantois, so that the müllerian and urinary orifices empty as separate orifices into the shallow remains of the urogenital sinus, now the vestibule of the vulva (Figs. 36-4 and 36-5).

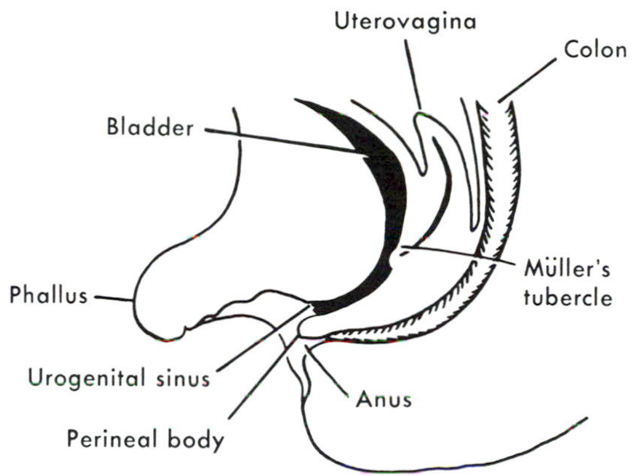

Fig. 36-4. Diagrammatic sagittal section showing relationship between urinary bladder, urogenital sinus, and Müller's tubercle. Age is approximately 10 weeks. (Redrawn from Arey, L.B.: Developmental anatomy, ed. 6, Philadelphia, 1954, W.B. Saunders Co.)

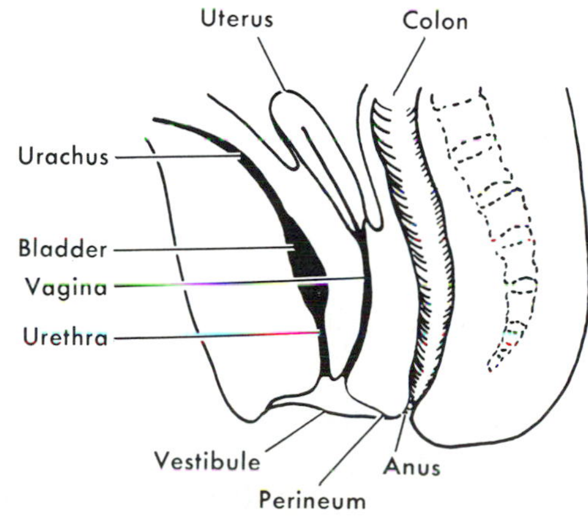

Fig. 36-5. Caudad growth of perineum and urovaginal septum separates bladder and vagina and enlarges separation between vulvar vestibule and anus. (Redrawn from Arey, L.B.: Developmental anatomy, ed. 6, Philadelphia, 1954, W.B. Saunders Co.)

The development of the vulva begins at a sexually indeterminate stage.[28] At about 36 days (9 mm) the external structures are represented by a genital tubercle (a conic anterior midline protuberance) and the labioscrotal swellings (two broad lateral elevations located just caudad to the genital tubercle on either side of the cloacal groove) (Fig. 36-6). The cloacal groove at first is closed by the cloacal membrane. After the urorectal septum grows down to meet it, the cloacal membrane becomes divided into an anterior urogenital groove, closed by the urogenital membrane, and a posterior anal membrane. The urogenital membrane disintegrates at about 42 days; a glans becomes evident on the genital tubercle in the 46-day-old (19 mm embryo). The urogenital groove extends anteriorly on the caudal aspect of the phallus thus formed. A sexual distinction is made evident by the urethral groove, which extends onto the phallus from the urogenital groove; the urethral groove extends distally onto the glans in the male but not in the female. This distinction is probably not a reliable indicator of sex until after the eleventh week (50 mm). The urethral folds lateral to the urethral groove fuse to form the male penile urethra; they persist as separate structures, the labia minora, in the female. The labioscrotal swellings enlarge to form the labia majora; they fuse posteriorly at the posterior commissure at about 50 mm. In the 4-month-old (100 mm) embryo the prepuce forms around the glans of the clitoris.

The most significant events in the embryology of the female genital tract are summarized in Table 36-1. This timetable of development is useful in relating malformations to possible teratogenic events such as maternal infection with a virus or exposure to a teratogenic drug.

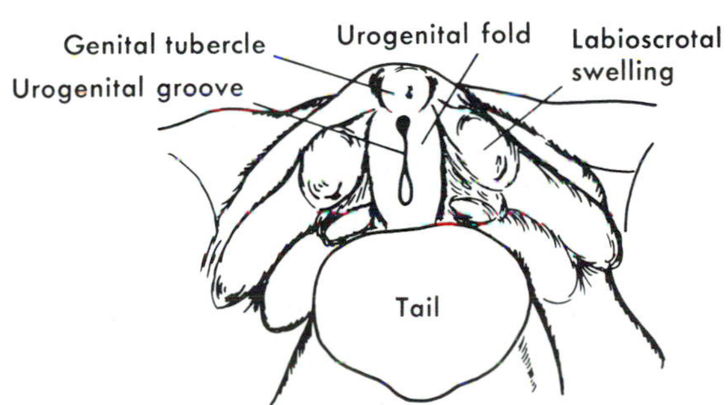

Fig. 36-6. External genitalia at about 7 weeks are sexually indeterminate. (Redrawn from Arey, L.B.: Developmental anatomy, ed. 6, Philadelphia, 1954, W.B. Saunders Co.)

Table 36-1. Correlation of age, size, and sequence of development of female urogenital organs

Age (approximately*)	Crown-rump length (mm)	Developmental levels in female urogenital tract
25 days	2.5	Pronephros formed; pronephric ducts grow caudad as blind tubes; cloaca and cloacal membrane present; embryo has 14 somites
32 days	5	Pronephros degenerated; mesonephric tubules forming; pronephric (now mesonephric) ducts reach cloaca; metanephric bud forms at distal end of mesonephric duct
35 days	8	Genital ridge bulges; ureteric and renal pelvic primordia formed
40 days	13	Urorectal septum begins to subdivide cloaca; genital tubercle and labioscrotal swellings evident; müllerian duct begins to form
7 weeks	22	Urogenital membrane dissolves; cloaca separated into urogenital sinus and rectum; glans of phallus is evident
8 weeks	30	Testis and ovary become recognizable as such; müllerian ducts approach urogenital sinus and begin to fuse (distal portion) to become uterovaginal primordium
10 weeks	46	Mesonephric ducts atrophy; glands of urogenital sinus (vulvourethral and vestibular glands) appear
12 weeks	56	Uterine horns absorbed; muscular walls appear in uterus, vagina, and fallopian tubes; distinction of sex from external genitalia becomes possible
16 weeks	112	Uterus and vagina become distinctive structures
5 months	150	Primary ovarian follicles are found; vagina develops lumen; urogenital sinus becomes shallow vestibule
7 months	230	Uterine glands appear

*There is no accurate way of determining embryonic age from the length; the figures given represent a composite or average and are based on the stages described by Hamilton, W.J., Boyd, J.D., and Mossman, H.W.: Human embryology, Baltimore, 1962, The Williams & Wilkins Co.; and by Van Wagenen, G., and Simpson, M.E.: Embryology of the ovary and testis, New Haven, 1965, Yale University Press.

Sexual differentiation: male and female

Female genital developmental anomalies often involve some degree of substitution of male-directed organogenesis. Therefore genital development in the male is basic to any understanding of the anatomy and physiology of intersex states in children or adults reared as females. The specific genes that determine testicular differentiation—hence "maleness"—are located on the Y chromosome and are expressed on the surface membrane of all male cells as a weak, sex-specific histocompatibility antigen, the H-Y antigen.[1] In the absence of a Y chromosome the embryo develops (at least transiently) ovaries, müllerian ducts and their derivatives, vagina, vulva, and a basically female phenotype. Full expression of all female secondary sexual characteristics and development of a functional ovary require a second X chromosome.

The gonadal blastemas begin similarly in both sexes and at first are morphologically indistinguishable from one another. The definitive ovary and testis have been identified by Van Wagenen and Simpson[33] in 23 mm embryos after the age of 42 days. In the female the müllerian ducts and vulva develop appropriately, but this progression is *not* dependent on the presence of one or both ovaries. In males, however, the persistence and development of the mesonephric (wolffian) ductal system, together with atrophy of the müllerian ducts and the structures that form from them, are dependent on two factors: a local-acting müllerian regression factor and circulating testosterone, both produced by the testis.[15]

Testosterone induces the formation of epididymis, vas deferens, and seminal vesicle from the mesonephric duct. Dihydrotestosterone, produced from testosterone by the action of 5-alpha-reductase within the cells of the perineal tissues, stimulates fusion of labioscrotal folds and growth of the glans and shaft of the penis, enclosed penile urethra, and scrotum. Male structures fail to develop when the somatic cells of a fetus are unresponsive to testosterone, which occurs in androgen-insensitivity (resistance) syndromes.

Because the müllerian regression factor acts locally, it must be produced in adequate amounts by both testes to prevent completely the development of both tubes, uterus, and upper vagina. Therefore an individual with a testis on one side and a streak (no gonad), an ovary, or ovotestis on the other usually will have a uterus and upper vagina and possibly a tube on the side opposite the testis.

In the strongly estrogenic maternal environment, genital development is female independent of the presence of a fetal ovary. Therefore at birth a fetus with no gonadal tissue on either side (bilateral streaks or bilateral agenesis) will have a uterus, vagina, tubes, and the female pattern of external genitalia. Individuals with abnormal (dysgenetic) testes, which may not produce either müllerian regression factor or testosterone in adequate amounts, will have some degree of müllerian tract development and either female external genitalia or incompletely formed male external genitalia. A single testis might be expected to inhibit müllerian development on the same side but not to inhibit that on the opposite side or the entire uterus; however, it could generate enough dihydrotestosterone to masculinize the external genitalia.

Genital anomalies

Because of the importance of sex in social development, genital anomalies have a devastating impact. Any classification of female genital tract anomalies must reflect the incomplete knowledge of genetics and of teratogenic factors such as viruses and toxic chemicals or drugs. At present it is convenient to divide genital malformations into two broad groups: (1) those related to intersex states, in which a genetic abnormality of a sex chromosome is demonstrable or suspected and (2) those more simply structural and localized developmental abnormalities in which one of the processes of the growth, fusion, canalization, or separation of developing tubular structures is incomplete. A detailed classification in relation to biochemical and cytogenetic anomalies has been prepared by Park, Aimakhu, and Jones.[20]

Intersex states and cytogenetic abnormalities

Normal sexual development is determined first of all by the presence in the zygote of a normal set of sex chromosomes, XX for a female and XY for a male. The initial factor in many genital anomalies is the contribution of abnormal or deficient genetic material by one of the gametes. Alternatively, during the first division of the zygote some genetic material may be lost or unevenly distributed in the daughter cells (nondisjunction), resulting in a mixture (mosaic) of two or more types of cells as the organism develops further. Although the loss, severe alteration, or duplication of an autosome is usually lethal, most sex chromosomal abnormalities exert their most notable effects in the form of altered genital structure and function.

A significant chromosomal abnormality can be detected in about 50% of spontaneous abortions when the fetus is either absent or morphologically abnormal,[27] and 5% of perinatal deaths or stillbirths involve chromosomal anomaly.[16] Among 50 women who failed to begin to menstruate (primary amenorrhea), Sarto[23] found chromosomal anomalies in 19.

A bewildering array of intersex states has been described, together with associated cytogenetic analyses and deranged endocrine physiology. Extensive clinical descriptions and genetic studies are available in monographs such as those by Federman[6] and Mittwoch.[18] This discussion is limited to a summary of the usual findings in a few of the more common intersex syndromes, with Table 36-2 for comparison. This table is a generalization. There is no perfect correspondence between phenotype, karyotype, and other features of these syndromes at the present state of the art: many patients will not fit the chart.

Certain commonly used terms require definition, as follows.

hermaphrodite An inexact term indicating that an individual has some kind of mixture of both male and female gonads, external genitalia, and sexual characteristics. A true hermaphrodite has both ovarian and testicular tissue, either or both of which may be functional.

pseudohermaphrodite An inexact, confusing, and often unnecessary general term for an individual with gonads and genotype of one sex and external genitalia more consistent with the opposite sex. A male pseudohermaphrodite has testes but otherwise appears to be female (typically represented by the androgen-insensitivity syndrome). A female pseudohermaphrodite has ovaries, but the external genitalia are masculinized (typically represented by congenital adrenal hyperplasia). It is nearly always possible, desirable, and sufficient to name the specific condition or syndrome.

genotype An expression of the genetic characteristics of an individual cell as determined by analysis of the number and morphologic characteristics of the chromosomes examined at metaphase; for example, 46XX indicates that the individual has 44 normal autosomes and two normal X chromosomes, the genotype of a normal female; 46XY is the normal male genotype; and 45XO indicates 44 autosomes, one X, and deletion of the second sex chromosome, as seen in Turner's syndrome.

phenotype The external habitus and general appearance of the individual. In intersex states, it refers more specifically to the appearance of the external genitalia (male or female). In the postpubertal individual it generally also includes secondary sexual characteristics such as hair distribution, wide or narrow hips, laryngeal enlargement.

dysgenetic gonad An ovary or testis that has been abnormal from the beginning, usually as the result of the absence or other abnormality of a sex chromosome complement of the cells. The streak gonad (as in Turner's syndrome) can be regarded as a dysgenetic ovary. Neoplasms, especially gonadoblastoma, are likely to occur in dysgenetic gonads.[26]

gonadal dysgenesis The gonads are streaks composed of fibrous ovarian stroma with no follicles and no ova (Fig. 36-7). The phenotype is female, and fallopian tubes, uterus, and vagina are present. Patients with associated short stature, webbing of the neck, widely spaced nipples, and, less frequently, coarctation of the aorta and red-green color blindness are said to have Turner's syndrome. Those with the gonadal lesion only are classified as having pure gonadal dysgenesis. The cytogenetic lesion is some kind of abnormality—usually absence—of the second sex chromosome in at least some of the cells—typically 45XO.

Hilus cells, mesonephric duct remnants, and a fibrous stroma reminiscent of ovarian stroma usually are identifiable. The presence of a few ova suggests that the patient is a mosaic: the XO karyotype has been leavened with a few XX (or other karyotype with a second X) cells. Cordlike structures

Table 36-2. Intersex syndromes affecting females, apparent females, or female genitalia

Syndrome	Gonads	Karyotype (genotype)	Inheritance	Internal genitalia	External genitalia	Habitus (phenotype)	Comment
Pure gonadal dysgenesis	Bilateral streaks	XX, mosaics	Autosomal recessive	Vagina, uterus, and tubes	Female	Female	Nerve deafness
Swyer's syndrome	Bilateral streaks	XY	X-linked recessive or autosomal dominant	Vagina, uterus, and tubes	Female	Female	Gonadal neoplasms; virilization
Turner's syndrome	Bilateral streaks	XO, mosaics	No	Vagina, uterus, and tubes	Female	Female	Multiple malformations
Gonadal agenesis	Absent	XY	Uncertain	Rudimentary tubular structures; no uterus or vagina	Ambiguous or female	Female	Minor malformations in some cases
Mixed gonadal dysgenesis	Streak and dysgenetic testis	XO/XY	No	May be uterus and tubes	Variable male-female	Female	Gonadal neoplasms; virilization
True hermaphrodite	Ovary and testis Ovotestis Ovotestis with ovary or testis	Majority XX Some XY Many mosaics	No	Usually vagina, uterus, and tubes	Ambiguous, variable	Variable male-female	
Female pseudohermaphrodite (chiefly adrenogenital syndrome)	Ovaries	XX	Autosomal recessive	Vagina, uterus, and tubes	Ambiguous	Female	Some infants virilized by iatrogenic androgens
Male pseudohermaphrodite (chiefly androgen-insensitivity syndrome, partial or complete)	Testes	XY	X-linked recessive or sex-limited autosomal dominant	Partial vagina; no uterus or tubes	Female	Female	Testes in inguinal hernias; less pubic and axillary hair
47XXX syndromes	Ovaries	XXX, XXXX, and a variety of mosaics	No	Uterus, vagina, and tubes	Female	Female	Some have been mentally retarded
Male XX	Testes	XX	No	Male	Male		Similar to Klinefelter's syndrome (see Chapter 21)

Courtesy Dr. Robert H. Shikes, Denver.

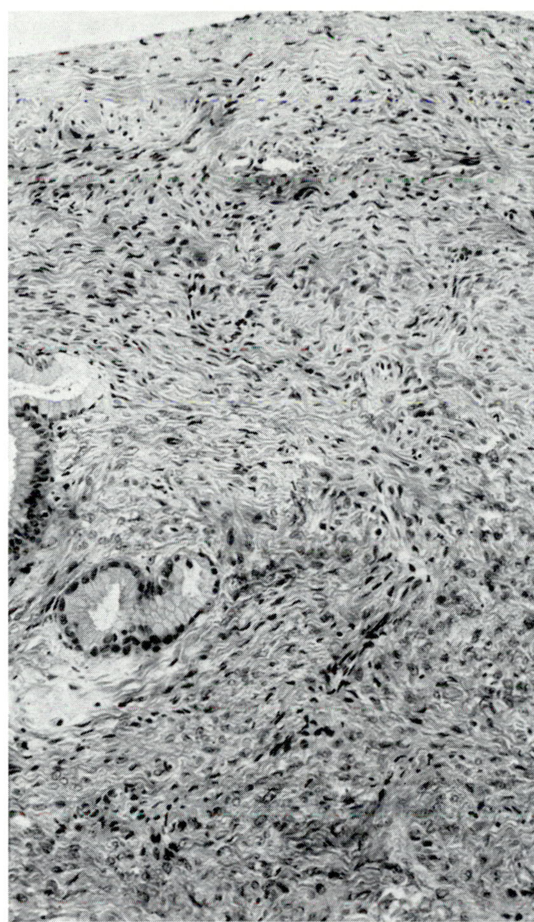

Fig. 36-7. Streak gonad from patient with Turner's syndrome. Tiny müllerian cysts *(lower left)* and hilar Leydig cells are occasionally evident, but germ cells and follicles are absent after birth. (150×.)

similar to an immature testis support the existence of at least a few Y chromosomes.[17]

mixed gonadal dysgenesis One gonad is a fibrous streak, as in Turner's syndrome, and the other is a testis, usually an immature or rudimentary testis, but occasionally the dysgenetic gonad opposite the streak is replaced by a tumor. The internal genitalia include a uterus, upper vagina, and, despite the influence of the testis, usually two fallopian tubes. The phenotype varies considerably, from normal male to normal female with variable degrees of ambiguity in many instances; a few have the appearance of those with Turner's syndrome. The chromosomal lesion varies but commonly includes mosaicism with both XO and XY stem lines.

gonadal agenesis Gonads and internal genitalia are completely absent. Phenotype is female; genotype is XY. This is an extremely rare condition; the absence of müllerian duct derivatives is unexplained.[6]

True hermaphroditism. Recognizable ovarian and testicular tissues are both present, together in the same gonad (an ovotestis), on opposite sides, or in combinations such as ovotestis on one side with ovary or testis on the other. There is nearly always a uterus. The side with a testis has a vas deferens; the side with an ovary has a tube. A wide variety of internal genitalia combinations occurs and the phenotypes and external genitalia are also extremely variable. Most patients have a 46XX karyotype, but 46XY and a variety of mosaics have been reported. Some testes (but not ovotestes) have produced spermatozoa; there have been rare pregnancies.[30]

Androgen-insensitivity (resistance) syndromes and other male pseudohermaphroditism. Androgen-insensitivity syndromes are the most common cause of male pseudohermaphroditism; there are three groups, all with XY genotypes and testes.[9] In the first group, absence of the intracellular enzyme 5-alpha-reductase blocks formation of dihydrotestosterone, on which development of external genitalia depends: the external genitalia appear to be female. At puberty testicular androgens induce masculine habitus and phallus enlargement. The second category, testicular feminization, is a generalized insensitivity to all androgens; not only are the external genitalia female, but also at puberty the breasts enlarge and a typical general female body habitus with normal female self-image develops. The vagina is short and ends blindly. A comparable syndrome exists in rats.[3] The third, somewhat variable group may be lumped together as Reifenstein's syndrome. The predominant phenotype is male, and external genitalia appear male but with defects, notably hypospadias. Gynecomastia occurs at puberty. The testes are small and immature, spermatogenesis is defective, and infertility is the rule. Rare instances of deficient testosterone synthesis result in incomplete development of wolffian duct derivatives and female or ambiguous external genitalia. Finally, ineffective müllerian-inhibitory factor results in a phenotypic male with testes (often cryptorchid), male internal and external genitalia, and uterus and fallopian tubes.

Congenital adrenal hyperplasia and other hormonally induced causes of female pseudohermaphroditism. Congenital adrenal hyperplasia is fundamentally an adrenal abnormality in which defective hydrocortisone synthesis leads to androgen excess (see p. 1431). The gonads are normal ovaries; the uterus and tubes are likewise normal. The morphologic genital defect involves the external genitalia only and is the result of excessive androgen production by hyperplastic adrenal glands. This is the most common cause of ambiguous genitalia; it is also the most effectively treatable so that fertility and all other aspects of a normal sex role can usually be achieved. Because of the hydrocortisone deficiency, it is also likely to be fatal if unrecognized and is therefore the most important abnormality of sexual development to recognize at birth.

Rarely a similar masculinization of the external genitalia has been caused by the androgenic effect of progestogens administered to pregnant women in the hope of preventing abortion.

Other chromosomal syndromes. Other cytogenetic abnormalities affecting the sex chromosomes are less likely to be seen as malformations of female genitalia. The female with one or more extra X chromosomes (such as 47XXX) is phenotypically normal; some have mental retardation. Klinefelter's syndrome (usually 47XXY) involves a malformation of the male genitalia.

Localized developmental anomalies

Ovary. An ovary may be absent. The tube and uterine horn on the same side usually are also absent, and, of great clinical significance, the kidney and ureter on the affected side may be absent as well. Supernumerary ovaries and accessory ovarian tissue are most commonly found adjacent to a normally situated ovary and should be distinguished from lobulation of a single ovary. In rare instances ovarian tissue has been identified in the retroperitoneum, posterior bladder wall, and omentum and sigmoid mesentery.[22,34] Occasionally a cystic teratoma has arisen at such a site; the rare finding of other neoplasms of ovarian type that seem to have arisen in the pelvic retroperitoneum may in some instances be explained on a similar basis.

Fallopian tube. Duplication and atresia of the fallopian tubes occur rarely. Occasionally tiny accessory ostia, like miniature representatives of the fimbriated end, sprout from the side of the fallopian tube, especially the distal half.[36] Small patches of mucinous and endometrial epithelium may occur, especially when there is inflammation or endometriosis, so that it may not be clear whether this change in the tubal lining is congenital or acquired by metaplasia.

Unilateral absence of a tube is uncommon and is associated with ureteral and renal abnormalities, including absence of ipsilateral kidney and ureter.

Uterus, vagina, and vulva. The most common anomaly of the uterus, vagina, and vulva is the result of failure of fusion of some or all of the lower müllerian ducts. All gradations may occur, from complete separation causing the development of two complete genital tracts, to minimum failure with an incomplete sagittal septum at the uterine fundus. In the presence of a complete double vagina a double cervix and uterus are usual, but duplication of a distal structure such as the cervix does not invariably indicate that the uterine corpus is duplicated. Pregnancy may occur in either side or both. Both elements of a duplicated structure may not be of equal size. Development of one side may be discontinuous; a semidetached uterine horn may form a muscular walled cyst connected to the cervix by a fibrous cord.

Anomalies involving failure of fusion or establishment of patency in the lower müllerian system are often associated with urinary tract anomalies, including unilateral renal agenesis and misplaced ureters that discharge into the bladder at an abnormal site such as the uterus or vagina.

Transverse septa and atresias in the vagina probably result from the failure of canalization of the distal end of the müllerian duct. Retention of fluid (hydrocolpos or hematocolpos) is usually caused by a transverse septum situated proximal to a patent hymen.

Nearly all patients with congenital absence of the vagina have no uterus; however, when the vagina is apparently absent and accumulated menstrual blood forms a bulging cystic mass, the obstruction is almost always below the cervical level.

An extreme degree of hypoplasia of the cervix—or apparent absence or atresia of the cervix—occasionally also causes a cystic accumulation of menstrual blood in the normally formed uterine corpus; successful term pregnancy is possible after surgical reconstruction.[5]

Associated with internal duplications, there may be even more rarely a duplication of the external genitalia, including both labia, the clitoris, and the urethra. Congenital fistulas between the anus or rectum and vestibule, anterior displacement of the anus, and vestibular location of the anus have been described in detail by Stephens.[29] These anomalies depend chiefly on the extent of the contribution by the uroanal septum to the formation of the perineum.

VULVA

Anatomy

The vulva is composed of the labia majora, labia minora, mons veneris, clitoris, vestibule, hymen, Bartholin's glands, and minor vestibular glands. The mons veneris and labia majora are covered externally by skin with hair follicles, sebaceous glands, and sweat glands, including apocrine sweat glands. The inner surfaces of the labia majora, labia minora, and vestibule have sebaceous glands but no hair and are covered by a less keratinized epidermis. The vulva is profusely permeated by lymphatics that cross the midline extensively so that a lesion on one side is very likely to affect the lymph nodes on the opposite side. Lymph from the labia flows to the superficial inguinal nodes; lymph from the vestibule and clitoris may flow directly to the deep femoral nodes. An inconspicuous layer of specific stroma similar to that beneath the epithelium of the vagina and cervix also extends beneath the vulvar epithelium.

The vulvar epithelium is subject to all of the dermatoses that affect the body skin generally, as well as specific dystrophic conditions that may also affect the perineum and perianal skin. Reactive changes expressed as atrophy and inflammation with pruritus that occur in women with diabetes mellitus and pernicious anemia are relieved by control of the primary disease.

Inflammation

The vulva represents the portal of entry and the site of destructive results of most venereal infections. Many inflammatory lesions are ulcerated and painful or pruritic. The most common cause in a large series of women with vulvar ulcers was herpes simplex.[115] The inflammatory patterns vary considerably; although none is entirely specific, the pathologic changes are often sufficiently distinctive to suggest the agent responsible. Confirmation by culture or serologic techniques usually is possible.

The specific pathologic features of venereal diseases and other specific infectious diseases of the vulva are described in the chapters devoted to bacterial diseases (Chapter 7), viral diseases (Chapter 11), and fungal diseases (Chapter 10). Crohn's disease of the intestinal tract (p. 1065) may produce destructive vulvar granulomas and abscesses.[52] Amebiasis may simulate carcinoma grossly and microscopically.[89]

Bartholin's gland cyst and abscess

Bartholin's glands may be invaded by any bacterial agent; the ducts may become dilated behind an obstruction, so that an abscess, which may be acutely swollen and painful, is produced. A less severe chronic bacterial infection may evolve more slowly into a fluid-filled cyst. The most common cause of Bartholin's gland abscesses and cysts is gonorrhea, but other pathogenic bacteria can cause the same reactions. The mass must be distinguished from a neoplasm, and therefore a biopsy at the time of drainage is desirable, especially in the absence of any prior symptoms of acute inflammation.

Herpes simplex

Herpes simplex infection of the vulva deserves special attention. There has been a remarkable increase in the incidence of genital herpes. A distinctly specific strain of virus (herpesvirus, type 2) that is indigenous to the genital tract has emerged.[81]

Vulvar herpetic lesions begin as painful vesicles, ulcerate, and heal in about 2 weeks (Fig. 36-8). The lesions are more numerous and slightly larger in primary infections.

The virus can be inactivated by photodynamic dyes applied topically, although the clinical effectiveness of this approach has been disputed.[92] A relationship between genital herpes simplex and vulvar cancer is supported by association and by analogy with more systematic studies of cervical cancer.[77] Active vulvar herpes infections are especially threatening during pregnancy because transmission to the newborn at parturition is usually fatal.[40]

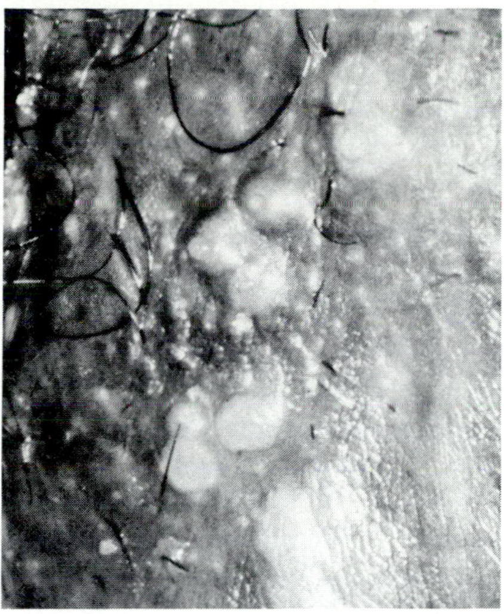

Fig. 36-8. Herpes simplex of vulva. Ulcers have yellow shaggy necrotic base and surrounding erythema. (Courtesy Dr. Ernst R. Friedrich, St. Louis, Mo.)

Cells with viral inclusions are easily identifiable in vaginocervical smears (see p. 1466).

Dystrophies, keratoses, and atrophy

Terminology

The vulvar epithelium is subject to a group of chronic conditions of unknown origin, chiefly affecting older women. The skin appears white, mottled red and white, or, less commonly, red. There are variable degrees of atrophy of the subcutaneous tissue so that at an advanced stage the labia are obliterated and the introitus is stenotic. Pruritus is common and may be severe and unremitting. The perineum and perianal skin may also be affected.

The term "leukoplakia" often is used by clinicians to describe the patchy areas of whitened skin. Similarly, the term "kraurosis" indicates that the atrophy and shrinkage are advanced. As the result of extremely varied usage in the past, both terms have no specific pathologic diagnostic meaning at this time. Their use by a pathologist now is undesirable.

The following lesions of the vulvar skin have the appearance and symptoms just noted:

1. Hyperplastic dystrophy (hyperkeratosis)
2. Lichen sclerosus et atrophicus
3. Specific intraepithelial neoplasms: carcinoma in situ, Bowen's disease, Paget's disease
4. Specific dermatoses, especially psoriasis, neurodermatitis, allergic or contact dermatitis, and lichen planus (see Chapter 35)
5. Systemic diseases such as pernicious anemia and diabetes with or without candidiasis

The spectrum of clinical significance varies from

benign to malignant; the treatment varies from excision to insulin injections. Biopsy of the lesions must be performed to identify them correctly and treat them appropriately.

Hyperplastic dystrophy

The combination of a thick layer of surface keratin, hyperplastic but cytologically benign squamous epithelium, and a mixture of chronic inflammatory cells distributed through the underlying dermis (Fig. 36-9) causes the vulva to appear thickened and white and usually to itch unremittingly. Scratching adds trauma and chronic inflammation and thereby probably reinforces the pruritus. Areas where the keratin layer is lacking appear red. The epidermis is usually hyperplastic; elongation of rete ridges in obliquely oriented microscopic sections may falsely suggest an invasive lesion. Either hyperkeratosis or parakeratosis may occur at the surface.

The cause is unknown. Symptomatic relief has resulted from use of topical creams containing hydrocortisone or other corticoid hormone preparations.[80] Occasionally (in about 10% of cases) some of the squamous epithelial cells appear slightly dysplastic; the added significance, if any, of hyperplastic dystrophy with atypia is not established.

Lichen sclerosus et atrophicus

Lichen sclerosus et atrophicus is not confined to the vulva and may affect both sexes at any age. However, the majority of patients who consult a gynecologist about this are postmenopausal women whose lesion and symptoms are either confined to the vulva or associated with perianal and perineal involvement.

The lesions appear first as small coalescent macules, which may have central pits resulting from follicular plugging. There is progressive shrinkage of the vulvar connective tissues so that the skin becomes smooth, shiny, and thin. Eventually the atrophic connective tissue changes obliterate the labia and produce stenosis of the introitus. Although usually white and opaque, the skin may appear mottled red and white.

The microscopic appearance is specific and characteristic: the epidermis in cross section is a thin atrophic band without rete ridges. The surface layer is hyperkeratotic. The most distinctive feature is the amorphous homogeneous degenerative change in the dermal collagen, usually in a wide band beneath the epidermis. Elastic fibers are absent; the collagen that remains may stain densely or faintly and is relatively acellular, except for scattered lymphocytes. A band of lymphocytes with a few plasma cells lies beneath, in the middermis. There is often separation at the epidermal-dermal junction, at least in focal areas (Fig. 36-10). Kaufman and associates[80] have reported considerable success with topical application of ointments containing testosterone or other andro-

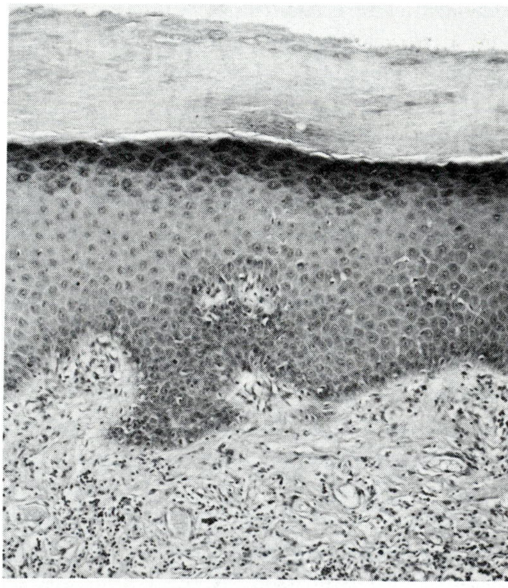

Fig. 36-9. Hyperplastic dystrophy (hyperkeratosis). Note dense keratin layer at surface and fibrosis and chronic inflammation in underlying dermis. Cytologic pattern is benign. (85×.)

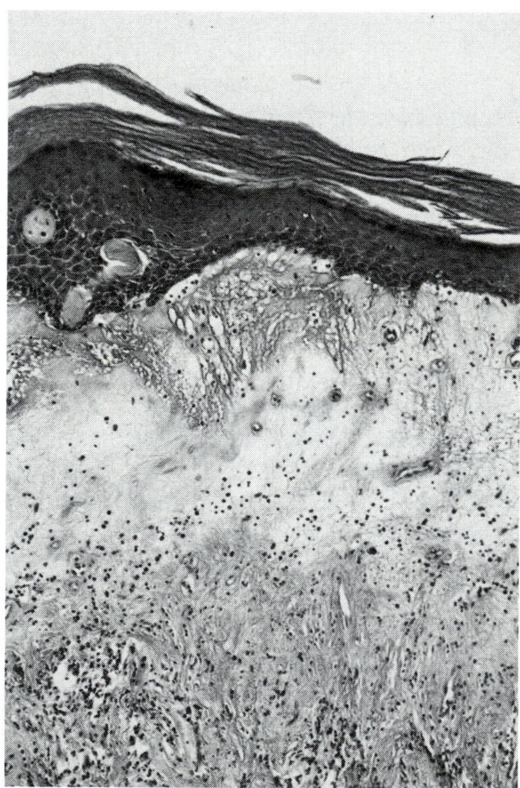

Fig. 36-10. Lichen sclerosus. Epidermis is thin and atrophic; underlying dermal collagen is hyalinized and edematous. Beneath this area of degenerative change is moderate chronic inflammation. There is surface hyperkeratosis. (85×.)

genic steroids; response to vulvectomy is poor, since the lesions recur consistently.

Clinicopathologic correlation

Lichen sclerosus and hyperplastic dystrophy may occur together, and other more threatening lesions may also be present. Multiple biopsies are necessary to evaluate an extensive lesion, especially if its appearance varies from place to place.

The frequency of subsequent malignant change has been much debated. In the few large series of patients whose original lesion was a benign dystrophy, subsequent malignant change has been uncommon, in the range of 1% to 3%[75,80] even after follow-up periods of many years. Detailed pathologic studies have failed to show any evidence that lichen sclerosus et atrophicus predisposes vulvar epithelium to the development of cancer.[67]

It is important to emphasize that vulvectomy for a chronic vulvar dystrophy is not likely to relieve the symptoms, remedy the disease, or change the small possibility of subsequent cancer.[75] The best results to date have occurred after topical treatment with corticosteroids for hyperplastic dystrophy and androgens for lichen sclerosus et atrophicus; none of the treated patients has developed a carcinoma.[80]

Neoplasms

Benign tumors and tumorlike conditions

Hidradenoma (hidradenoma papilliferum). Hidradenoma is a small papillary neoplasm that forms a nodule in the subcutaneous tissue of the vulva. The papillary fronds are covered by a double layer of epithelial cells, supported by a delicate fibrovascular stalk, an arrangement that resembles papilloma of the breast (Fig. 36-11). As in the breast, clusters of pink apocrine cells may form a part of the pattern. Most are located in the labia; about one fifth of the cases reported[91] occurred in the perianal region.

Granular cell tumor. Although it is more commonly found in other sites such as tongue, breast, and respiratory tract, granular cell tumor occasionally produces a poorly circumscribed indurated gray or yellow solid mass in the subcutaneous tissue of the vulva. The tumor cells are large, with abundant pink granular cytoplasm and benign, uniform, round nuclei. Ultrastructural studies show a varied appearance that suggests a cell full of secondary lysosomes. Some of the cells contain larger granular structures, called angulate bodies, that are packed with fibrillar material and sometimes lipid.[105]

Because the general pattern suggests organelles and membrane arrangements found in Schwann cells, especially the degenerative changes found in Schwann cells during wallerian degeneration, it is likely that most granular cell tumors are of Schwann cell origin. However, similar cytoplasmic changes have been described in smooth muscle cells of the appendix,[105] in the irradiated myometrium, and in one tumor of the urinary bladder.[45] The characteristic histologic and cytologic features probably represent one type of cellular response to injury that may occur in a variety of neoplastic or nonneoplastic cells.

All vulvar lesions, and virtually all those located elsewhere as well, have been benign.

Fibroadenoma. The vulva is at the caudal end of the embryonic milk line, and nodular masses of breast tissue measuring as much as 10 cm in diameter have been reported. Sometimes the lesion first becomes evident during lactation as the result of rapid and alarming enlargement. The various patterns associated with

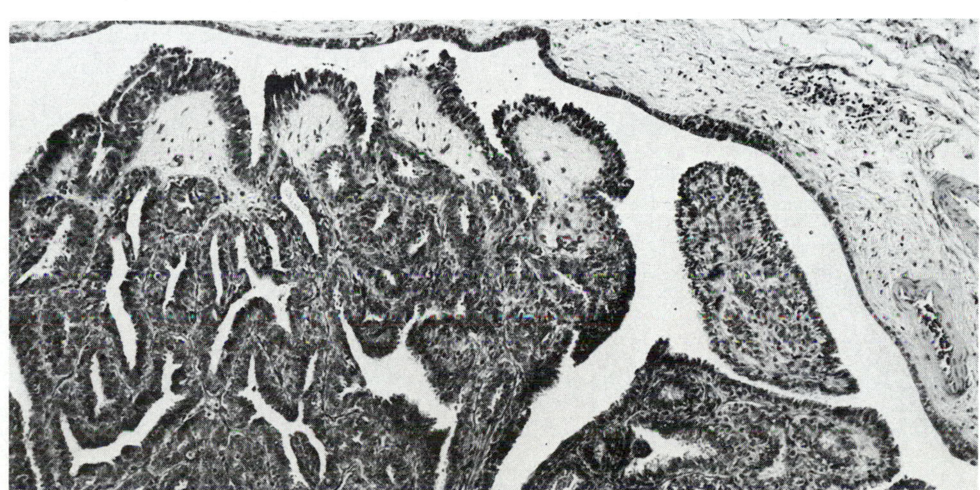

Fig. 36-11. Hidradenoma papilliferum. All the papillary processes have a delicate fibrovascular support, and there is a double layer of epithelial cells covering each of the papillary processes. (90×.)

chronic cystic disease of the breast also occur in vulvar breast tissue. Fibroadenomas in the vulva resemble breast fibroadenomas. A primary adenocarcinoma of the vulva with the patterns of breast adenocarcinoma has actually occurred[65] but is most unusual; the finding of such a lesion in the vulva strongly suggests metastatic and disseminated breast adenocarcinoma.[51]

Stromal polyps. Cutaneous polyps are invested externally by an orderly epidermis that covers a loose fibrous connective tissue stroma with a variable component of adipose tissue and vessels; most polyps of the vulva have this pattern.

Rarely a stromal polyp may include scattered large giant cells of the type encountered more commonly in the vagina (see p. 1469). The specific subepithelial stroma of the cervix and vagina also extends beneath the epithelium of the vulva.

Condyloma acuminatum. Condyloma acuminatum is a papillary lesion of squamous epithelium that occurs chiefly as multiple soft warty masses. They may be large or small and can be distributed about the anus, perineum, vaginal wall, and cervix, as well as the vulva (Fig. 36-12).

The squamous epithelium that covers the papillary fronds is histologically benign and is supported by a uniformly distributed fibrovascular stroma that ramifies into all the papillary projections (Fig. 36-13). Perinuclear vacuolation, called koilocytosis, is common and characteristic. Scattered cells may have enlarged, darkly stained, dysplastic nuclei related to polyploidy and arrested mitoses, especially after podophyllin treatment and sometimes in pregnant women.

The etiologic agent is a papovavirus closely related to the virus of the ordinary cutaneous wart. Most lesions respond to podophyllin, cautery, excision, or freezing. The surprising effectiveness of an autogenous vaccine in eradicating large or resistant condylomas is at present unexplained.[99]

Malignant change in a typical condyloma acuminatum rarely, if ever, has been documented convincingly. The condyloma virus sometimes is demonstrable in the cells of genital carcinoma in situ (see p. 1464), and some vulvar carcinomas have arisen adjacent to condylomas.[77] The role of condyloma virus as a carcinogen is not settled.

Miscellaneous benign neoplasms. Benign mucinous cysts lined by a single layer of columnar cells are more common than is generally appreciated. Most have appeared in the vicinity of the vestibule. The tissue of origin is the urogenital sinus vestiges.[59]

A collection of 34 benign vulvar neoplasms studied by Lovelady, McDonald, and Waugh[87] included 16 fibromas, seven lipomas, five hemangiomas, two neurofibromas, two leiomyomas, one ganglioneuroma, and one lymphangioma. Infiltrating margins and numerous mitoses are the most reliable indicators of aggressive behavior of smooth muscle tumors.[106] Rare instances of salivary gland pleomorphic adenomas have been reported.[112] Cutaneous lesions such as pyogenic granuloma, seborrheic keratosis, nevi of various types, and single squamous papillomas have no distinctive features when encountered in the vulva and are discussed in Chapter 38.

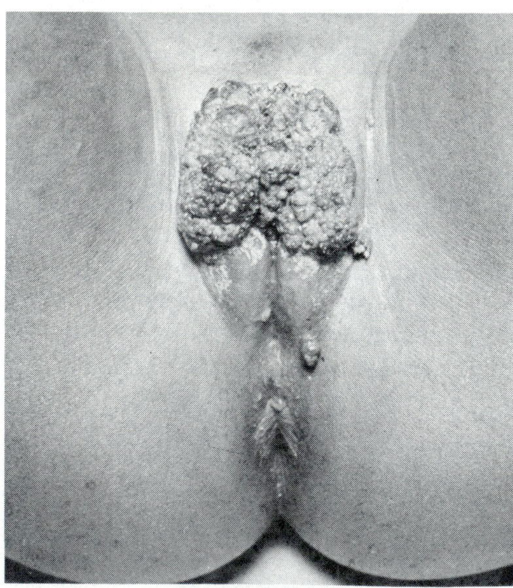

Fig. 36-12. Condyloma acuminatum. Exuberant keratotic papillary processes may cover and obliterate large areas of vulva.

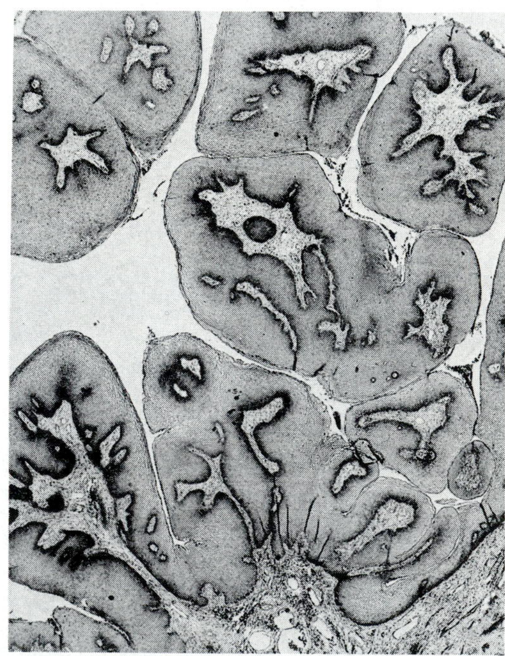

Fig. 36-13. Condyloma acuminatum. Papillary processes are covered by orderly squamous epithelium, each supported by a fibrovascular connective tissue stalk. (20×.)

Endometriosis occurs in the vulva usually as the result of implantation of endometrial tissue in minor operative wounds, notably episiotomy scars.

Malignant tumors

The predominant malignant tumor of the vulva is epidermoid carcinoma (at least 96%). Malignant melanomas make up another 2%, and the rest are a mixture of rare adenocarcinomas, soft tissue sarcomas, and an occasional basal cell carcinoma. Vulvar carcinomas comprise less than 1% of all cancers and 5% of genital tract cancers in women.

Epidermoid carcinoma. Invasive epidermoid carcinoma is chiefly a disease of postmenopausal women. Smaller lesions are usually elevated and superficial with an irregular granular, nodular, or ulcerated surface. Larger lesions tend to protrude as an outward-growing warty mass with a weeping ulcerated surface and a mottled red-gray or yellow surface (Fig. 36-14). More aggressive, poorly differentiated, infiltrating tumors have ulcerated surfaces with elevated, undermined margins.

Associated carcinoma in situ or dystrophic changes in the adjacent skin are commonly present. Women with vulvar carcinoma are likely to have diabetes mellitus, obesity, hypertension, early menopause, and other neoplasms.[62] The usual location is the labia majora, especially the inner aspect, and most carcinomas begin on the anterior two thirds of the vulva.

Most vulvar epidermoid carcinomas are well differentiated, produce keratin, and have well-circumscribed margins (Fig. 36-15). Lesions with this pattern are more likely to remain localized and have a better prognosis. Poorly differentiated carcinomas have a more diffusely infiltrating pattern, invade nerve sheaths and lymphatics, grow in narrow strands, and have a more aggressive natural history. The loose fibroblastic stroma in such cases is usually relatively abundant, and the tumor margin is indistinct.

It is important to emphasize that a physical examination is an unreliable indicator of metastatic spread; even an experienced examiner is likely to miss metastases or overdiagnose their presence in about 40% of patients.[110] The presence of a hyperkeratotic dysplastic lesion in the adjacent skin is associated with a significantly better prognosis.[61]

The size of the primary tumor is not a reliable indicator of metastasis; in the experience of Green, Ulfelder, and Meigs[63,64] one third of the lesions 1 cm in maximum diameter or smaller and half of the well-differentiated grade I epidermoid carcinomas were associated with

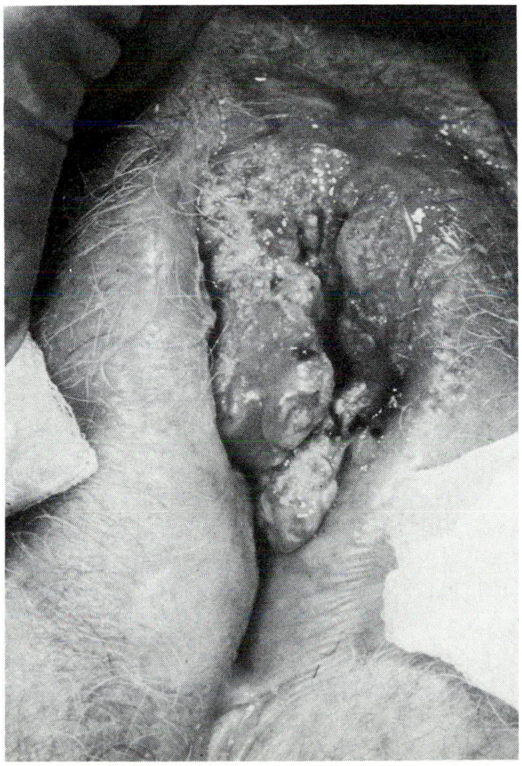

Fig. 36-14. Carcinoma of vulva. Tumor forms nodular erythematous mass with ulceration and erythema. Adjacent labia are edematous.

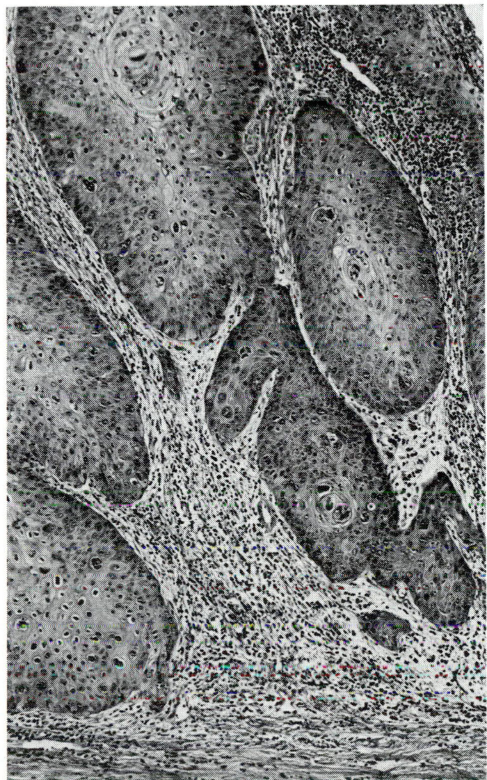

Fig. 36-15. Epidermoid carcinoma of vulva. Irregular rounded masses of well-differentiated keratinizing epidermoid carcinoma with well-circumscribed margin and associated inflammatory changes. (80×.)

lymph node metastases. Even the earliest microinvasive changes may occasionally be the source of lymph node metastasis.[95] On the other hand, it appears that the risk of lymph node metastases is limited if the primary cancer invades no deeper than 5 mm.[111] Barnes and associates[41] found that the tiny lesions with metastases were less differentiated, confluent, and usually not associated with overlying carcinoma in situ. Lymph node metastases commonly appear in the opposite side of the vulva so that bilateral inguinal lymph node dissections are necessary. Lesions located anteriorly or on the clitoris are more likely to spread to deeper (pelvic, iliac) lymph nodes. Frozen-section evaluation of Cloquet's node may be a logical way to select the patients who will require bilateral iliac and pelvic lymph node dissection, in addition to bilateral inguinal node dissection.

There is a distinct association with other areas of carcinoma of the lower genital tract, notably the cervix[38,50] and upper vagina, as well as the anus and perineum.

Earlier diagnosis has resulted in increased effectiveness of surgical treatment, fewer women with lymph node metastases, and improved survival.[62]

Verrucous carcinoma. Verrucous carcinoma is an extremely well-differentiated form of epidermoid carcinoma first described by Ackerman as a lesion occurring primarily in the oral cavity. It may become quite large and expands inexorably into adjacent tissues. The vulva is the most common site of genital verrucous carcinoma, but it also occurs in the vagina and cervix.[71]

Although the histologic and cytologic pattern appears benign, it is possible to distinguish verrucous carcinoma from condyloma acuminatum by the uneven distribution of the fibrovascular stromal support in the former.

Lymph node metastases occur only rarely, but any tissue, including lymph nodes and nerve sheaths, may be involved by direct extension. A satisfactory response to radiotherapy is unusual.[84]

Epidermoid carcinoma in situ and Bowen's disease. Epidermoid carcinomas are white or mottled red and white patches that often form plaquelike elevations. Some lesions have a warty papillomatous appearance (papillary carcinoma in situ). Pruritus is common. Distinction between benign dystrophy and carcinoma in situ is impossible without biopsy.

Before 1970 the typical patient was a postmenopausal woman, and the condition was uncommon. In a more recent series 40% of the women were under 40 years of age.[43] Many had prior or concomitant condyloma acuminatum,[78,108] and even more common was a history of vulvar herpes simplex infection.[81] The presence of virus-specific markers was demonstrated in the lesions of many women by both immunocytochemistry[81] and in situ hybridization,[46] strongly suggesting that herpes simplex virus is an important etiologic factor. The relative importance of these two common viral infections individually or in concert is not established, but both viruses seem to be strongly associated with the increasing incidence of vulvar neoplasms in young women.

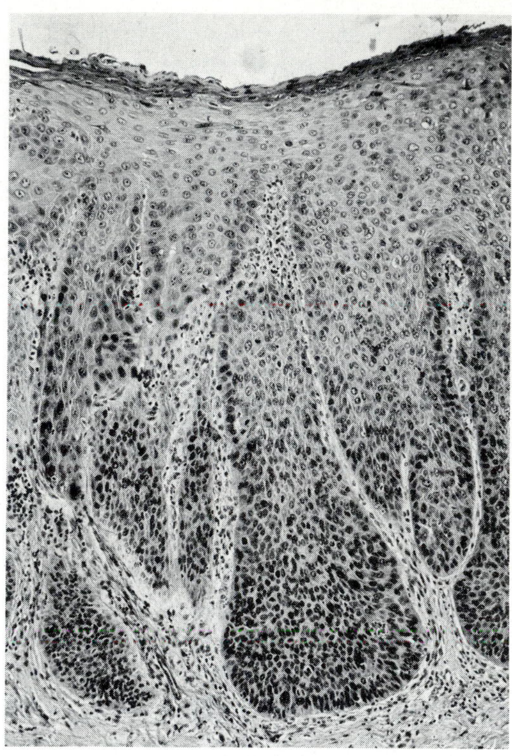

Fig. 36-16. Vulvar carcinoma in situ. Note hyperchromatic dysplastic nuclei, mitoses, and disorderly pattern in comparison with hyperkeratosis. (140×.)

The affected epithelium is composed almost entirely of small, relatively uniform dysplastic or anaplastic squamous epithelial cells that lie typically beneath a keratotic surface of variable thickness (Fig. 36-16). It is important to identify invasion if it is present.

A variant, more pleomorphic pattern called Bowen's disease now occurs with increasing frequency in young women. The lesions are brown papules, usually multiple, and often extend to involve the anus (Fig. 36-17, *A*). The histologic pattern is heterogeneous with a scattering of large bizarre cells, dyskeratotic cells, and bizarre mitoses distributed through a background of smaller uniform dysplastic cells (Fig. 36-17, *B*). Ulbright and colleagues[109] found a lesser risk of invasive cancer among younger women whose lesions were more uniform and did not involve the pilosebaceous apparatus. The histologic pattern sometimes includes koilocytosis and other features of condyloma acuminatum. Although the same type of lesion may recur in an adjacent area, invasive carcinoma has not developed in most young women with this condition, prompting a consensus in favor of conser-

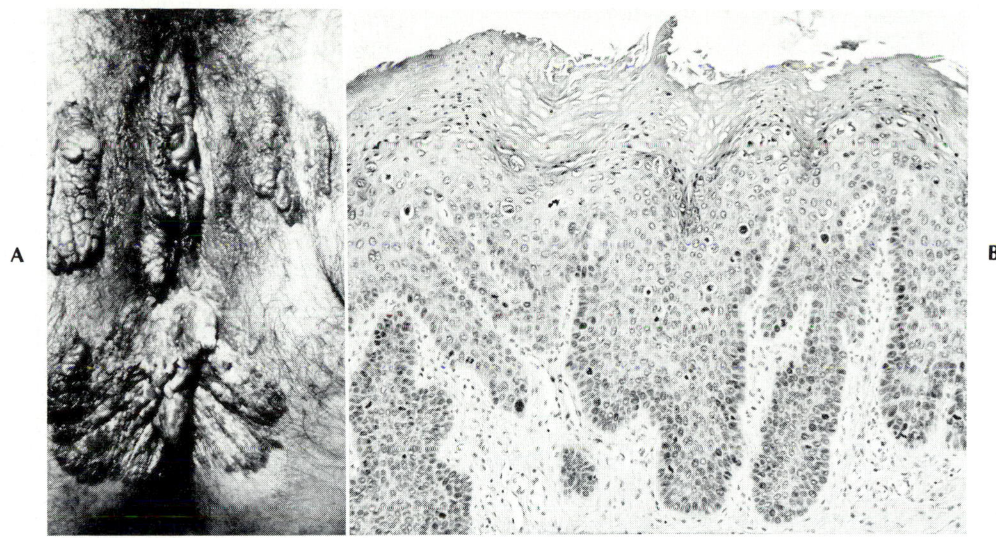

Fig. 36-17. A, Vulva with carcinoma in situ, Bowen's disease type. Elevated red-brown plaques composed of warty, sometimes papillary, anaplastic epithelium. There was no invasion in this extensive lesion. **B,** Vulva with carcinoma in situ, Bowen's disease type. Large, multinucleated, anaplastic cells and isolated dyskeratotic cells, are distinguishing histologic features of this variant pattern of carcinoma in situ. Perinuclear vacuolation (koilocytosis) suggests condyloma virus infection. (150×.)

vative treatment and close follow-up study when possible.[43,72,78,109] Lesions that appear during pregnancy may regress spontaneously in the postpartum period.[56,104]

Extramammary Paget's disease. Vulvar Paget's disease begins as an intraepidermal, noninvasive adenocarcinoma. The affected skin is mottled red and white, scaling, elevated, and slightly indurated. Characteristically there are small, white, keratotic patches separated by red fissures of irregular bands from which the superficial epidermis has exfoliated. The neoplastic cells infiltrate into adjacent epidermis. Extensive lesions may eventually spread onto the pubic area, thighs, or sacral region.

The epidermis is infiltrated by large pale adenocarcinoma cells, scattered between compressed but normal-appearing squamous epithelial cells (Fig. 36-18). The epithelium of hair follicles and apocrine sweat glands is characteristically involved. Many of the Paget cells contain stainable epithelial mucin. In ultrastructural studies various patterns of cytologic differentiation, resembling eccrine, apocrine, and squamous cell patterns, have been described. Probably the cell of origin is primitive and capable of differentiation into any cell type specific to the epidermis and its appendages.

If there is no invasion, the prognosis is good. Margins are difficult to see, and local recurrence is therefore common. The colposcope may refine the planning of surgical margins.

Approximately one patient in three has an underlying tumor mass composed of infiltrating adenocarcinoma,

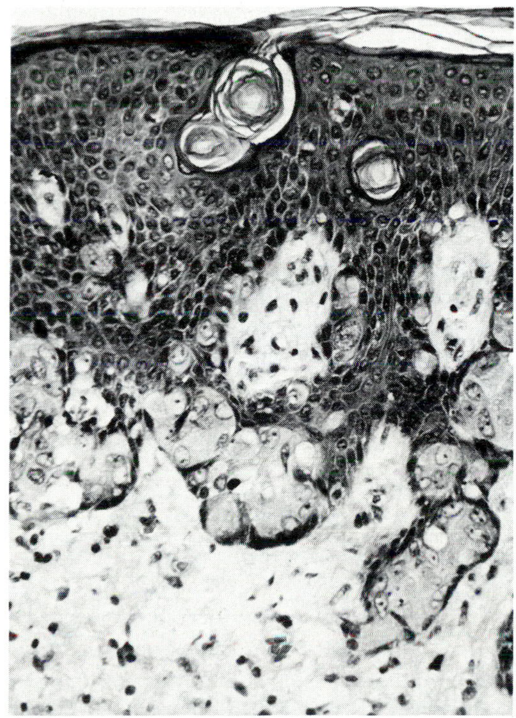

Fig. 36-18. Vulvar Paget's disease. Neoplastic cells infiltrate epidermis individually and in small clumps. Squamous cells of epidermis itself are histologically benign and compressed by tumor. There is no infiltration of underlying dermis. (260×.)

usually poorly differentiated; foci of squamous differentiation are commonly present. In the presence of invasion, metastases are likely, and the prognosis is very poor.

Adenocarcinoma and Bartholin's gland carcinoma. Adenocarcinomas of the vulva are uncommon; they may arise in Bartholin's gland or the minor vestibular glands. The initial appearance is a subcutaneous lump. The microscopic pattern may be that of an adenoid cystic adenocarcinoma, papillary adenocarcinoma, mucoepidermoid carcinoma, or mucinous adenocarcinoma. About one third of Bartholin's gland carcinomas are epidermoid carcinomas.

The principles of treatment are the same as for other vulvar carcinomas. Many patients are premenopausal: half of the lesions studied by Chamlian and Taylor[44] were originally underestimated as Bartholin's gland cysts. Adenoid cystic adenocarcinomas characteristically do not metastasize to lymph nodes but invade widely along nerve sheaths.

Malignant melanoma. Most malignant melanomas are located anteriorly near the midline. The prognosis in recent years (30% 5-year survival) is less bleak than formerly. Local recurrence is usually at vaginal and urethral margins where the impulse to temporize is greatest. The bilateral distribution of lymph node metastases and surgical approach are the same as for epidermoid carcinoma.

Metastatic carcinoma. Metastatic carcinoma was the third most common malignant tumor encountered in a study by Dehner,[51] comprising 22 of 262 primary malignant neoplasms (8%). The most common primary sources are cervix and endometrium. Metastatic cancers from the colon, breast, and ovary also are found in the vulva and should not be mistaken for primary vulvar cancer.

Rare malignant neoplasms. Malignant fibrous histiocytoma, epithelioid sarcoma,[49] leiomyosarcoma, rhabdomyosarcoma, and malignant lymphoma may occur in the soft tissues of the vulva.[49] Basal cell carcinomas of the vulvar skin[48] resemble those ocurring in more common cutaneous locations (see Chapter 38).

VAGINA

Anatomy and physiology

The vagina is a collapsed cylinder situated between the vestibule externally and the cervix internally. It has an inner lining of nonkeratinized squamous epithelium surrounded by a layer of connective tissue stroma, all supported by a double layer of smooth muscle. There are no named glands, but small glandular remnants of the mesonephric ducts occasionally persist and may form cysts.

The histologic and cytologic features of the squamous epithelium are affected by hormonal stimuli. During the reproductive years estrogens increase the thickness of the epithelium and the amount of cytoplasmic glycogen. The epithelium is thin in childhood and atrophic after menopause, when estrogen stimulation is minimal.

Cytologic patterns, as seen in the vaginal smear, vary with age and undergo cyclic changes with the menstrual cycle. During the first 14 days of the menstrual cycle, a period of estrogen predominance, the exfoliated cells, called superficial cells, are large and flattened and have pyknotic nuclei. After ovulation, under the superimposed influence of progesterone, the nuclei are larger and vesicular, and the cell margins are folded; these are called intermediate cells (Fig. 36-19). The amount of cytoplasmic glycogen is greatly increased and cytoplasmic margins are dense and accentuated in pregnancy. In childhood, after menopause, and after childbirth the mucosa is atrophic and the predominant exfoliated cells are small, round or oval, parabasal cells that have little glycogen. Small amounts of estrogen administered at these times induce maturation to the estrogenic pattern of superficial cell predominance.

Knowledge of the normal cytologic variations is important in the identification of neoplastic cells and other pathologic states.

Cytologic manifestations of pathologic states

Endocrine disturbances

The vaginal cell population in precocious puberty shows pronounced maturation with superficial cell predominance as the result of estrogen stimulation. Exposure to any estrogenic drug, including estrogen-containing face creams, will have a similar effect. Digitalis is said to have an estrogenic effect on the vaginal smear of some postmenopausal women. Death of a fetus with inevitable abortion results in a reversion of the pregnancy pattern to the superficial cell smear of estrogen predominance.

Women taking artificial progestogens cyclically (the contraceptive pill) may have increased numbers of large parabasal cells or intermediate cells with large but cytologically benign nuclei. Syndromes of ovarian dysfunction such as the Stein-Leventhal syndrome are associated with continuous exfoliation of intermediate cells, without any sort of cyclic change.

Vaginal inflammation

The vaginal smears of women with active gonorrhea contain the typical intracellular diplococci of *Neisseria gonorrhoeae* located in the cytoplasm of polymorphonuclear leukocytes. Streptococci, staphylococci, and *Escherichia coli*, as well as a number of other bacteria, may cause vulvovaginitis. Vaginitis caused by *Gardnerella vaginalis* is associated with malodorous leukorrhea.

The most common causes of symptomatic vaginitis are a fungus, *Candida albicans*, and a protozoan, *Trichomonas vaginalis*. Hyphae of *Candida* species and trichomo-

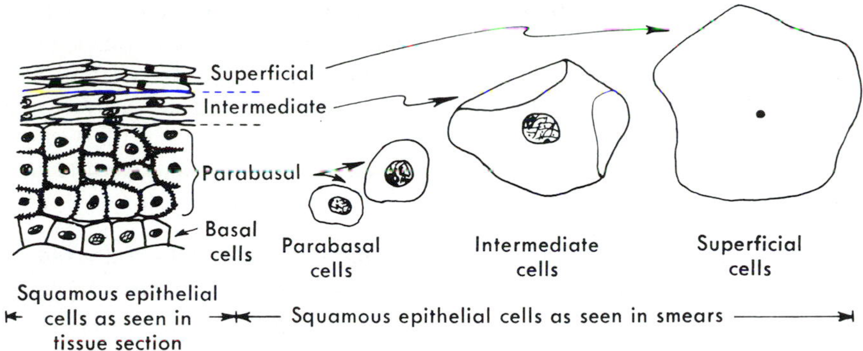

Fig. 36-19. Diagram of relationship between squamous mucosa of vagina and ectocervix, and parabasal, intermediate, and superficial cells exfoliated and seen in smears. Superficial cells predominate in estrogenic smears of first 2 weeks of menstrual cycle, and intermediate cells predominate in second 2 weeks after ovulation under influence of progesterone. (Redrawn from Frost, J.K.: Concepts basic to general cytopathology, Baltimore, Md., 1972, The Johns Hopkins Press.)

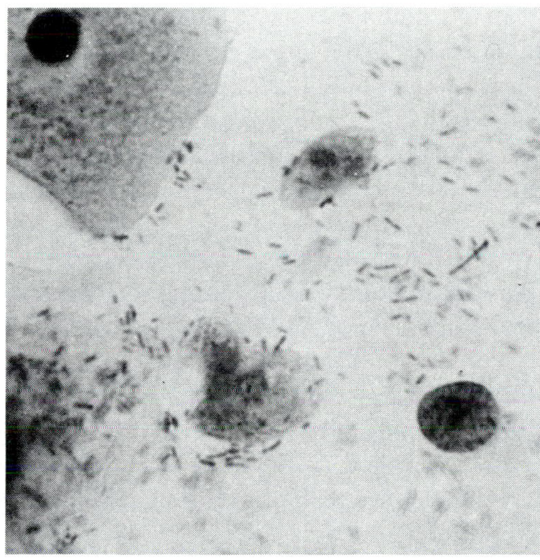

Fig. 36-20. *Trichomonas* organisms in cervicovaginal smear. Organisms are above and below the center. Portion of superficial squamous cell is present at top left, indicating relative size. (1000×.)

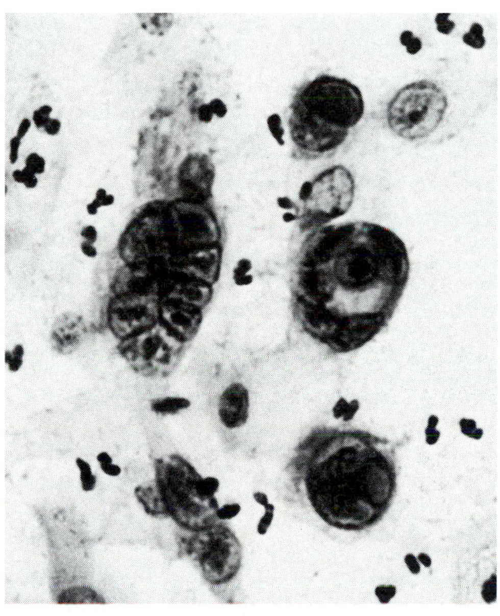

Fig. 36-21. Vaginal smears showing epithelial cells containing typical herpes simplex viral inclusions. Note syncytial clustering of nuclei. (600×.)

nads are easily identified in smears (Fig. 36-20). In *Trichomonas* infections the vagina has a red punctate appearance with abundant frothy discharge. Candidiasis is associated in typical cases with white patches of mycelia attached to an inflamed mucosa and is more common in pregnant and diabetic women.[130] The vulva and cervix are usually involved simultaneously.

The most important viral disease identifiable by vaginal cytology is herpes simplex. The infected epithelial cells form a multinucleated syncytium, like a cluster of bubbles. Ng, Reagan, and Lindner[143] have described two types of intranuclear inclusions and have found that one type with a homogeneous ground-glass appearance is more common in primary infections, whereas the typical eosinophilic inclusions surrounded by a clear zone are seen more frequently in secondary or recurrent infections (Fig. 36-21).

Cysts and nonneoplastic growths

Subepithelial cysts

Vaginitis emphysematosa is a remarkable process characterized by the presence of numerous subepithelial gas-filled cysts, which may pop audibly when traumatized (Fig. 36-22). They are essentially stromal bubbles with no epithelial lining, associated with a slight inflammatory response, including scattered giant cells. Many patients are pregnant, and a significant association with *Trichomonas* infection has been suggested.[129]

Epithelial cysts

Gartner's duct cysts of the lateral vaginal wall are lined with cuboid glandular epithelium without cytoplasmic mucin; they are considered to arise from dilated vestiges of the mesonephric ducts. Mucinous cysts, considered to be of urogenital sinus origin, seem to be more commonly situated near the vestibule[127] and are actually more common.[123] An occasional paramesonephric cyst contains ciliated cells.

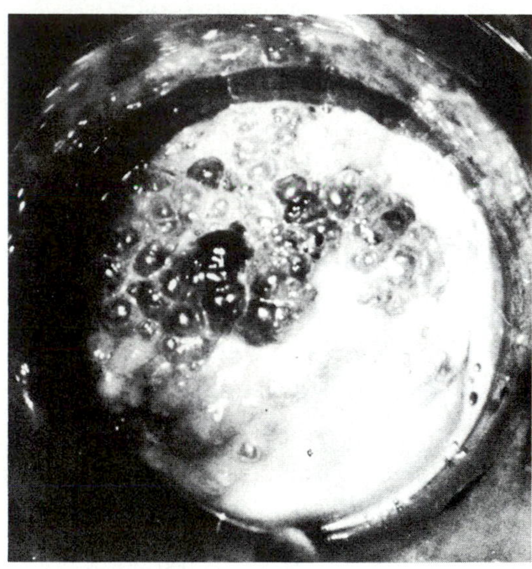

Fig. 36-22. Vaginitis emphysematosa. Vesicles and vaginal discharge as photographed through a cylindrical speculum. (From Close, J.M., and Jesurun, H.M.: Obstet. Gynecol. **19:**513, 1962.)

Squamous epithelial inclusion cysts, lined by squamous epithelium and filled with keratin, occur in the vaginal mucosa, as they do in the skin. Endometriosis of the vagina forms multiple blue mucosal cysts, which may rupture and bleed during menses. The usual cause is implantation of endometrium in an incision, especially an episiotomy.

Adenosis, clear cell carcinoma, and in utero diethylstilbestrol exposure

Adenosis in the context of vaginal pathologic conditions refers to the presence of histologically benign mucinous epithelium of typical endocervical pattern in an area that is normally covered by stratified squamous vaginal mucosa. The extent ranges from tiny foci 1 or 2 mm in greatest diameter to a virtual conversion of the entire vaginal lining to a surface of columnar mucous epithelium.

The affected mucosa has a reddened, velvety appearance, in contrast to the more opaque pale pink of the normal squamous mucosa (Fig. 36-23, *A*). Focal lesions require a colposcope for identification; larger patches are visible in ordinary physical examination.

The epithelium in areas of adenosis is composed of a single layer of mucinous columnar epithelial cells, but glandular crypts and slight papillary projections produce a more complicated pattern in some areas (Fig. 36-23, *B*). Occasional patches of epithelium are composed of ciliated columnar cells without mucin vacuoles, resembling tubal mucosa.[152] Some degree of squamous metaplasia is often present, beginning as a proliferation of reserve cells beneath the gland cell layer, as in the cervix; a complete conversion to a squamous epithelial lining probably occurs eventually in most cases.

Adenosis in adolescent girls received considerable

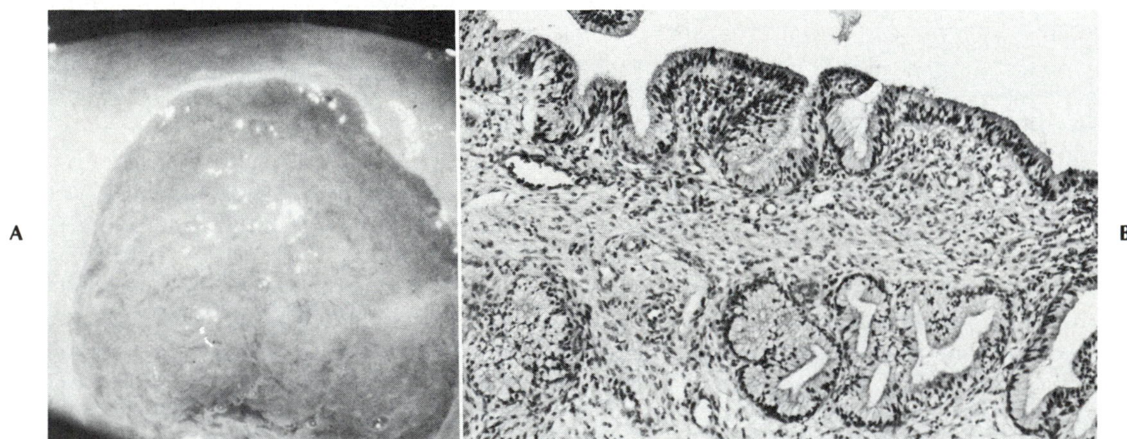

Fig. 36-23. Vaginal adenosis. **A,** Glandular mucosa covers ectocervix and adjacent vaginal mucosa in place of normal squamous epithelium. **B,** Photomicrograph of abnormal epithelium shown in **A.** Epithelial surface is covered by columnar mucinous epithelium, thrown into tiny clefts and folds. (**B,** 150×; **A** and **B,** courtesy Dr. James G. Blythe, St. Louis, Mo.)

notoriety after the demonstration of a causal relationship with exposure in utero to diethylstilbestrol ingested by the mother. It has been shown that the crucial period of exposure is before the eighteenth week of gestation. After this time formation of the vagina is completed, and susceptibility to the effects of diethylstilbestrol is apparently lost. Diethylstibestrol-induced adenosis may also occur in the mucosa of the portio vaginalis of the cervix. About one third of the patients have an anomalous ridge or "hood" of muscular connective tissue surrounding the cervix. Forsberg[126] has experimentally produced identical lesions with diethylstilbestrol in neonatal mice.

The incidence of adenosis in diethylstilbestrol-exposed infants is probably very high, if minute areas are searched for carefully with a colposcope. A much more significant but fortunately less common association is clear cell adenocarcinoma of the vagina and cervix.[134,135] Both the mucinous epithelium of adenosis and the clear cell adenocarcinomas are probably of müllerian duct origin.

Neoplasms

Benign tumors

Fibroepithelial polyp (stromal polyp). The subepithelial connective tissue of the vagina may form single or multiple polypoid masses, covered by orderly vaginal squamous mucosa. This stroma characteristically has a loose myxoid appearance, interspersed with giant cells (Fig 36-24). Benign polyps lack the subepithelial crowded zone of proliferating immature cells found in sarcoma botryoides, and they occur in young women, especially during pregnancy.[124,145] Rarely there is a component of mucinous epithelial glands intermixed with the stroma. Bleeding and awareness of a mass are the common initial symptoms.[120]

Leiomyoma. The most common benign connective tumor of the vagina is leiomyoma, and even these are rare. The morphologic features are like those of more common uterine leiomyomas. Tavassoli and Norris[156] found that recurrence and metastasis occurred in large tumors, with more than five mitoses per 10 high-power microscopic fields and infiltrating margins. Only five of 60 smooth muscle tumors recurred; only one metastasized.

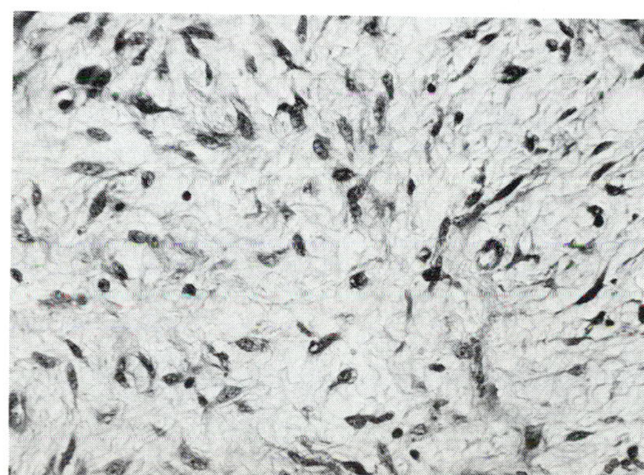

Fig. 36-24. Connective tissue of stromal polyp of vagina has loose myxoid appearance. Cells are spindle shaped or stellate and may be multinucleated. (260×.)

Other benign tumors. Other benign tumors include neurofibroma and neurilemoma. Kurman and Prabha[140] identified ectopic parathyroid and thyroid tissue in a vaginal nodule and reviewed six reported cases of vaginal teratoma. Rare benign mixed tumors are composed of islands of squamous or mucinous epithelium scattered through a stroma of spindle cells that resembles endometrial stroma.[154] Ulbright and I[158] have encountered endometrial-type stromal nodules in the perivaginal connective tissue. A glandular papilloma of the vaginal wall of a child studied ultrastructurally had morphologic features suggesting müllerian origin.[157]

Occasionally after a hysterectomy the tubal fimbria may herniate into the vaginal apex, simulating a neoplasm.[153] Granulation tissue, which may contain rapidly proliferating blood vessel sprouts, can produce sizable lumps at the vaginal apex after surgery.

Malignant tumors

Most cancers encountered in the vaginal wall are metastatic. According to the definition adopted by the International Federation of Gynecology and Obstetrics,[117] a lesion that extends to the cervical os is classified as a cancer of the cervix, and a lesion that extends to the vulva is a vulvar carcinoma. The remaining true primary vaginal carcinomas comprise slightly less than 1% of female genital cancers.

Over 95% of vaginal cancers are epidermoid carcinomas; of these, 10% have not invaded the vaginal wall and are called in situ carcinomas. The remaining 5% are adenocarcinomas, malignant melanomas, and sarcomas.

Epidermoid carcinoma in situ. It is uncommon to first find a carcinoma in situ in the vagina. In most instances there has been a prior or concurrent, in situ or invasive carcinoma in the cervix or vulva.

The histologic and colposcopic features are identical to those of an epidermoid carcinoma of the cervix. If there is no invasion, local excision of involved areas is adequate treatment; the use of a colposcope is a valuable and important way to identify all areas of involvement and their margins. An associated carcinoma of the vulva, cervix, or both is highly probable and must be excluded before therapy is planned.

Vaginal carcinoma in situ may appear 10 or more years after treatment of a carcinoma in situ of the cervix or vulva. The prognosis for in situ lesions is good even if superficial invasion is present, which emphasizes the importance of continued cytologic follow-up study of women treated for carcinoma of the cervix or vulva.

Invasive epidermoid carcinoma. Most invasive vaginal epidermoid carcinomas are indurated, ulcerated nodules; a few are elevated, soft, and papillary. The histologic pattern is commonly (about 50%) moderately differentiated, without keratinization. Well- and moderately differentiated carcinomas with keratinization account for about 15% each, and the rest are poorly differentiated without keratinization. Moderately differentiated keratinizing lesions with large anaplastic nuclei seemed to be more aggressive in the series studied by Perez and associates.[146] Most patients are elderly postmenopausal women; the usual location is the upper posterior vaginal wall. Significant etiologic factors have not been identified. Lesions of the distal aspect of the vagina may metastasize to inguinal lymph nodes.

For evaluating the prognosis and comparing the results of treatment, the extent of spread is classified by stages according to criteria agreed on by the International Federation of Gynecology and Obstetrics, as follows:

Stage 0	Carcinoma in situ
Stage I	Limited to vaginal wall
Stage II	Involving subvaginal tissue without extension to pelvic wall
Stage III	Extension to pelvic wall
Stage IV	Extension beyond true pelvis or to mucosa of bladder or rectum
	a. Spread to adjacent organs
	b. Spread to distant organs

Radiotherapy has been selected for most patients; about 75% of those with stage I disease survive for 5 years. Unfortunately, less than one third of the patients have stage I lesions; overall, less than half the patients survive for 5 years.

Metastatic cancer. The most frequent primary source of metastatic carcinoma in the vagina is the uterine cervix, often by direct extension. Carcinomas of the urinary bladder, rectum, vulva, urethra, or anus may infiltrate directly into the vagina. Embolic metastases from the endometrium, ovary, kidney, breast, or intestinal tract occur less frequently. The first evidence of a choriocarcinoma may be a vaginal metastasis.

Adenocarcinoma. Adenocarcinomas of the vagina are rare. Clear cell adenocarcinoma associated with adenosis in adolescent girls exposed in utero to diethylstilbestrol or its derivatives (as discussed previously) is currently the most frequently encountered pattern. The occurrence of an adenocarcinoma is estimated to be between 0.14 and 1.4 per 1000 diethylstilbestrol-exposed women through the age of 24 years; the incidence appears to have peaked in 1975.[136] Similar tumors also occur rarely in older women not exposed to diethylstilbestrol. The tumors are usually superficial and either papillary or nodular (Fig. 36-25). Most have been located in the upper or middle third of the vagina, primarily on the anterior wall.

The histologic pattern, like that of clear cell carcinomas found elsewhere in the female genitalia, consists of tubules or small cysts with inconspicuous stroma (Fig. 36-26). The tumor cells are large with variable degrees of nuclear anaplasia. There is abundant clear cytoplasm, containing much glycogen and no mucin; there may be some intraluminal mucin. The nuclei of cells lining cystic spaces may protrude into the lumina; the cells are separated and produce a pattern that is said to resemble hobnails in a boot.

Vaginal adenosis has been found in almost all patients with adenocarcinoma. Factors associated with recurrence and poor prognosis are large size, proximity to resection margins, and penetration more than 3 mm into the wall of the vagina. Girls under 15 years of age have a less favorable prognosis than those over 19. The use of oral contraceptives does not seem to influence tumor behavior.[136] The entire subject of diethylstibestrol-associated lesions has been reviewed extensively in a large cooperative study edited by Herbst.[133]

Mucinous adenocarcinomas also occur in the vagina. Although usually well differentiated, they are characteristically aggressive and may metastasize widely. Some tumors of this type have been associated with adenosis[151]; these lesions occurred in older women whose birth dates precluded any possibility of diethylstilbestrol exposure in utero.

Embryonal rhabdomyosarcoma (sarcoma botryoides). Embryonal rhabdomyosarcoma is a malignant tumor of

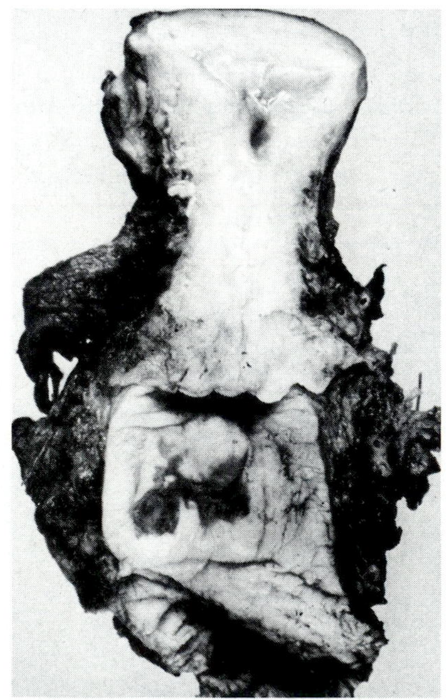

Fig. 36-25. Vagina with clear cell adenocarcinoma subsequent to in utero exposure to diethylstilbestrol. Carcinoma forms elevated nodule in vagina just below cervix *(center)*. Dark patches of adenosis are contiguous, just below tumor.

undifferentiated muscle cells. It tends to produce ovoid masses that protrude into the vagina, covered by normal epithelium (Fig. 36-27). There is a cambium zone of immature round or spindle cells crowded beneath the epithelium; this contrasts with the looser, more myxoid pattern of the central core. The cambium layer is seen best in smaller polyps.

Most of the patients are infants; 90% are under 5 years of age. After puberty there is an overwhelming probability that a polypoid lesion with myxoid-appearing stroma is a benign stromal polyp (p. 1469). Embryonal rhabdomyosarcoma has a predilection for the anterior vaginal wall and tends to invade extensively in the pelvis and metastasize to regional lymph nodes and distant sites such as lung and liver.[137] Most instances of successful treatment have resulted from early diagnosis and radical surgery. Similar tumors may arise also in the orbit, urinary bladder, external auditory canal, and biliary tract. There is probably no relationship to malignant mixed müllerian tumor; glandular components have been absent in nearly all cases reported.[137]

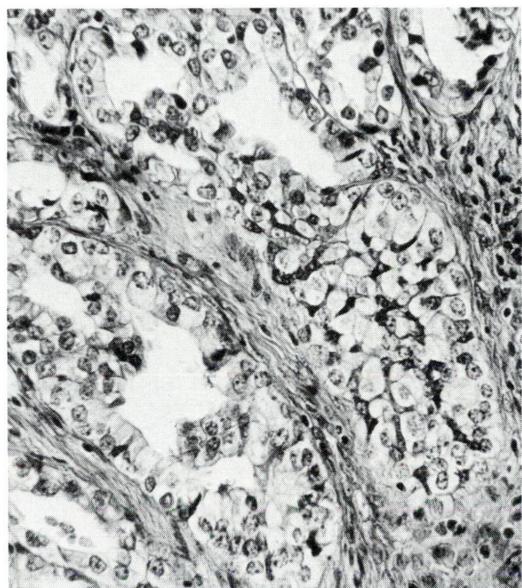

Fig. 36-26. Clear cell carcinoma arising in adenosis of vagina of young woman exposed to diethylstilbestrol in utero. Tumor cells contain glycogen but not mucin. (300×; courtesy Dr. Robert E. Scully, Boston, Mass.)

Distinctive adenocarcinoma of infant vagina (endodermal sinus tumor). Distinctive vaginal adenocarcinoma in infants arises as multiple polypoid masses, resembling the botryoid gross appearance of embryonal rhabdomyosarcoma. The histologic pattern is identical to that of a type of germ cell carcinoma that has been called the endodermal sinus tumor, arising in the ovary (see Fig. 36-77) or infant testis.[144] The tumor cells produce alphafetoprotein, which circulates in the blood and serves as a tumor marker to monitor therapy. The prognosis has been poor, although promising results have been reported with chemotherapy.[116]

Other neoplasms. Rare instances of leiomyosarcoma[141] and malignant melanoma[145] have been reported. The pathologic features do not differ significantly from those of similar lesions in more common locations.

CERVIX

Anatomy and physiology

The distal third of the adult uterus is channeled by a central endocervical canal that communicates superiorly with the endometrial cavity at an ill-defined internal os and inferiorly with the vagina through an equally ill-defined external os. The endocervical canal is lined by a single layer of tall columnar mucin-producing cells. The endocervical mucosa is thrown into redundant, longitu-

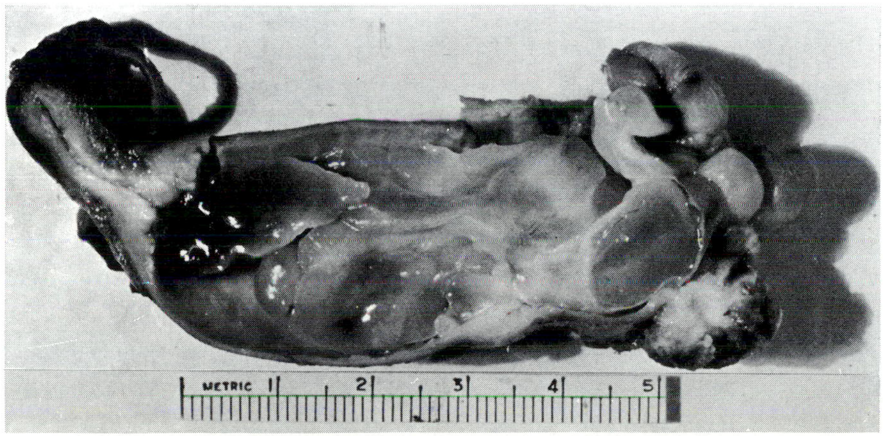

Fig. 36-27. Embryonal rhabdomyosarcoma of vagina (sarcoma botryoides) in sagittal section. Tumor arose in and filled vagina of 16-month-old infant and invaded adjacent pelvic tissues including base of urinary bladder. (Courtesy Dr. Sidney Farber, Boston, Mass.)

dinally oriented folds, separated by clefts. Opposing walls of clefts tend to fuse irregularly to form irregular tunnels that may reenter the endocervical canal or end blindly. These grooves and tunnels may produce an intricate pattern on cross section and commonly are referred to as glands; in fact, they represent extensions of the endocervical mucosa.

The physical properties of the cervical mucus vary during the menstrual cycle. After menses the mucus is at first viscous and sticky; under the influence of estrogen it becomes thin, glossy, and permeable to spermatozoa; when it dries on a glass slide, the sodium chloride crystallizes in delicate arborizing patterns (fern test). After ovulation and in pregnancy, when progesterone predominates, this crystallization is inhibited.

The portio vaginalis is part of the cervical mucosa exposed to the vagina; these surfaces are covered by stratified squamous epithelium, which is resistant to infection. Variable areas of exposed cervical mucosa may be covered with glandular endocervical mucosa at birth (congenital erosion). Of greater significance is the fact that cervical reconstitution and healing after parturition leave variable areas of endocervical glandular surfaces everted into the vagina and exposed to its contents. Such areas of eversion appear red and have been called erosions. This expression is misleading because the mucosal layer is actually intact; glandular mucosa is transparent, and the visible underlying vessels give a red color.

The exposed glandular surfaces are less resistant to infections of all kinds; a discharge is common, and the subepithelial layers are infiltrated by chronic inflammatory cells. The resulting chronic cervicitis is the invariable morphologic finding in the cervix of women with a normal reproductive life.

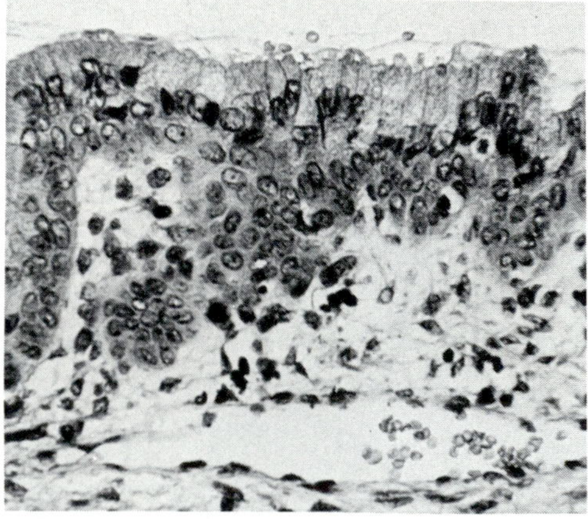

Fig. 36-28. Squamous metaplasia of cervix begins by proliferation of reserve cells beneath columnar epithelium. This new layer thickens, keratinizes, and will become a squamous mucosal surface when surface gland cells ultimately are sloughed away. (300×.)

Squamous metaplasia (squamous prosoplasia)

The normal response to eversion is the gradual conversion of exposed glandular epithelium to squamous epithelium. Local factors such as pH and estrogen[196] stimulate the proliferation of an underlying layer of reserve cells that eventually forms a multilayered covering several cells thick (Fig. 36-28). The surface gland cells slough away to leave mature stratified squamous epithelium. The area involved in these changes is called the transition zone.

Hyperkeratosis

The squamous epithelium of the portio vaginalis may develop a thick surface layer of keratin, especially in patients with uterine prolapse. Biopsy is important, especially if the process is patchy, since some well-differentiated carcinomas may have a similar appearance. The keratotic process is itself benign, as in the vulva.

Microglandular hyperplasia

A very characteristic pattern of gland cell hyperplasia occurs in young women taking oral contraceptives.[213,257] The larger lesions are polypoid. They are formed of masses of small endocervical gland cells intermixed with reserve cells in an early stage of squamous metaplasia, producing an intricate but recognizable pattern (Fig. 36-29) that should never be confused with carcinoma. Similar changes occur in pregnancy. Less commonly, gland

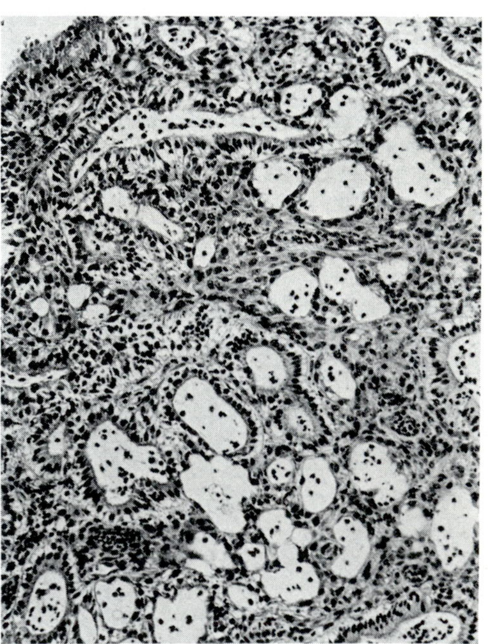

Fig. 36-29. Microglandular hyperplasia of cervix has complicated pattern produced by many small glandular spaces surrounded by immature proliferating reserve cells and squamous epithelial cells intermixed with inflammatory cells and strands of fibrous stroma. This pattern should not be confused with a neoplasm. (150×.)

cells with large, dark, but cytologically benign polyploid nuclei may be found. This change is analogous to the secretory gestational hyperplasia described in the endometrium by Arias-Stella[270] (see p. 1480). There is no evidence that birth control pills have any direct carcinogenic effect on the cervix.[264]

Vestigial and heterotopic structures

Vestiges of the mesonephric ducts commonly persist in the lateral walls of the cervix and occasionally produce sizable collections. These are distinguished from well-differentiated cervical adenocarcinoma by the absence of cytoplasmic mucin and benign cytologic pattern. A few mesonephric cysts have been large enough to produce a mass.[245]

Roth and Taylor[238] described heterotopic hyaline cartilage in the cervix. Benign stromal polyps containing well-differentiated skeletal muscle, like those in the vagina,[178] also occur on the cervix. In most instances it is possible to show that apparent heterotopic tissues are the result of implantation of aborted fetal tissues.[170,223] Endometriosis of the cervix may appear as one or more blue hemorrhagic nodules or blisters on the portio vaginalis.

The startling occurrence of sebaceous glands, hair, and sweat glands[262] is harder to explain in this mesodermal organ. Lesions with a similar appearance, called Fordyce's spots, occurred simultaneously in the mouth of the patient described by Watson and Cochran.[259]

Inflammation

Acute cervicitis may be associated with an acute gonococcal infection or puerperal sepsis. Caustic substances used as abortifacients, such as potassium permanganate, produce extensive ulceration and hemorrhage. Occasionally biopsy of a primary chancre will be performed to exclude carcinoma. Acute cervicitis occurs also with herpes simplex infection; the characteristic multinucleated cells and intranuclear viral inclusions are demonstrated infrequently. Ulcerated lesions may resemble cancer on visual inspection. The clinical and pathologic features have been well illustrated by Kaufman and associates[204] and Naib and associates.[221] The relationship between herpes simplex infections and cervical cancer is discussed on p. 1476.

Cervical infection caused by *Chlamydia trachomatis* has been identified with increasing frequency as cultural techniques become more widely available. Although not all infected women are symptomatic, approximately 45% have extensive inflammation in the transitional zone, as seen with the colposcope, and severe histologic changes, including intraepithelial microabscesses, epithelial necrosis, and ulceration.[227] Some also have had cervical dysplasia, a possible relationship that deserves further study.

"Chronic cervicitis" is so common in sexually active women that the term is essentially useless as an informative pathologic diagnosis. Characteristically the everted endocervical mucosa may have a slightly papillary appearance, and the stroma is infiltrated by lymphocytes and plasma cells. The epithelium is intact, and usually some degree of squamous metaplasia is in progress, at least focally.

Exotic inflammatory lesions

Amebiasis may cause painful ulcerative lesions in the cervix and vagina.[184] Schistosomiasis is common in some parts of Africa[173]; the finding of calcified ova in the stroma is characteristic. The tiny vessels in which they are lodged may be difficult to identify in most histologic preparations.

Polyps and papillomas

Endocervical polyps represent the growth of redundant folds of endocervical mucosa, including both stroma and epithelium. There is often squamous metaplasia of the epithelium, especially at the tip. Much of the substance of the polyp may be the result of cystic dilatation of endocervical glands. Stromal polyps of the cervix resemble those in the vagina, described previously (p. 1462).

Condyloma acuminatum may occur as a typical papilloma in the cervix, but flattened keratotic papules with cytologic features of condyloma are more common and have been recognized with increasing frequency.[235] The cytologic hallmark in cervical scrapings or histologic sections is koilocytic atypia: nuclei are enlarged, appear wrinkled, stain densely but evenly, and are surrounded by a clear halo. This pattern probably is frequently misinterpreted as dysplasia.[218] Particles resembling human papilloma virus organisms appear in affected cells studied by electron microscopic[230] and immunohistochemical[263] techniques. Coxcomb polyp, a rare lesion of pregnancy, and true papilloma, with more dysplastic-looking epithelium, are difficult to distinguish from condyloma acuminatum.[232] The possibility of a relationship to each other and to carcinoma deserves further study.

Neoplasms

Benign tumors

Leiomyomas of the cervix resemble those in the myometrium, described later. They may cause cervical stenosis with secondary pyometra or hematometra. The occasional polypoid smooth muscle mass with an admixture of endocervical or endometrial glands and stroma is an adenomyoma.

Rarely a glandular papilloma, said to be of mesonephric duct origin, has been described in children.[202] The stroma is inconspicuous, and the epithelial component is cytologically benign. Hemangiomas include the cervix in their ubiquitous distribution; the cervix itself is very vascular, and many reported "hemangiomas" are nothing more than a conspicuous demonstration of local vascularity.

Dysplasia, carcinoma in situ, cervical intraepithelial neoplasia, microinvasion, and pathogenesis of epidermoid carcinoma of cervix

In some women the sequence of repair by squamous metaplasia in the transition zone does not proceed in an orderly manner to form mature stratified squamous epithelium. Instead the proliferating epithelial surface contains many cells that resemble carcinoma cells. These abnormal cells are confined to the surface epithelium and do not invade the stroma. The progressively more anaplastic-appearing lesions that result seem to evolve from dysplasia, which can be graded as slight, moderate, or severe, into carcinoma in situ. An alternative classification widely used to represent the same basic concept is cervical intraepithelial neoplasia (CIN), which is similarly graded from I to III. According to this scheme, CIN I is the equivalent of slight dysplasia, and CIN III is equivalent to carcinoma in situ.[236] Currently there is a consensus that carcinoma in situ (CIN III) is an important stage in the development of invasive epidermoid carcinoma of the cervix. An estimated 40,000 women with carcinoma in situ are treated annually in the United States.[248]

Definitions. The term *dysplasia* (CIN I and II) indicates that many but not all the cells of an epithelial surface resemble cancer cells; it is possible to recognize a sequence of maturation from basal layer to surface, although it may be disorderly (Fig. 36-30).

The term *carcinoma in situ* indicates that all the cells in the affected area from basement membrane to surface resemble cancer cells (Fig. 36-31), and they tend to resemble one another. Both dysplasia and carcinoma in situ occur within endocervical glandular crypts; such a locus may represent a separate focus of involvement but is not evidence of invasion or that the process is more aggressive.

Although there is general agreement about the definitions of dysplasia and carcinoma in situ,[195] the histologic distinctions are necessarily subjective. Complete agreement among a group of pathologists will occur in about 65% of the cases they examine.[207]

A microinvasive carcinoma is a small carcinoma that has invaded the cervical stroma to a limited extent. The maximum allowable depth of penetration and how to measure it are debated; a majority of reports favor a limit of 3 mm.[190a] Measurement from the surface of the lesion to the point of maximum penetration gives the most reproducible figure in most cases.

The earliest invasive changes have the appearance of tiny irregular sprouts of neoplastic epithelial cells projecting into the cervical stroma, usually beneath an area of carcinoma in situ (Fig. 36-32). The cells at the interface between infiltrating epithelium and stroma appear more differentiated, have more cytoplasm, and are often degenerated. The adjacent stroma is infiltrated by lymphocytes and plasma cells. No metastases or deaths from such lesions have been reliably documented. These early changes, including the stromal reaction and cytologic features at the stromal interface, were described and discussed in an interesting early account by Stoddard[256] in 1952.

Small confluent growths composed of nests of invasive epidermoid carcinoma cells in the cervical stroma are classified as occult invasive carcinomas, if they are more than 3 mm in diameter, because metastases to lymph nodes have been demonstrated, rarely with a fatal outcome.[190a] The presence of histologically apparent involvement of lymphatic spaces did not correlate with demonstrable lymph node metastases in 30 cases of microinvasive carcinoma studied by Roche and Norris.[237] It is rare to find lymph node metastases in radical hysterectomy specimens that include nodes, and long-term follow-up study after simple hysterectomy has shown favorable results in over 98% of women with microinvasive carcinoma.

Pathogenesis. Studies of epidemiology, viral culture, cytogenetics, marker enzymes, and tumor-specific immune response have added many dimensions to the understanding of the biology of carcinoma in situ and its relationship to invasive carcinoma of the cervix.

Cytogenetic studies have shown that dysplastic cells not only look different but also have profoundly altered chromosomes. A relatively small proportion of cells from dysplasia of the cervix show this change.[206] Both the number of chromosomes and their appearance vary widely among the abnormal cells; there is no consistent pattern in the genetic derangement.

In contrast, many or most of the cells from an area of carcinoma in situ are cytogenetically abnormal, and furthermore the abnormal genetic patterns, although not identical, tend to be similar in a sizable proportion of the cells. Apparently an aggressive strain of cells (modal group) has emerged and managed to proliferate more rapidly than do other cell types.

One or more modal groups are characteristically present in carcinoma in situ; in microinvasive carcinoma there is usually a single modal group. Marker chromosomes having a distinctive and recognizable shape are also often present in early invasive lesions.[253] This suggests that all the affected cells are closely related, possibly members of a clone originating from a single cell.

Radioautographic studies of epithelium incubated with tritiated thymidine confirm increased DNA replication in large numbers of cells scattered throughout the epithelium.[242] Replication normally occurs only in the parabasal cells in the nonneoplastic cervical epithelium.

The most striking increases in DNA replication occur in early "budding" areas of microinvasion.[240]

The ultrastructure of the cells of dysplasia and carcinoma in situ is similar. Mitochondria remain numerous even in surface layers, there are many free ribosomes, and the glycogen accumulation normally found in surface cells does not occur. These changes together reflect increased metabolic activities in the individual cells and decreased organization and surface maturation of the epithelium as a whole.[246]

Epidemiologic analyses of large populations of women with carcinoma of the cervix indicate that a considerable increase in risk is associated with early sexual activity, especially with multiple partners.[172,239] This observation prompted a search for a venereally transmissible etiologic factor. A variety of possible pathogenic agents have been investigated, including spermatozoa, mycoplasma, and various other organisms.[165] An interesting study of the potential role of the male as a carrier found that the subsequent wives of men whose first spouse had cervical

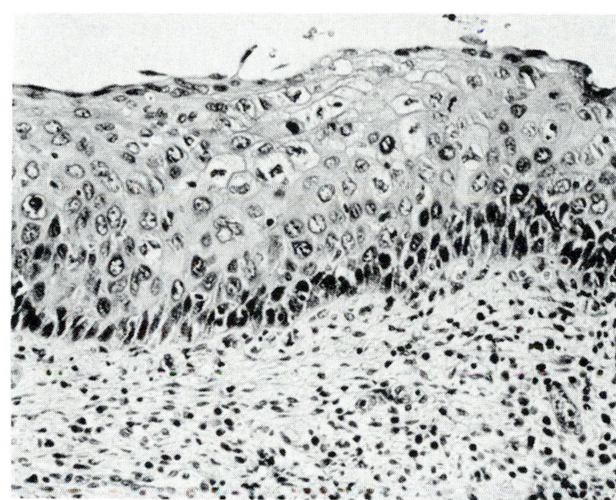

Fig. 36-30. Dysplasia (CIN II) of cervix. Abnormal squamous epithelial cells appear anaplastic, but they vary considerably in size and shape and have a relative abundance of cytoplasm. Sequence of maturation is evident as the surface is approached. (150×.)

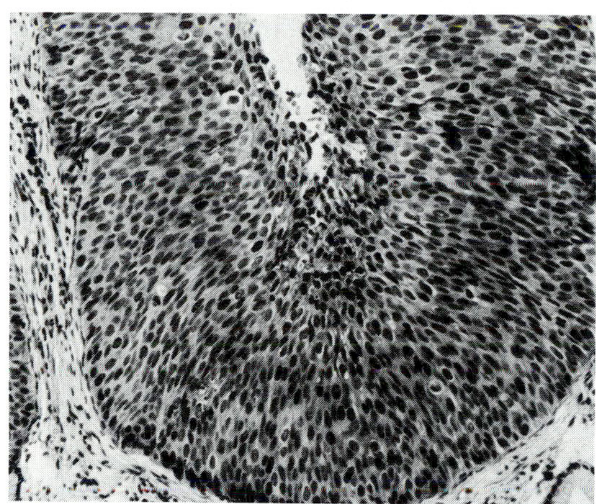

Fig. 36-31. Carcinoma in situ (CIN III) of cervix. Abnormal cells have a more uniform size and shape and relatively scant cytoplasm, and sequence of maturation is lost. (130×.)

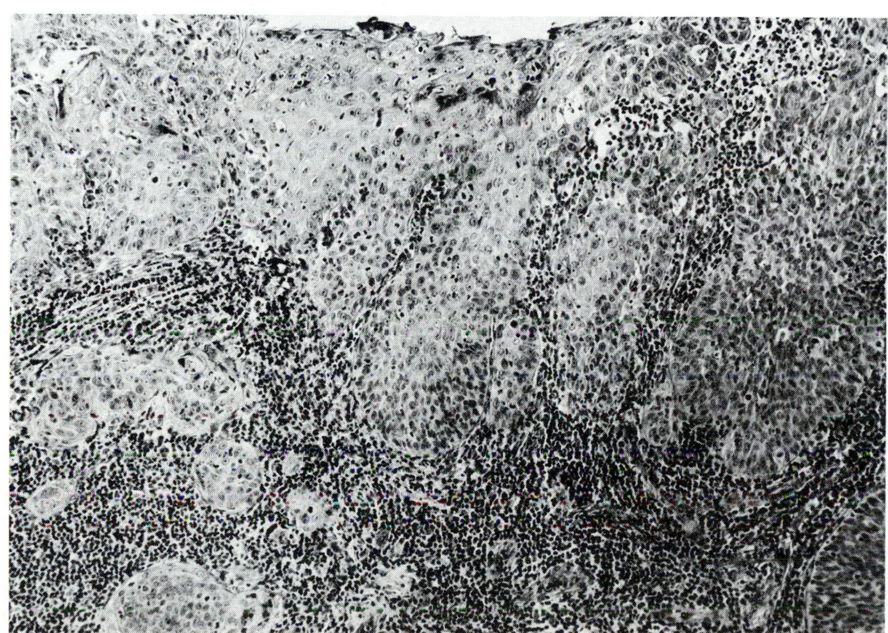

Fig. 36-32. Carcinoma in situ (CIN III) with microinvasion. Early invasive clumps have a more differentiated appearance with more abundant cytoplasm. Prominent inflammatory infiltrate in adjacent stroma is characteristic. (130×.)

carcinoma are themselves at greater risk of developing cervical carcinoma.[205]

Virologic and immunologic studies of women with in situ and invasive cervical cancer implicate herpesvirus 2 as the most promising etiologic agent. Antibodies to herpesvirus 2 are present in the sera of women with cervical carcinoma more often than in control subjects; furthermore, the titers are higher, and the high titers appear at an earlier age.[234] Membrane antigens extracted from cervical carcinoma cells seem to be specific markers for the presence of the virus genome in the tumor cells.[201] Latent virus can be unmasked from cultured cervical cancer cells, and 90% of patients with cervical cancer have antibody to a virus-specific antigen (AG-4) that is not found in control subjects or in successfully treated patients; many other virus-associated proteins have been identified in tumor cells and patient sera.[169] Tumor cells also contain messenger RNA with sequences corresponding to those of viral RNA.[217] Even inactivated herpesvirus is carcinogenic in mice.[261]

A less obvious association between condyloma acuminatum and dysplastic lesions in the cervix has prompted study of human papilloma (condyloma) virus in the genesis of cervical cancer.[216] Only a minority of the cervical cancers studied contain identifiable condyloma virus.[230,263] Dysplastic lesions consistently contain viral antigens,[212a] however, prompting the hypothesis that some cervical carcinomas are the result of synergistic action by both herpes simplex and human papilloma viruses.[264a]

Immunopathology. Epidermoid carcinoma of the cervix, like other cancers, produces circulating tumor-specific antigens, and patients form antibodies to them. Circulating antigens appear before invasion occurs. Cell-mediated immune response is unimpaired,[180] and lymphocytes of patients with cervical carcinoma are sensitized to epidermoid carcinoma cells and can destroy them in vitro.[189] Using a specific erythrocyte absorption test, Davidsohn and associates[186] have shown that A, B, and H blood group surface antigens normally also found in squamous epithelium are lost or masked in invasive and metastatic epidermoid carcinomas.

Colposcopy. The use of a magnifying instrument, the colposcope, has remarkably improved the accuracy of physical diagnosis of lesions of the cervix.[185,209] Based chiefly on differences in vascular pattern, distinctions can be made between squamous metaplasia, dysplasia, carcinoma in situ, and early invasive carcinoma (Figs. 36-33 and 36-34). Used in conjunction with cytology, biopsy, and conization, the colposcope has significantly improved the accuracy of diagnosis and the effectiveness of local treatment.[179,185,258]

Clinical significance of dysplasia and carcinoma in situ of cervix. Opinions about the significance of carcinoma in situ of the cervix vary widely. The name implies a threat of death, poised, yet momentarily held in check. The usual management, hysterectomy, usually is applied swiftly.

Dysplasia, left undisturbed, may progress to carcinoma in situ.[236] If there is no intervention of any sort, the observed conversion of dysplasia and carcinoma in situ to invasive carcinoma is nearly constant: 21% in 5 years, 28% in 10 years, 33% in 15 years, and 38% in 20 years.[252]

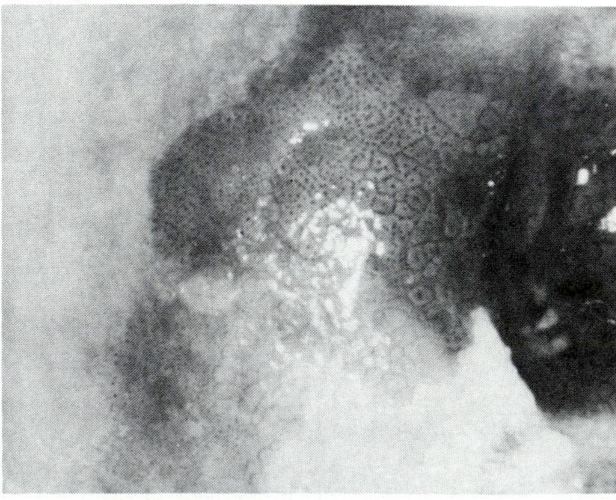

Fig. 36-33. Colposcopic photograph of carcinoma in situ of cervix. This mosaic pattern and accentuated punctate vessels emphasized against a background of opaque whitened epithelium are characteristic. (Courtesy Dr. James G. Blythe, St. Louis, Mo.)

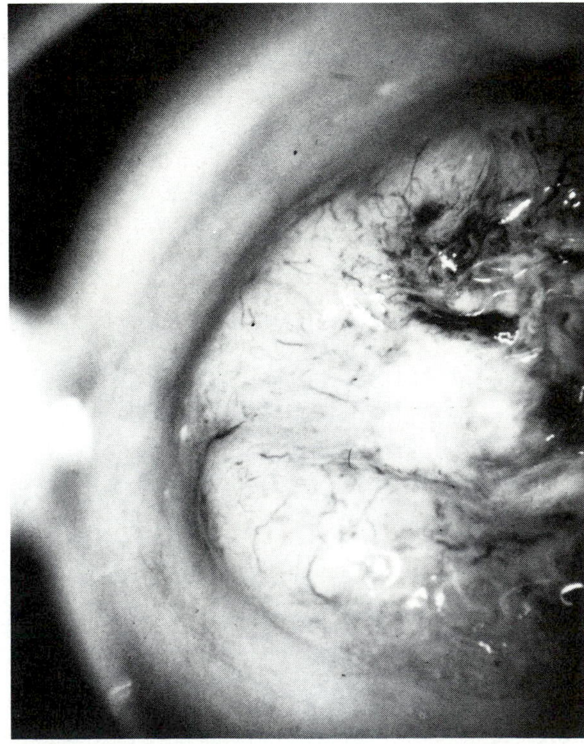

Fig. 36-34. Invasive carcinoma of cervix. Protruding mass and irregular tortuous blood vessels running over surface of lesion are features of invasive process. (Courtesy Dr. James G. Blythe, St. Louis, Mo.)

However, local treatment in the form of conization or cautery effectively interrupts the process in a high percentage of patients.[179,197,212,258] Residual in situ carcinoma has been identified in as much as one third of hysterectomy specimens obtained after cervical conization.[244] Those patients who require more extensive treatment can be identified by colposcopy and cytologic studies, if one assumes that meticulous follow-up examinations will be carried out. Prospective studies designed to show the best form of treatment have not been carried out.[207] In a carefully conducted long-term study of 1121 women with carcinoma in situ, subsequent invasive carcinoma was found in 2.1% of those treated by hysterectomy and in 0.9% of those treated only by conization.[208] The popularity of hysterectomy may be related to the fact that it solves other problems.

The screening of large populations of women has identified hundreds of women with carcinoma in situ, as well as early invasive carcinomas. Treatment of the lesion at this stage has considerably reduced the number of women with advanced cervical cancer, for which treatment is much less effective, and improved survival. The desirability of annual mass screening of women has been debated.[215] Success has been notable only in programs that include groups at greatest risk.[175,183] Various factors influence the frequency of false-negative and false-positive interpretation of smears. One of the most important and least defensible is the high frequency (88.2%) of failure of cytologists to identify and report technically inadequate specimens, as documented in surveys conducted by the College of American Pathologists.[188]

There is a definite but apparently small group of invasive cervical carcinomas that originate from the basal layer of histologically normal squamous epithelium. There may be no detectable surface abnormality at any point in the cervix, until (presumably) the lesion ulcerates, sloughing the surface and exposing the cancer beneath.[222] Approximately 10% of cervical carcinomas may arise in this manner.[161]

Adenocarcinoma in situ. Adenocarcinoma in situ is a rare lesion characterized by replacement of the gland cells of endocervical mucosa and its crypts by cytologically malignant gland cells. The columnar pattern is usually retained, but the basal polarity of the nuclei is lost, the cytoplasmic mucin is replaced by amphophilic cytoplasm, and the nuclei have malignant cytologic features. If involved gland-space outlines resemble those lined by normal epithelium in the same cervix, and if only part of the gland-space lining is affected, it is reasonable to conclude that stromal invasion has not occurred. Associated epidermoid carcinoma in situ is often present. The histologic pattern has been extensively illustrated by Burghardt.[177] In nearly every case the lesion is discovered when malignant gland cells are found in the cervical cytologic smear.[232]

Christopherson, Nealon, and Gray[181] concluded that adenocarcinoma in situ is a precursor to invasive adenocarcinoma because it was invariably found with very small (microinvasive) adenocarcinomas. Adenocarcinoma in situ is also located higher in the endocervix; a residual lesion remains in the resected uterus after conization in 66% of cases, which implies that conization for this lesion is probably an inadequate treatment.

Invasive carcinoma of cervix

In contrast to the remarkable increase in the numbers of women treated for carcinoma in situ of the cervix, it was estimated that the number of patients with invasive cervical carcinoma had decreased to 16,000 in 1980 from 19,000 in 1975 and 20,000 in 1970. After several decades as the most common gynecologic cancer, cervical carcinoma is now encountered less often than endometrial carcinoma, which has increased to first place in many institutions in the United States.

Gross appearance. Cervical carcinomas large enough to be visible and palpable have one of three growth patterns, sometimes in combination. The ulcerating type has an infiltrative pattern of growth and eventually becomes necrotic in the center and sloughs, leaving a cavity surrounded by invasive cancer. The exophytic type is often papillary and may form a bulky mass of considerable size while still confined to the superficial portions of the cervix. The nodular type originates typically in the endocervix, forming multiple firm masses that expand the cervix and isthmus. The mass may be large, and when it is distributed circumferentially, it has been called the barrel-shaped cervix. The gross relationships are important clinically because they affect the placement of radioactive sources used in treatment.

Clinical stages. The extent of involvement of the cervix and pelvic tissues is determined by physical examination. The clinical staging of the extent of disease must be determined before beginning treatment. It is in part the basis of selection of the best treatment for the patient and forms the standard for comparing the results of treatment of large groups of patients.

Definitions of the different clinical stages in carcinoma of the cervix uteri, as established by the Cancer Committee of the International Federation of Gynecology and Obstetrics,[117] are as follows:

Stage 0 Carcinoma in situ, intraepithelial carcinoma

Stage I Carcinoma strictly confined to the cervix (extension to the corpus should be disregarded)

- a. Microinvasive carcinoma (early stromal invasion)
- b. All other cases of stage I (occult cancer should be marked *Occ*)

Stage II The carcinoma extends beyond the cervix but has not extended to the pelvic wall. The carcinoma involves the vagina, but not the lower third.

a. No obvious parametrial involvement
b. Obvious parametrial involvement

Stage III The carcinoma has extended to the pelvic wall. On rectal examination there is no cancer-free space between the tumor and the pelvic wall. The tumor involves the lower third of the vagina. There is presence of hydronephrosis or nonfunctioning kidney.
a. No extension to the pelvic wall
b. Extension to the pelvic wall and/or hydronephrosis or nonfunctioning kidney

Stage IV The carcinoma has extended beyond the true pelvis or has involved the mucosa of the bladder or rectum. A bullous edema as such does not permit a case to be classified as stage IV.
a. Spread to adjacent organs
b. Spread to distant organs

Microscopic appearance. The majority of invasive cervical carcinomas, about 80%, are epidermoid carcinomas; adenocarcinomas comprise about 10%, and the remainder is a variety of unusual adenocarcinoma patterns or mixtures.[161]

Epidermoid carcinoma. A moderately differentiated, nonkeratinizing, large cell epidermoid carcinoma is the most common pattern (70%) and in some series, at least, has the best prognosis (Fig. 36-35). Well-differentiated keratinizing epidermoid carcinoma occurs less frequently (25%); small cell undifferentiated carcinoma is uncommon (about 5%) and has a distinctly poor prognosis.[224]

Adenocarcinoma. Although they are much less common than epidermoid carcinomas, the proportion of cervical carcinomas arising from gland cells doubled in the decade from 1960 to 1970.[161,162] The patterns vary from a well-differentiated mucinous adenocarcinoma (Fig. 36-36), sometimes papillary, to a clear cell pattern containing glycogen but no mucin. A mixed adenosquamous carcinoma apparently arises from subcolumnar reserve cells capable of both squamous and gland cell differentiation.

Spread of carcinoma of cervix. It is important to recognize simultaneous involvement of the cervix and endometrium because this distribution affects principles of treatment; the prognosis is not as good as that for carcinoma limited to the cervix. Hysterectomy with radiotherapy improves the results, probably because the more extensive distribution of some lesions interferes with the spatial arrangement of intrauterine radiation sources.

Carcinoma of the cervix spreads by direct extension into contiguous tissues, through lymphatics to regional lymph nodes, and less often by blood vessel invasion to embolize throughout the body. Because of their close anatomic relationship to the cervix, the ureters may be obstructed; secondary hydronephrosis, pyelonephritis, and renal failure remain the most common causes of death.[171] Distant metastases to lungs and liver are found in about 25% of fatal cases at autopsy. In patients dying of cancer of the cervix, central pelvic recurrences are more common after surgery, and distant metastases are more common after radiotherapy.[171] Less than 2% of patients with stage I or IIa carcinoma of the cervix treated by megavoltage radiotherapy with adequate dosage and distribution of the radiation will have a central pelvic recurrence.[228]

Local recurrence occurs in 5% of patients with stage IIb disease, 7.5% with stage IIIa, and 17% with stage IIIb. Over half the distant metastases become evident within the first year after treatment, and 95% appear by the end of the fifth year after treatment. Because most of the patients without evidence of cancer 5 years after treatment die of unrelated causes, this follow-up period is customarily used in evaluating the effectiveness of therapy.

Rare tumors. Verrucous carcinoma, an extremely well-differentiated form of epidermoid carcinoma, resembles and behaves like the same lesion in the vulva. Clear cell adenocarcinomas identical to those in the vagina (p. 1470) also occur occasionally in the cervix after in utero exposure to diethylstilbestrol. This pattern of adenocarcinoma also has been called "mesonephroma"; in fact, origin from mesonephric remnants is rarely if ever demonstrable. Rarely a cervical adenocarcinoma may have a histologic pattern identical to that of adenoid cystic carcinoma, which is highly specific and more common in the salivary gland. This lesion in the cervix is highly aggressive, occurs in older women, and nearly always is associated with a more conventional epidermoid carcinoma or adenosquamous carcinoma pattern.[219]

An extremely well-differentiated mucinous adenocarcinoma may be difficult to recognize because the epithelial pattern closely resembles that of benign endocervical epithelium, even in metastases. With adequate treatment the prognosis is probably the same as that of any adenocarcinoma at the same stage.[250]

Malignant mixed müllerian tumors, carcinosarcomas, and leiomyosarcomas of the cervix resemble those occurring in the endometrium (p. 1489) and share the same unfavorable prognosis.[163] Carcinoid tumors occur in the cervix as distinctly aggressive neoplasms. Like other tumors of the diffuse endocrine (APUD) system, they contain argyrophil and neurosecretory granules.[164] The less-differentiated cases resemble oat cell carcinoma in the lung; one cervical carcinoma of this type produced ACTH, causing Cushing's syndrome.[203] Melanin is rarely evident in basal cells of the cervix. Blue nevi and primary malignant melanomas are rare; Hall[199] has reported a dramatic example that produced fatal metastases.

Metastatic adenocarcinoma in the cervix is not common, but one should not mistake it for a primary lesion, thereby exposing the patient to a lengthy, painful, and expensive treatment that would be inappropriate. A cervical metastasis is usually the harbinger of rapid dissemination and death. The most common primary sites have been the ovary, colon, and breast.[162,187]

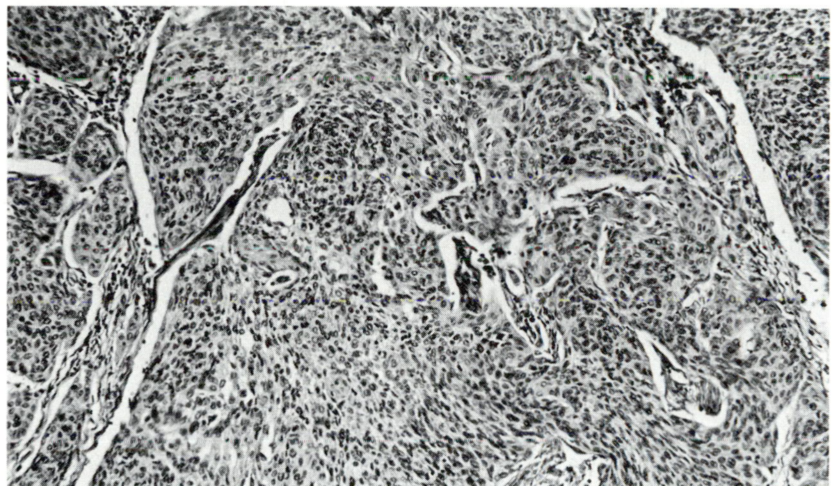

Fig. 36-35. Epidermoid carcinoma of cervix. This poorly differentiated, nonkeratinizing pattern is most common histologic type. (150×.)

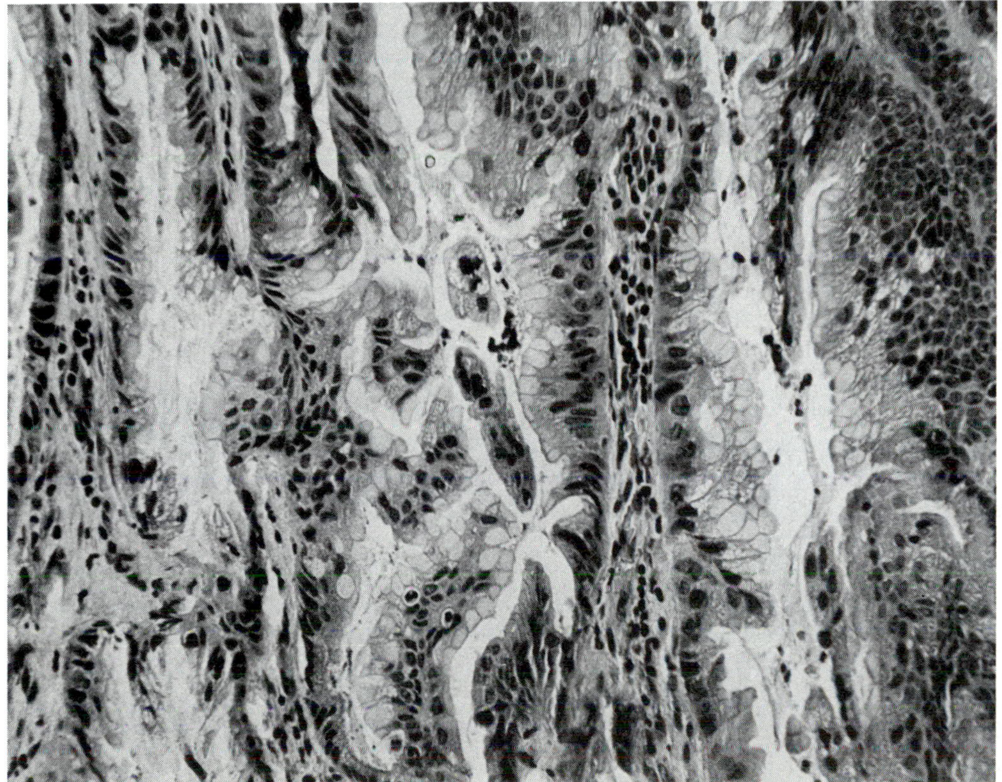

Fig. 36-36. Well-differentiated adenocarcinoma of cervix. Cytologic pattern appears deceptively benign, but bridges formed by epithelial cells without stromal support identify lesion as a carcinoma. (275×.)

ENDOMETRIUM

The function of the normal endometrium is to produce a satisfactory substrate in which a healthy blastocyst may implant and flourish. Many of the pathologic changes that occur in the endometrium reflect its responsiveness to either hormonal stimulation or the lack of it.

Normal cyclic changes

The endometrial cycle starts with a phase of proliferation for about 14 days under the influence of estrogen. If ovulation occurs, the endometrium then undergoes prominent secretory changes for the next 7 days, in time for implantation if the ovum has been fertilized. If not, the secretion wanes slowly during the following 7 days, after which the endometrium sloughs away, and the whole cycle begins anew.

The histologic, ultrastructural, and histochemical changes of the endometrial cycle have been reviewed in detail by Noyes,[331] Ferenczy and Richart,[298] and Boutselis,[280] respectively. By convention, the first day of a cycle begins with the onset of menstrual flow, which results from ischemic necrosis of the inner layer of the endometrial stroma. The denuded surface heals after about 4 days. Under the influence of estrogen the stromal cells and endometrial gland cells proliferate rapidly (Fig. 36-37, *A*). The associated histochemical events are related chiefly to protein synthesis; RNA, glucose-6-phosphatase, alkaline phosphatase, beta-glucuronidase, and nonspecific esterase are especially abundant.

After ovulation, under the influence of progesterone, there is a rise in enzymes related to carbohydrate synthesis. Lactic dehydrogenase, glucose-6-phosphate dehydrogenase, and isocitric, succinic, and malic dehydrogenases are active as increasing amounts of glycogen become evident in the gland cells.

The morphologic changes related to secretion follow a distinctive sequence. Thirty-six hours after ovulation, prominent basal vacuolation appears in the glandular epithelial cells, representing an accumulation of glycogen (Fig. 36-37, *B*). Ultrastructural studies have related the appearance of a unique and specific nucleolar channel system to ovulation. It is seen in endometrium on the sixteenth day and for several days thereafter.[298,352] Giant mitochondria with tubular cristae also appear and increase in numbers in step with the secretory process.[273] During the next 3 days secretion increases, occupying the entire cytoplasmic mass. Coincident with the time of implantation (day 20 or 21) abundant edema is present in the stroma (Fig. 36-37, *C*). If implantation does not occur, there follows a progressive decrease in secretion and stromal edema, as the activity of the corpus luteum wanes. During the 2 or 3 days before menses, cytoplasmic secretion is exhausted, and stromal cells undergo a predecidual reaction, that is, become progressively plump and prominent, especially around the spiral arterioles and beneath the surface epithelium (Fig. 36-37, *D*). On the twenty-eighth day of a typical cycle the spiral arterioles contract, the stroma crumbles, and menstrual bleeding and expulsion of the functional endometrial lining occur.

If implantation occurs, the presence of gestation is reflected in the endometrial pattern by the twenty-fifth day, 3 days before the next period of bleeding is expected to begin. Hertig[307] has shown that this early gestational hyperplastic pattern is a highly characteristic combination of recrudescence of glandular secretion and accentuation of stromal edema, together with normal predecidual reaction and increased vascular prominence. A distinctive pattern of gestational glandular hyperplasia, emphasized by Arias-Stella,[270] especially in ectopic pregnancy and in abortions, is formed by masses of enlarged gland cells with abundant clear cytoplasm and large bizarre nuclei; there is no decidual reaction in the intervening stroma.

The importance of relative proportions of estrogen to progesterone in producing the normal sequence of menstrual patterns has been shown by Good and Moyer[302] in a study of endometrial biopsies in *Macaca mulatta* monkeys.

Pathologists vary in their willingness to ascribe a specific day in the cycle to an endometrial biopsy; physicians vary in their request for and acceptance of a specific date supplied by a pathologist.[342] In the course of infertility investigations, endometrial biopsy may be used to confirm that ovulation has occurred and that the morphologic development of the endometrium is sufficiently normal to support implantation. In general, a pathologic process such as atrophy or hyperplasia indicates that the prospects for pregnancy are poor.[349] Some patients who are unable to develop an adequate secretory response may be helped by hormonal therapy.[294]

Effects of hormones

Physicians treat women with estrogens or progestogens or both, most frequently to alleviate the symptoms of estrogen deficiency (especially after menopause) and to control conception. The morphologic changes that result in the endometrium vary with the dosage and the sequence with which different combined preparations are used.

Estrogens

The characteristic changes of the proliferative phase are produced by estrogen. The estradiol produced by the ovarian follicle and synthetic estrogens have similar effects. Unremitting estrogen stimulation may occur with approximately physiologic estrogen concentrations at the time of menopause, in postmenopausal women treated with estrogen, or in younger women after multiple anovulatory cycles, as in the Stein-Leventhal syn-

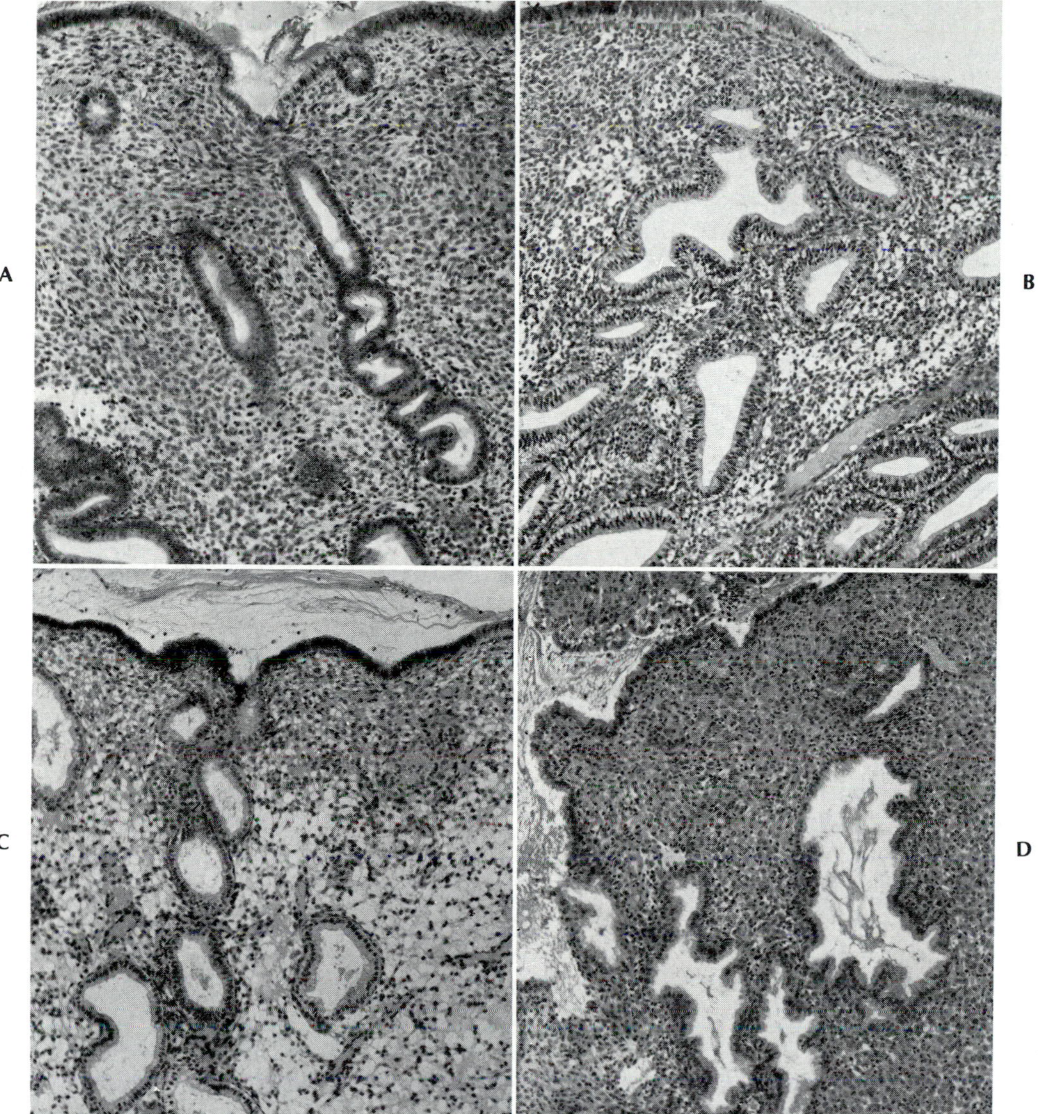

Fig. 36-37. A, Late proliferative endometrium at or about time of ovulation. Tortuous, pseudostratified glands with many mitoses are characteristic. Stroma, without predecidual reaction, may have variable degree of edema. **B,** Sixteen-day secretory endometrium. This early postovulatory endometrium is characterized by tortuous growing glands with irregular vacuolization caused by accumulation of glycogen in cytoplasm beneath nuclei. **C,** Twenty-two-day secretory endometrium. Significant features of this stage are massive stromal edema, tortuosity of glands nearing secretory exhaustion, thin-walled blood vessels, and absence of predecidua. This coincides with peak of corpus luteum activity during which time ovum is in process of implanting. **D,** Premenstrual endometrium. This phase is characterized by nearly complete predecidual transformation of stroma, secretory exhaustion of glands (which have serrated pattern), and inspissation of secretion. There is also leukocytic infiltration—both polymorphonuclear and monocytic. (150×; from Noyes, R.W., Hertig, A.T., and Rock, J.: Fertil. Steril. **1:**3, 1950.)

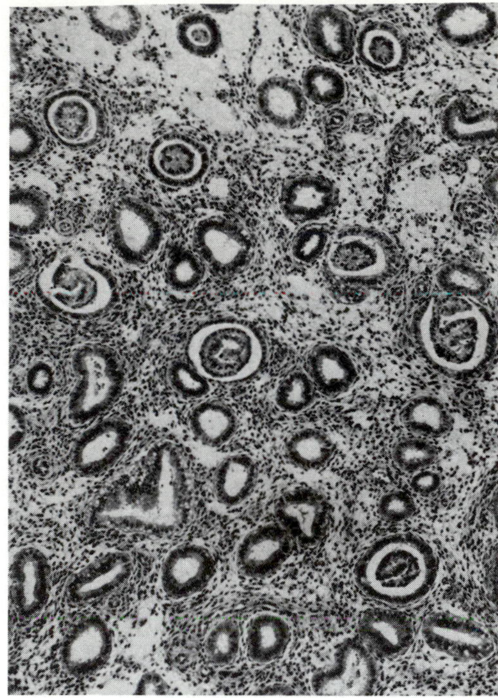

Fig. 36-38. Anovulatory endometrium. Irregular gland outlines and intraglandular epithelial protrusions are frequently found after anovulatory cycles, especially at time of menopause. (85×.)

drome. In such cases proliferative activity continues, producing a characteristic anovulatory pattern with intraglandular protrusions of redundant epithelium and a compact stroma (Fig. 36-38). After longer periods or with higher degrees of estrogen stimulation the endometrium may become hyperplastic. The pattern in some cases may resemble atypical hyperplasia. High doses of estrogen in animal experiments actually cause endometrial atrophy.

Progestogens

The therapeutic addition of progesterone or artificial progestogens causes estrogen-primed endometrial gland cells to differentiate into a secretory pattern, and further growth is inhibited. This effect is produced if the endometrium has become hyperplastic, even in the case of atypical hyperplasia or carcinoma in situ.[317] The secretory changes induced are followed by regression, gland cell atrophy, and a decidua-like reaction in the stroma.

Estrogens and progestogens

If dosages and sequences are regulated carefully, it is possible to reproduce physiologically normal cycles with a normal morphologic sequence in the endometrium. This fact has had some application in treatment of functional bleeding, dysmenorrhea, endometriosis, menopausal symptoms, infertility, and some intersex states.

Unquestionably the most common application of hormonal therapy in gynecology is in conception control. Estrogen-progestogen combination regimens produce secretion at an early point in the cycle, arresting the proliferative stimulus of estrogen at an incompletely developed stage. Continuation of the same stimulus leads to further gland atrophy, with a relatively pronounced decidua-like stromal reaction at the end of the cycle. Estrogen-progestogen sequential regimens operate in a different manner. The estrogen stimulus is carried past the time of ovulation and implantation so that secretion is delayed until about the twenty-fifth day and does not exceed the early secretory pattern of endometrium of the eighteenth day. Predecidual stromal changes do not appear.

After several months of cyclic therapy with combination agents the endometrial lining becomes thin and atrophic. Stromal cells are plump, with abundant cytoplasm. Vessels are small. The glands are generally small and lined with small, low columnar cells with traces of cytoplasmic secretion (Fig. 36-39).

The atrophy is less pronounced after long-term exposure to sequential agents. Perhaps because of the stimulative effects of estrogen, hyperplasia and even carcinoma have developed in occasional patients at a relatively young age after long-term exposure to sequential agents.[346]

Luteal phase defect

Infrequently, perhaps in 3% of infertile women, the endometrium fails to produce a fully developed secretory reaction, apparently because an inadequate corpus luteum fails to produce enough progesterone.[269,311] Early abortion has also been attributed to this condition. In a large proportion of women the basic disorder may be pituitary overproduction of prolactin, which in excess seems to diminish progesterone production. Rarely the endometrium lacks progesterone receptors. The diagnosis is customarily based on endometrial biopsy, which shows a lag in development of more than 2 days according to the dating scheme described previously. The syndrome is ill defined, appears to have many causes, and responds variably to progesterone replacement.

Metaplasia

Squamous metaplasia occasionally appears in the endometrium much the same as in the endocervix. Small clusters of cells proliferate beneath the glandular epithelium and eventually replace it. Actual keratinization is unusual. Chronic inflammation from various causes has been the most common associated factor; squamous metaplasia may occur after long-term estrogen therapy and in patients with hyperplasia. The rounded masses, or morules,[295] usually are easily recognized. Extensive squamous metaplasia produces a more complicated pattern that has been confused with carcinoma because the confluent masses of metaplastic cells resemble the epithelial bridging of carcinoma.[290] Most patients are obese

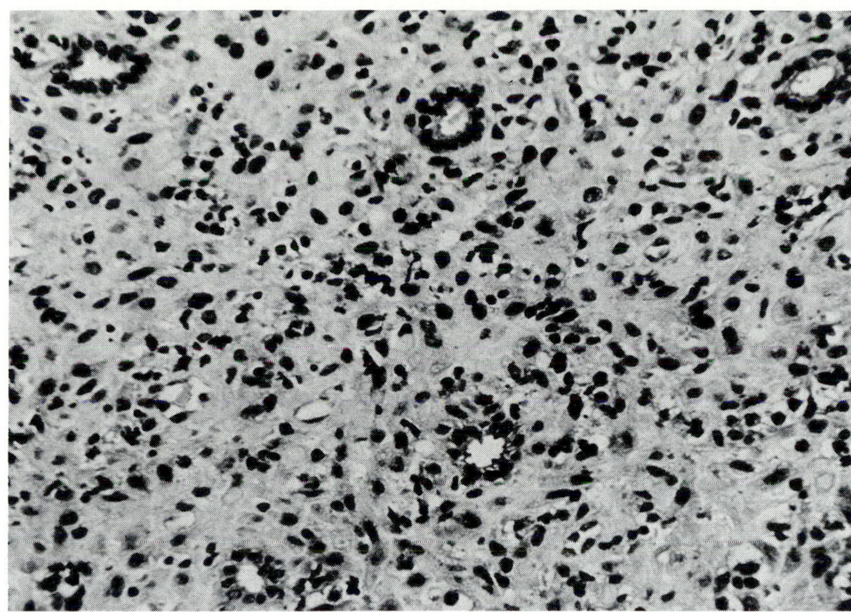

Fig. 36-39. Secretory atrophic pattern after long-term exposure to combination type of contraceptive hormonal preparation. Stromal cells are large and decidua like; glands are small and atrophic with faint traces of secretion. (350×.)

young women with the polycystic ovary syndrome. The cytologic pattern confirms the benign prognosis. Other, less common epithelial metaplasias include mucinous patterns (like those in the endocervix), ciliated cells (like those in the fallopian tube), eosinophilic cells, and papillary metaplasia, all extensively illustrated by Hendrickson and Kempson.[306]

More exotic tissues such as cartilage,[339] bone,[300] and glial tissue[364] probably also arise as metaplastic foci sometimes, but implanted aborted fetal tissue may be the most common cause. It is also possible that the endometrial stroma may react to organizing substances produced by an aborted embryo.

Hysterectomy and normal uterus

The uterus is one of the most commonly resected organs in any institution in which major surgical procedures are performed on women. There is surprisingly little objective data or discussion on the measurements, appearance, and significance of the "normal" uterus, which accounts for some pointless disagreement in hospital tissue committees.

Langlois[321] has reviewed sizes and weights of a series of 461 uteri considered to have normal gross appearance in that there was no detectable lesion known to have an effect on uterine size. The principal factor determining uterine weight in this population was parity. In general, it was found that the weight above which a uterus is *probably* abnormal was 130 g for the nulliparous woman, 210 g for parity of one to three, and 250 g for parity of four and more.

As a practical matter, objective pathologic data about the uterus frequently have little relevance to the reason for hysterectomy. Nearly half the "normal" uteri in the series reported by Langlois[321] were resected for relief of symptoms related to prolapse or abnormal bleeding. Assuming that the associated symptoms and abnormal physical findings are truthfully reported, hysterectomy is an extremely valuable means of providing relief for these patients. The uterus itself, however, usually shows no morphologic changes commensurate with the degree of preoperative symptoms. Review of the pathologists' reports alone in these circumstances does not provide the data required to audit the desirability of the surgical procedure. The endometrium examined by prior curettage either is normal, especially in the case of prolapse, or has one of the types of benign anovulatory or mixed patterns discussed subsequently.

A more controversial basis for hysterectomy is that it is undeniably an effective form of contraception. In certain ethnic and religious groups it may actually be the only available approach to contraception, although other diagnoses and symptoms are necessarily and even sincerely offered and believed by both patient and physician.

The estimated hysterectomy rate for women 15 to 44 years of age in the United States between 1970 and 1975 rose from 7.2 to 9.1 per 1000 women.[284] Estimated costs, potential benefits, and ultimate reasons for hysterectomy are perceived differently and still debated.[281]

Dysfunctional uterine bleeding

Uterine bleeding that occurs at irregular intervals in excessive or scant amounts, especially when prolonged, is said to be dysfunctional when there is no easily assign-

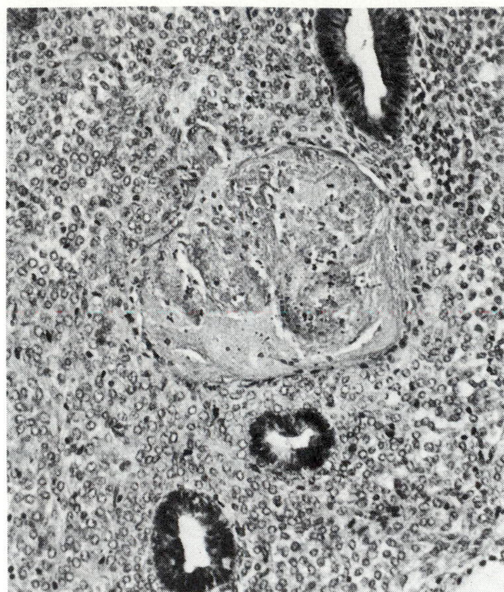

Fig. 36-40. This large fibrin thrombus distending a thin-walled vessel, with irregular proliferative phase gland outlines, indicates anovulatory endometrial bleeding. (150×.)

able cause such as hyperplasia, neoplasm, polyps, trauma, blood dyscrasia, pregnancy, or hormone administration.

The morphologic findings are variable. The presence of a mixed proliferative and secretory pattern (irregular shedding) is believed to be the result of continued progesterone secretion from a corpus luteum that fails to involute. Another common pattern is irregular nonsecretory glands with intraluminal protrusions of epithelial folds, a somewhat disorganized proliferative pattern that is common after a series of anovulatory cycles. Pathologic findings that confirm the history of bleeding include fragmentation of the stroma into compact ball-like masses, stromal fibrin accumulations, hemosiderin, and scattered tiny fragments of nuclear material sometimes called nuclear dust (Fig. 36-40). The histologic abnormality can be readily identified in curettings and is best classified as "anovulatory bleeding pattern."

A majority of the patients are in the perimenopausal period, have elevated follicle-stimulating hormone levels, and tend to have anovulatory cycles. A second group is young perimenarcheal women with the Stein-Leventhal syndrome, obesity, stress, or ovarian anomalies; most have abnormal luteinizing hormone levels, either elevated or prolonged.[267] A detailed classification has been presented by Arronet and Arrata.[274]

Inflammation

Chronic endometritis

The finding of an infiltrate of plasma cells in the endometrial stroma is the pathologic basis for the diagnosis of chronic endometritis. Most patients have menstrual disturbances, and about half may have pelvic pain or tenderness. The most common etiologic factors are recent abortion or recent delivery, coexisting pelvic inflammatory disease, and the presence of an intrauterine contraceptive device (IUD).[282]

The finding of hyalinized thick-walled stromal vessels and stellate glands with moderate secretory changes is sufficiently characteristic to identify a recent abortion as the most likely cause, even in the absence of villi.[333] Although the endometrium seems to be sterile in the presence of most IUDs, serious infections do occur, some of which have been fatal.[312]

Tuberculous endometritis is rare in the United States in comparison with other countries; the disparity so far is unexplained by factors such as variations in sophistication of treatment or public health control.[310] Granulomas are usually small, sparse, and without caseation. Patients are usually sterile; tubal infection typically occurs first.

Organisms implicated as possible causes of endometritis that deserve more study include *Mycoplasma*[293] *and Listeria*[268] species, especially with respect to chronic endometrial infection and infertility or repeated abortion. Rare causes of endometritis have been reviewed by Dallenbach-Hellweg.[292]

Acute endometritis

The most significant form of acute endometritis is postpartum bacterial sepsis originating in the endometrium. The pathologic lesion is an acute invasive suppurative infection with progressive infiltration of the endometrium, myometrium, and parametrium by polymorphonuclear leukocytes. The portal of entry is the vagina. The classic agent is the streptococcus, but anaerobic bacteria, notably *Bacteroides* species, have more recently been implicated.[279] The precise role of anaerobes is controversial. Because of the prevalence of these organisms in the lower genital tract, the significance of a positive culture may be difficult to interpret.

Hyperplasia

Abnormally prolonged, profuse, and irregular uterine bleeding in the menopausal or postmenopausal woman is commonly associated with proliferative glandular and stromal patterns called hyperplasia. Hyperplastic endometrial patterns vary, and the diagnostic terms used are confusing because their usage by different writers has varied widely. The following terminology is recommended by the World Health Organization[335] and employed in widely used textbooks of gynecologic pathology.[301]

Cystic hyperplasia is characterized by large dilated gland spaces with rounded profiles lined by relatively atrophic epithelium, separated by edematous, sparsely cellular stroma. Cystic atrophy would be a more apt designation.

Adenomatous hyperplasia is represented by a more distinctly proliferative pattern; the glands are lined by tall columnar epithelial cells with large nuclei often dis-

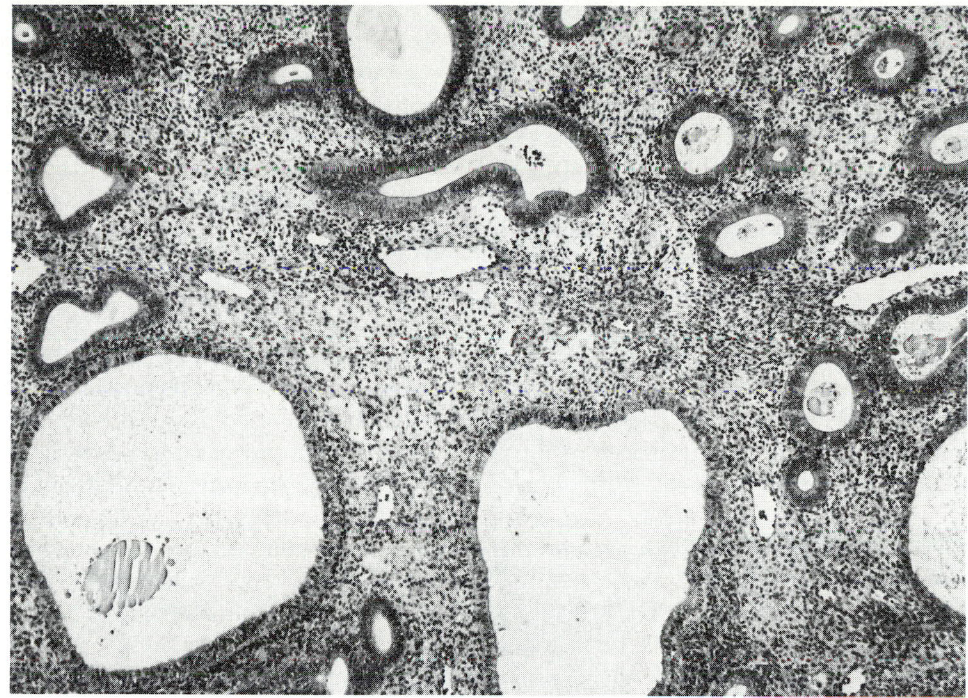

Fig. 36-41. Adenomatous hyperplasia. Dilated glands with irregular outlines and abundant stroma. (150x; from Kraus, F.T.: Gynecologic pathology, St. Louis, 1967, The C.V. Mosby Co.)

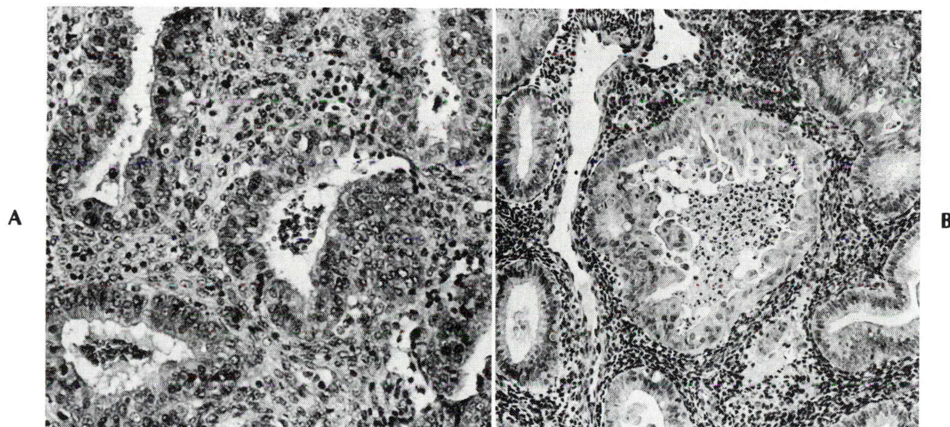

Fig. 36-42. Atypical hyperplasia. **A,** Epithelium two or three cells thick, loss of polarity, and atypical cytologic pattern (not evident at this magnification, 175×). **B,** Piled-up masses of large cells with abundant dense pink cytoplasm, small round nuclei, and loss of polarity. (75×.)

tributed at different levels, but basal polarity of nuclei is generally maintained. The gland outlines are irregular because of outpouchings and papillary infoldings of glandular epithelium. The stroma is dense, cellular, and compact. There are numerous mitoses in both glands and stroma (Fig. 36-41).

Atypical hyperplasia is more controversial as a concept and in terms of the histologic pattern it represents. There is general agreement that the cytologic features—large cells and large irregular nuclei and nucleoli—are more like those of adenocarcinoma. The cells that line the glands lose columnar orientation; cytoplasm often has a dense eosinophilic staining character (Fig. 36-42). As reported by Tavassoli and Kraus,[350] leukocytes may or may not be present. The terms *anaplasia* and *carcinoma in situ* are frequently used as synonyms. In the original description[308] carcinoma in situ designated glands lined by enlarged irregularly heaped cells with abundant homogeneous eosinophilic cytoplasm, pale nuclei, and, notably, an absence of leukocytes. Two benign conditions with large eosinophilic cells and consistent leukocytic infiltrate—but no neoplastic connotations—are eosinophilic metaplasia and some postabortal gestational endometrial glands, which also often have large polyploid nuclei.

Small foci of well-differentiated adenocarcinoma can be identified in about one fourth of uteri resected as treatment for atypical hyperplasia.[350] The significance of this observation is uncertain; carcinoma seldom develops in women with atypical hyperplasia whose uteri are not resected, if they are treated with progestogens. The minimal criteria for diagnosis of adenocarcinoma developing in endometrial hyperplasia are not as clear or settled as most textbooks imply.[306a]

The etiology and significance of hyperplastic lesions is debated, and the varied use of terms has not clarified understanding of the subject. Unquestionably, estrogen administration produces hyperplasia.[318] Prolonged periods of anovulation with steady estrogen secretion that omit the periodic differentiating stimulus of progesterone have a similar effect, even in young women.[285,303,356] Atypical hyperplastic patterns may occur after prolonged anovulation in the Stein-Leventhal syndrome and will regress after therapeutic induction of ovulation.[313]

Actual progression of hyperplastic lesions to carcinomas has been observed, as reviewed by Gore and Hertig[304] and by Vellios,[356] but not frequently; most patients have been treated with progestogens or by hysterectomy, usually to control bleeding within a few months or years of the diagnosis of hyperplasia. The lesions classified here as atypical hyperplasia and carcinoma in situ apparently respond completely to the differentiating effect of progestogens.[317] For this reason the term "carcinoma in situ" as applied to the endometrium may be semantically confusing. Despite reversal of the morphologic lesion, abnormal bleeding often resumes and eventually is the basis for hysterectomy in many women treated for endometrial hyperplasia.

Benign polypoid lesions

Endometrial polyps are composed of a mixture of endometrial glands and stroma organized into a circumscribed mass that protrudes into the endometrial cavity. The histologic pattern usually resembles that of so-called cystic hyperplasia, as described previously. There may be variable degrees of stromal fibrosis, traces of smooth muscle are commonly present, and stromal vessels are disproportionately large. When smooth muscle is abundant, the lesion is classified as a pedunculated adenomyoma. Squamous metaplasia in a polypoid adenomyoma produces a complex pattern that is easily confused with cancer.[324] Follow-up data currently indicate a benign course.

Endometrial polyps may be a source of abnormal uterine bleeding. An isolated carcinoma arising in an endometrial polyp is rare; the patients who had a focal carcinoma in a polyp, described by Salm,[341] also had a focal carcinoma elsewhere in the endometrium. Armenia[271] found that 17 of 482 women with endometrial polyps subsequently were shown to have carcinoma of the endometrium. This is a greater incidence than expected in all women of the same age, but such an association is not commonly demonstrable.

Neoplasms

Adenocarcinoma

Carcinoma of the endometrium is primarily a disease of menopausal and postmenopausal women. The patients are more commonly nulliparous and as a group are more likely to be obese, diabetic, and hypertensive than a comparable group of women with a normal endometrium. Although endometrial carcinoma occurred with one-tenth the frequency of cervical carcinoma 40 years ago, it has become increasingly common and has finally surpassed the incidence of cervical carcinoma.[327]

The etiology is unknown, but long-continued noncyclic endometrial stimulation by estrogen, even at normally occurring concentrations, seems to be an important factor, especially when unopposed by the periodic differentiating stimulus provided by progestogen.

Estrone appears to be the most significant estrogenic hormone in this postulated relationship to cancer. Estrone is produced by conversion from adrenal (or ovarian) androstenedione in women who are menopausal, have polycystic ovary syndrome, or are obese. Conversion apparently occurs in peripheral adipose tissue. Statistical studies indicate that endometrial carcinoma is four to eight times more likely to develop in the postmenopausal woman who takes estrogens than in a group of matched control subjects,[348] especially with estrogens composed principally of estrone. The carcinomas identified in estrogen users differ from those occurring without estrogen use; they are well differentiated, superficial, and identified at a younger age and appear to behave less aggressively.[336,347] Also, in contrast to less-differentiated cancers in women who did not take estrogens, there is often an associated hyperplasia in adjacent endometrium. The addition of a progestogen on a cyclic dosage schedule seems to eliminate the risk of cancer among women taking estrogens in the perimenopausal period.[305,353] This is fortunate because estrogens are effective in delaying osteoporosis and the consequent debilitating fractures that may occur in postmenopausal women.[357]

Hyperstimulation by high levels of estrogen may produce an extremely hyperplastic pattern that may be difficult to distinguish from that of a well-differentiated carcinoma. Such a pattern also has been produced by exogenous estrogens and by endogenous estrogen from ovarian neoplasms, especially granulosa-theca cell tumors. Lesions of this type seem to be estrogen depen-

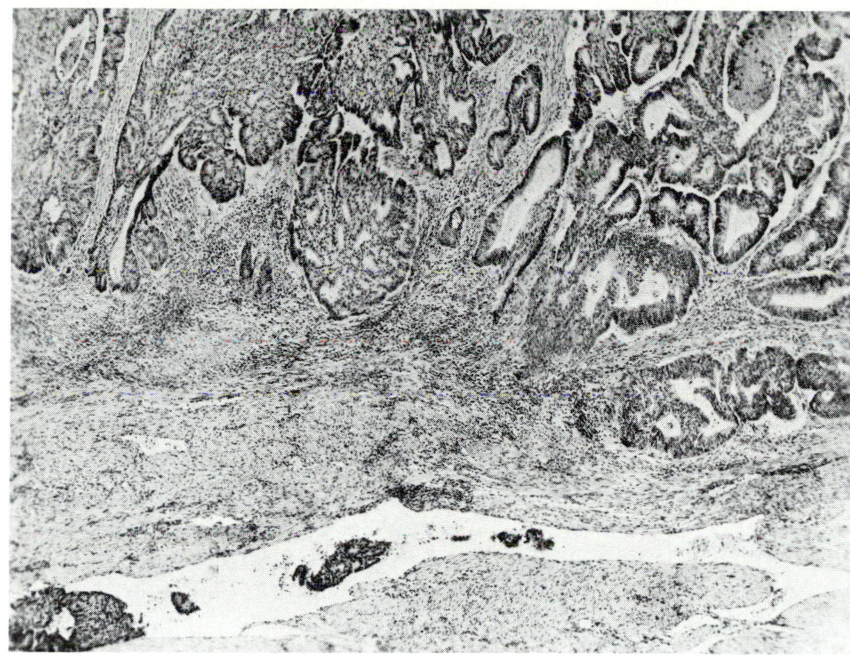

Fig. 36-43. Endometrial adenocarcinoma, moderately differentiated, invading myometrium and dilated lymphatic. (46×; AFIP 264087-2.)

dent, since they may regress when the stimulus is removed, and there are few documented reports of death or metastases. More recently a relationship between the use of the sequential type of contraceptive hormone preparation and endometrial cancer has been suggested. The relatively extended exposure to estrogen may be responsible. Some kind of constitutional predisposition may also be necessary; few cases have been identified.[346]

Gross appearance. Endometrial adenocarcinoma forms large irregular masses of friable, granular, gray-tan tissue that protrude into the endometrial cavity. Extension into the muscular wall of the uterus is identified in cut sections by the presence of softer bulging masses of lighter gray granular tissue that replaces the myometrium.

Microscopic appearance. Most endometrial adenocarcinomas are well differentiated and composed of festoons and ribbons of columnar epithelium, forming multiglandular masses. The gland spaces are typically bridged by strands of epithelium that lack stromal support (Fig. 36-43). Nuclei are large and have irregular outlines, clumped chromatin, and prominent nucleoli. Focal histologically benign squamous metaplasia is common especially in well-differentiated tumors, a pattern that is designated adenoacanthoma (Fig. 36-44). Ng and associates[327] recommended that the term *adenosquamous carcinoma* be used to identify mixed carcinomas in which the squamous and glandular elements both are malignant. Rarely an endometrial carcinoma is composed of large clear cells that produce abundant glycogen; these clear cell adenocarcinomas resemble the endometrial

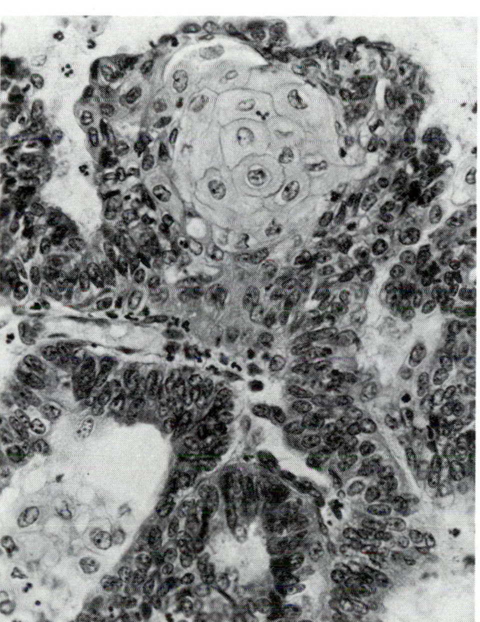

Fig. 36-44. Adenocarcinoma with squamous metaplasia (adenoacanthoma). Benign squamous epithelial pattern distinguishes this from adenosquamous carcinoma in which squamous component is malignant. (235×; AFIP 264048-1.)

hypersecretory pattern seen during pregnancy. Ultrastructural studies indicate a müllerian histogenesis; there is no evidence for a relationship to mesonephric structures.[345]

Many endometrial carcinomas include a few cells that produce vacuoles of mucin, and occasionally adenocarcinomas limited to the fundus may be composed chiefly of typical mucinous epithelium of the cervical type. For this reason histochemical stains for mucin are of little use in identifying the precise location of an adenocarcinoma; one must examine tissue from the endocervix and endometrium specifically and separately to localize the extent of an adenocarcinoma of the uterus. There are occasional reports of endometrial epidermoid carcinoma.[314]

Factors affecting prognosis. Nearly 90% of women with endometrial cancer limited to the endometrium survive 5 years. As invasion extends to the inner half of the myometrium, survival falls to 70%, and with cancer spread outside the uterus, survival is less than 15%. Endometrial carcinomas that involve the cervix are more likely to metastasize to pelvic lymph nodes, with a similar distribution to that of cervical carcinoma. For this reason cervical involvement must be determined before treatment can be planned on a rational basis. Survival is good (85%) when the cancer is well differentiated and bad (30%) when it is poorly differentiated.[326] Carcinomas with a mixed adenosquamous pattern are usually poorly differentiated and have a poor prognosis.[327,344]

Endometrial stromal neoplasms

Benign endometrial stromal nodules form single, well-circumscribed masses that can often be distinguished grossly from leiomyomas by their yellow color and softer consistency. Most are in the myometrium, but some protrude into the endometrial cavity. The histologic appearance closely resembles that of normal endometrial stroma, with numerous evenly distributed small vessels forming a distinctive part of the pattern. Stromal lesions of similar origin that have a distinct trabecular pattern have also been called plexiform tumorlets.[322] The endometrial stroma can form a variety of glandlike structures, some of which mimic ovarian stromal tumor patterns, including sex cords and Call-Exner bodies.[325]

Endolymphatic stromal myosis forms multiple bulging masses of variable size, although there is often a single

A

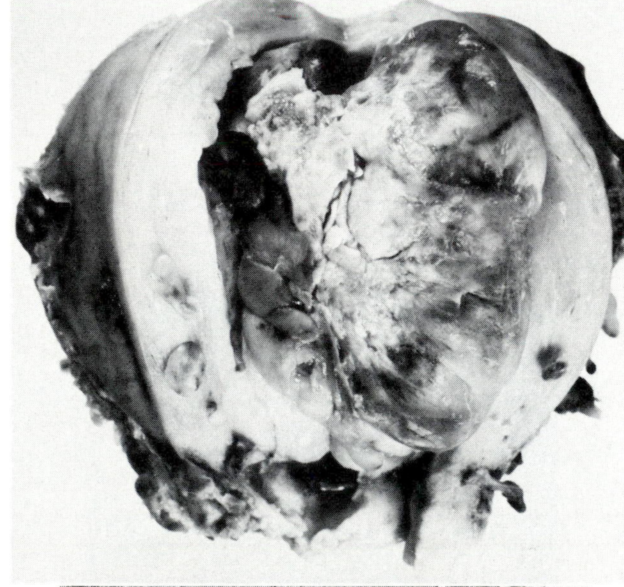

B

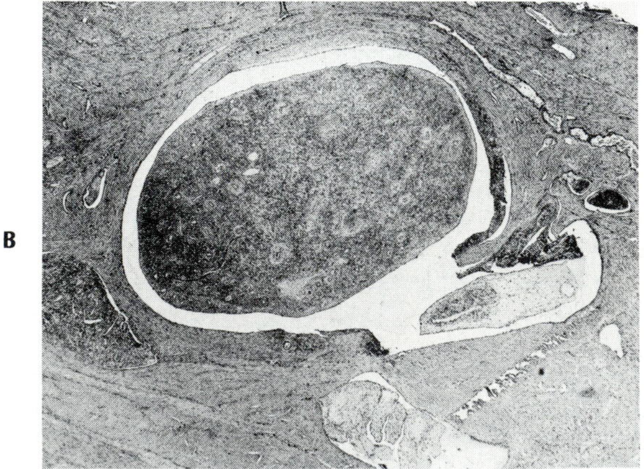

Fig. 36-45. Endolymphatic stromal myosis. **A,** Large, soft, polypoid mass distends endometrial cavity; extensions of mass protrude wormlike from dilated vascular spaces in sectioned uterine wall. **B,** Photomicrograph of neoplastic stroma extending through vascular space in uterine wall. Myometrium is not infiltrated.

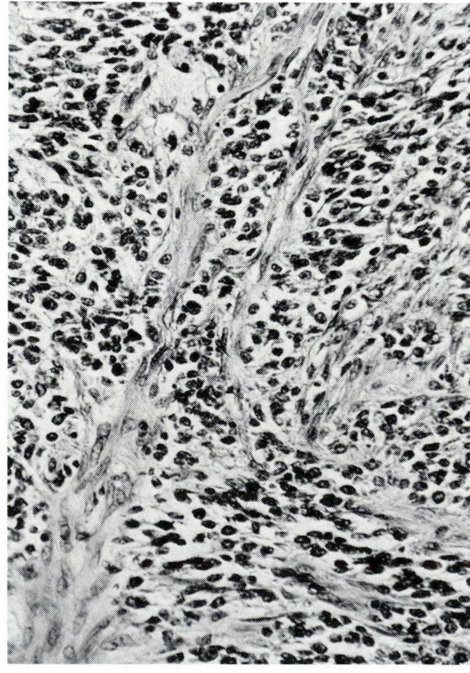

Fig. 36-46. Endometrial stromal sarcoma. Myometrial fibers are separated by infiltrating anaplastic endometrial stromal cells. (150×.)

dominant endometrial mass. The most dramatic and characteristic feature is the presence of numerous wormlike masses of stromal tissue that extrude from vascular channels when the uterine wall is cut (Fig. 36-45). Margins of stromal growths are well circumscribed; mitoses are infrequent. The clinical course is usually benign, but incompletely resected lesions may recur slowly in the pelvis, and in an occasional patient a pulmonary metastasis has developed. One of the 19 patients reported by Norris and Taylor[330] died of the tumor 12 years after the initial resection. Some metastatic lesions have regressed after progestogen therapy.[320] Similar stromal lesions may arise in the pelvic retroperitoneum.[355]

Endometrial stromal sarcoma is a highly malignant tumor that characteristically forms one or more polypoid endometrial masses. Margins are indistinct as the result of diffuse infiltration of the myometrium by poorly differentiated small cells (Fig. 36-46). Mitoses are numerous; more than 10 per 10 high-power microscopic fields indicate a poor prognosis.[330]

Malignant mixed müllerian tumor (carcinosarcoma; mixed mesodermal tumor)

An uncommon and highly malignant group of endometrial cancers is composed of a mixture of carcinoma and sarcoma patterns. The patients are usually elderly and postmenopausal. A surprisingly large proportion have had prior radiotherapy.[329]

Abnormal bleeding is the most common symptom; the tumor may appear as a polyp protruding through the cervical canal. The carcinoma component includes the full range of patterns seen in endometrial carcinoma. Poorly differentiated endometrial adenocarcinoma is usually predominant. Focal components of clear cell adenocarcinoma, epidermoid carcinoma, and even papillary serous adenocarcinoma like that in the ovary also are common, and occasional embryonic-appearing gland structures are characteristic. If the stromal component is an undifferentiated sarcoma, the tumor is said to be homologous mixed müllerian tumor or carcinosarcoma (Fig. 36-47). Heterologous mixed müllerian tumors are those that also contain chondrosarcoma, osteosarcoma, or rhabdomyosarcoma.

The prognosis is extremely poor. Metastases occur early. The few survivors have had small lesions confined to the uterus, but even with such limited involvement the tumor often may disseminate widely, rapidly, and fatally.[276] The presence or absence of heterologous elements has not affected the prognosis significantly in most series. Radiotherapy may control localized lesions.[332] My experience and some reports[277] indicate improved results with chemotherapy.

An uncommon variant with a benign epithelial component mixed with a sarcomatous stroma has been called adenosarcoma by Clement and Scully.[288] Mitoses among the stromal cells exceed 4 per 10 high-powered microscopic fields; the most aggressive lesions are those that invade the uterine wall.[363]

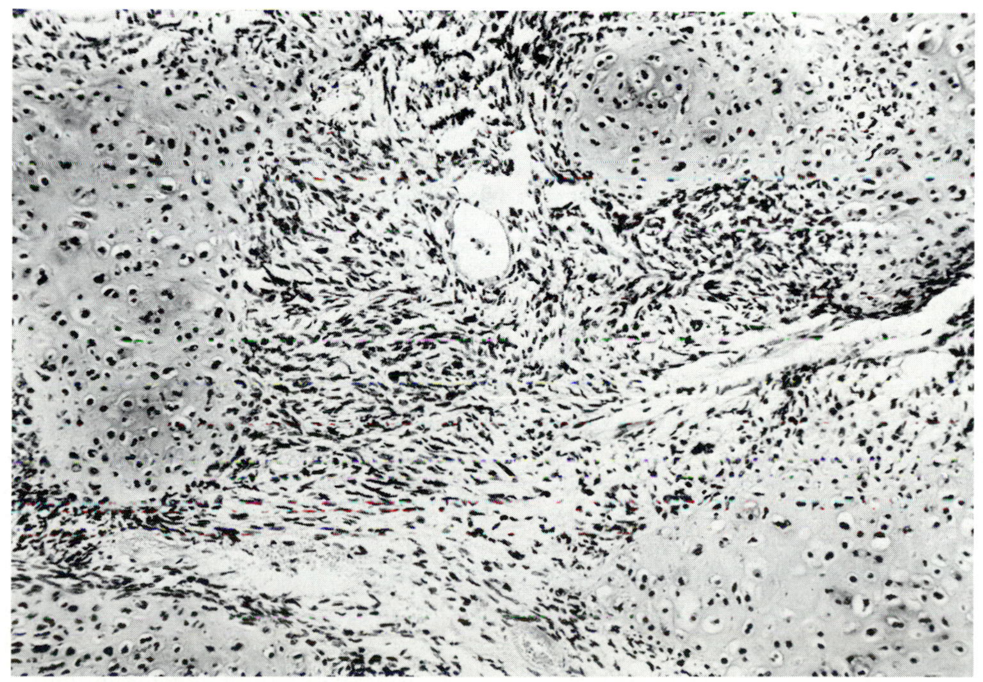

Fig. 36-47. Malignant mixed müllerian tumor. Sarcoma pattern, undifferentiated at center, with chondrosarcoma at margins. (150×; from Kraus, F.T.: Gynecologic pathology, St. Louis, 1967, The C.V. Mosby Co.)

Adenofibroma, the benign extreme in the spectrum of mixed müllerian tumors of the uterus, is distinguished by its circumscribed growth pattern and fewer than 4 mitoses per 10 high-power microscopic fields among the stromal cells. The histologic pattern resembles that of the more common ovarian adenofibroma.[363]

Metastatic carcinoma

Carcinoma metastatic from distant primary sites is rare in the endometrium. The most common origin noted is usually breast cancer identified at autopsy.[319] Gastrointestinal cancer has also been reported and may be identified in endometrial curettage. The simultaneous finding of areas of neoplastic change in the endometrium together with cancer of the tube, cervix, or ovary occasionally may represent a metastasis, but in most instances it probably has a multifocal origin.[361]

Primary malignant lymphomas originating in the cervix and body of the uterus have a relatively good prognosis when confined to the uterus. Chorlton and associates[286] found lymphocytic lymphomas, both nodular and diffuse (eight cases), histiocytic lymphoma (four), granulocytic sarcomas (two), and only one instance of Hodgkin's disease.

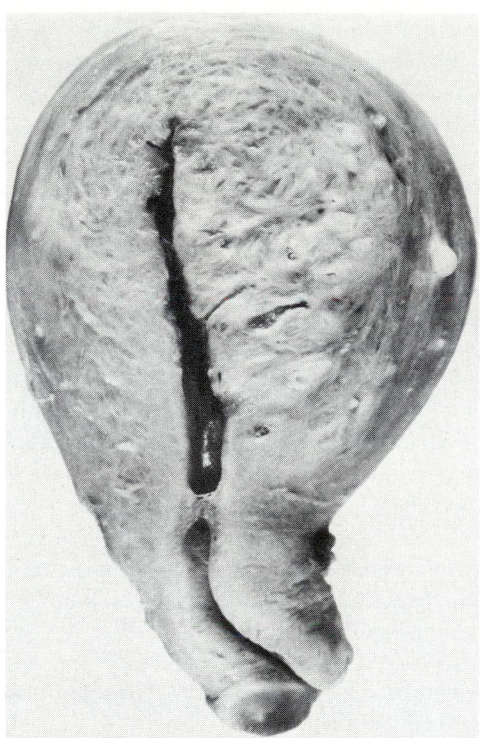

Fig. 36-48. Adenomyosis. Uterus has globular shape. In sagittal section, myometrial mass is poorly circumscribed. Soft depressions are composed of heterotopic endometrium; some are hemorrhagic.

MYOMETRIUM

The myometrium provides a tough envelope for the developing fetus and propels it into independent life at parturition. It is painful when ischemic, as in the case of prolonged contraction and perhaps with infarction of a smooth muscle neoplasm.

Adenomyosis

The abnormal distribution of nests of histologically benign endometrial tissue within the myometrium is adenomyosis. It may be focal or diffuse. The involved portions of myometrial smooth muscle are hypertrophied.

The typical uterus is enlarged and globular, often with lateral humps at the horns. The posterior wall is most commonly affected and is more extensively involved when the process is diffuse. The cut surface of areas of adenomyosis bulges and has ill-defined margins and a coarse trabecular appearance. The scattered foci of endometrial tissue appear depressed, soft, and occasionally hemorrhagic (Fig. 36-48).

The islands of ectopic endometrium appear normal on histologic examination, except that orientation of glands is lacking. Both glands and stroma are present. Recent hemorrhage and hemosiderin in macrophages, indicating past hemorrhage, are usually found only in occasional areas. Both glands and stroma may respond to hormonal stimulation, but not in all cases or in all parts of the same lesion.

The minimum criteria for diagnosis are vague. Most texts refer to the depth of more than 1 low-power microscopic field as the borderline beyond which endometrium qualifies for the diagnosis of adenomyosis. Microscopes vary. It is probable that the occasional superficial foci of endometrial growth that retain cystic accumulation of old blood are symptomatic and significant even if they do not qualify as adenomyosis by this criterion. The presence of associated muscle hypertrophy, as detected by bulges on the fresh-cut surface, also probably indicates a pathologic process. The common extensions of endometrium that retain continuity with the surface but reach a depth of 1 to 2 mm are probably not significant. Some judgment is required in evaluating the possibility that a superficial process may have been the cause of symptoms; rigid criteria of measurement alone probably will never enable one to classify all cases reliably.

The symptoms ascribed to adenomyosis are pain, especially with menstrual periods, cramps, and abnormally prolonged and profuse menstrual bleeding. Correlation of the degree of symptoms with the extent of the pathologic process is frequently poor. Occasionally a uterus is found to be extensively involved, with no history of menstrual difficulty. Just as often, an enlarged uterus is removed for all the appropriate reasons, but no adenomyosis can be demonstrated by the pathologist to justify the symptoms or the hysterectomy.[371]

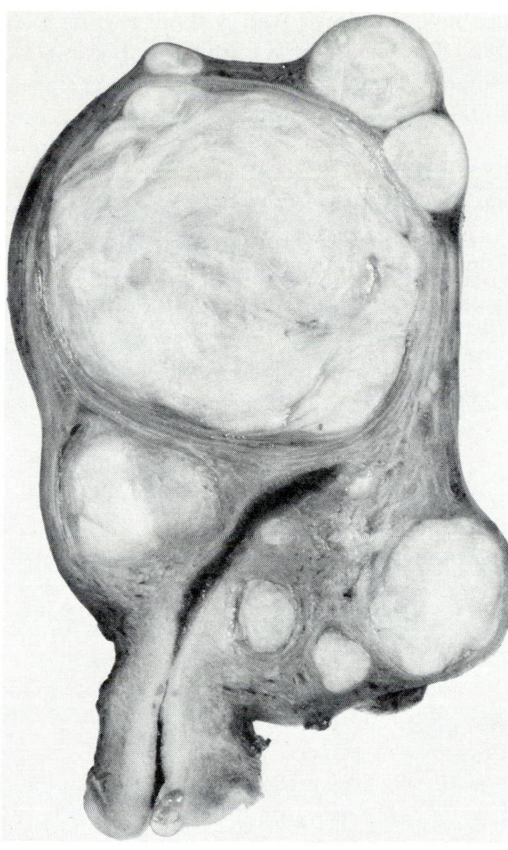

Fig. 36-49. Multiple leiomyomas in sagittal section. Typical, well-circumscribed, solid, light gray nodules distort uterus.

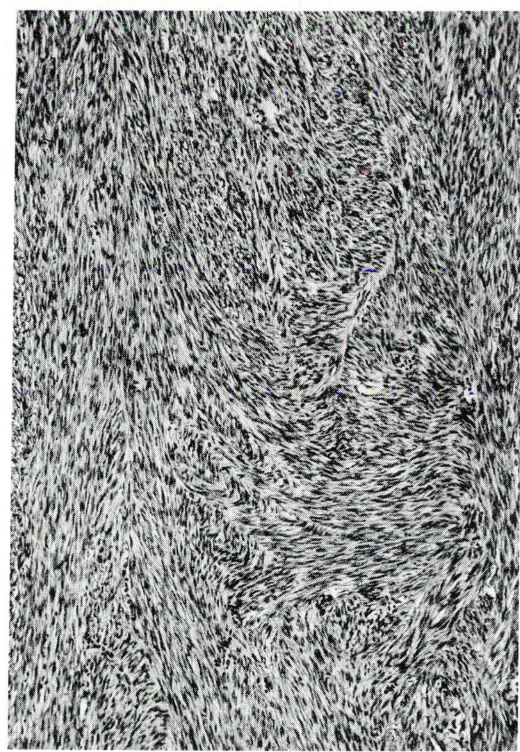

Fig. 36-50. Leiomyoma. Typical interlacing pattern. (140×; from Kraus, F.T.: Gynecologic pathology, St. Louis, 1967, The C.V. Mosby Co.)

The pathogenesis is unexplained. Adenomyosis is not seen in children and is much less common in young women, a finding suggesting that it is unlikely to be a congenital malformation. The most popular concept is that the endometrium extends into the myometrium; a metaplasia of the myometrium is equally tenable. Estrogen stimulation may be an important etiologic factor. Adenomyosis is not usually associated with endometriosis, even when the endometriosis is extensive. It does seem to occur more frequently in women with endometrial hyperplasia or endometrial carcinoma.[379] In such cases the foci of adenomyosis may occasionally also appear hyperplastic or neoplastic, in step with the endometrial lesion.

Neoplasms of smooth muscle

Leiomyoma

The most common lesion of the myometrium is a benign neoplasm composed of smooth muscle with a variable fibrous tissue component. Leiomyomas are well-circumscribed, rounded, firm or hard rubbery masses of gray-white tissue with a characteristic whorled appearance on cut surface. They are often multiple and vary considerably in size (Fig. 36-49). Most occur during the years of active reproductive life; growth may be stimulated by pregnancy or hormonal therapy.

Symptoms vary with location. Subserosal leiomyomas may impinge on the bladder or the sacral plexus, for instance, causing urinary frequency or pain. Submucous leiomyomas that protrude into the endometrial cavity cause abnormal bleeding. Rarely very large leiomyomas have been associated with polycythemia[383,386]; whether the leiomyoma secretes an erythropoietic factor itself or stimulates the kidney to do so remains to be shown. Leiomyomas undergoing infarction or hemorrhage may be painful. Hysterography may amplify physical findings in establishing the diagnosis and sites of involvement with considerable accuracy.[385]

The histologic pattern is familiar, with streaming masses of smooth muscle separated by strands or masses of collagen (Fig. 36-50). Some remarkable variations occur, with pronounced edema or massive calcification or hyalinization. Leiomyomas that have a sizable adipose tissue component have been called lipoleiomyomas.[377]

Cellular leiomyomas have a threatening histologic appearance because of the absence of fibrotic areas and the large size of the individual cells and their nuclei. They are distinguished from leiomyosarcoma by the absence of mitoses.[369]

Bizarre leiomyomas have an even more frightening

microscopic appearance because of the many large giant cells with very large, cytologically malignant-looking nuclei, which may be multiple. These lesions also lack the mitoses that characterize leiomyosarcoma and have proved to be benign after many years of follow-up study.[369] Fechner[372] has described bizarre leiomyomas in a few younger women who were using oral contraceptives. A direct relationship has not been established; the prognosis has been good.

Clear cell leiomyomas (leiomyoblastomas) are rare uterine counterparts of a similar tumor found in the stomach,[393] characterized histologically by abundant clear cytoplasm. Nearly all are benign; the few aggressive lesions have had more numerous mitoses.

Borderline smooth muscle lesions

Rarely proliferating masses of smooth muscle may behave in an aggressive manner that belies their benign microscopic appearance.

Peritoneal leiomyomatosis. Peritoneal leiomyomatosis refers to the extensive spread of histologically benign masses of smooth muscle about the peritoneal surfaces but limited to the peritoneal cavity. There seems to be a close relationship to pregnancy; it is probable that the origin is metaplastic rather than metastatic from the uterus.[384,394]

Metastasizing leiomyoma. Rarely a histologically benign leiomyoma may seem to be the source of lymph nodal or pulmonary metastases.[376] Mitoses are not seen. In some cases progression seems related to hormonal factors, including pregnancy.[368] Intravenous extensions of the uterine tumor are absent.

Cramer and associates[370] identified estrogen receptors in an aggressive metastasizing leiomyoma and noted regression after termination of pregnancy. Other smooth muscle lesions (pulmonary lymphangiomyomatosis) have appeared to respond to endocrine manipulation.[365] Wolff, Silva, and Kay[360] argue cogently that most or all "multiple pulmonary fibroleiomyomas" are actually metastatic uterine smooth muscle tumors, despite admixed (entrapped) glandular components.

Intravenous leiomyomatosis. Intravenous leiomyomatosis is a benign smooth muscle neoplasm that produces fleshy outgrowths of histologically benign smooth muscle into pelvic veins. Mitoses are absent. The prognosis is good even if all the intravenous extensions cannot be resected.[382,390] The changes are dramatic when extensive; less obvious cases are probably often overlooked.

Leiomyomas of uncertain malignant potential. Rarely an otherwise orderly, circumscribed, cytologically benign leiomyoma in a young woman turns out to have a surprisingly large number of cells in mitosis, in the range of 5 to 9 per 10 high-powered microscopic fields. A few patients have been pregnant; in most the leiomyoma was resected by enucleation (myomectomy) only. These patients have remained well without further treatment. Whether some or any may ultimately become examples of "benign metastasizing leiomyoma" remains to be determined by extended follow-up study.

Leiomyosarcoma

Leiomyosarcoma, the most common of uterine sarcomas, arises from the muscular wall of the uterus; although origin from a leiomyoma is possible and associated leiomyomas are present in a minority of cases, it is unusual to be able to prove such an occurrence.[315,369,382,391] The incidence is approximately 0.6 per 100,000 women over 20 years.[369,388] The mean age of patients at the time of diagnosis in most series is over 50, with a range of 40 to 80 years. Nonspecific symptoms related to uterine enlargement and abnormal uterine bleeding form the usual basis for exploration; only occasionally does tissue obtained by curettage establish a preoperative diagnosis.

Most leiomyosarcomas are large and soft; the yellow or tan color, lack of a trabeculated pattern, at least in some areas, and poorly circumscribed margins may suggest the diagnosis on gross inspection.

The histologic pattern nearly always includes areas with typical swirling masses of spindle-shaped smooth muscle cells containing identifiable myofibrils (Fig. 36-

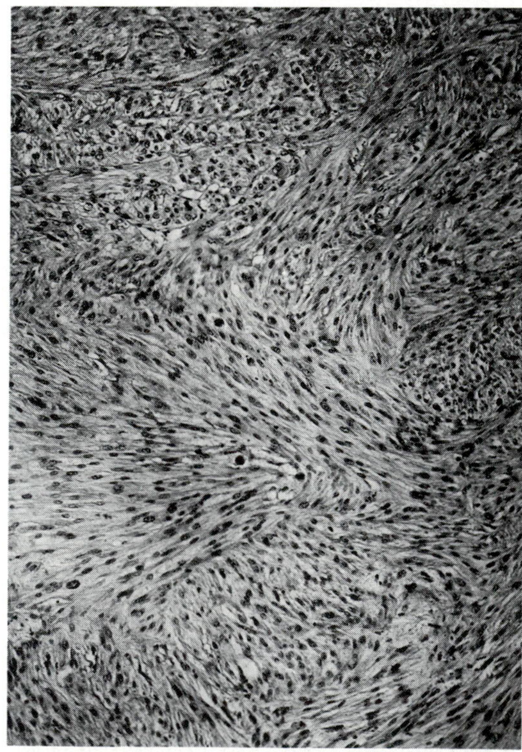

Fig. 36-51. Leiomyosarcoma, well differentiated. Tumor cells are only moderately pleomorphic, but mitoses are numerous. (150×; from Kraus, F.T.: Gynecologic pathology, St. Louis, 1967, The C.V. Mosby Co.)

51). Nuclei are large and hyperchromatic with irregularly clumped chromatin. Most leiomyosarcomas include a few areas with large pleomorphic or anaplastic tumor cells. The most significant indicator of malignant behavior is the number of mitoses found in microscopic sections. Lesions that contain areas with more than 10 mitoses per 10 high-power fields are classified as sarcomas.[369,396] Lesions with less than 5 mitoses per 10 high-power fields have been associated with a good prognosis.[315,369,388,391] Those lesions in which the numbers of mitoses lie between 5 and 10 per high-power fields constitute a borderline group; most of these patients will survive, at least for 5 years, but several reports have recorded a few deaths in this category. The most significant clinical prognostic factor is age. Over half the premenopausal patients studied by Vardi and Tovell[397] survived 5 years; in contrast, only 1 of 18 postmenopausal women with leiomyosarcoma survived.

Extension beyond the uterus is associated uniformly with a fatal prognosis. Chemotherapy with doxorubicin (Adriamycin) has seemed to produce a transient antitumor effect in a few patients.[366]

Other neoplasms. Lipomas, composed entirely of adipose tissue, are rare and probably result from metaplasia in smooth muscle or stromal cells.[389] Adenomatoid tumor is an uncommon benign nodular mass that resembles a leiomyoma grossly but microscopically has a microcystic honeycomb appearance caused by numerous small spaces lined by vacuolated cells.[398] Similar lesions occur in the fallopian tube. Ultrastructural and histochemical studies support a mesothelial origin.[373,395]

Uterine hemangiopericytoma is another rare benign nodular tumor. It resembles an endometrial stromal nodule grossly and microscopically; the photomicrographs of many reported cases appear more consistent with a stromal nodule. Reticulin stains accentuate the pericapillary growth of plump, spindle-shaped pericytes that make up the tumor. This histogenetic concept is supported by ultrastructural study.[392]

FALLOPIAN TUBE

Anatomy and physiology

The paired fallopian tubes are divided into specific regions, each of which has somewhat different functions. The interstitial portion is a narrow channel through the cornual wall of the uterine fundus. The isthmic portion, about 2 to 3 cm long, is immediately distal to the tubouterine junction. The muscular wall, both longitudinal and circular, is especially prominent in this portion and probably functions as a sphincter. The ampullary portion, about 5 to 8 cm long, has a much wider lumen and an extensive mucosa as the result of the complex folds, or plicae, which greatly increase its surface and secretory capacity. The infundibulum is the trumpetlike distal portion that terminates in the tubal fimbriae. The infundibular muscle also has the capacity to act as a sphincter.

The tubal mucosa is composed of three types of cells. The ciliated cells have an obvious function in transport through the tube. The secretory cells are columnar; they become especially tall and actively secreting during the secretory half of the menstrual cycle. Also present are narrow, dark intercalated cells, which apparently represent secretory cells at an inactive or exhausted stage. Both scanning and transmission electron microscopy have contributed considerably to current concepts of tubal mucosal morphology.[402]

The outer serosal covering is a mesothelial structure; tiny nodular masses of mesothelial proliferation may glisten like dewdrops on the outer surface of the tube; these so-called Walthard's cell rests should not be confused with tumor implants. The ultrastructural pattern is similar to that of urinary transitional epithelium, apparently involving a metaplastic change in mesothelial cells.

The fallopian tubes are complex structures that represent considerably more than conduits from ovary to endometrial cavity. The fringelike fimbriae are actively approximated to the ovary at ovulation by a fold of smooth muscle.

Coordination of muscular activity, epithelial proliferation, ciliary activity, and mucosal secretion is under endocrine control and varies with the phases of the menstrual cycle. Muscular activity also is probably affected by coitus. Mitochondria are greatly increased in both ciliated and secretory cells during the secretory half of the menstrual cycle; granular endoplasmic reticulum and secretion granules appear in the secretory cells at this time.

The circular smooth muscle layer can have a peristaltic effect under appropriate stimulation; spermatozoa are conveyed to the ampullary portion of the tube, where fertilization takes place faster than can be achieved with their unaided locomotive powers. The secretions of the tubal epithelium are indispensable for capacitation of both spermatozoa and ova, without which fertilization cannot take place. The transport of the zygote cannot be unduly accelerated or retarded if the blastocyst is to develop and implant properly.

Inflammation

Acute salpingitis and pelvic inflammatory disease

Acute inflammation of the fallopian tube originates chiefly as a complication of venereally transmitted infections of the lower genital tract. Puerperal or postabortal salpingitis occurs especially after intrauterine instrumentation. Intra-abdominal infections such as appendicitis with peritonitis may secondarily affect the tube. Hematogenous spread is important in the pathogenesis of tuberculosis of the tube and some cases of pneumococcal salpingitis occurring in children.

The most common agent, at least initially, is *Neisseria*

gonorrhoeae; gonococcal salpingitis develops in about 10% of women with gonorrhea of the lower genital tract.[412] Subsequently, with the formation of more extensive pelvic tubo-ovarian abscess, numerous other organisms, notably anaerobes, have been cultured. IUDs may increase the potential for salpingitis and more extended pelvic infection after lower genital tract infections, including gonorrhea.[423]

Meticulous culture techniques are important because the most common anaerobes identified have been *Bacteroides* species, which are not sensitive to penicillin[418] and pose a considerable threat to the patient if inadequately controlled. Mycoplasmas also represent important organisms that will not be cultured by "routine" bacteriologic cultural techniques in most laboratories unless the possibility is specifically stressed by the physician performing the culture.[408] *Chlamydia trachomatis* infections, an increasingly common form of nongonococcal urethritis, have been implicated also as a cause of salpingitis.[408] Laparoscopic examinations are especially effective in establishing an accurate diagnosis.[405]

The fallopian tubes are nearly always affected bilaterally. The fimbriated ends are sealed by organizing inflammatory exudate, and the lumina are dilated, especially the ampullary portion, producing a retort-shaped deformation (Fig. 36-52). The serosa is red and covered with purulent exudate, which extends to the ovaries and pelvic wall. Loculated pockets of pus may accumulate, producing a tubo-ovarian abscess, with the tube, uterus, broad ligament, and ovary forming parts of the surrounding abscess wall.

Microscopically the lumen of the tube is filled with polymorphonuclear leukocytes, which also extensively infiltrate the tubal mucosa and wall. The mucosal epithelium may be focally ulcerated but generally remains intact.

Chronic salpingitis

After approximately 10 days plasma cells, macrophages, and lymphocytes begin to dominate the inflammatory cell pattern. Fibrosis becomes progressively more apparent as the exudate organizes. The tubal plicae form adhesions in many areas, sometimes producing a complicated multiglandular pattern. As the inflammatory process finally resolves, this arrangement persists. The epithelium lining the spaces thus formed by inflammatory entrapment produces secretions, eventually forming small cysts, which in aggregate form a multicystic structure sometimes termed follicular salpingitis.

It must be emphasized that active inflammation is not a self-perpetuating process, and the expression "sterile pus" is a fallacy. The causative organisms, often anaerobes, may be difficult to culture, but they are there and can be identified and treated effectively.[419] Anaerobes are especially likely to be present in the most serious and life-threatening pelvic infections.

Granulomatous salpingitis

Granulomatous salpingitis is most commonly caused by *Mycobacterium tuberculosis*. The tube is dilated, with a thickened wall. The exudate within the lumen usually appears purulent rather than caseous. Typical caseating granulomas are identified in microscopic sections, however. The glandlike pattern produced by the combination of adhesions of plicae and epithelial hyperplasia may be remarkably proliferative and has been mistaken for adenocarcinoma (Fig. 36-53). In a very large clinicopathologic study researchers[410] found that tubal tuberculosis was invariably present when any part of the female genital tract was affected; two thirds of the women were between 25 and 35 years of age, and the most common initial complaint was infertility (94%).

Foreign body granulomas in the tube may occur after

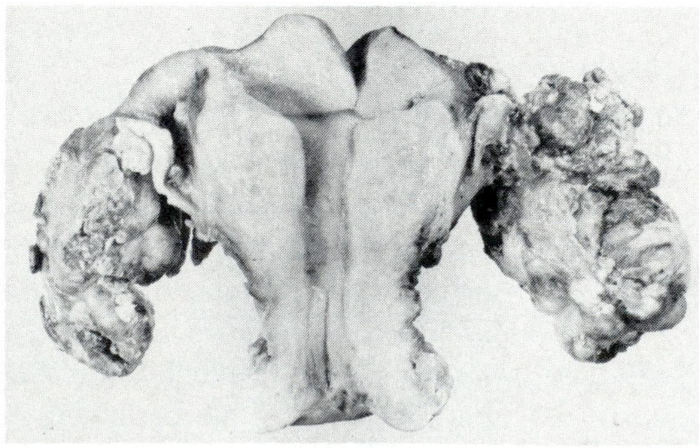

Fig. 36-52. Note bilateral retort-shaped, swollen, sealed tubes and adhesions of ovaries, typical of salpingitis.

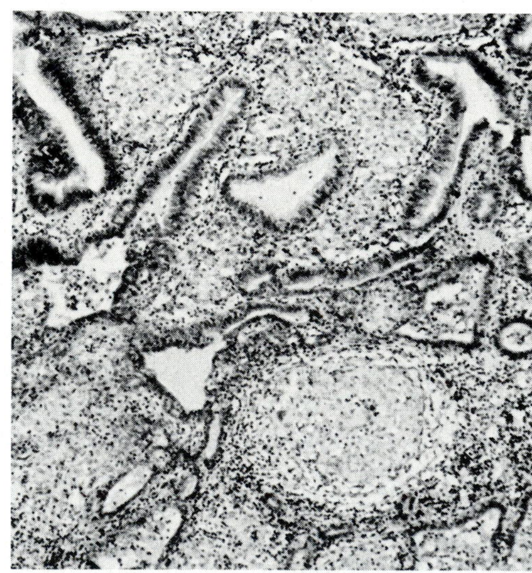

Fig. 36-53. Tuberculous salpingitis. Severe chronic inflammation, inconspicuous granulomas, and exuberant glandular epithelial proliferation (90×.)

instillation of oily contrast media used in hysterosalpingography, and talc granulomas have occurred after laparotomy. Rare instances of sarcoidosis, actinomycosis, and schistosomiasis have been reported.[422]

Endometriosis

Ectopic growth of endometrial glands and stroma can occur in all parts of the tube. Serosal implants appear as small red or red-brown patches or nodules with hemorrhage and fibrous adhesions. They are most common as a part of more generalized pelvic endometriosis. Involvement of the muscular wall stimulates muscle proliferation, and a nodular enlargement results. In about 10% of cases the tubal mucosa is replaced by endometrial glandular epithelium and stroma.[413]

In pregnancy focal decidual reaction may involve the serosa or mucosal stroma, especially in the plicae of the ampullary portion of the tube. The cells are large with refractile borders and closely resemble endometrial decidual cells; they must not be confused with granulomas or metastatic carcinoma.

Salpingitis isthmica nodosa

The characteristically bilateral nodular enlargements of salpingitis isthmica nodosa are located in the tubal isthmus and may be multiple. They vary from a few millimeters to a few centimeters in diameter, are firm, and appear gray, yellow, or brown on the cut surface.

Microscopically the nodules are composed of channels or spaces, lined by benign tubal epithelium separated by bundles of smooth muscle, which forms the major component of the mass. Inflammatory changes are inconspicuous or absent. The glandular channels communicate with the tubal lumen and therefore can be demonstrated by hysterosalpingography.[420]

The lesions apparently are acquired, but the pathogenesis is unknown. Benjamin and Beaver[400] considered inflammation to be an unlikely cause and suggested that the process is analogous to that of adenomyosis. Most patients are sterile.

Ectopic pregnancy

Implantation of a fertilized ovum may occur in the tube, especially when tubal structure or function has been altered or impaired by inflammation. The muscular wall is weakened by trophoblastic infiltration and attenuated because the lumen is distended by hemorrhage (Fig. 36-54). Vascular invasion by trophoblast is invariably present.

The diagnosis is not always easy because only a minority of the patients report the typical clinical picture of amenorrhea, pain, and vaginal bleeding, and at least half will have negative pregnancy test results.[422] Salpingectomy is done to control the massive hemorrhage that often results from rupture of the tube. Repeat tubal pregnancy occurs in about 10% of patients.

Attempts to enhance future fertility by a more conservative procedure than salpingectomy have been disappointing; although the prospects for future pregnancy are somewhat greater, the higher incidence of abortion and repeat tubal pregnancy tends to cancel any gains.[421] On the other hand, when only one functional tube remains, repair and conservation attempts have been followed by successful intrauterine pregnancy about one time in four, which certainly exceeds the results following loss of both tubes.[416]

Benign tumors and cysts

Hydatids of Morgagni are unilocular, thin-walled cysts that hang from the tubal fimbriae. Ferenczy and Rich-

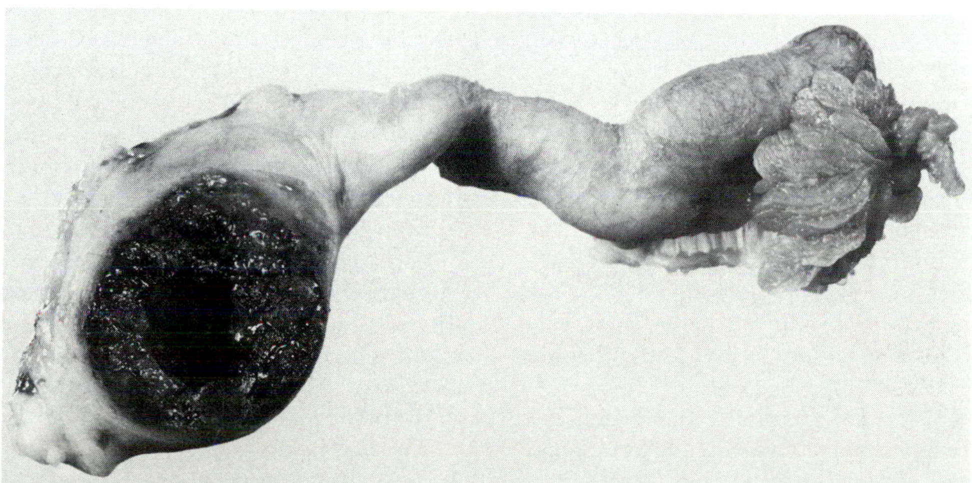

Fig. 36-54. Tubal ectopic pregnancy. Placental villi and trophoblast have infiltrated muscular wall, forming a hemorrhagic mass.

art[402] have shown that the epithelium is like that of the tube and undergoes cyclic changes in step with tubal epithelium; these are true tubal cysts.

Mesonephric (paratubal or parovarian) cysts are also unilocular thin-walled cysts filled with clear straw-colored fluid. The epithelium of these cysts resembles that of the mesonephric duct remnants of the mesovarium and does not undergo cyclic changes as does tubal epithelium.[402] The larger cysts spread to the mesovarium and mesosalpinx so that the tube often is compressed and attenuated into a longer structure.

Adenomatoid tumors of the tube are histologically identical to those in the uterine wall (p. 1492). In the tube they form a small nodular mass that compresses the tubal lumen to one side. It is important to recognize the pseudoglandular pattern to avoid a mistaken diagnosis of adenocarcinoma.[424]

Leiomyomas of the tube are surprisingly rare in view of their common occurrence in the adjacent uterus and the smooth muscle origin of both organs. Of the 60 or 80 cases reported, a few have been remarkably large.[422]

Teratomas in rare instances have originated from within the tube.[409] Most have been intraluminal and cystic and have resembled ovarian cystic teratomas (dermoid cysts). A few have been solid. A single instance of malignant teratoma is recorded.[417]

The histogenesis of these lesions is much debated. I have seen one instance of ovarian tissue, including ova and typical ovarian stroma, within tubal mucosa. The patient had been subjected to pelvic surgery, but the wall of the tube appeared to be intact. Such a finding also may explain the unique report of a Sertoli-Leydig cell tumor of the tube,[401] but a satisfactory explanation for the ovarian tissue itself at this location is still lacking.

Malignant tumors

Adenocarcinoma

Adenocarcinoma, the least common of female genital tract carcinomas, is also one of the most aggressive. The symptoms of pain and vaginal discharge are more characteristic of tubal inflammation, which commonly is also present. The inflammatory changes usually affect only the tube containing the neoplasm, which suggests that the neoplasm appears first; primary inflammation of the tube usually affects both sides at the same time. The often mentioned symptom of sudden copious watery discharge accompanied by relief of pain, dignified by the Latin term *hydrops tubae profluens,* is not commonly encountered. In about one patient in five, both tubes are affected.

Because of the nonspecific symptoms, the diagnosis is rarely made before laparotomy. Cancer cells were found in the vaginal smears of 24 of the 40 patients by Sedlis,[415] but a lower incidence is found in most series.

The affected tube resembles a distorted sausage and tends to feel firm instead of fluctuant (Fig. 36-55). The appearance of the tumor in the opened tube is usually papillary but may be soft or solid. Simultaneous involvement of tube and ovary may occur, in which case the lesion is considered by convention to be of ovarian origin.

The histologic appearance closely resembles the various patterns of papillary serous adenocarcinoma of the ovary (Fig. 36-56). Better-differentiated lesions may contain psammoma bodies. It is common to see invasion of the tubal stroma and muscle.

The prognosis is poor; about one patient in five lives for 5 years after the diagnosis is established. The few survivors have tended to have well-differentiated lesions confined to the tubal mucosa, situated within a sealed tube.

Malignant mixed müllerian tumor of the tube is extremely rare. It has no gross distinguishing features. The histologic patterns and clinical correlations are similar to those described for carcinosarcoma and malignant mixed müllerian tumors of the endometrium.[399] The prognosis is very poor.

Metastatic carcinoma involving the tube is more common than primary carcinoma. The most frequent primary site is from one of the more common female genital tract carcinomas, but breast and gastric adenocarcinoma are also encountered. The conspicuous lymphatic involvement and lack of neoplastic change in the tubal epithelium easily distinguish metastatic from primary carcinomas in most instances.

OVARY

The ovary has a complex structure and operates on a multiphasic schedule. Its function is to produce eggs to implant after fertilization in the endometrium, whose preparation is coordinated afresh each time by the ovarian hormones. To do this, the ovary must react appropriately to a set of trophic substances (hormones, prostaglandins) whose stimulation schedules these activities.

The disarray of body structure and function that can occur when the ovarian hormonal stimuli appear inappropriately is often devastating and in many cases still incompletely explained. The bizarre collection of neoplasms and their fascinating effects on the patient rival the repertory of any other organ.

Both the disorders of physiology and the tumors are more easily understood when the morphology and activities of the cellular components of the ovary have been explained.

Anatomy and physiology

The two bean-shaped ovaries hang from either tube posterior to the broad ligament, attached to the tube by a mesentery, the mesovarium. The blood vessels and lymphatics enter and leave through the lateral suspensory

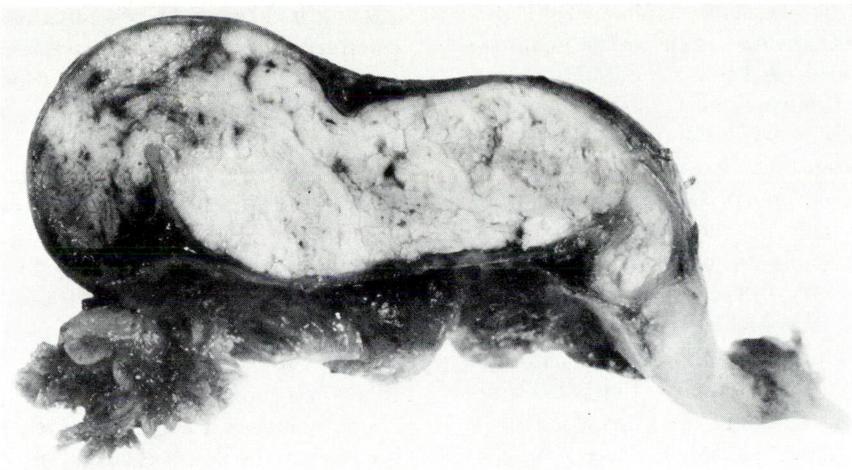

Fig. 36-55. Adenocarcinoma of fallopian tube, distending tubal lumen with soft gray tissue.

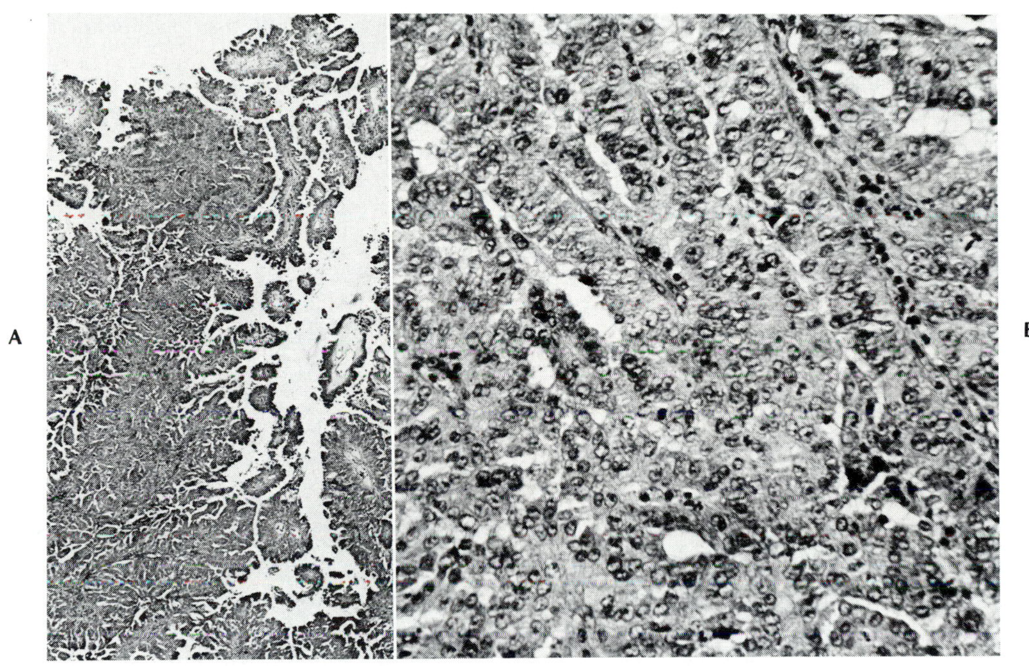

Fig. 36-56. Adenocarcinoma of fallopian tube. **A,** Typical papillary pattern. **B,** Higher magnification showing poorly differentiated adenocarcinoma. (**A,** 40×; **B,** 350×; from Kraus, F.T.: Gynecologic pathology, St. Louis, 1967, The C.V. Mosby Co.)

ligaments and thence through long channels to terminate at the level of the kidneys. The first order of lymph nodes that drain the ovaries is therefore in the aortic chain at the level of the kidneys, which must be remembered when the possible extent of an ovarian neoplasm is being investigated.

Cells of ovary

Germ cells. At birth the germ cells are represented by oocytes, in a resting stage of the first meiotic division, a process that will not be completed until ovulation occurs and fertilization is in process. Ultrastructural features of these events have been compiled by Ferenczy and Richart.[402] Germ cells have the potential for reproducing tissues of all germ layers and are considered to be the cell of origin of teratomas. They do not themselves produce ovarian hormones but organize the cells that do; adjacent ovarian stromal cells are induced to specialize and form the granulosa and theca cells that produce estrogens and progestogens.

Specialized gonadal stroma cells

Granulosa cells. In the primary follicle of an infant the granulosa cells lie in a single layer around the oocyte. Under the influence of follicle-stimulating hormone they proliferate, forming a fluid that contains the precursor of the zona pellucida, a dense capsule that surrounds the maturing oocyte. Cytoplasmic projections of granulosa cells extend through the zona pellucida and abut on the oocyte cell membrane. As the graafian follicle enlarges, a fluid-filled space, the antrum, forms. The oocyte, surrounded by a hillock of granulosa cells, lies eccentrically near the wall of the follicle (Fig. 36-57). Small round masses of dense pink material surrounded by a rosette of granulosa cells are usually evident in sections; these Call-Exner bodies are a specific product of granulosa cells, normal and neoplastic. The granulosa layer is avascular until ovulation.

Granulosa cells can synthesize estrogen (estrone) and various intermediates, including dehydroepiandrosterone.[520] At the time of ovulation they enlarge and form the corpus luteum, described subsequently.

Theca cells. As the maturing graafian follicle enlarges, the immediately surrounding stromal cells also enlarge and become rounded and plump. This change in an ovarian stromal cell is called luteinization. The luteinized theca layer becomes noticeably more vascular than the adjacent stroma. Follicle-associated theca cells thus activated produce estrogen (both estrone and estradiol) and are considered to be the primary source of estrogen in the preovulatory stage of the menstrual cycle.

Corpus luteum. In response to the midcycle peak of pituitary luteinizing hormone (and with local help from prostaglandins[438]), the graafian follicle ruptures, expels the oocyte, and rapidly becomes a corpus luteum. The granulosa layer becomes vascularized, and the granulosa cells enlarge to accommodate a massive accumulation of cytoplasm; they are then said to be luteinized (Fig. 36-58). This transformation probably results from luteinizing hormone stimulation alone.[478] Electron micrographs show abundant cytoplasmic agranular reticulum and mitochondria with tubular cristae typical of steroid hormone–producing cells. The corpus luteum is the principal source of progesterone (which stimulates the secretory endometrial pattern) and estrone and estradiol as well. If a pregnancy does not occur, the corpus luteum rapidly regresses. The morphologic changes attending the growth and decline of the corpus luteum have been extensively discussed by Adams and Hertig.[427] The roles of gonadotropins in the rise, and prostaglandins in the fall, of the corpus luteum have been reviewed by Hammerstein.[468]

Unspecialized ovarian stroma. The unspecialized ovarian stroma is a deceptively innocent-appearing mass of spindle-shaped cells. They produce collagen and also are capable of responding to gonadotropic stimuli to

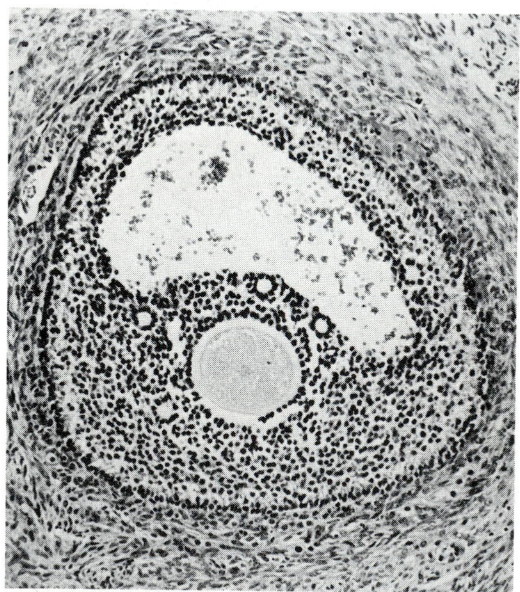

Fig. 36-57. Ovarian follicle. Large ovum is surrounded by mass of granulosa cells in which four Call-Exner bodies can be seen. Concentrically surrounding plump spindle cells compose theca externa. (150×.)

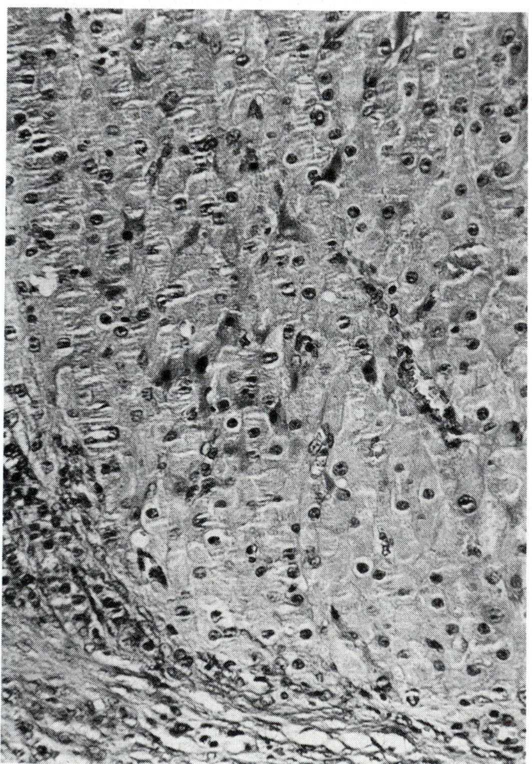

Fig. 36-58. Corpus luteum late in menstrual cycle. Luteinized granulosa cells are large and pale. Luteinized theca cells are smaller, intermixed with stromal cells at peripheral margin *(lower left).* (275×.)

become luteinized producers of steroid hormones. They are considered to be the cells of origin from which hyperplastic and stromal tumors (such as granulosa-theca cell and Sertoli-Leydig cell) arise. The ovarian stroma also contains smooth muscle fibers, which respond to prostaglandins, cholinergic agents, and oxytocin; contractile responses to drugs vary with the stage of the menstrual cycle.[451]

Surface mesothelium. The ovary is invested with a mesothelial covering, like other organs of the abdominal cavity (Fig. 36-59). It is the mesothelium of the urogenital ridge from which the müllerian ducts arise; the surface covering of the ovary seems to share or retain some specialized potential for differentiation with the related müllerian cells that form the lining of tube, endometrium, cervix, and upper part of the vagina. This relationship seems to be the basis for the close similarity between the epithelial cell types found in hyperplastic, metaplastic, and neoplastic growths that occur in or on the ovary.

Focal decidual reaction is regularly present on the surface of the ovaries in pregnancy and may be extensive on peritoneal surfaces generally. These areas look like tiny pink patches of serosal thickening. Rarely a similar change is seen in postmenopausal women[503] (Fig. 36-60).

Hilum cells (hilar Leydig cells). Clusters of large cells with abundant pink cytoplasm commonly are associated with nonmyelinated nerve fibers in the hilum of the ovary at the insertion of the mesovarium. Hilum cells regularly contain proteinaceous crystalloids of Reinke, a feature shared with testicular Leydig (interstitial) cells but not with luteinized stromal cells in the ovary. The physiologic significance of hilum cells in the ovary has not been demonstrated; they are increased in the newborn in association with pregnancy complications such as toxemia, diabetes, and multiple pregnancy, perhaps as a response to increased amounts of placental chorionic gonadotropin.[552]

Vestigial structures. Traces of the mesonephros persist as isolated small ducts in the mesovarium; a more plexiform glandular structure, the rete ovarii, is situated at the margin of the ovarian-hilar junction. It is homologous with the rete testis; confusion with focal neoplastic change is to be avoided.

Tiny nodules of heterotopic adrenocortical tissue occur in the ovarian suspensory ligament, broad ligament, and mesovarium. They are common if carefully sought, especially in children.[455] Although there is some potential for neoplastic change in any cell, no important type of neoplasm has been consistently related to either mesonephric or adrenal rests.

Ovarian senescence, failure, and atrophy

The ovary at birth contains about a half million oocytes.[441] Between 300 and 400 oocytes may mature as potential gametes. Some of the rest form small follicles, which undergo atresia, but the majority lyse and disappear without a trace.

As the age of menopause approaches, the number of oocytes diminishes, and the number of anovulatory

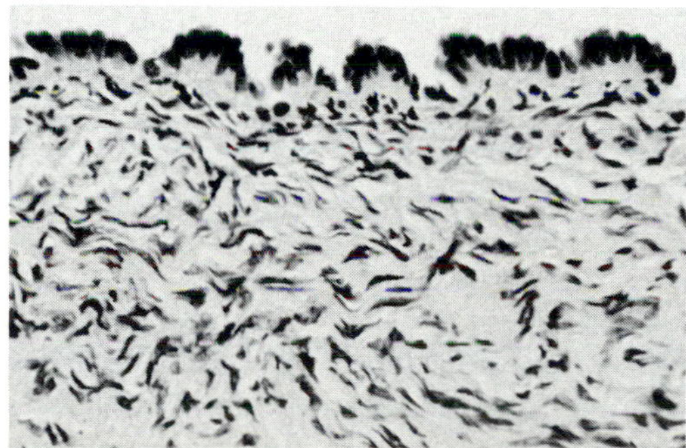

Fig. 36-59. Ovarian surface, covered by low columnar or cuboid coelomic epithelium; cortical stroma immediately below has fibrotic appearance. (300×.)

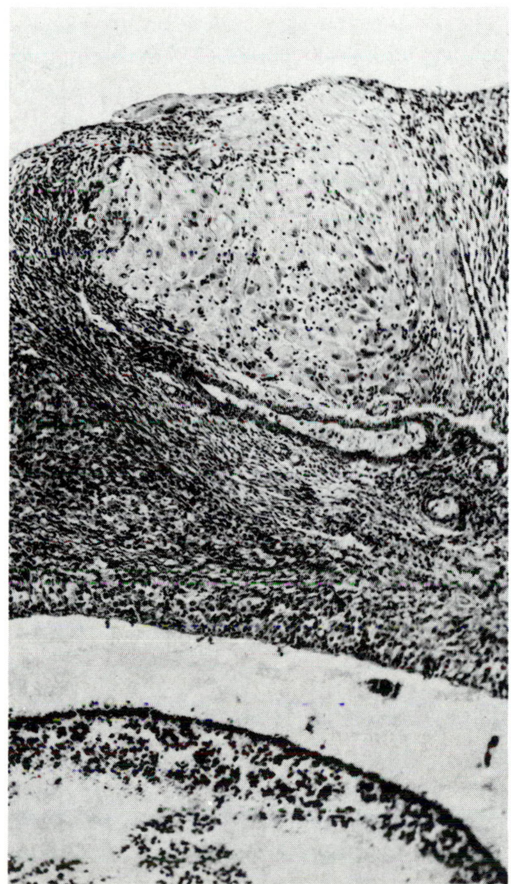

Fig. 36-60. Decidual change at ovarian surface. Multiple foci are found in ovaries of all pregnant women and rarely in postmenopausal women. (100×; AFIP 294919-17074.)

cycles increases. The follicles undergoing atresia leave behind a thin convoluted skein of hyalinized tissue. A few residual oocytes can be identified during the sixth decade in about 25% of ovaries studied; functional corpora lutea with secretory endometrial changes are present in about 10%.[502]

The postmenopausal ovary is composed chiefly of stroma, which remains biochemically active and may be slightly or moderately hyperplastic. It produces chiefly the androgenic steroids dehydroepiandrosterone, androstenedione, and testosterone; it does not aromatize androgens to estrogen.[493]

Menopausal changes may occur prematurely in young women from 15 to 25 years of age. The ovaries are small and atrophic and usually contain no follicles. A few or no oocytes are present.[535] Gonadotropin titers are characteristically elevated, and the ovaries do not respond to gonadotropin therapy.

The basis of premature ovarian atrophy has not been explained by morphologic study, except in some instances of autoimmune ovarian failure. Thus far the patients with autoimmune ovarian destruction have had other well-recognized forms of autoimmune disease, notably Addison's disease and Hashimoto's thyroiditis.[450] At an active stage of the antiovarian immune response, the follicles are infiltrated by lymphocytes and plasma cells.

A form of ovarian atrophy that usually is reversible is caused by prolonged use of contraceptive progestogen-estrogen drugs. The ovaries are small and contain essentially no graafian follicles, but numerous oocytes persist.[492]

Nonneoplastic cysts and hyperplasia

Surface inclusion cysts

The ovary gradually develops a convoluted surface, perhaps as the result of contraction after ovulation, when the stigma of rupture heals, leaving a crevice with buried epithelium and delicate surface adhesions.[546] The buried epithelium may proliferate and often undergoes metaplastic changes, typically to a tubal epithelial pattern.[374] With accumulation of fluid, small cysts result. The resulting surface-inclusion cysts usually remain tiny; an occasional large unilocular cyst may also originate in this fashion.

Follicle cyst, corpus luteum cyst

Follicles and corpora lutea generally do not exceed 2 cm in diameter; when either exceeds a diameter of 3 cm, it may be regarded as cystic, that is, larger than usual. Symptoms that can be related to such a cyst usually do not occur, although menstrual irregularities have been attributed to corpus luteum cysts in some reports.[508] Rarely a large follicle cyst may be a source of excessive estrogen secretion; such a lesion in a child has been reported as a cause of sexual precocity.[537] Severe hemorrhage may originate from the site of rupture in an early corpus luteum.[425]

Luteoma of pregnancy and other luteinized cysts and nodules

Luteoma of pregnancy. Nodular masses of theca-lutein hyperplasia have been discovered chiefly as incidental findings during cesarean section.[538] They are solid and orange-brown and may be bilateral or multiple within the same ovary.

The cells are large and uniform, about half the diameter of a luteinized granulosa cell, and form solid masses or, less commonly, microcystic follicle-like structures. Mitoses may be numerous (Fig. 36-61).

A minority of women and a few female infants have been virilized; testosterone levels may be elevated.[509] Luteomas of pregnancy regress when the pregnancy terminates.

Theca lutein cysts. Hyperplasia of luteinized theca cells regularly occurs in pregnancy, usually without significant disturbance in the gross morphologic traits of the ovary. Occasionally the process is greatly accentuated, producing multiple large cysts with prominent luteinization of theca cells but not of granulosa cells. This change, sometimes called hyperreactio luteinalis, is seen in association with hydatidiform mole, multiple pregnancy, erythroblastosis fetalis, and conditions in which chorionic gonadotropin titers are increased.[463] Occasional cases have been associated with otherwise uncomplicated pregnancy.[449] A remarkable degree of theca-lutein cystic hyperplasia can be produced when clomiphene or gonadotropin is administered to stimulate ovulation.[523]

Stromal luteoma. Scully[524] has described nodular theca-lutein proliferation of the ovarian stroma, chiefly in postmenopausal women. Associated endometrial changes suggested estrogen or progesterone production. In view of the somewhat elevated gonadotropin secrection at this age, the pathogenesis may be analogous to that of pregnancy luteoma; the original lesions were considered to be neoplastic. The lesions reported have been small and benign.

Polycystic ovary (Stein-Leventhal) syndrome

The syndrome described by Stein and Leventhal[536] in 1935 included infertility, secondary amenorrhea, hirsutism, and obesity in a group of young women whose only notable endocrine lesion was enlarged, pale, cystic ovaries. Actual masculinization with clitoral hypertrophy, frontal balding, a deep voice, and changes of body habitus does *not* occur. Since that time a great many facts have been accumulated, but a fully satisfactory explanation remains to be found. In any series there is a general

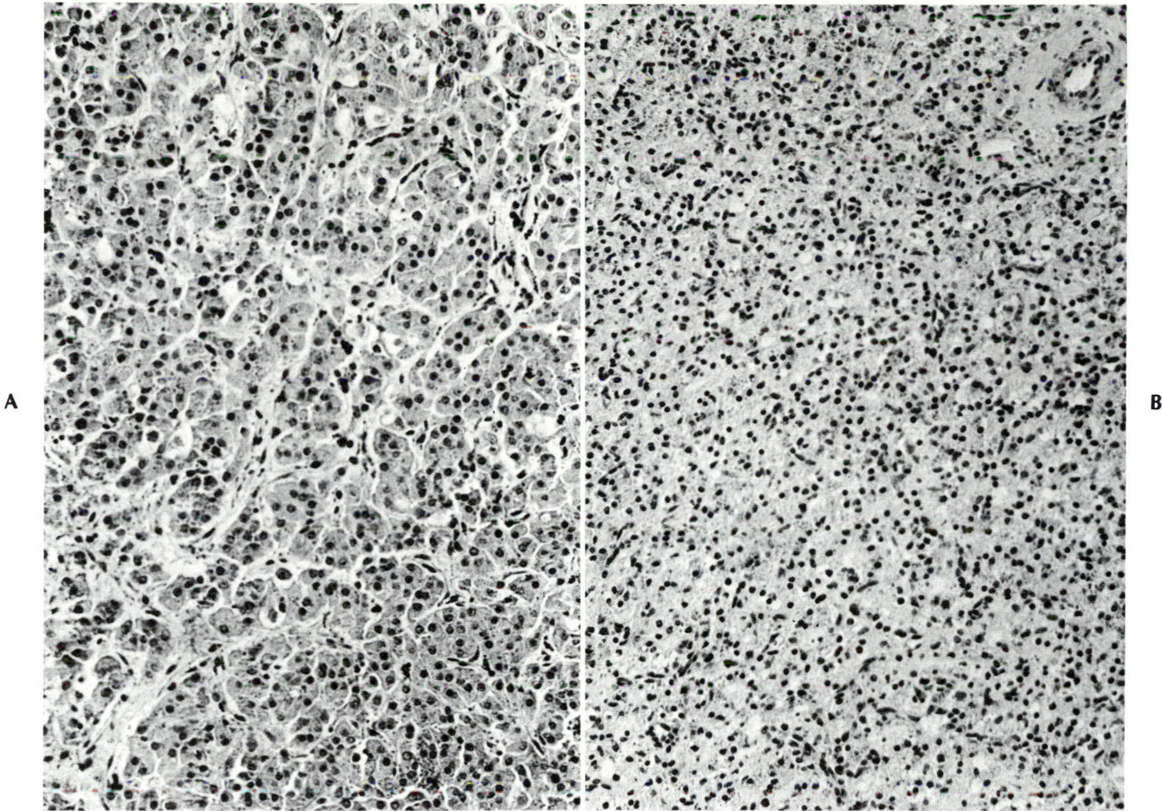

Fig. 36-61. A, Pregnancy luteoma composed of large luteinized stromal cells occurred as multiple red-brown nodules, identified at cesarean section. Female infant was temporarily masculinized. **B,** Section from ill-defined yellow area in opposite ovary 2 months later. (Courtesy Drs. L.R. Malmak and George V. Miller.)

similarity in the endocrine problems, but only a minority of patients have all the criteria just listed. The condition is sometimes hereditary.[446]

The ovarian lesion is not specific; it is almost certainly just a reactive change like the other features of the syndrome. The appearance is essentially that of an anovulatory ovary. Numerous follicles are present; typically they form a layer beneath the thickened white cortex. The medullary stroma that forms the central core is solid, gray, and somewhat edematous (Fig. 36-62). Microscopically the follicles and atretic follicles are all surrounded by a relatively prominent luteinized theca cell layer. The stromal cells themselves may be focally luteinized. Except in rare cases there is no corpus luteum. The ovaries usually are enlarged, sometimes more than 6 cm in diameter, but may be of normal size.

Unquestionably more than one basic physiologic defect triggers the entire symptom complex and physical changes, including those in the ovary. For instance, androgens from adrenal hyperplasia or neoplasm can do it; a similar syndrome has resulted from use of contraceptive steroids.[430,545] A common thread seems to be con-

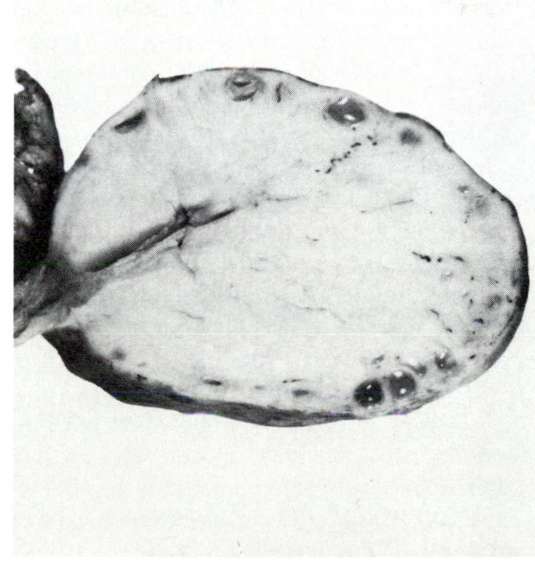

Fig. 36-62. Enlarged ovary from young woman with polycystic ovary (Stein-Leventhal) syndrome. Note abundant central stroma and peripheral subcapsular follicles.

sistently elevated secretion of androgen, especially testosterone. It is necessary to identify the concentration of the protein-bound testosterone component, as well as the total, because only the unbound component reacts biologically; women with the polycystic ovary syndrome have low levels of testosterone-binding protein, which rises as they respond to treatment.[452]

Greenblatt and Mahesh[466] note that the pituitary follicle-stimulating hormone is inhibited to low levels by testosterone, but luteinizing hormone is not always so affected. The levels of luteinizing hormone are sufficient to stimulate the ovarian theca and stromal cells to luteinize[460]; they may then secrete androgens inappropriately because of the abnormal pattern of initial gonadotropin stimulation, perpetuating the abnormal anovulatory state.

Any intervention that elicits a surge of follicle-stimulating hormone sufficient to stimulate maturation of a follicle and ovulation will correct this abnormal state, at least temporarily. This has been done by direct injection of gonadotropins, by stimulation of their production with hypothalamic follicle-stimulating and luteinizing hormone–releasing factors,[447,541,551] and by reduction of ovarian steroid feedback effect through ovarian injury (chiefly wedge resection), clomiphene,[519] or suppression with corticoids.

Hyperthecosis and stromal hyperplasia

The amount of ovarian stroma varies, and it may be abundant even at menopause and thereafter. When stromal proliferation is excessive, it is said to be hyperplastic.

In some young women stromal hyperplasia is sufficiently pronounced to cause enlargement or displacement of follicles and other structures. Variable degrees of stromal luteinization may occur. The abnormal stromal cells produce androgens, especially testosterone; in some patients masculinization may be severe. The ovaries may be solid or partly cystic. The clinical and pathologic features tend to overlap with those of the polycystic ovary syndrome, except that hyperthecosis produces masculinization. This condition is harder to treat than the polycystic ovary syndrome. Some patients have responded to oophorectomy.[436]

Massive edema

Massive edema is a rare form of ovarian enlargement that usually occurs in young women who are initially seen either with severe abdominal pain or with severe masculinization. The ovarian enlargement may be unilateral or bilateral. There often seems to be some degree of torsion, especially in patients who have pain. The masculinizing lesions have histologic evidence of stromal luteinization that resembles hyperthecosis. Both types of ovaries are massively edematous so the water leaks copiously from the cut surface. The pathogenesis is unknown; it has been suggested that torsion is responsible.[516] Total ovariectomy is probably unnecessary for this benign condition; resection to a normal-sized remnant has been recommended.[527]

Endometriosis

Ectopic endometrium in the ovary is troublesome because it forms fibrous adhesions and hemorrhagic cysts, which are painful and a cause of infertility. Accumulated hemorrhage results from stromal breakdown at the time of menstrual bleeding. Cysts may become large and typically are filled with semisolid, dark brown, altered blood. Endometrial tissue usually can be found somewhere in the fibrous wall, but a search may be necessary. Smaller foci of hemorrhage organize and contract, leaving a characteristic puckered scar tinged yellow-brown with hemosiderin (Fig. 36-63).

The pathogenesis has been debated. Implants from a reflux of menstrual blood have been shown to occur, and implants have been observed growing from such material. Serosal metaplasia is another possibility and almost certainly has been the cause in some cases. In a given case it is usually impossible to demonstrate the origin of the lesion.

Heterotopic ovarian tissue

Misplaced ovarian tissue is rare. The usual sites lie near the migratory route of the germ cells, in the pelvic retroperitoneum and mesosigmoid[547]; unquestionable nodules of ovarian stroma with oocytes have been encountered beneath the uterine serosa.[428] Heterotopic ovarian tissue has been the site of neoplasm (see discussion of fallopian tubes) and a source of unexpected ovarian function after bilateral ovariectomy.[482]

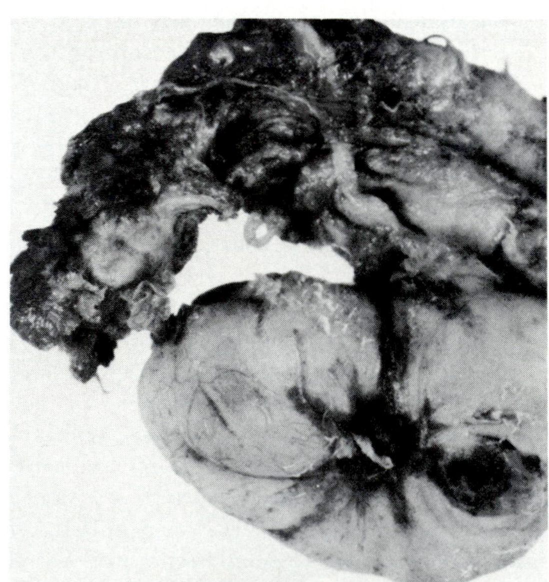

Fig. 36-63. Ovarian endometriosis forming characteristic puckered hemorrhagic scar and extensive tubal adhesions.

Neoplasms

Classification

Because of their remarkable diversity, ovarian tumors may be bewildering. Natural history and response to treatment vary considerably from one group of tumors to another. Especially in the area of chemotherapy and radiotherapy, the best therapeutic approach may be highly specific for a single type of neoplasm; accordingly, accurate histologic diagnosis is often a critical factor in achieving an optimum treatment response. It is extremely important therefore that the pathologist responsible for diagnosis and the physician responsible for therapy communicate clearly. Similarly, the classification used in any discussion of new therapeutic techniques must be understandable, or the pathologist's report is useless.

Neoplasms arise from and tend to resemble any of the normally occurring cellular components of the ovary described at the beginning of this section. This classification is based on histogenesis: the cell or tissue of origin. It is essentially the classification presented by the World Health Organization[530] with minor abridgments in the interest of clarity for this introduction to the subject.

- I. Tumors of surface epithelium
  - A. Serous tumors
    1. Benign cystadenoma, cystadenofibroma, and papillary cystadenoma
    2. Borderline serous tumors
    3. Malignant serous cystadenocarcinomas, papillary carcinomas
  - B. Mucinous tumors
    1. Benign mucinous cystadenoma
    2. Borderline mucinous tumors
    3. Malignant mucinous carcinomas
  - C. Endometrioid tumors
    1. Benign (cystic endometriosis?)
    2. Borderline; rare lesions resembling atypical endometrial hyperplasia
    3. Malignant
       - a. Adenocarcinomas, well differentiated and poorly differentiated, and adenosquamous carcinoma
       - b. Endometrioid stromal sarcoma
       - c. Malignant mixed müllerian tumor
  - D. Clear cell tumors
    1. Benign clear cell tumor (chiefly cystadenofibroma)
    2. Borderline clear cell tumors
    3. Malignant clear cell adenocarcinoma
  - E. Brenner tumor
    1. Benign
    2. Borderline (proliferating Brenner tumor)
    3. Malignant
  - F. Mixed (such as serous and mucinous)
  - G. Undifferentiated carcinoma (always malignant)
- II. Sex cord stromal tumors
  - A. Granulosa-theca cell tumors
    1. Granulosa cell tumor
    2. Thecoma
    3. Fibroma
    4. Mixed and indeterminate types
  - B. Sertoli-Leydig cell tumors (androblastomas, "arrhenoblastomas")
    1. Well differentiated; tubular and Leydig cell types
    2. Intermediate differentiation
    3. Poorly differentiated (sarcomatoid)
  - C. Gynandroblastoma
- III. Lipid cell tumors (such as hilum cell tumor, "adrenal rest" tumor)
- IV. Germ cell tumors
  - A. Dysgerminoma
  - B. Endodermal sinus tumor
  - C. Embryonal carcinoma, polyembryoma
  - D. Choriocarcinoma
  - E. Teratomas
    1. Mature: chiefly benign cystic teratoma (dermoid cyst)
    2. Immature (malignant teratoma)
    3. Specialized (such as struma, carcinoid)
  - F. Mixed forms
- V. Gonadoblastoma

It was estimated that about 18,300 women in the United States would be found to have ovarian cancer in 1984, and that in the same year about 11,500 would die of ovarian cancer.[247] The yearly death rate from ovarian cancer remained about 8.5 per 100,000 women from 1950 to 1975.[248]

Table 36-3. General classification of primary ovarian neoplasms

Cell of origin (representative tumor types)	Relative proportion of all ovarian neoplasms (%)*	Relative proportion of malignant neoplasms only (%)
Surface epithelium (serous, mucinous, endometrioid, clear cell, etc.)	65	95
Germ cells (immature ova) (cystic teratoma, solid teratoma, dysgerminoma, etc.)	20	1
Stromal cells (sex cords) (granulosa-theca cells, Sertoli–Leydig cells, lipid cells, fibroma, etc.)	12	2
Tumors in dysgenetic gonads (gonadoblastoma)	1	—
Unclassified (chiefly undifferentiated carcinoma)	2	2

*The relative proportion of figures noted here represents an approximation.

The relative frequency with which different types of ovarian neoplasms occur is summarized in Table 36-3. The proportions indicated are approximate and represent a synthesis of numerous reports. This is necessary because older studies use uncertain criteria for malignancy and do not distinguish important tumor categories, especially endometrioid carcinoma. More recent reports from cancer treatment centers do not reflect the true incidence of common benign neoplasms, which are usually treated in less specialized institutions.

Tumors of surface epithelium

Tumors of the surface epithelium form the most common group of ovarian neoplasms and include the majority of ovarian carcinomas (Table 36-3). The tissue of origin is considered to be the surface celomic mesothelium that covers the ovary (Fig. 36-64); it seems to retain, in neoplasms, the capacity to recapitulate tumor patterns that resemble the epithelial components of the müllerian ducts. For example, the epithelium of serous tumors resembles that lining the tube; the cells that line mucinous cystadenomas resemble endocervical mucosa. These neoplasms usually have a prominent cystic component with single or multiple loculations, often a variable amount of fibrous stroma, and an epithelial lining that often is thrown into papillary tufts.

It is necessary to recognize a spectrum of aggressiveness that is divided into benign, malignant, and borderline categories. Clearly benign cystic tumors are lined by a single layer of well-oriented columnar epithelial cells; papillary projections, if present, are supported by fibrovascular stromal stalks and covered by the same type of epithelium. Obviously malignant tumors have an anaplastic epithelial component that invades the stroma of the tumor or other structures, in addition to forming the epithelial lining. The epithelial cells are often several layers thick and have anaplastic nuclei, with a loss of polarity. The prognosis is very poor; about 15% of patients survive for 5 years, regardless of treatment.

The important intermediate, or borderline, group is identified chiefly by the absence of invasion in an otherwise highly proliferative neoplasm. A complex papillary pattern is often present, and the epithelium may be two or three cells thick. The epithelial cells generally appear only moderately dysplastic and maintain some degree of columnar orientation in most areas. Even proliferative epithelial masses with an anaplastic cytologic pattern do not signify a carcinoma in the absence of stromal invasion; the clinical behavior is still that of a borderline tumor.[476]

Although the behavior of borderline tumors is unpredictable in individual cases, as a group they have a much better prognosis than do malignant tumors of the ovary. More than 80% of patients survive 5 years, and almost as

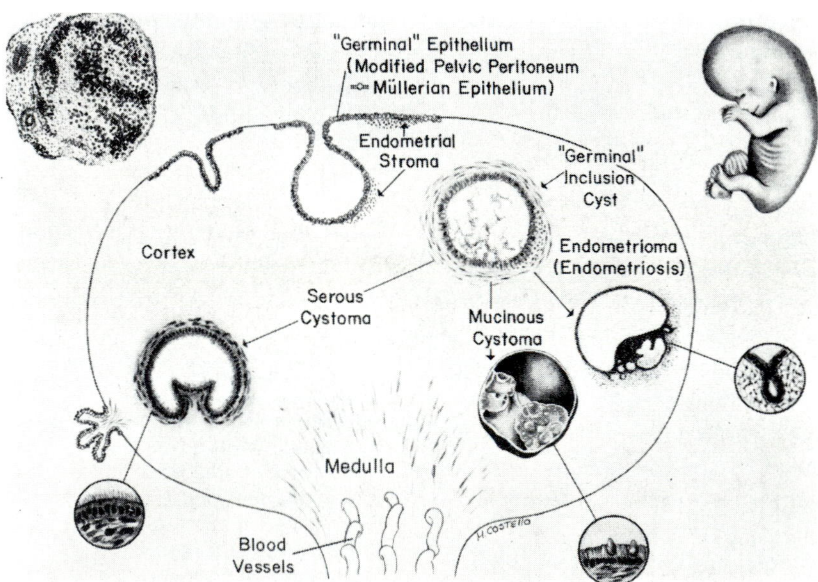

Fig. 36-64. Semidiagrammatic drawing of ovary to illustrate origin and types of cystomas derived from "germinal" epithelium. Note papillary growth on surface and various types of cystic tumors derived from infolding of this type of epithelium. Embryonic ovary and müllerian duct *(top left)* are drawn from 35 mm embryo *(top right)* and illustrate embryonic similarity of müllerian duct to germinal epithelium. The three types of cystomas (and their malignant counterparts) derived from "germinal" inclusion cysts are serous, endometrial, and mucinous—all recapitulating müllerian system, to which germinal epithelium is embryologically closely related. Low- and high-power drawings are from actual specimens. (From Hertig, A.T., and Gore, H.M.: Rocky Mountain Med. J. **55**:47, 1958.)

many survive 10 years, even in the presence of implants on peritoneal surfaces.[521] Recurrences typically appear after several years, if at all; the minority of tumors that have a malignant course tend to progress slowly. Radical therapy has not improved survival. It is important therefore to avoid radical or extensive therapeutic methods that carry a significant risk of morbidity and mortality for patients in this group unless it can be shown that the prospective benefits outweigh the risks.[481]

Serous tumors. Benign serous cysts and cystadenomas may form single or multiple loculations, lined by low columnar epithelium, which is sometimes ciliated, often distinctly resembling tubal epithelium (Fig. 36-65). The cyst fluid is watery or viscous and clear and contains a variety of mucins; however, the epithelial cells that secrete the fluid do not have the characteristic vacuolated pattern of mucinous epithelium. Papillary processes are common and may be numerous and complicated. The epithelial component of serous tumors, unlike other neoplasms of surface epithelium, may appear on the external surfaces; occasional lesions are composed entirely of a surface papillary growth with no cystic component. It is common to find tiny round laminated calcific concretions called psammoma bodies in the stroma of the papillary processes.

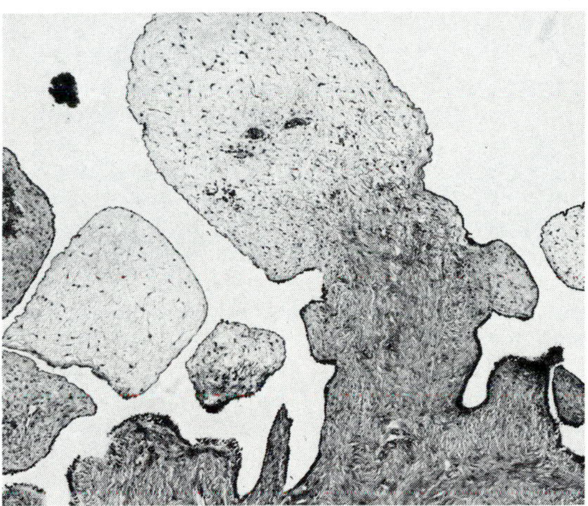

Fig. 36-65. Benign papillary serous tumor, with abundant fibrous stroma covered by single layer of small flattened epithelial cells. (85×.)

A relatively prominent or abundant fibrous tissue stroma produces plump papillae and large solid fibrous masses, as well as cysts. The resulting growths are papillary adenofibromas and cystadenofibromas.

Borderline serous tumors are often multilocular (Fig. 36-66) and have a more complex papillary pattern; fine papillae, closely packed, may resemble solid epithelial proliferation. Variable degrees of dysplastic nuclear change and mitotic activity are present (Fig. 36-67).

The presence of stromal invasion is the basis for identifying a serous tumor as a serous carcinoma[476] (Fig. 36-68). Bilateral ovarian involvement occurs in about two thirds of both borderline and malignant serous tumors and in one third of tumors that have not spread beyond the uterus, tubes, and ovaries. Because microscopic foci of cancer may lurk in an apparently normal ovary when serous carcinoma is present on the opposite side, Kottmeier[481] favors bilateral oophorectomy in every case.

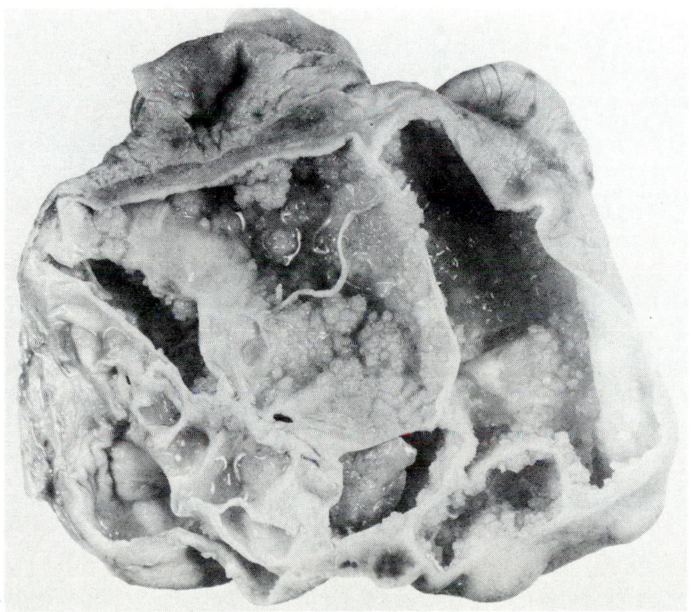

Fig. 36-66. Borderline serous tumor of ovary, a multilocular cystic mass with spaces lined by papillary epithelial masses.

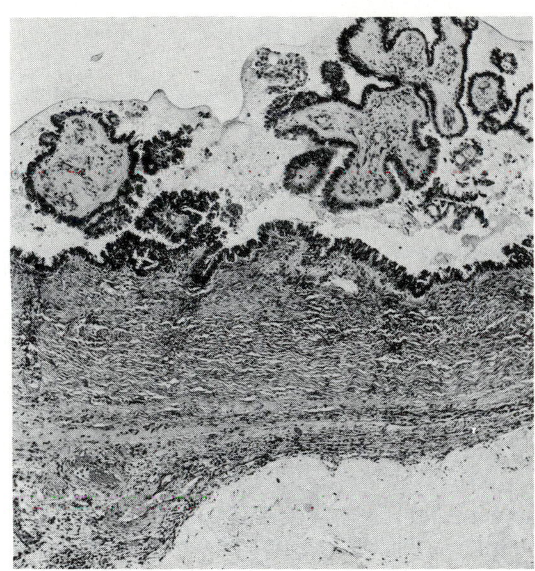

Fig. 36-67. Borderline serous cystadenoma of ovary without invasion. Epithelium is pleomorphic and forms small papillary processes. (46×; AFIP 264082-1.)

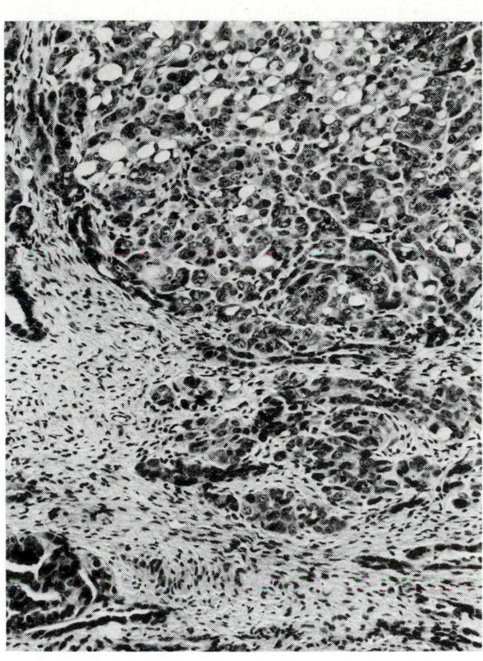

Fig. 36-68. Serous carcinoma of ovary showing invasion of stroma by strands and small clusters of adenocarcinoma cells. (100×.)

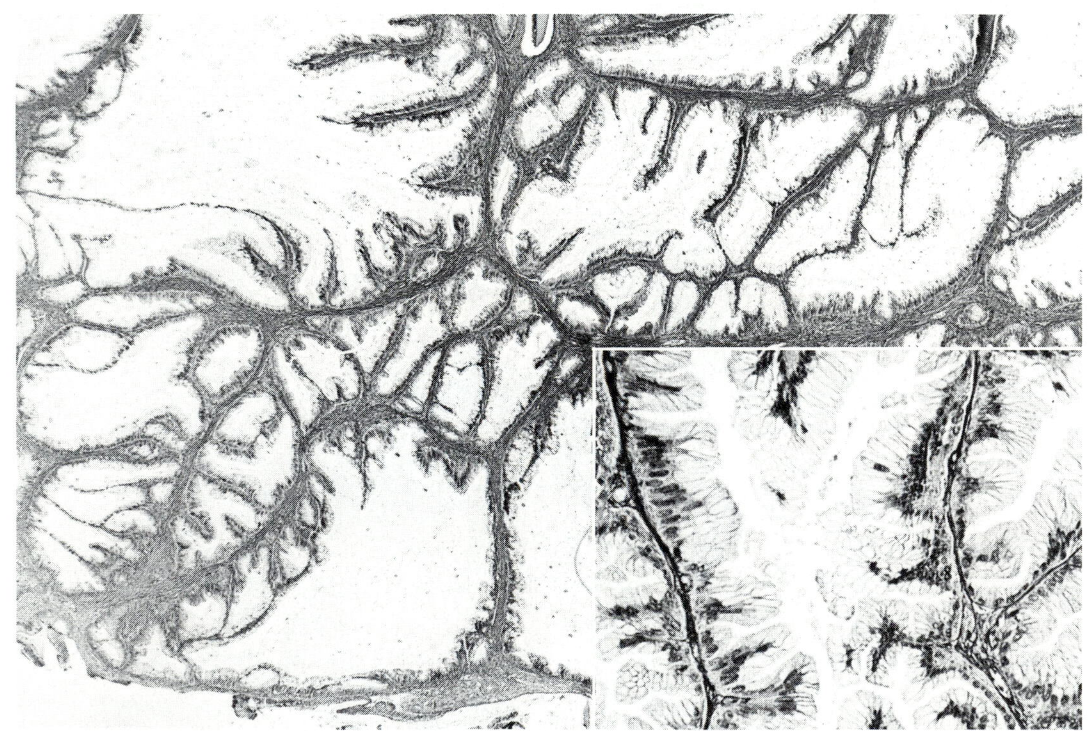

Fig. 36-69. Mucinous cystadenoma of ovary. Gland spaces are lined with tall columnar cells with basal nuclei and large apical mucin vacuoles. Note resemblance to cervical mucosa. (40×; *inset,* 300×.)

Mucinous tumors. Mucinous tumors are also typically unilocular or multilocular cystic masses. The epithelium that lines the cysts is composed of tall columnar goblet cells with basal nuclei and prominent mucin vacuoles; it resembles endocervical mucosa (Fig. 36-69). In some instances the pattern appears even more like intestinal epithelium, including argentaffin cells and even Paneth's cells.[526] Rarely a mucinous tumor has produced enough gastrin to cause Zollinger-Ellison syndrome.[445] Since about 5% of mucinous tumors are associated with cystic teratomas, it has been suggested that some, at least, originate from germ cells; an intestinal metaplasia of these exotic cell types seems more likely, despite the apparent production of endodermal derivatives by mesodermal cells.[457] A larger number, however, may have endometrioid or serous elements, which supports their classification with surface epithelial tumors. Since the biologic activity of mucinous tumors is more like the biologic activity of other surface epithelial tumors, their inclusion in this section has a solid practical basis, which outweighs the potential quibble over histogenesis.

In carcinomas the mucin vacuoles are less prominent, and nuclear polarity is lost, but the typical pattern is usually evident in better differentiated parts of the tumor. Stromal invasion is sometimes considerably more difficult to evaluate in mucinous tumors when small glandular spaces are distributed through fibrous stroma. Hart and Norris[469] have noted that a multilayered epithelial proliferation more than three cells thick also correlates well with malignant behavior. Borderline mucinous tumors, then, are defined as mucinous tumors in which there is no stromal invasion, and the epithelial proliferation, although sometimes cytologically atypical, remains no more than two or three cells thick.[469] In cases selected by these criteria more than 90% of women with borderline tumors survived for 10 years; in the same report 59% of patients with mucinous carcinoma (all stage I) survived for 10 years. Survival at 10 years in mucinous carcinoma (all stages) is 34%.[522]

Bilateral ovarian involvement occurs in about one fifth of both borderline and malignant mucinous tumors but in only 10% of cases in which there is no spread beyond the uterus, tubes, and ovaries. Kottmeier[481] found no instance of microscopic involvement of an apparently normal ovary on the side opposite a mucinous carcinoma.

Mucinous ascites (pseudomyxoma peritonei) occasionally occurs in association with a well-differentiated borderline mucinous tumor. The ovarian tumor characteristically contains mucin-filled cystic spaces that dissect the ovarian stroma. The neoplastic epithelium in the ovary and in the peritoneal lesion is sparse and well differentiated.[469] Chemotherapy with alkylating agents has provided symptomatic improvement and prolonged survival in some patients.[489]

Endometrioid tumors. Endometrioid carcinomas are so named because the histologic pattern closely resembles that of uterine endometrial adenocarcinoma. The distinction is most easily made in well-differentiated carcinomas (Fig. 36-70). Less-differentiated lesions may have a typical endometrioid pattern only in focal areas or a few patches of squamous metaplasia as the only clues to

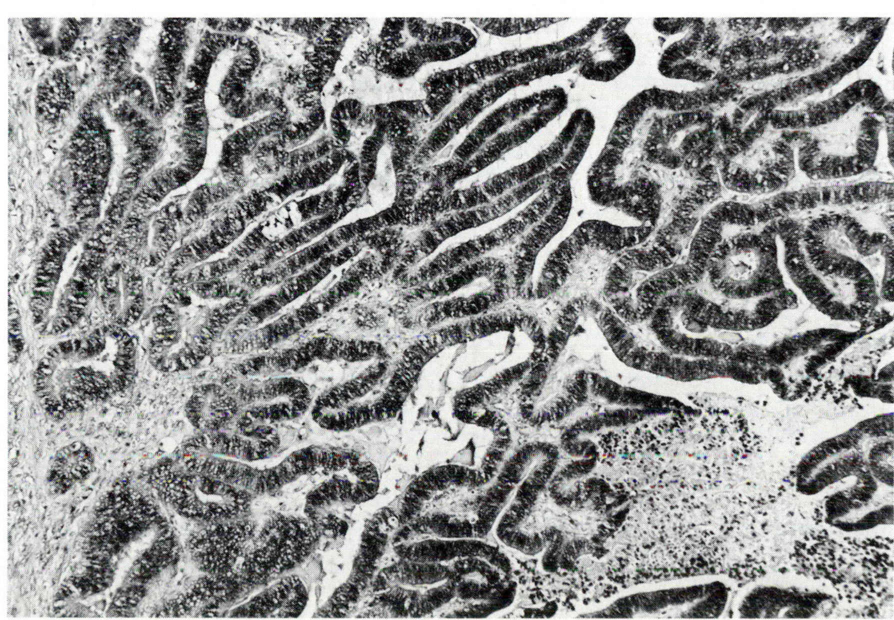

Fig. 36-70. Well-differentiated endometrioid adenocarcinoma of ovary. Pattern is identical to that of uterine endometrial adenocarcinoma. (150×.)

their identity, which accounts for some of the variation in the frequency with which they are reported. They probably comprise between 15% and 20% of ovarian cancers.

The benign counterpart is probably represented by some cases of cystic endometriosis of the ovary. A clearly defined concept of the borderline endometrioid tumor is lacking; certainly such lesions are rare.

Endometrioid carcinomas are often partly cystic, frequently with prominent solid areas; the cyst fluid is often brown or bloody. The cyst lining has a velvety or papillary appearance. Association with endometriosis is demonstrable in about one third of cases,[522] but the presence of endometriosis is not the basis for inclusion of a tumor within this group. Endometriosis is a common lesion of the ovary and occurs with other ovarian neoplasms, especially clear cell tumors.

The prognosis for well-differentiated carcinomas is good; about 60% of patients survive for 5 years, compared with 23% survival for poorly differentiated carcinomas.[522]

In about one third of the patients there is a coexistent adenocarcinoma of the endometrium. It is generally accepted that both lesions are separate primary cancers because the survival rate in the presence of endometrial involvement is not appreciably lower.[481] Furthermore, the two lesions commonly occur together without evidence of any other metastatic lesion; the common presence of multiple foci of dysplastic endometrial change is further evidence of a multifocal process.

Other endometrioid neoplasms such as stromal sarcoma, malignant mixed müllerian tumor, and adenosarcoma have been reported rarely as primary tumors of the ovary. The histologic features and prognosis (poor) do not differ significantly from those of similar lesions occurring in the endometrium.

Clear cell tumors. The gross appearance of clear cell tumors is often a combination of solid and cystic components much like that of endometrioid carcinoma. The cyst is usually unilocular; the fluid is commonly brown, and the solid areas form nodular masses that protrude into the lumen.

The histologic pattern is characterized by masses of large epithelial cells with abundant clear cytoplasm, supported by delicate fibrous trabeculae (Fig. 36-71). The cytoplasm contains abundant glycogen. A variation in this pattern is the presence of small cystic spaces lined by a single layer of large cuboid cells that are somewhat separated from one another; the nuclei may be oriented toward the cyst lumen rather than the basal area, producing a hobnail pattern.

Less than 10% are bilateral. Benign, borderline, and malignant varieties occur, but the malignant variety is much more common. Association with endometriosis is six times as great as with ovarian carcinoma in general.[526]

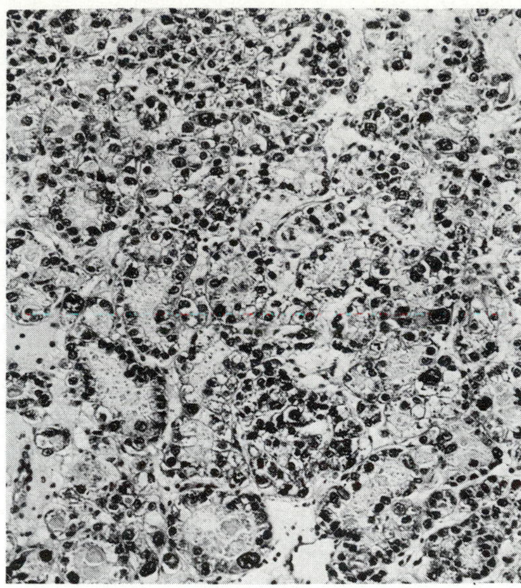

Fig. 36-71. Clear cell adenocarcinoma. There is abundant cytoplasmic glycogen; mucin is found only in extracellular secretions. (100×.)

Because the clear cell histologic pattern resembles that of renal adenocarcinoma and because of the proximity of adjacent mesonephric structures, the term *mesonephroma* has also been used to designate this type of neoplasm. There is no convincing evidence to support the concept of mesonephric origin.[528] On the other hand, ovarian clear cell carcinomas and identical neoplasms of the endometrium, cervix, and vagina seem to be related to tumors of müllerian epithelial type, especially endometrioid tumors. Endometrioid and clear cell patterns occur together in ovarian and endometrial carcinomas, and clear cell tumors have been shown to arise in patients with endometriosis.[528] Clear cell carcinoma patterns also occur in many malignant mixed müllerian tumors. Survival rates are in an intermediate range; 37% survive 5 years.[521]

Brenner tumor. Brenner tumors are solid gray or yellow-gray masses of fibrous tissue; occasionally it is possible to find scattered tiny cysts on cut section. The external serosal surface is smooth and shiny.

The microscopic appearance of scattered epithelial masses on a field of fibrous stroma is distinctive (Fig. 36-72). The epithelial component is composed of ovoid cells with clear cytoplasm, vesicular nuclei, and a characteristic nuclear groove. Mucinous epithelial cells form tiny cysts in the epithelial masses in about one third of the tumors, and one fifth have a conspicuous cystic mucinous component.

In the borderline variety of Brenner tumor (called proliferating Brenner tumor) the epithelial masses form larger cysts with a redundant, sometimes papillary lining of cells that look identical to transitional cell papilloma of the urinary bladder. Malignant Brenner tumors have an

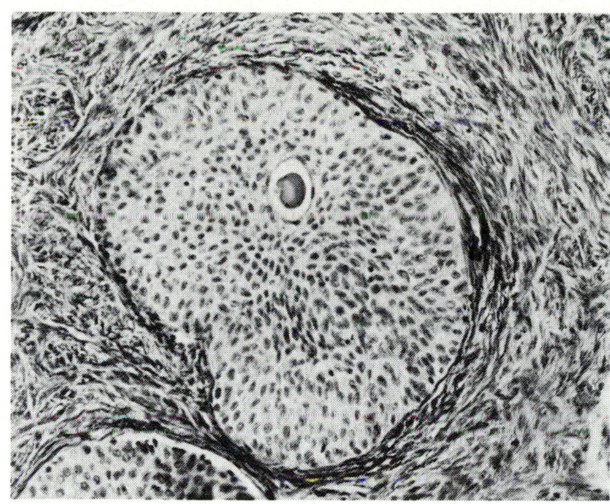

Fig. 36-72. Brenner tumor. Typical sharply circumscribed nest of uniform cytologically benign cells surrounded by dense fibrous stroma. (140×; AFIP 305334-1-4-2.)

anaplastic epithelial component that resembles poorly differentiated transitional cell carcinoma or epidermoid carcinoma and invades the stroma of the tumor. Borderline and malignant Brenner tumors are both extremely rare; one needs to identify a well-differentiated Brenner tumor pattern in some part of the lesion to establish the diagnosis.

Arey's wax model reconstructions[429] have shown that the epithelial islands are actually anastomosing cords of epithelial cells, in continuity with the covering serosal epithelium of the ovary. The ultrastructural appearance of Brenner epithelial cells resembles that of urinary bladder transitional epithelium and the Walthard's cell nests of the tubal serosa. On the basis of these studies it is generally accepted that Brenner tumors probably represent a neoplastic proliferation of ovarian surface epithelial cells that further differentiate into urinary transitional epithelium.[448,514,532]

Less than 10% are bilateral. The stromal component is not always inert. In occasional cases the stromal cells appear luteinized and contain birefringent lipid; associated endometrial hyperplasia has indicated secretion of estrogen by the tumor.[453]

Mixed forms. Surface epithelial tumors often include a combination of the foregoing types. Unless two or more patterns form a distinct and prominent component, the neoplasm is usually and most reasonably classified after the predominant cell type represented.

Cystadenofibromas combine any of the cystic epithelial patterns described previously with a prominent solid fibrous tissue component. Epithelial atypia, even when pronounced, has not been associated with aggressive behavior in the few instances described by Kao and Norris.[475] Malignant mixed müllerian tumor, histologically identical to its uterine counterpart (see p. 1489), occurs rarely as a highly aggressive ovarian primary neoplasm.[437]

Undifferentiated carcinoma. Nearly all adenocarcinomas too undifferentiated for subclassification probably belong to the group of tumors originating from surface epithelium. About 54% are bilateral; they comprise about 4% of ovarian carcinomas.[481] The prognosis is extremely poor. Many are composed of small cells of nearly uniform size. Mitoses are numerous; nuclei are anaplastic. It is a mistake to classify such lesions as granulosa cell carcinomas. Confusion of this highly malignant group of neoplasms with granulosa cell tumors only blurs the distinct clinical correlation associated with these two different neoplastic diseases.

Extragenital tumors with müllerian histologic patterns. The peritoneal and retroperitoneal tissues of the female pelvis occasionally generate primary neoplasms resembling any of the foregoing tumor types without necessarily involving any part of the uterus, tubes, or ovaries. Thus serous tumors with psammoma bodies,[459] mucinous tumors,[517] adenosarcomas,[444] and even endometrial stromal tumors[355] may be found on or beneath the peritoneal surface of any part of the pelvis. Various metaplastic changes also occur; Lauchlan[486] refers to this versatile tissue as the secondary müllerian system.

Sex cord stromal tumors (sex cord–mesenchyme tumors)

The sex cord stromal tumors arise from specialized ovarian stromal cells. The general designation of sex cord–mesenchyme tumors is favored by Scully[526] because the assumption that the embryonic sex cords and their derivatives are mesenchymal or stromal derivatives (rather than celomic epithelium) remains unproved. It is the specialized stromal cells that produce ovarian steroid hormones. The tumors that arise from them produce the full range of the ovarian and testicular steroid hormonal repertory, including intermediates, and occasionally adrenal steroids as well.

Granulosa-theca cell tumors. About half the granulosa-theca cell tumors are thecomas, a fourth are composed only of granulosa cells, and the remaining fourth are a mixture of both.

Granulosa cell tumors are often partly cystic, and multiple areas of hemorrhage are common. Solid areas are yellow-brown. Thecomas are solid, firm, and yellow or yellow-white with dense streaks and patches of hyalinized white tissue. Mixed granulosa-theca tumors are made firm and solid by the fibrotic thecal component.

Granulosa cells have uniform, small, oval or rounded nuclei, with a fold or cleft in the nuclear membrane. The cells are distributed in masses with little intervening stroma. Ultrastructural studies support and extend the resemblance to normal granulosa cells.[506] Characteristic rosettelike structures, or Call-Exner bodies, are nearly always present; they are rounded masses of pink inspissated material surrounded by a circular row of typical granulosa cells and resemble structures found in the normal graafian follicle (Fig. 36-73). Unlike acini, with

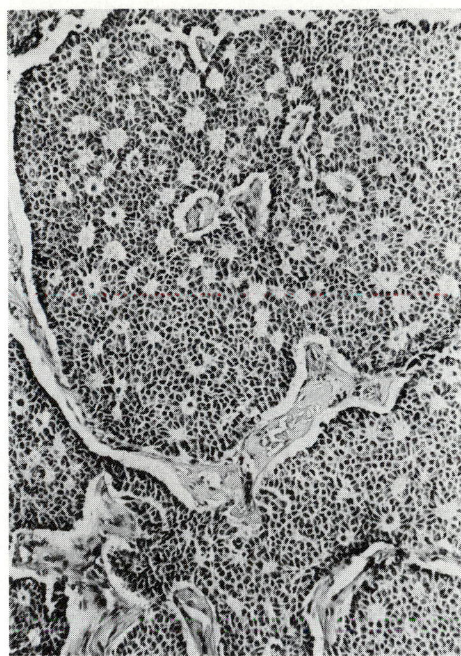

Fig. 36-73. Granulosa cell tumor. Many rounded spaces (Call-Exner bodies) containing amorphous eosinophilic material are scattered among uniform small cells with compressed-appearing nuclei. Compare with Fig. 36-57. Strands of hyalinized stroma are characteristic feature. (70×.)

which they are often confused, the central cytoplasmic margins are indistinct, there is no stainable mucin, and the nuclei tend to lie adjacent to the inner rim of the space.

A variety of microscopic patterns occur; microfollicular and macrofollicular tumors resemble clusters of small or large graafian follicles. The descriptive terms *trabecular, insular, gyriform, solid tubular*, and *diffuse* are often applied, without significant clinical correlations. Paradoxically the cystic macrofollicular tumors produce androgenic effects.[500] The so-called sarcomatoid variety, in which large masses of granulosa cells tend to form swirling patterns of somewhat spindle-shaped cells, may have a more aggressive natural history.[488] Scully[527] has identified a distinctive juvenile pattern, chiefly prepubertal, in which both granulosa and thecal components are strikingly luteinized.

The most consistent indicator of aggressive behavior has been the presence of metastases or invasion of structures outside the ovary at the time of diagnosis.[439,454,458,499] Also unfavorable but less significant factors are large tumor size, increasing age, abdominal symptoms, and tumor rupture. Frequent mitoses correlate poorly with prognosis in my experience and that reported by Norris and Taylor.[499]

Thecomas are solid fibrotic masses in which some of the spindle-shaped cells that form the tumor are plump and rounded and contain abundant cytoplasm that reacts with lipid stains. Another characteristic feature is the presence of hyaline plaques.

Granulosa-theca cell tumors characteristically produce estrogenic hormones, but they are occasionally androgenic. Using immunohistochemical techniques Kurman, Goebelsmann, and Taylor[483] found that granulosa and theca cells both produce a wide range of steroid hormones, but the chief product of granulosa cells is estradiol, and luteinized theca cells make progesterone.

The most common symptom is uterine bleeding. Women with estrogen-secreting granulosa-theca cell tumors often have endometrial hyperplasia. Well-differentiated endometrial adenocarcinoma occurs in 9%[499] to 24%[491] of cases in postmenopausal women. Although the morphologic features of these adenocarcinomas meet the criteria of a well-differentiated adenocarcinoma, they have a remarkably good prognosis; reports of death or metastasis related to these cancers are very difficult to find. It is possible that some of these endometrial carcinomas are highly estrogen dependent and therefore fail to progress when the source of estrogen is withdrawn.

Less than 5% of granulosa cell tumors are bilateral. Over 90% of the patients studied by Norris and Taylor[499] survived for 10 years, and some had residual tumor. Recurrences continued to appear as late as 25 years after original treatment. Studies that report a less favorable prognosis[439,458] include a larger proportion of poorly differentiated tumors with a high mitotic rate than I have encountered. It is reasonable to conserve the opposite ovary and uterus of a young woman with a small tumor confined to one ovary. Thecomas can be regarded as invariably benign.

Fibroma. Large fibrous tumors of the ovary without clinical or morphologic evidence of endocrine activity are relatively common, forming about 5% of all ovarian tumors in most large series. Densely collagenized fibrous tissue forms a monotonous histologic pattern, broken by areas of calcification in some cases. Occasionally there may be an associated benign ascites and pleural effusion, which disappear when the tumor is resected (Meigs' syndrome).

Fibrosarcoma is extremely rare.

Sertoli-Leydig cell tumors (arrhenoblastoma, androblastoma). Although Sertoli-Leydig cell tumors often produce androgens and masculinize the patient, many are hormonally inert, and some even have estrogenic effects.[494] Testosterone and a variety of androgenic precursors may be secreted in variable proportions. In an immunohistochemical study Kurman and associates[485] demonstrated both testosterone and estradiol in Sertoli cells, in Leydig cells, and also in less-differentiated stromal cells. Although their histologic patterns resemble those of developing male gonadal structures, Sertoli-Leydig cell tumors arise from the same female sex cord

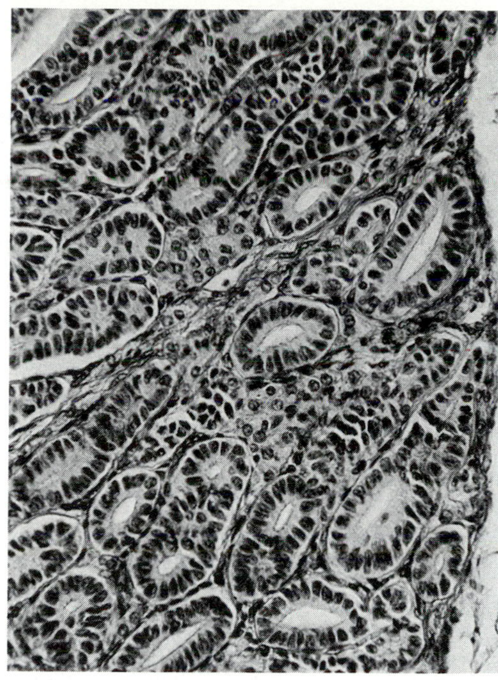

Fig. 36-74. Well-differentiated Sertoli-Leydig cell tumor, forming small tubules composed of Sertoli cells. Leydig cells are scattered through stroma *(center)*. (250×.)

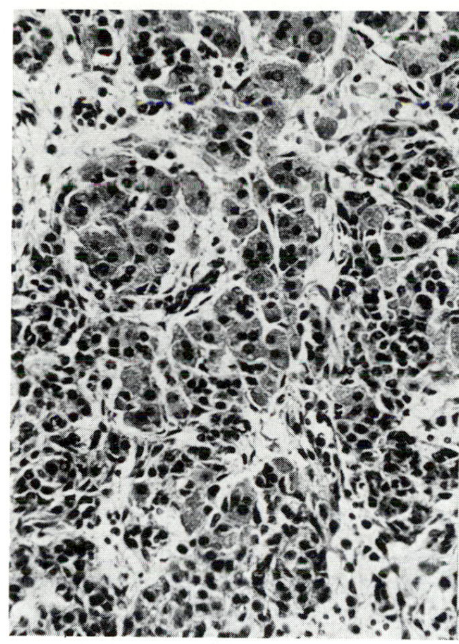

Fig. 36-75. Moderately differentiated intermediate type of Sertoli-Leydig cell tumor. Large, dense, eosinophilic Leydig cells are intermixed with cordlike strands of smaller Sertoli cells in a loose, sparsely cellular stroma. (275×.)

stromal cells as granulosa-theca cell tumors and consistently contain female sex chromatin.[504] Some ultrastructural studies confirm a closer relationship to ovarian stroma than to the testis[471,477]; however, the finding of cilia and other structures[473] leaves the subject unsettled.

Three histologic types are distinguishable. Well-differentiated tumors form tubular structures composed of Sertoli cells, separated by a fibrous stroma, intermixed with large round Leydig cells in poorly circumscribed clumps (Fig. 36-74). Tumors of intermediate differentiation have a biphasic pattern in which large pink Leydig cells are prominent, separated by a spindly stroma in which the abortive tubule formation resembles early sex cords of the embryonic testis (Fig. 36-75). A few tumors contain unexpected heterologous elements such as neoplastic mucinous glands, cartilage, and rhabdomyoblasts.[527]

Least differentiated is the sarcomatoid variety, composed of spindle cells that condense focally into a vague trabecular arrangement, separated by a looser myxoid component composed of the same type of cell. Leydig cells may or may not be present.

About half the well-differentiated tumors, three fourths of intermediate tumors, and all sarcomatoid tumors are androgenic. Sertoli cell tumors in children, however, are estrogenic and cause precocious puberty.[426] Nearly all Sertoli-Leydig cell tumors are benign, despite reports indicating malignant behavior in more than 20%; it has been suggested that the higher figures resulted from inclusion of other kinds of adenocarcinoma, primary and metastatic, with functioning stroma.[504] Malignant behavior takes the form of intraabdominal implantation, ordinarily without distant metastases.

Gynandroblastoma. Rarely, a sex cord stromal tumor may include both granulosatheca cell and Sertoli-Leydig cell patterns.[501] Most have been benign. Those with hormonal function have produced androgens. Authentic examples are extremely rare.

Lipid cell tumors

Lipid cell tumors are a distinctive group of neoplasms that occur in the form of soft yellow or yellow-brown nodules. Examples are hilum cell tumors, "adrenal rest" tumors, and luteomas. The cells that compose them may be relatively small and rounded with dense pink cytoplasm or larger with foamy or clear cytoplasm. Occasionally the smaller cells may contain crystalloids of Reinke, as in testicular Leydig cells and ovarian hilum cells. Both types of cells may occur in the same tumor. The ultrastructure is consistent with ovarian stromal origin; the cytoplasmic organelles resemble those of steroid-secreting cells,[477] such as the cells of the adrenal cortex. Crystalloids of Reinke must be identified to support classification as hilar Leydig cell or hilum cell tumor.

Most are benign. The few that behave aggressively are likely to be larger and to invade contiguous structures and may have atypical cytologic features.[540] The most common endocrine abnormality is virilization; a few have caused Cushing's syndrome.

Germ cell tumors

Ovarian germ cells are those that produce the female gametes—ova. They retain the capacity to produce an extremely diverse group of tissues in tumors. Most are benign cystic teratomas and occur chiefly in the young; malignant teratomas nearly always occur in children and young women. Optimum therapy depends on accurate identification and knowledge of the natural history of each type of neoplasm; various combinations of the different types are likely to occur.

Dysgerminoma. Dysgerminomas are large, solid, encapsulated masses of soft, gray-white tissue, often with foci of hemorrhage and necrosis. They are composed of large vesicular cells indistinguishable from the primordial germ cells of the embryonic gonad, distributed in large clumps and masses separated by fibrous trabeculae (Fig. 36-76). The fibrous stroma is almost always infiltrated by lymphocytes and may contain sarcoidosis-like granulomas. This pattern is indistinguishable from that of testicular seminoma. About 10% are bilateral.[431] The opposite ovary may contain microscopic foci of dysgerminoma even when it appears grossly normal (Table 36-4); if it is to be preserved, biopsy with frozen-section examination is desirable.

Dysgerminoma is extremely radiosensitive and curable with radiotherapy even in the presence of metastases. Thus, since most patients are young, unilateral oophorectomy is desirable and sufficient when the opposite ovary is normal. The 5-year survival rate is between 70% and 90%. For pure dysgerminoma limited to one ovary, the 5-year survival rate in one large series[465] was 94% for patients whose treatment was limited to resection of the affected ovary. The occasional dysgerminoma that contains syncytiotrophoblastic giant cells looks worse but does not behave more aggressively.[550] These tumors may produce human chorionic gonadotropin (HCG); all patients should be tested for it by radioimmunoassay of serum or urine, since HCG can serve as a tumor marker for early detection of recurrence.

Endodermal sinus tumor. Teilum[542] has established endodermal sinus tumor as a morphologically distinct entity. The most specific feature of this rare neoplasm is the presence of isolated papillary projections with a central blood vessel and peripheral sleeve of malignant embryonic epithelial cells (Fig. 36-77). Cross sections of this structure once were erroneously compared with immature glomeruli. In fact, they closely resemble invaginations of yolk sac endoderm, as seen best in the rat placenta, forming the endodermal sinuses of Duval.[542] Another distinctive feature is the presence of periodic acid–Schiff–positive, diastase-resistant hyaline globules partly composed of alpha-fetoprotein.[543] Some tumors contain multiple gland spaces with an hourglass constriction resembling yolk sac vesicles, a pattern that Teilum has designated polyvesicular vitelline tumor.

The gross appearance is much like that of dysgerminoma except for the more extensive yellow and red areas of hemorrhage and necrosis and the often present cystic areas. Endodermal sinus tumors consistently produce alpha-fetoprotein, which can be demonstrated in tissue sections by immunohistochemical techniques[543] and in the patient's serum.[434] This substance is produced in the yolk sac of the developing embryo and may serve as a tumor marker in evaluating the course of the patient after treatment. All the patients have been children or young adults. The prognosis is very poor; remissions have occurred in some patients treated postoperatively with multiple chemotherapeutic agents. Bilateral involvement in stage I is unlikely (Table 36-4).

Embryonal carcinoma. Embryonal carcinoma is an uncommon germ cell tumor that has been confused with endodermal sinus tumor, which it resembles. The patients are young, have an abdominal mass, and consistently have positive pregnancy test results because the tumors produce HCG. Premenarchal girls undergo precocious puberty. The histologic pattern resembles that of testicular embryonal carcinoma: large primitive anaplastic cells form solid masses interspersed with glandlike clefts and scattered giant cells. The multinucleated giant cells of syncytiotrophoblastic type are common, and immunohistochemical studies have shown that they contain HCG.[484] Similarly, mononuclear embryonal cells contain alpha-fetoprotein. Both substances can and

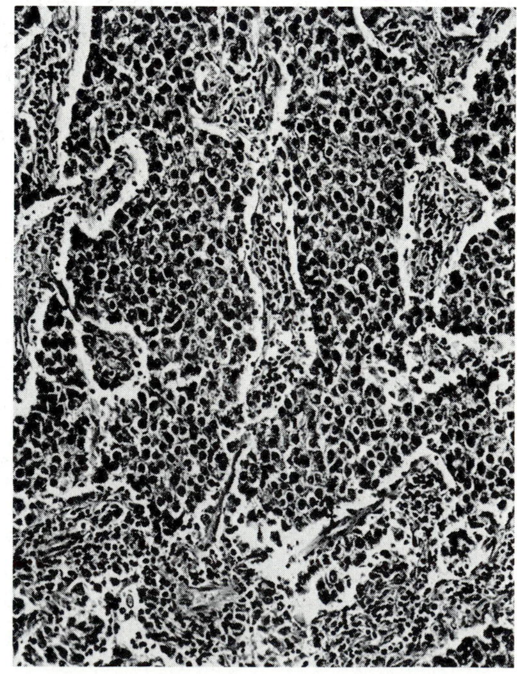

Fig. 36-76. Dysgerminoma. Masses of large uniform germ cells are separated by fibrous trabeculae that are infiltrated by lymphocytes. (130×.)

should be used as tumor markers to evaluate therapeutic response and detect recurrence early.

Although these tumors are highly malignant, chemotherapy has resulted in some long-term survivors. There is little to gain from resecting a normal-appearing opposite ovary (tested by biopsy), since most tumors are unilateral, and occult metastases probably lie elsewhere.

Polyembryoma. Some germ cell tumors contain large numbers of embryoid bodies that closely resemble an early embryo, typically distributed in a primitive mesenchymal stroma.

Choriocarcinoma. Nongestational primary choriocarcinoma of the ovary is rare and malignant. The histologic pattern and clinical correlations are similar to those of gestational choriocarcinoma (p. 1532), except that the remarkable response to chemotherapy usually does not occur. There have been occasional survivors.[470]

Teratomas. Teratomas are composed of recognizable tissues of ectodermal, mesodermal, and endodermal origin, in any combination. They are common and usually benign and inert but rarely produce remarkably bizarre and varied syndromes, reflecting the diverse potentials of the germ cell.

Benign cystic teratoma (dermoid cyst). Cystic teratomas are composed of mature somatic tissues of almost every description. Most cysts are unilocular, and the tissue that forms the lining is usually skin (Fig. 36-78). The dequamated keratin and secretions, notably from sebaceous glands, accumulate with masses of hair to fill the lumen of the cyst. This disagreeable mixture is liquid at body temperature but solidifies when chilled. Other common components are salivary gland; bronchus; fat; smooth muscle; cartilage; bone; neural tissue, including ganglia, glia, and choroid plexus; retina; pancreas; thyroid; and teeth. Characteristically a protuberance from the inner surface is the locus of growth of most of the hair and the richest depository of odd tissues. Uncommon tissues are skeletal and cardiac muscle, kidney, and liver.

In collected series bilateral teratomas occurred in 8% to 15% of cases. Cystic teratomas comprise 20% of all ovarian tumors in adults and 50% of all ovarian tumors in

Table 36-4. Status of contralateral ovary in patients with stage I germ cell tumors of ovary

Tumor	Number of patients		Number of stage Ia patients with microscopic involvement of opposite ovary	
	Stage Ia	Stage Ib	Number examined microscopically	Number positive
Dysgerminoma	71	7	21	4
Endodermal sinus tumor	51	0	24	0
Immature teratoma	40	0	6	0
Embryonal carcinoma	9	0	0	0
Mixed germ cell tumor	20	0	5	1

Courtesy Drs. Robert J. Kurman and Henry J. Norris, Washington, D.C.

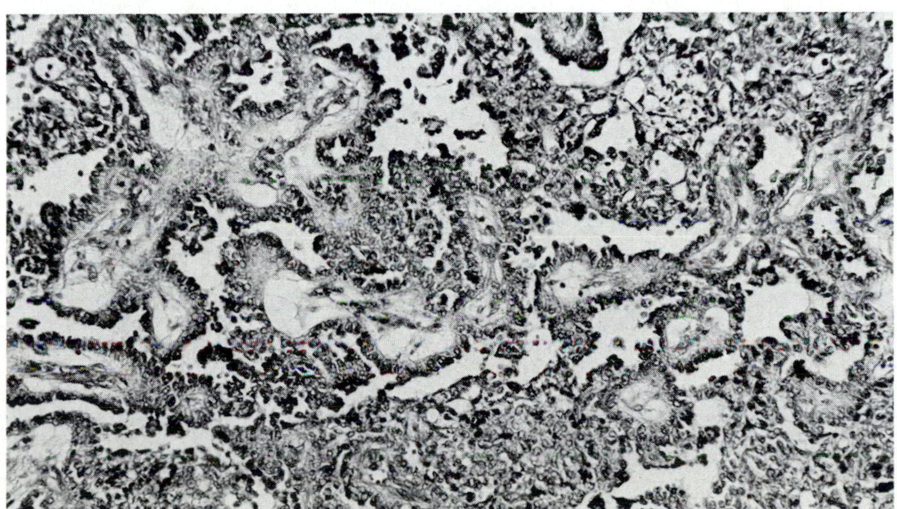

Fig. 36-77. Endodermal sinus tumor. There is a tangle of papillary processes with central blood vessel, usually covered by single layer of anaplastic germ cells; stroma is inconspicuous. (150×.)

children. Most patients are between 20 and 40 years, but the tumors occur at all ages. Roentgenograms often are diagnostic, especially when teeth or bone is present. Most patients are operated on because a mass was discovered during a physical examination.

The pathogenesis of teratomas has always excited speculation because of their exotic composition; Blackwell and associates[440] have made an interesting historical review of this subject. Analysis of more recent cytogenetic studies using chromosome-banding techniques indicates that ovarian teratomas are parthenogenetic tumors that must originate from a single germ cell after its first meiotic division.[487]

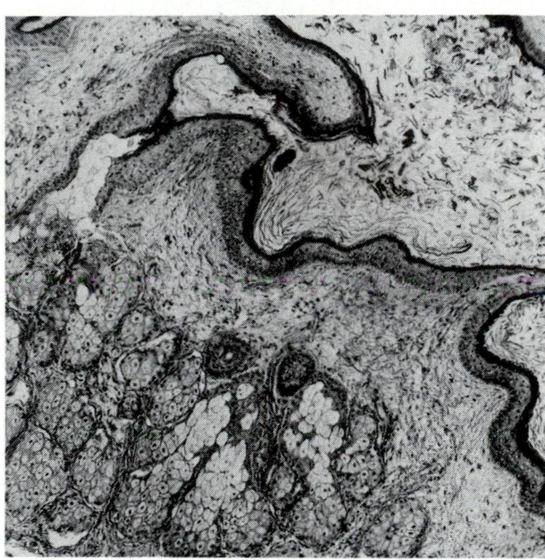

Fig. 36-78. Lining of typical benign cystic teratoma (dermoid cyst) is composed chiefly of skin with sebaceous glands, hair follicles, and sweat glands. (75×; AFIP 510588-07023.)

Malignant change in a cystic teratoma is certainly less frequent than the 1.8% of cases reported[507] because most benign teratomas are not reported. Almost any component may become malignant; epidermoid carcinoma is most common, but sweat gland carcinoma, thyroid carcinoma, malignant melanoma, and various sarcomas, including osteosarcoma, occur rarely.

Solid teratomas (teratomas with abundant solid tissue and relatively small cysts) are nearly all malignant (as discussed subsequently), but a few benign solid teratomas have been reported.[544] All the tissue components of a benign solid teratoma are as mature as the other tissues of the patient in whom they occur.

Immature teratoma (malignant teratoma). Malignant teratoma is a unilateral solid mass with a heterogeneous appearance on cut surface. The histologic pattern is also extremely variable; many tissues have an embryonic appearance, with numerous mitoses. Islands of immature cartilage, bone, and glandular structures are distributed through a poorly differentiated stroma of actively growing spindle-shaped myxoid or undifferentiated sarcoma cells (Fig. 36-79). Bilateral involvement in patients with stage I malignant teratoma is rare (Table 36-4).

Relatively mature (grade I) malignant teratomas have a good prognosis, whereas immature teratomas (grade III) have an extremely poor prognosis.[484,511] The relative amount of primitive neuroepithelial tissue is an important factor in grading and determining the prognosis.[484]

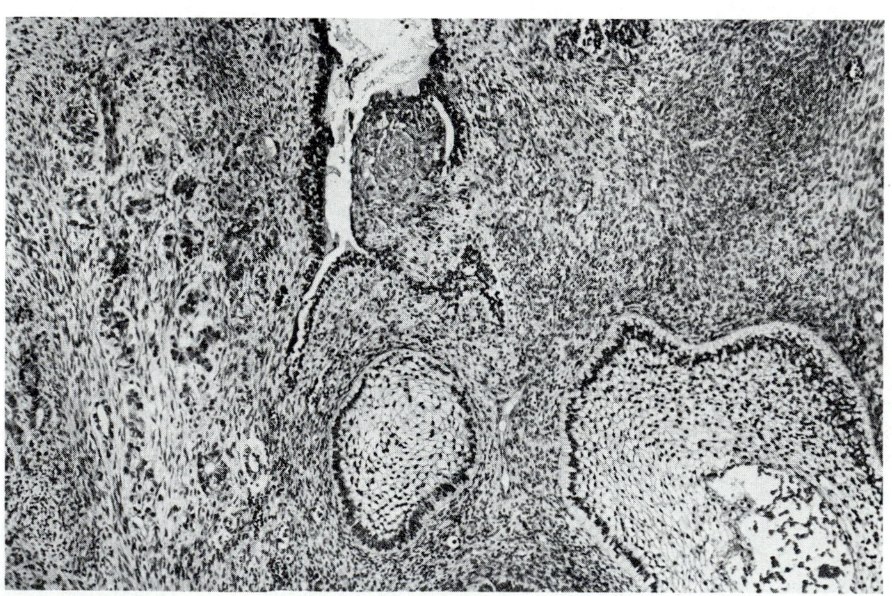

Fig. 36-79. Malignant teratoma. In addition to differentiated structures, there is an embryonic stroma resembling sarcoma *(upper right)*. (80×.)

Areas of endodermal sinus tumor, embryonal carcinoma, and choriocarcinoma are extremely unfavorable. Tumors that lack these structures but have an abundant neural component—resembling ganglioneuroblastoma—are more unpredictable; nearly half these patients survive for 2 years. The neural component, even in peritoneal implants, may mature, leaving well-differentiated glial vestiges on the peritoneal surfaces. Although they may persist for many years, mature glial implants are innocuous and not a basis for radical treatment.[511] Therefore the grading of metastases, once they have occurred, is also prognostically important.[484]

Specialized teratomas. Rare teratomas composed solely of thyroid tissue are usually benign but may function and even cause thyrotoxicosis.[496] Carcinoid tumors with the insular pattern typical of midgut derivatives[510] and trabecular carcinoids of the foregut and hindgut type also occur as primary ovarian tumors. The latter type may be mixed with thyroid tissue. Both are nearly always unilateral and benign; insular carcinoids, especially if large, may cause the carcinoid syndrome. On the other hand, intestinal carcinoids metastatic to the ovary are usually bilateral and have a poor prognosis. It is especially important to distinguish them from granulosa cell tumors and Sertoli-Leydig cell tumors, as well as from primary ovarian carcinoids.[510]

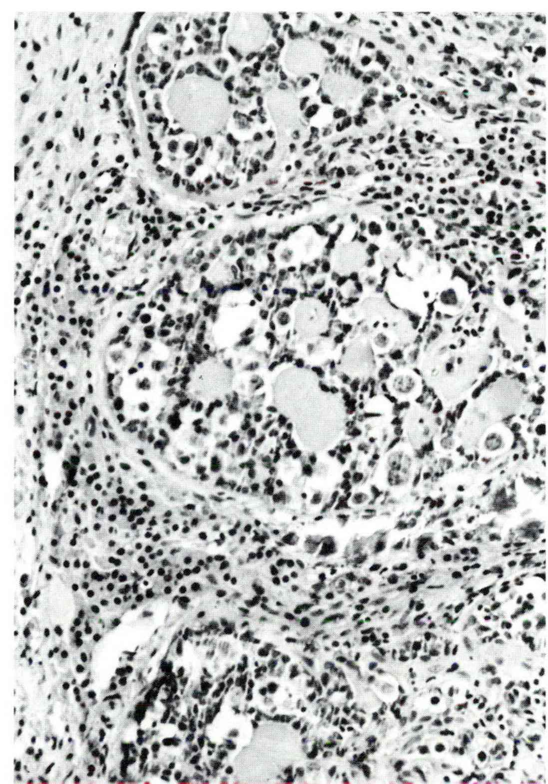

Fig. 36-80. Gonadoblastoma. Large germ cells and hyaline globules are intermixed with smaller granulosa cells, forming islands or nests. Clumps of Leydig cells are scattered through intervening stroma. (160×; courtesy Dr. Jerzy Teter, Warsaw, Poland; from Scully, R.E.: Androgenic lesions of the ovary. In Grady, H.G., and Smith, D.E., editors: The ovary, Baltimore, 1963, The Williams & Wilkins Co.)

Mixed forms. Germ cell tumors occur in various combinations. Solid areas in the wall of a cystic teratoma deserve careful study, since they may represent a locus of endodermal sinus tumor or other malignant category with a greatly different prognosis and implications for further treatment.

Malignant mixed germ cell tumors (stage I) have a poor prognosis if more than one third of the tumor consists of endodermal sinus tumor, choriocarcinoma, or stage III teratoma. Tumors that contain less than one third of these components or contain combinations of dysgerminoma, embryonal carcinoma, or stage I or II teratoma have a good prognosis. Patients with tumors less than 10 cm in diameter are more likely to survive regardless of tumor composition.[484]

Gonadoblastoma. Gonadoblastoma is a rare tumor that may arise in a dysgenetic gonad. The patients are usually phenotypic females, but nearly all are genotypic males (that is, have a Y chromosome). The tumor contains both immature germ cells and sex cord–stromal cells, which resemble granulosa or Sertoli cells, growing in small islands, intermixed with rounded pink hyaline bodies. Leydig cells or lutein cells are distributed through the intervening stroma in about two thirds of the cases (Fig. 36-80). Small calcifications may be extensive and have a distinctive roentgenographic pattern. Most are benign, but dysgerminomas and other malignant germ cell tumors develop occasionally.[525]

Metastatic carcinoma

Metastatic carcinomas represent 6% of ovarian cancers encountered in the course of surgical exploration of the abdomen.[521] The primary site in most instances is the colon, stomach, or breast; it may be small and difficult to locate, even when the ovarian metastases are large.

The characteristic pattern of growth is diffuse infiltration of the ovarian stroma by strands and small nests of poorly differentiated carcinoma cells, forming a solid mass. The external surface is knobby and smooth. The eponymic designation of "Krukenberg's tumor" is usually reserved for this typical presentation when the tumor cells have large eccentric mucin vacuoles (signet-ring cells) and the primary site is the stomach (Fig. 36-81). The same pattern rarely occurs in a lesion that seems to be primary in the ovary after a thorough search for extraovarian primary carcinoma.[472] Because of wide variation in the use of this name, it is essentially useless; since Krukenberg's original paper erroneously concluded that the tumors were primary in the ovary, there is

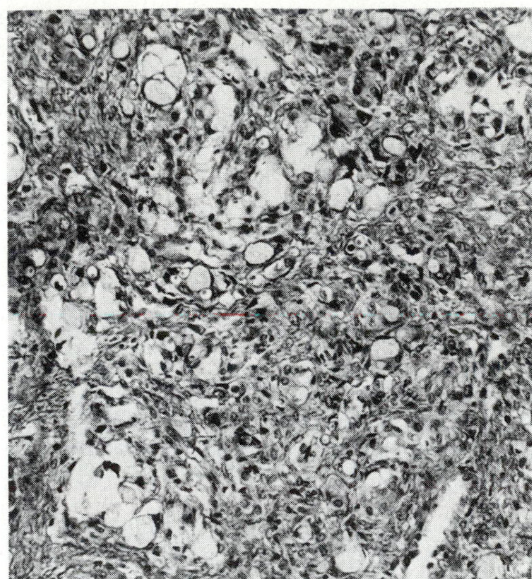

Fig. 36-81. Metastatic adenocarcinoma to ovary from stomach. Signet-ring cells and small acini are present. Stromal cells are hyperplastic. (150×.)

little point in clamoring for a rigorous use of this term for metastatic carcinoma. Colon cancers metastatic to the ovary may secrete enough mucin to produce cystic cavities; distinction in these cases from primary mucinous carcinoma of the ovary may be difficult.

The most important clinical correlation is the surprising fact that the ovarian metastases are often the only metastases apparent, and if they and the primary lesion are resected, the patient may live without symptoms for several years. For this reason ovarian metastases should generally be resected.

The basis for the selective enhancement of growth of certain adenocarcinoma cells in the ovary is unexplained. It is of interest that most of the patients are premenopausal, about a decade younger than those with primary ovarian adenocarcinoma; the phenomenon may be hormone dependent.

The ovarian stroma may be stimulated to secrete both androgenic and estrogenic hormones in the presence of metastatic carcinoma, especially colon carcinoma.

Malignant lymphoma

Like any other tissue, the ovaries may be involved by leukemic and lymphomatous infiltrate in patients with systemic disease. They rarely represent the primary locus of lymphoma, especially the poorly differentiated lymphocytic form of non-Hodgkin's lymphoma.[443] The ovaries, like the facial bones and orbital tissue, are preferential sites of involvement in Burkitt's lymphoma, including the American variety. An occasional instance of granulocytic leukemia has initially appeared as an ovarian tumor (so-called granulocytic sarcoma).[435]

Pathologic factors affecting prognosis

The foregoing discussion has emphasized that each different type of ovarian neoplasm is in fact a separate disease. There are other general characteristics that also affect the outcome of treatment.

Clinical stage. The extent of disease at the time of diagnosis is an important determinant of the outcome of therapy and must be stated in any comparison of effectiveness of different therapeutic techniques. The following internationally recognized criteria for staging primary ovarian carcinoma have been established by the International Federation of Gynecology and Obstetrics,[117] based on findings at clinical examination and surgical exploration. The histology is to be considered in the staging, as is cytology as far as effusions are concerned.

Stage I Growth limited to the ovaries
- a. Growth limited to *one* ovary; no ascites
  - i. No tumor on the external surface; capsule intact
  - ii. Tumor present on the external surface and/or capsule ruptured
- b. Growth limited to *both* ovaries; no ascites
  - i. No tumor on the external surface; capsules intact
  - ii. Tumor present on the external surface and/or capsule(s) ruptured
- c. Tumor either stage Ia or stage Ib, but with obvious ascites present or positive peritoneal washings

Stage II Growth involving one or both ovaries with pelvic extension
- a. Extension and/or metastases to the uterus and/or tubes
- b. Extension to other pelvic tissues, including the peritoneum and uterus
- c. Tumor either stage IIa or stage IIb, but with obvious ascites present or positive peritoneal washings

Stage III Growth involving one or both ovaries with intraperitoneal metastases outside the pelvis and/or positive retroperitoneal nodes; tumor limited to the true pelvis with histologically proved malignant extension to small bowel or omentum

Stage IV Growth involving one or both ovaries with distant metastases; if pleural effusion is present, there must be positive cytologic tests to allot a case to stage IV; parenchymal liver metastasis equals stage IV

Implants. The significance of implants depends on the nature of the primary lesion. The prognosis is good, even in the presence of omental or other peritoneal implants, if the primary tumor is borderline.[526] It is extremely important to examine the undersurface of the diaphragm for distant metastases in establishing the stage of an ovarian cancer because this may be the only area with grossly evident metastases.[456]

Ascites. The significance of effusions depends on the nature of the primary lesion. Effusions associated with fibromas or Brenner tumors (Meigs' syndrome) are benign and do not recur after the tumor has been resected. Effusions that contain cancer cells, originating from an invasive ovarian cancer, indicate an average survival of 7.2 months.[480]

Rupture. The significance of rupture depends on the nature of the neoplasm. It has no demonstrable effect in the case of benign or borderline tumors. The prognosis of an invasive carcinoma, which is poor in any case, may be adversely affected, but it is difficult to demonstrate such a change convincingly.[467]

Metastases. The lymphatic drainage of the ovaries is directly to the aortic lymph nodes at the level of the renal veins. Biopsies inferior to this site are generally useless. From a study of aortic lymph node biopsies it is clear that many ovarian cancers believed to be confined to the ovaries have actually produced lymph node metastases at the time of diagnosis.[479]

Role of pathologic study in management of apparently normal opposite ovary in young women. Preservation of an apparently normal ovary is extremely important in young women. A comparison of the results of ovarian conservation in the presence of apparently unilateral invasive carcinoma with a similar group of patients treated by bilateral ovariectomy shows no significant difference in survival.[495,513] On the other hand, Kottmeier[481] found that invasive serous carcinomas produced microscopic metastases that were grossly undetectable in a third of the patients in his series of 71 cases and recommended bilateral oophorectomy for this specific neoplasm in all cases.

PLACENTA*

Examination of placenta

The placenta is best examined fresh. The decisions to prepare for electron microscopy and to culture viruses, bacteria, or tissues for cytogenetic study must be made immediately after delivery, based on historical data, physical examination of mother and infant, and gross inspection of the placenta itself. Subsequent examination of the placenta by a pathologist is not impeded seriously by refrigeration for a few hours.

The first step is to reconstruct the relationships of the membranous sac, noting the width of the narrowest margin between the site of rupture and the placental margin. Any margin at all excludes placenta previa.

After an inspection the membranes are cut away from the placental margin, rolled into a sausage-shaped structure, and held thus by transfixation with a pin; after fixation a cross section of this roll is submitted for microscopic study.

The cord is next examined and measured; the number of vessels is recorded. The cord is separated by a cut near the placenta, and the placenta is weighed. The surfaces are inspected for disruption or exudate. A whole mount of the amnion may be examined immediately for the presence of bacteria or sex chromatin. The placenta is then sliced in cross section like a loaf of bread, and representative blocks are cut for microscopic study. A detailed protocol prepared for the National Institutes of Health collaboration study has been described with further comments about more specialized techniques.[612]

Development: anatomy and physiology

Significant stages in the formation of the placenta are as follows:

1. Implantation of the 6- to 7-day blastocyst occurs, with formation of solid trophoblast from its wall at the point of contact with the endometrium (Fig. 36-82, *A*).
2. Gradual peripheral orientation of the syncytiotrophoblast, in which vacuoles appear and then coalesce to form the intervillous space, occurs, with central orientation of the cytotrophoblast, which proliferates as isolated masses, forerunners of the primordial villi; these changes occur from the ninth to thirteenth day of development (Fig. 36-82, *B*).
3. Conversion of the cytotrophoblastic masses covered by syncytiotrophoblast to primordial villi occurs from the fourteenth to seventeenth day (Figs. 36-82, *C*, and 36-83, *D*).
4. Branching of primordial villi occurs from the eighteenth day through the first trimester; each primordial villus with its derivatives constitutes a cotyledon of the mature placenta (Fig. 36-83).
5. Gradual enlargement of the entire ovum occurs from the twentieth day to the twentieth week, resulting in the following.
   a. Obliteration of the entire uterine cavity by fusion of decidua capsularis and decidua vera
   b. Progressive thinning of the abembryonic chorion to become the chorion laeve
   c. Progressive growth of the amnion with gradual obliteration of the chorion cavity by fusion of chorionic and amniotic fibrous tissue
   d. Progressive growth of the chorion frondosum, forming eight to 15 cotyledons, constituting the placenta (Fig. 36-84)

*Although this entire chapter on pathology of the female genitalia derives heavily from the towering work of Arthur T. Hertig, the debt is nowhere as immense and obvious as in this section on the placenta. These illustrations and the words to describe them will be recognized by anyone who has so much as glanced at the subject, since they are unique and have been published necessarily by every writer who sets out to review the morphology of the early conceptus. The best and only completely original review of the subject is the monograph in which Hertig[612] summarizes earlier work done by himself and in collaboration with others.

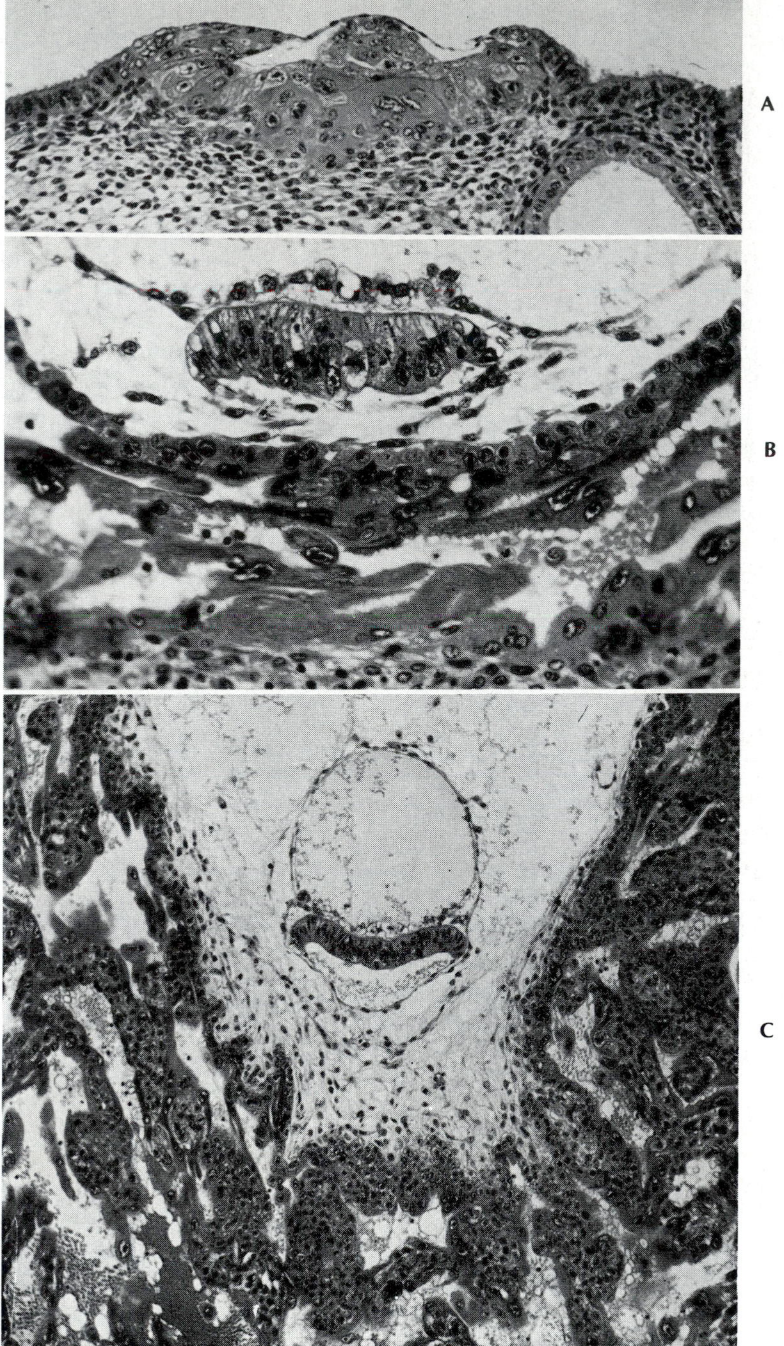

Fig. 36-82. **A,** Human 7½-day ovum superficially implanted for 36 hours on edematous 22-day secretory endometrium. Note solid trophoblast, derived from blastocyst wall at its contact with endometrium and composed of pale cytotrophoblast and darker syncytiotrophoblast. **B,** Human 12½-day ovum showing embryonic disc *(above)* and adjacent trophoblast in contact *(below)* with predecidual stroma of 26-day secretory endometrium. Note inner cytotrophoblast, beginning to form primordial chorionic villi, and outer syncytiotrophoblast, whose lacunar spaces contain maternal blood, beginning of uteroplacental circulation. **C,** Human 14-day ovum showing embryo *(upper center)* surrounded by early chorion frondosum. Note simple unbranched primordial villi composed largely of central cytotrophoblastic core, beginning to form mesenchymal core and surrounded by syncytium, which lines intervillous space. (**A,** 150×; **B,** 250×; **C,** 100×; **A** to **C,** courtesy Department of Embryology, Carnegie Institution of Washington; **A** and **C,** Carnegie No. 7801; from Heuser, C.H., Rock, J., and Hertig, A.T.: Contrib. Embryol. **31:**85, 1945; **B,** Carnegie No. 7700; from Hertig, A.T., and Rock, J.: Contrib. Embryol. **29:**127, 1941.)

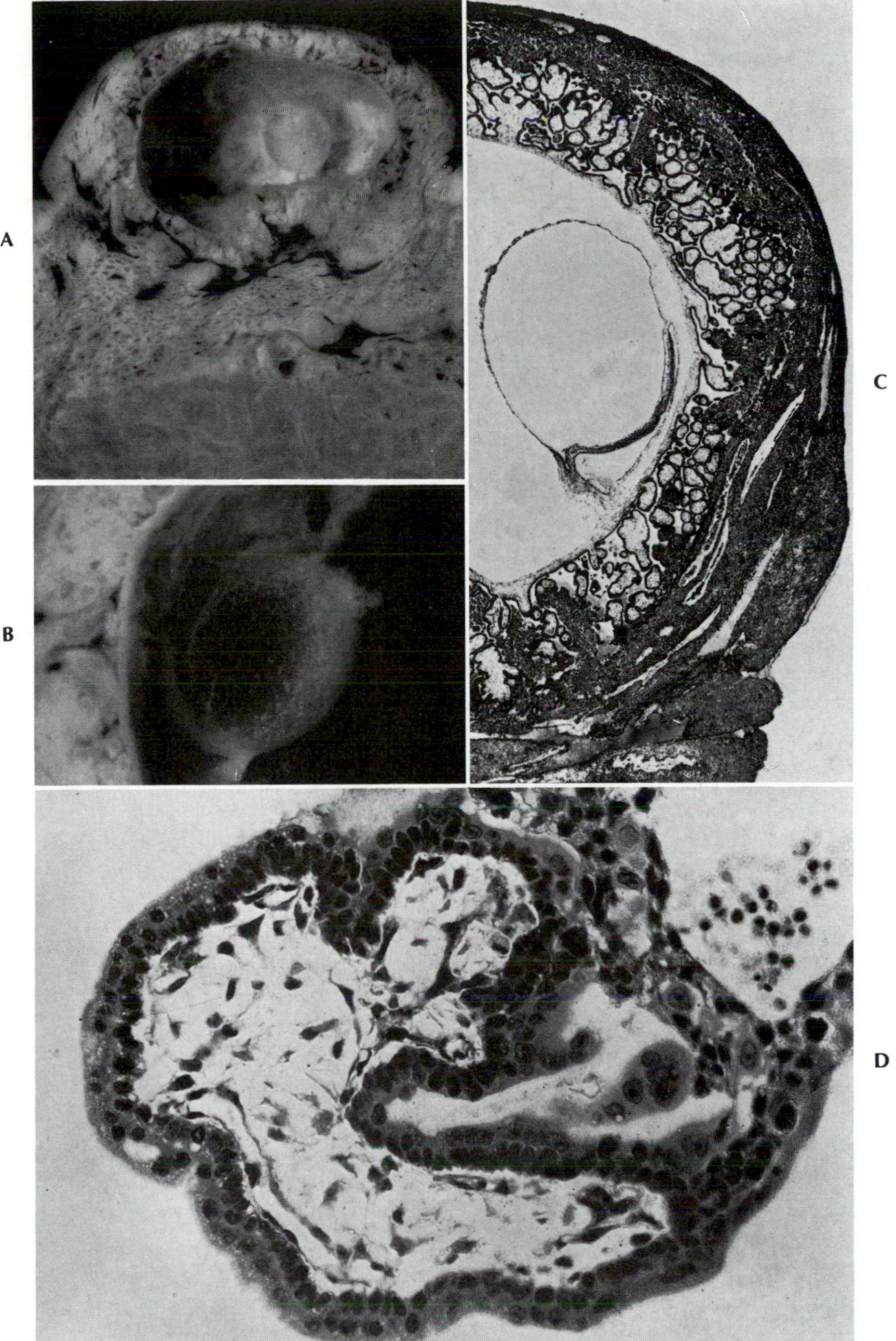

Fig. 36-83. Gross and microscopic aspects of chorionic, embryonic, and body stalk development at developmental age of 19 days (menstrual age of 33 days). **A,** Ovisac and implantation site bisected to show embryo, chorionic cavity, and chorionic villi around entire circumference. Thin decidua capsularis above, decidua vera laterally, and decidua basalis below, but above myometrium. For gross details of embryo viewed at right angles, see **B. B,** Embryo showing yolk sac with blood islands *(right),* curved germ disc *(left),* and crescent-shaped amniotic cavity between chorionic membrane *(extreme left)* and body stalk *(below).* For microscopic details (in mirror image), see **C. C,** Midsagittal section of embryo, body stalk, and adjacent chorion, the last representing one half of chorion and including both chorion laeve *(top)* and chorion frondosum *(bottom).* **D,** Detail of chorionic villus from pregnancy comparable to that shown in **A** to **C.** Note immature stroma containing developing blood vessels. Trophoblast consists of outer syncytium and inner Langhans' epithelium. Between streamers of solid trophoblast *(upper right)* are maternal blood cells within intervillous space (**A,** 4×; **B** and **C,** 12×; **D,** 300×. **A** to **D,** Courtesy Department of Embryology, Carnegie Institution of Washington; Carnegie Numbers: **A,** 8671, seq. 2; **B,** 8671, seq. 6; **C,** 8671, sect. 10-4-2; **D,** 5960, sect. 5-2-1; **D,** from Hertig, A.T.: Contrib. Embryol. **25:**37, 1935.)

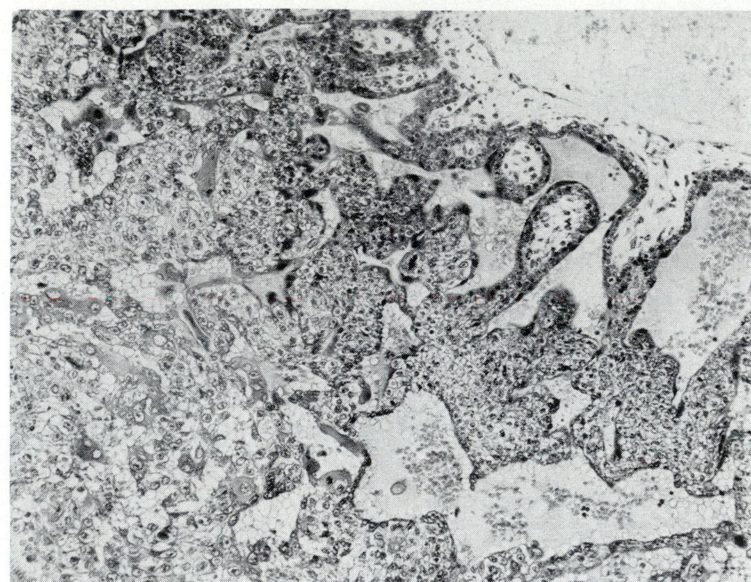

Fig. 36-84. Primordial chorionic villi from normal human ovary of approximately 15 days' gestation. These villi *(upper right)* are comparable to that shown in Fig. 36-83, *D,* and are continuous with cytotrophoblast of cell column and placental floor. The latter is contiguous with decidua basalis *(left margin)*. Remnants of peripheral syncytiotrophoblast appear as giant cells *(center)* from which placental site giant cells will be derived. (150×.)

Amnion

Significant phases in the formation of the amnion are as follows:

1. Its in situ delamination from the adjacent cytotrophoblast of the implanting ovum during the seventh to ninth day of development
2. Resulting formation of a veil-like membrane over and attached to the periphery of the circular concave germ disc during the ninth to thirteenth day of development (Fig. 36-82, *B*)
3. Gradual transformation of this membrane to amniotic epithelium during the fourteenth to twenty-fifth day of development (Fig. 36-82, *C*)
4. Simultaneous accumulation of a second mesoblastic layer
5. Progressive distension of the amniotic cavity, growth of the embryo, and its prolapse into the amniotic cavity
6. Gradual obliteration of the chorionic cavity by fusion of connective tissue of amnion and chorion

Umbilical cord

Significant stages in the formation of the umbilical cord are as follows:

1. Its origin as a mass of chorionically derived mesoblast at the caudal end of the embryonic disc when the latter develops its longitudinal axis during the fourteenth to sixteenth day (Fig. 36-83, *C*)
2. Gradual shifting of the caudally located body stalk to a more ventrally situated umbilical cord as the embryo grows caudally
3. Gradual prolapse of the embryo accompanied by its cord into the amniotic cavity and simultaneous covering of the cord by amniotic epithelium

Chorionic villi

The immature villi are covered by an outer layer of syncytiotrophoblast and an inner layer of cytotrophoblast cells (Fig. 36-83, *D*). The latter divide, mature, and become incorporated into the growing syncytiotrophoblast layer, a process that is virtually completed by the sixteenth week. Only syncytiotrophoblast is evident thereafter. The capillary vessels are very small. The stromal core contains fibroblasts, collagen, and Hofbauer cells, which are macrophages with very large vacuoles that apparently result from the imbibition of large amounts of water.[596] In mature placental villi the cytotrophoblast cells have disappeared, the stroma is scant, capillaries are multiple with thin walls, and the immensely active syncytiotrophoblast layer is thin, except where nuclei accumulate into clusters or knots. The morphology of placental anatomy and development has been described in detail in the beautifully illustrated monographs by Hertig[612] and Boyd and Hamilton.[571]

The syncytiotrophoblast cells of the villi are responsible for sorting and distributing nutrients to the fetus and fetal metabolic by-products back to the mother and for synthesizing a remarkable variety of hormones. Placental functions are so numerous and placental products so varied that a completely satisfactory clinical test of placental function remains to be elaborated. The steroid hormones include estrogens, progesterone, androgens, adrenocorticosteroids, and aldosterone. The placental peptide hormones include HCG, chorionic somatomammotropin (HCS), also called human placental lactogen (HPL), chorionic thyrotropin, and adrenocorticotropic hormone. These placental activities have been summarized in monographs by Jaffe[622] and Gruenwald.[606] When the exact cell origin of substances identified in the mother during gestation involves fetal and placental tissues together, the metabolic products are considered to define the functional status of the fetoplacental unit; for example, the amount of estriol in maternal urine is dependent on fetal adrenal glands and liver, as well as the placenta, and a decline indicates a threat to survival of the fetus, although the site of the lesion responsible may not have been determined.

HCG alters the maternal immune response and is probably an important factor in the survival of the placental allograft. Trophoblast is antigenic.[567,619] Circulating HCG levels throughout pregnancy are not as high as those required for complete in vitro inhibition of lymphocyte transformation[554] or mixed lymphocyte culture reaction. However, local concentrations in the syncytiotrophoblast layer are very high in comparison with those in other tissues.[587,591] There seems to be an important electronegative barrier of sialic acid (an HCG moiety) at the syncytiotrophoblast surface.[639] This surface is the interface between maternal and fetal tissues and ultimately the locus at which accommodation between the two must be settled. Of great interest is the apparent paradox that maternal sensitization to trophoblast, which must be blocked for the placenta to survive, actually enhances implantation and subsequent fetal growth.[563]

One postulated protective factor active soon after implantation is uteroglobin, a protein activated locally in the uterus by transglutaminase. Uteroglobin appears to cross-link with embryonic transplantation antigens, masking them from maternal immune response. In addition, an immunologic blocking antibody, present in maternal serum, is necessary for successful pregnancy; women without it abort repeatedly.[655] It is actually genetic compatibility between parents that seems to mediate this cause of habitual abortion.

One important line of cancer research is based on the similarity between cancer cells and trophoblast: cancers produce HCG and other placental hormones[671]; they also recapitulate the placental capacity for immunologic hiding.[603]

The dynamics of placental circulation are unique. Maternal blood from the uterine arteries works its way through the uterine wall into the spiral arterioles of the maternal endometrium (now decidua vera) and empties in spurts into the intervillous space of the placenta. The openings of the spiral arterioles are distributed about the placental floor; between them are the openings of the decidual veins, through which blood from the intervillous space returns into the maternal venous system.

In the early weeks of pregnancy an extremely important sequence of changes enlarges the flow capacity of the decidual spiral arteries. The cytotrophoblast cells of the outer margin of the conceptus invade opened ends of these small arteries, replace the endothelium, and infiltrate the muscular walls; the muscular layer and elastic tissue are destroyed (Fig. 36-85). By the middle of the second trimester this change has extended to involve the myometrial segments of the spiral arteries. The result is a group of 100 to 150 tortuous, greatly widened, funnel-shaped arterial channels—the true uteroplacental arteries—with walls composed of fibrinoid material and a lining of trophoblast. Thus the placenta must structure its vascular supply line.

The fetal circulation begins with the umbilical arteries, which come to the placenta through the umbilical cord. The umbilical arteries divide and redivide in the placenta, ultimately into small capillaries of the villi, and return through tributaries of the umbilical vein into the umbilical cord.

The intervillous space is a single vast pool of maternal blood in which the placental villi dangle, rootlike, with margins sealed by tight contact between decidua and placental membranes. There is no "marginal sinus" in the sense of an anatomic walled structure to collect maternal blood before its return to the uterus. A premature separation at this margin may allow maternal blood to leak out rapidly, an alarming event that is still called marginal sinus tear.

Anomalies

Abnormal shapes

The umbilical cord usually inserts near the center of the placenta, but in about 10% of cases it may insert at the placental margin (battledore placenta). Less frequent (1%), but of greater potential importance, is velamentous insertion, in which the cord runs for variable distances through the membranes before reaching the placenta. This fixes the location of the cord and may result in compression or even rupture if the area involved passes over the cervical outlet.

A placenta divided into two parts is bipartite; a small accessory succenturiate lobe is important as a cause of bleeding if left behind, an event that can be detected because the vessels that extend to it end abruptly at a tear in the membranes.

Single umbilical artery

In a series of 39,773 white and black single births, 0.9% of umbilical cords contained a single umbilical

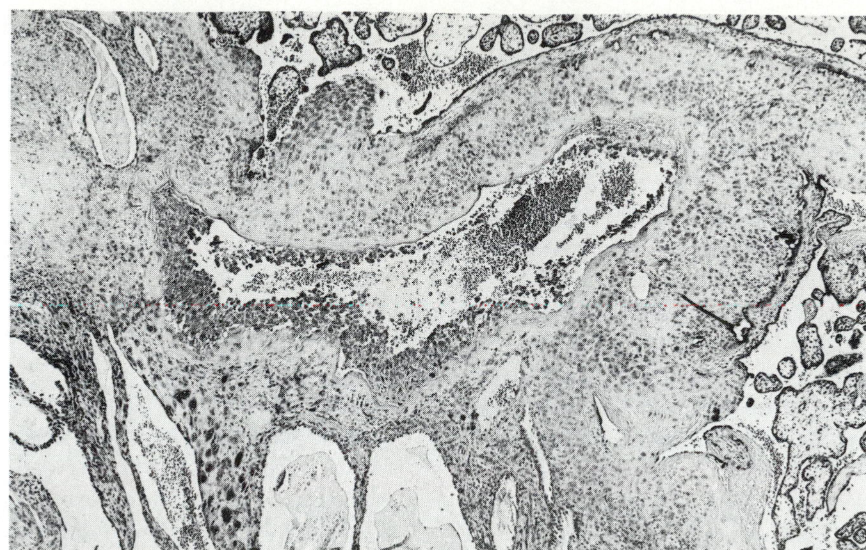

Fig. 36-85. Decidual spiral arteriole *(center)* during fifth month, showing dilatation, replacement of endothelium by cytotrophoblast, and hyalinization of vessel wall. Decidua is infiltrated by syncytiotrophoblast cells at lower left. Placental villi are at top, and dilated decidual glands are at bottom center. (40×.)

artery.[600] Fourteen percent of the infants so affected were stillborn or died in the neonatal period; of those on whom autopsies were performed, half were found to have significant congenital anomalies, chiefly affecting the cardiovascular or genitourinary system. Although the presence of a single umbilical artery implies a 10- to 20-fold increase in serious congenital malformations, affected infants who survive the perinatal period have normal prospects, except for a 1 in 20 chance of developing an inguinal hernia.

Placenta membranacea

Persistence of villi surrounding the entire conceptus is called placenta membranacea; the situation is comparable to placenta previa, including the threat of severe hemorrhage.[599] Arteriographic studies may be misleading.[585]

Amnion nodosum

Amnion nodosum occurs with any condition resulting in extreme oligohydramnios, such as renal agenesis. Clusters of squamous cells, fibrin, and other amorphous debris become inspissated and form loosely attached plaques on the amnionic surfaces.[569] It should be distinguished from focal squamous metaplasia of the amnion, which is common around the insertion of the cord and has no known significance.

Multiple gestation

The question of genetic relationship in multiple pregnancy has increased importance because of the potential need for organ transplantation and because of the threatening implications of circulatory connections in monochorionic placentas. The relationships of the membranes are diagramed in Fig. 36-86.

Dichorionic diamnionic twin placenta

If two separate zygotes implant concurrently, the placentas may fuse; the twins in this case are fraternal (not identical). Separate placentas (chorions) also result if a single zygote divides and the two daughter cells separate completely and implant; each will mature, producing identical twins. The fused placentas will be recognizable by a persistent ridge of chorion at the base of the septum between the two amnions after the amniotic membranes are stripped away. Histologic section of the septum shows two amnions and an intervening layer of chorion. It appears that about 20% of twins with this type of placenta are monozygotic (identical), and 80% are dizygotic (fraternal).[565]

Monochorionic diamnionic twin placentas

If two germ discs form after implantation of a single zygote, the twins (always identical) will share a single placenta. Vascular connections are large and easily demonstrated, and no chorionic ridge is present when the amnions are stripped away.[570] There is no layer of chorion (trophoblast) between the two amnions that fuse to form the septum between the amnionic cavities.

Monochorionic monoamnionic twin placentas

When there is no intervening septum, the twins (always identical) share the same amnionic cavity. The prospects for entanglement are great, and mortality is high.

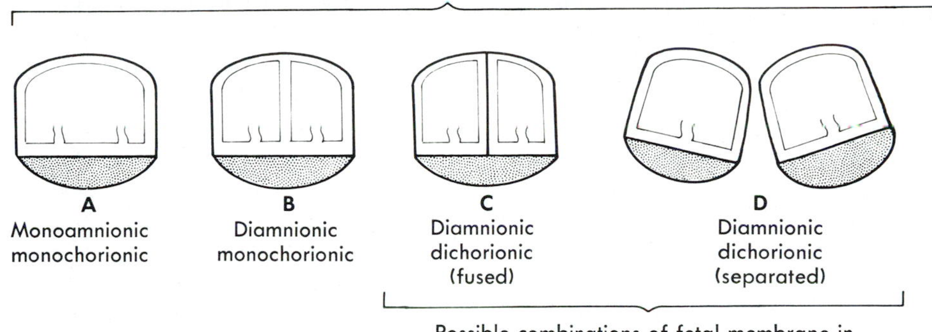

Fig. 36-86. Diagram of common morphologic variations in twin placentation. Types **A** and **B** occur only in identical twins; types **C** and **D** are common to both. (From Kraus, F.T.: Gynecologic pathology, St. Louis, 1967, The C.V. Mosby Co.)

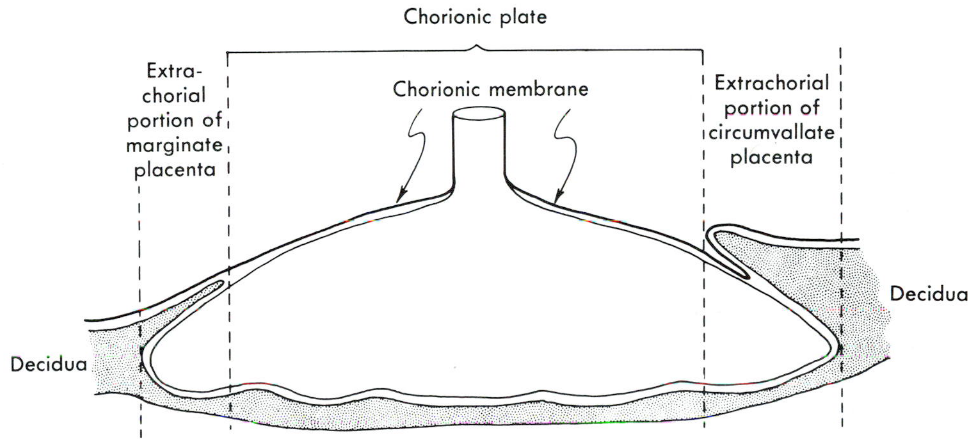

Fig. 36-87. Diagrams of placenta-uterus relationships in extrachorial placenta. (Modified from Scott, J.S.: J. Obstet. Gynaecol. Br. Cwlth. **67**:904, 1960.)

Clinicopathologic correlation

In a series of 250 twin placentas carefully correlated by all possible factors to confirm zygosity (fraternal versus identical), 56% of placentas were dizygotic and 44% were monozygotic. Thirty percent of the monozygotic twins had dichorionic placentas, and 70% had monochorionic placentas; 3% of the latter had monochorionic monoamnionic placentas. Eighty percent of twins with dichorionic placentas are dizygotic. Thus, by examination of a twin placenta, one can conclude that the twins are definitely identical in the case of a monochorionic placenta and probably fraternal (four chances in five) in the case of a dichorionic placenta.[565]

Twins are exposed to greater risks of many kinds; both morbidity and mortality are increased. Malformations are more common than in single births; monozygotic twins sharing the same circulation both may be injured by unequal distribution, and prematurity is much more common. The abnormal relationships, causes, and pathologic physiology of multiple gestations have been comprehensively presented by Benirschke and Kim.[566]

Higher orders of multiple pregnancy

The same criteria of zygosity may be applied by examination of the septal membranes between adjacent amnionic cavities.

Abnormal implantation

Extrachorial implantation

In about 18% of deliveries the margins of the placenta lie submerged beneath the decidua. If the amnionic membrane extends to the placental rim and is reflected back toward the center, it is called a circumvallate placenta (Fig. 36-87). The amnion of a marginate placenta does not follow the placental rim beneath the decidua but continues out over the decidual surface. Scott[659] found no significant risk to mother or infant attributable to this relationship; there may be a slight increase in vaginal bleeding.

Placenta accreta

Placental separation at parturition occurs by cleavage through the decidua. If there is no intervening decidua, the villi become attached to the myometrium and will not separate. The condition may be complete over the entire base of the placenta or, more commonly, only partial; the villi may extend into the myometrium (placenta increta) or entirely through it, resulting in rupture (placenta percreta).[574] In all cases the placenta cannot be delivered, the uterus cannot contract, and hemorrhage is usually brisk. In most cases hysterectomy is necessary to control bleeding.

Ectopic pregnancy

Implantation may occur outside the uterine cavity. The most common site is the uterine tube. Less frequent sites include the interstitial part of the tube, the cervix, the ovary, and the intra-abdominal peritoneal surface.[573]

Tubal ectopic pregnancy usually occurs in a tube altered by prior inflammation, which apparently interferes with transport of the ovum. Fetal abnormalities also probably contribute to ectopic gestation; Poland, Dill, and Styblo[648] found embryos with gross abnormalities, apparently genetically induced, in about one fourth of a series of carefully examined ectopic pregnancies. In all sites there is a threat of rupture attended by severe hemorrhage. Maternal death, sudden, unexpected, and always a calamity, continues to challenge obstetricians and threaten their patients.[573,658]

The endometrium may or may not show gestational histologic changes, depending on the extent to which the gestation has progressed and the length of time between fetal death and onset of bleeding. An occasional abdominal pregnancy is successfully terminated by cesarean section, but the fetal mortality exceeds 90%[562]; attempts at placental removal at delivery (laparotomy) may lead to serious hemorrhage.[618]

Placenta previa

After low implantation of a normal ovum the enlarging placenta may come to lie over the internal os of the cervix. Even before onset of labor the exposed maternal surface may be a source of bleeding, and with the onset of labor the certainty of massive hemorrhage necessitates cesarean section. Variable degrees of placenta accreta often accompany placenta previa, probably because of the generally deficient endometrium in the lower uterine segment.[612]

Spontaneous abortion (miscarriage)

The termination of a pregnancy, regardless of the mechanism, before the fetus can survive (if it is present) is called an abortion. Spontaneous abortion is usually the result of a pathologic ovum, infection, or maternal disease. Missed abortion is retention of a dead fetus longer than 2 months.

By far the most common abnormality leading to spontaneous abortion is a genetic defect of the conceptus. In about half of all spontaneous abortions the fetus is either absent or grossly malformed. Hertig[612] has written a detailed description and classification of various gross abnormalities. Cytogenetic studies have shown a chromosomal abnormality in about a third of the cases,[580] but the incidence was nearly 60% in a small series using more refined chromosome-banding techniques.[632] The most common chromosomal anomalies demonstrated have been triploidy, 45XO karyotype, and single autosomal trisomy.[564]

The decidua associated with spontaneous abortion shows hemorrhage, necrosis, and leukocytic infiltration. The endometrium away from the implantation site often shows the pattern of secretory gestational hyperplasia described by Arias-Stella.[270]

The chorionic villi may appear nearly normal or be surrounded by dense deposits of intervillous fibrin clot. In a majority of the cases in which the embryo is absent, the villous stroma is swollen and hydropic as the result of fluid accumulation. This is the hallmark of a "blighted" ovum and probably a result of continued trophoblast function in the absence of a vascular transport to carry the accumulated fluid, since there is no fetus. Hydropic villi have no direct significance for the mother and especially should not be confused with hydatidiform mole.

Phillippe[645] has correlated cytogenetic studies of spontaneous abortions with histologic patterns. Invagination of the surface trophoblast into the core of the villus was found chiefly in instances of triploidy (Fig. 36-88). The marked hydropic change in the villi of triploid abortions has prompted the designation of "partial hydatidiform mole"[666]; it is important to recognize that hydatidiform mole is clinically, grossly, microscopically, and cytogenetically very different (as discussed later). Choriocarcinoma as a complication of a triploid abortion remains a remote possibility that has never been convincingly demonstrated.[564] Cases with autosomal trisomy show migration of occasional large cytotrophoblast cells into the villous stroma. Occasional abortuses with large edematous winglike projections from the posterior neck suggesting hygromas have been shown to have a 45XO karyotype.[646]

Maternal factors in abortion include induced abortion and its complications, often related to infection. Infectious diseases generally have been considered to be an

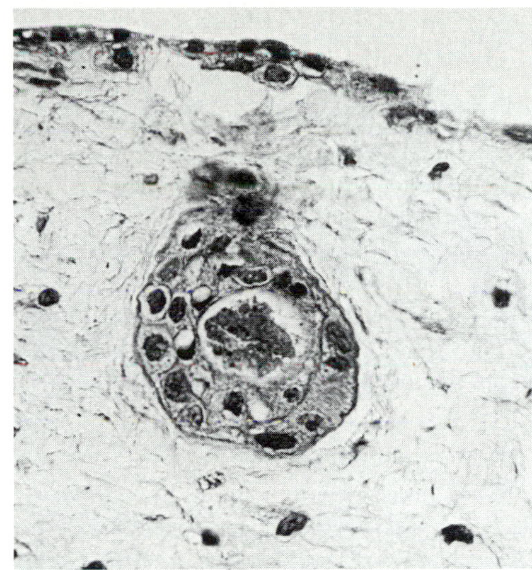

Fig. 36-88. Trophoblastic invagination in villus, shown in cross section. Chromosomal analysis of cultured cells showed a 69XXX triploid karyotype, which correlates consistently with this morphologic abnormality. (Courtesy Dr. Emile Philippe, Strasbourg, France.)

uncommon primary cause of spontaneous abortion. With the increased use of sophisticated microbiologic techniques, infections have been detected in increasing numbers; their role in abortion and fetal loss will have to be reevaluated. The organisms that have been implicated include herpesvirus,[601,637] cytomegalic inclusion virus,[586,636] virus of rubella,[640] *Listeria monocytogenes,*[646] *Toxoplasma gondii,*[558,589] and mycoplasmas.[609,617] Anaerobic bacteria are especially important in the pathogenesis of septic abortion and its maternal complications.[656] When compared with the pain and vast expense incurred by disabled living children injured by intrauterine infection, abortion may be one of the least problematic outcomes.

Toxemia of pregnancy (eclampsia and preeclampsia)

Toward the end of pregnancy, salt retention, edema, albuminuria, and hypertension develop in about 6% of women. This syndrome is called toxemia of pregnancy or preeclampsia. The most severe manifestation, eclampsia, is accompanied by convulsions; there is extensive intravascular coagulation with fibrin thrombi and focal necrosis in the liver, kidneys, and brain.

The pathogenesis of toxemia of pregnancy has been extensively studied but remains unexplained; theories are numerous.[641] The most significant pathologic lesion seems to be in the uterine spiral arteries. As described originally by Hertig,[611] there is fibrinoid necrosis of the walls of the terminal ends of the spiral arteries in the decidua. The myometrial segments of the uteroplacental arteries of the placental bed and the basal arteries that supply the decidua are also affected. In addition, there is an accumulation of foamy lipophages in the necrotic vessel walls and an infiltrate of small mononuclear cells in and around the vessels. These changes, called acute atherosis, begin with lipid accumulation in smooth muscle cells, necrosis of smooth muscle, exudation of fibrin into the vessel wall, and infiltration of the vessel wall by phagocytic macrophages that become swollen with accumulated lipid. They are often accompanied by thrombosis.[653]

Brosens, Dixon, and Robertson[576] have found that the physiologic trophoblastic invasion of placental bed spiral arteries (see p. 1521) does not extend into the myometrial segments of these vessels. These segments cannot expand and therefore represent a constriction between the proximal radial arteries and the distended distal segments in the decidua. It is in these areas that acute atherosis occurs. The similarity between acute atherosis and vascular changes in rejected renal allografts suggests that this placental vascular lesion may be the result of a local immunologic attack, which ordinarily is blocked by the physiologic invasion of trophoblast. Immunofluorescence studies provide some support for this.[627]

Regardless of how they are produced, the lesions of acute atherosis impair blood flow to the placenta and to the decidua itself. In this ischemic background, placental infarction, retroplacental hematoma, premature placental separation, fetal distress, and the small fetus appear.

In experimental models of eclampsia McKay[634] has emphasized the similar features of the generalized Shwartzman reaction and the degenerative changes in the placental trophoblast. The placental lesions are not specific, but the ischemia and accentuation of degenerative changes produce a very abnormal pattern. Syncytiotrophoblast nuclei form tight clusters. Some are necrotic. The cytoplasm of the syncytiotrophoblast becomes vacuolated. The amount of intervillous fibrin material—always present at term—is increased. Infarcts are common and may be extensive.

Circulatory lesions

In addition to the changes more clearly related to toxemia, there are other disturbances in the vascular supply of the placenta and its decidual support. These include infarcts, hematomas, and vascular lesions resulting from systemic maternal disease and unrelated to pregnancy.

Infarcts

The blood supply that supports the placenta comes from the maternal circulation. Impaired maternal circulation in local areas produces placental infarcts; impaired fetal circulation does not.

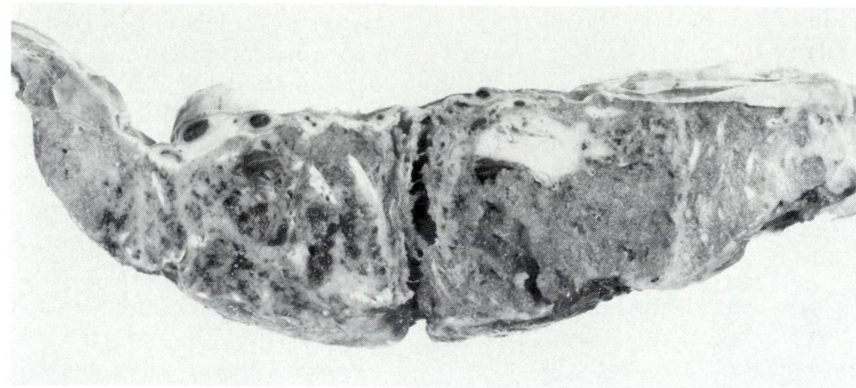

Fig. 36-89. Placental infarcts. Note granular cut surface, mottled white and red of old and recent lesions, and irregular margins. The mother had severe toxemia.

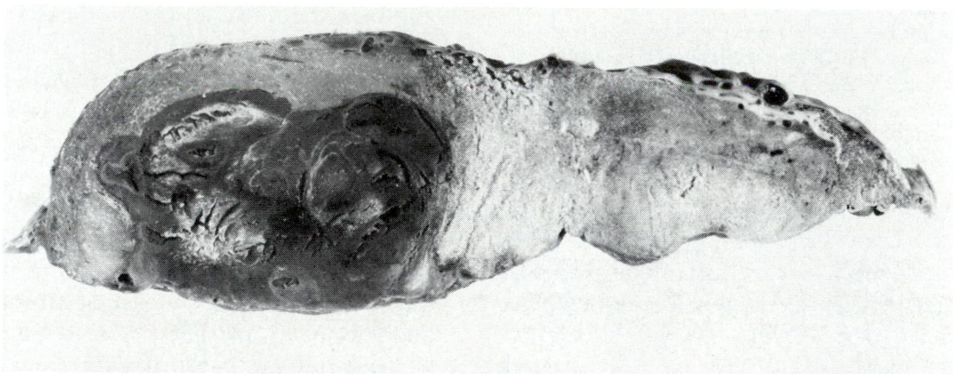

Fig. 36-90. Premature separation (abruptio placentae) with large hematoma that compresses overlying placenta.

The lesion responsible may be thrombosis of a group of decidual spiral arteries or atherosclerotic changes in branches of the uterine artery. A recent infarct appears red and granular. As the blood pigment is broken down and carried away, the infarct becomes progressively lighter, eventually achieving a pale yellow color (Fig. 36-89).

Intraplacental hematoma

Clots that develop in the intervillous space have a characteristic laminated pattern. They are red if recent and pale yellow if old. Since the villi are pushed aside as the hematoma forms, there are no villi in it, and the granularity of an infarct is not seen. The blood is of maternal origin.

A specific type of placental hematoma forms in the subchorionic area, producing a large tuberous mass. It usually but not always is associated with missed abortion and is called a Breus mole; there is no relationship to hydatidiform mole.[662]

Premature separation

The normally implanted placenta may become detached before the onset of labor. The bland decidual necrosis that disrupts the normal attachment may be the result of vascular disease, such as toxemia, or possibly poor nutrition, especially folic acid deficiency.[615]

The placenta is compressed by the clot that forms behind it (Fig. 36-90). As the result of consumption of clotting factors in this large hematoma, the circulating blood is depleted; thus there is a severe bleeding diathesis in at least one fifth of the patients. The uterine bleeding often leads to shock. The subsequent disseminated intravascular coagulation may be associated with bilateral renocortical necrosis and pituitary infarction. Any delay in delivery of the fetus results in prolonged anoxia and fetal death; the perinatal mortality is high.

Premature separation carries an increased risk of amniotic fluid embolism, a grave complication with a high mortality found also in women of high parity, with intrauterine fetal death or hypertonic labor, or with symptoms such as sudden onset of dyspnea, shock, or disseminated intravascular coagulation.[644] The presence of amniotic fluid is not always easily identified at autopsy with standard histologic sections but is readily demonstrated with the colloidal iron stain for acid mucopolysaccharide.[654]

Atherosclerosis: essential hypertension and diabetes mellitus

Young women with essential hypertension who also happen to become pregnant have hyperplastic intimal atherosclerotic lesions affecting the myometrial segments of the spiral arteries of the placental bed. The lesions here are often disproportionately severe in comparison with similar vessels elsewhere in the body. If the arterial physiologic changes of pregnancy (p. 1521) progress normally, the prognosis for the fetus is good.[653] Decidual arterioles in diabetes mellitus may be thick walled with hyalinized media.[565] Either situation may be further complicated by lesions of atherosis if toxemia develops; the consequences are usually severe.

Haust[608] has illustrated in great detail the morphologic changes in the placenta and implantation site of diabetic mothers. The placentas are often large, and the edematous cords have increased diameter. The villi are large and appear immature with abundant stroma, increased numbers of Hofbauer cells, and prominent, sometimes continuous cytotrophoblast cells. Arterioles of the implantation site may have thickened walls and hyalinized media.

Infectious diseases

Intrauterine infection may be transplacental or may ascend from the vagina. Unquestionably infection is an underestimated cause of spontaneous abortion. Many birth defects once considered to be "acts of God" are now reliably ascribed to a specific infectious organism, notably viruses. The extent to which the cytogenetic alterations described in the section on abortions might be virus induced is essentially unexplored. Midtrimester abortion is especially likely to be the result of chorioamnionitis.[555] About one fourth of placentas of small-for-gestational-age infants show nonspecific villitis; the mortality for this group is 16%.[556]

Bacterial infections

Rupture of the fetal membranes before the onset of labor provides a path for ascending bacterial infection. If the infection is well developed by the time of delivery, purulent exudate may be obvious on gross inspection of the fetal surfaces of the placenta and membranes, and similar advanced infection may be presumed to exist in the infant's lungs. Microscopically a dense infiltrate of neutrophils obliterates the amniotic epithelium; bacterial colonies may or may not be present. In many instances an infiltrate of leukocytes and fibrin in the subchorionic plate of the placenta is the only histologic evidence of infection. The most common species of organisms are those that inhabit the vagina in pregnancy, including *Escherichia coli* and *Streptococcus*, *Proteus*, and *Pseudomonas* species and highly virulent anaerobes such as *Bacteroides* and *Peptostreptococcus* species.

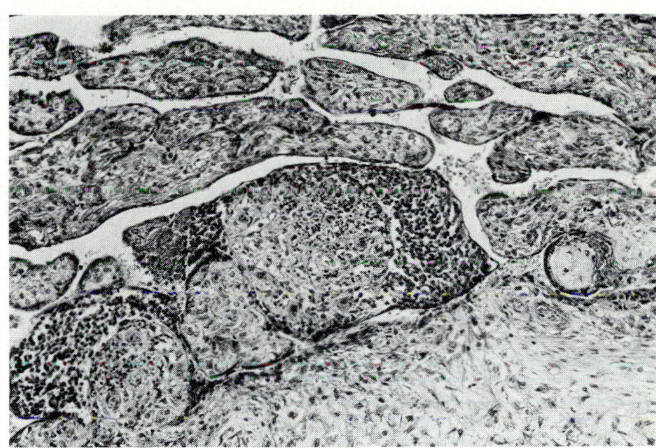

Fig. 36-91. Placental villitis associated with *Listeria monocytogenes* infection. Inflammatory cells expand villus, but thin envelope of attenuated trophoblast persists. (130×.)

Placental tuberculosis occurs rarely as a complication of miliary spread in the mother. Syphilis may cause villitis and fetal endovasculitis, but none of the gross or microscopic changes is specific for *Treponema pallidum* infection. Group B streptococcus, which is rarely a human pathogen, colonizes the vagina of 3% to 25% of pregnant women. Transmission to the fetus, which can cause pneumonia and meningitis, takes place only if maternal antibodies fail to develop. Vaginal colonization is detected by culture, since the women are asymptomatic; antibiotic coverage may not be necessary in the presence of adequate antibody response.[559]

Listeria monocytogenes produces a severe placentitis characterized by miliary abscesses and is one of the less recognized causes of septic abortion, especially repeated abortion.[650] The histologic appearance of the abscesses is a characteristic collection of polymorphonuclear leukocytes and mononuclear cells at the tip of a villus, enveloped by an attenuated layer of trophoblast (Fig. 36-91). The organism is better known as a cause of fetal wastage in animals, especially cattle; the basis for its selective pathogenicity in pregnancy is unknown.[565] The newborn is also susceptible, developing a distinctive disseminated infection called granulomatosis infantiseptica, in which the liver, lungs, spleen, and adrenal glands are riddled with miliary abscesses; the cause of death in the few born alive is acute meningitis.[635] The organism is a small gram-positive rod, which must not be hastily classified as a diphtheroid. Maternal endometrial infection may be chronic and should be treated even though it is asymptomatic.

Viral infections

Transmission of viruses to the fetus may be hematogenous and transplacental or by contact at the time of delivery. Smallpox, varicella, herpes simplex, and cytomegalic inclusion virus[636] cause necrotizing villitis with typical intranuclear inclusions. Placental lesions in congenital rubella infection include acute necrotizing villitis, older fibrotic areas, and cytoplasmic viral inclusions. Ornoy and associates[640] found a close correlation between severe fetal anomalies and placental inflammation (including cytoplasmic inclusions) in pregnancies complicated by rubella infection. They suggested that evaluation of placental biopsies would aid in the decision of whether to continue a pregnancy in the face of maternal rubella exposure or infection.

Perinatal infection with cytomegalovirus in term infants born alive is apparently transmitted by contact with recently contracted active cervical infection in the mother.[652] First and second trimester abortion caused by necrotizing villitis and deciduitis has also been reported, but its numerical significance is uncertain. The immature nervous system is most susceptible to intrauterine infection. Mental retardation, deafness, impaired vision, low birth weight, and microcephaly are the more devastating disabilities that follow. The social costs are incalculable. The total cost for 5000 infants affected annually by cytomegalovirus certainly is comparable to the $161,000 direct cost estimated for each rubella-affected child; cytomegalovirus is clearly a billion dollar problem.

Protozoal infections

Toxoplasmosis is transmitted to the infant through the placenta. Mothers who have antibodies before pregnancy do not have infected infants. The most serious fetal lesions are produced when maternal exposure occurs during the first two trimesters of pregnancy. The encysted organisms can be demonstrated histologically, but often with difficulty; more consistent identification is obtained by intraperitoneal injection in mice.[589] The placental lesion is focal necrosis and villitis, with a mononuclear infiltrate. Cysts without inflammation may be found in the placentas of neonates who develop severe disease months later.[569] The injuries are not rare and include deafness, blindness, and mental retardation.[676] The accumulated direct costs from each year's total of 3300 disabled infants exceed $200 million in the United States alone.[675] The toll in misery and frustration is impossible to calculate. Effective control in the form of simple hygienic measures should be available to everyone.[675]

When infection is severe, fetal hydrops occurs, and the placental appearance mimics erythroblastosis grossly and microscopically.[558]

Malarial parasites have been identified in maternal erythrocytes in the intervillous space.

Fungous infections

The most common fungous infection of the placenta is that caused by *Candida* organisms that invade transvaginally after premature rupture of the membranes. Associated bacterial infection is common. Fungal hyphae may infiltrate the umbilical cord. Instances of *Coccidioides* infection have been reported.[565]

Mycoplasma infection

Mycoplasma organisms have been implicated in infertility[617] and abortion,[635] and organisms have been cultured in cases of chorioamnionitis. The lesions resemble those produced by bacteria, with a polymorphonuclear leukocytic infiltrate. Correlation between placental lesions caused by T mycoplasmas and any sort of fetal disease seems to be poor.[664]

Hemorrhagic endovasculitis

Sander[657] has described a distinctive form of focal intravillous hemorrhage; fragmented and intact erythrocytes are scattered through the vessel walls and villous stroma. The infants are often stillborn. The cause is undetermined. There was chronic villitis in a majority of cases; viral inclusions occurred in 10%.

Erythroblastosis fetalis

The placenta in erythroblastosis fetalis is greatly enlarged, from two to four times the normal size and weight. The fetal membranes are pale gray when associated with fetal hydrops. The cut surface is pale, spongy, and granular. The microscopic appearance represents a recapitulation of the immature state, with prominent cytotrophoblast cells, abundant villous stroma, and many Hofbauer cells.[610] Nucleated red blood cells in clusters may fill and distend capillary spaces.

Trophoblastic hyperplasia and neoplasia

The aggressive overgrowth of trophoblast, benign or malignant, is an unusual but always dramatic complication of pregnancy. All the lesions described subsequently are frequently discussed together as forms of "trophoblastic disease."

Hydatidiform mole

Hydatidiform mole is a form of pathologic pregnancy that is uncommon in the United States (about 1 per 2000 pregnancies) but for reasons still unknown occurs with about 10 times that frequency in various parts of Asia and Central America.[642] There is a rapid increase in uterine size, often with symptoms of toxemia and vaginal bleed-

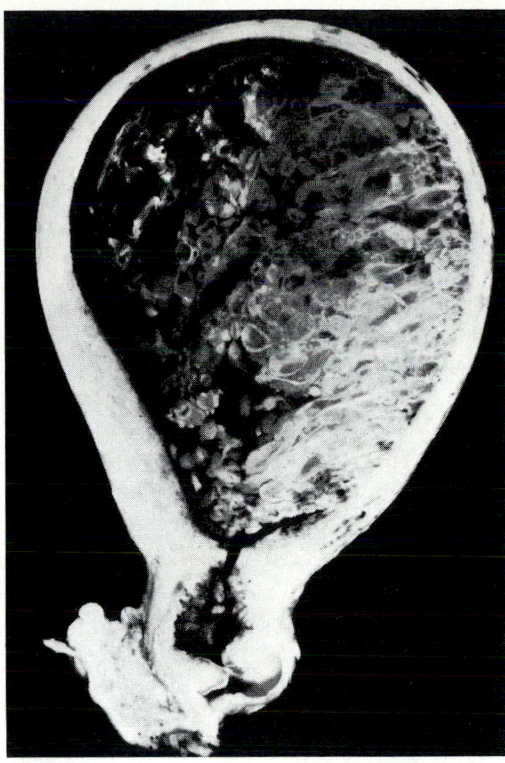

Fig. 36-92. Midsagittal section of typical molar uterus approaching term size, although of gestational age of only about 20 weeks. Uterine cavity is greatly distended, but small, oval, centrally located chorionic sac may still be identified. (Courtesy Dr. H. Sheehan, Armed Forces Institute of Pathology.)

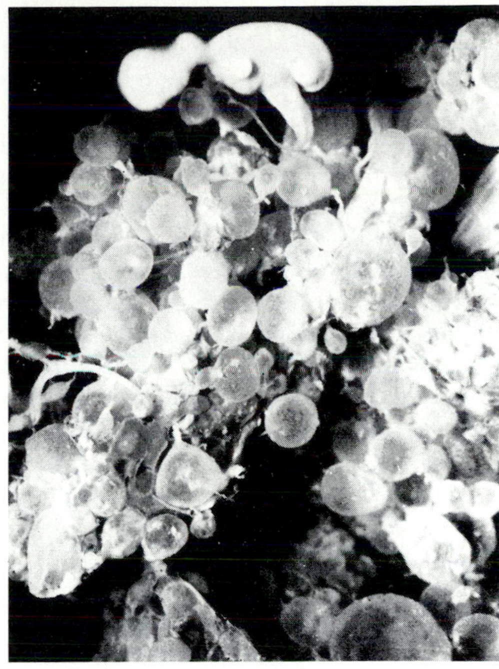

Fig. 36-93. Grapelike vesicles of varying size constituting hydatidiform mole. Stunted, macerated fetus at menstrual age of approximately 6 weeks was within intact chorionic sac (not shown here) when mole was delivered at hysterectomy. This is unusual, since chorionic sac is usually empty. (2×; Carnegie No. 8723, seq. 1; from Hertig, A.T: Hydatidiform mole and chorionepithelioma. In Meigs, J.V., and Sturgis, S.H., editors: Progress in gynecology, vol. II, New York, 1963, Grune & Stratton, Inc.; by permission.)

ing. Ultrasonography can be used to confirm the absence of the fetus. By the middle of the second trimester the uterus may approach the size of a uterus at term; bleeding begins at this time, if not before.

A hydatidiform mole itself is actually a placenta composed entirely or almost entirely of immensely swollen villi. The volume varies from about 1 to 3 liters (Fig. 36-92). There is usually an abundance of hyperplastic trophoblast covering some or all of the villi and infiltrating the decidua at the implantation site. It is possible but rare to find a fetus (Fig. 36-93). In the presence of a fetus, or in smaller abortions composed of a mixture of normal and hydropic villi, subsequent choriocarcinoma is extremely unlikely. The term "hydatidiform mole" should be avoided in such cases, which are usually triploid abortions, as described previously.[666]

The pathogenesis is unknown. The considerably higher incidence in the lowest socioeconomic populations suggests a nutritional factor that remains undefined. The cytogenetics of hydatidiform mole are startling. The karyotype is consistently 46XX and occasionally 46XY; in either case *both* sets of chromosomes are paternally derived.[624] The mechanism is not certain; it appears, however, that the female nucleus is expelled, and the genetic complement of a single sperm usually replicates by endoreduplication. The 46XY karyotype would appear to require two sperm.

The histologic pattern of the villous core varies little; the jellylike edematous stroma is nearly clear and traversed by thin strands of connective tissue, most of which are ruptured (Fig. 36-94). Capillary structures are not apparent in ordinary microscopic examination but can be demonstrated by electron microscopy. The most significant component is the trophoblast that covers the villi and infiltrates the implantation site. There is considerable variation, from thin layers of atrophic degenerated attenuated syncytiotrophoblast cells with pyknotic nuclei to piled-up hyperplastic masses of syncytiotrophoblast, cytotrophoblast, or both. Large anaplastic-looking nuclei often have the appearance of a malignant neoplasm (Fig. 36-95, *A*). In fact, the manner in which cytotrophoblast and syncytiotrophoblast remain segregated is characteristic and resembles the trophoblast pattern in the area of the cytotrophoblast shell of a 10- to 12-day implantation.

Extreme degrees of dysplastic and anaplastic nuclear change undeniably have an ominous appearance when present. As a practical matter, the presence of the villi, even hydropic villi, serves to classify the lesion in question as benign. Grading of moles on the basis of degrees of anaplastic change in the trophoblast has little prognostic significance in an individual case.[565,612,642]

The most important factor in the decision to treat the patient is the demonstration of a rise in HCG titers after the fall attending the removal of the mole. Since it is extremely important to detect this rise early, a suitably sensitive assay is absolutely necessary. The radioimmunoassay of serum or urine samples for the presence of the beta subunit of HCG is specific and sufficiently sensitive to detect minute amounts and capable of showing changes in ranges at which the ordinary immunoassay of standard pregnancy tests will not react.[671]

Invasive mole (destructive mole). In addition to the threat that attends severe bleeding and the possibility of infection, hydatidiform mole may invade the wall of the uterus (Fig. 36-96), and molar tissue may be deported to other sites. Invasion of the uterine wall is a source of hemorrhage after the mole has been passed or removed. Molar trophoblast cells, like normal trophoblast,[557] are constantly embolizing the general circulation. Molar tissue may be deported to the lungs[560] or vaginal wall and produce local nodular lesions, which are usually hemorrhagic because of the vascular destructiveness of trophoblasts. Such a lesion is regarded as benign in the sense that it is not a malignant neoplasm, but the potential for hemorrhage is a strong inducement for treatment. Before the availability of chemotherapy it was generally recognized that such lesions regressed and could usually be managed conservatively.

The most devastating complication of hydatidiform mole is the subsequent occurrence of choriocarcinoma (as discussed later) in about 2.5% of patients. The morphologic findings are not as important a factor in the decision to treat the patient as continued HCG production. Demonstration of a rising HCG titer after delivery of the mole is the basis for starting chemotherapy, regardless of the presence of a demonstrable lesion. The production of HCG is a constant and consistent property of trophoblast and is generally proportional to the amount of trophoblast present in a given patient. Rising titers mean growing trophoblast. If the location of proliferating trophoblast is uncertain or inaccessible, it is not necessary or desirable to identify it morphologically before instituting chemotherapy. A detailed plan for the follow-up care of patients after passage of a mole is obviously important; the protocols at the regional centers for treatment of trophoblastic disease are similar.[605,607] The drugs used successfully have been methotrexate and actinomycin D.

Having emphasized the overriding significance of HCG in management of clinical problems, we should give attention to some interesting morphologic correlations. Hydatidiform mole in the presence of a fetus is often associated with unusually severe toxemia and hypertension; subsequent choriocarcinoma is most unlikely.[643] Transitional (partial) moles (abortions of small size with a high proportion of vesicular villi) are followed rarely if ever by choriocarcinoma. Women who have had one mole are somewhat more likely to have another than are women who have not. The trophoblast cells of the molar implantation site occasionally persist for several months, with slowly *declining* HCG titers, and may be a source of bleeding. The histologic pattern is not that of choriocarcinoma, and demonstration of trophoblast cells at the implantation site of a mole does not mean that the patient has or ever will have a choriocarcinoma, but it is a reasonable basis for extending the period of follow-up study.

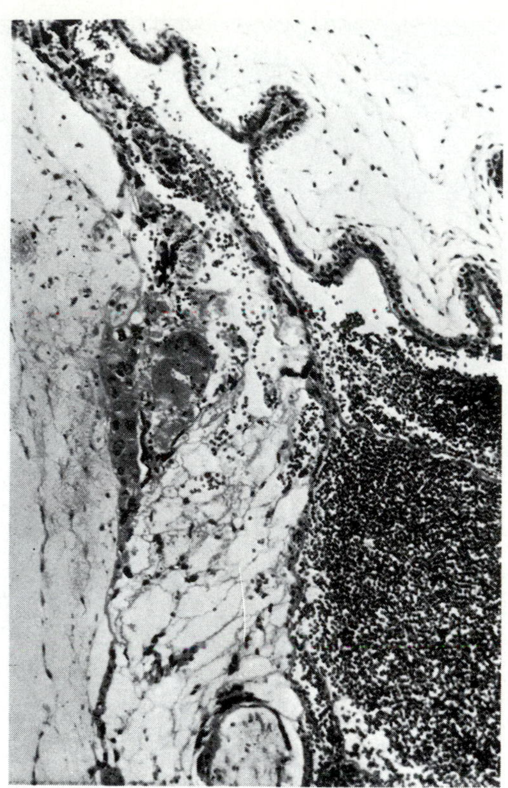

Fig. 36-94. Group II mole (probably benign). Despite benign appearance, clinically invasive mole (chorioadenoma destruens) developed 5 weeks after evacuation of mole. These portions of two villi show normal double-layered trophoblast on upper right and pleomorphism of Langhans' epithelium and vacuolization of syncytiotrophoblast on other villus. (110×; from Hertig, A.T., and Sheldon, W.H.: Am. J. Obstet. Gynecol. **53:**1, 1947.)

Trophoblastic pseudotumor

Cytotrophoblastic placental site cells rarely proliferate sufficiently to produce a uterine mass. The trophoblastic cells infiltrate the uterine wall individually; the plexiform biphasic pattern of choriocarcinoma (see next section) is absent. There is persistent HCG secretion. Some lesions treated only by curettage have regressed, prompting the

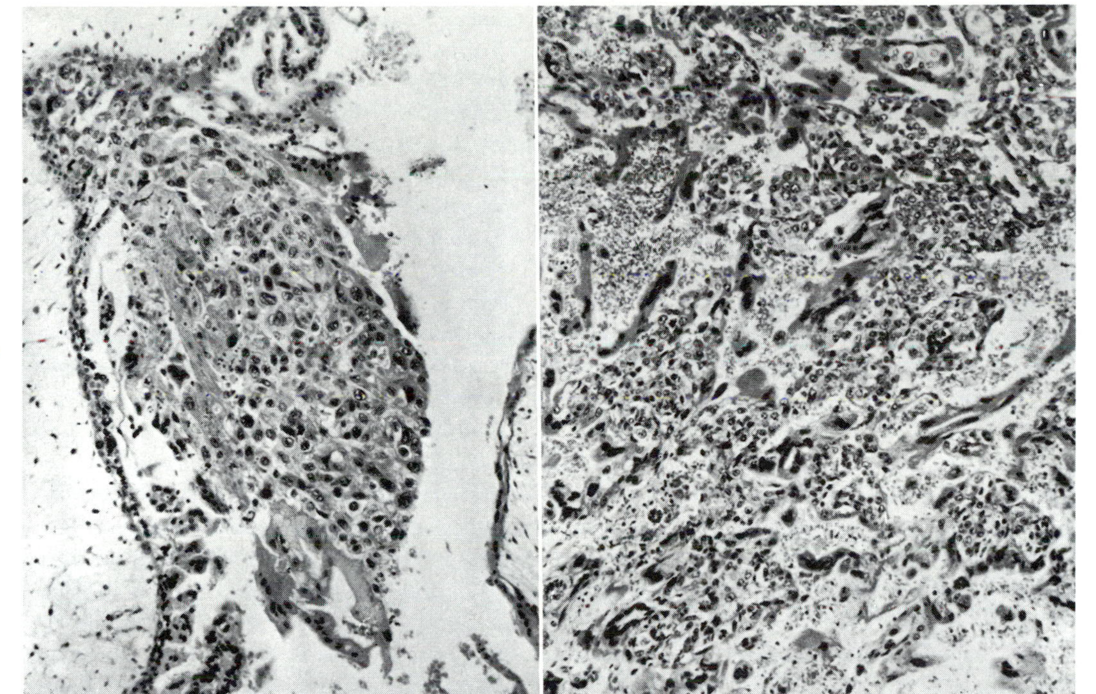

Fig. 36-95. A, Mass of molar trophoblast with pronounced anaplasia attached to villus while remainder of trophoblast is not unusually active. Although mole gave rise to choriocarcinoma, this trophoblast does not resemble that of tumor shown in **B. B,** Renal metastasis of typical choriocarcinoma in patient whose original mole is shown in **A.** Patient died 16 months after delivery of hydatidiform mole. (110×; courtesy Rhode Island Hospital, Providence; AFIP 218754-562 and 218754-563.)

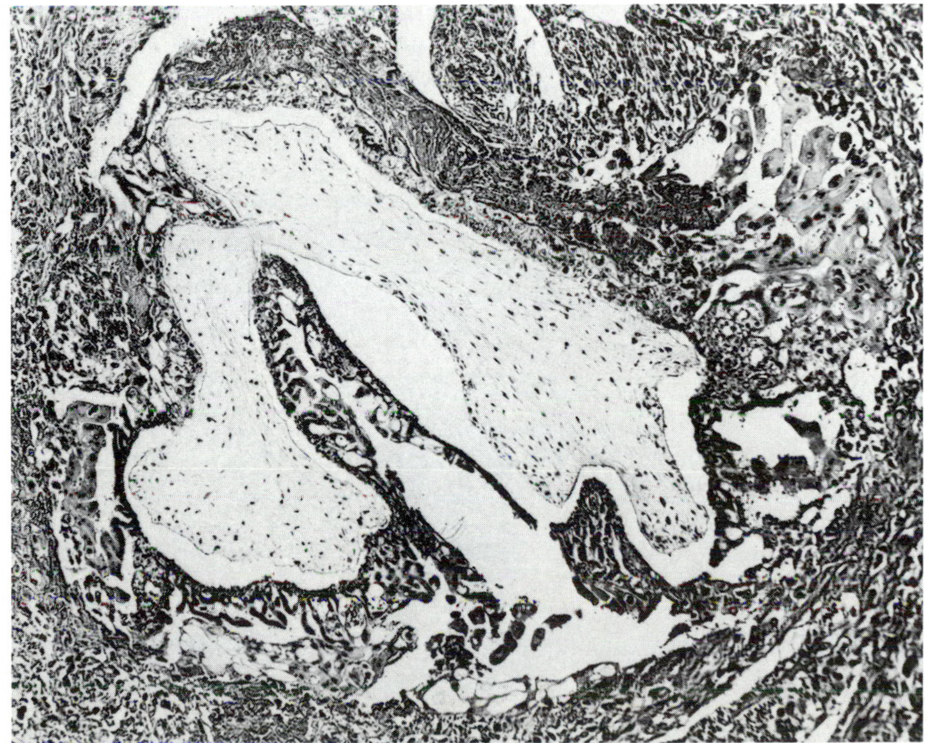

Fig. 36-96. Single hydatidiform villus invading myometrium, pathognomonic of invasive mole (48×; AFIP 298593-2.)

concept that the lesion is a hyperplasia, not a neoplasm.[628] Reports of metastasis in rare instances indicate that some lesions may be aggressive. The full range of expression and basic nature of this condition remain to be delineated.[660]

Choriocarcinoma

Gestational choriocarcinoma is a malignant neoplasm of trophoblast; it may occur after hydatidiform mole (50%), spontaneous abortion (25%), normal pregnancy (22.5%), and even rarely an ectopic pregnancy (Fig. 36-97).

Intravascular metastases occur early and disseminate widely. They are found chiefly in the lung (60%), vagina (40%), brain (12%), liver (16%), and kidney (13%), but virtually any site perfused by blood vessels is possible. The uterine lesion may be small, and often no uterine lesion can be identified.

The tumor masses are soft, necrotic, and hemorrhagic wherever they are found. The bulk of a nodular lesion is often a blood clot, and the trophoblastic tissue is occasionally difficult to find.

The histologic pattern varies only slightly. Plexiform masses of syncytiotrophoblast and cytotrophoblast are intimately intermixed, forming a distinctive biphasic pattern (Fig. 36-95, *B*). Nuclei of both cell types may be bizarre and anaplastic; mitoses occur in the cytotrophoblast cells. Unlike other malignant neoplasms of all types, choriocarcinoma has no stroma and no vascular supply of its own. In a study of treated patients, Mazur, Lurain, and Brewer[631] found an unexpected change in histologic pattern among four women whose tumors were resistant to treatment after multiple courses of chemotherapy. Instead of the typical biphasic pattern, these tumors were characterized by a significant predominance of cytotrophoblast growing in masses and infiltrating strands producing a histologic pattern that is more like that of a conventional carcinoma.

Choriocarcinoma is the best example of a malignant tumor that responds to chemotherapy. Nearly always fatal in the past, it has now become nearly always curable; many of the patients go on to have children. The drugs used most successfully have been actinomycin D and methotrexate. It is important to monitor therapy with serial HCG determinations. The drugs themselves can be dangerous, and the protocol for treatment can be

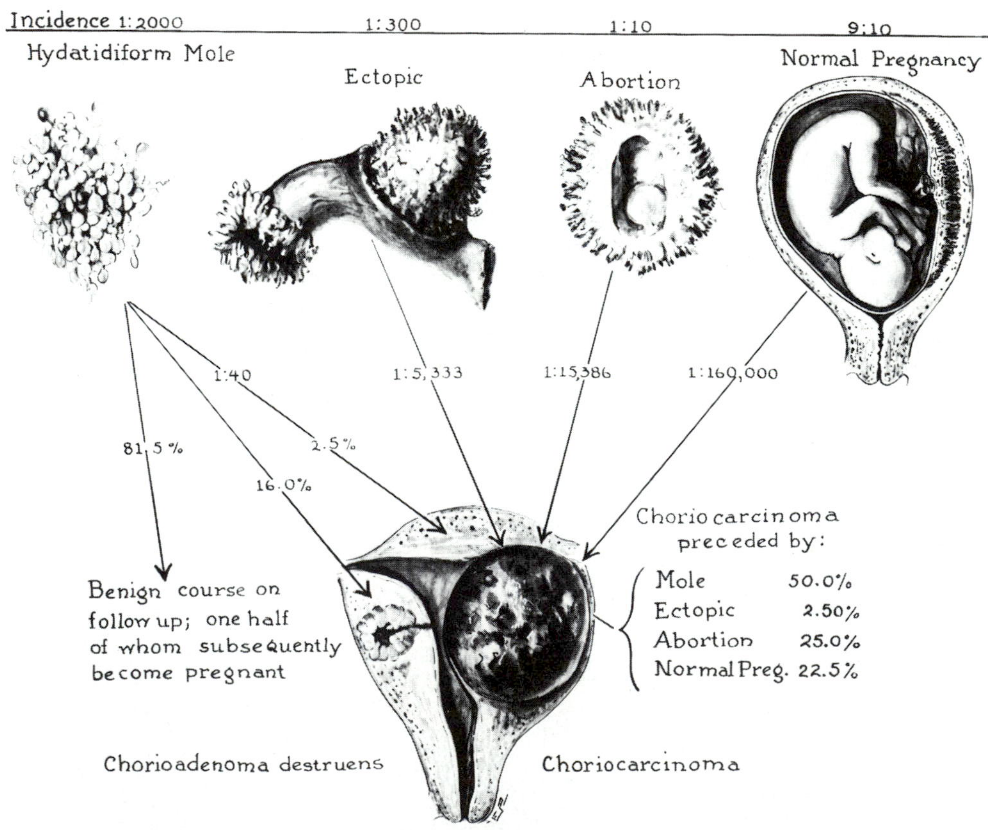

Fig. 36-97. Schematic representation of relationship between various types of pregnancy and chorioadenoma destruens and choriocarcinoma. (Adapted from Hertig, A.T.: Hydatidiform mole and chorionepithelioma. In Meigs, J.V., and Sturgis, S.H., editors: Progress in gynecology, vol. II, New York, 1963, Grune & Stratton, Inc.; by permission.)

extremely complicated. The results in the regional centers for treatment of trophoblastic disease have been excellent.[605,607] Their consultation and support are generally available on request and should be sought, since the results without highly specialized clinical and laboratory facilites can be disastrous.

The prognosis for the patient with cerebral or liver metastases is poor. Very high HCG titers are also an unfavorable finding; the inhibition of the immune response by large amounts of HCG could be the responsible factor. It would be interesting to know if its removal, for example, by plasmapheresis, would help in these grave circumstances. Gestational choriocarcinoma after an otherwise normal pregnancy has an unfavorable prognosis, probably because the diagnosis is delayed. In rare instances it has been possible to identify a small focus of choriocarcinoma in such a placenta.[575] In each case the patient was seen first with evidence of metastases while carrying a normally developing fetus. The primary tumors were inconspicuous, often requiring an extensive search.

Chorioangioma is a small and insignificant hemangioma that has been reported in 0.5% to 7% of placentas. Large lesions may be associated with hydramnios, toxemia, prematurity, and even a hydrops fetalis syndrome unrelated to Rh sensitization. Metastatic malignant tumors of maternal origin, notably breast and malignant melanoma, occur occasionally but usually do not cross the placental barrier to the fetus.[651] Rarely, malignant lesions of the fetus affect the placenta (leukemia, neuroblastoma), and instances of congenital giant nevus with placental metastasis have occurred.[583]

ACKNOWLEDGMENT: The continued use of Figs. 22, 27, 37, 43, 44, 60, 61, 64, 67, 72, 78, 80, 82, 83, and 92 to 97 in this chapter, originally prepared by Dr. Arthur T. Hertig, is gratefully acknowledged.

REFERENCES

Embryology and congenital malformations

1. Bernstein, R.: The Y chromosome and primary sexual differentiation, J.A.M.A. **245**:1953, 1981.
2. Boczkowski, K.: Abnormal sex determination and differentiation in man, Obstet. Gynecol. **41**:310, 1973.
3. Bullock, L.P., and Bardin, C.W.: *In vivo* and *in vitro* testosterone metabolism by the androgen insensitive rat, J. Steroid Biochem. **4**:139, 1973.
4. Dewhurst, C.J.: Congenital malformations of the genital tract in childhood, J. Obstet. Gynaecol. Br. Cwlth. **75**:377, 1968.
5. Farber, M., and Marchant, D.J.: Congenital absence of the uterine cervix, Am. J. Obstet. Gynecol. **121**:414, 1975.
6. Federman, D.: Abnormal sexual development, Philadelphia, 1967, W.B. Saunders Co.
7. Forsberg, J.G.: Origin of vaginal epithelium, Obstet. Gynecol. **25**:687, 1965.
8. Green, L.K., and Harris, R.E.: Uterine anomalies: frequency of diagnosis and associated obstetric complications, Obstet. Gynecol. **47**:427, 1976.
9. Griffin, J.E.: The syndromes of androgen resistance, N. Engl. J. Med. **302**:198, 1980.
10. Hamilton, W.J., Boyd, J.D., and Mossman, H.W.: Human embryology, ed. 4, Baltimore, 1972, The Williams & Wilkins Co.
11. Holmes, L.B.: Current concepts in congenital malformations, N. Engl. J. Med. **295**:204, 1976.
12. Jacobs, P.A., Melville, M., and Ratcliffe, S.: A cytogenetic survey of 11,680 newborn infants, Ann. Hum. Genet. **37**:359, 1974.
13. Jost, A.: Problems of fetal endocrinology, Recent Prog. Horm. Res. **8**:379, 1953.
14. Jost, A.: Hormonal factors in the development of the fetus, Cold Spring Harbor Symp. Quant. Biol. **19**:167, 1954.
15. Jost, A., et al.: Studies on sex differentiation in mammals, Recent Prog. Horm. Res. **29**:1, 1973.
16. Machin, G.A.: Chromosome abnormality and perinatal death, Lancet **1**:549, 1974.
17. Marquez-Monter, H., et al.: Histopathologic study with cytologic correlation in 20 cases of gonadal dysgenesis, Am. J. Clin. Pathol. **57**:449, 1972.
18. Mittwoch, U.: The genetics of sexual differentiation, New York, 1973, Academic Press, Inc.
19. Naftolin, F., and Judd, H.L.: Testicular feminization, Obstet. Gynecol. Annu. **2**:25, 1973.
20. Park, I.J., Aimakhu, V.E., and Jones, H.W., Jr.: An etiologic and pathogenic classification of male hermaphroditism, Am. J. Obstet. Gynecol. **123**:505, 1975.
21. Pinkerton, J.H.M., et al.: Development of the human ovary—a study using histochemical techniques, Obstet. Gynecol. **18**:152, 1961.
22. Prinz, J.L., et al.: The embryology of supernumerary ovaries, Obstet. Gynecol. **41**:246, 1973.
23. Sarto, G.E.: Cytogenetics of 50 patients with primary amenorrhea, Am. J. Obstet. Gynecol. **119**:14, 1974.
24. Sarto, G.E., and Opitz, J.M.: The XY gonadal agenesis syndrome, J. Med. Genet. **10**:288, 1973.
25. Schellhas, H.F.: Malignant potential of the dysgenetic gonad, Obstet. Gynecol. **44**:298, 1974.
26. Scully, R.E.: Gonadoblastoma: a review of 74 cases, Cancer **25**:1340, 1970.
27. Singh, R.P., and Carr, D.H.: Anatomic findings in human abortions of known chromosomal constitution, Obstet. Gynecol. **29**:806, 1967.
28. Spaulding, M.H.: The development of the external genitalia in the human embryo, Contrib. Embryol. **13**:67, 1921.
29. Stephens, F.D.: The female anus, perineum, and vestibule: embryogenesis and deformities, Aust. N.Z. J. Obstet. Gynaecol. **8**:55, 1968.
30. Tegenkamp, T.R., et al.: Pregnancy without benefit of surgery in a bisexually active true hermaphrodite, Am. J. Obstet. Gynecol. **135**:427, 1979.
31. Ulbright, T.M., and Kraus, F.T.: Endometrial stromal tumors of the extra-uterine tissue, Am. J. Clin. Pathol. **76**:371, 1981.
32. Van Niekerk, W.A.: True hermaphroditism: an analytic review with a report of three cases, Am. J. Obstet. Gynecol. **126**:890, 1976.
33. Van Wagenen, G., and Simpson, M.E.: Embryology of the ovary and testis: *Homo sapiens* and *Macaca mulatta*, New Haven, Conn., 1965, Yale University Press.
34. Wharton, L.R.: Two cases of supernumerary ovary and one of accessory ovary, with an analysis of previously reported cases, Am. J. Obstet. Gynecol. **78**:1101, 1959.
35. Wilson, J.D., et al.: Familial incomplete male pseudohermaphroditism, type I: evidence for androgen resistance and variable clinical manifestations in a family with the Reifenstein syndrome, N. Engl. J. Med. **290**:1097, 1974.
36. Woodruff, J.D., and Pauerstein, C.J.: The fallopian tubes, structure, function, pathology, and management, Baltimore, 1969, The Williams & Wilkins Co.
37. Woolf, R.M., and Allen, W.M.: Concomitant malformations: the frequent, simultaneous occurrence of congenital malformations of the reproductive and urinary tracts, Obstet. Gynecol. **2**:236, 1953.

Vulva

38. Abell, M.R.: Adenocystic (pseudoadenomatous) basal cell carcinoma of the vestibular glands of the vulva, Am. J. Obstet. Gynecol. **86**:470, 1963.

39. Abell, M.R., and Gosling, J.R.G.: Intraepithelial and infiltrative carcinoma of vulva: Bowen's type, Cancer **14**:318, 1961.
40. Amstey, M.S., et al.: Cesarean section and genital herpes infection, Obstet. Gynecol. **53**:641, 1979.
41. Barnes, A.E., et al.: Microinvasive carcinoma of the vulva: a clinicopathologic evaluation, Obstet. Gynecol. **56**:234, 1980.
42. Burger, R.A., and Marcuse, P.M.: Fibroadenoma of the vulva, Am. J. Clin. Pathol. **24**:965, 1954.
43. Buscema, J., et al.: Carcinoma in situ of the vulva, Obstet. Gynecol. **55**:225, 1980.
44. Chamlian, D.L., and Taylor, H.B.: Primary carcinoma of Bartholin's gland: a report of 24 patients, Obstet. Gynecol. **39**:489, 1972.
45. Christ, M.L., and Ozzello, L.: Myogenous origin of granular cell tumor of the urinary bladder, Am. J. Clin. Pathol. **56**:736, 1971.
46. Crum, C.P., et al.: Intraepithelial neoplasia of the vulva and vagina: an analysis for herpes simplex-2 by *in-situ* hybridization techniques (abstract), Lab. Invest. **44**:13A, 1981.
47. Crum, C.P., et al.: Vulvar intraepithelial neoplasia; correlations of nuclear DNA content and the presence of a human papillomavirus structural antigen (abstract), Lab. Invest. **44**:13A, 1981.
48. Cruz-Jimenez, P.R., and Abell, M.R.: Cutaneous basal cell carcinoma of the vulva, Cancer **36**:1860, 1975.
49. Davos, I., and Abell, M.R.: Soft tissue sarcomas of vulva, Gynecol. Oncol. **4**:70, 1976.
50. Dean, R.E., et al.: The treatment of premalignant and malignant lesions of the vulva, Am. J. Obstet. Gynecol. **119**:59, 1974.
51. Dehner, L.C.: Metastatic and secondary tumors of the vulva, Obstet. Gynecol. **42**:47, 1973.
52. Devroede, G., et al.: Crohn's disease of the vulva, Am. J. Clin. Pathol. **63**:348, 1975.
53. Dgani, R., et al.: Granular cell myoblastoma of the vulva: report of four cases, Acta Obstet. Gynecol. Scand. **57**:385, 1978.
54. Edsmyr, F.: Carcinoma of the vulva: an analysis of 560 patients with histologically verified squamous cell carcinoma, Acta Radiol. **217**(suppl.):1, 1963.
55. Franklin, E.W., and Rutledge, F.D.: Epidemiology of epidermoid carcinoma of the vulva, Obstet. Gynecol. **39**:165, 1972.
56. Friedrich, E.G.: Reversible vulvar atypia, Obstet. Gynecol. **39**:173, 1972.
57. Friedrich, E.G.: Vulvar disease, Philadelphia, 1976, W.B. Saunders Co.
58. Friedrich, E.G., Cole, W., and Middlekamp, J.N.: Herpes simplex, Am. J. Obstet. Gynecol. **104**:758, 1969.
59. Friedrich, E.G., and Wilkinson, E.J.: Mucous cysts of the vulvar vestibule, Obstet. Gynecol. **42**:407, 1973.
60. Gardner, H.L., and Kaufman, R.H.: Benign diseases of the vulva and vagina, St. Louis, 1969, The C.V. Mosby Co.
61. Gosling, J.R.G., et al.: Infiltrative squamous cell (epidermoid) carcinoma of the vulva, Cancer **14**:330, 1961.
62. Green, T.H.: Carcinoma of the vulva: a reassessment, Obstet. Gynecol. **52**:462, 1978.
63. Green, T.H., Ulfelder, H., and Meigs, J.V.: Epidermoid carcinoma of vulva: analysis of 238 cases. I. Etiology and diagnosis, Am. J. Obstet. Gynecol. **75**:834, 1958.
64. Green, T.H., Ulfelder, H., and Meigs, J.V.: Epidermoid carcinoma of the vulva: analysis of 238 cases. II. Therapy and end results, Am. J. Obstet. Gynecol. **75**:848, 1958.
65. Guerry, R.L., and Pratt-Thomas, H.R.: Carcinoma of supernumerary breast of vulva with bilateral mammary cancer, Cancer **38**:2570, 1976.
66. Hart, W.R.: Paramesonephric mucinous cysts of the vulva, Am. J. Obstet. Gynecol. **107**:1079, 1970.
67. Hart, W.R., Norris, H.J., and Helwig, E.B.: Relationship of lichen sclerosus et atrophicus of the vulva to development of carcinoma, Obstet. Gynecol. **45**:369, 1975.
68. Hassim, A.M.: Bilateral fibroadenoma in supernumerary breasts of the vulva, J. Obstet. Gynaecol. Br. Cwlth. **76**:275, 1969.
69. Helwig, E.B., and Graham, J.H.: Anogenital (extramammary) Paget's disease: a clinicopathological study, Cancer **16**:387, 1963.
70. Hertig, A.T., and Gore, H.: Tumors of the female sex organs. II. Tumors of the vulva, vagina, and uterus. In Atlas of tumor pathology, Section IX, Fascicle 33, Washington, D.C., 1970, Armed Forces Institute of Pathology.
71. Isaacs, J.H.: Verrucous carcinoma of the female genital tract, Gynecol. Oncol. **4**:259, 1976.
72. Iverson, T., Abeler, V., and Kolstad, P.: Squamous cell carcinoma in situ of the vulva: a clinical and histopathological study, Gynecol. Oncol. **11**:224, 1982.
73. Janovski, N.A., and Ames, S.: Lichen sclerosus et atrophicus of the vulva: a poorly understood disease entity, Obstet. Gynecol. **22**:2697, 1963.
74. Japaze, H., Garcia-Bunuel, R., and Woodruff, J.D.: Primary vulvar neoplasia: a review of *in situ* and invasive carcinoma 1935-1972, Obstet. Gynecol. **49**:404, 1977.
75. Jeffcoate, T.N.A.: Chronic vulval dystrophies, Am. J. Obstet. Gynecol. **95**:61, 1966.
76. Jimerson, G.K., and Merrill, J.A.: Multicentric squamous malignancy involving both cervix and vulva, Cancer **26**:150, 1970.
77. Josey, W.E., Nahmias, A.J., and Naib, Z.M.: Viruses and cancer of the lower genital tract, Cancer **38**:526, 1976.
78. Kaplan, A.L., et al.: Intraepithelial carcinoma of the vulva with extension to the anal canal, Obstet. Gynecol. **58**:368, 1981.
79. Kaufman, R.H., et al.: Herpes genitalis treated by photodynamic inactivation of the virus, Am. J. Obstet. Gynecol. **117**:1144, 1973.
80. Kaufman, R.H., et al.: Vulvar dystrophies: an evaluation, Am. J. Obstet. Gynecol. **120**:363, 1974.
81. Kaufman, R.H., et al.: Herpes-induced antigens in squamous cell carcinoma in situ of the vulva, N. Engl. J. Med. **305**:483, 1981.
82. Kelly, J.: Malignant disease of the vulva, J. Obstet. Gynaecol. Br. Cwlth. **79**:265, 1972.
83. Kolstad, P., and Stafl, A.: Atlas of colposcopy, Baltimore, 1972, University Park Press.
84. Kraus, F.T., and Perez-Mesa, C.: Verrucous carcinoma: a clinical and pathologic study of 105 cases involving oral cavity, larynx, and genitalia, Cancer **19**:26, 1966.
85. Kurman, R.J., et al.: Immunoperoxidase localization of papillomavirus antigens in cervical dysplasia and vulvar condylomas, Am. J. Obstet. Gynecol. **140**:931, 1981.
86. Lee, S.C., et al.: Extramammary Paget's disease of the vulva: a clinicopathologic study of 13 cases, Cancer **39**:2540, 1977.
87. Lovelady, S.B., McDonald, J.R., and Waugh, J.M.: Benign tumors of the vulva, Am. J. Obstet. Gynecol. **42**:309, 1941.
88. Lukas, W.F., Benirschke, K., and Lebherz, T.B.: Verrucous carcinoma of the female genital tract, Am. J. Obstet. Gynecol. **119**:435, 1974.
89. Majmudar, B., Chaikeu, M.L., and Lee, K.U.: Amebiasis of clitoris mimicking carcinoma, J.A.M.A. **236**:1145, 1976.
90. Medenica, M., and Sahihi, T.: Ultrastructural study of a case of extramammary Paget's disease of the vulva, Arch. Dermatol. **105**:236, 1972.
91. Meeker, J.H., Neubecker, R.D., and Helwig, E.B.: Hidradenoma papilliferum, Am. J. Clin. Pathol. **37**:182, 1962.
92. Meyers, M.G., et al.: Failure of neutral red photodynamic inactivation in recurrent herpes simplex infections, N. Engl. J. Med. **293**:945, 1975.
93. Morrow, C.P., and DiSaia, P.S.: Malignant melanoma of the female genitalia: a clinical analysis, Obstet. Gynecol. Surv. **31**:233, 1976.
94. Morrow, C.P., and Rutledge, F.N.: Melanoma of the vulva, Obstet. Gynecol. **39**:745, 1972.
95. Nakao, C.Y., et al.: "Microinvasive" epidermoid carcinoma of the vulva with an unexpected natural history, Am. J. Obstet. Gynecol. **120**:1122, 1974.
96. Neilson, D., and Woodruff, J.D.: Electron microscopy of in situ and invasive vulvar Paget's disease, Am. J. Obstet. Gynecol. **113**:719, 1972.
97. Ng, A.B.P., Reagan, J.W., and Lindner, E.: The cellular manifestations of primary and recurrent herpes genitalis, Acta Cytol. **14**:124, 1970.
98. Palladino, V.S., Duffy, J.L., and Bures, G.J.: Basal cell carcinoma of the vulva, Cancer **24**:460, 1969.

99. Powell, L.C., Jr.: Condyloma acuminatum, Clin. Obstet. Gynecol. **15**:948, 1972.
100. Ragni, M.V., and Tobaon, H.: Primary malignant melanoma of the vagina and vulva, Obstet. Gynecol. **43**:658, 1974.
101. Robboy, S.J., et al.: Urogenital sinus origin of mucinous and ciliated cysts of the vulva, Obstet. Gynecol. **51**:3447, 1978.
102. Roth, L.M., Lee, S.C., and Erlich, C.E.: Paget's disease of the vulva: a histogenetic study of five cases including ultrastructural observations and a review of the literature, Am. J. Surg. Pathol. **1**:193, 1977.
103. Rutledge, F., Smith, J.P., and Franklin, E.W.: Carcinoma of the vulva, Am. J. Obstet. Gynecol. **106**:1117, 1970.
104. Skinner, M.S., et al.: Spontaneous regression of Bowenoid atypia of the vulva, Obstet. Gynecol. **42**:40, 1973.
105. Sobel, H.J., Schwarz, R., and Marquet, E.: Light and electron microscope study of the origin of granular cell myoblastoma, J. Pathol. **109**:101, 1973.
106. Tavassoli, F.A., and Norris, H.J.: Smooth muscle tumors of the vulva, Obstet. Gynecol. **53**:213, 1979.
107. Tsukada, Y., et al.: Paget's disease of the vulva: clinicopathologic study of eight cases. Obstet. Gynecol. **45**:78, 1975.
108. Tuthill, R.J., and Wheeler, J.E.: Simple condylomata acuminata of vulva with focal squamous carcinoma (abstract), Lab. Invest. **44**:69A, 1981.
109. Ulbright, T.M., et al.: Bowenoid dysplasia of the vulva, Cancer **50**:2910, 1982.
110. Way, S., and Benedet, J.L.: Involvement of inguinal lymph nodes in carcinoma of the vulva: a comparison of clinical assessment with histological examination, Gynecol. Oncol. **1**:119, 1973.
111. Wharton, J.T., Gallager, S., and Rutledge, F.N.: Microinvasive carcinoma of the vulva, Am. J. Obstet. Gynecol. **118**:159, 1974.
112. Wilson, D., and Woodger, B.A.: Pleomorphic adenoma of the vulva, J. Obstet. Gynaecol. Br. Cwlth. **81**:1000, 1974.
113. Woodworth, H.J., et al.: Papillary hidradenoma of the vulva: clinicopathologic study of 69 cases, Am. J. Obstet. Gynecol. **110**:501, 1971.
114. Yackel, D.B., Symmonds, R.E., and Kempers, R.D.: Melanoma of the vulva, Obstet. Gynecol. **35**:625, 1970.
115. Young, A.W., Tovell, H.M.M., and Sadri, K.: Erosions and ulcers of the vulva: diagnosis, incidence, and management, Obstet. Gynecol. **50**:35, 1977.

Vagina

116. Allyn, D.L., Silverberg, S.G., and Salzberg, A.M.: Endodermal sinus tumor of the vagina: report of a case with 7-year survival and literature review of so-called "mesonephromas," Cancer **17**:1231, 1971.
117. Annual reports on the results of treatment in carcinoma of the uterus, vagina, and ovary, vol. 17, Editorial Office, Stockholm, 1979, Radiumhemmet.
118. Bennet, H.G., and Ehrlich, M.M.: Myoma of the vagina, Am. J. Obstet. Gynecol. **42**:314, 1941.
119. Berry, A.: A cytopathological and histopathological study of bilharziasis of the female genital tract, J. Pathol. Bacteriol. **91**:325, 1966.
120. Chirayil, S.J., and Tobon, H.: Polyps of the vagina: a clinicopathologic study of 18 cases, Cancer **47**:290, 1981.
121. Davis, B.A.: Vaginal moniliasis in private practice, Obstet. Gynecol. **34**:40, 1969.
122. Davos, I., and Abell, M.R.: Sarcomas of the vagina, Obstet. Gynecol. **47**:342, 1976.
123. Deppisch, L.M.: Cysts of the vagina: classification and clinical correlations, Obstet. Gynecol. **45**:632, 1975.
124. Elliot, G.B., and Elliot, J.D.A.: Superficial stromal reactions of lower genital tract, Arch. Pathol. **95**:100, 1973.
125. Fentanes de Torres, E., and Benitez-Bribiesca, L.: Cytologic detection of vaginal parasitosis, Acta Cytol. **17**:252, 1973.
126. Forsberg, J.G.: Late effects in the vaginal and cervical epithelia after injections of diethylstilbestrol into neonatal mice, Am. J. Obstet. Gynecol. **121**:101, 1975.
127. Friedrich, E.G., and Wilkinson, E.J.: Mucous cysts of the vulvar vestibule, Obstet. Gynecol. **42**:407, 1973.
128. Frost, J.K.: Concepts basic to general cytopathology, Baltimore, 1972, Johns Hopkins Press.
129. Gardner, H.L., and Fernet, P.: Etiology of vaginitis emphysematosa, Am. J. Obstet. Gynecol. **88**:680, 1964.
130. Gardner, H.L., and Kaufman, R.H.: Benign diseases of the vulva and vagina, St. Louis, 1969, The C.V. Mosby Co.
131. Gray, L.A., and Christopherson, W.W.: In-situ and early invasive carcinoma of the vagina, Obstet. Gynecol. **34**:226, 1969.
132. Hart, W.R.: Paramesonephric mucinous cysts of the vulva, Am. J. Obstet. Gynecol. **107**:1079, 1970.
133. Herbst, A.L., editor: Intrauterine exposure to diethylstilbestrol in the human, Proceedings of Symposium on DES, 1977, Chicago, 1978, American College of Obstetricians and Gynecologists.
134. Herbst, A.L., Green, T.H., Jr., and Ulfelder, H.: Primary carcinoma of the vagina: an analysis of 68 cases, Am. J. Obstet. Gynecol. **106**:210, 1970.
135. Herbst, A.L., et al.: Clear cell adenocarcinoma of the vagina and cervix in girls: analysis of 170 registry cases, Am. J. Obstet. Gynecol. **119**:713, 1974.
136. Herbst, A.L., et al.: Epidemiologic aspects and factors related to survival in 384 registry cases of clear-cell adenocarcinoma of the vagina and cervix, Am. J. Obstet. Gynecol. **135**:876, 1979.
137. Hilgers, R.D., Malkasian, G.D., Jr., and Soule, E.H.: Embryonal rhabdomyosarcoma (botryoid type) of the vagina: a clinicopathologic review, Am. J. Obstet. Gynecol. **107**:484, 1970.
138. Hummer, W.K., et al.: Carcinoma in-situ of the vagina, Am. J. Obstet. Gynecol. **108**:1109, 1970.
139. Koss, L.G.: Diagnostic cytology and its histopathologic bases, ed. 2, Philadelphia, 1968, J.B. Lippincott Co.
140. Kurman, R.J., and Prabha, A.C.: Thyroid and parathyroid glands in the vaginal wall: report of a case, Am. J. Clin. Pathol. **59**:503, 1973.
141. Malkasian, G.D., Welch, J.S., and Soule, E.H.: Primary leiomyosarcoma of the vagina: report of eight cases, Am. J. Obstet. Gynecol. **86**:730, 1963.
142. McIndoe, W.A., and Green, G.H.: Vaginal carcinoma in situ following hysterectomy, Acta Cytol. **13**:158, 1969.
143. Ng, A.B.P., Reagan, J.W., and Lindner, E.: The cellular manifestations of primary and recurrent herpes genitalis, Acta Cytol. **14**:124, 1970.
144. Norris, H.J., Bagley, G.P., and Taylor, H.B.: Carcinoma of the infant vagina: a distinctive tumor, Arch. Pathol. **90**:473, 1970.
145. Norris, H.J., and Taylor, H.B.: Polyps of the vagina; a benign lesion resembling sarcoma botryoides, Cancer **19**:227, 1966.
146. Perez, C.A., et al.: Prognostic significance of endometrial extension from primary carcinoma of the uterine cervix, Cancer **35**:1493, 1975.
147. Prempree, T., et al.: Radiation management in primary carcinoma of the vagina, Cancer **40**:109, 1977.
148. Pride, G.L., et al.: Primary invasive squamous carcinoma of the vagina, Obstet. Gynecol. **53**:218, 1979.
149. Robboy, S.J., Herbst, A.L., and Scully, R.E.: Clear cell adenocarcinoma of the vagina and cervix in young females: analysis of 37 tumors that persisted or recurred after primary therapy, Cancer **34**:606, 1974.
150. Robboy, S.J., et al.: Intrauterine diethylstilbestrol exposure and its consequences, Arch. Pathol. Lab. Med. **101**:1, 1977.
151. Sandberg, E.C., et al.: Adenosis vaginae, Am. J. Obstet. Gynecol. **93**:209, 1965.
152. Scully, R.E., Robboy, S.J., and Herbst, A.L.: Vaginal and cervical abnormalities, including clear cell adenocarcinoma, related to prenatal exposure to diethylstilbestrol, Am. Clin. Lab. Sci. **4**:222, 1974.
153. Silverberg, S.G., and Frable, W.J.: Prolapse of fallopian tube into vaginal vault after hysterectomy, Arch. Pathol. **97**:100, 1974.
154. Sirota, R.L., Dickersin, G.R., and Scully, R.E.: Mixed tumors of the vagina: a clinicopathological analysis of eight cases, Am. J. Surg. Pathol. **5**:413, 1981.
155. Stabler, F.: The treatment of adenosis (adenomatosis) vaginae, J. Obstet. Gynaecol. Br. Cwlth. **74**:493, 1967.
156. Tavassoli, F.A., and Norris, H.J.: Smooth muscle tumors of the vagina, Obstet. Gynecol. **53**:689, 1979.

157. Ulbright, T.M., Alexander, R.W., and Kraus, F.T.: Intramural papilloma of the vagina: evidence of Müllerian histogenesis, Cancer **48**:2260, 1981.
158. Ulbright, T.M., and Kraus, F.T.: Endometrial stromal tumors of extrauterine tissue, Am. J. Clin. Pathol. **76**:371, 1981.
159. Underwood, P.B., Jr., and Smith, R.: Carcinoma of the vagina, J.A.M.A. **217**:46, 1971.
160. Vooijs, P.G., Ng, A.B.P., and Wentz, W.B.: The detection of vaginal adenosis and clear cell carcinoma, Acta Cytol. **17**:59, 1973.

Cervix

161. Abell, M.R.: Invasive carcinomas of the cervix. In Norris, H.J., Hertig, A.T., and Abell, M.R., editors: The uterus, Baltimore, 1973, The Williams & Wilkins Co.
162. Abell, M.R., and Gosling, J.R.G.: Gland cell carcinoma (adenocarcinoma) of the uterine cervix, Am. J. Obstet. Gynecol. **83**:729, 1962.
163. Abell, M.R., and Ramirez, J.A.: Sarcomas and carcinosarcomas of the uterine cervix, Cancer **31**:1176, 1973.
164. Albores-Saavedra, J., et al.: Carcinoid of the uterine cervix, Cancer **38**:2328, 1976.
165. Alexander, E.R.: Possible etiologies of cancer of the cervix other than herpesvirus, Cancer Res. **33**:1485, 1973.
166. Ashley, D.J.B.: The biologic status of carcinoma in situ of the uterine cervix, J. Obstet. Gynaecol. Br. Cwlth. **73**:372, 1966.
167. Aurelian, L.: Virions and antigens of herpes virus type 2 in cervical carcinoma, Cancer Res. **33**:1539, 1973.
168. Aurelian, L., et al.: Antibody to HSV-2 induced tumor specific antigens in serums from patients with cervical carcinoma, Science **181**:161, 1973.
169. Aurelian, L., et al.: Viruses and gynecologic cancers: herpesvirus protein (ICP 10/AG-4), a cervical tumor antigen that fulfills the criteria for a marker of carcinogenicity, Cancer **48**:455, 1981.
170. Ayers, L.R., Drosman, S., and Saltzstein, S.L.: Iatrogenic paracervical implantation of fetal tissue during therapeutic abortion: a case report, Obstet. Gynecol. **37**:755, 1971.
171. Badib, A.O., et al.: Metastasis to organs in carcinoma of the uterine cervix, Cancer **21**:434, 1968.
172. Beral, V.: Cancer of the cervix: a sexually transmitted infection? Lancet **1**:1037, 1974.
173. Berry, A.: A cytopathological and histopathological study of bilharziasis of the female genital tract, J. Pathol. Bacteriol. **91**:325, 1966.
174. Boyes, D.A.: The value of a pap smear program and suggestions for its implementation, Cancer **48**:613, 1981.
175. Boyes, D.A., Worth, A.J., and Fidler, H.K.: The results of treatment of 4389 cases of pre-clinical cervical squamous carcinoma, J. Obstet. Gynaecol. Br. Cwlth. **77**:769, 1970.
176. Brudnell, J.M., Cox, B., and Taylor, C.: The Royal College of Obstetricians and Gynaecologists' carcinoma in situ survey, J. Obstet. Gynaecol. Br. Cwlth. **80**:673, 1973.
177. Burghardt, E.: Early histological diagnosis of cervical cancer, Philadelphia, 1973, W.B. Saunders Co.
178. Ceremsak, R.J.: Benign rhabdomyoma of the vagina, Am. J. Clin. Pathol. **52**:604, 1969.
179. Chanen, W., and Hollyock, V.E.: Colposcopy and the conservative management of cervical dysplasia and carcinoma in situ, Obstet. Gynecol. **43**:527, 1974.
180. Chen, S.S., Koffler, D., and Cohen, C.J.: Cellular hypersensitivity in patients with squamous cell carcinoma of the cervix, Am. J. Obstet. Gynecol. **121**:91, 1975.
181. Christopherson, W.M., Nealon, N., and Gray, L.A., Sr.: Noninvasive precursor lesions of adenocarcinoma and mixed adenosquamous carcinoma of the cervix uteri, Cancer **44**:975, 1979.
182. Christopherson, W.M., and Parker, J.E.: Control of cervix cancer in women of low income in a community, Cancer **24**:64, 1969.
183. Christopherson, W.M., and Scott, M.A.: Trends in mortality from uterine cancer in relation to mass screening, Acta Cytol. **21**:5, 1977.
184. Cohen, C.: Three cases of amoebiasis of the cervix uteri, J. Obstet. Gynaecol. Br. Cwlth. **80**:476, 1973.
185. Coppleson, M., Pixley, E., and Reid, B.: Colposcopy: a scientific and practical approach to the cervix in health and disease, Springfield, Ill., 1971, Charles C Thomas, Publisher.
186. Davidsohn, I., et al.: Metastatic squamous cell carcinoma of the cervix: the role of immunology in its pathogenesis, Arch. Pathol. **95**:132, 1973.
187. Daw, E.: Extragenital adenocarcinoma metastatic to the cervix uteri, Am. J. Obstet. Gynecol. **114**:1104, 1972.
188. Derman, H., et al.: Cervical cytopathology. I. Peers compare performance, Pathologist **35**:317, 1981.
189. DiSaia, P.J., et al.: Cell mediated immunity to human malignant cells: a brief review and further studies with two gynecologic lesions, Am. J. Obstet. Gynecol. **114**:979, 1972.
190. Ehrmann, R.L.: Sebaceous metaplasia of the human cervix, Am. J. Obstet. Gynecol. **105**:1284, 1969.
190a. Ferenczy, A.: Carcinoma and other malignant tumors of the cervix. In Blaustein, A., editor: Pathology of the female genital tract, ed. 2, New York, 1982, Springer-Verlag.
191. Fluhmann, C.F.: The cervix and its diseases, Philadelphia, 1961, W.B. Saunders Co.
192. Friederich, E.R.: The normal morphology and ultrastructure of the cervix. In Blandau, R.J., editor: The biology of the cervix, Chicago, 1973, University of Chicago Press.
193. Gallagher, H.S., Simpson, C.B., and Ayala, A.G.: Adenoid cystic carcinoma of the uterine cervix: report of four cases, Cancer **27**:1398, 1971.
194. Goodheart, C.R.: Nucleic acid by hydridization and the relationship between cervical cancer and herpes simplex virus type 2, Cancer Res. **33**:1548, 1973.
195. Govan, A.D.T., et al.: The histology and cytology of changes in the epithelium of the cervix uteri, J. Clin. Pathol. **22**:383, 1969.
196. Graham, C.E.: Uterine cervical epithelium of fetal and immature females in relation to estrogenic stimulation, Am. J. Obstet. Gynecol. **97**:1033, 1967.
197. Green, G.H., and Donovan, J.W.: Natural history of carcinoma in situ of the cervix, J. Obstet. Gynaecol. Br. Cwlth. **77**:1, 1970.
198. Gunderson, L.L., et al.: Correlation of histopathology with clinical results following radiation therapy for carcinoma of the cervix, Am. J. Roentgenol. **120**:74, 1974.
199. Hall, D.J., et al.: Primary malignant melanoma of the uterine cervix, Obstet. Gynecol. **56**:525, 1980.
200. Hertig, A.T., and Gore, H.: Tumors of the female sex organ. II. Tumors of the vulva, vagina and uterus. In Atlas of tumor pathology, Section IX, Fascicle 33, Washington, D.C., 1960, Armed Forces Institute of Pathology.
201. Hollinshead, A.C., and Tarro, G.: Soluble membrane antigens of lip and cervical carcinomas: reactivity with antibody for herpesvirus nonvirion antigens, Science **179**:698, 1973.
202. Janovski, N.A., and Kasdon, E.J.: Benign mesonephric papillary and polypoid tumors of the cervix in childhood, J. Pediatr. **63**:211, 1963.
203. Jones, H.W., III, et al.: Small cell non-keratinizing carcinoma of the cervix associated with ACTH production, Cancer **38**:1629, 1976.
204. Kaufman, R.H., et al.: Clinical features of herpes genitalis, Cancer Res. **33**:1446, 1973.
205. Kessler, I.I.: Etiologic concepts in cervical carcinogenesis, Gynecol. Oncol. **12**(suppl.):7, 1981.
206. Kirkland, J.A., Stanley, M.A., and Cellier, K.M.: Comparative study of histologic and chromosomal abnormalities in cervical neoplasia, Cancer **20**:1934, 1967.
207. Knapp, R.C., and Feldman, G.B.: The problem of optimal management of cervical carcinoma in-situ, Clin. Obstet. Gynecol. **13**:889, 1970.
208. Kolstad, P., and Klem, V.: Long-term followup of 1121 cases of carcinoma in situ, Obstet. Gynecol. **48**:125, 1976.
209. Kolstad, P., and Stafl, A.: Atlas of colposcopy, Baltimore, 1972, University Park Press.
210. Kraus, F.T.: The biology of carcinoma in situ and microinvasive carcinoma of the cervix. In Norris, H.J., Hertig, A.T., and Abell, M.R., editors: The uterus, Baltimore, 1973, The Williams & Wilkins Co.

211. Kraus, F.T.: Irradiation changes in the uterus. In Norris, H.J., Hertig, A.T., and Abell, M.R., editors: The uterus, Baltimore, 1973, The Williams & Wilkins Co.
212. Krieger, J.S., and McCormack, L.J.: Graded treatment for *in situ* carcinoma of the uterine cervix, Am. J. Obstet. Gynecol. **101**:171, 1968.
212a. Kurman, R.J., Jenson, A.B., and Lancaster, W.D.: Papillomavirus infection of the cervix, Am. J. Surg. Pathol. **7**:39, 1983.
213. Kyriakos, M., Kempson, R.L., and Konikov, N.F.: A clinical and pathologic study of endocervical lesions associated with oral contraceptives, Cancer **22**:99, 1968.
214. Levi, M.: Autogenicity of ovarian and cervical malignancies with a view toward possible immunodiagnosis, Am. J. Obstet. Gynecol. **109**:686, 1971.
215. Love, R.R., and Camilli, A.E.: The value of screening, Cancer **48**:489, 1981.
216. Ludwig, M.E., Lowell, D.M., and Livolsi, V.A.: Cervical condylomatous atypia and its relationship to cervical neoplasia, Am. J. Clin. Pathol. **76**:255, 1981.
217. McDougall, J.K., Galloway, D.A., and Fenoglio, C.M.: Cervical carcinoma: detection of herpes simplex virus RNA in cells undergoing neoplastic change, Int. J. Cancer **25**:1, 1980.
218. Meisels, A., Fortin, R., and Roy, M.: Condylomatous lesions of the cervix. II. Cytologic, colposcopic, and histopathologic study, Acta Cytol. **21**:379, 1977.
219. Miles, P.A., and Norris, H.J.: Adenoid cystic carcinoma of the cervix: an analysis of 12 cases, Obstet. Gynecol. **38**:103, 1971.
220. Mussey, E., Soule, E.H., and Welch, J.S.: Microinvasive carcinoma of the cervix: late results of operative treatment in 91 cases, Am. J. Obstet. Gynecol. **104**:738, 1969.
221. Naib, Z.M., et al.: Relation of cytohistopathology of genital herpesvirus infection to cervical anaplasia, Cancer Res. **33**:1452, 1973.
222. Nangle, R., Berger, M., and Levin, M.: Variations in the morphogenesis of squamous carcinoma of the cervix, Cancer **16**:1151, 1963.
223. Newton, C.W., and Abell, M.R.: Iatrogenic fetal implants, Obstet. Gynecol. **40**:686, 1972.
224. Ng, A.B.P., and Atkin, N.B.: Histological cell type and DNA value in the prognosis of squamous cell cancer of the uterine cervix. Br. J. Cancer **28**:322, 1973.
225. Ng, A.B.P., and Reagan, J.W.: Microinvasive carcinoma of the cervix, Am. J. Clin. Pathol. **52**:511, 1969.
226. Niven, P.A.R., and Stansfield, A.G.: Glioma of the uterus: a fetal homograft, Am. J. Obstet. Gynecol. **115**:534, 1973.
227. Paavonen, J., et al.: Colposcopic and histological findings in cervical chlamydial infection, Lancet **2**:320, 1980.
228. Paunier, J.P., Delclos, L., and Fletcher, G.H.: Causes, time of death, and sites of failure in squamous cell carcinoma of the uterine cervix on intact uterus, Radiology **88**:555, 1967.
229. Perez, C.A., et al.: Prognostic significance of endometrial extension from primary carcinoma of the uterine cervix, Cancer **35**:1493, 1975.
230. Pilotti, S., et al.: Condylomata of the uterine cervix and koilocytosis of cervical intraepithelial neoplasia, J. Clin. Pathol. **34**:532, 1981.
231. Quizilbash, A.H.: Papillary squamous tumors of the uterine cervix: a clinical and pathologic study of 21 cases, Am. J. Clin. Pathol. **61**:508, 1974.
232. Quizilbash, A.H.: *In situ* and microinvasive adenocarcinoma of the uterine cervix: a clinical, cytologic, and histologic study of 14 cases, Am. J. Clin. Pathol. **64**:155, 1975.
233. Rapp, F., and Duff, R.: Transformation of hamster embryofibroblasts by herpes simplex viruses types 1 and 2, Cancer Res. **33**:1527, 1973.
234. Rawls, W.E., Adam, E., and Melnick, J.L.: An analysis of seroepidemiological studies of herpesvirus type-2 and carcinoma of the cervix, Cancer Res. **33**:1477, 1973.
235. Reid, R., et al.: Noncondylomatous cervical wart virus infection, Obstet. Gynecol. **55**:476, 1980.
236. Richart, R.M., and Barron, B.A.: A followup study of patients with cervical dysplasia, Am. J. Obstet. Gynecol. **105**:386, 1969.
237. Roche, W.D., and Norris, H.J.: Microinvasive carcinoma of the cervix: the significance of lymphatic invasion and confluent patterns of stromal growth, Cancer **36**:180, 1975.
238. Roth, E., and Taylor, H.B.: Heterotopic cartilage in the uterus, Obstet. Gynecol. **27**:838, 1966.
239. Rotkin, I.D., and Cameron, J.R.: Clusters of variables influencing risk of cervical cancer, Cancer **21**:663, 1968.
240. Rubio, C.A., and Lagerlof, B.: Autoradiographic studies of dysplasia and carcinoma *in situ* in cervical cones, Acta Pathol. Microbiol. Scand. **82**:411, 1974.
241. Rutledge, F.N., et al.: Adenocarcinoma of the uterine cervix, Am. J. Obstet. Gynecol. **122**:236, 1975.
242. Schellhas, H.F., and Heath, G.: Cell renewal in the human cervix uteri: a radioautographic study of DNA, RNA, and protein synthesis, Am. J. Obstet. Gynecol. **104**:617, 1969.
243. Scully, R.E.: Definition of precursors of gynecologic cancer, Cancer **48**:531, 1981.
244. Selim, M.A., So-Bosita, J., and Neuman, M.R.: Carcinoma in situ of cervix uteri, Surg. Gynecol. Obstet. **139**:697, 1974.
245. Sherrick, J.C., and Vega, J.G.: Congenital intramural cysts of uterus, Obstet. Gynecol. **19**:486, 1962.
246. Shingleton, H.M., et al.: Human cervical intraepithelial neoplasia: fine structure of dysplasia and carcinoma in situ, Cancer Res. **18**:695, 1968.
247. Silverberg, E.: Cancer statistics, 1984, Cancer **34**:7, 1984.
248. Silverberg, E., and Holleb, A.I.: Major trends in cancer: 25 year survey, CA **25**:2, 1975.
249. Silverberg, S.G.: Adenomyomatosis of the endometrium, Am. J. Clin. Pathol. **64**:192, 1975.
250. Silverberg, S.G., and Hurt, G.W.: Minimal deviation adenocarcinoma ("adenoma malignum") of the cervix: a reappraisal, Am. J. Obstet. Gynacol. **121**:971, 1975.
251. Singer, A.: The uterine cervix from adolescence to the menopause, Br. J. Obstet. Gynaecol. **82**:81, 1975.
252. Sorensen, H.M., et al.: The spontaneous course of premalignant lesions on the vaginal portion of the uterus, Acta Obstet. Gynecol. Scand. **43**(suppl. 7):103, 1964.
253. Spriggs, A.I., Bowey, E., and Cowdell, R.H.: Chromosomes of precancerous lesions of the cervix, Cancer **27**:1239, 1971.
254. Stamler, T., Fields, C., and Andelman, S.L.: Epidemiology of cancer of the cervix. I. The dimensions of the problem: mortality and morbidity from cancer of the cervix, Am. J. Pub. Health **57**:791, 1967.
255. Steiner, G., and Friedell, G.H.: Adenosquamous carcinoma *in situ* of the cervix, Cancer **18**:807, 1965.
256. Stoddard, L.D.: The problem of carcinoma in situ with reference to the human cervix uteri. In McManus, J.F.A., editor: Progress in fundamental medicine, Philadelphia, 1952, Lea & Febiger.
257. Taylor, H.B., Irey, N.S., and Norris, H.J.: Atypical endocervical hyperplasia in women taking oral contraceptives, J.A.M.A. **202**:637, 1967.
258. Thompson, B.H., et al.: Cytopathology, histopathology, and colposcopy in the management of cervical neoplasia, Am. J. Obstet. Gynecol. **114**:329, 1972.
259. Watson, A.A., and Cochran, A.J.: Sebaceous glands of the cervix uteri and buccal mucosa, J. Pathol. Bacteriol. **98**:87, 1969.
260. Wentz, W.B., and Reagan, J.W.: Survival in cervical cancer with respect to cell type, Cancer **12**:384, 1959.
261. Wentz, W.B., et al.: Experimental studies of carcinogenesis of the uterine cervix in mice, Gynecol. Oncol. **12**(suppl.):90, 1981.
262. Willis, R.A.: The borderland of embryology and pathology, ed. 2, Washington, D.C., 1962, Butterworth, Inc.
263. Woodruff, J.D., et al.: Immunological identification of papillomavirus antigen in paraffin-processed condyloma tissue from the female genital tract, Obstet. Gynecol. **56**:727, 1980.
264. Worth, A.J., and Boyes, D.A.: A case control study of the possible effects of birth control pills on pre-clinical carcinoma of the cervix, J. Obstet. Gynaecol. Br. Cwlth. **79**:673, 1972.
264a. zurHausen, H.: Human genital cancer: synergism between two virus infections or between a virus infection and initiating events, Lancet **2**:1370, 1982.

Endometrium

265. Ackerman, L.V., and Rosai, J.: Surgical pathology, St. Louis, 1974, The C.V. Mosby Co.

266. Aikawa, M., and Ng, A.B.P.: Mixed (adenosquamous) carcinoma of the endometrium: electron microscopic observations, Cancer **31**:385, 1973.
267. Aksel, S., and Jones, G.S.: Etiology and treatment of dysfunctional uterine bleeding, Obstet. Gynecol. **44**:1, 1974.
268. Anderson, G.D.: *Listeria monocytogenes* septicemia in pregnancy, Obstet. Gynecol. **46**:102, 1975.
269. Andrews, W.C.: Luteal phase defects, Fertil. Steril. **32**:501, 1979.
270. Arias-Stella, J.: Gestational endometrium. In Norris, H.J., Hertig, A.T., and Abell, M.R., editors: The uterus, Baltimore, 1973, The Williams & Wilkins Co.
271. Armenia, C.S.: Sequential relationship between endometrial polyps and carcinoma of the endometrium, Obstet. Gynecol. **30**:524, 1967.
272. Armstrong, E.M., et al.: The giant mitochondrion–endoplasmic reticulin unit of the endometrial glandular cell, J. Anat. **116**:375, 1973.
273. Armstrong, E.M., et al.: Reappraisal of the ultrastructure of the human endometrial glandular cell, J. Obstet. Gynaecol. Br. Cwlth. **80**:446, 1973.
274. Arronet, G.H., and Arrata, W.S.M.: Dysfunctional uterine bleeding: a classification, Obstet. Gynecol. **29**:97, 1967.
275. Baggish, M.D., and Woodruff, J.D.: The occurrence of squamous epithelium in the endometrium, Obstet. Gynecol. Surv. **22**:69, 1967.
276. Barwick, K.W., and LiVolsi, V.S.: Malignant mixed müllerian tumors of the uterus: a clinicopathologic assessment of 34 cases, Am. J. Surg. Pathol. **3**:125, 1979.
277. Blum, R.H., et al.: Successful treatment of metastatic sarcomas with cyclophosphamide, Adriamycin, and DTIC, Cancer **46**:1722, 1980.
278. Blythe, J.G., and Ali, Z.: Endometrial adenocarcinoma: in estrogen, oral contraceptive, and nonhormone users, Gynecol. Oncol. **7**:199, 1979.
279. Bosio, B.B., and Taylor, E.S.: *Bacteroides* and puerperal infections, Obstet. Gynecol. **42**:271, 1973.
280. Boutselis, J.G.: Histochemistry of the normal endometrium. In Norris, H.J., Hertig, A.T., and Abell, M.R., editors: The uterus, Baltimore, 1973, The Williams & Wilkins Co.
281. Braun, P., and Druckman, E.: Public health rounds at the Harvard School of Public Health, N. Engl. J. Med. **295**:264, 1976.
282. Cadenz, D., et al.: Chronic endometritis: a comparative clinicopathologic study, Obstet. Gynecol. **41**:733, 1973.
283. Cavazos, F., and Lucas, F.V.: Ultrastructure of the endometrium. In Norris, H.J., Hertig, A.T., and Abell, M.R., editors: The uterus, Baltimore, 1973, The Williams & Wilkins Co.
284. Center for Disease Control: Surgical sterilization surveillance: hysterectomy in women aged 15-44, 1970-1975, Atlanta, 1980.
285. Chamlian, D.L., and Taylor, H.B.: Endometrial hyperplasia in young women, Obstet. Gynecol. **36**:659, 1970.
286. Chorlton, I., et al.: Primary malignant reticuloendothelial disease involving the vagina, cervix, and corpus uteri, Obstet. Gynecol. **44**:735, 1974.
287. Chuang, J.T., Van Velden, D.J.J., and Graham, J.B.: Carcinosarcoma and mixed mesodermal tumor of the uterine corpus: review of 49 cases, Obstet. Gynecol. **35**:769, 1970.
288. Clement, R.B., and Scully, R.E.: Müllerian adenosarcoma of the uterus, Cancer **34**:1138, 1975.
289. Craig, J.M.: The pathology of birth control, Arch. Pathol. **99**:233, 1975.
290. Crum, C.P., Richart, R.M., and Fenoglio, C.M.: Adenoacanthosis of the endometrium: a clinicopathologic study in premenopausal women, Am. J. Surg. Pathol. **5**:15, 1981.
291. Czernobilsky, B., et al.: Endocervical-type epithelium in endometrial carcinoma: a report of 10 cases with emphasis on histochemical methods for differential diagnosis, Am. J. Surg. Pathol. **4**:481, 1980.
292. Dallenbach-Hellweg, G.: Histopathology of the endometrium, New York, 1975, Springer-Verlag, New York, Inc.
293. deLouvois, J., et al.: Frequency of mycoplasma in fertile and infertile couples, Lancet **1**:1073, 1974.
294. deMoraes-Ruehsen, M.D., et al.: The aluteal cycle: a severe form of the luteal phase defect, Am. J. Obstet. Gynecol. **103**:1059, 1969.
295. Dutra, F.R.: Intraglandular morules of the endometrium, Am. J. Clin. Pathol. **31**:60, 1959.
296. Fechner, R.E.: Endometrium with the pattern of mesonephroma: report of a case, Obstet. Gynecol. **31**:485, 1960.
297. Fechner, R.E., and Kaufman, R.H.: Endometrial adenocarcinoma in Stein-Leventhal syndrome, Cancer **34**:444, 1974.
298. Ferenczy, A., and Richart, R.M.: Female reproductive system: dynamics of scan and transmission electron microscopy, New York, 1974, John Wiley & Sons, Inc.
299. Friederich, E.R.: Effects of contraceptive hormone preparations on the fine structure of the endometrium, Obstet. Gynecol. **30**:201, 1967.
300. Ganem, K.J., Parsons, L., and Friedell, G.H.: Endometrial ossification, Am. J. Obstet. Gynecol. **83**:1592, 1962.
301. Gompel, C., and Silverberg, S.G.: Pathology in gynecology and obstetrics, ed. 2, Philadelphia, 1977, J.B. Lippincott Co.
302. Good, R.G., and Moyer, D.L.: Estrogen progesterone relationships in the development of secretory endometrium, Fertil. Steril. **19**:37, 1968.
303. Gore, H.: Hyperplasia of the endometrium. In Norris, H.J., Hertig, A.T., and Abell, M.R., editors: The uterus, Baltimore, 1973, The Williams & Wilkins Co.
304. Gore, H., and Hertig, A.T.: Carcinoma in situ of the endometrium, Am. J. Obstet. Gynecol. **94**:134, 1966.
305. Hammond, C.B., et al.: Effects of long-term estrogen replacement therapy. II. Neoplasia, Am. J. Obstet. Gynecol. **133**:537, 1979.
306. Hendrickson, M.R., and Kempson, R.L.: Endometrial epithelial metaplasias: proliferations frequently misdiagnosed as adenocarcinoma: report of 89 cases and proposed classification, Am. J. Surg. Pathol. **4**:525, 1980.
306a. Hendrickson, M.R., Ross, J.C., and Kempson, R.L.: Toward the development of morphologic criteria for well-differentiated adenocarcinoma of the endometrium, Am. J. Surg. Pathol. **7**:819, 1983.
307. Hertig, A.T.: Gestational hyperplasia of endometrium: a morphologic correlation of ova, endometrium, and corpora lutea during early pregnancy, Lab. Invest. **13**:1153, 1964.
308. Hertig, A.T., Sommers, S.C., and Bengloff, A.: Genesis of endometrial carcinoma. III. Carcinoma in situ, Cancer **2**:964, 1949.
309. Horwitz, R.I., et al.: Histopathologic distinctions in the relationship of estrogens and endometrial cancer, J.A.M.A. **246**:1425, 1981.
310. Israel, S.L., Roitman, H.B., and Clancy, E.: Infrequency of unsuspected endometrial tuberculosis, histologic and bacteriologic study, J.A.M.A. **183**:63, 1963.
311. Jones, G.S.: The luteal phase defect, Fertil. Steril. **27**:351, 1976.
312. Kahn, H.S., and Tyler, C.W.: Mortality associated with use of IUD's, J.A.M.A. **234**:57, 1975.
313. Kaufman, R.H., Abbot, J.P., and Wall, J.A.: The endometrium before and after wedge resection of the ovaries in the Stein-Leventhal syndrome, Am. J. Obstet. Gynecol. **77**:1271, 1959.
314. Kay, S.: Squamous cell carcinoma of the endometrium, Am. J. Clin. Pathol. **61**:264, 1974.
315. Kempson, R.L., and Bari, W.: Uterine sarcomas: classification, diagnosis, and prognosis, Hum. Pathol. **1**:331, 1970.
316. Kempson, R.L., and Pokorny, G.E.: Adenocarcinoma of the endometrium in women aged 40 and younger, Cancer **21**:650, 1968.
317. Kistner, R.W.: Endometrial alterations associated with estrogen and estrogen-progestin combinations. In Norris, H.J., Hertig, A.T., and Abell, M.R., editors: The uterus, Baltimore, 1973, The Williams & Wilkins Co.
318. Kistner, R.W., Duncan, C.J., and Mansell, H.: Suppression of ovulation by tri-*p*-anisylchloroethelyne (TACE), Obstet. Gynecol. **8**:399, 1956.
319. Klaer, W., and Holm-Jensen, S.: Metastases to the uterus, Acta Pathol. Microbiol. Scand. **80**:835, 1972.

320. Krumholz, B.A., Lobovsky, F.Y., and Hahtsky, V.: Endolymphatic stromal myosis with pulmonary metastases: remission with progestin therapy; report of a case, J. Reprod. Med. **10**:85, 1973.
321. Langlois, P.L.: The size of the normal uterus, J. Reprod. Med. **4**:220, 1970.
322. Larbig, G.G., et al.: Plexiform tumorlets of endometrial stromal origin, Am. J. Clin. Pathol. **44**:32, 1965.
323. Laros, R.K., and Work, B.A.: Female sterilization. II. A comparison of methods, Obstet. Gynecol. **46**:215, 1975.
324. Mazur, M.T.: Atypical polypoid adenomyomas of the endometrium, Am. J. Surg. Pathol. **5**:473, 1981.
325. Mazur, M.T., and Kraus, F.T.: Histogenesis of morphologic variations in tumors of the uterine wall, Am. J. Surg. Pathol. **4**:59, 1980.
326. Ng, A.B.P., and Reagan, J.W.: Incidence and prognosis of endometrial carcinoma by histologic grade and extent, Obstet. Gynecol. **35**:437, 1970.
327. Ng, A.B.P., et al.: Mixed adenosquamous carcinoma of the endometrium, Am. J. Clin. Pathol. **59**:765, 1973.
328. Nogales, F., Beato, M., and Martinez, H.: Funktionelle Veranderungen des tuberculosen Endometriums, Arch. Gynecol. **203**:45, 1966.
329. Norris, H.J., Roth, E., and Taylor, H.B.: Mesenchymal tumors of the uterus. II. A clinical and pathological study of 31 mixed mesodermal tumors, Obstet. Gynecol. **28**:57, 1966.
330. Norris, H.J., and Taylor, H.B.: Mesenchymal tumors of the uterus. I. A clinical and pathological study of 53 endometrial stromal tumors, Cancer **19**:755, 1966.
331. Noyes, R.W.: Normal phases of the endometrium. In Norris, H.J., Hertig, A.T., and Abell, M.R., editors: The uterus, Baltimore, 1973, The Williams & Wilkins Co.
332. Perez, C.A., et al.: Effects of radiation on mixed müllerian tumors of the uterus, Cancer **43**:1274, 1979.
333. Philippe, E.: Endometre et sequelles d'avortement, Rev. Fr. Gynecol. **65**:413, 1970.
334. Picoff, R.C., and Luginbuhl, W.H.: Fibrin in the endometrial stroma: its relation to uterine bleeding, Am. J. Obstet. Gynecol. **88**:642, 1964.
335. Poulsen, H.E., Taylor, C.W., and Subin, L.H.: Histological typing of female genital tract tumors, Geneva, 1975, World Health Organization.
336. Robboy, S.J., and Bradley, R.: Changing trends and prognostic features in endometrial cancer associated with exogenous estrogen therapy, Obstet. Gynecol. **54**:269, 1979.
337. Rorat, E., Ferenczy, A., and Richart, R.M.: The ultrastructure of clear cell adenocarcinoma of the endometrium, Cancer **33**:880, 1974.
338. Rosai, J.: Ackerman's surgical pathology, ed. 6, St. Louis, 1981, The C.V. Mosby Co.
339. Roth, E., and Taylor, H.B.: Heterotopic cartilage in the uterus, Obstet. Gynecol. **27**:838, 1966.
340. Ryan, G.M., Jr., Craig, J., and Reid, D.E.: Histology of the uterus and ovaries after long-term cyclic norethynodrel therapy, Am. J. Obstet. Gynecol. **90**:715, 1964.
341. Salm, R.: The incidence and significance of early carcinomas in endometrial polyps, J. Pathol. **108**:47, 1972.
342. Shanklin, D.R.: Histologic dating of the endometrium: an invitational symposium, J. Reprod. Med. **3**:179, 1969.
343. Sheffield, W.H., Soule, S.D., and Herzog, G.M.: Cyclic endometrial changes in response to monthly injections of an estrogen-progestogen contraceptive drug: a histologic study, Am. J. Obstet. Gynecol. **103**:828, 1969.
344. Silverberg, S.G., Bolin, M.G., and DeGeorgi, L.S.: Adenoacanthoma and mixed adenosquamous carcinoma of the endometrium: a clinicopathologic study, Cancer **30**:1307, 1972.
345. Silverberg, S.G., and DiGeorgi, L.S.: Clear cell carcinoma of the endometrium, Cancer **31**:1127, 1973.
346. Silverberg, S.G., and Makowski, E.L.: Endometrial carcinoma in young women taking oral contraceptive agents, Obstet. Gynecol. **46**:503, 1975.
347. Silverberg, S.G., et al.: Endometrial carcinoma: clinical-pathologic comparison of cases in post-menopausal women receiving and not receiving exogenous estrogens, Cancer **45**:3018, 1980.
348. Smith, D.C., et al.: Association of exogenous estrogen and endometrial carcinoma, N. Engl. J. Med. **293**:1164, 1975.
349. Stevenson, C.S.: The endometrium in infertile women: prognostic significance of the initial study biopsy, Fertil. Steril. **16**:208, 1965.
350. Tavassoli, F.A., and Kraus, F.T.: Endometrial lesions in uteri resected for atypical endometrial hyperplasia, Am. J. Clin. Pathol. **70**:770, 1978.
351. Tavassoli, F.A., and Norris, H.J.: Mesenchymal tumors of the uterus. VII. A clinicopathological study of 60 endometrial stromal nodules, Histopathology **5**:1, 1981.
352. Terzakis, J.A.: The nucleolar channel system of human endometrium, J. Cell. Biol. **27**:293, 1965.
353. Thom, M.H., et al.: Prevention and treatment of endometrial disease in climacteric women receiving estrogen therapy, Lancet **2**:455, 1979.
354. Tiltman, A.J.: Mucinous carcinoma of the endometrium, Obstet. Gynecol. **55**:244, 1980.
355. Ulbright, T.M., and Kraus, F.T.: Endometrial stromal tumors of extra-uterine tissue, Am. J. Clin. Pathol. **76**:371, 1981.
356. Vellios, F.: Endometrial hyperplasias, precursors of endometrial carcinoma. In Sommers, S.C., editor: Pathology annual, vol. 7, New York, 1972, Appleton-Century-Crofts.
357. Weiss, N.S., et al.: Decreased risk of fractures of the hip and lower forearm with post-menopausal use of estrogen, N. Engl. J. Med. **303**:1195, 1980.
358. Wienke, E.C., et al.: Ultrastructural effects of norethynodrel and mestranol on human endometrial stromal cell, Am. J. Obstet. Gynecol. **103**:102, 1969.
359. Williamson, E.O., and Christopherson, W.M.: Malignant mixed müllerian tumors of the uterus, Cancer **29**:585, 1972.
360. Wolff, M., Silva, F., and Kaye, G.: Pulmonary metastases (with admixed epithelial elements) from smooth muscle neoplasms: report of nine cases, including three males, Am. J. Surg. Pathol. **3**:325, 1979.
361. Woodruff, J.D., and Julian, C.G.: Multiple malignancy in the upper genital canal, Am. J. Obstet. Gynecol. **103**:810, 1969.
362. Young, R.H., Kleinman, G.M., and Scully, R.E.: Glioma of the uterus, Am. J. Surg. Pathol. **5**:695, 1981.
363. Zaloudek, C.J., and Norris, H.J.: Adenofibroma of the uterus: a clinicopathologic study of 35 cases, Cancer **48**:354, 1981.
364. Zettergren, L.: Glial tissue in the uterus, Am. J. Pathol. **71**:419, 1973.

Myometrium

365. Banner, A.S., et al.: Efficacy of oophorectomy in lymphangiomyomatosis and benign metastasizing leiomyoma, N. Engl. J. Med. **305**:204, 1981.
366. Barlow, J.J., et al.: Adriamycin and bleomycin, alone and in combination, in gynecologic cancers, Cancer **32**:735, 1973.
367. Bartsich, E.G., Bowe, E.T., and Moore, J.G.: Leiomyosarcomas of the uterus: a 50 year review of 42 cases, Obstet. Gynecol. **32**:101, 1968.
368. Boyce, C.R., and Buddhdev, H.N.: Pregnancy complicated by metastasizing leiomyoma of the uterus, Obstet. Gynecol. **42**:252, 1973.
369. Christopherson, W.M., Williamson, E.O., and Gray, L.A.: Leiomyosarcoma of the uterus, Cancer **29**:1512, 1972.
370. Cramer, S.F., et al.: Metastasizing leiomyoma of the uterus: S-phase, fraction, estrogen receptor, and ultrastructure, Cancer **45**:932, 1980.
371. Emge, L.A.: The elusive adenomyosis of the uterus: its historical past and its present state of recognition, Am. J. Obstet. Gynecol. **83**:1541, 1962.
372. Fechner, R.E.: Atypical leiomyomas and synthetic progestin therapy, Am. J. Clin. Pathol. **49**:697, 1968.
373. Ferenczy, A., Fenoglio, J., and Richart, R.M.: Observations on benign mesothelioma of the genital tract (adenomatoid tumor): a comparative ultrastructural study, Cancer **30**:244, 1972.
374. Ferenczy, A., Richart, R.M., and Okagaki, T.: A comparative ultrastructural study of leiomyosarcoma, cellular leiomyoma, and leiomyoma of the uterus, Cancer **28**:1004, 1971.
375. Goodhue, W.W., Susin, M., and Kramer, E.E.: Smooth muscle origin of uterine plexiform tumors, Arch. Pathol. **71**:263, 1974.

376. Idelson, M.G., and Dairds, A.W.: Metastasis of uterine fibromyomata, Obstet. Gynecol. **21**:78, 1963.
377. Jacobs, D.S., Cohen, H., and Johnson, J.S.: Lipoleiomyomas of the uterus, Am. J. Clin. Pathol. **44**:45, 1965.
378. Konis, E.E., and Belsky, R.D.: Metastasizing leiomyoma of the uterus: report of a case, Obstet. Gynecol. **27**:442, 1966.
379. Marcus, C.C.: Relationship of adenomyosis uteri to endometrial hyperplasia and endometrial carcinoma, Am. J. Obstet. Gynecol. **82**:408, 1961.
380. Mathur, B.B.L., Shah, B.S., and Bhende, Y.M.: Adenomyosis uteri, Am. J. Obstet. Gynecol. **84**:1820, 1962.
381. Murphy, E.: Diffuse myometrial sclerosis, Am. J. Obstet. Gynecol. **103**:403, 1969.
382. Norris, H.J., and Parmley, T.: Mesenchymal tumors of the uterus. V. Intravenous leiomyomatosis: a report of 14 cases, Cancer **36**:2164, 1975.
383. Paranjothy, D., and Vaish, S.K.: Polycythemia associated with leiomyoma of the uterus, J. Obstet. Gynaecol. Br. Cwlth. **74**:603, 1967.
384. Parmley, T.H., et al.: Histogenesis of leiomyomatosis peritonealis disseminata (disseminated fibrosing deciduosis), Obstet. Gynecol. **46**:511, 1975.
385. Pietila, K.: Hysterography in the diagnosis of uterine myoma: roentgen findings in 829 cases compared with operative findings, Acta Obstet. Gynecol. Scand. **48**(suppl. 5): 1, 1969.
386. Rothman, D., and Rennard, M.: Myoma erythrocytosis syndrome: report of a case, Obstet. Gynecol **21**:102, 1963.
387. Rywlin, A.M., Rechner, L., and Benson, J.: Clear cell leiomyoma of the uterus: report of two cases of a previously undescribed entity, Cancer **17**:100, 1964.
388. Saksela, E., Lampinen, V., and Procope, B.J.: Malignant mesenchymal tumors of the uterine corpus, Am. J. Obstet. Gynecol. **120**:452, 1974.
389. Salm, R.: The histogenesis of uterine lipomas, Beitr. Pathol. **149**:284, 1973.
390. Scharfenberg, J.C., and Geary, W.L.: Intravenous leiomyomatosis, Obstet. Gynecol. **43**:909, 1974.
391. Silverberg, S.G.: Leiomyosarcoma of the uterus: a clinicopathologic study, Obstet. Gynecol. **38**:613, 1971.
392. Silverberg, S.G., Willson, M.A., and Board, J.A.: Hemangiopericytoma of the uterus: an ultrastructural study, Am. J. Obstet. Gynecol. **110**:297, 1971.
393. Stout, A.P.: Bizarre smooth muscle tumors of the stomach, Cancer **15**:400, 1962.
394. Taubert, H.-D., Wissner, S.E., and Haskins, A.L.: Leiomyomatosis peritonealis disseminata: an unusual complication of genital leiomyomata, Obstet. Gynecol. **25**:561, 1965.
395. Taxy, J.B., Battifora, H., and Oyasu, R.: Adenomatoid tumors: a light microscopic, histochemical, and ultrastructural study, Cancer **34**:306, 1974.
396. Taylor, H.B., and Norris, H.J.: Mesenchymal tumors of the uterus. IV. Diagnosis and prognosis of leiomyosarcomas, Arch. Pathol. **82**:40, 1966.
397. Vardi, J.R., and Tovell, H.M.M.: Leiomyosarcoma of the uterus: clinicopathologic study, Obstet. Gynecol. **56**:428, 1980.
398. Youngs, L.A., and Taylor, H.B.: Adenomatoid tumors of the uterus and fallopian tube, Am. J. Clin. Pathol. **48**:537, 1967.

Fallopian tube

399. Acosta, A.A., Kaplan, A.L., and Kaufman, R.H.: Mixed müllerian tumors of the oviduct, Obstet. Gynecol. **44**:84, 1974.
400. Benjamin, C.L., and Beaver, D.C.: Pathogenesis of salpingitis isthmica nodosa, Am. J. Clin. Pathol. **21**:212, 1951.
401. Dokumov, S., and Dekov, D.: A rare case of precocious pseudopuberty due to a Sertoli–Leydig cell tumor originating from the left fallopian tube, J. Clin. Endocrinol. Metab. **23**:1262, 1963.
402. Ferenczy, A., and Richart, R.M.: Female reproductive system: dynamics of scan and transmission electron microscopy, New York, 1974, John Wiley & Sons, Inc.
403. Flege, J.B.: Ruptured tubal pregnancy with elevated serum amylase levels, Arch. Surg. **92**:397, 1966.
404. Fogh, I.: Primary carcinoma of the fallopian tube, Cancer **23**:1332, 1969.
405. Jacobson, L., and Westrom, L.: Objectivized diagnoses of acute pelvic inflammatory disease, Am. J. Obstet. Gynecol. **105**:1088, 1969.
406. Manes, J.L., and Taylor, H.B.: Carcinosarcoma and mixed müllerian tumors of the fallopian tube, Cancer **38**:1687, 1976.
407. Mardh, P.A., and Westrom, L.: Tubal and cervical cultures in acute salpingitis with special reference to *Mycoplasma hominis* and T-strain mycoplasmas, Br. J. Vener. Dis. **46**:179, 1970.
408. Mardh, P.A., et al.: *Chlamydia trachomatis* infection in patients with acute salpingitis, N. Engl. J. Med. **296**:1377, 1977.
409. Mazzarella, P., Okagaki, T., and Richart, R.M.: Teratoma of the uterine tube: a case report and review of the literature, Obstet. Gynecol. **39**:381, 1972.
410. Nogales-Ortiz, F., Tarancon, I., and Nogales, F.F.: The pathology of female genital tuberculosis: a 31 year study of 1436 cases, Obstet. Gynecol. **53**:422, 1979.
411. Palladino, V.S., and Trousdell, M.: Extrauterine müllerian tumors, Cancer **23**:1413, 1969.
412. Rees, E., and Annels, E.H.: Gonococcal salpingitis, Br. J. Vener. Dis. **45**:205, 1969.
413. Rubin, I.C., Lisa, J.R., and Trinidad, S.: Further observations of ectopic endometrium of fallopian tube, Surg. Gynecol. Obstet. **103**:469, 1956.
414. Schiller, H.M., and Silverberg, S.G.: Staging and prognosis in primary carcinoma of the fallopian tube, Cancer **28**:389, 1971.
415. Sedlis, A.: Primary carcinoma of the fallopian tube, Obstet. Gynecol. Surv. **16**:209, 1961.
416. Siegler, A.M., Wang, C.F., and Westhoff, C.: Management of unruptured tubal pregnancy, Obstet. Gynecol. Surv. **36**:599, 1981.
417. Sweet, R.I., Selinger, H.E., and McKay, D.G.: Malignant teratoma of the uterine tube, Obstet. Gynecol. **45**:553, 1975.
418. Swenson, R.M., et al.: Anaerobic bacterial infections of the female genital tract, Obstet. Gynecol. **42**:538, 1973.
419. Thadepalli, H., Gorbach, S.L., and Keith, L.: Anaerobic infections of the female genital tract: bacteriologic and therapeutic aspects, Am. J. Obstet. Gynecol. **117**:1034, 1973.
420. Thomas, M.L., and Rose, D.H.: Salpingitis isthmica nodosa demonstrated by hysterosalpingography, Acta Radiol. **14**:295, 1973.
421. Timonen, S., and Nieminen, U.: Tubal pregnancy: choice of operative method of treatment, Acta Obstet. Gynecol. Scand. **46**:337, 1967.
422. Woodruff, J.D., and Pauerstein, C.J.: The fallopian tube, Baltimore, 1969, The Williams & Wilkins Co.
423. Wright, N.H., and Laemmle, P.: Acute pelvic inflammatory disease in an indigent population, Am. J. Obstet. Gynecol. **101**:979, 1968.
424. Youngs, L.A., and Taylor, H.B.: Adenomatoid tumors of the uterus and fallopian tube, Am. J. Clin. Pathol. **48**:537, 1967.

Ovary

425. Abel, K.P.: Ovarian apoplexy, Lancet **1**:136, 1964.
426. Abell, M.R., and Holtz, F.: Ovarian neoplasms in childhood and adolescence. II. Tumors of non–germ cell origin, Am. J. Obstet. Gynecol. **93**:850, 1965.
427. Adams, E.C., and Hertig, A.T.: Studies on the human corpus luteum. II. Observation on the ultrastructure of luteal cells during pregnancy, J. Cell Biol. **41**:716, 1969.
428. Angervall, L., and Knutson, H.: Heterotopic ovarian tissue, Acta Obstet. Gynecol. Scand. **38**:275, 1959.
429. Arey, L.B.: The origin and form of the Brenner tumor, Am. J. Obstet. Gynecol. **81**:743, 1961.
430. Arrata, W.S.M., and deAlvarez, R.R.: Oversuppression syndrome, Am. J. Obstet. Gynecol. **112**:1025, 1972.
431. Asadourian, L.A., and Taylor, H.B.: Dysgerminoma: an analysis of 105 cases, Obstet. Gynecol. **33**:370, 1969.
432. Aure, J.C., Hoeg, K., and Kolstad, P.: Clinical and histologic studies of ovarian carcinoma: long-term follow up of 990 cases, Obstet. Gynecol. **37**:1, 1971.
433. Aure, J.C., Hoeg, K., and Kolstad, D.: Psammoma bodies in serous carcinoma of the ovary: a prognostic study, Am. J. Obstet. Gynecol. **109**:113, 1971.

434. Ballas, M.: The significance of alpha-fetoprotein in the serum of patients with malignant teratomas and related germinal neoplasms, Ann. Clin. Lab. Sci. **4**:267, 1974.
435. Ballon, S.C., et al.: Myeloblastoma (granulocytic sarcoma) of the ovary, Arch. Pathol. Lab. Med. **102**:474, 1978.
436. Bardin, C.W., et al.: Studies of testosterone metabolism in a patient with masculinization due to stromal hyperthecosis, N. Engl. J. Med. **277**:399, 1967.
437. Barwick, K.W., and LiVolsi, V.A.: Malignant mixed mesodermal tumors of the ovary: a clinicopathologic assessment of 12 cases, Am. J. Surg. Pathol. **4**:37, 1980.
438. Behrman, H.R., and Caldwell, B.V.: Role of prostaglandins in reproduction. In Greep, R.O., editor: Reproductive physiology, M.T.P. International Review of Science, vol. 8, Baltimore, 1974, University Park Press.
439. Bjorkholm, E., and Silfverswärd, C.: Prognostic factors in granulosa-cell tumors, Gynecol. Oncol. **11**:261, 1981.
440. Blackwell, W.J., et al.: Dermoid cysts of the ovary; their clinical and pathologic significance, Am. J. Obstet. Gynecol. **51**:151, 1946.
441. Block, E.: A quantitative morphological investigation of the follicular system in newborn female infants, Acta Anat. **17**:201, 1953.
442. Case records of the Massachusetts General Hospital: Ovarian hyperthecosis with massive edema, case 24-1971, N. Engl. J. Med. **284**:1369, 1971.
443. Chorlton, I., Norris, H.J., and King, F.M.: Malignant reticuloendothelial disease of the ovary as a primary manifestation: a series of 19 lymphomas and 1 granulocytic sarcoma, Cancer **34**:397, 1974.
444. Clement, P.B., and Scully, R.E.: Extrauterine mesodermal (müllerian) adenosarcoma: a clinicopathologic analysis of five cases, Am. J. Clin. Pathol. **69**:276, 1978.
445. Cocco, A.E., and Conway, S.J.: Zollinger-Ellison syndrome associated with ovarian mucinous cystadenocarcinoma, N. Engl. J. Med. **293**:485, 1975.
446. Cooper, H.E., et al.: Hereditary factors in the Stein-Leventhal syndrome, Am. J. Obstet. Gynecol. **100**:371, 1968.
447. Crosignani, P.G., et al.: Hormonal profiles in anovulatory patients treated with gonadotropins and synthetic luteinizing hormone releasing hormone, Obstet. Gynecol. **46**:15, 1975.
448. Cummins, P., Fox, H., and Langley, F.A.: An ultrastructural study of the nature and origin of the Brenner tumor of the ovary, J. Pathol. **110**:167, 1973.
449. Daane, T.A., Lurie, A.D., and Barton, R.K.: Ovarian lutein cysts associated with an otherwise normal pregnancy, Obstet. Gynecol. **34**:655, 1969.
450. deMoraes-Ruehsen, M., et al.: Autoimmunity and ovarian failure, Am. J. Obstet. Gynecol. **112**:693, 1972.
451. Diaz-Infante, A., et al.: *In vitro* studies of human ovarian contractility, Obstet. Gynecol. **44**:830, 1974.
452. Easterling, W.E., Talbert, L.M., and Potter, H.D.: Serum testosterone in the polycystic ovary syndrome: effect of an estrogen-progestin on protein binding of testosterone, Am. J. Obstet. Gynecol. **120**:385, 1974.
453. Ehrlich, C.E., and Roth, L.M.: The Brenner tumor: a clinicopathologic study of 57 cases, Cancer **27**:332, 1971.
454. Evans, A.T., III, et al.: Clinicopathologic review of 118 granulosa and 82 theca cell tumors, Obstet. Gynecol. **55**:231, 1980.
455. Falls, J.L.: Accessory adrenal cortex in the broad ligament: incidence and functional significance, Cancer **8**:143, 1955.
456. Feldman, G.B., and Knapp, R.C.: Lymphatic drainage of the peritoneal cavity and its significance in ovarian cancer, Am. J. Obstet. Gynecol. **119**:991, 1974.
457. Fenoglio, C.M., Ferenczy, A., and Richart, R.M.: Mucinous tumors of the ovary: ultrastructural studies of mucinous cystadenomas with histogenetic considerations, Cancer **36**:1709, 1975.
458. Fox, H., Agrawal, K., and Langley, F.A.: A clinicopathologic study of 92 cases of granulosa cell tumor of the ovary with special reference to the factors influencing prognosis, Cancer **35**:231, 1975.
459. Foyle, A., Al-Jabi, M., and McCaughey, W.T.: Papillary peritoneal tumors in women, Am. J. Surg. Pathol. **5**:241, 1981.
460. Gambrell, R.D., Greenblatt, R.B., and Mahesh, V.B.: Inappropriate secretion of LH in the Stein-Leventhal syndrome, Obstet. Gynecol. **42**:429, 1973.
461. Garcia-Bunuel, R., and Morris, B.: Histochemical observations on mucins in human ovarian neoplasms, Cancer **17**:1108, 1964.
462. Gillim, S.W., Christensen, A.K., and McLennan, C.E.: Fine structure of the human menstrual corpus luteum at its stage of maximum secretory activity, Am. J. Anat. **126**:409, 1969.
463. Girouard, D.P., Barclay, D.L., and Collins, C.G.: Hyperreactio luteinalis: a review of the literature and report of two cases, Obstet. Gynecol. **23**:513, 1964.
464. Givens, J.R., Wiser, W.L., and Coleman, S.A.: Familial ovarian hyperthecosis: a study of two families, Am. J. Obstet. Gynecol. **110**:955, 1971.
465. Gordon, H., Lipton, D., and Woodruff, J.D.: Dysgerminoma: a review of 158 cases from the Emil Novak Ovarian Tumor Registry, Obstet. Gynecol. **58**:497, 1981.
466. Greenblatt, R.B., and Mahesh, V.B.: Some new thoughts on the Stein-Leventhal syndrome, J. Reprod. Med. **13**:85, 1974.
467. Grogan, R.H.: Accidental rupture of malignant ovarian cysts during surgical removal, Obstet. Gynecol. **30**:716, 1967.
468. Hammerstein, J.: Regulation of ovarian steroidogenesis: gonadotropins, enzymes, prostaglandins, cyclic-AMP, luteolysins. In Greep, R.O., editor: Reproductive physiology, M.T.P. International Review of Science, vol. 8, Baltimore, 1974, University Park Press.
469. Hart, W.R., and Norris, H.J.: Borderline and malignant mucinous tumors of the ovary, Cancer **31**:1031, 1973.
470. Hay, D.M., and Stewart, D.B.: Primary ovarian carcinoma, J. Obstet. Gynaecol. Br. Cwlth. **76**:941, 1969.
471. Jensen, A.B., and Fechener, R.E.: Ultrastructure of an intermediate Sertoli–Leydig cell tumor: a histogenetic misnomer, Lab. Invest. **21**:527, 1969.
472. Joshi, V.V.: Primary Krukenberg tumor of the ovary: review of the literature and case report, Cancer **22**:1199, 1968.
473. Kalderon, A.E., and Tucci, J.R.: Ultrastructure of a human chorionic gonadotropin and adrenocorticotropin-responsive functioning Sertoli-Leydig cell tumor (type I), Lab. Invest. **29**:81, 1973.
474. Kalstone, C.E., Jaffe, R.B., and Abell, M.R.: Massive edema of the ovary simulating fibroma, Obstet. Gynecol. **34**:564, 1969.
475. Kao, G.F., and Norris, H.J.: Cystadenofibromas of the ovary with epithelial atypia, Am. J. Surg. Pathol. **2**:357, 1978.
476. Katzenstein, A.-L., et al.: Proliferative serous tumors of the ovary: histologic features and prognosis, Am. J. Surg. Pathol. **2**:339, 1978.
477. Kempson, R.L.: Ultrastructure of ovarian stromal cell tumors: Sertoli–Leydig cell tumor and lipid cell tumor, Arch. Pathol. **86**:492, 1968.
478. Keyes, P.L.: Luteinizing hormone: action on the Graafian follicle in vitro, Science **164**:846, 1969.
479. Knapp, R.C., and Friedman, E.A.: Aortic lymph node metastases in early ovarian cancer, Am. J. Obstet. Gynecol. **119**:1013, 1974.
480. Konikov, N., Bleisch, V., and Piskie, V.: Prognostic significance of cytologic diagnosis of effusions, Acta Cytol. **10**:335, 1966.
481. Kottmeier, H.-L.: Surgical management—conservative surgery. In Gentil, F., and Junqueira, A.C.: Ovarian cancer, U.I.C.C. monograph series, vol. II, New York, 1968, Springer-Verlag New York, Inc.
482. Kriss, B.R.: Neoplasms of a supernumerary ovary: report of two cases, J. Mt. Sinai Hosp. **14**:798, 1947.
483. Kurman, R.J., Goebelsmann, U., and Taylor, C.R.: Steroid localization in granulosa–theca cell tumors of the ovary, Cancer **43**:2377, 1979.
484. Kurman, R.J., and Norris, H.J.: Malignant germ cell tumors of the ovary, Hum. Pathol. **8**:551, 1977.
485. Kurman, R.J., et al.: An immunohistological study of steroid localization in Sertoli–Leydig cell tumors of the ovary and testis, Cancer **43**:1772, 1978.
486. Lauchlan, S.C.: The secondary Müllerian system, Obstet. Gynecol. Surv. **27**:133, 1972.
487. Lindner, D., McCaw, B.K., and Hecht, F.: Pathogenic origin of benign ovarian teratomas, N. Engl. J. Med. **292**:63, 1975.

488. Long, M.F., and Taylor, H.C.: Endometrioid carcinoma of the ovary, Am. J. Obstet. Gynecol. **90**:936, 1964.
489. Long, R.T.L., Spratt, J.S., and Dowling, E.: Pseudomyxoma peritonei, Am. J. Surg. **117**:162, 1969.
490. Malkasian, G.D., Dockerty, M.D., and Symmonds, R.E.: Benign cystic teratomas, Obstet. Gynecol. **29**:719, 1967.
491. Mansell, H., and Hertig, A.T.: Granulosa–theca cell tumors and endometrial carcinoma: a study of their relationship and a survey of 80 cases, Obstet. Gynecol. **6**:385, 1955.
492. Maques, M., et al.: Ovarian morphology after prolonged use of steroid contraceptive agents, Contraception **5**:177, 1972.
493. Mattingly, R.F., and Huang, W.Y.: Steroidogenesis of the menopausal and postmenopausal ovary, Am. J. Obstet. Gynecol. **103**:679, 1969.
494. Morris, J.M., and Scully, R.E.: Endocrine pathology of the ovary, St. Louis, 1958, The C.V. Mosby Co.
495. Munnell, E.W.: Is conservative therapy ever justified in stage I (IA) cancer of the ovary? Am. J. Obstet. Gynecol. **103**:641, 1969.
496. Nieminen, I., von Numers, C., and Widholm, O.: Struma ovarii, Acta Obstet. Gynecol. Scand. **42**:399, 1964.
497. Nikrui, N.: Survey of clinical behavior of patients with borderline epithelial tumors of the ovary, Gynecol. Oncol. **12**:107, 1981.
498. Norris, H.J., and Taylor, H.B.: Nodular theca-lutein hyperplasia of pregnancy (so-called pregnancy luteoma), Am. J. Clin. Pathol. **47**:557, 1967.
499. Norris, H.J., and Taylor, H.B.: Prognosis of granulosa-theca tumors of the ovary, Cancer **21**:255, 1968.
500. Norris, H.J., and Taylor, H.B.: Virilization associated with cystic granulosa cell tumors, Obstet. Gynecol. **34**:624, 1969.
501. Novak, E.R.: Gynandroblastoma of the ovary: review of eight cases from the tumor ovarian registry, Obstet. Gynecol. **30**:709, 1967.
502. Novak, E.R.: Ovulation after 50, Obstet. Gynecol. **36**:903, 1970.
503. Ober, W.B., Grady, H.G., and Schoenbucher, A.K.: Ectopic ovarian decidua without pregnancy, Am. J. Pathol. **33**:199, 1957.
504. O'Hern, T.M., and Neubecker, R.D.: Arrhenoblastoma, Obstet. Gynecol. **19**:758, 1962.
505. Pearl, M., and Plotz, E.J.: Supernumerary ovary: report of a case, Obstet. Gynecol. **21**:253, 1963.
506. Pedersen, P.H., and Larsen, J.F.: Ultrastructure of a granulosa cell tumour, Acta Obstet. Gynecol. Scand. **49**:105, 1970.
507. Peterson, W.F.: Malignant degeneration of benign cystic teratomas of the ovary: a collective review of the literature, Obstet. Gynecol. Surv. **12**:793, 1957.
508. Piver, M.S., Williams, L.J., and Marcuse, P.M.: Influence of luteal cysts on menstrual function, Obstet. Gynecol. **35**:740, 1970.
509. Polansky, S., dePapp, E.W., and Ogden, E.B.: Virilization associated with bilateral luteomas of pregnancy, Obstet. Gynecol. **45**:516, 1975.
510. Robboy, S.J., Norris, H.J., and Scully, R.E.: Insular carcinoid primary in the ovary: a clinicopathologic analysis of 48 cases, Cancer **36**:404, 1975.
511. Robboy, S.J., and Scully, R.E.: Ovarian teratoma with glial implants on the peritoneum, Hum. Pathol. **1**:643, 1970.
512. Robboy, S.J., Scully, R.E., and Norris, H.J.: Carcinoid metastatic to the ovary—a clinicopathologic analysis of 35 cases, Cancer **33**:798, 1974.
513. Roberts, D.W.T., and Haines, M.: Conserving ovarian tissue in treatment of ovarian neoplasms, Br. Med. J. **2**:917, 1965.
514. Roth, L.M.: Fine structure of the Brenner tumor, Cancer **27**:1482, 1971.
515. Roth, L.M.: The Brenner tumor and the Walthard cell nest: an electron microscopic study, Lab. Invest. **31**:15, 1974.
516. Roth, L.M., Deaton, R.L., and Sternberg, W.H.: Massive ovarian edema: a clinicopathologic study of five cases including ultrastructural observations and review of the literature, Am. J. Surg. Pathol. **3**:11, 1979.
517. Roth, L.M., and Ehrlich, C.E.: Mucinous cystadenocarcinoma of the retroperitoneum, Obstet. Gynecol. **49**:486, 1977.
518. Roth, L.M., and Sternberg, W.H.: Proliferating Brenner tumors, Cancer **27**:687, 1971.
519. Rust, L.A., Israel, R., and Mishell, D.R., Jr.: Individualized graduated therapeutic regimen for clomiphene citrate, Am. J. Obstet. Gynecol. **120**:785, 1974.
520. Ryan, K.J., Petro, Z., and Kaiser, J.: Steroid formation by isolated and recombined ovarian granulosa and thecal cells, J. Clin. Endocrinol. **28**:355, 1968.
521. Santesson, L.: Cited by Kraus, F.T.: Gynecologic pathology, St. Louis, 1967, The C.V. Mosby Co.
522. Santesson, L., and Kottmeier, H.L.: General classification of ovarian tumors. In Gentil, F., and Junqueira, A.C.: Ovarian cancer, U.I.C.C. monograph series, vol. 11, New York, 1968, Springer-Verlag, New York, Inc.
523. Schenker, J.G., and Polishuk, W.Z.: Ovarian hyperstimulation syndrome, Obstet. Gynecol. **46**:23, 1975.
524. Scully, R.E.: Stromal luteoma of the ovary: a distinctive type of lipoid cell tumor, Cancer **17**:769, 1964.
525. Scully, R.E.: Gonadoblastoma: a review of 74 cases, Cancer **25**:1340, 1970.
526. Scully, R.E.: Recent progress in ovarian cancer, Hum. Pathol. **1**:73, 1970.
527. Scully, R.E.: Tumors of the ovary and maldeveloped gonads, Washington, D.C., 1979, Armed Forces Institute of Pathology.
528. Scully, R.E., and Barlow, J.F.: "Mesonephroma" of the ovary: tumor of müllerian nature related to the endometrioid carcinoma, Cancer **20**:1405, 1967.
529. Scully, R.E., and Richardson, G.S.: Luteinization of the stroma of metastatic cancer involving the ovary and its endocrine significance, Cancer **14**:827, 1961.
530. Serov, S.F., Scully, R.E., and Sobin, L.H.: Histological typing of ovarian tumours, Geneva, 1973, World Health Organization.
531. Silverberg, E., and Holleb, A.I.: Major trends in cancer: 25 year survey, CA **25**:2, 1975.
532. Silverberg, S.G.: Brenner tumor of the ovary: a clinicopathologic study of 60 tumors in 54 women, Cancer **28**:588, 1971.
533. Silverberg, S.G., and Nogales-Fernandez, F.: Endolymphatic stromal myosis of the ovary: a report of three cases and literature review, Gynecol. Oncol. **12**:129, 1981.
534. Sjostedt, S., and Wahlen, T.: Prognosis of granulosa cell tumors, Acta Obstet. Gynecol. Scand. **40**(suppl. 6):1, 1961.
535. Starup, J., and Sele, V.: Premature ovarian failure, Acta Obstet. Gynecol. Scand. **52**:259, 1973.
536. Stein, I.F., Sr., and Leventhal, M.L.: Amenorrhea associated with bilateral polycystic ovaries, Am. J. Obstet. Gynecol. **21**:181, 1935.
537. Steiner, M.M., and Hadawi, S.A.: Sexual precocity: association with follicular cysts of ovary, Am. J. Dis. Child. **108**:28, 1964.
538. Sternberg, W.H., and Barclay, D.L.: Luteoma of pregnancy, Am. J. Obstet. Gynecol. **95**:165, 1966.
539. Stevens, V.C.: Comparison of FSH and LH patterns in plasma, urine, and urinary extracts during the menstrual cycle, J. Clin. Endocrinol. **29**:904, 1969.
540. Taylor, H.B., and Norris, H.J.: Lipid cell tumors of the ovary, Cancer **20**:1953, 1967.
541. Taymor, M.L., et al.: Hormone factors in human ovulation, Am. J. Obstet. Gynecol. **114**:445, 1972.
542. Teilum, G.: Classification of endodermal sinus tumour (mesoblastoma vitellinum) and so-called "embryonal carcinoma of the ovary," Acta Pathol. Microbiol. Scand. **64**:407, 1965.
543. Teilum, G., Albrechtsen, R., and Norgaard-Pedersen, J.: Immunofluorescent localization of alpha-fetoprotein in endodermal sinus tumor, Acta Pathol. Microbiol. Scand. **82**:586, 1974.
544. Thurlbeck, W.M., and Scully, R.E.: Solid teratoma of the ovary; a clinicopathological analysis of nine cases, Cancer **13**:804, 1960.
545. Tyson, J.E., et al.: Neuro-endocrine dysfunction in galactorrhea-amenorrhea after oral contraceptive use, Obstet. Gynecol. **46**:1, 1975.
546. van Wagenen, G., and Simpson, M.E.: Postnatal development of the ovary, in *Homo sapiens* and *Macaca mulatta*, and induction of ovulation in the macaque, New Haven, 1973, Yale University Press.

547. Wharton, L.R.: Two cases of supernumerary ovary and one of accessory ovary, with an analysis of previously reported cases, Am. J. Obstet. Gynecol. **78**:1101, 1959.
548. Woodruff, J.D., Protos, P., and Peterson, W.F.: Ovarian teratomas: relationship of histologic and ontogenetic factors to prognosis, Am. J. Obstet. Gynecol. **102**:702, 1968.
549. Woodruff, J.D., et al.: Metastatic ovarian tumors, Am. J. Obstet. Gynecol. **107**:202, 1970.
550. Zaloudek, C.J., Tavassoli, F.A., and Norris, H.J.: Dysgerminoma with syncytiotrophoblastic giant cells: a histologically and clinically distinctive subtype of dysgerminoma, Am. J. Surg. Pathol. **5**:361, 1981.
551. Zanartu, J., et al.: Induction of ovulation with synthetic gonadotropin-releasing hormone in women with constant anovulation induced by contraceptive steroids, Br. Med. J. **1**:605, 1974.
552. Zondek, L.H., and Zondek, T.: Leydig cells of the foetus and newborn in various complications of pregnancy, Acta Obstet. Gynecol. Scand. **46**:392, 1967.

Placenta

553. Acosta-Sison, H.: Changing attitudes in the management of hydatidiform mole: a report on 196 patients admitted to the Philippine General Hospital from April 10, 1959, to March 27, 1963, Am. J. Obstet. Gynecol. **88**:634, 1964.
554. Adock, Eugene W., II, et al.: Human chorionic gonadotropin: its possible role in maternal lymphocyte suppression, Science **181**:845, 1973.
555. Altshuler, G., and McAdams, A.J.: The role of the placenta in fetal and perinatal pathology, Am. J. Obstet. Gynecol. **113**:616, 1972.
556. Altshuler, G., Russell, P., and Ermocilla, R.: The placental pathology of small-for-gestational age infants, Am. J. Obstet. Gynecol. **121**:351, 1975.
557. Attwood, H.D., and Park, W.W.: Trophoblast (benign) in lung, J. Obstet. Gynaecol. Br. Cwlth. **68**:611, 1963.
558. Bain, A.D., et al.: Congenital toxoplasmosis simulating hemolytic disease of the newborn, J. Obstet. Gynaecol. Br. Emp. **63**:826, 1956.
559. Baker, C.J., and Casper, D.L.: Correlations of maternal antibody deficiency and susceptibility to neonatal group B streptococcal infection, N. Engl. J. Med. **294**:753, 1976.
560. Band, P.R., et al.: Hydatidiform mole metastasizing to the lung, Can. Med. Assoc. J. **114**:813, 1976.
561. Banti, D., et al.: Significance of placental pathology in transplacental haemorrhage, J. Clin. Pathol. **21**:322, 1968.
562. Beacham, W.D., et al.: Abdominal pregnancy at Charity Hospital in New Orleans, Am. J. Obstet. Gynecol. **84**:1257, 1962.
563. Beer, A.E.: Immunogenetic determinants of the size of the fetoplacental unit and their modus operandi. In Brosens, I.A., Dixon, G., and Robertson, W.B.: Human placentation, Amsterdam, 1975, Excerpta Medica.
564. Benirschke, K.: Abortions and moles. In Naeye, R.L., Kissane, J.M., and Kaufman, N., editors: Perinatal diseases, Baltimore, 1981, The Williams & Wilkins Co.
565. Benirschke, K., and Driscoll, S.G.: The pathology of the human placenta, New York, 1967, Springer-Verlag New York, Inc.
566. Benirschke, K., and Kim, C.K.: Multiple pregnancy, N. Engl. J. Med. **288**:1276, 1973.
567. Billington, W.D.: Immunologic aspects of normal and abnormal pregnancy. In Brosens, I.A., Dixon, G., and Robertson, W.B.: Human placentation, Amsterdam, 1975, Excerpta Medica.
568. Blanc, W.A.: Vernix granulomatosis of amnion (amnion nodosum) in oligohydramnios, N.Y. J. Med. **61**:1492, 1961.
569. Blanc, W.A.: Pathology of the placenta, membranes, and umbilical cord in bacterial, fungal, and viral infections in man. In Naeye, R.L., Kissane, J.M., and Kaufman, N., editors: Perinatal diseases, Baltimore, 1981, The Williams & Wilkins Co.
570. Bleisch, V.R.: The diagnosis of monochorionic placenta, Am. J. Clin. Pathol. **42**:277, 1964.
571. Boyd, J.D., and Hamilton, W.J.: The human placenta, Cambridge, 1970, W. Heffer & Sons.
572. Braunstein, G.D., et al.: Secretory rates of human chorionic gonadotropin by normal trophoblast, Am. J. Obstet. Gynecol. **115**:447, 1973.
573. Breen, J.L.: A 21 year survey of 654 ectopic pregnancies, Am. J. Obstet. Gynecol. **106**:1004, 1970.
574. Breen, J.L., et al.: Placenta accreta, increta and percreta: a survey of 40 cases, Obstet. Gynecol. **49**:43, 1977.
575. Brewer, J.I., and Mazur, M.T.: Gestational choriocarcinoma: its origin in the placenta during seemingly normal pregnancy, Am. J. Surg. Pathol. **5**:267, 1981.
576. Brosens, I.A., Dixon, G., and Robertson, W.B., editors: Human placentation, Amsterdam, 1975, Excerpta Medica.
577. Brosens, I.A., Robertson, W.B., and Dixon, H.G.: The role of the spiral arteries in the pathogenesis of pre-eclampsia. In Wynn, R.M., editor: Obstetrics and gynecology annual, New York, 1972, Appleton-Century-Crofts.
578. Burrows, S., et al.: Giant chorioangiomas, Am. J. Obstet. Gynecol. **115**:579, 1973.
579. Cameron, A.H.: The Birmingham twin survey, Proc. R. Soc. Med. **61**:229, 1968.
580. Carr, D.H.: Chromosome studies in selected spontaneous abortion. III. Early pregnancy loss, Obstet. Gynecol. **37**:750, 1971.
581. Carter, B.: Premature separation of the normally implanted placenta, Obstet. Gynecol. **29**:30, 1967.
582. Carter, J.E., Vellios, F., and Huber, C.P.: Histologic classification and incidence of circulatory lesions of the human placenta, with a review of the literature, Am. J. Clin. Pathol. **40**:374, 1963.
583. Clark, P.B., Gusdon, J.P., and Burt, R.L.: Hydatidiform mole with co-existent fetus: discussion and review of diagnostic methods, Obstet. Gynecol. **35**:597, 1970.
584. Craig, J.M.: The pathology of birth control, Arch. Pathol. **99**:233, 1975.
585. Culp, W.C., et al.: Placenta membranacea: a case report with arteriographic findings, Radiology **108**:309, 1973.
586. Dehner, L.P., and Askin, F.B.: Cytomegalovirus endometritis: report of a case associated with spontaneous abortion, Obstet. Gynecol. **45**:211, 1975.
587. de Ikonicoff, L., and Cedard, L.: Localization of human chorionic gonadotropic and somatomammotropic hormones by peroxidase immunohistoenzymologic method in villi and amniotic epithelium of human placentas (from 6 weeks to term), Am. J. Obstet. Gynecol. **116**:1124, 1973.
588. Demian, S.D.E., et al.: Placental lesions in congenital giant pigmented nevi, Am. J. Clin. Pathol. **61**:438, 1974.
589. Desmonts, G., and Couvreur, J.: Congenital toxoplasmosis: a prospective study of 378 pregnancies, N. Engl. J. Med. **290**:1110, 1974.
590. Douthwaite, R.M., and Urbach, G.I.: In vitro antigenicity of trophoplast, Am. J. Obstet. Gynecol. **109**:1023, 1971.
591. Dreskin, R.B., Spicer, S.S., and Greene, W.B.: Ultrastructural localization of chorionic gonadotropin in human term placenta, J. Histochem. Cytochem. **18**:862, 1970.
592. Driscoll, S.G.: Histopathology of gestational rubella, Am. J. Dis. Child. **118**:49, 1969.
593. Dyke, P.C., and Fink, L.M.: Latent choriocarcinoma, Cancer **20**:150, 1967.
594. Elston, C.W.: Cellular reaction to choriocarcinoma, J. Pathol. **97**:261, 1969.
595. Elston, C.W., and Bagshawe, K.D.: The value of histological grading in the management of hydatidiform mole, J. Obstet. Gynaecol. Br. Cwlth. **79**:717, 1972.
596. Enders, A.C., and King, B.F.: The cytology of Hofbauer cells, Anat. Rec. **167**:231, 1970.
597. Faulk, W.P., et al.: Immunological studies of the human placenta: characterization of immunoglobulins on trophoblastic basement membranes, J. Clin. Invest. **54**:1011, 1974.
598. Ferenczy, A., and Richart, R.M.: Scanning electron microscopic study of normal and molar trophoblast, Gynecol. Oncol. **1**:95, 1972.
599. Finn, J.L.: Placenta membranacea, Obstet. Gynecol. **3**:438, 1954.
600. Froehlich, L.A., and Fujikura, T.: Follow-up of infants with single umbilical artery, Pediatrics **52**:6, 1973.
601. Gagnon, R.A.: Transplacental inoculation of fatal herpes simplex in the newborn: report of two cases, Obstet. Gynecol. **31**:682, 1968.

602. Gartner, A., Larsson, L.-I., and Sjoberg, N.-O.: Immunohistochemical demonstration of chorionic gonadotropin in trophoblastic tumors, Acta Obstet. Gynecol. Scand. **54**:161, 1975.
603. Gleicher, X., et al.: Common aspects of immunologic tolerance in pregnancy and malignancy, Obstet. Gynecol. **54**:335, 1979.
604. Goldstein, D.P.: Prophylactic chemotherapy of patients with molar pregnancy, Obstet. Gynecol. **38**:817, 1971.
605. Goldstein, D.P., et al.: Rapid solid-phase radioimmunoassay specific for human chorionic gonadotropin in gestational trophoblastic disease, Obstet. Gynecol. **45**:527, 1975.
606. Gruenwald, P.: The placenta and its maternal supply line, Baltimore, 1975, University Park Press.
607. Hammond, C.B., et al.: Treatment of metastatic trophoblastic disease: good and poor prognosis, Am. J. Obstet. Gynecol. **115**:451, 1973.
608. Haust, M.D.: Maternal diabetes mellitus: effects on the fetus and placenta. In Naeye, R.L., Kissane, J.M., and Kaufman, N., editors: Perinatal diseases, Baltimore, 1981, The Williams & Wilkins Co.
609. Hawick, H.J., et al.: *Mycoplasma hominis* septicemia associated with abortion, Am. J. Obstet. Gynecol. **99**:715, 1967.
610. Hellman, L.M., and Hertig, A.T.: Pathologic changes in the placenta associated with erythroblastosis of the fetus, Am. J. Pathol. **14**:111, 1938.
611. Hertig, A.T.: Vascular pathology on the hypertensive albuminuric toxemias of pregnancy, Clinics **4**:602, 1945 (quoted by Robertson, Brosens, and Dixon[653]).
612. Hertig, A.T.: Human trophoblast, Springfield, Ill. 1968, Charles C Thomas, Publisher.
613. Herva, R., et al.: Cluster of severe amniotic adhesion malformations in Finland, Lancet **1**:818, 1980.
614. Heyderman, E., Gibbons, A.R., and Rosen, S.W.: Immunoperoxidase localization of human placental lactogen: a marker for the placental origin of the giant cells in "syncytial endometritis" of pregnancy, J. Clin. Pathol. **34**:303, 1981.
615. Hibbard, B.M., and Jeffcoate, T.N.A.: Abruptio placentae, Obstet. Gynecol. **27**:155, 1966.
616. Higginbottom, M.C., et al.: The amniotic band disruption complex: timing of amniotic rupture, and variable spectra of consequent defects, J. Pediatr. **95**:544, 1977.
617. Horne, H.W., et al.: Subclinical endometrial inflammation and T-mycoplasma: a possible cause of human reproductive failure, Int. J. Fertil. **18**:226, 1973.
618. Hreschchyshyn, M.M., Bozen, B., and Loughran, C.H.: What is actual present-day management of the placenta in late abdominal pregnancy? Analysis of 101 cases, Am. J. Obstet. Gynecol. **81**:302, 1961.
619. Hulka, J., and Mohr, K.: Trophoblast antigenicity as demonstrated by altered challene graft survival, Science **161**:696, 1968.
620. Irving, F.C., and Hertig, A.T.: A study of placenta accreta, Surg. Gynecol. Obstet. **64**:178, 1937.
621. Jacobson, F.J., and Enzen, N.: Hydatidiform mole with "benign" metastasis to lung: histological evidence of regressing lesion in lung, Am. J. Obstet. Gynecol. **78**:868, 1959.
622. Jaffe, R.B.: The endocrinology of pregnancy. In Yen, S.C., and Jaffe, R.B., editors: Reproductive endocrinology, Philadelphia, 1978, W.B. Saunders Co.
623. Jaffe, R.B., Lee, P.A., and Midgley, A.R.: Serum gonadotropins before, at the inception of, and following human pregnancy, J. Clin. Endocrinol. **29**:1281, 1969.
624. Kajii, T., and Oyama, K.: Androgenic origin of hydatidiform mole, Nature **268**:633, 1977.
625. Kaye, M.D., and Jones, W.R.: Effect of human chorionic gonadotropin on in vitro lymphocyte transformation, Am. J. Obstet. Gynecol. **109**:1029, 1971.
626. Khudr, G., et al.: Trophoblastic origin of the X cell and the placental site giant cell, Am. J. Obstet. Gynecol. **115**:530, 1973.
627. Kitzmiller, J.L., and Benirschke, K.: Immunofluorescent study of placental bed vessels in pre-eclampsia of pregnancy, Am. J. Obstet. Gynecol. **115**:248, 1973.
628. Kurman, R.J., Scully, R.E., and Norris, H.J.: Trophoblastic pseudotumor of the uterus: an exaggerated form of "syncytial endometritis" simulating a malignant tumor, Cancer **38**:1214, 1976.
629. Luke, R.K., Sharpe, J.W., and Greene, R.R.: Placenta accreta: the adherent or invasive placenta, Am. J. Obstet. Gynecol. **95**:660, 1966.
630. Marshall, J.R., et al.: Plasma and urinary chorionic gonadotropin during early human pregnancy, Obstet. Gynecol. **32**:760, 1968.
631. Mazur, M.T., Lurain, J.R., and Brewer, J.I.: Fatal gestational choriocarcinoma: clinicopathologic study of patients treated at a trophoblastic disease center, Cancer **50**:1833, 1982.
632. McConnell, H.D., and Carr, D.H.: Recent advances in the cytogenetic study of human spontaneous abortions, Obstet. Gynecol. **45**:547, 1975.
633. McCord, J.R.: Syphilis of the placenta; the histologic examination of 1,085 placentas of mothers with strongly positive blood Wassermann reactions, Am. J. Obstet. Gynecol. **28**:743, 1934.
634. McKay, D.G., et al.: Experimental eclampsia: an electron microscope study and review, Arch. Pathol. **84**:557, 1967.
635. Monif, G.R.G.: Infectious diseases in obstetrics and gynecology, New York, 1974, Harper & Row, Publishers, Inc.
636. Monif, G.R.G., and Dische, R.M.: Viral placentitis in congenital cytomegalovirus infections, Am. J. Clin. Pathol. **58**:445, 1972.
637. Naib, Z.M., et al.: Association of maternal genital herpetic infection with spontaneous abortion, Obstet. Gynecol. **35**:260, 1970.
638. Naughton, M.A., et al.: Localization of the B chain of human chorionic gonadotropin on human tumor cells and placental cells, Cancer Res. **35**:1887, 1975.
639. Nelson, D.M., et al.: The non-uniform distribution of acidic components on the human placental syncytial trophoblast surface membrane: a cytochemical and analytical study, Anat. Rec. **184**:15, 1976.
640. Ornoy, A., et al.: Fetal and placental pathology in gestational rubella, Am. J. Obstet. Gynecol. **116**:949, 1973.
641. Page, E.W.: The pathogenesis of pre-eclampsia and eclampsia, J. Obstet. Gynaecol. Br. Cwlth. **9**:883, 1972.
642. Park, W.W.: Choriocarcinoma, Philadelphia, 1971, F.A. Davis Co.
643. Park, W.W.: Possible function of nonvillous trophoblast. In Brosens, I.A., Dixon, G., and Robertson, W.B., editors: Human placentation, Amsterdam, 1975, Excerpta Medica.
644. Peterson, E.P., and Taylor, H.B.: Amniotic fluid embolism; an analysis of 40 cases, Obstet. Gynecol. **35**:787, 1970.
645. Philippe, E.: Morphologic et morphometrie des placentas d'abberation chromosomique lethale, Rev. Fr. Gynecol. **68**:645, 1973.
646. Philippe, E.: Histopathologie placentaire, Paris, 1974, Masson et Cie.
647. Philippe, E., et al.: Endometre et sequelles d'avortement, Rev. Fr. Gynecol. **65**:413, 1970.
648. Poland, B.J., Dill, F.J., and Styblo, C.: Embryonic development in ectopic human pregnancy, Teratology **14**:315, 1976.
649. Ramsey, E.M., Corner, G.W., and Donner, M.W.: Serial and cineradiographic visualization of maternal circulation in the primate (hemochorial) placenta, Am. J. Obstet. Gynecol. **86**:213, 1963.
650. Rappaport, F., et al.: Genital listeriosis as a cause of repeated abortion, Lancet **1**:1273, 1960.
651. Rewell, R.E., and Whitehouse, W.L.: Malignant metastasis to the placenta from carcinoma of the breast, J. Pathol. **91**:255, 1966.
652. Reynolds, D.W., et al.: Maternal cytomegalovirus excretion and perinatal infection, N. Engl. J. Med. **289**:1, 1973.
653. Robertson, W.B., Brosens, I.A., and Dixon, G.: Uteroplacental vascular pathology. In Brosens, I.A., Dixon, G., and Robertson, W.B., editors: Human placentation, Amsterdam, 1975, Excerpta Medica.
654. Roche, W.D., Jr., and Norris, H.J.: Detection and significance of maternal pulmonary amniotic fluid embolism, Obstet. Gynecol. **43**:729, 1974.
655. Rocklin, E., et al.: Absence of an immunologic blocking factor from the serum of women with chronic abortions, N. Engl. J. Med. **295**:1209, 1976.
656. Rotheram, E.B., and Schick, S.F.: Nonclostridial anaerobic bacteria in septic abortion, Am. J. Med. **46**:80, 1969.
657. Sander, C.: Hemorrhagic endovasculitis and hemorrhagic villitis of the placenta, Arch. Pathol. Lab. Med. **104**:371, 1980.

658. Schneider, J., Berger, C.J., and Cattell, C.: Maternal mortality due to ectopic pregnancy: a review of 102 deaths, Obstet. Gynecol. **49**:557, 1977.
659. Scott, J.S.: Placenta extrachorialis (placenta marginata and placenta circumvallata); a factor in antepartum hemorrhage, J. Obstet. Gynaecol. Br. Cwlth. **67**:904, 1960.
660. Scully, R.E., and Young, R.H.: Trophoblastic pseudotumor: a reappraisal, Am. J. Surg. Pathol. **5**:75, 1981.
661. Seeliger, H.P.R.: Some new aspects of human listeriosis. In Human listeriosis: its nature and diagnosis, Atlanta, 1957, U.S. Department of Health, Education, and Welfare, Communicable Disease Center.
662. Shanklin, D.R., and Scott, J.S.: Massive subchorial thrombohaematoma (Breus' mole), Br. J. Obstet. Gynecol. **82**:476, 1975.
663. Shanklin, D.R., and Sotel-Avila, C.: The pathogenesis and significance of placenta extrachorialis, Lab. Invest. **15**:1111, 1966.
664. Shurin, P.A., et al.: Chorioamnionitis and colonization of the newborn infant with genital mycoplasma, N. Engl. J. Med. **293**:5, 1975.
665. Steigrad, S.J., James, R.W., and Osborn, R.A.: Choriocarcinoma with intact pregnancy, Aust. N.Z. J. Obstet. Gynaecol. **8**:79, 1968.
666. Szulman, A.E., et al.: Human triploidy: association with partial hydatidiform moles and nonmolar conceptuses, Hum. Pathol. **12**:1016, 1981.
667. Taylor, H.B., and Peterson, E.P.: Amniotic fluid embolism: an analysis of 40 cases, Obstet. Gynecol. **35**:787, 1970.
668. Teteris, N.J., Lina, A.A., and Holaday, W.J.: Placenta percreta, Obstet. Gynecol. **47**(suppl.):15s, 1976.
669. Thomson, A.M., et al.: The weight of placenta in relation to birthweight, J. Obstet. Gynaecol. Br. Cwlth. **76**:865, 1969.
670. Tominaga, T., and Page, E.W.: Sex chromatin of trophoblastic tumors, Am. J. Obstet. Gynecol. **96**:305, 1966.
671. Vaitukaitis, J.L.: Human chorionic gonadotropin as a tumor marker, Ann. Clin. Lab. Sci. **4**:276, 1974.
672. Vaitukaitis, J.L., Braunstain, G.D., and Ross, G.T.: A radioimmunoassay which specifically measures human chorionic gonadotropin in the presence of human luteinizing hormone, Am. J. Obstet. Gynecol. **113**:751, 1972.
673. Villee, D.B.: Development of endocrine function in the human placenta and fetus, N. Engl. J. Med. **281**:473, 1969.
674. Wallenburg, H.C.S.: Chorioangioma of the placenta: 13 new cases and a review of the literature from 1939 to 1970 with special reference to the clinical complications, Obstet. Gynecol. Surv. **26**:411, 1971.
675. Wilson, C.B., and Remington, J.S.: What can be done to prevent congenital toxoplasmosis? Am. J. Obstet. Gynecol. **138**:357, 1980.
676. Wilson, C.B., et al.: Development of adverse sequelae in children born with subclinical congenital *Toxoplasma* infection, Pediatrics **66**:767, 1980.
677. Wynn, R.M.: Noncellular components of the placenta, Am. J. Obstet. Gynecol. **103**:723, 1969.
678. Wynn, R.M.: Cytotrophoblastic specializations: an ultrastructural study of the human placenta, Am. J. Obstet. Gynecol. **114**:339, 1972.
679. Wynn, R.M., and Harris, J.A.: Ultrastructure of trophoblast and endometrium in invasive hydatidiform mole (chorioadenoma destruens), Am. J. Obstet. Gynecol. **99**:1125, 1967.

CHAPTER 37 Breast

ROBERT W. McDIVITT

Breast disease is less varied than diseases of many other organs in that it is predominantly neoplastic. Congenital anomalies of the breast are uncommon and usually only of cosmetic interest. Inflammatory disease for the most part is limited to mastitis caused by staphylococci or streptococci during pregnancy and lactation. Metabolic disease consists primarily of secondary changes in the breast produced by estrogen and androgen therapy or by abnormalities in the production of these hormones. The symptomatology of breast disease also tends to be uncomplicated. Most breast disease produces a palpable mass unaccompanied by other symptoms.

In view of these facts, one may conclude that were neoplastic disease of the breast not so important both as a public health problem and in providing day-to-day medical care, little attention would be devoted to diseases of the breast in relation to other medical subjects. However, breast disease is extremely common. It is estimated that breast cancer will develop in 1 of every 22 women in the United States and that it accounts for approximately 30,000 deaths in this country each year.[49] Therefore breast disease is an important aspect of every physician's life, regardless of the specialty he or she practices.

This chapter presents an introductory view of the pathology of breast disease and its importance in patient care. Although morphology is emphasized, no attempt to be encyclopedic has been made, since several excellent texts describing the pathology of breast disease are available.[8,44] Instead, the role of morphology as it is related to the epidemiology, natural history, and treatment of breast diseases is emphasized.

STRUCTURE AND FUNCTION

The breast is a modified skin appendage that lies superficial to the deep pectoral fascia and the pectoralis major and minor muscles. Its major lymphatic drainage is into the lymph nodes of the ipsilateral axilla. Secondary lymphatic drainage is medial into lymph nodes of the internal mammary chain that lies subjacent to the sternum. The breast is divided into a dozen or more poorly defined lobes, each having its own ramifying collecting duct system that empties into a lactiferous sinus subjacent to the nipple. As the collecting ducts extend out into the breast lobe from the lactiferous sinus, they branch several times, each branching producing ducts of progressively smaller diameter. The collecting duct system terminates peripherally in a myriad of breast lobules, the secretory units of the breast during lactation (Fig. 37-1). Each lobule is comprised of between six and 20 small terminal ducts invested in loose areolar connective tissue.

The breast lobules and the collecting duct system comprise the epithelial portion of the breast, which in the mature breast accounts for less than 10% of its total volume. The lobules and collecting ducts are surrounded and supported by large quantities of connective tissue that give the breast its form and shape. In young women this connective tissue is predominantly fibrous, but as women age, it is gradually replaced by fat. The terminal ducts comprising breast lobules are lined by a single layer of low cuboidal epithelium, as are many of the smaller ramifications of the collecting duct system. Larger collecting ducts at times appear to have a double-layered epithelial lining, as do the lactiferous sinuses. The portion of lactiferous sinuses nearest the surface of the nipple is lined by squamous epithelium. In addition to epithelial cells, myoepithelial cells may occasionally be seen in histologic sections of collecting ducts of intermediate size. These elongated cells with small, flattened nuclei are immediately adjacent to the duct basement membrane. They are arranged around intermediate-sized ducts in a spiral fashion and are thought to assist in the propulsion of milk to the external surface of the nipple.

The various operative procedures performed on the breast are best understood in terms of breast anatomy. In a simple or total mastectomy the breast is removed along with the nipple, overlying skin, and subcutaneous tissue,

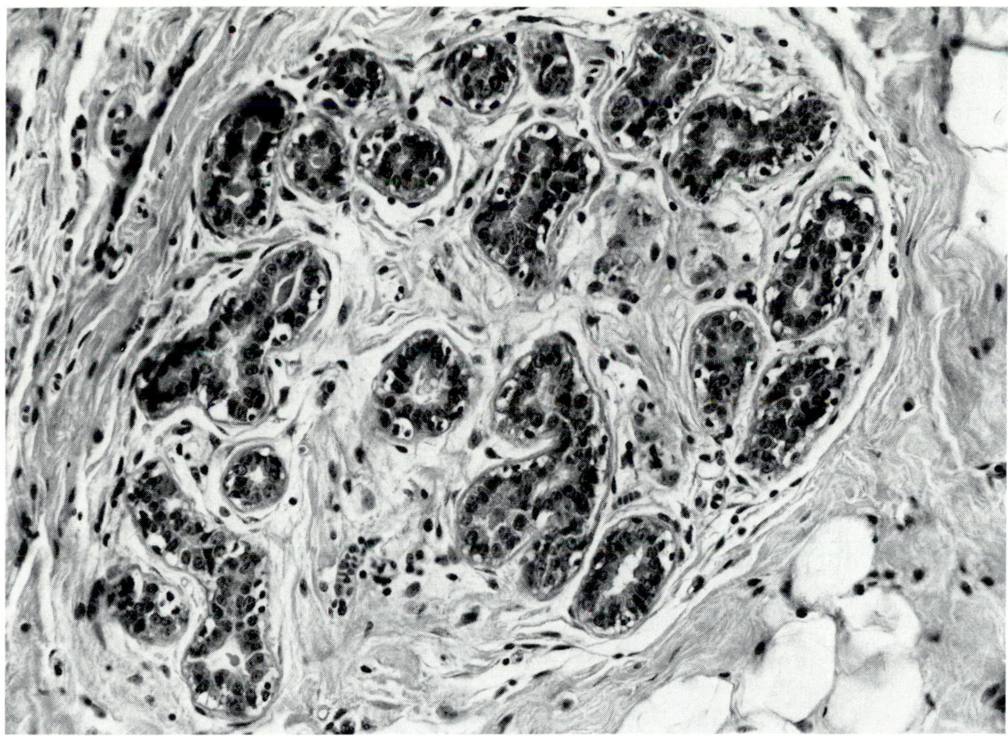

Fig. 37-1. Normal breast lobule. Terminal ducts are surrounded by loose areolar connective tissue demarcating lobule from adjacent stroma. Terminal ducts are lined by single layer of cuboidal epithelium.

but the axilla or underlying pectoral muscles and fascia are not disturbed. In a subcutaneous mastectomy the breast is removed, and an attempt is made to preserve the overlying skin, subcutaneous tissue, and nipple. However, in subcutaneous mastectomy, residual breast tissue usually is left behind. In a modified radical mastectomy removal of ipsilateral axillary lymph nodes is accomplished in combination with simple mastectomy. The number of axillary lymph nodes removed in a modified radical mastectomy and the extent of the axillary dissection depend on the operative approach and vary in accordance with the disease being treated and the philosophy of the surgeon. In a radical mastectomy the breast along with overlying skin and nipple, the underlying pectoralis muscles, fascia, and ipsilateral axillary lymph nodes are removed. In an extended radical mastectomy a portion of the chest wall and the subjacent internal mammary lymph nodes are removed in combination with radical mastectomy. An operation that removes a palpable breast lesion along with a margin of grossly normal surrounding breast tissue is referred to as an excisional biopsy. An operation that removes an entire breast quadrant is called a quadrantectomy.

BENIGN BREAST DISEASE

The following outline lists the common benign diseases of the breast:

1. Common benign breast lesions
   a. Cystic disease
   b. Sclerosing adenosis
   c. Fibroadenoma
   d. Mammary duct ectasia
   e. Intraductal papilloma
   f. Epithelial hyperplasia involving lobules
   g. Epithelial hyperplasia involving larger ducts
2. Less common benign breast lesions
   a. Granular cell tumor
   b. Gynecomastia (male)
   c. Juvenile mammary hypertrophy
   d. Lactational mastitis

Although breast disease in children and adult men is much less common than in adult women, a similar spectrum of benign disease is observed, with the exception of epithelial proliferative lesions involving lobules. (In children and in men the lobular apparatus is undeveloped except under unusual circumstances.) Both benign breast disease and carcinoma may occur in adult women of all ages, but benign breast disease tends to occur more commonly in younger women and carcinoma in women who are somewhat older, that is, in the fourth decade extending through the menopausal era. However, there is sufficient overlap in the age distribution of benign and malignant diseases of the breast that age alone cannot be used to predict the nature of any given lesion. Although the incidence of benign breast disease in different populations throughout the world is difficult to estimate, in teaching hospitals in the United States approximately 70% of all breast biopsies performed are interpreted as benign and the remainder are malignant.

Cystic disease

Cystic disease is the most frequent benign breast disease of adult women. Haagensen[28] estimates that about 10% of adult women in the United States have symptomatic fibrocystic disease. Franz and associates[24] in an autopsy study of women with no history of breast disease have found grossly visible cystic disease in about 20%. Although cystic disease in women in the third and fourth decades of life is not unusual, its peak incidence is in women in the fifth decade. The incidence drops dramatically with menopause, suggesting that the cause of cystic disease may somehow be related to estrogen production. Women with this disease usually have a freely movable, palpable mass unassociated with other physical findings or symptoms. However, at times it may cause pain, particularly when women are in the premenstrual phase of the menstrual cycle. The palpable lesion may appear to increase and decrease in size cyclically, usually achieving its maximum size in the premenstrual phase of the menstrual cycle.

Pathologic findings

The characteristic gross pathologic finding is cysts of varying size that are filled with clear or serosanguineous fluid (Plate 6, *A*). The cysts may be solitary or multiple, discrete or multiloculated, and so small as to be almost invisible grossly or 5 to 6 cm in diameter. Ordinarily these cysts are surrounded by rather dense fibrous connective tissue, the normal stromal component of younger women's breasts. The cysts usually are lined with a single or double layer of cuboidal epithelium, although the epithelial lining of larger cysts may be somewhat atrophic and less conspicuous (Fig. 37-2). At times the basement membrane is focally disrupted by dissection of cyst contents out into the adjacent breast stroma, inducing a chronic inflammatory reaction. This may be accompanied by cholesterol clefts and multinucleated giant cells.

Pathogenesis

Although these cysts ordinarily are thought to arise from obstructed collecting ducts, some authors have suggested that smaller cysts may be of lobular origin.[8,62,82] The mechanism of duct obstruction is not clearly understood. Some authors have suggested that localized epithelial hyperplasia may produce duct obstruction, although this is difficult to document in histologic sections.[25] Others suggest that duct obstruction is caused by periductal fibrosis resulting from inspissation and extrusion of duct contents into the adjacent stroma with secondary inflammation and fibrosis. Some suggest that it is caused by an overgrowth of connective tissue produced by estrogen stimulation.[28] Although most cysts are surrounded by varying amounts of dense fibrous connective tissue, this is a normal stromal component of the mature breast.

Natural history

Most women who have one or more cysts excised from their breasts may expect that additional cysts will appear from time to time until menopause, when the process appears to abate. The question of whether cystic disease increases the risk of subsequent breast cancer has attracted considerable interest. Although some articles have reported an increased breast cancer risk associated with fibrocystic disease, this is probably a false conclusion based on misuse of the pathologic term.[39,46] Cystic disease is frequently accompanied by varying degrees of epithelial hyperplasia in adjacent ducts and lobules. In the past pathologists tended to lump together these two dissimilar disease processes under the single designation "cystic disease", not realizing the precancerous significance of epithelial hyperplastic lesions of the breast. However, several recent pathologic studies have shown that, whereas some types of epithelial hyperplasia are associated with a significant increase in subsequent breast cancer risk, cystic disease itself is not.[14,36,58]

Sclerosing adenosis

Sclerosing adenosis is a benign overgrowth of lobular epithelium, myoepithelium, and stromal connective tissue. Its main importance is that it may be confused with carcinoma by both surgeons and pathologists. It is a common lesion in women during the reproductive years. In most cases involving sclerosing adenosis, a nonpalpable microscopic finding is identified in breast tissue excised for some other reason, usually cystic disease. However, at times sclerosing adenosis may become florid and produce a palpable mass that may mimic carcinoma of the breast both clinically and grossly. On gross pathologic examination, sclerosing adenosis may be firm, white, and stellate although usually not as rock hard as the ordinary scirrhous carcinoma. It rarely exceeds 2 cm in maximum diameter. The pathologist's problems with identifying sclerosing adenosis are compounded because it also may resemble infiltrating carcinoma of the breast microscopically. However, it differs from carcinoma in that its overall pattern as viewed under the scanning lens is whorled and circumferential, whereas carcinoma tends to be linear and stellate (Fig. 37-3). In addition, in adenosis the epithelium lining the small glands often appears somewhat atrophic, being compressed by overgrowth of adjacent myoepithelium and fibrous breast stroma. Often in sclerosing adenosis, myoepithelial hyperplasia

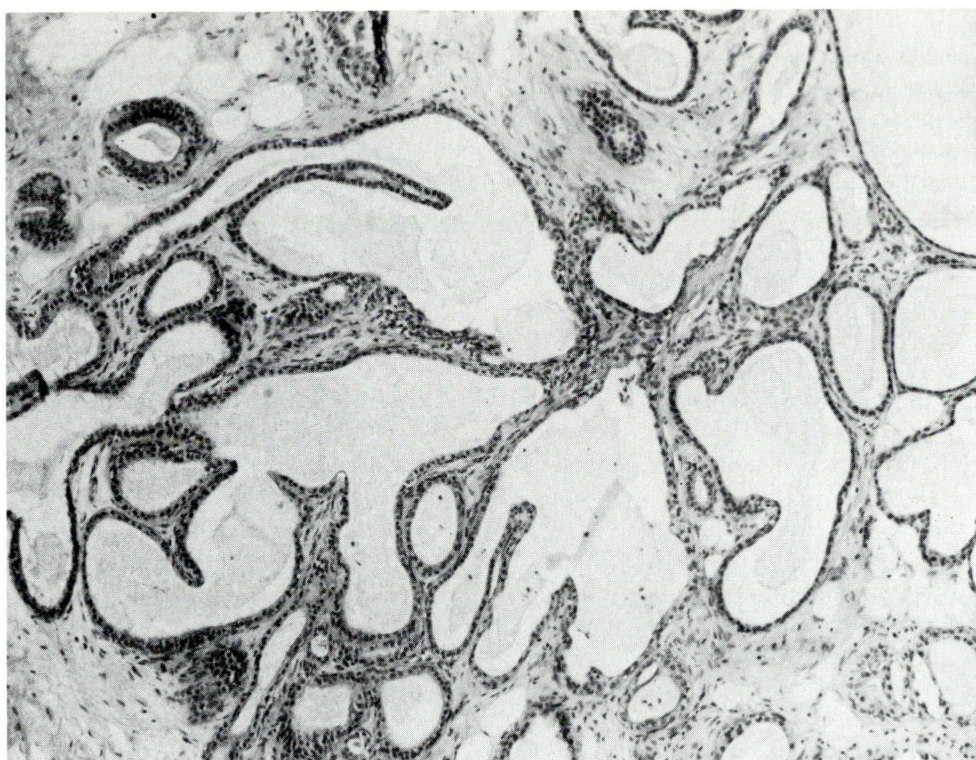

Fig. 37-2. Cystic disease. Numerous ducts are cystically dilated, presumably because of obstruction. They are lined by single layer of flattened, somewhat atrophic epithelium. There is no associated epithelial hyperplasia.

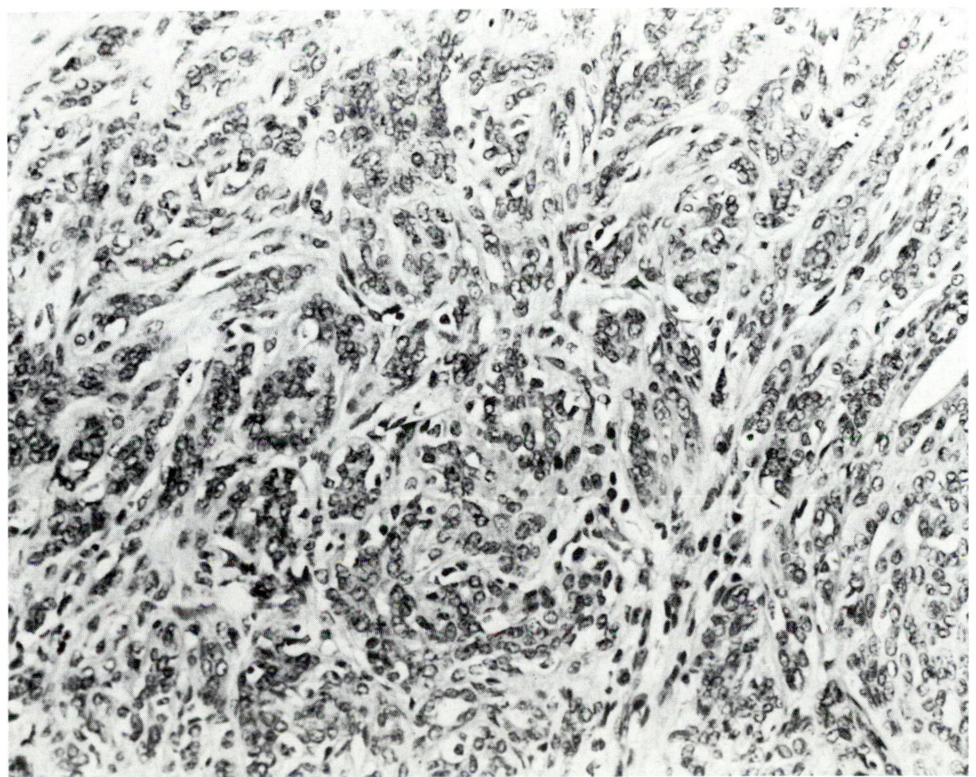

Fig. 37-3. Sclerosing adenosis. Overall pattern is concentric and whorled in contrast to more stellate pattern produced by infiltrating carcinoma. Epithelium appears compressed, and lumina for the most part are absent. Surrounding myoepithelium, which appears homogeneous and dark gray, is prominent.

is exuberant, and identification of the rather intensely eosinophilic myoepithelium also aids in differential diagnosis. The cause of sclerosing adenosis is unknown. It is of no known clinical significance, except for its propensity to be confused with breast carcinoma.

Fibroadenoma

Fibroadenoma is a benign overgrowth of periductal stromal connective tissue that tends to compress the entrapped ducts and produce a well-circumscribed or encapsulated mass. Its incidence is less evenly distributed throughout the reproductive years than that of either sclerosing adenosis or cystic disease. It is a disease predominantly of young women and is the most common cause of a palpable breast mass in women younger than 30 years of age.[28] Clinically, fibroadenomas usually are well circumscribed, freely movable lesions that in most patients are correctly identified preoperatively. In addition, their mammographic appearance is usually quite distinct.

Pathologic findings

On gross pathologic examination fibroadenomas appear as well-circumscribed, spherical lesions that are well demarcated from the surrounding breast stroma (Plate 6, *B*). They vary in size from barely perceptible gross lesions to lesions 15 cm or more in diameter. Their size depends both on their growth rate and on their duration before excision. Blunt dissection may be used to "shell out" fibroadenomas from the adjacent breast tissue. However, they often have small irregular bosselated projections on their external surface that may be amputated by the enucleation procedure. This explains why fibroadenomas may recur locally if enucleated rather than being excised with an adequate margin of adjacent breast tissue. The cut surface of fibroadenomas is firm, rubbery, and light gray. Often the slitlike spaces formed by compressed ducts are obvious grossly. Microscopically, fibroadenomas are easily recognized. Long, attenuated, and compressed ducts lined by a single or double layer of epithelium are surrounded by fibrous connective tissue and stroma (Fig. 37-4).

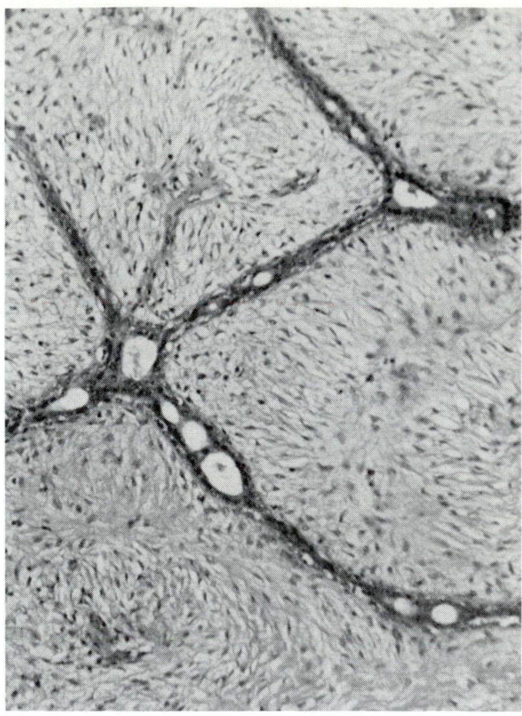

Fig. 37-4. Fibroadenoma. Anastomosing, epithelium-lined intralobar ducts are compressed into slitlike spaces by proliferation of surrounding stromal connective tissue. Stromal cells show no pleomorphism and few mitoses.

Fibroadenoma in pregnancy

During pregnancy fibroadenomas may grow rapidly and become relatively large over a short period of time, perhaps because of hormone stimulation. At times during a rapid growth phase they may partially or totally infarct, causing acute localized pain in the breast. Infarcted fibroadenomas not removed at this time usually become densely hyalinized and irregularly calcified, producing a distinct mammographic and histologic appearance. During pregnancy fibroadenomas also may assume a histologic appearance different from that of the ordinary fibroadenoma. The lobular epithelium may be sufficiently overgrown to produce a fibroadenoma that appears densely glandular. This epithelium also usually participates in the secretory activity that occurs elsewhere in the breast, giving the fibroadenoma a distinct appearance. Fibroadenomas of this type at times have been designated lactational adenomas.

Carcinoma in fibroadenomas

Rarely do fibroadenomas contain either in situ or invasive carcinoma of duct or lobular origin.[43] At times carcinomas arise from the epithelium contained in the fibroadenoma; in other cases carcinoma is found to have invaded the fibroadenoma from a primary site in the adjacent breast.

Cystosarcoma phyllodes

The term *cystosarcoma phyllodes* was introduced by Muller in 1838 to describe fibroadenoma-like lesions that pursue an aggressive clinical course with local chest wall recurrence or distant metastases.[48] On microscopic examination the stroma of these aggressive tumors appears histologically malignant, explaining the clinical course. In the past, some confusion has been caused by the use of the term *cystosarcoma phyllodes* to describe benign fibroadenomas that are unusually large or that have stroma displaying a modest increase in cellularity. Preferably such lesions are designated *giant fibroadeno-*

ma and *cellular fibroadenoma,* respectively, reserving the term *cystosarcoma phyllodes* to describe lesions with the potential for aggressive behavior. Cystosarcoma phyllodes is an uncommon tumor of the breast. Treves and Sunderland[77] found only 18 malignant cystosarcomas during a 20-year breast clinic experience at Memorial Hospital in New York. Haagensen[28] states that they comprise about 2% to 3% of fibroadenoma-like lesions seen in the breast clinic at Columbia Presbyterian Hospital in New York. Their clinical presentation is much like that of fibroadenoma. They tend to be totally or partially encapsulated and vary in size from less than 1 cm in diameter to giant lesions that occupy most of the breast.[44] When large, they may ulcerate the skin and become fixed to the underlying chest wall.

Pathologic findings. On gross inspection cystosarcoma phyllodes differs little from fibroadenoma except that it has a greater tendency to show local hemorrhage and necrosis and to become cystic. In addition, the lesion may appear less fully encapsulated with focal areas where the tumor appears to invade the adjacent breast stroma. Microscopically cystosarcoma phyllodes differs from fibroadenoma in that the stroma is more cellular, it displays more cellular pleomorphism, and the stromal cells have an increased mitotic rate. The epithelial portion of the tumor is benign and similar to that of fibroadenoma. In current pathologic practice cystosarcoma phyllodes is divided into two types, those that histologically appear fully malignant (capable of metastasis) and those assigned to a borderline malignant category because it is less clear from histologic examination of the stroma whether the tumor will pursue an aggressive course.[30,31] The stroma of tumors assigned to the fully malignant category displays the characteristics of some other recognized type of sarcoma, such as fibrosarcoma or liposarcoma; in addition eight or more mitotic figures per 10 high-power fields are usually seen. Lesions assigned to the borderline category have less pleomorphism, are less cellular, and have lower mitotic rates. The tendency for malignant cystosarcoma to metastasize appears to depend on size. Overall, approximately 10% of malignant cystosarcomas produce metastases. Metastases usually are first observed in the lungs, although bone and visceral metastases also occur.[35] Regional lymph node metastases also may occur, but this usually happens relatively late in the course of the disease subsequent to or concurrent with pulmonary metastasis. Metastatic lesions show only sarcomatous stroma, not the benign epithelial component of cystosarcoma phyllodes. Cystosarcomas of the borderline histologic type rarely metastasize and usually do so only after having recurred locally one or more times. It is difficult for pathologists to predict from histologic examination which borderline cystosarcomas will produce distant metastases.

Mammary duct ectasia

Mammary duct ecstasia is important primarily because it may be confused clinically with carcinoma. It is cured by simple excision. A disease of older women, it is most common among multiparous women who have nursed their children. It affects the larger collecting ducts subjacent to the nipple and may produce a palpable mass and nipple discharge. The pathogenesis of the lesion is not clearly understood. On gross examination, multiple dilated ducts containing inspissated secretions are seen surrounded by varying amounts of dense fibrous connective tissue. By compressing the gross specimen, inspissated secretion may be expressed from the ducts, a feature that led to the older designation "comedomastitis." Microscopically the ectatic ducts appear to be lined by atrophic epithelium, and their lumina are filled with amorphous debris. The periductal tissue may show rather intense chronic inflammation with scattered foreign body–type giant cells that have phagocytosed cholesterol debris. In addition, the periductal stroma often shows dense fibrosis. This periductal chronic inflammation and fibrosis are thought to be a reaction to leakage of the inspissated duct secretion into the adjacent tissues.

Benign intraductal papilloma

Pedunculated papillary proliferations comprised of a branching central fibrovascular core that is covered externally by one or more layers of epithelium may extend out from the duct walls into the duct lumen. Intraductal papillomas usually are solitary, most frequently are located in larger ducts near the nipple, and produce serous or serosanguineous nipple discharge as their most common symptom. They vary in size from lesions that are barely perceptible grossly to those measuring 5 cm or more in diameter. When large, they may partially or totally occlude the duct in which they are located and produce a palpable clinical mass. They occur in women of all ages but are most common in the third and fourth decades of life.

Pathologic findings

Large papillomas and their relationship to the duct wall usually are apparent on inspection of the gross specimen. Small papillomas may be more difficult to locate by random sectioning unless the surgeon has marked the duct in which the papilloma is located. If this is done, the duct can be opened along its course and the anatomic relationship between the papilloma and the duct wall is preserved. Small intraductal papillomas usually appear delicate and friable and are attached to the duct wall by a narrow stalk. As papillomas become larger, they tend to become more broadly based, and their anatomic relationship to the duct wall becomes more distorted by fibrosis. Large papillomas frequently contain focal areas

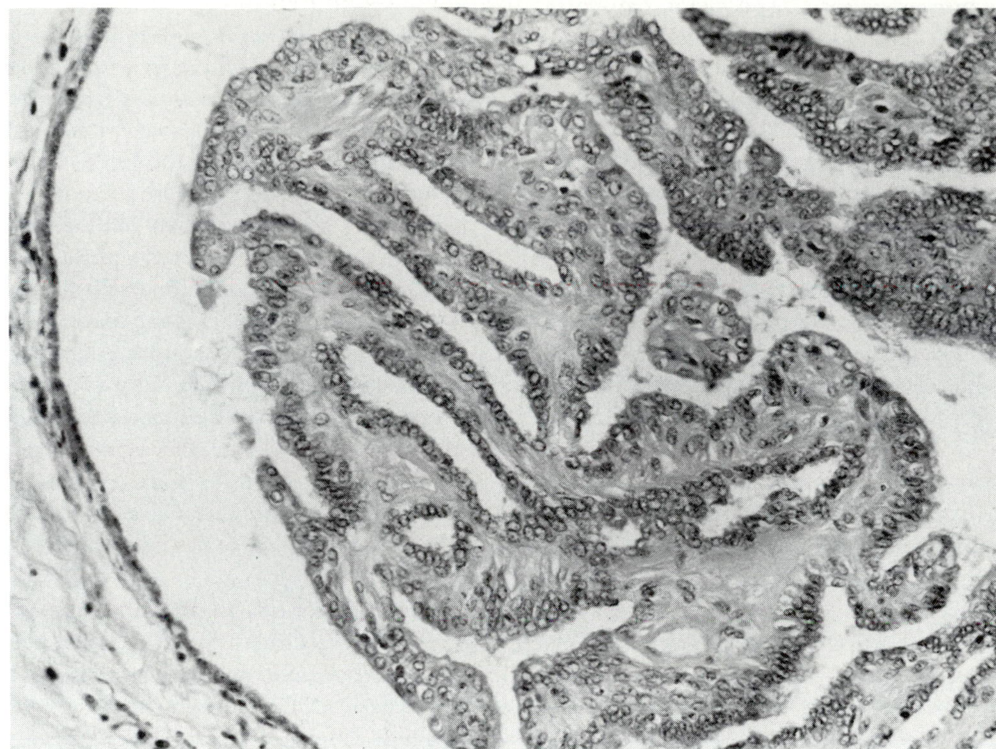

Fig. 37-5. Intraductal papilloma. Central branching fibrovascular stalk is covered by single or double layer of orderly epithelium. Cell polarity is maintained, and there is no epithelial hyperplasia.

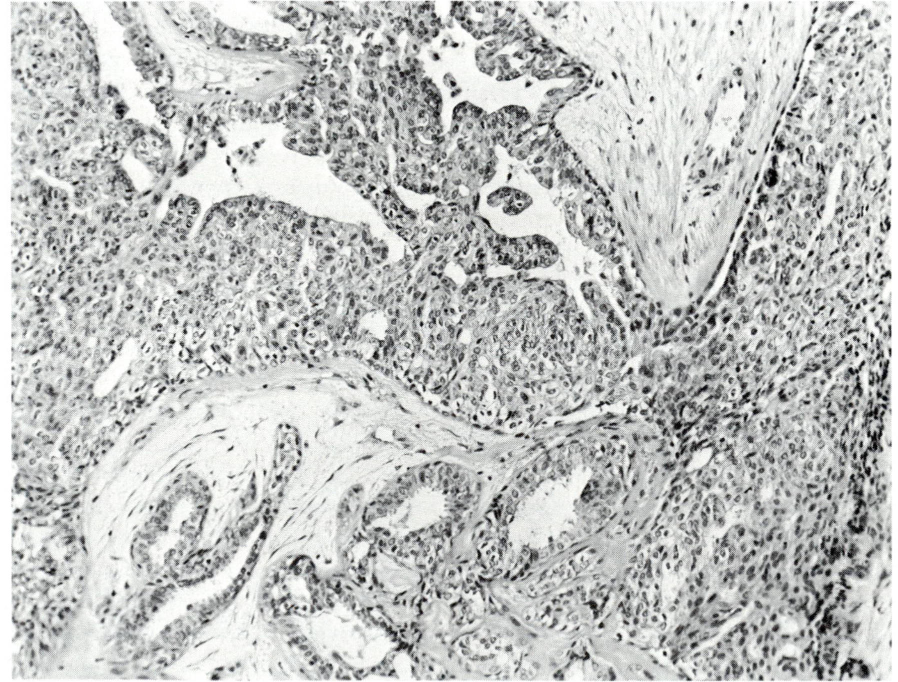

Fig. 37-6. Sclerotic intraductal papilloma. Normal configuration of benign intraductal papilloma has been distorted by dense hyaline connective tissue, trapping small islands of epithelium to produce pseudoinfiltrative appearance.

of hemorrhage and infarction. Intraductal papillomas that occur in the lactiferous sinuses immediately subjacent to the nipple, sometimes referred to as adenomas of the nipple, are often multicentric and may be so distorted by fibrosis that their papillary nature and the relationship of the lesion to the sinuses is not obvious on gross examination.[61,74] Lesions of this type produce a firm, poorly circumscribed mass that may resemble carcinoma grossly. Although fibrosis is most often seen with papillomas in the subareolar location, it may occur with papillomas of the more peripheral portions of the duct system, distorting the relationship of the papilloma with the surrounding tissues in such a way as to suggest carcinoma grossly. As mentioned previously, on microscopic examination the typical benign intraductal papilloma is seen to have a central connective tissue core made up of loose areolar connective tissue and small blood vessels (Fig. 37-5). This central stalk branches in treelike fashion to give the papilloma its characteristic structure. The external surface of this central stalk is covered by epithelium that usually is only one or two layers thick and is arranged along the basement membrane in an orderly fashion. However, at times this relationship is distorted by fibrosis that may result from trauma to the papilloma or from partial duct obstruction with subsequent leakage of duct contents into the adjacent stroma. When this occurs, small nests of epithelium trapped in dense connective tissue give the papilloma a pseudoinfiltrative appearance (Fig. 37-6).

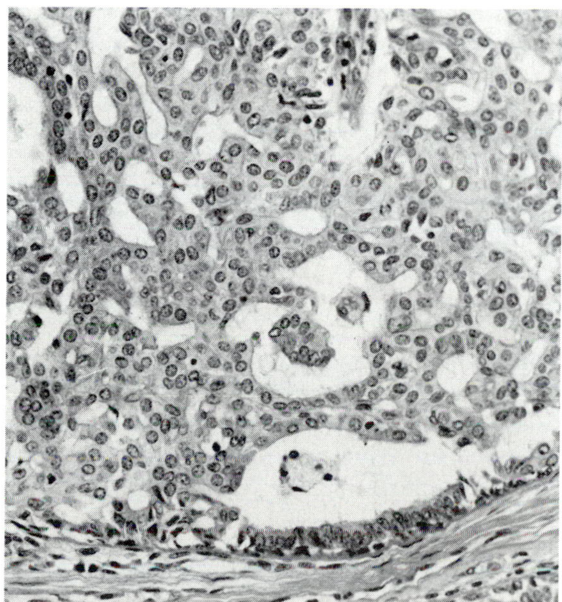

Fig. 37-7. Atypical intraductal epithelial hyperplasia. Proliferating epithelial cells partially fill duct lumen and produce small microglandular spaces that are more irregular in shape than those of intraductal carcinoma. No fibrovascular stroma supports proliferating epithelium. Cell polarity is disrupted, cytoplasmic margins are indistinct, and nuclei are somewhat elongated.

Epithelial proliferative lesions

The epithelium lining the duct system and breast lobules may become hyperplastic independent of any known physiologic stimulus. Epithelial hyperplasia may display varying degrees of atypia (dysplastic changes) such as those described in Chapter 13. Epithelial hyperplasia and dysplasia seem to occur more commonly in the segmental ducts, subsegmental ducts, and terminal ducts comprising lobules than in the larger ramifications of the duct system, although the epithelium that lines all portions of the duct system may participate in these changes.

Although epithelial hyperplasia and dysplasia may occur in women of all ages, including prepubertal girls, its incidence increases in the decades when women are at highest risk of breast cancer.[36,58] Most breast biopsy specimens that contain atypical epithelial hyperplasia are taken from women in the fourth through the sixth decades of life.

The ability of epithelial hyperplasias to produce a mass that can be palpated or appreciated on gross inspection depends primarily on the extent of the proliferative change and secondarily on the portion of the duct system that is involved. Generally, the more peripheral the portion of the duct system involved, the less likely the lesion will be palpable or grossly visible. Because of this, many epithelial hyperplasias and dysplasias are detected first microscopically in the breast biopsy specimens obtained for some other purpose, most commonly because of cystic disease. The microscopic appearance of epithelial hyperplasia and dysplasia also depends to some extent on the portion of the duct system involved. As epithelium proliferates in the small terminal ducts comprising lobules, it may rapidly obliterate their lumina with a solid, sheetlike growth of cells that may distend these small ducts. In larger ducts the solid, sheetlike growth pattern may prevail, or the proliferation may be only partly solid, containing microlumina of varying size and shape (Fig. 37-7). At times in larger ducts the pattern may be more papillary, forming small, cellular projections that extend out from various points along the duct wall. This process differs from benign intraductal papilloma in that a central fibrovascular stalk is absent. In larger ducts the epithelium that covers benign intraductal papillomas may undergo epithelial hyperplastic change, producing a composite pattern of papilloma and epithelial hyperplasia.

The more closely epithelial hyperplasia of the breast resemble in situ carcinoma, the more atypical they are considered. Therefore in terminal ducts the greater the tendency for cells to lose their basilar orientation, develop indistinct cytoplasmic margins, become loosely cohesive, and develop rounded, monomorphous nuclei, the more they are considered atypical (dysplastic). Similar criteria are usually applied to hyperplastic lesions of larger ducts. In this instance, however, credence also is given to the extent to which the overall configuration of the proliferative lesion resembles one of the recognized patterns of in situ carcinoma. Several recent studies have shown that the risk of subsequent breast cancer is two to six times greater in patients whose breast biopsy specimens contained atypical epithelial hyperplastic (dysplastic) lesions than in comparable women.[14,36,58] Epithelial hyperplastic lesions are the only type of benign breast disease that is associated with a significant increase in subsequent breast cancer risk.

Less common benign breast lesions

Granular cell tumor

Granular cell tumor is an uncommon benign breast lesion that nevertheless represents a bête noire for pathologists because it is easily confused with carcinoma on both gross and microscopic examination. In our review of 110 granular cell tumors, six (5%) were located in the breast.[72] In the world literature an additional 100 granular cell tumors of the breast have been reported, but some of these appear to have been located in the overlying skin rather than in the breast itself.[79] Granular cell tumor may produce skin or deep fascial fixation and may otherwise closely simulate the clinical presentation of carcinoma of the breast. Also, the gross appearance of the tumor often is indistinguishable from scirrhous carcinoma. Microscopically about 50% of granular cell tumors appear arranged in a nodular, solid, sheetlike pattern; the remainder more diffusely infiltrate the breast and induce a stromal response similar to that of scirrhous carcinoma. Diffusely infiltrating granular cell tumors are distinguished from carcinoma cytologically. Their cytoplasm contains coarse, intensely eosinophilic granules, and the nuclei are small, round, and densely basophilic.

Gynecomastia

Gynecomastia may produce either a well-circumscribed breast nodule or diffuse enlargement of one or both breasts. The majority of gynecomastia is idiopathic, transient, and seen in pubertal boys and in men in the fifth and sixth decades of life.[76] Most cases of idiopathic gynecomastia are characterized by a disc-shaped, well-localized subareolar mass. Gynecomastia may also result from diseases that alter endocrine function. The most common of these are testicular neoplasms, hepatic cirrhosis, metastatic lung carcinoma, starvation, adrenocortical neoplasms, and exogenous estrogen or androgen therapy. Microscopically the breast ducts show varying degrees of papillary epithelial hyperplasia and are surrounded by a halo of edematous, loose areolar connective tissue. Beyond this halo zone, the intervening breast stroma is densely sclerotic.

Juvenile mammary hypertrophy

Juvenile mammary hypertrophy, which resembles gynecomastia in microscopic appearance, usually affects girls between 10 and 15 years of age.[42] Like gynecomastia, it may be characterized by a localized nodule, usually subareolar, or by diffuse enlargement of one or both breasts. The disease almost always is idiopathic and self-limited, being corrected by further breast development. When the localized form of the disease occurs in a young girl who has not yet undergone breast development, considerable damage may be done to the subareolar breast bud if an attempt is made to excise it. The damage may result later in a malformed, misshapen breast.

CARCINOMA OF THE BREAST

Factors influencing the risk of developing breast carcinoma

About one of every 11 women in the United States will have breast cancer sometime during her lifetime.[49] Breast cancer is diagnosed in approximately 100,000 women in this country each year, accounting for approximately 30% of all cancers in females.[50]

The incidence of breast cancer varies markedly among geographic regions (Fig. 37-8). Many Western European countries and Canada, Australia, and New Zealand have high breast cancer incidence rates similar to those of the United States, some six times greater than those observed in Asia or among black Africans.[81] The rates in South America and Eastern Europe are intermediate between these two extremes. These geographic differences in breast cancer incidence do not appear to be determined by genetic susceptibility. Black American women have incidence rates similar to those of U.S. white women; and Japanese women who have emigrated to Hawaii and California within a generation or two develop the high incidence rates characteristic of American women.[29] Although at present these geographic differences in breast cancer incidence are not fully understood, evidence suggests that they may be related to nutritional differences, particularly to animal fat and cholesterol consumption.[33]

In addition to these geographic differences, other factors within a given population are associated with increased breast cancer risk. Women who have menarche at an early age,[32] who have menopause relatively late in life,[75] who have their first full-term delivery at a late age, or who are nulliparous[38] have an increased breast cancer risk. It is also increased among women who consume large amounts of fat and high-calorie foods,[6,21] women who use exogenous estrogens for a prolonged period of time at menopause,[34] and women who have a family history of breast cancer.[2,4] For example, women who have menarche before 12 years of age have been estimated to have a 2.8-fold increased risk compared with those who have menarche at 14 years or older.[32] Women who have their first full-term delivery before 20 years of age have about one half the breast cancer risk of nulliparous women.[38] The familial effect on breast cancer incidence is particularly striking in women whose breast cancer occurs at an early age or who have had bilateral

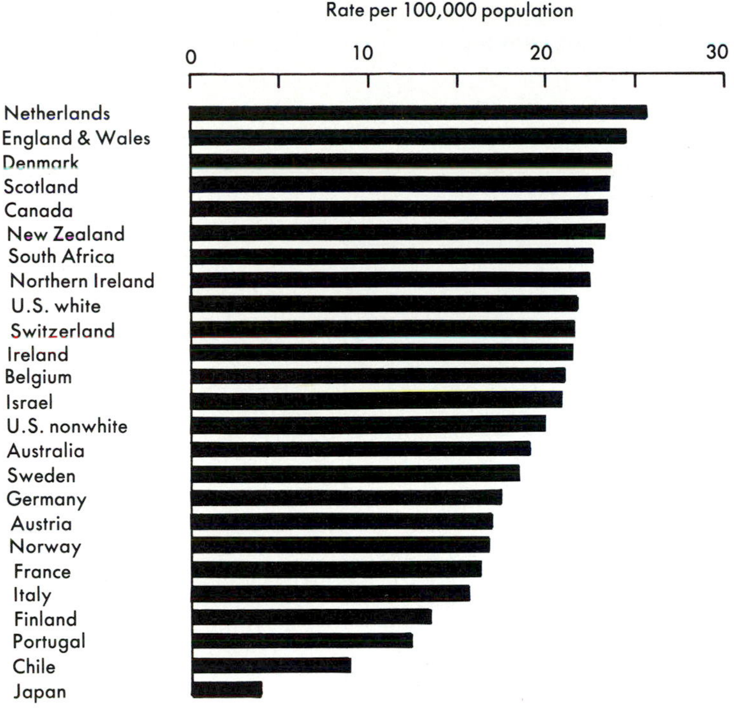

Fig. 37-8. Variation in age-adjusted death rates for breast cancer by country (1964-1965). (Modified from Segi, M. In Haagensen, C.D.: Diseases of the breast, Philadelphia, 1971, W.B. Saunders Co.)

breast cancer.[4] Overall there is approximately a twofold to threefold increase in breast cancer risk among first-degree relatives of women who have had breast cancer; however, among first-degree relatives who have had breast cancer before menopause or who have had bilateral breast cancer, the increase in risk is ninefold. Also, as has been mentioned, women who have had atypical epithelial hyperplastic lesions excised from their breast have a twofold to sixfold increase in subsequent breast cancer risk.[15,36,59]

In situ carcinoma

In situ carcinoma may develop in any portion of the epithelial lining of the duct system of the breast, including the terminal ducts comprising lobules. Because certain clinical and pathologic features of in situ carcinoma involving breast lobules differ from those of in situ carcinoma involving larger ducts, the processes are usually separately designated in situ lobular carcinoma and intraductal carcinoma.

In situ lobular carcinoma

In situ lobular carcinoma does not produce a palpable or grossly visible breast lesion.[42] In the past, it usually was detected microscopically in breast biopsy specimens obtained because of some palpable breast lesion, usually cystic disease. More recently, with the perfection of the mammographic x-ray technique, an appreciable number of in situ lobular carcinomas are being detected by this modality in breasts that contain no palpable abnormality. For example, in a recent breast cancer screening project, 38 of 50 in situ lobular breast cancers were detected by mammography alone.[10]

Pathologic findings. Since in situ lobular carcinoma is not palpable or grossly visible, the gross pathologic findings of breasts found on biopsy to contain this lesion are those produced by an accompanying palpable breast disease. As is seen in Fig. 37-9, *A*, the microscopic characteristics of in situ lobular carcinoma are easily recognized. The terminal ducts are filled and expanded by rather monomorphous, loosely cohesive tumor cells that have indistinct cytoplasmic margins and small, spherical nuclei. Central terminal duct lumina are obliterated by this epithelial proliferative process.

Natural history. The usual method for studying the natural history of in situ carcinoma of the breast is to observe the clinical course of patients in whom in situ carcinoma has been found by means of biopsy and in whom further treatment has not been attempted. This of course is an imperfect method, since pathologic study of mastectomy specimens obtained subsequent to biopsy indicates that the biopsy removes all the in situ carcinoma in 30% to 40% of patients.[19] Fig. 37-10 shows the results of a long-term prospective follow-up study of 42 patients in whom in situ lobular carcinoma was discovered by excisional biopsy and no further treatment was given.[45] Approximately 8% of patients had returned with invasive cancer of the ipsilateral breast at 5 years, 15%

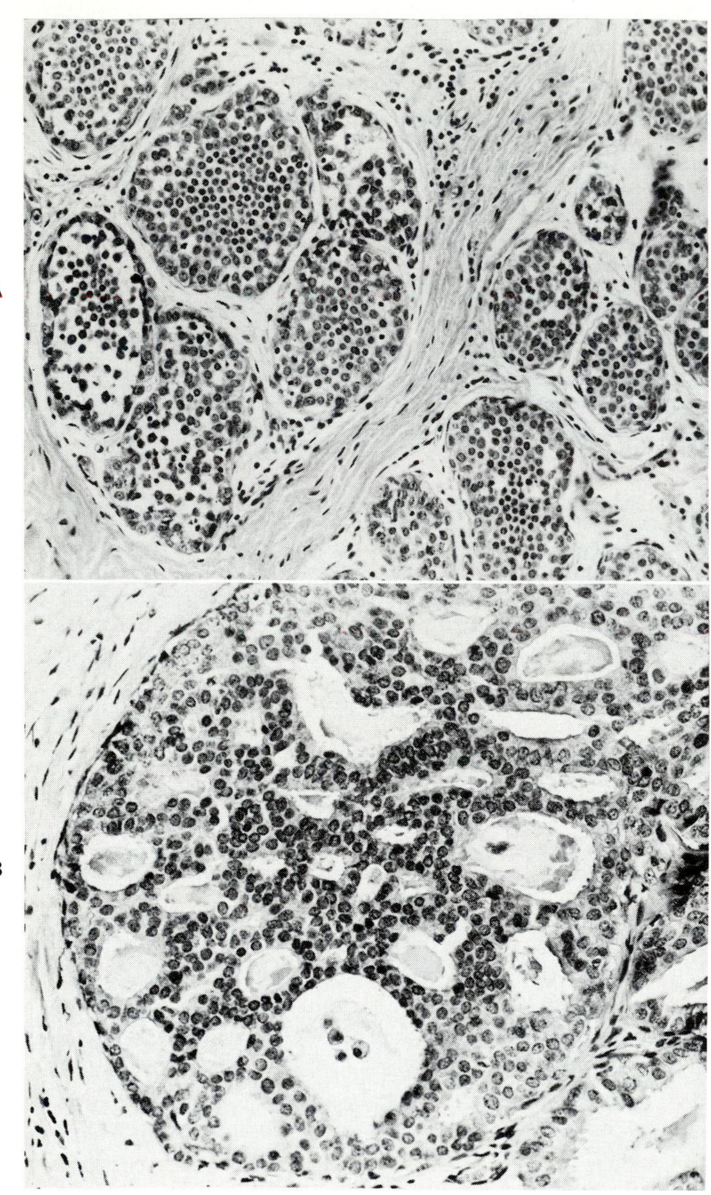

Fig. 37-9. A, In situ lobular carcinoma. Terminal ducts are distended, and their central lumina are obliterated by loosely cohesive tumor cells that have round, monomorphous nuclei and indistinct cytoplasmic margins. No tumor penetration of terminal duct basement membranes is seen. **B,** Cribriform intraductal carcinoma. Proliferating tumor cells produce spherical, smooth-walled microluminal spaces. Nuclei are round, monomorphous, and deeply basophilic. Cytoplasmic margins are indistinct.

after 10 years, and 27% after 15 years. Rosen and associates[64] in studying a series of 99 patients similarly treated concluded that patients in whom in situ lobular carcinoma is diagnosed by excisional biopsy have approximately 12 times the subsequent ipsilateral invasive breast cancer risk that would be expected in an otherwise comparable population. They also found the risk of subsequent invasive breast cancer to be approximately equal for the ipsilateral and contralateral breasts (Fig. 37-11).

Intraductal carcinoma

Unlike in situ lobular carcinoma, intraductal carcinoma produces a palpable breast mass in 30% to 75% of cases.[83] Ability to produce a mass is related to the bulk of the lesion at the time of discovery and to the portion of the duct system in which the intraductal carcinoma is located. Intraductal carcinoma of the more proximal, larger ducts may expand these ducts and produce a sizable mass before it invades the adjacent stroma; intraductal carcinoma of the smaller, more peripheral portions of the duct system is more likely to be nonpalpable and multicentric. Modern mammographic techniques have proved to be an effective means for detecting nonpalpable intraductal carcinomas, particularly those that produce a partially calcified, central detritus.[10,66] Nipple discharge accompanies intraductal carcinoma in approximately 30% of cases.[28]

Pathologic findings. Gross pathologic findings also depend on the bulk of the lesion and on the portion of the duct system in which the intraductal carcinoma is locat-

C

D

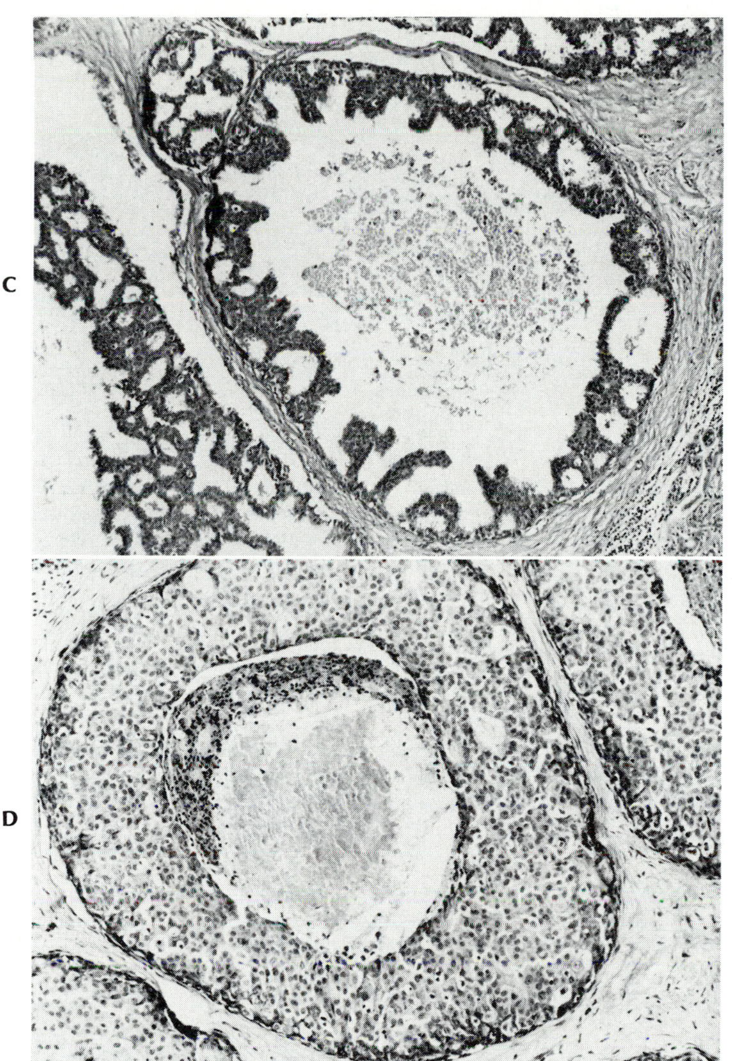

Fig. 37-9, cont'd. C, Micropapillary intraductal carcinoma. Delicate fronds of tumor cells bridge out from duct basement membrane without supporting stroma. **D,** Comedo intraductal carcinoma. Copious central detritus is surrounded by rim of loosely cohesive tumor cells that show no appreciable tendency toward gland formation.

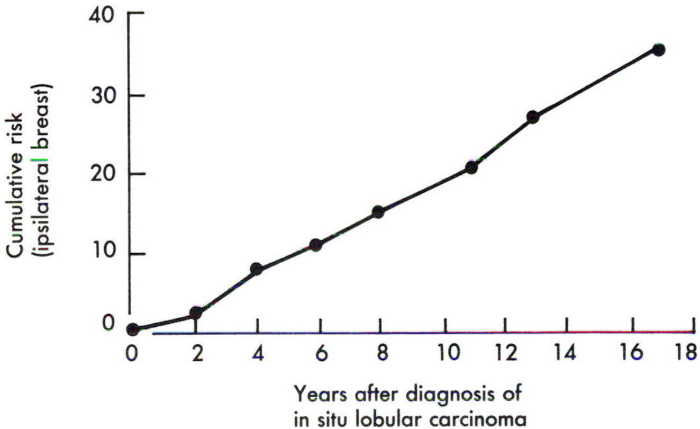

Fig. 37-10. Cumulative risk of ipsilateral invasive breast cancer by year subsequent to excision of in situ lobular carcinoma. (From McDivitt, R.W., et al.: In situ lobular carcinoma, J.A.M.A. **201**:94, 1967. Copyright 1967, American Medical Association.)

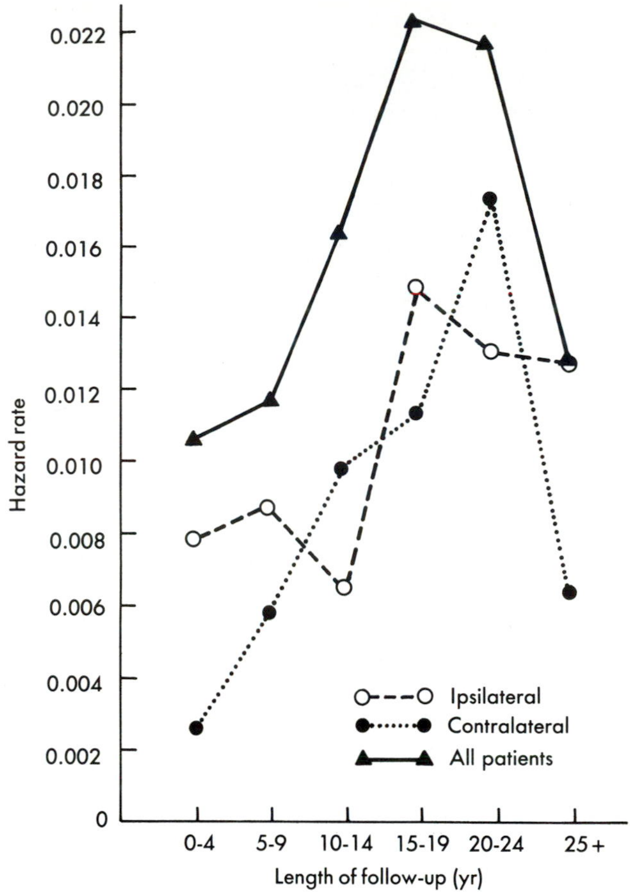

Fig. 37-11. Hazard rates for subsequent carcinoma related to length of follow-up monitoring after excision of in situ lobular carcinoma. Hazard rate indicates risk that subsequent cancer will develop as patient enters given follow-up interval. (From Rosen, P.P., et al.: Am. J. Surg. Pathol. **2**:233, 1978.)

ed. Large intraductal carcinomas in the 3 to 5 cm diameter range often produce gross findings similar to those of large benign intraductal papillomas. They tend to be polypoid and friable and often contain areas of necrosis and scarring. The cystically dilated portion of the duct system that surrounds the intraductal carcinoma usually is easily identified. Intraductal carcinomas that occur in the more peripheral portions of the duct system produce more subtle gross findings that are difficult to distinguish from those of cystic disease and benign epithelial hyperplasia. These smaller ducts may appear dilated and partially filled with friable, gray material. If extensive necrosis has occurred, the gross findings will be similar to those of mammary duct ectasia. Three different microscopic varieties of intraductal carcinoma are recognized: cribriform, micropapillary, and comedo.[36] (Pathologists find these terms useful in describing the varying histologies of intraductal carcinoma; their use is not meant to imply that there are important differences in behavior.) The cribriform and micropapillary types of intraductal carcinoma occur so often in combination and contain cells that are cytologically so similar that they probably represent variations of a single pattern. Comedo intraductal carcinoma occurs less commonly in combination with the other types and is comprised of cells that are cytologically somewhat different. Fig. 37-9, *B*, illustrates the cribriform type of intraductal carcinoma. In contrast to the epithelial hyperplasias, the microlumina formed by the cribriform type of intraductal carcinoma are round and regular and the epithelial cells have lost their polar orientation in relation to the basement membrane. Cytologically the cells are similar in many respects to those of in situ lobular carcinoma, although they may be somewhat larger. Nuclei are round and monomorphous, and cytoplasmic boundaries are indistinct. Fig. 37-9, *C*, illustrates the micropapillary type of intraductal carcinoma, so named because of the marked papillarity of the lesion as viewed microscopically. Cytologically the cells are indistinguishable from those of the cribriform type of intraductal carcinoma. Small anastomosing cellular fronds without obvious supporting stroma extend out into the duct lumen. When cut perpendicular to their long axis, these fronds seem to float unattached in the luminal space. A characteristic histologic feature of the comedo type of intraductal carcinoma, as is seen in Fig. 37-9, *D*, is copious necrotic detritus in the center of the duct lumen. Detritus formation of this type and magnitude is of diagnostic importance because it almost never is produced by benign epithelial hyperplasias. In comedo intraductal carcinoma the tumor cells are arranged circumferentially around the central detritus, nearer the duct basement membrane. They are loosely cohesive and may display significantly more cytologic atypia than those of cribriform and micropapillary types of intraductal carcinoma.

Natural history. The natural history of intraductal carcinoma is less well understood than that of in situ lobular carcinoma because no large prospective follow-up study of patients treated by excisional biopsy has been conducted. However, the literature does contain several reports of small numbers of patients with intraductal carcinoma followed in this manner. When information from these reports is pieced together to arrive at some sort of composite picture, the impression given is that the chance of invasive carcinoma occurring subsequent to the excision of intraductal carcinoma is similar to or slightly greater than the chance of invasive cancer occurring subsequent to the excision of in situ lobular carcinoma. For example, in a recent series reported from Memorial Hospital in New York, seven of 25 patients who had intraductal carcinoma initially treated by excisional biopsy developed recurrent ipsilateral carcinoma during a follow-up period that averaged just under 10 years.[13] Intraductal carcinoma differs from in situ lobular carcinoma in another important respect. The risk of contralateral breast cancer developing in patients with cribriform or micropapillary intraductal carcinoma is far less than that associated with in situ lobular carcinoma.[13] In contrast, the contralateral breast cancer risk for patients who have comedo type of intraductal carcinoma is approximately equal to that of patients who have in situ lobular carcinoma.[1]

Invasive breast cancer

Pathologic parameters useful in predicting invasive breast cancer prognosis

The clinical course of breast cancer varies considerably from patient to patient; some women have recurrent cancer and die within a year of mastectomy, others are cured by mastectomy, and still others survive for 10 or 15 years after mastectomy with proven metastatic disease. Although it is not possible to predict with certainty how a particular breast cancer will behave in a particular patient, certain parameters are useful in predicting the chance of a woman's being cured or dying of the disease. In discussing these parameters, one must remember that breast cancer is a disease in which total mortality accrues relatively slowly. With some cancers, such as carcinoma of the lung and melanoma, almost all patients who die of the disease will do so within the first few years after primary treatment. In contrast, the mortality from breast cancer accrues steadily during the tenth, fifteenth, and even twenty-fifth postoperative year. Therefore it is possible for a woman to have no clinical evidence of recurrent or metastatic breast cancer for 10 or 15 years after mastectomy and still subsequently die of carcinoma of the breast. Another generalization of equal importance is that the more favorable breast cancer appears in terms of pathologic stage, the more slowly total mortality from the disease will accrue.[1] Therefore the more successful we become in discovering and treating breast cancers of a favorable pathologic stage, the longer we will have to wait to determine the efficacy of our treatment methods.

The median survival of women with untreated breast cancer is 2.7 years, and the 10-year survival subsequent to the onset of symptoms is 3.6%.[16] Overall approximately half of all women who received primary surgical therapy for breast cancer survive for 10 years postoperatively; the remainder die of disease during this interval.[12] If one becomes slightly more sophisticated in characterizing breast cancers according to pathologic stage, one may predict that about 75% of women who have no evidence of regional metastatic disease at the time of primary surgical therapy will be 10-year survivors, whereas only 35% of those whose cancer has spread to axillary lymph nodes will survive for a similar period of time.[12] The chance of 10-year survival of women who have distant metastases at the time of primary treatment is similar to that of untreated breast cancer. Pathologists can make certain additional observations that help characterize the chance of an individual patient's surviving breast cancer. These assume importance in part because they define women at high risk to whom we might wish to give adjuvant chemotherapy. The most important are as follows.

Histologic type of tumor. The rationale for subclassifying breast cancers into various different histologic types lies in the fact that this has an important influence on prognosis (Table 37-1). In a recent analysis of 30-year survivors of invasive breast cancers treated by mastectomy, it was found that 29% of women who had poorly differentiated scirrhous duct cancers and 34% of women who had lobular carcinomas survived for this period of time.[1] In contrast, the chance of 30-year survival among women whose breast cancer was of colloid type was 55% and among women who had medullary type of breast cancer, 58%.[1] Women who had papillary breast cancer had the most favorable 30-year survival of any of the major histologic subtypes, 65%.

Histologic grade. Breast cancers may be characterized in terms of histologic grade as well as histologic type. The most popular method of grading uses three histologic grades of ascending pleomorphism based on degree of gland formation, nuclear atypia, degree of hyperchromatism, and mitotic rate. Twenty-year survival of patients with grade I breast cancers is approximately 40%; 20-year survival for patients with grade II and grade III breast cancers is only 29% and 21%, respectively.

Tumor size. Fig. 37-12 demonstrates an inverse relationship between primary breast cancer diameter at the time of mastectomy and chance of long-term survival. Approximately 60% of patients whose breast cancers measured less than 2 cm in diameter were long-term survivors, whereas fewer than half as many patients whose primary tumors measured greater than 3 cm in diameter survived for a similar period of time.[1] Although this relationship between tumor size and survival was particularly noteworthy among patients who had axillary metastases, it was evident among node-negative patients as well.

Table 37-1. Long-term survival of patients with infiltrating breast cancer treated by radical mastectomy

Tumor type	Actuarial survival		
	5 years	10 years	20 years
Scirrhous	59%	47%	38%
Lobular	57%	42%	34%
Medullary	69%	68%	62%
Colloid	76%	72%	62%
Papillary	89%	65%	65%

Modified from McDivitt, R.W., Stewart, F.W., and Berg, J.W.: Tumors of the breast. In Atlas of tumor pathology, Washington, D.C., 1967, Armed Forces Institute of Pathology Press.

Similarly, in an analysis of 5-year survival of 2000 women with operable breast cancers treated by radical mastectomy, Fisher and associates[23] observed an inverse relationship between tumor size and survival. For tumors less than 1 cm in diameter, 5-year mortality was 18%. For tumors between 1 and 1.9 cm in diameter, it was 22%. The 5-year mortality for tumors measuring between 3 and 6 cm in diameter varied from 37% to 43%. In this study tumor size was also related to probability of axillary metastasis and to extent of axillary nodal involvement by metastatic tumor. The median tumor size of patients who had no axillary lymph node metastases was 2.7 cm; for patients who had between one and three axillary lymph nodes involved by metastatic cancer, the median tumor size was 2.9 cm, and for patients who had more extensive axillary metastatic disease the median tumor size was 3.3 cm.

Axillary lymph node status. In the course of performing mastectomies for breast carcinoma, most often the pathologist removes and examines the axillary lymph nodes. During the course of a complete axillary dissection 20 to 30 lymph nodes may be removed. Lymph nodes that lie near the breast medial to the insertion of the pectoralis minor muscle customarily are designated level I; those under the pectoralis muscle, level II; and those nodes deepest in the axilla, level III. Twenty years after mastectomy, the survival for patients with no axillary metastases is reported by Berg and Robbins[11] as 65%; for patients with metastases at level I only, 38%; for patients with metastases at level II, 30%; and for patients with level III metastases, 12%. Chance of survival also may be calculated according to the number of lymph

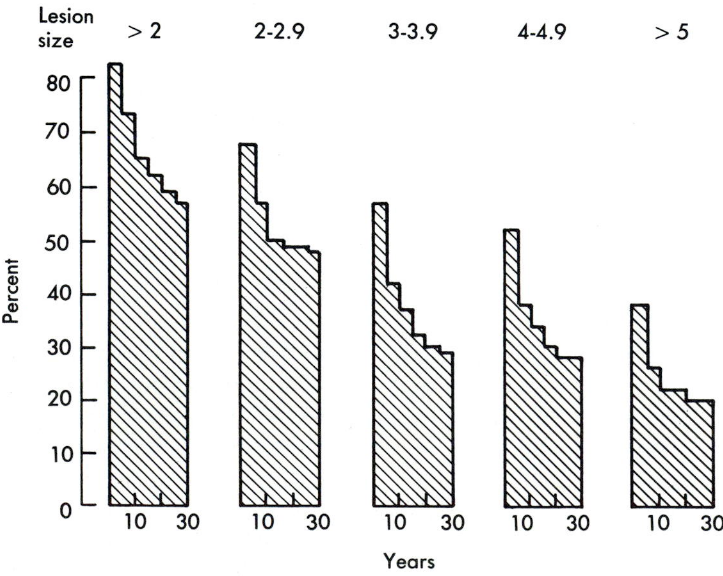

Fig. 37-12. Relationship between primary tumor size and long-term survival. (From Adair, F., et al.: Cancer **33**:1147, 1974.)

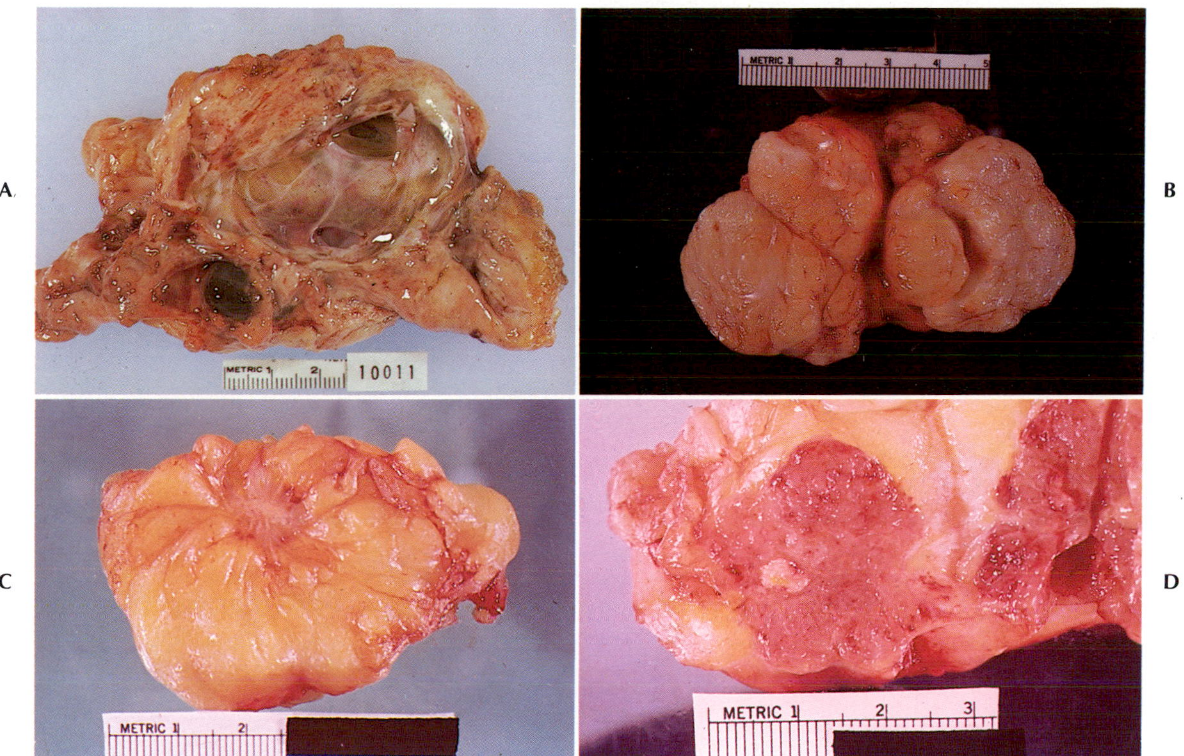

Plate 6

A, Cystic disease. Large cyst, measuring approximately 4 cm in diameter, appears in upper portion of specimen. Anterior cyst wall has been removed to reveal its multiloculation and smooth internal surface. Numerous smaller cysts are seen in lower right-hand portion of specimen. One appears dark red because of its serosanguineous contents.

B, Fibroadenoma. External surface appears well circumscribed. Compressed ducts, which help characterize the lesion microscopically, appear as slitlike spaces on lesion's cut surface.

C, Scirrhous carcinoma. Cut surface is light gray, stellate, and depressed beneath surface of surrounding fat. Note linear depressions in surrounding fat that radiate out from carcinoma.

D, Medullary carcinoma. In contrast to scirrhous carcinoma in **C,** external surface of this tumor is smooth and convex and appears to push against rather than infiltrate adjacent fat. Cut surface is soft and on the same plane as surrounding fat.

nodes involved by metastatic disease. About 60% of patients with between one and three lymph nodes involved by metastatic tumor survive 10 years; only 20% of patients with four or more lymph nodes involved by metastatic tumor have a 10-year survival.[65] Survival figures based on counting involved lymph nodes correlate well with survival figures based on level of involvement because metastatic breast cancer usually spreads from the proximal to the distal axilla, progressively involving more lymph nodes.

Other potentially useful parameters. Breast cancers also may be characterized according to whether the tumor cells contain a cytoplasmic protein that binds estrogen, designated estrogen receptor (ERP). Although the presence or absence of ERP has been used primarily to predict which breast cancers will respond to endocrine therapy, evidence suggests that the presence or absence of ERP may correlate with prognosis. Osborne and McGuire[56] have reported that ERP-negative tumors have a higher rate of short-term recurrence after mastectomy than ERP-positive carcinomas. ERP status, however, has not yet been correlated with chance of long-term breast cancer survival. ERP status correlates to some degree with tumor histology. Invasive lobular carcinomas have a high frequency of ERP positivity (71% to 89%), whereas for medullary carcinomas the rate of ERP positivity is much lower (18%).[67] Meyer and associates[47] also have studied the relationship between ERP status, histologic grade, and breast cancer kinetics, using a tritiated thymidine labeling index to measure the proportion of cells engaged in DNA synthesis at any given time. They report that tumors of higher histologic grade are more likely to be ERP negative and have higher labeling indices, indicating more rapid cell proliferation. No correlation has been found between ERP status and tumor size or axillary lymph node status.

Interrelationship of prognostic parameters. Alderson and associates[3] in a recent computer-assisted multiple regression analysis of 258 infiltrating breast cancers found axillary lymph node status, tumor size, and histologic grade to be of decreasing order of influence in predicting long-term survival. Other factors such as histologic type were not included in this study, although they are obviously important, in part to predict chance of axillary metastasis. There is also some evidence to suggest that breast cancer cell kinetics may offer the single most useful parameter in predicting chance of breast cancer survival, although these studies are still incomplete.[46]

Common histologic types of invasive breast carcinoma

The following outline lists the five most common histologic types of invasive breast carcinoma, which in aggregate comprise 90% to 98% of all breast cancers seen in the day-to-day practice of surgical pathology.

A. Common histological types
   1. Invasive lobular carcinoma
   2. Invasive duct carcinoma
      a. Scirrhous
      b. Colloid
      c. Medullary
      d. Papillary
B. Less common favorable histologic types
   1. Tubular
   2. Secretory
   3. Adenoid cystic
C. Unusual presentations
   1. Paget's disease
   2. Inflammatory carcinoma

Of these, approximately 10% are of lobular origin and the remaining 90% arise from larger ducts.[42] Scirrhous carcinoma comprises approximately 90% of all cancers of duct origin; the remaining 10% are colloid, medullary, or papillary. Invasive breast cancers are subclassified by means of variations in their histologic appearance.

Invasive lobular carcinoma. As is seen in Fig. 37-13, *A*, invasive lobular carcinoma characteristically produces a linear or "Indian file" pattern of stromal infiltration with very little tendency toward gland formation. At times, infiltrating lobular carcinoma also may distribute itself circumferentially around ducts to produce a bull's-eye or targeting pattern. Individual tumor cells resemble those of in situ lobular carcinoma. They are relatively small, have round nuclei, and have very little pleomorphism. Mitoses are infrequent. Some invasive lobular carcinomas may accumulate considerable cytoplasmic mucus, resembling the signet-ring cells of poorly differentiated carcinomas of gastrointestinal tract origin.[27] This histologic variation appears to be of no prognostic significance.

Scirrhous duct carcinoma. As is seen in Fig. 37-13, *B*, scirrhous duct carcinoma looks somewhat different histologically from invasive lobular carcinoma. The infiltrating tumor produces small glandular spaces that vary in number and maturity of development in accordance with the pleomorphism of the tumor. In addition, in contrast to invasive lobular carcinoma, the invading ribbons in scirrhous carcinoma usually are several cells thick, and the cells are larger and more pleomorphic. Individual nests of tumor cells are surrounded by copious dense stromal collagen, a feature that gives scirrhous carcinoma its name.

Colloid carcinoma. Colloid carcinoma is characterized by abundant, tumor-produced, extracellular mucus, as is seen in Fig. 37-13, *C*. The mucus is produced by the tumor cells and subsequently extruded into the surrounding stroma. Mucus production may be so abundant that in some histologic sections tumor cells may be difficult to locate. They usually form small clusters and show

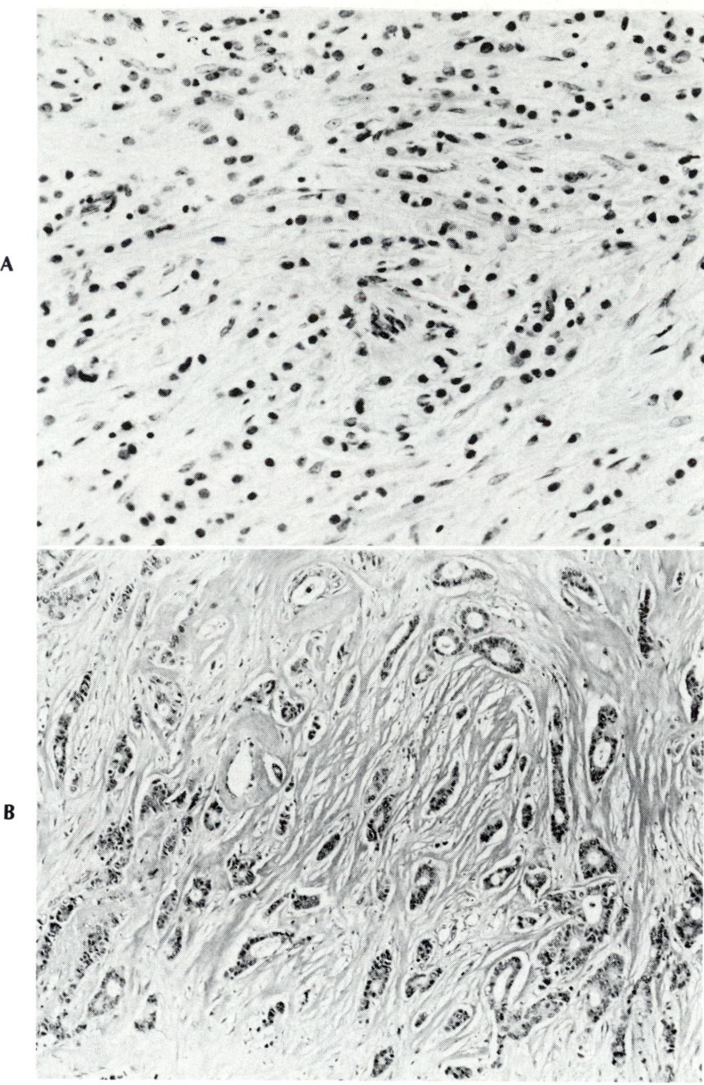

Fig. 37-13. A, Invasive lobular carcinoma. Individual tumor cells infiltrate stroma in linear arrangement without gland formation. **B,** Scirrhous carcinoma. Small clusters of cells, which often form rudimentary glands, infiltrate stroma in haphazard arrangement. Stromal sclerosis is prominent.

little pleomorphism. It is useful in the differential diagnosis of colloid carcinoma to remember that no benign breast tumor is capable of producing copious extracellular mucus.

Medullary carcinoma. Medullary carcinoma, as is seen in Fig. 37-13, *D*, is comprised of cells that are relatively large and pleomorphic. Mitoses are frequent and often bizarre. Medullary carcinoma produces a sheetlike growth pattern with no appreciable tendency toward gland formation. Desmoplastic stromal reaction is minimal or absent, and an abundant infiltration of mature plasma cells and lymphocytes accompanies approximately 50% of tumors. The presence or absence of mononuclear infiltration is of no prognostic significance.

Papillary carcinoma. Except for stromal invasion, infiltrating papillary carcinoma resembles papillary intraductal carcinoma. The infiltrating carcinoma is arranged in large papillary fronds with varying amounts of stromal fibrosis.

Gross pathology. Colloid, medullary, and papillary carcinomas produce soft, well-circumscribed, discrete masses that may be lobulated but are generally spherical in contour (Plate 6, *C*). They are sometimes described as having pushing rather than infiltrative margins. The cut surface usually is friable and has a mottled light and dark gray color. The cut surface of colloid carcinomas appears more glistening than the surface of tumors of the other two types and is somewhat sticky. These features help distinguish colloid carcinoma from the medullary and papillary varieties grossly. In contrast, the cut surface of scirrhous carcinoma appears stellate and its margins jagged because of the irregular infiltration of tumor into the

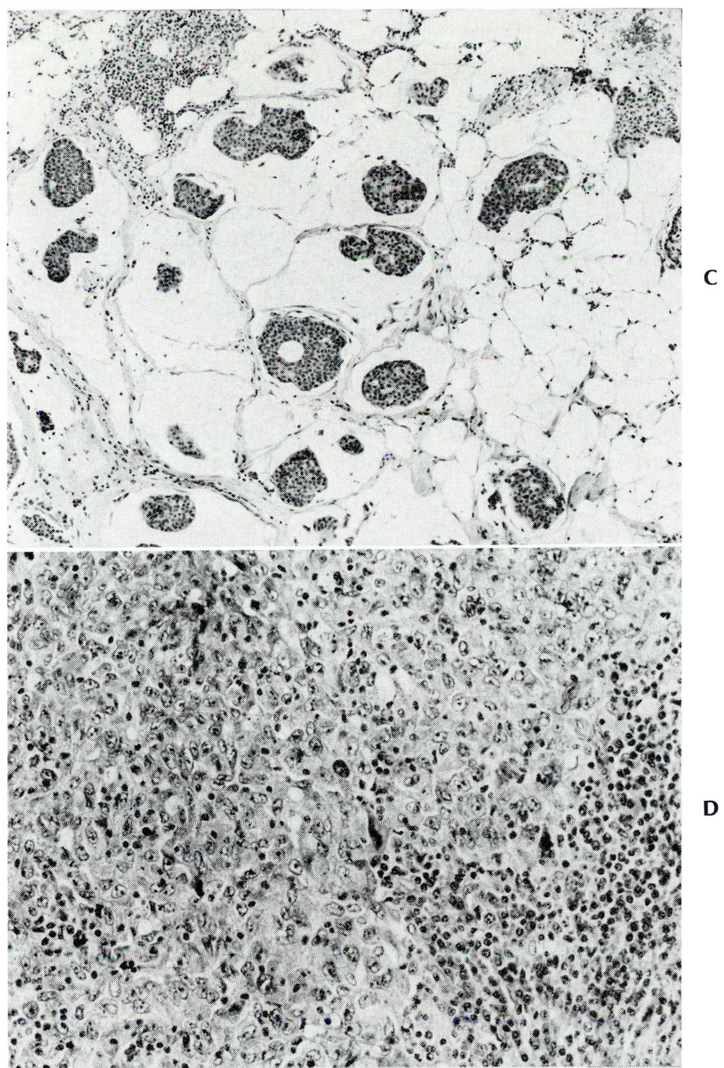

Fig. 37-13, cont'd. C, Colloid carcinoma. Small clusters of tumor cells appear suspended in pool of mucus that is produced by tumor. **D,** Medullary carcinoma. Large pleomorphic tumor cells produce sheetlike growth pattern without obvious gland formation. Mitoses are frequent, and stroma sclerosis is minimal. Mixed infiltration of mature mononuclear cells, seen in the lower right-hand corner, often accompanies medullary carcinoma.

adjacent stroma (Plate 6, *D*). The tumor surface usually is depressed in relation to the surrounding breast stroma and is firm, at times rock hard, because of intense desmoplastic stromal collagen production. Radially arranged, dull yellow streaks produced by necrosis may interrupt the otherwise light gray or white appearance of the tumor. The gross appearance of infiltrating lobular carcinoma may be similar to that of scirrhous carcinoma. Alternatively, infiltrating lobular carcinoma may be more subtle, producing no visible gross lesion but only a poorly defined area of localized firmness. However, if one cuts across an area of this type and keeps the knife perpendicular to the cut surface of the specimen, the edges produced by the cut are firm and sharp rather than rounded and soft as they would be with benign breast disease.

Clinical presentation. The older literature describes the clinical presentation of breast cancer as a firm, palpable mass that is adherent to the surrounding breast tissue and often fixed to the underlying chest wall or overlying skin. Large cancers not infrequently produce dimpling of the overlying skin or nipple retraction and inversion, caused by increased tension on the suspensory ligaments of the breast. At times, skin or nipple ulcerations, caused by direct tumor extension, are observed. These findings are clinical signs of relatively advanced breast cancer. They occur less frequently today because women have learned to seek medical attention as soon as a breast mass is discovered, usually by the woman herself. Since smaller breast cancers may produce no clinical signs or symptoms other than a discrete mass, most surgeons excise any dominant, noncystic breast mass for histologic evaluation. Of course, if invasive breast cancers are sufficiently small, they may be nonpalpable. The diameter at which breast cancers become palpable depends to some degree on the consistency of the tumor and the size and consistency of the breast. However, most breast cancers smaller than 1 cm in diameter are nonpalpable. In a recent breast cancer screening program that employed both physical examination and mammography, 61 of 104 (59%) infiltrating breast cancers that measured less than 1 cm in diameter were detected by mammography only, not by physical examination.[10] Obviously mammography plays an important role in detecting small cancers of this type.

Prognosis. The rationale for subclassifying infiltrating breast cancers is to identify tumors that vary in their natural history. Table 37-1 shows a similar actuarial survival for patients with infiltrating lobular carcinoma and scirrhous carcinoma treated by radical mastectomy; approximately 45% at 10 years after mastectomy and 35% at 20 years after mastectomy.[44] Ten- and 20-year survival of similarly treated patients with colloid, medullary, and papillary carcinoma is considerably more favorable, varying from 65% to 72% at 10 years and from 62% to 65% at 20 years.[42] There also are marked differences in the chance that carcinoma of the contralateral breast will develop, depending on the histologic type of the first breast carcinoma. Fig. 37-14 shows that during a 30-year follow-up period approximately 25% of patients with infiltrating lobular and comedo types of carcinoma develop contralateral breast carcinoma; the contralateral breast cancer risk is significantly less for tumors of other histologic types.[1]

Less common, favorable histologic types of infiltrating carcinoma

Three additional types of infiltrating carcinoma are noteworthy because they carry a particularly favorable prognosis: tubular, secretory, and adenoid cystic carcinoma.

Tubular carcinoma. Tubular carcinoma is a very orderly type of infiltrating duct carcinoma in which small, nonanastomosing glands lined by a single layer of cells infiltrate the breast stroma (Fig. 37-15). In the majority of cases the infiltrating carcinoma is accompanied by cribriform or micropapillary intraductal carcinoma.[40] Tubular carcinomas tend to be small; in a recent study of 93 tubular carcinomas, tumors were found to vary in diameter from 0.2 to 2.5 cm, with a mean diameter of 0.8 cm.[40] (This small size has led to the speculation that tubular carcinoma may be an early infiltrative growth phase of cribriform and micropapillary intraductal carcinoma, a pattern that is later obliterated by scirrhous overgrowth.) Because tubular carcinomas are small, they are particularly amenable to mammographic detection. Axillary metastases were found in only two of the 93 patients with tubular carcinoma described above. No patient developed disseminated metastatic disease

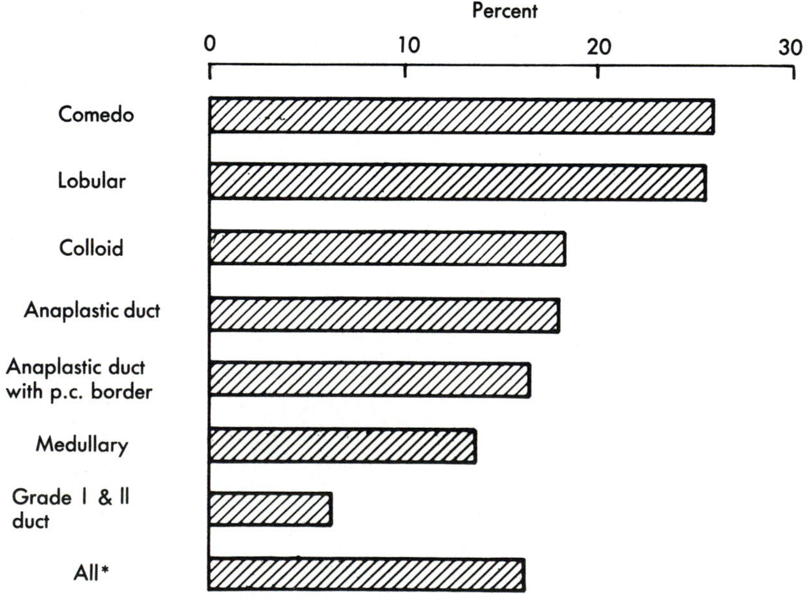

Fig. 37-14. Risk of contralateral breast cancer by histologic type of first breast cancer during 30-year postmastectomy follow-up period. (From Adair, F., et al.: Cancer **33**:1149, 1974.)

during the follow-up period. Only one patient, initially treated by excisional biopsy, had a local recurrence, and she is currently without evidence of disease subsequent to mastectomy. An additional 17 patients who were treated by procedures less extensive than mastectomy remained without evidence of disease. Although previous reports concerning infiltrating carcinomas of relatively large size listed tubular carcinoma as an infrequent variety, more recent studies of infiltrating carcinoma list tubular carcinoma as comprising between 8% to 10% of the total.[10,18]

Secretory carcinoma. Secretory carcinoma is an unusual type of infiltrating duct carcinoma that was first described in children.[41] Although it is the most frequent type of breast cancer seen in children, it comprises less than 1% of lesions excised from children's breasts.[22] Secretory carcinoma may occur in women of any age, but the mean age of patients with secretory carcinoma who seek treatment is only 25 years.[73] The lesion is easily recognized histologically because the tumor produces abundant secretions similar to those seen during lactation. This eosinophilic secretory product is seen both within the cytoplasm of tumor cells and within glandular spaces formed by the tumor. In a recent review of secretory carcinoma, only four of 19 patients were found to have axillary metastases.[73] One patient with axillary metastasis, treated initially by partial mastectomy, had a local recurrence after 8 months but subsequently has remained without evidence of disease following mastectomy. One additional 25-year-old patient in whom eight of 14 axillary lymph nodes were involved by metastatic tumor died of breast carcinoma 8 months later. The remaining 17 patients (90%) have shown no evidence of recurrent or metastatic disease.

Adenoid cystic carcinoma. Adenoid cystic carcinoma is an infrequent type of breast carcinoma comprising from 0.1% to 0.2% of infiltrating carcinomas.[26] The characteristic diphasic histologic growth pattern of the tumor is similar to that of adenoid cystic carcinoma of salivary gland origin (Chapter 29). Approximately 100 adenoid cystic carcinomas of the breast have been reported; none have had axillary metastases.[5] Although three deaths have been attributed to the disease, the details of these case reports are incomplete.[51,54]

Unusual clinical presentations of breast cancer

Paget's disease. In 1874 Sir James Paget observed that an eczematoid lesion of the nipple at times preceded carcinoma of the breast.[60] The nipple lesion that bears Paget's name is caused by tumor cells invading the basilar

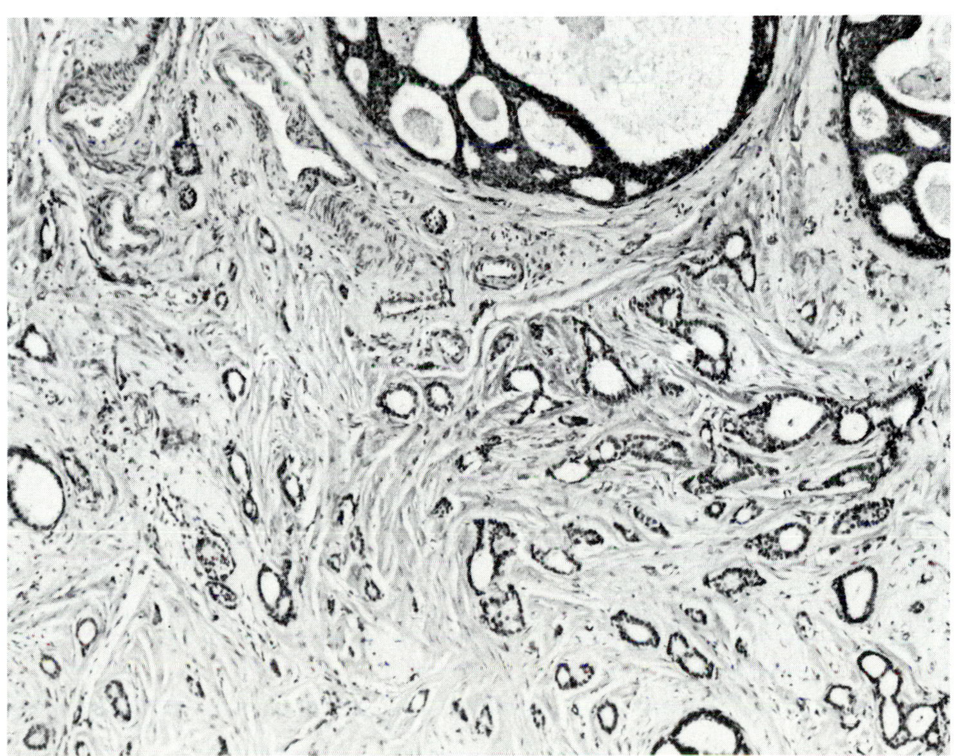

Fig. 37-15. Tubular carcinoma. Small, well-formed glands with patent lumina infiltrate breast stroma. These glands are lined by single layer of tumor cells whose polarity is well maintained. Cribriform type of intraductal carcinoma, seen in the upper right-hand corner, often accompanies tubular cancer.

layers of the epidermis of the nipple after having migrated through the lactiferous sinuses from an underlying carcinoma of the breast (Fig. 37-16). These cells, which are larger and more pleomorphic than the adjacent epidermal cells, form rudimentary glands and stain irregularly with mucicarmine. Most patients with Paget's disease have a crusted, scaling, eczematoid lesion of the nipple; about half have a palpable underlying subareolar mass. However, occasionally Paget's disease may be discovered by microscopic examination in instances in which gross nipple lesion is absent. Most patients in whom a breast mass is palpated are subsequently proved to have scirrhous carcinoma; however, occasionally an invasive lobular, medullary, or papillary carcinoma produces the nipple lesion. About 70% of patients in whom no breast mass is palpated have intraductal carcinoma; the remainder have small invasive carcinomas, usually scirrhous.[7] The presence of Paget's disease does not alter the excellent prognosis of intraductal carcinoma. The prognosis of patients who have invasive carcinoma accompanied by Paget's disease is slightly less favorable than that of other patients with breast cancer who do not have Paget's disease. The overall 10-year post-mastectomy survival of patients with Paget's disease is 60%.[7]

Inflammatory carcinoma. Inflammatory carcinoma is a diffuse erythema of the breast caused by packing of the dermal lymphatics with tumor emboli from an underlying carcinoma of the breast, usually of scirrhous type (Fig. 37-17). This phenomenon accompanies approximately 1% of invasive breast cancers.[63] The mean age of patients with inflammatory carcinoma is the same as that of other breast cancer patients.[71] Most patients have increased warmth and diffuse erythema of the breast, and about 60% have a palpable underlying mass. The prognosis of inflammatory carcinoma is so bleak that most surgeons do not consider it worthwhile to treat patients with this disease by mastectomy.[63] Almost all die within a short time. Occasionally dermal lymphatic emboli are observed microscopically in patients who do not have the clinical stigmata of inflammatory carcinoma. These patients have a similarly poor prognosis.

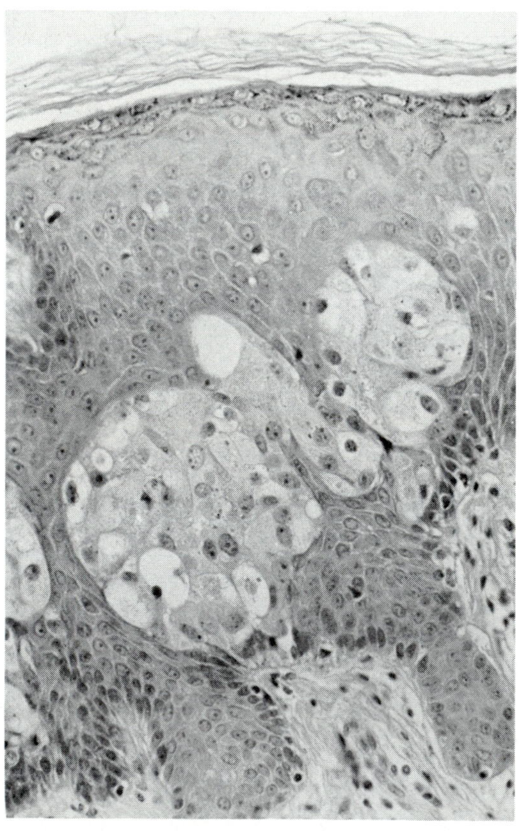

Fig. 37-16. Paget's disease. Small nests of pale-staining tumor cells in basilar region of the epidermis contrast with surrounding squamous epithelium. At times Paget's cells may form rudimentary glands and contain cytoplasmic mucus, behavior characteristics similar to those of underlying breast cancer from which they are derived.

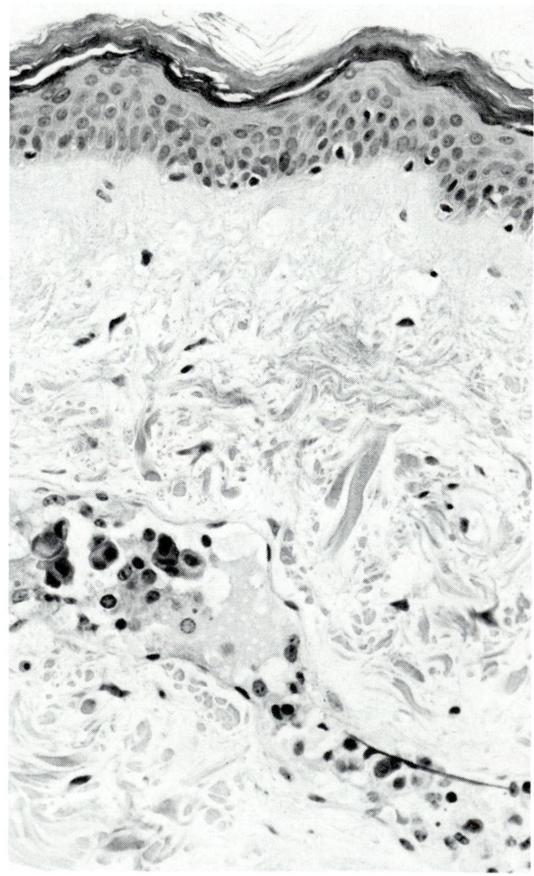

Fig. 37-17. Inflammatory carcinoma. Dermal lymphatics are distended with tumor cells from underlying breast carcinoma. (Note that there is no inflammatory reaction. "Inflammatory" refers to cutaneous erythema seen clinically.)

Breast carcinoma in unusual hosts

Although most discussions of breast carcinoma do not emphasize variations resulting from differences in the host, some special circumstances may modify patterns of breast carcinoma incidence and behavior.

Oral contraceptive users

Although the relationship between oral contraceptive use and breast cancer risk remains undetermined, recent studies suggest that long-term oral contraceptive use, particularly in women who have underlying benign breast disease, may increase the chance of subsequent breast carcinoma.[57] Interestingly, other studies have reported a decreased incidence of benign breast disease among long-term oral contraceptive users.[55] LiVolsi and associates[37] have refined this latter observation by showing that oral contraceptive use decreases the incidence of most types of benign breast disease but has no effect on the incidence of atypical epithelial hyperplastic lesions of the breast. It remains to be seen what effect, if any, long-term oral contraceptive use has on breast cancer risk among patients with atypical epithelial hyperplastic lesions.

Perimenopausal exogenous estrogen users

Although most studies investigating the relationship between exogenous estrogen use and breast cancer risk have been poorly controlled, Hoover and associates[34] in a carefully controlled case study showed a 25% excess breast cancer risk among (menopausal) exogenous estrogen users and an even greater risk among women taking high doses of exogenous estrogens for a prolonged period of time.

Males

Breast cancer accounts for 0.2% of male cancers and is approximately 100 times less frequent than carcinoma of the female breast. However, countries such as Australia, United States, and England that have high rates of breast cancer in women also have proportionally higher rates in men, and countries such as Japan that have low rates of breast cancer in women have proportionally lower rates in men.[69] Gynecomastia does not appear to increase the risk of male breast cancer, whereas Klinefelter's syndrome does by a magnitude of approximately 20 fold.[68,70] Since approximately 4% to 5% of males with breast cancer have Klinefelter's syndrome, appropriate chromosome studies should be done as part of the male breast cancer workup.

Men who seek treatment for breast cancer are on average 10 years older than women, and men delay approximately twice as long as women before seeking medical attention. Most breast cancers in men lie immediately below the areola, 25% are associated with nipple ulceration and retraction, and 10% have associated Paget's disease.[53] With the exception of lobular carcinoma, men develop the same histologic types of breast cancer as do women in approximately the same proportion of each histologic type. Since normally the male breast does not contain lobules, lobular carcinoma of the male breast is not ordinarily seen, except rarely after high doses of estrogen therapy that have induced lobular development.

Because of patient delay in seeking therapy, breast cancer in men tends to be more advanced at the time of primary surgical therapy than breast cancer in women. More than half of all male patients have metastatic carcinoma when first seen. (However, the prognosis of male breast cancer that is developed from studying the size and node is essentially the same as that of the female.) For this reason, the same types of surgical therapies are ordinarily employed. Aside from gynecomastia and carcinoma, breast lesions in men are infrequent.

Malignant mesenchymal tumors

Primary malignant mesenchymal tumors of the breast are infrequent in comparison with carcinoma. At Memorial Sloan Kettering Cancer Institute between 1926 and 1956, only 86 malignant mesenchymal tumors were indexed by the pathology department. Of these, 47% were diagnosed as malignant cystosarcoma, 29% as stromal sarcoma, 16% as malignant lymphoma, and 8% as angiosarcoma.[39] Aside from these types, an occasional tumor resembling pure liposarcoma or malignant fibrous histiocytoma is seen.

Malignant cystosarcoma

Malignant cystosarcoma is discussed in a previous section dealing with fibroadenoma.

Stromal sarcoma

Malignant mesenchymal tumors of the breast that do not contain the elongated ducts characteristic of a fibroadenoma are designated stromal sarcoma. Stromal sarcomas most often contain a mixture of malignant mesenchymal elements. A fibrosarcomatous component is most frequent; however, about one third also contain areas resembling liposarcoma. Less frequently, malignant bone and cartilage are seen, and areas resembling malignant giant cell tumor also may be present. In Barnes and Pietruszka's review of 100 cases collected from the literature, the average age of patients with stromal sarcoma at initial examination was 52 years, and the median tumor size was 5.3 cm.[9] Stromal sarcomas most often have diffusely infiltrative margins rather than being circumscribed. Their cut surface is usually light gray mottled with areas of hemorrhage and necrosis. At times cystic areas also are seen. Approximately 25% to 30% of patients with stromal sarcoma die of disease, most frequently from pulmonary metastases.[52] Since most

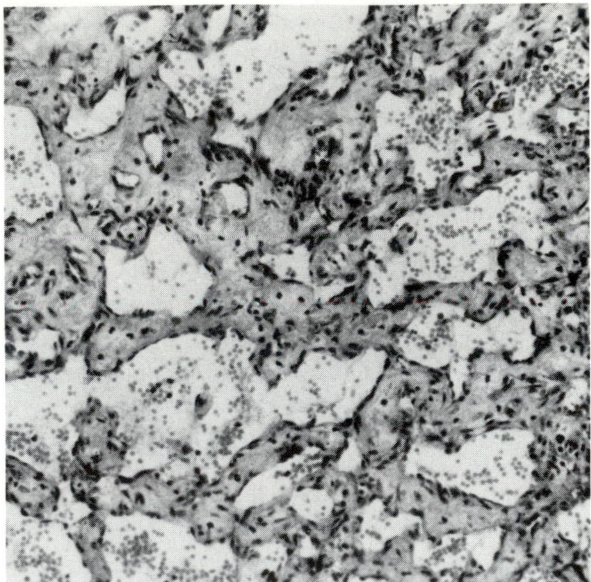

Fig. 37-18. Angiosarcoma. Anastomosing network of small, benign vascular clannets, similar to those in hemangioma, may be all that is seen microscopically.

patients treated by radical mastectomy who subsequently die of pulmonary metastases were not found to have axillary metastases, it is postulated that metastatic spread is via the bloodstream rather than lymphatic channels. Stromal sarcomas containing malignant bone and cartilage and those with a high mitotic rate (eight to 10 mitoses per each 10 high-power fields) are believed to have a particularly poor prognosis.[9,52]

Malignant lymphoma

Although breast involvement by malignant lymphoma most often is a sign of disseminated disease, at times patients have what appears to be primary lymphoma of the breast. The incidence of primary breast lymphoma is estimated to be in the range of 1:500 to 1:1000 malignant breast tumors.[42] The histiocytic type is most common, followed by poorly differentiated lymphocytic lymphoma.[42] Primary Hodgkin's disease of the breast has not been reported. Breast lymphoma is characterized by a well-circumscribed, soft, gray mass that usually is spherical, somewhat resembling the gross appearance of medullary carcinoma. In about 10% of cases there is bilateral breast involvement.[8] Ten-year survival of patients treated with local radiotherapy is about 50%.[20]

Angiosarcoma

Breast angiosarcoma almost always is a relentlessly fatal disease of young women. Although the disease occurs in women of all ages, as well as children, the majority of women are between 20 and 29 years of age at diagnosis. The tumor most frequently is initially seen as a poorly defined area of thickening. During the operation the surgeon may be confronted with little more than a diffusely bloody field that is difficult to control. Grossly the biopsy specimen appears hemorrhagic and firm. The histologic features of angiosarcoma often are deceptively bland, resembling those of benign cutaneous hemangioma (Fig. 37-18). In view of this, we hesitate to consider any grossly visible vascular tumor of the breast benign. The 5-year mortality from angiosarcoma of the breast approaches 100%; most patients die within a year of diagnosis. No therapy has proved effective.

REFERENCES

1. Adair, F., et al.: Long term followup of breast cancer patients: the 30-year report, Cancer **33**:1145, 1974.
2. Anderson, D.E.: A genetic study of human breast cancer, J. Natl. Cancer Inst. **48**:1029, 1972.
3. Alderson, M.R., et al.: Relative significance of prognostic factors in breast carcinoma, Br. J. Cancer **25**:646, 1971.
4. Anderson, D.E.: Genetic study of breast cancer: identification of a high risk group, Cancer **34**:1030, 1974.
5. Anthony, P.P., and James, P.D.: Adenoid cystic carcinoma of the breast: prevalence, diagnostic criteria, and histogenesis, J. Clin. Pathol. **28**:647, 1975.
6. Armstrong, B., and Dall, D.: Environmental factors and cancer incidence and mortality in different countries with special reference to dietary practices, Int. J. Cancer **15**:617, 1975.
7. Ashikari, R., et al.: Paget's disease of the breast, Cancer **26**:680, 1970.
8. Azzopardi, J.G., Ahmed, A., and Millis, R.R.: Problems in breast pathology, Philadelphia, 1979, W.B. Saunders Co.
9. Barnes, L., and Pietruszka, M.: Sarcomas of the breast, Cancer **40**:1577, 1977.
10. Beahrs, O.H., Smart, C., and Shapiro, S.: Report of the Working Group to Review the National Cancer Institute, American Cancer Society Breast Cancer Detection Demonstration Projects, J. Natl. Cancer Inst. **62**:640, 1969.
11. Berg, J.W., and Robbins, G.F.: Twenty year followups of breast cancer, Acta Un. Int. Cancr. **19**:1575, 1963.
12. Berg, J.W., et al.: Histology, epidemiology and end results: the Memorial Hospital Cancer Registry, New York, 1969, Memorial Hospital.
13. Betsill, W.L., et al.: Intraductal carcinoma, long term follow-up after treatment by biopsy alone, J.A.M.A. **239**:1863, 1978.
14. Black, M.M., Barclay, T.H.C., and Cutler, S.J.: Association of atypical characteristics of benign breast lesions with subsequent risk of breast cancer, Cancer **29**:338, 1972.
15. Block, M.M., et al.: Association of atypical characteristics of benign breast lesions with subsequent risk of breast cancer, Cancer **29**:338, 1972.
16. Bloom, H.J.G.: The natural history of untreated breast cancer, Ann. N.Y. Acad. Sci. **114**:747, 1964.
17. Bloom, H.J.G., and Field, J.R.: Impact of tumor grade and host resistance on survival of women with breast cancer, Cancer **28**:1580, 1971.
18. Carstens, P.H.B.: Tubular carcinoma of the breast, Am. J. Clin. Pathol. **70**:214, 1978.
19. Carter, D.L., and Smith, R.I.: Carcinoma in situ of the breast, Cancer **40**:1189, 1977.
20. Decosse, J.J., et al.: Primary lymphosarcoma of the breast, Cancer **15**:1264, 1962.
21. Eniq, M.G., Munn, R.J., and Keeney, M.: Dietary fat and cancer trends: a critique, Fed. Proc. **37**:2215, 1978.
22. Farrow, J.H., and Ashikari, H.: Breast lesions in young girls, Surg. Clin. North Am. **49**:261, 1969.
23. Fisher, B.F., et al.: Cancer of the breast: size of neoplasm and prognosis, **24**:1071, 1969.
24. Franz, V.K., et al.: Incidence of chronic cystic disease in so-called "normal breasts," Cancer **4**:762, 1951.

25. Franzas, F.: Uber die Mastopathia cystica latenta und andere bemerkenswerte Veränderungen in klinisch symptomfreien weiblichen Brüsten, Arb. a. d. path. Inst. d. Univ. Helsingfors **9**:401, 1936.
26. Friedman, B.A., and Oberman, H.A.: Adenoid cystic carcinoma of the breast, Am. J. Clin. Pathol. **54**:1, 1970.
27. Gad, A., and Azzopardi, J.G.: Lobular carcinoma of the breast: a special variant of mucin-secreting carcinoma, J. Clin. Pathol. **28**:711, 1975.
28. Haagensen, C.D.: Diseases of the breast, ed. 2, Philadelphia, 1971, W.B. Saunders Co.
29. Haenszel, W., and Kurihara, M.: Studies on Japanese migrants. I. Mortality from cancer and other diseases among Japanese in the United States, J. Natl. Cancer Inst. **40**:43, 1968.
30. Hajdu, S.I., Espinosa, M.H., and Robins, G.F.: Recurrent cystosarcoma phyllodes: a clinico-pathologic study of 32 cases, Cancer **38**:1402, 1976.
31. Hart, W.R., Bauer, R.C., and Oberman, H.A.: Cystosarcoma phyllodes: a clinicopathologic study of twenty-six hypercellular periductal stromal tumors of the breast, Am. J. Clin. Pathol. **70**:211, 1978.
32. Henderson, B., et al.: An epidemiological study of breast cancer, J. Natl. Cancer Inst. **53**:609, 1974.
33. Hirayama, T.: Epidemiology of breast cancer with special reference to the role of diet, Prev. Med. **7**:173, 1978.
34. Hoover, R., et al.: Menopausal estrogens and breast cancer, N. Engl. J. Med. **295**:401, 1976.
35. Kessinger, A., et al.: Metastatic cystosarcoma phyllodes: a case report and review of the literature, J. Surg. Oncol. **4**:131, 1972.
36. Kodlin, D., et al.: Chronic mastopathy and breast cancer, Cancer **39**:2603, 1977.
37. LiVolsi, V.A., et al.: Fibrocystic breast disease in oral-contraceptive users, N. Engl. J. Med. **299**:381, 1978.
38. MacMahon, B., et al.: Age at first birth and breast cancer risk, Bull. WHO **43**:209, 1970.
39. McDivitt, R.W.: unpublished data, 1981.
40. McDivitt, R.W., Gersell, D.J., and Boyce, W.H.: Tubular carcinoma of the breast, Lab. Invest. **44**:41, 1981.
41. McDivitt, R.W., and Stewart, F.W.: Breast carcinoma in children, J.A.M.A. **195**:388, 1966.
42. McDivitt, R.W., Stewart, F.W., and Berg, J.W.: Tumors of the breast. In Atlas of tumor pathology, Series 2, Fascicle 2, Washington, D.C., 1967, Armed Forces Institute of Pathology Press.
43. McDivitt, R.W., Stewart, F.W., and Farrow, J.H.: Breast carcinoma arising in solitary fibroadenomas, Surg. Gynecol. Obstet. **125**:572, 1967.
44. McDivitt, R.W., Urban, J.A., and Farrow, J.H.: Cystosarcoma phyllodes, Johns Hopkins Med. J. **120**:33, 1967.
45. McDivitt, R.W., et al.: In situ lobular carcinoma, J.A.M.A. **201**:96, 1967.
46. Meyer, J.S.: Personal communication.
47. Meyer, J.S., Bauer, W.G., and Rao, B.R.: Subpopulations of breast cancer defined by S-phase fraction, morphology, and estrogen receptor content, Lab. Invest. **39**:225, 1978.
48. Muller, J.: Uber den feinern Bau and die Farmen der kraukhaften Gerschwulste, Berlin, 1838, 6 Reiner.
49. National Cancer Institute Breast Cancer Digest, Pub. No. 80-1691, Bethesda, Md., 1980, National Institutes of Health.
50. National Cancer Institute Cancer Patient Survival Report No. 5 1976, Pub. No. NTH 77-992, Bethesda, Md., 1977, Department of Health, Education and Welfare.
51. Nayer, H.R.: Cylindroma of the breast with pulmonary metastases, Dis. Chest **31**:324, 1957.
52. Norris, H.J., and Taylor, H.B.: Sarcomas and related mesenchymal tumors of the breast, Cancer **22**:22, 1968.
53. Norris, H.J., and Taylor, H.B.: Carcinoma of the male breast, Cancer **23**:106, 1969.
54. O'Kell, R.T.: Adenoid cystic carcinoma of the breast, Mo. Med. **61**:855, 1964.
55. Ory, H., Cole, P., and MacMahon, B.: Oral contraceptives and reduced risk of benign breast diseases, N. Eng. J. Med. **294**:719, 1972.
56. Osborne, C.K., and McGuire, W.L.: Current use of steroid hormone receptor assay in the treatment of breast cancer, Surg. Clin. North Am. **58**:777, 1978.
57. Paffenbarger, R.S., et al.: Cancer risk as related to use of oral contraceptives during fertile years, Cancer **39**:1887, 1977.
58. Page, D., et al.: Relationship between component parts of fibrocystic disease complex and breast cancer, J. Natl. Cancer Inst. **61**:1055, 1979.
59. Page, D.L., et al.: Relation between component parts of fibrocystic disease complex and breast cancer, J. Natl. Cancer Inst. **61**:1055, 1978.
60. Paget, J.: On disease of the mammary areola preceding cancer of the mammary gland, St. Barth. Hosp. Rep. **10**:86, 1974.
61. Perzin, K.H., and Lattes, R.: Papillary adenoma of the nipple, Cancer **29**:996, 1972.
62. Pullinger, B.D.: Cystic disease of the breast: human and experimental, Lancet **2**:567, 1947.
63. Robbins, G.F., et al.: Inflammatory carcinoma of the breast, Surg. Clin. North Am. **54**:801, 1974.
64. Rosen, P.P., et al.: Lobular carcinoma in situ of the breast: detailed analysis of 99 patients with average follow-up of 24 years, Am. J. Surg. Pathol. **2**:225, 1978.
65. Rosen, P.P., and Mike, V.: Prognostic factors in breast cancer. In Hoogstraten, B., and McDivitt, R.W., editors: Breast cancer, Boca Raton, Fla., CRC Press, Inc. (In press.)
66. Rosen, P.P., and Snyder, R.E.: Non-palpable breast lesions detected by mammography and confirmed by specimen radiography, Breast **3**:13, 1977.
67. Rosen, P.P., et al.: Estrogen receptor protein (ERP) and the histopathology of human mammary carcinoma. In McGuire, W.L., editor: Hormones, receptors and breast cancer, New York, 1978, Raven Press.
68. Scheike, O., Visfeldt, J., and Peterson, B.: Male breast cancer, Acta Pathol. Microbiol. Scand. **81**:352, 1973.
69. Sergi, M., et al: An epidemiological study on cancer in Japan, Gan **48**(suppl.):1, 1957.
70. Sirtori, C., and Veronesi, U.: Gynecomastia: a review of 218 cases, Cancer **10**:645, 1957.
71. Stocks, L.H., and Simmons, F.M.: Inflammatory carcinoma of the breast, Surg. Gynecol. Obstet. **143**:885, 1976.
72. Strong, E.W., McDivitt, R.W., and Brasfield, R.D.: Granular cell myoblastoma, Cancer **25**:415, 1970.
73. Tavassoli, F.A., and Norris, H.J.: Secretory carcinoma, Cancer **45**:2404, 1980.
74. Taylor, H.B., and Robertson, A.G.: Adenomas of the nipple, Cancer **18**:995, 1965.
75. Treichopoulos, D., MacMahon, B., and Cole, P.: The menopause and breast cancer risk, J. Natl. Cancer Inst. **48**:605, 1972.
76. Treves, N.: Gynecomastia, Cancer **11**:1083, 1958.
77. Treves, N., and Sunderland, D.A.: Cystosarcoma phyllodes of the breast: a malignant and a benign tumor; a clinicopathological study of seventy-seven cases, Cancer **4**:1286, 1951.
78. Veronisi, U., and Pizzocaro, G.: Breast cancer in women subsequent to cystic disease of the breast, Surg. Gynecol. Obstet. **126**:529, 1968.
79. VonToth, J.: Das granularzellige myoblastom der mamma, Zentralbl. Allg. Pathol. **115**:366-371, 1972.
80. Warren, S.: The relation of "chronic mastitis" to carcinoma of the breast, Surg. Gynecol. Obstet. **71**:257, 1940.
81. Waterhouse, J., et al.: Cancer incidence in five continents. In International Agency for Research on Cancer, vol. 3, no. 15, Lyon, France, 1976, IARC Scientific Publications.
82. Wellings, S.R., Jensen, H.M., and Marcum, R.G.: An atlas of subgross pathology of the human breast with special reference to possible precancerous lesions, J. Natl. Cancer Inst. **55**:231, 1975.
83. Westbrook, K.D., and Gallager, H.S.: Intraductal carcinoma of the breast: a comparative study, Am. J. Surg. **130**:667, 1975.

CHAPTER 38

Skin

ARTHUR C. ALLEN

This text was the first to devote a comprehensive chapter to the pathology of the skin, an allocation soon followed by other editors. However, we must admit that our initial objective—to help develop among colleagues in general pathology a renewed interest and a practical expertise in dermatopathology—has not been realized. Because of increasing awareness of the dermatologic manifestations of systemic disease, this failure to elicit interest in this fascinating, highly informative aspect of pathology is regrettable.

In the interval between this and the previous edition, promising sophisticated methodology has been improved or initiated. This includes transmission and scanning electron microscopy, electron histochemistry, tissue cultures, fracture-freeze replication, diagnostic and pathogenetic fluorescent immunology, the determination of B and T cell markers, and the observation of defective DNA repair after ultraviolet irradiation. The inferences from these newer approaches do not always match the sophistication of the methodology. Nonetheless, hard data are useful, but they often must await maturation of interpretations.

There is a sizable group of dermatoses that have significant morphologic individuality. In many instances the distinguishing features are so clear cut that a diagnosis may be offered on examination merely of the histologic slide. In other cases a small range of diagnoses may be suggested by the section. In the remainder the microscopic changes give no diagnostic help in the absence of a clinical history. Although the size of the last group will obviously be determined by the experience of the examiner, the percentage of cases that falls into it can be made sufficiently low as to spark the lagging interest of the general pathologist. One of the major difficulties in the learning of dermatopathology is that the changes usually are not of the all-or-none or qualitatively distinct variety but are often a matter of weighted quantitative differences. The proper judgment of these differences depends on a knowledge of the normal histologic range of the structures of the skin, as well as on an ability to interrelate and interpret a whole series of aberrations in these structures.

Obviously, only a small segment of cutaneous pathology can be included in this chapter. Accordingly, it would seem to underscore the applicability of dermatopathology best if some of the many lesions diagnosable by histologic characteristics alone were given preference over those less easily recognizable.

Immunopathology of the skin actually adds another bridging dimension to several disciplines, including rheumatology, hematology, infectious diseases, and therapy. The direct and indirect fluorescent techniques depicting, as they do, the precise localization of antibodies, fibrin, and components of complement, allow a new dynamic insight into the pathogenesis of such dermatoses as the bullous disorders, systemic lupus erythematosus (SLE), porphyrias, psoriasis, vasculitic diseases, and others. Similarly, diagnostic and pathogenic vistas are being opened and rapidly widened by the analysis of HLA antigens (human leukocyte antigens) and their disease-linked genes. These are active in varying degrees in psoriasis, the bullous diseases, lupus erythematosus, atopic dermatitis, lichen planus, granuloma annulare, and many others. Additionally useful is the ability to distinguish in situ individual cells of an infiltrate from tissue homogenates. The indirect peroxidase labeling of anti-HTLA (heterologous human T [or B] cell antiserum) permits this.

STRUCTURE OF NORMAL SKIN

The skin normally varies in color, elasticity, thickness, blood supply, and texture depending on anatomic location, age, state of nutrition, endocrinologic status, and race of the individual. With the unaided eye, fine (Blaschko's) ridges are noted over the skin generally, and coarse folds, allowing for movement, are present, particularly over the joints. Between the ridges are sulci of Heidenhain. The ridges are further marked by delicate, crisscross, triangular or polygonal lines. In recent years there has been considerable interest in the science of dermatoglyphics, which deals with the interpretation of detailed patterns of sulci, furrows, and ridges of the palms. Dermatoglyphic abnormalities have been observed in patients with rubella, psoriasis, neurofibromatosis, anonychia, a variety of chromosomal abnormalities, and some disorders otherwise unassociated with cutaneous manifestations.

The ostia of sweat glands, the pores, open into the ridges. The hair also varies in texture, length, density, contour, and color depending on age, race, sex, and so on. The smooth, hairless skin, or the skin with fine vellus hairs, is known as glabrous skin. The epidermis varies from 0.07 to 0.12 mm over most of the body and from 0.8 to 1.4 mm or more on the palms and soles. The cutis has a corresponding range of thickness. The junction of the cutis and the subcutis or subcuticular fat is usually indistinct, except in certain regions such as the forehead, ear, perineum, and scrotum.

Fig. 38-1 is a diagram of normal skin. It is of diagnostic use to bear in mind how the skin varies in different parts of the body. For example, sebaceous glands are particularly prominent about the face, especially in the region of the nose, so diagnoses of hyperplasia or adenoma of sebaceous glands should take this feature into account. The epidermis is normally thin and the rete ridges are relatively inconspicuous over the tibia, the breasts, and the flexor surfaces of the forearms. This variant should not, therefore, be mistaken for atrophy. Similarly, the dermis over the lower legs is normally much thinner than it is in many other portions of the body, so that, again, the possibility of confusion with atrophy exists. The elastic tissue of the dermis shows such a large range in its quantity, as well as in the degree of fraying and splintering of the fibers, even in normal tissues, that considerable caution should be used in concluding that abnormalities of elastic tissue are present. Finally, the normally thick stratum corneum of the sole may prompt the diagnosis of keratoderma. These are a few of the examples of the variation

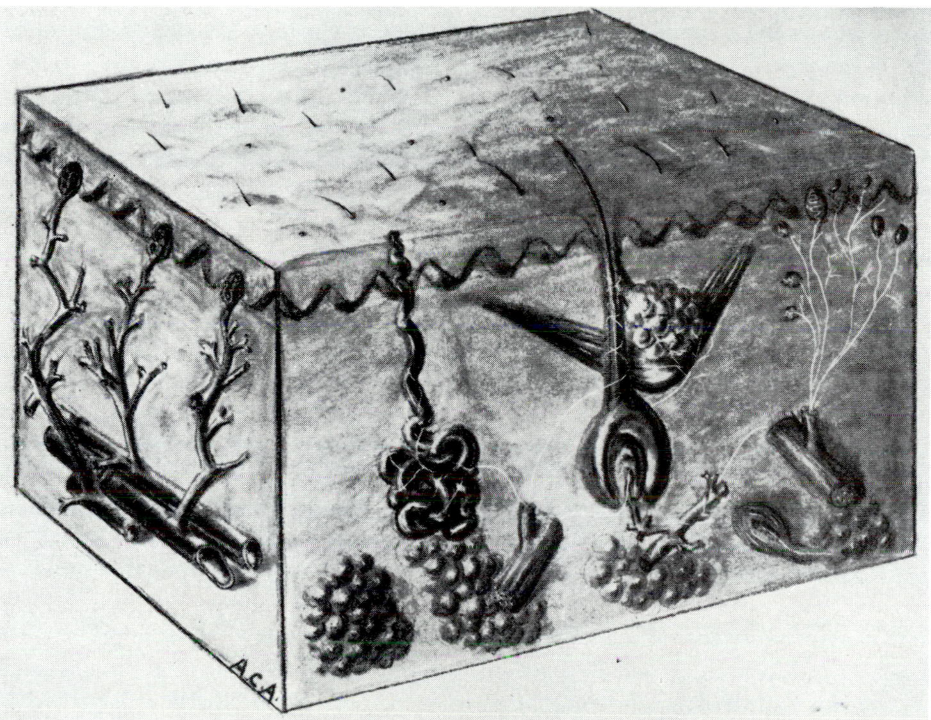

Fig. 38-1. In smaller panel at left are shown arteries, veins, and lymphatic vessels, along with their plexuses within papillae. In reality, plexuses of all three types of vessels overlap in same regions. In larger front panel are included appendages, nerves, and subcutaneous fat. Tubular sweat gland on left reaches surface through duct that, in its course through epidermis, maintains its own epithelial lining. Ductal ostium or sweat pore is independent of hair follicle. In center is pilosebaceous apparatus comprising hair follicle, sebaceous glands, and arrectores pilorum. Nerves and vessels supplying critical papillae are shown at deep portion of follicle. Sebaceous gland is intimately linked to hair follicle, into which its duct empties directly. Arrectores pilorum not only stiffen hair shaft but, as may be surmised from position illustrated, also help, by contraction, to expel contents of sebaceous gland and to constrict superficial vessels. On right are shown nerves and nerve endings—corpuscles of Merkel-Ranvier, Meissner, Ruffini, Krause, and Pacini. Nerve fibers entwined about appendages are also illustrated.

in cutaneous histology, an accurate evaluation of which is clearly essential for an appraisal of some of the qualitatively similar pathologic changes.

The objective of the pathologist is to match the dermatologist's clinical observation of erythema, scales, pigmentation, blisters, and patterns of lesions with the pathologist's observation of parakeratosis, acanthosis, edema, epidermal spongiosis or cleavages, vascular alterations, and type and location of inflammatory cells, along with several other ancillary histologic changes. One would hope that these factors, properly weighted and fed into the "clinical-histologic computer," would lead to the appropriate diagnosis. Undoubtedly, when the precise pattern and location of fluorescently revealed immunologic deposits, enzymatic abnormalities, and qualitative, quantitative, and topographic distribution of B and T lymphocytes are one day soon added to the input, the composite diagnoses will be refined.

Finally, the assessment of the intradermal cells depends on their patterns, their nature, their source, their correlation with similar cells in the peripheral blood and the regional lymph nodes, their content of immunoglobulins and complement, and their identification with categories, fulminance, and deflorescence of clinical lesions, in addition to the common antigenicity of these cells and other specific anatomic sites such as the various parts of the epidermis. These are the urgent problems that need to be resolved for better insight into currently vaguely understood cutaneous disorders. In addition, one of the great deficiencies in dermatopathology is the lack of animal models.

Epidermis

The epidermis is composed of the following layers:

1. Basal cell layer (stratum germinativum)
2. Prickle cell layers (stratum spinosum, rete mucosum, rete Malpighii)
3. Granular layers (stratum granulosum)
4. Stratum lucidum
5. Cornified layer (stratum corneum)

Basal cell layer

The basal cell layer is one cell thick and forms the junction between epidermis and dermis. The nuclei are relatively hyperchromatic, are arranged perpendicular to the epidermal basement membrane, and normally contain a few mitoses as evidence of the activity of a layer that serves in part as the progenitor of the remainder of the epidermis. Interspersed in the basal layer are cells with a clear zone separating and often compressing most of the cytoplasm and nucleus away from the cell wall (the so-called *cellule claire*). The cytoplasm may or may not contain melanin, but these cells are likely to be dopa positive and, accordingly, are melanocytes. Not all melanocytes of the basal layer are "clear cells." Ultrastructurally the melanocytes contain melanosomes, but most observers believe that they contain few or no desmosomes or tonofilaments. As a matter of fact, such structures may be noted, albeit often reduced in number, not only in many melanocytes but, more vividly and meaningfully, also in the marginal cells of melanocarcinomas in situ. The fairly universal insistence that keratinocytes lack lysosomes has contributed to the circular reasoning that melanocytes are ipso facto nonkeratinocytes inasmuch as they contain these organelles. A directly contrary observation has recently clearly indicated that keratinocytes are characterized by Odland bodies, which are membrane-coated granules, keratinosomes, or lysosomes.

For a long time it has been accepted, on debatable evidence, that melanocytes are really nerve endings that originated in the neural crest, became incorporated in the epidermis, and later constituted the source of normal pigment in skin as well as of pigmented nevi and melanocarcinomas. It is generally maintained that melanocytes are the same in number in both white and black skin and the pigment is transferred to neighboring keratinocytes, which "nip off" pieces of melanized dendrites attached to scattered, basally located melanocytes.

The simplistic notion that keratinocytes acquire melanosomes by "nipping off" and incorporating tips of dendrites is untenable. The objections to this hypothesis include the following:

1. That the keratinocytic melanosomes usually are not scattered haphazardly in their cytoplasm as they would be in histiocytes or melanophages, but usually are located supranuclearly as if produced in situ
2. That the pigmentation or melanosomes are often confined to a single (basal) layer, at times in conjunction with the spinous layer immediately above, unlike the scattered, multilayered distribution to be expected if the sequestration of hydralike dendrites were operative
3. That pigmentation or melanosomes may be uniformly incorporated into keratinocytes within hours after ultraviolet radiation or x-radiation, hardly the short time span compatible with the process of dendritic phagocytosis and pigmentary alignment. My opposing theory is that the development of pigment is normally inherent in many keratinocytes and modulated with certain provocations, such as radiation, drugs, or hormones, may be induced to express this function.

It is clearly important that these controversial matters be addressed rather than disregarded or presented in article after article as if proved.

Another question is how epidermis, regenerated after ulceration, develops basal melanocytes spaced every tenth cell or so. In my opinion the process of conversion of basal cells and keratinocytes into melanocytes normally takes place continuously and may be retarded (as in vitiligo) or accelerated (as in sunburn). Actually, as might be anticipated, the numbers of dopa-reactive epidermal melanocytes have been found to be increased after irradiation with ultraviolet light, although contrary results previously had been reported. In other words, the activation of basal cells and keratinocytes into melanocytes is an in situ conversion and varies in speed and extent with different age groups, races, and stimuli. However, it would be misleading to fail to acknowledge that the concept of neurogenesis of melanocytes, nevi, and melanocarcinomas is the popular one at the moment.

There has been a revival of interest in the nature of the controverted intraepidermal, aurophilic Langerhans cell. To some, it is a worn-out (effete) melanocyte with a possible capacity to manufacture or even to phagocytose melanin. To others, it is a form of intraepidermal neural element with a spectrum of neural enzymes, including adenosine triphosphatase (ATPase) and leucine aminopeptidase. To still others, it is a histiocyte that has wandered into the epidermis and is identical to the histiocytes of histiocytosis X. Ultrastructurally it has been forcefully emphasized that this cell possesses a specific racquet-shaped organelle but, as was to be expected, similar organelles have been observed in other organs, such as the thymus gland. More recently it has been admitted, in a refreshing reversal of opinion, that Langerhans cells are not related to melanocytes, that they are not derived from the neural crest, and that the whole question of their nature, derivation, and function must be regarded from a new perspective.

It now appears clear that this aurophilic, ATPase-positive, antigen-bearing cell with the characteristic racquet-shaped (Birbeck) granule is immunologically part of a very much alive migrating population that finds itself not fixed within the epidermis but essentially located wherever macrophages are to be seen. Reality would be better served if this Langerhans cell were regarded as a variety of hematic cell rather than an epidermally derived effete dendritic cell.

Prickle cell layer

The prickle cells are several layers thick, the number varying in different parts of the body. The cells are joined by cytoplasmic bridges (spines, prickles, desmosomes), which serve as the most easily recognizable identification of such cells, both in squamous cell neoplasms and in metaplastic processes. The intracellular cytoplasmic tonofilaments usually are regarded as the precursors of keratin. Glycogen is usually present. The generally accepted absence of lysosomes (keratinosomes) in keratinocytes has been disputed; thus the supposed differences between keratinocytes and melanocytes are narrowed.[33]

Stratum granulosum

The stratum granulosum averages about two layers thick and is composed of cells with blue, round cytoplasmic granules of keratohyalin. The chemical nature of the keratohyaline granules remains essentially obscure. Although superficially resembling nuclear material, they are Feulgen and periodic acid–Schiff negative and contain no protein-bound sulfhydryl groups. They appear as electron-dense bodies and apparently contain tonofilaments. The granules are also osmophilic, are digested with elastase, and are presumed to be closely related histogenetically to keratin. Lysosomes are present in abundance in the granular layers, in contrast to their sparse distribution in the basal and squamous cell layers. The stratum lucidum, which is practically confined to the palms and soles, is a clear, homogeneous, acidophilic, anuclear, thin layer of eleidin.

Stratum corneum

The stratum corneum, also normally without nuclei, is made up of various thicknesses of keratin. The stratum corneum, particularly its lower half, is important as the barrier in regulating the transfer of water through the skin. Fat globules may be present in the two uppermost layers.

Periodic acid–Schiff–positive, diastase-resistant mucopolysaccharides are present in the epidermis and are presumed to play a role in binding or cementing the epidermal cells together. Since keratinization normally takes place in the upper layers of epidermis, the acid mucopolysaccharides are presumably degraded, allowing the keratin to be discarded as invisible flakes. With incomplete degradation of the mucopolysaccharides, visible, coherent, parakeratotic scales occur, as in psoriasis.

Basement membrane

There is convincing histologic evidence that a true epidermal basement membrane, equivalent, for example, to the one surrounding glands, does not exist. Basement membranes in other locations, such as those about sweat glands and renal tubules, are argyrophilic. No such continuous epidermal basement membrane is demonstrable with silver stains, although an illusion of one occasionally is created by argyrophilic granules of melanin aligned in the basal layer. On the other hand, stains with the periodic acid–Schiff reagent do reveal what appear to be interrupted segments of a basement membrane. This simulation is caused by the presence of polysaccharides that have been irregularly concentrated by the varying densities of the subepidermal collagen, especially with edema of the upper cutis. In this connection one other fact should be mentioned again. Basal cells do have intercellular bridges (desmosomes) that bind them to the overlying cells of the stratum spinosum and, in their upper portions, to each other. To the corium they are attached by semidesmosomes to an ultrastructurally visible membrane called an adepidermal lamina, visible only electron microscopically and not equivalent to the argyrophilic structures readily detectable even in routine stains, as mentioned.

Dermis

The dermis, or corium, is divided into the superficial pars papillaris and the deeper pars reticularis. The papillae of the dermis alternate with projections of epidermis called rete ridges. The length of the papillae, the thickness of the overlying epidermal plate, the vascularity, the edema, and the direction and consistency of the collagenous fibers of the papillae are all of diagnostic value.

The thickness of the pars papillaris varies considerably, from several microns to hundreds of microns. In the papillary portion the fibers of collagen tend to run vertically. In the deeper part the fibers are rather loosely dispersed in a horizontal direction. Accuracy in evaluating changes in the consistency, tinctorial qualities, and cellularity of the collagen and elastic tissue of the dermis furnishes the basis for many diagnoses. With electron microscopy, elastic fibers show a fibrillar structure within an otherwise almost homogeneous matrix in which the characteristic periodicity of collagen is lacking.[62]

The cutaneous appendages include the sweat glands, sebaceous glands, hair follicles, arrectores pilorum, and nails. The sweat glands are coiled glands of two varieties: eccrine and apocrine.

The eccrine glands are universally distributed in the skin and are made up of several coils of tubular glands lying deep in the dermis. These glands empty their secretion into tubules traversing the dermis and epidermis, opening into the fine ridges of the skin as pores. The coils are lined by two principal layers of cells: (1) the more superficial, basophilic, dark, granular, mucopolysaccharide-containing cells and (2) the more basilar, acidophilic clear or chief cells. There may be some interdigitation between these cells. A flattened third type of cell, the myoepithelial or basket cell, is interposed between these secretory cells and the basement membrane. A large battery of enzymes is detectable in the eccrine glands, including oxidases, dehydrogenases, phosphorylases, alkaline phosphatases, and glucuronidases. Their presence has been used in defining certain of the neoplasms of sweat glands. The ducts are lined also by two layers of epithelial cells, but the myoepithelium is absent. The inner lining of the ducts of sweat glands is keratinized in their course through the epidermis, and indeed some of the neoplasms of sweat glands show evidence of squamous cell metaplasia. In any case, the inner hyaline membrane of the ducts often serves as a clue to the genesis of these neoplasms.

The apocrine glands occur in the axilla, groin, nipple, umbilicus, anus, and genital region. They are easily recognized by their large lumina, prominence of secretory cytoplasmic granules, and rows of myoepithelial cells longitudinally oriented below the cuboid or columnar secretory cells. The periglandular basement membrane is especially conspicuous. Light yellow, sudanophilic granules, as well as granules of hemosiderin and a minimum of glycogen, are commonly present. Mucin normally is noted within the lumen and cells of apocrine glands and is periodic acid–Schiff positive and diatase resistant. Desmosomes, similar to those of keratinocytes, have been noted. The ultrastructural observation of canaliculi, particularly, suggests that an eccrine type as well as an apocrine (that is, apically erosive) type of secretion occurs. Secretory activity varies with the menstrual cycle. The ducts of the apocrine glands usually open in close relationship to the hair follicles but may reach the surface independently, as do the eccrine glands.

The sebaceous or holocrine glands are racemose structures that serve mainly as appendages to the hair follicle to which they are attached. Each alveolus is rimmed by a basement membrane surrounding one or two layers of squamous cells, internal to which are the characteristic sebaceous cells with small round nuclei and abundant, finely latticed, fatty cytoplasm. The sebaceous cells are pushed toward the duct, wherein they finally rupture and release their fatty contents in the hair follicle. Modifications of sebaceous glands occur in the eyelids and ears, in the areolae of the nipples, and in the male and female genitalia (odoriferous glands). In these regions they are unconnected with hairs or hair follicles. The amount of sebum secreted is about the same in the adolescent boy and girl, shows no appreciable change in the aging woman, and decreases in the aging man. Ectopic sebaceous glands may be found in the salivary glands and in the glans penis. Such ectopic glands of the corona penis are often referred to as Tyson's glands. Actually, Tyson appears to have described a beaded rim of fibroepithelial pearly nodules about the corona.

The hair consists of a shaft that at its lower end enlarges into a bulb. The bulb embraces an invaginating dermal papilla, through which the hair receives its blood supply. The intracutaneous portion of the hair shaft and the bulb are enclosed in a hair follicle. The hair shaft is made up of a cuticle, a sheath, and a more or less pigmented cortex and medulla, the latter being absent in lanugo hairs.

The arrectores pilorum are bands of smooth muscle originating in or near the papillary layer of the dermis and inserting at several points into the outer layer of adjacent hair follicles just above their papillae. The direction of the muscle is at an angle to the hairs so that their contraction (gooseflesh) causes the hairs to be erected. At the same time, the superficial vessels are constricted to avoid cooling, and sebaceous secretion is expelled by the pressure of the contracting arrectores pilorum. However, there is some disagreement as to this last function.

The blood and lymphatic vessels of the skin are arranged in plexuses. The arterial vessels are derived from the subcutaneous arteries, which give off plexuses to the papillary layer, as well as to the reticular layer and the various appendages. It has been suggested that the selective localization of infiltrate to various components of the dermis is related to the pattern of these plexuses. In the skin of certain regions of the body, particularly the fingers, there are normally arteriovenous shunts or glomera that serve to regulate blood flow and surface temperature. The glomus is composed of an afferent arteriole, a shunt called the Sucquet-Hoyer canal, and an efferent vein. The canal is lined by layers of rounded glomus cells that have a contractile function. The veins also form plexuses in the papillary, subpapillary, and deep reticular layers, as well as about the appendages.

The lymphatic plexuses are localized principally in the papillae and at the juction of dermis and subcutaneous tissue. The deeper lymphatic vessels have valves.

The nerves of the skin are preponderantly medullated. A few are nonmedullated and lead to the blood vessels, smooth muscles, epidermis, hair follicles, and glands. The specialized nerve endings include the corpuscles of Vater-Pacini, which are found in the deep layers of the skin and subcutaneous tissue, in the mucous membranes, and in the conjunctiva and cornea. These structures are particularly numerous in the skin of the nipple and external genital organs. Other nerve endings are the Meissner corpuscles of the papillae of the skin of palms, soles, and tips of fingers and toes, the end bulbs of Krause, which are smaller than but structurally similar to the Meissner corpuscles and are found in the external genitalia, the elongated, dermal corpuscles of Ruffini, and the intraepidermal disclike, tactile Merkel-Ranvier corpuscles, which are identified with silver stains and are present in the epidermis and external root sheath of hairs. The endings are presumably receptors for touch (Merkel-Ranvier and Meissner corpuscles), pressure (pacinian corpuscles), heat (corpuscles of Ruffini), and cold (end bulbs of Krause).

DEFINITIONS

Clinical terms

macule Circumscribed flat area of altered coloration of skin; evanescent or permanent; varies in size from pinhead to several centimeters, in color from red (erythema), brown (ephelis), and the various colors of blood pigment (petechiae and ecchymoses) to white (vitiligo), and in shape from circular, polygonal, or linear to polymorphous varieties of erythema multiforme.

papule Circumscribed elevated area; varies in size from pinhead to about 5 mm, in surface contour from flat, conical, or pointed circular to umbilicated, in color from red, yellow, or white to violaceous, and in shape of base from round to more or less polygonal (such as the papules of lichen planus and psoriasis); the papule, as well as the macule, may provoke pruritus, burning sensation, anesthesia, and pain or may cause no symptoms; both macules and papules may be overlain by scales.

nodule An enlarged papule varying in size from about 0.5 to 2 cm, usually deep seated, involving the lower dermis and subcutaneous fat (for example, the nodules of rheumatoid arthritis and leprosy).

vesicle Circumscribed, single or grouped elevations of the epidermis, beneath which are collections containing serum, plasma, or blood; surface may be flat, globoid, or umbilicated (as in smallpox and eczema).

pustule Vesicle containing pus predominantly (for example, impetigo).

bulla (bleb) Similar to vesicle, except that the bullae are larger, varying from 0.5 to more than 8 cm (as in pemphigus).

scale Loosened, imperfectly cornified, parakeratotic superficial layer of skin that is shed as fine, branny, dirty white, yellowish keratinous dust or large pearly-white flakes; distribution may be focal or universal and usually is associated with inflammation of the skin (psoriasis and exfoliative dermatitis) but need not be (as in ichthyosis).

crust Residue of dried serum, blood, pus, and epithelial, keratinous, and bacterial debris; crusts vary in color from yellow to green to dark brown, depending on the admixture of the different ingredients, and in consistency from a thin superficial and watery (as in impetigo) to a thick, bulky and loosely or firmly attached covering of a rupioid syphiloderm; crusts occur after the oozing of serum, blood, or pus in a disrupted, eroded, or ulcerated epidermis (as in eczema, impetigo, smallpox, abrasions, and other conditions).

excoriation (erosion) Superficial erosion and ulceration produced mechanically, usually by the fingernails in scratching pruritic skin or in picking at various lesions (as in neurotic excoriations).

fissure (rhagade) Linear, often crusted, tender, painful defect in continuity of the skin, occurring usually at mucocutaneous junctions at sites where there is normally considerable elasticity of the skin (about the anus, mouth, fingers, palms, and soles) and also in certain diseases (such as syphilis, nonspecific anal fissures, keratoderma, intertrigo, and eczema).

ulcer Defect of the skin, deeper than an erosion or excoriation, extending at least into the dermis; the edges may be ragged, punched out in appearance, undermined, or everted; the floor may be glazed or granular, puriform or hemorrhagic, and shallow or deep; the outline of an ulcer may be circular, serpiginous, crescentic, ovoid, or irregular; ulcers may be painless or exquisitely sensitive; they heal generally by concentric scarring and epithelization (for example, tropical, diphtheritic, and varicose ulcers).

lichenification Thickening of the skin with exaggeration of its normal markings so that the striae form a crisscross pattern; occurs after chronic irritation of pruritic skin.

comedo Keratinous plug, sometimes admixed with bacteria and inflammatory cells, within ducts of sebaceous glands; characteristic of acne.

Histologic terms

acanthosis Thickening through hyperplasia of the rete Malpighi; may exist without hyperkeratosis (Fig. 38-13).

hyperkeratosis Thickening of the keratinized layer, the stratum corneum; generally is associated with a prominent stratum granulosum.

parakeratosis Persistence of nuclei in the stratum corneum, signifying the presence clinically of a loosely adherent scale (such as dandruff); characterized by the absence or striking diminution of the stratum granulosum, except in the stage of healing (Fig. 38-13); with fluorescence microscopy (with acridine orange, rhodamine B, and thioflavine S) hyperkeratosis is reflected by orthochromasia and brilliance, and parakeratosis is reflected by dullness and metachromatic color changes.

spongiosis Intercellular edema of the epidermis, which, when pronounced, progresses to vesiculation (as in eczema).

acantholysis Separation of individual cells from the stratum spinosum, with loss of prickle cells and consequent isolation within the fluid of a vesicle (for example, pemphigus).

ballooning degeneration One of the diagnostic morphologic phenomena leading to vesiculation in viral diseases; characterized by the isolation of a cell from its neighbors, especially in the lower layers of the epidermis, the withdrawing of its prickles after intracytoplasmic edema and vacuolization, and the amitotic division of its nucleus so as to form a multinucleated giant cell (as in variola, but particularly herpes and varicella).

reticular colliquation Another characteristic of the cutaneous vesicles caused by viruses; the cytoplasm of several cells becomes edematous, granular, coalescent, and partially disintegrated; the residual cytoplasm forms reticulated septa that separate multiloculated intraepidermal collections of fluid or vesicles; the nuclei become small, pyknotic, or completely karyorrhectic.

dyskeratosis Abnormality of development or distinctive alteration of epidermal cells; two types are distinguished: (1) benign dyskeratosis—such as the molluscum bodies of mulluscum contagiosum, represented by swollen brightly eosinophilic cells, mostly of the stratum granulosum, containing virus elementary bodies, or the corps ronds and grains of the stratum granulosum and stratum corneum, respectively, as noted in Darier's disease; in molluscum contagiosum, the dyskeratosis is caused by a virus; (2) malignant dyskeratosis—anaplastic changes such as hyperchromatism, changes in polarity, increase in mitotic figures, and enlargement of nuclei and nucleoli that signify potential or actual development of carcinoma.

pseudoepitheliomatous hyperplasia Pronounced acanthosis with extensive downgrowth of rete ridges as may occur at the periphery of an ulcer, in bromodermas, and after insect bites; occasionally the exuberant epidermal hyperplasia is mistaken for carcinoma, as in so-called molluscum sebaceum or keratoacanthoma (Fig. 38-33).

liquefaction degeneration Obliteration of the line of demarcation of epidermis and dermis by edema of the basal cells and subepidermal dermis, as well as by the presence of inflammatory cells at this junction (such as lichen planus and lupus erythematosus) (Figs. 38-13 and 38-17).

CUTANEOUS-VISCERAL DISEASE

The cutaneous reflection of visceral disease is finally coming to be accorded the significance it has long merited. Recent surveys show that, because of the increasing awareness of the importance of the association of visceral with cutaneous diseases, graduate students of dermatology are requesting more sophisticated training in internal medicine. A simple listing of some of the cutaneous manifestations of visceral lesions, many of which have become apparent within the past decade, will underscore this often vital relationship:

1. Pigmentations
   a. Acanthosis nigricans of adults ("malignant" type)—commonly associated with visceral adenocarcinoma
   b. Acanthosis nigricans (juvenile)—occasionally associated with congenital lipodystrophy and insulin-resistant diabetes or with Rud's syndrome (tetany, epilepsy, anemia, and mental retardation); also with ichthyosis hystrix
   c. Peutz-Jeghers syndrome—focal mucosal and cutaneous pigmentation with gastrointestinal polyps and, rarely, with carcinomas
   d. Hemochromatosis—with pigmentary cirrhosis of liver and diabetes mellitus
   e. Addison's disease
   f. Incontinentia pigmenti—with neurologic and cardiac abnormalities
   g. Ochronosis—with cardiac disease
   h. Phenylketonuria—with neurologic manifestations
   i. Pellagra
   j. Café-au-lait spots—with von Recklinghausen's disease and fibrous dysplasia
   k. Chediak-Higashi syndrome—with specific leukocytic inclusions and semialbinism
2. Miscellaneous nonbullous dermatoses
   a. Lupus erythematosus—with nephritis, carditis, arthritis, and hypersplenism
   b. Dermatomyositis in adults—with visceral cancer
   c. Ichthyosis in adults—with lymphomas
   d. Alopecia mucinosa—with mycosis fungoides
   e. Erythema annulare (gyratum)—with rheumatic fever and cancer
   f. Pyoderma gangrenosum—with ulcerative colitis
   g. Sarcoidosis and other granulomatous diseases—with visceral involvement
3. Vesiculobullous lesions
   a. Zoster—with malignant lymphomas (occasionally dermatitis herpetiformis, pemphigoid, and erythema multiforme bullosum are associated with visceral cancers)
   b. Acrodermatitis enteropathica
   c. Bullous lesions—with porphyrias
   d. Dermatitis herpetiformis—with intestinal disease (spruelike)
   e. Toxic epidermal necrolysis—several instances associated with malignant lymphomas
4. Urticaria
   a. Urticaria pigmentosum—with involvement of bones, liver, spleen, and lymph nodes
   b. Urticaria—with amyloidosis, nerve deafness, and renal disease
5. Diseases of collagen and elastic tissue
   a. Scleroderma—with renal, cardiac, and gastrointestinal lesions

b. Pseudoxanthoma elasticum—with ocular and cardiac lesions
c. Ehlers-Danlos syndrome—increased serum hexosamine; involvement of vessels, heart, and gastrointestinal tract
d. Cutis laxa
e. Necrobiosis lipoidica diabeticorum—with diabetes mellitus
f. Circumscribed myxedema—with exophthalmic goiter
g. Amyloidosis (primary and secondary)—with myeloma (primary amyloidosis), chronic infections (secondary amyloidosis)

6. Vascular diseases
   a. Angiokeratoma of Fabry—with renal and vascular lesions
   b. Allergic granulomatosis—with visceral angiitis
   c. Degos' syndrome—thromboangiitis of skin and intestines
   d. Blue rubber-bleb nevus—with intestinal angiomas
   e. Neurocutaneous-vascular syndromes
      (1) Sturge-Weber syndrome—cutaneous angiomatosis and epilepsy
      (2) Ataxia-telangiectasia
      (3) Rendu-Osler-Weber syndrome—with arteriovenous fistulas of lungs, brain
7. Metabolic disorders
   a. Xanthomatoses—with diabetes mellitus, von Gierke's disease, biliary cirrhosis, lipid nephrosis, and essential familial hypercholesterolemia
   b. Lipidoses with cutaneous infiltration—reticulohistiocytic granulomas (lipid dermatoarthritis); lipid proteinosis; gangliosidoses and other sphingolipidoses (Fabry's, Tay-Sachs, Gaucher's)
   c. Mucopolysaccharidoses—for example, Hurler's syndrome
   d. Dysproteinemias—including Waldenström's macroglobulinemia (with malignant lymphomas), cryoglobulinemias (with cutaneous infarcts), and multiple myeloma (with cutaneous infiltration)
8. Cutaneous tumors
   a. Arsenical lesions (keratoses, Bowen's disease)—with visceral cancers in limited percentage
   b. Kaposi's sarcoma—with malignant lymphomas
   c. Sebaceous adenomas—with tuberous sclerosis
   d. Basal cell nevus syndrome and other neurocutaneous syndromes

DERMATOSES

To be set up as what may possibly be a more workable and more orderly classification of the dermatoses than seems currently to exist for pathologists, the diseases of the skin have been divided primarily into histologic categories. Although some overlapping of criteria is present, it is hoped that the basis for the classification is sufficiently defined to be of practical value. The diseases discussed are not only those that the pathologist is most likely to encounter but also those that, with minor exceptions, are diagnosable on the basis of histologic changes alone.

Shave biopsy

The shave, or horizontal, biopsy is used commonly by dermatologists. This method is opposed to the vertical biopsy performed with a punch instrument or scalpel. A case for its use has been formally, but unconvincingly, made.[43] The advantages listed include the saving of time, supplies, and equipment, the preservation of dermal "hammock" for subsequent curettage, minimal hemorrhage, and good cosmetic results. However, the disadvantages are more serious than generally conceded. The precise histologic diagnosis of many lesions is jeopardized by a limited, superficial shaving, which of course also fails to disclose the involvement or clearance of the margins.

Diseases principally of epidermis

Hyperplasias

Darier's disease. Clinically, Darier's disease (keratosis follicularis, psorospermosis) is recognized by the early development of small, uniform, firm, reddish brown, greasy keratinous papules that subsequently become coalescent, papillomatous, and crusted and acquire an offensive odor. The lesions tend to be located about the face and neck and to spread to the chest, limbs, and loins. The palms and nails may be involved, as may the oral mucosa. The disease occurs predominantly in the second and third decades.

The histologic picture is so distinctive as to be pathognomonic and consists of the following (Fig. 38-2):

1. Focal, truncated masses of keratin, usually partially parakeratinized, especially near the surface, may be located over the ostia of hair follicles or over the interfollicular epidermis. For this reason the term "keratosis follicularis" is inaccurate.
2. Corps ronds, or dyskeratotic cells, practically limited to the stratum granulosum, contain nuclei that are rounded and encircled by a clear cytoplasmic halo.
3. The "grains" are cells basically similar to the corps ronds, but they occur in the lower portion of the overlying keratinous masses.
4. The suprabasilar cleavage of the epidermis at the junction of the basal layer and the lowermost layer of the stratum spinosum forms a lacuna or small vesicle with a papillary base (Fig. 38-2).

The lesions that may offer some difficulty in differentiation are the isolated keratosis follicularis and benign chronic familial pemphigus (bullous Darier's disease). Verrucal or isolated keratosis follicularis, originally recorded by me in 1948,[4] is histologically similar to Darier's disease, although the lesions of the latter appear more regular, smaller, and often multiple even in the same section.[4] This verrucal lesion is likely to be single and has a predilection for the scalp. Others have seen an identical histologic picture in the wall of the epidermal inclusion or pilosebaceous cysts.

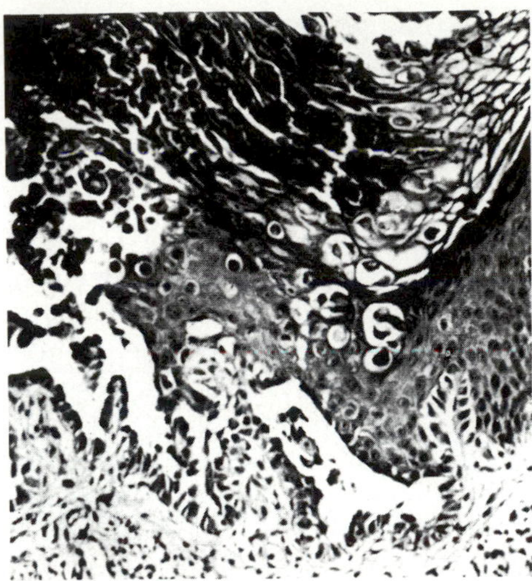

Fig. 38-2. Darier's disease (keratosis follicularis) showing suprabasilar cleavage, corps ronds, grains, and pronounced parakeratosis. (Hematoxylin and eosin.)

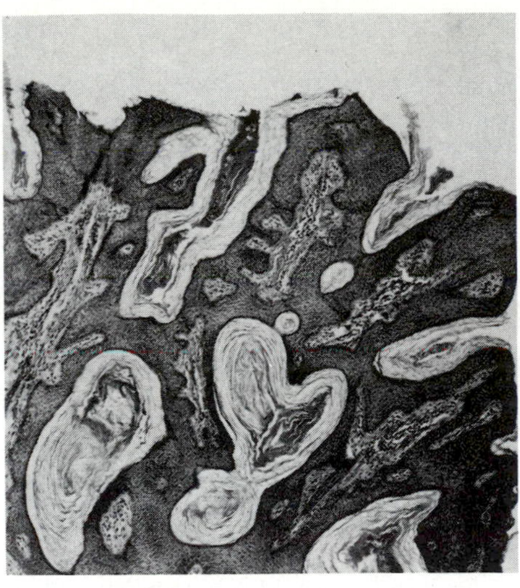

Fig. 38-3. Acanthosis nigricans with melanin pigmentation of basal layer. (Hematoxylin and eosin.)

Acanthosis nigricans. Acanthosis nigricans appears as patches of gray-black warty masses with a predilection for the axilla, groin, submammary region, elbows, knees, and occasionally the oral mucous membranes. Two types are recognized: juvenile and adult. The distinction is based on age rather than any difference in appearance of the lesions.

The juvenile type, unlike the adult form, is rarely associated with cancer, and in some instances it may accompany lipodystrophies and mental retardation.[22] The adult type is associated with visceral cancer in about 50% of patients, particularly in those beyond the fourth decade.[22] In about 65% of patients the associated cancer is a gastric adenocarcinoma. Adenocarcinomas of other viscera, such as the lung and infrequently the uterus, may be found. Occasionally the acanthosis nigricans may appear to antedate the visceral cancer. The association of acanthosis nigricans and abdominal cancer in elderly persons is a very real (if poorly understood) phenomenon. Acanthosis nigricans may also occur after the use of oral contraceptive drugs in the absence of visceral cancer.

The histologic picture of acanthosis nigricans is that of a papillary hyperkeratosis, in most areas disproportionately greater than the underlying acanthosis. The epidermis is thrown into folds by its excessive lateral growth and in sections often appears reticulated where rete ridges have joined. The basal layer is densely pigmented with fine argyrophilic melanin granules (Fig. 38-3), and a few chromatophores lie in the upper corium. This folding of a hyperkeratotic epidermis in which the basal layer is diffusely darkened as an almost solid line of melanin is characteristic of acanthosis nigricans. There is no anaplasia of the epidermis even in cases accompanied by abdominal neoplasms. Oral florid papillomatosis may be associated with acanthosis nigricans.

Molluscum contagiosum. Molluscum contagiosum is a mildly contagious autoinoculable disease of the skin, caused by a virus and characterized by pinhead- to pea-sized, waxy, firm, buttonlike, often pruritic papules occurring on the face, trunk, and genital regions particularly and on the feet rarely. The lesions develop slowly over a period of weeks and may remain indefinitely if untreated. The disease appears especially in children and may occur in epidemic proportions in institutions. Molluscum contagiosum may occur in deceptively giant forms and apparently may be transmitted venereally.

The histologic picture should be immediately recognizable. The connective tissue papillae between the lobules are compressed or altogether obliterated, so that the inwardly projecting lobules appear as a bulbous downgrowth. This lobulation of the epidermis is almost as suggestive of the diagnosis as is the pathognomonic feature, the molluscum bodies, and may help to differentiate this lesion from verrucae, particularly when the molluscum bodies are inconspicuous. The molluscum bodies are clustered cells, principally of the stratum granulosum but also of the stratum spinosum, which are enlarged, as are virus-infected cells generally, and contain homogeneously smooth, brightly eosinophilic cytoplasm. The nucleus is inconspicuously flattened to one side of the cell, and keratohyalin granules tend to disappear. The cytoplasm, when studied with vital stains, appears actually to contain many elementary bodies (Lipschütz) embedded in a mucoid matrix. These dyskeratotic cells are enclosed in an eosinophilic, keratin-like membrane that resembles the dense cell membranes of plants. The molluscum bodies have been confused with the brightly eosinophilic cells of the stratum granulosum that are often prominent in verrucae vulgares. The virus seen electron microscopically measures about 300 × 200 ×

100 nm, is characteristically brick shaped, and contains a dumbbell-shaped nucleoid. The virus replicates in the cytoplasm rather than in the nucleus.[47] Specific fluorescence staining of the inclusion bodies with tagged antibodies of serum from infected humans and rabbits has been demonstrated.

Vesicles

The vesicles of various diseases may closely simulate each other clinically. Inasmuch as the prognosis, even as to fatality, may depend on the exact diagnosis, it is important that the diagnostic histologic features be definitely evaluated. In general, three types of vesicles occur: (1) eczematous, (2) cleavage (such as dermatitis herpetiformis, pemphigus, epidermolysis bullosa, impetigo, and burns), and (3) viral (such as smallpox, chickenpox, and herpes).

Eczema. Eczema may begin as an erythema and evolve through the papular, vesicular, pustular, and exfoliative stages. Some cases of eczema remain in one of the phases (for example, eczema rubrum, eczema squamosum, eczema papulosum), but in most instances the disease passes through the stage of vesiculation. Histologically the vesicle of eczema, whatever the etiology, is basically the same whether caused by an external irritant, ingested food, or the product of superficial fungi, as in the epidermophytid. Moreover, the histologic picture of the eczematous vesicle differs sharply from that of pemphigus, dermatitis herpetiformis, and the viral lesions of smallpox, chickenpox, and herpes.

The vesicle of eczema begins as foci of spongiosis in the rete Malpighii. The intercellular edema progresses to form microvesicles that coalesce with adjacent vesicles similarly formed. The walls of such vesicles are the compressed epidermal cells that usually are arranged as septa in the large blisters. In addition to the spongiotic vesicles, there may be transepidermal migration of mononuclear cells, upper dermal edema, telangiectasia, and basophils in the acute stages of contact dermatitis. More chronic forms may show acanthosis, parakeratosis, and dermal melanophores.

Histologic changes of this sort occur also in the vesicles of pompholyx, dyshidrosis, acrodermatitis perstans, and other eruptions of unknown etiology that are localized chiefly to the hands, as well as in the vesicles of pustular bacterids. These bacterids are usually sterile pustules of the palms and soles and are assumed to be provoked by allergic reactions to bacterial products.

Cleavage vesicles. Some years ago the term *cleavage* was applied to those vesicles formed by the separation or cleavage of the epidermis or dermis through a single horizontal plane.[4] The cleavage may occur at any level of the epidermis and occasionally may split the upper dermis. The precise level of cleavage usually embodies a key diagnostic clue. The following discussion is of representative types of cleavage vesicles.

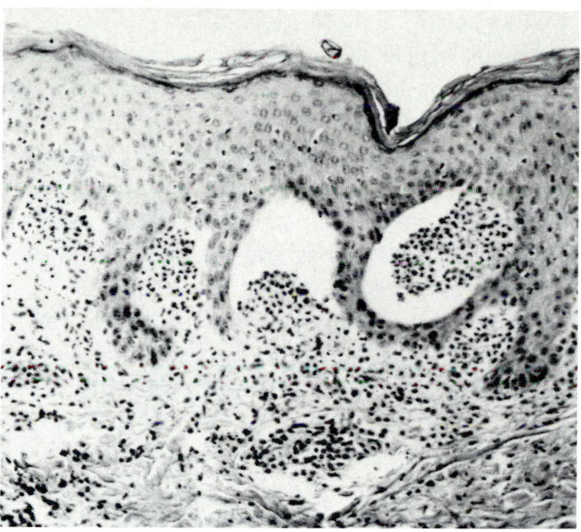

Fig. 38-4. Dermatitis herpetiformis in its early stage showing cleavage of epidermis from dermis by collections of leukocytes. (Hematoxylin and eosin.)

The lesions of dermatitis herpetiformis (Duhring's disease) are symmetrically distributed in groups in the scapular regions, on the buttocks, or on the extremities. The lesions may be erythematous macules or papules, but in most cases they are characterized by vesicles that may vary from those detectable only microscopically to large bullae. Oral lesions in dermatitis herpetiformis are more common than is generally indicated.[32] The disease may be accompanied by mild constitutional symptoms and signs. Itching, burning, and pricking sensations almost always are present. The disease is characterized by spontaneous remissions and relapses. The etiology is unknown. The lesions respond remarkably in most instances to penicillin and sulfapyridine but usually do not react satisfactorily to other sulfonamides.

Remarkably, the cutaneous lesions of dermatitis herpetiformis can be produced in the susceptible individual with topically applied potassium iodide. The mechanism is unknown.

The microscopic features of the vesicle of dermatitis herpetiformis consist of a collection of serum, fibrin, and a few neutrophilic and eosinophilic leukocytes that have cleaved and lifted the entire epidermis from the corium. The epidermis itself shows no other constant change. Of diagnostic importance is the change in the dermal base of the vesicle—particularly the flattened, edematous papillae that are infiltrated with cells of the same type found in the vesicle itself (Fig. 38-4). Eosinophilic leukocytes are often present in considerable numbers, but their absence by no means precludes the diagnosis of dermatitis herpetiformis.

It has been suggested that dermatitis herpetiformis is attributable to an immunologic disorder linked with gluten sensitivity. Both the cutaneous and intestinal lesions respond to the withdrawal of gluten. Immunofluorescence studies reveal IgA in granular or fibrillary form, rarely linear, at the dermoepidermal junction. By contrast, in pemphigoid the immunoglobulin is mostly IgG, but it appears in linear form.

Although IgG in the basement membrane zone characterizes bullous pemphigoid, and IgA in granular form in the basement membrane zone is a feature of dermatitis herpetiformis, the two may coexist (including IgA in linear form). This overlapping contribution has suggested to some a relationship between the two entities.[53] The histologic similarity in many instances also points in this direction. Dermatitis herpetiformis may be associated with the nephrotic syndrome, with IgA demonstrable both in the glomerular basement membranes and in the cutaneous basement membrane zone. So-called benign chronic bullous dermatosis of childhood appears to have the characteristics of dermatitis herpetiformis, except for the absence of circulating epithelial antibodies.

Pemphigus refers to a group of bullous diseases of unknown etiology that were generally fatal before corticosteroids were available. The prognosis has been dramatically improved with the use of steroids and immunosuppressive agents. The disease involves both sexes equally, affects mainly those between 40 and 70 years of age, and most frequently begins in the mucous membranes of the mouth. It may take about 5 months for involvement of the glabrous skin after the oral lesions appear.

Pemphigus occurs in more than one form. The several varieties include pemphigus vulgaris, pemphigus foliaceus, and pemphigus vegetans. These forms are entities primarily on the basis of the acuteness of the disease or the type of lesions accompanying the vesicles, for example, the foul-smelling scales of pemphigus foliaceus and the fungoid papillomatous masses of pemphigus vegetans. Pemphigus erythematodes (Senear-Usher syndrome) previously was regarded as a separate entity with a good prognosis. It is now believed that this condition is actually a variant of pemphigus in which the erythematous stage may be prolonged. The incidence of pemphigus vulgaris is about four times that of all other varieties combined. Bullae are observed at some time in the course of pemphigus foliaceus and pemphigus vegetans. The group name is applied also to benign chronic familial pemphigus (Hailey-Hailey disease), but there is reason to believe that this disease is quite distinct from the usually fatal varieties of pemphigus. The actual cause of death in pemphigus uncomplicated by sepsis is not clear, although the loss of proteins and electrolytes in the bullous fluid is probably a significant factor. The prognosis for patients with pemphigus is better if the disease develops before 40 years of age and is treated with steroids early in its course.

The triad of pemphigus, myasthenia gravis, and thymoma has been well documented, as has the association of pemphigus with neoplasms, especially lymphomas.

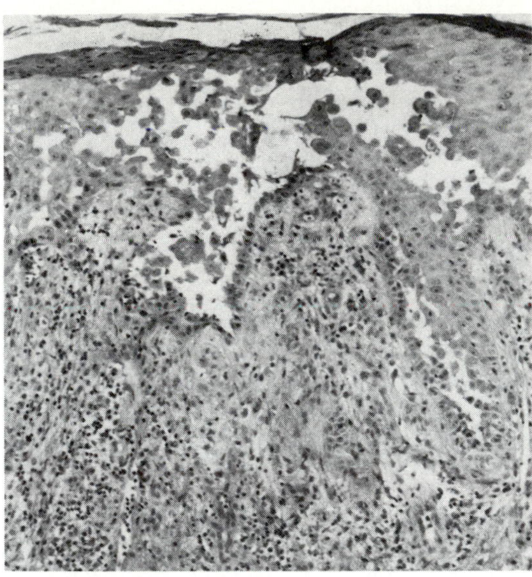

Fig. 38-5. Pemphigus vulgaris with suprabasilar cleavage and isolated clusters of epidermal cells within vesicle. These are acantholytic cells of Tzanck. (Hematoxylin and eosin.)

The histologic picture of the cutaneous lesion of pemphigus is as follows:

1. The typical vesicle or bulla consists of a collection of serous fluid, most often at the suprabasilar layer of the epidermis. As a rule there is little or no reaction in the dermis, although there are many exceptions in which the upper dermis or submucosa is crowded with polymorphonuclear leukocytes admixed with the various mononuclear cells (that is, lymphocytes, plasma cells, and histiocytes). Such a vesicle or bulla characterizes pemphigus vulgaris but may a part of the picture of other varieties of pemphigus (Fig. 38-5). In addition, rounded epidermal cells loosened by acantholysis (Tzanck cells) frequently are found in the vesicles of pemphigus, but they are not pathognomonic of this disease. These acantholytic cells may be recognized in smears of vesicles stained with hematoxylin and eosin and may be distinguished from cells of viral vesicles, for example. They are characterized by the disintegration of desmosomes and the separation, disorganization, and loss of tonofilaments, a sequence of events accompanying acantholysis not only in other dermatoses such as Darier's disease but also in some epidermal neoplasms, particularly melanocarcinomas. The vulnerability of the desmosomes is regarded as the principal pathogenic basis of pemphigus, a concept reinforced by immunofluorescence demonstration of the fixation of autoantibodies at these intercellular sites. As indicated, autoimmune antibodies may be demonstrated by fluorescence in the intercellular spaces of the epidermis of patients with pemphigus vulgaris.

In pemphigus of whatever variant an IgG antibody is

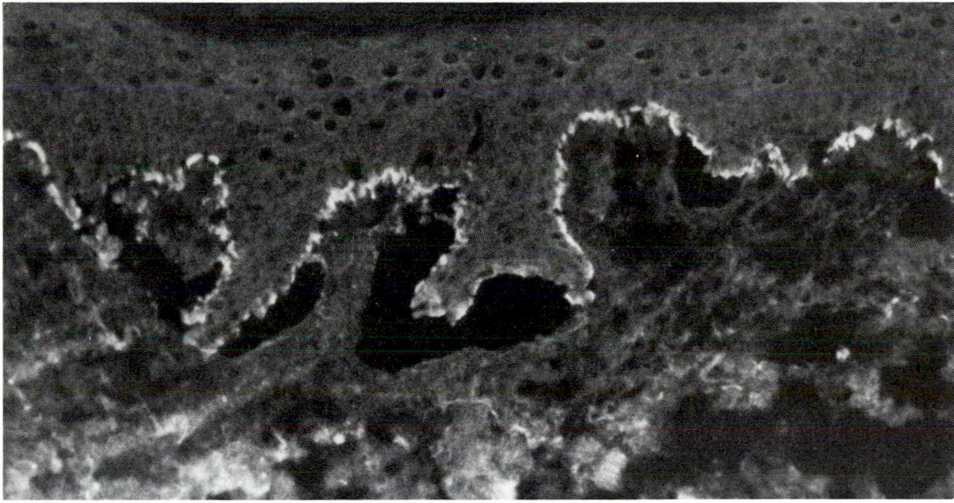

Fig. 38-6. Direct immunofluorescence of IgG in basement membrane zone of bullous pemphigoid. C3, C4, and beta$_{1H}$ globulin also are fixed in this zone in pemphigoid. (Courtesy Dr. L.P. Pertschuk.)

produced against the antigenic epidermal intercellular material. This critical antibody not only binds to the intercellular region but also is detectable in the sera.[1] In bullous pemphigoid the antibodies are localized to the position of the basement membrane zone (Fig. 38-6). Some investigators have noted that the immunoglobulins of bullous pemphigoid are localized between the epidermis and basal lamina, in contrast to the localization deep to the basal lamina in lupus erythematosus.[63]

The histologic differentiation of pemphigus vulgaris from bullous pemphigoid is often not as clear cut as was implied when the latter term was coined. The early mucosal involvement, the relative lack of inflammation, the abundance of acantholysis, and the suprabasilar (versus epidermal-dermal) cleavage are features indicative of pemphigus. The cleavage is attributed to pemphigus antibodies, which induce epidermal cells to activate cellular proteases, with resulting cellular dyshesion and acantholysis.[65] It has been suggested that the acantholysis is caused by an immunologic reaction between the epidermal cell and the pemphigus antibody, resulting in release of a "pemphigus acantholytic factor."[64] The agent initiating this reaction (such as a virus, toxin, or chemical) is yet to be discerned.

Benign mucosal pemphigoid may involve the conjunctivae, oronasal cavity, larynx, esophagus, and genitalia. The histology is like that of bullous pemphigoid except for the occurrence of cicatrization as a consequence of the submucosal inflammatory reaction. Probably pemphigoid is a variant of erythema multiforme bullosum, as is the Stevens-Johnson syndrome. Pemphigoid may, on occasion, be associated with visceral cancer (Fig. 38-7).

Features of dermatitis herpetiformis are granular IgA deposits in the dermal papillae about the bullae and no circulating antibodies. In contrast, bullous pemphigoid shows IgG and complement at the dermoepidermal zone and in the skin uninvolved by lesions, as well as specific antibodies in the serum. Bullae also may result from the use of anticoagulants. These bullae are subepidermal and histologically simulate erythema multiforme.

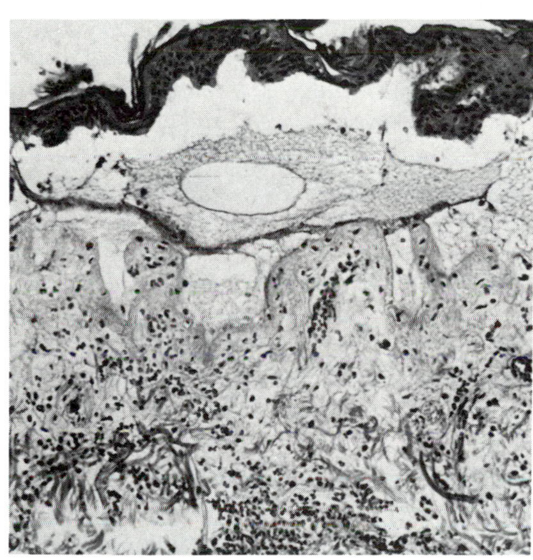

Fig. 38-7. Pemphigoid. Cleavage vesicle between epidermis and dermis with relatively sparse dermal reaction. Tzanck cells are absent. (Hematoxylin and eosin.)

2. In pemphigus vegetans, in addition to the bulla just described, there is an associated diagnostic lesion consisting of pronounced acanthosis with prominent prolongation of the rete ridges, between which are brightly dense collections of eosinophilic leukocytes. The eosinophils may migrate into the epidermis, which may

become ulcerated and be the seat of intraepidermal microabscesses. The ulcerations, the intraepidermal abscesses, and the extensive acanthosis with winding reticulated ridges may simulate a bromoderma or the reaction to deep fungal infections such as coccidioidomycosis.

3. In pemphigus foliaceus the typical bulla often is immediately adjacent to a unique acanthosis. Often the fluid accumulates between layers of the upper rete Malpighii. If the accumulation of fluid is minimal, the cleavage may be sufficient to separate the uppermost portion of the epidermis by crude pressure of the thumb on the patient's skin (Nikolsky's sign). The ridges are rounded and formed in congeries so that in a single section they may appear isolated in the deep dermis, as in early squamous cell carcinoma. This type of acanthosis resembles most the epidermal proliferation often seen overlying myoblastomas. The epidermal proliferation usually is accompanied by a polymorphous cellular infiltrate of neutrophilic leukocytes and mononuclear cells. Tzanck cells are present in pemphigus foliaceus and pemphigus vegetans and in lesser numbers in Hailey-Hailey disease and other vesicular dermatoses.

Circulating intercellular antibodies are demonstrable in the serum of patients with pemphigus, and their titers tend to parallel the severity of the disease. Indeed, reappearance of the antibodies may herald the recrudescence of the disease. Immunofluorescence studies of cutaneous biopsy specimens reveal a striking, diffuse, intercellular localization of immunoglobulins in a characteristic polygonal pattern about the keratinocytes. Pemphigus-like antibodies occur in patients with burns, toxic epidermal necrolysis, and several other drug-induced eruptions. In sharp contrast, the results of immunofluorescence studies are negative in Hailey-Hailey (bullous Darier's) disease, in which the acantholysis may present a differential diagnostic problem in routinely stained sections. In bullous and cicatricial pemphigoid, dermatitis herpetiformis, and lupus erythematosus, immunoglobulins may be demonstrated by fluoresceinated sera in the immediate subepidermal region.

Epidermolysis bullosa occurs soon after birth (congenital) or may first appear in the second or third decade (so-called acquired type). There are two varieties of epidermolysis bullosa; simple and dystrophic. In the simple type the lesions occur after slight trauma on any portion of the body and regress, leaving temporary pigmentation but no permanent changes. The dystrophic type is characterized by lesions of the extremities, provoked by minimal trauma and associated with pigmentation, milia (epidermal cysts) (Fig. 38-8), atrophy, destruction of nails, cicatrizations, hypoplasia of dental enamel, and syndactylism. It may be complicated by the development of epidermoid carcinomas both in the skin and in the mucosa of the mouth and esophagus. The pathogenesis may well be related to the associated desmoplasia or scarring as in other situations, such as burns and chronic osteomyelitis. It is known to precede the development of systemic lupus erythematosus, myeloma, diabetes mellitus, and enteritis and to follow penicillamine therapy.

Both the simple and dystrophic types may be congenital or acquired. The histologic features are those of a pressure vesicle with cleavage often at the junction of the stratum corneum and stratum granulosum or between the epidermis and dermis, especially in the dystrophic type (Fig. 38-8). The inflammatory reaction within both the vesicle and the underlying dermis is mild except in regions, such as the feet, that are easily traumatized and infected. Small epidermal inclusions lie in the dermis beneath or at the margins of the vesicles (Fig. 38-8). A congenital disturbance of the dermal elastic tissue is said to occur in the dystrophic type, but the evidence for this is not satisfactory. However, necrosis of upper dermal collagen and elastic tissue may occur in the dystrophic form and may result in severe contractures of the extremities, with bony absorption. Involvement of the conjunctiva, oral mucosa, and esophagus may develop, heralding a poor prognosis. The epidermal inclusion cysts are particularly prone to appear in the dystrophic form and reflect, in part, the dermal isolation of portions of sweat ducts and rete ridges that subsequently form the cysts. The relative lack of inflammatory cellular response within and beneath the vesicles is of diagnostic usefulness in differentiating them from other vesicles with cleavages at corresponding sites. The bullae of dystrophic epidermolysis bullosa have been attributed to the specifically higher local production of collagenase in contrast to pemphi-

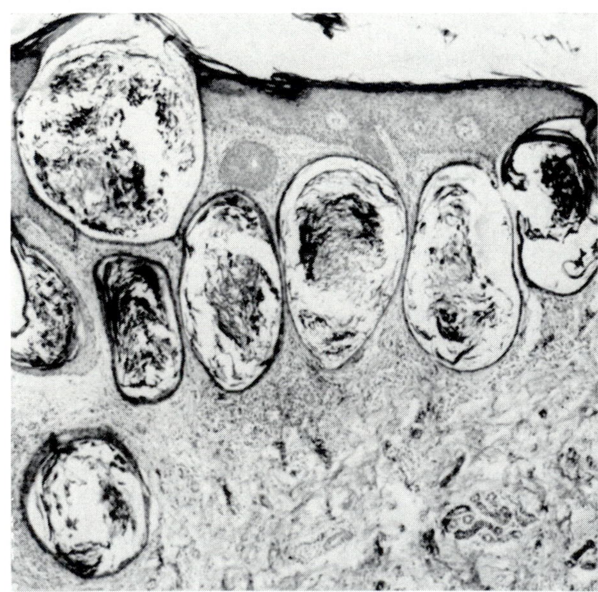

Fig. 38-8. Epidermolysis bullosa with milia (keratinous, sweat gland cysts).

gus vulgaris and bullous pemphigoid. A picture simulating epidermolysis bullosa may occur after the administration of penicillamine. Subepidermal cleavage vesicles (along with necrosis of the epithelium of sweat glands and ducts) may also occur, especially over traumatized pressure points, after carbon monoxide or barbiturate poisoning.[13] IgG is localized beneath the basal lamina rather than in the lamina lucida, as occurs in bullous pemphigoid.

Subcorneal pustular dermatosis is considered to be a special vesicular entity. The lesions, which tend to affect particularly middle-aged women, appear as minute gyrate or annular groups of erythematous, superficial vesiculopustules localized chiefly in the intertriginous areas about the breasts, axillae, and groin.

Histologically the changes consist of cleavage vesicles and pustules located immediately beneath the stratum corneum, as the name indicates. Eosinophils are not a part of the picture, although occasionally acantholytic cells may be present. The exudate is usually sterile—unlike that of impetigo contagiosa, which the lesion otherwise resembles histologically (Fig. 38-9). *Staphylococcus aureus* is the most common offender in impetigo contagiosa; it is often mixed with beta-hemolytic streptococci. Streptococci also may occur alone or in association with a variety of organisms. Diphtheroids *(Corynebacterium pyogenes)* are responsible for about 5% of cases.

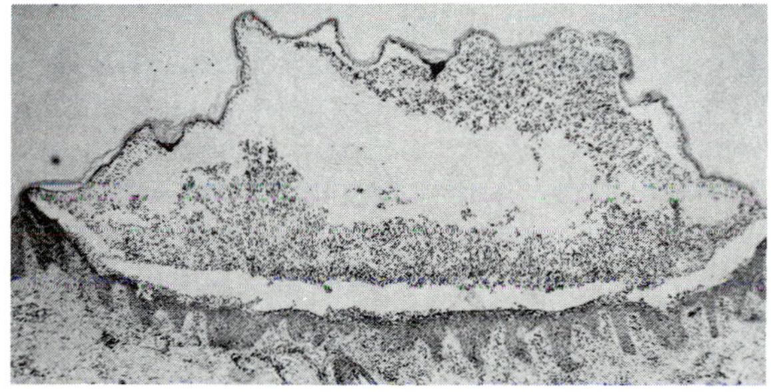

Fig. 38-9. Impetigo contagiosa. Superficial cleavage vesicle with purulent exudate. (Hematoxylin and eosin; AFIP 99848.)

Toxic epidermal necrolysis (Lyell's disease). Toxic epidermal necrolysis is characterized by a tender, painful rash resembling scalded skin, with rapid onset and recovery or rapid death.[49] The exotoxin of *Staphylococcus* organisms is implicated in most cases, but drugs, viruses, and vaccinations (such as those against poliomyelitis, diphtheria, and measles) have also been involved. The drugs linked to this fairly new entity include allopurinol, barbiturates, sulfonamides, penicillin, phenylbutazone, hydantoins, salicylates, and antihistamines.[25] In about 20% of cases no agent can be implicated.

Histologically the epidermal cleavage may develop at one of several levels: dermal-epidermal, as in erythema multiforme bullosum; suprabasilar, as in pemphigus; or the upper rete Malpighi. Scattered foci of necrotic keratinocytes are characteristically present, and some of these may occupy the vesicles as acantholytic cells (Fig. 38-10). Few or no dermal inflammatory cells appear unless secondary infection takes place, so the simulation of erythema multiforme may be striking. Indeed, some observers regard the disease as a variant of erythema multiforme bullosum. In both there has been occasional association with membranoproliferative glomerulonephritis. In sharp contrast to the good prognosis in small children, the mortality in adults is more than 40%, and recovery is often protracted for many months.

Herpes gestationis. Herpes gestationis is a vesiculobullous eruption that is prone to recur in succeeding pregnancies. This condition, unrelated to the herpesvirus, is a rare, cleavage type of vesicular rash that appears during or shortly after pregnancy. The differential diagnoses are principally bullous pemphigoid, erythema multiforme, and dermatitis herpetiformis. The immuno-

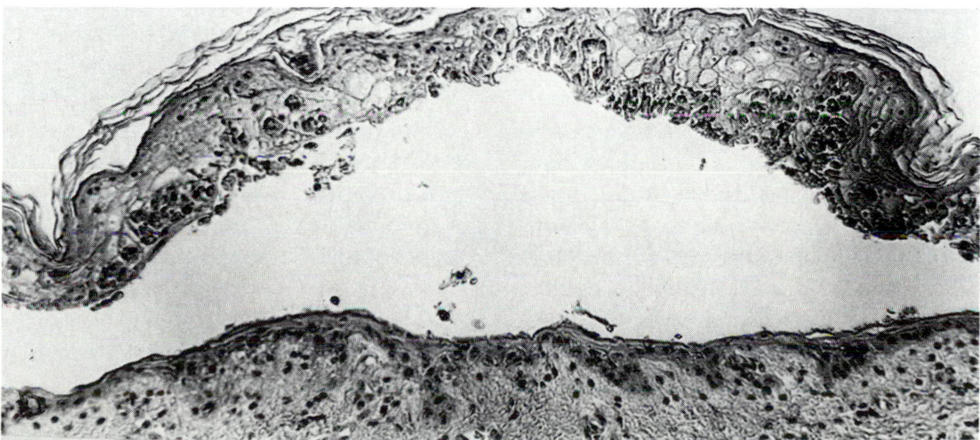

Fig. 38-10. Lyell's disease (toxic epidermal necrolysis) showing bulla with intraepidermal cleavage and necrosis of keratinocytes.

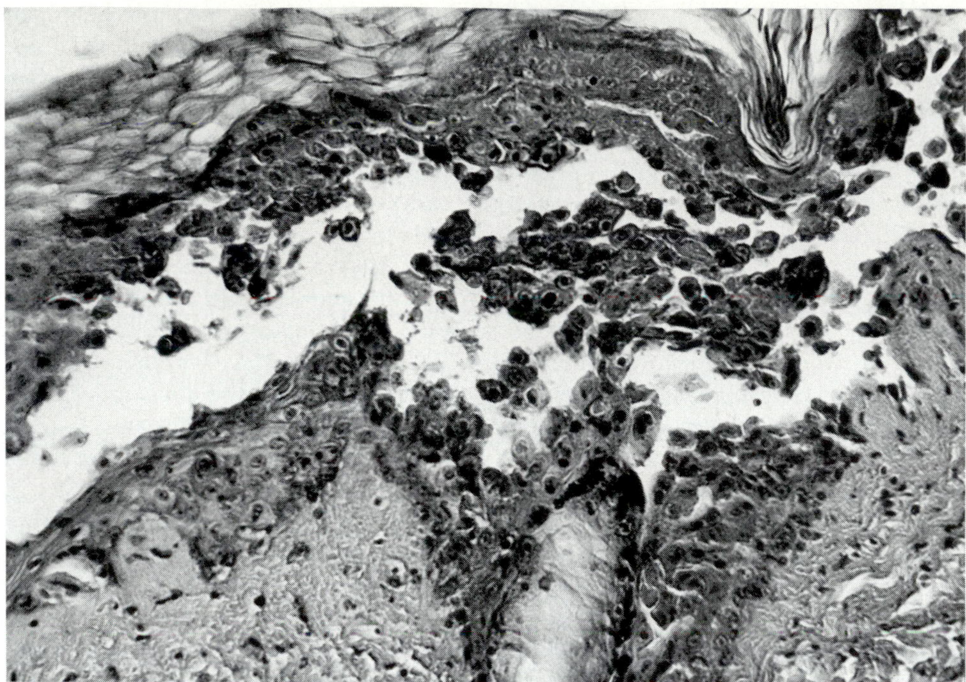

Fig. 38-11. Varicella illustrating intranuclear inclusion (type A) in vesicle. (Hematoxylin and eosin.)

logic and ultrastructural evidence favors a closer relationship to bullous pemphigoid than to the others. The histologic findings also suggest bullous pemphigoid, except for the conspicuous necrosis of cells of the basal layer, even in clinically uninvolved areas. Necrosis of the basal cells over the dermal papillae is said to be characteristic of herpes gestationis.

Pyoderma gangrenosum. Pyoderma gangrenosum refers to the ugly, large, purple-rimmed, undermined suppurative ulcerations occurring especially with ulcerative colitis but associated with other diseases, such as rheumatoid arthritis. Its etiology and pathogenesis are still problematic, although leukocytoclastic arteriolitis, perhaps as part of a Shwartzman phenomenon, has been suspected.

Viral vesicles. Smallpox (variola), chickenpox (varicella), alastrim, vaccinia (cowpox), herpangina, herpes simplex, and herpes zoster (shingles) are described in Chapter 10. In contrast to the ease with which most of the exanthemas can be differentiated clinically is the difficulty or impossibility of differentiating the vesicles histologically. Nevertheless, there are certain histologic features common to each of these vesicles that at least permit the recognition of each as a vesicle produced by a virus. These features include (1) reticular colliquation, by which the epidermis becomes transformed into multiple locules bounded by a reticulum of drawn-out, stringy, cytoplasmic septa, (2) ballooning degeneration, the formation of multinucleated giant cells in the lower layers of the rete Malpighi, and (3) intranuclear inclusions.

It is stated that in the vesicle of smallpox, reticular colliquation proceeds at a faster pace, particularly at the periphery of the lesion, than does ballooning degeneration, which accounts for the umbilication of this vesicle (Fig. 38-11). In smallpox, Guarnieri bodies are found as eosinophilic, varying-sized, round, cytoplasmic inclusions—especially in cells at the base of the vesicle, including those undergoing ballooning degeneration. In addition, eosinophilic intranuclear inclusions with margination of the nuclear chromatin are common in these cells. In the vesicles of herpes these intranuclear inclusions are referred to as zoster bodies of Lipschütz, although they are morphologically similar to the intranuclear inclusions of the other viral vesicles (Fig. 38-12).

The scarring that follows some of these vesicles (such as those of zoster and occasionally of smallpox) is an index of the prior inflammatory destruction of the upper corium. As a rule, edema and infiltrate of inflammatory cells are present in the upper dermis of most vesicles of the various viral diseases. The residual scarring, however, appears to reflect the greater intensity and destructiveness of the process. The virus of zoster appears capable of producing the clinical picture of varicella in susceptible persons. It is suggested that steroids increase this susceptibility.

Relatively recently an entity referred to as herpangina has been described. It is a benign, febrile, self-limited disease of viral etiology, affecting children chiefly and characterized by a sudden onset of grayish white, papulovesicular, oral or pharyngeal lesions with a surrounding

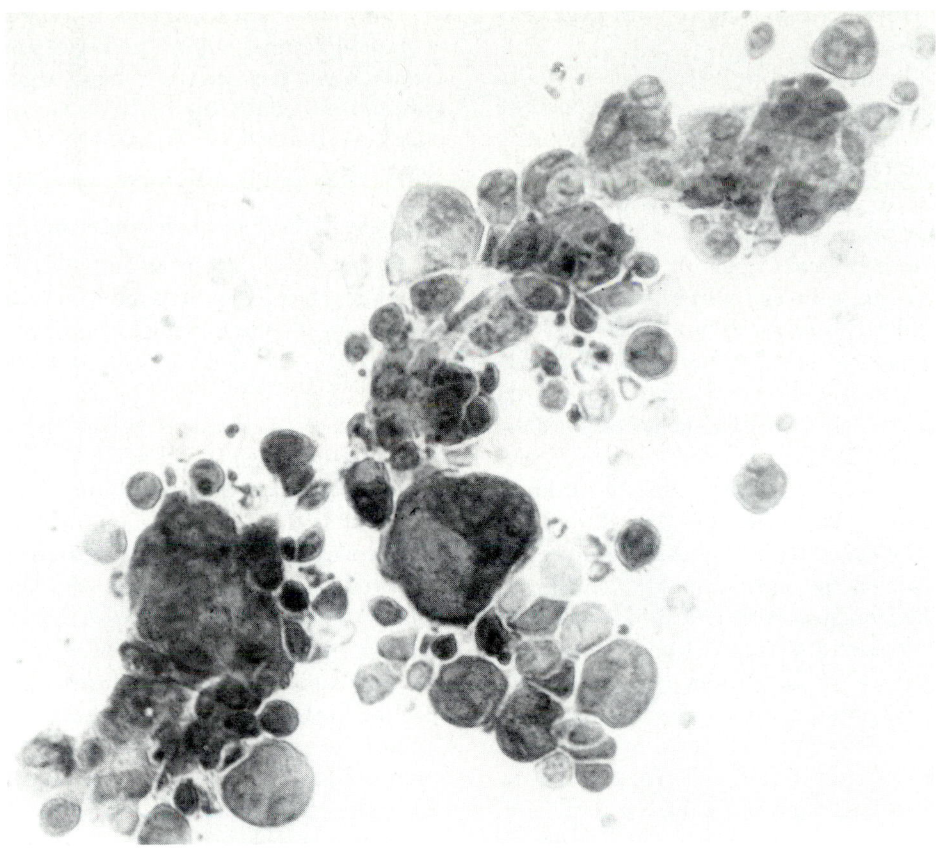

Fig. 38-12. Herpes simplex. Smear of contents of vesicle showing viral inclusions within nuclei of keratinocytes. (Hematoxylin and eosin.)

red areola. Histologic studies of the vesicles are not available, but probably they would resemble the vesicles of herpes.

Another controverted disease that now appears clearly virogenic is Kaposi's varicelliform eruption. This disease is actually either disseminated herpes simplex or generalized vaccinia, often inoculated in skin made receptive by a preceding dermatosis such as eczema or atopic dermatitis. The diagnosis of viral vesicles is expedited by the use of smears of the vesicular contents. This cytodiagnostic method is particularly useful with the viral vesicles; in other types excessive dependence may be placed on acantholytic cells. It is hypothesized that the virus of varicella-zoster remains latent in sensory ganglia after a preceding varicella and that hematogenous dissemination of the virus occurs with subsequent activation.

Herpesvirus type 2, unlike type 1, tends to disseminate. They may be differentiated by cultural or immunofluorescence studies and, it is said, morphologically by the greater tendency toward ballooning degeneration by type 2 virus.

Superficial mycoses

Superficial mycoses are included in this section because they principally involve the epidermis. The mycoses are separated into the superficial type (ringworm, tinea corporis, and favus) and the deep type (such as blastomycosis, coccidioidomycosis, and actinomycosis). Superficial mycoses are divided, according to the region affected, into tinea capitis, barbae, corporis, cruris, and pedis (or epidermophytosis). Several kinds of fungi may be responsible for the same clinical type of lesion. On the other hand, the form and chronicity of the ringworm may vary considerably with the causative fungus. For example, *Trichophyton* infection of the feet is characterized by a dry, scaly dermatosis, whereas *Epidermophyton* infection appears vesicular and moist. It has therefore been suggested that the etiology, as well as the anatomic region, be indicated in the name, such as tinea corporis trichophytica. However, usage sanctions the retention of additional names for varieties of ringworm infection that have distinguishing features of pattern, color, severity, or chronicity of lesions, for example, favus, kerion (ringworm of scalp complicated by abscesses), tinea imbricata, and tinea versicolor.

Botryomycosis is merely a bacterial infection histologically confused with actinomycosis because of the eosinophilic radiate or asteroid formation about the colonies of bacteria. The etiologic agent is usually a *Staphylococcus* organism, but streptococci and *Proteus* organisms also may produce this pattern. Gram stains on histologic sections facilitate the diagnosis.

The fungus may be observed in wet smears of scrapings soaked in sodium or potassium hydroxide, or they may be cultured on special media, such as Sabouraud's agar. However, with the exceptions of tinea versicolor and favus, it is rare to observe the fungus in a routine paraffin section of a lesion of ringworm. Generally, the histologic picture comprises merely the presence of scales or vesicles along with subepidermal hyperemia and slight perivascular cuffing by mononuclear cells. In tinea versicolor the spores and hyphae of *Pityrosporon furfur* are usually abundant and confined to the stratum corneum. In favus the large scutula, or matted scales, contain masses of fungus.

The vesicle of ringworm, no matter where the lesion is located, is eczematous, usually multiloculated, and the morphologic result of excessive spongiosis. This type of vesicle is the picture of the dermatophytid or allergic manifestation of the fungal infection. The dermatophytids are free of fungi and are caused by the cutaneous reaction to the products of fungi transported probably through the blood or lymph. For example, the dermatophytids after ringworm of the feet often occur on the hands. It has been suggested that sensitizing antibiotic therapy with preparations from fungi such as penicillin may be responsible in some measure for the dermatophytids after superficial mycoses. The deep mycoses are described in Chapter 11.

Scabies. Another lesion of the epidermis that is often recognizable in a fortunate histologic section is caused by *Acarus scabiei*. The disease is characterized by the occurrence of intensely pruritic papules, vesicles, pustules, and excoriations usually located in relation to the burrow, cuniculus, or gallery dug by the *Acarus* mite into the epidermis. These lesions tend to occur in the webs of the fingers, on the wrists, in the genital regions, and beneath the breast. The disease is contagious and in most instances is transmitted by direct body contact with an infected individual. The diagnosis may be made clinically by picking the female mite out of the burrow and identifying it with the low-power lens of the microscope.

Histologically, none of the lesions of scabies is diagnostic except the burrow with the tenant mite. However, the mite often may not be included in the section, but the presence of ova or fecal material of the *Acarus* within the burrow or merely the presence of the gallery itself is strongly presumptive evidence of scabies. The burrow is a superficial epidermal defect extending obliquely through the thickened stratum corneum, which serves as a roof to shelter the *Acarus*.

A form of scabies may be transmitted to man by mites that infest dogs, cats, birds, and monkeys. So-called Norwegian scabies appears to be merely a more fulminant form of ordinary scabies.

Infestation with *Demodex folliculorum*, the acarid commonly found within the keratinous follicular plugs of comedones, has generally been regarded as innocuous, but more recently the harmless nature of the infestation has been questioned. Blepharitis, for example, has been attributed to this arthropod.

Diseases affecting both epidermis and dermis

In this discussion are included those histologic entities in which changes in the epidermis and the dermis jointly contribute to the morphologic diagnosis.

Lupus erythematosus

Lupus erythematosus occurs in two principal forms: chronic, or discoid, and acute.

Discoid lupus erythematosus. The discoid variety is fortunately the more common, manifests itself by stationary or slowly progressive coalescent macules or plaques covered irregularly with fine, whitish or yellowish greasy scales, and is associated with focal gray patches of atrophy and keratotic plugging of follicles. The lesions usually are well defined (hence, discoid) and show a predilection for the malar areas and bridge of the nose distributed in the shape of a butterfly. The process is not limited to this area but may occur also on other parts of the face, the scalp, the neck, extremities, and elsewhere. In any location the lesions are aggravated by exposure to sunlight or other forms of irradiation. The lesions may regress completely, but usually there is residual, rather typical superficial scarring with pigmentation or leukoderma and alopecia. Acute changes also may be superimposed on the discoid lesions. Carcinomatous transformations (squamous cell) may occur in the chronic process, probably for nonspecific reasons similar to those that obtain in some other forms of chronic cicatrizing ulcerations.

The histologic features of the discoid variety of lupus erythematosus are easily recognizable in most cases. They include the following:

1. Alternating acanthosis and atrophy of the epidermis, with the process infrequently progressing to squamous cell carcinoma.
2. Liquefaction degeneration of the basal layer
3. Hyperemia or telangiectasis and edema of the papillary and subpapillary layers of the dermis
4. Dense collections of mononuclear cells, principally lymphocytes, in the upper and midportions of the dermis, most concentrated about the appendages, often with atrophy and consequent alopecia (Fig. 38-13)
5. Focal depigmentation of the basal layer along with clusters of melanophages resulting from the subepidermal inflammation

Basophilic "degeneration" of collagen in the upper dermis is a completely unreliable criterion of chronic lupus erythematosus, inasmuch as it is found normally in

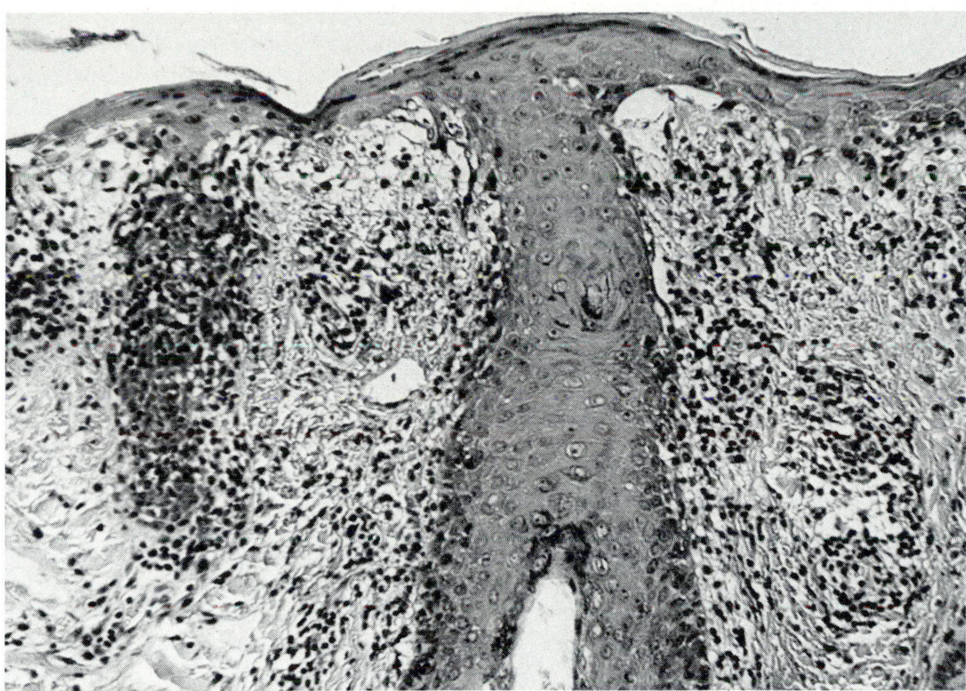

Fig. 38-13. Acute and chronic lupus erythematosus with early vesiculation.

the skin of the malar regions, especially in older age groups. Changes in vessels, other than telangiectasis, are not part of the picture of discoid lupus erythematosus. The lesions of rosacea may occasionally offer differential diagnostic difficulty because of the presence of keratotic plugs and erythema. The epidermal changes and mid-dermal masses of lymphocytes favor the diagnosis of lupus erythematosus. Occasionally the collections of lymphocytes extend into the underlying panniculus (lupus erythematosus profundus) and may be mistaken for Weber-Christian disease. Lupus erythematosus profundus (lupus erythematosus panniculitis) is characterized by nodular involvement of the subcutis with or without overlying dermal and epidermal involvement. This lesion, too, has been attributed to injury caused by immune complexes.[72] Similar dense masses of lymphocytes in the dermis may be confused with a malignant lymphoma, the benign dermal lymphocytosis of Jessner, or the potpourri of lesions labeled Spiegler-Fendt sarcoid.

Acute lupus erythematosus. The acute (or subacute) lupus erythematosus may occur as a focal, transient reaction to sunlight or may be part of the frequently fatal systemization of the disease. These acute lesions may be superimposed on the chronic process or may affect previously uninvolved skin. The chronic lesion is assumed to be complicated by the disseminated form in the rarest instances. However, although this may be the impression clinically, the histologic and recent clinical data belie this impression. Moreover, antinuclear antibodies are stated to be present in over 90% of patients with systemic lupus erythematosus and in 15% to 40% of those with discoid lupus erythematosus. Immunofluorescence studies reveal characteristic bands of immunoglobulins (IgG) and complement at the dermoepidermal junction in both systemic and discoid lupus erythematosus.[23,41] The immunofluorescence is said to be positive occasionally in rosacea and in a few other diseases in which, however, the differential histologic diagnosis may be achieved in sections stained routinely.

Immunoglobulin deposits may be found in clinically uninvolved skin. However, the generally accepted assumption that intact-appearing skin is necessarily normal histologically is not justified. Moreover, no conclusions can be drawn regarding the nature of the antigens or the pathogenesis of the junctional deposition of immunoglobulin. This same facile hypothesis embodying a direct cause-and-effect relationship between the presence of immunoglobulin and the pathogenesis of a lesion of given structures (such as glomeruli, renal tubules, or vessels) is far from proved. There does seem to be greater activity of the disease in patients with IgG at the junctional zone.

In acute cases the skin becomes reddened, edematous, and sometimes purpuric, with patchy macules that may coalesce into an erysipeloid, somewhat mottled malar flush. On the hands the lesions may be erythematous or purpuric and macular or papular. Elsewhere they may take other forms, such as vesicles, bullae, scaling macules, and telangiectases. When the acute process complicates the discoid lesion, fresh superficial or even moderately deep ulcerations may occur, in addition to

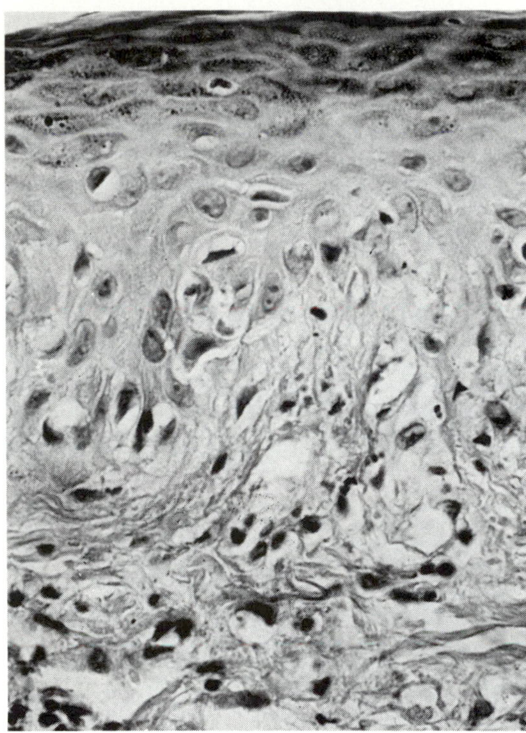

Fig. 38-14. Acute disseminated lupus erythematosus with pronounced liquefaction degeneration at dermoepidermal junction. (Hematoxylin and eosin.)

the other changes mentioned, particularly at the advancing periphery of the old lesion. As stated, the acute cutaneous alterations may be a localized reaction to sunlight without systemic complications. In the disseminated variety, which occurs particularly but by no means exclusively in young women, the constitutional signs and symptoms include fever, thrombocytopenia, leukopenia, excessive gammaglobulinemia, splenomegaly, arthralgias, valvular disease (Libman-Sacks disease), anorexia, vomiting, diarrhea, dysphagia, abdominal pain, and lymphadenitis. The principal causes of death are renal insufficiency, bacterial endocarditis, cardiac failure, sepsis, and pneumonia (see also pp. 611 and 883).

The acute histologic changes in the skin include an exaggeration of the liquefaction degeneration of the basal layer of the epidermis (Fig. 38-14) with eosinophilic swelling of the cytoplasm of the basal cells, edema of the papillary and subpapillary layers, necrobiosis with karyorrhexis and nuclear distortion of inflammatory cells in the upper dermis, telangiectasis, and occasionally fibrinoid degeneration of foci of collagen in this region, as well as in the walls of some of the arterioles. The last change, arteriolar involvement, is inconstant and is surely not responsible for the other cutaneous alterations.

By far the most diagnostically revealing histologic changes occur at the dermo-epidermal junction. They are the vacuolization of the basal cells (liquefaction degeneration) and the subepidermal edema with a linear condensation of periodic acid–Schiff–positive material simulating a basement membrane but differing by its discontinuity and nonargyrophilia in the absence of melanin. Direct immunofluorescence studies reveal in this zone an immunofluorescent band reflecting immunoglobulins (IgG, IgM), components of complement (C1q, C3), and fibrin and properdin in both clinically involved and clinically intact skin.[26,41] The presence of the immunofluorescent band in clinically uninvolved skin worsens the prognosis and has been found to be associated with renal disease.[34] Although such skin may appear clinically uninvolved, careful histologic evaluation of even routinely hematoxylin and eosin–stained sections is likely to reveal some evidence of edema in this zone. In patients who have an inherited deficiency of complement there are likely to be an absence of C3 at the dermoepidermal junction and low titers of antinuclear antibodies. Interestingly, systemic lupus erythematosus has been associated with porphyria in more than a fortuitous manner.

Characteristic histologic changes occur in other organs in the disseminated disease. These include the following:

1. Atypical verrucous endocarditis (Libman-Sacks disease)
2. Striking fibrinoid alteration of the interstitial collagen of the myocardium that may, but need not, be mistaken for Aschoff bodies
3. Concentric dense rings of collagen, apparently thickened reticulum, about the central splenic arterioles (Figs. 30-26 and 30-27)
4. Focal fibrinoid swelling of the walls of glomerular capillaries ("wire loops")

Viruslike, microtubular cytoplasmic inclusions have been noted in the skin, glomeruli, and other sites. These have provoked much interest, but their presence in patients without systemic lupus erythematosus and even in the vascular endothelium of patients with bullous pemphigoid has dampened the initial enthusiasm for the likelihood that they represent the etiologic virus.

Undoubtedly, one of the most provocative discoveries in the field of cutaneovisceral integration of the last few decades has been the phenomenon of the lupus erythematosus cell. Cytologically the phenomenon is manifested typically by a rosette of neutrophilic leukocytes about a mononuclear cell (apparently a lymphocyte) or, less typically, by a neutrophilic leukocyte with a cytoplasmic vacuole or a cytoplasmic inclusion of a nuclear fragment. Often there is excessive clumping of platelets. The essence of this phenomenon resides in the gamma globulin of the serum of patients with disseminated lupus erythematosus and may be observed not only with cells of the patient's marrow but with cells of the peripheral blood. It also may be observed with normal cells (human or animal) after mixture with the patient's serum. Similar cells are noted in a cantharides-induced blister in the skin of patients with disseminated lupus erythematosus. It is of interest, but by now not surprising, to see dramatic remissions initiated by cortisone and ACTH in profoundly ill patients. With this improvement the lupus erythematosus cells diminish and may completely disappear. Some instances of a positive lupus erythematosus phenomenon have been recorded in multiple myeloma, leukemia, Hodgkin's disease, rheumatoid arthritis, viral hepatitis, acquired hemolytic anemia, and reactions to drugs (phenylbutazone and hydralazine) and in association with infection or contamination of serum with *Aspergillus niger* or *Trichophyton gypseum*. The lupus erythematosus cell is generally absent in scleroderma and dermatomyositis, which, together with disseminated lupus erythematosus, have been gratuitously linked as diffuse vascular or diffuse collagen disease—notwithstanding this and other discrepancies. Moreover, there is adequate reason to conclude that none of these diseases is either a diffuse vascular disease or a generalized disease of collagen. Review of the histologic findings in even a small number of autopsies in such cases quickly reveals that the involvement of vessels or collagen is, as a rule, neither diffuse nor itself responsible for the clinical picture, with the exception of scleroderma.

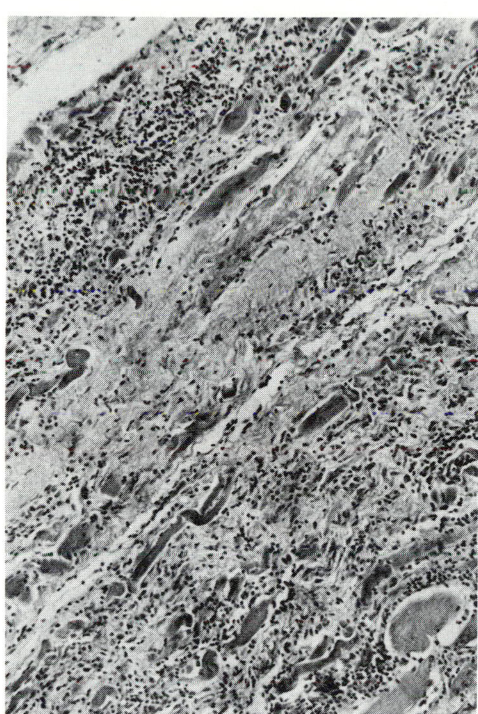

Fig. 38-15. Dermatomyositis with dense inflammatory cells interspersed among atrophic muscle fibers. (Hematoxylin and eosin.)

Mixed connective tissue disease

Mixed connective tissue disease is a designation applied to a mild form of systemic lupus erythematosus without renal involvement and with high titers of antinuclear antibodies exhibiting a speckled rather than membranous rim of homogeneous nuclear staining with indirect immunofluorescence tests. Features of systemic sclerosis and polymyositis are included.

Dermatomyositis

The purplish red, finely scaly edematous rash located principally about the upper face is fairly diagnostic; the histologic picture of the skin is not. It consists chiefly of spotty parakeratosis, some liquefaction degeneration at the dermoepidermal junction, and edema of the upper dermis. However, the vacuolar sarcolysis, coagulation necrosis, and acute inflammatory changes in the swollen muscle fibers may be strongly suggestive. As stated, the search for vascular alterations is generally fruitless (Fig. 38-15). Widespread calcinosis of the skin, subcutaneous and periarticular tissue, and muscles may occur, along with thickening of arterioles and venules of muscles.

The pathogenic and etiologic spectra of myositides are expanding rapidly and form an intriguing subject dealing with viruses, unresolved relationship to visceral cancer, and lesions of the thymus. It appears evident that some of the confusion related to dermatomyositis occurs because a variety of myositic disorders as well as systemic lupus erythematosus and scleroderma are mistakenly considered to be dermatomyositis. The presence of dermal mucin in a specimen with no specific pattern is stated to be suggestive of dermatomyositis. The cutaneous eruption of dermatomyositis may occur before involvement of muscle is evident clinically or histologically. Direct immunofluorescence studies usually show no abnormalities except globular deposits of IgG, IgM, and IgA in the upper dermis, which are of unknown significance.

Psoriasis

Psoriasis is characterized by reddish brown papules covered with silvery-white micaceous scales with a predilection for symmetric distribution on the extremities, especially on the knees and elbows. Lesions may occur also on the scalp, upper back, face, and genitalia and over the sacrum. The nails often are involved and become thickened, dirty white, irregularly laminated, rigid, and brittle. The disease is notoriously chronic, although remissions may occur spontaneously and after certain therapy, such as x-ray or ultraviolet-ray therapy.

The remarkable, if inconstant, resolution of psoriasis after plasmapheresis or dialysis, as well as its occurrence during dialysis and cardiac disease, must provide pathogenic clues.

Occasionally a widespread erythroderma or exfoliative dermatitis may complicate psoriasis, either spontaneous-

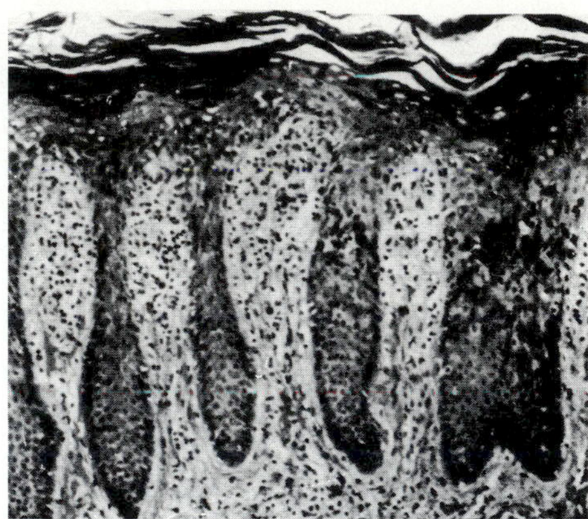

Fig. 38-16. Psoriasis with conspicuous parakeratosis, elongated, clubbed rete ridges, thinned suprapapillary epidermis, and rigid vessels in papillae. (Hematoxylin and eosin.)

ly or, more particularly, after vigorous therapy. Another complication of psoriasis is arthritis, occurring usually in association with the generalized erythroderma. Occasionally the arthritis is deforming and persistently ankylotic, as in rheumatoid arthritis. The association of psoriasis with hypertensive cardiovascular disease is of some note.

The use of various qualifying terms, such as psoriasis punctata, psoriasis guttata, psoriasis rupioides, psoriasis follicularis, and psoriasis nummularis, reflects simply the predominant clinical pattern of the lesions.

The histologic features of psoriasis (Fig. 38-16) are as follows:

1. Acanthosis with regular downgrowth of the rete ridges to about the same dermal level
2. Rounded tips of the rete ridges
3. Prolongation of the papillae, frequently with single vessels (venules) extending the length of the papillae as if rigid rather than tortuous
4. Thin epidermal plates over the elongated papillae, which offer so little covering for the dilated vessels of the papillae that bleeding occurs when a scale is lifted (Auspitz's sign)
5. Prominent parakeratosis, usually extending the length of the lesion rather than occurring focally
6. Absence or sparsity of stratum granulosum
7. Microabscesses (of Munro) in the upper rete Malpighi

In addition, there is usually an absence of spongiosis except in the immediate vicinity of the epidermal microabscesses. Intracellular edema in the rete Malpighi is common. The papillae are infiltrated chiefly with lymphocytes and histiocytes. In lesions in the early stage of development, some of these features, such as the rounding of the ridges and the elongation of the papillae with thin epidermal plates, may be absent. Furthermore, as in other dermatoses, recent therapy, trauma, or secondary infection obviously will modify the pattern. However, in patients who have had a superimposed exfoliative dermatitis the basic histologic picture of the psoriatic lesion tends to persist and thereby may help differentiate it from the exfoliative stage of mycosis fungoides, a problem that occasionally arises. Neurodermatitis may simulate psoriasis so closely as to be histologically indistinguishable. As a rule, however, the psoriasiform features listed previously are irregular or less developed in neurodermatitis, or individual changes are altogether lacking. Ultrastructurally the tonofibrils are abnormal, and a lack of secretion of the adhesive cell surface coat has been noted.

Parapsoriasis. Parapsoriasis, despite the name, is not related to psoriasis. The disease is characterized by erythematous macules covered with fine scales and distributed on the trunk and extremities. The lesions are extremely resistant to therapy.

The histologic changes of parapsoriasis are said to be nonspecific and to simulate psoriasis, seborrheic dermatitis, lichen planus, a macular syphiloderm, or the early stage of mycosis fungoides. Although the changes may simulate these other diseases, the specific diagnosis of parapsoriasis may be made with considerable assurance in many cases on the basis of the histologic changes alone. These changes include the spotty, thin areas of parakeratosis, slight to moderate acanthosis, vertical arrangement with some hyperchromatism of the basal layer along with slight liquefaction degeneration, and perhaps most revealing, the localization of inflammatory cells, mostly mononuclear, in the immediately subepidermal zone. The infiltrate hugs the epidermis tightly, and characteristically some of the inflammatory cells are located in the epidermis in their transepidermal migration. The presence of parakeratosis and a minimal stratum granulosum, as well as the shape of the ridges, easily distinguishes parapsoriasis from lichen planus. One of the serious errors of histologic diagnosis is mislabeling as parapsoriasis (en plaque) the early stage of mycosis fungoides. This error is also made clinically.

Lichen planus

Lichen planus is generally easily recognized clinically by the irregular, violaceous, glistening, flat-topped, pruritic papules covered with a thin, horny, adherent film and distributed symmetrically, particularly along the flexor aspects of the wrists, forearms, and legs. The usual form of lichen planus tends to resolve spontaneously after a year or so.

On careful examination minute whitish points and lines (Wickham's striae) are seen on the surface of the papules. The disease is chronic, may last from months to years, and is rarely associated with constitutional reac-

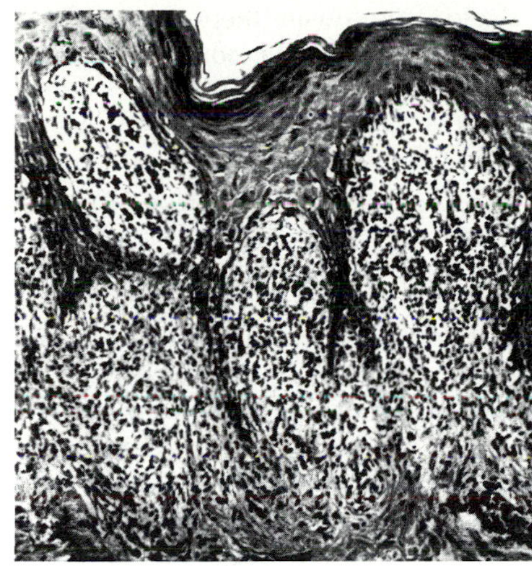

Fig. 38-17. Lichen planus with hyperkeratosis, acanthosis, pointed rete ridges, liquefaction degeneration, and dense subepidermal inflammatory zone. (Hematoxylin and eosin.)

tion except in some of the hyperacute cases. The varieties include lichen planus, lichen planus hypertrophicus, and lichen planus atrophicus.

The histologic features of lichen planus are strikingly characteristic and comprise the following:

1. Hyperkeratosis
2. Prominence of the stratum granulosum
3. Acanthosis, with elongated, saw-toothed rete ridges
4. Liquefaction degeneration of the basal layer
5. A mononuclear infiltrate consisting mostly of lymphocytes and histiocytes, sharply limited to the papillary and subpapillary layers of the dermis (Fig. 38-17)

Many of the subepidermal macrophages are laden with melanin from the basal cells, not because these cells are unable to unload their pigment into "damaged" unreceptive neighboring keratinocytes and so spill over into the dermis, but because the subepidermal infiltrate provokes not only the development of the epidermal pigmentation but also its release from the epidermis into dermal histiocytes. This same phenomenon is observed in other dermatoses, such as mycosis fungoides, Atabrine dermatitis, dermal postinflammatory pigmentation, and lupus erythematosus, in each of which a subepidermal inflammatory or cellular reaction occurs.

In the atrophic form the ridges are flattened, and the dermal infiltrate is sparse and replaced by an increased density of collagen containing somewhat thickened arterioles. Single foci of lesions histologically indistinguishable from the usual lichen planus are labeled benign lichenoid keratosis or solitary lichen planus.

Immunofluorescence reflecting the presence of immunoglobulins and complement is noted in the eosinophilic, clustered, subepidermal globular bodies (Civatte's bodies). Somewhat similar foci and necrotic keratinocytes are seen also in a variety of other dermatoses, but their diagnostic significance in these is inconsequential. Actually, the meaning of these deposits even in lichen planus is not understood. To suggest that they represent an autoimmune process is not warranted at this time. In ulcerated lichen planus of the feet, results of antinuclear-antibody tests may be positive and gamma globulin levels may be elevated, resulting in confusion with systemic lupus erythematosus.

Keratoderma blennorrhagica

Infrequently, perhaps in 1 in 5000 cases, an ugly eruption develops after the contraction of gonorrheal urethritis. This eruption is called keratoderma blennorrhagica or gonorrheal keratosis and is associated with a nonsuppurative migrating arthritis and gonorrheal urethritis that persist despite chemotherapy. The cutaneous lesions appear several weeks after the urethritis, do not contain gonococci according to most observers, and clear only after disappearance of the urethritis. The lesions of the skin are identical to those of Reiter's syndrome, which is associated with a presumed nonspecific urethritis, conjunctivitis, and nonsuppurative arthritis. In both the keratoderma and Reiter's syndrome, evolution of the disease is essentially similar. In both the arthritis clears, as a rule, without residual damage to the joints. In the few cases of Reiter's syndrome in which the complement fixation test for gonorrhea was used, results were negative. More recently *Chlamydia trachomatis* and the pleuropneumonia, or L, organisms have been considered responsible for Reiter's syndrome.

The histologic features of keratoderma blennorrhagica are as follows:

1. Prominent parakeratosis with excessive loosening of the scales so that they may be difficult to include in the histologic sections
2. Acanthosis with elongation and rounding of the ends of the rete ridges, much as in psoriasis, so that pustular psoriasis may be a difficult differential diagnostic problem
3. Elongation of the papillae, but generally not as strikingly as in psoriasis because the overlying epidermal plate usually is not as thinned as in the latter disease
4. Numerous polymorphonuclear leukocytes, particularly in the upper rete Malpighi and the scales

Diseases principally of dermis

Urticaria pigmentosa

Urticaria pigmentosa is a chronic disease of the skin that begins usually in the first year of life but may start shortly after puberty or in later adult life, particularly in males of light complexion. A significant number of patients with urticaria pigmentosa have a history of asthma or hay fever. The eruption characteristically is made up of oval, 0.5 to 2.5 cm, pigmented, yellowish brown to reddish brown, macular, papular, and even nodular lesions occurring on the back especially but also on the face, scalp, palms, and soles. Infrequently a patient has merely a solitary nodule of urticaria pigmentosa. Solitary mastocytomas generally are detected by the first month of life and comprise about 10% to 15% of all instances of cutaneous mastocytosis. The disseminated cutaneous form usually develops in the next few months. About 25% of cases appear in late teenage or adult life, between the ages of 15 and 40 years, and occur equally in males and females.

Occasionally the eruptions may be sufficiently yellow to simulate xanthomatosis. The lesions are often intensely pruritic and, when irritated, become reddened, swollen, and urticarial, that is, they show evidence of dermographism. They may persist for years and in many instances disappear spontaneously. When the lesions of urticaria pigmentosa appear in childhood and are confined to the skin, the likelihood of spontaneous resolution during adolescence is great. If the lesions first appear in adolescence or later, the likelihood of their persistence and systemization is considerable. Bullae are common in neonatal mastocytosis.

Systemic involvement (bones, liver, lymph nodes, spleen) occurs in about 10% of patients, mostly in adults, and in about one third of them the equivalent of a mast cell leukemia develops. Uncommonly a solitary nodule or mastocytoma is followed by dissemination to the viscera or to the remainder of the skin. Such dissemination is said not to occur if the nodule remains solitary for approximately 2 months.

The histologic picture of urticaria pigmentosa is distinctive. In the more striking examples the upper half or two thirds of the dermis is replaced by a compact zone of mast cells that obscure the dermal landmarks (Fig. 38-18). The mast cells should be recognized in sections stained with the routine hematoxylin and eosin, notwithstanding their simulation of ordinary histiocytes and of plasma cells. Frequently, under high magnification, even with this routine stain the cytoplasmic granules of mast cells may be discerned (Fig. 38-19). These granules are of course more clearly demonstrable in metachromatic stains, such as Giemsa's or toluidine blue.

Mast cells contain heparin, hyaluronic acid, serotonin, and histamine. Indeed, there are isolated reports that these agents are reflected in an increase in the level of serum mucopolysaccharides and in coagulation defects. In some cases mast cells are present in smaller numbers and are dispersed as clumps of 10 to 20 cells about the middermal vessels. In these instances fine judgment may be required to differentiate the presence of mast cells in normal and abnormal numbers. In addition to the mast cells, there often are subepidermal edema (urticaria), chromatophores containing melanin in the upper dermis, and eosinophilic leukocytes scattered among the mast cells. Melanosis of the basal layer of the epidermis also may be present. The full-blown picture of urticaria pigmentosa closely resembles the so-called mastocytoma of dogs. Systemic foci of infiltrations of mast cells are found also in the viscera, for example, in the spleen, liver, and lymph nodes. Routine histologic sections of urticaria pigmentosa are commonly mistaken for leukemia, nevi, malignant melanomas, and Letterer-Siwe disease. Acceptance of the teaching that mast cells cannot be

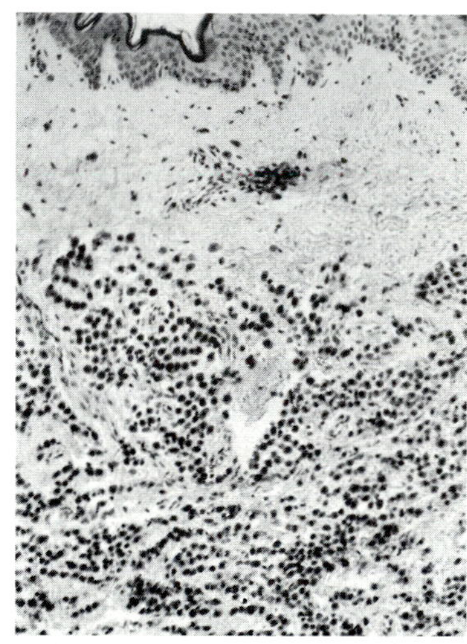

Fig. 38-18. Urticaria pigmentosa with superficial edema of cutis and extensive numbers of mast cells in remainder of dermis. (Hematoxylin and eosin.)

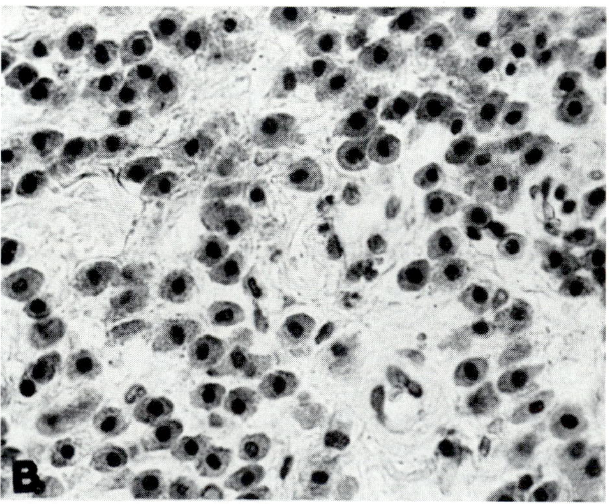

Fig. 38-19. Urticaria pigmentosa showing mast cells recognizable in routine stains of hematoxylin and eosin.

detected or strongly suspected with stains of hematoxylin and eosin is in large part responsible for these serious errors.

Simple urticaria may be caused in a variety of ways: by drugs, allergenic foods, infections (melioidosis), ultraviolet irradiation (urticaria solaris), and, fairly commonly, emotional disturbances. Urticaria solaris occurs immediately after exposure to light of sufficient intensity and of proper wavelength, usually in the violet or blue part of the spectrum. The essential histologic picture is that of bland subepidermal edema. In the inherited angioneurotic lesion the edema may extend into the subcutis. The evidence for a deficiency in plasma protease inhibitors (alpha-1-antitrypsin) in patients with chronic urticaria has been stressed recently.[24]

Urticarial vasculitis

Urticarial vasculitis appears to be a nonspecific spectrum of clinical, laboratory, and immunopathologic features caused by a variety of agents with variable degrees of severity.[54] The combination of hives and leukocytoclastic, fibrinoid dermal arteriolitis with immune complexes and complement, at times with hypocomplementemia, arthralgias, and glomerulonephritis, may form the background of a number of diseases, including systemic lupus erythematosus, viral hepatitis, and others.

Leukocytoclastic vasculitis (palpable purpura) represents an activated complement–induced inflammation of the small dermal vessels.

Erysipelas

Erysipelas is described in Chapter 7 (p. 292).

Diseases of collagen

Keloid. A keloid is a hypertrophic cutaneous scar that develops as a reaction to burns, incisions, insect bites, vaccinations, and other stimuli. Ulcerated keloids are prone to undergo carcinomatous transformation of the epidermis after a long interval, particularly those attributable to burns or associated with chronic sinuses, as in osteomyelitis. The dermal portion of a keloid is not more likely to become sarcomatous than the dermis elsewhere. Rarely, a keloid resolves spontaneously.

The histologic features of a keloid include thick, homogeneously eosinophilic bands of collagen admixed with thin collagenous fibers and large active fibroblasts. The sweat glands, sebaceous glands, follicles, and arrectores pilorum are atrophic, destroyed, or displaced by the scar. The epidermis may be atrophic or only slightly altered by fusion and an irregular pattern of the ridges. The ordinary scar of the skin is more cellular than a keloid and is composed of uniformly thinner collagenous fibers. In both instances elastic tissue is diminished or absent. The keloidal reaction of hypertrophic collagenous bundles and large fibroblasts is characteristic of dermatitis papillaris capillitii (keloidal acne), which occurs particularly in the nuchal region and with the associated extensive plasmacytic reaction, represents a type of response to folliculitis.

Balanitis xerotica obliterans. Balanitis xerotica obliterans is a disease of collagen that appears clinically as whitish, firm, coalescent papules or a sclerotic plaque of the glans penis and foreskin and often occurs after circumcision. The disease is of some importance because the process tends to extend to the urethral meatus, causing stenosis of the orifice. The lesion is to be differentiated clinically from erythroplasia of Queyrat and circumscribed scleroderma. Balanitis xerotica obliterans is probably a form of lichen sclerosus et atrophicus, which tends to occur on the vulva.

The histologic picture consists of:

1. Atrophic epidermis or epithelium with loss of rete ridges
2. Striking homogenization of the collagen affecting about one third of the upper dermis
3. A more or less dense zone of lymphocytes and histiocytes beneath the homogenized collagen (Fig. 38-20)

The small arteries and arterioles of the upper and middle dermis may show evidence of endarteritis obliterans, but this process is sufficiently inconstant as not to warrant the use of the qualification "obliterans" in the name of the disease. Furthermore, on the basis of other cutaneous atrophy there is reason to believe that the vascular change does not initiate the collagenous change but perhaps is an incidental secondary reaction as in other kinds of chronic inflammation (such as chronic gastric ulcer).

In lichen sclerosus et atrophicus the initial change is a subepidermal edema that subsequently progresses to the

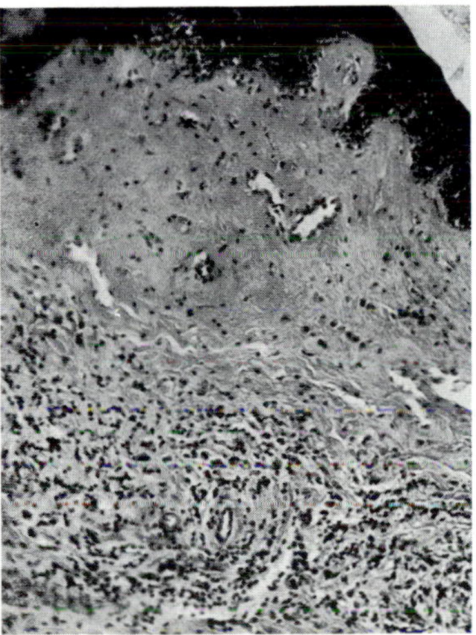

Fig. 38-20. Balanitis xerotica obliterans with homogenization of subepidermal collagen over zone of inflammatory cells. (Hematoxylin and eosin.)

characteristically homogenized densely sclerotic collagen in which the elastic fibers are diminished because of their displacement downward. The edema may be so great as to cause actual vesiculation at the dermoepidermal junction. Uncommonly an epidermoid carcinoma develops in the presence of lichen sclerosis et atrophicus. Even though the association is infrequent, the histologic appearance of transition of the two processes suggests that the carcinoma develops from the sclerosis on more than a chance basis.

Acrodermatitis chronica atrophicans. Acrodermatitis chronica atrophicans involves atrophy of the epidermis and a subepidermal homogenized zone of collagen beneath which is a dense zone of mononuclear cells. There are also loss of dermal elastic tissue and atrophy of appendages.

Acrodermatitis chronica atrophicans begins as erythematous, slightly edematous macules that later become wrinkled, atrophic, and sclerodermatoid. As the prefix *acro-* indicates, the disease tends to select the extremities, particularly the hands and feet and the extensor surfaces of the elbows and knees. The condition occurs predominantly in middle-aged women.

Granuloma annulare and rheumatoid nodules. Granuloma annulare is a chronic eruption made up of papules or nodules grouped in a ringed or circinate arrangement, with a tendency to occur on the dorsa of the fingers and hands and on the elbows, neck, feet, ankles, and buttocks, particularly of children and young adults. The lesions can be palpated intracutaneously rather than subcutaneously, in contrast to rheumatic nodules.

The etiology of the disease is unknown. The histologic findings suggest a rheumatic or rheumatoid basis for the disease, but clinical evidence is sparse. I have seen cases associated with disseminated allergic granulomatous arteritis. The histologic picture of granuloma annulare has been observed also as a reaction to *Culicoides furans*, a biting gnat.

Histologically granuloma annulare is characterized by an intradermal oval or circular focus of fibrinoid degeneration of collagen. The nodules may occasionally ulcerate and are then categorized as perforating granuloma annulare. These necrotic foci of dermal collagen suggest infarcts, although corresponding occlusion of adjacent vessels is not regularly noted. About such a focus are palisaded rows of epithelioid cells or histiocytes, some of which may be vacuolated by fat (Fig. 38-21). It is the combination of fibrinoid alteration of collagen and palisaded histiocytes that suggests a possible rheumatic etiology. In fact, the histologic features of granuloma annulare are identical to those of the rheumatic or rheumatoid nodule—the only difference, as indicated, being the location of the latter in the subcutaneous tissue, adjacent to or within synovial membranes. Certainly the histologic picture is not that of tuberculosis, although the characteristic fibrinoid degeneration of the collagen of granuloma annulare and the rheumatic nodule has been mistaken for the caseation of tuberculosis, a simulation that usually can be detected easily. There may be considerable difficulty, however, in recognizing early or small lesions of granuloma annulare in which the only clue may be a minimal smudgy fibrinoid swelling of collagen with clumps of a few histiocytes, some vacuolated and others partially palisaded. These minute lesions may be confused with xanthoses, necrobiosis lipoidica diabeticorum, or leprosy. Aschoff bodies are absent in granuloma annulare, as they are in the subcutaneous rheumatic nodule; they are confined to the heart. A protease and a collagenase similar to those of rheumatoid synovial enzymes have been isolated from rheumatoid nodules.

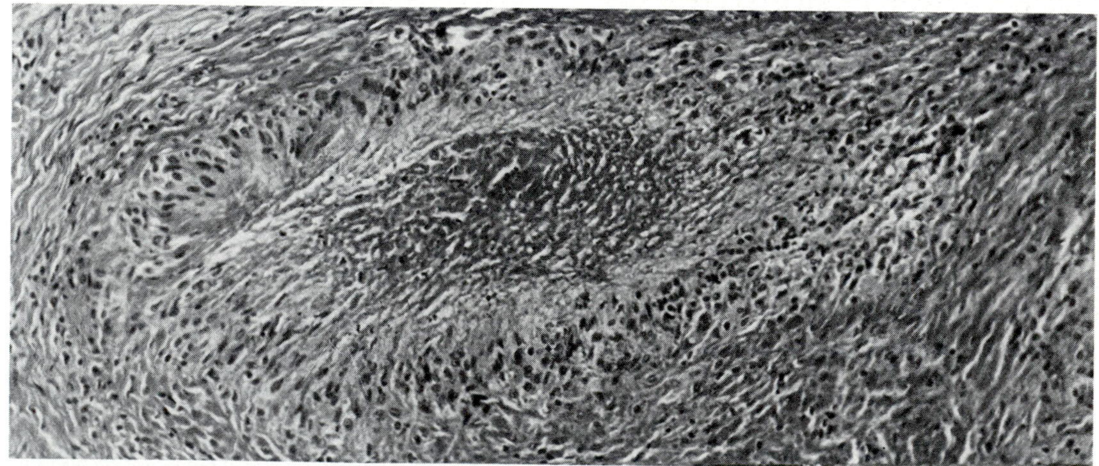

Fig. 38-21. Granuloma annulare with dermal lesion showing central necrosis bordered by histiocytes.

The necrosis has been attributed to these, but the greater likelihood is the primacy of vascular compromise as a cause of the infarctlike necrosis both in these nodules and in granuloma annulare. These necrotic foci may perforate the epidermis, as stated.

Necrobiosis lipoidica diabeticorum. Necrobiosis lipoidica diabeticorum is characterized by oval, circular, firm, sharply defined plaques with yellowish centers and violaceous peripheries, occurring predominantly on the legs but found also on the forearms, palms, soles, neck, and face. The centers of the lesions are prone to ulcerate. Trauma, often inconspicuous, may initiate the lesions. In about 50% to 80% of patients the disease is associated with diabetes. In about 10% the lesions precede the onset of diabetes. In the remainder, diabetes does not develop. Obviously, the recognition of necrobiosis lipoidica diabeticorum can be of prophetic importance.

Clinically the disease must be differentiated from other such focal diseases of collagen as granuloma annulare, amyloidosis, morphea, and lipid proteinosis, as well as the granulomas of sarcoid and erythema induratum, which also tend to occur on the extremities. The diabetic state in some instances of necrobiosis lipoidica diabeticorum may be missed with the standard glucose tolerance test and discovered with the cortisone glucose tolerance test.

The basic histologic change of necrobiosis diabeticorum consists of ischemia-like degeneration of collagen that occurs in irregular patches, especially in the upper dermis. In well-developed foci the altered collagen is swollen and somewhat granular, with loss of fibrils and a diminution in nuclei of fibrocytes. At the periphery of the collagenous alteration are small collections of histiocytes often arranged about Langhans giant cells and simulating sarcoid or tuberculosis (Fig. 38-22). This giant cell reaction occasionally may involve the walls of veins to produce a giant cell phlebitis reminiscent of the reaction in temporal arteritis. Vacuoles may be present in the cytoplasm of the giant cells and histiocytes, but fat is found infrequently within the cells of these lesions, although extracellular fat is detectable about the altered collagen.

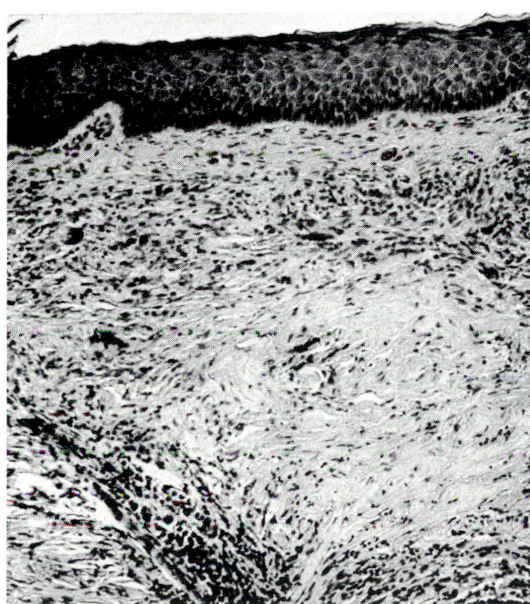

Fig. 38-22. Necrobiosis lipoidica diabeticorum with irregularly homogenized, degenerated dermal collagen and tuberculoid granulomas at periphery. (Hematoxylin and eosin.)

Scleroderma. There are two basic varieties of scleroderma, the differentiation of which is of great importance prognostically: (1) morphea, or circumscribed scleroderma, and (2) diffuse scleroderma.

Circumscribed scleroderma occurs as well-delimited, round or oval plaques with whitish, yellowish, or ivory-colored centers and violaceous peripheries. Occasionally the plaques correspond in distribution to the innervation of a cutaneous nerve, so a trophic origin has been suggested. Degeneration and regeneration of dermal nerves are said to occur with characteristic patterns in scleroderma and acrosclerosis. Morphea guttata or white-spot disease is a modification of circumscribed scleroderma characterized by varying-sized chalky-white patches on the chest and neck. Rarely does circumscribed scleroderma progress into the often fatal diffuse scleroderma. Usually the lesions clear, with a barely noticeable thin atrophic area as a residuum. Linear scleroderma of an extremity may be associated with melorheostosis or linear hyperostosis of the underlying bone.

Diffuse scleroderma, which affects women twice as often as men, begins insidiously—usually as edema of the hands, other parts of the extremities, or neck—and extends inexorably on to sclerosis that stiffens, binds, and limits the mobility of the affected part. Ulcerations may occur over bony prominences. Calcareous cutaneous deposits and pigmentation, the latter of such a degree as to simulate Addison's disease, are frequent. The normal cutaneous lines become obliterated. Diminution in sweating, hyperesthesias, and pruritus may occur. Sclerosis limited to the hands in association with the vasospastic symptoms of Raynaud's disease is called acrosclerosis or sclerodactylia. In actuality this symptom complex presents a phase of diffuse scleroderma, although the progress to the fatal disease is not invariable.

Systemic sclerosis refers to diffuse scleroderma with visceral involvement. Dense fibrosis may affect the myocardium and the esophagus and other portions of the gastrointestinal tract. The lungs may be affected with cystic fibrosis, particularly at the bases. Renal vessels may present the histologic picture of accelerated nephroscle-

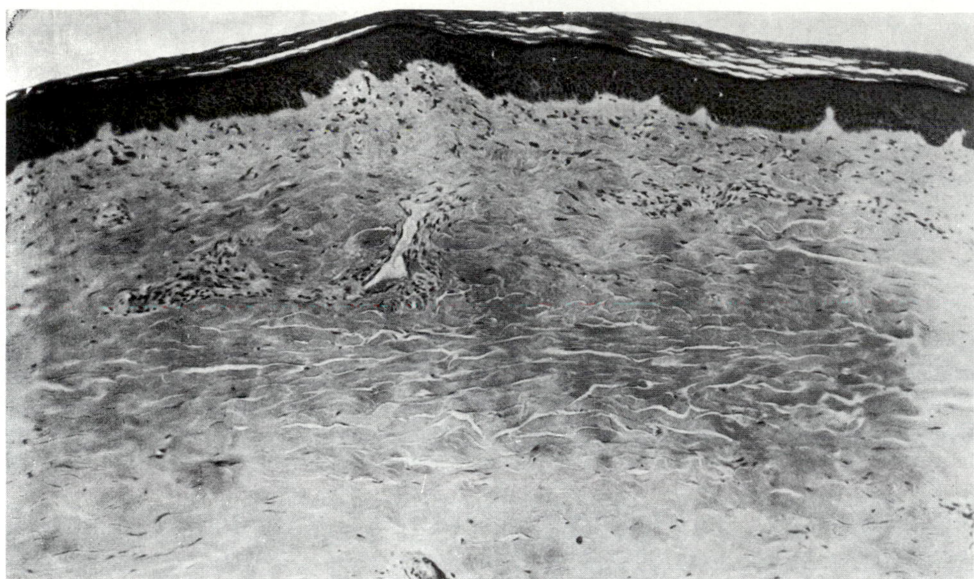

Fig. 38-23. Scleroderma with dense and thickened dermal fibers, atrophy of appendages and epidermis, and melanin pigmentation of basal layer. (Hematoxylin and eosin.)

rosis and, if widespread, will indeed be associated with malignant hypertension. The glomeruli may show conspicuous diffuse membranous glomerulonephritis. The cardiac fibrosis or the cystic pulmonary changes may lead to myocardial failure.

The histologic sections of morphea cannot be differentiated from those of diffuse scleroderma. The principal changes involve the collagenous fibers, which become hypertrophied through edema and then atrophy. The atrophic fibers are no longer loosely disposed as in the normal dermis but are compressed into dense, compact collagenous masses, with diminution of fibrocytic nuclei and obliteration of spaces between collagenous bundles so that the thickness of the dermis may be decreased (Fig. 38-23). Inflammatory reaction tends to be absent, except in the early stages, when focal collections of mononuclear cells may be disposed about appendages. The appendages (hair, sweat glands, and sebaceous glands) are atrophic. Elastic fibers may be diminished or distorted, but they represent the least informative alteration and are unduly emphasized in the literature. The epidermis may be normal, but usually it is atrophic, with flattened rete ridges and a hyperpigmented basal layer. Subepidermal melanin-containing chromatophores may be increased. In conjunction with the collagenous change, small arteries and arterioles may become secondarily sclerotic. Calcific or even ossified foci (osteoma cutis) may replace the altered collagen of the dermis and subcutaneous septa. The deposits of calcium may be so extensive as to camouflage the primary diagnosis and be dismissed as calcinosis. Superficial dermal telangiectasia is common, possibly as a consequence of sclerosis of deeper vessels. The dermis of patients in the indurative phase has been found by actual measurement to be thicker and heavier than normal.[60]

Eosinophilic fasciitis and subcutaneous morphea are considered subsets of scleroderma. In these there are varying degrees of edema, eosinophilia, and sclerosis of the subcutis and fascia. Atrophic myositis may accompany the cutaneous lesions, although uncommonly to the degree found in dermatomyositis or poikilodermatomyositis, in which the inflammatory reaction in the skeletal muscles may be extreme, despite the usual nondescript subepidermal edema and focal liquefaction degeneration in the latter diseases. Here again it is emphasized that neither diffuse vascular nor diffuse visceral collagenous changes occur in dermatomyositis or poikilodermatomyositis any more than they do in the majority of cases of diffuse lupus erythematosus.

CRST refers to a tetrad of findings consisting of calcinosis, Raynaud's phenomenon, sclerodactyly, and telangiectasia. Most patients with CRST eventually develop visceral involvement.

In view of the association between sclerosis of skin and lung (systemic sclerosis, burns, healed infarcts, and so on) on the one hand and carcinoma on the other, it may be anticipated that carcinoma of the skin would be a complication of diffuse scleroderma. This latter association is rare and may be a reflection of the duration of the sclerosis.

Scleredema. Scleredema (Buschke's disease) is to be distinguished from scleroderma. Although the entity is commonly known as scleredema adultorum, it does involve children in an appreciable percentage of cases.

Scleredema is usually a self-limited disease characterized by a tough, nonpitting, uniform edema of the head and neck, producing a masklike expression and restricted motion that simulates scleroderma. The periphery of the process is readily palpable. The disease generally runs its course in several months to a year and a half, leaving no residuum. Recurrences have been recorded.

The lesion differs from scleroderma in the absence of pigmentation, the rarity of involvement of the hands and feet, and complete resolution with very rare exceptions. The usually self-limited scleredema of Buschke is distinguished from the long-lasting, often extensive scleredema associated with diabetes mellitus.

The histologic picture of scleredema is that of striking edema and hypertrophy of tight collagenous bundles so that, despite the compactness of the bundles, the thickness of the dermis is distinctly increased over normal. The epidermis, vessels, elastic tissue, and muscle show no changes. The changes of sclerema neonatorum are altogether different from those of scleredema or scleroderma and consist of the precipitation of fatty acid crystals and foreign body reaction in the subcutaneous fat, possibly because of a deficiency of olein in the fat, with consequent raising of its melting point. The localized, nodular sclerema, which some believe may result from birth trauma, is also self-limited. The diffuse form, which may involve also visceral (such as periadrenal and perirenal) fat, is a fatal disease. Scleredema and scleroderma are to be differentiated also from myxedema of either the circumscribed or the diffuse type.

Lipid proteinosis. Lipid proteinosis (hyalinosis cutis et mucosae) is another remarkable disease affecting dermal collagen and its vessels. The disorder generally manifests itself in infancy and is characterized by verrucous yellowish plaques, especially on the hands, feet, elbows, and face. The lesions may involve also the mouth and larynx. In the latter location the woody consistency of the lesions may cause a stenosis severe enough to require tracheotomy. Persistent hoarseness is a common symptom. Disturbances in phospholipids are inconstant. A familial tendency toward diabetes mellitus is occasionally present. It does not now appear that the entity is a primary lipidosis but rather that the lipid is normal in composition incidental to other tissue changes, especially those of collagen. One form of lipid proteinosis is light sensitive and occurs with erythropoietic porphyria.

The histologic features of lipid proteinosis are a hyperkeratotic and acanthotic epidermis overlying eosinophilic homogenized collagen in the upper dermis. The walls of arterioles and small arteries of this region are thickened. A fat stain reveals dense sudanophilic deposits in and about their walls, as well as in the stroma. No foam cells are present such as are found in Fabry's disease (angiokeratoma corporis diffusum). The serum lipids are normal as a rule. It is stated that the fat is combined with the protein of the collagen and therefore resists ordinary fat solvents. This property was not borne out in two cases I observed. As might be expected, the hyalinized collagen is periodic acid–Schiff positive and diastase resistant. Accordingly the entity has been designated a lipoglycoproteinosis.

Amyloidosis. Amyloidosis may be confined to the skin, or the cutaneous lesions may represent part of a systemic process. The eruption is characterized by pruritus and brownish papules, nodules, or plaques occurring particularly on the legs. Histologically there are focal areas of bland homogenization of dense collagen, occasionally scattered in the dermis but often located as subepidermal round masses (lichen amyloidosis) that stain metachromatically with the ordinary stains for amyloid.

The subepidermal nodules of amyloidosis (lichen amyloidosis) tend to be restricted to the skin. The nodular, para-articular masses of amyloid, along with amyloidotic macroglossia, are likely to be a manifestation of primary amyloidosis (para-amyloidosis) and to be associated with myeloma or related plasmacytosis and globulinemias. The cutaneous manifestations of amyloidosis resulting from leprosy, tuberculosis, rheumatoid arthritis, Hodgkin's disease, and chronic suppuration may be detectable only microscopically. The amyloid of primary amyloidosis tends to resist metachromatic stains, in contrast to amyloid of secondary amyloidosis. Rarely, epidermolysis bullosa may overlie secondary amyloidosis of the skin.

The histologic picture of lichen amyloidosis may closely simulate colloid milium, in which there is also a homogeneous alteration, with swelling into nodular masses of the subepidermal collagen (Fig. 38-24). However, the collagen of colloid milium does not stain metachromatically, and the fibers in this disease appear looser, more edematous, and more friable than do those of amyloidosis (Fig. 38-25).

Clinically colloid milium appears as small translucent papules from 1 to 5 mm in diameter, occurring commonly on the exposed areas, particularly the face, of fair-skinned persons, more commonly men.

Circumscribed myxedema. Circumscribed or localized myxedema occurs in association with exophthalmic Graves' disease. It appears as a fairly demarcated nonpitting, solidly edematous, usually bilateral plaque of the pretibial region, at times extending to the dorsa of the feet.

Persistently elevated serum levels of long-acting thyroid stimulator (LATS) are the rule in patients with pretibial myxedema. In some instances LATS has been detected in homogenates of tissue from the affected areas in concentrations significantly higher than in unaffected tissue. It is hypothesized that LATS acts as a specific antibody that, when fixed in tissue, elicits the characteristic local edematous reaction.

Histologically, abundant basophilic mucin is found

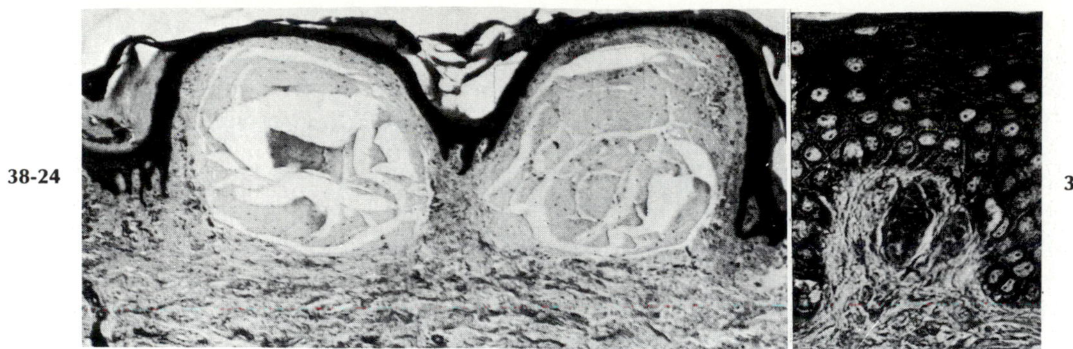

Fig. 38-24. Colloid milium with characteristic nodules of altered collagen. (Hematoxylin and eosin.)
Fig. 38-25. Amyloidosis showing metachromatic focus in papilla. (Toluidine blue stain.)

separating and fragmenting dermal collagenous bundles, without inflammatory reaction other than an occasional increase of mast cells. The diffuse myxedema of hypothyroidism is characterized by swelling of the collagenous bundles by interfibrillary mucin, which in some instances is demonstrable with Alcian or toluidine blue. There is less disruption of the collagenous bundles in diffuse myxedema than in circumscribed myxedema of hyperthyroidism. These lesions are to be distinguished from the nonendocrinogenic subepidermal mucinous papules of lichen myxedematosis or papular mucinosis.

Mucinous cysts

Mucinous dermal cysts, often loosely referred to as synovial cysts or myxoid cysts, are single, smooth, firm, 5 to 6 mm nodules at the bases of distal phalanges. The overlying epidermis is likely to be slightly thinned but not otherwise significantly altered. The cyst contains a mucinous, clear material quite like that of synovial cysts, and the similarity extends to the histologic structure. The mucin is periodic acid–Schiff negative but contains large amounts of hyaluronic acid as reflected in the positive Alcian blue stain. There is no communication of these cysts with bursae or joint cavities.

Microscopically the cyst is found to be unilocular or multilocular and to be derived from a simple liquefaction of the dermal collagen, so no mesothelial or endothelial lining is present. Such a lining may be simulated by compressed fibrocytes of the dermal collagenous fibers. Essentially this picture is analogous to that found in what are also loosely called synovial cysts of tendons or ganglions. These, too, do not represent cysts of expanded synovial walls with mesothelial lining but rather foci of mucinous degeneration of collagen of tendon or synovia. The mucinous dermal cyst may become obliterated by fibrosis and calcification.

Diseases of elastic tissue

Although alterations in elastic tissue, especially diminution and fraying, occur in many dermatoses, there are several principal, primary disorders of elastic tissue: (1) cutis hyperelastica (Ehlers-Danlos syndrome), (2) pseudoxanthoma elasticum, (3) senile elastosis, (4) elastoma dorsi, (5) elastosis perforans serpiginosa, and (6) dermatolysis (cutis laxa).

Cutis hyperelastica. Cutis hyperelastica (Ehlers-Danlos syndrome) is a familial disease characterized by hyperelastic velvety skin (rubber skin) associated with hyperlaxity and hyperextensibility of the joints and the tendency of the skin to bleed, tear, and scar after slight trauma. There are at least 10 varieties of this disorder, depending principally on the biochemical defects of both collagen and elastin and possibly also on platelets and on fibronectin, the adhesive glycoprotein that cross-links fibrin and glues it to collagen. The fibronectins are concerned also with the normal aggregation of platelets. The disorder may be associated with skeletal deformities, including arachnodactyly, blue sclerae (as in Löbstein's syndrome), dilatation of viscera (trachea, esophagus, and colon), pulmonary blebs, dissecting aneurysms, scoliosis, and easy bruisability that may be mistaken for battering.

Histologically, abundant compact masses of elastic fibers throughout the dermis are demonstrable by Weigert's stain for elastic tissue (Fig. 38-26). The suggestion that the increase in elastic fibers is illusionary rather than real has not been borne out by my observations. There appears to be no qualitative alteration in these or in the collagenous fibers. The tendency for calcification, as observed in elastic fibers in pseudoxanthoma elasticum and in degenerative arterial diseases, is not apparent in the elastic fibers of Ehlers-Danlos syndrome. Edema of the superficial dermis, with disruption of the normal wavy pattern of the dermal collagenous fibers, may be

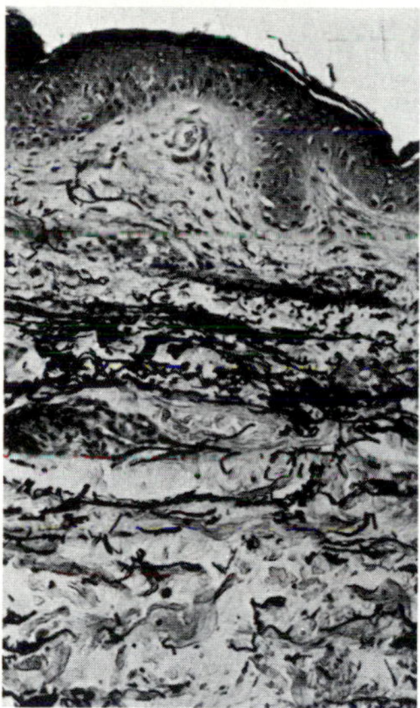

Fig. 38-26. Hyperelastosis cutis. (Weigert–van Gieson.)

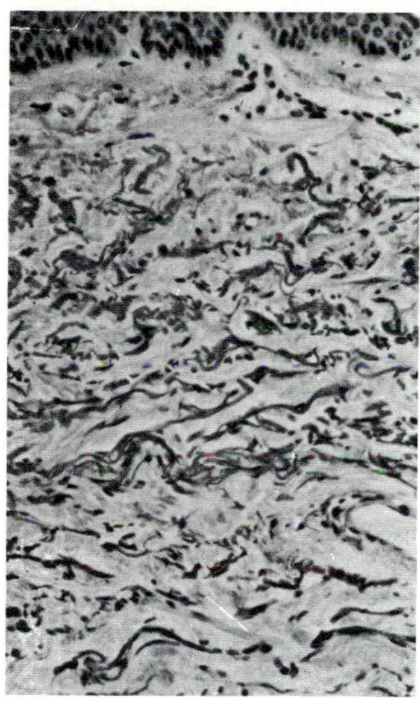

Fig. 38-27. Senile or degenerative elastosis. (Hematoxylin and eosin.)

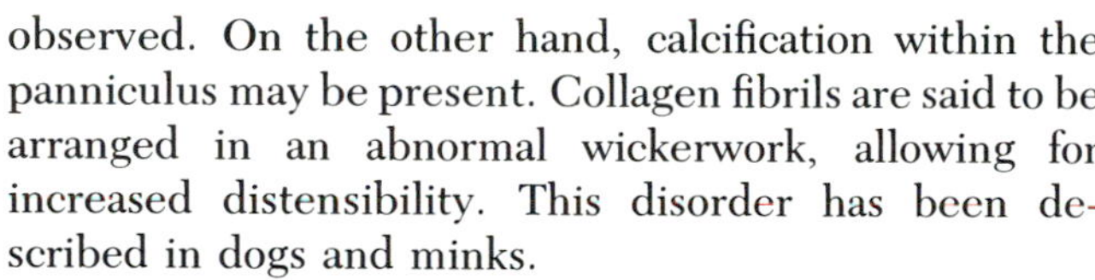

observed. On the other hand, calcification within the panniculus may be present. Collagen fibrils are said to be arranged in an abnormal wickerwork, allowing for increased distensibility. This disorder has been described in dogs and minks.

Pseudoxanthoma elasticum. Pseudoxanthoma elasticum is a hereditary disease in which yellowish papules and plaques are symmetrically distributed in abnormally lax skin of the neck, axilla, groin, and cubital and popliteal spaces. Other parts of the body are less frequently involved.

In histologic sections the elastic fibers are easily detectable, even in routine preparations stained with hematoxylin and eosin, as masses of basophilic, curved, small, partially calcified fragmented curlicues, with a tendency toward concentration near the mid-dermis. Occasionally there are associated disorganized granulomas of the foreign body type. About 50% of patients with pseudoxanthoma elasticum have ophthalmoscopically visible angioid streaks in the retina that are said to be similar to the dermal changes histologically and are attributed to cracking of Bruch's elastic membrane of the choroid. The histologic evidence, however, is limited.

Ultrastructurally an elastic fiber appears as a central amorphous core of elastin surrounded by microfibrils. Abnormal fibers show changes in size, shape, and granularity. The presence of calcium and polyanions such as sulfates or pyrophosphates is reported.

Pseudoxanthoma elasticum may be associated with changes in the cardiovascular system, including arterial aneurysms, mitral valve prolapse, and calcification and degeneration of elastic tissue of arteries. Other congenital cardiovascular, gastrointestinal, and genitourinary defects may occur with the syndrome. Rarely, it is associated with cutis hyperelastica and osteitis deformans.

Senile elastosis. Senile elastosis is the loss of elasticity of the skin of elderly people, particularly on the exposed portions of the body such as the face and the dorsum of the hands. In microscopic sections the change is represented by a subpapillary zone of basophilic alteration of swollen elastic fibers. This form of elastosis may or may not be associated with atrophy of the epidermis and appendages (Fig. 38-27). Despite the increase in elastic tissue, such skin is characterized by a loss of elasticity as if the physical properties of these fibers had been altered or as if collagenous fibers had acquired the staining properties of elastic tissue.

A subject of paramount importance, albeit seriously neglected, is dermatogerontology in all of its parameters, morphology not the least. There is neither the space nor authenticated information to document the changes that accompany aging within this chapter.

Elastofibroma dorsi. Elastofibroma dorsi is an apparently reactive fibrous tumefaction that is localized preponderantly to the scapula but occurs also near the ischial tuberosity and greater trochanter. It is firm, varies in size from about 2 to 10 cm, and develops over a period of years. The surprising histologic finding is the presence of numerous clusters of thick and fragmented elastic fibers, readily recognizable by their eosinophilia even in sections stained with hematoxylin and eosin. Although these fibers lack the periodicity of collagen and are digested with elastase, there are reasons to suggest origin from denatured collagen. These fibers, which do not contain fat or calcium, exhibit differences from those of the elastic laminae of arteries, elastotic degeneration of the skin, and pseudoxanthoma elasticum.

Elastofibroma dorsi is to be distinguished from the familial fibromas or collagenomas recently described, in which no change in the elastic tissue is noted.

Elastosis perforans serpiginosa. There is a group of disorders that have in common the gross and histologic features of transepidermal extrusion of plugs of keratin, collagen, and elastic tissue. These entities, which are commonly mistaken for one another, are known as reactive perforating collagenosis (RPC), perforating folliculitis, elastosis perforans serpiginosa, and Kyrle's disease. Elastosis perforans serpiginosa is characterized by groups of arciform or circinate, erythematous, acuminate keratotic papules, usually on the face and neck. It has been noted to develop after long courses of penicillamine therapy.

The characteristic histologic feature is compact packets of curled, frayed, thickened basophilic elastic fibers over which the epidermis is acanthotic and hyperkeratotic. The papule or plug is attributable chiefly to the penetration and extrusion of masses of elastic fibers through the epidermis.[51] Lymphocytes and foreign body–type giant cells surround the lesion. The pattern simulates that of Kyrle's disease (hyperkeratosis follicularis in cutem penetrans), in which the extruded plugs are keratinous rather than elastic tissue. Furthermore, in Kyrle's disease the parakeratotic plug penetrates the dermis through invaginated epidermis. The lesion is not confined to follicles, is not accompanied by pseudoepitheliomatous hyperplasia, and may show a giant cell granulomatous reaction.

Specific granulomas

Of the specific granulomas of the skin the following should be mentioned: those caused by tuberculosis, sarcoidosis, berylliosis, leprosy, brucellosis, leishmaniasis, syphilis, and granuloma inguinale, those caused by atypical acid-fast bacilli, and those from deep fungi, such as sporotrichosis, blastomycosis, coccidioidomycosis, and histoplasmosis.

Tuberculosis cutis. Tuberculosis cutis may assume a large variety of clinical forms of which lupus vulgaris, scrofuloderma, tuberculosis cutis verrucosa, miliary cutaneous tuberculosis, and many kinds of tuberculids are a few examples. Although differing prognostic implications usually make the precise diagnosis of tuberculosis significant, the important service the pathologist is expected to render is to name the overall tuberculous process. In this the problem is complicated by the difficulty with which the sparse tubercle bacilli are demonstrable in paraffin sections of the skin, so that the tubercle is usually the chief basis for the diagnosis. Unfortunately, many agents other than tubercle bacilli are capable of producing tubercles. Moreover, the tubercle often is incompletely formed, and reliance is then placed on such suggestions as epithelioid cells clustered or palisaded in the vicinity or in a matrix of caseated tissue, with or without giant cells. The cutaneous reaction of leishmaniasis, as well as of histoplasmosis and other fungi, is often tuberculoid, but the detection of the respective organisms in histiocytes and giant cells establishes the diagnosis.

Of increasing interest are the cutaneous granulomas produced by atypical acid-fast bacilli or, more accurately, bacilli that although acid fast are basically different from *Myocobacterium tuberculosis* in drug sensitivity as well as in cultural and pathogenic respects. Runyon's classification of these strains into four groups—photochromogens (for example, *Mycobacterium balnei*), scotochromogens, Battey strain, and rapid growers—is a workable one. Not all of the granulomas produced by these organisms have a tuberculoid structure histologically. Some appear quite nonspecific.

Sarcoidosis. The histologic diagnosis of Boeck's sarcoid is based on the finding of dermal hyperplastic tubercles, with or without giant cells and Schaumann's or asteroid bodies but in the absence of caseation. Usually the tubercules are surrounded by dense bands of collagenous stroma. No tubercle bacilli are detectable. The term *Darier-Roussy sarcoid* is reserved for an essentially similar histologic process occurring in the deep dermis and subcutaneous fat, thereby resembling erythema induratum. Confusion arises from the simulation of the tuberculous process by the tissue reaction in the tuberculoid form of leprosy, in the syphilitic gumma, and by the tissue response in blastomycosis, coccidioidomycosis, leishmaniasis, and sporotrichosis. Moreover, in some instances of sarcoid a form of fibrinoid degeneration simulating caseation may occur (p. 883).

A diagnostic test for sarcoidosis, called the Kveim test, consists of injecting intradermally a brei of tissue known to be involved with Boeck's sarcoid and observing the delayed clinical and tuberculoid histologic reaction to the injection several weeks later. Sarcoidosis is rare in children.

Berylliosis and brucellosis. The granulomas of berylliosis (usually acquired by inoculation of the beryllium phosphors from broken fluorescent lamps) and those of brucellosis may be histologically indistinguishable from those of sarcoidosis or tuberculosis. Silica granulomas are distinguished by the presence of birefringent silica crystals within giant cells. Zirconium in stick deodorants may also cause giant cell granulomas.

Other granulomas. The remainder of the granulomatous lesions, including those of leprosy, syphilis and other venereal diseases, the deep mycoses, and parasitic infestation, are discussed in other chapters.

PIGMENTATIONS

The abnormalities of cutaneous pigmentation may be considered under two principal categories: metallic and nonmetallic.

Metallic abnormalities of cutaneous pigmentation

The exogenous pigmentations are chiefly those from metals introduced into the body in a variety of ways, including ingestion, parenteral administration, inunction, and intradermal injection. In general, the metallic pigmentations provoke at least an increased deposition of melanin in the basal layer and in dermal chromatophores. The brown arsenic pigmentation caused particularly by the ingestion of trivalent arsenicals (in Fowler's solution, sodium cacodylate, or arsenic trioxide) often is associated with keratosis of the palms and soles. Histologically there is relative hyperkeratosis with atrophy of the remainder of the epidermis, hyperchromatism, and a tendency toward palisading of the basal cells and increased melanin deposits in these cells as well as in the chromatophores of the upper dermis, which usually is edematous. Late complications include Bowen's disease and squamous and basal cell carcinomas.

Argyria, in which the skin is discolored bluish gray, may occur after the ingestion of silver nitrate, formerly used in the treatment of peptic ulcers, or the application of this drug as well as colloidal silver compounds (Argyrol and Neo-Silvol) to mucous membranes. The pigmentation is particularly noticeable in areas of the skin exposed to light. The black granules of silver are noted especially in the argyrophilic basement membrane of the sweat glands but also in the connective tissue about sebaceous glands and hair follicles and just beneath the epidermis.

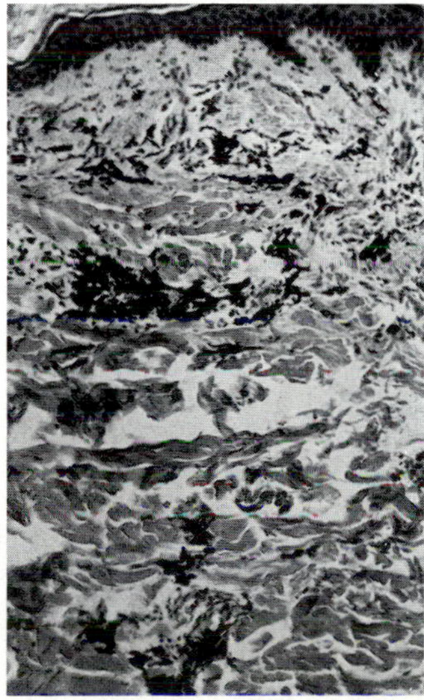

Fig. 38-28. Tattoo with irregular deposits of black-appearing pigment. (Hematoxylin and eosin.)

Chrysiasis, from the parenteral use of gold preparations, causes an ash-gray or mauve pigmentation characterized histologically by irregular, large granules located chiefly in chromatophores and in the walls of blood vessels. A somewhat similar histologic picture is caused by pigmentation from bismuth and mercury.

In tattoos the pigmentation is the result of the deposition of various metallic and vegetable pigments (such as cinnabar or red mercuric sulfide) both within chromatophores and extracellularly in irregularly large clumps sometimes surrounded by foreign body reaction (Fig. 38-28). Discoid lupus erythematosus may selectively involve the red areas of tattoos (mercuric sulfide) and spare the blue. Similarly, persons sensitive to mercury may show allergic reactions in the red portions. Conversely, syphilitic lesions may spare these mercury-impregnated red components of tattoos.

Nonmetallic abnormalities of cutaneous pigmentation

The nonmetallic abnormalities of cutaneous pigmentation include those attributable to hemochromatosis, Addison's disease, pellagra, Peutz-Jeghers syndrome, acanthosis nigricans, chloasma, melanosis of Riehl, ephelides (freckles), sunburn, purpuras, tinea versicolor, and pinta. Several of these entities illustrate once again the cutaneous reflection of visceral disease.

In hemochromatosis (bronze diabetes) hemosiderin and, less noticeably, hemofuscin are deposited as brownish granules in melanophores, principally and diagnostically about sweat glands. In addition there is increased melanin in the epidermis and adjacent chromatophores. This cutaneous lesion is commonly associated with deposits of the pigments in the pancreas, liver, and lymph nodes and the development of diabetes mellitus and cirrhosis of the liver. The mostly deeply pigmented areas are the exposed surfaces but may include also the genital regions and mucous membranes in 10% to 15% of cases.

In Wilson's disease (hepatolenticular degeneration) the pigmentation takes the form of epidermal melanosis favoring the anterior portions of the legs.

In Addison's disease there is an excessive deposit of melanin in the basal layer of the epidermis and in underlying melanophores. A similar histologic picture is found in the ordinary freckle (ephelis), sunburn, and chloasma (the latter especially during pregnancy).

Melanosis of Riehl, often associated with malnutrition, is characterized by brown macular discoloration of the face, neck, and occasionally hands. Histologically there is irregular pigmentation by melanin of the basal layer and chromatophores, in addition to telangiectasis, varying degrees of hyperkeratosis, liquefaction degeneration of the basal layer, and partial obliteration of the rete ridges. a similar picture is seen in tar melanosis, an occupational dermatosis probably concerned with photosensitization.

The Peutz-Jeghers syndrome consists of melanosis of the lips, oral mucosa, and digits in patients with gastrointestinal polyposis and occasional carcinomas.

The association of dermatoses with intestinal disorders is a facet of dermatology that is as intriguing as it is puzzling. A partial list of such dermatoses includes, in addition to the Peutz-Jeghers syndrome, acrodermatitis enteropathica, dermatitis herpetiformis, Fabry's disease, and pyoderma gangrenosum (with idiopathic ulcerative colitis), systemic lupus erythematosus, and systemic sclerosis. In some of the diseases the nature of the relationship is clear but variable for obvious reasons; in others the connection is enigmatic.

Increased pigmentation of the skin follows a variety of cutaneous purpuras: purpura annularis telangiectodes (Majocchi's disease), Schamberg's disease, and pigmented purpuric lichenoid dermatitis of Gougerot and Blum. Each of these disorders occurs selectively on the lower extremities. The pigment in these cases is hemosiderin, which is deposited in chromatophores in the upper dermis. Angioma serpiginosum, which is also rather loosely included in the category of cutaneous purpuras, is really an inflammatory telangiectasia and usually shows little or no hemosiderin. In all of these purpuras, which are unassociated with systemic disorders, there are inflammatory cells (principally lymphocytes and histiocytes) localized in the upper dermis, especially about arterioles and capillaries, which may have swollen, prominent endothelium. This latter finding is particularly true of Majocchi's disease. There is some question as to whether these conditions are actually different phases of the same basic vascular disease. Occasionally these purpuric lesions, particularly those of Majocchi's disease, may be confused histologically with the vascular changes of polyteritis nodosa or bacterial and rickettsial arteritis. The changes of thrombophlebitis migrans and of thromboangiitis obliterans are discussed elsewhere (pp. 705 and 716).

Achromia should be mentioned among the abnormalities of cutaneous pigmentation. The congenital absence of pigment is referred to as partial or complete albinism or leukoderma. Vitiligo or acquired leukoderma is usually of unknown etiology. The depigmented patches may be rimmed by hyperpigmented borders, and the histologic sections reveal the depigmented and hyperpigmented basal layers in the respective portions. Vitiliginous areas may occur also in any lesion in which there are considerable liquefaction degeneration of the basal layer and encroachment onto this layer by inflammatory cells. Pinta and lichen planus are cases in point. In both the melanin is extracted from the basal layer, phagocytosed by chromatophores, and carried away to regional lymph nodes. Vitiliginous patches occur in patients with tinea versicolor, partly because the areas affected by the fungus prevent absorption of ultraviolet irradiation and partly because the fungus itself actively causes a degree of depigmentation. In skin that has been planed for scars of acne there is a tendency for the unabraded skin to become hyperpigmented and for the abraded epidermis to regenerate with less pigmentation than the original.

DISEASES OF APPENDAGES

Limitations of space permit no more than a brief mention of the nonneoplastic diseases of the cutaneous appendages.

Sweat glands

The disorders of the sweat glands include hyperhidrosis, congenital or acquired hypohidrosis, miliaria (prickly heat and tropical or thermogenic hypohidrosis with plugging of the sweat ducts by hydropic edematous epithelium), bromhidrosis (fetid sweat), chromhidrosis (colored sweat), hidradenitis suppurativa of the apocrine glands, and Fox-Fordyce disease (pruritic papular chronic adenitis of the sweat glands of the axillae, nipples, and pubic and perineal regions).

Sebaceous glands

The diseases of the sebaceous glands include varieties of seborrhea, hyposteatosis or diminished secretion, comedones, acne in its several forms, and rhinophyma.

Hair

The abnormal conditions of the hair are many. Hypertrichosis, the alopecias of the cicatricial types (pseudopelade, folliculitis decalvans, and chronic lupus erythematosus of the scalp) and the noncicatricial types (alopecia

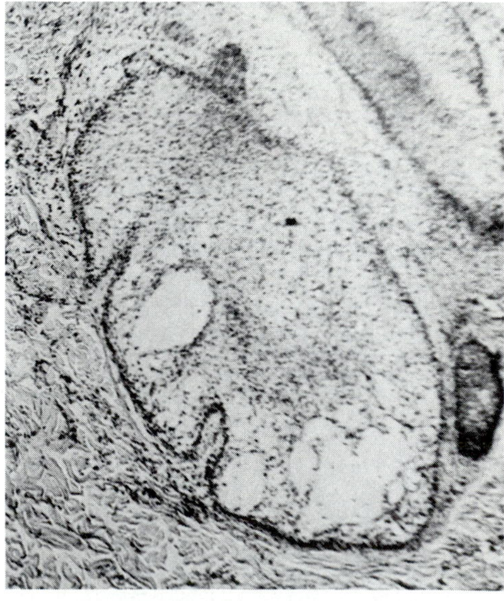

Fig. 38-29. Follicular mucinosis from patient with mycosis fungoides. (Hematoxylin and eosin.)

areata, ordinary male baldness, fungal infections), fragile hairs (fragilitas crinium), trichorrhexis nodosa, pili torti (twisted hairs), fungal infections such as piedra and trichomycosis nodosa, and trichostasis spinulosa (multiple lanugo hairs in a single follicle) constitute a few of the problems.

One of the more interesting disorders of hair follicles is alopecia mucinosa or follicular mucinosis (Fig. 38-29). Histologically it is characterized initially by intracellular and subsequently extracellular mucin within the hair sheaths, perifollicular inflammatory cells, and loss of hair shafts. The mucin stains with Alcian blue and is periodic acid–Schiff negative. The significant fact concerning this lesion is that in persons over 40 years of age it is strong presumptive evidence of the early stage of mycosis fungoides.[6,9]

Nails

The diseases of the nails are of particular interest not only for the involvement of the nails themselves but for the accessory information they reflect on systemic disorders. Beau's lines are transverse furrows in the nail that date periods of arrested function of the matrix resulting from severe acute illnesses or inflammations near the nail folds.

The discoloration and the thickening of the nail from psoriasis, eczema, or fungi; the spoon nails (koilonychia) associated with trauma, eczema, and the Plummer-Vinson syndrome; the brittleness (onychorrhexis) after the use of certain chemicals or in vitamin A deficiency; the loss of nails (onycholysis) after trauma or systemic diseases such as hypothyroidism; and the whitening of nails (leukonychia) are some of the possible changes.

The yellow nail syndrome is associated with lymphedema and pleural effusions and at times with ascites. The nails not only are discolored yellow but show transverse ridging, onycholysis, curving, and defective cuticles.

PANNICULITIS

Several diseases of the subcutaneous fat closely simulate each other histologically but have different prognostic and etiologic implications.

Erythema induratum

Erythema induratum appears as chronic, recurring, often ulcerated, bluish red nodules (of the calves of the legs particularly). The lesions generally are found in patients with frank tuberculosis elsewhere. Histologically tubercles, usually of an incomplete or atypical variety, are found in the subcutaneous fat. Caseation may be present. Fat necrosis and fat atrophy associated with nonspecific inflammation of the fibrous septa, fat, and lower dermis are present. Endarterial and endophlebitic inflammation and proliferation are seen commonly. Tubercle bacilli are rarely found in these lesions, although positive results have been reported from guinea pig inoculation of the tissue.

Subacute nodular migratory panniculitis

Subacute nodular migratory panniculitis, which may follow acute infections such as tonsillitis, appears similar to erythema induratum histologically.

Nodular, nonsuppurative, febrile, relapsing panniculitis (Weber-Christian disease)

Nodular, nonsuppurative, febrile, relapsing panniculitis is observed preponderantly in women and is characterized by bluish discoloration of the skin over firm subcutaneous nodules on the extremities and trunk, usually associated with otherwise unexplained fever. Isolated cases have responded to chemotherapy (sulfapyridine and penicillin). Fatalities have occurred in several cases, but autopsy findings were not especially enlightening except for the steatitis in the pretracheal, mediastinal, and retroperitoneal regions. The recently recorded instances of mesenteric panniculitis appear unrelated.

In sections from patients with what are regarded as typical cases, the fat itself is infiltrated chiefly with lymphocytes and histiocytes, but the septa are relatively spared. Wucher atrophy of fat (replacement of atrophied fat by fat-laden histiocytes), foreign body giant cell reaction, and endophlebitis and endarteritis are also present. However, the septa, although relatively spared, often are infiltrated and edematous. Therefore the involvement of the septa cannot be used as a criterion for excluding the possibility of Weber-Christian disease. If they are free, the evidence is considerable that the panniculitis belongs to this category.

Although "nonsuppurative" is included in the name of the entity, the fact is that sterile abscesses occasionally are noted along with cystic liquefaction necrosis and focal calcification. It has been suggested that Weber-Christian disease is of diverse etiology and in some instances is attributable to pancreatitis.

Erythema nodosum

Erythema nodosum occurs clinically as tender, pale red to livid blue nodules, principally on the anterior aspect of the lower extremities. These lesions, unlike those of erythema induratum, do not ulcerate, are transient, lasting only for several weeks on an average, and are not necessarily associated with a tuberculous process elsewhere. The disease may be one manifestation of a variety of unrelated infections, including coccidioidomycosis, leprosy, syphilis, viral diseases (measles, cat-scratch fever), and ringworm, or it may follow lymphomas, the ingestion of drugs, or the administration of a vaccine.

The histologic picture of erythema nodosum is much like that of erythema induratum with the addition that there is a greater tendency in erythema nodosum for nonspecific inflammation of the middle and lower dermis, which is usually spared in erythema induratum.

Nodular vasculitis

Nodular vasculitis occurs chiefly in older women and refers to the often recurrent nodosities that are more painful, are of shorter duration, and have less tendency to ulcerate than the lesions of erythema induratum. The histologic picture of nodular vasculitis is the same as that of Bazin's disease.

Erythema pernio

Erythema pernio occurs usually on the hands and feet as tender, red, pruritic macules provoked by cold. The histologic picture may closely simulate that of erythema induratum, as may the lesions produced in response to cold allergy.

Miscellaneous forms

Miscellaneous forms of panniculitis include those resulting from trauma, insulin injections, pancreatitis, allergic reactions (including those occurring after insect bites), angiitis, cold agglutinins, and sclerosing lipogranulomas.

Actually the sharp artificial segregation of the panniculitides characteristic of the bulk of the dermatologic literature appears unwarranted by the histologic evidence of transitional merging of supposedly definitive criteria. This statement of confluence of diagnosis applies particularly to acute and chronic erythema nodosum, erythema nodosum migrans, nodular vasculitis, and often erythema induratum. This is so because tuberculoid or foreign body type of granulomas, phlebitis and arteritis, involvement or lack of involvement of septa or lobules, and the presence of microabscesses may characterize any of these entities. Otherwise, it is the weight given to one or other features, integrated with the clinical details, that leads to more informative diagnoses.

VASCULAR DISORDERS

There is a broad spectrum of vascular disorders in which the skin plays a prominent clinical, and at times diagnostic, role. A few of these are mentioned in Chapter 18. Additional ones, with probable or clear-cut vascular involvement, include the cutaneous lesions of rheumatic fever, subacute bacterial endocarditis, typhus fevers and other infections, Degos' syndrome, allergenic vasculitides, necrobiosis lipoidica diabeticorum, the vascular changes of diabetes mellitus and hypertension, granuloma annulare, rheumatoid granuloma, Mucha-Habermann disease, urticaria, and the purpuric dermatoses.

Acute, often necrotizing arteriolitis with karyorrhexis of polymorphonuclear neutrophil leukocytes (leukocytoclasis), deposition of immune complexes, hypocomplementemia, cryoglobulinemia, and arthralgia have been linked as a syndrome. Immunoglobulins and complement were demonstrable in the vessels of the skin before the infiltration of leukocytes and the development of clinical lesions.[54] Moreover, IgA has been demonstrated in the acutely inflamed dermal arterioles in purpuric hyperglobulinemia of Waldenström. This local finding was associated with elevated circulating levels of IgA and suggests the immunologic pathogenesis.

Immunofluorescence studies of dermal vasculitis promise diagnostic and pathogenic clues. At present IgG, IgM, IgA, and several components of complement have been demonstrated in and about vessels (for example, in Henoch-Schönlein purpura), but their full significance remains to be determined.

Angiolymphoid hyperplasia with eosinophilia (Kimura's disease)

The lesion termed angiolymphoid hyperplasia with eosinophilia usually starts as a papule or a cluster of papules in the skin of the head and neck of adults. This lesion is as extraordinary in its behavior as it is in its histologic features. On occasion the lesions may recur after excision or may spread uncontrollably to cover much of the face in the manner of a fulminant angiosarcoma. Histologically the characteristic features include dilated dermal thin-walled vascular sprouts with conspicuously hypertrophic, practically diagnostic endothelial cells with vesicular nuclei and abundant eosinophilic cytoplasm (Fig. 38-30). Often the endothelial cells appear clustered beside or at one end of a vessel that has been cut obliquely and in this pattern simulate masses of histiocytes. The stroma also is characteristically structured with loosely disposed eosinophilic leukocytes, histiocytes, lymphocytes, and mast cells. These cells are strongly positive for adenosine triphosphatase, indoxyl esterase, and nicotinamide adenine dinucleotide and negative for alkaline phosphatase, a pattern characteristic of endothelial cells.[16]

A form of superficial, subcutaneous thrombophlebitis known as Mondor's disease is characterized clinically by a linear, cordlike induration with an overlying cutaneous groove extending usually from the axilla toward the nipple. The lesion may be mistaken for a neoplasm clinically.

Thrombocytopenic verrucal angionecrosis (thrombotic thrombocytopenic purpura, TTP)

Of great interest is another truly diffuse vascular disease characterized by thrombocytopenia, purpura, a usually fulminant, fatal course (although rare protracted cases have occurred), and a specific histologic picture of fibrinoid necrosis and platelet-like verrucal thickening of the walls of dilated arterioles and capillaries. In the past

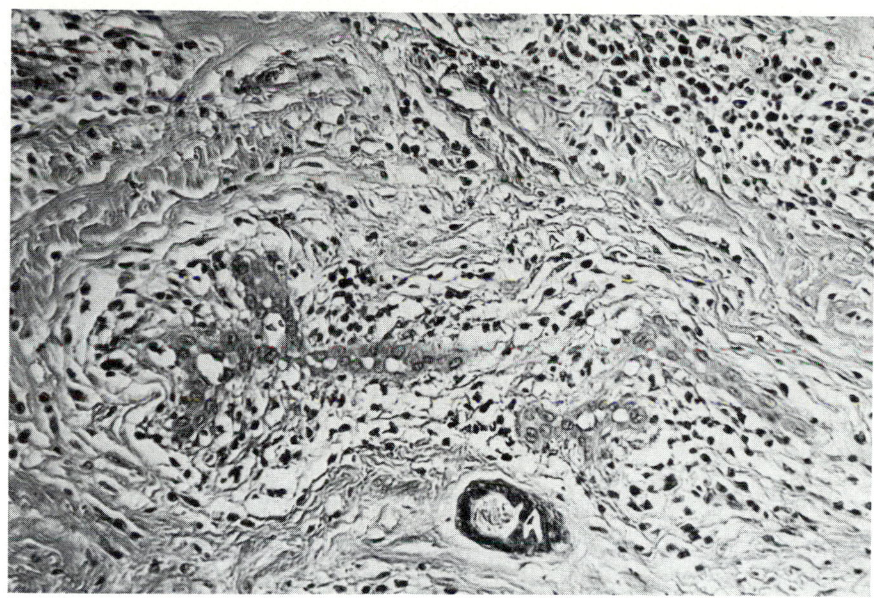

Fig. 38-30. Angiolymphoid hyperplasia with eosinophilia (Kimura's disease). Prominence of endothelium is evident. (Hematoxylin and eosin.)

the disease has been called generalized platelet thrombosis or some variant of this term. However, the histogenesis of the entire lesion from the vascular walls would seem to make the designation *thrombocytopenic verrucal angionecrosis*[4,6,9] more appropriate, as was long ago suggested. These cases are rarely diagnosed clinically. Inasmuch as the vascular necrosis occurs in the skin as well as the viscera, a skin, mucosal, marrow, or muscle biopsy is called for in obscure instances of thrombocytopenic purpura. There is strongly suggestive clinical and histologic evidence of a factor of hypersensitivity in this primarily diffuse vascular disease. Accordingly, it should be attributed to an allergic response rather than to depletion by so-called generalized thrombosis, which, as already indicated and despite certain immunofluorescence studies, does not occur.

In the syndrome called disseminated intravascular coagulation (DIC) the coagulating factors normally residing in the blood are assumed to be depleted by universally distributed clots in small vessels. The widespread presence of such clots has simply not been documented.

XANTHOSES

The xanthoses may be classified as follows:

1. Normolipemic
   a. Juvenile xanthoma (or xanthogranuloma)
   b. Xanthoma disseminatum
2. Hyperlipemic
   a. Xanthoma diabeticorum
   b. Xanthoma tuberosum multiplex (Fig. 38-31)
   c. Xanthoma eruptiva (in association with lipid nephrosis, von Gierke's disease, diabetes mellitus, biliary cirrhosis, hypothyroidism, idiopathic hyperlipemia)
   d. Xanthelasma (approximately 50% with hyperlipemia) (Fig. 38-32)
   e. Xanthoma planum (approximately 50% with hyperlipemia) (in association with biliary cirrhosis, diabetes mellitus, myeloma, and other dysproteinemias)

Other dermatoses characterized by the presence of lipid include lipid proteinosis, angiokeratoma of Fabry, necrobiosis lipoidica diabeticorum, lipid dermatoarthritis (reticulohistiocytoma), Hand-Schüller-Christian disease, and Neimann-Pick disease. These are described elsewhere in this book.

Many of the lesions included in this classification are often classified with neoplasms. Actually, none is really a neoplasm in the usual sense of neoplasia. Most are obviously a reflection of disordered metabolism of lipids or lipoproteins, but it would constitute no major contribution to discard the term *xanthoma*. The differentiation of these various xanthoses is often important from the prognostic and therapeutic viewpoints, although in many instances the distinction cannot be made on the basis of histology alone. Moreover, several of these types of lesions often are combined in the same patient.

RETICULOHISTIOCYTOMA (RETICULOHISTIOCYTIC GRANULOMA)

The entity *reticulohistiocytoma*, which was so named in 1948, produces remarkable lesions, the extent and nature of which are still being investigated.[2,4,6,9] Because of the association with arthritis, it has more

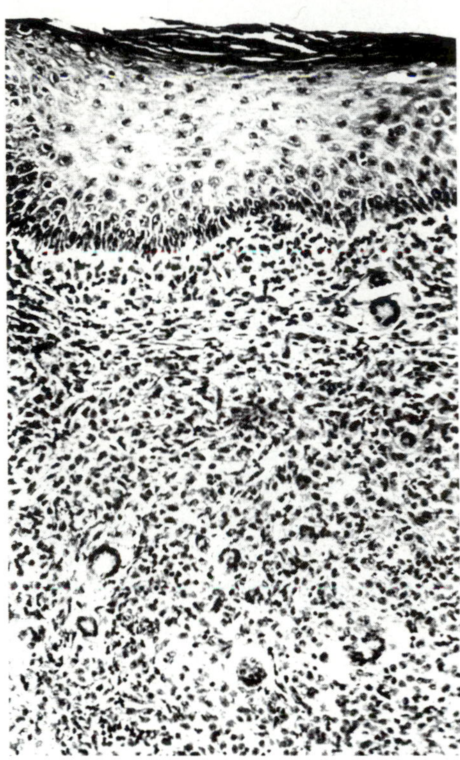

Fig. 38-31. Xanthoma tuberosum with numerous lipid histiocytes, some of which are congregated as Touton giant cells. (Hematoxylin and eosin.)

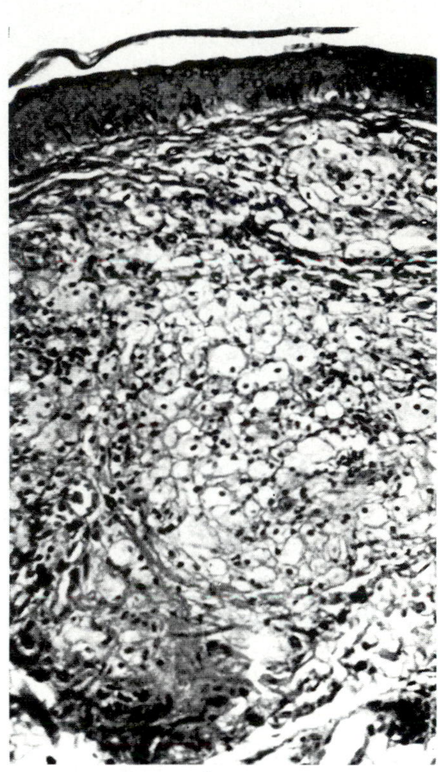

Fig. 38-32. Xanthelasma of eyelid with lipid-filled histiocytes. (Hematoxylin and eosin.)

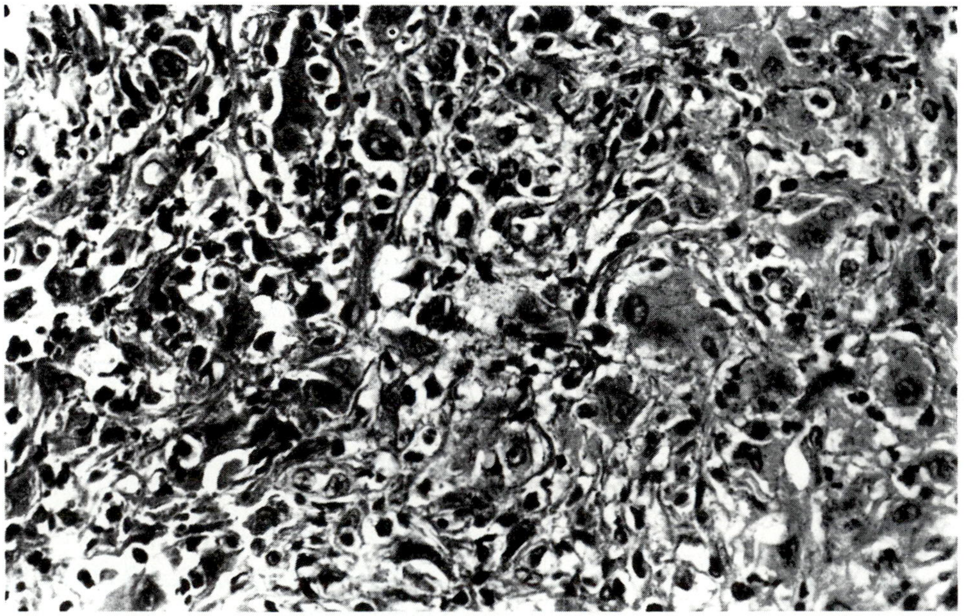

Fig. 38-33. Reticulohistiocytoma, illustrating histiocytes with abundant homogeneous cytoplasm loosely admixed with few lymphocytes and eosinophilic leukocytes. (Hematoxylin and eosin.)

recently been designated lipid dermatoarthritis. Originally this condition was believed to be limited to the skin and was regarded as a form of ganglioneuroma because of the superficial simulation of ganglion cells by the histiocytes.

Clinically the disease is characterized by cutaneous papules and nodules (rarely solitary) and often by an associated disabling polyarthritis. The nodules may resemble xanthomas, and indeed xanthelasma is present in about one fourth of the patients.

Histologically the cutaneous lesions are characterized by histiocytes with abundant basophilic cytoplasm intermingled with lymphocytes and occasionally scattered eosinophilic leukocytes (Fig. 38-33). The infiltrate tends to be confined to the upper dermis, with resulting moderate atrophy of the overlying epidermis. The cytoplasm of the histiocytes reacts positively with Sudan black B and periodic acid–Schiff stains and is presumed to contain a glycolipid.

ANGIOLIPOMA

There are two types of angiolipomas: (1) noninfiltrating or encapsulated and (2) infiltrating. In both there is likely to be associated pain or tenderness. The infiltrating angiolipomas tend to occur on the extremities and to ramify into the skeletal muscle. They may occur also in the spinal region and cause erosion of portions of vertebrae with resulting neurologic problems. Unlike liposarcomas, the infiltrating angiolipomas lack atypia of the fat cells. Fibrolipomas of infancy commonly show deceptive atypia.

ATYPICAL FIBROXANTHOMA

There has been considerable interest in the past few years in an ulceronodular lesion of the exposed skin (chiefly the ears and cheeks) of elderly people. The lesion has been called atypical fibroxanthoma and resembles an anaplastic sarcoma with spindle cells and multinucleated giant cells, as well as bizarre cells with single, large hyperchromatic nuclei, mitoses (often abnormal tripolar), and some intracellular lipid. The striking feature is the disparity between the histologic anaplasia and the benign course in most instances. Some of these are undoubtedly nonpigmented spindle cell melanocarcinomas. Fat may be present in melanocarcinomas.[6,9]

Although these lesions were originally considered benign, instances of metastasis are accumulating. Undoubtedly more such instances will follow and, in my judgment, for the reason that they represent either spindle cell epidermoid carcinomas or malignant melanomas. The origin from the overlying epidermis may be easily missed because this pivotal evidence is often obscure or minimal in spindle cell epidermoid carcinomas and melanocarcinomas of the ear.

NEOPLASMS OF SKIN

The following classification of neoplasms of the skin is based on the segregation of cutaneous neoplasms with respect to their location and histogenesis from epidermis, dermis and appendages. In the ensuing discussion several of the lesions are taken out of the order of the outline for purposes of clarity of presentation.

- I. Epidermis
  - A. Benign
    - 1. Verruca (including vulgaris, digitata, filiformis, plantaris, and juvenilis)
    - 2. Seborrheic keratosis
    - 3. Condyloma acuminatum
    - 4. Keratoacanthoma
    - 5. Junctional nevus
  - B. Precancerous
    - 1. Senile keratosis
    - 2. Leukoplakia (with atypia)
    - 3. Xeroderma pigmentosum
    - 4. Bowen's disease
    - 5. Erythroplasia of Queyrat
  - C. Malignant
    - 1. Basal cell carcinoma
    - 2. Squamous cell carcinoma
    - 3. Melanocarcinoma (malignant melanoma)
- II. Dermis
  - A. Nevus
    - 1. Intradermal nevus (common mole)
    - 2. Compound nevus (dermis and epidermis)
    - 3. Juvenile melanoma (dermis and epidermis)
    - 4. Blue nevus (Jadassohn-Tièche)
  - B. Tumors of vessels
    - 1. Lymphangioma
    - 2. Hemangioma
    - 3. Angiokeratoma (dermis and epidermis)
    - 4. Glomus tumor
    - 5. Hemangiopericytoma
    - 6. Kaposi's idiopathic hemorrhagic sarcoma
    - 7. Postmastectomy lymphangiosarcoma
    - 8. Sclerosing hemangioma (dermatofibroma lenticulare)
    - 9. Dermatofibrosarcoma protuberans
    - 10. Angiosarcoma
  - C. Fibroma and fibrosarcoma
  - D. Neurofibroma and neurofibrosarcoma
  - E. Tumors of muscle
    - 1. Leiomyoma (arrectores pilorum)
    - 2. Angiomyoma
    - 3. Myoblastoma (genesis?)
  - F. Osteoma
  - G. Xanthomas (discussed in previous section)
  - H. Lymphomas and allied diseases
  - I. Metastatic neoplasms
- III. Appendages
  - A. Sweat glands
    - 1. Adenoma or epithelioma
      - a. Ductal
      - b. Glandular
    - 2. Carcinoma

B. Sebaceous glands
   1. Adenoma
   2. Carcinoma
C. Hair follicles
   1. Brooke's tumor—trichoepithelioma or epithelioma adenoides cysticum
D. Miscellaneous cysts
   1. Dermoid
   2. Epidermoid
   3. Pilosebaceous
   4. Calcifying epithelioma (pilomatrixoma)

Benign lesions of epidermis

Verruca (wart)

The verrucae, or warts, represent thickenings or projections of epidermis to which are traditionally, if inconsistently, applied one of several adjectives in accordance with the shape, location, or other clinical feature of the lesion: verruca vulgaris, verruca plantaris, verruca digitata, verruca filiformis, verruca plana juvenilis, and verruca senilis.

The verruca vulgaris is the papillary wart common in children and found especially on the fingers, palms, and forearms. They occur singly or in groups. There is some question as to whether these tumors merit inclusion under neoplasms, inasmuch as they may disappear spontaneously or, as in some reported cases, under psychotherapy or with placebos. The possibility that these lesions are caused by viruses is still strongly considered and fortified by evidence from electron microscopy of viral particles. Wart-virus antibodies, measured by immunodiffusion and complement-fixation techniques, are detectable in a high percentage of cases. The warts associated with complement-fixing antibodies seem to disappear more quickly than those with antibodies determined by immunodiffusion techniques. The titers of such antibodies as well as the effects of cell-mediated immunity may be factors in the "spontaneous" regression of warts. The prevention and resolution of warts have been attributed also to cell-mediated immunity.[55]

Butchers' warts are infected with several kinds of papilloma viruses associated with somewhat varying histologic pictures.

Histologically the verruca vulgaris is characterized by a papillary acanthosis surmounted by friable keratotic material. The cells of the stratum granulosum are often acidophilic and vacuolated. The basophilic intranuclear inclusions of the verrucae are related to the viral particles rather than the osmophilic intranuclear eosinophilic material, which is related to keratin. A loose infiltration of various mononuclear cells may be present in the papillae. Carcinomatous transformation of these lesions occurs rarely, if ever, although occasionally a verrucal form of senile keratosis or a squamous cell carcinoma with a prominent papillary hyperkeratotic surface is erroneously regarded as having arisen from a verruca vulgaris.

Oral florid papillomatosis comprises benign condylomatoid verrucal masses covering large portions of the buccal mucosa. These presumably are of viral origin.

An oral and genital lesion histologically similar to condyloma occurs with the entity called dyskeratosis congenita, which may be associated with a variety of ectodermal and mesodermal changes, including hyperpigmentation of the skin, reticulated poikilodermatous changes, dystrophic nails, deforming atrophic arthritic changes, dental dystrophies, cardiovascular changes, testicular atrophy, and hyperplenism.

Seborrheic keratosis

The seborrheic keratosis is labeled also verruca senilis or pigmented papilloma. The term "verruca senilis" is not well chosen because the lesions often appear in young people and acanthosis is the feature of note. "Seborrheic keratosis" is used by the dermatologists and emphasizes the greasy feeling to the touch imparted by the abundant fatty keratinous nests within the lesion. These lesions occur particularly on the trunk and forehead and are usually dark brown, elevated, and sharply delimited. The sudden appearance of seborrheic keratoses, along with rapid increase in their size and number, may herald the presence of a visceral carcinoma, usually an adenocarcinoma. This phenomenon is known as the sign of Leser-Trélat.

The histologic picture is that of abruptly thickened epidermis that encloses nests of laminated keratin resulting from focal, irregular maturation of epidermis partially inverted within the core of the lesion. In places the central pearls are incompletely developed and present large mature squamous cells without the keratinous nests (Fig. 38-34). The surrounding cells are usually focally pigmented with fine brown granules of melanin and superficially resemble basal cells. However, close examination often reveals residual intercellular bridges that help identify them as squamous cells, despite statements to the contrary. Many of these epithelial cells are dopa positive. In my judgment the pigment is produced by the tumor cells (that is, the keratinocytes). Others assume, on evidence not easily acceptable, that the pigment is inoculated into the tumor cells by nonneoplastic melanocytes carried along with the tumor. This same judgment applies to the condylomatous, so-called melanoacanthoma. Rare cases of malignant transformation of the seborrheic keratosis have been recorded.[6,9,10] These have included basal cell carcinomas and malignant melanomas. Of interest is the high concentration of zinc in seborrheic keratoses.

A lesion that has many of the cellular characteristics of the verruca pigmentosum is the so-called inverted papilloma, which grows downward rather than outward from the epidermal surface. The inverted papilloma often is associated with an inflammatory reaction of mononuclear cells at its base, much as are the senile karatoses. The

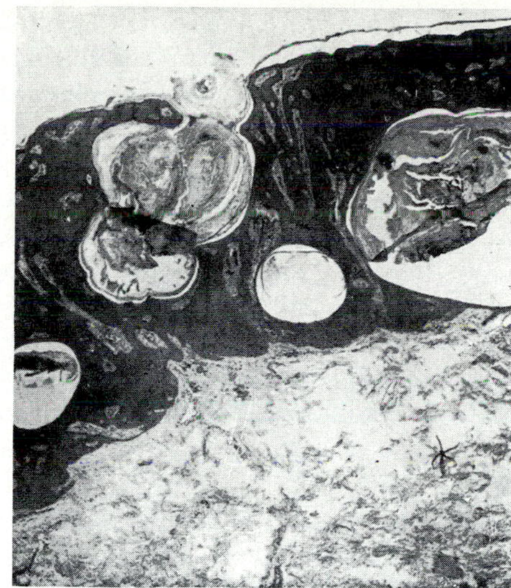

Fig. 38-34. Seborrheic keratosis. (Hematoxylin and eosin.)

lesion referred to as eccrine porothelioma or acrosyringoma closely resembles the earliest stage of seborrheic keratosis. The Degos' or clear cell acanthoma also is reminiscent of an initial stage in the development of seborrheic keratosis. Glycogen is present in the clear cells.

A disorder of keratinization, disseminated spiked hyperkeratosis, consists of bland, nonfollicular, nonviral keratosis with minimal underlying acanthosis.[31]

As with the generally benign seborrheic keratosis, other lesions such as linear epidermal nevi and eccrine poromas rarely may lead to basal or squamous cell carcinomas.

Keratoacanthoma

The problem of pseudoepitheliomatous hyperplasia is directly related to the histologically difficult subject of so-called self-healing squamous cell carcinomas, also more or less equivalently labeled molluscum sebaceum and molluscum pseudocarcinomatosum. Most commonly these occur in elderly men, although even adolescents may be affected, especially if there has been contact with oils. The lesions appear as single or multiple nodules that are smooth except for the characteristic umbilication of the central keratin. The nodules often regress spontaneously in about 2 months, leaving little or no scar. Recurrences have been recorded.

Histologically, as already implied, the nodules are not really carcinomas but rather are coalescent comedones or keratinous masses with prominent pseudoepitheliomatous hyperplasia at their bases (Fig. 38-35). Giant keratoacanthomas may become incredibly large, particularly on the face, and may recur after incomplete excision. The well-differentiated, keratoacanthomatous pattern in the rapid recurrence supports the original diagnosis, although considerable self-confidence may be required

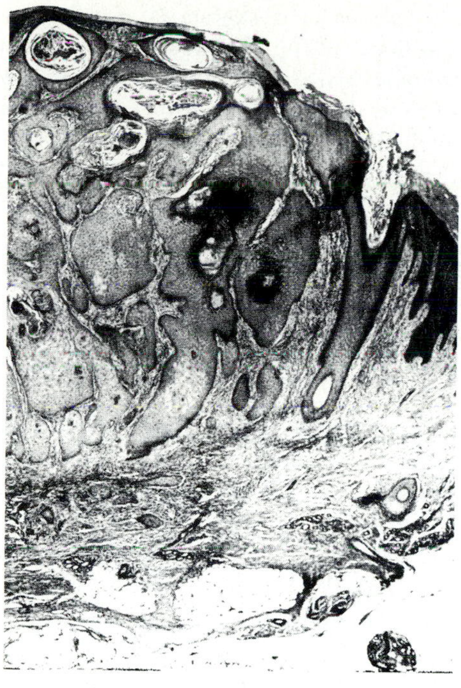

Fig. 38-35. Keratoacanthoma simulating squamous cell carcinoma. (Hematoxylin and eosin.)

to maintain it. An important clue is the absence of significant atypia in the epidermis at the margins of the keratoacanthomas. Perineural involvement in keratoacanthomas has been noted without corresponding evidence of malignant biologic behavior.[44]

Despite the occasional recurrences after incomplete removal, these lesions are benign. The attention that has been focused on keratoacanthomas has perforce led to misdiagnosis of squamous cell carcinomas as keratoacanthomas. An analogous problem exists in the erroneous diagnosis of melanocarcinomas as juvenile melanomas.

A variety of the lesion has been designated generalized eruptive keratoacanthoma. These may be so numerous as to cover most of the body and involve even the oral mucosa.

It is becoming obvious from reports in the literature that prior confidence is being replaced by considerable uncertainty regarding the differential diagnosis between keratoacanthoma and verrucal, keratinizing squamous cell carcinoma. This diagnostic difficulty is expressed in both directions, that is, unnecessarily radical surgical operations for giant keratoacanthomas, including leg amputation, and injudiciously delayed therapy for squamous cell carcinomas mistaken for keratoacanthomas.

Precancerous lesions

The precancerous lesions of the skin include senile keratosis, Bowen's disease, erythroplasia of Queyrat, and the active junctional nevus. Each of these entities is characterized by atypia or dyskeratosis of cells that is confined to the limits of the epidermis. To such lesions the term *carcinoma in situ* is often applied. *Precancerous* as applied to these lesions connotes, in a crude measure, the relatively high probability that they will undergo malignant degeneration rather than the inevitability of such a complication. Kraurosis vulvae, a term that has become unpopular in recent years, had been used diversely either in place of vulval lichen sclerosis et atrophicus, on the one hand, or as equivalent to epidermoid carcinoma in situ on the other.

Senile keratosis

The senile keratoses are irregular brownish patches of epidermis roughened by horny scales, occurring characteristically on the dorsa of the hands of aged people. Histologically similar lesions may occur after irradiation and exposure to arsenic or to the elements of the weather. They may be single or several, or they may occur in great numbers over many parts of the body.

Microscopically they are characterized chiefly by dyskeratosis of the cells of the basal layer and adjacent layers of the rete Malpighi. These cells show hyperchromatism, loss of polarity, increased numbers of mitotic figures, and irregularity of size and shape of nuclei. Hyperkeratosis and parakeratosis of varying degrees are responsible for the roughened surface. Inflammatory cells, principally mononuclear, are present in the subepidermal tissue. These cells often encroach onto the epidermis, obscuring the integrity of the basement membrane and occasionally prompting the premature and erroneous diagnosis of infiltrating carcinoma. The cutaneous horn in many instances represents a senile keratosis with an accumulation of keratinous material in the form of a projecting spur. The same type of horny projection may be superimposed also on verrucae.

Leukoplakia

Leukoplakia is a term that merits discussion of its usage. As applied clinically, or grossly, it refers to whitish patches of mucosa that encompass not only cancerous or precancerous foci, but also those benign patches of mucosa thickened and whitened by mycoses, lichen planus, reaction to dentures, and smoking. Nevertheless, to many (probably most) surgeons and pathologists, leukoplakia connotes a carcinoma in situ or a lesion morphologically approaching an intraepithelial carcinoma. The difficulty is that the diagnosis often is rendered as merely leukoplakia when the pathologist is not certain whether there is sufficient atypia to warrant a designation of leukokeratosis or of carcinoma in situ. This is the situation with lesions of the cervix, when the diagnosis is hedged with such terms as basal cell hyperplasia or dyskaryosis—to the bewilderment of the clinician. Surely there are instances in which the pathologist may not be certain of the malignant potential of such a whitish patch, but it would appear more informative if this uncertainty were indicated rather than concealed euphemistically.

Xeroderma pigmentosum

Xeroderma pigmentosum is a potentially cancerous familial disease of the skin, usually first manifested early in childhood. It is characterized clinically by areas of atrophy, as well as isolated and coalescent scaly patches of keratosis showing varying amounts of pigmentation. A hyper-alpha-2-globulinemia has been found consistently in patients with xeroderma pigmentosum, and it has been hypothesized that this abnormality is related to ceruloplasmin.

Histologically the changes in xeroderma pigmentosum are those of irregular atrophy, acanthosis, and hyperkeratosis, with excessive deposits of melanin in the basal layer and lowermost layers of the stratum spinosum, as well as in chromatophores in the upper dermis. Xeroderma pigmentosum may be complicated by junctional nevi, basal cell or squamous cell carcinomas, and melanocarcinomas.

The diagnosis of xeroderma pigmentosum may be established even before the characteristic cutaneous lesions appear, by estimation of the deoxyribonucleic acid excision repair level in cutaneous fibroblasts (after irradiation by ultraviolet light).[57] This defect in repair of DNA damaged by ultraviolet light has been detected prenatally by the use of amniotic cells cultured in vitro.[57]

Bowen's disease

Bowen's disease occurs as irregular, scaly, slowly progressive, usually brownish patches on the trunk, buttocks, and extremities. It was estimated that evidence of visceral cancer develops in approximately one third of patients within 6 to 10 years after the initial diagnosis of Bowen's disease. Here again, what was regarded as a proven relationship a few years ago must now be considered moot on the basis of more recent analyses.[12]

Microscopically the principal feature of the lesions is the presence of isolated dyskeratotic cells scattered haphazardly in all layers of the epidermis. These cells often have large, hyperchromatic single or double nuclei surrounded by cytoplasmic halos. Mitotic figures are numerous in these altered cells. Hyperkeratosis or parakeratosis may be pronounced. The acanthosis is usually uniform, but irregular thickening may be present.

Electron microscopic study of the dyskeratotic cells discloses displaced cytoplasmic fascicular aggregations of tonofilaments and separation of the desmosomal-tonofilament attachments. This desmosomal-tonafilament dissociation would be anticipated not only from the acantholytic appearance of Bowen's cells as seen under light microscopy, but also from the ultrastructural studies of acantholytic cells in other lesions such as Darier's disease and pemphigus vulgaris.[17] In my judgment, as previously stated, a basically similar retraction of tonofilaments and loss of desmosomes occur in the conversion of keratinocytes to neval and melanocarcinomatous cells.

Erythroplasia of Queyrat

Erythroplasia of Queyrat is the precancerous lesion occurring principally on the glans penis but also on the vulva and on oral mucous membranes.[35] In addition, the acanthotic thickening associated with erythroplasia is often characterized by long rete ridges that are psoriasiform or attached to each other in a reticulated pattern. A cytologic pattern somewhat similar to that of Bowen's disease occurs in the nipple and adjacent areas of the female breast on Paget's disease. However, unlike the lesions just described, Paget's disease is associated with carcinoma of the underlying mammary ducts. As indicated elsewhere, I find the evidence for the conclusion that so-called extramammary Paget's disease is associated with underlying adenocarcinoma of apocrine or eccrine glands somewhat less than convincing.[6,9] The majority of such lesions are pagetoid melanocarcinomas. The small group of remaining lesions includes epidermoid carcinomas and metastatic mucin-producing carcinomas, principally from the bowel and occasionally from other organs such as the ovaries.[9]

The much emphasized presence of mucopolysaccharides within epidermal cells hardly precludes the possibility that they are keratinocytes. Among several kinds of evidence is the clear fact that under the influence of an excess of vitamin A, keratinocytes are modulated into mucus-secreting cells.[39]

Bowenoid papulosis of the penis

Bowenoid papulosis of the penis refers to the presence of multiple macules and flat papules on the glans with an atypicality reminiscent of condyloma acuminata or carcinoma in situ. Infrequently virus particles have been noted by electron microscopy. Similar lesions, some with spontaneous regression, have been observed on the vulva.

Malignant lesions of epidermis

The malignant lesions of the epidermis include basal cell carcinoma, squamous cell carcinoma, Paget's disease, and melanocarcinoma.

Basal cell carcinoma

The term *carcinoma* is preferred to *epithelioma* in connection with the basal cell tumors that belong to the general group of rodent ulcers. If left untreated, these neoplasms progress, erode, and infiltrate neighboring bone and cartilage in a manner that would seem to merit the designation *cancer* despite the infrequency of metastasis. Over 100 instances of metastasizing basal cell carcinoma have been recorded.[19,28] The term *epithelioma* might best be reserved for the form of basal cell proliferation that does not show these invasive characteristics, that is, the trichoepithelioma, otherwise known as epithelioma adenoides cysticum or Brooke's tumor (see p. 1638).

Basal cell carcinomas occur predominantly in blond, fair-skinned people in the region of the face bounded by the hairline, ears, and upper lip. A tumor of the skin of the tip of the nose, however, is more likely to be a squamous carcinoma, provided that it is not a keratoacanthoma. Basal cell tumors are not confined to the face but in small numbers may occur in the skin of any part of the body, although there is a tendency to desmoplasia in those located away from the face. Squamous cell carcinomas of the anal canal, which are aggressive, particularly if they are located above the anal verge, may appear deceptively similar to basal cell carcinomas. Indeed, some of them are labeled basaloid—to the surgeon's confusion.

The basal cell carcinoma begins as a smooth, slightly elevated papule that may be scaly at first but tends soon to ulcerate centrally as the lesion spreads peripherally beneath the epidermis. Characteristically the ulcer is rimmed by a waxy, smooth, firm, rolled border representing the intact epidermis, which is wrapped over but not yet invaded by the underlying and undermining neoplastic nests. If neglected, the tumor may advance to a grotesque erosion of large portions of the soft tissue, as well as the cartilage and bone of the face. Early treatment by irradiation, excision, or the various other means of local destruction is usually adequate. The advantage of treatment of neoplasms by excision is that it then becomes possible to know by histologic examination not only the precise type of tumor present, but also whether the excised tumor is bounded by normal tissue.

Histologically, although there is considerable variability to the pattern of the basal cell carcinomas, there are sufficient characteristics in common to make them recognizable with relative ease. They are made up of nests of closely packed cells of uniform size and oval shape, with dark nuclei separated by a small amount of spineless cytoplasm. The nests often are rimmed by a single layer of similar cells arranged, however, in a neat radial pattern and strongly reminiscent of the more or less vertically arranged basal cells forming the lowermost layer of the normal epidermis or of the hair shafts. Mitotic figures are usually fairly common. Such nests may be observed arising not only from the basal portion of the epidermis but also from the corresponding layer of the hair shaft or from both sources in the same tumor. The presence in these tumors of cells of the same type as those that line both the epidermis and the hair follicle would appear to account for the origin of these neoplasms from either of these structures. This is by no means equivalent to maintaining that embryonic rests of hair matrix, in one or another phase of its development, are the source of basal cell carcinomas. The basal cells of adult epidermis do have a limited range of reaction to carcinogenic stimulation. One major form such a reaction takes is the production of hair matrices in the disheveled manner of a basal cell carcinoma, just as the basal cells in response to normal growth stimuli produce the orderly components of hair. In other words, when carcinogenic agents such as arsenic or x-irradiation produce basal cell carcinomas, they do so not by activating embryonic rests of hair follicles but by provoking neoplastic change in previously normally situated adult basal cells. The origin of basal cell carcinomas from any part of the mature pilary complex is demonstrable also in the skin of rats to which anthramine and methylcholanthrene have been applied.

The histologic features of basal cell carcinomas may vary in the following ways:

1. By the presence of edematous stroma rimmed by neoplastic cells to form the alveolar or cystic type
2. By excessive, dense, hyalinized stroma between nests of basal cells to give the morphea type
3. By the presence of foci of squamous cells or pearls, occasionally calcified, in the centers of nests of basal cells

This last modification has been called basosquamous cell (transitional or metatypical cell) carcinoma. It is stated that the keratin produced by basal cell carcinomas differs from that produced by squamous cell carcinomas in the histochemically demonstrable presence of cystine (hair follicle keratin) in the basal cell cancers. There is, in addition, the comedo type of basal cell carcinoma in which the cores of the masses of basal cells are necrotic.

Basal cell carcinomas, like squamous cell carcinomas, may exhibit focal sebaceous gland differentiation. This process can be distinguished from an original sebaceous gland carcinoma by the presence of abundant alpha-glycerophosphate dehydrase in the latter.

From time to time attempts are made to revive the notion that basal cell carcinomas with foci of squamous cell differentiation represent an intermediate phase in the aggressive deterioration to squamous cell carcinomas. These demonstrations still lack conviction, notwithstanding the invocation of some of the potentials of the basal cells. Despite general belief to the contrary, it has yet to be shown that there is any significant difference in the prognosis of these types. In particular, it is commonly stated that a basal cell carcinoma with areas of squamous cells has a more precarious prognosis than the ordinary basal cell carcinoma.

Superficial epitheliomatosis, or multicentric basal cell carcinoma, is a special variety of the basal cell tumors. These lesions occur predominantly on the trunk as either dry and scaly or moist and eczematous, slowly enlarging plaques. Histologically the lesions are small basal cell carcinomas arising from multiple foci in the basal layers of epidermis. The lesion is differentiated from the Jadassohn type of intraepidermal basal cell carcinoma, in which the neoplastic cells appear to be growing upward toward the surface from the basal cell layer instead of into the dermis. In the superficial lesions, as well as in other cutaneous carcinomas in situ, arsenic should be suspected as a possible etiologic factor (Fig. 38-36).

The so-called premalignant fibroepithelial tumor is really part of the spectrum of variants of basal cell carcinomas and hardly merits such segregation.

In situ and, infrequently, superficially invasive basal

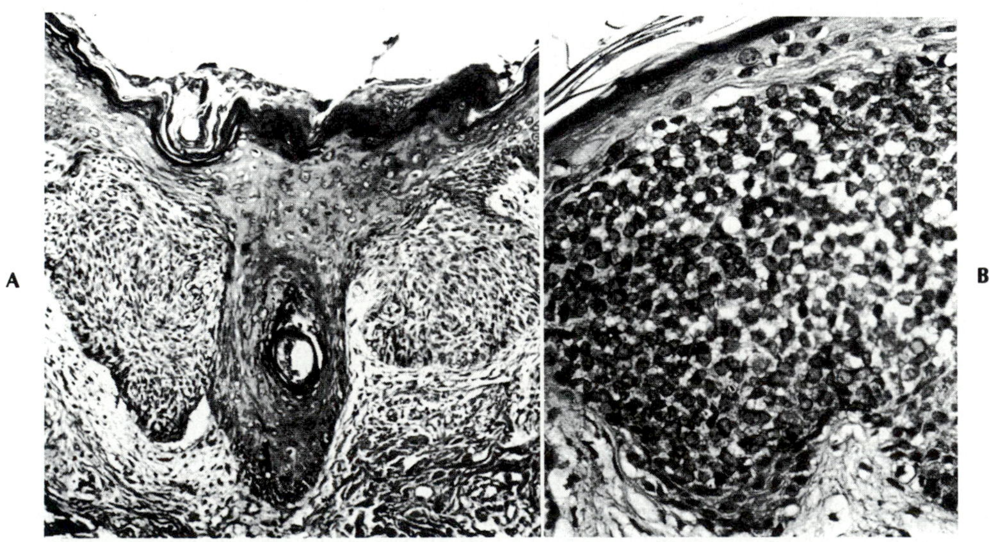

Fig. 38-36. A, Basal cell carcinoma (superficial epitheliomatosis, multicentric basal cell carcinoma). **B,** Intraepidermal basal cell carcinoma (Jadassohn type). (Hematoxylin and eosin.)

cell carcinomas may complicate sclerosing angiomas.[36] The existence of these fairly innocuous lesions has been disputed; they are indistinguishable from superficial epitheliomatosis and I believe they would be so diagnosed if seen without the underlying angioma.

Basal cell nevus syndrome

Basal cell carcinomas, along with a variety of adnexal hamartomas, may occur as a congenital hereditary phenomenon known as the basal cell nevus syndrome. These lesions may vary from several on the face to hundreds on the trunk and extremities. The associated lesions or symptom complexes may include pseudohypoparathyroidism, ovarian fibromas, mesenteric cysts, dental cysts, bifid ribs, spina bifida, hypertelorism, broad nasal root, bridging of the sella turcica, calcification of the falx cerebri, and agenesis of the corpus callosum. Occasionally granulomatous or ulcerative colitis may be present.

Isolated basal cell carcinomas in children occur more often than is generally suspected. As with the tumors of adults, they are present chiefly on the face.[52]

Squamous cell carcinoma

The squamous cell carcinoma may occur in the skin of any part of the body, but there is a predilection for the exposed areas, particularly the face and hands. Certain sources of chronic irritation definitely predispose to squamous cell carcinoma. These include pipe smoking, particularly clay pipes, irritation to the scrotum as incurred by chimney sweeps, the exposure to arsenic, tar, and carcinogenic oils that soak the clothes and abdomen of the mule spinner (in the textile industry), the constant contact of the abdomen with the small charcoal heaters causing the so-called kangri cancers observed in the Kashmir region, the exposure of susceptible blond skins to actinic rays and other elements of the weather, the unexplained cancerous irritant that is present in old scars as from burns or osteomyelitis, the vague irritant of syphilitic leukoplakia, and a variety of others.

The sources of the arsenic include that used therapeutically (Fowler's solution, arsphenamine), orchard sprays, and contaminated water from artesian wells (for example, of Taiwan). In the latter instance the cutaneous manifestations may be endemic and include a broad spectrum comprising benign-appearing keratoses, keratoses with fronds or ridges of early basal cell carcinoma, multicentric in situ and invasive basal cell carcinomas, Bowen's disease in its many variations, epidermoid carcinomas, and combinations of any of these lesions. Scars after vaccination may be complicated infrequently by basal cell carcinomas, squamous cell carcinomas, and melanocarcinomas. The basal and squamous cell carcinomas tend to occur in individuals with the type of skin vulnerable to damage from exposure to ultraviolet light. However, in most instances of squamous cell carcinoma the source of irritation or stimulation is not apparent.

Clinically the lesion begins as a superficially scaly, slightly indurated area that bleeds, crusts, and resists casual therapy. With growth the surface becomes ulcerated or cornified and the base indurated. The ulceration may extend to a deforming depth. The sectioned surface is granular and is grayish white flecked with yellow. Usually the limits of the neoplasm may be determined even by gross inspection of the cut surface.

Microscopically these carcinomas are characterized by irregular nests of epidermal cells that have infiltrated the dermis for varying depths. The nests of a squamous cell carcinoma may include cells representing any layer of the epidermis from the basal layer to the stratum corneum. In well-differentiated lesions the intercellular spines and the central keratinous nests, or the epithelial pearls, easily identify the origin of the tumor from squamous epithelium. In highly anaplastic lesions these elements may be altogether lacking. Indeed, the anaplasia may be so extreme in occasional squamous cell carcinomas that they may be almost indistinguishable from spindle cell sarcomas. These spindle cell carcinomas commonly follow irradiation and are controlled with difficulty. They are not to be confused with the unimportant, focal areas of spindle cells occurring in many basal cell carcinomas or with the spindle cell melanocarcinomas. Another variety characterized by intracellular edema, particularly affecting the central cells of the neoplastic nests that are rimmed by basilar cells, is occasionally mistaken for sebaceous or sweat gland carcinomas, even adamantinomas, or clear cell carcinomas.

Often of greater practical importance than determining the precise type of carcinoma is the decision as to whether an isolated nest of cells represents actual carcinomatous invasion or is merely an obliquely cut rete ridge in an area of pseudoepitheliomatous hyperplasia. In some instances the decision may be most difficult to make. However, the cells of a ridge in hyperplastic epidermis are quite differentiated and tend to resemble very closely the cells of the neighboring, obviously benign ridges and epidermis. The neighboring ridges—elongated, curved, and yet attached to the epidermis and cut perpendicularly—help to indicate that the isolated nest of cells actually represents an obliquely cut ridge rather than cancer. Another problem arises when abundant subepidermal inflammatory cells are present, some of which may have migrated across the basement membrane and lower epidermis, thereby obscuring the integrity of or even actually interrupting the basement membrane. Since disruption of the basement membrane is one of the standard (if reliable) criteria for provoking at least the suspicion of carcinoma, it becomes of some limited importance to judge, particularly by the anaplasia of the epidermal cells involved, whether the disruption is attributed merely to inflammation or to early cancer (Fig. 38-35).

The squamous cell carcinomas of the skin are, as a rule, not as anaplastic as the corresponding lesions of mucous membranes such as the lip or uterine cervix. Accordingly, metastases are considerably more common after squamous cell carcinoma of the mucous membranes than of the skin. Although this difference is the rule, there are conspicuous exceptions. One of the most anaplastic squamous cell carcinomas of my experience occurred in a scar after a burn of the skin of the leg. The tumor metastasized widely to the viscera.

Effects of ionizing radiation on skin

Ionizing radiation is used therapeutically for a great variety of inflammatory diseases, including acne, psoriasis, eczema, and plantar warts. Such treatment is usually at least temporarily effective for the dermatosis, but sequelae in the form of acute and chronic radiodermatitis occur often enough to warrant serious concern. It is estimated that carcinomas complicate approximately 20% of instances of chronic radiodermatitis.[27] This complication may occur over a wide span of years, from 3 to more than 50, with a median of 12 to 18 years. Because of the great time interval between the induction of therapy and the onset of complications, the frequency of such complications may be underestimated by therapists.

The usual type of cutaneous cancer occurring after radiotherapy is the squamous cell carcinoma, but basal cell carcinomas also may occur, particularly in areas about the face where such tumors are prone to arise spontaneously. As previously mentioned, spindle cell carcinomas are an especially anaplastic variety of squamous cell cancers produced by irradiation (see Fig. 15-34).

Merkel cell tumor

Recently enthusiasm has been aroused in support of the existence of a Merkel cell, neuroendocrine, or trabecular carcinoma of the skin. These are said to occur in various anatomic sites, to be composed of small anaplastic cells, some with neurosecretory granules capable of aggressive metastatic action, and to be differentiated, often with great difficulty, from metastatic carcinomas and epidermoid carcinomas, including melanocarcinomas. The presumed derivation of these tumors from Merkel cells and the presence of neurosecretory granules have persuaded observers that these tumors are individualistic and belong to the APUD system. The finding of neurosecretory granules in a variety of nonneural tumors, such as epidermoid carcinomas and carcinomas of the cervix, prostate, lung, and intestinal tract, as well as the aggressiveness of the Merkel cell tumor, uncharacteristic for a neoplasm of nerve endings, would seem to warrant some reconsideration of the derivation of this neoplasm.

Pigmented nevi

The term *nevus* is often used by dermatologists to refer to any congenital blemish. Therefore they refer not only to pigmented nevi but also to vascular nevi, sebaceous gland nevi, sweat gland nevi, and others. However, to most, nevus denotes a neoplasm derived from pigmented or at least dopa-positive cells. We have classified these nevi and their malignant counterparts as follows*:

- A. Benign
  1. Junctional nevus (Fig. 38-36)
  2. Intradermal nevus (Fig. 38-37)
  3. Compound nevus (including halo nevus) (Fig. 38-38)
  4. Juvenile melanoma (Fig. 38-39)
  5. Blue nevus—cellular blue nevus
- B. Malignant
  1. Melanocarcinoma (Figs. 38-42 and 38-44, *C*)
     - a. In situ
     - b. Superficial (including melanotic freckle of Hutchinson)
     - c. Deep
  2. Malignant blue nevus

*From Allen, A.C.: Cancer **2**:28, 1949, and Allen, A.C., and Spitz, S.: Cancer **6**:1, 1953.

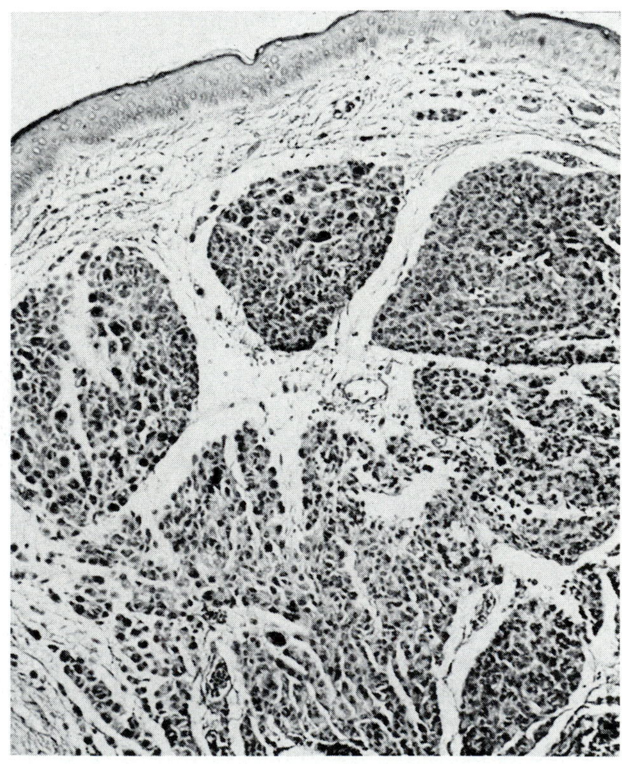

Fig. 38-37. Intradermal nevus showing intact epidermis, that is, without junctional change.

Junctional nevus

The junctional nevus, also known as dermoepidermal or marginal nevus, is of concern because in its active form it is a direct forerunner of the melanocarcinoma. Happily, this malignant transformation of junctional nevi occurs relatively infrequently.

The uncomplicated (quiescent versus active) junctional nevus appears as a flat, smooth, generally hairless, light brown to dark brown mole. The lesions may be single or multiple. Their smooth appearance may be altered by their combination with an underlying intradermal nevus (compound). *Unfortunately, it is not always possible to diagnose them accurately clinically*. However, one may assume that pigmented moles on the ventral surface of the hands and the feet and on the genitalia are usually junctional nevi or, at least, have a junctional component in the form of a compound nevus.[4-6,9,10]

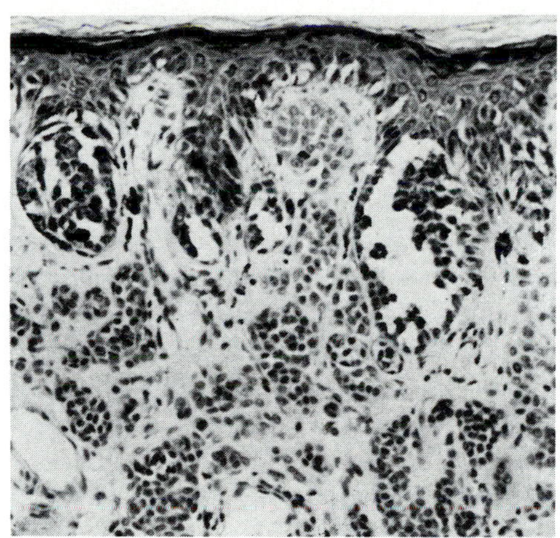

Fig. 38-38. Compound nevus showing junctional and intradermal components. (Hematoxylin and eosin.)

Histologically the junctional nevus is easily recognized by the clusters of enlarged, rounded, loosened cells of the basal and adjacent prickle cells of the epidermis. In addition, these cells lose their prickles and cohesion with neighboring cells, and many become powdered with fine granules of melanin. This acantholysis is reflected ultrastructurally in the partial to complete loss of desmosomes and tonofilaments, although residua of these structures are readily noted at the periphery of the junctional or acantholytic focus. If mitotic figures are present and the nuclei show any noteworthy anaplasia, the lesion may be assumed to have been on the verge of melanocarcinomatous transformation. Accordingly, depending on the extent of the atypia, these lesions are designated active junctional nevi or melanocarcinomas in situ.[10] The process may be diffuse along a strip of epidermis or it may be focal, with normal or skipped areas of epidermis intervening between involved portions. The limitation of junctional change or junctional nevus to acantholytic aggregates or nests of intraepidermal nevus cells in the rete ridges is arbitrary. It misses the equivalent contri-

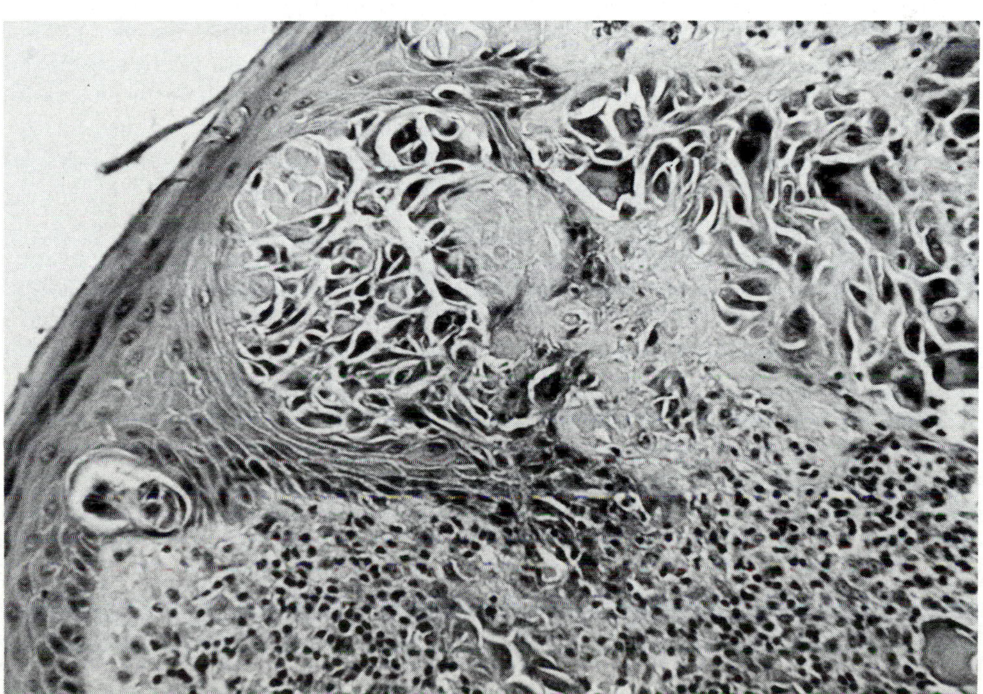

Fig. 38-39. Juvenile melanoma of Spitz showing the compound nevus with characteristic syncytial and myogenous-like nevus cells, necrobiotic nevus, eosinophilic cells, focally homogenized stroma, and a sparsity of melanin.

bution of the more diffuse lower epidermal acantholysis between the ridges, as in the Hutchinson freckle. Judgment as to the adequacy of normal margin bordering the lesion must be made with caution, inasmuch as the section may be removed through one of the intervening, unaltered areas (Fig. 38-36).

It is generally believed that the cells of the junctional nevus are derived from specialized nerve endings intercalated in the basal layer as clear cells. However, it seems that such a restricted view disregards the occurrence of cells of the junctional nevus (many dopa positive) not only in a continuous row in the basal layer, but also as isolated cells high in the prickle cell layers, in the stratum granulosum, and even well into the stratum corneum. This phenomenon I believe to occur not by proliferation of neurogenic cells within the epidermis, as many believe, but rather by the alteration in situ of the preexisting basal and spinous keratinocytes, as a few formerly believed (Fig. 38-44,*C*).

It was long ago clearly shown that dendrites, which to many seem automatically to connote neurogenesis, may be entirely absent in many of these cells. Actually, when the dendrites of melanocytes are seen with silver stains, they are made evident not because of an intrinsic argyrophilia such as is possessed by cells of true neurons but because of the argyrophilia of the contained granules of melanin. The supranuclear localization of pigment within the prickle cells is, in itself, indicative of an in situ origin rather than by a nipped-off dendrite belonging to a neighboring cell or by the diffusion of tyrosinase from a clear cell.[45] In the latter instance one would expect the granules of pigment to be diffusely or haphazardly deposited as in melanophores or histiocytes.

It is of course well established that the pigment of skin, hair, and feathers may be controlled by the transposition of the embryonic cells of the neural crest. That neural control of many varieties of pigmentation exists is obvious. However, to infer from this that the cells of the neural crest are incorporated in the epidermis as melanocytes is to fail, in effect, to distinguish the artist from his pigments.[9,10]

The addition of these facts, supplemented by evidence from the direct examination of many junctional nevi and melanocarcinomas, indicates that basal cells principally, but also prickle cells or keratinocytes, may become converted to melanocytes and that the junctional nevi are derived from these cells.

Intradermal nevus

The intradermal nevus, or common mole, is the ordinary pigmented spot that few people are altogether spared. The mole may be flat or raised, with or without hairs, papillary and keratotic. Intradermal nevi may be present at birth or may develop in later years. They tend to become more prominent at puberty.

Histologically the tumor is composed of nests and cords of cells with round, moderately chromatic nuclei surrounded by an even, easily seen rim of cytoplasm. Melanin pigment, when present, usually is limited to the superficial cells in the upper dermis. Similarly, the cells in the upper part of the lesion are more likely to be dopa positive than are the deeper ones.* Mitotic figures are seen rarely in these nevi in adults. Occasionally hyperchromatism and enlargement of nuclei are simulated by mere agglutination of neval cells. The neval cells characteristically trail off into the depths of the dermis, and rarely into the subcutis, without sharp limitation. The overlying epidermis usually is thinned and may be flat or papillary, with or without hyperkeratosis.

There is impressive histologic basis for the conclusion that the ordinary intradermal mole that is not overlain by a junctional nevus rarely becomes malignant.

The origin of the cells of the common mole is still unsettled. The possibilities include epidermal cells, specialized nerve endings similar to the Merkel-Ranvier corpuscles, and dermal nerves. Those who subscribe to the epidermal origin of the intradermal nevus assume, as Unna[73] did, that the altered epidermal cells drop off *(Abtropfung)* and migrate into the dermis. Those who believe in the neurogenesis of pigmented nevi suggest that the neval cells arise from dermal nerves or their sheaths, as well as from the intraepidermal nerve endings or cells that migrated from the neural crest. The frequency with which intradermal nevi are associated with loosened nests of epidermal cells that appear about to drop off (junctional changes) makes the epidermal origin of the common mole (as well as the junctional nevus) the likeliest possibility. This frequent association of the junctional change with the intradermal nevus can hardly be fortuitous, inasmuch as the change is rarely seen with blue nevi and yet is infrequently absent in the moles of children, normally diminishing in frequency and prominence after puberty.

Balloon cell nevus

Occasional intradermal nevi, called balloon cell nevi, are characterized by large, coalescent vacuoles within the cytoplasm of nevus cells. These have been shown ultrastructurally to represent altered melanosomes rather than lipid.[37]

Compound nevus

In about 98% of the intradermal nevi occurring before puberty and in about 12% of nevi of adults there is an associated junctional change (Fig. 38-38).[5,10] For lesions

*Melanophores are merely phagocytes that engulf and transport melanin. Melanophores are dopa negative. A pigmented neval cell or melanoblast may be dopa negative because its enzyme has been completely utilized at a given time or has never developed. The cells of a nonpigmented (amelanotic) melanoma may be dopa positive. However, not all cells of a pigmented or nonpigmented melanocarcinoma are necessarily dopa positive.

with this combination of features the term *compound nevus* was originally applied by me in 1949.[10] It was introduced (1) to underscore the morphogenic interplay between epidermal and dermal neval components and (2) to create a diagnostically usable classification. It recently has been stated that silver stains are of appreciable help in distinguishing compound nevi from malignant melanomas. This, unfortunately, is not correct.

Clinically, as stated, there is no way to be certain whether an intradermal nevus is compounded with a junctional nevus. This fact emphasizes the importance of histologic examination of all excised nevi. As is indicated in the discussion of melanocarcinomas, the compound nevus has the capacity for undergoing malignant transformation by virtue of its junctional component. This conversion takes place relatively infrequently. The possibility exists that an intradermal nevus may on occasion develop overlying junctional change.

Juvenile melanoma

Juvenile melanoma is the name applied to a special form of compound nevus occurring predominantly in children. In the past these lesions were considered to be histologically malignant but clinically benign. In other words, if the patient was prepubertal, these moles were arbitrarily labeled benign.

It was not until the basic histologic definition of these was first published in 1948 by the late Dr. Sophie Spitz that the morphologic distinction between the juvenile melanomas and true melanocarcinomas began to become evident.[10,11,67,68] It is now reasonably apparent that this much needed definition has served in a most practical way to clarify portions of a tortuously confused problem.[6,9]

Briefly, the distinguishing features of the juvenile melanomas are those of the compound nevi, with the addition of myogenous-appearing, occasionally spindled, single and multinucleated giant cells with abundant basophilic cytoplasm, often loosely dispersed in an edematous upper cutis. These giant cells are derived from overlying epidermal cells. There is no basis for believing that the juvenile melanoma, which as indicated is really a special form of compound nevus, is any more likely to become malignant than is the ordinary compound nevus. The juvenile melanomas undergo involutional fibrosis or desmoplasia, as do other types of nevi.[7,8]

The desmoplastic variant of the Spitz nevus has been mistaken for a variety of fibrohistiocytic entities, including the fibrous nodule of the tip of the nose.[14] The detection of residual foci of junctional change or clustering, however sparse, may be the most revealing clue. Giant cells, single nucleated or multinucleated—some with conspicuous intranuclear inclusions, offer additional diagnostic support. These are the same inclusions that others regard as cytoplasmic in origin through a process of intranuclear invagination. The collagenization has been variously attributed to involution,[7,9] active desmoplasia in response to provocation by the nevus cells,[14] and trauma. The pattern of the stroma in relation to the tumor cells, particularly their frequent relative sparsity in a loose stroma, as well as the progressive stromal increase with age, suggest the involutional nature of the process. On the other hand, the dense desmoplasia inherently invoked by certain cancers, such as prostatic and some mammary carcinomas, occurs pari passu with the extension of neoplastic cells.

With increasing experience, it has become possible to recognize the juvenile melanomas by the interpretation of the histologic picture alone (Fig. 38-40). On this basis the scope of the significance of the juvenile melanoma has been extended by my own and later confirmed discovery that this lesion may be found in adults, preponderantly in the second, third, and fourth decades but occasionally in older patients.[10] The practical importance of this observation is obvious when it is realized that benign juvenile melanomas of adults were previously treated as cancers.

Currently there is unfortunately an increasing tendency to submit for histologic examination the shaved top of a pigmented lesion. Such a superficial biopsy not only complicates the problems of histologic diagnosis and the determination of cleared margins, but also leads to local recurrences of incompletely removed lesions. These local recurrences may be difficult to diagnose correctly.

There has been a good deal of objection to our use of *juvenile melanoma* (rather than spindle cell nevus, for example) for a lesion that is benign and occurs occasionally in adults. Actually, we have always used the term in a descriptive, histologic sense, much as the terms *embryonal rhabdomyosarcoma*, *fetal adenoma of the thyroid gland*, *juvenile cirrhosis*, *juvenile nasopharyngeal angiofibroma*, and *juvenile carcinoma of the breast* are used.

The lesion has come to be known as Spitz's melanoma or Spitz's nevus. The use of *juvenile melanoma* or *Spitz's nevus* serves the important practical purpose of viewing with added caution the acceptance of a given evaluation of a lesion so diagnosed. Sometimes it seems to have been forgotten that it was not many years ago that no one claimed to be able to distinguish the juvenile melanoma from the malignant melanoma, and in a great many laboratories this problem has obviously been far from resolved.

Eosinophilic globules in juvenile melanomas

Eosinophilic, diffusely hyalinized, inconsistently periodic acid–Schiff–positive globules or masses have been noted in juvenile melanomas and have been assigned diagnostic significance. Actually these occur not only in juvenile melanomas but also in ordinary compound nevi and infrequently in malignant melanomas. They tend to

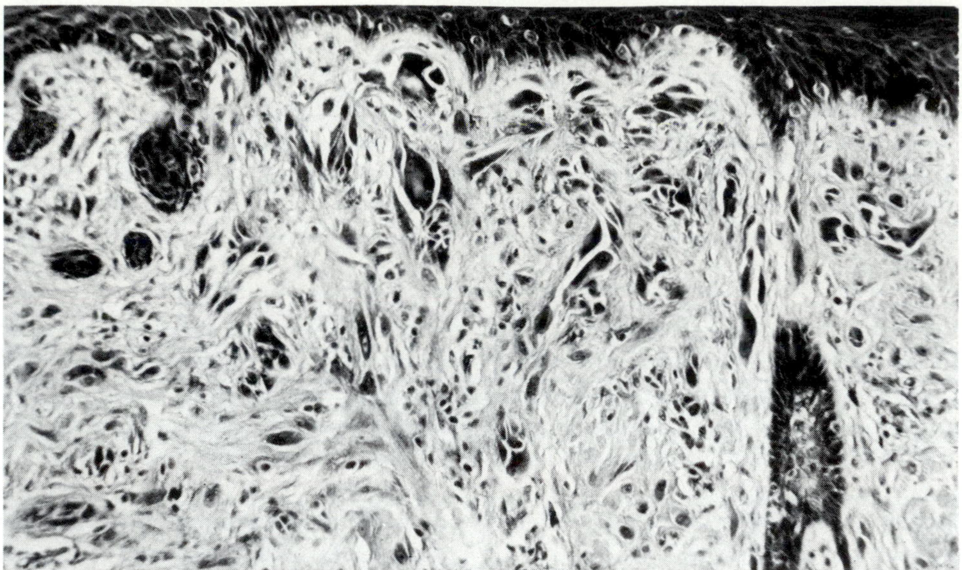

Fig. 38-40. Juvenile melanoma of Spitz. This is from an adult, as reflected by the fibrosis.

be located at the dermoepidermal junction, both in the lower epidermis and in the clusters of nevus cells in the upper dermis. When present in conspicuous numbers, as others have stated, they represent one of a number of parameters diagnostically weighted toward Spitz's nevus. To me they suggest a form of coagulative necrosis that may involve both nucleus and cytoplasm. Indeed, it may produce the necrosis of an almost complete loss of a nest of nevus cells, leaving a space simulating a diluted dermal lymphatic or venule (Fig. 38-39). I have previously referred to these as necrobiotic cells. As I wrote in 1967*:

The simulation of subepidermal lymphatic may be created by the dissolution of clusters of tumor cells so that eosinophilic debris closely approximates lymph in histologic appearance. A study of the transitional stages in the development of this pattern, particularly of the progressive lysis of these spongiotic clumps of cells, effectively suggests its histogenesis and provides a useful clue in the recognition of the juvenile melanoma.

Blue nevus

The blue or Jadassohn-Tièche nevus appears as a flat or slightly elevated blue or bluish black lesion, occurring particularly on the trunk and extremities and often mistaken clinically for a malignant melanoma. It is structurally essentially the same as the mongolian spot or the nevus of Ota. The former is found in the sacral region. The nevus of Ota occurs in the eye and on the skin of the face. Showers of blue nevi (eruptive) have been observed during pregnancy, at puberty, and in association with bullous dermatoses.

Histologically these nevi are composed of interlacing fasciculi of spindle cells with long cytoplasmic processes and oval fibrocytoid nuclei. The cells are usually much more loosely disposed than those of the blue nevus. If the pigment were not present, the histologic picture of the blue nevus would resemble that of a dermal neurofibroma, and indeed it is possible that the basic morphogenesis of the two is similar. However, many of the cells of the blue nevus and the mongolian spot are dopa positive. Abundant melanin pigment may obliterate the details of most of the cells of the blue nevus. In addition, the neoplastic cells are interspersed with numerous pigment-laden chromatophores. Usually the neval cells lie deep in the dermis, or occasionally they are directly apposed to the epidermis. The color of the nevus is, of course, dependent not only on the amount of pigment present but also on the distance of the lesion from the epidermis. Infrequently the blue nevus is combined with the ordinary intradermal nevus (common mole) and with the junctional nevus.

Cellular blue nevus. There is a striking variant of the blue nevus that is frequently incorrectly diagnosed as melanosarcoma. Some years ago I termed this lesion "cellular blue nevus."[5,6,9] It occurs in about 50% of cases in the skin of the buttocks and the dorsum of the hands or feet. The epidermis is unchanged. The cells of this tumor show no significant anaplasia, and mitotic figures almost always are absent. Fused nuclei often simulate the hyperchromasia of activity. One of the features that characterize the lesion is the cross sections of fasciculi surrounded by clear zones, giving the illusion that the

*From Allen, A.C.: The skin: a clinicopathologic treatise, ed. 2, New York, 1967, Grune & Stratton, Inc.

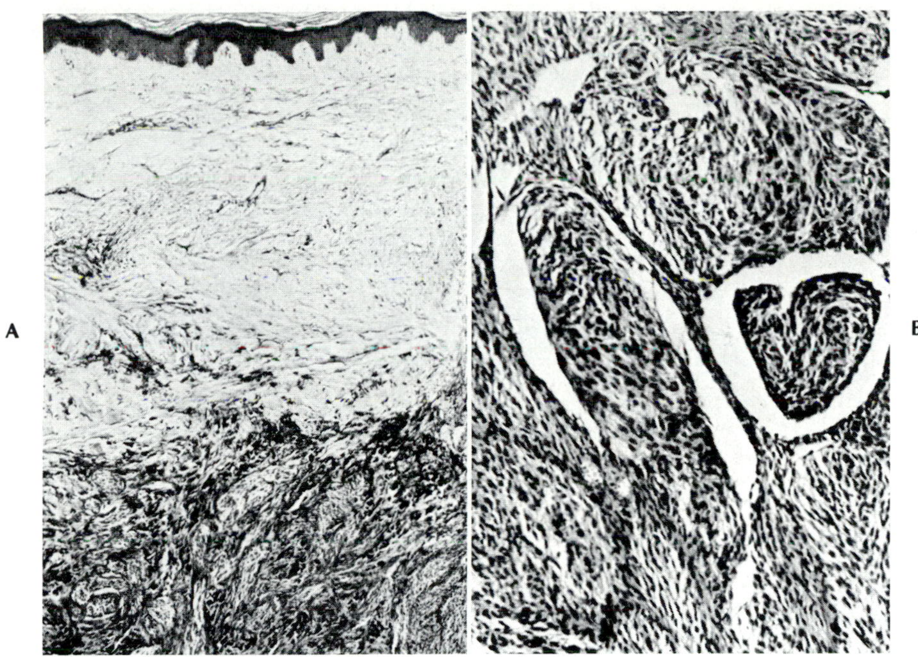

Fig. 38-41. Cellular blue nevus. **A,** Epidermis is intact. **B,** Appearance of invasion of lymphatics is an illusion characteristic of this lesion and results from artifactual shrinkage. (Hematoxylin and eosin.)

whorls are metastases in lymphatics when they actually represent artifactitious shrinkage and cleavage of the fasciculi (Fig. 38-41). The melanosomes of the cellular blue nevus are stated to have a distinctive ultrastructure.

Blue nevi undergo malignant change with consoling rarity. I have seen 53 examples of malignant blue nevi arising generally from cellular blue nevi. Although it appears obvious that the diagnosis of sarcomatous transformation of a blue nevus is often made unjustifiably, such cancers do occur, although rarely.

Senile lentigo

The senile lentigo is a common lesion occurring on exposed surfaces in approximately one third of individuals past middle age. It is characterized histologically by hyperkeratosis and parakeratosis and fringelike elongation of the hyperpigmented rete ridges, often showing an increase in basilar clear cells or minimal junctional change (Fig. 38-42).

Melanotic freckle of Hutchinson

Much attention has been given recently to essentially restatements of information concerning the melanotic freckle of Hutchinson, also known as *la mélanose circonscrite précancéreuse de Dubreuilh*, senile or malignant freckle, precancerous or acquired melanosis, premalignant lentigo, and lentigo maligna. Actually this lesion is characteristically a relatively slow-growing lesion of the face, generally of elderly patients, which evolves from epidermal melanosis to a junctional nevus with varying degrees of activity and finally, if the patient lives long enough, to a superficial and then deep (or nodular) melanocarcinoma. As long ago documented, the melanocarcinomas of the face, especially those of women, tend to be associated with a better prognosis than those of most other regions of the body.[10] Their histogenesis, however, is no different from that of any other junctional nevus or from the melanocarcinoma derived therefrom.

Halo nevus

Halo nevus (leukoderma acquisitum centrifugum, Sutton's nevus) is the progressive centripetal extension of a zone of depigmentation about a nevus. This perilesional depigmentation may encircle not only benign nevi (intradermal, compound, and blue) but also malignant melanomas, as well as cutaneous metastases. Accordingly, this leukodermatous reaction gives no hint as to whether a given lesion is benign or malignant.

It has been hypothesized that the destruction of the nevus cells may represent an immune response to the antigens of the nevus cells or, on occasion, melanocarcinomatous cells. The disintegration of nevus cells that has been noted in juvenile melanomas may reflect a similar immunologic self-destruction. In the instance of juvenile melanomas this reaction may occur in the absence of nearby lymphocytes. The distortion generated by this reaction in both instances—halo nevi and juvenile melanomas—may lead to the mistaken diagnosis of malignant melanomas.

As stated, a spectrum of hypotheses ranging from anti-

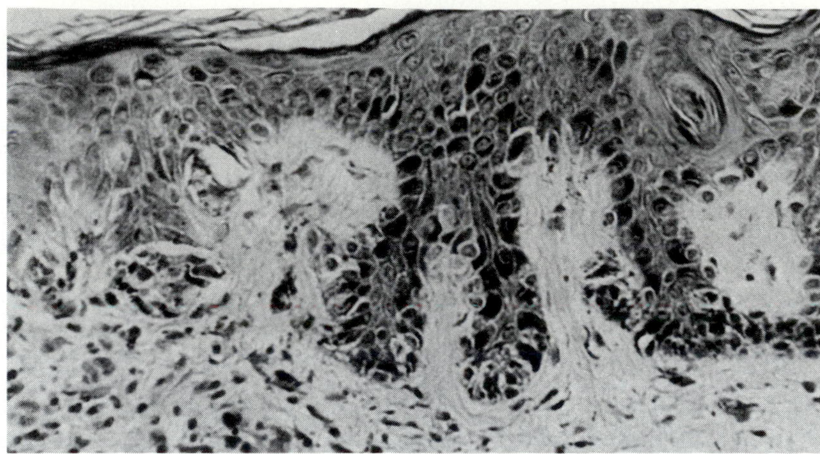

Fig. 38-42. Lentigo with pigmented rete ridges associated with junctional change. (Hematoxylin and eosin.)

gen-antibody reaction to neurotropic disturbance has been suggested to explain the local vitiligo or leukoderma. The most reasonable is that the depigmentation results from the underlying inflammatory reaction similar to the depigmentation that may occur with lichen planus, for example.

Malignant melanomas

In 1953 malignant melanomas were classified as indicated below.[10] Almost two decades later others modified this classification by the addition in effect of more subdivisions indicated by the levels in parentheses[18]:

1. Melanocarcinoma from active junctional nevus (or junctional component of compound nevus)
   a. Melanocarcinoma in situ (level I)
   b. Superficial (level II, some in level III)
   c. Deep (those deeper in level III; IV, reticular; and V, subcuticular)
2. Malignant blue nevus

The essential modification of the parallel classifications involves the subdivision of the deep level into levels III, IV, and V. Actually melanocarcinomas so advanced and neglected as to have directly invaded the panniculus (level V) are rarely seen these days, mostly on the soles where the dermis is especially thin. The debatable contribution therefore centers on deeper levels III and IV.[15] In one large series this subdivision has not proved informative[38] although others disagree somewhat.[74] However, there are several overlooked sources of error inherent in the classification by dermal levels, as follows:

1. Because of the pseudoepitheliomatous hyperplasia frequently associated with malignant melanomas, the rete ridges may extend illusorily deep into the reticular layer (level IV) and still function as a superficial melanocarcinoma.
2. The malignant melanomas have a remarkable propensity for growing outward, or exophytically. Accordingly, the nodular melanocarcinomas may behave the worst and yet not extend below the papillary layer of the dermis. This same nodular lesion eventually complicates or originates from superficially spreading or lentiginous melanocarcinomas (Fig. 38-43).
3. The dermal papillary layer varies considerably in different parts of the body, being particularly thin and superficial in the skin of many areas of the extremities.

In other words, the very premise on which the use of these levels rests is factitious, if only for their great variation in depth in different parts of the body. Hence the arbitrary use of the level of the interface between papillary and reticular layers as a measure of depth of invasion of lesion in various areas is grossly inaccurate. To imply further that the reticular layer is inherently a barrier to spread of the tumor is baseless. Finally, to state that the subdivision of melanoma into five anatomic levels of invasion permits the accurate assignment of prognosis to each case is patently hyperbolic. The behavior of these capriciously aggressive tumors cannot be measured predictably by boundaries of highly variable thicknesses, even if they are speciously drawn to the second decimal place. Therefore I believe that divisions of dermal invasion other than superficial and deep lend little substance to the analysis of these cancers. The hard fact is that the least invasive superficial melanocarcinoma in individual instances may be as devastatingly lethal as one that has reached the panniculus. Metastasis to lymph nodes and death may in fact result from melanocarcinomas merely 0.4 to 0.6 mm in depth.[74]

The lack of a relationship between histologic pattern and prognosis is demonstrated frequently in vulval and subungual malignant melanomas, for example. The so-called levels of extension are similarly uninformative in these areas.

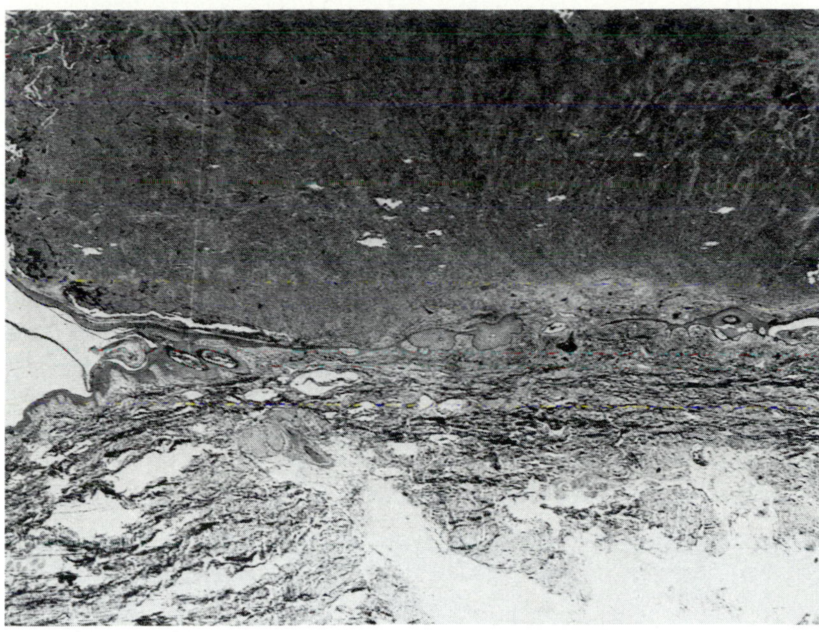

Fig. 38-43. Nodular malignant melanoma. This aggressive lesion does not extend beyond the papillary dermis, or so-called level II.

Directly more consonant with the original categorization of malignant melanomas into superficial and deep types[11] is the popular one of Breslow's derived from the direct measurement of the depth of dermal invasion by the tumor.[15] The critical dermal levels were to be 0.76 mm and 1.51 mm, and these were made the pivotal determinants for surgical therapy (excision of lymph nodes) and prognosis. For a cancer as virulent and as unpredictable as the melanocarcinoma, this tissue-thin line of transition would seem to be arbitrarily drawn. Aggressive neoplasms cannot be trusted to follow linearly the behavioral pattern dictated by a finely incremental graduation of the depth of invasion, except crudely as groups of superficial and deep tumors. The prognostic pattern is commonly not sustained in individual melanocarcinomas, not in the prognostically poor nodular melanomas with minimal dermal invasion, nor in the occasional instance of lethal superficially infiltrating melanoma at level II.

There is no perceptible advantage to labeling a melanocarcinoma in situ either *superficial spreading melanoma* or *lentigo maligna melanoma*. The pivotal point is the presence or absence of dermal invasion and, if present, whether it is superficial or deep. One of the disquieting consequences of the term *superficial spreading melanoma* is its increasingly facile use as an unwarranted substitute for junctional nevus, active junctional nevus, or melanocarcinoma in situ.

Clinically the malignant melanoma is preceded usually by a flat, hairless mole, pigmented light to dark brown. When such a mole, which may have appeared the same for years, begins to darken, it probably has already undergone at least local malignant transformation. The changes of ulceration, increase in size, and bleeding obviously worsen the prognosis.[5,10] The recently promoted notion that, with few exceptions, mainly congenital, malignant melanomas arise anew, fails to reckon with the duration of the lesions and their histologic composition. These establish the frequent superimposition of malignant melanomas onto long-standing junctional or compound nevi.

A mole that is hairy, elevated, and papillary is uncommonly the site of cancer, although the insurance is by no means absolute—for the histologic reasons to be explained. In some instances the neoplasm appears to arise anew, especially on the scrotum, palms, and soles. In these regions the common (intradermal) mole rarely occurs, but the small, flat, often unnoticed, frecklelike junctional or compound nevus frequently is present. Because the lesions of the soles and genitalia are likely to have a junctional component, tend to escape inspection, and are located in areas that appear to have a proportionately higher incidence of malignant melanomas than other anatomic sites, it would seem reasonable to have such nevi removed electively from these sites when feasible. Some years ago we suggested that the better prognosis for women with malignant melanomas of the face (which we documented statistically) might be related to their greater likelihood of having the unsightly lesions removed earlier than would men.[10] Therefore the lesions would be removed before they had penetrated as deeply as those in men.

In many instances the benign deeply pigmented blue nevus is mistaken for a developing malignant melanoma. As stated, metastasizing melanomas are uncommon before puberty, although a number of such cases have been recorded. In each of these instances the histologic picture could be distinguished from that of the juvenile melanomas but not from the melanocarcinomas of adults.[10]

Histology and histogenesis. There is considerable variation in the cellular pattern of the melanocarcinomas. The primary lesion may simulate a squamous cell carcinoma, a spindle or basal cell carcinoma, an adenocarcinoma, a neurofibrosarcoma, or other neoplasms. The usual melanocarcinoma is composed of cells arranged as compact masses with some cords and alveoli. The cells are likely to be more or less uniform in size and shape. The nuclei of the primary lesion commonly do not exhibit the classic evidence of anaplasia. Mitotic figures may not be numerous, despite the aggressiveness of the neoplasm. Often the nuclei are vacuolated and contain large acidophilic nucleoli resembling inclusion bodies, sometimes containing melanin. Melanin pigment may be present or absent without prognostic influence. In the neoplastic cells the pigment tends to be of a uniform, fine granularity, whereas in the chromatophores the pigment granules are likely to be more irregular in size and shape.

One of the most helpful histologic aids in diagnosis is the active junctional change overlying and continuous with the dermal portion of the cancer. The cells of the

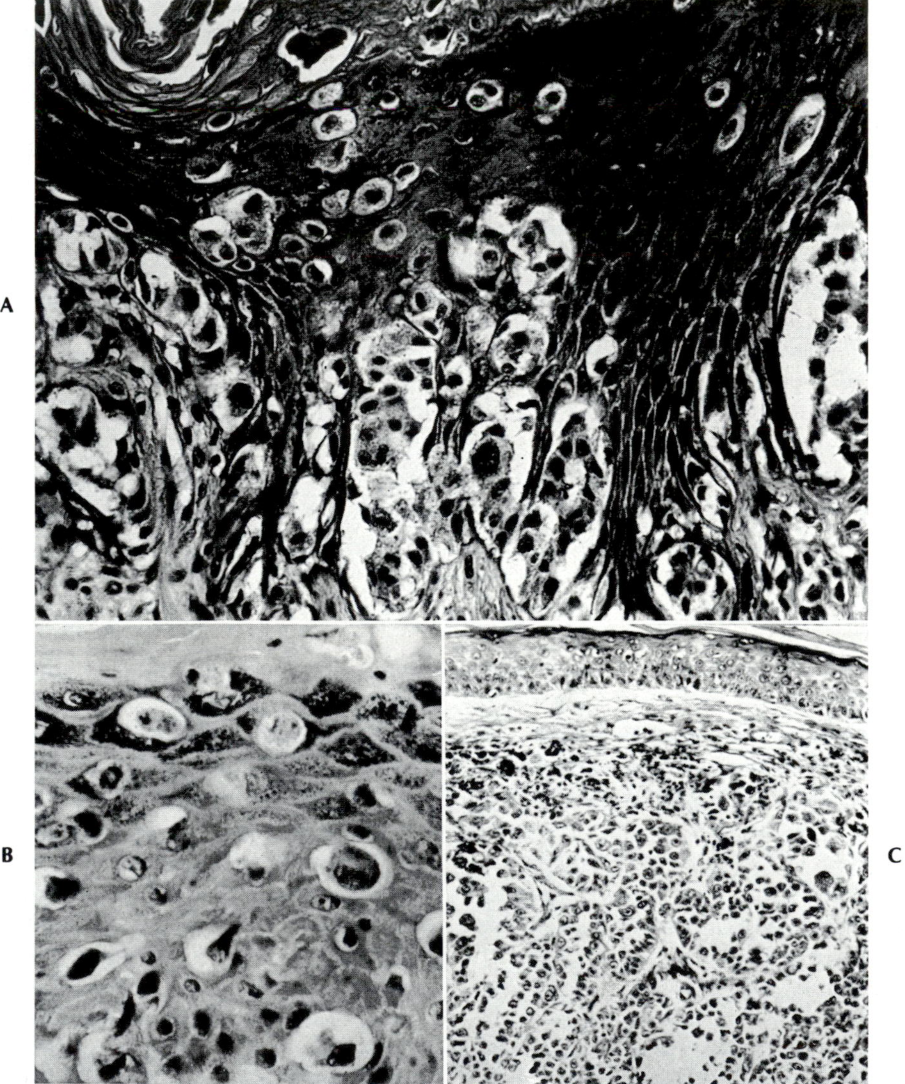

Fig. 38-44. Melanocarcinoma. **A,** Conversion of epidermal cells of pagetoid melanoma into melanocarcinomatous cells. **B,** In situ transformation of epidermal cells into melanocarcinomatous cells. **C,** Metastatic melanocarcinoma to skin showing overlying intact epidermis—criterion for primary versus metastatic melanocarcinoma. (Hematoxylin and eosin.)

rete ridges may be so loosened as to be incorporated in the dermal neoplasm, with consequent partial dissolution of the ridges. Isolated, spherical, haloed cells, often powdered with fine melanin granules, may be found as far up as the stratum corneum (Fig. 38-44, *A*). Such intraepithelial cells are in my opinion the source of practically all melanocarcinomas of the skin and mucous membranes (blue nevi excepted) (Fig. 38-44, *B*). These cancerous cells are not related to Langerhans cells or Merkel-Ranvier corpuscles but actually seem to have been originally cells derived from various layers of the epidermis. Nor is it true, as some believe, that these cells within the epidermis are metastatic from the underlying tumor within the dermis. Evidence for the autochthonous epidermal origin is found not only in the occurrence of such cells within the epidermis alone in early junctional nevi or superficial malignant melanomas but also in their absence in the epidermis overlying a snugly apposed dermal metastasis of a melanoma (Fig. 38-44, *C*), a criterion that distinguishes the primary from the metastatic melanocarcinoma (Fig. 38-45).

Active junctional nevus (melanocarcinoma in situ). It is now apparent that when a malignant melanoma appears to be superimposed on a benign intradermal nevus, originally a clinically obvious or latent junctional nevus was present that itself was the source of the malignant melanoma. Routine studies of the epidermis of the primary melanocarcinomas of skin (and mucous membranes, including conjunctivae) demonstrate this junctional change. In other words, the melanocarcinoma arising in the skin would actually seem to be a peculiarly virulent variant of an epidermogenic carcinoma, a view originally expressed by Unna in 1893.[73] Why the malignant melanoma usually behaves more aggressively than other epidermal carcinomas is not yet known. Occasionally it becomes a problem to decide if a given lesion is still in the stage of junctional nevus or has become a melanocarcinoma in situ. The histologic diagnosis of a superficial melanocarcinoma must, in the last analysis, depend on finding evidence of invasion of the upper dermis by the cells of the active junctional nevus (Fig. 38-44, *A*).[10]

Actually, all junctional nevi by definition exhibit a kind of activity or dynamics in the form of varying stages of acantholysis of the intraepidermal cells. However, with this reservation I have in the past applied the term *active junctional nevus* to the one with nuclear atypia and mitotic figures and often with large, pagetoid cells scattered singly or in clumps to various levels of the epidermis.[9-11] Such a lesion is equivalent to melanocarcinoma in situ. The presence of such an active junctional nevus should lead to a painstaking search for dermal invasion with the help of multiple sections. The histologic criteria for the distinction of a superficial melanocarcinoma—from an active junctional nevus on one hand or a deep melanocarcinoma on the other—are essentially similar to

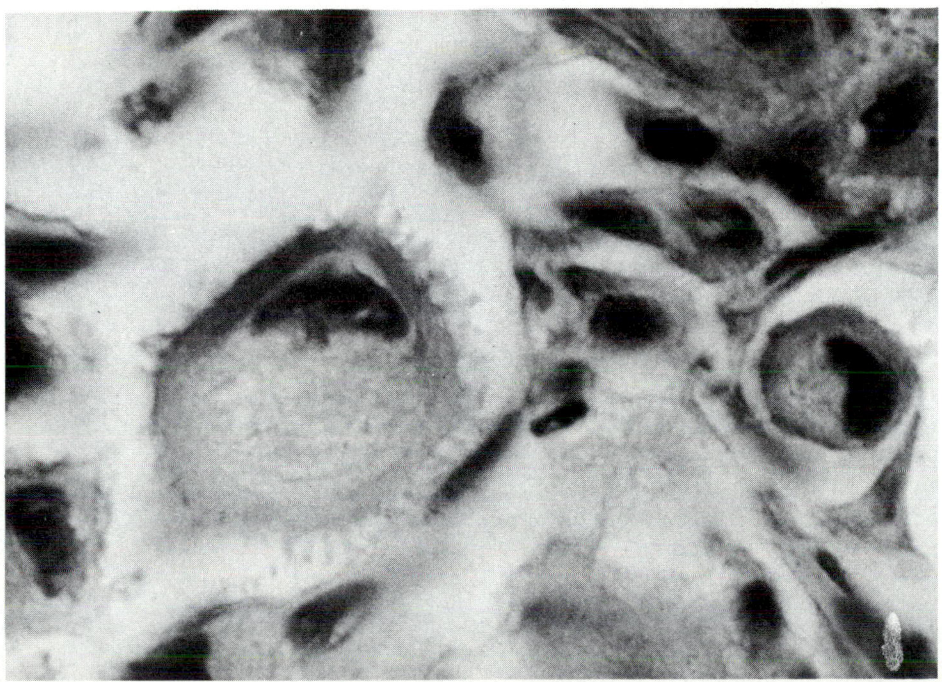

Fig. 38-45. Melanocarcinoma in situ showing histogenesis of neoplastic cells from keratinocytes. Residue of identifying "prickles" and atypical neoplastic nuclei are evident. (Hematoxylin and eosin; 1000×.)

those used for distinguishing a superficial squamous cell carcinoma from leukoplakia and from a deeply infiltrating carcinoma. Incidentally, the high degree of pseudoepitheliomatous hyperplasia so commonly associated with melanocarcinomas is largely responsible for mistaking these neoplasms for squamous cell carcinomas.[10] Patients with a melanocarcinoma appear to have a systemic diathesis for activation of junctional nevi, which in a percentage of cases (3.5%) leads to multiple primary melanocarcinomas. The activation of nevi in patients with malignant melanoma, first noted in 1953,[10] has been recently confirmed and its significance appreciated.[71]

Regression. Focal, piecemeal, incomplete regression of malignant melanomas has been repeatedly noted. However, complete regression of the local malignancy may occur.[66] We have recently seen a patient with inguinal node metastases from a primary melanocarcinoma of the heel of the foot with local residuum only of melanophores and focal minimal junctional change. The humoral attack on melanomas has thus far not proved fruitful, although their spontaneous regression, albeit rare, suggests further study. Cell-mediated and humoral antitumor reactions have been noted in patients with melanomas, but their effect on the clinical course has not been shown.[70] Malignant melanoma assays may exhibit positive estrogen receptors.

Bathing trunk nevi. These giant congenital nevi may be associated with leptomeningeal melanocytosis and often take the pattern of complex hamartomatous and choristomatous malformations. In addition to all varieties of pigmented nevi and malignant melanomas, they may develop neoplasms of lipoblastic, rhabdomyoblastic, and frankly neural origin (neurofibroma, schwannoma). It is in this type of lesion that the rare malignant melanoma unaccompanied by overlying junctional changes may be found. It is estimated that malignant melanomas develop in approximately 5% to 15% of patients with giant nevi.

Melanocarcinomas of mucous membranes. Melanocarcinomas of the mucous membranes of the oronasopharynx, larynx, bronchus, esophagus, gallbladder, and genitalia, including the cervix and anorectal region, are almost uniformly fatal. Undoubtedly some of the contributory reasons for their grave prognosis are the delay in detection and in accurate histologic diagnosis, the frequent injudicious therapy, the difficulties in adequate operative removal, and possibly such extraneous factors as chronic infection and repeated trauma. In approximately 15% of 337 patients in one study the tumors arose in these various mucous membranes (exclusive of the conjunctiva).[10] The ulceration of the junctional change and the absence of appreciable amounts of pigment in about 50% of the melanomas of mucous membranes increase the difficulties of histologic diagnosis. Melanocarcinomas of mucous membranes may arise in any mucosa lined by either normally present or metaplastic stratified squamous epithelium (Fig. 38-46).[6,9,10]

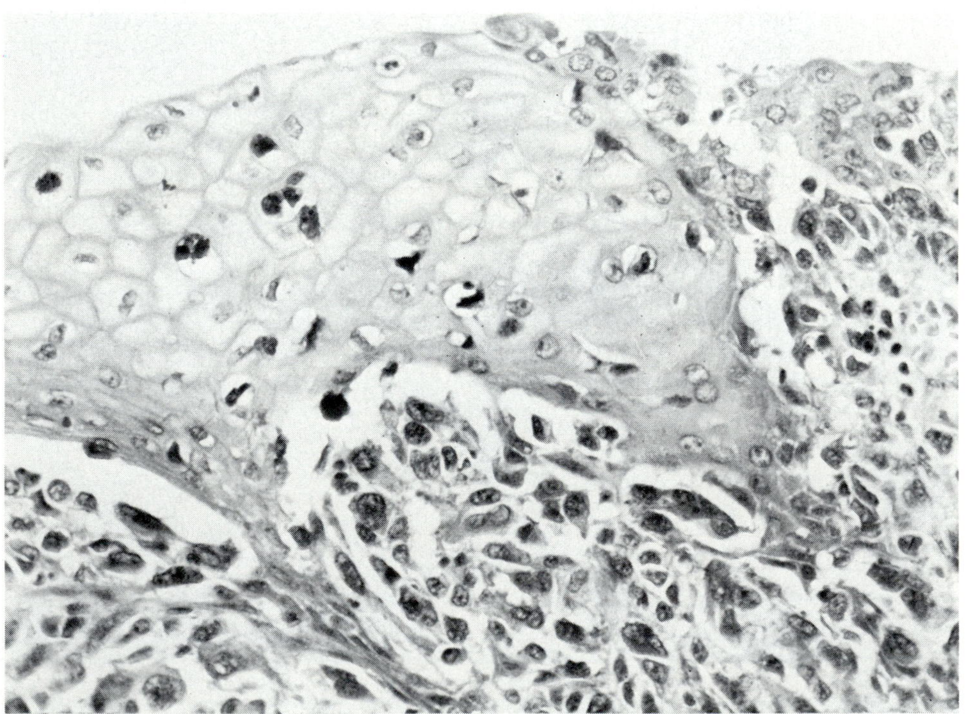

Fig. 38-46. Primary melanocarcinoma of bronchus illustrating the junctional change in the squamous epithelium, diagnostic of the primary site. (Hematoxylin and eosin.)

Tumors of vessels

Lymphangioma

The number of histologic and clinical variants, as well as the difficulty in distinguishing neoplasia of lymphatic vessels from ectasias, anomalies, and proliferations attributable to stasis, has led to the application of needlessly confusing names. The same situation exists with respect to the angiomas, but in both instances it has existed so long that scrapping of terminology at this point would add to the confusion.

The lymphangioma simplex is a soft, compressible, grayish pink nodule. The nodules are often multiple and grouped irregularly. Although the skin of the genitalia is the common site for these tumors, they are found also on the lips and tongue and may be associated with macroglossia or macrocheilia. They are composed of varying-sized, endothelium-lined, thin-walled vessels, either empty or containing lymph with occasional leukocytes. Some of the channels may contain a few red blood cells. There is an abundant proliferation of endothelial cells in a proportion of tumors, to which the designation *lymphangioma tuberosum multiplex* or *lymphangioendothelioma* has been applied.

Lymphangioma cutis circumscriptum occurs in the skin of the face, chest, or extremities in the form of a single tumor or multiple projecting, somewhat papillary, verrucose nodules. They may resemble opalescent vesicles, and there may be an associated telangiectasis. Histologically they are composed of dilated lymphatic vessels in the upper dermis and are so closely linked to the epidermis as to appear incorporated in it. The overlying epidermis may be irregularly atrophied and acanthotic as well as hyperkeratotic in a papillary manner so as to simulate the angiokeratomas (see also p. 1627).

The lymphangioma cavernosum may be small and circumscribed, or it may extend diffusely over an extensive area, causing macrodactylia, for example. Histologically the lymphatic channels are greatly dilated and may extend into fat and muscle, as do the so-called infiltrating angiomas. The unencapsulated extensions are in neither instance evidence of malignant transformation, but they do complicate local removal.

The lymphangioma cysticum coli or hygroma is a congenital lesion that arises usually in the neck and submaxillary regions and is histologically similar to the lymphangioma cavernosum in both structure and extension. The hygroma may ramify widely upward to the parotid area, downward as far as the mediastinum, and inward to lie precariously close to the trachea and adjacent structures. The lymphangioma cysticum may occur also in the region of the sacrum (p. 726).

Hemangioma

The problems of the pathogenesis and terminology of tumors of blood vessels are even more complicated than those of lymphangiomas. Theoretically a true hemangioma is to be differentiated from a simple dilatation of blood vessels by its independence from the adjacent normal circulatory channels. A hemangioma enlarges, therefore, by growth of its own elements rather than by incorporation of nearby vessels. In practice, however, these criteria are seldom applied, and accordingly many ectasias, hyperemias, and hyperplasias are included as neoplasias. The hemangiomas may be classified simply as capillary, cavernous, or mixed (p. 721).

The capillary angioma corresponds clinically to the familiar port-wine stain on the face and neck, but it exists also as simple small vascular nevi or birthmarks. In infants, such angiomas may be composed of compact masses of endothelial cells in which the capillary lumina are obscured in many areas. These proliferations often extend from the dermis into the subcutaneous tissue. The extension of the lesion beyond the dermis and its rich cellularity may provoke the erroneous diagnosis of angiosarcoma.[68] However, such angiomatous formations are usually sufficiently characteristic to make possible the diagnosis of benign infantile angioma on the basis of histologic appearance alone. The capillary angioma may be confused histologically also with granuloma pyogenicum, particularly if the former is ulcerated and inflamed, as the latter usually is. The granuloma pyogenicum, however, is characteristically polypoid, generally has been present for no longer than 1 to 3 months, and bleeds easily and repeatedly. The histologic features of the granuloma pyogenicum are identical with those of the so-called pregnancy tumor that occurs in the oral mucosa during gestation. Thrombocytopenia may be associated with giant vascular tumors. The remission of the thrombocytopenia after removal of the hemangioma suggests that the tumor may occasionally serve as a reservoir for the platelets.

The sclerosing hemangioma appears to be a special variety of capillary angioma, although few dermatologists subscribe to this interpretation. They prefer to regard the lesion as a dermatofibroma lenticulare, histiocytoma, or merely subepidermal fibrosis. The lesions occur chiefly on the extremities and appear clinically as single, firm, and slightly elevated intracutaneous nodules, averaging several millimeters to a centimeter in diameter. Their sectioned surface is smooth and yellow.

Histologically, more or less of the dermis is replaced by spindle cells, arranged generally in tight curlicues, although in some areas these cells appear to enclose tiny spaces suggestive of the lumina of capillaries.

Occasionally the vascular luminal component is predominant, and the cavernous channels are characteristically associated with abundant hemosiderin and numerous lipid-filled macrophages. This aneurysmal feature has no signficance other than reflecting the vascular histogenesis of the lesion variously termed *fibrosis histiocytoma*, *dermatofibroma*, *fibroma dura*, and others. It may also be associated with pain and tenderness. This histologic variability matches that of the glomangioma, which also may range from a cellular to a cavernous pattern.

Usually the cells are vacuolated by lipid, and in some cases the fat content is the most striking feature. Dark brown granules of hemosiderin are often present in many of the cells. At times the iron pigment may be so abundant that some observers, confusing the pigment with melanin, have made the serious error of labeling the lesion a malignant melanoma. The overlying epidermis may be normal, atrophied, moderately acanthotic, or the site of a superimposed basal cell carcinoma[36] (Fig. 38-47). In some instances a sharply delimited subepidermal zone of the dermis is spared. A similar free zone is seen in the dermal neurofibroma, although perhaps not so frequently. The sclerosing hemangioma may sometimes be justifiably confused with the neurofibroma when, as not infrequently occurs, the deeper portion of the lesion is composed of fasciculi of spindle cells such as characterize the neurofibroma. The impression gained by light microscopy of the hemangiomatous origin of these lesions is confirmed by the observation of We,bel-Palade bodies with the electron microscope. These are intracytoplasmic tubular structures, presumably derived from the Golgi apparatus and apparently specific for endothelial cells.

Occasionally a fibrotic tumor resembling the sclerosing hemangioma, particularly of the trunk, recurs locally with formation of satellite nodules. Usually such tumors originally extended into the subcutaneous fat and were removed incompletely. These tumors, called dermatofibrosarcoma protuberans, give rise to distant metastases in rare instances.

The cavernous hemangiomas are histologically similar to the cavernous lymphangiomas except for the presence of blood in the congeries of vessels. The vessels may ramify progressively in the subcutaneous fat, fascia, and intermuscular septa. The extensions may be so wide and inaccessible as to make surgical removal exceedingly difficult. The term *infiltrating angioma* is more aptly applied to such tumors than is *angiosarcoma*.

Clinically the cavernous hemangiomas appear on the skin surface as purple, single, globular or multilobular tumors or as the flat or slightly elevated strawberry nevus of infants. The angiomas may be multiple and may cause, or at least be associated with, enlargement and distortion of an area of the body in the vicinity of the tumors. The distortion from edema and hypertrophy of an arm (Weber syndrome) may be so great as to require amputation because of the sheer weight of the extremity.

Other syndromes associated with anomalies of blood vessels include the Sturge-Weber syndrome (nevus flammeus of the face, cerebral angiomatosis, hemiplegia, and mental retardation), Maffucci's syndrome (angiomas with dyschondroplasia), and heredofamilial angiomatosis (Rendu-Osler-Weber disease). Cutaneous angiomas also may be part of the complex of multiple congenital angiomas found in the viscera, particularly in the cerebellum and retina, and known as Hippel's disease. The blue rubber-bleb nevus appears to be a form of venous hamartoma involving both skin and gastrointestinal tract. It is

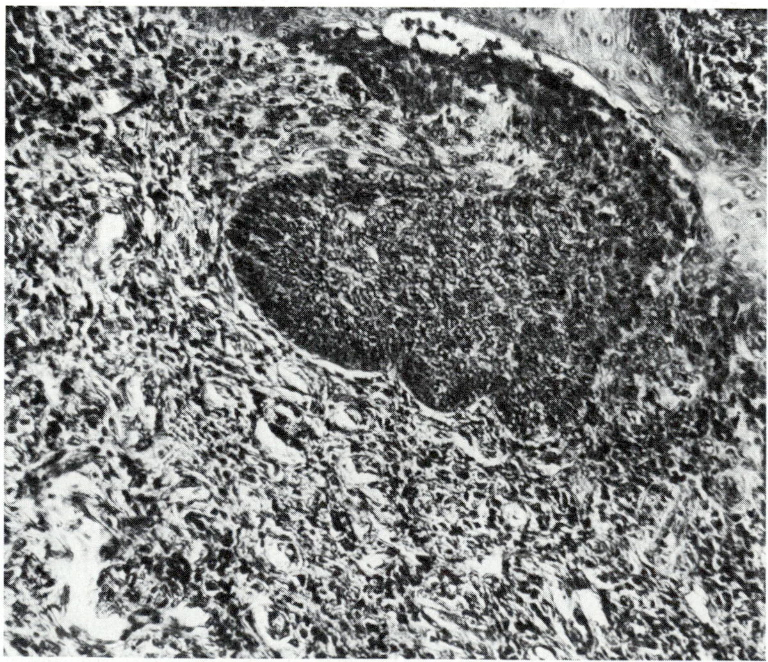

Fig. 38-47. Sclerosing angioma with overlying nest of basal cell carcinoma in situ. (Hematoxylin and eosin.)

characterized by pain, sweating, and a sensation of dermal herniation.[59]

The angiokeratoma or telangiectatic wart represents a variety of cavernous hemangioma that is structurally similar to the lymphangioma cutis circumscriptum. The dilated blood channels are high in the papillae and are so intimately associated with the epidermis as to appear actually within it in many places. The overlying epidermis is usually papillary, acanthotic, and hyperkeratotic. Clinically the lesions are dark purplish red, firm, the size of a pinhead or split pea, and located in the scrotum, ears, fingers, and toes. The lesions often are associated with some circulatory disturbance such as might follow chilblains and varicosites. This type that tends to occur on the extensor surface of the extremities is known as the Mibelli type of angiokeratoma as opposed to Fordyce's type without associated pernio. The angiokeratoma of Fabry may be associated with lesions of viscera, particularly the kidneys and vessels, with characteristic foam cells. Patients with angiokeratoma of Fabry may excrete increased amounts of the glycoproteins ceramide trihexoside and dihexoside. Examination of the urine for these glycoproteins may aid in the detection of the disorder in members of the families of patients.

Spider angiomas, which are really small telangiectases, possibly with arteriovenous shunts, occur with chronic hepatic damage as in Laennec's cirrhosis, as well as in pregnancy. They are believed to be an effect of excess of estrogenic hormones.

The term "hemangioendothelioma," as previously indicated, is hedgingly applied to hemangiomas in which there is a relative prominence of endothelial cells with or without atypia. The implication in its use is that the neoplasm shows greater activity and therefore presents more likelihood of local recurrence than the ordinary hemangioma. The evidence for this presumption is questionable. A similar situation exists with respect to the use of "lymphangioendothelioma." Unfortunately, the name "hemangioendothelioma," rather than "angiosarcoma," is sometimes applied to the frankly malignant tumor.

Cutaneous meningioma

The cutaneous meningioma occurs as an isolated dysembryogenetic subcutaneous nodule with occasional dermal involvement, or as an ectopic extension into soft tissue corresponding in distribution to cranial and spinal nerves. The latter may cause signs and symptoms reflective of the associated nerves or those of a tumor mass such as proptosis, nasal polyp, or soft tissue mass. The histologic picture is that of a meningothelial cell tumor or sclerosing angioma with characteristic psammoma bodies.[46]

Angiosarcoma

Primary solitary angiosarcoma of the skin, exclusive of Kaposi's hemorrhagic sarcoma, is rare. However, several cases have been recorded in which visceral metastases have occurred. The metastases tend to be more cellular and anaplastic than the original growth. Others have been reported as malignant vascular tumors of skin under the title *hemangioendothelioma*, but in most instances evidence of origin from dermis, as well as of the cancerous characteristics, is not convincingly presented. Knowledge of the rarity of such tumors is of practical importance because of its tempering effect on the tendency to call sarcomatous those nonmetastasizing angiomas with abundant endothelial cells or those that have infiltrated into the subcutaneous fat and beyond into the muscles. The Kaposi sarcoma, on the other hand, represents a process of vastly different significance.

Kaposi's idiopathic hemorrhagic sarcoma

Kaposi's sarcoma begins as reddish to purplish brown, discrete or grouped, painful, tender nodules varying from 1 to 2 mm in size to about 1 cm. They occur particularly on the hands and feet, although they may start in the skin of any part of the body. The incidence is about 10 times greater in men than in women, and the disease is seen especially in elderly patients, although it has been described in children. The surface of the nodules may be telangiectatic, but often it is verrucose. Local purpura and bullae may be associated with the lesions. Lymphatic blockage with elephantiasis of the extremities is common and is reminiscent of the edema associated with postmastectomy lymphangiosarcoma. The course of the disease is slow, the nodules often involuting, with resultant atrophic scarring and pigmentation. The condition may last from 1 to fully 25 years, although the average duration is from 5 to 10 years. The disease is found chiefly in Italian and Jewish people.

The lesions may involve extensive areas of the skin and nearly every organ of the body. The gastrointestinal tract, mesenteric nodes, liver, and lungs are the most common sites, although even the osseous and central nervous systems may be affected. The question is unsettled as to whether these lesions are truly metastases or actually multicentric foci of a neoplasm. The intestinal lesions of Kaposi's sarcoma, unlike most other metastatic lesions, have a predilection for the inner coats rather than the serosa. In this location the tumors give rise to profuse hemorrhage. This difference in location in the intestinal tract between the Kaposi's sarcoma and other metastatic tumors is evidence in favor of the multicentric origin of the former. Visceral tumors histologically identical to Kaposi's sarcoma have been found infrequently without cutaneous involvement. Patients with Kaposi's sarcoma die of hemorrhage from an intestinal lesion, intercurrent infection, extensive visceral involvement, or complicating malignant lymphomas.

Kaposi's sarcoma is a form of angiosarcoma that is so varied histologically that there is frequently difficulty in the interpretation of a given slide. In one phase, perhaps the earliest, the picture is that of a simple hemangioma or of foci of hyperemic, nonspecific granulation tissue characterized by clusters of capillaries placed close together, with or without a sprinkling of mononuclear cells and histiocytes containing hemosiderin in the intervening and often edematous stroma. At this stage the endothelial cells may be quite regular, without mitotic figures or other evidence of anaplasia. The important histologic clue is the disposition of these vascular foci not only near the epidermis, but also isolated about appendages in the deeper layers of the dermis. The presence of such vascular foci at a distance from the surface of the skin is suspiciously unlike the ordinary pattern of the response of skin to inflammation. In more advanced lesions there occurs proliferation of spindle cells and fibroblasts in association with scattered lymphocytes and histiocytes. The cells appear to form abortive capillaries, and in the actively growing lesions these cells are large and hyperchromatic and contain mitotic figures. In the later stages there is a tendency toward focal necrosis of the neoplastic tissue and subsequent fibrosis. These variegated pictures may be observed not only at different stages of the disease but often within a single lesion.

There is an increasing number of reports in the literature of the simultaneous occurrence of Kaposi's sarcoma with one or another of the malignant lymphomas, including Hodgkin's disease, lymphatic leukemia, lymphosarcoma, and mycosis fungoides. For both statistical and histologic reasons (the latter comprising evidence of transition of the two processes within the same lesion), the association is not considered coincidental.[6,9]

Acquired immune deficiency syndrome

In 1980 the United States, and later the world, was jolted by the outbreak of hundreds of instances of a dreaded form of Kaposi's sarcoma with a fulminance previously unknown, as part of a symptom complex now known as AIDS (acquired immune deficiency syndrome). Kaposi's sarcoma occurs in about one third of the cases. As of this writing approximately 1500 cases have been recorded, with a mortality close to 40% within 2 years and almost twice that rate beyond 2 years. The patients have been concentrated in New York City, with a predilection among male homosexuals, users of intravenous drugs, hemophiliacs and other blood recipients, and possibly Haitian immigrants. Adding a frightening new epidemiologic dimension are the recent discoveries that the disease may be transmitted heterosexually and among prison populations. Fear of the unknown has caused landlords to evict tenants with this disease.

The incubation period is highly variable, and the etiology thus far is unknown. In these immunologically deficient individuals, complication by rampaging opportunistic organisms (for example, *Pneumocystis carinii*, cytomegalovirus) is naturally frequent and often lethal. The histologic characteristics of the cutaneous Kaposi's sarcoma parallel the spectrum of the more slowly evolving counterpart. Although no causative organisms have yet been implicated in these nodules themselves, it is of ancillary interest that verruga peruana, the cutaneous form of bartonellosis, appears histologically as an angiomatoid lesion in which the tiny organisms are harbored within the endothelial cytoplasm, much as are rickettsiae. To date the etiologic agent of AIDS in these immunosuppressed persons is unknown.

The more than fortuitous relationship of the indolent, rare, old form of Kaposi's sarcoma to various types of malignant lymphomas may be related to the immunologic problem in AIDS. For example, in AIDS the normal 2:1 ratio of helper/suppressive T cells is reversed. The helper cells are also misshapen, further supporting the concept of immunologic compromise. Lymph nodes and spleens show a depletion of lymphocytes. The Kaposi's sarcoma of equatorial Africa (Kenya, Zaire, Tanzania) is more akin to that of AIDS in that it is virulent and attacks the young. But evidence of immunologic deficiency in the traditional form of torpid Kaposi's sarcoma has not been forthcoming (Fig. 38-48).

Postmastectomy lymphangiosarcoma

In 1948 an entity described as lymphangiosarcoma was recorded[69] as a complication of postmastectomy lymphedema of the upper extremity.[63] The lymphangiosarcoma in the skin of the edematous arm developed 6 to 24 years after the mastectomy, with the lymphedema having existed during the entire latent period. In one instance the tumor of the breast was benign. There was no relationship between the use of radiation and the development of the lymphangiosarcoma. As originally suspected, lymphangiosarcoma may complicate chronic edema, including congenital lymphedema of extremities unassociated with mammary carcinoma or its treatment.

Histologically the sarcoma has a range of variation quite equal to that of Kaposi's sarcoma, and indeed in many sections one cannot be certain that the neoplastic elements are lymphatic vessels rather than blood sinuses. The tumor is capable of metastasizing. Rare instances of lymphangiosarcoma as a complication of the lymphedema of filariasis have been recorded. The mechanism of cancerogenesis in the cases of lymphedema is obscure.

Glomus tumor

In the corium of the skin of the fingertips, particularly in the nail beds, around the joints of the extremities, and over the scapulae and coccyx, there are normally arteriovenous shunts or glomera. These are composed of an afferent artery, the Sucquet-Hoyer canal or shunt, and

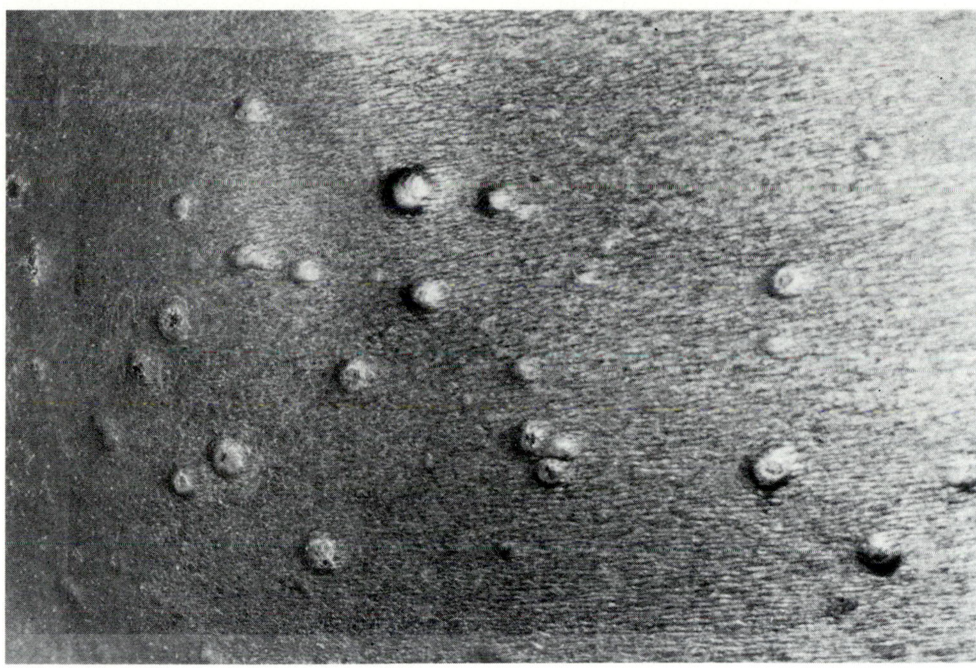

Fig. 38-48. Acquired immune deficiency syndrome. Nodules of cryptococcosis on back.

an efferent vein. The artery is surrounded by several layers of small, spherical uniform glomus cells that superficially resemble the cells of the intradermal nevus and that are presumed to control the flow of blood by their contractility. Nonmedullated nerves and bundles of smooth muscle are intimately associated with the shunt. Tumors of this structure are called glomangiomas, angiomyoneuromas, glomus tumors, or neuromyoarterial aneurysms. They are most common in the nail bed but occur elsewhere on the extremities and trunk and even beneath the skin in muscles and joints, as well as in viscera. No instance of tumor occurring in the coccygeal glomus has been observed.

Glomus tumors appear as purplish red spots several millimeters in diameter, which are often clinically diagnosable by a characteristically lancinating pain, remarkably severe in view of the small size of the tumors. Not all glomangiomas, however, are associated with this characteristic symptom, which occasionally is simulated by dermal angiomyomas.

Histologically the glomus tumors range from compact masses of uniform glomus cells with few vascular channels to cavernous skeins of vessels cuffed by these cells. The vessels of the tumors tend to be small, especially in the nail bed. The identifying features are the several rows of peritheliomatously arranged glomus cells in which mitotic figures are rare or absent. These cells may be so numerous as to obliterate vascular lumina and to resemble a basal cell tumor or a variety of sweat gland adenoma. Nonmedullated nerves usually are discerned, but there appears to be no apparent relationship between the pain and the number or location of these nerves. Occasionally, glomus tumors are called simply hemangiomas or glomangioid tumors because of the presence of only two or three perivascular rows of glomus cells. However, such tumors have been observed with the typical symptoms of glomangiomas. Ultrastructural studies reveal masses of cytoplasmic fibers suggestive of a transition from smooth muscle cells.

Tumors of muscle

Two varieties of tumors of dermal muscle are described: leiomyoma (arising from arrectores pilorum) and angiomyoma. What are called granular cell myoblastomas are lesions that were believed to have been myogenic.

Leiomyoma cutis

The leiomyoma cutis occurs singly or in groups of as many as dozens of firm, usually pea-sized nodules, which are often tender and painful. Histologically they are composed of interlacing sheets of smooth muscle that may resemble a haphazard compact collection of arrectores pilorum. Infrequently the nuclei are large, irregular in size and shape, and hyperchromatic so as to merit the terms *leiomyosarcoma cutis* or *dermatomyosarcoma*.

Leiomyosarcomas, primarily originating in the skin and less frequently in the subcutaneous tissue, occur rarely; approximately 80 such cases have been documented.[29] In these persons they appeared as painful or tender nodules, most commonly on the extremities of middle-aged individuals. None of the cutaneous leiomyosarcomas metastasized, whereas almost 50% of the subcutaneous lesions, even though initially circumscribed, metastasized or behaved aggressively.

The cutaneous leiomyosarcomas arise chiefly from arrectores pilorum, directly or via leiomyomas; the subcutaneous leiomyosarcomas arise from the media of blood vessels.

Angiomyoma

The angiomyoma is a small nondescript nodule that, microscopically, is made up of circular masses of smooth muscle strongly reminiscent of the media of arteries. The residual arterial lumen is discernible in the core of many of the masses of muscle. These lesions remain benign. Occasionally they may be found in the subcutaneous fat or even more deeply in the fascia or intermuscular septa of the extremities. As stated, they may cause the sharp pain generally associated with glomangiomas.

Myoblastoma

The granular cell myoblastoma is found as a nodule in the skin of various parts of the body, as well as on the mucous membranes, particularly of the tongue and isolated sites such as the larynx, thyroid gland, breast, gallbladder, esophagus, stomach, appendix, pituitary gland, and uvea.

Histologically the tumors are composed of nests and alveoli of large cells with small, centrally placed nuclei in cytoplasm loosely stippled with eosinophilic granules, occasionally replaced by polyhedral crystalloids. These periodic acid–Schiff–positive granules appear to contain lipoprotein or glycolipid and ultrastructurally may be amorphous, vesicular, vacuolar, or particulate. The cells closely resemble those of a xanthoma, but fat stains are negative. Close examination shows that the cytoplasm is not actually vacuolated, as are lipid histiocytes. The loose dispersion of granules that simulate vacuoles has been believed to represent embryonic fibrils of striated muscle cells. Such a hypothesis is open to question, inasmuch as these tumors are present in the corium and other sites where striated muscle does not occur. The same objection may be leveled at the hypothesis that these cells represent degenerated adult striated fibers, although in sites where striated muscle is normally present, such as the tongue, this kind of transition occasionally is suggested. In my opinion the evidence for the neurogenesis is not adequate. The concept of a fibroplastic origin has been advanced and appears far more convincing. In any event, whether or not these tumors are proved eventually to be fibroblastic, it is clear that they are easily recognizable histologic entities that rarely if ever metastasize. Some of the so-called malignant granular cell myoblastomas are, in reality, unrelated rhabdomyosarcomas in which a few of the cells happen to be granular.

One of the remarkable and distinctive features of many of the myoblastomas is the characteristic epithelial or epidermal acanthosis that overlies the lesion. This feature is not present in association with frank cutaneous leiomyomas. As a rule, dermal neoplasms leave the epidermis essentially unaltered or cause its atrophy through compression. The myoblastomas, on the other hand, appear to provoke a degree of acanthosis that may simulate squamous cell carcinoma. It is as if some epidermal irritant were present in the cells of the myoblastoma (Fig. 38-49). An analogous epidermal proliferation over-

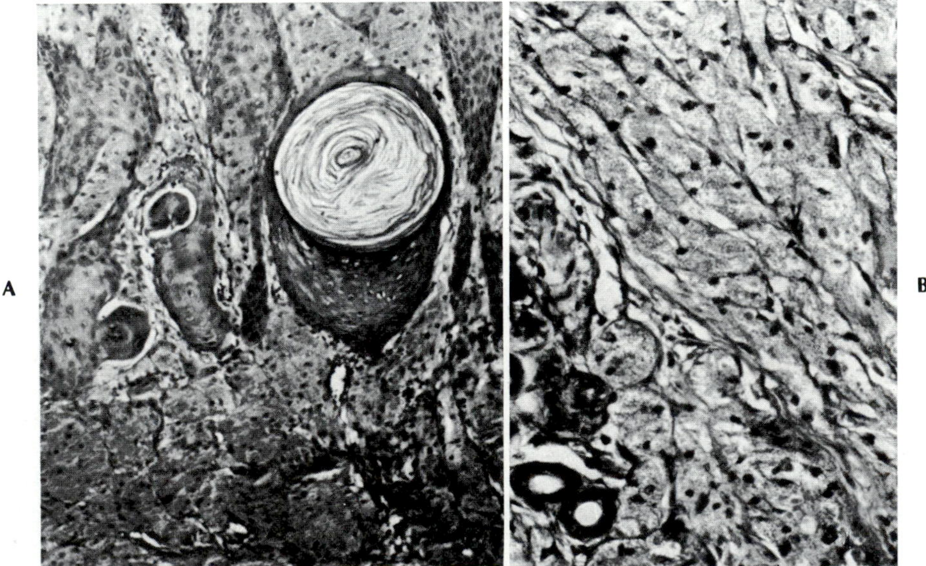

Fig. 38-49. Myoblastoma. **A,** Characteristic pseudoepitheliomatous hyperplasia. **B,** Granular cytoplasm and uniform small nuclei. (Hematoxylin and eosin.)

lies many of the sclerosing angiomas, as previously mentioned.

Cutaneous fibroma

The diagnosis of cutaneous fibroma is usually found on careful review to include dermatofibroma lenticulare or sclerosing hemangioma, neurofibroma, leiomyoma, keloids, and other scars. This confusion does not apply to the pedunculated soft lipofibromas (fibroma molle) in which the fibrous component closely simulates the normal dermal collagen. Undoubtedly some of the spindle-shaped squamous cell carcinomas and melanocarcinomas have been mistaken for fibrosarcomas and atypical fibroxanthomas of the skin.

Digital fibrous tumors of childhood

A form of well-differentiated, occasionally locally recurrent fibroma of childhood occurs on all digits but the thumb and great toe. Histologically they appear to be cellular fascial or dermal fibromas. They are characterized by a single, paranuclear, eosinophilic cytoplasmic inclusion attributed to a metabolic derangement.[21]

Neurofibroma

Neurofibroma may occur in the skin as a single tumor or as multiple nodules. In the latter condition the entity is classified as neurofibromatosis or von Recklinghausen's disease and may be associated with café au lait pigmented spots and neurofibromas of the sympathetic system, as well as of motor and sensory nerve trunks. The tumors of the skin may be so numerous as to cover almost the entire body from scalp to feet.

The histogenesis of the tumors is complex. The axons, as well as the nerve sheaths (neurilemma) and endoneurium, participate to a varying extent, so that the histologic picture may be altered accordingly. The tumor derived predominantly from nerve sheaths (neurilemoma) tends to manifest more obvious palisading of cells (Antoni A structure), degenerating, edematous microcystic foci (Antoni B), and hyaline Verocay bodies. Occasionally the neurilemoma presents pronounced central necrosis and such excessive telangiectasis that it can be mistaken for an angioma. An examination of the periphery of these degenerated tumors usually reveals the telltale palisading of the neurilemoma. A small percentage of the cutaneous neurofibromas show sufficient hyperchromatism and irregularity in size and shape of nuclei to suggest sarcomatous degeneration. Here, too, however, metastases from these neoplasms of the skin are rare, although local recurrence is fairly frequent. On the other hand, malignant changes in the visceral neurofibromas are common and may take the form of extensive, fatal, local infiltrations or metastases (p. 1925). The benign neurilemoma (schwannoma) undergoes malignant change with extreme rarity. However, malignant neurilemomas do occur. These are presumed not to have developed from a benign neurilemoma but to have been malignant from the start. These, too, are uncommon.

Osteoma

Osteoma cutis, an example merely of heterotopic bone, represents a metaplastic change of dermal collagen rather than true neoplasia. The lesion occurs as small nodules, as a rule, in scleroderma or syphilis, in association with acne or intradermal nevi, with hyperparathyroidism, and after trauma or cystotomies—the latter because of the osteogenic potentialities of urinary tract epithelium or without apparent reason.

The histologic picture may include fat and even marrow cells in addition to the bony trabeculae.

Lymphomas and allied diseases

The lymphomas and allied diseases of the skin include mycosis fungoides, Hodgkin's disease, lymphosarcoma, and leukemia.

Mycosis fungoides

There has been renewed interest in the histogenesis, histology, and natural history of the entity long ago and still unhappily labeled mycosis fungoides. It is a lymphomatous disease in which the cutaneous component is characterized clinically by three stages: (1) premycotic, (2) infiltrative, and (3) fungoid tumefaction.

The premycotic stage is characterized by eczematoid, severely pruritic, erythrodermic, scaly, well-defined patches or by a generalized erythroderma. The eruption in this phase may simulate eczema, psoriasis, parapsoriasis, seborrheic dermatitis, or a nonspecific exfoliative dermatitis. This stage may persist for months or years and may be impossible to diagnose with assurance either clinically or microscopically. In the second or infiltrative stage, firm, slightly elevated, bluish red plaques arise in both the previously involved and the uninvolved areas. Partial or incomplete loss of hair from the scalp and other regions may occur. The last or fungoid stage follows the infiltrative period by several months.

The tumors vary in diameter up to 10 cm or larger and are prone to ulcerate. In each of the stages spontaneous remissions may be noted, but these are temporary. Of interest in this respect is the regression—albeit temporary—of cutaneous lesions of mycosis fungoides occurring after reactions of delayed hypersensitivity provoked directly in the lesions. The diagnosis in the few reported instances of cure must be questioned. In some cases the preliminary two stages do not develop. This form is called mycosis fungoides d'emblée. True instances of mycosis fungoides d'emblée must be exceedingly rare. Undoubtedly, most of the recorded cases are, in reality, examples of Hodgkin's disease, reticulum cell sarcoma, or leukemia.

Sézary syndrome or reticulosis is a variant of mycosis fungoides consisting of erythroderma and Sézary cells in the peripheral blood, marrow, and lymphocytes. The likelihood is that the Sézary cells and the atypical cells of mycosis fungoides, with indented, convoluted, or cerebriform nuclei, are identical and represent T lymphocytes.[48] Similar cells have been noted in normal individuals, in patients with benign dermatoses, and after stimulation of lymphocytes with mitogens.[76] Actually, mycosis fungoides is being regarded as a response to antigenic persistence with malignant lymphoma developing as a consequence of immunologic imbalance. Perhaps related in principle is the occurrence of reticulum cell sarcoma in recipients of renal transplants with immunosuppressive therapy, as others have suggested.

The histologic picture of the first or premycotic stage of mycosis fungoides is usually not diagnostic and may resemble one of the many conditions simulated clinically. However, even in this phase of the disease there is a tendency for the infiltrate to be confined as a zone in the upper dermis and for the epidermis to appear psoriasiform. Occasionally, large single or binucleated hyperchromatic cells are observed, as well as a rare infiltrative cell in mitosis, affording a clue. In the subsequent stages the infiltrate, still selecting the upper dermis principally, becomes dense and polymorphous. In this variegated infiltrate the presence of eosinophilic leukocytes and cells that simulate the Reed-Sternberg cell of Hodgkin's disease and often an abundance of small and large (Marschalko) plasma cells constitutes the evidence for mycosis fungoides. In addition, there is a tendency toward scattered clumping of cells of the infiltrate. The epidermis tends to be moderately acanthotic and hyperkeratotic with focal spongiosis and small intraepidermal "microabscesses" of Darier-Pautrier. These "microabscesses" are actually foci of tumor cells that have extended into the epidermis. Their absence does not preclude the diagnosis (Fig. 38-50). The quality of the infiltrate may be indistinguishable from that of Hodgkin's disease. The cutaneous infiltrate of Hodgkin's disease tends to be irregularly distributed in parts of the dermis. The critical point is that the histologic changes even in the premycotic erythrodermatous stage are usually of the pattern and quality that, if properly evaluated, permit the diagnosis to be made.

Potentially the most revealing and yet most disputed morphologic clues to the nature of mycosis fungoides are the findings at autopsy. Recent reports indicate visceral involvement in abut 70% of cases in contrast with our finding some years ago of approximately 20%.[58] However, a good deal of this involvement consists of scattered microscopic foci of atypical cells. This applies especially to the lung, which may be involved microscopically in about two thirds of cases.[75] It has been suggested that the lower incidence in our material may reflect the longer survival in later series because of supportive measures not previously available. The peripheral lymph nodes often are enlarged because of their drainage of pigment and other material from the infiltrated skin. Such nodes—now called dermatopathic lymphadenopathy—

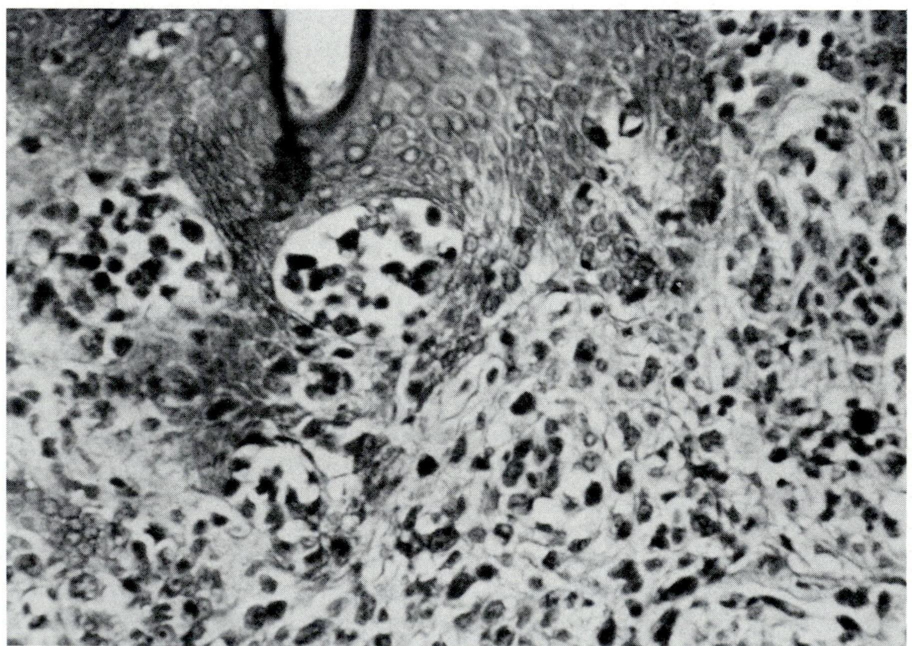

Fig. 38-50. Mycosis fungoides with Pautrier-Darier abscesses and characteristic subepidermal infiltrate. (Hematoxylin and eosin.)

show partial obliteration of their architecture by reticulum cell hyperplasia, deposits of melanin and fat, and—an especially common and presumptive clue in mycosis fungoides—numerous plasma cells. Similar plasma cells are generally in the bone marrow and spleen and occasionally even contain Russell bodies. These nonspecifically altered lymph nodes of Pautrier and Woringer may be mistaken for those of Hodgkin's disease.

Pagetoid reticulosis

Pagetoid reticulosis (Woringer-Kolopp disease) is regarded by some as an epidermotrophic variant of mycosis fungoides, but the absence of focal Pautrier microabscesses and of abnormal Lutzner-like cells in the dermis in pagetoid reticulosis has served to distinguish it from mycosis fungoides.

Hodgkin's disease, lymphosarcoma, leukemia

The criteria for the histologic recognition in the skin of Hodgkin's disease, lymphosarcoma, and the various leukemias are the same as those used for the visceral lesions. Additional clues are offered by the almost constant denseness of the infiltrate, immediately noted with low-power magnification, and the selectivity of the infiltrate for the upper dermis in some instances of leukemia (Fig. 38-50). An important deceptive feature of the lymphomas is the occurrence also of quite nonspecific cutaneous reactions in which neoplastic cells are absent. These reactions may take the clinical form of toxic erythema, excoriated pruritic exfoliative erythroderma, generalized pigmentation, urticaria, and herpes zoster. Severe nonspecific cutaneous reactions lead to dermatopathic lymphadenopathy, changes in the regional lymph nodes, which may become so enlarged as to be clinically indistinguishable from lymphomas. Among the most difficult neoplasms to evaluate from a biopsy specimen of skin are Letterer-Siwe disease of infancy and the related malignant histiocytoses of childhood, that is, the so-called reticuloendothelioses, histiocytosis X, or lipid and nonlipid histiocytoses. The crux of the problem is the decision as to whether the cutaneous lesion indicates visceral involvement and a fatal prognosis or merely a local histiocytosis or variant of xanthomatosis. In general, the degree of anaplasia and the compactness of the infiltrate of the monocytoid cells in the upper dermis are of great importance in suggesting the grave nature of the disease. However, remarkable disparities have been noted by Spitz.[68]

Another source of clinical and histologic confusion is the entity known as Spiegler-Fendt sarcoid, which is characterized by grouped, local or disseminated, bright red nodules. The histologic diagnosis is based principally on the finding of mature lymphocytes, as well as reticulum cells either scattered or as germinal centers of follicles. Anaplasia of the infiltrate or histologic evidence of appreciable activity is lacking. It is obvious that differentiation of this lesion from lymphosarcoma must, at times, require a great nicety of judgment. Indeed, some of the cases originally but erroneously considered to be Spiegler-Fendt sarcoid have been recorded as having terminated in lymphosarcoma. Further confusion results from the use of the term *benign lymphocytoma*, which is popular in dermatologic literature. This lesion, which may be single or multiple, resembles Boeck's sarcoid, leukemic infiltration, or discoid lupus erythematosus clinically. Histologically it consists essentially of dense masses of mature lymphocytes that may be arranged in follicles with germinal centers. As might be anticipated, the lesions are highly radiosensitive.

Lymphomatoid granulomatosis

Lymphomatoid granulomatosis is a focal, scattered, largely lymphocytic infiltration of the lung concentrated about vessels, both adventitially and intramurally. Since this disorder was first described in 1972, there has been confusion as to the malignant potential of the process. The nature of the lymphocytic infiltrate made it seem likely that the disease might develop in other organs. Indeed, the skin has been found to be involved by a similar infiltrate in about 40% of patients.[40]

The dispersed nodular dermal and subcutaneous infiltrate may include rare multinucleated giant cells and polymorphonuclear leukocytes as well as plasma cells, eosinophils, mature lymphocytes, and distinctly atypical lymphoreticular cells or histiocytes. In one series malignant lymphoma developed in eight of 44 patients within months after the initial diagnosis, often similar to the class of immunoblastic sarcoma.[40] The specific diagnosis of cutaneous lymphomatoid granulomatosis is largely dependent on the association with systemic signs such as neuropathy, arthropathy, and pulmonary diseases.

Lymphomatoid papulosis

Lymphomatoid papulosis is another disease made nosologically enigmatic because of the confusion regarding whether it is inflammatory or neoplastic.[50] As with the reactions to arthropod bites, it has two components: epidermal and dermal. The epidermal reaction commonly, but not always, consists of acanthosis, spongiosis with microvesiculation and neutrophilic crusting, and the transepidermal migration of cells from the dermal infiltrate. The latter consists prototypically of small and large lymphocytes and histiocytes, with a variable admixture of neutrophils and, at times, eosinophils. The infiltrate tends to hug the epidermis in lichenoid fashion and to extend diminishingly toward the subcutis. The disturbing feature is the large hyperchromatic lymphocytes, occasionally in mitosis, that encourage the diagnosis of malignant lymphoma. Indeed, at this point approximately 10% of patients appear actually to develop malignant lymphoma; in the remainder the lesions tend to appear in crops and defloresce with fibrosis. In my opinion the epidermal changes are not an integral part of the lesion. Rather, they appear ischemogenic, possibly related to the common endarteritis and phlebitis of the appertaining upper dermal vessels. Similar epidermal reactions are seen as a result of primary vascular diseases, including microembolization.

Diagnostically the most impressive cell is the atypical large lymphocyte, which suggests that there is a relationship between lymphomatoid papulosis and the eventual development of a malignant lymphoma. Accompanying cells include small lymphocytes, eosinophils, and intradermal, intravascular, and intraepidermal neutrophils. This lesion, along with mycosis fungoides and Sézary syndrome, is of T cell nature.[77]

Lymphomatoid papulosis has been observed with glomerulonephritis, rheumatoid arthritis, a mycosis fungoides–like picture, and in immunosuppressed patients. The papules develop in crops over a period of weeks on the extremities and trunk. The mononuclear cell infiltrate may be concentrated about blood vessels throughout the dermis along with lower epidermal necrosis and scattered atypical large T lymphocytes so atypical as to make it difficult to believe that the process will not eventuate as a malignant lymphoma.[20,26] The benign lymphocytic infiltrates tend preferentially to include the upper dermis, and the solitary lymphomatoid papule is likely to have a prominent intraepidermal component. Germinal centers within the dermal infiltrates favor hyperplasia.

Graft versus host disease

Graft versus host disease follows the increasing use of allogeneic bone marrow transplantation as therapy for aplastic anemia, leukemia, and genetic dysfunction of the marrow. The skin and other organs, such as the liver and gastrointestinal tract, may participate in the reaction. The skin shows an angry liquefaction degeneration at the dermoepidermal junction, with infiltration of lymphocytes and piecemeal eosinophilic necrosis of keratinocytes (Fig. 38-51). Sclerodermatous changes may develop in the more chronic reactions.

Reactions to arthropods

In 1948 I called attention to the remarkable diagnostically troublesome biphasic cutaneous reactions to the arthropods, or insect bites.[3] These reactions involve the epidermis and the dermis. The dermal lesion is commonly mistaken for one of the lymphomas. The reaction usually consists of eosinophilic leukocytes, histiocytes, plasma cells, and reticulum cells, with the last occasionally binucleated and even in mitosis. In some lesions there are also prominent lymphoid follicles with germinal centers. Often such an innocuous reaction has been given

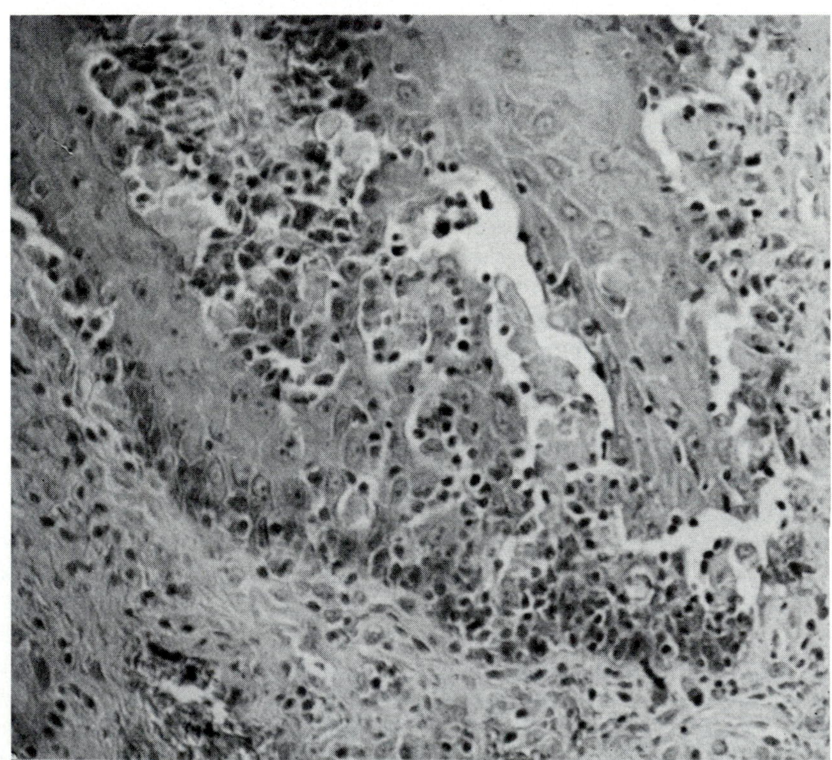

Fig. 38-51. Graft versus host reaction showing transepidermal migration of lymphocytes, liquefactive separation of dermoepidermal junction, and eosinophilic degeneration of keratinocytes.

the grave diagnosis of Hodgkin's disease, mycosis fungoides, or lymphosarcoma. Part of the reason for the error is that it is not generally appreciated that the reaction to arthopods may persist for many months. The presence of only a single lesion is suggestive evidence, in doubtful cases, of an insect bite. However, an isolated lesion may occur also in the neoplastic conditions.

A similar pseudolymphomatous cutaneous reaction may occur after injection of antigens for hyposensitization. The other deceptive reaction to the venom of insects and ticks is the pseudoepitheliomatous hyperplasias that may be mistaken for squamous cell carcinoma (Fig. 38-52).[4]

Eosinophilic granulomas and Jessner's lymphocytosis of the skin of the face also may be erroneously misinterpreted as forms of malignant lymphomas. Lethal midline granuloma refers to a fulminant, destructive ulceration of the nose and paranasal tissues often resulting from Wegener's granulomatosis or one of the malignant lymphomas. The abundant necrosis, along with secondary vascular involvement, commonly obscures the precise histologic diagnosis.

Kawasaki disease

Kawasaki disease (mucocutaneous lymph node syndrome) occurs in children under 10 years of age and is characterized by fever, pharyngitis, an exanthem, edema, and erythema of the hands followed by desquamation of the fingertips, and nonpurulent cervical lymphadenopathy. Death in 1% to 2% of instances is predominantly the result of coronary arteritis.[42] The cause is unknown.

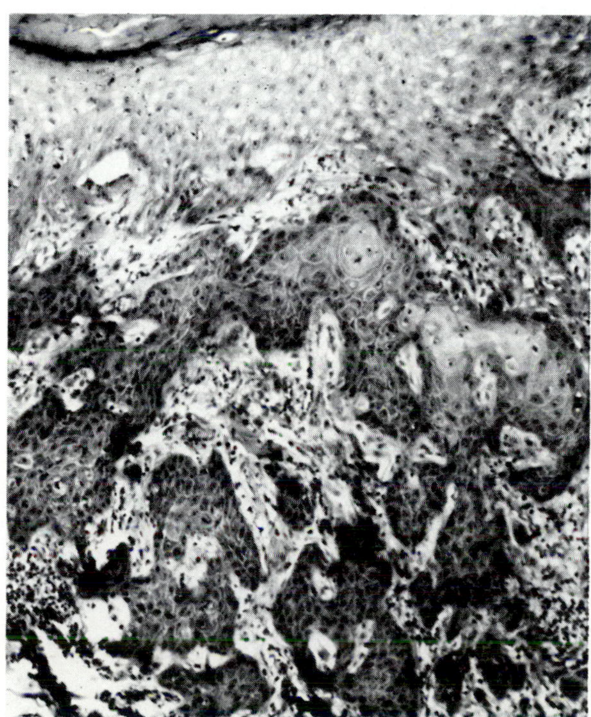

Fig. 38-52. Tick bite with pseudoepitheliomatous hyperplasia simulating squamous cell carcinoma. (Hematoxylin and eosin.)

Metastatic neoplasms

Cancerous metastases reach the skin by direct invasion or through the lymphatics or blood vessels. The most common metastases include those from carcinomas of the breast, uterus, lung, gastrointestinal tract, pancreas, thyroid gland, and prostate gland, in addition to those from melanocarcinomas, epidermoid carcinomas and lymphomas, and sarcomas of bone, muscle, and fascia.

There is generally little difficulty in recognizing the metastatic character of a tumor in the skin except of course in the case of the lymphomas and in Kaposi's sarcoma. In both of these instances the possibility of autochthonous multicentric origin is to be considered. Plasma cell myeloma occasionally involves skin. A nodule of malignant melanoma usually may be recognized as metastatic by the presence of an overlying intact epidermis showing no evidence of junctional change. Occasionally a metastatic focus of adenocarcinoma is mistaken for a primary cutaneous carcinoma of sweat gland origin, or extramammary Paget's disease.[9]

Tumors of dermal appendages

Following is a classification of benign tumors of the sweat apparatus:

A. Ductal (syringal)
   1. Eccrine
      a. Inverted, papillary syringoma (eccrine poroma, intraepidermal or dermal or both)
      b. Lobular syringoma (eccrine spiradenoma)
      c. Lobular hyalinized syringoma (cylindroma)
      d. Diffuse syringoma
   2. Apocrine
      a. Syringocystadenoma papilliferum
B. Glandular
   1. Eccrine cystadenoma with chondral metaplasia
   2. Apocrine cystoma or cystadenoma
   3. Hamartoma

Sweat glands

There is obviously an abundance of histologic variants of tumors of sweat gland or duct origin. As a result, a great number of terms have arisen that often are used ambiguously and applied inconsistently. It would seem that no practical purpose would be denied if all the neoplasms of sweat glands were labeled simply as solid or cystic syringadenoma or syringocarcinoma. However, the range of histologic variation is so great as to lead not infrequently to serious diagnostic errors—such as the mistaking of a sweat gland adenoma for a basal or a squamous cell carcinoma, malignant melanoma, or even synovioma. It may be worthwhile, therefore, at least to

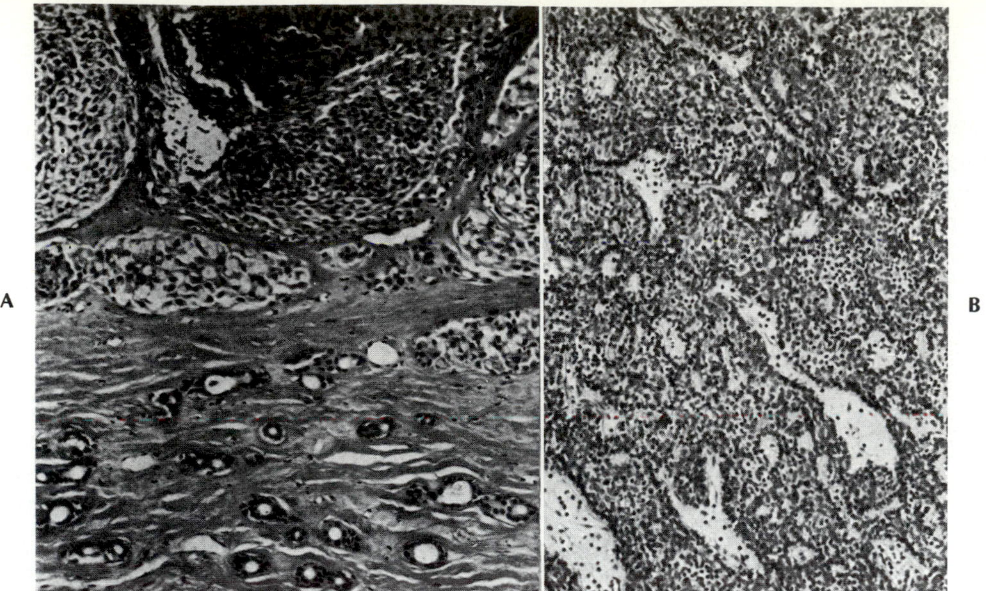

Fig. 38-53. A, Syringadenoma—usually labeled myoepithelioma on questionable evidence. **B,** Lobular syringadenoma (so-called eccrine spiradenoma). (Hematoxylin and eosin.)

Fig. 38-54 A, Syringadenoma (hidrocystoma). **B,** Diffuse syringoma (spiradenoma). **C,** Syringadenoma with chondral metaplasia (mixed tumor) such as occurs in salivary and lacrimal glands. **D,** Syringocystadenoma. (Hematoxylin and eosin.)

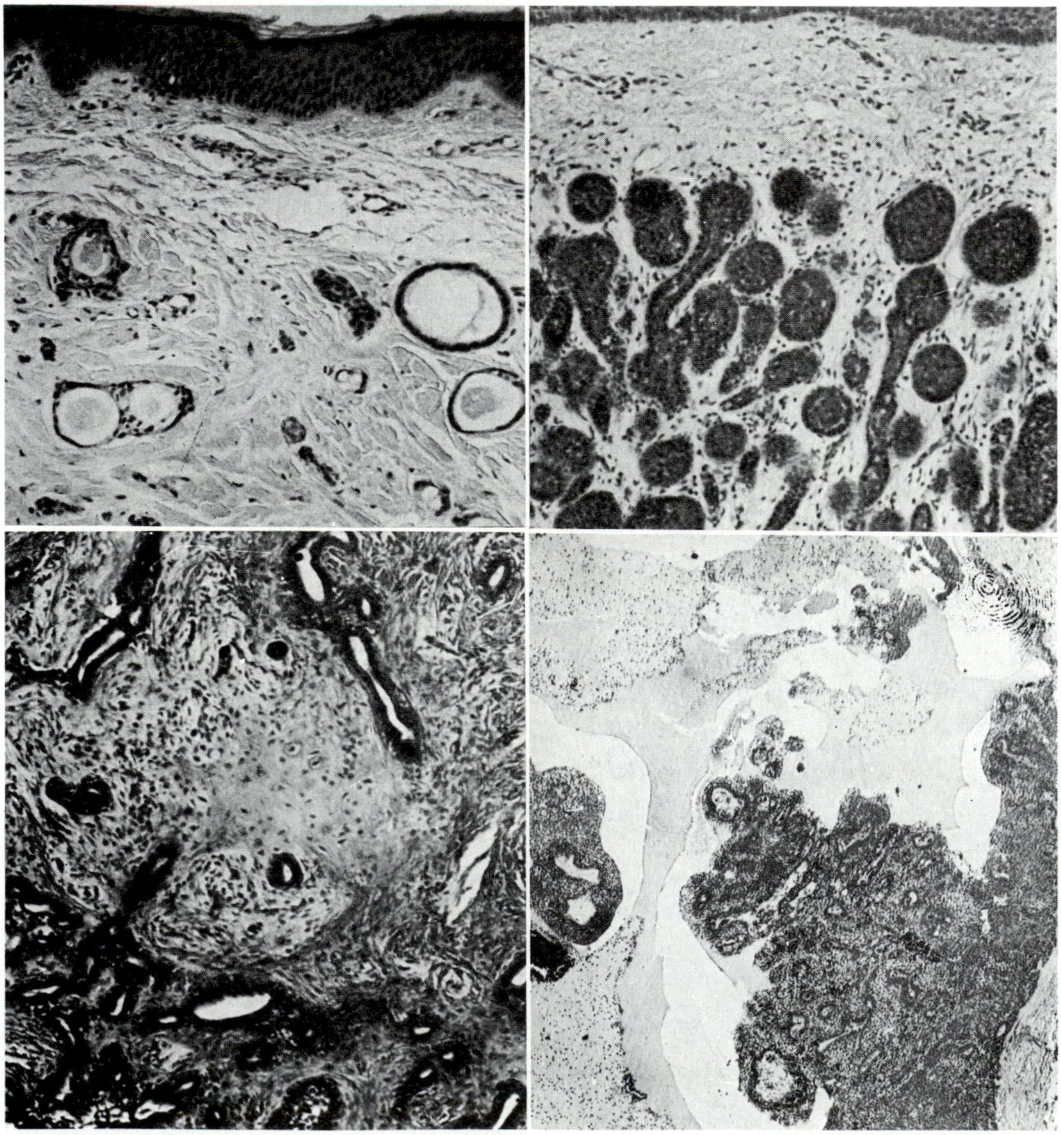

mention and illustrate the various sweat gland tumors. Despite their histologic variations, in almost all instances there are foci of cells that indicate their source by their resemblance to sweat glands or ducts. In many instances of the solid syringadenoma the hard, smooth, hyalinized, collagenous stroma is a clue to the nature of the tumor. In others, large cells with abundant acidophilic cytoplasm—cells that some observers (on insecure evidence) believe to be myoepithelial—suggest origin from sweat ducts (Fig. 38-53). In a considerable number of the cystic syringadenomas the stratified epithelium is papillated and the individual cells are vacuolated with glycogen (Fig. 38-54, *D*).

The inverted papillary syringoma (eccrine poroma) occurs as a single, slightly raised or pedunculated tumor predominantly on the soles, insteps, and palms.[56] The lesion extends downward into the dermis from the stratum corneum as papillary, reticulated bands of compact, uniform, rarely pigmented, nonkeratinizing, phosphorylase-positive cells suggestive of origin from the sweat duct. Often there is a fairly sharp demarcation from the adjacent epidermis. A similar lesion, comprised apparently of thickened, winding masses of ductal origin, may be confined to the dermis. The so-called clear cell hidroadenoma—the lesion that was once labeled myoepithelioma—is probably a partially cystic variant of the papillary syringoma in which abundant glycogen is present in the proliferating ductal cells. One might anticipate that the underlying sweat glands would be dilated as a consequence of these presumably obstructive lesions. I have, in fact, seen a single instance of grossly visible cyst formation in the sweat glands subtending this type of syringoma. Rarely do eccrine poromas undergo malignant change.

The terms *eccrine poroepithelioma* and *acrospiroma* also have been applied to what are believed to be intraepidermal proliferations of sweat duct origin (acrosyringium) of patterns somewhat different from the syringoma.

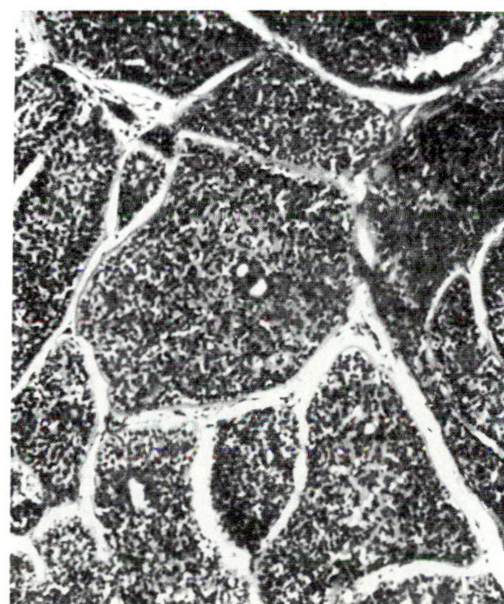

Fig. 38-55. Lobular hyalinized syringoma (turban tumor). (Hematoxylin and eosin.)

The lobular syringoma (eccrine spiradenoma) is usually a solitary firm nodule that is occasionally painful. The tumor is characteristically lobulated and composed of compact acini with predominant proliferation of the outer darker, lymphocytoid-appearing epithelial cells, as distinct from the lighter, larger inner cells that often lie beneath a residual cuticle-like structure. The origin of these tumors from the sweat duct is vividly demonstrable in the early or incompletely developed lesion.

A variant of the lobular syringoma is characterized by conspicuous, hyalinized bands of collagen surrounding and intertwining among the lobules and its cells (Fig. 38-55). This lesion (turban tumor, cylindroma) tends to be multiple and may be so extensive as to cover the scalp. Both types of lobular syringoma remain benign.

The diffuse syringoma usually occurs as multiple, small, soft yellowish papules on the chest, back, and face. The overlying epidermis is intact or may appear glistening. Histologically the lesion is composed of minute cysts scattered through the upper dermis (hence diffuse rather than lobular syringoma). The cysts are dilated sweat ducts containing inspissated secretion and occasionally keratin and characterized by epithelial spurs coming off the outer walls.

The syringocystadenoma papilliferum tends to occur as a solitary lesion of the scalp or forehead in patients of all ages. The overlying epidermis may be smooth or ulcerated. The histologic picture is easily recognizable by the cystic, papillary lesion projecting onto the surface from the upper dermis. The papillary components are lined by two layers of cells, a deeper layer of small cuboid cells and an outer layer of tall columnar cells. The luminal secretion of the latter at times is mistaken for cilia, and such tumors in the cervical region have been mistaken for odd branchiogenic fistulas. Frequently the lining is altered focally by squamous cell metaplasia that extends into underlying sweat ducts and glands. There is often considerable surrounding inflammatory reaction and a common association with hamartomas of sebaceous glands, pilary structures, and small basal cell carcinomas.

The term *hidradenoma papilliferum* is applied to the corresponding tumor of the labia majora or adjacent region that also simulates the papilloma of the subareolar mammary ducts.

The eccrine and apocrine cystadenomas occur on the face as solitary small translucent nodules and are easily identified by their lining epithelium. Some of these are regarded as retention cysts and are called hidrocystomas. Chondral metaplasia may occur in eccrine or apocrine cystadenomas. As I indicated many years ago, the genesis of such cartilage is epithelial, as it is in corresponding tumors of the salivary, lacrimal, and mammary glands.[6,9] These chondroid syringomas may also contain pilary components.

Cystic syringadenoma. The clear cell, solid, or partially cystic syringadenoma or hidradenoma (unsupportably labeled myoepithelioma) tends to be single, with a predilection for middle-aged and older women, and to occur in any region of the body. The tumors are likely to be sharply delimited and usually occur in the dermis but occasionally extend to the subcutis. In some instances the lesions are in direct contact with the epidermis, often thickened by pseudoepitheliomatous hyperplasia. The tumor cells are arranged in solid or cystic masses, the latter lined by stratified or papillary epithelium of characteristically clear, grossly vacuolated, large polyhedral cells. These cells contain abundant glycogen.

In some instances there are tubular lumina lined by cuboid cells and scattered through the lesion. Portions of the walls of the cysts may be lined by double layers of cuboid cells, which also suggest their origin from sweat glands. These tumors contain abundant phosphorylase, esterases, and respiratory enzymes characteristic of tissue derived from sweat glands. The stroma commonly is focally homogenized and, as long emphasized, is in itself suggestive of the syringadenomatous nature of these tumors.

Syringocarcinoma. There is a tendency to diagnose sweat gland adenomas as malignant not because of anaplasia of the cells but because of the irregular ramification of nests of cells into adjacent dermis. On the other hand, some of the basal and squamous cell carcinomas characterized by small, discrete nests of cells are mistaken for sweat gland tumors—as are adenocarcinomas metastatic to skin, as well as melanocarcinomas. As a rule the uncommon sweat gland carcinomas are of a low grade of virulence, as are carcinomas of appendages generally. There have been notable exceptions.

Diagnosis. The diagnosis of tumors of the sweat ducts or glands is usually made without difficulty with the light microscope. Electron microscopic and histochemical studies offer supplementary information. However, electron microscopic and histochemical criteria that appear decisive in the recognition of normal structures of the sweat apparatus are apparently not always applicable to neoplasms. The widely prevalent notion that the validity of conclusions parallels the magnification needs reexamination. In general, amylophorylase, branching enzyme, succinic dehydrogenase, and leucine aminopeptidase are regarded as indicative of eccrine ducts and glands, whereas acid phosphatase and beta-glucuronidase are said to be characteristic of apocrine glands. And yet, the lobular hyalinized syringoma (cylindroma), for example, which is clearly of eccrine origin, has been found by some investigators histochemically to suggest apocrine rather than eccrine origin.

Sebaceous glands

Adenomas of sebaceous glands occur as small yellowish papules principally on and beside the nose, cheeks, and forehead. In many cases of multiple adenomas, there are associated verrucae, neurofibromas, subungual fibrosis, and shagreen patches. These lumbosacral patches of tuberous sclerosis are nodules or elevated masses of skin produced by the proliferation and sclerosis of dermal collagen. This sclerosis may easily be mistaken histologically for scleroderma. The overlying epidermis may be normal or acanthotically reticulated. In some cases the patients develop tuberous sclerosis of the cerebral cortex and present the triad of sebaceous adenoma, mental deficiency, and epilepsy (see p. 1875). These patients also may have visceral tumors, such as renal angiolipomas. Poliosis, café au lait spots, fibroepithelial tags, and hemangiomas also may be associated with this entity. The sebaceous adenomas are likely to have developed during the first few years of life.

The histologic picture is that of an overgrowth of sebaceous glands without apparent linkage to the hair apparatus. Often it is difficult to be sure that the process is not simple hyperplasia rather than neoplasia. There is another histologic form of sebaceous adenoma, characterized by a proliferation of the basal cells lining the sebaceous glands interspersed with isolated sebaceous cells. Rarely a metastasizing sebaceous gland carcinoma develops in which at least a few scattered sebaceous cells help to identify the source.

The term *nevus sebaceus of Jadassohn* is applied to hamartomatous or dysembryogenetic papular or nodular tumefactions of sebaceous glands or the pilosebaceous apparatus. Such malformations may be associated with other ectodermal or mesodermal malformations. Overlying or adjacent verrucal epidermal hyperplasia, a variety of sweat or lacrimal gland adenomas, focal alopecia, dermoids, dermal lipomas, angiomas, or basal cell carcinomas may accompany the lesion. Occasionally it may be combined with ocular and cerebral lesions, with mental retardation and convulsions, as a form of neurocutaneous syndrome. Sebaceous gland hyperplasia, adenomas, and carcinomas have been reported in association with multiple visceral carcinomas.

Hair follicles

There is a divergence of opinion as to the types of neoplasms that may arise from hair follicles. Many observers believe that basal cell carcinomas are derived from embryonic hair follicles. However, as previously stated, the histologic evidence favors the view that basal cell carcinomas arise from the mature basal cells wherever they lie—at the base of the epidermis, at the periphery of sebaceous glands, or in the outermost layer of the hair follicles. However, the tumor that probably does arise from hair follicles is known synonymously as trichoepithelioma, Brooke's tumor, or epithelioma ade-

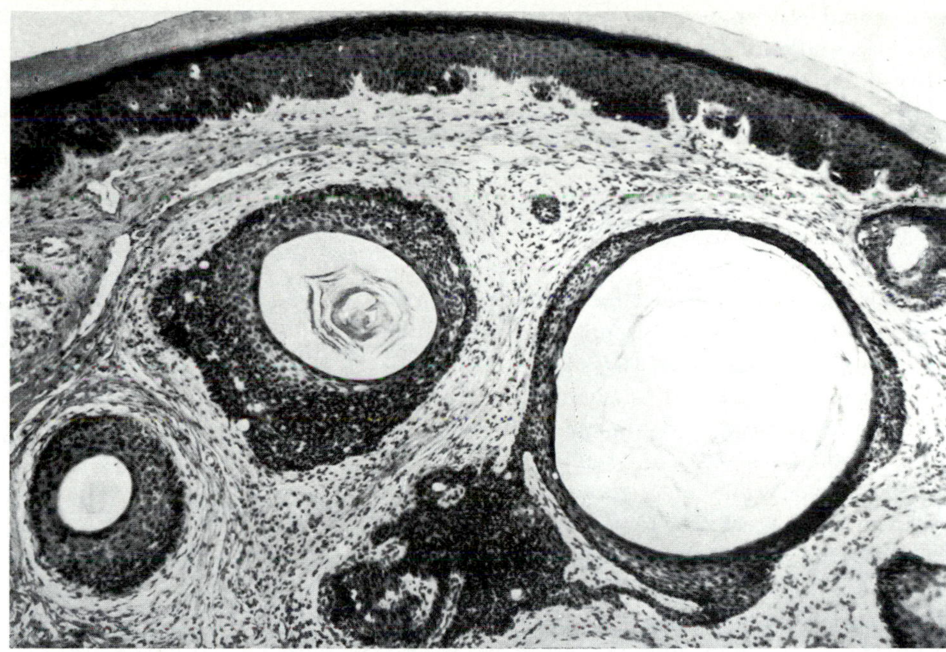

Fig. 38-56. Trichoepithelioma (Brooke's tumor, epithelioma adenoides cysticum). (Hematoxylin and eosin.)

noides cysticum (Fig. 38-56). Some observers believe that the origin of this tumor from sweat or sebaceous glands is a possibility. The lesion tends to be familial and appears as multiple smooth nodules on the face and chest.

Histologically, unlike most basal cell carcinomas, the tumor is overlain by intact epidermis. The lesion is made up of varying-sized units of cysts filled with keratin and lined with stratified squamous epithelium, from which nests of basal cells proliferate. The trichoepithelioma is benign, unlike the basal cell epithelioma.

Trichilemmoma

Trichilemmoma is an acanthosis of lobulated clear cells (glycogenated) often oriented about a hair follicle and reminiscent of the outer root sheath. A follicle may be present near the center of the lesion, which may contain whorled squamous eddies. The periphery of the lobules is sharply delimited by a vitreous zone of polarized basaloid cells and, indeed, the lesions may be mistaken for basal cell carcinomas. A few observers regard the trichilemmoma as a clear cell variant of a verruca. This may well be true of a few trichilemmomas. Multiple focal trichilemmomas are known as Cowden's syndrome.

Cysts

The dermoid cyst is a congenital cutaneous inclusion occurring usually in the skin of the forehead, especially in the supraorbital region or midline. Epidermoid cysts also may be congenital and familial, particularly steatocystoma multiplex, but commonly they are the result of trauma (including insect bites) or inflammatory downgrowth, with separation and eventual isolation and encystment of a fragment of epidermis. A number originate from obstructed sweat ducts or hair follicles rather than from implantation by trauma. As previously indicated, *sebaceous cyst* is the term loosely applied to cysts that are derived from the entire pilary or pilosebaceous apparatus rather than from the sebaceous gland alone.[6] These keratinous cysts are lined by ordinary stratified squamous epithelium with, rarely, some residual sebaceous cells in one segment of the lining. Usually the sebaceous cells have been obliterated in the mature cyst. Accordingly, they are labeled pilosebaceous cysts, although pilary cysts might be even more appropriate.

Grossly the dermoid cysts cannot be differentiated from pilosebaceous and epidermoid cysts. Histologically the wall of the cyst is actually skin with all of its appendages, often with a prominence of sebaceous glands. The epidermoid and sebaceous cysts differ from the dermoid cysts in that the former lack the appendages and their walls are made up of stratified squamous epidermis surrounded by fibrous tissue. As a rule it is impossible to distinguish the epidermoid from the pilosebaceous cyst. Infrequently, evidence of the relation of the cyst to a contiguous sebaceous gland may persist. The criteria that have been set up for the differentiation are unreliable. The epithelium of both tends to be nonpigmented.

The contents of each of the cysts are predominantly a beige greasy keratin, representing the stratum corneum, which in these instances cannot be shed but accumulates in the epidermal enclosures. There is also much fat within the laminated keratin, which either may not be demonstrable in routine sections or may be seen as cholesterin slits. In the dermoid cysts, hairs may be included. Occasionally the lining epithelium may proliferate as papillary buds, either externally or inward toward the lumen of the cyst. Because of the irregularity of these proliferations and perhaps because of their superficial resemblance to the carcinomas of epidermis, there is a tendency to classify these hyperplasias or benign proliferations as cancer—a tendency not warranted by their behavior.

The calcifying epithelioma is an exaggeration of this process of proliferation, which frequently is misinterpreted as cancer. Histologically this lesion is usually a sharply circumscribed mass of disheveled fragments of epithelium, many of which are necrotic and often partially calcified. The epithelial cells have a basaloid character, although it is likely that they are predominantly of prickle cell origin. This pattern has suggested to some observers an attempt of cells with the ever-invoked pluripotentiality to form abortive hair and so has been labeled the etymologically unlikely term *pilomatrixoma*.

Actual cancerous transformation of the lining of cysts is an infrequent occurrence. The incidence of 1% to 6% quoted in the literature is probably high. A figure of about 0.5% would appear to be more representative.

REFERENCES

1. Ahmed, R.A.: Pemphigus: current concepts, Ann. Intern. Med. **92**:396, 1980.
2. Albert, J., Bruce, W., and Allen, A.C.: Lipoid dermato-arthritis, Am. J. Med. **28**:661, 1960.
3. Allen, A.C.: Reaction to arthropods, Am. J. Pathol. **24**:367, 1948.
4. Allen, A.C.: Survey of pathology of cutaneous disease of World War II, Arch. Dermatol. **57**:19, 1948.
5. Allen, A.C.: Reorientation on histogenesis of nevi and malignant melanomas, Cancer **2**:28, 1949.
6. Allen, A.C.: The skin: a clinicopathologic treatise, ed. 1, St. Louis, 1954, The C.V. Mosby Co.
7. Allen, A.C.: Juvenile melanomas (editorial), Surg. Gynecol. Obstet. **104**:753, 1957.
8. Allen, A.C.: Juvenile melanomas, Ann. N.Y. Acad. Sci. **100**:29, 1963.
9. Allen, A.C.: The skin: a clinicopathologic treatise, ed. 2, New York, 1967, Grune & Stratton, Inc.
10. Allen, A.C., and Spitz, S.: Malignant melanomas: criteria for diagnosis and prognosis, Cancer **6**:1, 1953.
11. Allen, A.C., and Spitz, S.: Clinico-pathologic correlation of nevi and malignant melanomas, Arch. Dermatol. **69**:150, 1954.
12. Anderson, S., et al.: Bowen's disease and visceral cancer, Arch. Dermatol. **108**:367, 1973.
13. Bandy, S., and Ackerman, G.B.: Cutaneous lesions in drug-induced coma, J.A.M.A. **213**:253, 1970.
14. Barr, R.J., Morales, R.V., and Graham, J.H.: Desmoplastic nevus, Cancer **46**:557, 1980.
15. Breslow, A.: Thickness, cross-section areas, and depth of invasion in the prognosis of cutaneous melanomas, Ann. Surg. **172**:902, 1970.
16. Castro, G., and Winkelmann, R.K.: Angiolymphoid hyperplasia, Cancer **34**:1696, 1974.
17. Caulfield, J.B., and Wilgram, G.F.: Ultrastructure of acantholysis, J. Invest. Dermatol. **41**:57, 1963.
18. Clark, W.H., Jr.: Melanomas, Cancer Res. **29**:705, 1969.
19. Coleta, D.F., et al.: Metastasizing basal cell carcinomas, Cancer **22**:879, 1968.
20. Cormane, R.H., et al.: B and T lymphocytes, Ann. N.Y. Acad. Sci. **254**:592, 1975.
21. Cruz, T.S., and Reiner, C.B.: Recurrent digital fibroma of children, J. Cutan. Pathol. **5**:339, 1978.
22. Curth, H.O., et al.: Acanthosis nigricans, Cancer **15**:364, 1962.
23. Davis, P., Atkins, B., and Hughes, G.R.V.: Antibodies to DNA in discoid lupus erythematosus, Br. J. Dermatol. **91**:175, 1974.
24. Douglas, H.M.G., and Bleumink, E.: Lymphosarcoma and congenital lymphedema, Arch. Dermatol. **11**:608, 1974.
25. Ellman, M.A., et al.: Toxic epidermal necrolysis and allopurinol, Arch. Dermatol. **111**:986, 1975.
26. Evans, H.L., and Winkelmann, R.K.: Differential diagnosis of malignant and benign cutaneous infiltrates, Cancer **44**:699, 1979.
27. Fajardo, L.F., and Berthrong, M.: Radiation injury in surgical pathology, Am. J. Surg. Pathol. **5**:279, 1981.
28. Farmer, E.R., and Helwig, E.B.: Metastatic basal cell carcinoma, Cancer **46**:748, 1980.
29. Fields, J.P., and Helwig, E.B.: Leiomyosarcoma of the skin and subcutaneous tissue, Cancer **47**:156, 1981.
30. Flaxman, S.A., and Maderson, P.E.A.: Growth and differentiation of skin, J. Invest. Dermatol. **67**:8, 1976.
31. Frank, E., Mevorah, B., and Leu, F.: Disseminated spiked hyperkeratosis, Arch. Dermatol. **117**:412, 1981.
32. Fraser, N.G., Kerry, N.W., and Donald, D.: Oral lesions in dermatitis herpetiformis, Br. J. Dermatol. **89**:439, 1973.
33. Gazzolo, L., and Prunieras, M.: Lysosomes and keratinocytes, J. Invest. Dermatol. **51**:186, 1968.
34. Gilliam, J.N., et al.: Immunofluorescent band and renal disease in S.L.E., J. Clin. Invest. **53**:1434, 1974.
35. Graham, J.H., and Helwig, E.B.: Erythroplasia of Queyrat, Cancer **32**:1396, 1973.
36. Halpryn, H.J., and Allen, A.C.: Epidermal changes overlying sclerosing angiomas, Arch. Dermatol. **80**:160, 1959.
37. Hashimoto, K., and Bale, G.F.: Balloon cell nevi, Cancer **30**:530, 1973.
38. Huvos, A., et al.: Melanomas, Am. J. Pathol. **71**:33, 1973.
39. Jackson, S.F., and Fell, H.B.: Mucus-producing keratinocytes, Dev. Biol. **7**:394, 1963.
40. James, W.D., Odom, R.B., and Katzenstein, A.A.: Cutaneous manifestations of lymphomatoid granulomatosis, Arch. Dermatol. **117**:196, 1981.
41. Jordon, R.E., et al.: Dermoepidermal deposition of complement components and properdin in S.L.E., Br. J. Dermatol. **92**:263, 1975.
42. Kahn, G.: Mucocutaneous lymph node syndrome (Kawasaki's disease), Arch. Dermatol. **114**:948, 1978.
43. Kopf, A.W., and Popkin, G.L.: Shave biopsies, Arch. Dermatol. **110**:637, 1974.
44. Lapins, W.A., and Helwig, E.B.: Perineural invasion by keratoacanthoma, Arch. Dermatol. **116**:791, 1980.
45. Lever, W.F., and Schaumberg-Lever, G.: Histopathology of skin, ed. 5, Philadelphia, 1975, J.B. Lippincott Co.
46. Lopez, M.R.: Cutaneous meningiomas, Cancer **34**:728, 1974.
47. Lutzner, M.A.: Molluscum bodies, Arch. Dermatol. **87**:436, 1963.
48. Lutzner, M.A.: Sezary cells, J. Natl. Cancer Inst. **50**:1145, 1973.
49. Lyell, A.: Toxic epidermal necrolysis, Br. J. Dermatol. **68**:355, 1956.
50. MacCauley, W.L.: Lymphomatoid papulosis, Arch. Dermatol. **97**:23, 1968.
51. Mehregan, A.H.: Perforating elastosis, Arch. Dermatol. **97**:381, 1968.
52. Milston, E.B., and Helwig, E.B.: Basal cell carcinomas in children, Arch. Dermatol. **108**:523, 1973.
53. Miyagawa, S., et al.: Chronic bullous disease with coexistent circulating IgG and IgA antibasement membrane zone antibodies, Arch. Dermatol. **117**:349, 1981.
54. Monroe, E.W.: Urticarial vasculitis: an updated review, J. Am. Acad. Dermatol. **5**:88, 1981.
55. Morrison, W.L.: Viral warts and immunity, Br. J. Dermatol. **92**:625, 1975.
56. Pinkus, H., et al.: Eccrine poromas, Arch. Dermatol. **74**:51, 1956.

57. Ramsay, C.A., and Gianelli, F.: Erythemal action spectrum and DNA repair synthesis in xeroderma pigmentosum, Br. J. Dermatol. **92**:49, 1975.
58. Rappaport, H., and Thomas, L.B.: Mycosis fungoides: the pathology of extracutaneous involvement, Cancer **34**:1198, 1974.
59. Rice, J.S., and Fischer, D.S.: Blue rubber-bleb nevus, Arch. Dermatol. **86**:503, 1962.
60. Rodman, G.P., Lipinski, E., and Luksick, L., Jr.: Skin thickness and collagen content in progressive systemic sclerosis, Arthritis Rheum. **22**:130, 1979.
61. Sams, W.B., Jr.: Immunofluorescence in dermatology, yearbook of dermatology, Chicago, 1973, Year Book Medical Publishers, Inc.
62. Sandberg, L.B., Soskel, N.T., and Leslie, J.G.: Elastin structure, biosynthesis, and relation to disease states, N. Engl. J. Med. **304**:566, 1981.
63. Schaumberg-Lever, G., et al.: Immunoglobulins in pemphigoid and lupus erythematosus, J. Invest. Dermatol. **64**:74, 1975.
64. Shiltz, J.R., Michel, B., and Papay, R.: Appearance of "pemphigus, acantholysis factor" in human skin cultured with pemphigus, antibody, J. Invest. Dermatol. **73**:575, 1979.
65. Singer, H., et al.: Protease activation: a mechanism for cellular dyshesion in pemphigus, J. Invest. Dermatol. **74**:363, 1980.
66. Smith, J.L., and Stehlen, J.S., Jr.: Spontaneous regression of primary malignant melanomas with regional metastases, Cancer **18**:1399, 1965.
67. Spitz, S.: Melanomas of childhood, Am. J. Pathol. **24**:591, 1948.
68. Spitz, S.: Cutaneous tumors of childhood, J. Am. Med. Wom. Assoc. **6**:209, 1951.
69. Stewart, F.W., and Treves, N.: Postmastectomy lymphangiosarcoma, Cancer **1**:64, 1948.
70. Suter, L., et al.: Human malignant melanoma: assay of tumor-associated antigens, J. Invest. Dermatol. **75**:235, 1980.
71. Tucker, S.B., et al.: Activation of nevi in patients with malignant melanoma, Cancer **46**:822, 1980.
72. Tufanelli, D.L.: Lupus erythematosus panniculitis, Arch. Dermatol. **103**:231, 1971.
73. Unna, P.: Epithelial origin of melanocarcinomas, Berl. Blin. Wochenschr. **30**:14, 1893.
74. Wanebo, H.J., et al.: Clinicopathologic analysis of malignant melanomas, Cancer **35**:666, 1975.
75. Wolfe, J.D., Trevor, E.D., and Kjeldsberg, C.R.: Pulmonary manifestation of mycosis fungoides, Cancer **46**:2648, 1980.
76. Yeckley, J.A., et al.: Production of Sezary cells from normal lymphocytes, Arch. Dermatol. **111**:29, 1975.
77. Zackheim, H.S.: Cutaneous T-cell lymphomas, Arch. Dermatol. **117**:295, 1981.

CHAPTER 39 Tumors and Tumorlike Conditions of Soft Tissues

MICHAEL L. KYRIAKOS

In this chapter a diverse and fascinating group of lesions that arise from the supporting soft tissues of the body is discussed. These soft tissues include all the nonepithelial extraskeletal tissues with the exception of the central nervous system glia and the components of the reticuloendothelial system.[7,20] Included are lesions composed of or derived from fat, fibrous tissue, smooth muscle, skeletal muscle, blood vessels, and lymphatics, all of which originate in embryonic mesoderm. Tumors of peripheral nerve, the components of which are derived from the neuroectoderm, are also included because of their frequent occurrence in the superficial soft tissues. All the tumors that arise in soft tissue may also be found within the organs of the body, but these represent specific problems and are discussed in the appropriate chapters of this textbook.

Perhaps in no other field of diagnostic pathology has there been such a proliferation of newly described histologic entities as there has been in the area of soft tissue pathology within the past 10 years. The student of pathology is now faced with a host of diagnostic entities that number well over 100 and for which there are about 300 synonyms.[7,7a,10] However, many are so rare that they fall outside the experience not only of most general physicians but also of most pathologists. Even large referral centers may have only one or two examples of many of these soft tissue lesions in their files. This chapter, then, should not be considered an encyclopedic survey of the entire field of soft tissue tumor pathology. Only the more common lesions, or those of special interest, are presented. Reference should be made to the more general and encompassing publications given in the bibliography for lesions not discussed and for which greater detail is sought.*

Soft tissue tumors and tumorlike conditions are uncommon.[8,20,31] Data on the incidence of the benign tumors are difficult to come by because the emphasis in the literature has been on the malignant tumors. Some idea of their relative frequency, however, is given in data from the Laboratory of Surgical Pathology, Columbia University, where over a 45-year period only 8700 soft tissue tumors were accessioned, the benign outnumbering the malignant in a ratio of about 5:1 (7300 benign and 1400 malignant).[27] In 1981 the American Cancer Society placed the estimated number of new soft tissue cancers in the United States at approximately 4700 out of a total of 815,000 new cancers in all sites. Approximately 1600 deaths per year are caused by these tumors out of a total of more than 400,000 cancer deaths.[1]

It is the rarity of these tumors, however, that creates both their fascination and their problems. The wide variation in their histopathologic patterns extends the pathologist's diagnostic ability to the limit. However, since few pathologists come in contact with many of these lesions, the fortuitous encounter frequently leads to misdiagnosis. In a survey of cases in the Swedish Tumor Registry 10% of the lesions diagnosed as some form of sarcoma were, on review, benign reactive proliferative lesions.[6]

A more important reason for the interest that sarcomas have generated is that many of them affect children and young adults. Indeed, they are currently the fifth leading form of cancer in children.[31,33] Their anatomic location, frequently in the extremities, and the radical and at times mutilating surgical procedures required for their removal have created a natural interest in them that belies both their prevalence and clinical significance as a major cause of cancer deaths. Finally, recent advances in the use of adjuvant chemotherapy and radiotherapy have made dramatic inroads in the mortality of some of these sarcomas to the point that patients with tumors previously almost uniformly fatal are now being cured.[31]

The clinical appearance of most soft tissue lesions is nonspecific. Most develop as enlarging, painless masses, frequently located in an extremity. Sarcomas are usually deeply situated, rarely arising in the dermis or superfi-

*References 2, 6a, 6b, 7, 7a, 10, 14, 23, 27.

cial soft tissue. They may grow slowly, being present for months or even years, or show rapid growth within days to a few weeks. Those in areas such as the retroperitoneum or the thigh may grow to a large size before becoming clinically evident. Clinical inspection of the mass, or even its gross pathologic appearance, usually fails to provide any clue about its nature. Benign lesions, although frequently well circumscribed or even encapsulated, may have an infiltrative pattern, as in nodular fasciitis or any of the various fibromatoses. Similarly, it is the rule for sarcomas to appear grossly well circumscribed or even encapsulated.[7,7a,9] Microscopic examination, however, shows that they always infiltrate the surrounding normal tissue and that no true capsule exists. Furthermore, the gross appearance is, with few exceptions, not helpful in distinguishing among the various types of sarcomas. Areas of cystic degeneration, necrosis, and hemorrhage are frequently found, especially in the larger sarcomas, but such areas may also be seen in perfectly benign tumors.

Since the clinical appearance of a lesion cannot be used as a definitive guideline for distinguishing benign from malignant lesions, the clinician should consider a deep-seated soft tissue mass to be malignant until proved otherwise. Because the therapy to be used depends on the histologic nature of the lesion, a well-planned biopsy is a basic requirement in the management of these lesions. The plans for such a biopsy should take into consideration the possible need for future radiotherapy, and the placement of the biopsy should be such so as to avoid creating anatomic problems for the radiotherapist.[28] Specimens should always be taken from the growing edge of the tumor, avoiding any central necrotic zones.

Although sarcomas occur at all sites and in patients of all ages, most of the major types have a predilection for certain anatomic regions and age groups.[7,7a] For instance, embyronal rhabdomyosarcoma frequently occurs in the head or neck of young children and is rarely found in adults. In contrast, liposarcoma frequently occurs in the lower extremity of adults and is rarely found in children. Hence the clinician should supply, and the pathologist should demand, all pertinent clinical information.

Many tumors or tumorlike conditions of soft tissue have a fibroblastic component, and if the lesion is not properly sampled, it may be misdiagnosed as a fibrosarcoma. Further confusing the histologic situation is the variety of cellular constituents and histomorphologic patterns in many malignant lesions. At times the histologic pattern may even vary from section to section or area to area within a single tumor.[7,7a] Therefore proper sampling with numerous sections may be required before specific diagnostic features are found.

Most sarcomas grow by spreading along fascial planes, nerve trunks, and tendon sheaths and metastasize through the bloodstream, with the lungs, bones, liver, and skin the common sites for metastases.[20,27] Most metastases develop within 2 years of therapy, although in some varieties of sarcoma 10 to 20 years may elapse before metastases become manifest.[9,15,20] As a rule, lymph nodes are not involved, although certain sarcomas such as embryonal rhabdomyosarcoma and synovial sarcoma do metastasize to regional lymph nodes.[9]

Today surgical management is the treatment of choice for both benign and malignant soft tissue tumors.[5] The type of surgical excision, however, greatly influences the local recurrence rate. Local excision results in a recurrence in from 75% to 90% of cases, and even radical excision or amputation is followed by local recurrence in from 20% to 30% of cases.[15,20] Newer therapeutic techniques involving a combination of less radical operative procedures with postoperative radiotherapy have sharply reduced this local recurrence rate.[15,28-30] However, in approximately 25% to 30% of patients distant metastases develop that are unassociated with local recurrence. Hence microscopic foci of tumor must exist in such patients, requiring the use of adjuvant chemotherapy to eradicate distant foci of tumor. However, effective chemotherapeutic agents for the treatment of most soft tissue sarcomas, with some notable exceptions, have not been developed.[3,4,22,23a,31]

The previous statements are generalizations; sarcomas cannot be lumped together in terms of their behavior any more than can the various carcinomas. Hence the need exists for an adequate understanding of individual tumor types. The classification of the various lesions, benign and malignant, is based on the type of tissue that they contain.[7,7a,27] For instance, a tumor composed of benign smooth muscle cells is called a leiomyoma and its malignant counterpart a leiomyosarcoma. This does not imply, however, that leiomyosarcoma arises from a previous benign leiomyoma. Indeed, with few exceptions, sarcomas of soft tissue arise de novo and not from malignant transformation of their benign counterparts.[7,7a] Current dogma implicates a primitive, undifferentiated mesenchymal cell having the capacity to differentiate along a variety of cell pathways, as the mother cell of most sarcomas. Whether true or not, this is a convenient way of explaining the wide variety of histopathologic patterns in some of the more pleomorphic sarcomas, as well as the overlap in the type of cells present in the various sarcomas at the fine structure level.[17,32]

Most sarcomas may be easily diagnosed by light microscopy. However, as a malignant tumor becomes less differentiated, its cellular origin also becomes less clear until few if any clues remain that allow one to classify the tumor by light or electron microscopy.[11] Thus, even when examined by an experienced pathologist, 10% to 15% of sarcomas will remain "unclassified" in light of today's knowledge.[7,7a,20] Finally, the student should be warned not to place too much faith in histogenetic conclusions drawn on the basis of the electron microscopic examination of a single example of a particular sarcoma. With the known problems in the accurate light microscopic diagnosis of any particular sarcoma, combined with the inherent sampling problems of electron microscopy, errors in interpretation can easily be made.

A staging system has been proposed for soft tissue sarcomas that depends on the pathologist's evaluation of the grade or differentiation of the tumor. The proposed system has so many deficiencies, not the least of which is that well-established grading criteria do not exist for most sarcomas, that we do not believe it is of practical use in its present form.[24] A more recent grading system has been reported in which the presence or absence of tumor necrosis has correlated well with patient survival.[5a]

The myofibroblast, and its occurrence within benign and malignant soft tissue lesions, has recently been examined.[13,14,25] Although myofibroblasts apparently occur in a variety of tumors having extensive collagen formation, they do not comprise the major cellular component in soft tissue lesions, with the exception of pseudosarcomas, such as nodular fasciitis, and the fibromatoses. There has also been recent interest in the types of collagen composing the stroma of various sarcomas and the use of antibodies against these stromal components as possible diagnostic tools.[26] The type of mucosubstances produced by soft tissue tumors, which are mainly acid mucopolysaccharides, may also be helpful in distinguishing between some of the sarcomas.[12,18] The application of newer immunoperoxidase methods for the diagnosis of tumors of all types, including soft tissue tumors, is only now becoming widespread and offers exciting possibilities for the future.*

FIBROUS TISSUE LESIONS

Fibrosarcoma

Despite electron microscopic studies that have shown occasional myofibroblasts in fibrosarcoma,[35,39] it remains the prototypical tumor of fibroblasts. Although fibrosarcoma was formerly considered the most common of the sarcomas, the number of cases now included in this category has been dramatically reduced by the exclusion of other tumors and tumorlike conditions that have recently been better defined, such as malignant fibrous histiocytoma, nodular fasciitis, and the benign fibromatoses. Indeed, in some series approximately one third to one half of cases previously classified as fibrosarcoma were reassigned to other diagnostic categories based on current classifications.[37,40] Today fibrosarcomas comprise only 5% to 10% of all sarcomas.[36,38,40]

*References 4a, 7b, 20a, 21, 21a, 21b.

Fibrosarcoma occurs in all age groups, from infants to the very elderly, but it most commonly affects adults between the ages of 40 and 70 years.[34,37,40,42] Approximately 60% of cases are in men.[34,40] Childhood fibrosarcomas are usually found during the first year of life, 40% to 50% being congenital.[14,34,42]

The tumor usually develops as a slowly growing mass that is present for about 2 to 3 years, although some patients report having a mass for up to 25 years.[37,40] Pain is not a prominent symptom, although in one report slightly more than one half of the patients had pain.[40] Large tumors may be tender and cause pressure symptoms. Fibrosarcomas tend to arise in the external soft tissue, only rarely being found in the retroperitoneum, mesentery, omentum, or mediastinum.[27] They originate from the fascial connective tissues or deep subcutaneous tissue.[40] In adults 90% occur in the extremities, most (50% to 60%) in the lower extremity where the thigh is by far the most common site.[40] Less common locations include the upper extremity, trunk, and head and neck.[37] In children the anatomic location varies somewhat, with the distal portions of the lower extremity, the ankle and foot, more frequently involved than the thigh; a higher proportion of the tumors are in the shoulder and pelvic girdles.[34,42]

Grossly fibrosarcomas are grayish white, firm, lobulated masses that have such good circumscription that they may appear encapsulated.[40] Tumors in children are often more friable and less well circumscribed.[34,37] Foci of necrosis and hemorrhage are present in the more poorly differentiated tumors. Tumors average about 3 to 4 cm, but in some sites tumors larger than 10 cm are not uncommon.[34,37,40,42] In infantile cases the tumor may involve the entire distal portion of the extremity.

Histologically, fibrosarcomas are composed of spindle-shaped fibroblasts arranged in intersecting fascicles, which produces the typical "herringbone" pattern of fibrosarcoma (Fig. 39-1).[37,40,42] Nuclei are usually uniform, with tapered rather than rounded ends. The cytoplasm tends to be ill defined, with poorly formed cell borders. Reticulin and collagen production is best seen in well-differentiated lesions, where the reticulin fibers surround and run parallel to the long axis of each cell.[37,42] In less differentiated tumors there is an increase in the overall cellularity, with plumper and rounder nuclei that vary more in size and shape. There are also increased mitotic activity and less reticulin and collagen.[37,42] Foci of necrosis, degeneration, and hemorrhage are common in the more poorly differentiated tumors. This basic microscopic pattern also holds true for infantile fibrosarcomas, although there is a tendency for such tumors to be less differentiated, with loss of the herringbone pattern, and to be more vascular.[34,37] They also may contain areas of primitive-appearing mesenchymal cells.[34]

Fibrosarcoma is a sarcoma that lends itself well to a

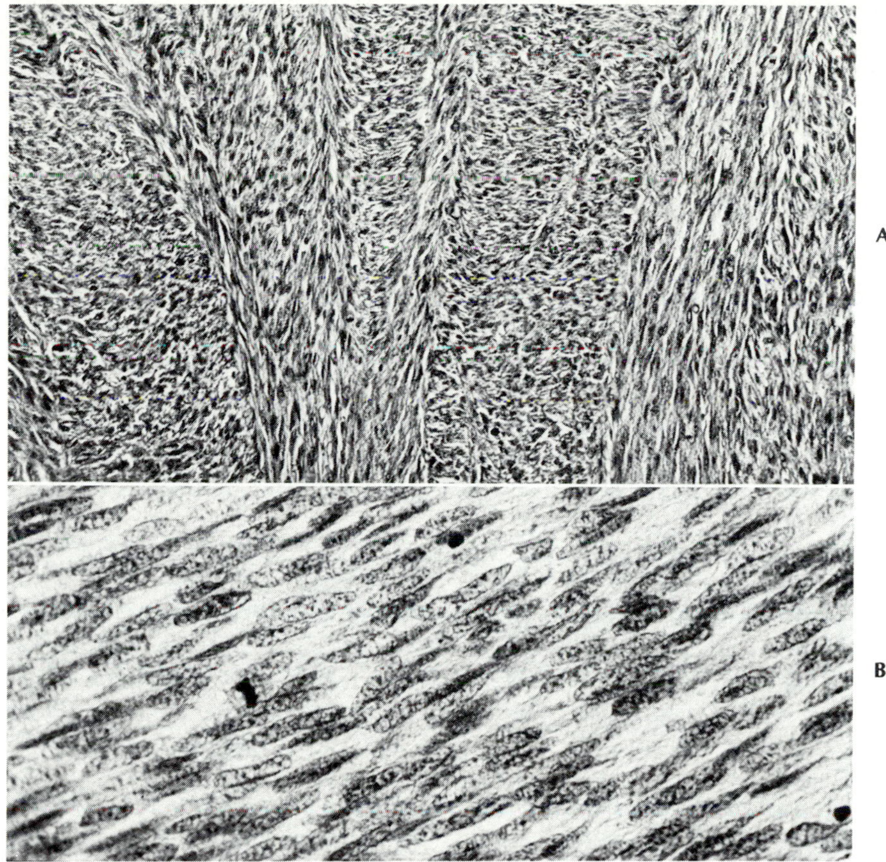

Fig. 39-1. A, Fibrosarcoma. Interlacing fascicles of spindle-shaped fibroblasts produce typical herringbone pattern of well-differentiated fibrosarcoma. **B,** Closely packed fibroblasts with ill-defined cytoplasmic borders. Mitotic figure is present to left of center. (**A,** 120×; **B,** 480×.)

grading system based on the differentiation of the tumor. The tumors may either be described as well differentiated, moderately differentiated, or poorly differentiated or be assigned a numerical grade of I to IV, with IV being the least differentiated. This grading system has prognostic significance because it correlates well with survival in adults; the better differentiated the tumor, the better the long-term survival rate.[23,40] Most fibrosarcomas tend to be moderately differentiated (grades II and III) and lack the pleomorphism of other sarcomas.[37,40,42] Indeed, the finding of many large, bizarre tumor giant cells excludes the diagnosis of fibrosarcoma.[23,40] It is important to remember that spindle cell fibroblastic areas may be found in a variety of soft tissue sarcomas such as synovial sarcoma, malignant fibrous histiocytoma, neurosarcoma, and rhabdomyosarcoma, and small specimens from these sarcomas may be misinterpreted as fibrosarcoma.

A further problem in the histologic diagnosis is distinguishing some of the benign fibromatoses from fibrosarcoma. A gray area exists between a cellular fibromatosis and a well-differentiated fibrosarcoma, especially in fibrous lesions of young children. Whether a lesion is too cellular and has too many mitotic figures to be considered benign becomes a matter of subjective opinion.

Fibrosarcomas are treated surgically by either wide local excision or, if necessary, amputation. In adults there is a good correlation between the tumor histology and rates of local recurrence, metastases, and survival. Recurrences after local excision have been noted in 60% of patients. Approximately 50% of patients develop distant metastases that are virtually all bloodborne. Regional lymph nodes are only rarely involved.[40] Current 5- and 10-year survival rates of 50% to 60% are reported, with few tumor deaths occurring after this time.[40]

The clinical course of childhood fibrosarcoma, unlike that in adults, cannot be predicted on the basis of histologic features.[34,52] In general, childhood fibrosarcoma has a more favorable outlook than the adult forms,[14,27,34] with survival rates greater than 85% being reported despite local recurrence rates of close to 50% after wide local excision.[34,42] Few patients with a diagnosis of childhood fibrosarcoma have died of metastatic disease.[27,34,41,42] It appears that children younger than 5 years of age may be treated less radically than adults and still have an excellent prognosis.[42] This may reflect the possibility that some childhood fibrosarcomas are in reality benign, locally aggressive, nonmetastasizing fibromatoses that cannot be histologically distinguished from true fibrosarcoma. Older children have the less favorable survival rate of adults.[42]

Fibromatoses

The fibromatoses are a group of lesions, each specific in its own right but all sharing common histologic features. A fibromatosis has been defined as "an infiltrating fibroblastic proliferation showing none of the features of an inflammatory response and no features of unequivocal neoplasia,"[55] or more broadly, "a group of non-metastasizing fibroblastic tumors which tend to invade locally and recur after attempted surgical excision."[43] Neither of these definitions is totally accurate, since inflammatory cells can be seen in some lesions, although in minimal degree, and some have little or no tendency to recur. In addition, these fibroblastic lesions have been found to be composed not only of fibroblasts but also of cells with both fibroblastic and smooth muscle features, the myofibroblasts.[16] However, both definitions characterize the general nature of all of these lesions and emphasize their salient feature, namely, that while in rare instances they may prove fatal because of local aggressiveness, they do not metastasize.

The fibromatoses occur in a wide variety of anatomic locations and in all age groups, although some are found exclusively or predominantly in infants and young children. These latter are broadly grouped as juvenile or infantile fibromatoses and include fibrous hamartoma of infancy, fibromatosis colli, diffuse infantile fibromatosis, aggressive infantile fibromatosis (congenital fibrosarcoma-like fibromatosis), juvenile aponeurotic fibroma, digital fibrous tumor of childhood, congenital generalized fibromatosis, congenital solitary fibromatosis, hereditary gingival fibromatosis, juvenile nasopharyngeal angiofibroma, and fibromatosis hyalinica multiplex juvenilis.[43,49,59] Several of these lesions are quite cellular, have primitive-type mesenchymal cells, and grow with an infiltrative pattern to such a degree that they may be worrisome to the pathologist and even be diagnosed as some form of sarcoma. Indeed, the histologic distinction between the so-called aggressive fibromatosis of children and a true fibrosarcoma may be impossible in some cases, the final truth being determined only by the patient's clinical course.[59] In most fibromatoses, however, careful attention to histologic detail will permit ready recognition of the entity.

In the adult category of fibromatoses, namely those seen primarily in older patients, are the various forms of Dupuytren's-type fibromatoses, which include palmar and plantar fibromatosis and Peyronie's disease, and the various types of desmoid fibromatoses.[43] As a group, the adult lesions are more common than the juvenile forms, some of which are so exceedingly rare that they are outside the experience of most pathologists. In this section only a few of these conditions will be discussed; the reader is referred to several of the excellent reviews of the subject given in the bibliography for more extensive coverage.

We agree with those who caution against the use of the term "fibroma" as a designation for any of these lesions or for any other fibroblastic lesion in the deep soft tissues.[54] Such a diagnosis implies a well-circumscribed and encapsulated lesion, composed of bland, well-differentiated fibroblasts, which will not recur or become aggressive following surgical removal. The experiences of many diagnostic pathologists have proved that such is not the case, and lesions fitting this description may, despite their gross and microscopic appearance, prove locally aggressive. For lesions in the deep soft tissues we do not use the term "fibroma."

Palmar and plantar fibromatoses

Palmar and plantar fibromatoses, occurring on the palm of the hand and the sole of the foot, respectively, are the most common and the best known of the fibromatoses.[43] Although each has certain specific characteristics, they share a common histomorphology and are considered together. They are members of what has been termed the Dupuytren's-like fibromatoses, which also includes such entities as knuckle pads and Peyronie's disease.[43]

They affect patients over a broad age range, but in general the palmar lesions are seen in older patients and are uncommon in children, whereas plantar lesions are more frequent in younger patients and children.[43,59] Palmar lesions are up to eight times more frequent in females than males, whereas plantar lesions occur in the sexes about equally.[43,54,56,59] Both forms may be multiple, may be bilateral, and have a familial tendency.[43,54,59] There is a higher incidence of these fibromatoses among patients with alcoholism and chronic lung disease and those receiving long-term drug therapy for epilepsy.[43,56]

These fibromatoses are initially seen as nodules or plaques that invade the dermis and underlying fascia but not muscle or tendons.[43,56,59] The palmar lesion frequently progresses to produce a scarlike band that causes a contracture, known as Dupuytren's contracture. Plantar lesions do not usually produce contractures.[43]

The evolution of the individual lesion is divided into three stages: proliferative, involutional, and residual. The diagnostic pattern noted in the proliferative phase consists of fibrovascular nodules that involve the fascia. They are composed of plump, tightly packed fibroblasts, with a high mitotic rate, surrounding a central small blood vessel. As the lesion ages or involutes, there is a progressive increase in the amount of collagen, and the fibroblasts align themselves into fascicles along lines of stress. In the residual phase one may see only a dense collagenized stroma containing only a few fibroblasts. This fibrosis may extend into the soft tissue of the palm, thus creating the contracture that is histologically nonspecific scar tissue.[43,54,59] Electron microscopic studies have shown the presence of myofibroblasts in both palmar and plantar lesions.[16,59]

Patients with Dupuytren's contracture may also have plantar lesions or penile lesions with similar histologic features (Peyronie's disease).[43] Both plantar and palmar lesions may remain stationary at the nodular or plaque stage, or they may progress or even spontaneously regress. Following operative procedures, both types may recur, with recurrences more common in younger patients. Plantar lesions are particularly prone to recur after local excision, with recurrence rates as high as 60% to 85% reported.[43] Radical excision for their complete removal, however, is contraindicated, since they may involute spontaneously.

Desmoid fibromatoses

Historically the desmoid fibromatoses (desmoids) have been divided into those in the soft tissue of the abdominal wall—the abdominal wall desmoids—and those elsewhere—the extra-abdominal desmoids.[43,54] The latter lesions are also known as musculoaponeurotic fibromatoses.[50] This is an arbitrary division, since the lesions are histopathologically similar.

Extra-abdominal lesions are more common than the abdominal wall types. Most abdominal wall desmoids occur in parous women,[55] raising the conjecture that they develop secondary to a resolving hematoma caused by the trauma of delivery. They also arise in surgical scars.[43,47] A history of trauma is reported in 30% to 60% of extra-abdominal lesions.[50]

Desmoids occur at all ages but are more frequent in the third and fourth decades of life.[43,50,54] It is rare to find abdominal desmoids in patients younger than 20 years, but extra-abdominal lesions do occur in young children.[43,47,55] Desmoids are more frequent in female than male patients, although in the extra-abdominal forms this sexual difference is not as great as it is in the abdominal type.[43,50,54,55]

Desmoids are slowly growing, firm to hard masses that may be tender or painful.[50] An increased incidence of desmoid tumors is found in patients with Gardner's syndrome (familial intestinal polyposis associated with osteomas and cutaneous keratinous cysts), and they may precede or follow the clinical appearance of the intestinal polyps.[43,47,55] Whereas abdominal wall desmoids occur primarily in the rectus sheath, extra-abdominal desmoids occur in the lower extremities, upper arm, shoulder girdle, and neck.[43,47,54,55] Intra-abdominal desmoids are also recorded.[43] On gross inspection desmoids are large (some exceeding 20 cm), infiltrative lesions that involve muscle and adjacent soft tissue and have a distinctive whorled, grayish white gross appearance that is unlike the more homogeneous appearance of a fibrosarcoma.[50] In the soft tissue it may be impossible to distinguish between scar tissue and tumor tissue. This situation is especially difficult in patients operated on for recurrences, since it causes severe problems for surgeons in their attempt to define the actual anatomic limits of the lesions. It is not uncommon for the surgeon to believe that the resection had completely removed the tumor, only to have the surgical margins later reported as involved.

Microscopic sections show a uniform appearance of long, slender, spindle-shaped fibroblasts arranged in bands and fascicles and surrounded by varying amounts of collagen. The cells characteristically lack pleomorphism.[43,50] Electron microscopic studies have shown the presence of myofibroblasts, which in some cases may be the dominant cells present.[51] The degree of cellularity varies from area to area, with hypocellular hyalinized foci alternating with compact cellular areas. Mitoses are notably scarce or absent. Typically invasion of muscle and tendons (Fig. 39-2) is seen.[43,50] Although the absence of pleomorphism and mitotic activity are features that distinguish desmoids from fibrosarcomas, this distinction is easier on paper than it is in actual practice. The difference between a very cellular fibromatosis having an occasional mitotic figure and a well-differentiated fibrosarcoma with only minimal cellular atypia may be blurred. This distinction is further clouded by the high rate of local recurrence exhibited by desmoids, which has varied from 19% to 77%, with multiple recurrences not infrequent.[43,47,50,55] The recurrence rate apparently depends on the adequacy of the primary resection. Abdominal wall lesions may have a lower rate of recurrence, but younger patients and those with large lesions have a higher incidence of local recurrence.[43,50] It should be remembered, however, that with a wide and adequate excision, these patients can be cured.[47,50,55] Despite desmoids' inability to metastasize, they have caused great morbidity with their tendency to invade neurovascular bundles, and they have even caused death by virtue of their local aggressiveness and involvement of vital structures, especially by lesions in the head and neck.[43] Amputation may be required because of a useless or painful limb. Such a therapeutic procedure, however, should be a last resort, since these lesions may stabilize in their growth and some have even regressed, although this is unusual.[43,50]

Fibrous hamartoma of infancy

Fibrous hamartoma of infancy is a distinctive histopathologic entity that is seen almost entirely in infants and young children, with almost all lesions appearing during the first 2 years of life.[43,48] To date, it has not been reported in adults. Boys are more commonly affect-

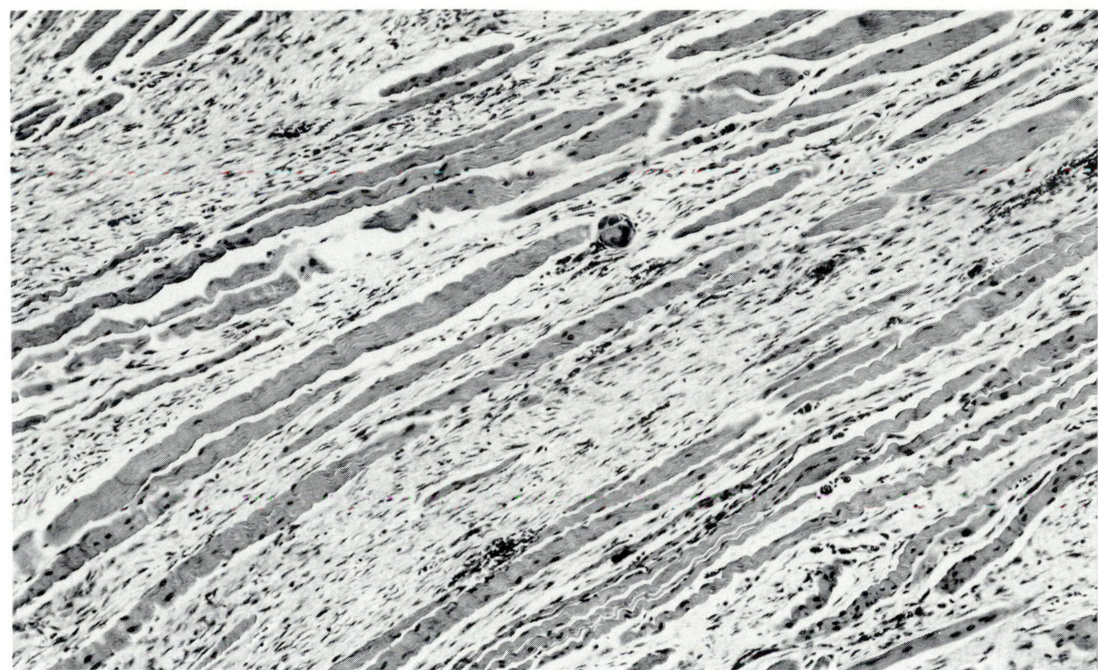

Fig. 39-2. Desmoid fibromatosis. Diffuse infiltration of skeletal muscle by bands of well-formed slender fibroblasts. (90×.)

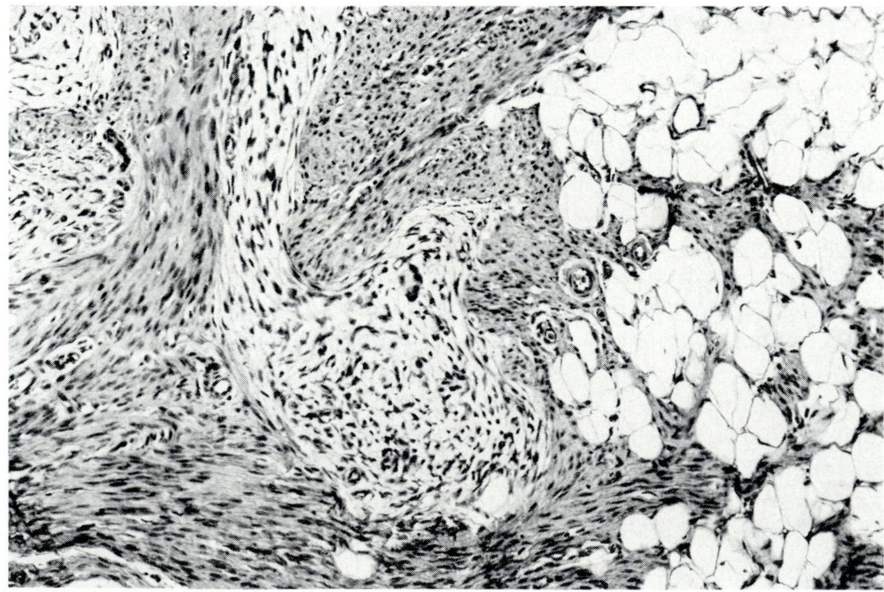

Fig. 39-3. Fibrous hamartoma. Mixture of fat, bundles of mature fibroblasts, and pale edematous-appearing nodules of primitive mesenchymal cells. (120×.)

ed than girls in a ratio of 2:1 or 3:1.[48] The lesions occur as palpable masses beneath the skin, with two thirds located in the region of the axilla, shoulder, or upper arm, the axillary fold being the most common site.[43,48] Other reported locations have included the forearm, abdomen, neck, scalp, chest wall, inguinal region, and vulva.[55a,59] The hands and feet appear to be spared.[43]

These lesions, as their original designation of "subdermal 'fibromatous tumors' of infancy"[57] suggests, occur in the lower dermis or the subcutaneous tissue as round or bosselated masses that may be as large as 8 cm. They are usually unencapsulated and blend into the subcutaneous fat or are attached to the superficial fascia.[48] The cut surface shows a mixture of white fibrous bands and yellow fat.

Fibrous hamartoma has a highly characteristic microscopic appearance.[57] The diagnosis depends on finding a mixture of mature fat cells, mature fibroblasts arranged in fibrocollagenous bundles, and foci of immature-appearing round, oval, or stellate cells embedded in a loose myxoid matrix. These latter cells are considered to be primitive mesenchymal cells. The proportions of the three elements vary, but they are always intimately mixed with one another (Fig. 39-3). The mesenchymal foci stand out as paler, edematous, ball-like areas within or surrounded by the denser fibrocollagenous bands. Occasionally, dense hyalinized areas that appear keloid-like are present. The fibrous bundles with their myxoid areas may at times simulate the appearance of a neurofibroma, but the presence of the fat cells helps to differentiate the two lesions. Electron microscopic studies have demonstrated the presence of both fibroblasts and myofibroblasts.[55a,59] Despite its well-accepted name, fibrous hamartoma is considered by most authors as a fibromatosis and included within the broad category of congenital or juvenile fibromatoses.[43,55,59]

The ultimate clinical evolution of these lesions if untreated is unknown, since they are all locally excised. Although a few have recurred, requiring a reexcision, they have no aggressive potential.[48,59]

Juvenile aponeurotic fibroma

Juvenile aponeurotic fibroma, also variously called calcifying juvenile aponeurotic fibroma or calcifying fibroma,[52] occurs principally in patients younger than 20 years,[44,55] with over half the lesions in one series occurring during the first 10 years of life, some being congenital.[59] Despite the name, rare examples are recorded in adults even in the sixth decade of life.[43,53] They are more than twice as common in male as in female patients.[59]

Juvenile aponeurotic fibroma is first seen as an essentially asymptomatic, firm, poorly circumscribed mass beneath unremarkable skin. About two thirds occur in the hand, with the majority in the palm about the thenar and hypothenar eminences.[44,55,59] Other frequent sites include the wrist and fingers, with recorded instances in the forearm, thigh, popliteal fossa, back, foot, and knee area. They are usually small lesions, rarely exceeding 3 cm, and are almost always located in the subcutaneous tissue in close relation to a tendon or joint capsule.[53,55,59] Grossly they appear as sharply demarcated nodular masses, or they have a distinct infiltrative pattern.[44,53] Histologically one finds a cellular lesion that infiltrates fat, connective tissue, and muscle. It is composed of plump to round, immature-appearing fibroblasts having ill-defined cytoplasmic borders that produce a syncytial appearance. Mitoses are scarce. The cells typically orient themselves in the same direction and appear to flow out into the adjacent normal tissue to form nodular aggregates. These nodules frequently have central foci of dense calcification. The cells immediately adjacent to these calcified foci assume a chondroid appearance, lying in lacunae, and appear to differentiate toward fibrocartilage.[44,52,53,55,59] This cartilaginous appearance has caused the lesion to be considered as the cartilage analog of the fibromatoses even though the component cells are plumper, smaller, and more irregular than the spindle cells of the usual fibromatosis.[53]

Following local excision, these lesions have recurred in about one half of the patients, with some having multiple recurrences.[44,59] Younger patients appear more prone to local recurrences.[44] There is no metastatic potential, and conservative management is indicated.[43]

Congenital generalized fibromatoses

Congenital generalized fibromatosis is a rare condition, with probably fewer than 50 well-documented cases reported in the English literature.[59,60] Unlike most of the fibromatoses, visceral involvement is frequent, and when this occurs, the disease is often fatal.[49,60] Authors have used different terms such as *multiple*, *diffuse*, or *generalized* to refer to either involvement of the viscera or the number of lesions present. In this chapter *multiple* refers to lesions that affect the skin, subcutaneous tissue, muscle, or bone and *visceral* to those that also involve other organs.[59] These lesions have recently been described under the term *infantile myofibromatosis*.[46]

These fibromatoses are almost always congenital, but new lesions may continue to develop after birth.[45,59] Boys are more commonly affected than girls in a ratio of 3:1.[59] The superficial lesions involve the skin and subcutaneous tissue and are firm to rubbery nodules that number from a few to as many as 100.[43,59] They are usually small, less than 3 cm. They may involve the underlying muscle and appear in bone, where they produce osteolytic lesions.[43,46,59]

Osseous lesions are seen in both forms of the disease, occurring in 63% of those with multiple and 47% with visceral lesions. Any bone may be involved, and spontaneous fractures may occur.[59] In those with visceral lesions any organ outside the central nervous system may be involved, including the heart, lungs, intestinal tract, tongue, liver, and pancreas.[43,59] In an addendum to a recent report, however, involvement of the central nervous system was found in a single patient.[46] Even in patients with visceral lesions, the skin and subcutaneous tissues are still the most frequent sites of involvement.[59] To date the number of patients reported with and without visceral lesions has been about equal.[59]

Grossly the nodules may appear well circumscribed and even shell out easily, but at times they infiltrate the soft tissue and have ill-defined margins. Unlike the desmoid fibromatoses, cells of this lesion have an immature appearance, with plump cells having abundant eosinophilic cytoplasm. Depending on their anatomic location, cells are arranged in bands, fascicles, or ball-like clusters, with the last very common in pulmonary lesions.[59] Cells frequently have the appearance of smooth muscle cells, and they may be seen to merge with the smooth muscle of adjacent blood vessels.[43,45,46,49,59] The resemblance to smooth muscle may be such that some consider these to be smooth muscle lesions. They have an abundant vascular component with numerous irregular vascular spaces. Well-formed blood vessels may show luminal occlusion by either fibrous tissue or cellular tumor tissue.[43,49,59] Dense collagenized areas may be present that alternate with the cellular areas, and central areas of necrosis containing stippled calcification may be found.[43,45] Such necrosis is unique in the fibromatoses. Some have noted that visceral lesions are more cellular with less collagen formation.[59] In the lungs the lesion either has a pattern of a diffuse infiltrate or centers on the pulmonary arteries and veins with florid proliferation of the tumor tissue into the vascular lumina.[59] Mitoses are scarce.

Most infants with the visceral form of the disease die soon after birth, although survivals for as long as 4 months are recorded. The cause of death is attributed to complications produced by the anatomic location of the lesion. However, examples of spontaneous regression have been reported.[43,59] Patients with pulmonary involvement have an extremely poor prognosis.[58] The prognosis in infants without visceral involvement is good. A recent review of the literature found only one death among 16 patients without visceral involvement.[59] The osseous lesions frequently regress within the first year of life.

Recently cases of solitary lesions having histopathologic features similar to those seen in the multiple or visceral forms have been reported.[45,46] The prognosis for patients with such lesions is excellent, since simple excision is curative.

PSEUDOSARCOMATOUS FIBROUS LESIONS

Many benign soft tissue lesions may, because of their cellularity or the presence of atypical-appearing cells, be mistaken for sarcomas and in that sense be considered "pseudosarcomas." However, in this section we restrict our discussion to reactive lesions whose main feature is a proliferation of fibrous elements, namely nodular fasciitis, proliferative fasciitis, and proliferative myositis.

Although these lesions have been well defined, with some excellent descriptions of their histologic appearance, we still receive consultation cases that carry the diagnosis of some form of sarcoma for which radical surgery is contemplated, but that on review represent one of these reactive conditions. The magnitude of the problem is illustrated by the fact that in one large cancer registry slightly over 10% of the lesions diagnosed as sarcoma were, on review, reclassified as benign.[64] In this latter group about 60% of the cases represented one of these pseudosarcomatous fibrous lesions. Because of their cellularity, rapid growth, gross infiltrative growth pattern, and high mitotic index, the pathologist considers them to be some form of fibrosarcoma, myxoid malignant fibrous histiocytoma, sclerosing liposarcoma, or neurofibrosarcoma. It should be remembered that rapid growth and an infiltrative gross pattern are not features of most sarcomas.

Nodular fasciitis

Since its original description as subcutaneous pseudosarcomatous fibromatosis,[70] nodular fasciitis has been known by a variety of synonyms, including infiltrative fasciitis, pseudosarcomatous fasciitis, and proliferative fasciitis.[61,69,72] The last term has recently been applied to another type of pseudosarcoma,[63] and we prefer the term *nodular fasciitis* for the lesion discussed here. Over 80% of the "sarcomas" reclassified as benign conditions in the study just mentioned were examples of nodular fasciitis.[64]

Nodular fasciitis occurs at all ages, with reports of patients ranging in age from 2 weeks to 74 years.[66,69,72] However, the usual patients are young adults with a mean age between 30 and 40 years.[64,66,68,72] Male patients are slightly more commonly affected than female patients.[72] Typically these are rapidly growing lesions, with over one half of the patients having symptoms for less than 1 month.[61,66,72]

Although originally described in the subcutaneous tissue, nodular fasciitis also occurs in the deep somatic soft tissues and has been reported in the parotid gland, breast, esophagus, trachea, vagina, and labia.[61] However, one half of cases are found in the upper extremity, where the forearm is by far the most common site. The trunk and head and neck region each account for about 20% of cases, with the lower extremity less commonly involved.* In children the head and neck region accounts for about one half of cases.[66] Small to medium-sized arteries and veins may also be sites of origin.[74]

The lesion grows from the superficial fascia into the

*References 61, 66, 68, 69, 71, 72.

subcutaneous tissue as a round to oval nodule that is usually well circumscribed but may also appear poorly delimited and infiltrative. Lesions tend to be small, rarely exceeding 5 cm, with most between 1 and 3 cm.[61,72] Occasionally lesions extend along the fascia and downward into the muscle.[66] Microscopically, nodular fasciitis has a wide range of morphologic patterns; one paper mentioned 11 histologic variants.[61] Fortunately, however, most lesions have mixed patterns, and all share a common set of features. Spindle-shaped, fibroblast-like cells are arranged in long fascicles described as having curved, whorled, or S-shaped patterns. The fascicles are loosely arranged, separated by a myxoid stroma that gives the lesion a characteristic edematous appearance.[61,62,66] Cells may vary from the usual spindle forms to plumper forms with prominent nucleoli (Fig. 39-4). Although some cellular atypia occurs, bizarre pleomorphic cells are not present, and mitoses, although numerous, are not atypical.[14,61,62,66] Electron microscopic studies have shown that the spindle cells are myofibroblasts.[75] Another frequent finding is the presence of extravasated red blood cells either infiltrating between stromal cells or located in clusters within microcystic spaces or clefts.[14,61,72] In hematoxylin and eosin sections these spaces have a blue-gray appearance and, along with the myxoid stroma, contain a hyaluronidase-sensitive acid mucopolysaccharide.[7a,14,66] Although its name implies inflammation, inflammatory cells, chiefly lymphocytes, are never very numerous. Osteoclastic-type giant cells are often found. At times the myxoid stroma is less prominent, and the cells are more compact and arranged in a storiform pattern similar to fibrous histiocytoma.[14] Another lesion that may be simulated by the compact regions is a cellular desmoid fibromatosis. Nodular fasciitis is quite vascular, with capillaries arranged in fanlike or radial arrays especially at the periphery of the nodules.[61] Areas with the histomorphology of nodular fasciitis are also found in the other two pseudosarcomas, proliferative myositis and proliferative fasciitis.[65]

Local excision is curative in almost all cases of nodular fasciitis, even when the lesion is incompletely excised. Recurrences are reported, but this happens in less than 5% of cases.[61,72] In many these recurrent cases, examination of the original tumor has shown it not to be nodular fasciitis.[61a]

Proliferative myositis and proliferative fasciitis

Proliferative myositis and proliferative fasciitis are discussed together because their histologic features frequently overlap. They are both less common than nodu-

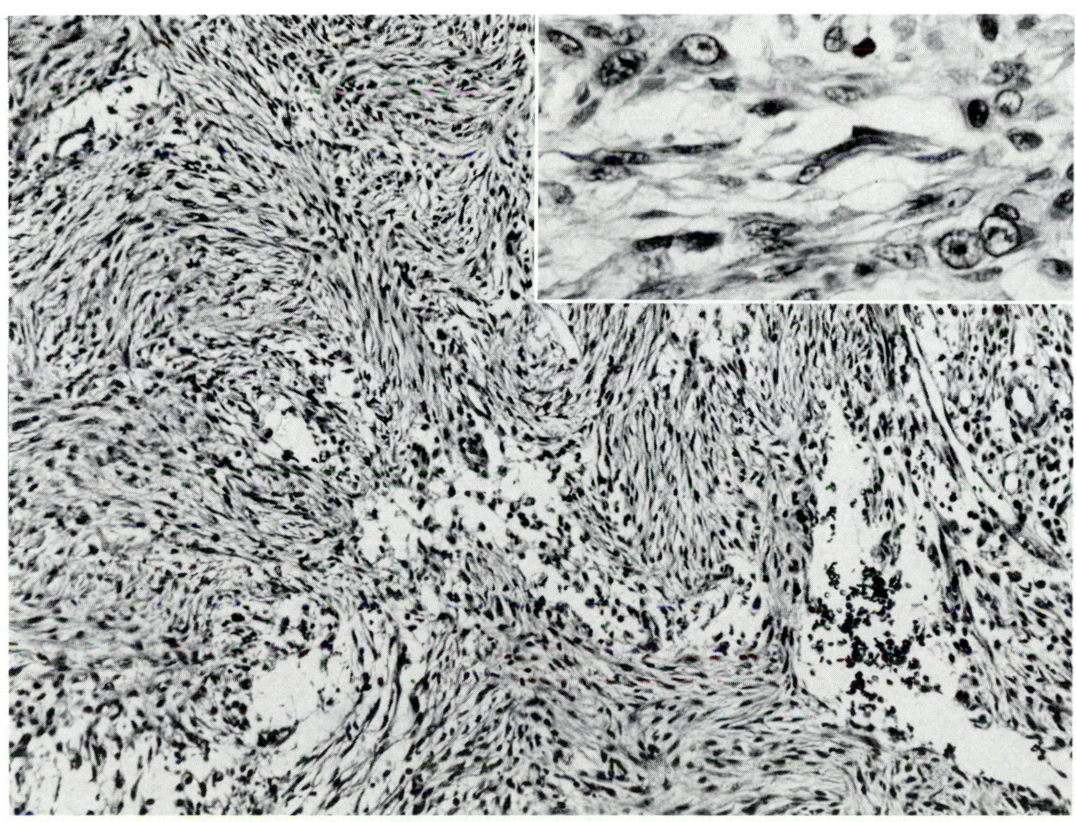

Fig. 39-4. Nodular fasciitis. Whorled pattern of fibroblasts with microcystic spaces containing red blood cells. (150×.) *Inset,* Mild nuclear atypia is present in some cells with round nuclei having prominent nucleoli. (600×.)

lar fasciitis. It should be noted that the term *proliferative fasciitis* was used in the past as a synonym for nodular fasciitis.

Unlike nodular fasciitis, which is found in children and young adults, both these lesions appear in older patients with an average age of from 50 to 55 years, and they do not occur in children.[63,65,67] Both are more frequent in men.[63,65] They are characterized by a rapid clinical evolution over a period of only a few weeks. Tenderness or pain is found in two thirds of patients.[63,67] Proliferative myositis is located within muscles, usually of the upper arm and shoulder, but also in the thigh, neck, and chest wall.[65,67] It is a poorly demarcated lesion and gives the appearance of scarlike tissue within the muscle. It varies in size from 1 to 6 cm.[67] Proliferative fasciitis involves the extremities in three fourths of cases, with the forearm and thigh being the most common sites.[63] The lesion exists in the region between the muscle and the subcutis where it runs along the superficial fascia in an infiltrative pattern. Mixed forms between proliferative myositis and proliferative fasciitis may be found where there is involvement of both muscle and the adjacent fascia and subcutis.[65]

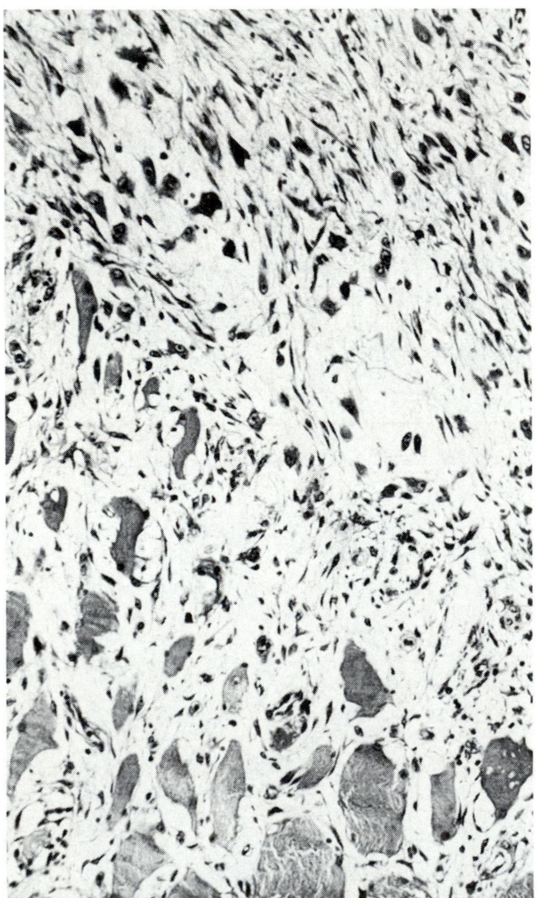

Fig. 39-5. Proliferative myositis. Fibroblasts and ganglion-like cells, embedded in a pale myxoid stroma, infiltrate between skeletal muscle fibers. (150×.)

Histologically, proliferative myositis shows a proliferation of spindle-shaped fibroblast-like cells that separate the muscle into bundles and infiltrate between individual muscle fibers (Fig. 39-5). Characteristically the muscle does not show necrosis or regenerative phenomena. Associated with these spindle cells are prominent large cells having an abundant basophilic cytoplasm and one or two prominent basophilic nucleoli.[65,67] These cells frequently have a ganglion cell–like appearance or resemble rhabdomyoblasts.[63] The giant cells, which lack cross striations, have been interpreted as modified fibroblasts. Such giant cells are also found in proliferative fasciitis, as are the fibroblast-like spindle cells that proliferate along the fascia and the fibrous septa in the subcutaneous tissue. A myxoid stroma surrounds the cells, giving the lesion an edematous appearance. Osteoid, mature bone, and cartilage may occur in both lesions.[65] Since areas of nodular fasciitis may be found in both proliferative fasciitis and proliferative myositis, all three lesions may be variants of the same disorder.[64,65,73] Despite their histologic appearance, these lesions are benign and self-limited, with no tendency to recur after local excision.

FIBROHISTIOCYTIC TUMORS

Over the last several years lesions of fibrohistiocytic differentiation, especially the malignant varieties, have held the center stage in the field of soft tissue tumor pathology. These malignant tumors, which were not even mentioned in the lists of the common sarcomas 10 to 20 years ago,[19,86] now comprise from 10% to 20% of all sarcomas, being somewhat less frequent than rhabdomyosarcoma and liposarcoma.[10,28,38,83] However, at the Armed Forces Institute of Pathology malignant fibrohistiocytic tumors are the most common sarcomas found in older adults,[84,115] and in some institutions they represent the most common soft tissue sarcoma.[83]

Fibrohistiocytic tumors, both benign and malignant, share common light microscopic features marked by the presence, in varying proportions, of cells with histiocytic and fibroblastic characteristics. There is a histomorphologic spectrum within the group, with some tumors exhibiting a predominantly histiocytic pattern, others a predominantly fibroblastic pattern, and more commonly those with a mixed composition. This had led to a multitude of designations for both the benign and malignant forms of these lesions, including fibroxanthoma, fibrous xanthoma, histiocytoma, malignant histiocytoma, malignant fibrous xanthoma, malignant fibrous histiocytoma, fibroxanthosarcoma, and xanthosarcoma. The general term *fibrous histiocytoma* is used to designate any of the tumors within this group, with individual and more specific names applied to the various morphologic subtypes.[92] Many lesions now considered to be fibrohistiocytic carry well-established and ingrained names by which they are known to clinicians and which are best not changed. To diagnose the common giant cell tumor of tendon sheath as a fibrous histiocytoma may cause more confusion than illumination.

As the concept of and diagnostic criteria for these tumors have evolved,[91,92,110,115] it has become evident that many pleomorphic soft tissue tumors previously diagnosed as pleomorphic fibrosarcoma, pleomorphic liposarcoma, or pleomorphic rhabdomyosarcoma are in reality malignant fibrohistiocytomas.[84,91] Caution should be exercised, however, in the use of malignant fibrous histiocytoma as a diagnosis. The current frequency of these tumors may reflect the increasing use of less stringent criteria by pathologists for the diagnosis of these tumors. The term is now, unfortunately, being used with such frequency that it is in danger of becoming a "wastebasket" diagnosis for every strange spindle cell or pleomorphic soft tissue sarcoma. Such indiscriminate use detracts from its clinical and pathologic significance. It is important to remember that some sarcomas cannot be definitively classified, and to diagnose such tumors as fibrous histiocytomas does harm to the criteria established for their diagnosis.[91,92,110,114]

Benign fibrous histiocytomas include such diverse entities as subepidermal nodular fibrosis (sclerosing hemangioma, dermatofibroma), atypical fibroxanthoma of skin, juvenile xanthogranuloma (nevoxanthoendothelioma), giant cell tumor of tendon sheath (nodular tenosynovitis), pigmented villonodular synovitis, xanthogranuloma, and plasma cell granuloma.[92] The low-grade malignant cutaneous tumor, dermatofibrosarcoma protuberans, is also accepted as a fibrohistiocytic lesion. These lesions are described elsewhere in this text. Discussed here are the malignant soft tissue fibrohistiocytic tumors. Giant cell tumor of soft parts and epithelioid sarcoma, both suggested by some as malignant fibrohistiocytic tumors, are detailed elsewhere in this chapter.

Malignant fibrohistiocytic tumors

Although malignant fibrohistiocytic tumors occur in children and young adults,[89,102] they are most common in patients in the fifth to seventh decades of life.* The recently described angiomatoid variety, however, does occur in a significantly younger age group, with most patients less than 30 years of age, the mean age being 13 years.[85] Fibrohistiocytic malignancies occur more commonly in males than in females in an approximately 1.5:1 ratio.[96,102,110,114,115]

The histologic classification of these tumors is still in a state of flux, since several authors have used slightly different terminologies and classifications.† However, with the increased recognition of these tumors, a variety of subtypes have been culled from the more general occurring forms. They are known as the myxoid, inflammatory, pleomorphic, and angiomatoid variants of malignant fibrous histiocytoma. Not only do these subtypes have specific histomorphologic patterns, but some have specific clinical manifestations and different prognoses.

Two thirds to three fourths of these tumors occur in the extremities, most commonly the lower extremity, where the thigh is the most common site, accounting for one third of cases.[84,91,92,97,110] Distal portions of the extremities, the hands and feet, are only rarely involved.[115] Other frequent locations include the trunk, shoulder region, and retroperitoneum.[84,88,91,115] The tumors are usually deep seated, arising in muscle and the deep fascia, although about 20% to 30% arise in the subcutaneous tissue or lower dermis.[91,110,114,115] They have also been reported in such diverse locations as the nose, paranasal sinuses, orbit, larynx, meninges, bone, lung, vagina, ovary, and submandibular gland.[80,86a,104]

The superficially located tumors tend to be small (2 to 4 cm), but deeply situated tumors frequently are greater than 5 cm and may reach a very large size in the retroperitoneum.[92,110,115] They have a nonspecific gross appearance as either a nodular or multinodular, well-circumscribed, fleshy mass. Depending on their cellular composition, they are gray or white or have a yellow cast caused by a high cellular fat content. Myxoid tumors have a translucent or mucoid appearance.[114] Unlike the other malignant fibrous histiocytomas, the angiomatoid lesions are almost all located in the subcutaneous tissue and on gross inspection contain irregular blood-filled cystic spaces.[85]

Most malignant fibrohistiocytomas are initially seen as painless enlarging masses present for less than 1 year,[91,115] although approximately one fourth of patients have some pain associated with the mass.[91,92] The angiomatoid variety has a bluish tint and may clinically resemble a cutaneous hemangioma or a hematoma. Patients with this variant may have associated systemic effects with weight loss, anemia, and fever.[85] Those with the inflammatory variant may have an elevation of their peripheral white blood cell count, producing a leukemoid reaction.[94]

The histomorphology of the fibrohistiocytomas is marked by their extreme cellular variability not only from tumor to tumor but also from area to area within the same tumor.[84,92,97] A small biopsy specimen or the examination of only one or two sections from one of these tumors is insufficient to appreciate their overall pattern. Usually there is an admixture of spindle-shaped fibroblasts and mononuclear, round to oval, histiocytic cells. Evidence of nuclear atypia in both types of cells varies from tumors in which this is found in only a few cells, the majority having bland cytologic features, to tumors with

*References 91, 92, 97, 99, 110, 115.

†References 23, 84, 91, 92, 95a, 99, 113a, 115.

extensive cellular pleomorphism, bizarre multinucleated tumor cells, hyperchromasia, and frequent and abnormal mitotic figures. This pleomorphic pattern is more common.[115] Fibrosis may be minimal or quite extensive, producing broad hyalinized regions. Islands of bland-appearing foam cells (xanthoma cells) may be found among the tumor cells, as are lymphocytes, plasma cells, and eosinophils. Focal hemangiopericytomatous areas may be found in some tumors.[84,91,92,110,115] Metaplastic bone and cartilage may be present to such a degree that a myositis ossificans–like pattern is suggested roentgenographically.[82a]

A further histologic characteristic of the fibrohistiocytic tumors, both benign and malignant, is the presence of a storiform pattern, best seen in tumors composed principally of spindle-shaped fibroblasts. First well described in what were considered to be neurofibromas,[79] it consists of a cartwheel or nebula arrangement of the cells around a central focus with bands of spindle cells radiating or spinning outward from this central region (Fig. 39-6). Three-dimensional analysis of this pattern has shown that it is formed by the junction of the peripheral portions of adjacent groups of proliferating cells. The centers apparently do not have a consistent relationship with blood vessels as was previously thought.[98] This storiform pattern is found in more than 80% of malignant fibrous histiocytomas, although at times it is only focally present and found only after an extensive search.[92,97a,99,110] As the histiocytic cell component increases, along with the degree of cellular anaplasia, the storiform pattern becomes less obvious and may be absent in the primary tumor. However, not infrequently metastases from such tumors have a storiform pattern. The storiform pattern is not diagnostic of fibrous histiocytoma. We have seen it in epithelial tumors such as melanomas, epidermoid carcinomas, and sarcomatoid renal cell carcinomas and in benign conditions such as nodular fasciitis. It may also appear focally in other sarcomas such as osteosarcoma, leiomyosarcoma, and neurosarcoma. Purely reactive lesions may also have prominent storiform regions.[109,116]

From this general category of malignant fibrous histio-

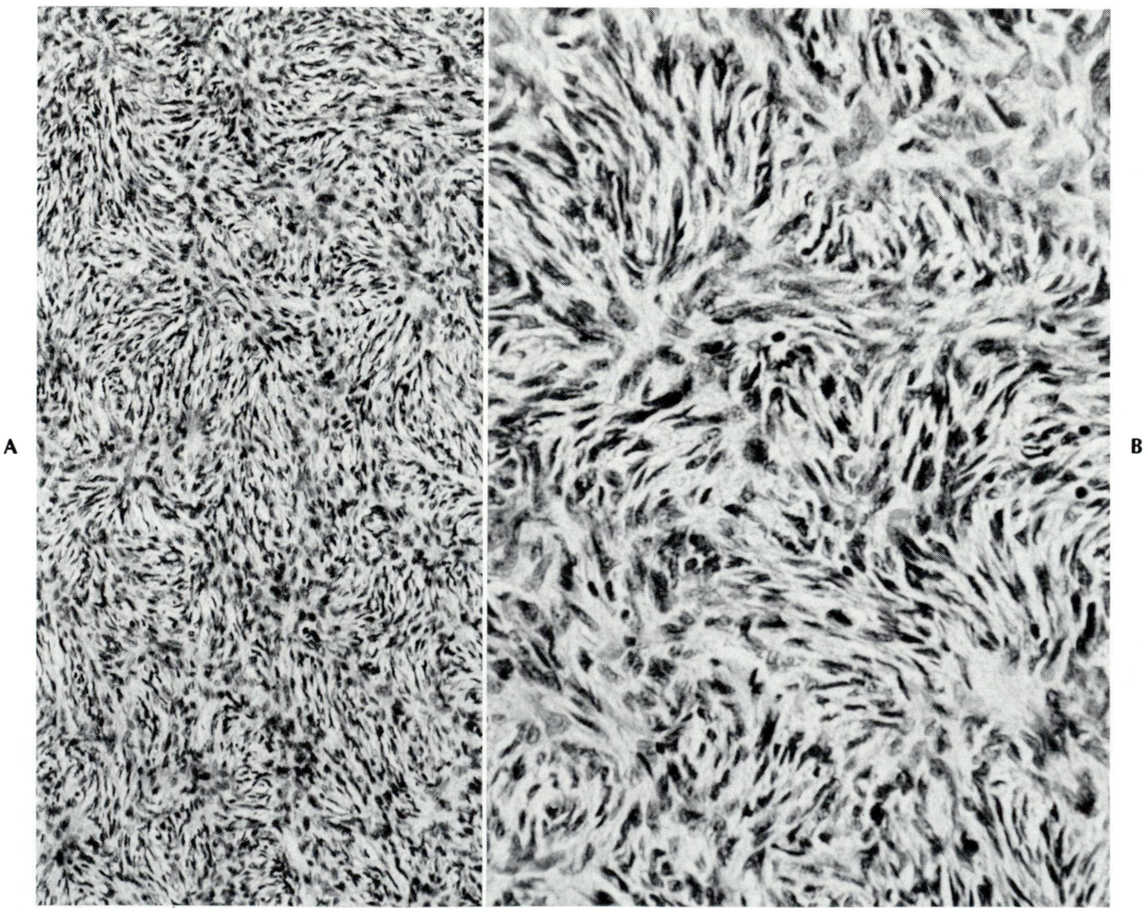

Fig. 39-6. A, Storiform pattern in fibrous histiocytoma. **B,** Spindle-shaped fibroblasts arranged in a whorling cartwheel fashion. This storiform pattern is characteristic but not diagnostic of fibrous histiocytoma. (**A,** 150×; **B,** 350×.)

cytoma can be identified some tumors that have either specific cellular constituents or are marked by an exaggeration of the normal histopathologic pattern. Rarely, light microscopy shows a tumor composed solely of polygonal histiocytes. These cells may have distinct cytoplasmic borders and be arranged in compact nodules, or their cytoplasm may merge into a syncytium. The cells have large vesicular nuclei with an irregular chromatin distribution and one or two prominent nucleoli. The tumor lacks a storiform pattern. This "malignant histiocytoma" histologically mimics a histiocytic lymphoma but differs from the latter by the absence of reticulin fibers around the cells.[82,89,103,110]

The pleomorphic variety of malignant fibrous histiocytoma, known as fibroxanthosarcoma,[92] is noted for its marked degree of cellular anaplasia with numerous large, bizarre tumor giant cells, many of which are multinucleated (Fig. 39-7). These cells have an abundant glassy eosinophilic cytoplasm and may show phagocytic activity. Malignant-appearing spindle cells and mononuclear histiocytes are also present. Necrosis may be marked. It is this variety of malignant fibrous histiocytoma that in the past has been diagnosed as pleomorphic fibrosarcoma, liposarcoma, or rhabdomyosarcoma. However, cross striations are absent, and lipoblasts are not found in the majority of these tumors. Occasionally, however, cells are present that do have lipoblastic features, and the distinction between pleomorphic liposarcoma and fibroxanthosarcoma may be blurred.[108,115] In the presence of a storiform pattern and only a few lipoblast-like cells we arbitrarily assign such cases to the malignant fibrous histiocytoma category.

The inflammatory variant of malignant fibrous histiocytoma has, in addition to atypical anaplastic histiocytes and fibroblasts, an intense polymorphonuclear cell infiltrate that is unassociated with tissue necrosis.[90,94,100] Reed-Sternberg–like cells and histiocytic cells that resemble ganglion cells are present. Although chronic inflammatory cells are also found, sometimes in abundance, it should be remembered that any of the malignant fibrohistiocytic tumors may contain chronic inflammatory cells, and it is only tumors that demonstrate a diffuse acute inflammatory component that satisfy the definition of inflammatory fibrous histiocytoma.[94] Most of these tumors have histiocytic-like cells as their major cell component. In their early stages they are composed of bland-appearing fibroblasts, histiocytes, and many foam cells, with only a few cells showing nuclear atypia. This, combined with the acute inflammation, may cause them to be considered benign reactive lesions (Fig. 39-8).

Areas of myxoid change are not uncommon in the usual malignant fibrous histiocytoma. When the myxoid component comprises at least one half of the lesion, however, it is separately classified as a myxoid malignant fibrous histiocytoma.[114] This tumor has also been described under the designation of myxofibrosarcoma.[78,93,99a] It is composed of hypocellular areas in which the tumor cells, both histiocytes and fibroblasts, are separated by a clear to basophilic mucinous matrix having a high content of hyaluronic acid. The cells may vary from well differentiated to highly pleomorphic, and lipoblast-like cells may be found. Compact cellular areas are found adjacent to the myxoid foci (Fig. 39-9). Mitotic figures are common and are frequently abnormal. Within the myxoid areas is a prominent capillary network that in some foci may be arranged in a plexiform pattern. These myxoid fibrous histiocytomas may be confused with myxoid liposarcoma. However, myxoid liposarcoma lacks the cellular pleomorphism, mitotic activity, and storiform pattern of the fibrous histiocytoma. The mucin pools of

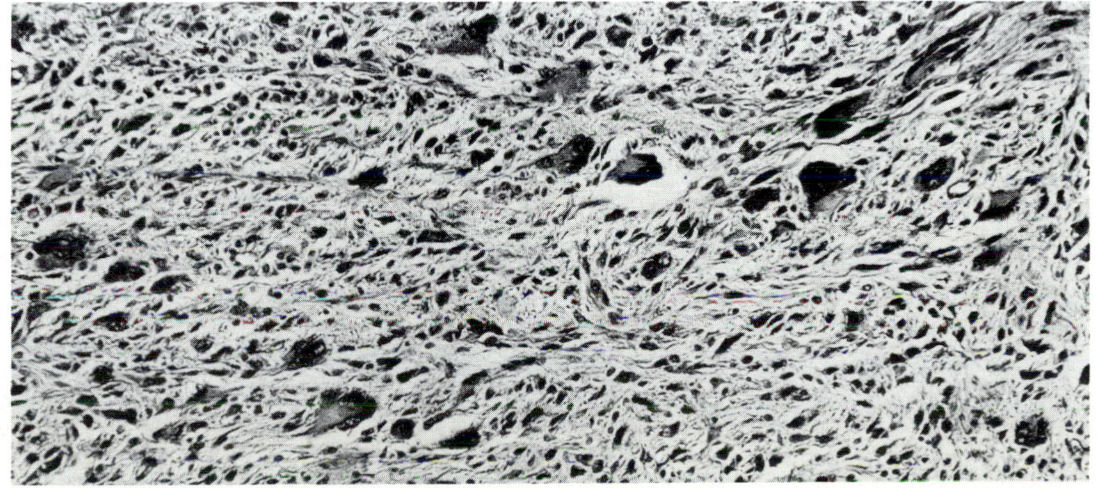

Fig. 39-7. Fibroxanthosarcoma. Bizarre, pleomorphic, multinucleated tumor giant cells with abundant eosinophilic cytoplasm within a fibrous stroma. (150×.)

myxoid liposarcoma are also not found in the myxoid malignant fibrous histiocytoma.[77]

Angiomatoid malignant fibrous histiocytoma, only recently described, is characterized by solid nodular masses of fibroblastic and histiocytic-like cells that surround hemorrhagic foci or blood-filled cystlike spaces.[85] There is a marked lymphocytic and plasmacytic infiltrate around the nodules. Histiocytic cells may contain abundant hemosiderin pigment, but foam cells and a storiform pattern are rare. Dense, hyalinized, fibrous areas exist between the nodules. Cellular pleomorphism is apparently not a marked feature of these tumors. A closely related benign cutaneous counterpart of this tumor, although lacking nodularity and the inflammatory component, has recently been described.[107]

Several electron microscopic studies have been conducted on the fibrohistiocytic tumors.* Basically three types of cells have been found: fibroblastic, histiocytic, and primitive mesenchymal-type cells. Transitional forms between histiocytes and fibroblasts are also found, as are some myofibroblasts.[14,76,81,105] Overlap between the electron microscopic features of liposarcoma and those of malignant fibrous histiocytoma are found, supporting those who believe that these two tumors are closely related.[17,108,115]

Originally believed to be primarily histiocytic tumors whose cells had the capacity to act as facultative fibroblasts,[89,103] these tumors are currently thought to develop from primitive mesenchymal cells that are able to differentiate along both histiocytic and fibroblastic pathways.[76,87,111] Significantly, Langerhans granules, peculiar to histiocytes, have not been found in these studies,[32,111] except in a single case of a radiation-induced malignant fibrous histiocytoma.[112]

Few histologic criteria permit one to predict the clinical course of these malignant tumors.[92,102] Indeed, metastases may develop in fibrohistiocytic tumors that show no cellular atypia in either the primary tumor or the metastases.[106] We do not apply the term "benign" to any fibrohistiocytic tumor in the deep soft tissue, since

*References 32, 76, 87, 95, 97, 101, 105, 111.

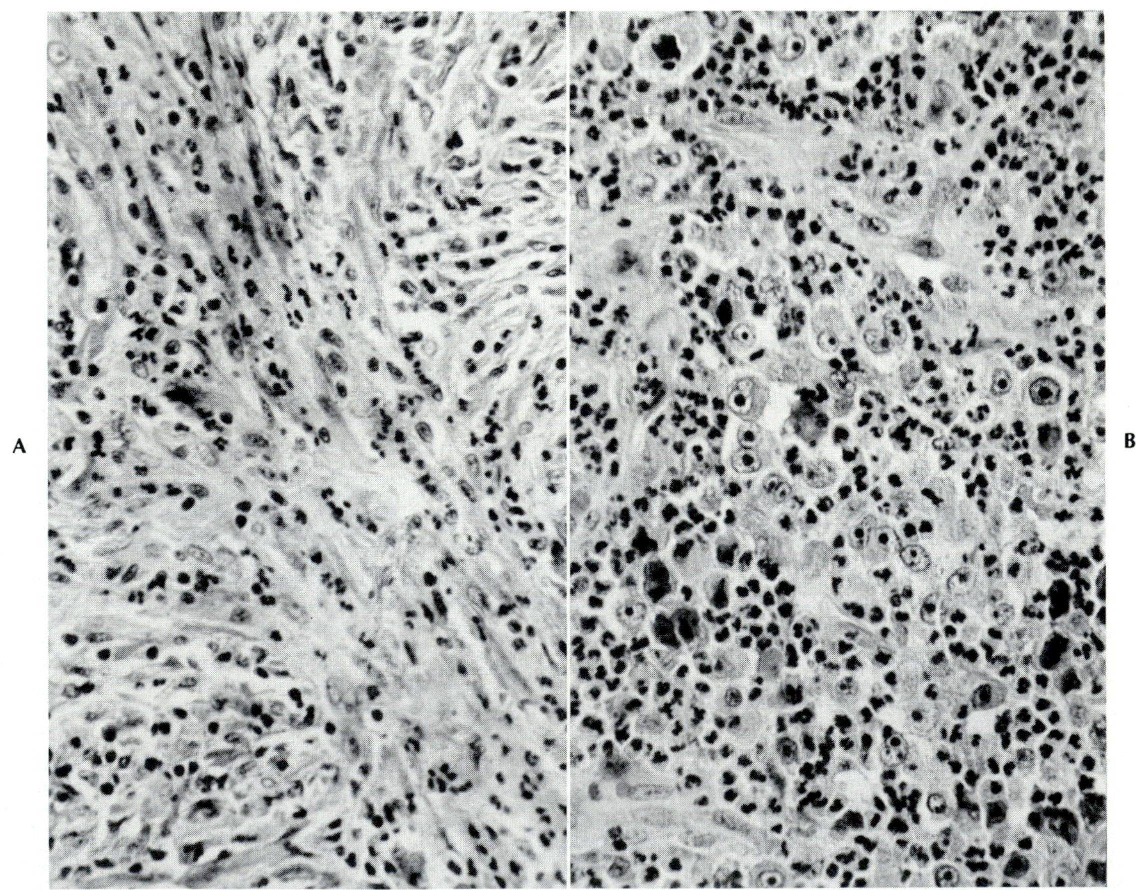

Fig. 39-8. A, Inflammatory fibrous histiocytoma, fibrous pattern. Portion of storiform area showing diffuse infiltration by polymorphonuclear leukocytes. **B,** Inflammatory fibrous histiocytoma, histiocytic pattern. Malignant-appearing histiocytic-like cells, with prominent nucleoli, surrounded by polymorphonuclear leukocytes. (350×.)

we believe that they are all capable of producing metastases. When no cellular atypia is present, they are simply reported as fibrous histiocytomas with an explanation of the potential for aggressive behavior. We reserve the designation "malignant" for those with clear cellular anaplasia.

As a group, roughly one half of these tumors recur following excision, and distant metastases develop in 20% to 50% of patients.* Five-year survival figures range from 30% to 55%.[15,83,91] Metastases are usually blood borne, with the lungs the most commonly involved site. The incidence of lymph node involvement has varied, with some claiming that nodes are frequently involved[27,84] and others placing the overall incidence at around 10%.[115] Tumors with a predominantly myxoid pattern apparently have a better overall prognosis,[114] although some disagree.[91] The inflammatory variant appears to be more aggressive than the usual malignant fibrous histiocytoma,[90,94,100] whereas the angiomatoid variety, reported in only one large series to date, appears to be less aggressive.[85] In patients with malignant fibrous histiocytoma, recurrences or metastases may develop more than 5 years after treatment, but most do so within 2 years of therapy. Recurrences and metastases appear to be related to the size and location of the primary lesions; deep-seated tumors have a higher rate of recurrence and subsequent metastases than tumors in the subcutaneous soft tissue.[114,115] Patients with large tumors also have poor prognoses,[115] as do those with tumors located proximally in the trunk, proximal aspect of the extremities, or retroperitoneum.[91]

*References 84, 96, 99, 110, 113, 115.

SMOOTH MUSCLE TUMORS

Neoplasms that differentiate toward cells with smooth muscle characteristics may be either benign (leiomyoma) or malignant (leiomyosarcoma). Although this is easily said, in practice differentiating clearly between these tumors may be among a diagnostic pathologist's most difficult and frustrating tasks. Indeed, in some cases the pathologist must be resigned to awaiting the decision of

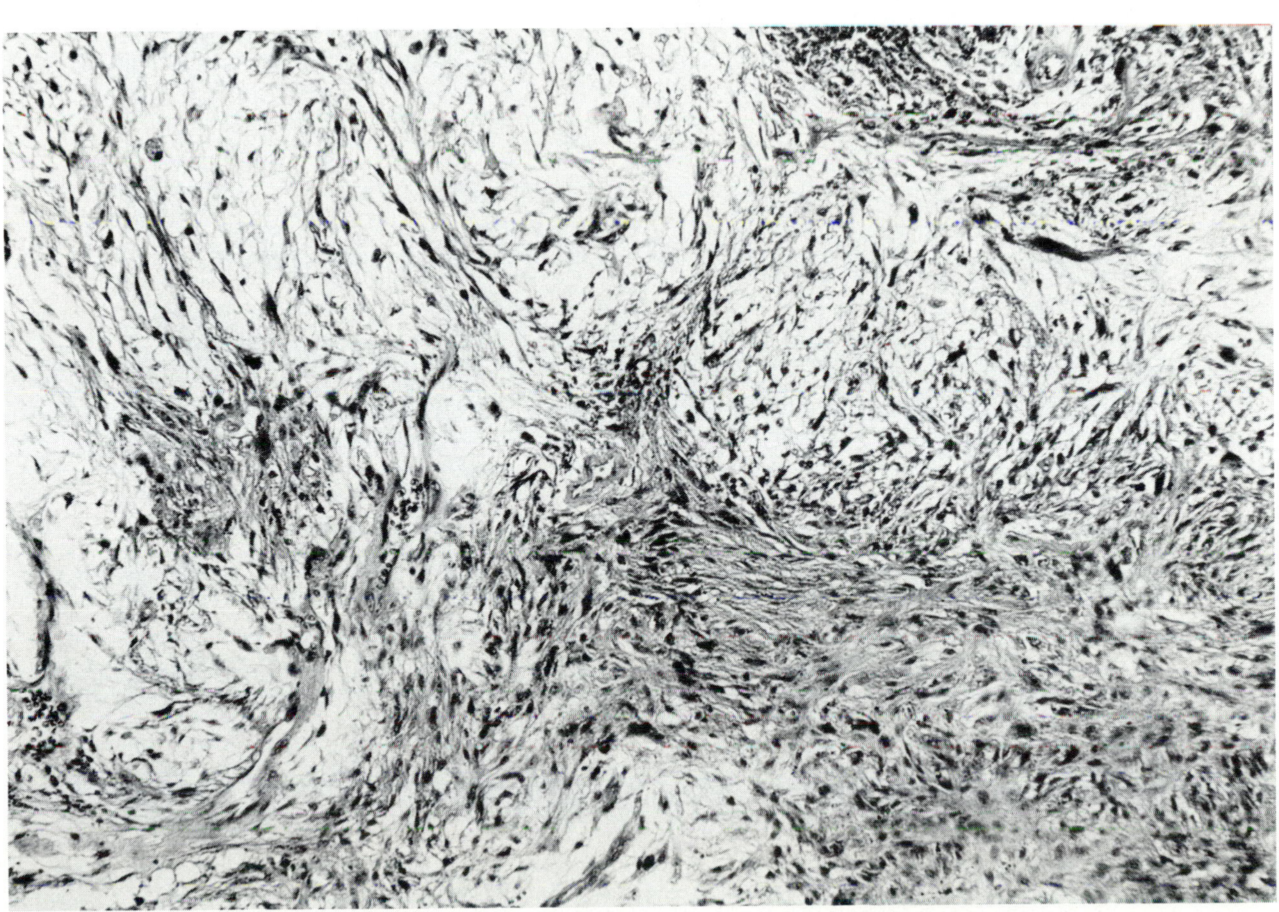

Fig. 39-9. Malignant fibrous histiocytoma, myxoid variant. Hypocellular myxoid area with atypical stromal cells is seen adjacent to a more compact cellular focus at lower right. (150×.)

time on whether the tumor is benign or malignant.

Smooth muscle tumors are far more frequent in organ systems, such as the gastrointestinal tract and female genital system, than in the somatic soft tissues.[27] Visceral lesions present special clinical and pathologic features and are described in the appropriate chapters of this book. The basic histopathologic characteristics of smooth muscle tumors are, however, similar regardless of anatomic location.

Leiomyoma

Within the soft tissue, leiomyomas are usually confined to the superficial subcutaneous tissue and skin, only rarely occurring in the deeper tissues. They arise from structures in these areas that normally contain smooth muscle, such as the arrectores pilorum, the tunica dartos, the erector muscles of the nipple, and the media of large and small blood vessels.[133,138] They occur almost exclusively in adults, rarely being found in children,[119,143] and show no sex predominance.[138] Leiomyomas in the skin and subcutaneous tissue may be quite vascular and well innervated and produce paroxysms of pain.[27,138] Otherwise, they are initially seen as a nonspecific mass of usually less than 5 cm. Superficial lesions are found anywhere in the extremities, trunk, and head and neck region.[138] In the deeper soft tissues, the retroperitoneum, omentum, mesentery, round and broad ligaments of the uterus, and the walls of large blood vessels are the common sites of origin.[27,137,140,144] An intrathoracic location in the mediastinum is rare, with most of the lesions reported as examples of smooth muscle tumors probably being neurogenous.[131]

Microscopically one finds interlacing bands and bundles of elongate spindle-shaped cells whose nuclei, in contrast to the tapered nuclei of fibroblasts, are usually blunt ended, giving them the cigar shape so frequently mentioned (Fig. 39-10). The nuclei are usually bland without obvious nucleoli. It is not uncommon to find some cells with two or three nuclei, as well as some that exhibit nuclear hyperchromasia and irregular shapes.

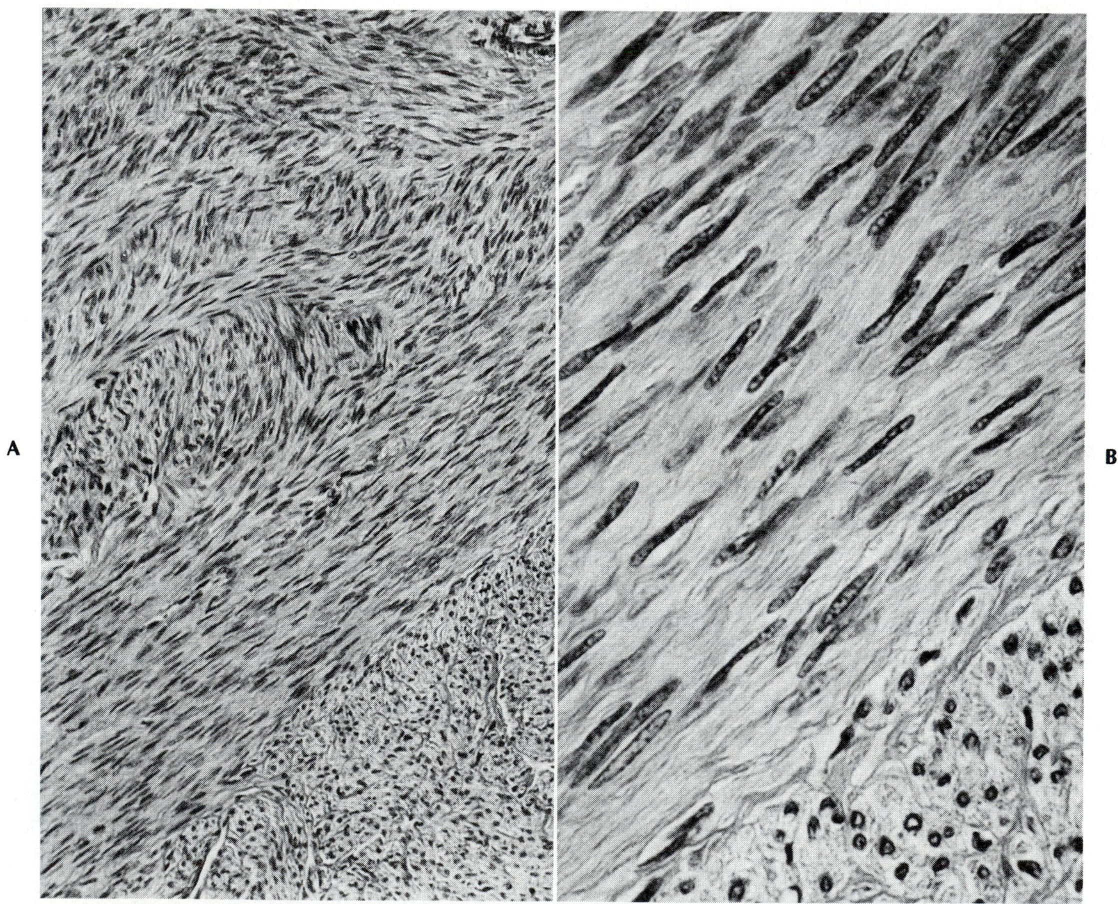

Fig. 39-10. A, Leiomyoma. Bands of smooth muscle cells seen in longitudinal and cross section. **B,** Higher magnification of area seen in Fig. 39-10, *A*. Cigar-shaped, bland-appearing nuclei of smooth muscle cells are seen in longitudinal array. At lower right cells are seen in cross section. (**A,** 150×; **B,** 600×.)

This should not be taken as evidence of malignancy when there is no associated increased mitotic activity.

Fine myofibrils, best seen with the use of phosphotungstic acid–hematoxylin stains, may be seen coursing the length of the cytoplasm. Adjacent cells may so arrange themselves that their nuclei are aligned in rows creating palisades. This may cause some diagnostic confusion with neurilemomas whose constituent cell nuclei also palisade.[27,123,138]

There is an abundant network of reticulin fibers that individually surround and run parallel to the long axis of each cell. Many leiomyomas are quite vascular and may, in focal regions, take on the appearance of a glomus tumor or a hemangiopericytoma. Necrosis in a leiomyoma is rare, and its presence should suggest the possibility of a leiomyosarcoma and stimulate the submission of further sections for study.[27,138]

By electron microscopy the cells of leiomyomas have the same features as normal smooth muscle cells: intracytoplasmic bundles of thin filaments considered to be actin, dense bodies distributed among these myofilaments, pinocytotic vesicles, condensation plaques on the cytoplasmic side of the cellular membrane, and the presence of basement membranes around the cells. Unlike the cells of leiomyosarcoma, these fine structural details usually are easily found in each cell.[128,129]

A histologic variant of leiomyoma is the epithelioid leiomyoma, also called bizarre leiomyoma, round cell leiomyoma, and leiomyoblastoma. Originally described in the stomach,[136] its most common location, it has been found in a variety of extragastric sites, including the uterus, mesentery, omentum, and retroperitoneum.[127,137,140,144] Rather than being elongate, the cells of this tumor are round or polygonal and frequently have a cytoplasmic clear zone around the nucleus.[27,136] These clear cells may so dominate the histologic pattern that the question of an epithelial neoplasm is raised. The clear zones do not contain glycogen, fat, or mucin.[134] Transitions between these epithelioid cells and the usual spindle-shaped smooth muscle cells can be found in some tumors, and electron microscopy has confirmed their smooth muscle nature.[120,134] It has been demonstrated that the clear areas are actually fixation artifacts, since they are not seen in tumors rapidly fixed for electron microscopy or when frozen sections are used for diagnosis.[134] Despite the common presence of these clear cells, the diagnosis of epithelioid leiomyoma may be made in their absence when only numerous round or polygonal cells are found.[120] Malignant forms of this tumor (epithelioid leiomyosarcoma) also occur.[117]

A peculiar condition, leiomyomatosis peritonealis disseminata, occurs in pregnant women or those recently pregnant and consists of intraperitoneal submesothelial nodules of smooth muscle. On examination at operation these nodules may appear to represent intraperitoneal metastases. They are, however, benign and may spontaneously regress.[142]

When a smooth muscle tumor lacks mitotic activity, it will in almost every case act in a benign fashion.[119,138] However, most pathologists have encountered large, deep-seated smooth muscle tumors that have pursued an aggressive course with metastases, despite the lack of significant mitotic activity.[27,119] Fortunately, this circumstance is rare. The use of mitotic counts as an aid in the differential diagnosis between benign and malignant smooth muscle tumors is discussed in the next section.

Leiomyosarcoma

Leiomyosarcomas account for 2% to 8% of soft tissue sarcomas, and are one fourth to one fifth as common as leiomyomas.[36,38,121,122,136] Their anatomic distribution is as varied as that of their benign counterparts, and like the latter they are rare in the somatic soft tissues, being more prevalent in the gastrointestinal and female genital tracts.[27,121,133] When they occur in the soft tissue, they are most commonly found in the superficial subcutaneous tissue and skin.[121,133,138] Here over 85% arise in the proximal aspect of the extremities, most frequently the lower extremity. Other sites include the head and neck region and trunk.[138] In the deep soft tissues the retroperitoneum is the most frequent site, with other sites including the mesentery, the omentum, the deep soft tissues of the neck, and between large muscle groups.[27,119,132,137,144] Major arteries and veins are also sites of origin. Veins are approximately five times more frequently involved than arteries, with the inferior vena cava accounting for over one half of the cases.[118,126,139] It should be emphasized that deep-seated leiomyosarcomas are rare tumors.

Although patients of all ages, including infants, are reported,[119,138] these tumors are rare in children. The highest incidence is in adults in the fifth and sixth decades of life.[121,122,141] The male/female ratio apparently depends on tumor location. Retroperitoneal lesions and those arising from major blood vessels are more common in female patients,[118,126,141] whereas those in the skin and subcutaneous tissue are more common in male patients.[121,122,141] Symptoms also depend on tumor location, with superficial lesions occurring as slowly growing nodules. It is usually stated that, unlike leiomyomas, superficial leiomyosarcomas are not painful.[138] However, a recent report of a large number of patients indicated that spontaneous pain, or pain on pressure, was present in close to 90% of cutaneous and 77% of subcutaneous tumors.[122] Pressure symptoms and abdominal distension are frequent findings in patients with retroperitoneal tumors. Tumors of the inferior vena cava produce symptoms of venous obstruction, the pattern of which reflects the level along the vessel where the tumor is located.[118,126]

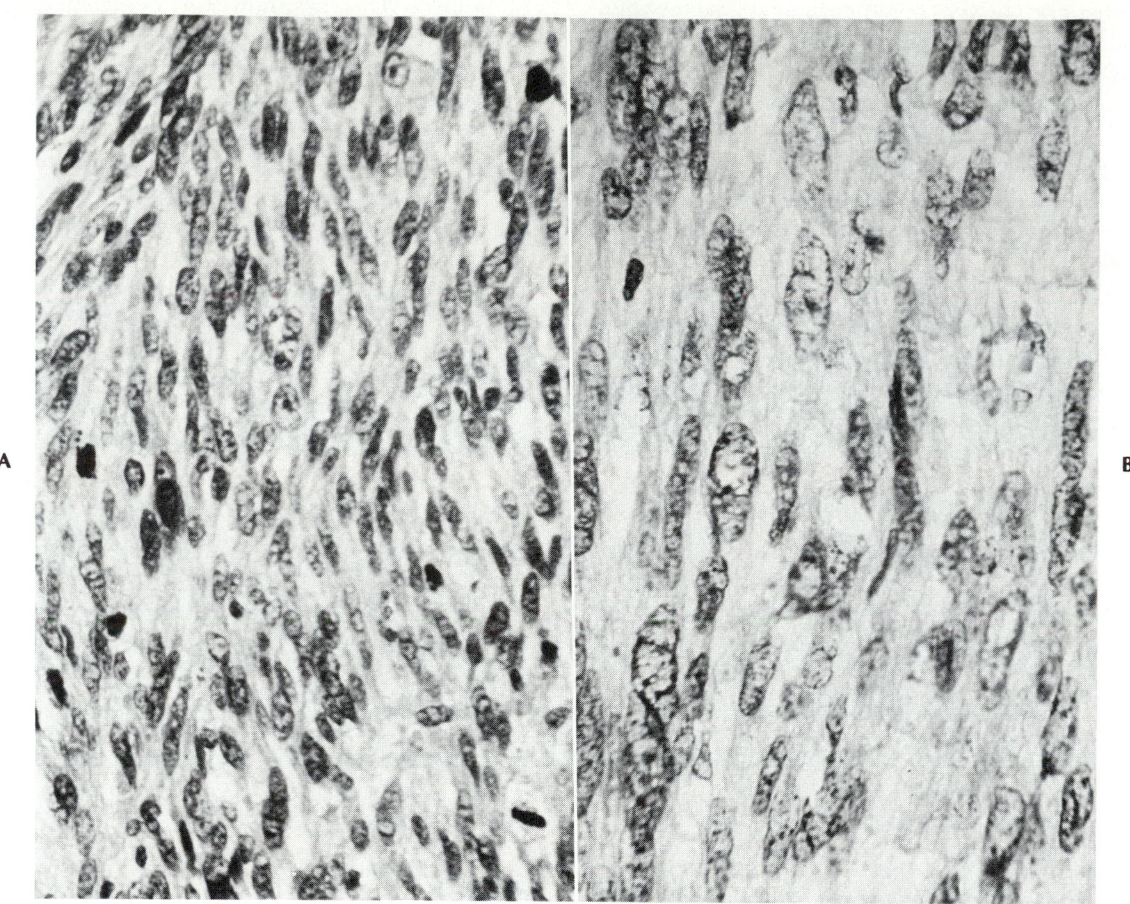

Fig. 39-11. **A,** Leiomyosarcoma. Spindle and oval cells with vesicular nuclei and some hyperchromasia. Several mitotic figures are present. **B,** Plump vesicular nuclei of leiomyosarcoma. Some cells are multinucleated. (**A,** 350×; **B,** 600×.)

Grossly, leiomyosarcomas appear well circumscribed and may even "shell out," but, as is usual with sarcomas, microscopically they are always infiltrative.[27] The superficial tumors tend to be small, usually less than 2 cm, with a progressive increase in tumor size for the deeper tumors, the retroperitoneal tumors frequently being greater than 10 cm.[122,132,141]

The histologic features that establish a diagnosis of leiomyosarcoma are not clear cut. Essentially the microscopic pattern parallels that seen in leiomyomas, with intersecting bundles of spindle-shaped cells having a fibrillar cytoplasm and blunt-ended nuclei (Fig. 39-11). Leiomyosarcomas tend to be more cellular, with a conspicuous increase in the number of cells showing bizarre nuclear characteristics and hyperchromasia.[27,132,138,141] Multinucleation is also common. The cells may round up and assume epithelioid or clear cell patterns (Fig. 39-12).[127] The tumors may vary from those composed almost entirely of well-differentiated spindle cells to those with many atypical cells, only a few of which have features suggestive of smooth muscle. Unlike its rarity in leiomyoma, necrosis is frequent in leiomyosarcoma, and such a finding is important in differentiating benign from malignant smooth muscle tumors.[132] Hyalinized areas and edematous myxoid regions may also be present.[141]

The principal difference between leiomyoma and leiomyosarcoma is the occurrence of a high mitotic rate in the latter. The use of mitotic counts as a means to diagnose leiomyosarcoma evolved from studies on uterine smooth muscle tumors in which mitotic indices have proved prognostically accurate.[123] However, these same criteria may not be directly applicable to extrauterine smooth muscle tumors.[125,132] Indeed, the reliability of mitotic counting has itself been called into question, since there may be a marked variability in the results of mitotic counts made by different pathologists on the same tumor.[135] Atypical hyperchromatic nuclei in poorly prepared sections may be misinterpreted as mitotic figures.[130] In addition, the cellularity and the frequency of the mitoses vary in different regions of the same tumor. Hence, failure to obtain enough sections and to perform the counts in areas containing the greatest number of

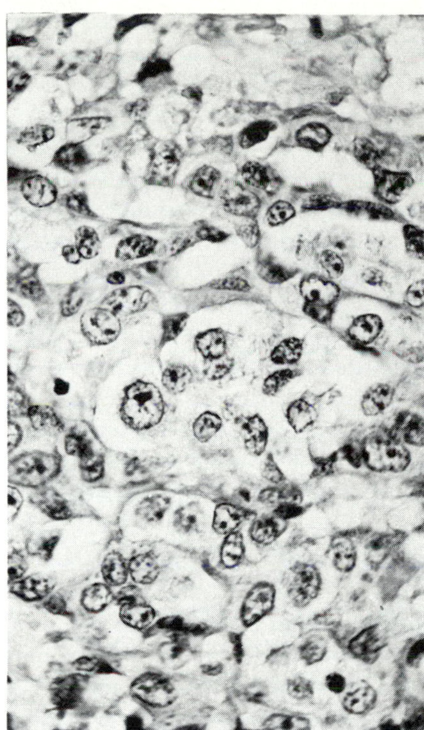

Fig. 39-12. Epithelioid (clear cell) leiomyosarcoma. Atypical nuclei are surrounded by clear zones or halos, which are fixation artifacts. (480×.)

mitoses will lead to dramatically different results.[135] In large, deeply placed tumors a rule of thumb should be that one section is taken for every centimeter of tumor size.[132] All pathologists with experience have encountered smooth muscle tumors that lack the usual parameters of malignancy but that behave aggressively.[119,124,132] Fortunately, these are rare, and a smooth muscle tumor without mitoses, necrosis, or cellular atypia is benign in the great majority of cases.[27,138] Those with high mitotic rates (five or more per 10 high-power fields), necrosis, and significant anaplasia may be expected to behave aggressively.[132,138] This leaves an undefined zone in which the course of the tumor cannot be predicted with assurance. Large tumors, with or without nuclear atypia, in which no necrosis is present and for which mitotic figures are absent or infrequent (one or two per 10 high-power fields) present such a problem. These tumors of indeterminate nature should be simply diagnosed as being of smooth muscle type with an explanation to the clinician of the pathology problem and the need for close clinical follow-up of the patient.

Electron microscopy has not been very rewarding in confirming that a pleomorphic spindle cell tumor is of smooth muscle origin. Unlike leiomyomas, all the fine structural characteristics of smooth muscle cells may be absent or incompletely developed in leiomyosarcomas, and those that are present are found in only some cells.[128,129] In one study only two thirds of cases considered to be leiomyosarcomas by light microscopy could be confirmed as such by electron microscopy.[129]

From what has been said concerning the difficulties in distinguishing between benign and malignant smooth muscle tumors, it is obvious that survival statistics are influenced by the inclusion of what are actually leiomyomas among those considered leiomyosarcomas. With this in mind, recurrences have been reported in from 40% to 60% of all leiomyosarcomas, with blood-borne metastases, most commonly to the lungs and liver, developing in approximately 30% to 60% of patients.[121,122,138,141] One recent report on somatic soft tissue leiomyosarcoma put the 5-year survival rate at 35%.[141] Retroperitoneal leiomyosarcomas have a poor prognosis, with over 90% of patients dying of either metastases or local invasion of adjacent structures.[132,141] Despite a 40% local recurrence rate, patients with cutaneous tumors do very well following wide excision without the development of metastases. In contrast, subcutaneous tumors are fully malignant and have a high rate of local recurrence and metastases.[122] Large (greater than 5 cm) and deep tumors also have a poor prognosis.[121,137,141,144] Extragastric epithelioid leiomyosarcomas behave in an aggressive fashion, with more than one half of patients dying of their tumor.[127] There is some difference of opinion in the assessment of outcome in children. Whereas some authors deny that the usual criteria of malignancy in smooth muscle tumors are applicable to tumors in children, claiming that these patients do well,[143] others believe that no difference exists in the outcome in children and adults.[119]

SKELETAL MUSCLE TUMORS

Rhabdomyosarcoma

Of all the sarcomas, rhabdomyosarcoma has in recent years attracted the most clinical interest and study. The reasons are easy to understand. Rhabdomyosarcoma is a highly aggressive tumor that predominantly affects young children. It is also the sarcoma that has responded best to improvements in radiotherapy and chemotherapy to such an extent that this disease, formerly almost uniformly fatal, now has a reasonable chance of being cured.[165]

Rhabdomyosarcoma is the most common sarcoma in childhood, representing more than half of all such cases.[145,165,167] It accounts for between 4% and 8% of all malignant disease in children under 15 years of age.[159] Among the soft tissue sarcomas, its incidence has ranged from 8% to 20%, with most reported figures in the 10% to 15% range.*

Rhabdomyosarcomas are divided into four principal histologic categories—embryonal, alveolar, pleomor-

*References 38, 83, 154, 155, 159, 164, 165.

phic, and botryoid—with the last essentially an embryonal rhabdomyosarcoma having a characteristic gross appearance.[152] Since the embryonal, alveolar, and botryoid types occur predominantly in young children, some use the general term *juvenile rhabdomyosarcoma* for these and reserve *adult rhabdomyosarcoma* for pleomorphic rhabdomyosarcoma, the form seen almost exclusively in adults.[27] However, these various tumor types exhibit enough clinical and pathologic differences to justify their retention and discussion as separate entities.

Approximately two thirds of patients with childhood rhabdomyosarcomas are under 10 years of age.[165] Boys are affected more commonly than girls in a ratio of approximately 1.5:1.[145,159,163,165] Among the childhood cases accessioned by the Intergroup Rhabdomyosarcoma Study Group,[159] the embryonal variety accounted for 57% of the cases, the alveolar type 19%, the botryoid form 6%, and the pleomorphic variety 1%. A special group of tumors was also found in which the cells resembled extraskeletal Ewing's sarcoma. These tumors accounted for 7% of the total accessioned cases. Another 10% of the lesions consisted of undifferentiated mesenchymal-type cells and could not be satisfactorily placed into one of the other categories. These were classed as "type indeterminate." This latter category, also called "sarcoma of undetermined histogenesis," has in some reports represented slightly more than one fourth of all the childhood cases originally diagnosed as rhabdomyosarcoma.[151] This indicates the difficulty, and inappropriateness, of classifying all small cell malignant tumors in childhood as rhabdomyosarcomas. The distribution of the major cell types in childhood is only slightly different from the distribution noted in a study from the Armed Forces Institute of Pathology on rhabdomyosarcomas in patients of all ages. Here embryonal tumors made up 69%, alveolar 19%, and pleomorphic 11% of the total cases.[171]

In general, each histologic type of rhabdomyosarcoma has a predilection for certain anatomic locations. Within the broad range of the common childhood cases, the head and neck region accounts for from 30% to 35% of all cases, with the orbit involved in 10% to 20% of these cases, while the genitourinary tract and the extremities each account for about 20% of the total.[145,159,165,166]

Understanding the histology and evolution of these malignant skeletal muscle tumors is aided by a knowledge of normal myogenesis.[146,161,163] At 1 to 9 weeks of embryonic development, small, primitive-appearing, stellate mesenchymal cells proliferate, elongate, and accumulate cytoplasm in which microfilaments develop. These microfilament-containing mononuclear cells are called myoblasts. They soon fuse to form a syncytium around a hollow core, and their nuclei move to the periphery to form the hollow myotube stage. The cytoplasm then begins to fill in, and there is an increasing accumulation of cytoplasmic filaments that soon split into thick (120 to 150 Å) filaments of myosin and thin (60 to 80 Å) filaments of actin. Together these filaments form the myofibrils of skeletal muscle. The position of the filaments relative to each other creates the banded pattern of skeletal muscle seen by light microscopy. These cross striations first make their appearance at about 10 weeks of embryonic development but are not prominent until 14 weeks of gestation. The Z bands are the first of the various bands to develop. The developing myogenic cells cannot be distinguished by electron microscopy from cells that are destined to differentiate into other cell types, and that may also contain cytoplasmic microfilaments, until the stage is reached in which both actin and myosin filaments are present. From this highly simplified version of myogenesis, it is clear that skeletal muscle cells originate from a proliferation of undifferentiated mesenchymal cells. Such cells may be located anywhere in the soft tissues, and this helps explain the occurrence of rhabdomyosarcomas in such areas as the middle ear, bile ducts, and bladder, where skeletal muscle is not present. It further emphasizes the point that the presence of unequivocal cross striations in an otherwise malignant-appearing small cell tumor of soft tissue is sufficient evidence to diagnose the tumor as a rhabdomyosarcoma. The finding by electron microscopy of specific thick and thin myofilaments or Z band material is also specific and diagnostic of skeletal muscle cells.[145a,146,153,160,161] It should be made clear, however, that at least in the embryonal, alveolar, and botryoid tumors, cross striations are not required for the diagnosis of rhabdomyosarcoma by light microscopy as long as the correct tumor pattern is present. Furthermore, the failure to find the specific myofilaments by electron microscopy should also not deter one from the diagnosis.[32,151,161] The sampling problems inherent in electron microscopy may yield such features in only about one half of the cases in which the light microscopic cellular morphology is consistent with rhabdomyosarcoma.[161] Newer immunologic techniques for the specific staining of myosin, myoglobin, and desmin offer hope for improving diagnostic certainty in such cases.[155,160a,162,166a]

Embryonal rhabdomyosarcoma

The most common of the rhabdomyosarcomas, the embryonal form, occurs predominantly in children usually under 12 years of age, with the mean age being about 5 years.[157,158a,165,166] However, adults 70 to 80 years of age are occasionally affected. In one series of head and neck rhabdomyosarcomas about 10% of the patients were over 30 years of age.[147] The most common locations in children are in the head and neck, where the orbit is the most frequent single location; the urogenital tract; and the retroperitoneum.[147,149,165,166] Most authors consider rhabdomyosarcomas in the extremities to be uncommon, although in one series the extremities and limb girdles accounted for 20% to 25% of cases.[164] Patients with extremity lesions tend to be older, with average ages between 25 and 30 years. In general, adults with embryonal rhabdomyosarcoma more frequently have the tumor in the extremities or trunk than in the head and neck.[158a]

Nothing distinguishes the gross appearance of most embryonal rhabdomyosarcomas from that of other soft tissue malignancies, except for the botryoid variety. This form grows close to the mucosal surfaces of hollow viscera or body cavities and produces edematous, smooth-appearing polypoid masses that protrude into the hollow cavities.[27,152] This form is most commonly found in the urogenital tract, pharynx, nasal cavity, common bile duct, and auditory canal. The remainder of the embryonal tumors frequently have no direct relation to skeletal muscle, growing instead between muscle groups or in deep subcutaneous tissue. They produce bulging masses that characteristically grow rapidly so that symptoms are usually present for less than a year before medical attention is sought.[147,157,164]

The histomorphology of these tumors varies.[27,151,152,163,164] They usually consist of a mixture of small, spindle-shaped cells, with tapering bipolar cytoplasmic extensions, and small round to oval cells about the size of lymphocytes or small monocytes with little cytoplasm (Fig. 39-13). The latter cells may accumulate more cytoplasm, which is usually intensely eosinophilic, and the finding of such rhabdomyoblasts scattered within the tumor is a clue to the diagnosis (Fig. 39-14). The cells frequently reside in a loose myxoid stroma, and mitoses are frequent. The spindle cells may be arranged in broad fascicles or bands and resemble the pattern of leiomyosarcoma or fibrosarcoma.[145] At times the cells are more uniformly round and compact, and since they also contain glycogen, they may resemble the cells of extraskeletal Ewing's sarcoma. Cross striations are found in only 30% to 40% of cases.[152,157,163]

The botryoid variant represents an exaggeration of the myxoid matrix. It has a hypocellular to acellular central region, with most of the tumor cells, which are small and round to oval, located in a narrow band beneath the overlying mucosa of the affected viscus. This cambium layer is characteristic of this tumor variant (Fig. 39-15).[27,152] The histologic pattern in embryonal rhabdomyosarcoma has been likened to the embryonic stage of muscle devel-

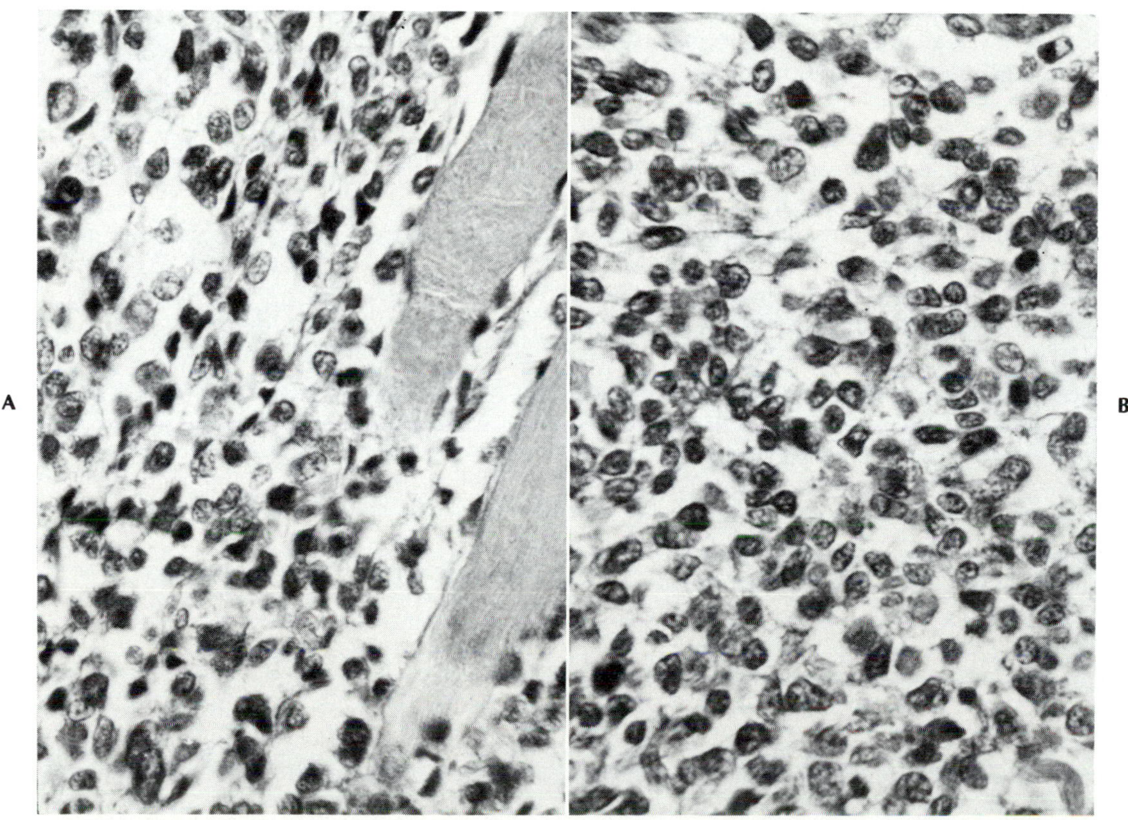

Fig. 39-13. A, Embryonal rhabdomyosarcoma. Small, undifferentiated tumor cells with little or no visible cytoplasm. Two skeletal muscle fibers are shown infiltrated by tumor cells. **B,** Embryonal rhabdomyosarcoma tumor cells with little variation in size or shape of their nuclei. (**A** and **B,** 600×.)

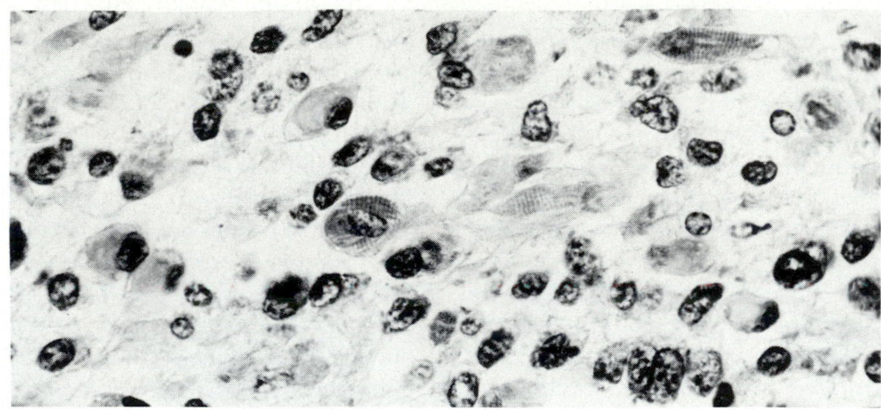

Fig. 39-14. Embryonal rhabdomyosarcoma. In addition to undifferentiated tumor cells, more mature rhabdomyoblasts are present with distinct cross striations. Large, round cells with abundant eosinophilic cytoplasm, but without striations, are also present. Such cells are a helpful guide to the diagnosis of rhabdomyosarcoma. (480×.)

opment noted between the third and tenth weeks of gestation.

Alveolar rhabdomyosarcoma

Alveolar rhabdomyosarcoma is more common in older children, teenagers, and young adults than is embryonal rhabdomyosarcoma. The mean patient age is between 15 and 20 years, and although the tumor has occasionally been found in older adults, it is rare after the age of 50.[14,148,150,163]

Unlike embryonal rhabdomyosarcoma, the alveolar form is commonly located in an extremity (60% to 70% of cases), where it is first seen as a rapidly growing mass that may reach 20 cm.[150,164] Also, unlike the embryonal form, it grossly appears to arise from within the muscle. The forearm, hand, and trunk are common sites, but unlike the embryonal form, less than 20% of cases occur in the head and neck region.[14,150]

In its classic form alveolar rhabdomyosarcoma has a characteristic histologic pattern with the cells arranged in ill-defined groups and nests in which the central cells are loosely cohesive, forming alveolar spaces (Fig. 39-16).[148,150,151] Fibrous trabeculae form the periphery of the cell nests, and the adjacent cells attach themselves to these trabeculae by a tapered cytoplasmic strand with their nuclei oriented toward the lumen of the spaces. Cells in the alveolar spaces vary in shape, are from 15 to 30 μm in size, and are frequently seen floating free within the spaces. Smaller cells, resembling those of the embryonal form, are also present, as may be round cells with eccentric nuclei and abundant bright eosinophilic cytoplasm. Multinucleated giant cells up to 200 μm in diameter, with their nuclei in a wreathlike arrangement within an eosinophilic granular cytoplasm, are also commonly found free within the alveolar spaces. These giant cells do not show cross striations.[150] Solid areas com-

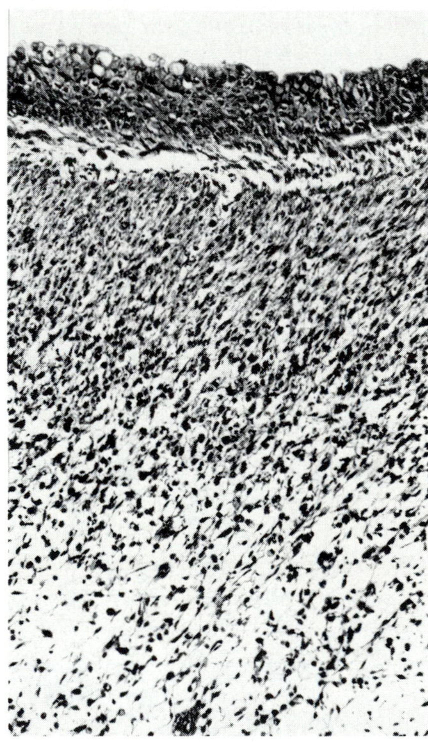

Fig. 39-15. Botryoid rhabdomyosarcoma of vagina. Concentration of tumor cells beneath vaginal mucosa creates cambium layer characteristic of this tumor. (120×.)

posed of cells that lack an alveolar arrangement are commonly noted at the growing edge of the tumor. These cells are similar to the small cells of embryonal rhabdomyosarcoma. Larger strap- and tadpole-shaped rhabdomyoblasts with bright eosinophilic cytoplasm are also seen within this tumor. Some of the larger round cells have peripheral vacuolization of their cytoplasm, giving them a spiderweb appearance. The occurrence of cross

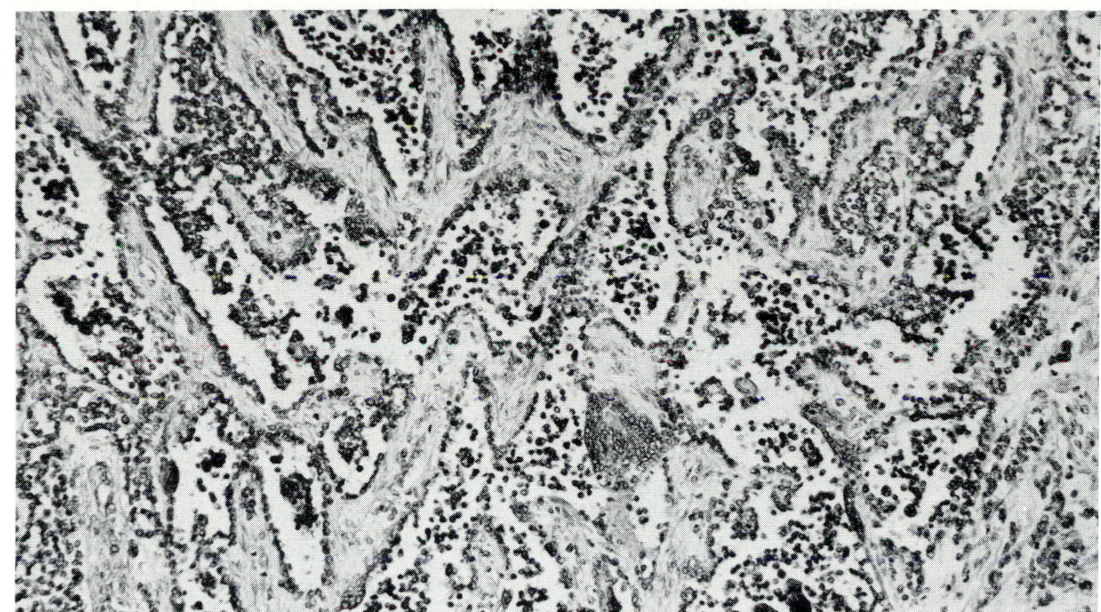

Fig. 39-16. Alveolar rhabdomyosarcoma. Fibrous septa are lined by tumor cells. Central cells are loosely cohesive and appear to float within alveolar spaces. A large multinucleated giant cell is present. (150×.)

striations depends on the diligence with which they are sought.[14,148] About 30% of the tumors have striated cells, but they may be sparse.[150] Mitoses are easily found.

In the past the alveolar pattern suggested to some the myotube stage of myogenesis, in which the cells form a cytoplasmic syncytium around a hollow core. Recently, however, electron microscopic study of a single case showed that cells lining the alveolar spaces are not in a syncytium but possess a basement membrane between the fibrous septa and the cell cytoplasm. If confirmed, this finding would negate the myotube hypothesis.[146]

Tumors are found that contain various proportions of both embryonal and alveolar rhabdomyosarcoma and are either diagnosed as mixed rhabdomyosarcoma or designated by the most dominant pattern.

Pleomorphic rhabdomyosarcoma

The very existence of pleomorphic rhabdomyosarcoma has recently been brought into question, since most cases so diagnosed are in reality malignant fibrous histiocytomas.[14,84,91,115] Others are more successful in diagnosing these tumors.[9] Since they often arise within the substance of the muscle, it is at times difficult to distinguish degenerative muscle cells, which may have quite atypical-appearing nuclei and may retain their cross striations, from actual tumor cells. If this tumor type does exist, it is an extremely rare neoplasm. The data presented here, which are based on older studies, should be viewed with some skepticism, since at a minimum they probably reflect the inclusion of other tumor types.

Pleomorphic rhabdomyosarcoma, in contrast to the other forms of rhabdomyosarcoma, is seen overwhelmingly in older adults, with probably less than 10% of cases occurring in children. The mean patient age is between 50 and 55 years.[154,158,163] Nearly all of these tumors arise within large muscles as circumscribed soft masses.[27,149] They are most common in the extremities, the lower extremity accounting for about half the cases, with the thigh the most common site. The upper extremity, trunk, and head and neck region account for most of the remainder, with some tumors also found in the retroperitoneum and the viscera. Pain is associated with these tumor masses in up to one fourth of patients.[154,158]

Histologically the tumors are composed of anaplastic cells that assume various configurations. Numerous large, multinucleated tumor cells with deeply eosinophilic cytoplasm are present (Fig. 39-17). The cells may assume racquet or tadpole shapes with a single large nucleus at one end and a tapering cytoplasmic tail or form large strap or ribbon shapes with several nuclei in tandem. Small round cells with eccentric nuclei and bright eosinophilic cytoplasm are also common. Cross striations have been reported in 7% to 62% of cases.[152,154,158] Mitoses are common and are frequently abnormal. Areas of necrosis are also common. We believe that the diagnosis of pleomorphic rhabdomyosarcoma should be restricted to lesions that show clear cross striations in tumor cells or that have either thick and thin myofilaments or Z band material by electron microscopy.

Most of the recent advances in the therapy of rhabdomyosarcoma have been confined to the childhood form of the disease, which was formerly almost uniformly fatal.[165] In the past, alveolar rhabdomyosarcoma had the worst prognosis, with lymph node metastases present in 75% to 80% of patients and a 5-year survival rate of only about 5%.[148,150,164] Most patients died within a year of diagnosis.[166] Embryonal rhabdomyosarcoma had 5-year survival rates that ranged from 10% to 20%, with lymph node metastases present in up to 30% of patients. Tumors of the extremities and urogenital tract produced the highest incidence of lymph node metastases,[156,159,165] whereas orbital tumors had the lowest incidence of nodal metastases and the best 5-year survival rates.[147,159,166] Tumors in regions of the head and neck other than the orbit had a very poor prognosis. Approximately one fifth of all childhood cases are initially seen with distant metastases most commonly involving the lungs, liver, bone, and lymph nodes.[159,165]

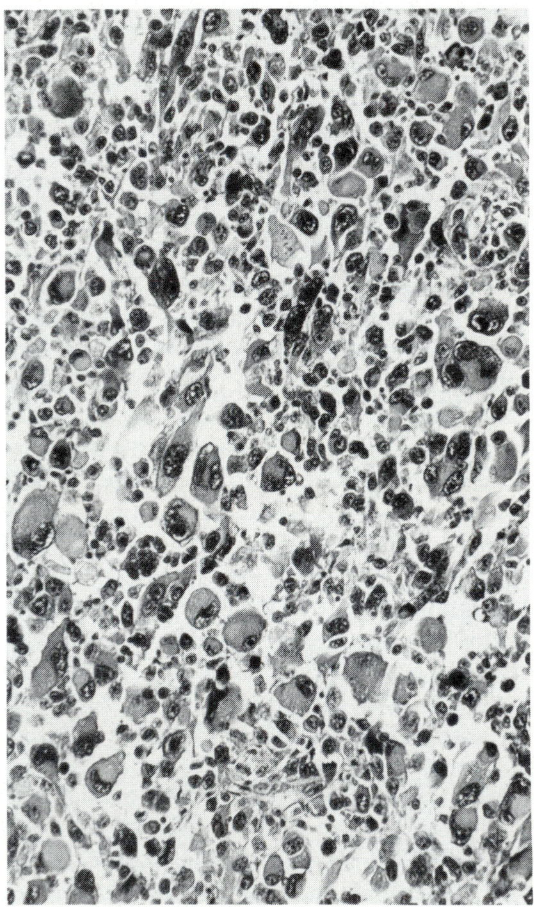

Fig. 39-17. Pleomorphic rhabdomyosarcoma. Anaplastic tumor cells with variety of shapes. Larger cells have abundant densely eosinophilic cytoplasm. Similar cells may be found in other pleomorphic sarcomas such as liposarcoma and malignant fibrous histiocytoma. (150×.)

The adult pleomorphic tumors had a better prognosis than the childhood cases, with 5-year survival rates of approximately 30% to 35%.[149,154,158] Lymph node metastases occurred in 10% to 15% of pleomorphic cases.[154] Recurrences following local excision in all forms of rhabdomyosarcoma were seen in about 60% of patients.

Today, with the use of surgery, radiotherapy, and adjuvant chemotherapy, 2-year survival rates in the 70% to 90% range are being reported, and one recent report indicated an overall 86% 5-year survival rate in childhood cases.[165] Even patients with distant metastases now survive in about 30% of cases. Survival still depends on factors such as the location and extent of the tumor at initial examination, with orbital tumors having the best prognosis and extremity lesions, most of which are of the alveolar type, having the worst prognosis. Children under 7 years of age appear to have a better survival rate than older children.[165] There is debate as to whether tumor type influences prognosis, since some investigators have found no difference in survival among the various childhood rhabdomyosarcomas.[145] A recent "solid" variant of alveolar rhabdomyosarcoma has been proposed. This may histologically mimic embryonal rhabdomyosarcoma but has a worse prognosis.[166b]

Rhabdomyoma

Rhabdomyoma of soft tissue origin is a totally benign, nonaggressive tumor that accounts for probably no more than 1% to 2% of all skeletal muscle tumors, the remainder being rhabdomyosarcomas.[171] The soft tissue rhabdomyoma should not be confused with the glycogen-containing lesion of the heart, also designated as rhabdomyoma, which is probably a hamartoma and not a true tumor. It is this cardiac lesion and not the soft tissue tumor that is associated with the tuberous sclerosis syndrome.[175]

Rhabdomyomas are divided histologically into adult and fetal types, with roughly equal numbers of each having been reported. Despite the fact that these tumors are in most cases histologically clearly distinct from rhabdomyosarcoma, they are still occasionally misdiagnosed as the latter, with horrendous consequences.

The adult rhabdomyoma occurs almost exclusively in older patients with a mean age of approximately 50 years and are only rarely found in children.[172,173,176] The fetal form affects patients over a broader age range from newborns to older adults, with the mean patient age being 20 to 30 years younger than in the adult type. The adult form is four to five times more frequent in male than in female patients, whereas the fetal type has an approximately equal sex distribution.[172,173,176]

Adult rhabdomyomas have a propensity for localization in the head and neck area, with the larynx and pharynx the most common sites involved.[172] Other locations include the oral cavity, lip, orbit, and nasopharynx. Rare tumors of multicentric origin are reported.[174,176] Fetal rhabdomyomas are also principally found in the head and neck region, with the posterior auricular region being the most common site.[14,171,176] Other reported locations include the tongue, orbit, larynx, nose, nasopharynx, axilla, and chest wall. They also occur in the female genital tract, arising in the vulva, vagina, or ectocervix.[172]

Histologically the adult forms are the more easily recognized. They consist of large oval to round cells having abundant, distinctly granular, eosinophilic cytoplasm that is frequently vacuolated.[169,172,174,175] Nuclei are uniform and either central or eccentric (Fig. 39-18). Cross striations, although uncommon, can be found in at least some cells. Stains for cytoplasmic glycogen are strongly positive.[169,175] Cytoplasmic crystalline-like granules or particles are also present and are best seen with phosphotungstic acid–hematohylin stains.[169,173,175] Adult rhabdomyomas may be confused with granular cell tumors, whose cells have a similar-appearing cytoplasm. However, the latter lack cross striations; contain cytoplasmic material that is periodic acid–Schiff positive and diastase resistant; and by electron microscopy lack the mixture of actin and myosin myofilaments seen in skeletal muscle cells.[168,169,175]

Fetal rhabdomyomas are histologically more heterogeneous, composed of immature-appearing skeletal muscle fibers in various stages of differentiation, admixed with mesenchymal-type cells that vary from small oval to round cells to large cells with bipolar tapering cytoplasmic extensions.[170-172,176a] The muscle cells have easily seen myofibrils, and in most cases cross striations can be found in some cells. Both cellular components are loosely arranged in bundles that run haphazardly throughout the lesion. They reside in a loose myxoid stroma, containing hyaluronic acid, that gives the lesion an edematous appearance. Significantly, the cells lack pleomorphism, and mitoses are scarce. In lesions of the female genital tract the stroma is more abundant, and the muscle cells appear more mature.[173] A "cellular" variant of fetal rhabdomyoma has also been described in which the stroma is sparse and there is a predominance of thin, elongate spindle cells arranged in a herringbone or palisading pattern.[172] Occasional ribbon and strap cells are also present, but cross striations are difficult to find. Despite nuclear atypism in occasional cells, mitoses are not present. Electron microscopy shows myofilaments in both adult and fetal lesions.[168,169,173,176a] The crystalline-like material seen in the adult form represents hypertrophic-appearing Z band myofilaments. This is not present in cells of the fetal rhabdomyoma.[172,174a]

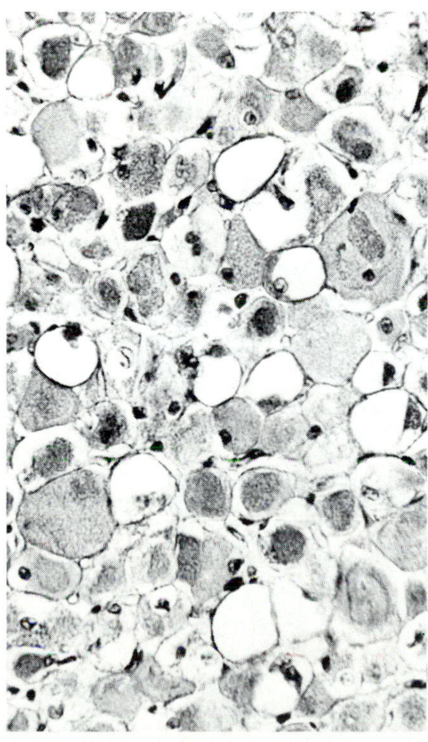

Fig. 39-18. Adult rhabdomyoma. Large cells with abundant granular eosinophilic cytoplasm mixed with cells having vacuolated cytoplasm. Nuclei are bland and central or eccentric in location. (280×.)

Although adult rhabdomyoma is easily differentiated from rhabdomyosarcoma, fetal rhabdomyoma may easily be confused with embryonal rhabdomyosarcoma.[174a] Indeed, as suggested, this latter distinction may be subtle.[171] The lack of necrosis, cellular pleomorphism, hyperchromasia, and significant mitotic activity, as well as its circumscription, support the diagnosis of fetal rhabdomyoma.[170-172]

Occasional local recurrences, even some multiple recurrences, have been reported in patients with adult rhabdomyomas. To date only one example of the fetal form has recurred.[174a] In neither variety has there been evidence of local aggressiveness or metastases.[171,175]

The nature of these lesions is still unclear, and some have suggested that they may be hamartomas.[170,171] Since some of the lesions occur in locations such as the vocal cord, ectocervix, and stomach,[172] where skeletal muscle is not normally found, they do not fit the usual definition of a hamartoma.

TUMORS OF ADIPOSE TISSUE

Liposarcoma

Liposarcoma is one of the most common of the adult soft tissue sarcomas, although its reported incidence varies greatly from institution to institution.[14] It has been reported to comprise anywhere from 5% to 30% of all soft tissue sarcomas.[38,83,186] In recent years, with the recognition of malignant fibrous histiocytoma as an entity and the application of this diagnosis to some lesions previously designated pleomorphic liposarcoma, malignant fibrous histiocytoma has equaled or surpassed liposarcoma as the most common sarcoma in some institutions.[83] Furthermore, with the recent recognition of spindle cell lipoma and pleomorphic (atypical) lipoma, some tumors previously designated well-differentiated or sclerosing liposarcoma will probably, on review, fit into these benign categories.[187] That the diagnosis of liposarcoma is not sacrosanct is evidenced by the fact that in some series close to one half of the lesions so designated were, on review, reassigned to other categories.[186,189] Despite their frequency among the sarcomas, it should be remembered that liposarcomas are still rare tumors, being about 100 times less common than benign lipomas.[177]

Liposarcoma is classically considered to be a tumor of lipoblasts. However, the number of lipoblasts present varies greatly among the various histologic subtypes of this tumor, and they may in fact be quite scarce. Lipoblasts, or cells that by light microscopy are indistinguishable from lipoblasts, are also found in reactive conditions involving fat, as well as in some benign adipose tumors such as lipoblastomas.[177] In addition, some pleomorphic sarcomas, such as malignant fibrous histiocytoma and osteosarcoma, also contain cells that resemble lipoblasts. Hence the presence of lipoblasts or lipoblast-like cells is not per se an indication of liposarcoma, since the diagnosis depends equally on the overall histologic pattern of the lesion. This having been stated, it must be admitted that what constitutes a lipoblast by light microscopy is still open to some debate, since what to one pathologist is a lipoblast may be a multivacuolated histiocyte to another.[177] It is at times easier to describe a lipoblast than to point one out, with assurance, under the microscope.

Depending on the number of fat vacuoles in their cytoplasm, lipoblasts are divided into univacuolated and multivacuolated varieties (Fig. 39-19).[177] In the univacuolated form the cells are smaller than mature fat cells and assume a signet-ring appearance caused by the presence of a single, large, sharply delimited cytoplasmic vacuole that pushes the nucleus to one side, giving it a demilune shape.[14,177] The cells may resemble the signet-ring cells of a mucin-producing adenocarcinoma. Although the nucleus may be hyperchromatic and bizarre, this is usually not the case, and mitotic figures are rarely found in these cells.

In contrast, multivacuolated lipoblasts have a centrally

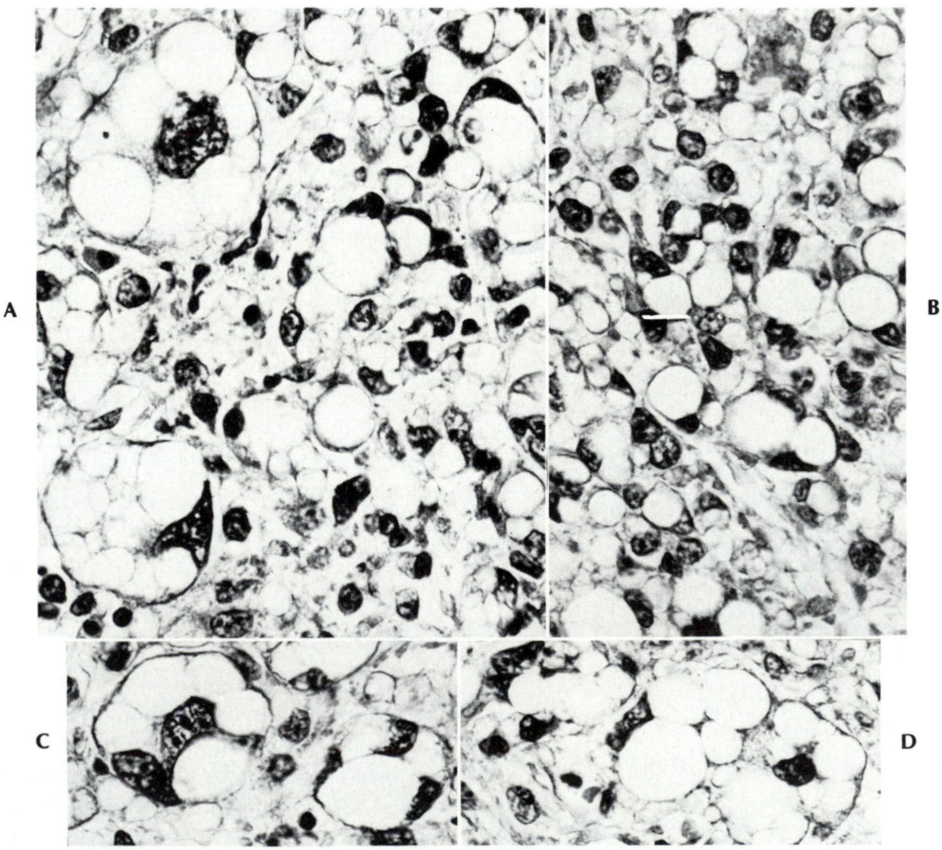

Fig. 39-19. A, Liposarcoma. Univacuolated and multivacuolated lipoblasts. Note compression of nuclei by fat vacuoles. **B,** Signet-ring lipoblasts are shown. **C,** Multinucleated, multivacuolated lipoblasts. **D,** Single-nucleated, multivacuolated lipoblasts. (480×.)

placed nucleus that is frequently large, bizarre in shape, and hyperchromatic. They vary greatly in size and may reach 300 to 400 μm in diameter. The cytoplasmic vacuoles may be large or small, are characteristically sharply defined, and indent the margins of the nucleus, giving it a scalloped appearance. Frequent and abnormal mitotic figures are commonly found in these cells. Both univacuolated and multivacuolated lipoblasts may be multinucleated, although this is more common among the multivacuolated cells.

Histologically, liposarcomas have been divided into four major types: well differentiated, which is further subclassified into a lipoma-like and a sclerosing form; myxoid; round cell; and pleomorphic.[185,189] Mixed forms occur in various combinations, that is, well-differentiated areas mixed with pleomorphic areas or myxoid forms with round cell areas. Recently a "dedifferentiated" tumor category has been proposed. These latter tumors consist of well-differentiated liposarcoma in combination with an undifferentiated spindle cell sarcoma.[186]

In contrast to what might be expected, fat stains are of little help in the diagnosis of liposarcoma. Many liposarcomas lack significant fat content, whereas other pleomorphic tumors may stain positively for fat because their tumor cells undergo degeneration and accumulate cytoplasmic lipid.

Myxoid liposarcoma is the most common histologic type and accounts for 35% to 50% of all cases.[177,185,186] It is composed of widely separated, monomorphic fusiform or stellate cells with indistinct borders, lying in a mucoid stroma rich in hyaluronic acid. Hypocellular pools or lakes of this mucoid matrix are frequently present (Fig. 39-20). When abundant, these pools may lead to diagnostic confusion with myxoma. However, another component not found in myxoma is always present and obvious, that is, a delicate plexiform capillary network. The cells

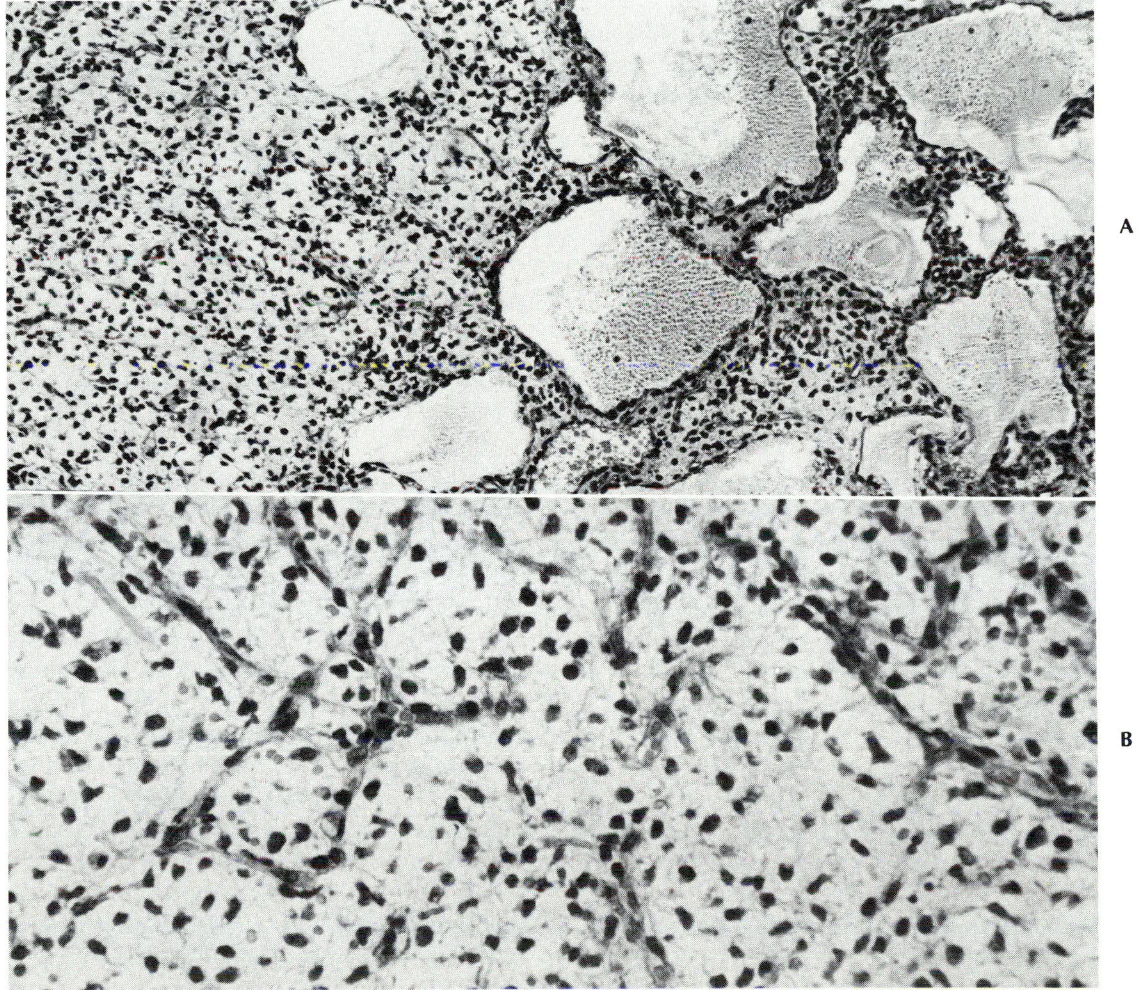

Fig. 39-20. A, Myxoid liposarcoma. Hypocellular pools of mucinous matrix within stellate cellular stroma. **B,** Widely separated round and stellate cells embedded in myxoid stroma. Cells are fairly uniform without pleomorphism. Note abundant plexiform capillary network. (**A,** 150×; **B,** 600×.)

of myxoid liposarcoma are not especially hyperchromatic or atypical. Indeed, pleomorphism and significant mitotic activity are not part of this tumor, and such findings eliminate it from the pure myxoid category.[177,185,186] Lipoblasts may be scarce and are usually univacuolated. This tumor is diagnosed on the basis of its pattern more than on the finding of numerous lipoblasts.

Well-differentiated liposarcoma comprises 20% to 30% of all cases[177,186,189] and can be found in two histologic forms that frequently occur together.[185] The lipoma-like variety is, as its name implies, composed principally of mature-appearing fat cells but has focal regions where hyperchromatic and bizarre lipoblasts are found. These lipoblasts tend to be multivacuolated and multinucleated. It is this variety of liposarcoma that can be mistaken for a benign lipoma if sufficient sections are not examined, since the atypical cellular foci may be few and far between (Fig. 39-21). In deeply situated fatty tumors, sections should be taken from areas having increased firmness with white discoloration or from any regions with obvious necrosis. The sclerosing type of well-differentiated liposarcoma is more common than the lipoma-like form and is characterized by fibrous tissue bands containing atypical and bizarre lipoblasts, frequently multivacuolated, alternating with areas of mature adipose tissue (Fig. 39-22). In neither of these subtypes is mitotic activity prominent.[177,189]

Pleomorphic liposarcoma is the most anaplastic of the liposarcomas and accounts for 10% to 25% of cases.[177,185,189] It is characterized by an abundance of large tumor giant cells, many having a dense eosinophilic cytoplasm, and bizarre lipoblasts with frequent and abnormal mitotic figures (Fig. 39-23). Spindle cell areas are frequent, to such a degree that distinction from fibroxanthosarcoma or pleomorphic rhabdomyosarcoma may be difficult.[14,185,186] The tumor giant cells lack the cross striations of rhabdomyosarcoma, and the storiform pattern of malignant fibrous histiocytoma is not usually present in liposarcoma. However, cases are found that have features of both liposarcoma and malignant fibrous histiocytoma, so that distinction between them at the light microscopic level may be impossible.[14,184]

Round cell liposarcoma is considered by some to be a variant of the myxoid type rather than a distinct cell type, although myxoid foci are seen in less than half the cases.[186] Microscopically one sees uniform round to oval cells with a fine multivacuolated cytoplasm and a central round nucleus that may be hyperchromatic but is not usually markedly atypical (Fig. 39-24). Such cells may resemble those of a hibernoma. Signet-ring lipoblasts are found but not in great numbers. The number of mitotic figures varies, but they are usually not common. Round cell liposarcoma may resemble a signet-ring adenocarcinoma but can be distinguished from it by means of mucin stains. The round cell tumor comprises approximately 10% to 15% of all liposarcomas.[177,185,189]

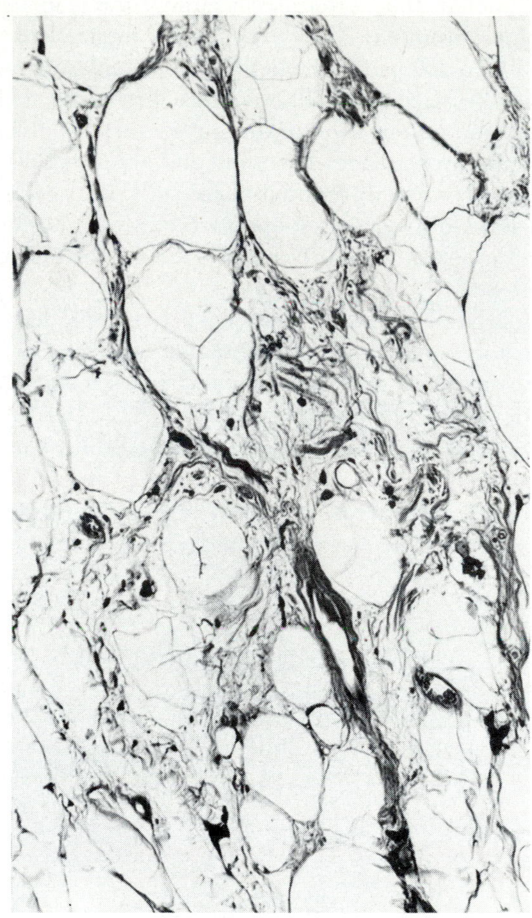

Fig. 39-21. Lipoma-like liposarcoma. Focal region with increased fibrous tissue in which fat cells with atypical nuclei are present. Multinucleated lipoblast is at right center of the field. Superficial tumors with this pattern have been termed pleomorphic lipomas. (150×.)

Liposarcoma is a disease of adults, with most cases occurring between the fourth and sixth decades and a mean patient age of about 50 years.[27,180,185,189] Patients with myxoid liposarcomas tend to be about 10 years younger than those with pleomorphic or round cell types, whereas those with well-differentiated tumors, especially retroperitoneal tumors, tend to be among the most elderly of patients.[14,177,186,189] Liposarcomas occur slightly more frequently in male patients.[27,180,185,189] Although liposarcomas have been reported in young children,[191b] most of these probably represent benign lipoblastomas.[14,182] A diagnosis of liposarcoma in a child less than 5 years of age should be viewed with skepticism.[14,177,185] A multinodular myxoid lesion that affects the omentum and mesentery of infants and that may be confused with myxoid liposarcoma has been reported. These lesions have been termed myxoid hamartomas.[188a]

Unlike lipomas, liposarcomas usually arise from deep soft tissue and only rarely from the subcutaneous tissue.[177,191a] In addition, with very rare exceptions, lipo-

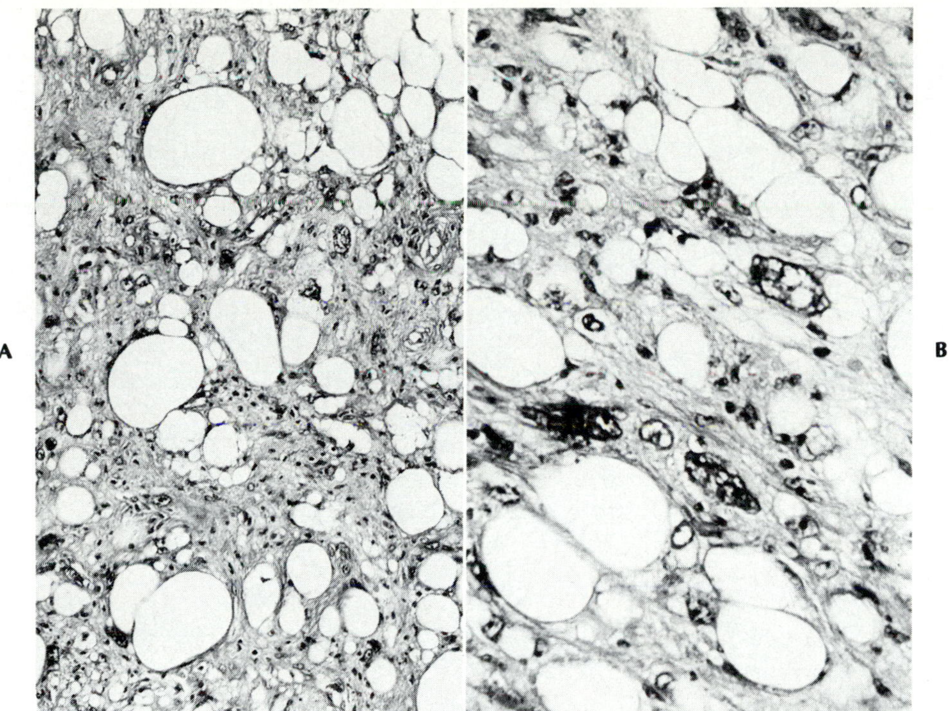

Fig. 39-22. A, Sclerosing liposarcoma. Dense fibrous tissue contains anaplastic tumor cells and lipoblasts. **B,** Higher magnification showing hyperchromatic malignant stromal cells. A few signet-ring lipoblasts are also present. (**A,** 120×; **B,** 280×.)

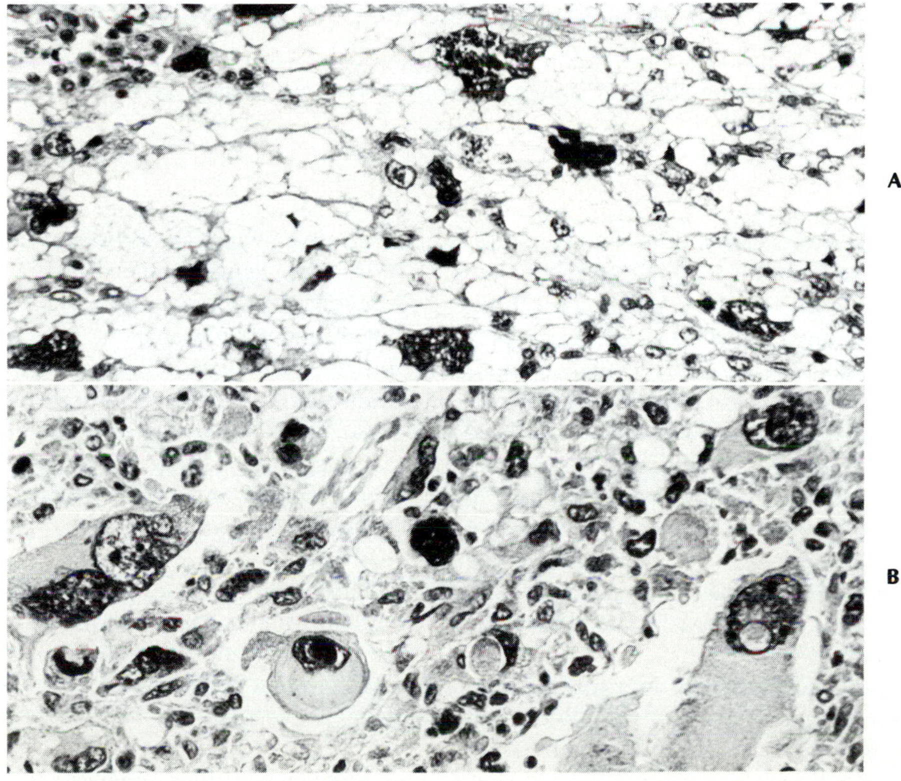

Fig. 39-23. A, Pleomorphic liposarcoma. Numerous multivacuolated lipoblasts with bizarre nuclei are shown. **B,** Another region from pleomorphic liposarcoma shows large bizarre tumor giant cells with abundant, densely eosinophilic cytoplasm. A few signet-ring lipoblasts are at upper right. (280×.)

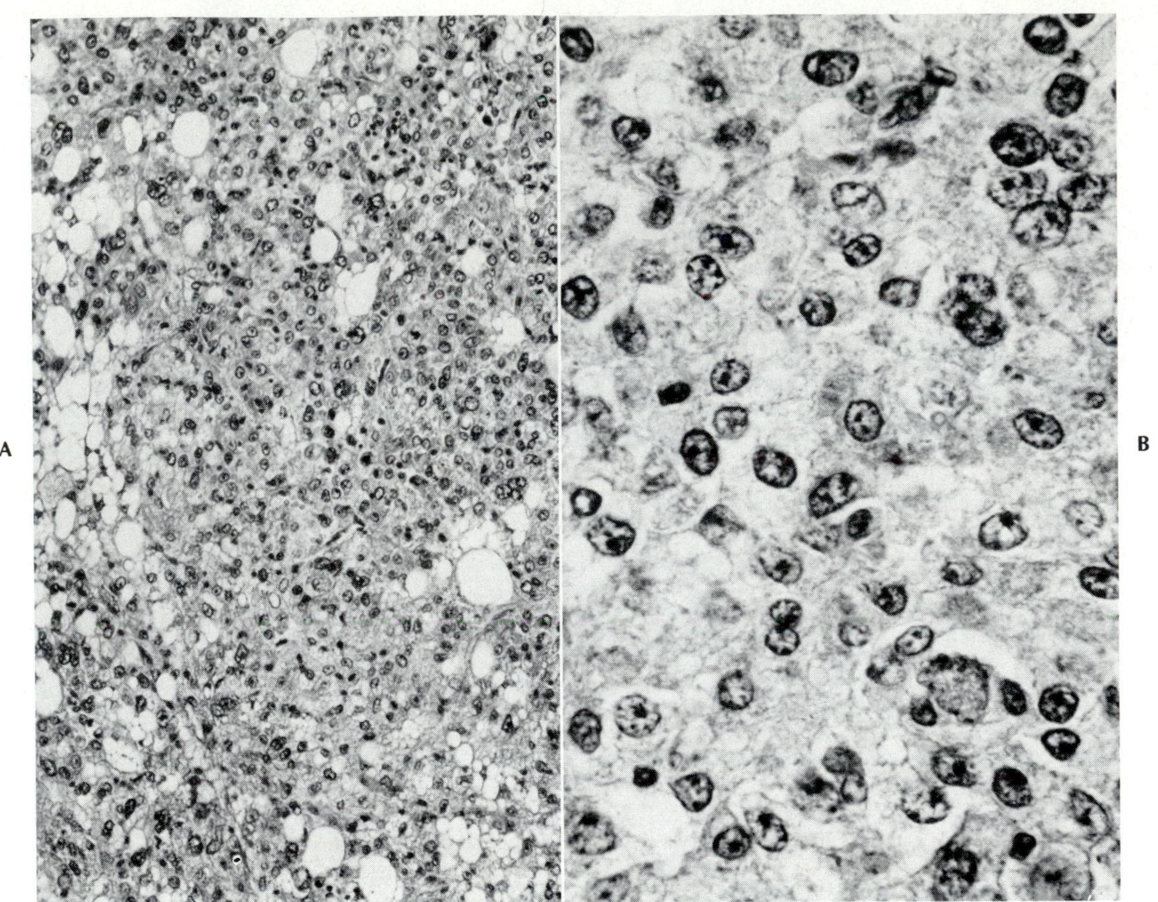

Fig. 39-24. A, Round cell liposarcoma. A few lipoblasts are mingled with uniform round cells. **B,** Higher magnification shows cells with mildly atypical nuclei and finely vacuolated granular cytoplasm. (**A,** 150×; **B,** 600×.)

sarcomas arise de novo and not from preexisting lipomas. Liposarcomas are usually found in the spaces between major muscle groups, with the most frequent locations being the medial thigh and popliteal fossa; the retroperitoneum, especially about the kidney; the shoulder region; the buttocks; and the inguinal and paratesticular areas. They are extremely rare in the hands and feet.[14,27,180,185] Whereas the myxoid and round cell tumors are most frequent in the lower extremities, the well-differentiated and pleomorphic varieties are more common in the retroperitoneum,[14,186,189] although some authors have noted some variation in this general scheme.[190] Paratesticular tumors tend to be of the sclerosing form.[177]

Depending on their anatomic location, liposarcomas are usually first seen as painless masses.[177,185] Retroperitoneal tumors cause abdominal distension or pressure symptoms.[189]

On gross inspection liposarcomas are large nodular masses that appear well circumscribed but are always infiltrative. The retroperitoneal tumors may reach enormous size, weighing many kilograms.[27,185] The well-differentiated variety may grossly resemble a benign lipoma but frequently has areas of increased firmness or foci of necrosis. The myxoid variety may be brainlike in consistency with a grayish white translucent surface that feels slimy.[177,189] They may drip mucoid material from small cystic spaces on their cut surface. The round cell and pleomorphic tumors have no distinguishing characteristics that differentiate them from other soft tissue sarcomas.

Most electron microscopic studies have dealt with the myxoid tumors. Here the prevailing opinion appears to be that the tumor roughly recapitulates the embryonic development of white fat,[178,179,181,188,192] although some have suggested that such tumors arise from brown fat.[191]

Prognosis in liposarcoma depends on several factors, paramount of which are the histologic type and the location of the tumor.[159,177,185] In general, myxoid and well-differentiated liposarcomas have excellent 5-year survival rates that have ranged from 75% to 100% with the 10-year survival rates about 10% to 15% less.[185,186,189] Pleomorphic liposarcoma has a significantly poorer prognosis with 5-year survival rates of 21% or less with still further decline in survival at 10 years. Survival with round cell liposarcoma has varied from 18% to 27% at 5 years and less than 10% at 10 years.[177,185,186,189]

Despite their overall good survival rates, both myxoid and well-differentiated liposarcomas have high local recurrence rates that have ranged from 50% to 100% in some series.[177,185,186,189] As one would expect, the more aggressive round cell and pleomorphic liposarcomas also yield high local recurrence rates of from 75% to 80%.[185,186,189] Metastatic rates for these latter two sarcomas are also higher than the others.[14,186,189] Well-differentiated tumors tend to recur locally before there is evidence of distant spread. Metastases from liposarcomas are almost all blood borne, usually to the lungs, with only rare involvement of the regional lymph nodes. Retroperitoneal lesions have a lower survival rate, type for type, than do tumors located in the extremities.[177,189,190] This probably reflects the adequacy of the type of surgical resection that can be done. Radiotherapy may benefit survival, with the myxoid and well-differentiated tumors responding best.[180,183] Recurrent liposarcomas may develop histologic patterns that mimic other sarcomas.

Lipoma

Perhaps because familiarity tends to breed contempt, lipoma of soft tissue, despite its position as the most common soft tissue tumor,[7a,10,193] has been neglected by pathologists. Usually interest is aroused only when the lipoma occurs in some esoteric location outside the soft tissue, such as the brain. It is, after all, difficult for diagnostic pathologists to get excited over a histologic expanse of mature fat cells. However, with the recent publication of an excellent monograph describing more than 40 varieties of benign mesenchymal lesions in which adipose tissue is a prominent or major component, as well as reports dealing with lipomas having histologic features that can mimic malignant tumors, there has been a renewed interest in lesions of adipose tissue, including the once prosaic lipoma.

Lipomas usually occur as a single, painless mass that may be present for many years. They either become stationary after achieving their usual size of 1 to 5 cm or continue to grow slowly, with tumors up to 50 to 60 cm having been reported.[177] Most patients seek medical treatment for cosmetic reasons rather than for any specific symptoms, with female patients accounting for 60% to 70% of cases.[177,193] It has been claimed that the fat within a lipoma is not metabolically available to the body, since in starvation states lipomas do not disappear and may actually increase in size.[27]

Lipomas are soft, freely movable masses that are most frequently located in the neck, shoulder, arm, and trunk. The hands, legs, and feet are rarely involved.[177,193,203] The tumor has a peak incidence in the fourth and sixth decades of life and occurs only rarely in young children.[27,177,193] Grossly, lipomas are smooth, encapsulated, round to oval, well-circumscribed masses that on cut section are soft, yellow, and greasy to the touch. They almost always arise superficially in the subcutaneous tissue, although deeper intramuscular lipomas do occur. This superficial location is unlike the usual deep-seated location of liposarcoma.

Microscopically one sees lobules of well-developed, mature adipose cells separated by thin, delicate, fibrous septa. The tumor is surrounded by a thin fibrous capsule that serves to distinguish the lipoma from a simple aggregation of fat. At times myxoid areas replace some of the fat lobules, and there may be some evidence of fat necrosis resulting from trauma.[193] Electron microscopy has demonstrated that the cells of the lipoma are morphologically the same as the cells of normal mature white adipose tissue.[188,195a] In deeply located fatty tumors, such as those in the retroperitoneum, atypical-appearing foci should be assiduously sought on gross inspection, and many sections should be taken from such a lesion before accepting the diagnosis of benign lipoma, since some of these tumors prove to be well-differentiated liposarcomas. It is such cases, inadequately sampled perhaps, that result in reports of malignant degeneration in benign lipomas. As a general rule, liposarcomas arise de novo and not from lipomas.

If not totally removed, lipomas may recur, probably in less than 1% of all cases.[177]

Multiple lipomas have been reported in patients with neurofibromatosis and in those with the multiple endocrine adenoma syndrome.[177,193] Some of these tumors may be angiolipomas rather than simple lipomas. Although multiple simple subcutaneous lipomas have been reported, they are rare.[177]

Infiltrating lipoma

Unlike their more common subcutaneous counterparts, infiltrating lipomas arise in and infiltrate the deeper soft tissues either between large muscle groups (intermuscular lipoma) or within muscle (intramuscular lipoma). Although patients in all age groups are affected, with some congenital examples reported, this is largely a tumor of adults, usually occurring in the fifth to seventh decades of life, with 80% of patients over the age of 40.[177,194-196] Also unlike subcutaneous lipomas, these tumors are more common in male patients.[177,195] They are painless masses that may become obvious only on contraction of the involved muscle when they may become round and firm.[177] Despite reaching very large size, at times up to 35 cm, they rarely produce actual

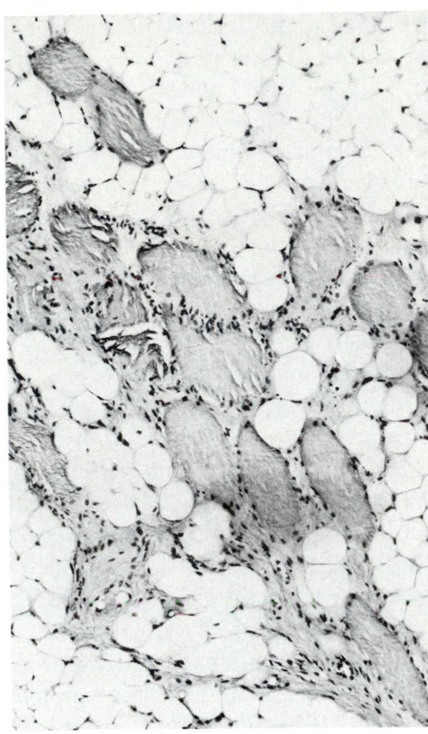

Fig. 39-25. Infiltrating intramuscular lipoma. Mature fat cells infiltrate around and between skeletal muscle fibers. (72×.)

dysfunction of the involved muscle.[194,196] Approximately two thirds are in the thigh and shoulder regions, and they occur less commonly in the upper arm, chest wall, and head and neck area.[177,195,196] Roentgenograms may show a sharply circumscribed radiolucent defect within the muscle, and, typically, angiographic studies show that these tumors, unlike soft tissue sarcomas, are poorly vascularized.[196]

On gross examination the tumor infiltrates and replaces large portions of muscle or infiltrates the tendons and fascia between muscles.[195] Histologically most tumors are composed of mature, normal-appearing fat cells lacking atypicality or mitotic activity.[195,196] The cells infiltrate between the muscle fibers, replacing them and causing pressure atrophy and degeneration (Fig. 39-25). Recently intramuscular lipomas have been described that have a significant degree of cytologic atypia. These pleomorphic or atypical lipomas are described separately in this chapter.

Recurrence rates following local excision have ranged widely from 3% to 62.5%,[177,194,195] with some patients having multiple recurrences. These recurrence rates probably reflect the adequacy of the initial excision rather than any inherent aggressive propensity of these tumors.[196] No metastases have been reported, and patients have remained well on extended follow-up study. As with any deep fatty tumor, the distinction from liposarcoma is important. The infiltrative growth pattern of the lipoma rather than the gross expansile pattern of liposarcoma, the absence of lipoblasts, and the bland nature of the fat cells in the lipoma serve to differentiate it from well-differentiated liposarcoma.

Spindle cell lipoma

A recently described histologic variant of lipoma,[199] spindle cell lipoma, unlike the usual lipoma, is far more frequent in men than in women. Over 90% of the reported cases have occurred in elderly men with a mean age of nearly 60 years. It is rarely found in patients under age 40.[197-199]

Almost all spindle cell lipomas are in the superficial subcutaneous tissue of the shoulder, upper back, or neck.[177,199] An example of this tumor in the perianal region has been reported.[199a] A few extend more deeply to involve the fascia and underlying muscle.[197] They range in size from 1 to 13 cm and either appear well demarcated or show an infiltrative pattern on gross inspection.[177,197]

Microscopic examination shows a varying proportion of four elements: bland-appearing, bipolar, elongate spindle cells; mature fat cells; bundles of birefringent collagen; and a myxoid stroma (Fig. 39-26).[177,199] In some tumors the spindle cells make up only a small portion of the lesion, with the fat cells dominating the picture; in others the fat cells are scarce, with the lesion composed almost solely of spindle cells.[197] The spindle cells are usually haphazardly arranged, but at times they are grouped in such a way as to produce a palisading pattern of their nuclei suggestive of neurilemoma. The myxoid matrix, in combination with the strands of collagen, may also produce a pattern suggestive of neurofibroma.[195,198] On the whole the vascular component is not prominent, but it may be so in the myxoid regions. Mast cells may be numerous.[195] Some cases contain focal areas in which multivacuolated cells have hyperchromatic and atypical nuclei similar to cells seen in pleomorphic (atypical) lipomas.[195] Mitotic figures, however, are rarely seen in these cases. Recurrences of spindle cell lipoma have not been reported following local excision.[195,197]

The distinction between spindle cell lipoma and the sclerosing and myxoid forms of liposarcoma is based on the absence of lipoblasts, mitotic activity, a diffuse plexiform capillary pattern, or pools of mucinous material. The superficial location of spindle cell lipoma is also in sharp contrast to the deep location of the typical liposarcomas.[177,197]

Although based on only a few cases that were studied by electron microscopy, one series concluded that the spindle cells of this tumor are fibroblasts or fibroblast-like cells.[199] A recent study, based on five cases, concluded that the spindle cells are independent of the fat cells and are analogous to the stellate mesenchymal cells seen in primitive fat lobules.[198]

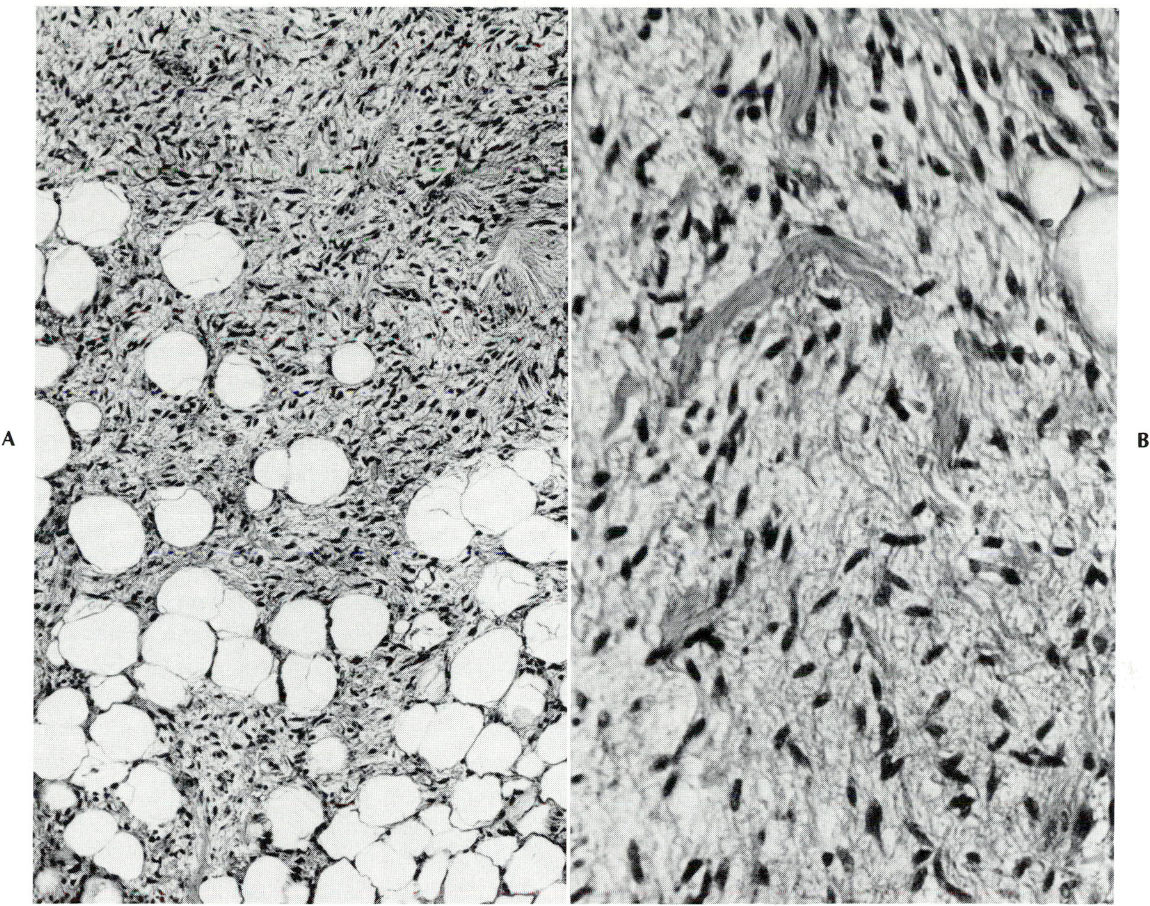

Fig. 39-26. A, Spindle cell lipoma. Mixture of mature fat cells and stellate spindle cells. **B,** Higher magnification shows spindle cells in myxoid stroma. Bundles of thick collagen fibers are present. (**A,** 90×; **B,** 350×.)

PLEOMORPHIC (ATYPICAL) LIPOMA

Fatty tumors histologically containing atypical multivacuolated lipoblasts have, in the past, all too often received the automatic diagnosis of liposarcoma, with all the consequences that such a diagnosis implies. With the recent recognition of subcutaneous and intramuscular fatty tumors having such cellular atypia, but a benign course,[195,200,200a,201] and for which the terms "pleomorphic" or "atypical lipoma" have been used, it is hoped that needless radical surgical procedures will now be performed less frequently as pathologists become cognizant of these tumors. Although some differences persist as to what type of lesion should be designated a pleomorphic or atypical lipoma, its general histologic features have been well described.[200,201]

As with liposarcoma, these tumors occur almost exclusively in older adults, usually between 50 and 70 years of age, with a mean age of about 60 years.[195,200,201] To date they have not been reported before 30 years of age.[200] Over 75% of the cases reported have been in men.[195] In most cases patients give a history of a slowly enlarging mass; it is not unusual for the mass to be present for 10 years or more. In others, however, the mass rapidly enlarges within a period of only a few weeks.[195,200] Approximately 80% are in the subcutaneous tissue of the neck, especially the posterior aspect, the shoulder, or the upper back, with a few tumors reported in the extremities.[200,201] In the few cases in which an intramuscular location has been reported, the thigh has been the most common site.[200] In the subcutaneous tissue the lesions are well circumscribed and partly or completely encapsulated, whereas the intramuscular lesion may be either well circumscribed or have an infiltrating pattern. Tumors in both sites may achieve a size of 10 cm or more, although the subcutaneous ones are usually smaller.[195,200]

As the name implies, these tumors are characterized by the presence of cellular pleomorphism consisting of multivacuolated lipoblasts with atypical nuclei, mixed with hyperchromatic multinucleated cells. The latter cells have an appearance described as "floretlike."[195,201] Their cytoplasm is eosinophilic, with or without vacuolization, and the nuclei are arranged in a wreathlike pattern at the periphery of the cytoplasm. The nuclei tend to overlap and may even be smudged together. The number of these floret cells varies, being abundant in some cases and rare in others.[201] Whereas some believe that their presence is essential to the diagnosis,[177] others report these cells in only one third of their cases.[200] In addition to floret cells, mononuclear cells of various sizes with hyperchromatic and atypical nuclei are also found. Interspersed between the atypical cells are mature fat cells and bands of thick, birefringent collagen (Fig. 39-27). Focal areas may be present with the characteristics of spindle cell lipoma, the latter reported in up to one fourth of cases.[201] Mast cells and scattered lymphocytes are also seen. Myxoid foci, either within the collagen bands or between the cells, are frequent. Mitotic figures are uncommon.

The differential diagnosis between these pleomorphic or atypical lipomas and sclerosing liposarcoma may be difficult. The location of the lesion in the subcutaneous tissue, its sharp circumscription and encapsulation, and the presence of thick collagen bundles and floret cells are indications of a benign lipoma rather than liposarcoma.[201] Before making a diagnosis of liposarcoma, one should always remember the extreme rarity of liposarcoma arising in a subcutaneous location.

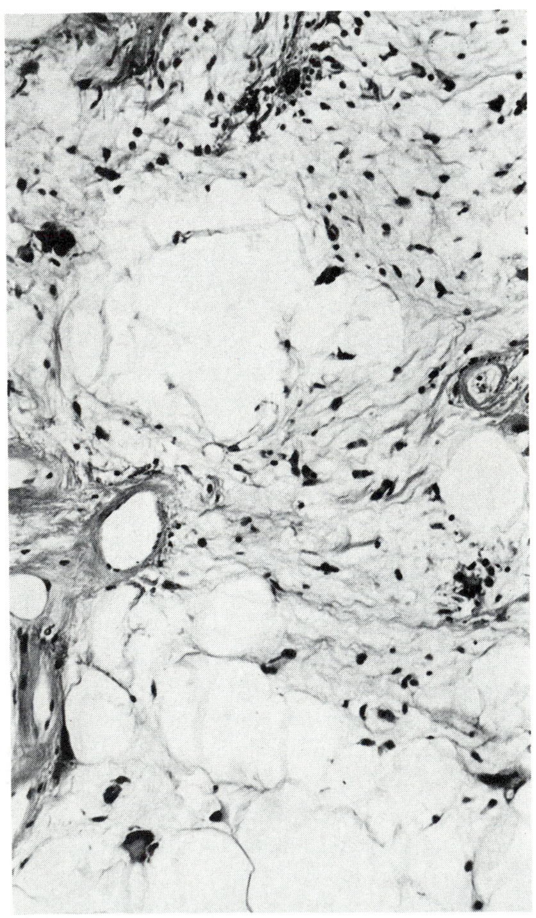

Fig. 39-27. Pleomorphic (atypical) lipoma. Hyperchromatic atypical cells within myxoid area. At lower left is floretlike cell. (150×.)

Follow-up studies of the subcutaneous tumors indicated only rare recurrences, with patients alive and well despite less than total excision of the tumor.[200,201] However, others have noted high recurrence rates even in subcutaneous tumors.[200a] Close to 70% of patients with the intramuscular variety have had a recurrence, but no tumor recurred that had been totally excised.[200] It is argued that this high local recurrence rate is similar to that noted in cases of the more typical intramuscular lipoma and should not be taken as an indication of aggressiveness of these tumors.[200] Others disagree, claiming that such recurrences may be less differentiated and fully malignant and that for this reason the intramuscular lesions should be called low-grade liposarcomas.[201] These differences await settlement by future reports of the tumors. It is apparently agreed that the subcutaneous lesions have a good prognosis. Deep-seated retroperitoneal fatty tumors with a similar cellular morphology behave in a locally aggressive manner and, despite their morphologic similarity to pleomorphic lipoma, should be considered liposarcomas.[200]

Angiolipoma

Angiolipoma, a histologic variant of lipoma, accounts for 5% to 17% of all benign fatty tumors.[205] Angiolipoma exists in two distinct forms: a subcutaneous, noninfiltrating, encapsulated tumor and a deeper, nonencapsulated, infiltrating lesion that involves muscle and adjacent fascia.[177,205] These two forms have different clinical features.

The noninfiltrating tumor almost never occurs before puberty. The average patient is between 17 and 21 years of age,[177, 204, 205] although in one series the average age was 41.7 years.[203] Men are more commonly affected than women, and a familial tendency has been noted.[177] Most patients seek treatment because of single or multiple, painful or tender nodules, usually less than 4 cm, located on the extremities in 70% of cases, most commonly the upper extremity. The abdomen and back are also common sites, accounting for 20% of cases.[177,204,205] The pain is usually not sharp or radiating, unlike that produced by glomus tumors.[204] The patient may continue to develop further nodules over a period of several years. The tumors are found in the subcutaneous tissue and appear as encapsulated red-yellow nodules.

Microscopically angiolipomas are composed of mature fat cells intermixed with a proliferation of delicate thin-walled capillaries (Fig. 39-28). The proportions of these two components vary somewhat; one may see lesions composed primarily of capillaries, with only a small amount of associated fat, or those with an abundance of fat and only a few foci of capillaries.[203,204] The vessels are predominantly located at the periphery of the tumor beneath the capsule and proliferate inward toward the center, accompanied by fine fibrous septa that extend from the capsule.[177,204,205] The fat cells lack atypia or mitotic activity. Fibrin thrombi are frequently present within the capillary lumina.[203,204] Foci of "undifferentiated" mesenchymal cells may be seen, but these are not numerous.[204] Simple excision is curative with no tendency for recurrence.[177,204,205]

Infiltrating angiolipoma is less common than its subcutaneous counterpart and affects patients over a broader age range. Patients vary in age from 2 to 67 years, with the average age being between 30 and 35 years.[202,205] Unlike the subcutaneous variety, infiltrating angiolipoma does occur in young children. There is no sex predilection.[202,205] The lesion involves the muscles of the lower extremity, neck, and shoulder region, and it is not usually painful.[202,205] The tumor histologically resembles an intramuscular hemangioma with its combination of

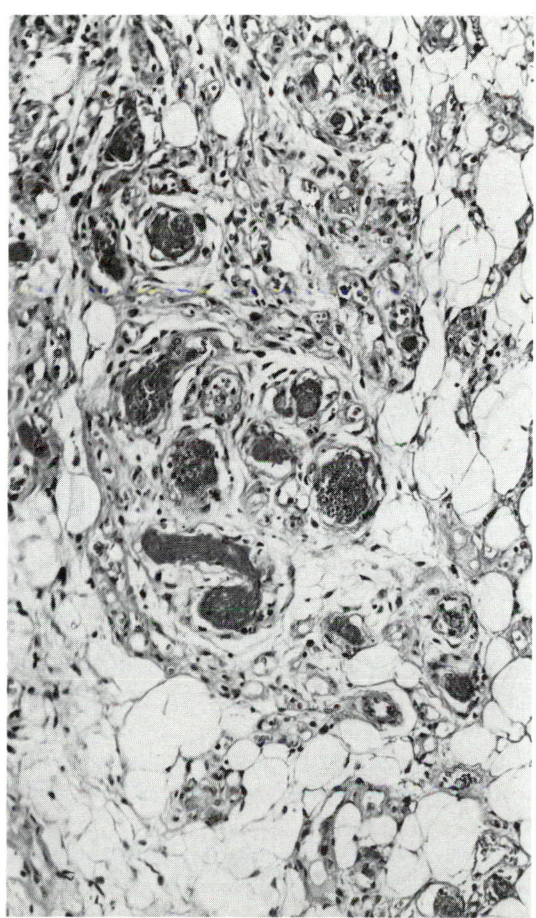

Fig. 39-28. Angiolipoma. Thin-walled blood vessels of capillary type are mixed with mature fat cells. Fibrin thrombi are visible in vessels just below center. (150×.)

blood vessels and fat. For this reason some suggest that the term "angiolipoma" be used to designate all infiltrating hemangiomas of the deep soft tissue and muscle.[177] A description of intramuscular hemangioma is given elsewhere in this chapter.

An electron microscopic study of angiolipoma found a decrease in the number of Weibel-Palade bodies present in the capillary endothelial cells. It was suggested that, since such a sparsity of Weibel-Palade bodies has also been noted in other vascular tumors, this reflects a possible relationship between these bodies and the functional state of the endothelial cell. The authors of the study also suggested that the fibrin thrombi so frequently found in angiolipomas may be caused by the occurrence of fibrinogen deposits that were found by immunofluorescence in the endothelial cells. These findings await confirmation.[203]

Lipoblastoma

To date, lipoblastoma has occurred exclusively in children, and its importance resides not in what it is but rather what it is not. Because of the presence of lipoblasts, a myxoid stroma, and occasionally an infiltrative growth pattern, it has been mistaken for myxoid liposarcoma with drastic consequences for the patient.[195,210]

Up to 90% of lipoblastomas are diagnosed before the age of 3, with the majority occurring within the first 2 years of life. The age range in one series was from 5 days to 7 years. Boys are involved more commonly than girls.[177,207] About three fourths of the tumors occur on the extremities, principally the lower extremity, but other locations include the neck, trunk, mediastinum, retroperitoneum, and labia.[177,195] Approximately two thirds of the lesions are circumscribed, encapsulated, lobular masses within the subcutaneous tissue.[195] The remaining one third are deeply situated, infiltrating lesions that grow between and into muscle and tend to be quite large.

The microscopic pattern is dominated by the presence of small lobules formed by fibrous connective tissue septa that may be quite thick. Within the lobules are monovacuolated and multivacuolated lipoblasts intermingled with immature-appearing stellate and spindle-shaped mesenchymal cells and mature fat cells. A myxoid stroma is present that is especially well seen at the periphery of the lobules and in areas where the cells are less mature. Some lobules are composed entirely of mature fat cells, whereas immediately adjacent lobules may consist entirely of lipoblasts and stellate cells. In lobules with a mixture of mature and immature cells, the central portions more commonly contain the mature fat cells, giving the impression of a maturation sequence from the periphery to the center (Fig. 39-29). Cells with central nuclei and a finely vacuolated cytoplasm, resembling brown fat cells, are also occasionally seen. The fibrous

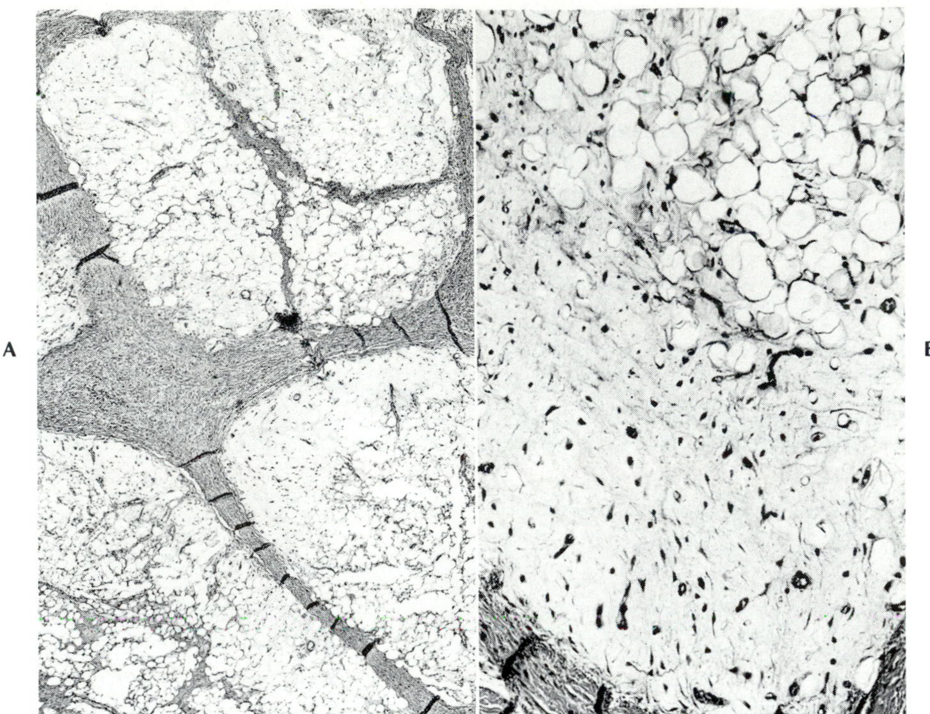

Fig. 39-29. A, Lipoblastoma. Lobules are formed by fibrous septa. Note myxoid foci adjacent to septa. **B,** Central portion of lobule, with mature fat cells, is at top. Foci containing a few signet-ring lipoblasts, as well as stellate cells embedded in myxoid stroma, are present toward periphery of field *(bottom)*. (**A,** 26×; **B,** 120×.)

septa contain numerous capillaries that extend into the lobules in a plexiform pattern. Mitoses are infrequent.[177,188,195,207,210]

Electron microscopic studies have shown a variety of cells including immature mesenchymal cells, fibroblasts, lipoblasts, mature fat cells, and transitional intermediate cell forms. The cells resemble those seen in the maturation phases of white adipose tissue and lack the fine structural features of brown fat.[188,206,209]

Although lipoblastoma has been confused with myxoid liposarcoma, its lobular character, apparent areas of maturation within the lobules, and absence of large mucinous pools are not the features of myxoid liposarcoma.[177,210] It is also important to remember the rarity of liposarcomas in a subcutaneous location and their virtual nonexistence in children under the age of 5 years.[207] Probably most of the liposarcomas previously reported in children in this age range were lipoblastomas.

Local recurrence following excision may occur in up to 20% of cases, but metastases are unknown.[195,207] It has been suggested that the term *lipoblastoma* be reserved for the superficial, well-circumscribed lesion and *lipoblastomatosis* be used for the more diffuse infiltrating lesion.[207] We prefer the single term *lipoblastoma* for both forms of the lesion. Some authors, unfortunately, still use "lipoblastoma" to refer to hibernoma, the tumor of brown fat.[208] This adds unnecessary confusion to the literature, and "lipoblastoma" should refer to this childhood tumor of white fat.

Hibernoma

Although tumors arising from white adipose tissue are among the most common of all soft tissue lesions, those originating from brown fat are among the rarest tumors, with only 21 case reports in the English literature as of 1972.[177,212] The name *hibernoma* derives from the tumor's histologic similarity to the brown fat of hibernating animals, but whether human brown fat is totally analogous to that of animals remains unclear.[212]

Brown fat occurs in only a few specific anatomic areas. In infants it is found in the interscapular areas, the axilla, mediastinum, neck, and posterior abdominal wall and around the kidneys, adrenals, and pancreas. In adults it persists in the neck, axilla, mediastinum, and periadrenal and perirenal areas.[213]

As one would expect, hibernomas have been reported to arise from most of these same areas, with the majority occurring in the interscapular region. However, they have also been found where brown fat is absent, such as the thigh, buttock, and popliteal fossa.[177,212,213] They

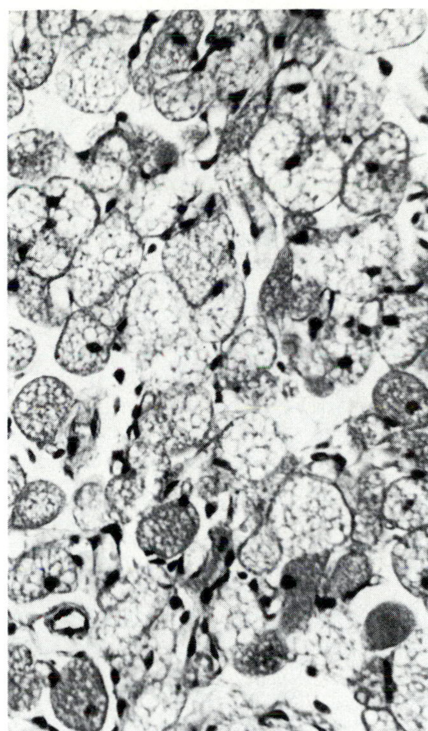

Fig. 39-30. Hibernoma. Cells with multivacuolated cytoplasm are mixed with cells having a less vacuolated, granular, darker, eosinophilic cytoplasm. (280×.)

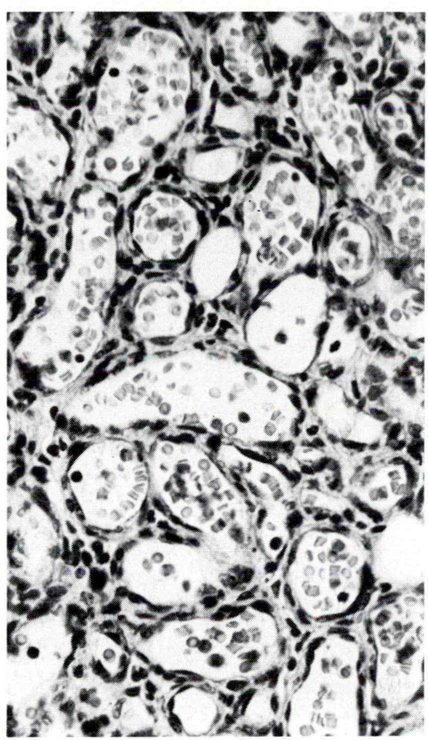

Fig. 39-31. Capillary hemangioma. Closely packed thin-walled blood vessels with small lumina containing red blood cells. (280×.)

have occurred in patients of all ages, from infants to adults in their sixties.[177,212,213] The tumor is a painless mass that usually grows slowly but occasionally enlarges rapidly.[177,212] Some patients have had their tumors for as long as 30 years. They are encapsulated, tan-brown, subcutaneous masses, although occasional tumors have involved muscle, where they may grow as large as 20 cm.[177,211,212]

Histologically a variety of cells are arranged in small lobules formed by delicate, well-vascularized, fibrous septa. The cells vary from those that are lipid free and have an eosinophilic granular cytoplasm to those that have monovacuolated and multivacuolated lipid containing cytoplasm (Fig. 39-30). In the multivacuolated cells, which are more common, the nucleus is either central or eccentric and has a bland appearance. The cytoplasmic vacuoles are small and delicate, giving the cells a foamy or bubbly appearance. Brown intracytoplasmic lipofuscin pigment is present in many cells. Mitoses and cellular pleomorphism are absent.[177,212] Electron microscopic studies have shown a similarity between hibernoma cells and those in animal brown fat.[213] A characteristic finding is the presence of moderately pleomorphic mitochondria having transverse cristae.[212]

Hibernomas apparently have no malignant potential and are cured by simple local excision.[177,212,213] Some consider the round cell liposarcoma to be the malignant counterpart of this tumor, but there is no good evidence to support this.[177]

VASCULAR TUMORS

Intramuscular hemangioma

The common benign vascular tumors, capillary and cavernous hemangioma, and benign hemangioendothelioma do occur in the soft tissue but more frequently are cutaneous lesions. Similarly, with rare exceptions such as in patients with long-standing lymphedema that follows radical mastectomy, the malignant vascular tumors—angiosarcoma and malignant hemangioendothelioma—also occur more commonly in the skin than in the soft tissues. These tumors are described in more detail in Chapter 18.

Briefly, capillary hemangioma consists of a proliferation of small thin-walled vessels with well-defined lumina.[7a,10,23,27] The endothelial cells are bland and usually flat (Fig. 39-31). At times, however, these cells round up and proliferate to such a degree, with obvious increased mitotic activity, that the vascular lumina are obscured, creating the impression of solid nests and sheets of cells. This is the pattern of benign hemangioendothelioma.[27]

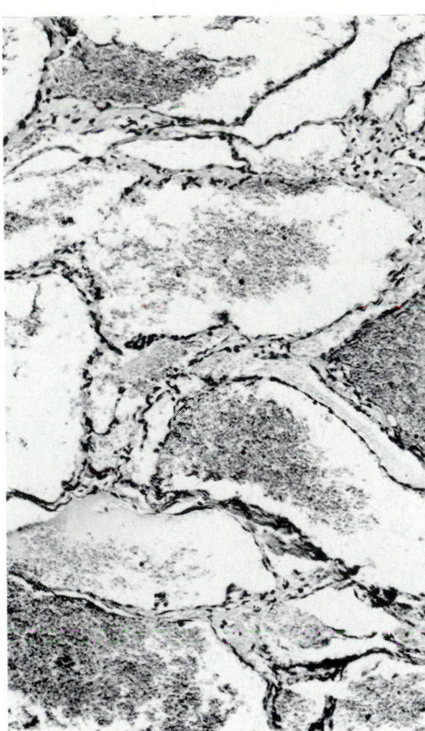

Fig. 39-32. Cavernous hemangioma. Widely dilated, thin-walled vessels containing red blood cells. (280×.)

The cavernous hemangioma is also composed of thin-walled vessels, but these are larger than in the capillary form and are quite dilated with gaping lumina filled with red blood cells (Fig. 39-32). Frequently both types of vessels are seen in the same lesion.

In the deep soft tissues, especially in skeletal muscle, such vascular tumors may occur as infiltrating lesions and be misdiagnosed as angiosarcoma. Histologically, few of these intramuscular lesions are of a pure type, and they are categorized as small vessel (capillary), large vessel (cavernous), or mixed types depending on which, if either, of the two types of vessels dominates the histologic pattern.[214]

Intramuscular hemangiomas occur in patients of all ages but are most frequent in young adults. Those predominantly of small vessel type occur with more or less equal frequency in the muscles of the trunk, head and neck region, and upper limbs and somewhat less frequently in the lower extremity. The large vessel type occurs more frequently in the muscles of the lower extremity. The mixed type has a propensity to occur in the trunk. However, any of these forms may occur in any muscle. When the small vessel type is present, it may take on the features of a hemangioendothelioma, leading to a consideration of angiosarcoma. This possibility is further enhanced by the frequent presence of mitoses and apparent invasion of perineural spaces. However, the lesion lacks the bizarre cells, necrosis, multilayering of cells, and extensive pattern of intercommunicating vascular channels of angiosarcoma.[214] Intramuscular angiosarcoma is an exceedingly rare neoplasm both in absolute terms and in comparison with occurrence of intramuscular hemangioma.

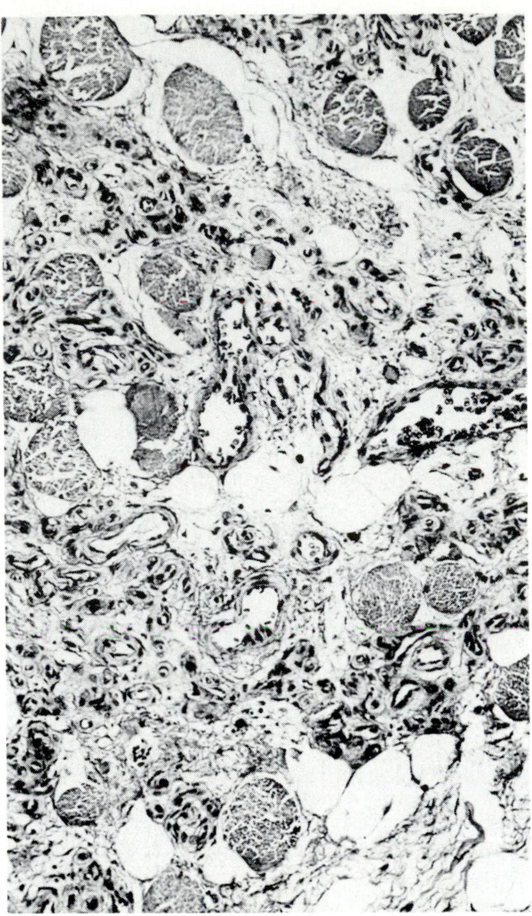

Fig. 39-33. Intramuscular hemangioma. Skeletal muscle infiltrated by blood vessels, mainly of small size. Scattered mature fat cells are present. Pattern is similar to an angiolipoma. (150×.)

In addition to the presence of blood vessels infiltrating between muscle fibers, there is frequently an abundance of adipose tissue, especially in the large vessel and mixed types (Fig. 39-33). The amount of fat may reach such a degree that it overshadows the vessels, and the lesion appears to be an angiolipoma. Indeed, because of the frequent presence of fat cells, angiolipoma is now preferred by some as the more appropriate designation for all intramuscular hemangiomas.[177]

As a group, intramuscular hemangiomas recur in about 20% of cases after local excision, with the mixed pattern having a slightly higher incidence of recurrence. The lesions do not metastasize.[214]

Hemangiopericytoma

Hemangiopericytoma is a much abused diagnosis frequently used as a convenient label for any vascular soft tissue tumor that does not easily fit into one of the other

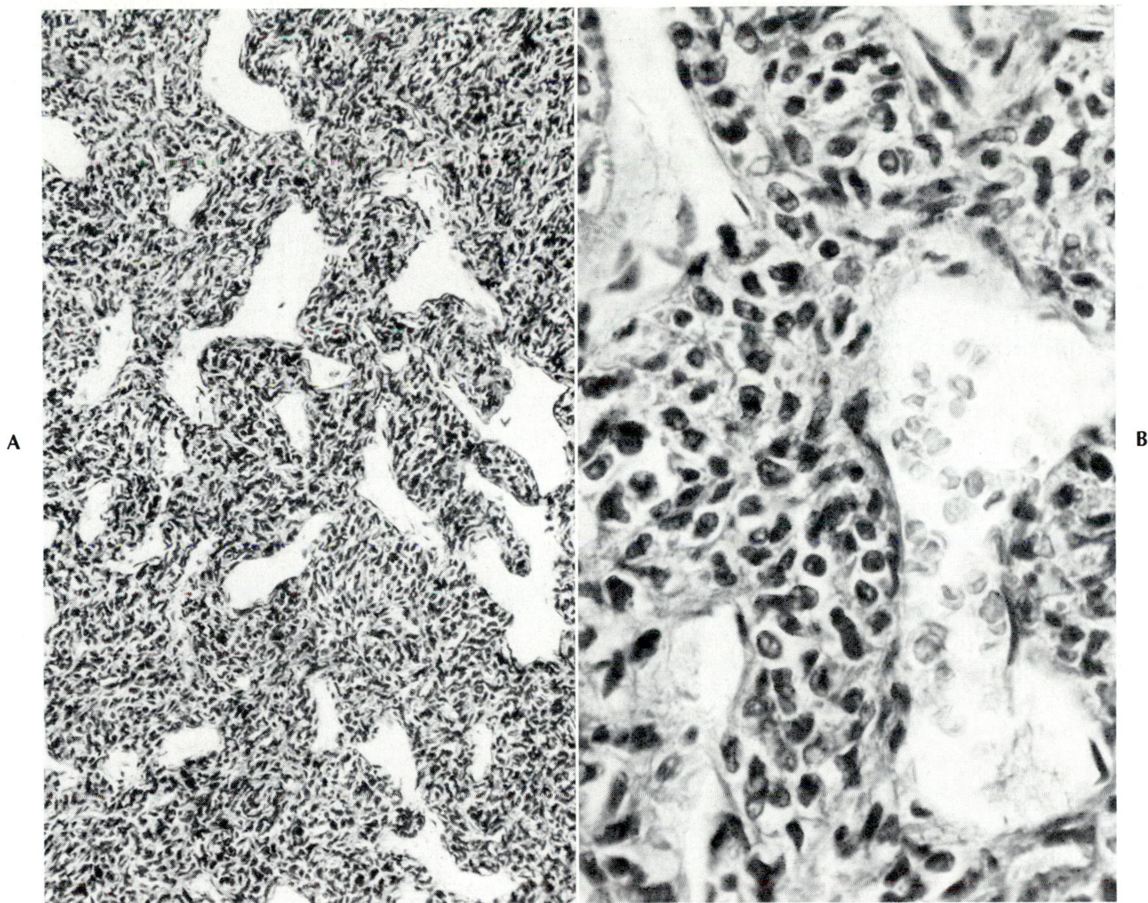

Fig. 39-34. A, Hemangiopericytoma. Vascular channels are surrounded by closely packed small cells. **B,** Higher magnification shows vessels, lined by flat endothelial cells, surrounded by pericytes. (**A,** 150×; **B,** 600×.)

major diagnostic categories. In one series from a cancer registry, only six of 42 cases diagnosed as hemangiopericytoma were acceptable as such on histologic review.[215]

Hemangiopericytoma is uncommon. In reports from two large referral institutions only 60 and 106 cases in the soft tissues were seen over periods of 57 and 43 years, respectively.[217,218] The tumor is found in all age groups, including infants and children, but it is principally a tumor of adults, 80% to 95% occurring in patients above the age of 20, with a peak in the fifth to sixth decades.[215,217,218] Male and female patients are approximately equally affected.[217,218]

Most patients seek treatment within a year of noting a lump or mass, which may be painful. The pain is typically described as dull, distinguishing it from the sharp pain produced by glomus tumors with which hemangiopericytoma may be confused histologically.[217,218] Hemangiopericytoma is found in a wide variety of locations, including the brain, various viscera, bones, and the soft tissues. In the last location the most common sites include the thigh, retroperitoneum and pelvic regions, the head and neck, and the trunk.[215a,217,218] Typically, with the exception of those in the subcutaneous tissue of infants, the tumors are located in the deep soft tissue either in muscle or along fascial planes.[217] When in the retroperitoneum or pelvis, not uncommonly lesions reach dimensions of 15 cm or more. Because of the vascularity of these tumors, the surgeon may encounter significant bleeding during attempts at resection.[217]

The histopathologic pattern is marked by ramifying blood vessels surrounded by closely packed, plump to spindle-shaped cells having indistinct cytoplasmic margins and oval to round vesicular nuclei.[217,218] The vascular channels, which are lined with flattened endothelial cells, vary in size from large sinusoidal spaces to narrow capillary-sized slits (Fig. 39-34). The angles at which the main vascular channels branch create a staghorn or antlerlike effect when viewed at low-power magnification.[217] In some cases the stromal cells compress the channels so that the tumor appears to be composed only of solidly packed cells without a vascular component. The vascular pattern, however, is dramatically brought out by reticulin stains that show an abundance of reticulin distributed around each vessel and surrounding each cell, being absent only around the lining endothelial cells. At times the stromal cells are arranged in a storiform pattern suggestive of fibrous histiocytoma.[14] Areas with this pattern may be so prominent that the distinction between hemangiopericytoma and fibrous histiocytoma cannot, with a reasonable degree of certainty, be made by light microscopy. A diagnosis of hemangiopericytoma should be made only tentatively when one is dealing with a small amount of biopsy material, since hemangiopericytoma-like areas are noted in other soft tissue tumors in addition to fibrous histiocytoma. Two of the more frequent of these are mesenchymal chondrosarcoma and synovial sarcoma.[14,217] The former is distinguished by the presence of islands of bland chondroid and cartilaginous tissue, whereas synovial sarcoma is easily distinguished from hemangiopericytoma if one insists on the presence of a biphasic histologic pattern in synovial sarcoma.

Based on electron microscopic evidence, it is now generally agreed that the cell of origin of hemangiopericytoma is the pericyte, which is normally found wrapped around capillaries and postcapillary vessels.[217,218] Pericytes are thought to serve a contractile function. Transitions between pericytes and smooth muscle cells in the walls of larger blood vessels have also been found. Pericytes have such fine structural features as basal lamina, pinocytotic vesicles, and cytoplasmic microfilaments.[219] Although some variation in the electron microscopic features of these cells has been noted in the different studies of hemangiopericytoma, electron microscopy may help confirm the diagnosis when the light microscopic pattern is suggestive of hemangiopericytoma.[219,220]

Tumors are placed into benign and malignant categories based on their cellularity, anaplasia, and mitotic rate and the presence or absence of necrosis. As one would expect, borderline lesions exist where a definite conclusion cannot be reached with regard to their benign or malignant character.[215,217,218]

An aggressive course with metastases has been reported in up to 57% of hemangiopericytomas.[217,218] The clinical course appears to correlate with the histologic pattern.[217,218] Tumors that are highly cellular, with or without anaplasia, and have a high mitotic rate have a poor prognosis. Similarly, tumors with a low mitotic rate but with a significant degree of cellular anaplasia or necrosis are also likely to pursue a malignant course. Patients with tumors that lack these features have 10-year survival rates of 80% to 90%; however, although most lesions that are composed of bland cells and lack mitoses or necrosis behave in a benign fashion, rare tumors with this pattern have recurred or metastasized.[215] Patients with malignant hemangiopericytomas have a survival rate of approximately 30%. Patients who have local recurrences after excision have a poor prognosis.[217] Recurrences and metastases, however, may be delayed for many years, and even a 15-year survival may not be indicative of a cure. Lesions of borderline or malignant histologic appearance may require radical resection or even amputation, since these tumors are for the most part radioresistant.[218]

Hemangiopericytomas in infants apparently behave differently from those in adults. Unlike the adult tumors, they occur superficially in the subcutaneous tissue as multilobulated lesions, often showing blood vessel invasion. Microscopically there is also a proliferation of endothelial cells such that transitions between the pattern of hemangiopericytomas and that of hemangioendothelioma are found. Despite the presence of necrosis and significant mitotic activity, these tumors are reported to follow a benign course. However, these conclusions are based on the results in only a small number of patients.[216,217]

NEUROGENOUS TUMORS

The terminology of the peripheral neurogenous tumors has been somewhat confused by the use of the term "schwannoma" as the appellation for both of the two major benign peripheral nerve tumors, neurofibroma and neurilemoma.[231] Although current opinion implicates the Schwann cell as the cell of origin for both of these tumors,[221,225,235,244] in most cases the two are sufficiently distinct to be easily differentiated. Although in practice the term *schwannoma* is used as a synonym for *neurilemoma*, only the latter will be used here to avoid any possibility of confusion. Tumors of the sympathetic nervous system are not discussed in this chapter.

Since Schwann cells are thought to be the major cellular component of these tumors, the tumors are considered to be neuroectodermal in origin. However, some believe that the mesodermally derived perineural fibroblasts are the actual cells of origin of these tumors or at least take part equally with Schwann cells in their formation.[221,225,237,238] Both cells are thought to have a pluripotential character capable of forming collagen, bone, cartilage, adipose tissue, and muscle.[221,246] This pluripotentiality is seen most clearly in some of the malignant neurogenous tumors, where a variety of malignant heterogeneous tissues are found. Electron microscopic studies have shown that the cells of these two peripheral nerve tumors are characterized by cytoplasmic extensions containing fine filaments and microtubules.[17,244] Practically all the benign nerve sheath tumors will yield positive results when stained for S-100 protein.[21a,244a]

Neurilemoma and neurofibroma must both be distinguished from the peripheral neuroma that is composed of a tangle of regenerating axons interwoven with Schwann cells within a fibrous stroma (Fig. 39-35).[221,225a,235,238a] These "traumatic" neuromas arise subsequent to some

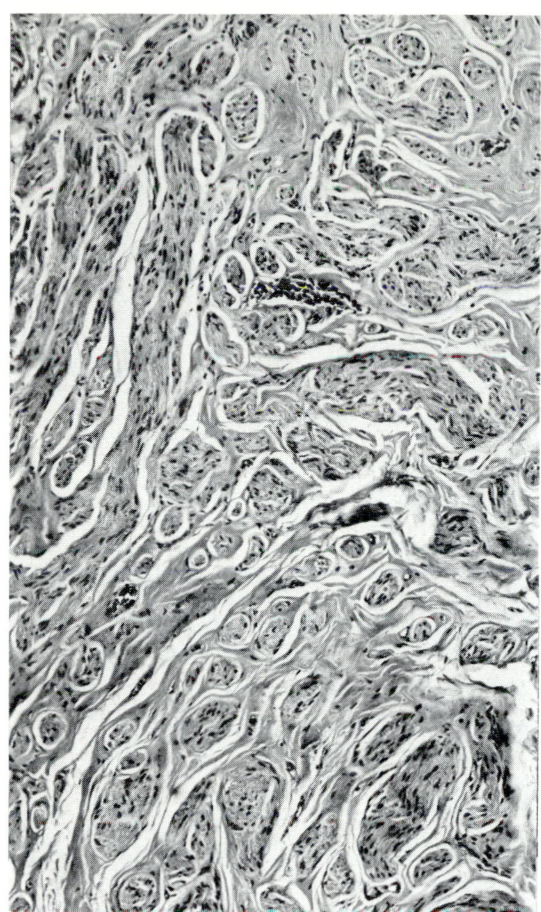

Fig. 39-35. Neuroma. Tangle of axons of various size within fibrous stroma. (90×.)

injury, such as surgical or blunt trauma, and develop as a firm, rubbery, and usually painful or tender mass at the site of injury. They are not true tumors but rather represent an exaggeration of the normal repair process in nerve regeneration, much like exuberant fracture callus following poor alignment of bone. They produce symptoms only after reaching large size. A variant of this process, Morton's neuroma, arises from one of the interdigital plantar nerves and forms an extremely painful mass near the heads of the metatarsal bones. Approximately 90% of these are between the third and fourth toes. They are most frequent in women between 30 and 60 years of age.[235] Morton's neuroma is probably caused by repeated trauma to this area, leading to reactive overgrowth of connective tissue that disrupts the nerves.[224a,234]

Neurilemoma

Neurilemomas arise from the neural sheaths of the peripheral motor, sensory, and cranial nerves, with the exception of the optic and olfactory nerves, which lack Schwann cell sheaths and are part of the central nervous system.[235] Neurilemomas are usually solitary painless lesions, but when large they can produce pressure symptoms with paresthesia or local tenderness.[224a,225,231,235] They occur in young to middle-aged adults, but no age group is exempt.[221,231] Women are affected twice as often as men.[225,231] The tumors may occur anywhere in the soft tissue or the viscera, but the more common locations include the soft tissue of the head and neck, especially the lateral aspect of the neck; the extremities; trunk; mediastinum; and retroperitoneum.[221,225,231] The acoustic nerve is the cranial nerve most commonly involved. Neurilemomas are fusiform, round or oval masses that are sharply circumscribed and encapsulated.[221,225,235] When on large nerve trunks, they may appear as pedunculated or bulbous masses. In the more superficial soft tissue one may not be able to recognize a nerve of origin. Neurilemomas are usually less than 5 cm, but those in the mediastinum or retroperitoneum may be as large as 20 cm.[231] On cut surface they are tan-gray to white and have a watery or slimy consistency. Larger lesions frequently have cystic and hemorrhagic foci.[225,235] In large nerve trunks it may be possible to clearly dissect the tumor from the nerve, since the nerve fibers do not course through the lesion but are confined to the capsule. Occasionally patients have multiple neurilemomas, and in the case of acoustic nerve tumors they may be bilateral. Such patients frequently have associated multiple neurofibromas (von Recklinghausen's disease) (see Chapter 44).[235]

The histologic appearance of neurilemoma alternates between compact cellular areas, which have historically been called Antoni A regions, and loosely arranged hypocellular areas known as Antoni B regions (Fig. 39-36).[221,225,235] The cells in the Antoni A areas are bipolar spindle cells having oval to elongate nuclei and an eosinophilic fibrillar cytoplasm. The cells are either aligned in interweaving fascicles or are arranged so that their nuclei line up to create a palisading pattern. Their long, tapering, fibrillar cytoplasmic processes may fuse into hyalin masses. Although nuclear palisades are a frequent finding in these neurogenous tumors, other tumors, especially those of smooth muscle origin, may also show prominent palisades, and hence their presence is not diagnostic of neural tumors. The spindle cells also occasionally are grouped in such a way as to create organoid structures similar in appearance to tactile corpuscles. These are called Verocay bodies. Mitotic figures are absent or only rarely present in neurilemomas. In the Antoni B areas the cells are widely separated by a loose, textured, watery matrix that stains poorly or not at all with stains for acid mucopolysaccharide, in contrast to the matrix of neurofibroma, which yields a strongly positive reaction. Microcystic spaces are also found in these Antoni B regions. Macrophages and lymphocytes are present in both A and B areas, but mast cells are infrequent. The proportions of A and B regions vary, and one

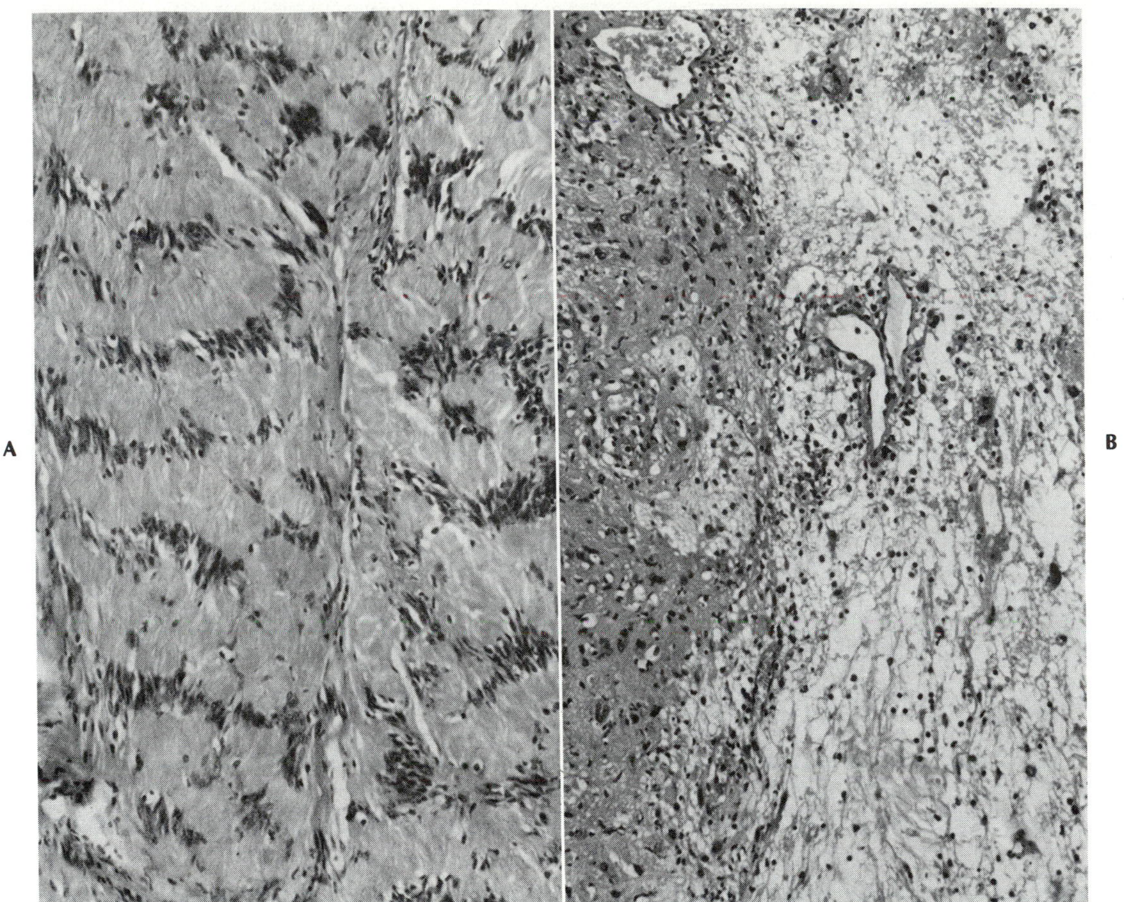

Fig. 39-36. A, Neurilemoma. Antoni A area is composed of spindle cells with tapering cytoplasmic extensions. Nuclei are aligned, creating characteristic palisading pattern. **B,** Antoni B area is present at far right with edematous stroma. More cellular Antoni A area is at left. Several blood vessels are present. (150×.)

or the other may dominate the pattern, but both are present in most neurilemomas. Another characteristic of these tumors is their abundant vascularity, with numerous small blood vessels. Larger vessels with dense hyalinized walls are common and characteristic of these tumors. Some vessels may have fibrous mural thrombi with associated evidence of recent and old hemorrhage in the adjacent stroma. Neurites are not found in the substance of neurilemomas.

The accepted dogma is that the major cell in a neurilemoma is the Schwann cell, but the role of the perineural fibroblast in the formation of the lesion has received considerable attention.[221,225,235] The relationship between the Schwann cell and the perineural fibroblast is still debated, with some believing that they are actually functional variants of the same cell. The issue is still unsettled.[238]

On excision, solitary neurilemomas only rarely recur and for all practical purposes never undergo malignant degeneration.[221,225] Occasional neurilemomas are found in which the cells are hyperchromatic and have bizarre nuclear configurations with some multinucleation. These "ancient" neurilemomas are totally benign, with cellular changes reflecting degenerative phenomena.[222,229] Cellular pleomorphism in neurogeneous tumors is not in itself evidence of malignancy. A type of neurilemoma has been described that, owing to its cellularity, may be confused with a variety of other tumors, including malignant nerve sheath lesions.[246a]

Neurofibroma

Neurofibromas are slightly more common than neurilemomas and tend to occur in younger patients.[223,239] Male and female patients are affected equally. Neurofibromas may be solitary or multiple and in the latter form are part of the von Recklinghausen's disease complex (see Chapter 44).[224a] They occur as small (2 to 4 cm) nodules in the skin and subcutaneous tissue of the extremities, trunk, and head and neck region but are also found in the deep soft tissues and viscera, where they

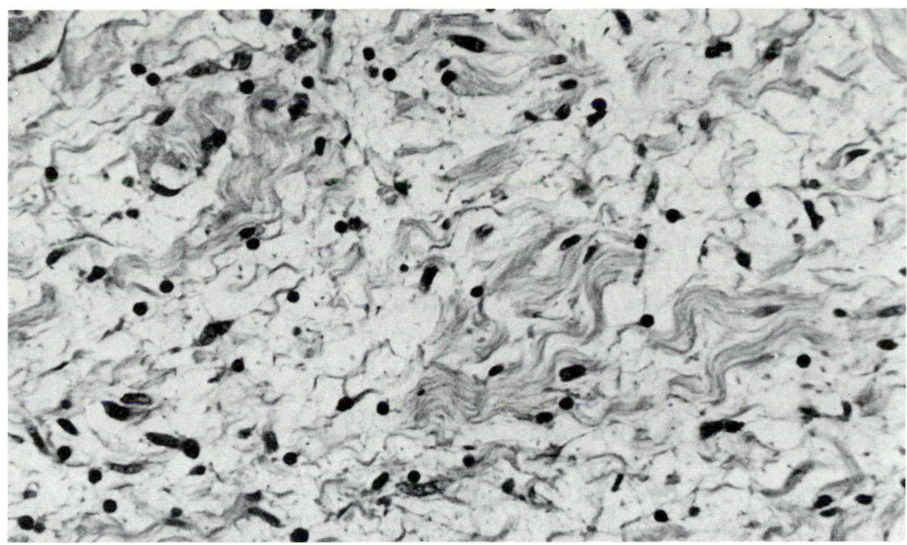

Fig. 39-37. Neurofibroma. Schwann cells within myxoid background intermixed with short, wavy collagen bundles. (350×.)

grow to a large size.[221,223,235] Neurofibromas also arise in areas that have received irradiation.[221] In some patients neurofibromas are associated with local subcutaneous tissue hypertrophy and even gigantism of all or part of an affected limb.[221] In the superficial tissues they are usually ill-defined unencapsulated lesions, whereas in the deeper soft tissues they are often better circumscribed and may be encapsulated.[221,225,235] When arising from large nerve trunks, they may produce multiple irregular fusiform swellings along the nerve, creating a tangled wormlike mass. The finding of this plexiform neurofibroma is tantamount to a diagnosis of von Recklinghausen's disease.[235]

On gross examination neurofibromas tend to be softer than neurilemomas and have a grayish-white glistening surface that has a distinctly gelatinous appearance and feels slimy.[223,235] This mucoid appearance may be so marked as to suggest a myxoma. If the tumor arises in a well-defined large nerve, the nerve runs through the lesion such that it cannot, as with a neurilemoma, be dissected free from the tumor.[225]

Microscopic examination shows a mixture of elements.[221,223,225,235] Spindle-shaped or stellate cells (Schwann cells or perineural cells) with elongate and at times wavy or twisted nuclei are associated with scattered lymphocytes and mast cells. Collagen fibers or bundles are present throughout the tumor, arranged in short lengths or in nodular arrays (Fig. 39-37). Unlike neurilemomas, neurofibromas contain neurites, although they are often difficult to find. The background stroma appears edematous, and the individual cells are widely separated. It stains strongly for acid mucopolysaccharide, unlike the weak or negative reaction noted in neurilemoma.[223,235] Plexiform neurofibromas show large areas of normal nerve mixed with spindle cells and myxoid stroma. Alternating Antoni A and B areas are usually absent, as are the conspicuous blood vessels seen in neurilemomas. However, areas that resemble neurilemoma may occur; indeed, some solitary neurofibromas have these foci to such a degree that a clear distinction between the two tumors is impossible.[223,235]

In the usual neurofibroma, mitoses are rare, and if more than an occasional mitotic figure is noted in several high-power fields, the possibility of malignant change should be considered. At times, as in neurilemoma, there are cells that show nuclear pleomorphism.[223,235] However, in the absence of mitotic figures and focal necrosis this finding is not an indication of malignancy.

Solitary neurofibromas have a low incidence of recurrence following local excision, as well as a low incidence of malignant degeneration, especially in those located superficially.[231,235] However, patients with multiple neurofibromas do have a significant risk of malignant neural tumors. This is discussed in the next section.

Neurosarcoma (malignant schwannoma)

The most common term used to designate malignant tumors of peripheral nerves is malignant schwannoma. This may create some confusion, since the term *schwannoma* is used as a synonym for *neurilemoma*, a tumor that virtually never undergoes malignant change.[231b] In addition, neurofibromas that become malignant frequently have histologic features resembling those of fibrosarcoma, and for that reason they are called neurofibrosarcomas.[241] Since many malignant tumors arising in peripheral nerves do not show definitive Schwann cell differentiation,[231b] being undifferentiated pleomorphic tumors, or contain metaplastic elements such as malignant osteoid, cartilage, fat, and even glands, we prefer the less specific but more encompassing term *neurosarcoma* to designate the malignant peripheral nerve tumors that have a sarcomatous pattern.

Unfortunately, regardless of the term used, the diagnosis of a soft tissue sarcoma as some form of neurogenic tumor has been used as a convenient "escape" for diagnostic pathologists faced with a spindle cell or pleomorphic sarcoma that does not obviously fit into a neat classification niche. We believe that the diagnosis of neurosarcoma should be restricted to tumors that can be identified as clearly arising within a nerve, have histologic areas of benign neurofibroma, or arise in a patient with von Recklinghausen's disease. If these criteria are used, neurosarcomas are not common, comprising between 5% and 10% of all sarcomas,[38,83] although these figures are probably high. They are also much less common than benign peripheral nerve tumors, making up about 2% of all nerve sheath tumors.[242] Neurosarcomas arise in patients with or without associated von Recklinghausen's disease.[227,228] Those arising in the absence of von Recklinghausen's disease are somewhat more common in any large series of neurosarcomas, although this depends on how stringently the criteria for the clinical diagnosis of von Recklinghausen's disease are applied. As a group, however, patients with von Recklinghausen's disease have a higher incidence of malignant neurogenous tumors than the general population. Estimates of this risk vary, since no long-term prospective study has been done to assess the true risk. However, series have been reported with incidence figures that range from 5% to 30%.[228,230] In one series malignancy developed in 19% of patients with von Recklinghausen's disease by 40 years of age. In 53% of patients whose neurofibromas appeared between the ages of 16 to 25, a malignant neurogenous tumor developed within 5 to 8 years of the appearance of the neurofibroma.[230]

Neurosarcomas in association with von Recklinghausen's disease usually develop in patients between 20 and 50 years of age (mean approximately 30 years), but patients who have spontaneously developing neurosarcoma are about 10 to 15 years older.[227,228,232,240,243] Women are more commonly affected than men.[232,240,243]

The most common initial symptom is a swelling or mass, which is painful in over half the cases.[227,228,233,243] Paresthesia, muscle atrophy, or weakness may be present if a major nerve trunk is involved.[227,228,233] Patients with von Recklinghausen's disease may have a clinical history of such a mass for many years. This probably reflects the presence of the previous neurofibroma rather than the actual tumor that develops.[228] The sudden onset of pain or rapid growth in a preexisting mass, or one that rapidly develops de novo, is highly indicative of malignancy in these patients.

Neurosarcomas are most commonly located in the extremities, the trunk, or paravertebral areas.[14,228,232,233,243] The head and neck region is not as frequent a site as it is for benign neurogenous tumors.[227] Patients with von Recklinghausen's disease have tumors that are centrally located, such as on the trunk, shoulder region, and pelvic area, with only a few located on the distal aspect of the extremities.[233,240] The tumors frequently involve major nerve trunks, where they form fusiform or nodular swellings that infiltrate the nerve proper and cannot be dissected from the nerve.[14,227,228,233,243] They commonly contain areas of necrosis and hemorrhage. In patients with von Recklinghausen's disease tumors may arise in the soft tissue adjacent to a major nerve or in an area where a major nerve cannot be grossly identified.[228] The tumors tend to be large, commonly exceeding 10 cm.[232,233]

Schwann cells or perineural cells are considered to have the ability to produce a variety of tissue elements including collagen.[226,236] It is not surprising therefore that most neurosarcomas have fibrosarcomatous foci composed of spindle cells arranged in interlacing fascicles with herringbone patterns.[227,233,234,243] The tumors may also mimic malignant fibrous histiocytosis.[235a] Nuclei vary from elongate to round and plump with hyperchromasia and various degrees of pleomorphism (Fig. 39-38). The stroma may be fibrotic or myxomatous. Mitoses are quite frequent (usually one or more per every high-power field), as are foci of hemorrhage and necrosis.[14,232-234,243] Without knowledge of direct origin within a nerve, these neurofibrosarcomas are indistinguishable from their soft tissue counterparts. Stains for S-100 protein yield positive results in about 50% of neurosarcomas, with only occasional cells staining in the positive cases.[244a] Electron microscopy may aid in the diagnosis of the better-differentiated tumors.[231b,241a] Undifferentiated pleomorphic sarcomas also arise within nerve, composed of bizarre giant cells and polygonal mononuclear tumor cells with irregular hyperchromatic nuclei.[228,232,240] Patients with von Recklinghausen's disease are reported to have a tendency to develop these pleomorphic tumors,[228,232] although some report that tumors in these patients are of the collagenous type, with the pleomorphic variety found in patients without von Recklinghausen's disease.[240] Neurosarcomas that arise in soft tissue that has been irradiated tend to be pleomorphic.[240]

Metaplastic malignant osteoid and cartilage may be found as components of these tumors, as well as areas of liposarcoma and rhabdomyosarcoma.[228,232,233,235] Tumors with rhabdomyosarcomatous differentiation have

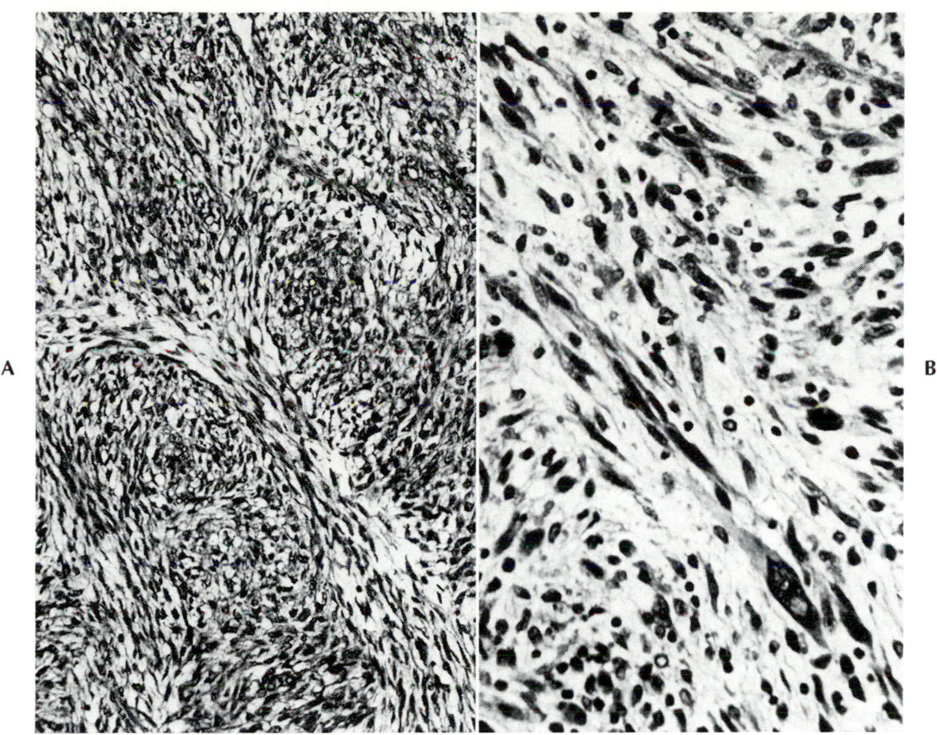

Fig. 39-38. A, Neurosarcoma. Cellular nodules of spindle cells. **B,** Higher magnification shows pleomorphic cells in elongate shapes. Mitotic figures are present at top and at left of center. Lymphocytes are scattered among the tumor cells. (**A,** 120×; **B,** 280×.)

been called malignant "triton" tumors.[225b,246] A benign variant of such lesions has recently been described.[225a,238a] Rarely, epithelial-like differentiation is found, with tumors resembling malignant melanoma, or tumors containing benign-appearing glands with goblet cell differentiation.[224,235,245]

Neurosarcomas are highly malignant lesions. Recurrences follow local excision in 50% to 80% of patients.[227,228,232,240,243] The prognosis is poor for patients with associated von Recklinghausen's disease, in whom 5-year survival rates range from 15% to 30% versus 50% to 75% for patients with spontaneously occurring neurosarcomas.* It is not uncommon, however, for recurrences and metastases to occur 5 to 10 years after therapy.[232,233] The development of local recurrence in patients with associated von Recklinghausen's disease indicates a grave prognosis, with almost all patients dying of their disease.[240] Small tumors (less than 5 cm) have a better prognosis than larger lesions.[231a] Centrally located tumors have a poorer prognosis than those on the distal aspect of the extremities. This may reflect the propensity for central tumors to grow to very large size. Malignant triton tumors and those with glandular differentiation also carry a very poor prognosis.[245,246] Radiation-induced neurosarcomas are almost uniformly fatal.[240]

*References 224a, 227, 228, 231a, 232, 233, 240.

MISCELLANEOUS TUMORS

Myxoma

Myxomas are benign tumors that occur in a variety of locations including the heart, bones, skin, subcutaneous and aponeurotic tissue, and skeletal muscle.[27,248,254] It is the skeletal muscle lesion that mostly concerns us here, since its frequent infiltrative pattern causes it to be occasionally misdiagnosed as one of the more myxoid-appearing sarcomas.[14,247,249] Several tumors and tumorlike conditions of the soft tissues have a mucinous stroma that may so dominate the histologic picture that they resemble myxomas.[247,249,253] Indeed, it is probable that some previously reported myxomas represent lesions other than true myxomas.[27,248]

Although myxomas have been reported in children, some even noted at birth,[248] the intramuscular myxoma is unusual in patients less than 20 years of age.[14,249-253] It most frequently occurs in adults between 40 and 60 years of age, with the sexes about equally affected.[251] Myxoma tends to grow slowly as a painless mass or to remain stationary for long periods of time before suddenly enlarging, although some are initially seen as a rapidly growing mass.[249,251,254] The average duration of symptoms is from 2 to 4 years, but some patients have reported lesions to be present for 10 to 40 years.[251,254] There is no apparent relationship between the size of the myxoma and the time it has been present.[250]

Intramuscular myxoma tends to involve large muscle groups such as those in the thigh, shoulder, upper arms, and buttocks, although some also occur in the head, neck, and chest wall.[14,247,249,252] Other myxomas tend to be subcutaneous or arise along fascial planes and neurovascular sheaths.[251] Grossly myxomas appear sharply circumscribed and in the superficial soft tissue they may be completely encapsulated.[249,251] Encapsulation in the intramuscular variety is, however, usually absent.[14,250-252] Although most range in size from 4 to 6 cm, large lesions (greater than 15 cm) may be found in the larger muscles. The cut surface has a grayish-white to snow-white, glistening, gelatinous appearance and is slimy to the touch. Millimeter-sized cysts may be found on the cut surface. The contained mucinous material may actually drip from the surface, resembling the luminal contents of the common ganglion cyst.[249,251]

As one might expect from this gross appearance, microscopic examinations shows a sea of loose myxoid substance in which reside widely separated stellate, oval, or spindle-shaped cells whose cytoplasm is ill defined. Although the cellularity of individual tumors varies, most are sparsely cellular.[14,249,251] Some cells seem to consist of only a hyperchromatic, degenerated nucleus embedded in the surrounding mucoid stroma (Fig. 39-39). Within this stroma are reticulin fibers that course in various directions.[248,249,254] Of significance, especially in the differential diagnosis of malignant myxoid tumors, is the fact that myxomas are poorly vascularized and have almost no mitotic activity.[14,248,249] The mucoid stroma gives only a weakly positive reaction for hyaluronidase-sensitive acid mucopolysaccharide, apparently having a high water content.[247,249] In muscle the tumor has an expansile and infiltrative pattern causing atrophy and necrosis of the normal muscle fibers.[249] It is this infiltrative character, combined with its myxoid stroma, that has caused myxoma to be confused with other malignant tumors, especially myxoid liposarcoma and myxoid malignant fibrous histiocytoma.[14,247,249,254] Myxoid liposarcoma, although having foci of hypocellular mucinous pools, is usually more cellular, contains lipoblasts, and most important, has a prominent and diffuse plexiform capillary network.[247] Myxoid malignant fibrous histiocytoma can be easily distinguished from myxoma because of its pleomorphic bizarre cells and numerous mitotic figures.

Myxomas are cured by simple local excision, and despite early reports of a fair number of recurrences,[248] they almost never recur and do not metastasize.[14,249-252] Current evidence favors the concept that myxomas orig-

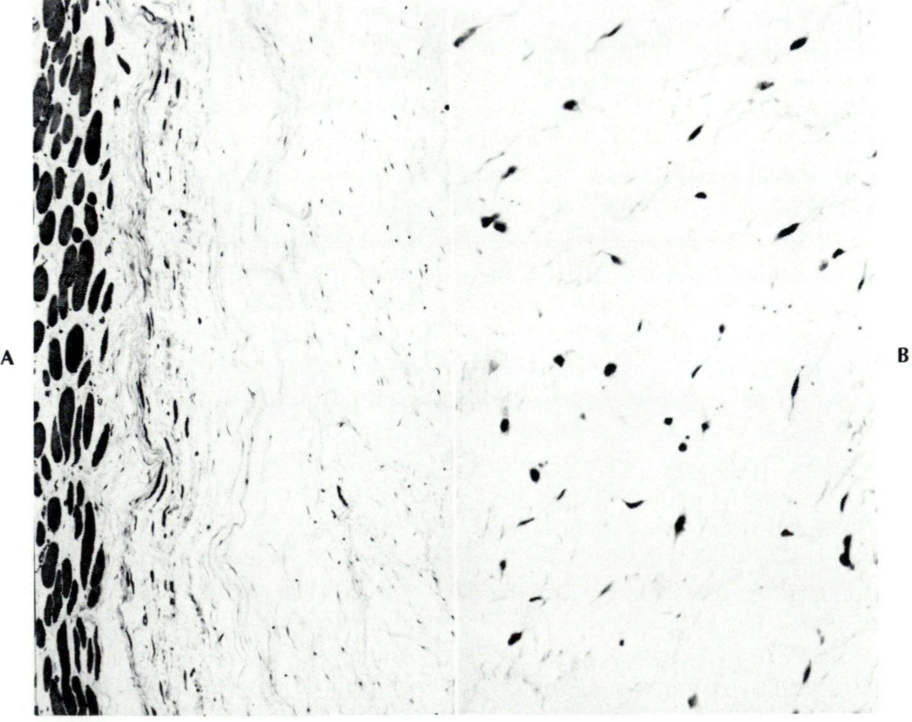

Fig. 39-39. A, Intramuscular myxoma. Pale, relatively hypocellular area, with pushing-type border, within skeletal muscle. **B,** Higher magnification shows small hyperchromatic oval to spindle-shaped nuclei in loose stroma. Note lack of blood vessels. (**A,** 72×; **B,** 280×.)

inate from primitive mesenchymal cells differentiating as fibroblasts that have lost their capacity to produce collagen and instead produce excess amounts of hyaluronic acid.[249-251]

Recently a locally aggressive myxoid tumor, affecting the soft tissue of the female pelvis and perineum, has been reported. It has histologic similarity to a myxoma but contains a prominent vascular pattern and has been termed angiomyxoma.[253a]

Rarely, multiple intramuscular myxomas develop, and such patients have a notable incidence of fibrous dysplasia of bone.[251,255] Myxomas develop years to decades after the appearance of bone lesions, most of which are polyostotic, and myxomas seem to occur in the vicinity of the most severely affected bones.[255] A high incidence of associated Albright's syndrome is also noted with this clinical combination.[247]

Synovial sarcoma

Synovial sarcoma is one of the more common soft tissue malignancies, accounting for approximately 3% to 10% of all sarcomas.[10,28,83,256,263] Although no age group is exempt, this is a tumor principally of young adults, two thirds of patients being less than 40 years old, with the average age in the low to middle thirties.[27,256,257,259] There is a predilection for men in ratios of from 2:1 to 3:2.[27,256,257,264]

From its name, one would expect that this tumor arises from synovial membranes. This, however, is the exception rather than the rule, with only 10% of the tumors actually involving joint spaces.[23,27,149,267] Rather, the tumor is usually found in the vicinity of large joints and in bursae. Approximately 75% to 95% are found in the extremities, with the lower extremity involved in 40% to 70% of cases. Principal locations include the thigh around the hip joints, the knee, the ankle, the shoulder, and the wrist.[14,27,256,257] The tumor is also found in regions where synovial tissue is not present, such as the anterior abdominal wall, the pelvis, the anterolateral aspect of the neck, the orofacial area, in the paravertebral connective tissue from the base of the skull to the hypopharynx, and the retroperitoneum.[256,266,267,267b,267c]

Unlike most soft tissue sarcomas, synovial sarcoma frequently is accompanied by pain that in about one fourth of cases is not associated with a definite mass. The pain, either localized or referred, may exist for several years before the appearance of a mass. In another one fourth of cases a painful mass is present; in the remaining cases a painless mass is the dominant feature.[257] The duration of symptoms is variable, averaging approximately 2½ years, but some patients have histories as long as 20 years.[27,256] It is not uncommon, however, for patients to be examined because of a mass that has been noted for only a few months.[257]

Roentgenographic examination shows tumor calcification in 30% to 40% of cases.[27,256,257] This unusual finding, combined with the presence of a painful mass near a major joint in a young person, is highly suggestive of synovial sarcoma.

Histologically, synovial sarcoma is characterized by a fibrosarcomatous-like proliferation of spindle cells, arranged in sheets or bands, in which are scattered paler epithelial-like cells that either line cleftlike spaces or are arranged in glandular formation (Fig. 39-40).[14,27,259a,264] The spindle cells may at times be plumper and have rounder nuclei than the usual fibroblast.[256,260,264] The epithelial-like cells may be cuboidal to tall and columnar in shape and may form papillary projections into the cleftlike spaces. At other times they form compact masses with no glandular spaces. These cells are set off from the spindle cell stroma by a basement membrane. Pleomorphism of either the spindle or epithelial-like cells is not a feature of these tumors.[256] The pseudoglandular areas combined with the spindle cell stroma represents the classic "biphasic" histologic pattern of synovial sarcoma.

Reticulin fibers are present in the fibrosarcomatous stroma but not within the glandular foci.[14] The glands contain a hyaluronidase-resistant mucinous material that stains positively with periodic acid–Schiff, mucicarmine, and Alcian blue stains.[259,262,267] The stromal cells also stain for acid mucopolysaccharide material, but this is abolished by pretreatment with hyaluronidase.[267]

The stroma may also contain broad hyalinized scarlike areas, and foci of calcification are present in 30% to 60% of cases.[256,267] In some instances mast cells are found in abundance.[259,267,267d] The tumor may be highly vascular, with spindle cells surrounding narrow vascular slits producing focal areas suggestive of hemangiopericytoma.[14,259,262]

The proportion of spindle and epithelial-like cells that are present varies not only from patient to patient but also within the same lesion.[264] The spindle cell areas usually so dominate the picture that many sections may be required before one finds both cellular elements. A biopsy may miss these epithelial-like areas, causing the lesion to be diagnosed as a fibrosarcoma. Some pathologists, however, claim that they can confidently diagnose synovial sarcoma based only on the finding of spindle cell areas, which, as noted, may contain cells that appear plumper than the fibroblasts of fibrosarcoma.[256] Furthermore, some insist that a "monophasic" form of this tumor exists, consisting entirely of either spindle cells or epithelial-like cells, and that the typical biphasic pattern is present in only a minority of cases.[259,262,263] Although competent pathologists vigorously defend these positions, we concur with those who believe that it is unwise to diagnose synovial sarcoma when a biphasic pattern is not seen, regardless of the obesity of the stromal cells.[14,27,260,264] Given the constellation of clinical find-

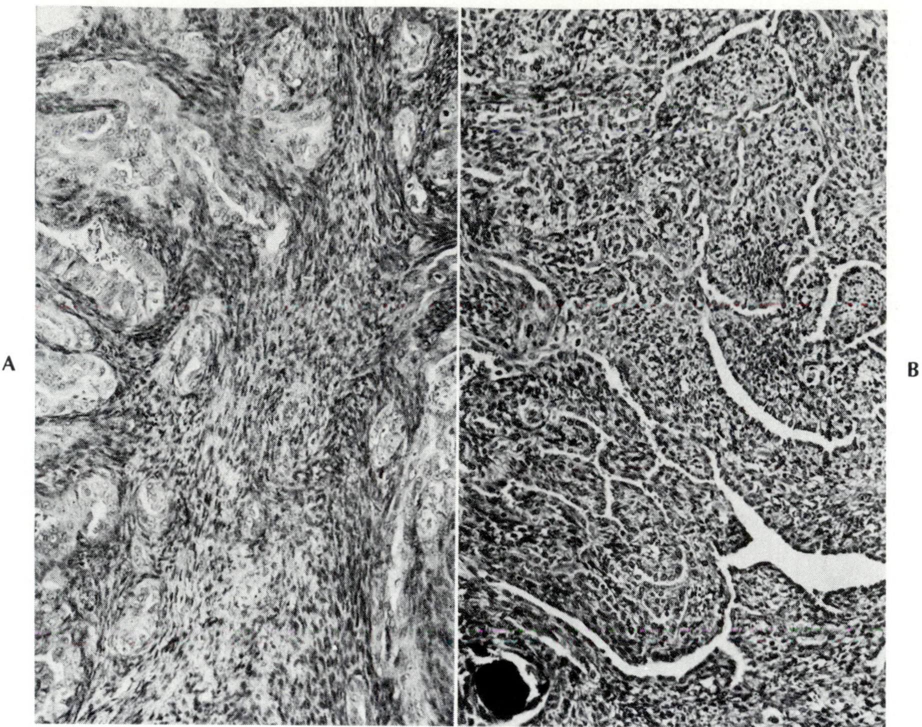

Fig. 39-40. A, Synovial sarcoma. Classic biphasic pattern is composed of glandlike spaces, formed by pale-staining cuboidal to columnar cells, residing in spindle cell stroma. **B,** Another synovial sarcoma. Here spaces are slitlike and resemble vascular channels. However, they are lined by cuboidal cells. Fragment of calcium is present at lower left. (150×.)

ings previously mentioned, a spindle cell tumor must be examined diligently for the presence of a biphasic pattern. If this is not found, we do not believe that one should read into sections more than is there.

Electron microscopic studies have also yielded conflicting data concerning whether or not the stromal cells resemble fibroblasts and can be distinguished from those of fibrosarcoma.[32,261,263,265] In any case the results of these studies, in which basement membranes and cellular junctions were found, are quite unlike what is found in normal synovial tissue. Nor do the cells resemble the type A and B cells of normal synovial membranes, adding further evidence that these sarcomas do not arise from synovial tissue.[258,265,267a] Current opinion falls back on the idea that these tumors originate from undifferentiated mesenchymal cells that differentiate as two different cell types. Whether true or not, this is a convenient explanation for the occurrence of synovial sarcomas in areas such as the abdominal wall, where synovial tissue is not present.[265-267] Stains for cytokeratin have been positive in the epithelial components of this tumor, while vimentin has been found in the stromal spindle cells. Some have also reported cytokeratin in these spindle cells.[257a,265a]

Prognostically, synovial sarcomas may pursue a protracted course, with metastases developing up to 20 years after treatment.[14,27,149,256,263] The average duration of survival is 5 to 6 years, and long survival is possible even in the presence of metastases.[14,256] Recurrences following local excisions are seen in 30% to 65% of patients.[257,259,263,264] There is a wide scatter in the reported 5-year survival rates, which range from 3% to 58%.* Ten-year survival figures are uniformly lower, some as low as 11%, reflecting the emergence of late metastases.[14,256,257,263] Some believe that metastases are to be expected in most patients if they are followed for a sufficient time.[27] Metastases develop primarily through bloodstream invasion, with the lungs, bones, and other soft tissue sites being commonly involved.[256,259] Synovial sarcoma, however, may also metastasize to regional lymph nodes, which have been involved in up to 20% of cases.[23,256]

With the exception of those who divide their cases into monophasic and biphasic categories, there does not appear to be any correlation between histologic features and survival.[256,264] However, tumors containing extensive calcification apparently have a better prognosis.[267d] In studies that do separate monophasic from biphasic tumors, the monophasic variety has an increased incidence of local recurrence and lower 5-year survival

*References 14, 149, 256, 257, 262-264, 267.

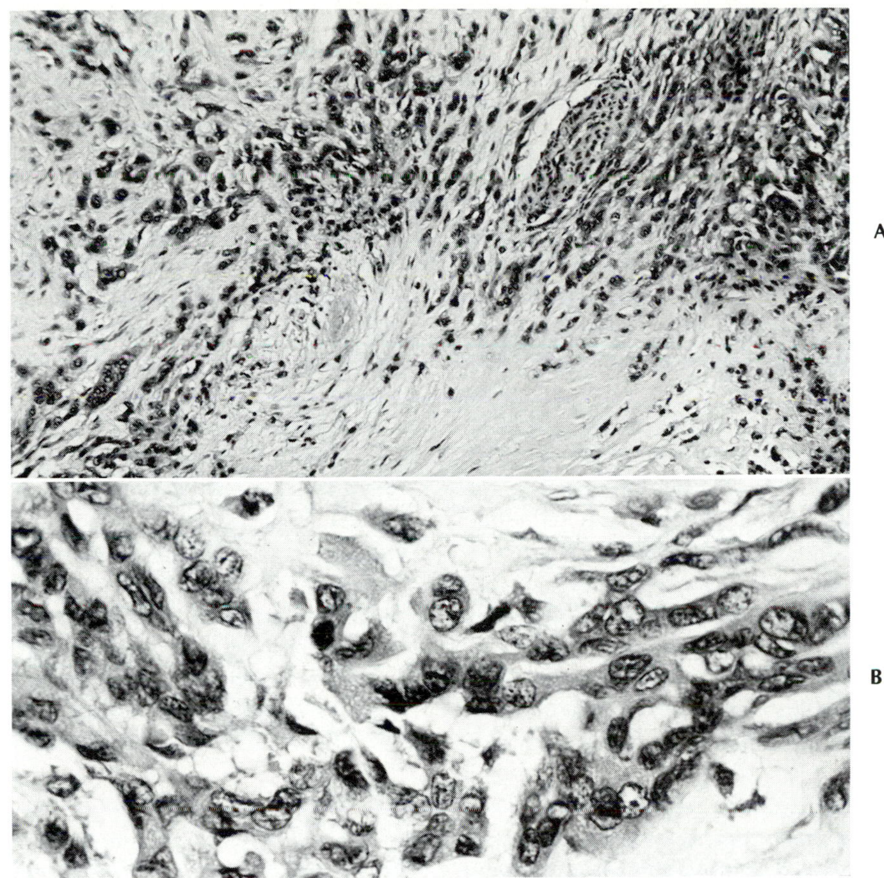

Fig. 39-41. A, Epithelioid sarcoma. Nodule with fibrotic center surrounded by strands and clusters of tumor cells. **B,** Higher magnification of tumor cells with epithelioid appearance. Cells have abundant eosinophilic cytoplasm. They may be arranged in long infiltrating strands. (**A,** 120×; **B,** 480×.)

rates.[262,263] Whereas metastases from biphasic tumors may have either a biphasic or a monophasic pattern, metastases from monophasic tumors are always monophasic.[259,262,263] The prognosis is better in patients with small tumors (less than 5 cm).[259,262,267] Children seem to have a poorer prognosis than adults.[256]

Epithelioid sarcoma

Epithelioid sarcoma has only recently been well defined as a specific tumor entity of the soft tissues.[270] It comprises less than 1% of sarcomas,[38,83] and to date there have probably been less than 200 cases reported in the English literature. The significance of this tumor is that in its early stages its clinical and histologic features may be confused with an inflammatory condition, and only after repeated recurrences is the suggestion of malignancy raised.[270] This time delay does nothing to improve the patient's chance for survival.

Epithelioid sarcoma occurs most often in male patients,[84,279] and although reported in those ranging in age from 2½ to 75 years, approximately 60% to 70% of patients are between the ages of 20 and 40.[84,110,270,277,279] The tumor is initially seen as a painless, subcutaneous or dermal nodule that slowly enlarges over months to years.[270,279] Although the average duration of symptoms is about 3 years, some patients have had lesions for more than 25 years.[277] The nodule may reach 5 to 6 cm, but it is usually less than 2 cm.[269,270,277] Because ulceration of the skin is frequent, the clinical diagnosis is almost always considered to be that of an inflammatory process. In some cases, especially after recurrences, multiple nodules occur.[269]

About 95% of epithelioid sarcomas arise in the extremities, with slightly over half in the hand and forearm, the most common sites being the volar aspect of the fingers, the palm, and the extensor surfaces of the forearm.[84,270,279] Another common location is the anterior surface of the leg over the tibia. Rare locations outside the extremities include the scalp, penis, vulva, buttocks, and abdominal wall.[268,274,275,279a] The tumor arises in the deep subcutaneous tissue and superficial fascia and occasionally from tendon and tendon sheaths.[84,269,270,278]

The more deeply located tumors tend to be larger than those in the hand or wrist.

Histologically the dominant cells are large, polygonal, and mononuclear, with vesicular nuclei and prominent nucleoli. The cytoplasm is characteristically abundant and deeply eosinophilic, giving the cells their epithelioid appearance.[84,270,278] Mixed with these cells, and showing transitional stages between them, are spindle-shaped, fibroblast-like cells producing fibrosarcomatous-like areas.[84,278,279] Occasional binucleated and multinucleated giant cells are present.[277] Mitoses are common. The cells are arranged into nodules that frequently show central areas of degeneration and necrosis (Fig. 39-41). This pattern, combined with the epithelioid-like appearance of the cells, has led to diagnostic confusion with granulomatous lesions, which is further enhanced by the frequent presence of marked chronic inflammation around the tumor.[279] Between the nodules is a prominent desmoplastic stroma composed of densely hyalinized collagen.[279] The collagen frequently infiltrates between the tumor cells, creating small nests and cords of cells that give the impression of an infiltrating carcinoma. Although the overlying skin may be ulcerated by tumor, it is otherwise normal. Despite this, the infiltrating tumor pattern has led to diagnoses of spindle cell epidermoid carcinoma or spindle cell melanoma.[278]

The tumor has a propensity to spread along the fascia, the tendon sheaths, and the periosteum of underlying bone, leading to local recurrences in 65% to 90% of patients.[270,277-279] Such recurrences usually occur within 6 months to a year after excision. Metastases have been noted in 30% to 50% of patients, usually, however, only after repeated local recurrences.[270,277,279] The distribution of the metastases is unusual, with a propensity for the tumor to spread to the skin, especially the scalp, as well as to involve lymph nodes.[84,270,277] In a review of 104 cases in the literature 24% of patients had died of their tumor, 11% were alive with recurrence and/or metastases, and 16% had recurrences alone.[279] Since the median time for metastases to appear has been 4 years, the reported 5-year survival rate of 50% to 60% can be expected to decline with time. There is no relationship between tumor size, mitotic rate, or degree of pleomorphism and prognosis, but lymph node involvement and vascular invasion indicate a poor prognosis.[277]

The histogenesis of this sarcoma remains cloaked with a variety of conflicting opinions based mostly on the electron microscopic evaluation of about a dozen cases. Whereas some claim that it originates from undifferentiated mesenchymal cells that differentiate along synovial or histiocytic lines, others believe that it is a variant of synovial sarcoma, malignant fibrous histiocytoma, or dermatofibrosarcoma.* One can say with assurance that the final word has not yet been received. Special studies have shown the presence of vimentin and cytokeratin proteins in the cells of this tumor.[269a,274a,274b]

*References 110, 268, 269a, 270-273, 274a, 276.

Clear cell sarcoma

Another rare soft tissue tumor, clear cell sarcoma, despite its infrequent appearance, has stimulated a great deal of interest among pathologists because of its unusual morphology and probable histogenesis.

In some series clear cell sarcoma accounts for less than 1% of all soft tissue sarcomas, but this may reflect its previous placement in other categories such as synovial sarcoma.[38,288] In a recent report it accounted for almost 3% of all sarcomas.[83]

Although patients varying in age from 7 to 83 years have been reported, this tumor primarily affects young adults, with a peak incidence in the third decade.[281-283] There is a slight preponderance in female patients.[282a,282b] As with most sarcomas, the presence of a slowly enlarging mass is the dominant symptom. Pain or tenderness is noted in up to one half of patients. Duration of symptoms has ranged from 3 months to 19 years, with an average of 3½ years, indicating the rather slow growth of most of these tumors.[281,283] The extremities are the most frequent sites involved, with up to three fourths of tumors located in the lower extremities.[282a,282b] Although tumors in the region of the knee or thigh occur, over one half of clear cell sarcomas have been located distally around the foot and ankle.[281,282a,283] Occasional examples have involved the fingers, hand, forearm, buttocks, and perineum.[282,288] The tumors are firm and nodular, unattached to skin, and usually fixed to underlying tendons and aponeuroses.[282,283] Although they are usually grayish white, it is not uncommon to see distinctive tan to black areas on the cut surface.[280,286,287]

In primary tumors the microscopic pattern is fairly distinctive.[281-283,288] There are nests and tight clusters of fairly uniform cells having a pale to clear cytoplasm that in about two thirds of cases stains positively for glycogen. At times the cytoplasm appears granular rather than clear. Nuclei are round and uniform, lacking any significant degree of pleomorphism. They characteristically have prominent nucleoli that may be highly basophilic. The cell nests are segregated from each other by delicate fibrous septa that appear continuous with the connective tissue of adjacent tendons and aponeurotic tissue to which these tumors attach themselves. With invasion of these structures the tumor cells line up in cordlike fashion and are surrounded by a dense desmoplastic stroma. Bland, multinucleated giant cells are also found in some tumors. Unlike primary tumors, recurrent or metastatic lesions may quickly assume such a pleomorphic appearance that no semblance of the primary tumor remains.[283,285]

The cells of clear cell sarcoma are also noted for their pigment content. In the original description of this tumor, iron stains were positive in all cases in which they were used, the iron pigment being both intracellular and extracellular. Melanin stains were also positive in about half of the cases in which they were used.[283] However, this positive melanin reaction was not abolished by melanin-bleaching procedures, and the same pigment also gave a weakly positive reaction for iron. This raised doubts as to whether the cells in fact contained true melanin. Subsequent reports, however, have found bleachable melanin in about 40% to 70% of cases, with or without associated iron pigment.* The distribution of both pigments may be irregular and found only focally. The presence or absence of the pigment also varies from recurrence to recurrence.[285] Stains for S-100 protein are positive in most cases.[282a,284a,285a]

Examination by electron microscopy has confirmed the presence of premelanosomes and melanosomes in these tumors.[280,281,284,287] Although some authors have suggested that some clear cell sarcomas are of synovial origin and that they are able to distinguish, by light microscopy, between tumors that are synovial and those that are melanotic,[288] this has not been confirmed by others. Most now agree that the tumor probably originates from the neural crest[284a,285a] and should be considered a "melanoma of soft parts" originating in misplaced melanocytes.[280-282,282a,287,288] Others believe that it could also represent a poorly differentiated or dedifferentiated melanotic malignant schwannoma.[286]

The clinical course is a progressive and aggressive one, with a 70% to 80% incidence of repeated local recurrences followed eventually by metastases in 50% to 70% of patients.[282,282a,282b,283,288] Short-term mortality appears to be within the 50% to 60% range, but metastatic lesions have developed after 10 years; hence 5-year survival rates, as with epithelioid sarcoma, alveolar soft part sarcoma, and synovial sarcoma, are of little significance as an indicator of long-term prognosis.[282,282a,282b,283,285]

Alveolar soft part sarcoma

Histologically, one of the most distinctive of all the soft tissue malignant tumors, alveolar soft part sarcoma, has unfortunately in the past been incorrectly labeled as malignant granular cell myeloblastoma, malignant granular cell tumor, and malignant nonchromaffin paraganglioma, lesions with which it has no relation.[297] The name "alveolar soft part sarcoma" was coined in 1952 as a purely descriptive term, since the histogenesis of this lesion was not understood.[289] To date our ignorance has withstood the test of time.[290,294a,294b] An understanding of this tumor is hampered by its infrequent occurrence; it accounts for probably less than 1% of all sarcomas.[38,83,291] Some institutions report no primary cases in over 20 years, and even cancer referral centers may have only one or two cases per year.[38,289] Hence few reports exist that deal with any appreciable number of patients.

From what has been published, the tumor primarily affects patients in their teens and early twenties; two thirds of the patients are between 10 and 40 years of age, with a median age of 21 years.[14,289,293] The tumor is also one of the few sarcomas that affect female patients more commonly, the female/male ratio being approximately 2:1.[293] Most alveolar soft part sarcomas arise in the deep tissues of the extremities, usually within skeletal muscle or along musculofascial planes.[14,27,289,293] They are most common in the lower extremity, with 60% located in the thigh. However, there is a wide distribution of anatomic sites, including the abdominal wall, retroperitoneum, vulva, perineum, nasal cavity, and orbit.[7a,27,292a] In children the tumor may be found in the head and neck region, including the tongue and orbit.[14]

Microscopically the tumor is characterized by round, ball-like aggregates of cells at the periphery of which are delicate thin-walled blood vessels and fine fibrous septa. The cells in the center of the clusters frequently lose their cohesiveness and fall away, leaving the more peripheral cells lining the fibrous septa. This produces the organoid or pseudoalveolar pattern characteristic of this tumor (Fig. 39-42).[289] The component cells are relatively bland in appearance and marked by a fine, granular, well-defined eosinophilic cytoplasm and a vesicular nucleus containing one or two distinct nucleoli.[14,27,289] Mitoses are infrequent. Tumor invasion into the fine vascular channels is common.[14,289] The most distinctive cytologic feature of these lesions is the intracytoplasmic presence of periodic acid–Schiff–positive, diastase-resistant granules and needlelike crystals arranged in sheaves and clusters. The crystals have been seen in 20% to 85% of cases.[14,27,293,295] These crystals, which by electron microscopy are rhomboid or rod shaped, are unique and have not been found in any other soft tissue sarcomas,[14,291,295,297] although similar crystals have recently been reported in a supposed gastric wall schwannoma (Fig. 39-42).[294] The tumor cells do not show definitive features of smooth muscle, skeletal muscle, or nerve, despite suggestions that the tumor represents some form of skeletal muscle tumor or that it arises from misplaced paraganglia.[291,292,295-297] The nature of the crystals and granules is also obscure, although a recent provocative report indicates that the granules stain with antibodies to renin and that, like renin-producing cells, the cells of alveolar soft part sarcoma incorporate zinc into the crystalline storage granules. It was claimed that the cells appear to be modified smooth muscle cells analogous to renal juxtaglomerular cells and the cells of juxtaglomeru-

*References 280-282, 282a, 284, 285, 287.

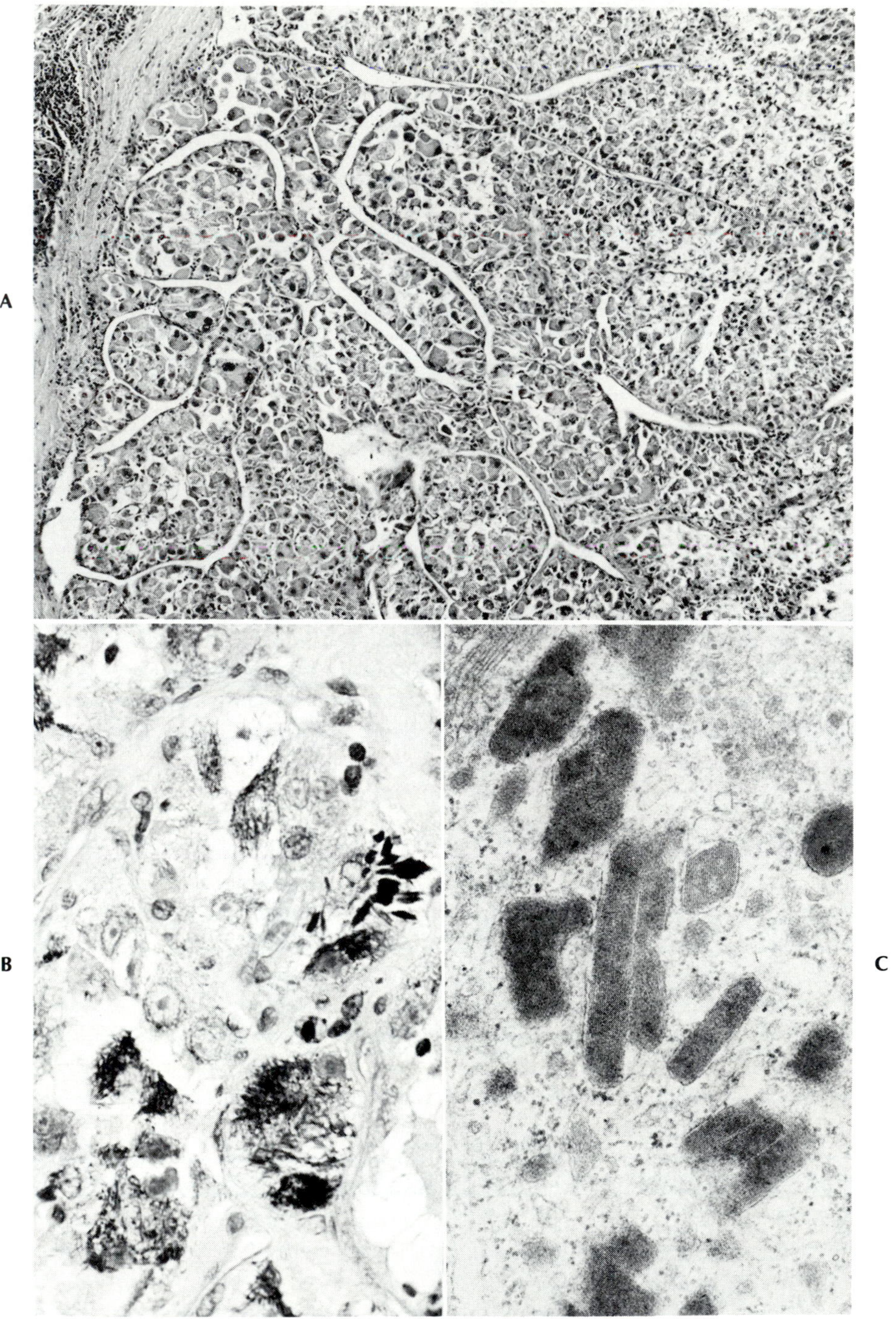

Fig. 39-42. Alveolar soft part sarcoma. Typical organoid pattern formed by ball-like clusters of cells having granular eosinophilic cytoplasm. Thin-walled vascular channels are present at periphery of clusters. Even at this low magnification, some nuclear atypia can be seen. **B,** Section shows thick intracytoplasmic crystals, as well as sheaves of needlelike crystals. **C,** Electron micrograph shows electron-dense, membrane-bound cytoplasmic structures of variable size and shape. Rhomboids have crystalline substructure of distinctive periodicity. (**A,** 72×; **B,** periodic acid–Schiff; 480×; **C,** 51,200×; courtesy Dr. Katherine DeSchryver-Kecskemeti, Washington University, St. Louis, Mo.)

lar tumors. Despite the authors' hypothesis that alveolar soft part sarcoma originates from metaplastic smooth muscle cells of the arterial musculature,[290] these results have recently been questioned.[294b]

Despite their bland histologic characteristics, alveolar soft part sarcomas are among the most malignant of all the soft tissue sarcomas. Most patients develop metastases and die of their tumor. The clinical course, however, may be protracted, since patients may live for several years even in the presence of known metastases. Although 5-year survival rates of approximately 60% are reported, the 10-year survival in one series was only 18%.[14] Furthermore, follow-up observation has indicated the occurrence of metastases as late as 20 years following therapy.[289,293] There appears to be a cumulative increase in the incidence of metastases over time and a corresponding cumulative decline in survival.[293] The most common sites for metastases are the lungs, bone, and brain, with only infrequent involvement of lymph nodes. The prognosis may be better in patients under 20 years of age and in those with head and neck lesions.[14,293]

Giant cell tumor of soft tissue

Giant cell tumor of soft tissue is a fairly recently described tumor whose histomorphology resembles that of giant cell tumor of bone (see Chapter 41).[300,301] However, considering the small number of patients reported to date, this lesion must await better clinical and histologic definition.

These tumors have been reported in patients ranging in age from 1 to 87 years,[299-301] but there may be some differences in the age of onset between the benign and malignant varieties. In the two reports dealing with the latter group[299,300] the mean patient ages were 56 and 68 years respectively, whereas in the report dealing with benign giant cell tumors the mean age was 46 years.[301] Whether an earlier age of onset for benign tumors is real must await further reports. Male patients were more common in the malignant group and female patients more common in the benign category.

Most patients relate a history of a painless mass that has been present for weeks to months, usually less than 1 year, and frequently less than 6 months. Some, however, have had a mass for periods of up to 15 years.[299-301]

Approximately 80% to 90% of the reported tumors have been in the extremities, with about 80% of these in the lower extremity, the thigh being the most common site. Other locations have included the face, abdominal wall, shoulders, neck, and retroperitoneum. The tumors are superficially located in the subcutaneous tissue and superficial fascia, deeply situated in muscle and the deep fascia or adherent to tendon sheaths.[298-300] Superficial tumors tend to be smaller than the deeply placed tumors, which may reach up to 15 cm.[299,300] The gross appearance is nonspecific, although in the malignant variety hemorrhage and necrosis are common.[299]

The microscopic pattern of the benign tumors is one of multiple nodules composed of a varied mixture of bland-appearing histiocytic, fibroblastic, and osteoclast type multinucleated giant cells. The nodules are separated by dense fibrous septa.[301] In the malignant tumors the cells demonstrate varying degrees of anaplasia and pleomorphism, with mononuclear pleomorphic giant cells present in most cases (Fig. 39-43). The fibroblastic cells produce fibrosarcomatous foci, especially at the periphery of the lesions.[299,300] In both types of tumor the osteoclast-like giant cells have bland, uniform nuclei, which may number up to 100, and a cytoplasm that may be vacuolated. Phagocytic activity is sometimes noted in these cells, as is the occasional presence of asteroid bodies, suggesting that they are histiocytic.[299] Significantly, in up to half the cases in the malignant group, malignant-appearing osteoid and, more rarely, malignant-appearing chondroid material have been found.[299,300,302] This finding raises semantic problems. A malignant tumor composed of a sarcomatous stroma that produces osteoid is, by definition, an osteosarcoma. Furthermore, conventional osteosarcomas of bone may also have areas of fibrohistiocytic proliferation, and in about 10% of cases they have a significant number of osteoclastic giant cells. One must conclude that at least some tumors categorized as malignant giant cell tumor of soft tissue may be extraskeletal osteosarcomas.

Electron microscopic studies have been limited to a few cases.[298,299,302] From these it has been concluded that the lesion resembles both the true giant cell tumor of bone and giant cell reparative granuloma.[298] Some believe that the lesion arises from primitive mesenchymal cells that differentiate along fibroblastic and histiocytic lines and therefore that the tumor is a variant of fibrous histiocytoma.[110,298,299] However, in one study the mononuclear cells were found to represent poorly differentiated mesenchymal cells, but other cells had chondroblastic and osteoblastic features.[302] It is our view that until further cases of this tumor are reported and clearly separated from osteosarcoma, the question of histogenesis should remain open and the tumor not be included in the fibrohistiocytic category.

The prognosis in these tumors has varied considerably. In the one report in which the histologic features of the lesions lacked any suggestion of malignancy, none of the 10 patients died of tumor and all but one were alive and well at the time of the report.[301] On the other hand, the malignant tumors have in most cases pursued an aggressive course, with 5-year survival rates of about 30%.[298-300] Patients with superficially located tumors that had minimal anaplasia had a better prognosis, with a

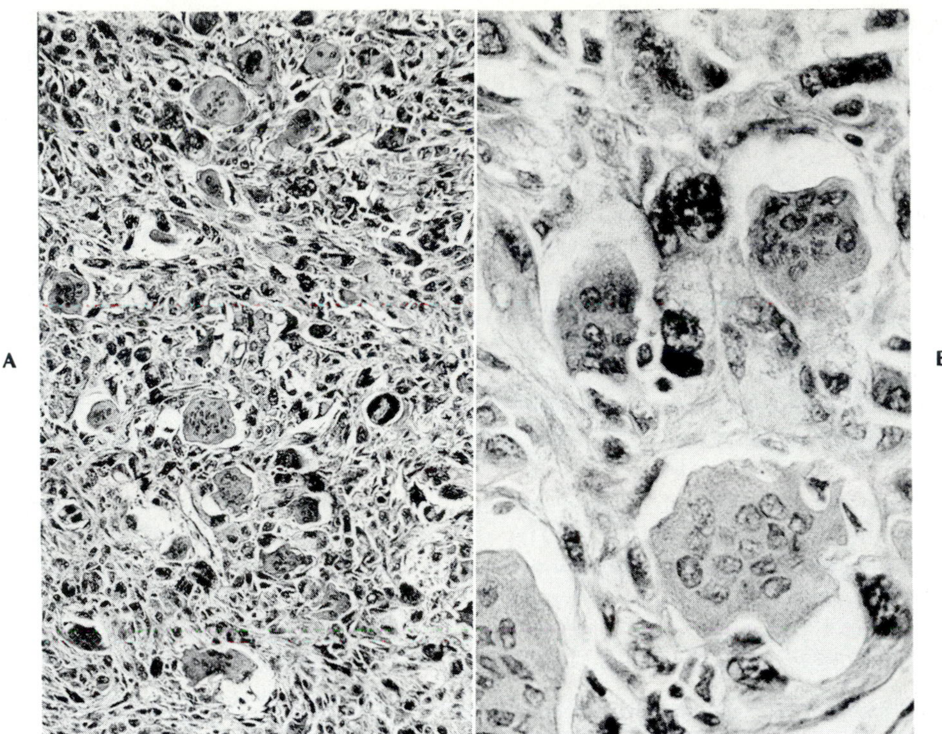

Fig. 39-43. A, Malignant giant cell tumor of soft tissue. Multinucleated, osteoclast-type giant cells within fibrous stroma containing anaplastic stromal cells. **B,** Higher magnification shows bland nuclei of the giant cells and atypical stromal cells. (**A,** 120×; **B,** 480×.)

50% 5-year survival rate reported.[300] These tumors must be clearly differentiated from the benign giant cell tumors of tendon sheath (see Chapter 42).

Extraskeletal Ewing's sarcoma

Ewing's sarcoma, an undifferentiated, presumably mesenchymal tumor, is one of the most aggressive and malignant intraosseous tumors and is found almost exclusively in children (see Chapter 40). It has only recently been recognized that tumors with similar morphology may originate within the soft tissues, where they may be difficult to distinguish from other small cell malignant tumors such as embryonal rhabdomyosarcoma, malignant lymphoma, metastatic small cell carcinoma, and neuroblastoma.[303]

The extraskeletal tumors have been reported in patients from infancy to over 60 years of age, but they are uncommon in patients over the age of 30.[303,305] As a rule, however, these patients are still somewhat older than those with osseous Ewing's sarcoma. In addition, although the number of reported patients is still few, there does not appear to be the same predilection for male patients as there is in Ewing's sarcoma of bone.[303]

The tumors grow rapidly, and pain or tenderness is present in about half the patients.[303] Most lesions are located in the deep soft tissues, although a few occur in the subcutaneous tissue. A wide variety of anatomic sites have been involved, with the extremities and paravertebral sites being the most common. Other areas include the axilla, chest wall, retroperitoneum, and pelvic regions.[303,305,307] As the rapid growth and undifferentiated nature of the cells would indicate, these tumors are usually soft and friable with frequent macroscopic areas of necrosis, hemorrhage, and degeneration.[303] The light microscopic pattern and positive staining for intracellular glycogen of these tumors are identical to those of their osseous counterparts. Electron microscopic studies, in about six cases, have shown no essential differences between the cells of this tumor and those of Ewing's sarcoma of bone.[305,306,308]

In the Intergroup Rhabdomyosarcoma Study, these extraskeletal lesions, which had been originally submitted as examples of rhabdomyosarcoma, have been separated into groups I and II, which differ from each other only in that the cells of group II are more irregular in shape, are slightly larger, and have a less hyperchromatic nucleus than the cells of group I.[307]

Although electron microscopic studies may aid in the differential diagnosis between these extraskeletal tumors and other small cell tumors, there may be cases in which the distinction from some of the less differentiated embryonal rhabdomyosarcomas is not possible.[305] To date, however, this has not been a practical problem because extraskeletal Ewing's tumors appear to respond in the same way to current chemotherapeutic agents as do rhabdomyosarcomas.[307] In the original report of these extraskeletal tumors over 60% of the patients died, usually within a year after diagnosis, with metastases to lungs and bone.[303] In contrast, 65% of the patients reported in the Intergroup Rhabdomyosarcoma Study were still alive (median survival 113 weeks), having responded well to radiotherapy and chemotherapy. No difference in response rate was found between the group I and group II cases.[307] However, it should be pointed out that the differences between these two studies may reflect either the more intensive therapy given in the latter study or some effect of age on prognosis, since the latter study involved children whereas most of the patients in the original study were over 16 years of age.

The relationship, if any, between extraskeletal Ewing's sarcoma and the recently described malignant, glycogen-negative, small cell tumor of the thoracopulmonary region that occurs in childhood is unclear at this time.[304] On the basis of electron microscopic studies and positive cell stains for neuron-specific enolase, a neural origin has been suggested for the latter tumor.[305a]

REFERENCES

General

1. American Cancer Society: Cancer statistics, 1981, CA **31**:13, 1981.
2. M.D. Anderson Hospital and Tumor Institute: Management of primary bone and soft tissue tumors, Chicago, 1977, Year Book Medical Publishers, Inc.
3. Benjamin, R.S., et al.: Advances in the chemotherapy of soft tissue sarcomas, Med. Clin. North Am. **61**:1039, 1977.
4. Benjamin, R.S., et al.: The chemotherapy of soft tissue sarcomas in adults. In M.D. Anderson Hospital and Tumor Institute: Management of primary bone and soft tissue tumors, Chicago, 1977, Year Book Medical Publishers, Inc.

4a. Brooks, J.J.: Immunohistochemistry of soft tissue tumors: progress and prospects, Hum. Pathol. **13**:969, 1982.

5. Chang, P.: Management of soft tissue sarcomas: current status, Am. J. Med. Sci. **273**:244, 1977.

5a. Costa, J., et al.: The grading of soft tissue sarcomas: results of a clinicohistopathologic correlation in a series of 163 cases, Cancer **53**:530, 1984.

6. Dahl, I., and Angervall, L.: Pseudosarcomatous lesions of the soft tissues reported as sarcoma during a 6-year period (1958-1963), Acta Pathol. Microbiol. Scand. **85A**:917, 1977.

6a. Das Gupta, T.K.: Tumors of the soft tissues, Norwalk, Conn., 1983, Appleton-Century-Crofts.

6b. Enterline, H.T.: Histopathology of sarcomas, Semin. Oncol. **8**:133, 1981.

7. Enzinger, F.M., Lattes, R., and Torloni, H.: Histological typing of soft tissue tumours, World Health Organization, International Histological Classification of Tumors, No. 3, Geneva, 1969, World Health Organization.

7a. Enzinger, F.M., and Weiss, S.W.: Soft tissue tumors, St. Louis, 1983, The C.V. Mosby Co.

7b. Falini, B., and Taylor, C.R.: New developments in immunoperoxidase techniques and their application, Arch. Pathol. Lab. Med. **107**:105, 1983.

8. Ferrell, H.W., and Frable, W.J.: Soft part sarcomas revisited, Cancer **30**:475, 1972.
9. Fine, G., Ohorodnik, J.M., and Horn, R.C., Jr.: Soft-tissue sarcomas: their clinical behavior and course and influencing factors, Proceedings of the Seventh National Cancer Conference, Philadelphia, 1973, J.B. Lippincott Co.
10. Hajdu, S.I.: Pathology of soft tissue tumors, Philadelphia, 1979, Lea & Febiger.
11. Kaye, G.I.: The futility of electron microscopy in determining the origin of poorly differentiated soft tissue tumors. In Fenoglio, C.M., and Wolff, M., editors: Progress in surgical pathology, vol. 3, New York, 1981, Masson Publishing USA, Inc.
12. Kindblom, L.-G., and Angervall, L.: Histochemical characterization of mucosubstances in bone and soft tissue tumors, Cancer **36**:985, 1975.
13. Lagacé, R., Schürch, W., and Seemayer, T.A.: Myofibroblasts in soft tissue sarcomas, Virchows Arch. (Pathol. Anat.) **389A**:1, 1980.
14. Lattes, R., and Enzinger, F.M.: Soft tissue tumors, Proceedings of the Thirty-Ninth Annual Anatomic Pathology Slide Seminar of the American Society of Clinical Pathologists, Chicago, 1973.
15. Lindberg, R.D., et al.: Conservative surgery and postoperative radiotherapy in 300 adults with soft-tissue sarcomas, Cancer **47**:2391, 1981.
16. Lipper, S., Kahn, L.B., and Reddick, R.L.: The myofibroblast, Pathol. Annu. **15**(Part 1):409, 1980.
17. Mackay, B.: Electron microscopy of soft tissue tumors. In M.D. Anderson Hospital and Tumor Institute: Management of primary bone and soft tissue tumors, Chicago, 1977, Year Book Medical Publishers, Inc.
18. Mackenzie, D.H.: The myxoid tumors of somatic soft tissues, Am. J. Surg. Pathol. **5**:443, 1981.
19. Martin, R.G., Butler, J.J., and Albores-Saavedra, J.: Soft tissue tumors: surgical treatment and results. In Tumors of bone and soft tissue, Chicago, 1965, Year Book Medical Publishers, Inc.
20. Martin, R.G., et al.: Soft tissue sarcomas. In Clark, R.L., and Howe, C.D., editors: Cancer patient care at M.D. Anderson Hospital and Tumor Institute, The University of Texas, Chicago, 1976, Year Book Medical Publishers, Inc.

20a. Miettinen, M., et al.: Expression of intermediate filaments in soft-tissue sarcomas, Int. J. Cancer **30**:541, 1982.

21. Mukai, K., and Rosai, J.: Applications of immunoperoxidase techniques in surgical pathology. In Fenoglio, C.M., and Wolff, M., editors: Progress in surgical pathology, vol. 1, New York, 1980, Masson Publishing USA, Inc.

21a. Nakajima, T., et al.: An immunoperoxidase study of S-100 protein distribution in normal and neoplastic tissues, Am. J. Surg. Pathol. **6**:715, 1982.

21b. Osborn, M., and Weber, K.: Biology of disease: tumor diagnosis by intermediate filament typing; a novel tool for surgical pathology, Lab. Invest. **48**:372, 1983.

22. Presant, C.A., et al.: Metastatic sarcomas: chemotherapy with Adriamycin, cyclophosphamide, and methotrexate alternating with actinomycin D, DTIC, and vincristine, Cancer **47**:457, 1981.
23. Rosai, J.: Ackerman's surgical pathology, ed. 6, St. Louis, 1981, The C.V. Mosby Co.

23a. Rosenberg, S.A., et al.: Prospective randomized evaluation of adjuvant chemotherapy in adults with soft tissue sarcomas of the extremities, Cancer **52**:424, 1983.

24. Russell, W.O., et al.: A clinical and pathological staging system for soft tissue sarcomas, Cancer **40**:1562, 1977.
25. Seemayer, T.A., et al.: The myofibroblast: biologic, pathologic, and theoretical considerations, Pathol. Annu. **15**(Part 1): 443, 1980.
26. Stern, R.: Current concepts in the diagnosis of human soft tissue sarcomas, Hum. Pathol. **12**:777, 1981.
27. Stout, A.P., and Lattes, R.: Tumors of the soft tissues. In Atlas of tumor pathology, Second Series, Fascicle 1, Washington, D.C., 1967, Armed Forces Institute of Pathology.
28. Suit, H.D.: Sarcoma of soft tissue, CA **28**:284, 1978.
29. Suit, H.D., Russell, W.O., and Martin, R.G.: Management of patients with sarcoma of soft tissue in an extremity, Cancer **31**:1247, 1973.

30. Suit, H.D., Russell, W.O., and Martin, R.G.: Sarcoma of soft tissue: clinical and histopathologic parameters and response to treatment, Cancer **35**:1478, 1975.
31. Sutow, W.W.: Malignant solid tumors in children: a review, New York, 1981, Raven Press.
32. van Haelst, U.J.G.M.: General considerations on electron microscopy of tumors of soft tissues. In Fenoglio, C.M., and Wolff, M., editors: Progress in surgical pathology, vol. 2, New York, 1980, Masson Publishing USA, Inc.
33. Young, J.L., Jr., and Miller, R.W.: Incidence of malignant tumors in U.S. children, J. Pediatr. **86**:254, 1975.

Fibrous tissue lesions

Fibrosarcoma

34. Chung, E.B., and Enzinger, F.M.: Infantile fibrosarcoma, Cancer **38**:729, 1976.
35. Churg, A.M., and Kahn, L.B.: Myofibroblasts and related cells in malignant fibrous and fibrohistiocytic tumors, Hum. Pathol. **8**:205, 1977.
36. Enjoji, M., et al.: Malignant fibrous histiocytoma: a clinicopathologic study of 130 cases, Acta Pathol. Jpn. **30**:727, 1980.
37. Iwasaki, H., and Enjoji, M.: Infantile and adult fibrosarcomas of the soft tissues, Acta Pathol. Jpn. **29**:377, 1979.
38. Krall, R.A., Kostianovsky, M., and Patchefsky, A.S.: Synovial sarcoma: a clinical, pathological, and ultrastructural study of 26 cases supporting the recognition of a monophasic variant, Am. J. Surg. Pathol. **5**:137, 1981.
39. Lagacé, R., Schürch, W., and Seemayer, T.A.: Myofibroblasts in soft tissue sarcomas, Virchows Arch. (Pathol. Anat.) **389A**:1, 1980.
40. Pritchard, D.J., et al.: Fibrosarcoma—a clinicopathologic and statistical study of 199 tumors of the soft tissues of the extremities and trunk, Cancer **33**:888, 1974.
41. Rosenberg, H.S., Stenback, W.A., and Spjut, H.J.: The fibromatoses of infancy and childhood. In Rosenberg, H.S., and Bolande, R.P., editors: Perspectives in pediatric pathology, vol. 4, Chicago, 1978, Year Book Medical Publishers, Inc.
42. Soule, E.H., and Pritchard, D.J.: Fibrosarcoma in infants and children, Cancer **40**:1711, 1977.

Fibromatoses

43. Allen, P.W.: The fibromatoses: a clinicopathologic classification based on 140 cases, Am. J. Surg. Pathol. **1**:255, 305, 1977.
44. Allen, P.W., and Enzinger, F.M.: Juvenile aponeurotic fibroma, Cancer **26**:857, 1970.
45. Briselli, M.F., Soule, E.H., and Gilchrist, G.S.: Congenital fibromatosis: report of 18 cases of solitary and 4 cases of multiple tumors, Mayo Clin. Proc. **55**:554, 1980.
46. Chung, E.B., and Enzinger, F.M.: Infantile myofibromatosis, Cancer **48**:1807, 1981.
47. Cole, N.M., and Guiss, L.W.: Extra-abdominal desmoid tumors, Arch. Surg. **98**:530, 1969.
48. Enzinger, F.M.: Fibrous hamartoma of infancy, Cancer **18**:241, 1965.
49. Enzinger, F.M.: Fibrous tumors of infancy. In Tumors of bone and soft tissue, Chicago, 1965, Year Book Medical Publishers, Inc.
50. Enzinger, F.M., and Shiraki, M.: Musculo-aponeurotic fibromatosis of the shoulder girdle (extra-abdominal desmoid): analysis of thirty cases followed up to ten or more years, Cancer **20**:1131, 1967.
51. Goellner, J.R., and Soule, E.H.: Desmoid tumors: an ultrastructural study of eight cases, Hum. Pathol. **11**:43, 1980.
52. Keasbey, L.E.: Juvenile aponeurotic fibroma (calcifying fibroma): a distinctive tumor arising in the palms and soles of young children, Cancer **6**:338, 1953.
53. Lichtenstein, L., and Goldman, R.L.: The cartilage analogue of fibromatosis: a reinterpretation of the condition called "juvenile aponeurotic fibroma," Cancer **17**:810, 1964.
54. Mackenzie, D.H.: The differential diagnosis of fibroblastic disorders, Oxford, Eng., 1970, Blackwell Scientific Publications.
55. Mackenzie, D.H.: The fibromatoses: a clinicopathological concept, Br. Med. J. **4**:277, 1972.
55a. Mitchell, M.L., di Sant'Agnese, P.A., and Gerber, J.E.: Fibrous hamartoma of infancy, Hum. Pathol. **13**:586, 1982.
56. Pojer, J., Radivojevic, M., and Williams, T.F.: Dupuytren's disease: its association with abnormal liver function in alcoholism and epilepsy, Arch. Intern. Med. **129**:561, 1972.
57. Reye, R.D.K.: A consideration of certain subdermal "fibromatous tumors" of infancy, J. Pathol. Bacteriol. **72**:149, 1956.
58. Roggli, V.L., Kim, H.-S., and Hawkins, E.: Congenital generalized fibromatosis with visceral involvement: a case report, Cancer **45**:954, 1980.
59. Rosenberg, H.S., Stenback, W.A., and Spjut, H.J.: The fibromatoses of infancy and childhood. In Rosenberg, H.S., and Bolande, R.P., editors: Perspectives in pediatric pathology, vol. 4, Chicago, 1978, Year Book Medical Publishers, Inc.
60. Shnitka, T.K., Asp, D.M., and Horner, R.H.: Congenital generalized fibromatosis, Cancer **11**:627, 1958.

Pseudosarcomatous fibrous lesions

61. Allen, P.W.: Nodular fasciitis, Pathology **4**:9, 1972.
61a. Bernstein, K.E., and Lattes, R.: Nodular (pseudosarcomatous) fasciitis, a nonrecurrent lesion: clinicopathologic study of 134 cases, Cancer **49**:1668, 1982.
62. Butler, J.J.: Fibrous tissue tumors: nodular fasciitis, dermatofibrosarcoma protuberans, and fibrosarcoma, grade 1, desmoid type. In Tumors of bone and soft tissue, Chicago, 1965, Year Book Medical Publishers, Inc.
63. Chung, E.B., and Enzinger, F.M.: Proliferative fasciitis, Cancer **36**:1450, 1975.
64. Dahl, I., and Angervall, L.: Pseudosarcomatous lesions of the soft tissues reported as sarcoma during a 6-year period (1958-1963), Acta Pathol. Microbiol. Scand. **85A**:917, 1977.
65. Dahl, I., and Angervall, L.: Pseudosarcomatous proliferative lesions of soft tissue with or without bone formation, Acta Pathol. Microbiol. Scand. **85A**:577, 1977.
66. Enzinger, F.M.: Recent trends in soft tissue pathology. In Tumors of bone and soft tissue, Chicago, 1965, Year Book Medical Publishers, Inc.
67. Enzinger, F.M., and Dulcey, F.: Proliferative myositis: report of thirty-three cases, Cancer **20**:2213, 1967.
68. Hutter, R.V.P., Stewart, F.W., and Foote, F.W., Jr.: Fasciitis: a report of 70 cases with follow-up proving the benignity of the lesion, Cancer **15**:992, 1962.
69. Kleinstiver, B.J., and Rodriquez, H.A.: Nodular fasciitis: a study of forty-five cases and review of the literature, J. Bone Joint Surg. (Am.) **50**:1204, 1968.
70. Konwaler, B.E., Keasbey, L., and Kaplan, L.: Subcutaneous pseudosarcomatous fibromatosis (fasciitis), Am. J. Clin. Pathol. **25**:241, 1955.
71. Lauer, D.H., and Enzinger, F.M.: Cranial fasciitis of childhood, Cancer **45**:401, 1980.
72. Meister, P., Buckmann, F.-W., and Konrad, E.: Nodular fasciitis (analysis of 100 cases and review of the literature), Pathol. Res. Pract. **162**:133, 1978.
73. Meister, P., Konrad, E.A., and Buckmann, F.W.: Nodular fasciitis and proliferative myositis as variants of one disease entity, Invest. Cell Pathol. **2**:277, 1979.
74. Patchefsky, A.S., and Enzinger, F.M.: Intravascular fasciitis: a report of 17 cases, Am. J. Surg. Pathol. **5**:29, 1981.
75. Wirman, J.A.: Nodular fasciitis, a lesion of myofibroblasts: an ultrastructural study, Cancer **38**:2378, 1976.

Fibrohistiocytic tumors

76. Alguacil-Garcia, A., Unni, K.K., and Goellner, J.R.: Malignant fibrous histiocytoma: an ultrastructural study of six cases, Am. J. Clin. Pathol. **69**:121, 1978.
77. Allen, P.W.: Myxoid tumors of soft tissues, Pathol Annu. **15** (Part 1):133, 1980.
78. Angervall, L., Kindblom, L.-G., and Merck, C.: Myxofibrosarcoma: a study of 30 cases, Acta Pathol. Microbiol. Scand. **85A**:127, 1977.
79. Bednář, B.: Storiform neurofibromas of the skin, pigmented and non-pigmented, Cancer **10**:368, 1957.

80. Blitzer, A., Lawson, W., and Biller, H.F.: Malignant fibrous histiocytoma of the head and neck, Laryngoscope **87**:1479, 1977.
81. Churg, A.M., and Kahn, L.B.: Myofibroblasts and related cells in malignant fibrous and fibrohistiocytic tumors, Hum. Pathol. **8**:205, 1977.
82. Cozzutto, C., et al.: Malignant monomorphic histiocytoma in children, Cancer **48**:2112, 1981.
82a. Dorfman, H.D., and Bhagavan, B.S.: Malignant fibrous histiocytoma of soft tissue with metaplastic bone and cartilage formation: a new radiologic sign, Skeletal Radiol. **8**:145, 1982.
83. Enjoji, M., et al.: Malignant fibrous histiocytoma: a clinicopathologic study of 130 cases, Acta Pathol. Jpn. **30**:727, 1980.
84. Enzinger, F.M.: Recent developments in the classification of soft tissue sarcomas. In M.D. Anderson Hospital and Tumor Institute: Management of primary bone and soft tissue tumors, Chicago, 1977, Year Book Medical Publishers, Inc.
85. Enzinger, F.M.: Angiomatoid malignant fibrous histiocytoma: a distinct fibrohistiocytic tumor of children and young adults simulating a vascular neoplasm, Cancer **44**:2147, 1979.
86. Ferrell, H.W., and Frable, W.J.: Soft part sarcomas revisited: review and comparison and a second series, Cancer **30**:475, 1972.
86a. Font, R.L., and Hidayat, A.A.: Fibrous histiocytoma of the orbit: a clinicopathologic study of 150 cases, Hum. Pathol. **13**:199, 1982.
87. Fu, Y.-S., et al.: Malignant soft tissue tumors of probable histiocytic origin (malignant fibrous histiocytomas): general considerations and electron microscopic and tissue culture studies, Cancer **35**:176, 1975.
88. Kahn, L.B.: Retroperitoneal xanthogranuloma and xanthosarcoma (malignant fibrous xanthoma), Cancer **31**:411, 1973.
89. Kauffman, S.L., and Stout, A.P.: Histiocytic tumors (fibrous xanthoma and histiocytoma) in children, Cancer **14**:469, 1961.
90. Kay, S.: Inflammatory fibrous histiocytoma (? xanthogranuloma): report of two cases with ultrastructural observations in one, Am. J. Surg. Pathol. **2**:313, 1978.
91. Kearney, M.M., Soule, E.H., and Ivins, J.C.: Malignant fibrous histiocytoma: a retrospective study of 167 cases, Cancer **45**:167, 1980.
92. Kempson, R.L., and Kyriakos, M.: Fibroxanthosarcoma of the soft tissues: a type of malignant fibrous histiocytoma, Cancer **29**:961, 1972.
93. Kindblom, L.-G., Merck, C., and Angervall, L.: The ultrastructure of myxofibrosarcoma: a study of 11 cases, Virchows Arch. (Pathol. Anat.) **381a**:121, 1979.
94. Kyriakos, M., and Kempson, R.L.: Inflammatory fibrous histiocytoma: an aggressive and lethal lesion, Cancer **37**:1584, 1976.
95. Lagacé, R., Delage, C., and Seemayer, T.A.: Myxoid variant of malignant fibrous histiocytoma: ultrastructural observations, Cancer **43**:526, 1979.
95a. Lattes, R.: Malignant fibrous histiocytoma: a review article, Am. J. Surg. Pathol. **6**:761, 1982.
96. Leite, C., et al.: Chemotherapy of malignant fibrous histiocytoma: a Southwest Oncology Group report, Cancer **40**:2010, 1977.
97. Limacher, J., Delage, C., and Lagacé, R.: Malignant fibrous histiocytoma: clinicopathologic and ultrastructural study of 12 cases, Am. J. Surg. Pathol. **2**:265, 1978.
97a. Meister, P., Konrad, E., and Höhne, N.: Incidence and histological structure of the storiform pattern in benign and malignant fibrous histiocytomas, Virchows Arch. (Pathol. Anat.) **393A**:93, 1981.
98. Meister, P., et al.: Fibrous histiocytoma: an analysis of the storiform pattern, Virchows Arch. (Pathol. Anat.) **383a**:31, 1979.
99. Meister, P., et al.: Malignant fibrous histiocytoma: histological patterns and cell types, Pathol. Res. Pract. **168**:193, 1980.
99a. Merck, C., Angervall, L., and Kindblom, L.-G.: Myxofibrosarcoma: a malignant soft tissue tumor of fibroblastic-histiocytic origin, Acta. Pathol. Microbiol. Immunol. Scand. A (suppl. 282) **91**:1, 1983.
100. Merino, M.J., and LiVolsi, V.A.: Inflammatory malignant fibrous histiocytoma, Am. J. Clin. Pathol. **73**:276, 1980.
101. Merkow, L.P., et al.: Ultrastructure of fibroxanthosarcoma (malignant fibroxanthoma), Cancer **28**:372, 1971.
102. O'Brien, J.E., and Stout, A.P.: Malignant fibrous xanthomas, Cancer **17**:1445, 1964.
103. Ozzello, L., Stout, A.P., and Murray, M.R.: Cultural characteristics of malignant histiocytomas and fibrous xanthomas, Cancer **16**:331, 1963.
104. Perzin, K.H., and Fu, Y.-S.: Non-epithelial tumors of the nasal cavity, paranasal sinuses and nasopharynx: a clinico-pathologic study. XI. Fibrous histiocytomas, Cancer **45**:2616, 1980.
105. Reddick, R.L., Michelitch, H., and Triche, T.J.: Malignant soft tissue tumors (malignant fibrous histiocytoma, pleomorphic liposarcoma, and pleomorphic rhabdomyosarcoma): an electron microscopic study, Hum. Pathol. **10**:327, 1979.
106. Rosas-Uribe, A., Ring, A.M., and Rappaport, H.: Metastasizing retroperitoneal fibroxanthoma (malignant fibroxanthoma), Cancer **26**:827, 1970.
107. Santa Cruz, D.J., and Kyriakos, M.: Aneurysmal ("angiomatoid") fibrous histiocytoma of the skin, Cancer **47**:2053, 1981.
108. Shimoda, T., et al.: Liposarcoma: a light and electron microscopic study with comments on their relation to malignant fibrous histiocytoma and angiosarcoma, Acta Pathol. Jpn. **30**:779, 1980.
109. Snover, D.C., Phillips, G., and Dehner, L.P.: Reactive fibrohistiocytic proliferation simulating fibrous histiocytoma, Am. J. Clin. Pathol. **76**:232, 1981.
110. Soule, E.H., and Enriquez, P.: Atypical fibrous histiocytoma, malignant fibrous histiocytoma, malignant histiocytoma, and epithelioid sarcoma, Cancer **30**:128, 1972.
111. Taxy, J.B., and Battifora, H.: Malignant fibrous histiocytoma: an electron microscopic study, Cancer **40**:254, 1977.
112. Tsuneyoshi, M., and Enjoji, M.: Postirradiation sarcoma (malignant fibrous histiocytoma) following breast carcinoma: an ultrastructural study of a case, Cancer **45**:1419, 1980.
113. Wasserman, T.H., and Stuard, I.D.: Malignant fibrous histiocytoma with widespread metastases: autopsy study, Cancer **33**:141, 1974.
113a. Weiss, S.W.: Malignant fibrous histiocytoma: a reaffirmation, Am. J. Surg. Pathol. **6**:773, 1982.
114. Weiss, S.W., and Enzinger, F.M.: Myxoid variant of malignant fibrous histiocytoma, Cancer **39**:1672, 1977.
115. Weiss, S.W., and Enzinger, F.M.: Malignant fibrous histiocytoma: an analysis of 200 cases, Cancer **41**:2250, 1978.
116. Weiss, S.W., Enzinger, F.M., and Johnson, F.B.: Silica reaction simulating fibrous histiocytoma, Cancer **42**:2738, 1978.

Smooth muscle tumors

117. Appelman, H.D., and Helwig, E.B.: Gastric epithelioid leiomyoma and leiomyosarcoma (leiomyoblastoma), Cancer **38**:708, 1976.
118. Bailey, R.V., et al.: Leiomyosarcoma of the inferior vena cava: report of a case and review of the literature, Ann. Surg. **184**:169, 1976.
119. Botting, A.J., Soule, E.H., and Brown, A.L., Jr.: Smooth muscle tumors in children, Cancer **18**:711, 1965.
120. Cornog, J.L.: Gastric leiomyoblastoma: a clinical and ultrastructural study, Cancer **34**:711, 1974.
121. Dahl, I., and Angervall, L.: Cutaneous and subcutaneous leiomyosarcoma: a clinicopathologic study of 47 patients, Pathol. Eur. **9**:307, 1974.
122. Fields, J.P., and Helwig, E.B.: Leiomyosarcoma of the skin and subcutaneous tissue, Cancer **47**:156, 1981.
123. Hendrickson, M.R., and Kempson, R.L.: Surgical pathology of the uterine corpus, Philadelphia, 1980, W.B. Saunders Co.
124. Ishikawa, O., et al.: Leiomyosarcoma of the pancreas: report of a case and review of the literature, Am. J. Surg. Pathol. **5**:597, 1981.
125. Kempson, R.I.: Mitosis counting—II (editorial), Hum. Pathol. **7**:482, 1976.
126. Kevorkian, J., and Cento, D.P.: Leiomyosarcoma of large arteries and veins, Surgery **73**:390, 1973.
127. Lavin, P., Hajdu, S.I., and Foote, F.W., Jr.: Gastric and extragastric leiomyoblastomas: clinicopathologic study of 44 cases, Cancer **29**:305, 1972.

128. Morales, A.R.: Electron microscopy of human tumors. In Fenoglio, C.M., and Wolff, M., editors: Progress in surgical pathology, vol. 1, New York, 1980, Masson Publishing USA, Inc.
129. Morales, A.R., et al.: The ultrastructure of smooth muscle tumors with a consideration of the possible relationship of glomangiomas, hemangiopericytomas, and cardiac myxomas, Pathol. Annu. **10**:65, 1975.
130. Norris, H.J.: Mitosis counting—III (editorial): Hum. Pathol. **7**:483, 1976.
131. Pachter, M.R., and Lattes, R.: Mesenchymal tumors of the mediastinum. I. Tumors of fibrous tissue, adipose tissue, smooth muscle, and striated muscle, Cancer **16**:74, 1963.
132. Ranchod, M., and Kempson, R.L.: Smooth muscle tumors of the gastrointestinal tract and retroperitoneum: a pathologic analysis of 100 cases, Cancer **39**:255, 1977.
133. Rosen, L., Payson, B.A., and Mori, K.: Leiomyosarcoma of the superficial soft tissues, Mt. Sinai J. Med. **46**:181, 1979.
134. Salazar, H., and Totten, R.S.: Leiomyoblastoma of the stomach: an ultrastructural study, Cancer **25**:176, 1970.
135. Silverberg, S.G.: Reproducibility of the mitosis count in the histologic diagnosis of smooth muscle tumors of the uterus, Hum. Pathol. **7**:451, 1976.
136. Stout, A.P.: Bizarre smooth muscle tumors of the stomach, Cancer **15**:400, 1962.
137. Stout, A.P., Hendry, J., and Purdie, F.J.: Primary solid tumors of the great omentum, Cancer **16**:231, 1963.
138. Stout, A.P., and Hill, W.T.: Leiomyosarcoma of the superficial soft tissues, Cancer **11**:844, 1958.
139. Varela-Duran, J., Oliva, H., and Rosai, J.: Vascular leiomyosarcoma: the malignant counterpart of vascular leiomyoma, Cancer **44**:1684, 1979.
140. Wellmann, K.F.: "Bizarre leiomyoblastoma" of the retroperitoneum: report of a case, J. Pathol. Bacteriol. **94**:447, 1967.
141. Wile, A.G., Evans, H.L., and Romsdahl, M.M.: Leiomyosarcoma of soft tissue: a clinicopathologic study, Cancer **48**:1022, 1981.
142. Williams, L.J., and Pavlick, F.J.: Leiomyomatosis peritonealis disseminata: two case reports and a review of the medical literature, Cancer **45**:1726, 1980.
143. Yannopoulos, K., and Stout, A.P.: Smooth muscle tumors in children, Cancer **15**:958, 1962.
144. Yannopoulos, K., and Stout, A.P.: Primary solid tumors of the mesentery, Cancer **16**:914, 1963.

Tumors of skeletal muscle

Rhabdomyosarcoma

145. Bale, P.M., and Reye, R.D.K.: Rhabdomyosarcoma in childhood, Pathology **7**:101, 1975.
145a. Bundtzen, J.L., and Norback, D.H.: The ultrastructure of poorly differentiated rhabdomyosarcomas: a case report and literature review, Hum. Pathol. **13**:301, 1982.
146. Churg, A., and Ringus, J.: Ultrastructural observations on the histogenesis of alveolar rhabdomyosarcoma, Cancer **41**:1355, 1978.
147. Dito, W.R., and Batsakis, J.G.: Rhabdomyosarcoma of the head and neck: an appraisal of the biologic behavior in 170 cases, Arch. Surg. **84**:582, 1962.
148. Enterline, H.T., and Horn, R.C., Jr.: Alveolar rhabdomyosarcoma: a distinctive tumor type, Am. J. Clin. Pathol. **29**:356, 1958.
149. Enzinger, F.M.: Recent trends in soft tissue pathology. In Tumors of bone and soft tissue, Chicago, 1965, Year Book Medical Publishers, Inc.
150. Enzinger, F.M., and Shiraki, M.: Alveolar rhabdomyosarcoma: an analysis of 110 cases, Cancer **24**:18, 1969.
151. Gonzalez-Crussi, F., and Black-Schaffer, S.: Rhabdomyosarcoma of infancy and childhood: problems of morphologic classification, Am. J. Surg. Pathol. **3**:157, 1979.
152. Horn, R.C., Jr., and Enterline, H.T.: Rhabdomyosarcoma: a clinicopathological study and classification of 39 cases, Cancer **11**:181, 1958.
153. Horvat, B.L., Caines, M., and Fisher, E.R.: The ultrastructure of rhabdomyosarcoma, Am. J. Clin. Pathol. **53**:555, 1970.
154. Keyhani, A., and Booher, R.J.: Pleomorphic rhabdomyosarcoma, Cancer **22**:956, 1968.
155. Koh, S.-J., and Johnson, W.W.: Antimyosin and antirhabdomyoblast sera: their use for the diagnosis of childhood rhabdomyosarcoma, Arch. Pathol. Lab. Med. **104**:118, 1980.
156. Lawrence, W., Jr., Hays, D.M., and Moon, T.E.: Lymphatic metastasis with childhood rhabdomyosarcoma, Cancer **39**:556, 1977.
157. Lawrence, W., Jr., Jegge, G., and Foote, F.W., Jr.: Embryonal rhabdomyosarcoma: a clinicopathological study, Cancer **17**:361, 1964.
158. Linscheid, R.L., Soule, E.H., and Henderson, E.D.: Pleomorphic rhabdomyosarcomata of the extremities and limb girdles: a clinicopathological study, J. Bone Joint Surg. **47**:715, 1965.
158a. Lloyd, R.V., Hajdu, S.I., and Knapper, W.H.: Embryonal rhabdomyosarcoma in adults, Cancer **51**:557, 1983.
159. Maurer, H.M., et al.: The Intergroup Rhabdomyosarcoma Study: a preliminary report, Cancer **40**:2015, 1977.
160. Mierau, G.W., and Favara, B.E.: Rhabdomyosarcoma in children: ultrastructural study of 31 cases, Cancer **46**:2035, 1980.
160a. Miettinen, M., et al.: Alveolar rhabdomyosarcoma: demonstration of the muscle type of intermediate filament protein, desmin, as a diagnostic aid, Am. J. Pathol. **108**:246, 1982.
161. Morales, A.R., Fine, G., and Horn, R.C., Jr.: Rhabdomyosarcoma: an ultrastructural appraisal, Pathol. Annu. **7**:81, 1972.
162. Mukai, K., Rosai, J., and Hallaway, B.E.: Localization of myoglobin in normal and neoplastic human skeletal muscle cells using an immunoperoxidase method, Am. J. Surg. Pathol. **3**:373, 1979.
163. Patton, R.B., and Horn, R.C., Jr.: Rhabdomyosarcoma: clinical and pathological features and comparison with human fetal and embryonal skeletal muscle, Surgery **52**:572, 1962.
164. Soule, E.H., Geitz, M., and Henderson, E.D.: Embryonal rhabdomyosarcoma of the limbs and limb-girdles: a clinicopathologic study of 61 cases, Cancer **23**:1336, 1969.
165. Sutow, W.W.: Childhood rhabdomyosarcoma. In Sutow, W.W., editor: Malignant solid tumors in children: a review, New York, 1981, Raven Press.
166. Sutow, W.W., et al.: Prognosis in childhood rhabdomyosarcoma, Cancer **25**:1384, 1970.
166a. Tsokos, M., Howard, R., and Costa, J.: Immunohistochemical study of alveolar and embryonal rhabdomyosarcoma, Lab. Invest. **48**:148, 1983.
166b. Tsokos, M., et al.: Histologic and cytologic characteristics of poor prognosis childhood rhabdomyosarcoma (abstract), Lab. Invest. **50**:61A, 1984.
167. Young, J.L., Jr., and Miller, R.W.: Incidence of malignant tumors in U.S. children, J. Pediatr. **86**:254, 1975.

Rhabdomyoma

168. Battifora, H.A., Eisenstein, R., and Schild, J.A.: Rhabdomyoma of larynx: ultrastructural study and comparison with granular cell tumors (myoblastoma), Cancer **23**:183, 1969.
169. Czernobilsky, B., Cornog, J.L., and Enterline, H.T.: Rhabdomyoma: report of a case with ultrastructural and histochemical studies, Am. J. Clin. Pathol. **49**:782, 1968.
170. Dahl, I., Angervall, L., and Säve-Söderbergh, J.: Foetal rhabdomyoma: case report of a patient with two tumors, Acta Pathol. Microbiol. Scand. **84A**:107, 1976.
171. Dehner, L.P., and Enzinger, F.M.: Fetal rhabdomyoma: an analysis of nine cases, Cancer **30**:160, 1972.
172. Di Sant'Agnese, P.A., and Knowles, D.M., II: Extracardiac rhabdomyoma: a clinicopathologic study and review of the literature, Cancer **46**:780, 1980.
173. Gold, J.H., and Bossen, E.H.: Benign vaginal rhabdomyoma: a light and electron microscopic study, Cancer **37**:2283, 1976.
174. Goldman, R.L.: Multicentric benign rhabdomyoma of skeletal muscle, Cancer **16**:1609, 1963.
174a. Konrad, E.A., Meister, P., and Hübner, G.: Extracardiac rhabdomyoma, Cancer **49**:898, 1982.
175. Moran, J.J., and Enterline, H.T.: Benign rhabdomyoma of the pharynx: a case report, review of the literature, and comparison with cardiac rhabdomyoma, Am. J. Clin. Pathol. **42**:174, 1964.

176. Scrivner, D., and Meyer, J.S.: Multifocal recurrent adult rhabdomyoma, Cancer **46**:790, 1980.

176a. Simha, M., et al.: Postauricular fetal rhabdomyoma: light and electron microscopic study, Hum. Pathol. **13**:673, 1982.

Tumors of adipose tissue

Liposarcoma

177. Allen, P.W.: Tumors and proliferations of adipose tissue: a clinicopathologic approach, New York, 1981, Masson Publishing USA, Inc.

178. Battifora, H., and Nunez-Alonso, C.: Myxoid liposarcoma: study of ten cases, Ultrastruct. Pathol. **1**:157, 1980.

179. Bolen, J.W., and Thorning, D.: Benign lipoblastoma and myxoid liposarcoma: a comparative light- and electron-microscopic study, Am. J. Surg. Pathol. **4**:163, 1980.

180. Brasfield, R.D., and Das Gupta, T.K.: Liposarcoma, CA **20**:3, 1970.

181. Chung, E.B., and Enzinger, F.M.: Benign lipoblastomatosis: an analysis of 35 cases, Cancer **32**:482, 1973.

182. Desai, U., Ramos, C.V., and Taylor, H.B.: Ultrastructural observations in pleomorphic liposarcoma, Cancer **42**:1284, 1978.

183. Edland, R.W.: Liposarcoma: a retrospective study of fifteen cases, a review of the literature and a discussion of radiosensitivity, Am. J. Roent. Rad. Therapy Nucl. Med. **103**:778, 1968.

184. Enzinger, F.: Management of primary bone and soft tissue tumors, Chicago, 1977, Year Book Medical Publishers, Inc.

185. Enzinger, F.M., and Winslow, D.J.: Liposarcoma: a study of 103 cases, Virchows Arch. **335**:367, 1962.

186. Evans, H.L.: Liposarcoma: a study of 55 cases with a reassessment of its classification, Am. J. Surg. Pathol. **3**:507, 1979.

187. Evans, H.L., Soule, E.H., and Winkelmann, R.K.: Atypical lipoma, atypical intramuscular lipoma, and well-differentiated retroperitoneal liposarcoma: a reappraisal of 30 cases formerly classified as well-differentiated liposarcoma, Cancer **43**:574, 1979.

188. Fu, Y.-S., et al.: Ultrastructure of benign and malignant adipose tissue tumors, Pathol. Annu. **15**(Part 1): 67, 1980.

188a. Gonzalez-Crussi, F., deMello, D.E., and Sotelo-Avila, C.: Omental-mesenteric myxoid hamartomas, Am. J. Surg. Pathol. **7**:567, 1983.

189. Kindblom, L.-G., Angervall, L., and Svendsen, P.: Liposarcoma: a clinicopathologic, radiographic and prognostic study, Acta Pathol. Microbiol. Scand **253** (suppl.):1, 1975.

190. Kinne, D.W., et. al.: Treatment of primary and recurrent retroperitoneal liposarcoma, Cancer **31**:53, 1973.

191. Lagacé, R., Jacob, S., and Seemayer, T.A.: Myxoid liposarcoma: an electron microscopic study; biologic and histogenetic considerations, Virchows Arch. (Pathol. Anat.) **384**:159, 1979.

191a. McKee, P.H., Lowe, D., and Shaw, M.: Subcutaneous liposarcoma, Clin. Exp. Dermatol. **8**:583, 1983.

191b. Shmookler, B.M., and Enzinger, F.M.: Liposarcoma occurring in children: an analysis of 17 cases and review of the literature, Cancer **52**:567, 1983.

191c. Snover, D.C., Sumner, H.W., and Dehner, L.P.: Variability of histologic pattern in recurrent soft tissue sarcomas originally diagnosed as liposarcoma, Cancer **49**:1005, 1982.

192. Wetzel, W., and Alexander, R.: Myxoid liposarcoma: an ultrastructural study of two cases, Am. J. Clin. Pathol. **72**:521, 1979.

Lipoma

193. Brasfield, R.D., and Das Gupta, T.K.: Soft tissue tumors: benign tumors of adipose tissue, CA **19**:3, 1969.

194. Dionne, G.P., and Seemayer, T.A.: Infiltrating lipomas and angiolipomas revisited, Cancer **33**:732, 1974.

195. Enzinger, F.M.: Benign lipomatous tumors simulating a sarcoma. In M.D. Anderson Hospital and Tumor Institute: Management of primary bone and soft tissue tumors, Chicago, 1977, Year Book Medical Publishers, Inc.

195a. Kim, Y.H., and Reiner, L.: Ultrastructure of lipoma, Cancer **50**:102, 1982.

196. Kindblom, L.-G., et al.: Intermuscular and intramuscular lipomas and hibernomas: a clinical, roentgenologic, histologic, and prognostic study of 46 cases, Cancer **33**:754, 1974.

Spindle cell lipoma

197. Angervall, L., et al.: Spindle cell lipoma, Acta Pathol. Microbiol. Scand. **84A**:477, 1976.

198. Bolen, J.W., and Thorning, D.: Spindle-cell lipoma: a clinical, light- and electron-microscopical study, Am. J. Surg. Pathol. **5**:435, 1981.

199. Enzinger, F.M., and Harvey, D.A.: Spindle cell lipoma, Cancer **36**:1852, 1975.

199a. Robb, J.A., and Jones, R.A.: Spindle cell lipoma in a perianal location, Hum. Pathol. **13**:1052, 1982.

Pleomorphic (atypical) lipoma

200. Evans, H.L., Soule, E.H., and Winkelmann, R.K.: Atypical lipoma, atypical intramuscular lipoma, and well differentiated retroperitoneal liposarcoma: a reappraisal of 30 cases formerly classified as well differentiated liposarcoma, Cancer **43**:574, 1979.

200a. Kindblom, L.-G., Angervall, L., and Fassina, A.S.: Atypical lipoma, Acta Pathol. Microbiol. Immunol. Scand. **90A**:27, 1982.

201. Shmookler, B.M., and Enzinger, F.M.: Pleomorphic lipoma: a benign tumor simulating liposarcoma; a clinicopathologic analysis of 48 cases, Cancer **47**:126, 1981.

Angiolipoma

202. Dionne, G.P., and Seemayer, T.: Infiltrating lipomas and angiolipomas revisited, Cancer **33**:732, 1974.

203. Dixon, A.Y., McGregor, D.H., and Lee, S.H.: Angiolipomas: an ultrastructural and clinicopathological study, Hum. Pathol. **12**:739, 1981.

204. Howard, W.R., and Helwig, E.B.: Angiolipoma, Arch. Dermatol. **82**:924, 1960.

205. Lin, J.J., and Lin, F.: Two entities in angiolipoma: a study of 459 cases of lipoma with review of literature on infiltrating angiolipoma, Cancer **34**:720, 1974.

Lipoblastoma

206. Bolen, J.W., and Thorning, D.: Benign lipoblastoma and myxoid liposarcoma: a comparative light- and electron-microscopic study, Am. J. Surg. Pathol. **4**:163, 1980.

207. Chung, E.B., and Enzinger, F.M.: Benign lipoblastomatosis: an analysis of 35 cases, Cancer **32**:482, 1973.

208. Gibbs, M.K., et al.: Lipoblastomatosis: a tumor of children, Pediatrics **60**:235, 1977.

209. Greco, M.A., Garcia, R.L., and Vuletin, J.C.: Benign lipoblastomatosis: ultrastructure and histogenesis, Cancer **45**:511, 1980.

210. Vellios, F., Baez, J., and Shumacker, H.B.: Lipoblastomatosis: a tumor of fetal fat different from hibernoma, Am. J. Pathol. **34**:1149, 1958.

Hibernoma

211. Kindblom, L.-G., et al.: Intermuscular and intramuscular lipomas and hibernomas: a clinical, roentgenologic, histologic, and prognostic study of 46 cases, Cancer **33**:754, 1974.

212. Levine, G.D.: Hibernoma: an electron microscopic study, Hum. Pathol. **3**:351, 1972.

213. Seemayer, T.A., et al.: On the ultrastructure of hibernoma, Cancer **36**:1785, 1975.

Tumors of vascular tissue

Intramuscular hemangioma

214. Allen, P.W., and Enzinger, F.M.: Hemangioma of skeletal muscle: an analysis of 89 cases, Cancer **29**:8, 1972.

Hemangiopericytoma

215. Angervall, L., et al.: Hemangiopericytoma: a clinicopathologic, angiographic and microangiographic study, Cancer **42**:2412, 1978.

215a. Croxatto, J.O., and Font, R.L.: Hemangiopericytoma of the orbit: a clinicopathologic study of 30 cases, Hum. Pathol. **13**:210, 1982.
216. Eimoto, T.: Ultrastructure of an infantile hemangiopericytoma, Cancer **40**:2161, 1977.
217. Enzinger, F.M., and Smith, B.H.: Hemangiopericytoma: an analysis of 106 cases, Hum. Pathol. **7**:61, 1976.
218. McMaster, M.J., Soule, E.H., and Ivins, J.C.: Hemangiopericytoma: a clinicopathologic study and long-term follow-up of 60 patients, Cancer **36**:2232, 1975.
219. Nunnery, E.W., et al.: Hemangiopericytoma: a light microscopic and ultrastructural study, Cancer **47**:906, 1981.
220. Waldo, E.D., Vuletin, J.C., and Kaye, G.I.: The ultrastructure of vascular tumors: additional observations and a review of the literature, Pathol. Annu. **12**(Part 2):279, 1977.

Neurogenous tumors

221. Abell, M.R., Hart, W.R., and Olson, J.R.: Tumors of the peripheral nervous system, Hum. Pathol. **1**:503, 1970.
222. Ackerman, L.V., and Taylor, F.H.: Neurogenous tumors within the thorax: a clinicopathological evaluation of forty-eight cases, Cancer **4**:669, 1951.
223. Allen, P.W.: Myxoid tumors of soft tissues, Pathol. Annu. **15** (Part 1):133, 1980.
224. Alvira, M.M., Mandybur, T.I., and Menefee, M.G.: Light microscopic and ultrastructural observations of a metastasizing malignant epithelioid schwannoma, Cancer **38**:1977, 1976.
224a. Ariel, I.M.: Tumors of the peripheral nervous system, CA **33**:282, 1983.
225. Asbury, A.K., and Johnson, P.C.: Pathology of peripheral nerve, Philadelphia, 1978, W.B. Saunders Co.
225a. Bonneau, R., and Brochu, P.: Neuromuscular choristoma: a clinicopathologic study of two cases, Am. J. Surg. Pathol. **7**:521, 1983.
225b. Brooks, J., et al.: Malignant "Triton" tumors: natural history of seven new cases with literature review (abstract), Lab. Invest. **48**:10A, 1983.
226. Chen, K.T.K., et al.: Malignant schwannoma: a light microscopic and ultrastructural study, Cancer **45**:1585, 1980.
227. D'Agostino, A.N., Soule, E.H., and Miller, R.H.: Primary malignant neoplasms of nerves (malignant neurilemomas) in patients without manifestations of multiple neurofibromatosis (von Recklinghausen's disease), Cancer **16**:1003, 1963.
228. D'Agostino, A.N., Soule, E.H., and Miller, R.H.: Sarcomas of the peripheral nerves and somatic soft tissues associated with multiple neurofibromatosis (von Recklinghausen's disease), Cancer **16**:1015, 1963.
229. Dahl, I.: Ancient neurilemmoma (schwannoma), Acta Pathol. Microbiol. Scand. **85**:812, 1977.
230. Das Gupta, T.K., and Brasfield, R.D.: Von Recklinghausen's disease, CA **21**:174, 1971.
231. Das Gupta, T.K., et. al.: Benign solitary schwannomas (neurilemomas), Cancer **24**:355, 1969.
231a. Ducatman, B.S., et al.: Malignant peripheral nerve sheath tumor: a clinicopathologic review of 120 cases (abstract), Lab. Invest. **50**:17A, 1984.
231b. Erlandson, R.A., and Woodruff, J.M.: Peripheral nerve sheath tumors: an electron microscopic study of 43 cases, Cancer **49**:273, 1982.
232. Ghosh, B.C., et. al.: Malignant schwannoma: clinicopathologic study, Cancer **31**:184,1973.
233. Guccion, J.G., and Enzinger, F.M.: Malignant schwannoma associated with von Recklinghausen's neurofibromatosis, Virchows Arch. (Pathol. Anat.) **383A**:43, 1979.
234. Ha'Eri, G.B., Fornasier, V.L., and Schatzker, J.: Morton's neuroma—pathogenesis and ultrastructure, Clin. Orthop. **141**:256, 1979.
235. Harkin, J.C., and Reed, R.J.: Tumors of the peripheral nervous system. In Atlas of tumor pathology, Second Series, Fascicle 3, Washington D.C., 1969, Armed Forces Institute of Pathology.
235a. Herrera, G.A., et al.: Malignant schwannomas presenting as malignant fibrous histiocytomas, Ultrastruct. Pathol. **3**:253, 1982.
236. Karcioglu, Z., Someren, A., and Mathes, S.J.: Ectomesenchymoma: a malignant tumor of migratory neural crest (ectomesenchyme) remnants showing ganglionic, schwannian, melanocytic and rhabdomyoblastic differentiation, Cancer **39**:2486, 1977.
237. Lassmann, H., et al.: Different types of benign nerve sheath tumors: light microscopy, electron microscopy and autoradiography, Virchows Arch. (Pathol. Anat.) **375A**:197, 1977.
238. Lazarus, S.S., and Trombetta, L.D.: Ultrastructural identification of a benign perineural cell tumor, Cancer **41**:1823, 1978.
238a. Markel, S.F., and Enzinger, F.M.: Neuromuscular hamartoma—a benign "Triton tumor" composed of mature neural and striated muscle elements, Cancer **49**:140, 1982.
239. Oberman, H.A., and Sullenger, G.: Neurogenous tumors of the head and neck, Cancer **20**:1992, 1967.
240. Sordillo, P.P., et. al.: Malignant schwannoma: clinical characteristics, survival, and response to therapy, Cancer **47**:2503, 1981.
241. Storm, F.K., et. al.: Neurofibrosarcoma, Cancer **45**:126, 1980.
241a. Taxy, J.B., et al.: Electron microscopy in the diagnosis of malignant schwannoma, Cancer **48**:1381, 1981.
242. Trojanowski, J.Q., Kleinman, G.M., and Proppe, K.H.: Malignant tumors of nerve sheath origin, Cancer **46**:1202, 1980.
243. Tsuneyoshi, M., and Enjoji, M.: Primary malignant peripheral nerve tumors (malignant schwannomas): a clinicopathologic and electron microscopic study, Acta Pathol. Jpn. **29**:363, 1979.
244. Waggener, J.D.: Ultrastructure of benign peripheral nerve sheath tumors, Cancer **19**:699, 1966.
244a. Weiss, S.W., Langloss, J.M., and Enzinger, F.M.: Value of S-100 protein in the diagnosis of soft tissue tumors with particular reference to benign and malignant Schwann cell tumors, Lab. Invest. **49**:299, 1983.
245. Woodruff, J.M.: Peripheral nerve tumors showing glandular differentiation (glandular schwannomas), Cancer **37**:2399, 1976.
246. Woodruff, J.M., et al.: Peripheral nerve tumors with rhabdomyosarcomatous differentiation (malignant "Triton" tumors), Cancer **32**:426,1973.
246a. Woodruff, J.M., et al.: Cellular schwannoma: a variety of schwannoma sometimes mistaken for a malignant tumor, Am. J. Surg. Pathol. **5**:733, 1981.

Miscellaneous tumors

Myxoma

247. Allen, P.W.: Myxoid tumors of soft tissues, Pathol. Annu. **15** (Part 1):133, 1980.
248. Dutz, W., and Stout, A.P.: The myxoma in childhood, Cancer **14**:629, 1961.
249. Enzinger, F.M.: Intramuscular myxoma: a review and follow-up study of 34 cases, Am. J. Clin. Pathol. **43**:104, 1965.
250. Feldman, P.S.: A comparative study including ultrastructure of intramuscular myxoma and myxoid liposarcoma, Cancer **43**:512, 1979.
251. Ireland, D.C.R., Soule, E.H., and Ivins, J.C.: Myxoma of somatic soft tissues: a report of 58 patients, 3 with multiple tumors and fibrous dysplasia of bone, Mayo Clin. Proc. **48**:401, 1973.
252. Kindblom, L.-G., Stener, B., and Angervall, L.: Intramuscular myxoma, Cancer **34**:1737,1974.
253. Mackenzie, D.H.: The myxoid tumors of somatic soft tissues, Am. J. Surg. Pathol. **5**:443,1981.
253a. Steeper, T.A., and Rosai, J.: Aggressive angiomyxoma of the female pelvis and perineum, Am. J. Surg. Pathol. **7**:463, 1983.
254. Stout, A.P.: Myxoma: the tumor of primitive mesenchyme, Ann. Surg. **127**:706, 1948.
255. Wirth, W.A., Leavitt, D., and Enzinger, F.M.: Multiple intramuscular myxomas: another extraskeletal manifestation of fibrous dysplasia, Cancer **27**:1167, 1971.

Synovial sarcoma

256. Cadman, N.L., Soule, E.H., and Kelly, P.J.: Synovial sarcoma: an analysis of 134 tumors, Cancer **18**:613, 1965.
257. Cameron, H.U., and Kostuik, J.P.: A long-term follow-up of synovial sarcoma, J. Bone Joint Surg. (Br.) **56**:613, 1974.
257a. Corson, J.M., et al.: Keratin proteins in synovial sarcomas: an immunohistochemical study of 24 cases (abstract), Lab. Invest. **48**:17A, 1983.

258. Dische, F.E., Darby, A.J., and Howard, E.R.: Malignant synovioma: electron microscopical findings in three patients and review of the literature, J. Pathol. **124**:149, 1978.
259. Evans, H.L.: Synovial sarcoma: a study of 23 biphasic and 17 probable monophasic examples, Pathol. Annu. **15**:309, 1980.
259a. Farris, K.B., and Reed, R.J.: Monophasic, glandular, synovial sarcomas and carcinomas of the soft tissues, Arch. Pathol. Lab. Med. **106**:129, 1982.
260. Fechner, R.E.: Neoplasms and neoplasm-like lesions of the synovium. In Ackerman, L.V., Spjut, H.J., and Abell, M.R., editors: Bones and joints, Baltimore, 1976, The Williams & Wilkins Co.
261. Gabbiani, G., et al.: Synovial sarcoma: electron microscopic study of a typical case, Cancer **28**:1031, 1971.
262. Hajdu, S.I., Shiu, M.H., and Fortner, J.G.: Tendosynovial sarcoma: a clinicopathological study of 136 cases, Cancer **39**:1201, 1977.
263. Krall, R.A., Kostianovsky, M., and Patchefsky, A.S.: Synovial sarcoma: a clinical, pathological, and ultrastructural study of 26 cases supporting the recognition of a monophasic variant, Am. J. Surg. Pathol. **5**:137, 1981.
264. Mackenzie, D.H.: Monophasic synovial sarcoma—a histological entity? Histopathology **1**:151, 1977.
265. Mickelson, M.R., et al.: Synovial sarcoma: an electron microscopic study of monophasic and biphasic forms, Cancer **45**:2109. 1980.
265a. Miettinen, M., Lehto, V.-P., and Virtanen, I.: Keratin in the epithelial-like cells of classical biphasic synovial sarcoma, Virchows Arch. (Cell Pathol.) **40B**:157, 1982.
266. Nunez-Alonso, C., Gashti, E.N., and Christ, M.L.: Maxillofacial synovial sarcoma: light- and electron-microscopic study of two cases, Am. J. Surg. Pathol. **3**:23, 1979.
267. Roth, J.A., Enzinger, F.M., and Tannenbaum, M.: Synovial sarcoma of the neck: a follow-up study of 24 cases, Cancer **35**:1243, 1975.
267a. Schmidt, D., and Mackay, B.: Ultrastructure of human tendon sheath and synovium: implications for tumor histogenesis, Ultrastruct. Pathol. **3**:269, 1982.
267b. Shmookler, B.M.: Retroperitoneal synovial sarcoma: a report of four cases, Am. J. Clin. Pathol. **77**:686, 1982.
267c. Shmookler, B.M., Enzinger, F.M., and Brannon, R.B.: Orofacial synovial sarcoma, Cancer **50**:269, 1982.
267d. Varela-Duran, J., and Enzinger, F.M.: Calcifying synovial sarcoma, Cancer **50**:345, 1982.

Epithelioid sarcoma

268. Bloustein, P.A., Silverberg, S.G., and Waddell, W.R.: Epithelioid sarcoma: case report with ultrastructural review, histogenetic discussion, and chemotherapeutic data, Cancer **38**:2390, 1976.
269. Bryan, R.S., et al.: Primary epithelioid sarcoma of the hand and forearm: a review of thirteen cases, J. Bone Joint Surg. (Am.) **56**:458, 1974.
269a. Chase, D., et al.: Keratin in epithelioid sarcoma: an immunohistochemical study (abstract), Lab. Invest. **50**:9A, 1984.
270. Enzinger, F.M.: Epithelioid sarcoma: a sarcoma simulating a granuloma or a carcinoma, Cancer **26**:1029, 1970.
271. Fisher, E.R., and Horvat, B.: The fibrocytic derivation of the so-called epithelioid sarcoma, Cancer **30**:1074, 1972.
272. Frable, W.J., et al.: Epithelioid sarcoma: an electron microscopic study, Arch. Pathol. **95**:8, 1973.
273. Gabbiani, G., et al.: Epithelioid sarcoma: a light and electron microscopic study suggesting a synovial origin, Cancer **30**:486,1972.
274. Gallup, D.G., Abell, M.R., and Morley, G.W.: Epithelioid sarcoma of the vulva, Obstet. Gynecol. **48**(suppl.):14s, 1976.
274a. Miettinen, M., et al.: Epithelioid sarcoma: ultrastructural and immunohistologic features suggesting a synovial origin, Arch. Pathol. Lab. Med. **106**:620, 1982.
274b. Mills, S.E., et al.: Intermediate filaments in eosinophilic cells of epithelioid sarcoma, Am. J. Surg. Pathol. **5**:195, 1981.
275. Moore, S.W., Wheeler, J.E., and Hefter, L.G.: Epithelioid sarcoma masquerading as Peyronie's disease, Cancer **35**:1706, 1975.
276. Patchefsky, A.S., Soriano, R., and Kostianovsky, M.: Epithelioid sarcoma: ultrastructural similarity to nodular synovitis, Cancer **39**:143, 1977.
277. Prat, J., Woodruff, J.M., and Marcove, R.C.: Epithelioid sarcoma: an analysis of 22 cases indicating the prognostic significance of vascular invasion and regional lymph node metastasis, Cancer **41**:1472, 1978.
278. Santiago, H., Feinerman, L.K., and Lattes, R.: Epithelioid sarcoma: a clinical and pathologic study of nine cases, Hum. Pathol. **3**:133, 1972.
279. Seemayer, T.A., Dionne, P.G., and Tabah, E.J.: Epithelioid sarcoma, Can. J. Surg. **17**:37, 1974.
279a. Ulbright, T.M., et al.: Epithelioid sarcoma of the vulva, Cancer **52**:1462, 1983.

Clear cell sarcoma

280. Bearman, R.M., Noe, J., and Kempson, R.L.: Clear cell sarcoma with melanin pigment, Cancer **36**:977, 1975.
281. Boudreaux, D., and Waisman, J.: Clear cell sarcoma with melanogenesis, Cancer **41**:1387, 1978.
282. Chung, E.B., and Enzinger, F.M.: Clear cell sarcoma of tendons and aponeuroses: further observation (abstract), Lab. Invest. **38**:338, 1978.
282a. Chung, E.B., and Enzinger, F.M.: Malignant melanoma of soft parts: a reassessment of clear cell sarcoma, Am. J. Surg. Pathol. **7**:405, 1983.
282b. Eckardt, J.J., Pritchard, D.J., and Soule, E.H.: Clear cell sarcoma: a clinicopathologic study of 27 cases, Cancer **52**:1482, 1983.
283. Enzinger, F.M.: Clear-cell sarcoma of tendons and aponeuroses: an analysis of 21 cases, Cancer **18**:1163, 1965.
284. Hoffman, G.J., and Carter, D.: Clear cell sarcoma of tendons and aponeuroses with melanin, Arch. Pathol. **95**:22, 1973.
284a. Kindblom, L.-G., Lodding, P., and Angervall, L.: Clear-cell sarcoma of tendons and aponeuroses: an immunohistochemical and electron microscopic analysis indicating neural crest origin, Virchows Arch. (Pathol. Anat.) **401A**:109, 1983.
285. Mackenzie, D.H.: Clear cell sarcoma of tendon and aponeuroses with melanin production, J. Pathol. **114**:231, 1974.
285a. Mukai, M., et al.: Histogenesis of clear cell sarcoma of tendons and aponeuroses, Am. J. Pathol. **114**:264, 1984.
286. Parker, J.B., Marcus, P.B., and Martin, J.H.: Spinal melanotic clear-cell sarcoma: a light and electron microscopic study, Cancer **46**:718, 1980.
287. Raynor, A.C., et al.: Clear-cell sarcoma with melanin pigment: a possible soft-tissue variant of malignant melanoma, J. Bone Joint Surg. (Am.) **61**:276, 1979.
288. Tsuneyoshi, M., Enjoji, M., and Kubo, T.: Clear cell sarcoma of tendons and aponeuroses: a comparative study of 13 cases with a provisional subgrouping into the melanotic and synovial types, Cancer **42**:243, 1978.

Alveolar soft part sarcoma

289. Christopherson, W.M., Foote, F.W., and Stewart, F.W.: Alveolar soft-part sarcomas: structurally characteristic tumors of uncertain histogenesis, Cancer **5**:100, 1952.
290. DeSchryver-Kecskemeti, K., et al.: Alveolar soft part sarcoma: a malignant angioreninoma, Am. J. Surg. Pathol. **6**:5, 1982.
291. Ekfors, T.O., et al.: Alveolar soft part sarcoma: a report of two cases with some histochemical and ultrastructural observations, Cancer **43**:1672, 1979.
292. Fisher, E.R., and Reidbord, H.: Electron microscopic evidence suggesting the myogenous derivation of the so-called alveolar soft part sarcoma, Cancer **27**:150, 1971.
292a. Font, R.L., Jurco, III, S., and Zimmerman, L.E.: Alveolar soft-part sarcoma of the orbit: a clinicopathologic analysis of seventeen cases and a review of the literature, Hum. Pathol. **13**:569, 1982.
293. Lieberman, P.H., et al.: Alveolar soft-part sarcoma, J.A.M.A. **198**:1047, 1966.

294. Marcus, P.B., Couch, W.D., and Martin, J.H.: Crystals in a gastric schwannoma, Ultrastruct. Pathol. **2**:139, 1981.

294a. Mathew, T.: Evidence supporting neural crest origin of an alveolar soft part sarcoma: an ultrastructural study, Cancer **50**:507, 1982.

294b. Mukai, M., et al.: Alveolar soft-part sarcoma: a review on its histogenesis and further studies based on electron microscopy, immunohistochemistry, and biochemistry, Am. J. Surg. Pathol. **7**:679, 1983.

295. Shipkey, F.H., et al.: Ultrastructure of alveolar soft part sarcoma, Cancer **17**:821, 1964.

296. Unni, K.K., and Soule, E.H.: Alveolar soft part sarcoma: an electron microscopic study, Mayo Clin. Proc. **50**:591, 1975.

297. Welsh, R.A., et al.: Histogenesis of alveolar soft part sarcoma, Cancer **29**:191, 1972.

Giant cell tumor of soft parts

298. Alguacil-Garcia, A., Unni, K.K., and Goellner, J.R.: Malignant giant cell tumor of soft parts: an ultrastructural study of four cases, Cancer **40**:244, 1977.

299. Angervall, L., et al.: Malignant giant cell tumor of soft tissues: a clinicopathologic, cytologic, ultrastructural, angiographic, and microangiographic study, Cancer **47**:736, 1981.

300. Guccion, J.G., and Enzinger, F.M.: Malignant giant cell tumor of soft parts: an analysis of 32 cases, Cancer **29**:1518, 1972.

301. Salm, R., and Sissons, H.A.: Giant-cell tumours of soft tissues, J. Pathol. **107**:27, 1972.

302. van Haelst, U.J.G.M., and de Haas van Dorsser, A.H.: Giant cell tumor of soft parts: an ultrastructural study, Virchows Arch. (Pathol. Anat.) **371A**:199, 1976.

Extraskeletal Ewing's sarcoma

303. Angervall, L., and Enzinger, F.M.: Extraskeletal neoplasm resembling Ewing's sarcoma, Cancer **36**:240, 1975.

304. Askin, F.B., et al.: Malignant small cell tumor of the thoracopulmonary region in childhood: a distinctive clinicopathologic entity of uncertain histogenesis, Cancer **43**:2438, 1979.

305. Gillespie, J.J., et al.,: Extraskeletal Ewing's sarcoma: histologic and ultrastructural observations in three cases, Am. J. Surg. Pathol. **3**:99, 1979.

305a. Linnoila, R.I., et al.: Evidence for neural origin and periodic acid-Schiff-positive variants of the malignant small cell tumor of thoracopulmonary region ("Askin tumor") (abstract), Lab. Invest. **48**:51A, 1983.

306. Mahoney, J.P., Ballinger, W.E., Jr., and Alexander, R.W.: So-called extraskeletal Ewing's sarcoma: report of a case with ultrastructural analysis, Am. J. Clin. Pathol. **70**:926, 1978.

307. Soule, E.H., et al.: Extraskeletal Ewing's sarcoma: a preliminary review of 26 cases encountered in the Intergroup Rhabdomyosarcoma Study, Cancer **42**:259, 1978.

308. Wigger, H.J., Salazar, G.H., and Blanc, W.A.: Extraskeletal Ewing sarcoma: an ultrastructural study, Arch. Pathol. Lab. Med. **101**:446, 1977.

CHAPTER 40 **Metabolic and Other Nontumorous Disorders of Bone**

STEVEN L. TEITELBAUM

*Bone is power. It is bone to which the soft parts cling; from which they are helpless, strung and held aloft to the sun, lest man be but another slithering earth-noser.**

COMPOSITION AND STRUCTURE OF BONE

Bone is a heterogeneous tissue that not only has structural importance but also plays the central role in mineral homeostasis.[7] It may be functionally divided into its cortical (compact) and trabecular (cancellous) components. Structural stability is provided by cortical bone, which comprises approximately 80% of the skeleton. Within the cortex are haversian canals, through which longitudinally oriented blood vessels pass, and horizontally arranged Volkmann's canals containing vascular offshoots. Surrounding each haversian canal is a series of concentric, lamellar, mineralized collagen bundles forming an osteon, which is the remodeling unit of cortical bone. Separating osteons are basophilic, metachromatic markers known as cement lines (Fig. 40-1).

Trabecular bone consists of a meshwork of spicules between which are the marrow elements (Fig. 40-2). These spicules are generally oriented along lines of stress. The surface area of trabecular bone is much greater than that of cortical bone, and therefore its primary role is metabolic rather than structural.

As demonstrated by Frost,[3] bone surfaces are lined by three cellular envelopes. These envelopes, which respectively cover the periosteum, haversian canals, and endosteum, function independent of each other. Hence it is possible, as in states of glucocorticoid excess, to have relative sparing of cortical bone and aggravated loss of cancellous bone.[5]

The four morphologically distinguishable cellular activities of bone are growth, modeling, remodeling, and repair.[4] Growth and modeling occur only before closure of the growth plate (physis). Growth refers to increasing skeletal mass, whereas modeling is the sculpting of bone

*From Silzer, R.: Mortal lessons, New York, 1976, Simon & Schuster.

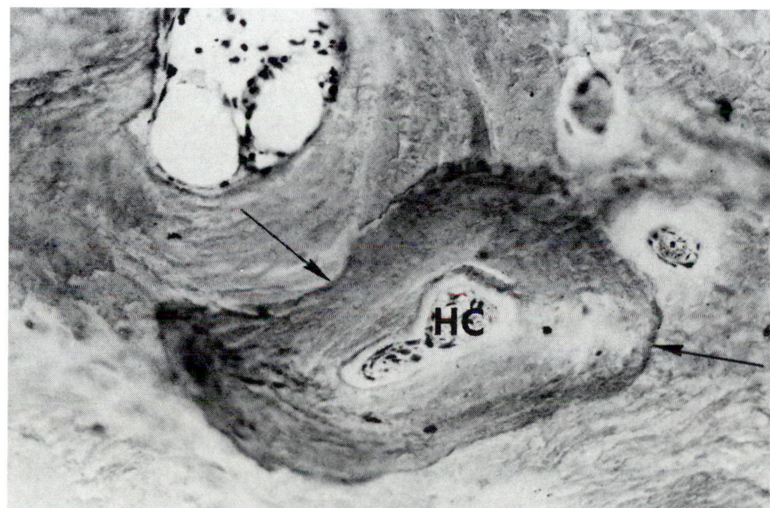

Fig. 40-1. Osteon enclosed by cement line *(arrows)*. Within center of osteon is haversian canal *(HC)*. (Undecalcified, toluidine blue; 100×.)

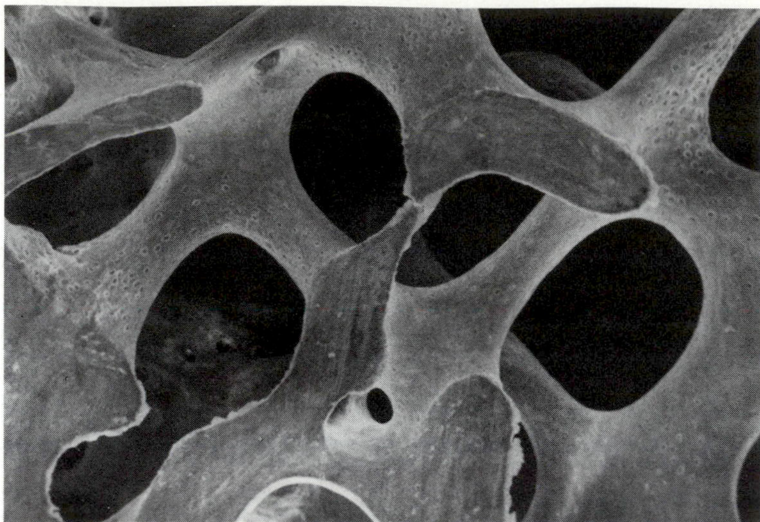

Fig. 40-2. Scanning electron micrograph of trabecular bone after removal of marrow. All trabeculae are joined in complicated meshwork. Small holes on surface are osteocytic lacunae. (57×.)

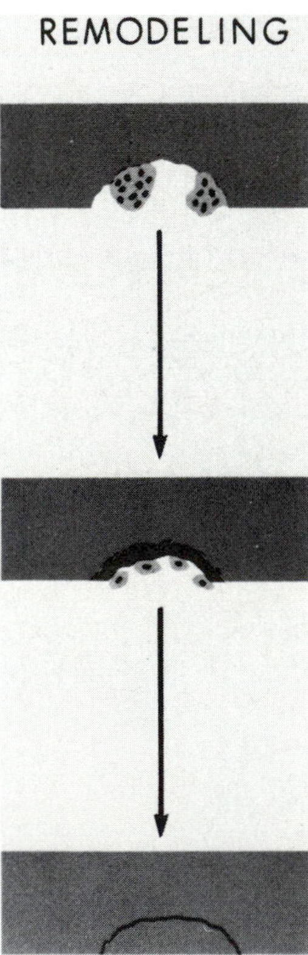

Fig. 40-3. Remodeling is initiated by osteoclastic resorption of packet of bone followed by osteoblastic bone formation in same location. Completed remodeling unit is permanently circumscribed by cement line.

and its movement through space. Both of these processes are responsible for the development of small fetal bones into the much larger, yet identically shaped bones of adults.

Despite the close association of growth and modeling they are independent processes. For example, the hypopituitary midget has normally modeled bones in a setting of growth arrest. Similarly, a variety of skeletal dysplasias, such as Engelmann's disease, are characterized by abnormally shaped, yet fully elongated bones.[1]

Remodeling occurs throughout life and is intimately related to mineral homeostasis. The histologic manifestations of remodeling, such as changes in the numbers of osteoclasts and osteoblasts, probably represent long-term metabolic demands. Maintenance of minute-to-minute mineral homeostasis may not be reflected morphologically and is most likely accomplished by changing ionic fluxes.

The unique and distinctive feature of remodeling is the anatomic coupling of resorption and formation (Fig. 40-3). The process is initiated by osteoclasts, which resorb a quantity of bone forming a scalloped Howship's lacuna (resorption bay). The point of termination of remodeling osteoclasts is marked in the cortex and trabeculum by the cement line. Osteoblasts then appear at the remodeling site and deposit varying amounts of bone in the Howship's lacuna. The description of the linkage of precursor cell activation and bone resorption and formation by Frost[4] has laid the foundation for the quantitative evaluation of bone remodeling by morphologic techniques. Even in states of abnormal bone turnover, such as Paget's disease and hyperparathyroidism, this anatomic tethering of formation and resorption persists, although, as is obvious from the changing skeletal mass,

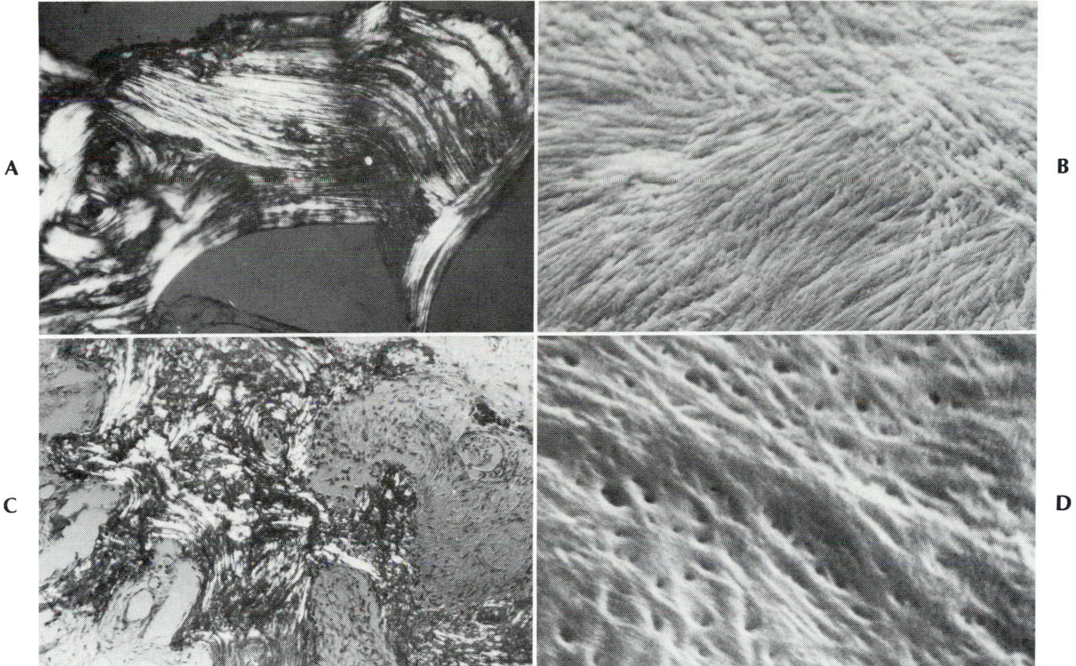

Fig. 40-4. A, Lamellar bone collagen as viewed under polarized light. Fibers are of uniform diameter and arranged in parallel fashion. **B,** Scanning electron micrograph of lamellar bone. **C,** Woven bone collagen viewed under polarized light. There is random directionality of fibers. **D,** Scanning electron micrograph of woven bone. Architectural arrangement and dimensions of collagen bundles are varied. (**A,** Decalcified; **A** and **C,** hematoxylin and eosin; 100×; **B** and **D,** 1000×.)

the rates of each of these functions generally differ. This association may be temporarily disrupted when the skeleton is perturbed by a new stimulus, such as a therapeutic agent. It is therefore extremely important to evaluate effects of a perturbation at a point past the transient time, which may be determined morphologically.[2] Undoubtedly many misconceptions concerning the effects of various drugs on the skeleton have arisen from evaluation of transient phenomena.

Repair is the fourth distinct functional activity of bone. Not only does this occur in a gross manner, but microfractures are probably always undergoing repair somewhere in the skeleton.

The importance of recognizing the distinction between these four processes relates not only to the appreciation of human skeletal dynamics but also to the choice of laboratory animals. Much work related to bone remodeling is of limited value because the studies were performed on rats. Since this animal continues to grow until death,[6] the processes of modeling and remodeling cannot be distinguished.

Matrical phase

Organic matrix

Bone consists of a relatively small number of cells undergoing metabolic activity in a vast organic and inorganic matrix. The organic component, of which 90% is collagen,[13] comprises approximately 25% of the dry weight of bone.[18] Bone collagen is produced by osteoblasts (and perhaps osteocytes) and is structurally and immunologically defined as exclusively type I, which is relatively insoluble in denaturing agents.[21] Because more than half of the body's collagen resides in bone,[9,10] and since collagen contains virtually all mammalian hydroxyproline and hydroxylysine,[20] urinary excretion of these two amino acids is a useful marker of skeletal resorption.[21]

The architecture of bone collagen reflects the rate at which it is synthesized. Nonfetal bone collagen is normally deposited in a lamellar fashion, characterized by parallel, relatively uniform bundles that are best appreciated by polarized or scanning electron microscopy. The architecture of fetal bone collagen, in contrast, is "woven." Its bundles vary in size and are randomly arranged. Woven bone is not formed in persons older than 4 years[8] except in states of accelerated bone synthesis, such as fracture repair or hyperparathyroidism. In normal skeletal development or repair, it serves as a scaffold for lamellar bone deposition and eventually undergoes osteoclastic resorption (Fig. 40-4).

The noncollagenous organic component of bone is the ground substance, which is particularly rich in glycosaminoglycans and proteoglycans.[15] These compounds contain abundant hexosamines,[16] particularly chondroitin sulfates,[15] and are therefore metachromatic. Glycosaminoglycans not only may play a role in mineralization but may also aggregate with collagen fibrils, perhaps increasing their stability.[12]

Recently an abundant noncollagenous protein containing the vitamin K–dependent amino acid, gamma-carboxyglutamate, has been described in bone.[11,14] This protein, known as osteocalcin or bone GLA-protein, avidly binds calcium. Hence it is incorporated in the mineral phase[17] and is therefore likely to be mobilized early in resorption. Circulating osteocalcin has been found to be elevated in a variety of conditions characterized by accelerated bone resorption.[19] Despite these interesting observations, the physiologic role of the protein is unknown.

Mineral phase

The mineral component of bone exists in at least two phases.[29,32,36] A few years ago it was commonly accepted that bone mineral is deposited in a roentgenographically amorphous form, [30,31] which within a short period of time transforms into crystalline hydroxyapatite. These conclusions were generally based on experiments involving synthetic materials. The ability to perform electron probe and x-ray diffraction analyses of mineralized tissues that have not been exposed to aqueous fixatives has resulted in serious challenge to the hypothesis.[26,29] Currently all that one may assume about the state of bone mineral is that it is deposited in one phase, which is probably not amorphous calcium phosphate, and with time it undergoes transformation to, or replacement by, another phase.

Although the mechanism by which mineralization occurs is in debate, there is little question that the relationship of the inorganic phase to its organic counterpart is of vital importance (Fig. 40-5). As with any structure, the strength of bone depends not only on the absolute quantities of its various components but also on the relationships of these components to one another. Hence, although pagetic bone may contain normal quantities of organic and inorganic material, because of its composition, it is relatively unstable. Therefore abnormalities of bone must be evaluated in qualitative as well as quantitative terms.

Bone cells undoubtedly play an active role in mineralization. One popular theory holds that intracellular granules of mineral are important in calcification. These particles may be transiently stored in the mitochondria of osteoblasts and osteocytes, from which they are passed into the cytoplasm and packaged and extruded into osteoid as trilaminar matrix vesicles (Fig. 40-6).[33,34,35]

Mineral deposition ultimately parallels the distribution of collagen fibrils. Whether the collagen fibril is the initial locus of calcification, however, remains in question. Glimcher and Krane[13] have shown that tropocollagen molecules are arranged in a quarter-stagger pattern, resulting in holes that reflect their 640 Å periodicity. They postulate that mineralization initially occurs within these cavities. In contrast, Bonucci[23] believes that matrix mineralization is initiated within the ground substance. If true, this process probably does not involve osteocalcin, since patients who have received long-term treatment with vitamin K antagonists have no evidence of bone disease.[11]

A major unresolved question is why collagen of bone and dentin mineralizes, whereas type I collagen in other locations fails to do so. That this is true casts serious doubt on the previously mentioned theory that the inter-

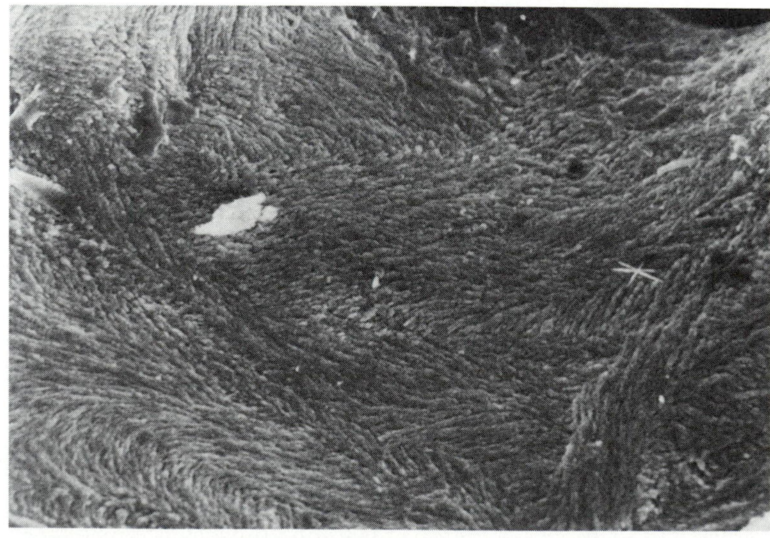

Fig. 40-5. Scanning electron micrograph of lamellar bone after extraction of all organic material. Arrangement of mineral phase of bone parallels that of bone collagen. (540×.)

fibrillar spaces initiate mineralization, since these holes are present in all collagens.[21] It is, however, possible that subtle architectural distinctions in molecular packing, perhaps in association with ground substance deposition, are responsible for the differences in propensity of various tissues to mineralize.[22]

It is believed that alkaline phosphatase plays a significant role in bone mineral deposition.[27,37] Recently, my co-workers and I have shown that stereospecific inhibition of this enzyme prevents mineralization.[24] The mechanism whereby alkaline phosphatase promotes bone calcification is unknown but may involve hydrolysis of pyrophosphate, which is thought to inhibit mineral deposition and maturation.[25,28]

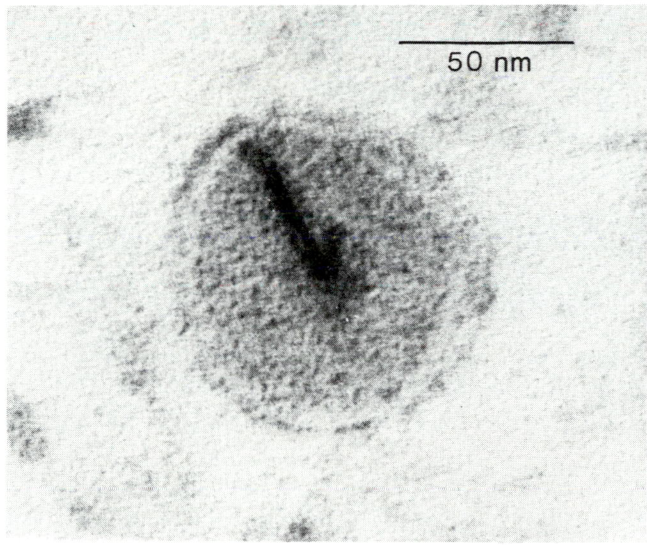

Fig. 40-6. Matrix vesicle in epiphyseal plate of rachitic rat. Vesicle contains single electron-dense crystal. (609,000×; courtesy Dr. H. Clarke Anderson, Kansas City, Kans.; from Anderson, H.C.: Calcium-accumulating vesicles in the intracellular matrix of bone. In Hard tissue growth, repair and remineralization, Ciba Foundation Symposium 11 [new series], Amsterdam, 1973, Elsevier/North Holland.)

Bone cells

Osteoblasts

Osteoblasts synthesize and mineralize bone matrix.[31] Consequently they contain abundant ribonuclear protein and are extremely basophilic. They also have a large Golgi apparatus, which appears histologically as a prominent perinuclear clear zone. When actively synthesizing bone, osteoblasts always line an osteoid seam (Fig. 40-7).

Although there are exceptions,[54] the microscopic appearance of osteoblasts generally reflects their relative bone-synthesizing activity.[45,49] Early in the formation of a cortical or trabecular osteon, synthesis of bone organic matrix is extremely rapid, and osteoblasts are cuboidal or columnar. As the osteon approaches completion, however, bone formation gradually slows. This change in kinetics is associated with a progressive flattening and attenuation of osteoblasts until they are transformed into a syncytium of fusiform cells that line the majority of bone surfaces, particularly those containing no osteoid seams (Fig. 40-8). These membranous-appearing cells generally do not synthesize bone[45,49,54] but may play an important role in calcium transport between the bone fluid compartment and general extracellular space.[40,47,51-53] Narrow spaces probably exist between these cells, which may function as channels of communication connecting the vascular system and bone surface.[47]

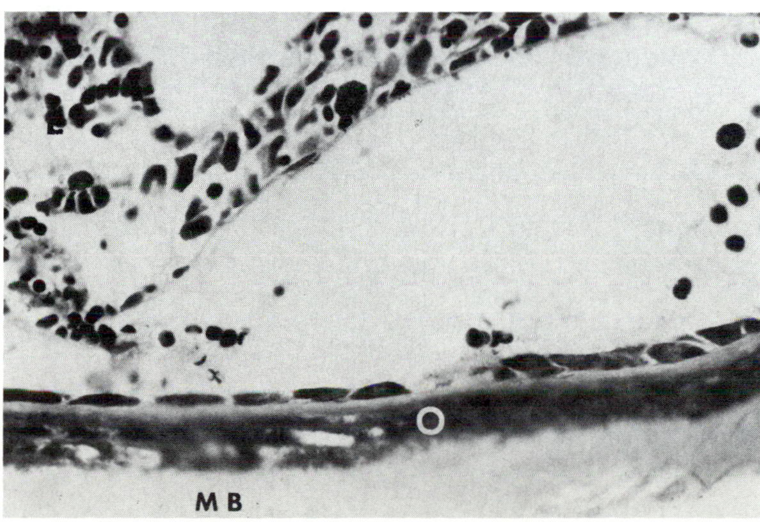

Fig. 40-7. Osteoblasts lining osteoid seam *(O)*. *MB,* Mineralized bone. (Undecalcified, Goldner's stain; 250×.)

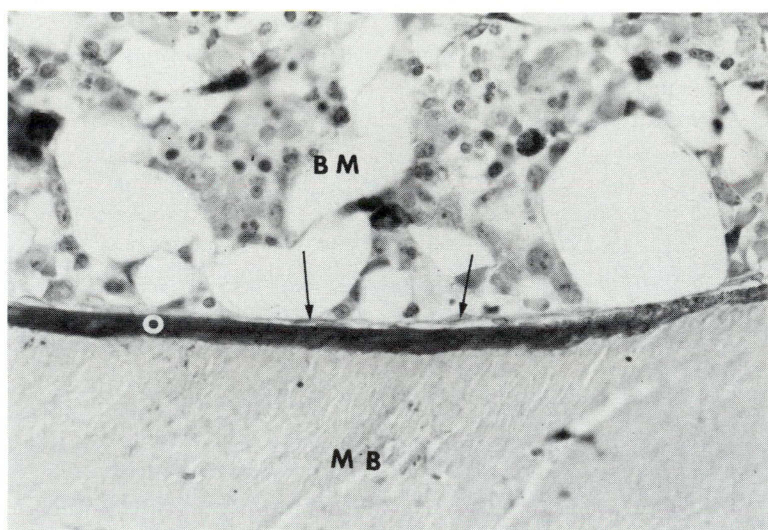

Fig. 40-8. Syncytium of fusiform cells *(arrows)* covering bone surface, which probably functionally separates bone from general extracellular fluid. *BM,* Bone marrow; *MB,* mineralized bone; *O,* osteoid. (Undecalcified, Goldner's stain; 250×.)

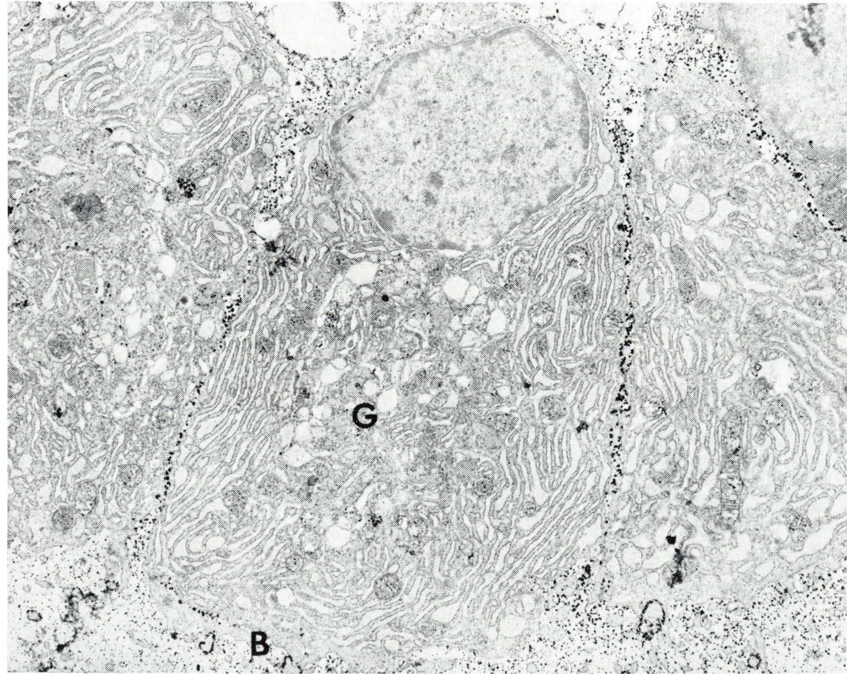

Fig. 40-9. Osteoblasts on bone matrix *(B).* Note abundant endoplasmic reticulum and prominent Golgi body *(G).* Black dots represent alkaline phosphatase reaction product. (7400×; courtesy Dr. Stephen Doty, New York, N.Y.)

Osteoblasts are also rich in alkaline phosphatase.[38,46] This enzyme is particularly important because its activity in the blood generally parallels the rate at which osteoblasts are producing bone (Fig. 40-9).[37,39,41,50]

Dramatic morphologic changes occur in osteoblasts in response to a variety of bone-related agents, such as parathyroid hormone[44] and calcitonin.[48] When examined by scanning electron microscopy, unstimulated osteoblasts appear as a mosaic of polygonal cells in a "flagstone" arrangement.[44,48] Following calcitonin exposure, the cells contract, separate from one another, and develop numerous blebs and craters.[48] Alternatively, parathyroid hormone rapidly leads to osteoblast elongation[44] and alignment of the cells in the direction of subjacent collagen fibers.[43] This parallelism of osteoblasts and matrix suggests that the formation of woven or lamellar bone is dictated by the geometry of osteoblasts.

Just how calcitonin and parathyroid hormone alter osteoblast shape remains a mystery. The cell, however, contains cytoskeletal proteins,[55] which are altered with change of osteoblast shape.[42] It is therefore possible that these hormone-induced morphologic changes of osteoblasts, which are tied to alterations of bone synthesis, may be mediated through the cytoskeleton.

Osteocytes

Following matrix deposition, most but not all osteoblasts are incorporated into osteoid as osteocytes.[61] They retain contact with their fellows and overlying osteoblasts via canaliculae through which cell processes extend and meet each other in tight junctions.[40] It is believed that this cell system regulates the transfer of calcium between the bone surface and extracellular fluid (Fig. 40-10).[47,51]

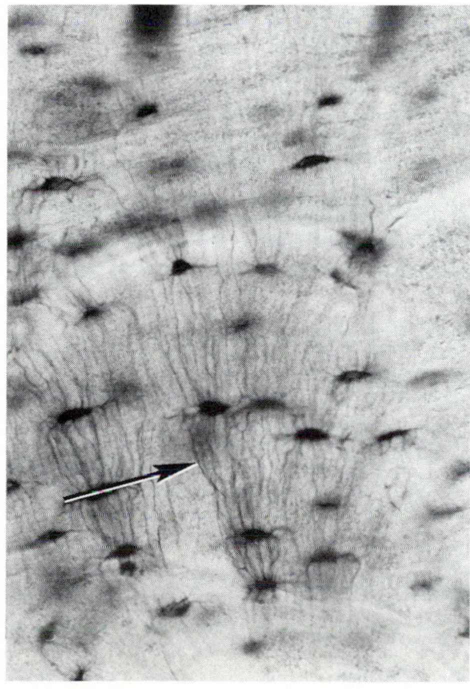

Fig. 40-10. Canaliculae *(arrow)* extending from osteocytic lacuna to osteocytic lacuna in fresh, unembedded ground section. (Villanueva bone stain; 250×.)

The number of osteocytes and the geometry of these cells are intimately related to collagen structure and the rate of bone formation. Specifically, the architecture of osteocytic lacunae is a reliable criterion for distinguishing lamellar from woven bone. Woven bone contains many more and larger lacunae than those present in its lamellar counterpart (Fig. 40-11). Moreover, as the long axes of osteocytic lacunae are oriented in the direction of collagen fibers,[63] these lacunae are parallel to each other in lamellar bone. In woven bone, however, the relative disarray of collagen fibers leads to a randomization of lacunar architecture.[64]

The size of osteocytic lacunae reflects the rate of bone formation. Consequently those in woven bone, which is always rapidly formed, are much larger than those in lamellar bone. Even within lamellar osteons the size of these lacunae varies greatly.[45] Because osteon formation is fastest at its inception, large osteocytic lacunae are found closest to cement lines. As the osteon approaches completion, formation gradually slows, resulting in relatively small lacunae closest to the haversian canal or trabecular bone surface. These differences in lacunar volume probably reflect the relationship of osteoblast size to its rate of bone formation.[49] As active cells are incorporated into bone matrix, larger lacunae are required for their accommodation.

The ability of osteocytes to mobilize bone is controversial. A body of literature is based on the assumption that these cells are capable of resorbing the walls of their lacunae, thereby playing a role in mineral homeostasis.[56,58,65,66] These conclusions result from the observation that osteocytic lacunae are larger in patients with a variety of conditions, such as primary hyperparathyroidism,[56,59] renal osteodystrophy,[60,62] or Paget's disease.[57] However, since these disorders are characterized by rapid bone formation, these large lacunae probably reflect large precursor osteoblasts rather than osteocyte-mediated resorption.

On the other hand, there is more convincing evidence that osteocytes are capable of bone deposition on their lacunar walls,[67] a conclusion that is teleologically consistent with their ontogeny. Consequently, enlarged lacunae may under certain circumstances represent deficient, osteocyte-mediated bone formation.

Osteoclasts

Osteoclasts are large, multinucleated cells that are the principal if not exclusive resorbers of bone. They differ histologically from megakaryocytes in that the nuclei of the latter are generally fused.

When engaged in resorptive activity, these cells are

juxtaposed to the bone surface in Howship's lacunae. Since there are no satisfactory methods of measuring osteoclastic activity in man, these lacunae merely inform the observer that resorption has taken place at that location and offer no information regarding the rate of matrix degradation (Fig. 40-12).

The osteoclast is the bone cell whose ultrastructural features have been most closely correlated with its activity. The ultrastructural sine qua non of the cell is the ruffled border. This complex of enfolded membrane is unique to the osteoclast and appears following exposure to resorption-promoting agents.[71] Resorption-inhibiting compounds, such as calcitonin, rapidly lead to its disappearance.[77]

Bone resorption, however, consists of two fundamental events: the attachment of osteoclasts to bone and its subsequent degradation. Binding of the cell to bone is accomplished by the ultrastructurally apparent "clear" or "ectoplasmic" zone. Unlike the ruffled border, this structure is not unique to this cell but may be seen in any member of the mononuclear phagocyte series when attaching to a subtrate.[76] This attachment is probably mediated by redistribution of the cytoskeletal protein actin, which is particularly abundant in the clear zone (Fig. 40-13).[78]

When osteoclasts are resorbing bone, the clear zone surrounds the ruffled border.[73] This circumferential isolation of the ruffled border is believed by Schenk, Spiro, and Weiner[87] to result in a microenvironment wherein biological events occur that may not be reflected in the general extracellular space.

In contrast to the ruffled border, the clear zone exists in both the resorbing and nonresorbing osteoclast.[72] In fact, treatment of parathyroid hormone–stimulated bone rudiments with resorption-inhibiting agents, such as calcitonin[77] or colchicine,[73] results in prompt disappear-

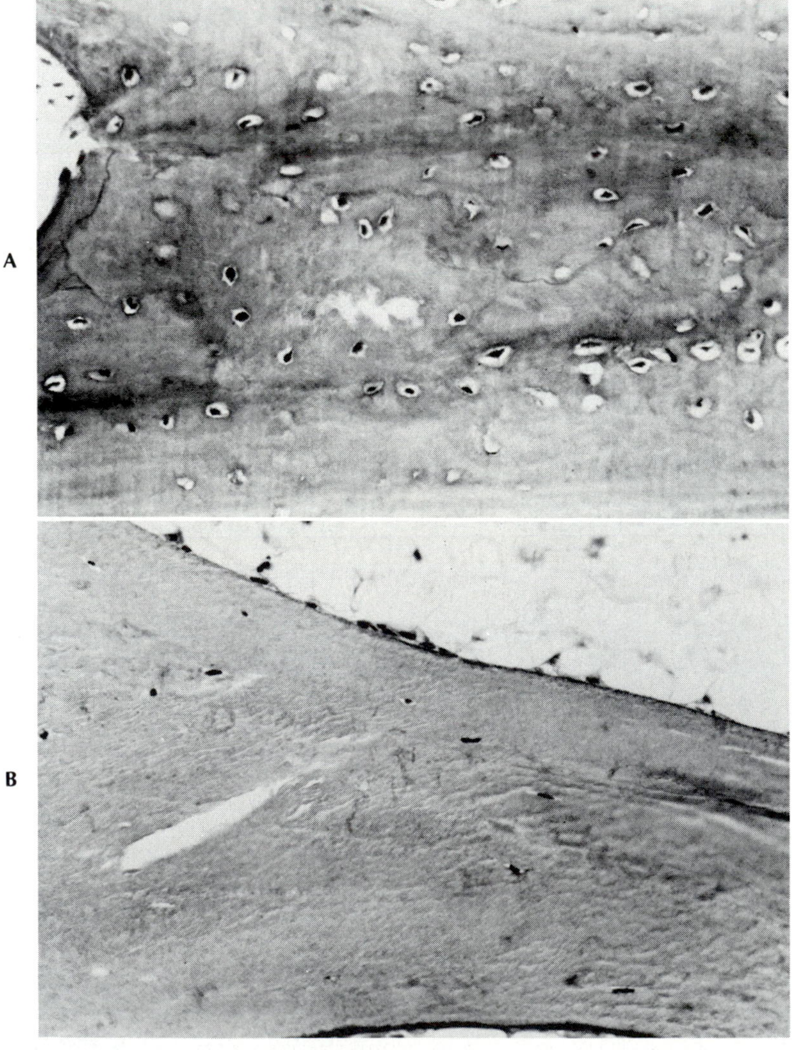

Fig. 40-11. A, Numerous, large osteocytic lacunae characterizing woven bone as compared with normal, lamellar bone, **B.** (Undecalcified, Goldner's stain; 250×.)

ance of the ruffled border and enlargement of the clear zone. These observations have lead Holtrop, Raisz, and Simmons[73] to postulate that with suppression of resorption the ruffled border is converted into clear zone.

The most potent known stimuli of bone resorption are parathyroid hormone, 1,25-dihydroxyvitamin D, and prostaglandins of the E series.[72] In addition, a lymphokine produced in vitro by plasmacytoma cells[83] or by mitogenically transformed lymphocytes[82] also promotes osteoclastic activity.[75] This peptide, known as osteoclast-activating factor, is probably responsible for the osteolysis of multiple myeloma.[83]

In considering stimulation of bone resorption, one must distinguish recruitment of additional osteoclasts from activation of those already present. It is clear that parathyroid hormone,[79] 1,25-dihydroxyvitamin D,[74] and prostaglandin E_2[86] lead to the rapid appearance of numerous "ruffled" osteoclasts and increased clear zone

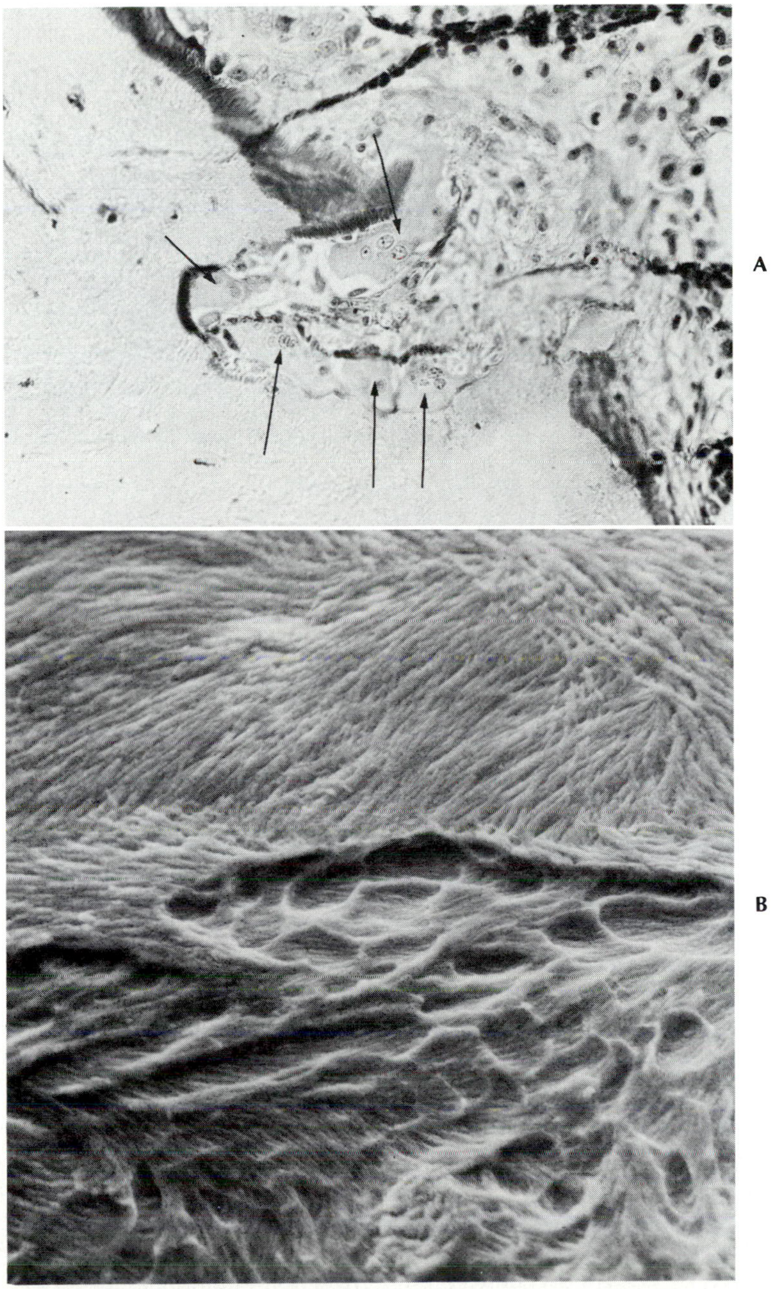

Fig. 40-12. A, Resorptive bay (Howship's lacuna) containing numerous osteoclasts *(arrows)*. **B,** Scanning electron micrograph of large resorptive bay. (**A,** Undecalcified, Goldner's stain; 250×; **B,** 750×.)

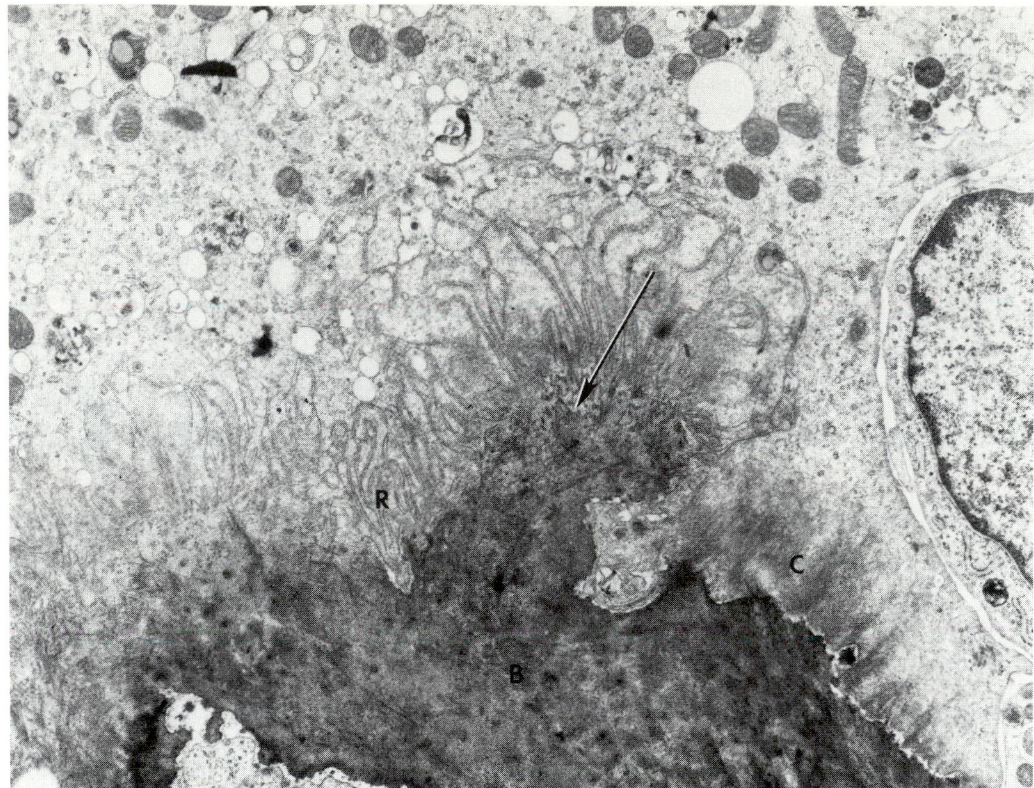

Fig. 40-13. Electron micrograph of osteoclast. Cell is attached to bone *(B)* via actin-rich clear zone *(C)*. Resorption is taking place at ruffled border *(R)* as evidenced by presence of demineralized collagen fibers *(arrow)*. (Nondecalcified; 2000×; from Teitelbaum, S.L., and Bullough, P.G.: The pathophysiology of bone and joint disease, Bethesda, Md., 1979, The American Association of Pathologists.)

and nuclear size. Additional osteoclasts are recruited many hours later. Because the morphologic features of early osteoclast activation are ultrastructural and not recognizable by light microscopy, one must avoid equating the normal delayed increase in cell number following a resorptive stimulus with a sluggish osteoclast response.

The ruffled border is undoubtedly the major site of bone matrix degradation. Its complexity and extent markedly increase the resorbing surface of the osteoclast that initially destroys the lamina limitans, the dense protein-rich line defining the border of a mineralized surface. There is also little question that, in bone resorption, mobilization of the inorganic phase and its associated noncollagenous proteins precede collagen digestion.[68] Moreover, the state of tissue calcification is central to osteoclast activity, since unmineralized matrix is resistant to resorption.[69]

Most investigators believe that bone mineral mobilization involves organic acid secretion,[88] perhaps mediated by carbonic anhydrase activity,[70,85] but this hypothesis is by no means confirmed.[81] At least part of the resorbed mineral is released in crystalline form and transported intracellularly by endocytosis via coated pits in the cell membrane.[80] Following engulfment, the particles are seen in cytoplasmic vacuoles and probably move to secondary lysosomes, where they undergo dissolution.[80]

The release of bone mineral during the initial phase of resorption results in exposure of frayed collagen bundles.[68] Significantly less is known about the means by which these fibers are digested than about how mineral is mobilized. The process probably involves extracellular digestion of the organic fibers by either acid hydrolases[89] or collagenase.[84]

Origin of bone cells

Few problems in the study of mineralized tissues have generated as much interest and controversy as the ontogeny of bone cells. Although not all of the issues have been resolved, significant insights into the origins of osteoblasts and osteoclasts have been gained.

Until recently there were two conflicting theories of bone cell ontogeny. The older theory held that both osteoblasts and osteoclasts are derived from a common marrow-residing precursor, which differentiated into either bone-forming or bone-resorbing cells, depending on the stimulus.[67,91] In 1973 Rasmussen and Bordier[65] modified this theory by hypothesizing that a common progenitor cell differentiates exclusively into osteoclasts, which subsequently undergo cytokinesis to form osteoblasts. There is little question, however, that osteoblasts and osteoclasts are derived from distinct precursors and that osteoclasts do not differentiate into osteoblasts.

Osteoblast origin. Much of the difficulty with determining osteoblast precursors has rested on the use of static morphologic techniques. These studies generally involved identification of a marrow-residing cell, usually located close to bone matrix, which the investigator subjectively labeled "osteoprogenitorial."[90] These techniques do not, however, permit direct identification of the transformation of such cells into osteoblasts, and therefore any such conclusions are at best intuitive.

In contrast, the work of Friedenstein[95] in the Soviet Union has been the most productive in confirming the presence of osteoprogenitor cells in the marrow. This investigator has cloned subpopulations of marrow-residing fibroblast-like cells and demonstrated that they form bone when implanted into the soft tissues of experimental animals. On the other hand, fibroblasts from other organs, such as spleen, do not form osseous tissue unless they are placed in contact with a substance that "induces" bone formation. The sum and substance of these experiments is that among fibroblasts there are at least two distinct populations of osteoblast precursors: (1) those that reside in bone marrow and can differentiate directly into bone-forming cells, and (2) those that exist in nonosseous tissues and can be induced into osteoblast differentiation. It is the latter population that is no doubt responsible for the development of heterotopic ossification.

Osteoclast origin. It has recently become clear that the osteoclast is derived from a cell of hemopoietic origin, probably a member of the monocyte-macrophage family. This concept is not new; it was proposed in 1949 by Hancox,[97] who noticed functional and morphologic similarities among osteoclasts, mononuclear phagocytes, and foreign body–type giant cells. Subsequently a number of investigators, using a variety of exogenously administered morphologic probes that can be followed from cell type to cell type, accumulated a host of circumstantial evidence that osteoclast formation occurs by fusion of mononuclear phagocytes.[92,94,96,98] Within the past few years a series of experiments performed in our laboratory has demonstrated that macrophages can resorb bone in an osteoclast-like manner[76,100,101] and that osteoclasts and osteoblasts are indeed derived from distinct precursors.[99] The most exciting such experiment involved bone marrow transplantation from a brother to a sister.[93] After transplantation, Y chromosomes were identified in the majority of osteoclast nuclei but were absent in osteoblasts.

Although it is clear that the osteoclast is derived from a hemopoietic precursor, its precise parentage has not been established. Specifically, direct transformation of macrophages to osteoclasts has never been observed. Moreover, the relationship between osteoclasts and macrophages is complex because it has been shown that under certain circumstances macrophages influence osteoclast function.[102] It is therefore probable that macrophages not only serve as osteoclast precursors but also as secondary effectors of bone resorption.

SKELETAL DEVELOPMENT

Skeletal development occurs by either endochondral or intramembranous ossification. The former entails partial replacement of a cartilaginous model by bone, with the residual cartilage serving as the growth plate and articular surface. Intramembranous ossification occurs by differentiation of primitive mesenchymal cells directly into osteoblasts that produce bone in the absence of cartilage.

Endochondral ossification

Cartilage is an avascular tissue that originates as clusters of primitive mesenchymal cells differentiating into chondroblasts, which in turn produce a matrix rich in mucopolysaccharides (Fig. 40-14). Like bone, cartilage can grow appositionally by development of perichondral cells into chondrocytes. The ability of cartilage to grow interstitially, however, enables it to serve as the skeletal growth plate. Interstitial growth implies duplication within the ground substances of chondrocytes, which in turn produce additional intracellular matrix and therefore expand the cartilaginous mass (Fig. 40-15).

Tubular bones develop predominantly but not exclusively by endochondral ossification. The transformation of cartilage to bone initially occurs at ossification centers within the cartilaginous model and at the perichondrium. As longitudinal growth occurs, the physis forms, consisting of four anatomically distinct zones. The zone of resting cartilage is firmly adherent to the overlying epiphyseal bone. The proliferating zone is characterized by vertical columns of chondrocytes, which expand the plate interstitially until they enter the hypertrophic zone, where they enlarge and polarize. It is in this zone that oxygen tension is lowest and the cellular metabolism is entirely anaerobic.[103] Alkaline phosphatase is produced by the hypertrophic cells closest to the metaphysis, presumably promoting formation of the zone of calcified cartilage (Fig. 40-16).

Just how growth plate cartilage mineralizes is unknown, but the geometry of the cells is probably important. Chondrocytes within the mineralized zone are arranged in orderly columns that are separated by well-mineralized, longitudinal septa. The matrix separating chondrocytes in the horizontal plane, however, is poorly mineralized.[87]

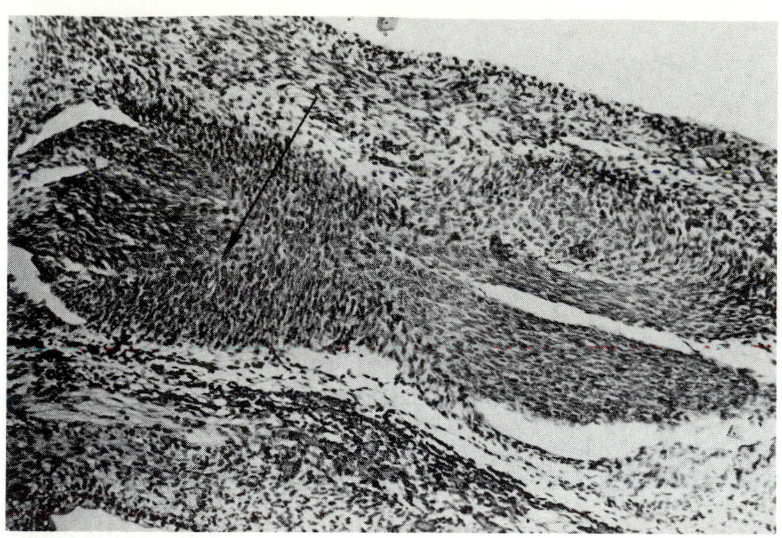

Fig. 40-14. Cluster of primitive mesenchymal cells *(arrow)* before differentiation into chondroblasts. (Hematoxylin and eosin; 80×.)

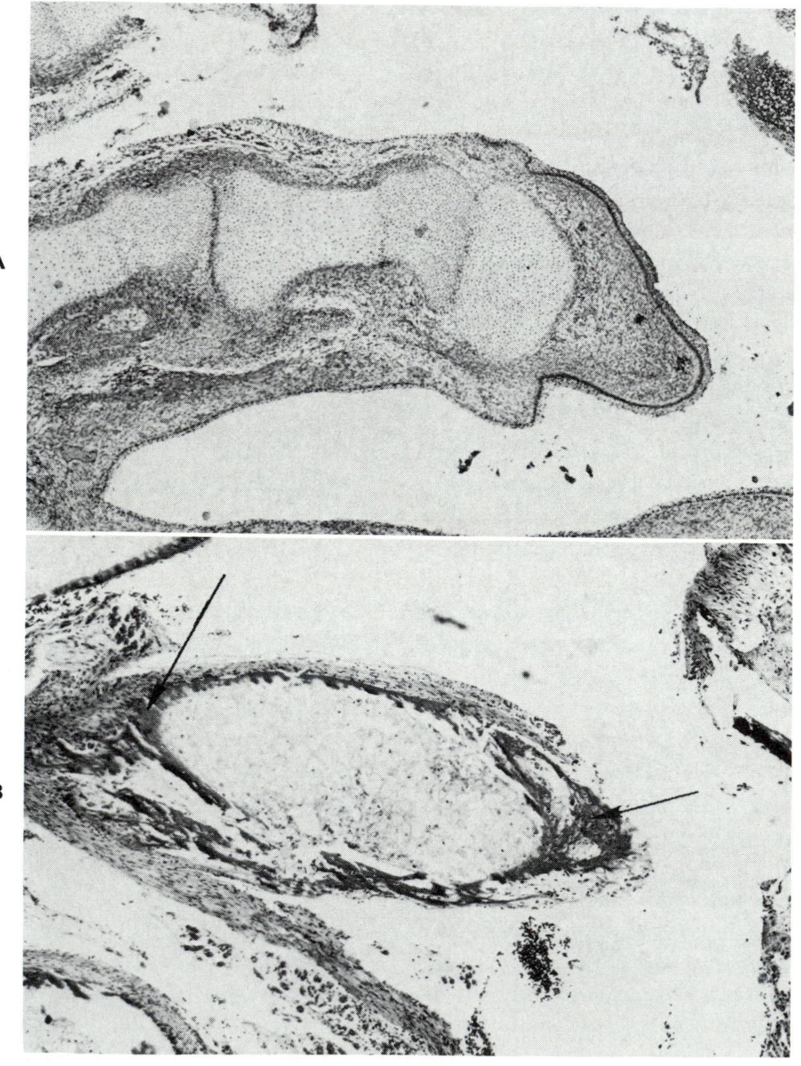

Fig. 40-15. A, Cartilaginous model of digit that will undergo endochondral ossification. **B,** Bone *(arrows)* forming in periphery of cartilaginous model in normal endochondral ossification. (Hematoxylin and eosin; **A,** 40×; **B,** 80×.)

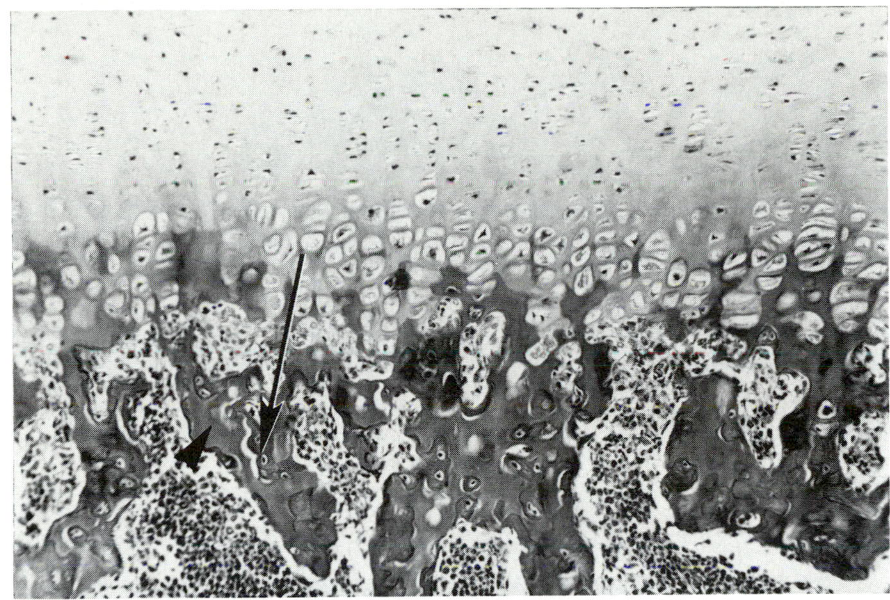

Fig. 40-16. Normal growth plate (physis). Chondrocytes enlarge as they approach metaphyseal bone. Cartilage subsequently undergoes mineralization, dies, and serves as lattice for deposition of bone. This complex of mineralized cartilage *(arrowhead)* and bone *(arrow)* is known as primary spongiosa. (Hematoxylin and eosin; 40×.)

Eventually both the horizontal and the longitudinal septa of the physis are resorbed, although much of the longitudinal septa persists for some time. Schenk, Spiro, and Weiner[87] have shown that, although the mineralized longitudinal trabeculae are degraded by chondroclasts (osteoclasts), resorption of unmineralized cartilage occurs by vascular invasion.

In any event the mineralized cartilage, which is temporarily spared, serves as a lattice for the deposition of bone in the primary spongiosa. This complex of mineralized cartilage and bone is eventually resorbed and replaced by lamellar bone, forming the metaphyseal trabeculae. Therefore, while the physis is expanded by interstitial growth of the proliferative zone, it is replaced by bone on the metaphyseal side, resulting in elongation of the shaft. As longitudinal bone growth occurs, it becomes necessary to expand and shape the bone to adult proportions. Structural modeling is accomplished by intramembranous ossification involving apposition and resorption at appropriate locations on the subperiosteal and endosteal surfaces. The cessation of interstitial expansion of the physeal plate results in its gradual obliteration and termination of growth.

Transformation of a cartilaginous model to bone may relate to vascular invasion from the metaphysis. The fact that osteoblasts and chondroblasts are probably ontogenetically related[104,105,112] may also be significant. In fact, not all chondrocytes in the hypertrophic zone of the growth plate die with its subsequent mineralization, but many appear to be converted into osteoblasts.[106,107,108] This conclusion is consistent with the observation that as chondrocytes pass through the mineralized zone, their collagen production shifts from type II, which is unique to cartilage, to type I of bone.[108,111] In addition, chondrocytes may induce other stromal cells to undergo osteoblastic differentiation.[109,110] Evidently there is a continuum of cellular activity between chondroblasts and osteoblasts eventuating in endochondral ossification.

Intramembranous ossification

Intramembranous ossification, the process responsible for development of the major part of the axial skeleton, differs from endochondral ossification in that no cartilaginous model is formed. Since bone cannot grow interstitially, intramembranous bone develops only by apposition.

The process originates with mesenchymal cells that cluster together in centers of ossification. These cells differentiate into large osteoblasts, which in turn produce the collagen matrix and ground substance. Coincidentally with secretion of alkaline phosphatase, mineralization occurs. This initial trabecula lined by osteoblasts branches into other trabeculae by apposition (Fig. 40-17). As the trabeculae widen, osteoblasts are included in the matrix as osteocytes. The trabeculae destined to form compact bone continue to expand, incorporating blood vessels into haversian canals. As the ossification center expands and joins its neighbors, structural modeling begins in a manner similar to that in endochondral ossification.

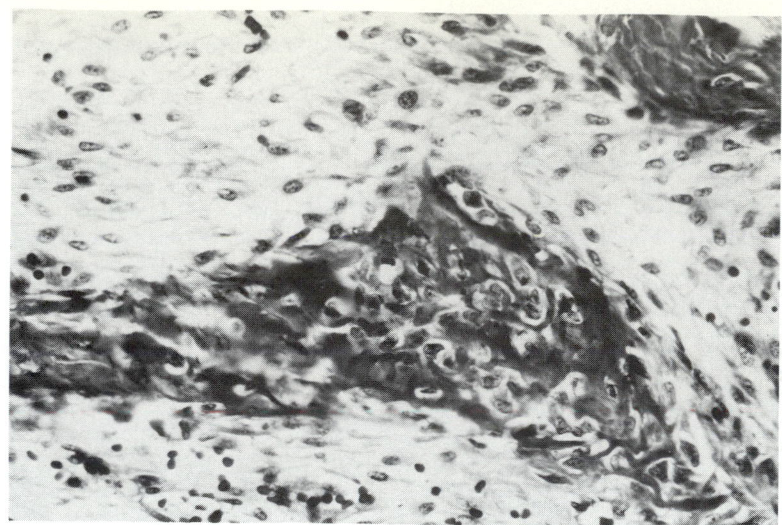

Fig. 40-17. Intramembranous ossification. Mesenchymal cells have differentiated directly into osteoblasts and are forming bone in absence of cartilaginous model. (Hematoxylin and eosin; 250×.)

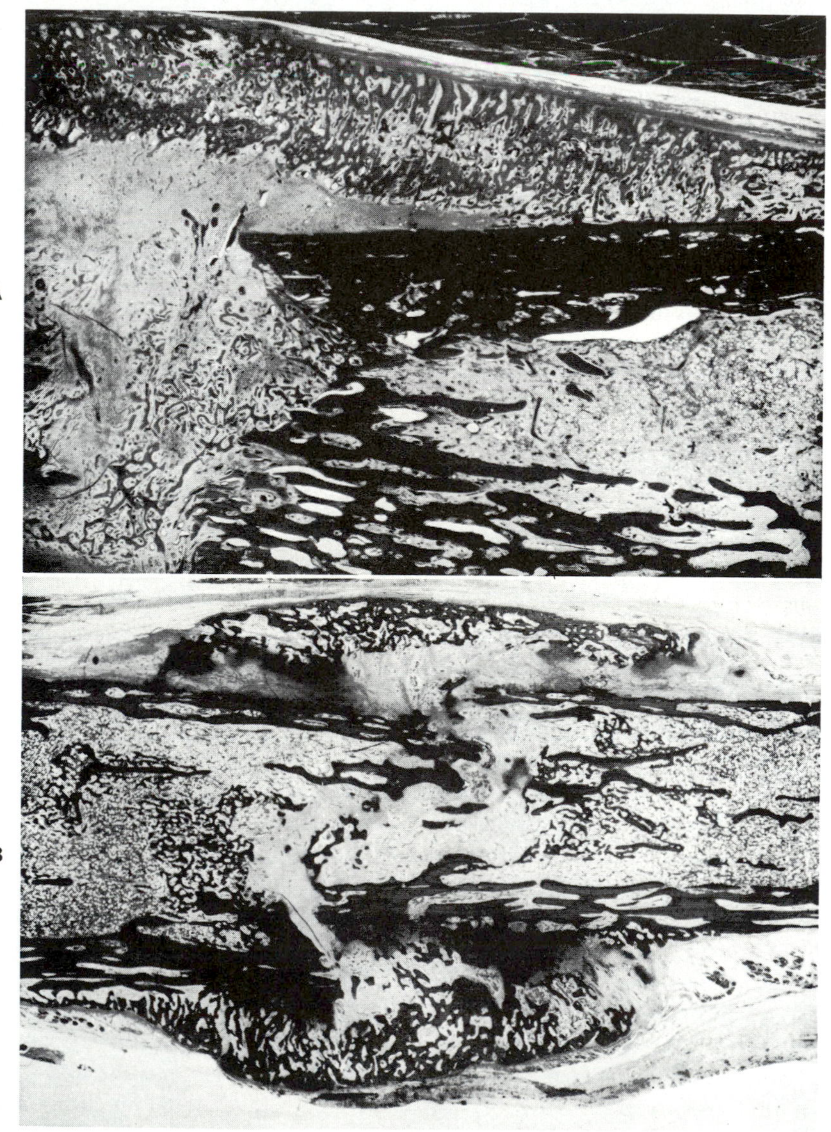

Fig. 40-18. A, Subperiosteal and intermediate callus in healing fracture of tibia of young child. **B,** Ten-month-old fracture site in rib of elderly woman. Interlocking ends of fractured bone are encased in abundant external and internal callus, which is in part cartilaginous and in part bony. (8×; from Bennett, G. A., and Bauer, W.: In Scudder, C.L., editor: The treatment of fractures, Philadelphia, 1938, W.B. Saunders Co.)

REPAIR

In a sense, repair is a microcosm of endochondral and intramembranous bone formation occurring in a tissue known as callus, which is deposited during fracture healing and is eventually modeled into normal bone. Analogous to growing bone, callus is dynamic and undergoes structural change much faster than mature osseous tissue. It is composed primarily of fibrous tissue, woven bone, and cartilage.[113] All of these components are derived from common endosteal or periosteal progenitor cells. Mechanical stress and oxygen tension are important in determining whether these cells differentiate into osteoblasts or chondroblasts. For example, intermittent stress favors cartilage formation.[118] Hence, immobilized fractures exhibit a predominance of intramembranous ossification, whereas endochondral ossification occurs in free fractures.[120] Similarly, low oxygen tension promotes chondroid rather than osteoid formation (Fig. 40-18).[123]

Shortly after fracture, periosteal osteoprogenitor cells proliferate along the entire shaft but particularly close to the break.[122] Locally these cells initiate formation of early external callus, collaring the ends of the bony fragments.[122] Endosteal progenitor cell recruitment promotes internal callus formation, which grows into the interfragmentary space. Probably resorption of dead spicules by osteoclasts and macrophages also enhances callus formation, since this devitalized tissue contains factors that promote the synthesis of cartilage and bone.[117,121] The clinical expression of these varied effects of fracture on bone formation is the propensity of a traumatized extremity of a child to grow longer than its contralateral partner.[115]

Because of its rapid growth and lack of proximity to blood vessels, external (superficial) callus is relatively avascular and anoxic, and its osteoprogenitor cells differentiate into chondroblasts rather than osteoblasts.[113] Hence early superficial callus is composed primarily of cartilage, whereas in the deep, more vascular location, woven bone is directly formed. With vascular encroachment the cartilaginous portion of callus is mineralized, dies, and is replaced by woven trabeculae. Active modeling of the mature callus occurs with replacement of woven bone by lamellae. Similar to intramembraous ossification, compaction of trabecular bone into cortex occurs where appropriate.

Fractures that are in poor alignment form exuberant callus. In contrast, those that are well aligned, particularly if internally immobilized, form little if any external callus. In addition, fracture repair entails modeling of haversian systems, which eventually cross the interfragmentary space. The speed with which this occurs depends on the degree of alignment.[119]

Nonunion is the condition wherein the repair process has stopped before complete healing. The space between the nonfused fragments of bone is generally filled with fibrous tissue and organizing hematoma (Fig. 40-19). Because repair is arrested, successful treatment of this condition necessitates recruitment or activation of bone cells. Great strides in this area have resulted from insights into the effect of electrical current on bone. Brighton and his colleagues[116] have shown that normally repairing bone exhibits electronegativity. Consequently, electrical currents have been applied to accelerate fracture repair[114] and heal nonunion.[116]

DISORDERS OF REMODELING

Morphologic methods of diagnosis

Metabolic bone diseases are generally disorders of remodeling and are characterized by involvement of the entire bony skeleton. That is not to say that the morphologic manifestations of any of these diseases may not vary in severity from one location to another. However, unlike neoplastic or inflammatory processes, which are focal or multifocal, metabolic bone diseases are diffuse. Therefore, with the realization that various bones have different quantities of cortex and trabecula and are subjected to distinct physical stresses, skeletal tissue from any site in a patient with a metabolic bone disease will exhibit some evidence of the disorder.

Perhaps the most important problem in diagnosing metabolic bone diseases is to distinguish diminished bone mass caused by osteoporosis (decreased mass of normally mineralized bone) from that caused by osteomalacia (defective mineralization). Roentgenographic studies are generally incapable of making this distinction, as are more sophisticated techniques of delineating abnormalities of skeletal mass, such as photon absorption bone densitometry and computerized axial tomography. The various types of deficient skeletal mass, indistinguishable by noninvasive techniques, should be classified under the generic term *osteopenia*.

Histologic examination of the skeleton is usually necessary to discriminate among the osteopenias. However, processing of bone by decalcification before paraffin embedding, as is practiced routinely in the histology laboratory, obscures the differences between mineralized and nonmineralized bone collagen (osteoid) (Fig. 40-20). Since osteomalacia is characterized by osteoid accumulation, its distinction from osteoporosis can be made only by studying nondecalcified bone sections (Fig. 40-21).

The application of histology to the diagnosis of generalized skeletal disorders rests on the ease with which bone biopsy samples can be obtained. Fortunately, a variety of trocars specifically designed to obtain large samples of the iliac crest are currently available. This procedure is relatively atraumatic even when performed with local anesthesia. My patients undergo multiple sequential biopsies on an outpatient basis, enabling me to follow the histologic progression of their disease as well as the effects of treatment.

The structural characteristics of bone lend themselves

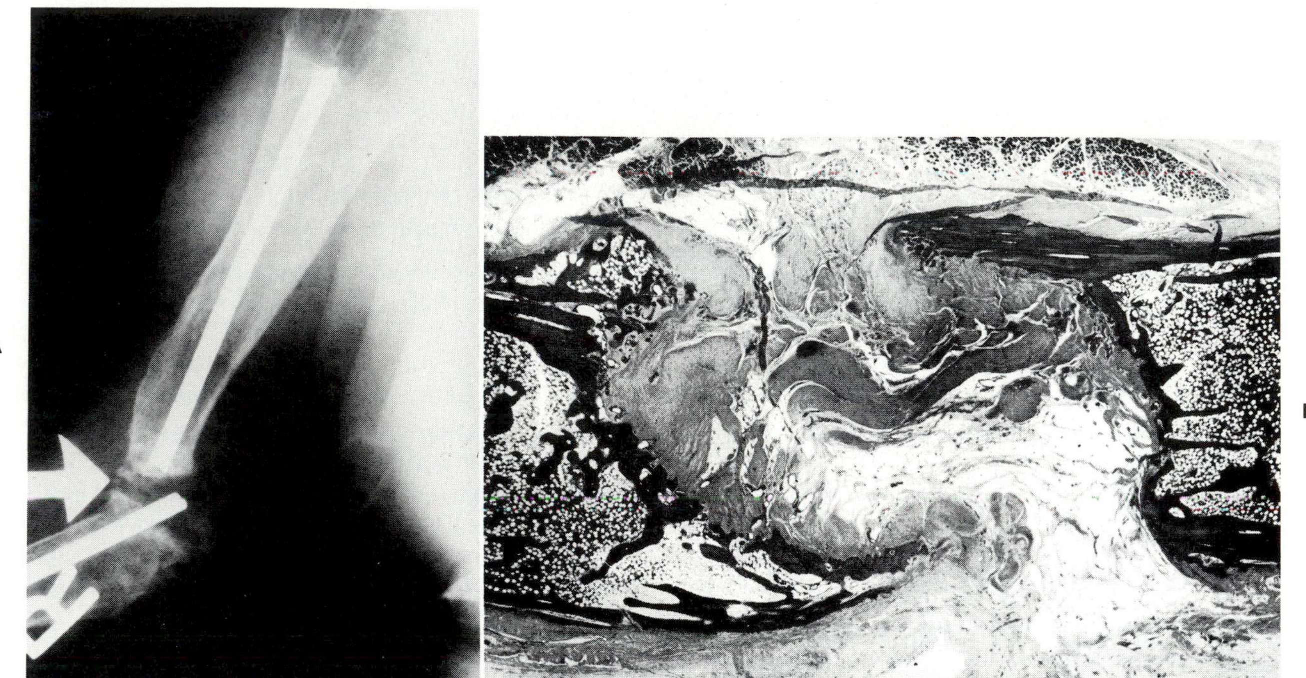

Fig. 40-19. A, Nonunion of fracture of humerus. **B,** Fracture site has resulted in fibrous union, and no evidence of reparative changes remains. Medulla of each fractured bone end is enclosed by osseous plate into which dense connective tissue bundles insert. (**A,** Courtesy Dr. Jerome Gilden, St. Louis, Mo.; **B,** 9×.)

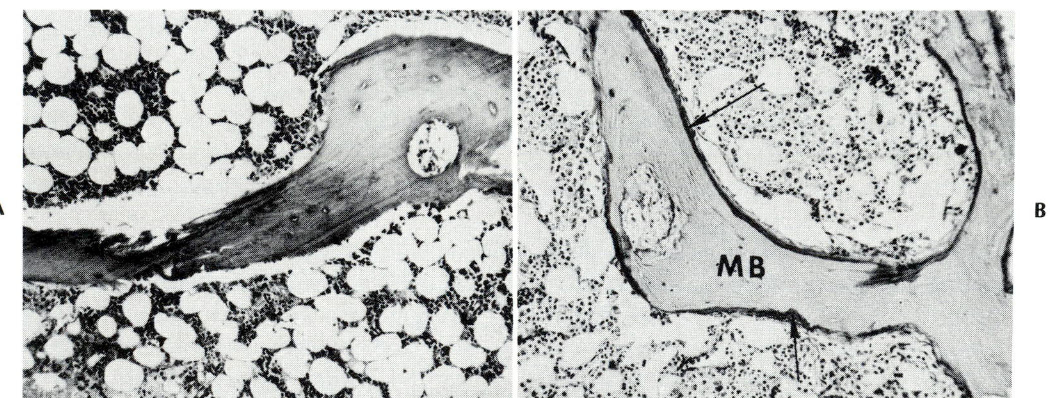

Fig. 40-20. A, Decalcified, paraffin-embedded bone biopsy specimen. It is not possible to distinguish mineralized from nonmineralized bone matrix by this technique. **B,** Nondecalcified, plastic-embedded section of bone taken simultaneously with **A.** Distinction between mineralized bone *(MB)* and nonmineralized bone matrix or osteoid *(arrows)* is easily made. In addition, there is superior preservation of bone architecture. (**A,** Hematoxylin and eosin; **B,** Goldner's stain; **A** and **B,** 100×.)

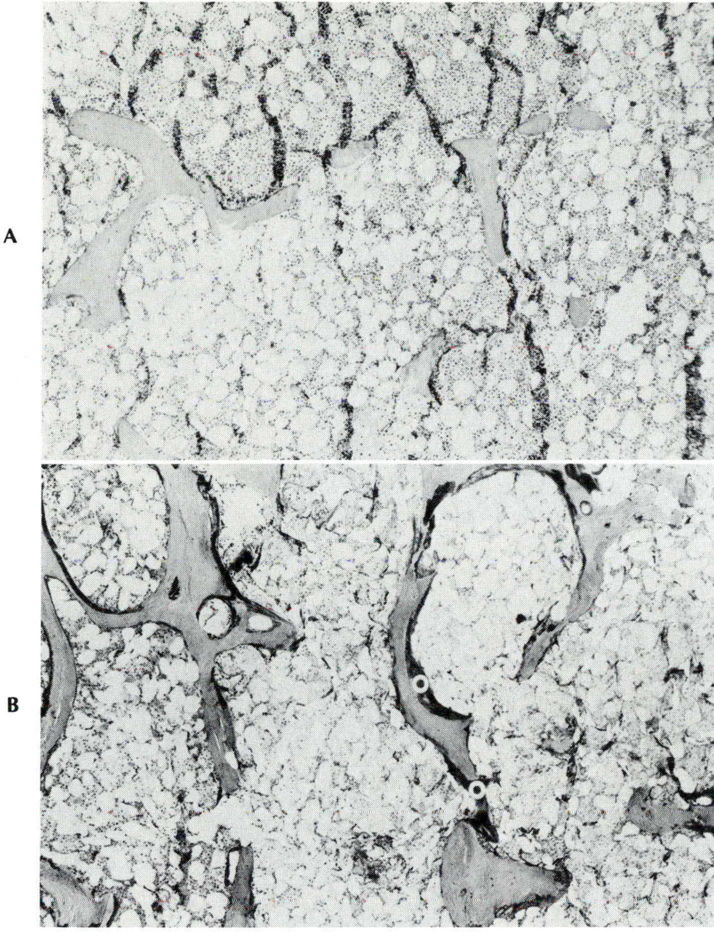

Fig. 40-21. A, Osteoporotic trabecular bone. Quantity of bone matrix is diminished but normally mineralized. **B,** Osteomalacic trabecular bone. Excess of osteoid *(O)* is present. Both **A** and **B** were taken from patients whose roentgenograms exhibited identical degree of osteopenia. (Undecalcified, Goldner's stain; 40×.)

to histologic quantitation. The amounts of mineralized and nonmineralized organic matrix are easily determined from nondecalcified sections. In addition, the cellular components of the skeleton may be quantitated with a high degree of precision.[127,133,135-137,141]

It is important to appreciate, however, that only static structural features of any tissue can be determined by examining a histologic section representing one point in time. For example, an abundance of osteoclasts and osteoblasts does not invariably mean that bone turnover is accelerated.[130,132] Similarly, osteoid accumulation does not always reflect defective mineralization (see discussion later in chapter). Fortunately, there are techniques, based on the use of tetracyclines, that permit the study of kinetic parameters in a single bone biopsy specimen.

Because of their fluorescent properties[129] and ability to complex with calcium,[131] tetracyclines are the most useful morphologic markers of mineralization.[145] In normal lamellar bone they are deposited exclusively at the calcification (mineralization) front at the interface between osteoid and mineralized lamellar bone (Fig. 40-22).[127,128] The predisposition of these antibiotics for this location is due to their stoichiometric binding to immature bone mineral.[36,138] Woven bone, which contains no calcification front, diffusely fluoresces when labeled with tetracycline, reflecting the predominance of immature mineral throughout this rapidly turning-over tissue (Fig. 40-23). Why tetracyclines bind only to immature hydroxyapatite in sufficient quantity to produce fluorescence is unknown, but it may be related to steric properties of the crystal.

Mineralization defects are often reflected by abnormalities in fluorescence of the calcification front. Although states of severe vitamin D[126] and phosphate deficiency[143] are associated with a decrease in the percentage of the mineralization front capable of assuming a fluorescent tetracycline label, more subtle abnormalities of calcification are characterized by wider and more diffuse patterns of fluorescence (Fig. 40-24).[7,138] This com-

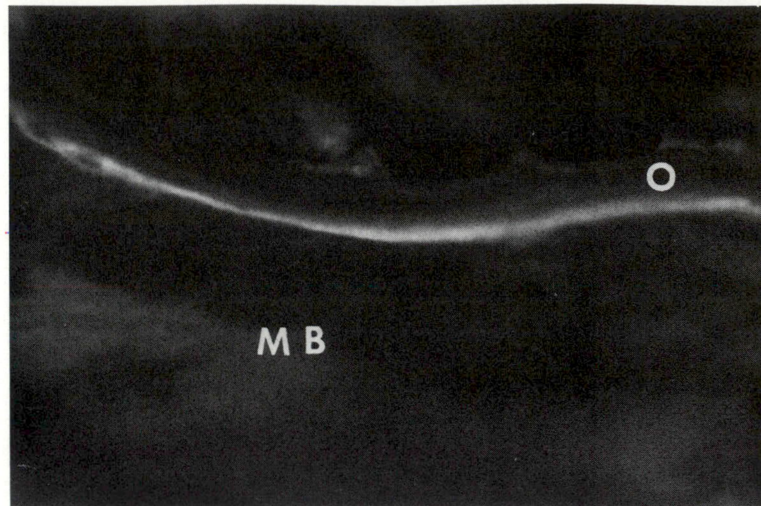

Fig. 40-22. Normal fluorescence of mineralization front following administration of tetracycline. Mineralization front is located at interface between osteoid *(O)* and mineralized bone *(MB)*. (Undecalcified, unstained; 250×.)

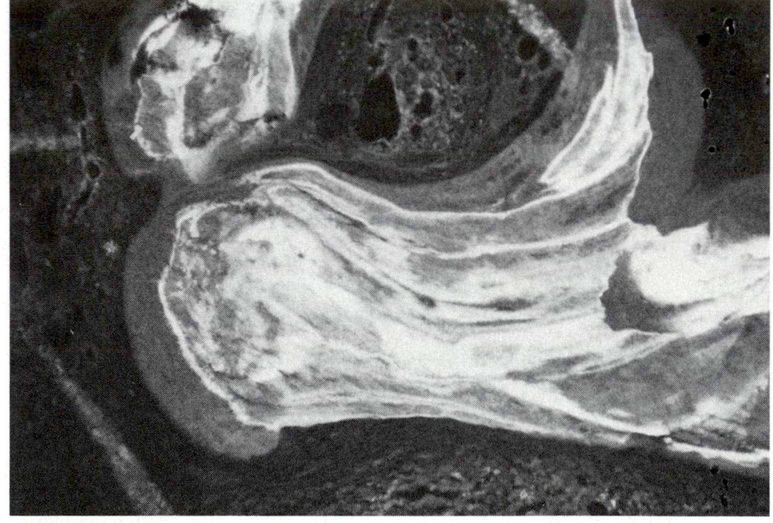

Fig. 40-23. Fluorescent micrograph of woven bone following administration of tetracycline. Bone diffusely fluoresces without distinct formation of calcification front formation. (Undecalcified, unstained; 100×.)

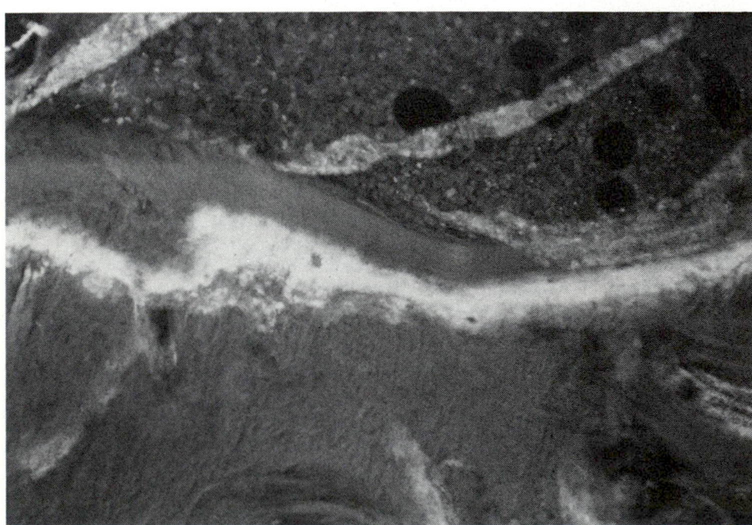

Fig. 40-24. Fluorescent micrograph of bone biopsy specimen from patient with osteomalacia. Compare with Fig. 40-22 and note wide diffuse appearance of fluorescent tables after administration of tetracycline. (Undecalcified, unstained; 250×.)

monly occurs in chronic renal failure,[124,144] Paget's disease, hypophosphatemic osteomalacia,[143] and experimentally in early vitamin D deprivation.[125] The diffuse fluorescence probably represents delayed maturation of calcium phosphate.[142] In addition, fluorescent antibiotics often diffuse through entire hypomineralized osteons in these diseases (Fig. 40-25). Since mineral maturation is retarded in human[140] and experimental renal failure,[39] the pattern of tetracycline fluorescence is probably the morphologic counterpart of this biophysically demonstrable abnormality.

The application of tetracyclines as kinetic markers of bone formation is based on administration of two time-spaced doses of the antibiotic.[129] This results in the development of two parallel fluorescent lines at sites of ongoing calcification (Fig. 40-26). The cellular rate of mineralization, which is the rate of mineralization at the average point on a bone-forming surface, is calculated by determining the mean distance between the two fluorescent labels and dividing this distance by the interval between doses.[134] The tissue-level bone mineralization rate, which is the total quantity of bone formed per unit of bone volume per unit of time, may then be calculated by multiplying the cellular rate by the absolute extent of bone surface containing fluorescent labels.

Distinction between cellular and tissue rates of bone mineralization is often fundamental to understanding the mechanisms of metabolic bone diseases. In certain circumstances, for example, the cellular and tissue rates differ from normal in opposite directions.[146] Specifically, parathyroid hormone, which recruits additional osteoblasts, may suppress the rate at which the average cell forms bone.[146] Hence, although tissue rate is increased in primary hyperparathyroidism, some patients have suppressed cellular level mineralization.[146]

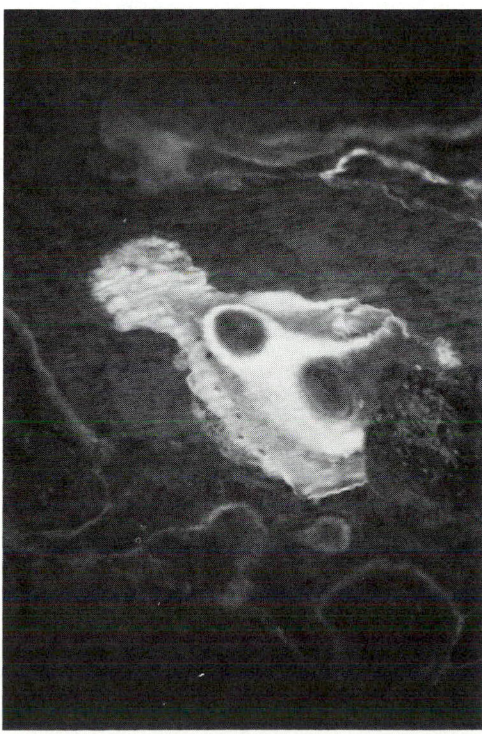

Fig. 40-25. Entire osteon fluorescing following administration of tetracycline to patient with chronic renal failure. (Undecalcified, unstained; 40×.)

These tetracycline-based techniques also permit identification of specific cellular mechanisms leading to osteoid accumulation. Osteoid may accumulate because of a decreased rate of mineralization (osteomalacia) or because of enhancement of its synthesis. If the cellular rate of mineralization is subnormal, the excess osteoid must be caused by osteomalacia. Conversely, abundant osteoid in the face of a normal or increased cellular rate of mineralization must reflect its accelerated deposition. This distinction is more than academic and has profound therapeutic implications, as discussed later in the chapter.

Physiologic effects of hormones, vitamins, inorganic compounds, enzymes, and viruses on bone, with attendant dysfunctions

Parathyroid hormone and vitamin D

Parathyroid hormone and vitamin D are probably the most important humoral determinants of skeletal activity. It is not surprising therefore that their metabolisms and biologic effects are interrelated (Fig. 40-27).

Parathyroid hormone. Parathyroid hormone is an 84 amino acid peptide[147] whose biologic activity resides in the first 26 to 34 residues.[156] Its secretion is primarily if not exclusively under the influence of circulating ionized calcium.[154] When the unbound fraction of this cation falls slightly, the parathyroid glands respond with enhanced secretion, which diminishes as the free calcium level rises. This exquisite tethering of circulating calcium and parathyroid hormone release is the cornerstone of normal mineral homeostasis.

The effects of parathyroid hormone are directed toward elevating serum calcium and are achieved via bone and kidneys. Although the hormone promotes recruitment of both osteoblasts[153] and osteoclasts,[79] its net effect on the skeleton is generally resorption.[148,150,152,155] This may be related to the fact that although additional osteoblasts appear,[79] in the uncomplicated state parathyroid hormone generally inhibits the individual activity of these bone-forming cells.[79,149] In contrast, the peptide not only recruits osteoclasts but also stimulates the activity of each cell.[153]

The renal effects of parathyroid hormone involve calcium, phosphorus, and vitamin D (see following discussion). The hormone enhances renal tubular resorption of calcium, which directly increases its serum levels.[151] In addition, there is a reciprocal relationship between cir-

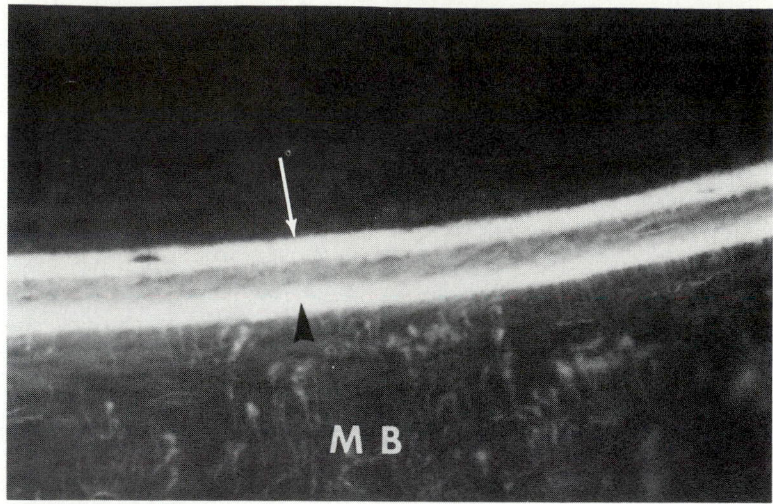

Fig. 40-26. Fluorescent micrograph of bone following administration of two courses of tetracycline. Label *(arrowhead)* deepest in mineralized bone *(MB)* represents first dose. Second label *(arrow)* represents dose administered 2 weeks later. Cellular rate of mineralization is determined by measuring distance between these labels and dividing that distance by interdose duration. (Undecalcified and unstained; 500×.)

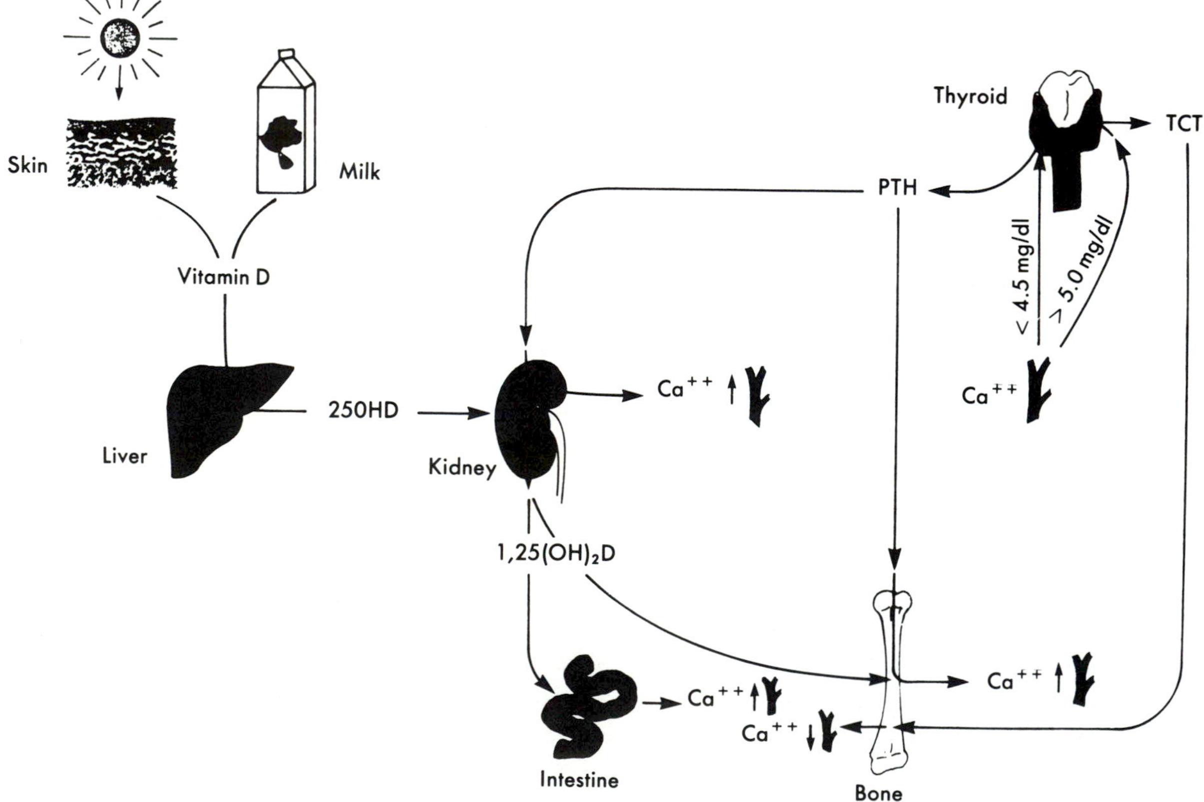

Fig. 40-27. Fundamental aspects of calcium homeostasis. Parathyroid hormone (PTH) secretion is stimulated by fall in blood ionized calcium *Ca^{++})*. PTH in turn directly mobilizes Ca^{++} from bone and promotes resorption of Ca^{++} from renal tubule. It also promotes conversion of 25-hydroxyvitamin D (25 OHD) to 1,25-dihydroxyvitamin D (1,25[OH]$_2$D). The latter enhances intestinal absorption of calcium and acts synergistically with PTH to stimulate bone resorption. Calcitonin (TCT), which inhibits bone resorption, is secreted when serum Ca^{++} increases.

culating calcium and phosphorus. Consequently, the hormone also raises the serum calcium level by its phosphaturic effect.[151]

Vitamin D. Within the past decade there have been great advances in defining the biochemistry and metabolism of vitamin D.[162] The steroid is obtained through diet or by ultraviolet irradiation of the skin.[162,166] The latter process, which contributes most of the vitamin D present in Americans, entails photoconversion of 7-dehydrocholesterol to the parent compound.[166]

Although other metabolites have been described, the two known important metabolic products of vitamin D are its 25-hydroxylated and 1,25-dihydroxylated compounds, which are synthesized in the liver[159,168] and kidney,[163] respectively. The concentrations of circulating 25-hydroxycholecalciferol, the major circulating metabolite of vitamin D, are directly related to dietary consumption of the vitamin and its photosynthesis.[164] The serum levels of this substance are highest in the summer,[165] when the incidence of osteomalacia in hip fractures is lowest.[157]

The production of 1,25-dihydroxyvitamin D, on the other hand, is humorally regulated. The process is initiated by activation of renal 25-hydroxyvitamin D–1-alpha-hydroxylase by parathyroid hormone.[169] As 1,25-dihydroxyvitamin D is synthesized, it raises serum calcium levels, which in turn reduce secretion of parathyroid hormone.[167] The increase in serum calcium is accomplished primarily by enhancement of its intestinal absorption, which is largely under the influence of the dihydroxylated metabolite.[161] Because of this classic feedback mechanism regulating the serum levels of 1,25-dihydroxyvitamin D, the steroid should be considered a hormone.

Vitamin D plays a critical role in bone mineralization. Circumstantial evidence suggests a direct physiologic action on the vitamin during skeletal calcification[171]; however, this has yet to be proved.[161] The mineralization of osteoid that follows administration of this compound to osteomalacic patients may theoretically be caused by stimulated intestinal absorption of calcium or bone resorption[161] leading to increased concentrations of calcium or phosphorus or both in the extracellular fluid.

The well-defined, direct role of vitamin D on bone relates to its osteolytic properties[160] in which the relative potencies of its metabolites differ greatly. Whereas the parent compound has no resorptive properties in vitro, 25-hydroxycholecalciferol has significant potency, which is superseded 100 fold by 1,25-dihydroxycholecalciferol.[170]

The direct effects of vitamin D on bone are best studied experimentally in the parathyroidectomized state. In this circumstance large doses of cholecalciferol induce osteoclastic and osteoblastic hyperplasia and proliferation of epiphyseal chondrocytes.[172] Bone alkaline phosphatase also increases.[172] These changes accompany hydroxyprolinuria and a rise in serum calcium to within the normal range.[172] On the other hand, physiologic doses of vitamin D administered to parathyroidectomized animals fail to induce these biochemical alterations and produce no distinctive morphologic changes.[172] It therefore appears that the physiologic effects of vitamin D on the skeleton are synergistically related to parathyroid hormone. Similarly, the skeletal manifestations of parathyroid hormone are blunted in the vitamin D–deficient state.[158]

Primary hyperparathyroidism. Primary hyperparathyroidism is the state of parathyroid hormone excess in a relatively uncomplicated milieu. It therefore is the pathologic condition that most accurately reflects experimental administration of the hormone.

The clinical manifestations of the disease are protean. In the past, patients usually had either renal or skeletal complications. Since the advent of multiphasic screening, however, most are asymptomatic,[186] and only 20% have roentgenographic skeletal changes.[180,185] On the other hand, approximately half of all patients retain increased quantities of bone-seeking tracers, making radionuclide scanning a sensitive method of detecting skeletal involvement.[178]

Bone disease when symptomatic may be striking. Not only do pain and fractures develop[175] but deformities—particularly those produced by cystic lesions—may be crippling.

The roentgenographic changes of primary hyperparathyroidism are usually first evident in the phalanges. Properly prepared hand films, particularly with magnification techniques, often show resorption of the subperiosteal bone of the radial aspect of the fingers. Intracortical striations, reflecting increased cortical porosity, also appear early but are a nonspecific sign of bone loss (Fig. 40-28). Roentgenographic evidence of more advanced skeletal involvement includes the cystic lesions of von Recklinghausen's disease of bone, loss of the lamina dura of the jaw, and resorption at sites of tendon insertion, resulting in avulsion.[184]

The net effect of primary hyperparathyroidism on skeletal mass is heterogeneous and controversial. Bone densitometry studies are consistent with the development of osteopenia,[148,155] whereas when histologically quantitated, cortical and trabecular bone volumes are normal.[183] In addition, the disease may occasionally be complicated by osteosclerosis.[179]

Virtually all patients with primary hyperparathyroidism have histologic evidence of the disease, the magnitude of which correlates with the degree of hypercalcemia.[188] There is generally an increase in the numbers of osteoclasts and osteoblasts and the percentage of trabecular surface covered by osteoid (Fig. 40-28). On the other

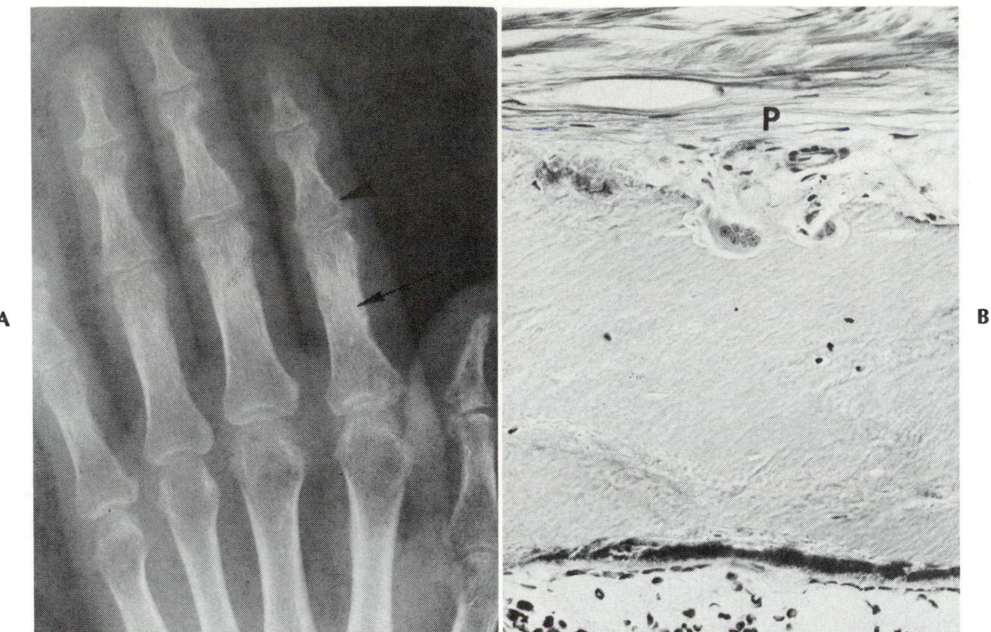

Fig. 40-28. A, Roentgenogram of hand of patient with severe skeletal disease caused by hyperparathyroidism. Intracortical striations *(arrow)* are present, as is subperiosteal resorption *(arrowhead)*. **B,** Osteoclasts resorbing subperiosteal bone in hyperparathyroidism. *P,* Periosteum. (**A,** Courtesy Dr. James W. Debnam, Jr., Chesterfield, Mo.; **B,** undecalcified, Goldner's stain; 100×.)

hand, the cellular rate of mineralization as determined by double tetracycline labeling is decreased,[183] indicating that although more osteoblasts than normal are present in primary hyperparathyroid bone, the rate of activity of each cell is diminished. The tissue rate of bone formation is enhanced, however, because many more osteoblasts are taking part in the process.[183]

In any event, it appears that primary hyperparathyroidism is characterized by the presence of increased numbers of remodeling sites and a diminished rate of individual osteoblastic activity. These data indicate that although the abundant osteoid and osteoclasts may be caused by recruitment of additional cells, there is also prolongation of the life span of remodeling units.

Precisely why osteoblast activity is diminished in primary hyperparathyroidism is unclear, but it is consistent with the suppressive effects of parathyroid hormone on bone formation in vitro.[149] Moreover, the hypophosphatemia[173] and increased[174,181] circulating 1,25-dihydroxyvitamin D levels[187] that attend the disorder also diminish bone formation in organ culture.

Osteitis fibrosa is the collective term often used to describe the microscopic features of hyperparathyroidism. However, osteitis fibrosa is a histologic entity that may occur in any state of accelerated bone turnover and in fact is significantly more frequent in a variety of other disorders, such as renal osteodystrophy, than in primary hyperparathyroidism.

Osteitis fibrosa is characterized by an abundance of osteoblasts, osteoid, and osteoclasts. The pathognomonic feature of the lesion, however, is fibrous tissue in a peritrabecular location within the marrow. In contrast, the fibrosis of idiopathic myelofibrosis is diffusely distributed throughout the marrow without respect to trabecular architecture (Fig. 40-29).

The cystic lesions of von Recklinghausen's disease of bone histologically resemble giant cell tumors (Fig. 40-30). There is osteoclast proliferation in a cellular, fibrous stroma, characteristically associated with hemosiderin deposition (brown tumor). Unlike giant cell tumors, these lesions generally occur in the diaphysis of long bones and the jaw and skull.[176] If a giant cell tumor appears in a location other than the paraepiphyseal portion of a long bone, hyperparathyroidism should be considered. In addition, fibrous dysplasia may occur with increased frequency in primary hyperparathyroidism.[177]

After parathyroidectomy of patients with primary hyperparathyroidism, the number of osteoclasts begins to decrease rapidly and returns to normal within a few hours.[182] Probably as a reflection of completion of the remodeling cycle, osteoblasts proliferate after surgery, reaching a peak within 2 weeks, after which they decline in number.[182] Within months, marrow fibrosis is markedly reduced or disappears (Fig. 40-31).

Hypoparathyroidism. Most of the available information regarding the effects of parathyroid hormone deficiency on bone is derived from experimental animals.[195,200] In the parathyroid-deprived state the rat skeleton grows poorly,[195] and osteoid formation and min-

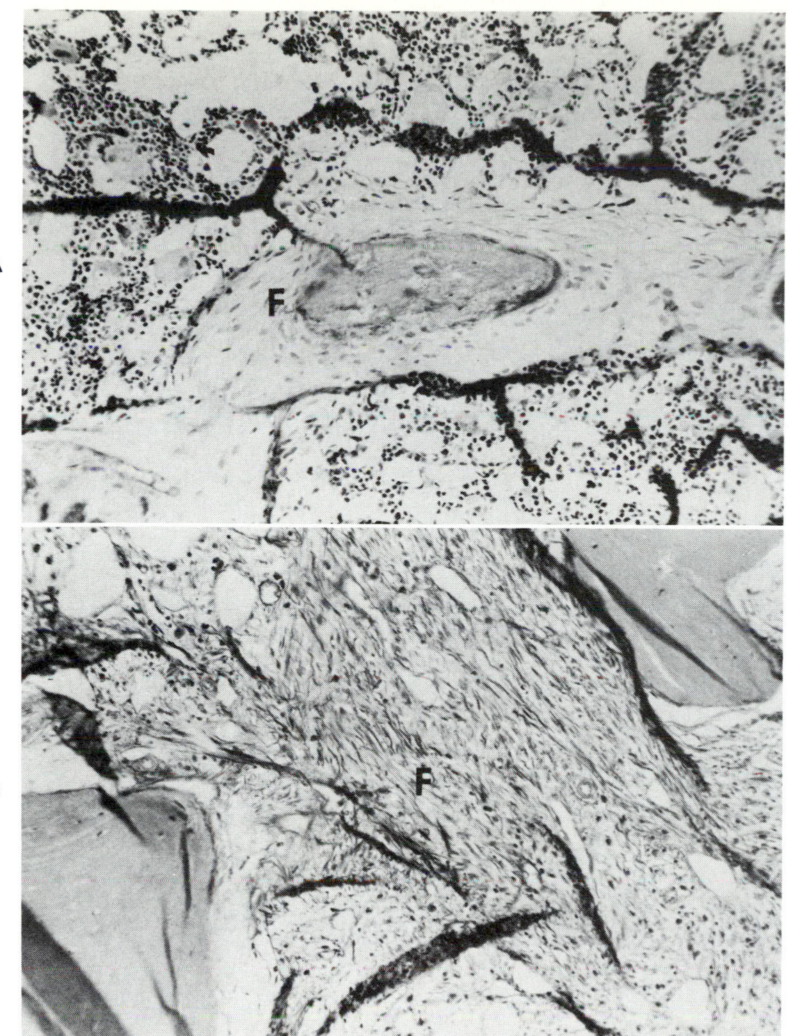

Fig. 40-29. A, Characteristic peritrabecular distribution of marrow fibrosis *(F)* of osteitis fibrosa. **B,** Distribution of fibrous tissue in idiopathic myelofibrosis. Distribution of fibrous tissue is not peritrabecular. (Undecalcified, Goldner's stain; 100×.)

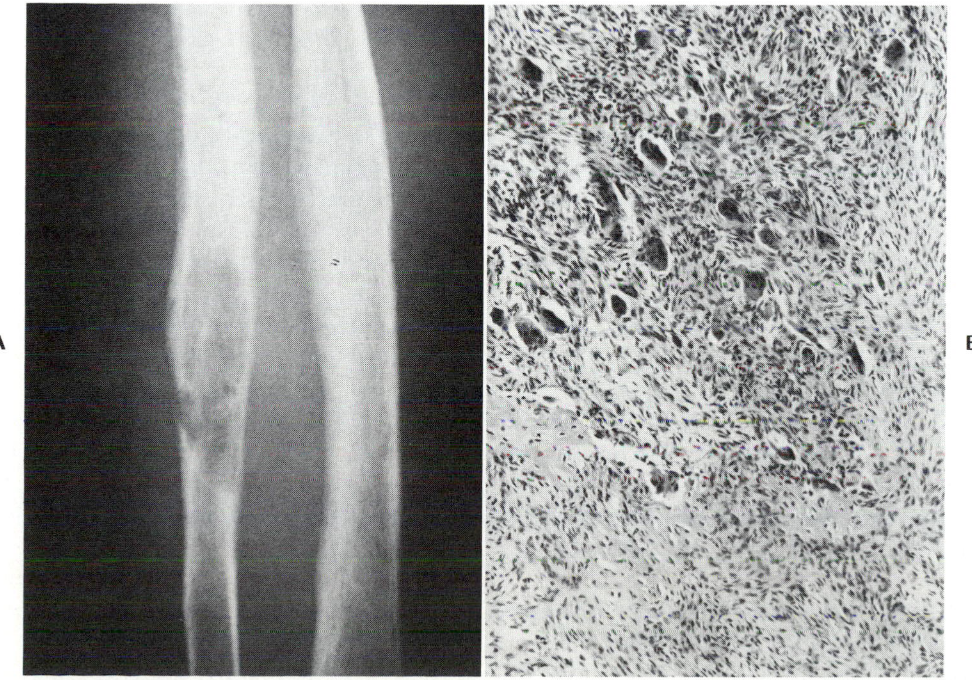

Fig. 40-30. A, Osteitis fibrosa cystica (brown tumor) of ulna. **B,** Osteitis fibrosa cystica (brown tumor). Numerous giant cells are present in cellular stroma. (**A,** Courtesy Dr. James W. Debnam, Jr., Chesterfield, Mo.; **B,** hematoxylin and eosin; 100×.)

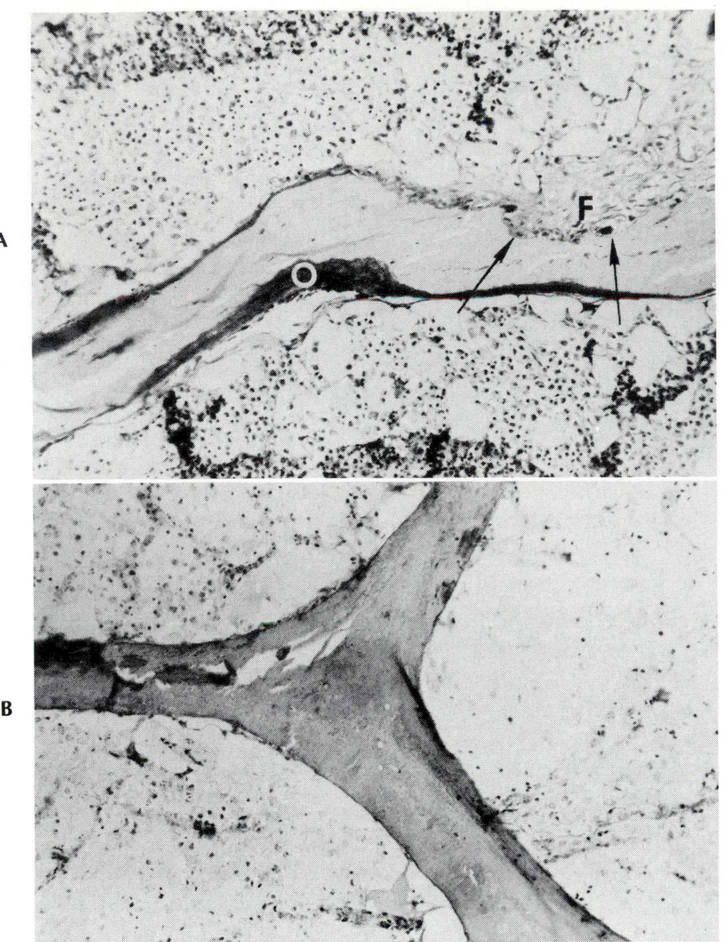

Fig. 40-31. A, Trabecular bone of patient with primary hyperparathyroidism from biopsy taken at time of parathyroidectomy. Osteitis fibrosa is present as manifested by peritrabecular fibrosis *(F)*, deep resorptive bays *(arrows)* containing osteoclasts, and wide osteoid seams *(O)*, lined by columnar osteoblasts. **B,** Bone biopsy specimen taken from same patient 1 year after parathyroidectomy. Histologic appearance of bone is now normal. (Undecalcified, Goldner's stain; 100×.)

eralization are slow.[200] As in other states of osteomalacia, defective mineralization is more pronounced than is the delay in matrix synthesis, resulting in osteoid accumulation and abnormal tetracycline labeling.[195]

It appears that hypoparathyroidism in humans also leads to osteomalacia.[189,191-193,199] The genesis of this lesion is, however, unclear. It is true that because of a lack of parathyroid hormone, circulating 1,25-dihydroxyvitamin D is diminished in hypoparathyroidism, but the magnitude of the decrease in blood levels of this metabolite is probably not sufficient to account for the attendant osteomalacia.[196] One must therefore consider the possibility that normal mineralization and matrix synthesis require a direct effect of parathyroid hormone on bone cells.

The skeletal lesion of hypoparathyroidism is similar to that of phosphate depletion, with an abundance of osteoid, poor mineralization front formation, and a paucity of osteoclasts and osteoblasts.[192] However, the majority of patients with surgical hypoparathyroidism, which is the most common form of the human parathyropyruvic state, have a spectrum of residual parathyroid tissue,[198] resulting in a variety of skeletal changes.

Patients with idiopathic hypoparathyroidism are more likely to exhibit clinical musculoskeletal abnormalities than are those with the iatrogenically induced disease. It is not uncommon to encounter changes usually associated with pseudohypoparathyroidism in these patients.[190,197] These features include soft tissue calcification and ossification,[194] abnormal dentition,[190] and osteosclerosis.[190] Intracranial calcification[190] and ankylosing spondylitis[189] also complicate idiopathic hypoparathyroidism.

Pseudohypoparathyroidism. The syndrome of pseudohypoparathyroidism consists of a multitude of phenotypic expressions. Affected patients are usually short and obese and have a characteristic moon facies. Their dentition is abnormal,[205] and the bones of the hands and

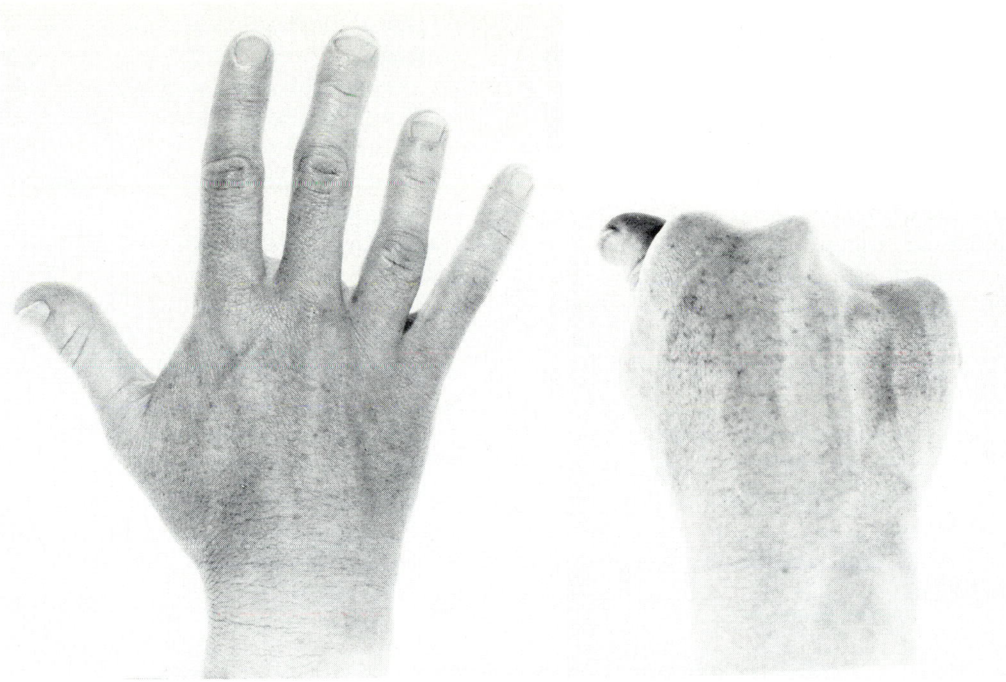

Fig. 40-32. Short fourth metacarpal of patient with pseudohyoparathyroidism. (Courtesy Dr. Susie Humphrey, Baltimore, Md.)

feet, particularly the fourth and fifth metacarpals and metatarsals, are short (Fig. 40-32).[208] The long bones are often curved, and soft tissue mineralization and ossification are common, as are cataracts and basal ganglia calcifications.[208,215] Consequently, these patients are often retarded and are prone to seizure disorders.[208]

The disease generally appears within the first decade and invariably by the end of the second.[190] Since the mode of inheritance is usually sex-linked dominant,[207,209] twice as many women as men are affected.[190] In some cases, however, the syndrome is transmitted as an autosomal recessive trait.[206,212]

The major physiologic defect in pseudohypoparathyroidism is the absence of renal excretion of phosphorus in response to parathyroid hormone. Most commonly (type I) this is associated with defective cyclic AMP generation by the kidney when exogenous parathyroid hormone is administered.[201] Patients with type II pseudohypoparathyroidism have the ability to synthesize nephrogenous cyclic AMP in response to parathyroid hormone, but like their type I counterparts, they do not generate a phosphaturia.[202]

Because of failure to excrete phosphorus, pseudohypoparathyroid patients are hyperphosphatemic and have secondary hyperparathyroidism.[208] Whether the attendant hypocalcemia is caused exclusively by hyperphosphatemia is unknown, but evidently the calcemic response to parathyroid hormone is blunted.[203] On the basis of this observation, skeletal resistance to parathyroid hormone is also a component of the syndrome.[203,208] In fact, there is a variant of the disease involving isolated bone resistance to the hormone.[210]

The poor calcemic response of these patients may be caused by abnormal vitamin D metabolism. Specifically, pseudohypoparathyroidism is generally associated with low serum levels of 1,25-dihydroxyvitamin D.[203,210,213] The calcium-mobilizing effect of parathyroid hormone is restored after normalization of circulating levels of the steroid.[203] This observation suggests that the skeletal resistance to parathyroid hormone is not caused by a primary defect in bone cells but reflects defective synthesis of 1,25-dihydroxyvitamin D.

The bone density of patients with pseudohypoparathyroidism is generally normal, although some may be osteopenic or osteosclerotic. Despite the relative infrequency with which radiologists diagnose subperiosteal resorption in this disease, most patients have histologic evidence of osteitis fibrosa. This situation is analogous to primary hyperparathyroidism and probably illustrates the relative insensitivity of standard roentgenographic techniques in detecting subtle skeletal changes.

Corresponding to the brachydactyly of pseudohypoparathyroidism,[208] the physes of tubular bones are histologically and biochemically abnormal.[214] They close prematurely and are narrow, and the chondrocytes are arranged in short columns.[209]

Idiopathic hypoparathyroidism, pseudohypoparathyroidism, and pseudo-pseudohypoparathyroidism represent a spectrum of morphologic and biochemical abnormalities.[197,204,211] Patients with idiopathic hypoparathyroidism frequently are physically similar to those with pseudohypoparathyroidism,[201] but some with the hormone-resistant disease appear normal.[204] Consequently, the diagnosis of pseudohypoparathyroidism should be reserved for hypocalcemic, hyperphosphatemic patients who, when challenged with parathyroid hormone, fail to generate a phosphaturic response.

Vitamin D deficiency. Because adequate stores of vitamin D are essential to normal calcification, its deficiency results in osteomalacia and, in the growing individual, rickets. Rickets (rachitis) refers exclusively to defective mineralization of the physis, whereas osteomalacia occurs in bony matrix. Consequently, rickets develops only before physeal closure, whereas osteomalacia may appear throughout life.

The rachitic growth plate is wide and irregular, and its architecture is in disarray. The columnar arrangement of the hypertrophic chondrocytes is lost, and the zone of provisional calcification disappears (Fig. 40-33). Cartilaginous cores extend deeply into the metaphysis, where they become surrounded by osteoid, which fails to mineralize. In affected children, cup-shaped growth plate indentations and bowed legs generally develop because of structural weakness of the widened physes and osteomalacic bone.

Secondary hyperparathyroidism and osteitis fibrosa usually accompany osteomalacia induced by vitamin D deficiency.[224] As opposed to primary hyperparathyroidism, which is the disorder of autonomous hyperfunctioning parathyroid glands, secondary hyperparathyroidism is a generic term encompassing the many conditions in which continuous parathyroid gland hyperactivity is stimulated by low levels of circulating ionized calcium. The most commonly diagnosed cause of secondary hyperparathyroidism in the United States is chronic renal failure. However, any form of vitamin D deficiency results in parathyroid gland stimulation. For example,

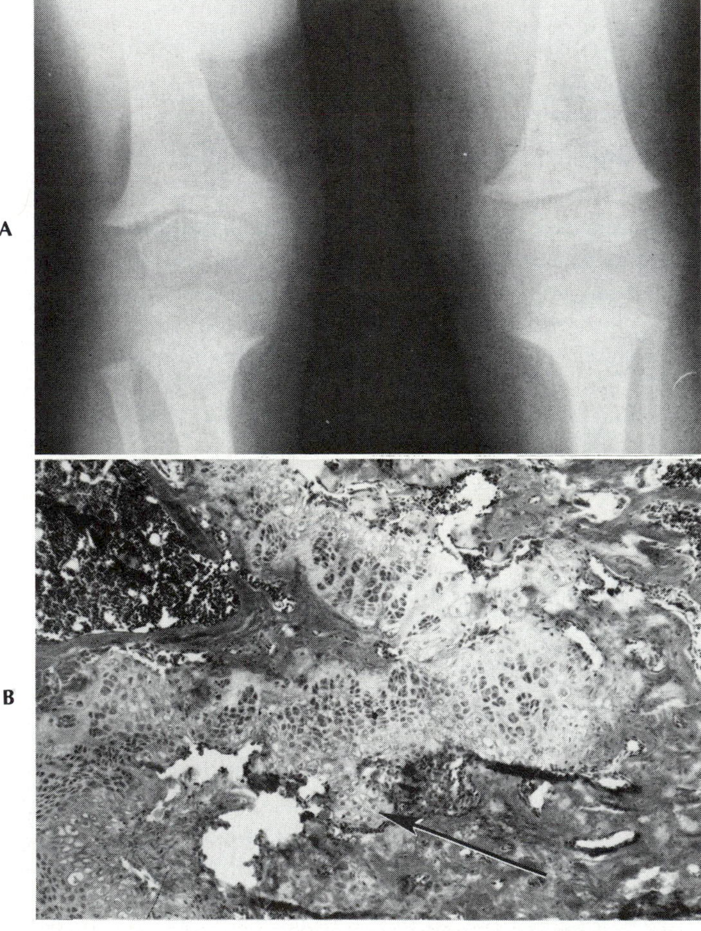

Fig. 40-33. A, Knees of rachitic child. Radiolucent growth plates are wide and irregular. **B,** Rachitic growth plate. As compared with normal physis in Fig. 40-16, gross architecture of rachitic growth plate is markedly distorted. In addition, note loss of polarity of chondrocytes and extensions of unmineralized cartilage *(arrow)* out of plane of growth plate. (Undecalcified, modified Masson's trichrome stain; 20×.)

this phenomenon almost universally accompanies severe malabsorption of the steroid, as is associated with biliary cirrhosis.[217,226] It also occurs in the large numbers of Asians with vitamin D–deficient osteomalacia who have emigrated to Great Britain. Vitamin D–deficient rickets and secondary hyperparathyroidism are also appearing in increasing numbers of American infants.[216,219] This resurgence of a historical disease is generally related to food faddism. Infants who are breast fed and receive no supplemental sources of calciferol are particularly at risk.

Within the past decade a variety of iatrogenically induced forms of vitamin D deficiency have appeared. Jejunoileal bypass surgery for morbid obesity probably has received the most attention in this regard.[229] The patients we studied had markedly reduced circulating levels of 25-hydroxyvitamin D immediately after surgery, but this defect was corrected with time.[232] However, the skeletal histology of postintestinal bypass patients varies[227] and often cannot be predicted on the basis of vitamin D stores.[227] In a number of patients classic osteomalacia develops[223,227] but there are also more subtle changes of suppressed osteoblast activity.[227] Osteoid volume is often normal, although narrow seams may cover an increased extent of trabecular surfaces.[227] The cellular rate of mineralization decreases,[227] and an increased percentage of seams fail to assume a tetracycline label.[153] One sees numerous Howship's lacunae, which contain no osteoclasts.[227] This phenomenon indicates a delay in the formation phase of the remodeling sequence and represents defective osteoblast recruitment.

This apparent histologic heterogeneity no doubt reflects the complex physiologic changes that follow intestinal bypass. The contribution that vitamin D deficiency may make is obvious, but functional caloric deprivation is perhaps more important. Rats that we have semistarved, for example, developed osteoblast dysfunction similar to that following jejunoileal bypass.[231]

The association of gastrectomy and bone loss has been long appreciated.[218,220,221] Osteomalacia eventually develops in approximately one fourth of gastrectomized patients.[218] The cause of postgastrectomy osteomalacia is unknown, but it may be due to decreased intestinal absorption of calcium[220,221] or inadequate dietary vitamin D.[222]

The bone disease following gastrectomy can be so severe that Looser's zones or pseudofractures develop (Fig. 40-34).[218] These linear cortical interruptions, which generally appear in the pelvis, represent callus that fails to mineralize. It is one of the few roentgenographic signs that are generally diagnostic of a metabolic bone disorder, although occasionally pseudofractures accompany inactive osteoporosis.[228]

Finally, total parenteral nutrition is associated with osteomalacia.[230] This lesion is probably caused by a

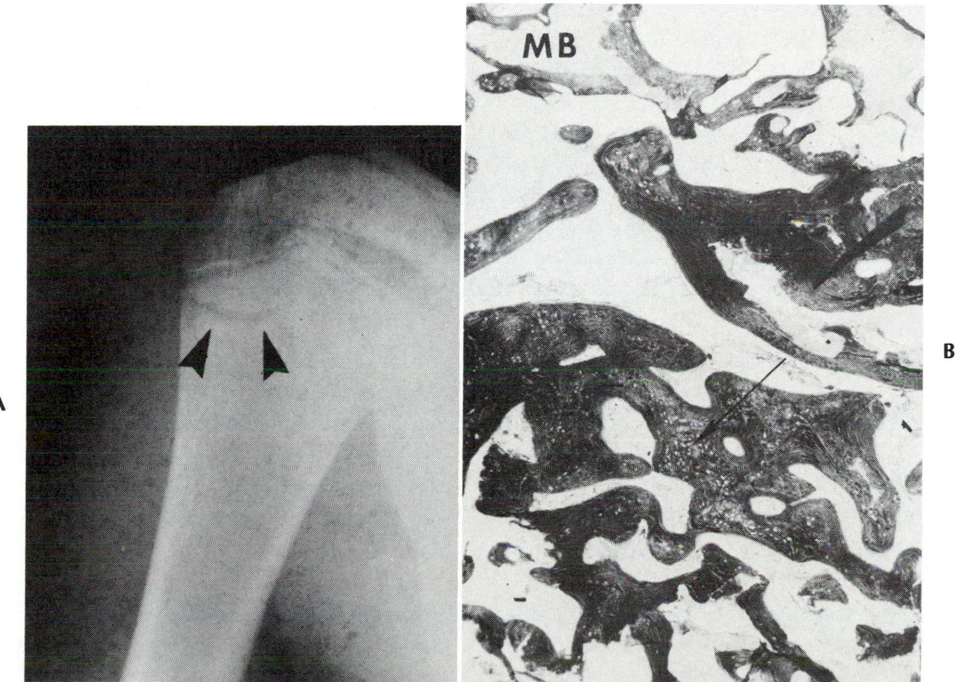

Fig. 40-34. A, Pseudofracture (Looser's zone) in proximal humerus of patient with osteomalacia. **B,** Biopsy specimen of pseudofracture (Looser's zone). Lesion is characterized by trabeculae consisting entirely of osteoid *(arrow)*. *MB,* Mineralized bone. (**B,** Undecalcified, Goldner's stain; 40×.)

marked reduction in serum levels of 1,25-dihydroxyvitamin D.[225]

Vitamin D–dependent rickets. Vitamin D–dependent rickets (pseudovitamin D–deficiency rickets) is a family of disorders that specifically involves defective metabolism of 1,25-dihydroxyvitamin D. The patients who were first identified (type I) have an osteomalacic and rachitic disease that is inherited as an autosomal recessive trait.[237] These children are hypocalcemic and hypophosphatemic and develop secondary hyperparathyroidism associated with decreased intestinal absorption of calcium.[240] Treatment with vitamin D or its 25-hydroxylated metabolite requires massive doses, but the disease can be completely cured by small amounts of 1,25-dihydroxyvitamin D.[237,240] Clearly, this form of vitamin D–dependent rickets is caused by defective conversion of 25-hydroxyvitamin D to 1,25-dihydroxyvitamin D.[237]

Recently, vitamin D–dependent rickets type II has been described by Brook and associates.[235] These patients may be siblings of those with the type I disorder,[239] and occasionally both defects exist simultaneously.[242] Type I and type II patients have similar degrees of osteomalacia and rickets and the same general biochemical abnormalities.[233,234,238,241] However, in contrast to the low serum content of 1,25-dihydroxyvitamin D that characterizes type I pseudovitamin D–deficient osteomalacia, patients with type II have extremly high circulating levels of the metabolite. The metabolic defect in these patients, therefore, lies in inadequate tissue responsivity to 1,25-dihydroxyvitamin D, and treatment requires massive doses of vitamin D, 25-hydroxyvitamin D, or 1,25-dihydroxyvitamin D. Hence it is not surprising that there is deficient receptor binding of 1,25-dihydroxyvitamin D by these patients' fibroblasts.[236]

Renal osteodystrophy. Chronic renal disease has profound and varied effects on bone metabolism and structure. In fact, uremic osteodystrophy is an excellent paradigm of the potential manifestations of most metabolic bone diseases.

Because of the profundity and speed with which skeletal disease accompanies renal failure, and the ease with which uremia may be induced in experimental animals, renal osteodystrophy is probably the generalized disorder of bone whose pathophysiology is best understood. For example, severe secondary hyperparathyroidism is one of the most consistent features of progressive uremia. It is clear that parathyroid gland stimulation initially occurs because of hypocalcemia resulting from phosphate retention.[275,278,279] With advancing renal insufficiency, the kidneys lose the ability to synthesize 1,25-dihydroxyvitamin D,[279] culminating in diminished intestinal absorption of calcium.[246] Impaired renal metabolism of parathyroid hormone also contributes to the marked elevations in circulating levels of this peptide.[253,266]

Renal osteodystrophy is a generic term referring to the variety of skeletal and biochemical changes that accompany chronic uremia. Before the advent of maintenance hemodialysis, the azotemic complications of renal failure overshadowed its skeletal effects.[252] Now, however, virtually all uremic patients maintained on life-support systems have histologic evidence of bone disease.[41]

The histologic manifestations of uremic osteodystrophy consist of osteitis fibrosa or osteomalacia or both in a setting of osteopenia, normal bone mass, or osteosclerosis. Since increased osteoid is almost universal,[41] osteoporosis rarely occurs in chronic uremia (Fig. 40-35).

Osteitis fibrosa is by far the most common manifestation of renal osteodystrophy in the United States. Its severity can generally be predicted by determinations of circulating parathyroid hormone and alkaline phosphatase.[252] Because the levels of immunoreactive parathyroid hormone are highest in chronic uremia, the degree of osteitis fibrosa is generally more pronounced than in other forms of secondary hyperparathyroidism or in primary hyperparathyroidism.[144] One frequently encounters abundant woven bone and peritrabecular marrow fibrosis. The latter may eventually become so extensive as to obliterate almost the entire marrow cavity, resulting in hemopoietic suppression and hypersplenism.[286]

Osteoid is also abundant in uremic osteitis fibrosa and most often does not reflect osteomalacia.[283] In fact, despite earlier claims to the contrary,[130] most of the hyperosteoidoses of uremic bone disease in the United States are caused by markedly accelerated organic matrix synthesis,[254,283] the degree of which also reflects the magnitude of secondary hyperparathyroidism.[252,283] Since the cellular and tissue level rates of mineralization are usually increased in end-stage renal failure,[41,254,283] both the mean productivity by osteoblasts and the frequency with which these cells are recruited are enhanced. That primary hyperparathyroidism is, in contrast, associated with a low cellular rate of mineralization[144] may reflect differences in circulating phosphorus levels in this state and chronic renal failure.

Although osteoclasts are also abundant in uremic hyperparathyroidism, they may individually resorb bone at a reduced rate.[132] Certainly the calcemic response to endogenous or exogenous parathyroid hormone is suppressed.[263,267,268] This relative inefficiency of osteoclastic activity may reflect the paucity of 1,25-dihydroxyvitamin D and an abundance of nonresorbable osteoid.[257]

Osteomalacia is usually a minor component of renal bone disease in the United States,[283,285] but in parts of England this form of osteodystrophy predominates.[272,285] Perhaps abnormalities of vitamin D metabolism contribute to its development,[250] but we have found that bone disease is not present in patients with the nephrotic syndrome who, through its urinary loss, have extremely low serum levels of 25-hydroxyvitamin D.[255,260,286] On the other hand, it is becoming increasingly evident that the high aluminum content in bone that occurs in uremia is important in the pathogenesis of osteomalacia.[249]

Chronically dialyzed patients frequently have a skeletal aluminum burden that is 40 or 50 times the normal.[243] The cation is largely accumulated through dialysis water,[259,261,271,284,285] although gastrointestinal absorption of phosphate-binding gels undoubtedly contributes.[258] Aluminum is deposited at the mineralization front (Fig. 40-36),[248] and the degree of osteomalacia[247] and the incidence of fracture in uremia[271] correlate well with the bone content of this ion. The elegant studies performed by Ellis, McCarthy, and Herrington[251] in Newcastle clearly implicate aluminum as the primary cause of renal osteomalacia in their patients. These investigators also produced severe osteomalacia in rats by systemic administration of the cation.[251]

Because of the overuse of phosphate-binding dietary

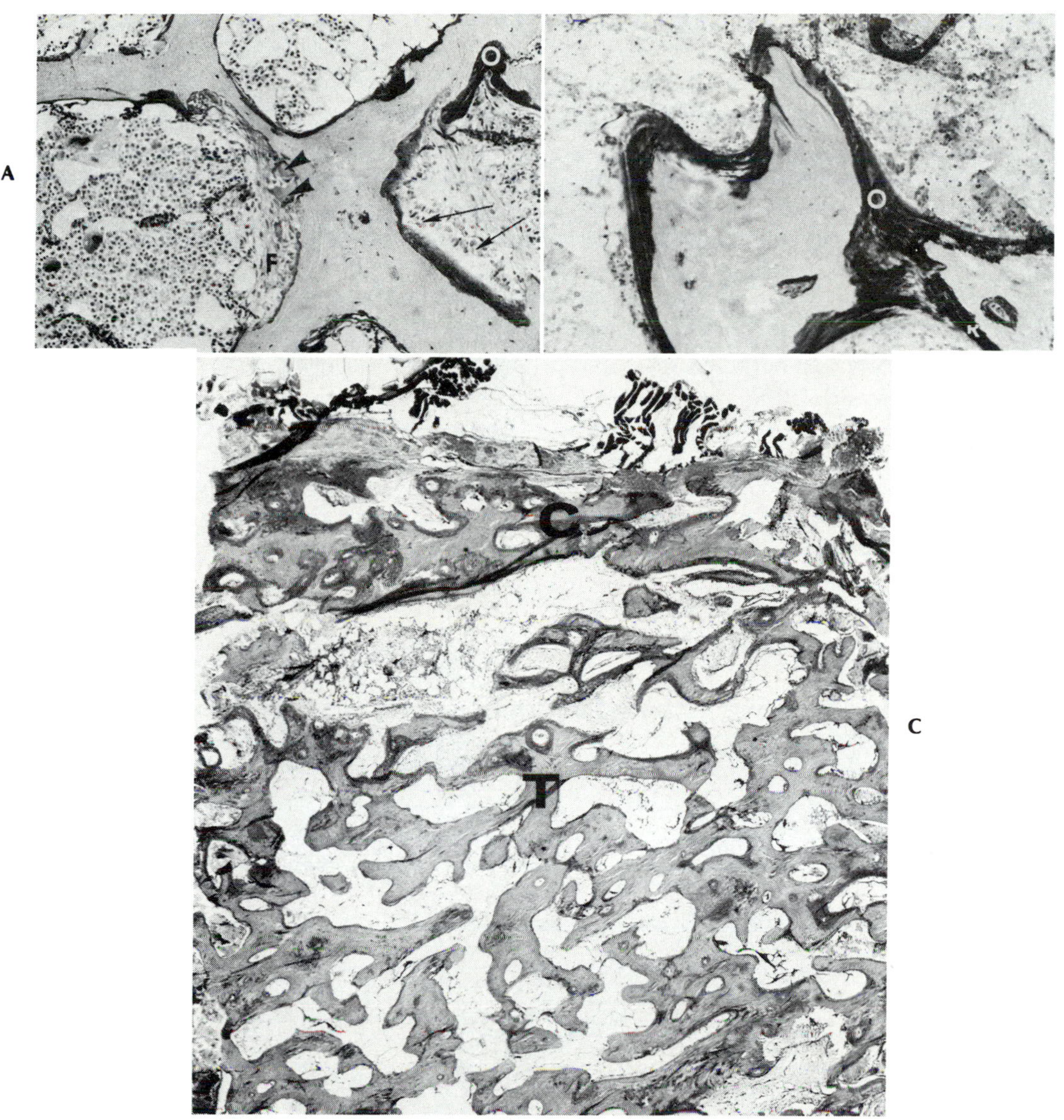

Fig. 40-35. Histologic spectrum of renal osteodystrophy. Combinations of the three basic lesions are usually found. **A,** Osteitis fibrosa is characterized by peritrabecular fibrosis *(F),* numerous osteoclasts *(arrowheads),* increased osteoid *(O),* and osteoblast proliferation *(arrows).* **B,** Osteomalacia exhibits predominance of wide osteoid seams *(O).* **C,** Osteosclerosis. Quantity of trabecular bone is markedly increased, and there is loss of distinction between cortical *(C)* and trabecular *(T)* bone. Osteoid is also increased. (Undecalcified, Goldner's stain; **A** and **B,** 40×; **C,** 30×; **C,** from Teitelbaum, S.L., and Bullough, P.G.: The pathophysiology of bone and joint disease, Bethesda, Md., 1979, The American Association of Pathologists.)

gels, some uremic patients have relatively low circulating phosphorus[264] and bone[282] phosphorus levels. Among the most clinically severe forms of renal osteomalacia develop in these patients. Similarly, uremic hypoparathyroidism is even worse than severe hyperparathyroidism. We have shown that a crippling form of osteomalacia develops in azotemic patients who have been totally parathyroidectomized.[283] Of greater concern is that similar changes have been noted by Weinstein[287] in subtotally parathyroidectomized uremic patients. Evidently some parathyroid hormone is essential for optimum skeletal homeostasis and therapeutic responsivity of the uremic skeleton. Unfortunately, the optimum levels of this hormone are unknown.

Patients with a predominance of osteomalacia have the most disabling form of uremic bone disease. They are also generally unresponsive to the newer forms of therapy, which are successful in the treatment of renal osteitis fibrosa.[254,256,281,283] Hodsman and associates[256] recently described a subset of American patients who had low circulating parathyroid hormone levels and a great propensity to fracture and whose skeletal changes consisted of "pure" osteomalacia. Such patients are relatively hypercalcemic, and when they are treated with 1,25-dihydroxyvitamin D, their blood calcium levels become dangerously high. This phenomenon probably represents marked resistance of bone to mineralize and serve as a repository for absorbed calcium.

Osteosclerosis, increased matrix volume per volume of whole bone, may be the most common form of renal osteodystrophy.[252] Since it does not commonly result in obvious deformities, the condition may escape clinical detection. On the other hand, osteosclerotic bone may fracture. This probably reflects qualitative abnormalities of the organic[274] and mineral[140,144] matrices of the uremic skeleton.

Roentgenographically the most severely osteosclerotic patients have a "rugger-jersey spine," a pathognomonic feature caused by alternating bands of increased and normal bone density (Fig. 40-37). Pathologically the trabeculae are wide and covered by thick osteoid seams. Large quantities of woven bone are present, and osteitis fibrosa progresses in tandem with osteosclerosis.[245]

Osteosclerosis is a disorder of trabecular bone and the axial skeleton. Increased trabecular mass is associated with progressive cortical porosity leading to histologic loss of distinction between compact and cancellous bone (Fig. 40-34, *C*). Probably because the appendicular skeleton is predominantly cortical, it tends to become increasingly osteopenic as vertebral osteosclerosis develops.

Enhanced bone formation paralleling the rise in circulating parathyroid hormone is responsible for the development of osteosclerosis.[41,283] This phenomenon appears early in the course of renal failure[265] because hyperparathyroidism may develop with modest reductions in glomerular function.[273]

Clinically significant bone disease is much more common in uremic children than in adults.[244,280] The growth failure that generally occurs is undoubtedly multifactori-

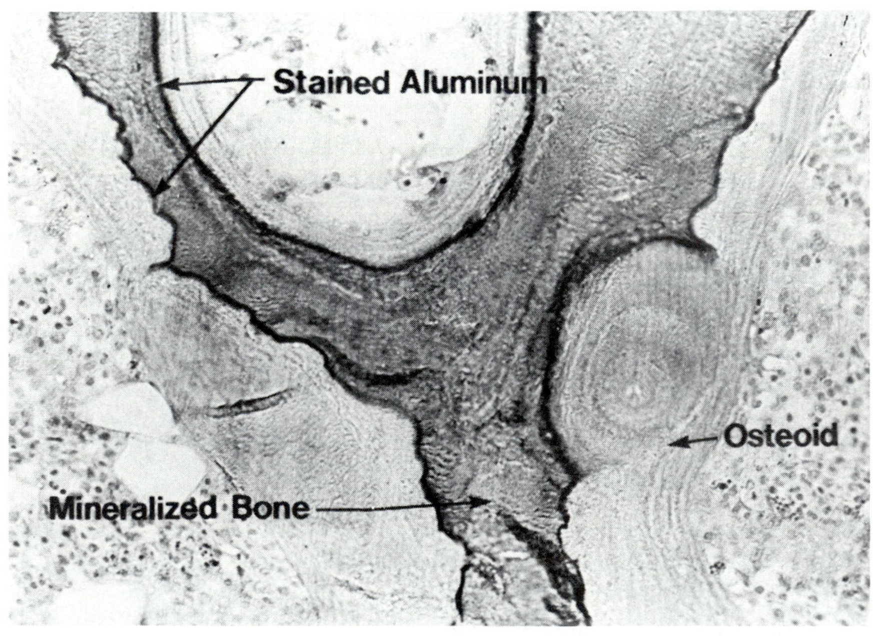

Fig. 40-36. Aluminum at mineralization front of uremic patient with pure osteomalacia. (Undecalcified, aluminum stain; 240×; courtesy Dr. Donald Sherrard, Seattle, Wash.; from Maloney, N.A., et al.: J. Lab. Clin. Med. **99**:206, 1982.)

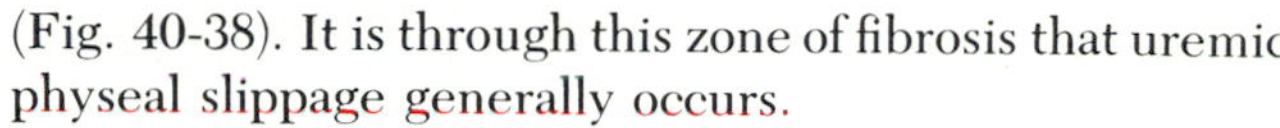

al, but clearly caloric deprivation is important.[269,270,277] These children also develop unique growth plate changes as contrasted with children with nutritional rickets.[262] Specifically the physes of both groups may be roentgenographically indistinguishable, but the cartilaginous plates of uremic children are narrower than normal. The radiolucency reflects extensive marrow fibrosis, which interrupts formation of the primary spongiosa and the attachment of the growth plate to the metaphysis (Fig. 40-38). It is through this zone of fibrosis that uremic physeal slippage generally occurs.

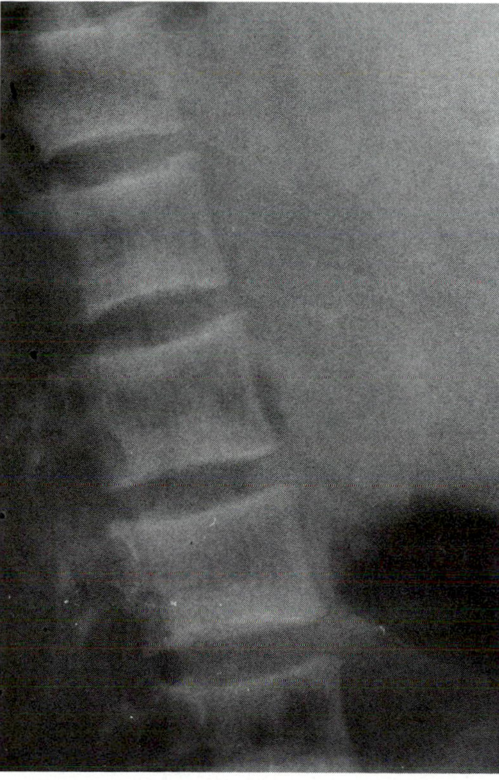

Fig. 40-37. Osteosclerosis of spine associated with long-standing renal failure. "Rugger jersey" appearance is due to alternating bands of sclerotic and normally dense bone.

Calcitonin

Calcitonin is a hypocalcemic, hypophosphatemic agent produced by the parafollicular cells of the thyroid.[289] Bone is the only tissue that this peptide is known to directly affect, and it does so primarily, if not exclusively, by inhibiting osteoclasts.[77,309] The direct action of calcitonin on bone has been confirmed by organ culture studies[293] and the presence of specific receptors in the skeleton.[300] The skeletal effects of this hormone in vivo can be appreciated only in parathyroidectomized animals because secondary hyperparathyroidism characteristically follows calcitonin administration.[297,301]

As manifested by alterations in serum calcium and hydroxyprolinuria, the hormone is most effective in states of osteoclastosis.[291] Consequently, osteoclast ultrastructure is the morphologic feature of bone most strikingly affected by calcitonin. Shortly after its administration and before the development of hypocalcemia,[291] osteoclasts leave the bone surface, decrease in number, and lose their ruffled border (Fig. 40-39).[77,309] Coincidentally a layer of osteoblasts often appears between osteoclasts and the trabecular surface.[309]

Curiously, despite its phylogenetic conservation, a biologic role for calcitonin in mammals is yet to be discovered. Talmage and associates[304] postulate that calcitonin functions primarily to inhibit the postprandial loss of calcium and phosphorus from the bone fluid compartment, which they believe to be principally under the influence of the osteocyte. They extend their hypothesis to the possibility that prolonged calcitonin lack, as would occur in the thyroidectomized patient, might result in enhanced urinary loss of calcium and hence contribute to the development of senile osteopenia.[304]

It is currently uncertain if calcitonin directly affects osteoblasts, although the hormone induces ultrastructur-

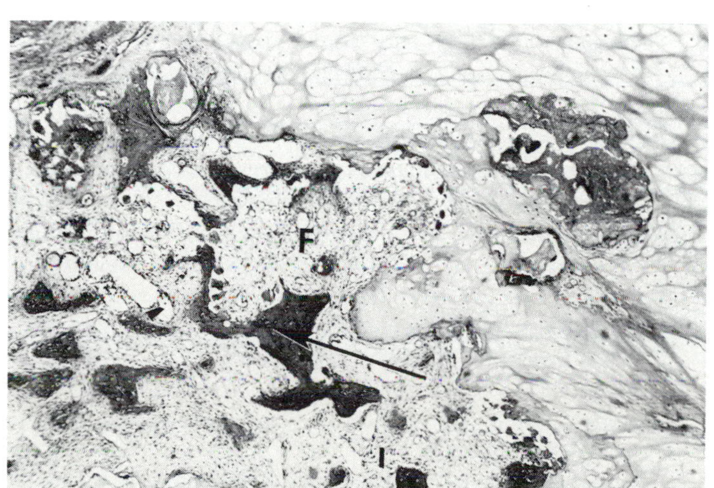

Fig. 40-38. Growth plate of child with chronic renal failure. Attachment of physis and metaphysis is interrupted by abundant fibrous tissue *(F)*. Metaphyseal bone *(arrow)* is forming intramembranously. Note architectural distortion of cartilage. (Hematoxylin and eosin; 40×; courtesy Dr. Ruth Silberberg, Jerusalem, Israel.)

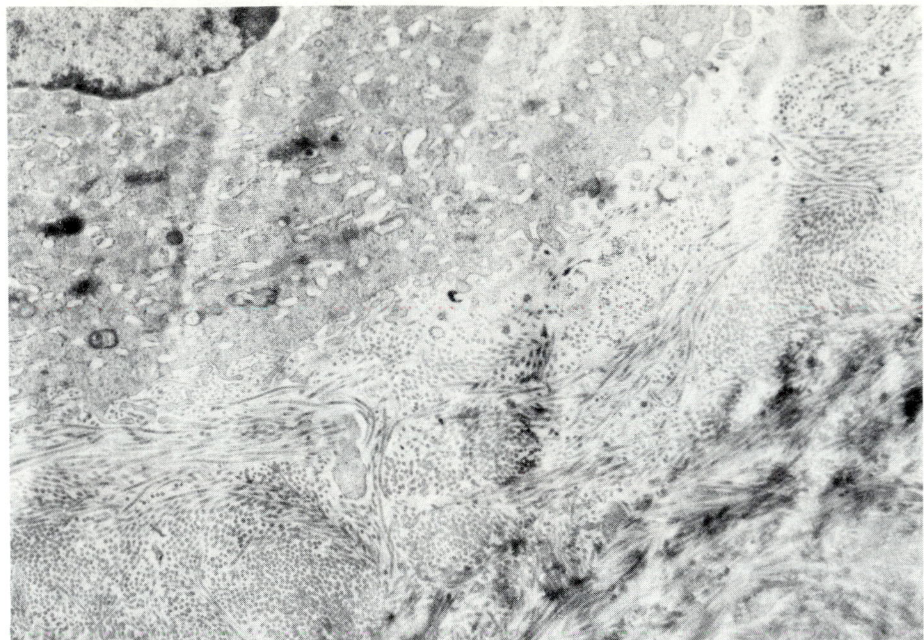

Fig. 40-39. Atrophy of ruffled border of osteoclast after administration of calcitonin. Compare with Fig. 40-13. (15,500×; courtesy Dr. Barbara Mills, San Marino, Calif.)

al changes in osteocytes.[302,304] Some believe that the hormone suppresses bone formation,[209,299] whereas others postulate that it promotes mineralization.[288,292]

The net effect of calcitonin on bone mass is also in dispute. Enhancement of fracture healing by the peptide has been noted,[294] but some investigators believe that it may delay repair.[303] Chronically administered calcitonin has also been reported to increase cortical mass in rats,[306] whereas such treatment may accelerate the progression of osteopenia in humans, presumably caused by parathyroid hormone–induced bone resorption.[297] Consequently, despite initial hopes for the use of the hormone in the treatment of osteopenia, little success has been achieved.[298] Paget's disease, in which the peptide retards the accelerated rate of remodeling, is the only pathologic entity that responds favorably with some regularity to calcitonin therapy.[295,296,307,308]

Patients with medullary carcinoma of the thyroid and many of their relatives are the only persons in whom chronic, endogenous hypercalcitoninemia occurs.[305] Associated hyperparathyroidism is unusual in these patients unless they have the familial form of the carcinoma.[301] Affected persons are not osteosclerotic and may be osteopenic.[301] Histologically the bones of the few patients with medullary carcinoma that have been studied appear inactive.[301]

Estrogens

Senile osteopenia. Loss of skeletal mass with age is the most common form of symptomatic osteopenia. Although men are occasionally affected, this is predominantly a disease of women. Moreover, since blacks develop greater bone mass than do whites, symptomatic osteopenia is distinctly rare in blacks, and when it occurs, causes other than senescence should be suspected.[332]

Although symptomatic osteopenia generally appears after menopause, loss of axial bone begins in early adulthood and progresses linearly throughout life.[327] Appendicular bone mass does not diminish until the sixth decade, when over 10 years it is rapidly lost.[327] Throughout her life, the average white woman loses 47% of her vertebral mass, 39% of her distal radius, and 30% of her midradius.[327]

The morbid consequences of senile osteopenia have great social implications. Of approximately 1 million fractures occurring annually in the United States in women at least 45 years of age, 700,000 are associated with osteopenia.[321] Although fractures of the distal radius and vertebral bodies occur commonly in osteopenic women[326] intertrochanteric hip fractures are responsible for the greatest attendant morbidity and mortality. Women with intertrochanteric hip fractures are significantly more osteopenic than age-matched controls, and the incidence of this fracture reflects severe skeletal demineralization (Fig. 40-40).[311,329]

The syndrome of postmenopausal osteopenia unquestionably represents a potpourri of pathogenic mechanisms. Obviously cessation of ovarian function is extremely important,[319,320] but the onset of bone loss in young adulthood[327] indicates that other factors are

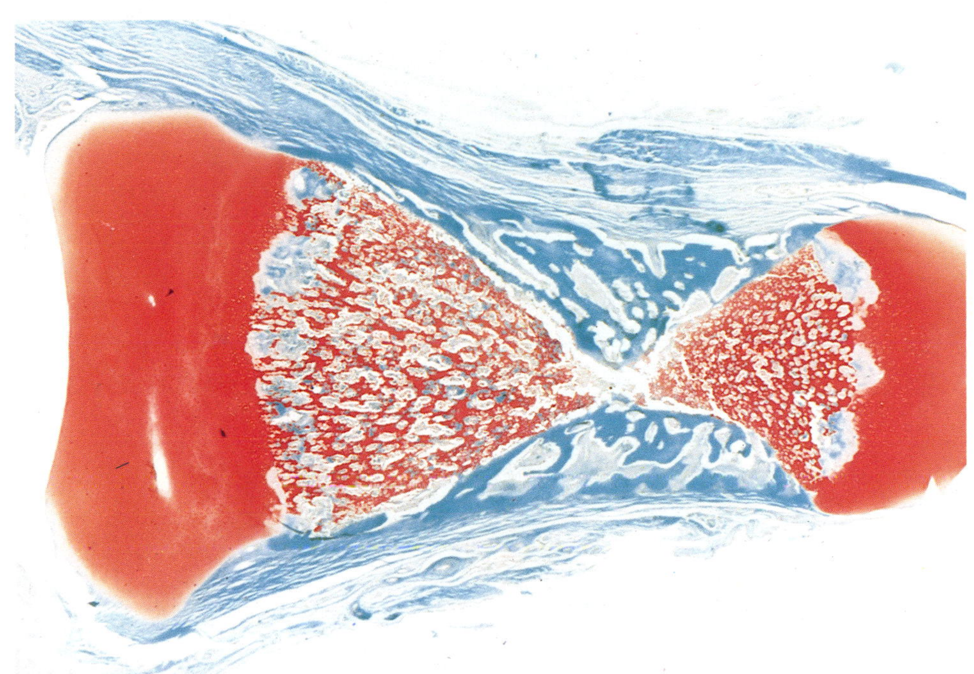

Plate 7. Phalanx of patient with malignant osteopetrosis. Red-staining cartilage, which is product of endochondral growth, fails to be resorbed and persists deep into metaphysis, forming characteristic cartilaginous bars. Bone formed intramembranously by periosteal apposition stains blue and contains no cartilaginous bars. (Safrinin O; 4×; courtesy Dr. Frederic Shapiro, Boston, Mass. From Shapiro, F., et al.: J. Bone Joint Surg. **62A:**384, 1980.)

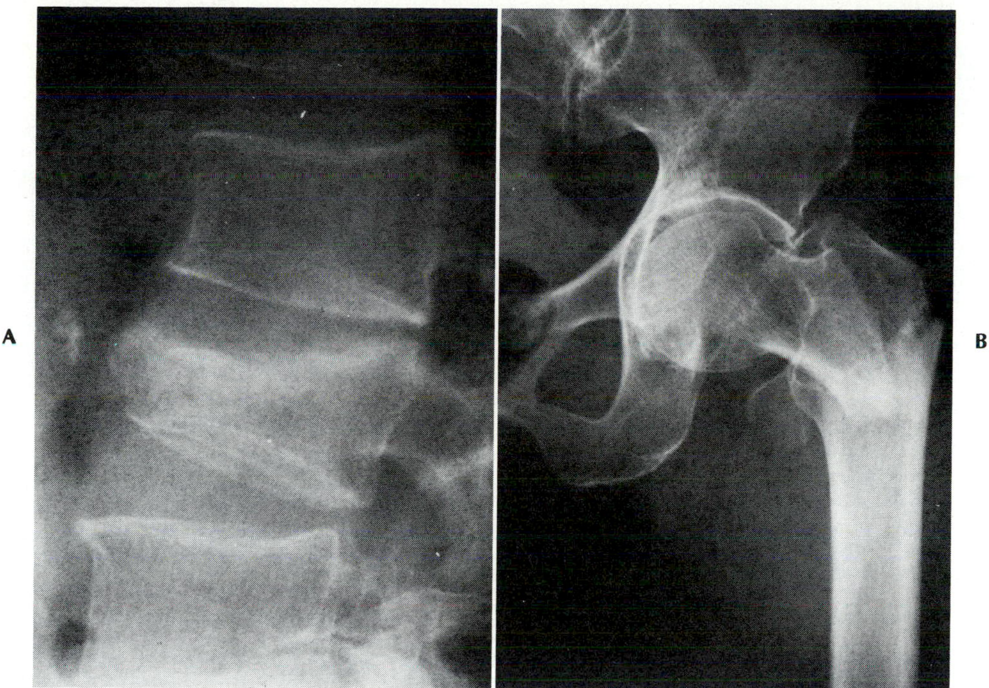

Fig. 40-40. A, Crush fracture of vertebral body of patient with senile osteopenia. **B,** Intertrochanteric hip fracture in elderly, osteopenic patient.

involved. These may include senescent reduction in intestinal absorption of calcium (perhaps mediated through alterations of 1,25-dihydroxyvitamin D synthesis),[315,326] modest increments in circulating parathyroid hormone levels,[317,30,331] and reduced calcitonin production.[328] The high acid residue[313] and the varying calcium[318] and phosphorus[323,324] content of the Western diet may also be elements of senile bone loss.

The histologic changes that occur in the skeleton of an aging woman include increased cortical porosity[322] and diminished trabecular mass.[325] Numerous small islands of cancellus are present in biopsy specimens from symptomatic osteopenic women. In fact, the cancellous mass of patients with vertebral crush fractures is invariably less than 16% of the total marrow space.[325]

The more detailed cellular histology of postmenopausal osteopenia is heterogeneous and probably reflects the variety of contributory events. My co-workers and I,[312,331,333] as well as others,[325] have found that bone biopsy specimens from postmenopausal osteopenic women may be divided into three categories. Approximately 30% have features of accelerated turnover, such as numerous osteoclasts, resorption bays, abundant osteoid, and occasionally peritrabecular marrow fibrosis. The cellular rate of mineralization is also enhanced in these patients. An additional 20% have histologic evidence of inactive remodeling. These patients have few bone cells and a paucity of osteoid and tetracycline uptake. The remaining half of osteopenic women have diminished bone mass in the face of normal indices of remodeling (Fig. 40-41).

The relationship of these histologic features to the mechanism of bone loss is still unclear, particularly since they are not predictable by biochemical changes.[331,333] However, it is probable that the first group (rapid turnover) represents a situation in which both resorption and formation are accelerated but the degradation of matrix is more rapid than its synthesis. Alternatively, "slow-turnover" (inactive) osteopenia probably reflects the hypothesis posited by Albright, Bloomberg, and Smith[310]: that postmenopausal osteoporosis is a disorder of osteoblast function. In these circumstances the rate of remodeling is reduced, but formation is slower than resorption.

The osteopenic patients with normal features of remodeling are more problematic. Perhaps these women develop less bone than normal at maturity, and although their rate of loss is not greater than that of nonosteopenic women, their skeletal mass enters the "fracture zone" earlier. However, the width of completed trabecular osteons diminishes with age, particularly in osteopenic women.[314] This suggests that despite a normal number of bone-forming units, the life span of each unit is diminished, resulting in a reduction in the amount of bone deposited during each remodeling cycle.

Ovarian dysgenesis. Ovarian dysgenesis is commonly associated with skeletal abnormalities. Affected patients are short, and bone maturation is frequently arrested at age 12 or 13.[338] They often have hypoplasia of the first

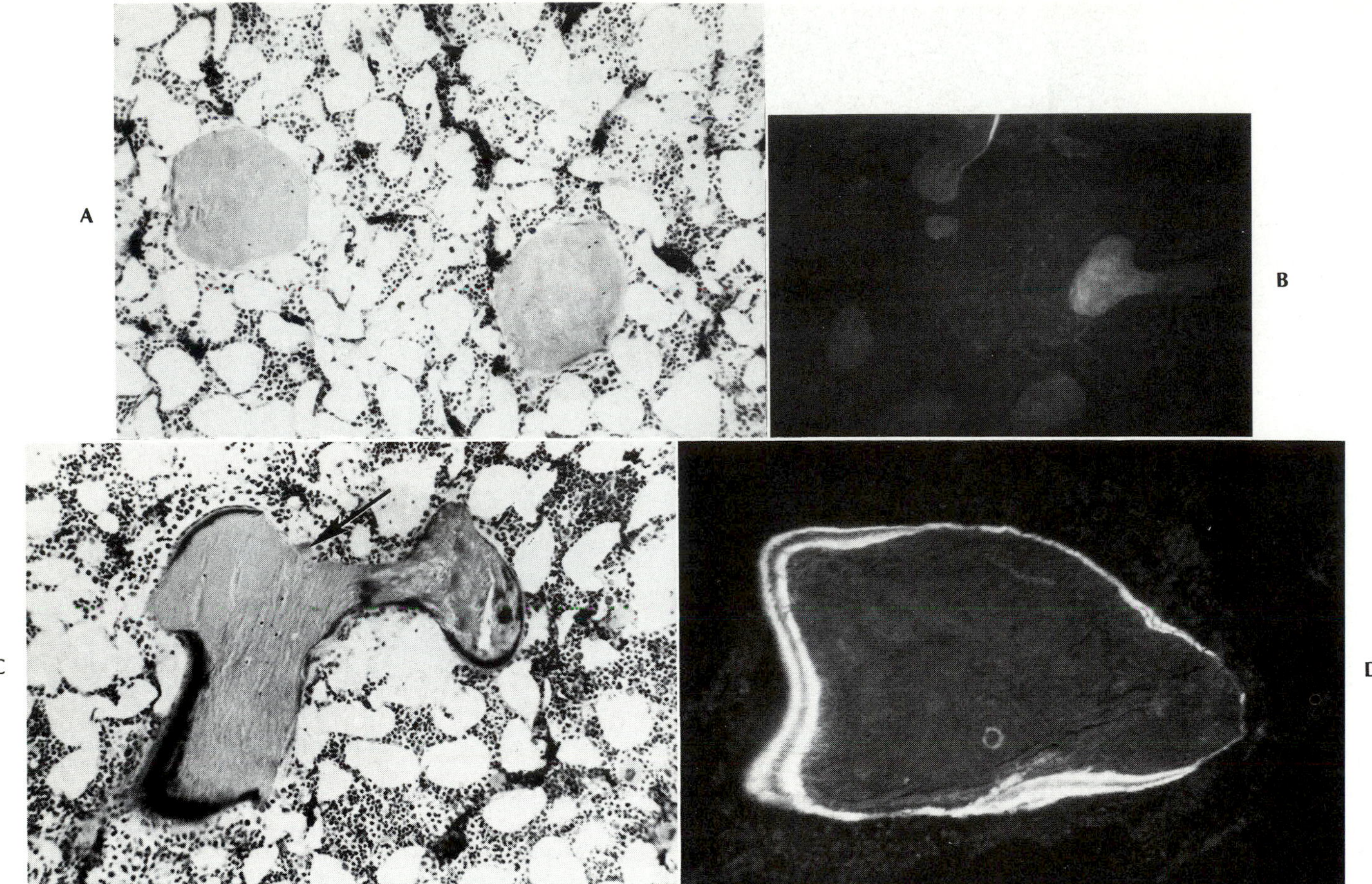

Fig. 40-41. Histologic spectrum of postmenopausal osteopenia. **A,** Inactive osteopenia characterized by scattered trabeculae exhibiting little evidence of osteoblastic or osteoclastic activity. **B,** Most trabecular surfaces do not assume tetracycline label, indicating low rate of bone turnover. **C,** Active osteopenia characterized by scattered trabeculae containing abundant osteoid and osteoclasts *(arrow)*. **D,** Double tetracycline label formation is abundant, indicating accelerated bone turnover. (Undecalcified; 100×; **A** and **C,** Goldner's stain; **B** and **D,** unstained, fluorescent.)

cervical vertebra[336] and fusion of adjacent bones throughout the skeleton.[338]

Patients with Turner's syndrome frequently resemble those with pseudohypoparathyroidism.[334] For example, both groups commonly have shortening of the fourth metacarpal.[334,338] Ovarian dysgenesis is not associated with renal resistance to parathyroid hormone.[334]

Osteopenia is common in Turner's syndrome.[335,338] Although its severity increases with age,[335] even young dysgenic females have significant bone loss. These patients may have accelerated rates of resorption,[335,337] but controversy exists as to whether formation is normal[335] or depressed.[337]

Not much is known about the bone histology in Turner's syndrome. Those few patients studied generally have inactive osteoporosis.[337] This is curious, since it is commonly believed that the primary effect of estrogens on bone is suppression of resorption.[339]

Growth hormone

Growth hormone is probably the agent most responsible for longitudinal skeletal development. Its growth-promoting properties are effected through somatomedin (sulfation factor), which stimulates sulfate uptake and mitogenesis in physeal cartilage.[343]

The influence of growth hormone on endochondral growth is best studied in the hypophysectomized state. In the absence of somatotropin the physis diminishes the width, the number of chondrocyte columns decreases, and cartilage matrix becomes relatively more abundant.[356] In addition, vascular invasion of the growth plate disappears, and a transverse bone seal forms between the metaphysis and physis.[356] Trabecular bone may be resorbed without replacement, resulting in osteopenia.[356]

Growth hormone administration to a hypophysectomized, growing animal leads to growth plate widening caused by chondrocyte proliferation and matrix synthe-

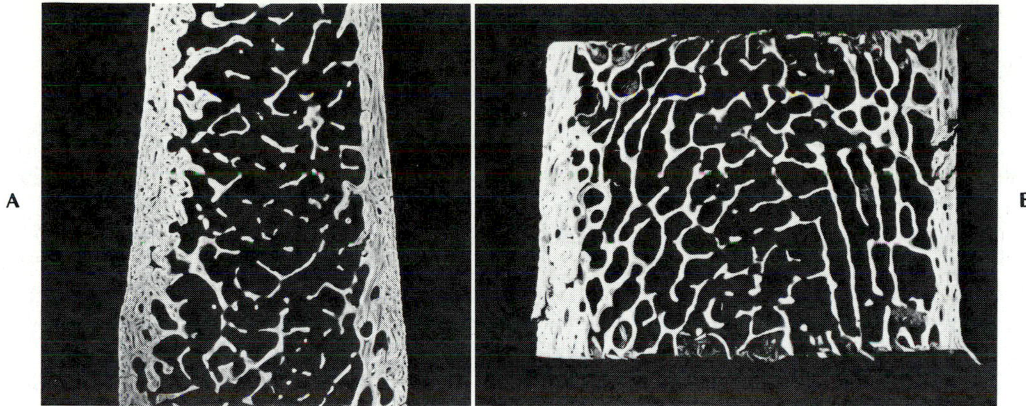

Fig. 40-42. Microroentgenographs of anterior iliac crest biopsies of normal 24-year-old man, **A,** and similarly aged acromegalic male, **B.** Note increased trabecular width in acromegalic bone. (Courtesy Dr. Jenifer Jowsey, Rochester, Minn.; from Aloia, J.F., et al.: J. Clin. Endocrinol. Metab. **35:**543, 1972.)

sis.[356] Vascular invasion from the metaphysis reappears, and the tranverse bone seal is resorbed.[356] Continued administration eventuates in gigantism caused by persistent endochondral growth. Under the circumstances, rapid proliferation of the growth plate can result in slipped physes.[345]

The effect of growth hormone on the skeleton appears to be stimulation of progenitor cell proliferation. Ramser, Frost, and Smith[353] maintain that increased bone turnover induced by excess somatotropin is caused by formation of additional bone remodeling sites, whereas the activity of individual cells remains unaltered. Regardless of the mechanism, the net result is acceleration of both formation and resorption, with the magnitude of these processes directly related to the circulating levels of immunoreactive growth hormone.[354]

The effects of somatotropin on bone metabolism are reflected in the skeletal manifestations of acromegaly. Acromegalic patients typically have enhanced periosteal bone formation and thick cortices.[349,354] There is also increased cortical porosity caused by activation of haversian remodeling.[354]

The acromegalic changes in trabecular bone are more controversial. It has been held that trabecular osteopenia develops in these patients,[354] but in a large series reported by Delling and Schulz[344] cancellous bone was noted to contain wide trabeculae, constituting a normal osseous mass. Moreover, the number of trabecular osteoblasts in these patients is significantly increased (Fig. 40-42).[344] These bone-proliferating effects of growth hormone are related to its ability to stimulate collagen formation.[356] In addition, this peptide results in retention of phosphorus,[347] an ion also capable of promoting osteoblastic activity.[173] Growth hormone also enhances interstitial absorption of calcium[340,351] via elevated levels of 1,25-dihydroxyvitamin D.[352] Perhaps this stimulation of vitamin D metabolism is caused by the hyperparathyroidism that frequently accompanies acromegaly.[347] Hypercalciuria is also common in the disease,[342,351] and loss of calcium generally equals its absorption from the intestine.[342]

Growth hormone deficiency in humans occurs in hypopituitary midgets, who may have an isolated defect in somatotropin synthesis. This deficiency can also be combined with that of other pituitary hormones. Since growth hormone is not necessary for in utero growth,[346] birth length is normal in infants with the monotropic deficit,[351] and growth retardation is not apparent until 6 months to 1 year of age.[355] With puberty, growth spurts are frequent.[355]

Because of its bone-forming properties, growth hormone has been proposed as a therapeutic agent in the treatment of senile osteopenia.[348] Perhaps related to loss of responsivity of the skeleton to sulfation factor with age,[350] and because of the bone-resorbing properties of somatotropin,[354] therapeutic trials have been largely unsuccessful.[341]

Thyroid hormone

Thyroid hormone stimulates bone remodeling[183,367,371,375] and mediates skeletal maturation.[377] When present in excess, the hormone often leads to osteopenia[357] and negative calcium balance.[364]

The net loss of calcium associated with hyperthyroidism reflects both decreased intestinal absorption of the cation[366,369] and enhanced skeletal resorption.[373] Thyrotoxic patients are deficient in 1,25-dihydroxyvitamin D,[360] which no doubt contributes to their hypoabsorptive state. Reflecting the tendency toward hypercalcemia,[370] hyperthyroidism is also generally attended by low levels of circulating parathyroid hormone.[359,362] This relative hypoparathyroidism certainly plays a role in the reduced renal 25-hydroxyvitamin D–1-alpha-hydroxylase activity.[169]

The incidence of thyrotoxicosis-induced osteopenia is proportional to the duration of thyroid dysfunction.[372] No such relationship exists, however, between the skeletal lesion and magnitude of hyperthyroidism.[372]

The genesis of hyperthyroid bone disease reflects the potency with which thyroxine enhances remodeling.[183,367,371,375] The hormone promotes the resorptive effects of 1,25-dihydroxyvitamin D[376] and parathyroid hormone[362] and experimentally induces the development of disuse osteopenia.[361] More important, thyroxine directly stimulates osteoclastic activity.[373] Consequently, hyperthyroid patients excrete supranormal quantities of urinary hydroxyproline and hydroxylysine.[363] The associated hypercalciuria may lead to nephrocalcinosis.[374]

Thyrotoxic bone contains an increased number of Howship's lacunae.[183,367,371,375] Although osteoclast proliferation occurs within the trabecula,[183] their prominence in the compacta is a distinguishing feature of the disease (Fig. 40-43).[183,367] This predilection is often manifest roentgenographically by the presence of flaky-appearing phalangeal cortices.[372]

Despite enhancement of initiation of remodeling sites in hyperthyroidism, most patients do not have an abundance of osteoid seams.[371,472] This observation reflects an increased cellular rate of mineralization, resulting in a decreased life span of each seam.[183,371] In other words, hyperthyroidism is a condition in which more osteoblasts are born per unit of time and rapidly complete their task. This increase in the rate of bone cell recruitment is reflected by occasional peritrabecular fibrosis.

The skeletal manifestations of hypothyroidism are often related to growth retardation, perhaps because thyroxine may act synergistically with somatotropin.[356] Therefore the growth-inhibiting effect of hypothyroidism is probably caused by abnormal chondrogenesis.[365] In affected children, physeal cell maturation is retarded and cartilaginous matrix calcifies irregularly.[378] Roentgenographically the growth plates are fragmented and have a stippled appearance.[378] Vascular penetration of the physis occurs prematurely, and there is abnormal accumulation of glycogen in chondrocytes. The depth of the growth plate is reduced, and metaphyseal development is retarded.[365]

Despite increased circulating parathyroid hormone in hypothyroidism,[359,362] the bones of adults with this disease appear generally inactive.[358,371] Trabecular mass is either normal or increased, and both osteoclasts and osteoblasts are rare. There is also a paucity of tetracycline uptake.[371] Skeletal mass does not appear affected, but there may be abnormalities in calcium balance caused by reduced bone turnover.[368]

Adrenal corticosteroids

The coexistence of hypercortisolism and loss of skeletal mass was noted 50 years ago by Cushing.[384] Subsequently it has become evident that varying degrees of osteo-

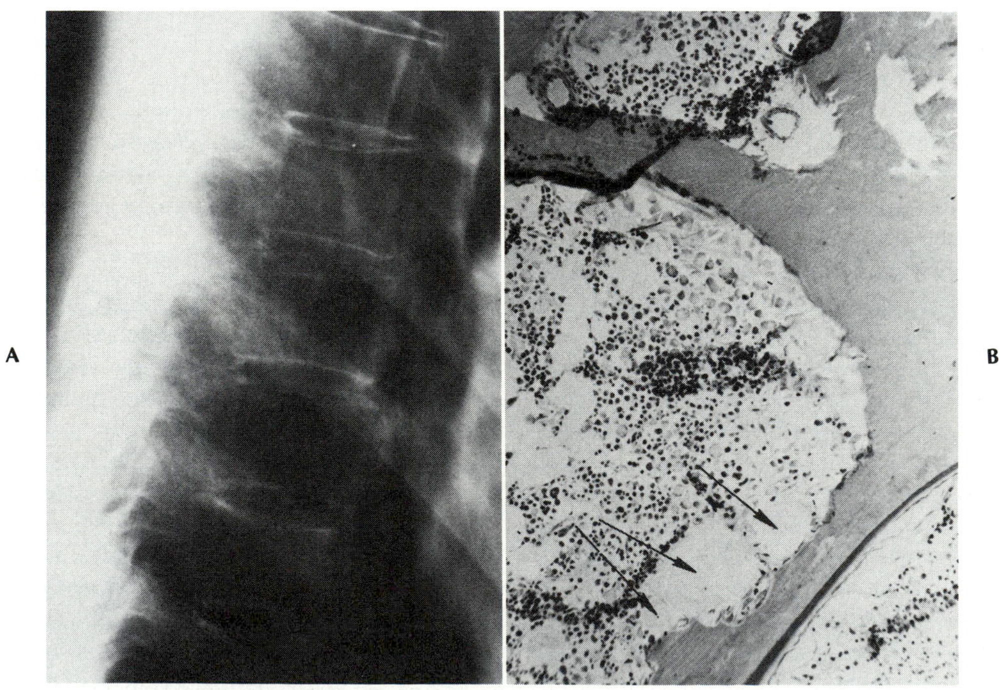

Fig. 40-43. A, Markedly osteopenic vertebrae of patient with hyperthyroidism. **B,** Bone biopsy specimen from hyperthyroid patient. There are numerous scalloped resorption bays and extensive osteoid seam formation. (Undecalcified, Goldner's stain; 100×.)

penia commonly develop in patients with adrenal hyperactivity or subjected to long-term glucocorticoid therapy.*

Because of the widespread use of glucocorticoid therapy, iatrogenically induced steroid osteopenia is common. In fact, more than 90% of patients who received these drugs on a long-term basis have diminished bone mass at autopsy.[394,407]

The genesis of osteopenia when caused by adrenal hyperactivity is more likely to escape detection. My coworkers and I,[464] as well as others,[404] have encountered young patients with severe skeletal demineralization caused by Cushing's syndrome who have no other signs of glucocorticoid excess. Endogenous hypercortisolism is also more commonly associated with postmenopausal osteopenia than is appreciated. I therefore recommend that the urinary excretion of cortisol be evaluated in all osteopenic patients.

Steroid-induced bone loss is generally most pronounced in the axial skeleton.[5,393] Furthermore, the rate of fracture repair is markedly reduced even though steroid-treated patients produce abundant callus.[379]

There is little question that glucocorticoids reduce the mean rate of osteoblastic activity in vivo and that the genesis of steroid-induced osteopenia is in a large part caused by diminished bone formation.[381,387,397,398] Hence, osteoid seams of patients chronically exposed to these drugs are narrower than normal, and the cellular rate of mineralization, as determined by double tetracycline labeling, is diminished.[381] Despite abundant evidence that corticosteroids inhibit bone formation in vivo, when added to bone organ culture they curiously enhance osteoblast-mediated collagen synthesis.[385]

The effects of glucocorticoids on bone resorption are more puzzling. Clearly, moderate cortisol excess may be associated with abundant osteoclasts[392] and numerous resorption bays.[381] However, it is uncertain if the osteoclast proliferation is caused by a direct effect of the steroid on bone cells or reflects a secondary, systemic influence. Some investigators have reported modest hyperparathyroidism[381,392] in glucocorticoid-treated patients, presumably caused by decreased intestinal absorption of calcium.[391,392] On the other hand, when bone cells are exposed to these agents, the longevity of 1,25-dihydroxyvitamin D cytosolic receptors is prolonged,[400] and production of cyclic AMP in response to parathyroid hormone is enhanced.[382,401] In addition, in our laboratory modest doses of cortisol stimulate bone resorption by putative osteoclast precursors in culture.[410] These observations must, however, be conditioned by the fact that glucocorticoids clearly suppress resorption of fetal bone rudiments in vitro.[403,409] This discrepancy may reflect inability to determine the rate of osteoclast activity in vivo, despite the abundance of these cells following corticosteroid treatment. It has been observed, for example, that despite numerous osteoclasts, the metaphyses of steroid-treated rats become sclerotic because of failure to resorb primary spongiosa.[380,395]

*References 5, 383, 390, 394, 404, 407.

Regardless of exacerbation of secondary hyperparathyroidism, large doses of glucocorticoids suppress bone cell recruitment, leading to paucity of osteoclasts and osteoblasts.[397] As the number of bone-remodeling units is markedly reduced, tetracycline uptake is minimal.[386] It is of interest that tetracycline sequestration may increase dramatically either with tapering of steroids from a therapeutic to a maintenance dose or following surgical treatment of Cushing's syndrome (Fig. 40-44).[381]

The universal growth-suppressive effects of glucocorticoids are probably largely caused by direct skeletal inhibition.[399,406] For example, when exposed to these agents, chondrocytes synthesize less mucopolysaccharide[400,406] and the RNA content of isolated bone cells declines.[402] Histologically the growth plates of cortisol-treated children are thin, the proliferative zone is atrophic, and the zones of hypertrophy and provisional calcification are in architectural disarray.[399] Although glucocorticoids inhibit growth hormone release,[388] somatotropin deficiency per se does not appear responsible for these changes.[408]

After correction of the hypercorticoid state the rate of growth increases, but normal height is rarely achieved.[389] Moreover, demineralized portions of the skeleton often persist, surrounded by normal bone.[396] Roentgenographically this phenomenon appears as a lucent core in a vertebral body.[396]

Insulin

The coexistence of diabetes mellitus and altered bone and mineral metabolism has been reported in humans and experimental animals. For example, both insulin-dependent and adult-onset diabetic patients have diminished bone mass whether measured by densitometric or by roentgenographic techniques.[413,417,418] Moreover, detectable osteopenia may appear within 5 years after the onset of glucose intolerance.[417,418]

The clinical sequelae of diabetic osteopenia are controversial. Although some investigators claim that the incidence of fractures is increased by diabetes,[422] others fail to confirm this observation.[415]

Untreated diabetes mellitus suppresses bone turnover. Microscopically there is a paucity of osteoid and bone cells, and tetracycline uptake is diminished.[416,421] In addition, the physeal plates of untreated diabetic animals are narrow, reflecting growth arrest.[412,418] All of these changes are prevented or dramatically reversed by insulin therapy.[412,418]

The inactivity of skeletal turnover in diabetes reflects abnormal calcium homeostasis. Diabetic patients have enhanced intestinal absorption of the cation,[419] probably related to mucosal hypertrophy.[423] Consequently blood

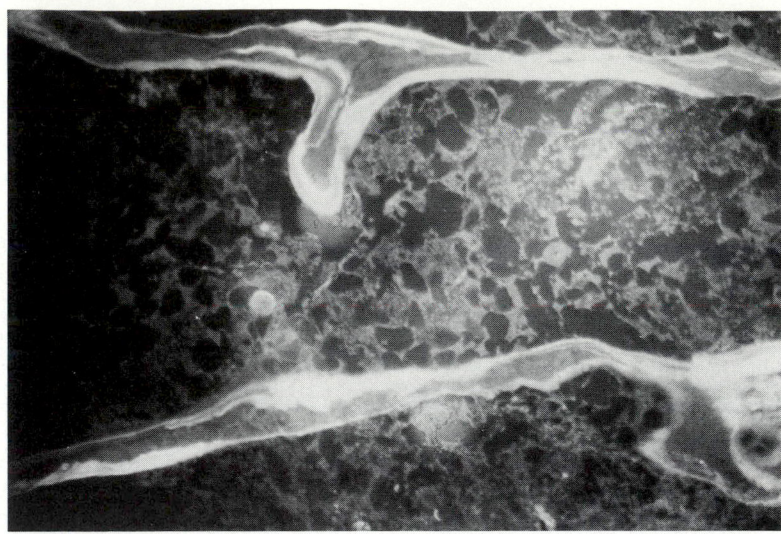

Fig. 40-44. Bone biopsy specimen from patient undergoing tapering of corticosteroid dosage following long-term administration. Virtually every trabecular surface assumes tetracycline label, indicating marked increase in rate of bone formation. (Undecalcified, unstained, fluorescent micrograph; 40×.)

levels of parathyroid hormone and 1,25-dihydroxyvitamin D, both of which activate bone remodeling, are reduced.[413,416,421,423]

Insulin deficiency may also directly contribute to skeletal abnormalities. In experimental diabetes, meticulous control normalizes the low parathyroid hormone and 1,25-dihydroxyvitamin D levels.[416] Insulin also stimulates bone collagen synthesis[411,414,425] and mucopolysaccharide production within cultured physes[420] and promotes endochondral bone formation in matrix implants in diabetic rats.[424] A paucity of two major activators of bone remodeling combined with diminished osteoblastic activity must certainly contribute to the skeletal inactivity of diabetics.

Vitamin C

Clinical scurvy rarely occurs in Western society and is largely a disease of historical interest. However, alcoholics do occasionally become scorbutic. In addition, because cellular uptake of ascorbic acid declines with age,[438] growing individuals are the most sensitive to its deficiency.

The essential role of vitamin C in skeletal metabolism is related to collagen formation. It promotes hydroxylation of both proline[433] and lysine,[426] and collagen synthesis ceases in its absence. The defective mineralization believed to accompany scurvy is therefore probably caused by altered organic matrix production.[428] Moreover, ascorbic acid induces ribosome aggregation on the endoplasmic reticulum of collagen-producing cells.[430] Consequently, scorbutic osteoblasts lose their characteristic ribonuclear protein–dependent basophilia.[440]

Because the skeletal pathology of scurvy primarily reflects defective collagen synthesis, hemorrhages, particularly in the periosteum, are common (Fig.40-45). These may later calcify[440] or, in the partially scorbutic animal, ossify.[439] This new periosteal bone is generally trabecular and poorly vascularized. It pushes between the cortex and the now easily elevated periosteum, and when associated with fracture, it may extend along the entire shaft.[439]

In the totally scorbutic animal complete failure of collagen synthesis results in cessation of periosteal apposition. Because endosteal resorption continues, the cortex becomes markedly attenuated.[431] Osteoblasts decrease in number and are shriveled and spindle shaped.[435] Trabecular bone mass diminishes, and when fracture occurs, a peculiar gelatinous area (gerüstmark), which contains mesenchymal cells juxtaposed to skeletal detritis, develops at the bone ends.[435] Since this area does not appear in immobilized limbs of scorbutic animals,[507] it probably represents the effects of trauma in poorly developing callus.[432]

Repair is greatly delayed in hypovitaminosis C.[429] The initial clot is slow to resorb,[432] and callus formation by both endosteum and periosteum is arrested.[442] Because lack of ascorbic acid does not affect previously synthesized collagen, healed fractures do not break down.[440] In addition, there is no evidence that additional vitamin C given to a nonscorbutic animal accelerates fracture repair.

Vitamin C also participates in cartilage metabolism as illustrated by defective uptake of labeled sulfate when this tissue is exposed to a scorbutic environment.[427,428,434] Both collagen and ground substance synthesis by chondrocytes is impaired, endochondral

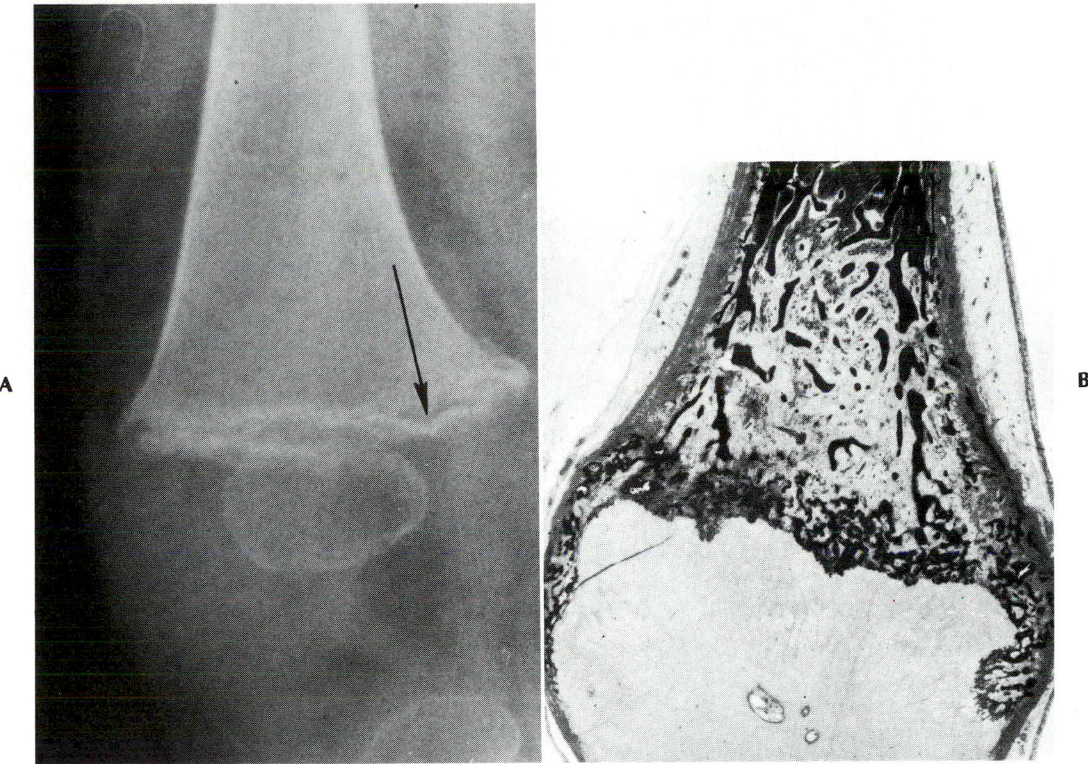

Fig. 40-45. A, Distal femur of child with scurvy. Characteristic roentgenographic features include relative sclerotic rimming of distal metaphyses. Area of radiolucency is present *(arrow)* close to metaphyseal sclerosis. **B,** Classic features of well-advanced scurvy in costochondral junction. Bone shows evidence of osteoporosis and marrow spaces filled with loosely textured and edematous connective tissue in which some hemorrhage has occurred. Metaphyseal end of bone is widened and made up of irregularly arranged spicules of heavily calcified matrix. (**A,** Courtesy Dr. William McAlister, St. Louis, Mo.; **B,** 10×.)

growth stops, cellularity of the growth plate diminishes, and there is disorientation of cellular architecture.[432,435] Ascorbic acid also inhibits lysosomal enzyme activity in human cartilage and therefore may be important in growth and the prevention of degenerative arthritis.[427,434]

Because of disruption of the synthesis of collagen and ground substance, growth plate slippage is common.[435] The physis and metaphysis also push into each other, resulting in irregularity of their junction and expansion of bone ends.[431,435] Therefore the chest wall of a scorbutic child may resemble a rachitic rosary.

During the past few years vitamin C has been ingested in large quantities in Western society. Little is known of the effects of hypervitaminosis C on the skeleton, although it appears to stimulate turnover.[441]

Vitamin A

Both excess and deficiency of vitamin A lead to pathologic changes in bone. Chronic hypervitaminosis A occurs in children ingesting large quantities of fish oil[444] or chicken liver[453] and in Eskimos eating polar bear liver.[457] Excess vitamin A stimulates osteoclasts, particularly those involved in modeling.[443] Because only those portions of the bone involved in this process are affected, there may be gross skeletal deformity.[460]

Osteoid proliferation juxtaposes resorption in vitamin A toxicity.[460] Whether this represents osteoblast stimulation or a mineralization defect is unclear. However, abundant, well-calcified callus commonly accompanies repair of the frequent fractures that occur in rats with vitamin A toxicity.[460] Moreover, periosteal mineralization[456] and abnormal bone formation[446] are usual manifestations of the disorder (Fig. 40-46).

Since this substance has degenerative effects on cartilaginous matrix and chondrocytes in vitro,[446] it is not surprising that endochondral growth is arrested by excess vitamin A.[445] Premature growth plate closure results from penetration of the physes by metaphyseal vessels and subsequent mineralization. Because of growth failure and accelerated resorption at modeling sites, the anterior-posterior diameter of the long bones of rats with vitamin A toxicity is decreased.[460]

The skeletal manifestations of hypervitaminosis A in humans differ somewhat from those in experimental animals. Although resorption is accelerated and thinning of

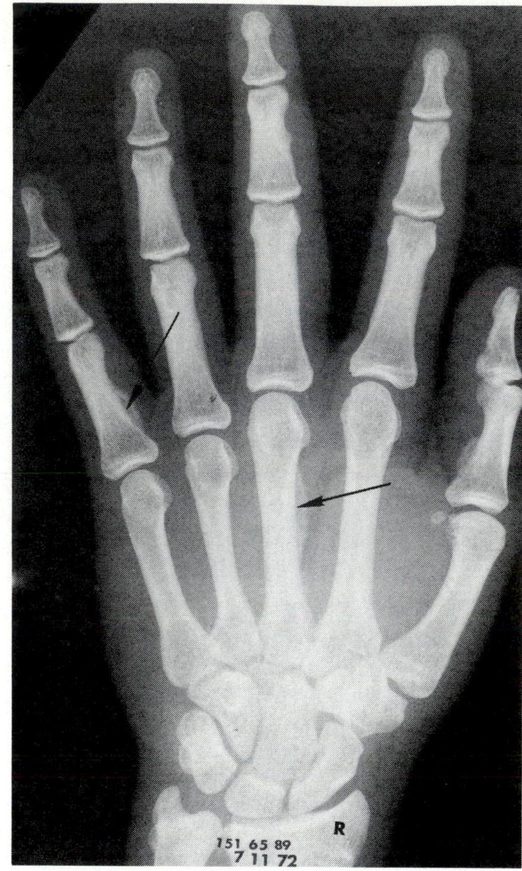

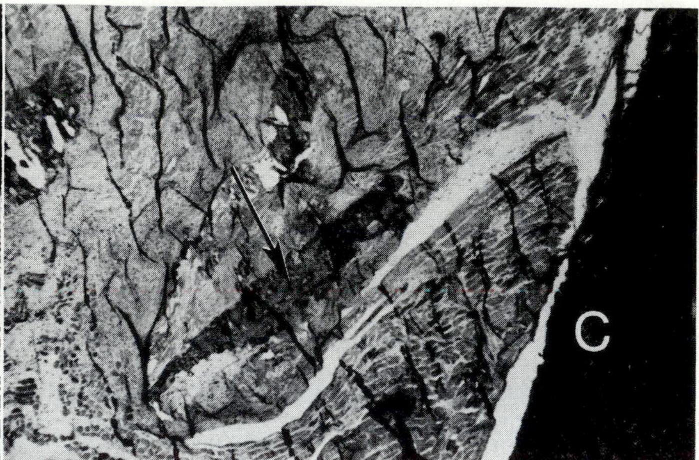

Fig. 40-46. A, Periosteal calcifications *(arrows)*, which characterize hypervitaminosis A. **B,** Histologic correlate of **A.** Bone *(arrow)* has formed within periosteal soft tissues in rat with vitamin A toxicity. **C,** Cortex of tibia. (**A,** Courtesy Dr. Boy Frame; from Frame, B., et al.: Ann. Intern. Med. **80:**44, 1974; with permission of publisher; **B,** undecalcified, modified Masson's trichrome stain; 40×.)

the cortex and long bones may occur, human osteopenia is not as common a complication.[455] Furthermore, in contrast to rats with vitamin A toxicity, fractures are unusual in humans.[428] The most common skeletal manifestation of toxicity in humans is proliferation of tender, moundlike periosteal calcifications and exostoses, almost invariably involving the ulna.[444] Histologically the periosteum is thick, and calcification of the tendons and ligaments may occur.[447]

The most devastating skeletal effects of excess vitamin A occur with growth. For example, vitamin A is teratogenic to rodent fetuses, in which it produces limb deformities[451] and cleft palates.[452] Moreover, when rat fetal maxillae are cultured in excess vitamin A, suppression of DNA, glycosaminoglycan, and collagen synthesis ensues.[459] The collagen that is produced contains a paucity of intermolecular cross links.[459]

In light of these observations one would expect childhood hypervitaminosis A to result in permanent skeletal deformities.[450] In fact the physes may be impressed into cup-shaped, wide metaphyses, particularly about the knees. Although premature growth plate closure occurs in these children,[445] infants less than 6 months of age who have vitamin A toxicity have wide physes.[455] Unlike those seen in rickets, these cartilaginous plates are sharply demarcated from the adjacent metaphyses.[455]

Vitamin A deficiency has received increased attention because of its association with total parenteral nutrition.[450] In hypovitaminosis A, remodeling virtually ceases,[460] osteoclastic activity disappears from the subperiosteal surface, and apposition of cancellous bone continues in that location, resulting in overgrowth of the entire skeleton.[454] This new periosteal bone may encroach on spaces containing neurologic tissues,[454] leading to symptoms such as loss of hearing.[448] However, because of failure of modeling of trabecular bone into cortex, the absolute quantity of cortical bone diminishes.[454]

Hypovitaminosis A also has profound cartilaginous effects. For example, glycosaminoglycan degradation is inhibited in vitro.[449] This may relate to the failure of physeal chondrocytes to proliferate, resulting in arrested endochondral growth.[460] A bone plate develops across the face of the cartilaginous disc, isolating it from the underlying metaphysis.[447] Therefore, because of the failure of both remodeling and growth combined with continuous periosteal apposition, the bones of vitamin A–deficient persons are short and thick, with a predominance of newly formed cancellous, periosteal bone.[460]

Phosphorus

Phosphorus probably promotes collagen formation and mineralization[468,471] and is essential to normal skeletal metabolism. It increases the tensile strength of bone,[470] accelerates fracture healing[480] and inhibits resorption in vitro.[188]

It is likely that phosphorus stimulates osteoblast-mediated calcification by influencing a variety of metabolic events.[31,478,479] For example, the presence of adequate stores of ATP[472] and the formation of collagen-orthophosphate bonds appear to be important in the mineralization of osteoid.[465,469] This is illustrated clinically by failure of normal calcification front formation in hypophosphatemic states despite adequate calcium[474] and vitamin D.[142,143] Moreover, since phosphorus is intimately linked to the cellular uptake and intracellular distribution of calcium, its presence is necessary for the cation to act as a second messenger, enabling bone cells to respond to hormonal stimuli.[481]

Phosphorus homeostasis may also indirectly influence bone metabolism through its effect on acid-base balance.[467] Depletion of the anion leads to bicarbonate wasting and acidosis, which can mobilize bone salts,[476] enhance resorption,[461] delay bone collagen maturation,[482] and disturb both vitamin D metabolism[475] and the skeletal response to parathyroid hormone.[477]

Because phosphate-binding gels are extensively used to relieve dyspepsia, phosphorus depletion is relatively common.[464,473] Low circulating levels are associated with increased intestinal absorption of calcium[463] and hypercalcemia.[474] Consequently, circulating parathyroid hormone levels are not elevated with iatrogenic hypophosphatemia.[466] Classic rickets and osteomalacia therefore develop without evidence of osteitis fibrosa.[464] Hypophosphatemic individuals may, however, have evidence of increased resorption,[143,462] which is probably related to enhanced synthesis of 1,25-dihydroxyvitamin D.[483]

Hypophosphatemic osteomalacia. Familial hypophosphatemia (vitamin D resistant) is the most common cause of rickets in Western society.[487] The disease is generally transmitted as an X-linked dominant trait, although approximately one third of the cases are sporadic.[502] The availability of the Hyp mouse, whose disorder appears identical to human X-linked hypophosphatemia, has resulted in many insights into the pathogenesis and appropriate treatment of this disease.[486,498,499,]

The fundamental abnormality of the disorder is defective renal conservation of phosphorus.[494] Hence the diagnosis is generally based on the presence of diminished tubular reabsorption of the anion, despite low circulating levels.

The clinical manifestations of familial hypophosphatemia often appear within the second year of life. Affected patients fail to grow and have bowed legs.[487] In contrast to other forms of rickets, muscle weakness is uncommon.[487] Roentgenographically, typical rachitic physes are present, particularly in the extremities, whereas the axial skeleton is relatively spared. With time, osteosclerosis may develop, and bony protuberances often appear at sites of tendon insertion.

Histologically the mass of mineralized cancellous bone is normal, and the quantity of osteoid is greatly increased (Fig. 40-47).[495,497] Unmineralized seams covered by fusiform cells line virtually all trabecular surfaces. Before treatment the number of osteoclasts is normal, but with phosphorus therapy, secondary hyperparathyroidism and osteitis fibrosa may develop.

Studies employing tetracycline labeling demonstrate the characteristic changes of osteomalacia.[497] Many seams fail to assume a fluorescent label, and the cellular rate of mineralization is diminished. Consequently the production of new remodeling foci is diminished. These data are also consistent with suppressed activity and increased longevity of osteoclasts.

Although these histologic changes may occur in any form of osteomalacia, there is one morphologic feature that is characteristic of X-linked hypophosphatemia. These patients have a peculiar halo effect about the osteocytic lacunae, which is best appreciated by microroentgenography[490] or in thick, hand-ground sections stained with basic fuchsin (Fig. 40-48).[491] This abnormality has been shown by scanning electron microscopy to be foci of hypomineralization, characteristically polarized toward the nearest free bone surface.[142] These zones are particularly prominent in the most recently deposited portions of osteons and probably represent a delay in osteocyte-mediated calcification.[484,490]

The major efforts in treating vitamin D–resistant rickets have centered on phosphorus and vitamin D or its metabolites.[489,495,501] Administration of phosphorus with the vitamin D heals the rickets but appears to have little effect on attendant osteomalacia.[495] There is, however, evidence that despite normal circulating levels, patients with X-linked hypophosphatemia have defective synthesis of 1,25-dihydroxyvitamin D.[489] Moreover, substitution of this metabolite for vitamin D results in healing of both rickets and osteomalacia.[485,495]

There are also a variety of non-X-linked forms of congenital hypophosphatemic osteomalacia.[487,492,500] These conditions generally do not become apparent until adolescence, and therefore there may be no history of rickets. Unlike patients with the X-linked type, those with the adult-onset forms often have muscle weakness and aminoaciduria. Both muscle weakness and bone lesions often respond dramatically to appropriate therapy.[143]

Urinary phosphorus wasting and osteomalacia are associated with a variety of benign and malignant neoplasms. For example, approximately one fifth of patients with carcinoma of the prostate are hypophosphatemic and often have osteomalacia.[496] Since this lesion is often painful, it is important to identify it and distinguish it from metastases. Like the X-linked form of hypophosphatemia, the tumor-induced form may be attended by low blood levels of 1,25-dihydroxyvitamin D.[488,493] Resection of the neoplasm may lead not only to cure of

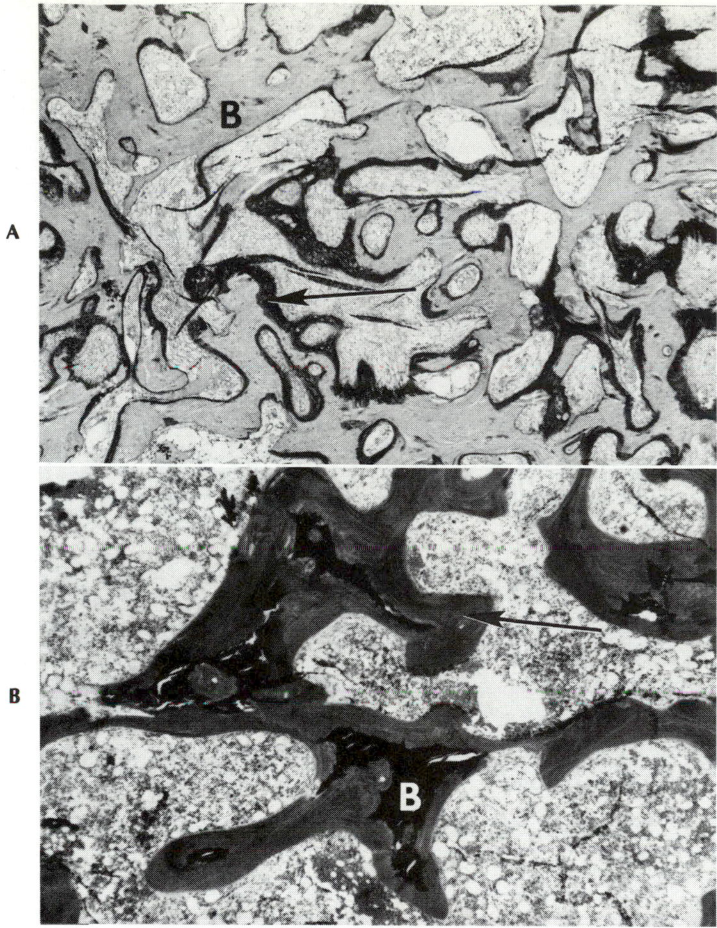

Fig. 40-47. A, Bone biopsy specimen from typical patient with X-linked hypophosphatemic osteomalacia. Trabecular mass is increased, and there are numerous wide osteoid seams *(arrow)*. If tetracyline were administered to patient, most of these seams would fail to assume fluorescent label. *B,* Mineralized bone. **B,** Bone biopsy specimen from patient with severe osteomalacia complicating X-linked hypophosphatemia. Most of bone consists of osteoid *(arrow)*. (*B,* Mineralized bone; undecalcified; **A,** Goldner's stain; **B,** modified Masson's trichrome stain; 40×.)

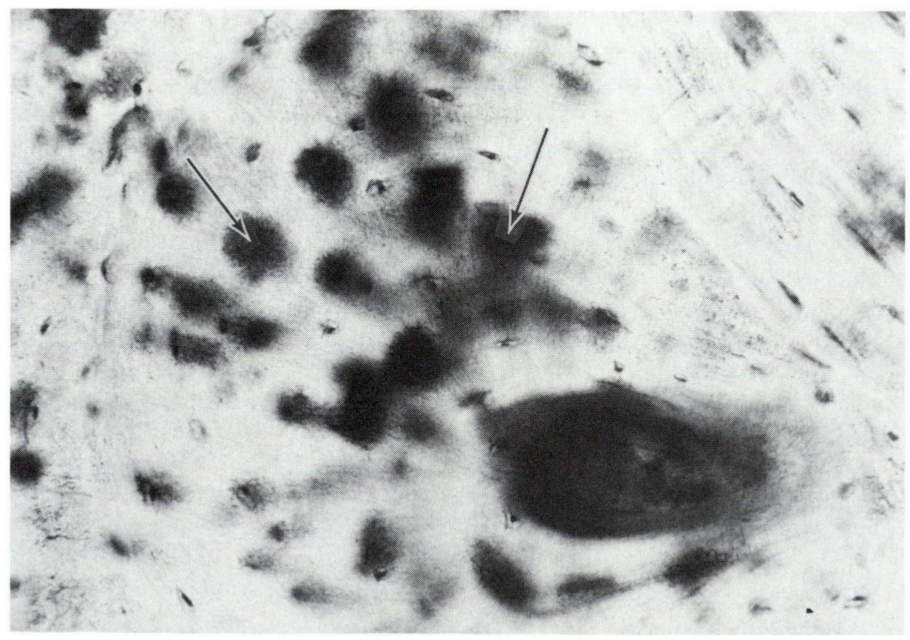

Fig. 40-48. "Halo effect" *(arrows)* surrounding osteocytes in vitamin D–resistant rickets. (Fresh, ground sections; Villanueva bone stain; 390×; courtesy Antonio R. Villanueva, Detroit, Mich.)

the bone lesion but also to normalization of circulating levels of the steroid.[493]

Fluoride

Ingested fluoride accumulates in hard tissues, and when present in toxic amounts, it has profound skeletal effects. Fluoritic bone forms in workers exposed to cryolite[510] and endemically in residents of areas such as India[521] and Qatar,[503] which have extremely high water concentrations of the ion.

Skeletal fluorosis produces bone pain and restricted spinal motion.[511] Roentgenographically there are severe osteosclerosis[511,521] and periosteal new bone formation.[511] There may be calcification of the interosseous membranes, ligaments, and tendons.[511] Grossly the bones have a yellow-brown discoloration.[505]

The primary physical effect of fluoride is displacement of hydroxyl ions from apatite to form fluorapatite.[509] This crystal is larger than its normal analog and hence less soluble.[510] Because the ion directly inhibits mineralization, osteomalacia and rickets attend fluorosis.[506] These factors, associated with suppression of intestinal absorption of calcium,[516] are responsible for the secondary hyperparathyroidism commonly accompanying ingestion of large quantities of fluoride.[521] The presence of subperiosteal resorption and cystic expansion of the small bones certainly suggests a hyperparathyroid effect.[511,521,522] Whether parathyroid hormone excess contributes to the manifestations of skeletal fluorosis is, however, controversial. For example, Liu and Baylink[514] noticed no difference between the bones of intact rats and parathyroidectomized, fluoride-fed rats.[514]

The most consistent histologic feature of fluoritic bone is abundant osteoid,[511,512,515,521,522] which is often associated with poor uptake of tetracycline.[505,515] There are often many osteoclasts, and occasionally marrow fibrosis develops. The number of haversian remodeling sites is increased, resulting in a porous cortex.[518] Osteocytic lacunae are enlarged, and osteoblasts are generally numerous, correlating with elevated serum alkaline phosphatase activity.[503,511] Woven bone is often abundant,[393,396,407] and microfractures are common.[505] Periosteal apposition may be associated with enhanced endosteal resorption, resulting in an increase in both the total transverse diameter of the bone and the size of the medullary cavity (Fig. 40-49).[504,514]

Ironically fluoride has become one of the most promising agents for the treatment of osteopenia.[513,514] Its therapeutic use was prompted by the demonstration of significantly fewer vertebral crush fractures among older women in areas with fluoridated water.[507] A series of clinical trials indicate that bone mass is increased by modest doses of the anion, particularly when administered concurrently with or followed by a course of vitamin D and calcium.[513,515] However, there is as yet no convincing evidence that this approach reduces the number of fractures. This paradox is perhaps a result of the abnormal structural features of fluoritic bone, which has not proved more resistant to breakage.[512,517,520,522]

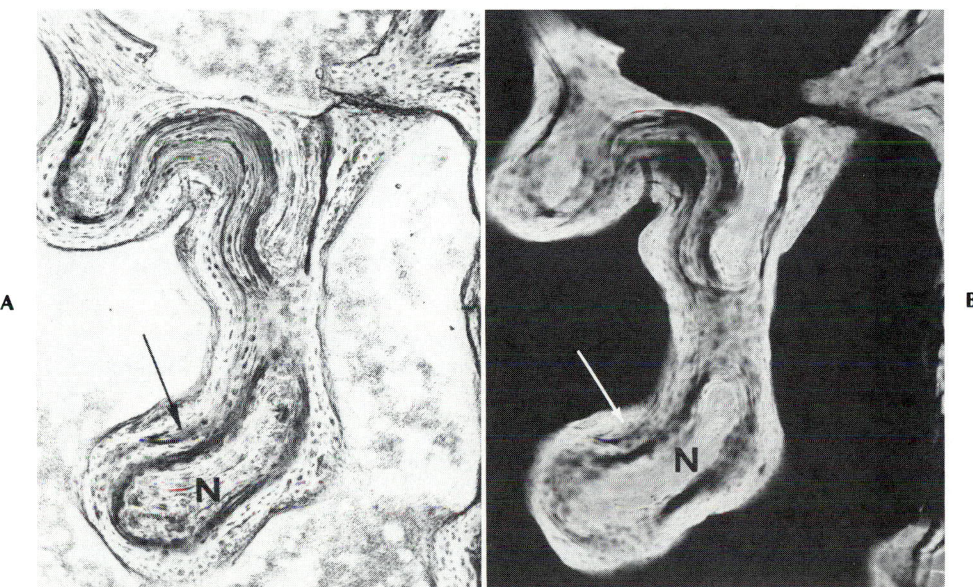

Fig. 40-49. Histologic section, **A,** and microradiograph, **B,** of bone of patient following 2 years of fluoride treatment. Abnormally calcified bone *(arrow)* has been deposited on normal trabeculae *(N)*. (Basic fuchsin; 50×; from Jowsey, J., Schenk, R.K., and Reutter, F.W.: J. Clin. Endocrinol. **28:**869, 1968.)

Alkaline phosphatase

Hypophosphatasia is a heritable disorder characterized by subnormal circulating alkaline phosphatase activity, osteomalacia, and increased urinary excretion of phosphoethanolamine and pyrophosphate.[37,527] The low blood level of the enzyme is reflected by its reduced activity in a variety of tissues, including bone and cartilage.[527] This observation and the failure of normal bone mineralization in this disease[37,530] offer convincing evidence of the fundamental role that alkaline phosphatase must play in skeletal calcification. However, it appears that the disorder is primary within the skeleton and is heralded by low levels of circulating alkaline phosphatase. For example, hypophosphatasemic sera are capable of mineralizing rachitic rat cartilage in vitro,[526] whereas costochondral tissue from affected patients fails to calcify in normal sera.[525]

Approximately half the patients who inherit hypophosphatasia as an autosomal recessive trait exhibit clinical evidence of the disorder at birth and usually die within a year.[524] Infants in whom the disease becomes evident after 6 months of age are less severely compromised and may eventually achieve significant recovery. Occasionally the diagnosis is made in adulthood (Fig. 40-50).[37,524,531] We have found that unaffected siblings of patients with the adult-onset form of hypophosphatasia may have low serum alkaline phosphatase activity and osteomalacia detectable on bone biopsy.[37]

The cardinal morphologic features of the infantile and childhood forms of the disease are rickets and poorly mineralized bone with particular involvement of the calvaria. Because of arrested calvarial growth, the fontanels bulge and are often associated with craniostenosis.[523] Endochondral growth is retarded, and the physes and bony matrix are usually histologically indistinguishable from those in phosphate-deficient rickets. However, the common occurrence of subperiosteal bone formation may on occasion distinguish the disease from other rachitic lesions.[357] In addition, early loss of anterior deciduous teeth caused by deficient alveolar bone synthesis or poor dental root development is a frequent and important diagnostic feature of hypophosphatasia.[529]

Immobilization osteopenia

Osteopenia in immobilized portions of the skeleton is a universal phenomenon. Not only does this occur with

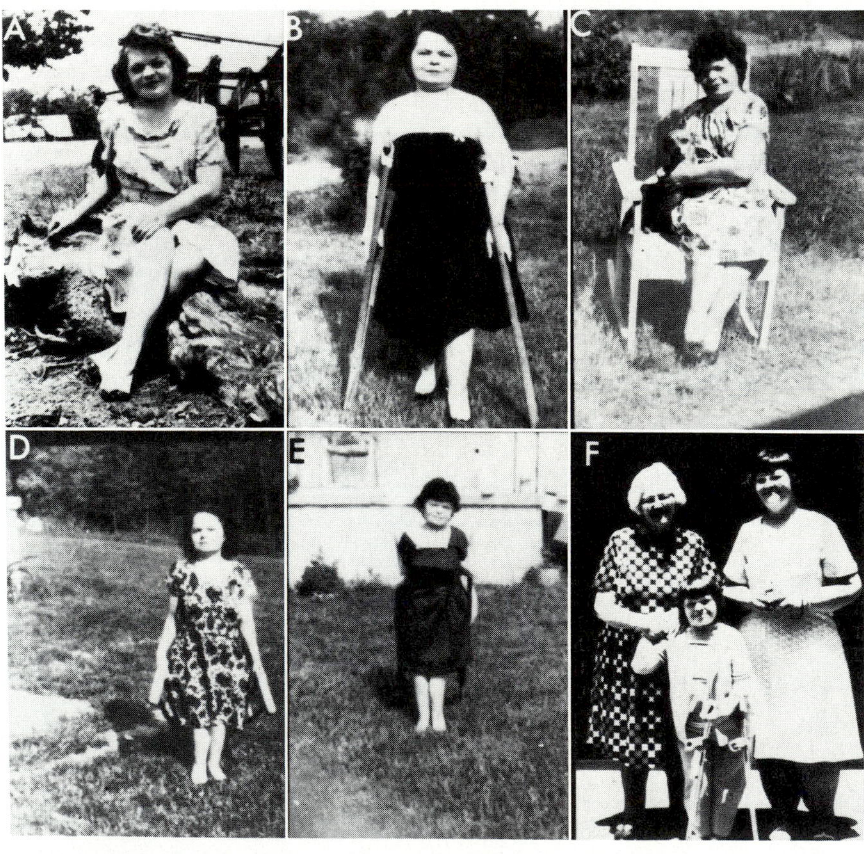

Fig. 40-50. Woman with adult-onset hypophosphatasia. There was progression of more than 13 inches of height with age. Patient was 18 years old in **A** and 56 years old when photographed with two normal-sized friends in **F.** (Courtesy Dr. Robert Weinstein, Augusta, Ga.; from Weinstein, R.S., and Whyte, M.P.: Arch. Intern. Med. **141**:727, 1981.)

bed rest,[534] paralysis,[533] and plaster casting,[542] but also in a weightless environment,[538,541] as observed with the advent of space travel. Astronauts, for example, lose 4 g of calcium per month during flight.[546] This remarkable degree of bone mobilization may be the limiting factor in prolonged space exploration.

Hypercalcemia and hypercalciuria may be so severe as to be life threatening in the immobilized patient.[536] Parathyroid hormone secretion may also be enhanced,[536] and, in fact, parathyroidectomy has an ameliorating effect on the development of osteopenia.[537,539] The absence of bone loss in the contralateral functional limb may be caused by local factors that increase the sensitivity of immobilized bone to normal circulating levels of the hormone.[539]

Growth may also be affected by immobilization. Perhaps the best example is the limb shortening that attends denervated states such as poliomyelitis.[549]

The pathogenesis of disuse osteopenia is controversial. Different patterns of bone loss appear in denervated (in contrast to nondenervated), immobilized limbs.[543] Moreover, compensation for the loss of weight on the vertebral column does not prevent the negative calcium balance induced by horizontal immobilization.[532] Therefore the lack of direct mechanical stress does not appear to be the primary inducer of immobilization osteopenia. On the other hand, application of electrical forces prevents loss of bone in an immobilized limb, indicating that alterations in piezoelectricity may be etiologically important.[539]

Clearly, disuse osteopenia develops primarily because of accelerated resorption without a compensatory increase in formation.[540,545] Bone loss is more rapid in the early stages and may be followed by a new steady state of formation and resorption in which the rate of diminution of skeletal mass is markedly slowed.[540,545]

Trabecular bone volume falls with immobilization,[544] but there appear to be striking differences in cell dynamics with age. In young dogs the greatest degree of bone loss is caused by enhanced subperiosteal resorption (Fig. 40-51),[545] whereas older, immobilized animals lose most bone via the endosteum.[535] Consequently, a bone subjected to prolonged immobilization is characterized by slightly increased medullary cavity size and a substantial decrement in its total transverse diameter (Fig. 40-52).[545]

Osteitis deformans (Paget's disease)

In 1877 Paget described a potentially deforming bone disease[566] that affects 3% to 4% of the population.[544,573]

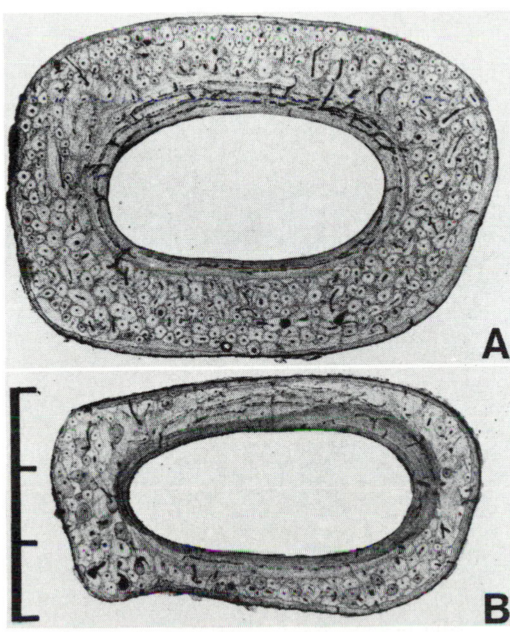

Fig. 40-51. Cross sections of, **A,** control and, **B,** immobilized metacarpal of young dog. Medullary cavity areas are the same, but cross-sectional area of immobilized bone is reduced. These findings indicate that loss of bone in immobilized young dogs is largely due to enhanced subperiosteal resorption. (From Uhthoff, H.K., and Jaworski, Z.F.G.: J. Bone Joint Surg. **60B:**420, 1978; with permission of publisher.)

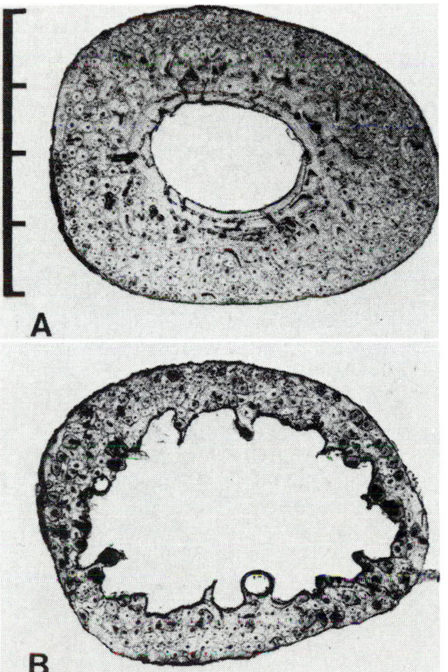

Fig. 40-52. Cross sections of, **A,** control and, **B,** immobilized metacarpal of old dog. Entire cross-sectional areas are the same, but medullary cavity of immobilized bone is enlarged. These findings indicate that loss of bone in immobilized old dogs is largely due to enhanced endosteal resorption. (From Jaworski, Z.F.G., et al.: J. Bone Joint Surg. **62B:**104, 1980; with permission of publisher.)

It is rarely encountered before the fourth decade[555] but can occur in children.[552] The disorder is the most frequent precursor of primary adult malignant bone tumors,[567] may be familial,[558] and is usually diagnosed at autopsy.[554]

Current evidence suggests that respiratory syncytial virus has an etiologic role in Paget's disease. Osteoclasts of all patients contain particles[569,574] that specifically bind antisera to this virus (Fig. 40-53).[564] It is therefore ironic that Paget proposed an infectious etiology when he initially described the disorder.[566]

The cardinal feature of osteitis deformans is focal acceleration of bone resorption and formation.[563,565] Although some view Paget's disease as a form of dysplasia or benign neoplasia,[568] the continued coupling of resorption and formation indicates that it is a form of abnormal remodeling.

The disease may be monostotic[554,555] but usually involves multiple portions of the skeleton, with predilection for the skull, pelvis, tibia, and femur. A single involved bone contains many stages of the process. Therefore osteitis deformans is not generalized and probably not of metabolic origin.[547] Since the disease is nonuniform within the skeleton, histologic examination of a biopsy specimen from a given individual is of little value in predicting changes in other bones or in following the effects of therapy. However, much can be learned by studying bone biopsy specimens from large numbers of pagetic patients.[563]

Reflecting the general phenomenon of bone remodeling, a focus of Paget's disease begins as active resorption. This lytic phase may progress rapidly and result in mechanical instability.[550] The tibia, femur, and humerus often fracture in a characteristic transverse pattern.[548] These fractures, when stressed, heal normally. However, since resorption is stimulated by immobilization, placing pagetic limbs in a restrictive cast frequently accelerates osteolysis.[557]

When involving a long bone, the process invariably begins at one end. Osteoporosis circumscripta cranii, which occurs in the frontal or occipital poles of the skull, is a manifestation of osteolytic Paget's disease.[548] In addition, platybasia, bowed back, curvatures of the femur and tibia, erosion of the lamina dura, and protrusion deformities of the acetabulum are caused by bone softening. On occasion there is cord compression resulting from vertebral collapse.[559]

Histologically the trabeculae in the osteolytic phase of Paget's disease are slender and extremely vascular. Because of osseous hyperperfusion, the skin over involved bone is warm, and in severe cases cardiac output is markedly elevated.[556] Although the long-hypothesized existence of arteriovenous shunts in pagetic bone has been disproved,[571] the diminished arteriovenous oxygen saturation gradient remains unexplained.

Giant osteoclasts, which may contain up to 100 nuclei, are the sine qua non of the lytic phase of osteitis deformans and a pathognomonic feature of Paget's disease. Whereas the nuclei of normal osteoclasts are adjacent to the free surface of the cell, those of pagetic osteoclasts are randomly distributed throughout the cytoplasm (Fig. 40-54).

The mixed phase of Paget's disease is characterized by accelerated formation as well as resorption. Roentgenographically this appears as a V-shaped advancing edge of osteolysis followed by a blastic zone. The proliferative

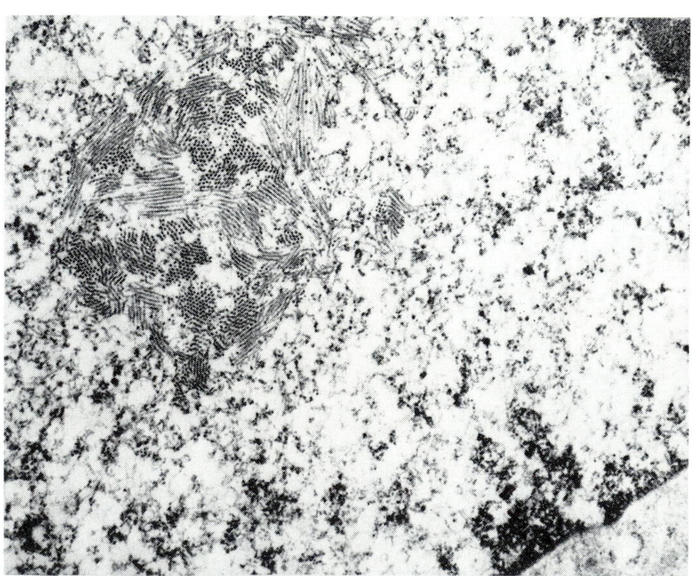

Fig. 40-53. Intranuclear viral-like inclusions in osteoclast of patient with Paget's disease. (31,000×; courtesy Dr. Barbara Mills, Los Angeles, Calif.)

region contains irregular, vascular trabeculae. Osteoclasts and Howship's lacunae are numerous, and there is a marked increase in the extent of osteoid-lined trabeculae.[563] Despite their abundance, however, these seams are narrower than normal (Fig. 40-55).[558]

The biochemical hallmark of active Paget's disease is elevation of serum alkaline phosphatase activity. Therefore it is not surprising that virtually all osteoid seams contain large osteoblasts and take up a tetracycline label (Fig. 40-56). The cellular rate of mineralization is also approximately twice normal.[563] Consequently, accelerated recruitment of remodeling units and enhanced osteoblastic activity are central components of the disorder. Because of brisk bone cell activation, woven collagen proliferates, as does fibrous tissue in the marrow. These changes may be confused with hyperparathyroidism, particularly since the lesions occasionally appear similar roentgenographically.[565] In this regard, Meunier and associates[563] have found increased circulating parathyroid hormone levels in 12% of their pagetic patients. In light of the accelerated remodeling found in the nonpagetic portions of these skeletons, the investigators postulate that a state of secondary hyperparathyroidism frequently exists in the disorder.[563] This hypothesis awaits confirmation.

Paradoxically the areas that roentgenographically are most characteristic of Paget's disease are the ones that are no longer active or symptomatic.[561] The bone of the

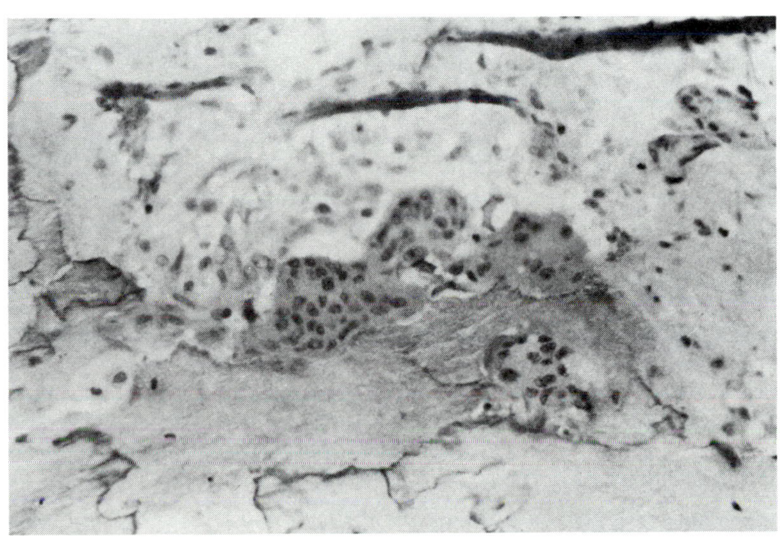

Fig. 40-54. Pagetic osteoclasts containing large numbers of nuclei distributed throughout cytoplasm. (Undecalcified, toluidine blue; 250×.)

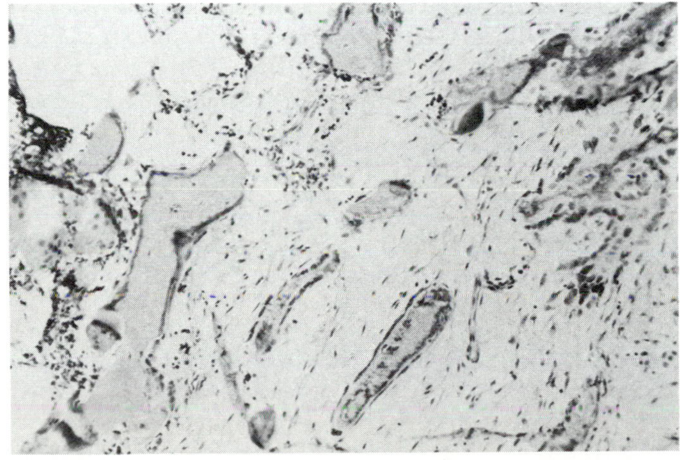

Fig. 40-55. Mixed phase of Paget's disease. There are numerous osteoclasts and osteoblasts. Marrow has myxomatous appearance, and woven bone is present. (Undecalcified, Goldner's stain; 100×.)

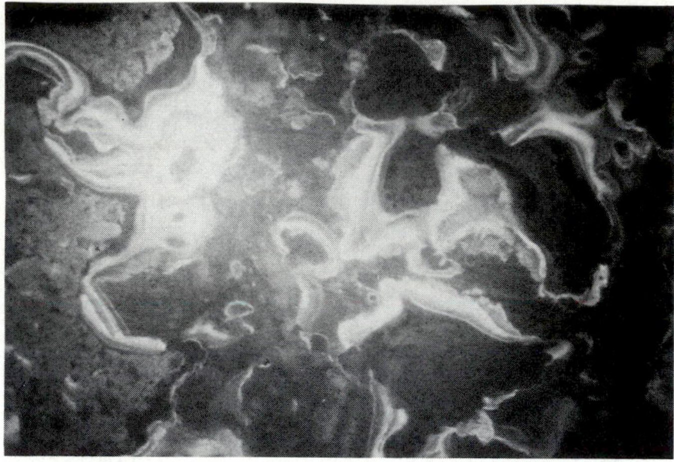

Fig. 40-56. Fluorescent micrograph of biopsy site of active Paget's disease. As seen by exuberant uptake of tetracycline, there is marked acceleration of bone turnover. (Fluorescent micrograph, undecalcified, unstained; 40×.)

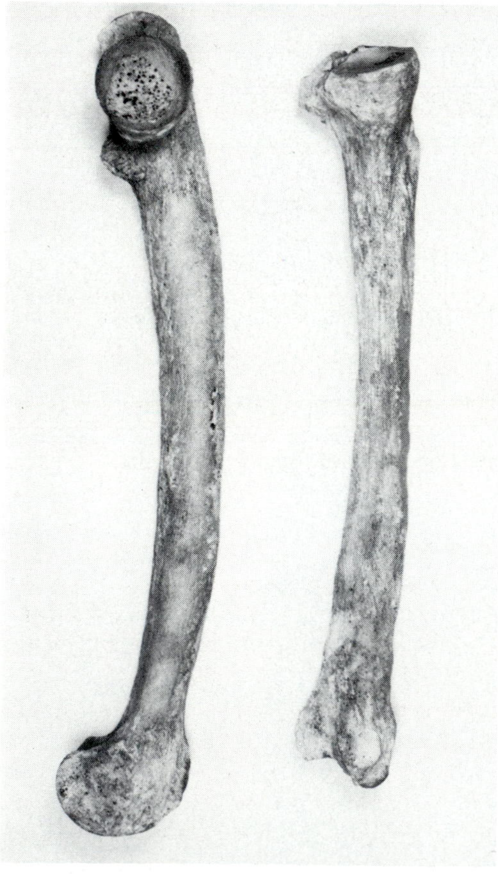

Fig. 40-57. Femur and tibia from severely pagetic skeleton. Note anterior bowing of both bones and marked periosteal reaction. (Courtesy Dr. Stephen Molnar, St. Louis, Mo.; WU 76-2964.)

sclerotic or "burned-out" phase is rock hard and difficult to cut. Its sclerotic nature may lead to neurosensory deafness caused by degeneration of auditory receptors within temporal bones.[562] Extremely active periosteal bone formation leads to rough, uneven surfaces (Fig. 40-57). The bone width is increased and the anatomic structure distorted, resulting in a characteristic roentgenographic cotton ball appearance of the skull and coarse trabecular striations (Fig. 40-58). Cortical and trabecular bone can no longer be distinguished, and osteonal architecture is distorted. Trabeculae are wide and disorganized, and vascular sinusoids are not as prominent as in the earlier stages of the process. Osteoclasts and osteoblasts are much fewer in number, but the striking histologic feature of this phase of the disease is a mosaic pattern of cement lines reflecting the previously rapid alternating processes of resorption and formation (Fig. 40-59).

The discovery of inhibitors of bone resorption, and therefore of remodeling, has resulted in effective treatment of Paget's disease. Calcitonin[295,307,308] is particularly useful, as are the diphosphonates.[549,551,553] The latter compounds, which are nonhydrolyzable analogs of pyrophosphate, bind to bone crystals and render them resistant to osteoclasts.[560,570,572]

SKELETAL DYSPLASIA

Osteogenesis imperfecta

Osteogenesis imperfecta, a hereditary disorder of connective tissue, usually becomes manifest by a predisposition toward multiple fractures. Although significant overlap occurs,[583,584] there are two general phenotypic expressions. Infants with osteogenesis imperfecta congenita, the most severe form, have multiple fractures at birth and subsequently develop crippling deformities. The mode of inheritance may be autosomal recessive,[578]

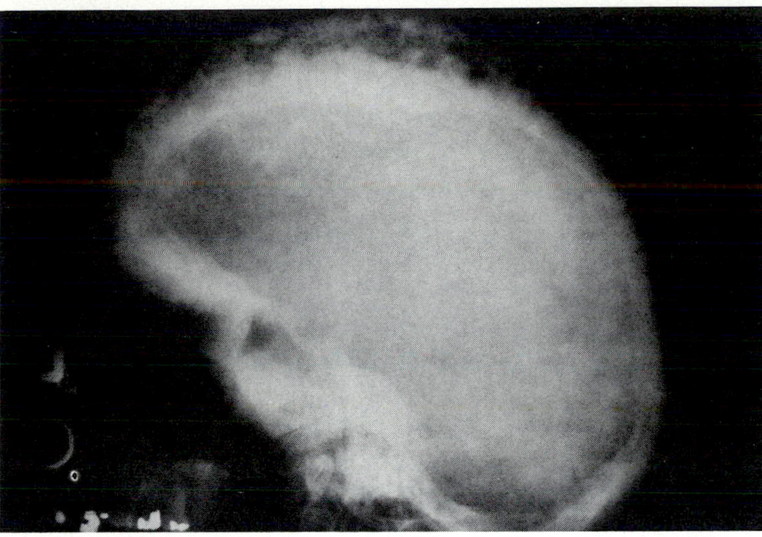

Fig. 40-58. Pagetic skull with characteristic "cotton-ball" appearance. (Courtesy Dr. James W. Debnam, Jr., Chesterfield, Mo.)

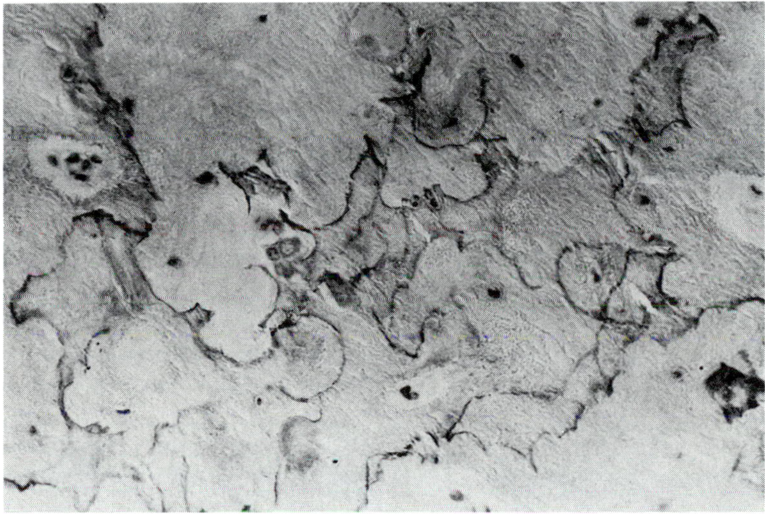

Fig. 40-59. Mosaic pattern of cement lines characteristic of sclerotic phase of Paget's disease. (Undecalcified, toluidine blue; 100×.)

but this remains uncertain because few patients are capable of reproduction.

Children with osteogenesis imperfecta tarda, which is less incapacitating and usually transmitted as an autosomal dominant,[582] may be born with fractures. However, clinical evidence of bone disease often does not appear until after the perinatal period. Bowing of the extremities is of particular diagnostic and prognostic significance.[576]

Regardless of the phenotypic expression of osteogenesis imperfecta, the mass of cortical and trabecular bone is reduced. There is failure of normal modeling of cancellous into compact bone, resulting in poorly demarcated, thick trabeculae and a porous cortex. The bones are often so distorted that the x-ray study is diagnostic. However, fractures, although frequent, heal normally with exuberant callus formation (Fig. 40-60).

It has become increasingly evident that the skeletal manifestations of osteogenesis imperfecta are caused by defective osteoblasts. One of the most conspicuous features, for example, is a striking increase in the number of osteocytes per unit volume of lamellar bone (Fig. 40-61).[8] This observation can be best explained by a decrease in the volume of bone synthesized by each osteoblast before its incorporation into matrix as an osteocyte. The presence of both osteopenia and

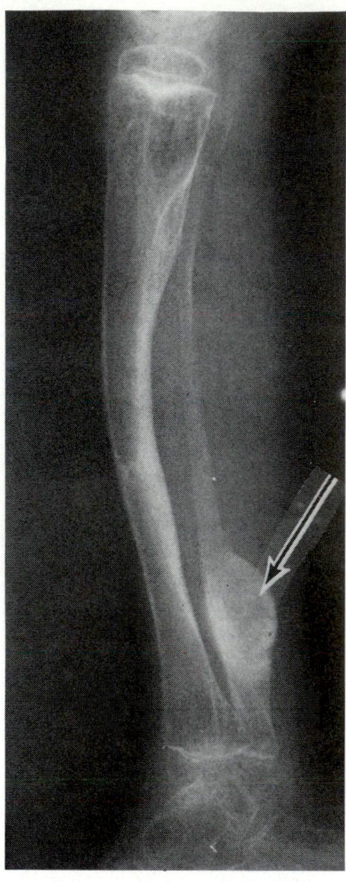

Fig. 40-60. Severely osteopenic and distorted tibia and fibula of child with osteogenesis imperfecta. Healing fracture exhibits abundant callus formation *(arrow)*. (Courtesy Dr. James W. Debnam, Jr., Chesterfield, Mo.)

increased osteocytes suggests that the absolute number of osteoblasts is normal despite their hypoactivity.

Although abnormal numbers of osteocytes are extremely helpful in diagnosing osteogenesis imperfecta, the most consistent microscopic skeletal abnormality is related to collagen structure. Falvo and Bullough[8] have shown that woven bone, which normally disappears by 4 years of age, is universally present in patients who undoubtedly have the disease. This finding is of great help in distinguishing them from those with juvenile osteoporosis.[579] In addition, we noted that patients with osteogenesis imperfecta congenita do not aggregate bone collagen into adequately thick fibers (Fig. 40-62).[586] These morphologic abnormalities may reflect the failure of normal bone collagen cross linking in this disease.[577,587]

Because of the ubiquity of collagen, osteogenesis imperfecta has varied extraskeletal manifestations. Patients frequently have ligamentous laxity, the severity of which appears to parallel skeletal dysfunction.[576] Many develop inguinal and umbilical hernias[576] and have fragile, easily bruised skin.[583] The most frequently noted extraskeletal manifestation is the presence of blue sclerae.[576,583]

In light of these many extraskeletal abnormalities, studies of skin fibroblast culture have afforded insights into the pathogenesis of osteogenesis imperfecta. A number of laboratories, for example, note a decrease in the ratio of type I/type III collagen production by cells derived from affected patients.[581,585] Since this phenomenon is caused by diminished synthesis of type I, which is the unique collagen of bone,[575] the abnormality may contribute to skeletal dysfunction. It is also of interest that whether or not abnormalities of collagen synthesis

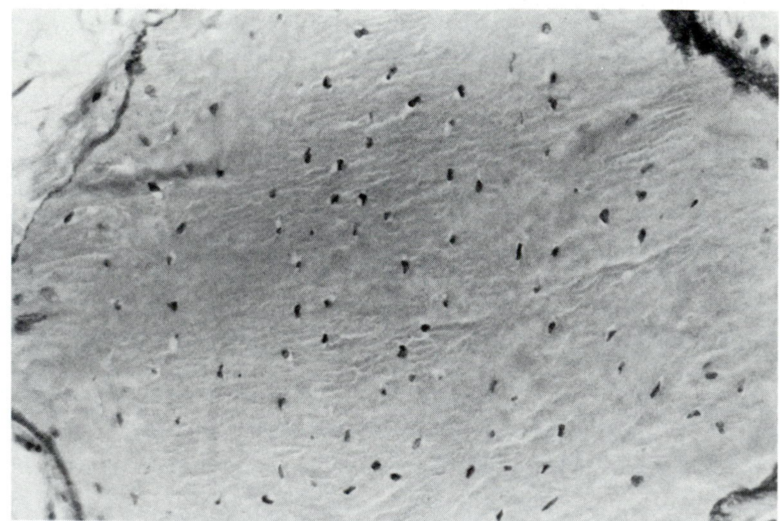

Fig. 40-61. Note marked increase in number of osteocytes in lamellar bone from patient with osteogenesis imperfecta as compared with Fig. 40-11, *B*. (Undecalcified, Goldner's stain; 100×.)

can be identified in fibroblasts of patients with osteogenesis imperfecta when cultured, the appearance and geometric packing of these cells are distinctly abnormal.[580]

Osteopetrosis

The osteopetroses consist of two phenotypically distinct diseases of increased skeletal mass caused by osteoclast dysfunction.[590,591] Autosomal recessive (malignant) osteopetrosis is almost invariably lethal within the first decade.[588,589] The more common form, which is transmitted as an autosomal dominant trait, is, however, not life threatening.[593,604]

Malignant osteopetrosis is generally diagnosed roentgenographically. The skeleton is opaque with loss of an identifiable medullary cavity.[597,598] Because of defective modeling, the tubular bones are truncated and broad. The physes, on the other hand, may appear rachitic (Fig. 40-63).[596,597]

The pathognomonic histologic feature of both forms of osteopetrosis is the presence of islands of mineralized cartilage deep in the metaphysis and diaphysis.[593,594] This abnormality is the result of failure of osteoclastic resorption of the primary spongiosa. Consequently, most of the radiopacity of this disease actually reflects excess mineralized cartilage. This abnormality of skeletal matrix is probably responsible for the numerous fractures that occur in these densely sclerotic bones (Fig. 40-64.)[597,604]

Intramembranous ossification also occurs in osteopetrotic bone.[604] Past the fetal stage, such ossification contributes greatly to the bone shaft via periosteal apposition. Consequently a significant portion of osteopetrotic long bones may not contain cartilaginous bars,[603] and the site of tissue sampling is extremely important in establishing the diagnosis (Plate 7).

Despite the failure of osteoclasts to resorb matrix, these cells are found in abundance in malignant osteopetrosis.[596-598] In fact, they are so numerous that they probably contribute to the associated marrow suppression (Fig. 40-64).[598] Marrow fibrosis, which progresses with age in this disease, also inhibits hemopoiesis.[596]

Probably reflecting a variety of pathogenetic mechanisms, osteoclast morphology is heterogeneous in malignant osteopetrosis. In some patients the cells appear nor-

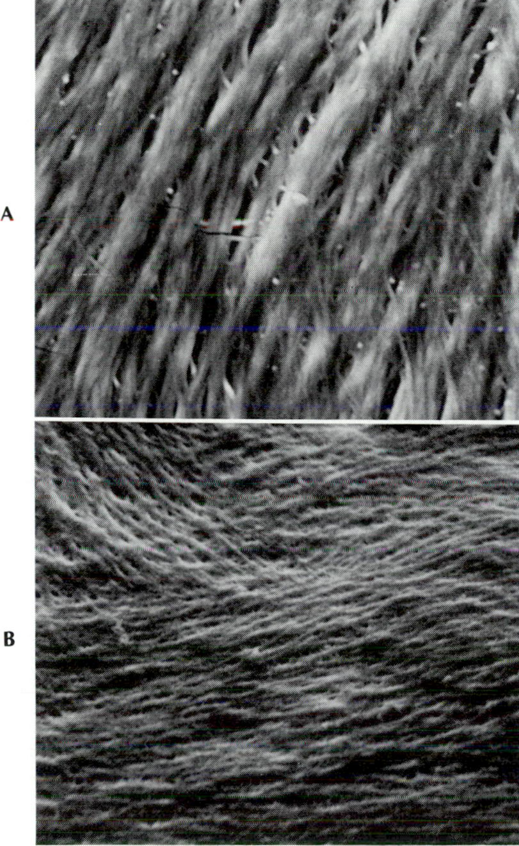

Fig. 40-62. A, Scanning electron micrograph of osteoid of normal 11-year-old child. Note thick interweaving fiber bundles. **B,** Scanning electron micrograph of 11-year-old patient with osteogenesis imperfecta. Fibers fail to aggregate into bundles of normal width. (2200×; from Teitelbaum, S.L., et al.: Calcif. Tissue Res. **17:**75, 1974.)

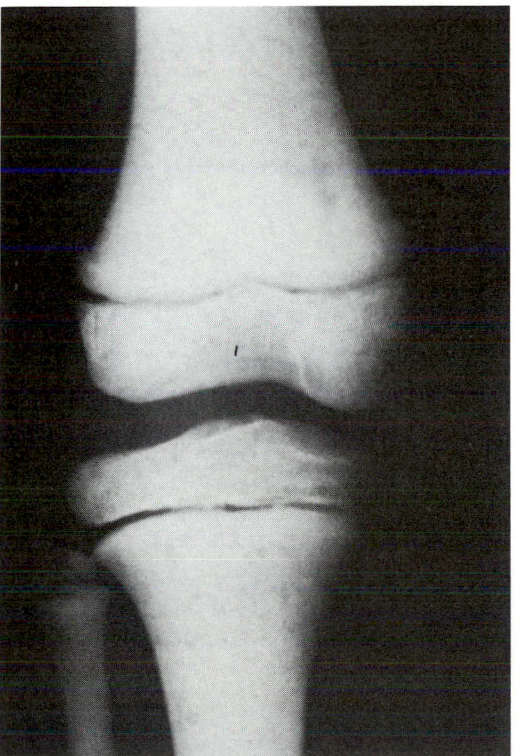

Fig. 40-63. Characteristic sclerotic appearance of osteopetrotic bones. Distinction between cortical and trabecular bone is lost. (Courtesy Dr. James W. Debnam, Jr., Chesterfield, Mo.)

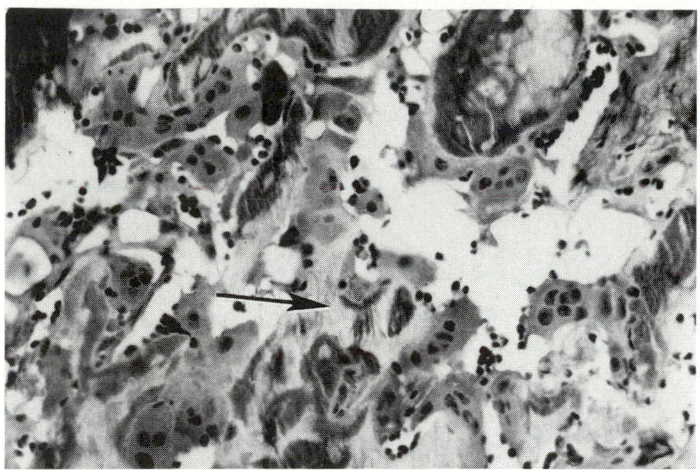

Fig. 40-64. Bone biopsy specimen from patient with malignant osteopetrosis. Note large numbers of osteoclasts and presence of cartilaginous bars *(arrow)*. (Undecalcified, Goldner's stain; 250×; reprinted with permission from Metabolic Bone Disease and Related Research, vol. 3, Teitelbaum, S.L., et al.: Copyright 1981, Pergamon Press, Ltd.)

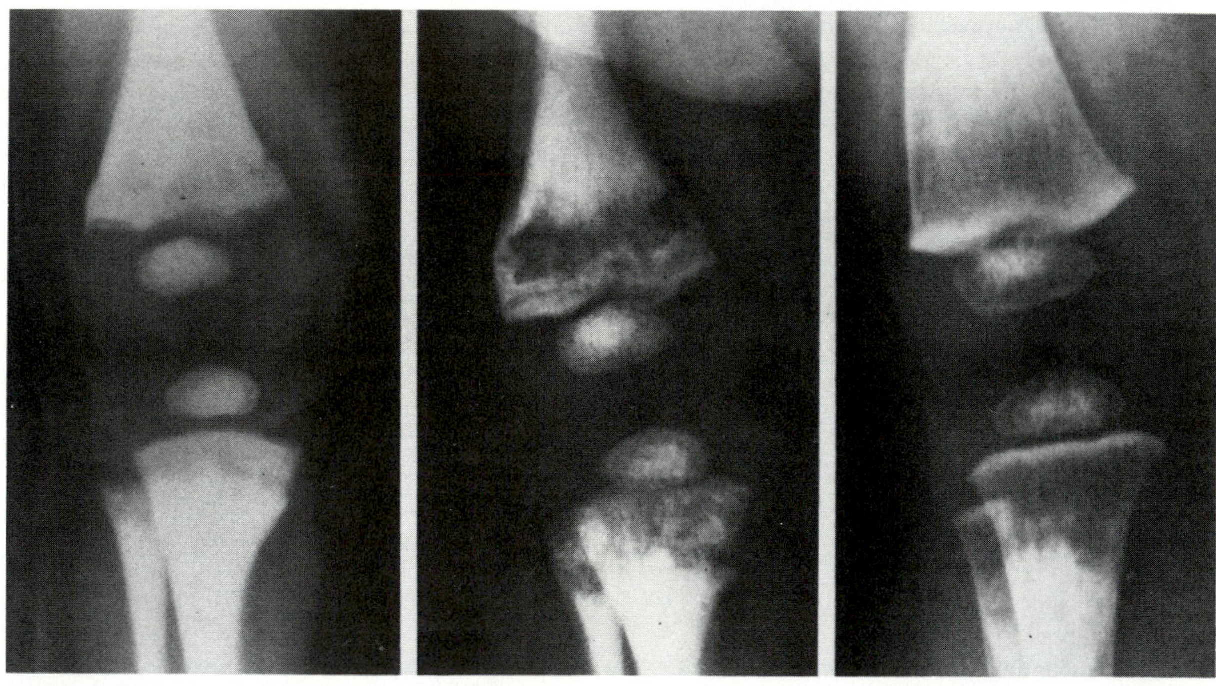

Pretransplant +7 weeks +22 weeks

Fig. 40-65. Roentgenograms of patient with malignant osteopetrosis before and 7 and 22 weeks after bone marrow transplantation. Note progressive resorption of osteopetrotic bone. (From Coccia, P., et al. Reprinted by permission of The New England Journal of Medicine **302:**701, 1980.)

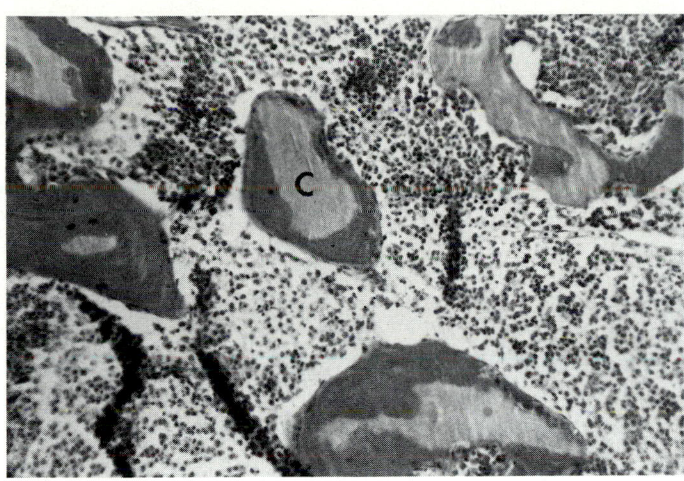

Fig. 40-66. Autosomal dominant osteopetrosis. As in malignant form, bars of mineralized cartilage *(C)* persist into metaphysis. However, bone marrow in benign form is normal. (Undecalcified, Goldner's stain; 100×.)

mal and may even have ruffled borders.[598] This observation calls into question the claim that membrane ruffling is invariably associated with resorption. In other patients the osteoclasts are bizarre, contain large numbers of nuclei, and have no evidence of a ruffled membrane.[596-598]

The predominant clinical manifestations of malignant osteopetrosis involve the central nervous system and hemopoiesis.[588,589,596] Skeletal overgrowth occurs in the cranial cavity and its foramina, resulting in blindness,[594] deafness, and severe mental retardation. Reduction in size of the nares leads to persistent nasal obstruction, which is the most common initial symptom.[594] Bone marrow failure results in a leukoerythroblastic anemia and hepatosplenomegaly. Death is usually caused by infection or severe neurologic dysfunction.

Virtually all insights into the pathogenesis and treatment of malignant osteopetrosis rest on the pioneering work of Walker.[599-601] This investigator was the first to cure osteopetrosis in rodents by temporary parabiosis to normal litter mates.[601] Such a cure can also be effected by transfusing normal marrow,[602] spleen,[602] or liver cells[595] into sick animals. Alternatively, osteopetrosis can be induced in healthy mice by injecting spleen cells from affected animals.[603] My co-workers and I[101] have recently extended these studies to humans: we cured the disease in a female infant by grafting bone marrow from her immunologically identical brother (Fig. 40-65).

The clinical manifestations of the autosomal dominant form of osteopetrosis are generally confined to the skeleton,[604] although a family with associated renal tubular acidosis and basal ganglia calcification has been studied.[604] These patients have abnormal bone modeling, which, curiously, may almost normalize with age.[604] However, the early influence of the disease leaves its mark in growth retardation.[604] The radiopacity of the skeleton with benign osteopetrosis is identical to that with the malignant variety.[604] The bone marrow, however, is normal, with no evidence of increased numbers of osteoclasts or fibrosis; herein lies its basic distinction from the malignant form (Fig. 40-66).[604]

Achondroplasia

Achondroplasia is the most common of the chondrodystrophies and the most frequent cause of disproportionate, short stature. It is inherited as an autosomal dominant trait,[607] but because of the physical and social difficulties of reproduction, 80% of cases are sporadic.[355]

The characteristic appearance of achondroplastic patients reflects the failure of normal endochondral ossification. They have short limbs, and although spinal abnormalities are common, truncal length is relatively normal (Fig. 40-67).[608,613] Because of decreased interpediculate distance and a narrow foramen magnum, the most serious complications of the disorder are cord and nerve root compression.[608] Achondroplastic persons have a saddle nose, are prominently lordotic, and have varus deformities of the knees. Wide spacing of the third and fourth fingers results in a trident appearance of the hand. Since intramembranous ossification is not affected, there is disproportionate growth of the calvaria, resulting in prominent frontal bossing and mild macrocephaly. Because the base of the skull develops largely in cartilage, it is relatively hypoplastic.

There is much debate concerning the appearance of achondroplastic cartilage. Rimoin and associates,[611] who view the chondrodystrophies as those with histologically well-ordered endochondral ossification or those in which enchondral ossification is histologically disordered,[611] believe that achondroplastic cartilage is well ordered and

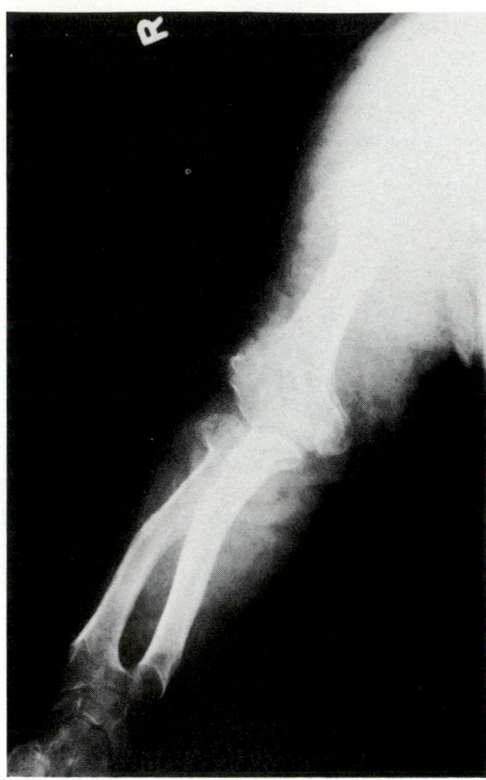

Fig. 40-67. Achondroplastic arm. Note marked attenuation of diaphyseal length with normal width. Metaphyses are characteristically flared. (Courtesy Dr. Hyman R. Senturia, St. Louis, Mo.)

that the dysfunctions of growth are probably rate related rather than caused by gross cartilaginous abnormalities. They state that the reports of disordered cartilage in achondroplasia are actually observations of other chondrodystrophies, particularly thanatophoric and metatropic dwarfism, as well as achondrogenesis.

In contrast, other investigators report striking abnormalities of achondroplastic growth plates.[606,610,614] The hypertrophic zone is markedly attenuated, and the number of chondrocytes is diminished. The cells that are present are located in short columns or clusters.[606]

The growth plate matrix may also appear abnormal in achondroplasia.[606,614] Proteoglycans are generally decreased in concentration and largely distributed around chondrocyte clusters. The remainder of the cartilage looks fibrotic and contains banded collagen fibrils.[606] The hypertrophic zone undergoes premature mineralization, which perhaps leads to the abundant chondroclasts present at the growth plate–metaphyseal junction.[606] This area also contains broad, horizontal trabeculae, particularly juxtaposed to clustered chondrocytes.[606]

Why endochondral ossification fails in this disorder is unknown. However, cartilaginous lysosomal enzymes and alkaline phosphatase may be deficient.[614] Particularly in older achondroplastic children, cartilaginous proteoglycans are less soluble than normal, and glucosamine is frequently increased.[609] These changes relate to curvilinear inclusion bodies composed of rough endoplasmic reticulum present in chondrocytes of hypochondroplastic dwarfs, a disorder similar to but less severe than achondroplasia.[605] Cooper, Ponseti, and Maynard[605] interpret these bodies as manifestations of the failure of chondrocytes to transfer synthesized protein from ergastoplasm to the Golgi apparatus.[605]

Regardless of the controversy surrounding the histologic appearance of their cartilage, there is little question that the growth plates of achondroplastic persons are grossly and roentgenographically abnormal. The physes are V shaped, and their apices point toward the metaphyses.[610] As a result of normal periosteal bone formation with retarded endochondral ossification, periosteal bone grows over and into the perichondrium, resulting in cup-shaped costochondral junctions.[612]

Mucopolysaccharidoses

The mucopolysaccharidoses are a group of disorders characterized by defective degradation of mucopolysaccharides. Identification of various specific enzyme defects has enabled McKusick[629] to classify these diseases into six categories.[629] Because of these enzyme defects, cultured fibroblasts from patients of each group exhibit abnormal metachromasia correctable by the addition of normal serum or serum of patients with other forms of mucopolysaccharidoses.[623] Although significant bone changes may exist in patients with any of the mucopolysaccharidoses, those with the Morquio's (MPS IV) or Maroteaux-Lamy (MPS VII) syndromes are the most strikingly affected.

Hurler's syndrome (MPS I H), the first of the mucopolysaccharidoses to be described, is caused by a deficiency of alpha-L-iduronidase.[616] It is associated with increased tissue stores and excretion of dermatan sulfate and heparan sulfate.[621] Gargoylism describes the characteristic troll-like appearance of these patients. The gross skeletal defects, which are also present in other mucopolysaccharidoses, represent a spectrum of changes called dysostosis multiplex.[619]

Hurler's syndrome patients are dwarfed, with saber-shaped, broad, flat ribs, clawed hands, and a characteristic shoe-shaped sella turcica.[619] Because of expansion of the marrow cavity the tubular bones are swollen. The proximal one third of the femur, however, is narrow.[619] Focally decreased anterior-posterior development and replacement of defective areas by radiolucent cartilage result in the hook-shaped roentgenographic appearance of some lumbar vertebral bodies.[626] These defectively developed vertebrae may be displaced posteriorly, resulting in spinal cord compression.[620]

Histologically there is arrest of endochondral growth in Hurler's syndrome.[620,626] The resting zone of the growth plate appears normal, whereas the proliferative zone is attenuated.[620] The cells of the hypertrophic zone are severely disarrayed. The chondrocytes are enlarged, contain abundant intracellular glycoprotein, and completely fill their lacunae.[617] An abnormal variant of mucopolysaccharide, which may appear focally fibrillar and birefringent,[617] is present in the cartilaginous matrix.[618]

Ultrastructurally the chondrocytes of patients with Hurler's syndrome contain numerous, often coalescing vacuoles, which push the endoplasmic reticulum to the periphery of the cells.[634] Since the mucopolysaccharidoses are diseases of enzyme deficiencies, these abnormal vacuoles may be derived from lysosomes. Presumably caused by discharge of cytoplasmic contents into the matrix, normal chondrocytes have scalloped cell membranes. These crenations, however, are not present in Hurler's syndrome patients.[634] Silberberg and associates[634] believe that this absence of scalloping represents deficient release of intracellular contents by chondrocytes (Fig. 40-68).

The thin cortices of bone in Hurler's syndrome are essentially unremarkable. However, a transverse bony plate commonly develops between the growth plate and the metaphysis.[626] Little osteoblastic activity is present, and the osteocytes may be enlarged.[626] Whereas "gargoyle cells" are common in cartilage and periosteum,[626] there is little evidence that they infiltrate osseous tissue.[620] Therefore the etiology of the associated osteopenia may be different from that of the abnormal endochondral growth.[620]

Hunter's syndrome (MPS II) is also associated with abnormal excretion of dermatan sulfate and heparan sulfate.[624] Patients with this disease may have skeletal changes similar to but less severe than those with Hurler's syndrome.[619,629]

Because of sulfamidase deficiency,[628] patients with Sanfilippo's syndrome (MPS III) have high urinary and tissue content of heparan sulfate.[625] Although this disorder is often characterized by slight dwarfism, the gross skeletal abnormalities tend to be the mildest of the mucopolysaccharidoses.[631] The chondrocytes of Sanfilippo's syndrome are distended with distinct types of vacuoles, which, as in Hurler's syndrome, may represent altered lysosomes.[634] Moreover, like Hurler chondrocytes, these cells exhibit a lack of cell membrane scalloping, again suggesting a failure in the egress of cytoplasmic contents (Fig. 40-69).

The skeletal changes of Morquio's syndrome (MPS IV) are among the most severe of the mucopolysaccharidoses.[632] These patients excrete excessive amounts of keratan sulfate.[630] They appear normal at birth, but clinical manifestations usually develop between the first and second years. Because of severe dysplasia of epiphyseal growth centers, virtually all bones other than those of the skull are affected.[632] Generalized osteopenia is present. The vertebral bodies are characteristically flat (platyspondylia),[630] and because of hypoplasia of the first cervical vertebra, high spinal cord compression is a complication of the disorder.[622] The ribs resemble paddles, and the physes are misshapen.[632] The hips are enlarged and irregular.[632]

The characteristic histologic alterations of Morquio's syndrome are confined to the skeleton, particularly the cartilage.[615,632,635] There are several abnormalities of the physes, such as short, disorganized zones of proliferative and hypertrophic cartilaginous cells. The chondrocytes are large, sparse, and clumped; they contain large amounts of metachromatic material.[635] Ultrastructurally they exhibit distended ergastoplasmic sacs.[633] Distinct areas of clumped, metachromatic granules juxtaposed with nonmetachromatic foci are common in Morquio cartilaginous matrix.[632] Not infrequently, areas of this cartilage have the birefringent qualities of fibrillar connective tissues such as collagen.[615,632,635] Fibrous tissue strands containing areas of intramembranous bone formation may be interposed between cartilage and bone in the growth plate.[635]

Although severe osteopenia is common in Morquio's syndrome, the bony abnormalities may be the result of cartilage dysfunction.[615,632] As in Hurler's syndrome, a transverse osseous plate forms across the face of metaphyseal-cartilaginous junction.[615] Osteoblastic and osteoclastic activity appears normal, but there is a disorderly array of sparse trabeculae.[635] Calcified cartilage persists in these trabeculae, but there are now foam cells in the bone.[615,632] It is therefore likely that deficient metaphyseal osteogenesis results from inadequate chondrocyte proliferation and maturation.[615]

Maroteaux-Lamy syndrome (MPS IV) is a rare mucopolysaccharidosis. It is associated with excessive excretion of dermatan sulfate,[627] and the skeletal changes are severe. However, no information regarding histologic changes in cases in which the diagnosis is certain is yet available.

Patients with Maroteaux-Lamy syndrome are markedly dwarfed and have severe dysostosis multiplex. Radiolucencies suggesting residual islands of cartilage are present in the tibial and distal femoral metaphyses.[627] Irregular ossification of the femoral head, which may be confused with Legg-Calvé-Perthes disease, is also present.[627] As in Morquio's syndrome, there is often hypoplasia of the odontoid process.[627]

OSTEONECROSIS

Osteonecrosis is a family of infarctive disorders of the skeleton that most commonly involves the femoral head. Although all forms have the common feature of bone death, the natural histories of these various entities and their pathologic expressions may differ greatly.

A

B

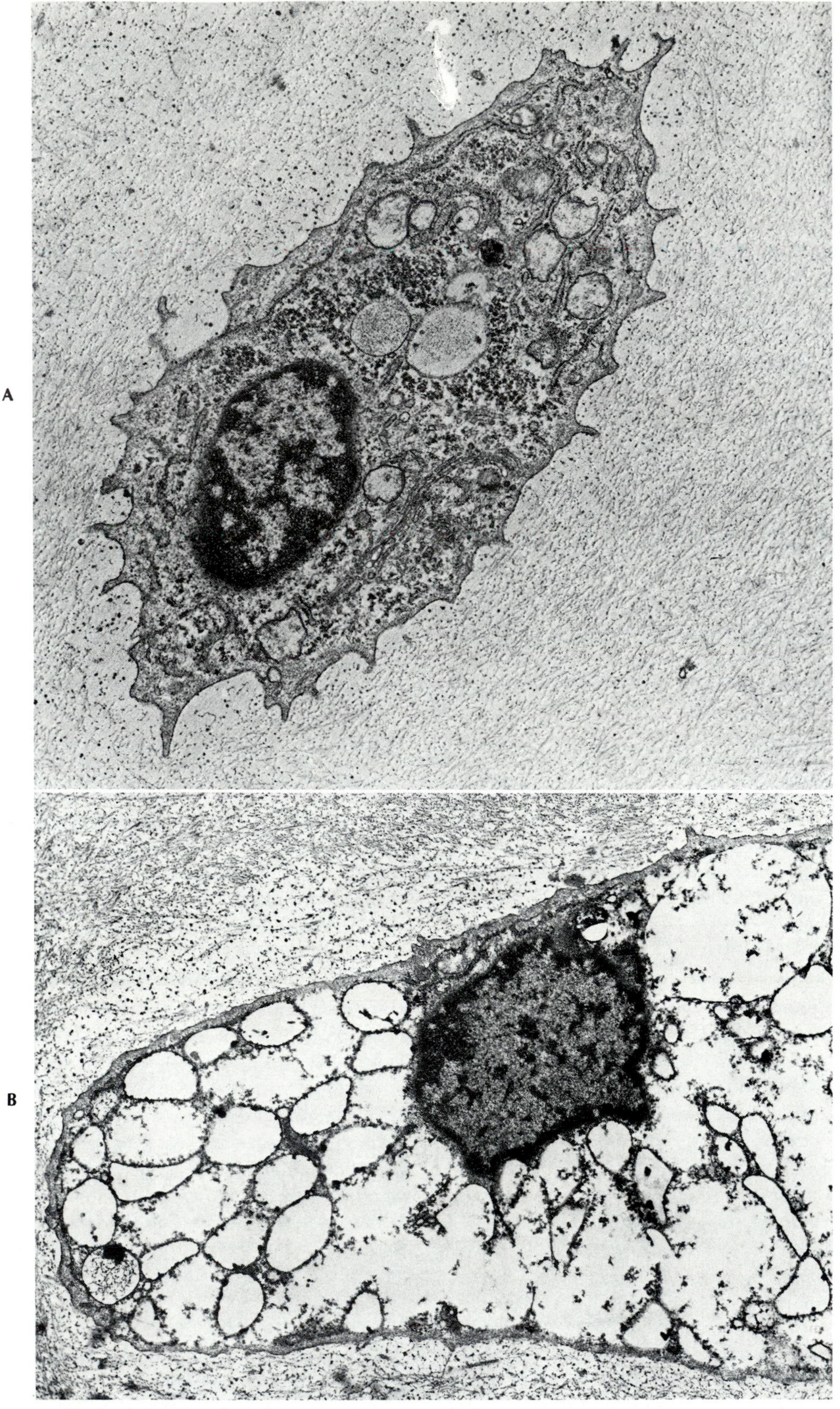

Fig. 40-68. A, Normal chondrocyte. Note scalloped cell membrane. **B,** Giant chondrocyte from patient with Hurler's syndrome. Note large, distended cytoplasmic vacuoles and absence of scalloping of cell membrane. (19,900×; courtesy Dr. Ruth Silberberg, Jerusalem, Israel.)

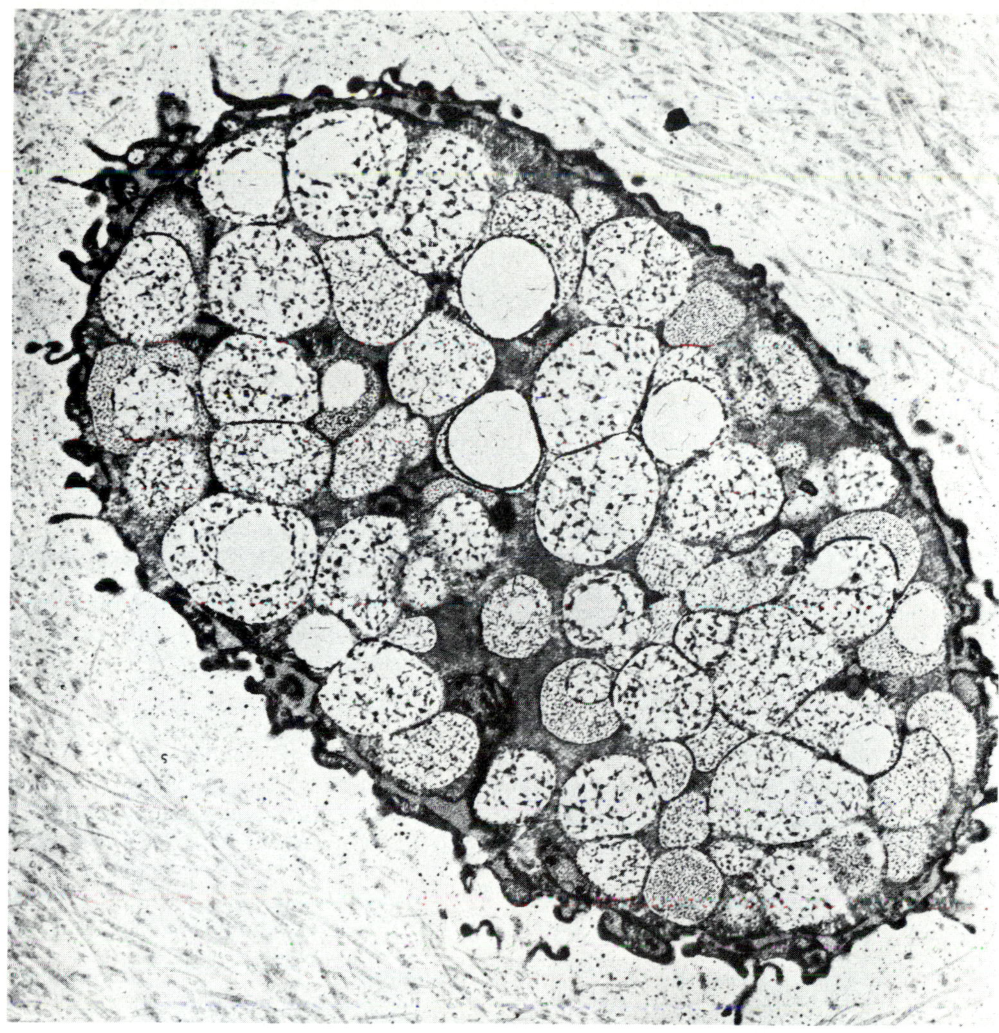

Fig. 40-69. Chondrocyte of patient with Sanfilippo's syndrome. Note distinctive cytoplasmic vacuoles. (19,900×; courtesy Dr. Ruth Silberberg, Jerusalem, Israel.)

There are three generic categories of osteonecrosis.[641-643] Most commonly the infarct follows fracture of the femoral neck[644] and in this setting may be referred to as avascular necrosis. Osteonecrosis is also sustained by a number of individuals who do not have vascular insufficiency and are not receiving immunosuppressive drugs. Although there is a significant incidence of associated systemic diseases, such as alcoholism[636] and hyperuricemia,[644,653] the cause of this condition is unknown; it is best described as *idiopathic osteonecrosis*. Finally, a number of patients taking immunosuppressive agents, particularly corticosteroids, sustain osteonecrosis.[658] Patients who have received renal transplants are particularly prone to this complication.[655]

The earliest histologic change occurring in any form of osteonecrosis is death of marrow cells and of their associated trabeculae, which lose their osteocytes.[641,645] Subsequently a fracture, which can be seen roentgenographically in the femoral head as the crescent line, develops through the necrotic bone.[641-643,654] This radiolucent, subchondral fissure is the first diagnostic hallmark of osteonecrosis of the femoral head.

All of the remaining pathologic changes reflect repair, and it is in the exuberance of these events that the various forms of osteonecrosis differ.[641] The most dramatic repair develops in avascular necrosis. Marrow fibroblasts differentiate into osteoblasts and deposit woven bone on dead cancellum. This complex is eventually resorbed and replaced by extremely wide lamellar trabeculae, which are of such dimensions as to resemble cortex. At this point the involved bone appears roentgengraphically sclerotic. It should be appreciated that this increased bone density may also represent collapse and compaction of necrotic trabeculae. Regardless of the mechanism, the wedge-shaped area of sclerosis in the femoral head is diagnostic of osteonecrosis (Fig. 40-70).

The most devastating event in the natural history of osteonecrosis involves subchondral cortical bone.[641-643] In contrast to the cancellum, the subchondral cortex is resorbed and hence becomes attenuated and structurally

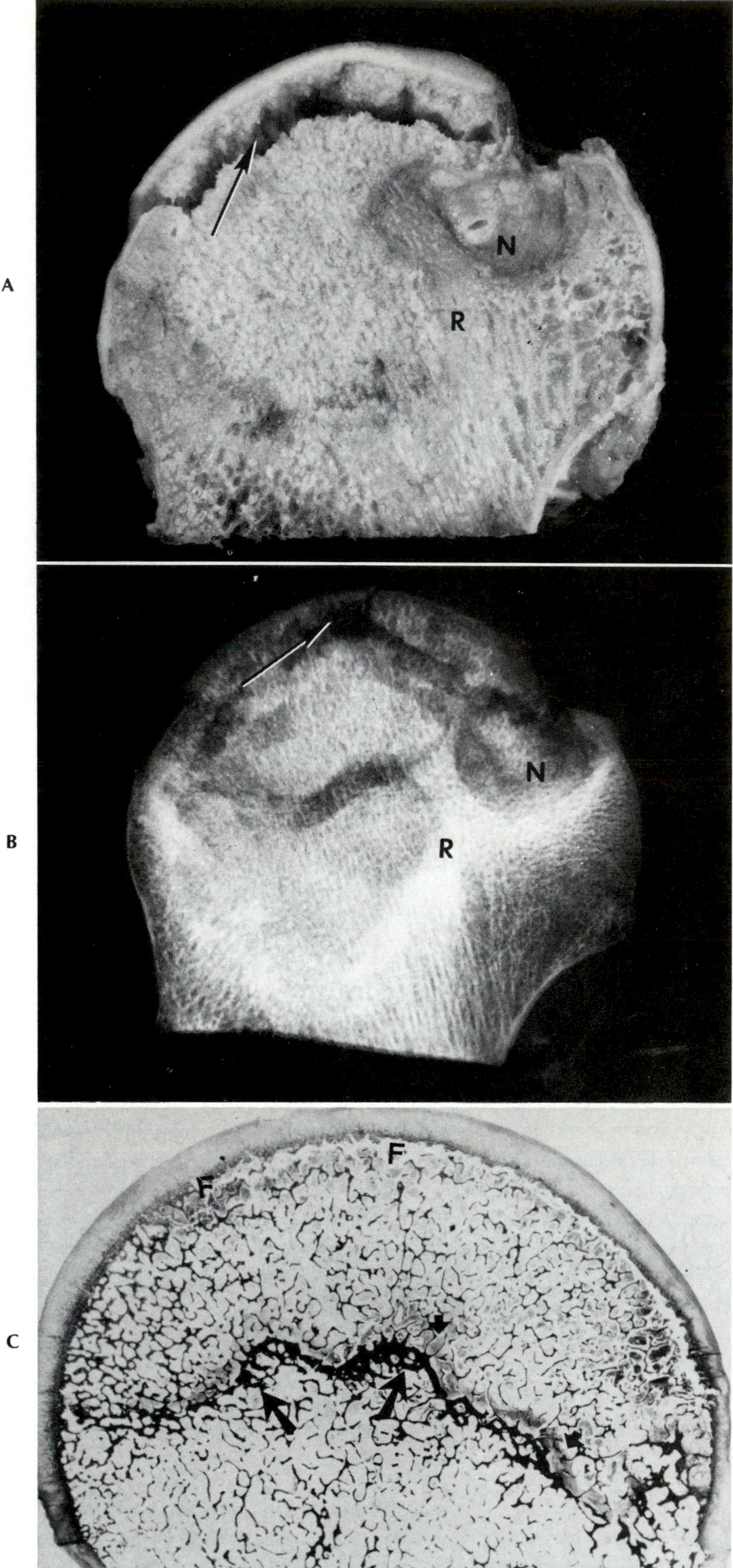

Fig. 40-70. A, Sagittal section and, **B,** roentgenogram of femoral head excised for advanced avascular necrosis. Note subchondral lucent zone *(arrow),* destruction and collapse of the articular cartilage, and sclerotic zone of repair *(R)* surrounding necrotic focus *(N).* **C,** Coronal section of femoral head from patient with idiopathic osteonecrosis. Note subchondral fracture *(F).* Thickened trabeculae *(large arrows)* reflect new bone synthesis. Mesenchymal cell and fibrous tissue proliferation *(small arrows)* are occurring just proximal to new bone. (**C,** Courtesy Dr. Melvin Glimcher, Boston, Mass.; from Glimcher, M.J., and Kenzora, J.E.: Clin. Orthop. **138**:284, 1971.)

unstable. This leads to femoral head collapse and laceration and marked distortion of articular cartilage, eventuating in degenerative arthritis. Consequently the major clinical and roentgenographic manifestations of avascular necrosis reflect the repair process rather than the initial lesion.

Idiopathic osteonecrosis, particularly that associated with immunosuppression, undergoes a less profound repair process.[641-643] Woven bone does not form about dead trabeculae, and the degree of sclerosis may not be great. Because of this seeming arrest of repair, these patients do not invariably have femoral head collapse.

Avascular necrosis develops in almost one half of patients after hip fracture; the incidence increases markedly with poor alignment.[640,647] The mechanisms underlying idiopathic osteonecrosis are, however, more elusive. A number of investigators indict embolization of hepatic fat, particularly in alcoholics or patients treated with corticosteroids.[637,639,649,659] These lipid globules are believed to lead to bone necrosis by vascular occlusion and increased intramarrow pressure.[659] However, the presence of lipid emboli in necrotic and nonnecrotic femoral heads alike[658] and the failure to produce bone infarcts in corticosteroid-treated rabbits despite the presence of these emboli[637,648] cast doubt on this hypothesis. A more reasonable proposal, particularly as regards steroid-associated osteonecrosis, is failure of microfracture repair.[652]

Although ischemic necrosis occurs in numerous locations in the growing skeleton, as in adults, the femoral head is most commonly involved. This childhood disorder, known as Legg-Calvé-Perthes disease, has many pathologic and roentgenographic similarities to idiopathic avascular necrosis of the adult femoral head. However, since it involves growing bone, some differences do exist.[638] The capital femoral physeal plate is open in patients with Legg-Calvé-Perthes disease and perhaps is the primary site of involvement.[656] Histologically the cartilage appears irregular and fragmented.[652] Ponseti and Cotton[656] postulate that the destroyed growth plate restricts blood flow to the portion of the bone that will undergo necrosis. In addition, repeated infarction may be necessary for the development of the pediatric disease.[646]

It was previously believed that the extent of femoral head involvement and the degree of subluxation are reasonable indicators of future hip function in children with Legg-Calvé-Perthes disease.[650] However, not only has this contention been disproved, but the incidence of degenerative arthritis after Legg-Calvé-Perthes disease appears much greater than suspected.[657]

OSTEOMYELITIS

Pyogenic osteomyelitis

Osteomyelitis, the generic term for bone infections, may be divided into cases of hematogenous origin, those caused by direct extension of an associated infection, and cases related to peripheral vascular disease.[672] Before growth plate closure, most osteomyelitis is of hematogenous origin.[662] However, this condition is appearing in increasing numbers of patients over 30 years of age,[672] particularly drug addicts.[667,671] Currently one third of adult cases of chronic osteomyelitis originate hematogenously.[673]

The bacterial spectrum responsible for hematogenous osteomyelitis has also changed in the last 2 decades.[665,668,672] In years past, *Staphylococcus aureus* was by far the most common offending organism. Recently the incidence of childhood and adult hematogenous osteomyelitis caused by gram-negative bacilli has dramatically increased.[664,672] Group B streptococci are also a frequent cause in children.[672] Sickle cell anemia is associated with a high incidence of *Salmonella*-induced osteomyelitis.[660]

Hematogenous osteomyelitis in children usually involves the tibial or femoral metaphyses.[669] In adults the spine is most commonly affected,[674] and cord compression may occur.[666] Despite the increase in adult hematogenous osteomyelitis, however, direct extension from soft tissue abscesses or more commonly from operative incision related to fracture repair is responsible for the majority of skeletal infections.[672] Peripheral vascular disease, particularly among diabetic patients, is associated with involvement of the small bones of the hands and feet.[672]

The skeletal vascularity and its relation to the growth plate appear responsible for the varied locations of hematogenous osteomyelitis within a given bone.[670] In the first year of life the metaphyseal branches of the nutrient artery penetrate the physis. Consequently infantile osteomyelitis spreads to epiphyseal bone, often with permanent growth plate damage. In childhood these vessels turn back on themselves proximal to the growth plate and enter large vascular channels, resulting in a relative stasis of blood flow. Since the pooling of blood and the presence of necrotic tissue are the factors commonly predisposing to osteomyelitis,[662] the metaphysis is where childhood infections localize. After physeal closure the metaphyseal vessels cross into epiphyseal bone. Hence adult osteomyelitis localizes subchondrally, often with extension into the joint space.

The rigid limits of the marrow cavity define the spread of purulent exudate. In a child pus is forced through haversian and Volkmann's canals, breaking into the subperiosteal space at points of cortical attenuation. By this dissection between the periosteum and cortex, periosteal vessels are torn, resulting in sequestration of the outer portion of cortical bone. This focus of necrosis may persist as a nidus of reinfection, and its complete excision is generally necessary for optimum treatment of chronic osteomyelitis.[661] The separated periosteum exuberantly synthesizes new bone some distance from the cortex, forming the involucrum. It is the formation of sequestra and a large involucrum that largely distinguishes childhood from adult hematogenous osteomyelitis. Because of exuberant periosteal new bone formation, the process is frequently confused with malignant skeletal tumors, particularly Ewing's sarcoma.[661] In the many cases of osteomyelitis in which roentgenographic studies are not diagnostic and blood cultures are negative, biopsy should be performed.[663]

In adults pus may break through the epiphyseal cortical bone and enter the joint space. Because of pressure atrophy, focal trabecular osteopenia occurs. Since the periosteum is now rigidly attached, it is unusual for cortical sequestration and involucrum formation to occur in the mature skeleton. Repair is more likely to follow the classic pattern of removal of necrotic tissue, osteogenesis, and fibrosis. Hence the roentgenographic appearance of hematogenous osteomyelitis often has both lytic and sclerotic features.

The clinical course and pathologic features of osteomyelitis have been drastically altered by the advent of antibiotics. Although one no longer encounters the marked deformities associated with chronicity, persistent disease does exist, particularly when associated with sequestration.[662] Brodie's abscess, a lytic process surrounded by a sclerotic margin usually in metaphyseal bone, represents a persistent, low-grade focus of chronic osteomyelitis that no longer contains purulent material.[662,663]

Skeletal tuberculosis

Following the virtual disappearance of the transmission of bovine tuberculosis to humans in Western society, the incidence of skeletal tuberculosis has markedly decreased.[672] However, bone remains the most common site of the extrapulmonary form of the disease, which is almost exclusively caused by *Mycobacterium tuberculosis*.[663] Skeletal complications develop in approximately 1% of patients with pulmonary tuberculosis.[675] Although half the patients with tuberculous osteomyelitis have or have had a pulmonary focus, an equal number have no such history.[672,675] Moreover, simultaneous active extraskeletal disease is present in only a minority of patients.[677]

The major sites of skeletal tuberculosis are the spine and hips.[672] The knees, ankles, and small bones of the hands and feet are also frequently involved.[672] Multiple skeletal foci are not unusual[675] and may be manifested as cystlike defects.[677] The basic lesion is often a combination of tuberculous osteomyelitis and arthritis.[675] The arthritis arises hematogenously or by extension from epiphyseal bone.[676]

Although varying degrees of a vertebral collapse may occur, tuberculous osteomyelitis usually does not produce the bone destruction and repair common in its pyogenic counterpart.[675] Since the quantity of purulent exudate is not great, sequestration and involucrum formation are unusual.[662] Histologically the classic changes of tuberculosis including caseation and granulomas are present.

REFERENCES

Composition and structure of bone

1. Fallon, M.D., Whyte, M.P., and Murphy, W.A.: Progressive diaphyseal dysplasia (Engelmann's disease): report of a sporadic case, J. Bone Joint Surg. **62A**:465, 1980.
2. Frost, H.M.: Bone dynamics in metabolic bone disease, J. Bone Joint Surg. **48A**:1192, 1966.
3. Frost, H.M.: The bone dynamics of osteoporosis and osteomalacia, Springfield, Ill., 1966, Charles C Thomas, Publisher.
4. Frost, H.M.: Tetracycline-based histological analysis of bone remodeling, Calcif. Tissue Res. **3**:211, 1969.
5. Hahn, T.J., Boisseau, V.C., and Avioli, L.V.: Effect of chronic corticosteroid administration on diaphyseal and metaphyseal bone mass, J. Clin. Endocrinol. Metab. **39**:274, 1974.
6. Jowsey, J.: Age and species differences in bone, Cornell Vet. 58(suppl.):74, 1968.
7. Teitelbaum, S.L., and Bullough, P.G.: The pathophysiology of bone and joint disease, Am. J. Pathol. **96**:283, 1979.

Matrical phase

Organic phase

8. Falvo, K.A., and Bullough, P.G.: Osteogenesis imperfecta: a histometric analysis, J. Bone Joint Surg. **55A**:275, 1973.
9. Forbes, R.M., Cooper, A.R., and Mitchell, H.H.: The composition of the adult human body as determined by chemical analysis, J. Biol. Chem. **203**:359, 1953.
10. Forbes, R.M., Mitchell, H.H., and Cooper, A.R.: Further studies on the gross composition and mineral elements in the adult human body, J. Biol. Chem. **223**:969, 1956.
11. Gallop, P.M., Lian, J.B., and Hauschka, P.V.: Carboxylated calcium-binding proteins and vitamin D, N. Engl. J. Med. **302**:1460, 1980.
12. Gelman, R.A., and Blackwell, J.: Interaction between collagen and chondroitin-6-sulfate, Connect. Tissue Res. **2**:311, 1973.
13. Glimcher, M.J., and Krane, S.M.: The organization and structure of bone and the mechanism of calcification. In Gould, B.S., editor: Treatise on collagen. Vol. 2, Biology of collagen, New York, 1968, Academic Press, Inc.
14. Hauschka, P.V., Lian, J.B., and Gallop, P.M.: Direct identification of the calcium-binding amino acid, γ-carboxyglutamate, in mineralized tissue, Proc. Natl. Acad. Sci. U.S.A. **72**:3925, 1975.
15. Herring, G.M.: The organic matrix of bone. In Bourne, G.H., editor: The biochemistry and physiology of bone. Vol. 1. Structure, ed. 2, New York, 1972, Academic Press, Inc.
16. Hjertquist, S.O., and Vejlens, L.: The glycosaminoglycans of dog compact bone and epiphyseal cartilage in the normal state and in experimental hyperparathyroidism, Calcif. Tissue Res. **2**:314, 1968.
17. Lian, J.B., Hauschka, P.V., and Gallop, P.M.: Properties and biosynthesis of a vitamin K–dependent calcium-binding protein in bone, Fed. Proc. **37**:2615, 1978.
18. Oldroyd, D., and Herring, G.M.: A method for the study of bone microsubstances by using collagenase, Biochem. J. **104**:20P, 1967.
19. Price, P.A., Parthemore, J.G., and Deftos, L.J.: New biochemical marker for bone metabolism: measurement by radioimmunoassay of bone GLA protein in the plasma of normal subjects and patients with bone disease, J. Clin. Invest. **66**:878, 1980.
20. Prockop, D.J., et al.: The biosynthesis of collagen and its disorders, (in two parts), N. Engl. J. Med. **301**:13, 77, 1979.
21. Smith, R.: Collagen and disorders of bone, Clin. Sci. **59**:215, 1980.

Mineral phase

22. Avioli, L.V.: Collagen metabolism, uremia and bone, Kidney Int. **4**:105, 1973.

23. Bonucci, E.: The locus of initial calcifications in cartilage and bone, Clin. Orthop. **78**:108, 1971.
24. Fallon, M.D., Whyte, M.P., and Teitelbaum, S.L.: Stereospecific inhibition of alkaline phosphatase by 1-tetramisole prevents in vitro cartilage calcification, Lab. Invest. **43**:489, 1980.
25. Fleisch, H., and Bisaz, S.: Mechanism of calcification: inhibitory role of pyrophosphate, Nature **195**:911, 1962.
26. Glimcher, M.J., et al.: Recent studies of bone mineral: is the amorphous calcium phosphate theory valid? J. Crystal Growth **53**:100, 1981.
27. Gomori, G.: Calcification and phosphatase, Am. J. Pathol. **19**:197, 1943.
28. Irving, J.T., and Wuthier, R.E.: Histochemistry and biochemistry of calcification with special reference to the role of lipids, Clin. Orthop. **56**:237, 1968.
29. Landis, W.J., and Glimcher, M.J.: Electron diffraction and electron probe microanalysis of the mineral phase of bone tissue prepared by anhydrous techniques, J. Ultrastruct. Res. **63**:188, 1978.
30. Luben, R.A., Sherman, J.K., and Wadkins, C.L.: Studies of the mechanisms of biological calcification. IV. Ultrastructural analysis of calcifying tendon matrix, Calcif. Tissue Res. **11**:39, 1973.
31. Martin, J.H., and Matthews, J.L.: Mitochondrial granules in chondrocytes, osteoblasts, and osteocytes: an ultrastructural and microincineration study, Clin. Orthop. **68**:273, 1970.
32. Posner, A.S.: Bone mineral on the molecular level, Fed. Proc. **32**:1933, 1973.
33. Rabinovitch, A.L., and Anderson, H.C.: Biogenesis of matrix vesicles in cartilage growth plates, Fed. Proc. **35**:112, 1976.
34. Sela, J., Bab, I.A., and Muhlrad, A.: A comparative study on the occurrence and activity of extracellular matrix vesicles in young and adult rat maxillary bone, Calcif. Tissue Int. **33**:129, 1981.
35. Slavkin, H.C., et al.: Matrix vesicle heterogeneity: possible morphogenetic functions for matrix vesicles, Fed. Proc. **35**:127, 1976.
36. Wergedal, J.E., and Baylink, D.J.: Electron microprobe measurements of bone mineralization rate in vivo, Am. J. Physiol. **226**:345, 1974.
37. Whyte, M.P., et al.: Adult hypophosphatasia: clinical, laboratory, and genetic investigation of a large kindred with review of the literature, Medicine **58**:329, 1979.

Bone cells

Osteoblasts

38. Bourne, G.H.: Phosphatase and calcification. In Bourne, G.H., editor: The biochemistry and physiology of bone, New York, 1972, Academic Press, Inc.
39. Doty, S.B., Robinson, R.A., and Schofield, B.H.: Morphology of bone and histochemical staining characteristics of bone cells. In Aurbach, G., editor: Handbook of physiology-endocrinology, vol. 7, Washington, D.C., 1976, American Physiological Society.
40. Holtrop, M.E., and Weinger, J.M.: Ultrastructural evidence for a transport system in bone. In Talmage, R.V., and Munson, P.L., editors: Calcium, parathyroid hormone, and the calcitonins, Int. Congr. Ser. No. 243, Amsterdam, 1972, Excerpta Medica Foundation.
41. Hruska, K.A., et al.: The predictability of the histological features of uremic bone disease by non-invasive techniques, Metab. Bone Dis. Rel. Res. **1**:39, 1978.
42. Jones, J.L., et al.: The effect of cytochalasin B on the endosteal lining cells of mammalian bone, Calcif. Tissue Res. **24**:1, 1977.
43. Jones, S.J., Boyde, A., and Pawley, J.B.: Osteoblasts and collagen orientation, Cell. Tissue Res. **159**:73, 1975.
44. Jones, S.J., Boyde, A., and Shapiro, I.M.: The response of osteoblasts to parathyroid hormone (PTH 1-34) in vitro, Metab. Bone Dis. Rel. Res. **2**:335, 1981.
45. Marotti, G.: Decrement in volume of osteoblasts during osteon formation and its effect on the size of the corresponding osteocytes. In Meunier, P., editor: Bone histomorphometry: Second International Workshop and Bone Morphology, Lyon, France, 1976, Armour-Montagu.
46. Martin, B.F., and Jacoby, F.: Diffusion phenomenon complicating the histochemical reaction for alkaline phosphatase, J. Anat. **83**:351, 1949.
47. Matthews, J.L., and Martin, J.H.: Intracellular transport of calcium and its relationship to homeostasis and mineralization, Am. J. Med. **50**:589, 1971.
48. Matthews, J.L., Talmage, R.V., and Doppelt, R.: Responses of the osteocyte lining cell complex: the bone cell unit to calcitonin, Metab. Bone Dis. Rel. Res. **2**:113, 1980.
49. Parfitt, A.M. et al.: Kinetics of matrix and mineral apposition in osteoporosis and renal osteodystrophy: relationship to rate of turnover and to cell morphology, Metab. Bone Dis. Rel. Res. **2S**:213, 1980.
50. Stepan, J., et al.: Relationship of the activity of the bone isoenzyme of serum alkaline phosphatase to urinary hydroxyproline excretion in metabolic and neoplastic bone diseases, Eur. J. Clin. Invest. **8**:373, 1978.
51. Talmage, R.V., and Grubb, S.A.: A laboratory model demonstrating osteocyte-osteoblast control of plasma calcium concentrations, Clin. Orthop. **122**:299, 1977.
52. Talmage, R.V., and Vander Wiel, C.J.: The influence of calcitonin on the plasma and urine phosphate changes produced by parathyroid hormone, Calcif. Tissue Int. **28**:113, 1979.
53. Talmage, R.V., et al.: The demand for bone calcium in maintenance of plasma calcium concentrations. In Horton, J.E., Tarpley, T.M., and Davis, W.F., editors: Proceedings, Mechanisms of Localized Bone Loss, Calcif. Tissue Abstracts Suppl. 73, Washington, D.C., 1978, Information Retrieval, Inc.
54. Teitelbaum, S.L., and Bates, M.: Relationships of static and kinetic histomorphometric features of bone, Clin. Orthop. **156**:239, 1980.
55. Weinger, J.M., and Holtrop, M.E.: An ultrastructural study of bone cells: the occurrence of microtubules, microfilaments, and tight junctions, Calcif. Tissue Res. **14**:15, 1973.

Osteocytes

56. Baud, C.A., and Boivin, G.: Effects of hormones on osteocyte function and perilacunar wall structure, Clin. Orthop. **136**:270, 1978.
57. Belanger, L.F.: Osteocytic osteolysis, Calcif. Tissue Res. **4**:1, 1969.
58. Belanger, L.F., et al.: Resorption without osteoclasts (osteolysis). In Sognnaes, R.F., editor: Mechanisms of hard tissue destruction, Pub. No. 75, Washington, D.C., 1963, American Association for the Advancement of Science.
59. Bernard, J., and Meunier, P.: L'analyse morphometrique et l'osteolyse periosteocytaire: son application au diagnostic des hyperparathyroidies, Ann. d'Anat. Path. **20**:367, 1975.
60. Bonucci, E., and Gheradi, G.: Electron microscope investigations of osteocytes in renal osteodystrophy. In Meunier, P., editor: Bone histomorphometry, Paris, 1977, Armour-Montagu.
61. Johnson, L.C.: Morphologic analysis in pathology: the kinetics of disease and general biology of bone. In Frost, H.M., editor: Bone dynamics, Boston, 1964, Little, Brown & Co.
62. Krempien, B., et al.: Osteocytes in chronic uremia: differential count of osteocytes in human femoral bone, Virchows Arch. (Pathol. Anat.) **360**:1, 1973.
63. Marotti, G.: Osteocyte orientation in human lamellar bone and its relevance to the morphometry of periosteocytic lacunae, Metab. Bone Dis. Rel. Res. **1**:325, 1979.
64. Marotti, G.: Three-dimensional study of osteocyte lacunae, Metab. Bone Dis. Rel. Res. **2S**:223, 1980.
65. Rasmussen, H., and Bordier, P.: The cellular basis of metabolic bone disease, N. Engl. J. Med. **289**:25, 1973.
66. Weisbrode, S.T., Capen, C.C., and Nagode, L.A.: Influence of parathyroid hormone on ultrastructural and enzymatic changes induced by vitamin D in bone of thyroparathyroidectomized rats, Lab. Invest. **30**:786, 1974.
67. Young, R.W.: Cell proliferation and specialization during endochondral osteogenesis in young rats, J. Cell Biol. **14**:357, 1962.

Osteoclasts

68. Bonucci, E.: The organic-inorganic relationship in bone matrix undergoing osteoclastic resorption, Calcif. Tissue Res. **16**:13, 1974.
69. Cameron, D.A.: The ultrastructure of bone. In Bourne, G.H., editor: The biochemistry and physiology of bone. Vol. 1. Structure, ed. 2, New York, 1972, Academic Press, Inc.

70. Gay, C.V., and Mueller, W.J.: Carbonic anhydrase and osteoclasts: localization by labeled inhibitor autoradiography, Science **195**:432, 1974.
71. Holtrop, M.E., and King, G.J.: The ultrastructure of the osteoclast and its functional implications, Clin. Orthop. **123**:177, 1977.
72. Holtrop, M.E., and Raisz, L.G.: Comparison of the effects of 1,25-dihydroxycholecalciferol, prostaglandin E_2, and osteoclast-activating factor with parathyroid hormone on the ultrastructure of osteoclasts in cultured long bones of fetal rats, Calcif. Tissue Int. **29**:201, 1979.
73. Holtrop, M.E., Raisz, L.G., and Simmons, H.A.: The effects of parathyroid hormone, colchicine, and calcitonin on the ultrastructure and the activity of osteoclasts in organ culture, J. Cell Biol. **60**:346, 1974.
74. Holtrop, M.E., et al.: 1,25-Dihydroxycholecalciferol stimulates osteoclasts in rat bones in absence of parathyroid hormone, Endocrinology **108**:2293, 1981.
75. Horton, J.E., et al.: Bone-resorbing activity in supernatant fluid from a cultured human peripheral blood leukocyte, Science **177**:793, 1972.
76. Kahn, A.J., Stewart, C.C., and Teitelbaum, S.L.: Contact-mediated bone resorption by human monocytes in vitro, Science **199**:988, 1978.
77. Kallio, D.M., Garant, P.R., and Minkin, C.: Ultrastructural effects of calcitonin on osteoclasts in tissue culture, J. Ultrastruct. Res. **9**:205, 1972.
78. King, G.J., and Holtrop, M.E.: Actin-like filaments in bone cells of cultured mouse calvaria as demonstrated by binding to heavy meromyosin, J. Cell Biol. **66**:445, 1975.
79. King, G.J., Holtrop, M.E., and Raisz, L.G.: The relation of ultrastructural changes in osteoclasts to resorption in bone cultures stimulated with parathyroid hormone, Metab. Bone Dis. Rel. Res. **1**:67, 1978.
80. Lucht, U.: Cytoplasmic vacuoles and bodies of the osteoclast, Z. Zell. Forsch. Mikrosk. Anat. **135**:229, 1972.
81. Malone, J.D., Kahn, A.J., and Teitelbaum, S.L.: Dissociation of organic acid secretion from macrophage-mediated bone resorption, Biochem. Biophys. Res. Commun. **108**:468, 1982.
82. Milhaud, G., and Labat, M.-L.: Osteopetrosis reconsidered as a curable immune disorder, Biomedicine **30**:71, 1979.
83. Mundy, G.R., et al.: Evidence for the secretion of an osteoclast-stimulating factor in myeloma, N. Engl. J. Med. **291**:1041, 1974.
84. Puzas, J.E., and Brand, J.S.: Collagenolytic activity from isolated bone cells, Biochem. Biophys. Acta **429**:969, 1976.
85. Robinson, R.A., and Elliot, S.R.: The water content of bone. I. The mass of water, inorganic crystals, organic matrix, and CO_2 space components in a unit volume of the dog bone, J. Bone Joint Surg. **39**:167, 1957.
86. Schelling, S.H., Wolfe, H.J., and Tashjian, A.H.: Role of the osteoclast in prostaglandin E_2–stimulated bone resorption: a correlative morphometric and biochemical analysis, Lab. Invest. **42**:290, 1980.
87. Schenk, R., Spiro, D., and Weiner, J.: Cartilage resorption in tibial epiphyseal plate of growing rats, J. Cell Biol. **34**:275, 1974.
88. Vaes, G.: On the mechanisms of bone resorption, J. Cell Biol. **39**:676, 1968.
89. Vaes, G.: Collagenase, lysosomes, and osteoclastic bone resorption. In Woolley, D.E., and Evanson, J.M., editors: Collagenase in normal and pathological connective tissues, New York, 1980, John Wiley & Sons, Ltd.

Origin of bone cells

90. Bloom, W., Bloom, M.A., and McLean, F.C.: Calcification and ossification: medullary bone changes in the reproductive cycle of female pigeons, Anat. Rec. **81**:443, 1941.
91. Bloom, W., and Fawcett, D.W.: A textbook of histology, ed. 10, Philadelphia, 1975, W.B. Saunders Co.
92. Buring, K.: On the origin of cells in heterotopic bone formation, Clin. Orthop. **110**:293, 1975.
93. Coccia, P.F., et al.: Successful bone marrow transplantation for infantile malignant osteopetrosis, N. Engl. J. Med. **302**:701, 1980.
94. Fischman, D.A., and Hay, E.D.: Origin of osteoclasts from mononuclear leukocytes in regenerating newt limbs, Anat. Rec. **143**:329, 1962.
95. Friedenstein, A.J.: Precursor cells of mechanocytes, Int. Rev. Cytol. **47**:327, 1976.
96. Gothlin, G., and Ericsson, J.L.E.: The osteoclast: review of ultrastructure, Clin. Orthop. **120**:201, 1976.
97. Hancox, N.M.: The osteoclast, Biol. Rev. **24**:448, 1949.
98. Jee, W.S.S., and Nolan, P.D.: Origin of osteoclasts from the fusion of phagocytes, Nature **200**:225, 1963.
99. Kahn, A.J., and Simmons, D.J.: Investigation of cell lineage in bone using a chimera of chick and quail embryonic tissue, Nature **258**:325, 1975.
100. Teitelbaum, S.L., and Kahn, A.J.: Mononuclear phagocytes, osteoclasts, and bone resorption, Min. Electrolyte Metab. **3**:2, 1980.
101. Teitelbaum, S.L., Stewart, C.C., and Kahn, A.J.: Rodent peritoneal macrophages as bone-resorbing cells, Calcif. Tissue Int. **27**:255, 1979.
102. Yoneda, T., and Mundy, G.R.: Monocytes regulate osteoclast-activating factor production by releasing prostaglandins, J. Exp. Med. **150**:338, 1979.

Skeletal development

Endochondral ossification

103. Brighton, C.T., and Heppenstall, R.B.: Oxygen tension in zones of the epiphyseal plate, the metaphysis and diaphysis, J. Bone Joint Surg. **53A**:719, 1971.
104. Hall, B.K.: Cellular differentiation in skeletal tissue, Biol. Rev. Phil. Soc. **45**:455, 1970.
105. Hall, B.K., and Jacobson, H.N.: The repair of fractured membrane bones in the newly hatched chick, Anat. Rec. **181**:55, 1975.
106. Holtrop, M.E.: The potencies of the epiphyseal cartilage in endochondral ossification, Proc. Kon. Nederl. Akad. Wet. (Biol. Med.) **70**:21, 1967.
107. Holtrop, M.E.: The ultrastructure of the epiphyseal plate. I. The flattened chondrocyte, Calcif. Tissue Res. **9**:131, 1972.
108. Holtrop, M.E.: The ultrastructure of the epiphyseal plate. II. The hypertrophic chondrocyte, Calcif. Tissue Res. **9**:140, 1972.
109. Shimomura, Y., Wezeman, F.H., and Ray, R.D.: The growth cartilage plate of the rat rib: cellular differentiation, Clin. Orthop. **90**:246, 1973.
110. Shimomura, Y., Yoneda, T., and Suzuki, F.: Osteogenesis by chondrocytes from growth cartilage of rat rib, Calcif. Tissue Res. **19**:179, 1975.
111. von der Mark, K., and von der Mark, H.: The role of three genetically distinct collagen types in endochondral ossification and calcification of cartilage, J. Bone Joint Surg. **59B**:458, 1977.
112. White, A.A., III: Fracture treatment: the still unsolved problem, Clin. Orthop. **106**:279, 1975.

Repair

113. Bassett, C.A.L., and Hermann, I.: Influence of oxygen concentration and mechanical factors on differentiation of connective tissues in vitro, Nature **190**:460, 1961.
114. Bassett, C.A.L., Pawluk, R.J., and Pilla, A.A.: Augmentation of bone repair by inductively coupled electromagnetic fields, Science **184**:575, 1974.
115. Bisgard, J.D.: Longitudinal overgrowth of large bones with special reference to fracture, Surg. Gynecol. Obstet. **62**:823, 1936.
116. Brighton, C.T., et al.: Treatment of nonunion with constant direct current, Clin. Orthop. **124**:106, 1977.
117. Glowacki, J., Altobelli, D., and Mulliken, J.B.: Fate of mineralized and demineralized osseous implants in cranial defects, Calcif. Tissue Int. **33**:71, 1981.
118. Hall, B.K.: Immobilization and cartilage transformation into bone in the embryonic chick, Anat. Rec. **173**:391, 1972.
119. Ham, A.W., and Harris, W.R.: Repair and transplantation of bone. In Bourne, G.H., editor: The biochemistry and physiology of bone. Vol. III, Development and growth, ed. 2, New York, 1971, Academic Press, Inc.
120. Jarry, L., and Uhthoff, H.K.: Differences in healing of metaphyseal and diaphyseal fractures, Can. J. Surg. **14**:127, 1971.

121. Reddi, A.H., and Anderson, W.A.: Collagenous bone-matrix–induced endochondral ossification and hemopoiesis, J. Cell Biol. **69**:557, 1976.
122. Tomna, E.A., and Cronkite, E.P.: Changes in the skeletal cell proliferative response to trauma concomitant with aging, J. Bone Joint Surg. **44A**:1557, 1962.
123. von der Mark, K., and Conrad, G.: Cartilage cell differentiation, Clin. Orthop. **139**:185, 1979.

Disorders of remodeling
Morphologic methods of diagnosis

124. Avioli, L.V., and Teitelbaum, S.L.: The renal osteodystrophies. In Brenner, B.M., and Rector, F.C., editors: The kidney, Philadelphia, 1976, W.B. Saunders Co.
125. Baylink, D., et al.: Formation, mineralization, and resorption of bone in vitamin D–deficient rats, J. Clin. Invest. **49**:1122, 1970.
126. Bordier, P., et al.: Vitamin D metabolites and bone mineralization in man, J. Clin. Endocrinol. Metab. **46**:284, 1978.
127. Evans, R.A., Dunstan, C.R., and Baylink, D.J.: Histochemical identification of osteoclasts in undecalcified sections of human bone, Min. Electrolyte Metab. **2**:179, 1979.
128. Frost, H.M.: Tetracycline labeling of bone and the zone of demarcation of osteoid seams, Can. J. Biochem. Pharmacol. **40**:485, 1962.
129. Frost, H.M.: Tetracycline-based histological analysis of bone remodeling, Calcif. Tissue Res. **3**:211, 1969.
130. Hitt, O., et al.: Tissue-level bone formation rates in chronic renal failure measured by means of tetracycline bone labeling, Can. J. Physiol. Pharmacol. **48**:824, 1970.
131. Ibsen, K.H., and Urist, M.R.: The biochemistry and the physiology of the tetracyclines, with special reference to mineralized tissue, Clin. Orthop. **32**:143, 1964.
132. Jaworski, Z.F.G., Lok, E., and Wellington, J.L.: Impaired osteoclastic function and linear bone erosion rate in secondary hyperparathyroidism associated with chronic renal failure, Clin. Orthop. **107**:298, 1975.
133. Lauffenburger, T., et al.: Bone remodeling and calcium metabolism: a correlated histomorphometric, calcium kinetic, and biochemical study in patients with osteoporosis and Paget's disease, Metabolism **26**:589, 1977.
134. Melsen, F., and Mosekilde, L.: Tetracycline double-labeling of iliac trabecular bone in 41 normal adults, Calcif. Tissue Res. **26**:99, 1978.
135. Melsen, F., et al.: Histomorphometric analysis of normal bone from the iliac crest, Acta Pathol. Microbiol. Scand. **86**:70, 1978.
136. Merz, W.A., and Schenk, R.K.: A quantitative histological study on bone formation in human cancellous bone, Acta Anat. **76**:1, 1970.
137. Merz, W.A., and Schenk, R.K.: Quantitative structural analysis of human cancellous bone, Acta Anat. **75**:54, 1970.
138. Rolle, G.K.: The distribution of calcium in normal and tetracycline modified bones of developing chick embryo, Calcif. Tissue Res. **3**:142, 1966.
139. Russell, J.E., Termine, J.D., and Avioli, L.V.: Abnormal bone maturation in the chronic uremic state, J. Clin. Invest. **52**:2848, 1973.
140. Russell, J.E., et al.: The therapeutic effects of 25-hydroxyvitamin D_3 on renal osteodystrophy: biochemical and morphometric analyses, Min. Electrolyte Metab. **1**:129, 1978.
141. Schenk, R.K., Merz, W.A., and Muller, J.: A quantitative histological study on bone resorption in human cancellous bone, Acta Anat. **74**:44, 1969.
142. Steendijk, R., and Boyde, A.: Scanning electron microscopic observations on bone from patients with hypophosphatemic (vitamin D–resistant) rickets, Calcif. Tissue Res. **11**:242, 1973.
143. Teitelbaum, S.L., et al.: The effects of phosphate and vitamin D therapy on osteopenic hypophosphatemic osteomalacia of childhood: a morphometric study, Clin. Orthop. **116**:38, 1976.
144. Teitelbaum, S.L., et al.: Tetracycline fluorescence in uremic and primary hyperparathyroid bone, Kidney Int. **12**:366, 1977.
145. Treharne, R.W., and Brighton, C.T.: The use and possible misuse of tetracycline as a vital stain, Clin. Orthop. **140**:240, 1979.
146. Wilde, C.D., et al.: Quantitative histological measurements of bone turnover in primary hyperparathyroidism, Calcif. Tissue Res. **12**:127, 1973.

Physiologic effects of hormones, vitamins, inorganic compounds, enzymes, and viruses on bone with attendant dysfunctions
Parathyroid hormone

147. Brewer, H.B., et al.: Recent studies on the chemistry of human, bovine, and porcine parathyroid hormones, Am. J. Med. **56**:759, 1974.
148. Dalen, N., and Hjern, B.: Bone mineral content in patients with primary hyperparathyroidism without radiological evidence of skeletal changes, Acta Endocrinol. **75**:297, 1974.
149. Dietrich, J.W., et al.: Hormonal control of bone collagen synthesis *in vitro*: effects of parathyroid hormone and calcitonin, Endocrinology **98**:943, 1976.
150. Forland, M., et al.: Bone density studies in primary hyperparathyroidism, Arch. Intern. Med. **122**:236, 1968.
151. Haas, H.G., et al.: Renal effects of calcitonin and parathyroid extract in man, J. Clin. Invest. **50**:2689, 1971.
152. Knop, J., et al.: Bone calcium exchange in primary hyperparathyroidism as measured by ^{47}calcium kinetics, Metabolism **29**:819, 1980.
153. Melsen, F., and Mosekilde, L.: Trabecular bone mineralization lag time determined by tetracycline double-labeling in normal and certain pathological conditions, Acta Pathol. Microbiol. Scand. **88**:83, 1980.
154. Sherwood, L.M., et al.: Regulation of parathyroid hormone secretion: proportional control by calcium, lack of effect of phosphate, Endocrinology **83**:1043, 1968.
155. Tougaard, L, et al.: Bone mineralization and bone mineral content in primary hyperparathyroidism, Acta Endocrinol. **84**:314, 1977.
156. Tregear, G.W., et al.: Bovine parathyroid hormone: minimum chain length of synthetic peptide required for biological activity, Endocrinology **93**:1349, 1973.

Vitamin D

157. Aaron, J.E., Gallagher, J.C., and Nordin, B.E.C.: Seasonal variation of histological osteomalacia in femoral neck fractures, Lancet **2**:84, 1974.
158. Arnaud, C., Rasmussen, H., and Anast, C.: Further studies on the interrelationship between parathyroid hormone and vitamin D, J. Clin. Invest. **45**:1955, 1966
159. Bhattacharyya, M.H., and DeLuca, H.F.: The regulation of rat liver calciferol-25-hydroxylase, J. Biol. Chem. **268**:2969, 1973.
160. Carlsson, A.: Tracer experiments on the effect of vitamin D on the skeletal metabolism of calcium and phosphorus, Acta Physiol. Scand. **26**:212, 1952.
161. DeLuca, H.F.: Vitamin D—1973, Am. J. Med. **57**:1, 1974.
162. DeLuca, H.F.: Vitamin D metabolism and function, Arch. Intern. Med. **138**:836, 1978.
163. Fraser, D.R., and Kodicek, E.: Unique biosynthesis by kidney of a biologically active vitamin D metabolite, Nature **228**:764, 1970.
164. Haddad, J.G., and Chyu, K.J.: Competitive protein-binding radioassay for 25-hydroxycholecalciferol, J. Clin. Endocrinol. **33**:992, 1972.
165. Haddad, J.G., and Stamp, T.C.B.: Circulating 25-hydroxyvitamin D in man, Am. J. Med. **57**:57, 1974.
166. Horlick, M.F., et al.: Photometabolism of 7-dihydrocholesterol to previtamin D_3 in skin, Biochem. Biophys. Res. Commun. **76**:107, 1977.
167. Miravet, L., et al.: Action of vitamin D metabolites on PTH secretion in man, Calcif. Tissue Int. **33**:191, 1981.
168. Olson, E.B., et al.: The effect of hepatectomy on the synthesis of 25-hydroxyvitamin D_3, J. Clin. Invest. **57**:1213, 1976.
169. Rasmussen, H., et al.: Hormonal control of the renal conversion of 25-hydroxycholecalciferol to 1,25-dihydroxycholecalciferol, J. Clin. Invest. **51**:2502, 1972.
170. Reynolds, J.J., Holnick, M.F., and DeLuca, H.F.: The role of vitamin D metabolites in bone resorption, Calcif. Tissue Res. **12**:295, 1973.

171. Teitelbaum, S.L.: Histological effects of vitamin D and its analogs on bone, Am. J. Clin. Nutr. **29**:1300, 1976.
172. Weisbrode, S.E., Capen, C.C., and Nagode, L.A.: Fine structural and enzymatic evaluation of bone in thyroparathyroidectomized rats receiving various levels of vitamin D, Lab. Invest. **28**:29, 1973.

Primary hyperparathyroidism

173. Bingham, P.J., and Raisz, L.G.: Bone growth in organ culture: effects of phosphate and other nutrients on bone and cartilage, Calcif. Tissue Res. **14**:31, 1974.
174. Broadus, A.E., et al.: The importance of circulating 1,25-dihydroxyvitamin D in the pathogenesis of hypercalciuria and renal-stone formation in primary hyperparathyroidism, N. Engl. J. Med. **302**:421, 1980.
175. Byers, P.D., and Smith, R.: Quantitative histology of bone in hyperparathyroidism: its relation to clinical features, x-ray and biochemistry, Q. J. Med. **40**:471, 1971.
176. Clark, O.H., and Taylor, S.: Osteoclastoma of the jaw and multiple parathyroid tumors, Surg. Gynecol. Obstet. **135**:188, 1972.
177. Ehrig, U., and Wilson, D.R.: Fibrous dysplasia of bone and primary hyperparathyroidism, Ann. Intern. Med. **77**:234, 1972.
178. Fogelman, I., et al.: Estimation of skeletal involvement in primary hyperparathyroidism, Ann. Intern. Med. **92**:65, 1980.
179. Genant, H.K., et al.: Osteosclerosis in primary hyperparathyroidism, Am. J. Med. **59**:104, 1975.
180. Gordon, G.S.D., et al.: Clinical endocrinology of parathyroid hormone excess., Recent Prog. Horm. Res. **18**:297, 1962.
181. Gray, R.W., et al.: The importance of phosphate in regulating plasma 1,25$(OH)_2$–vitamin D levels in humans: studies in healthy subjects, in calcium-stone formers, and in patients with primary hyperparathyroidism, J. Clin. Endocrinol. Metab. **45**:299, 1977.
182. Merz, W.A., et al.: Bone remodeling in primary hyperparathyroidism: preoperative and postoperative studies, Isr. J. Med. Sci. **7**:494, 1971.
183. Mosekilde, L., and Melsen, F.: A tetracycline-based histomorphometric evaluation of bone resorption and bone turnover in hyperthyroidism and hyperparathyroidism, Acta Med. Scand. **204**:97, 1978.
184. Preston, E.T.: Avulsion of both quadriceps tendons in hyperparathyroidism, J.A.M.A. **221**:406, 1972.
185. Purnell, D.C., et al.: Primary hyperparathyroidism: a prospective clinical study, Am. J. Med. **50**:670, 1971.
186. Purnell, D.C., et al.: Treatment of primary hyperparathyroidism, Am. J. Med. **56**:800, 1974.
187. Raisz, L.G., et al.: Comparison of the effects of vitamin D metabolites on collagen synthesis and resorption of fetal rat bone in organ culture, Calcif. Tissue Int. **32**:135, 1980.
188. Shieber, W., Bates, M., and Teitelbaum, S.L.: Histometric evaluation of nondecalcified thin sections of bone biopsies of patients with primary hyperparathyroidism: clinical-pathological correlations, Surg. Forum **26**:508, 1975.

Hypoparathyroidism

189. Albright, F.: Hypoparathyroidism as a cause of osteomalacia, J. Clin. Endocrinol. Metab. **16**:419, 1956.
190. Bronsky, D., et al.: Idiopathic hypoparathyroidism: case reports and review of the literature, Medicine **37**:317, 1958.
191. Cantor, M.M., and Scott, J.W.: Chronic idiopathic hypoparathyroidism, Can. Med. Assoc. J. **47**:551, 1942.
192. Drezner, M.K., et al.: Hypoparathyroidism: a possible cause of osteomalacia, J. Clin. Endocrinol. Metab. **45**:114, 1977.
193. Emerson, K., Jr., Walsh, F.B., and Howard, J.E.: Idiopathic hypoparathyroidism: a report of two cases, Ann. Intern. Med. **14**:1256, 1941.
194. Jimenea, C.V., et al.: Spondylitis of hypoparathyroidism, Clin. Orthop. **74**:84, 1971.
195. Keil, L.C., Evans, J.W., and Prinz, J.A.: Effect of parathyroidectomy on bone growth and composition in the young rat, Growth **38**:519, 1974.
196. Lund, B.J., et al.: Vitamin D metabolism in hypoparathyroidism, J. Clin. Endocrinol. Metab. **51**:606, 1980.
197. Moses, A.M., et al.: Parathyroid hormone deficiency with Albright's hereditary osteodystrophy, J. Clin. Endocrinol. Metab. **39**:496, 1974.
198. Parfitt, A.M.: The spectrum of hypoparathyroidism, J. Clin. Endocrinol. Metab. **34**:152, 1972.
199. Schulman, J.L., and Ratner, H.: Idiopathic hypoparathyroidism with bone demineralization and cardiac decompensation, Pediatrics **16**:848, 1955.
200. Wergedal, J., et al.: Inhibition of bone matrix formation, mineralization, and resorption in thyroparathyroidectomized rats, J. Clin. Invest. **52**:1052, 1973.

Pseudohypoparathyroidism

201. Chase, L.R., Melson, G.L., and Aurbach, G.D.: Pseudohypoparathyroidism: defective excretion of 3′5′-AMP in response to parathyroid hormone, J. Clin. Invest. **48**:1832, 1969.
202. Drezner, M., Neelon, F.A., and Lebovitz, H.E.: Psuedohypoparathyroidism type II: a possible defect in the reception of the cyclic AMP signal, N. Engl. J. Med. **289**:1056, 1973.
203. Drezner, M.K., et al.: 1,25-Dihydroxycholecalciferol deficiency: the probable cause of hypocalcemia and metabolic bone disease in pseudohypoparathyroidism, J. Clin. Endocrinol. Metab. **42**:621, 1976.
204. Frame, B., et al.: Renal resistance to parathyroid hormone with osteitis fibrosa: "pseudohypoparathyroidism," Am. J. Med. **52**:311, 1972.
205. Jensen, S.B., Illum, F., and Dupont, E.: Nature and frequency of dental changes in idiopathic hypoparathyroidism and pseudohypoparathyroidism, Scand. J. Dent. Res. **89**:26, 1981.
206. Kinard, R.E., Walton, J.E., and Buckwalter, J.A.: Pseudohypoparathyroidism: report on a family with four affected sisters, Arch. Intern. Med. **139**:204, 1979.
207. Lee, J.B., et al.: Familial pseudohypoparathyroidism: role of parathyroid hormone and thyrocalcitonin, N. Engl. J. Med. **279**:1179, 1968.
208. Lewin, I.G., et al.: Studies of hypoparathyroidism and pseudohypoparathyroidism, Q.J. Med. **47**:533, 1978.
209. Mann, J.B., Alterman, S., and Hills, A.G.: Albright's hereditary osteodystrophy comprising pseudohypoparathyroidism and pseudo-pseudohypoparathyroidism, with a report of two cases representing the complete syndrome occurring in successive generations, Ann. Intern. Med. **56**:315, 1962.
210. Metz, S.A., et al.: Selective deficiency of 1,25-dihydroxycholecalciferol: a cause of isolated skeletal resistance to parathyroid hormone, N. Engl. J. Med. **297**:1084, 1977.
211. Nusjnowitz, M.L., and Klein, M.H.: Pseudoidiopathic hypoparathyroidism: hypoparathyroidism with ineffective parathyroid hormone, Am. J. Med. **55**:677, 1973.
212. Reinhart, R., et al.: Studies in three generations of a kindred with pseudohypoparathyroidism, Clin. Res. **21**:255, 1973.
213. Sinha, T.K., DeLuca, H.F., and Bell, N.H.: Evidence for a defect in the formation of 1α,25-dihydroxyvitamin D in pseudohypoparathyroidism, Metabolism **26**:731, 1977.
214. Stanescu, V., Dona, C., and Ionescu, U.: Histochemical and histoenzymological investigations of growing cartilage in pseudohypoparathyroidism, Acta Endocrinol. **60**:433, 1969.
215. Steinbach, H.L., and Young, D.A.: The roentgen appearance of pseudohypoparathyroidism (PH) and pseudo-pseudohypoparathyroidism (PPH): differentiation from other syndromes associated with short metacarpals, metatarsals, and phalanges, Am. J. Roentgenol. **97**:49, 1966.

Vitamin D deficiency

216. Backrach, S., Fisher, J., and Parks, J.S.: An outbreak of vitamin D–deficiency rickets in a susceptible population, Pediatrics **64**:871, 1979.
217. Compston, J.E., Crowe, J.P., and Horton, L.W.L.: Treatment of osteomalacia associated with primary biliary cirrhosis with oral 1-alpha-hydroxyvitamin D_3, Br. Med. J. **2**:309, 1979.
218. Eddy, R.L.: Metabolic bone disease after gastrectomy, Am. J. Med. **50**:442, 1971.
219. Edidin, D.V., et al.: Resurgence of nutritional rickets associated with breast-feeding and special dietary practices, Pediatrics **65**:232, 1980.

220. Fujita, T., et al.: Age-dependent bone loss after gastrectomy, J. Am. Geriatr. Soc. **19**:840, 1971.
221. Garrick, R., Ireland, A.W., and Posen, S.: Bone abnormalities after gastric surgery: a prospective histological study, Ann. Intern. Med. **75**:221, 1971.
222. Gertner, J.M., Liliburn, M., and Domenech, M.: 25-Hydroxycholecalciferol absorption in steatorrhoea and postgastrectomy osteomalacia, Br. Med. J. **1**:1310, 1977.
223. Halverson, J.D., et al.: Skeletal abnormalities after jejunoileal bypass, Ann. Surg. **189**:785, 1979.
224. Jaffe, B.I., et al.: Parathyroid hormone concentrations in nutritional rickets, Clin. Sci. Mol. Med. **42**:113, 1972.
225. Klein, G.L., et al.: Reduced serum levels of 1α,25-dihydroxyvitamin D during long-term total parenteral nutrition, Ann. Intern. Med. **94**:638, 1981.
226. Long, R.G., et al.: Parenteral 1,25-dihydroxycholecalciferol in hepatic osteomalacia, Br. Med. J. **1**:75, 1978.
227. Parfitt, A.M., et al.: Metabolic bone disease after intestinal bypass for treatment of obesity, Ann. Intern. Med. **89**:193, 1978.
228. Perry, H.M., et al.: Pseudofractures in the absence of osteomalacia, Skel. Radiol. **8**:17, 1982.
229. Rickers, H., et al.: Bone mineral content before and after intestinal bypass operation in obese patients, Acta Med. Scand. **209**:203, 1981.
230. Shike, M., et al.: Metabolic bone disease in patients receiving long-term total-parenteral nutrition, Ann. Intern. Med. **92**:343, 1980.
231. Shires, R., et al.: Effects of semi-starvation on skeletal homeostasis, Endocrinology **107**:1530, 1980.
232. Teitelbaum, S.L., et al.: Abnormalities of circulating 25-hydroxyvitamin D following jejunal-ileal bypass for obesity: evidence of an adaptive response, Ann. Intern. Med. **86**:289, 1977.

Vitamin D–dependent rickets

233. Balsan, S., et al.: Serum 1,25-dihydroxyvitamin D concentration in two different types of pseudo-deficiency rickets. In Norman, A.W., et al., editors: Vitamin D: basic research and its clinical application, New York, 1979, Walter de Gruyter.
234. Bell, N.H.: Vitamin D-dependent rickets type II, Calcif. Tissue Int. **31**:89, 1980.
235. Brooks, M.H., et al.: Vitamin-D-dependent rickets type II: resistance of target organs to 1,25-dihydroxyvitamin D, N. Engl. J. Med. **298**:996, 1978.
236. Eil, C., et al.: A cellular defect in hereditary vitamin-D-dependent rickets type II: defective nuclear uptake of 1,25-dihydroxyvitamin D in cultured skin fibroblasts, N. Engl. J. Med. **304**:1588, 1981.
237. Fraser, D., et al.: Pathogenesis of hereditary vitamin-D-dependent rickets: an inborn error of vitamin D metabolism involving defective conversion of 25-hydroxyvitamin D to 1α,25-dihydroxyvitamin D, N. Engl. J. Med. **289**:817, 1973.
238. Liberman, J.A., et al.: End-organ resistance to 1,25-dihydroxycholecalciferol, Lancet **1**:504, 1980.
239. Marx, S.J., et al.: A familial syndrome of decrease in sensitivity to 1,25-dihydroxyvitamin D, J. Clin. Endocrinol. Metab. **47**:1303, 1978.
240. Scriver, C.R.: Rickets and the pathogenesis of impaired tubular transport of phosphate and other solutes, Am. J. Med. **57**:43, 1974.
241. Tsuchiya, Y., An unusual form of vitamin D-dependent rickets in a child: alopecia and marked end-organ hyposensitivity to biologically active vitamin D, J. Clin. Endocrinol. Metab. **51**:685, 1980.
242. Zerwekh, J.E., et al.: An unique form of osteomalacia associated with end organ refractoriness to 1,25-dihydroxyvitamin D and apparent defective synthesis of 25-hydroxyvitamin D, J. Clin. Endocrinol. Metab. **49**:171, 1979.

Renal osteodystrophy

243. Alfrey, A.C., LeGendre, G.R., and Kaehny, W.D.: The dialysis encephalopathy syndrome, N. Engl. J. Med. **294**:184, 1976.
244. Avioli, L.V., and Teitelbaum, S.L.: Renal osteodystrophy. In Edelman, C., editor: Pediatric kidney disease, vol. 1, Boston, 1978, Little, Brown & Co.
245. Campos, C., Arata, R.O., and Mautalen, C.A.: Parathyroid hormone and vertebral osteosclerosis in uremic patients, Metabolism **25**:495, 1976.
246. Colodro, I.H., et al.: Effect of 25-hydroxyvitamin D_3 on intestinal absorption of calcium in normal man and patients with renal failure, Metabolism **27**:745, 1978.
247. Cournot-Witmer, G., et al.: Aluminum and dialysis bone-disease, Lancet **2**:795, 1979.
248. Cournot-Witmer, G., et al.: Aluminum in bone from haemodialyzed patients: relationship to bone histology and localization by electron microprobe and secondary ion microscopy, Metab. Bone Dis. Rel. Res. **2S**:491, 1980.
249. Drueke, T.: Dialysis osteomalacia and aluminum intoxication, Nephron **26**:207, 1980.
250. Eastwood, J.B., et al.: Vitamin-D-deficiency in the osteomalacia of chronic renal failure, Lancet **2**:1209, 1976.
251. Ellis, H.A., McCarthy, J.H., and Herrington, J.: Bone aluminum in haemodialysed patients and in rats injected with aluminum chloride: relationship to impaired bone mineralisation, J. Clin. Pathol. **32**:832, 1979.
252. Ellis, H.A., and Peart, K.M.: Azotaemic renal osteodystrophy: a quantitative study on iliac bone, J. Clin. Pathol. **26**:83, 1973.
253. Freitag, J., et al.: Impaired parathyroid hormone metabolism in patients with chronic renal failure, N. Engl. J. Med. **298**:29, 1978.
254. Frost, H.M., et al.: Histomorphometric changes in trabecular bone of renal failure patients treated with calcifediol, Metab. Bone Dis. Rel. Res. **2**:285, 1981.
255. Goldstein, D.A., et al.: Blood levels of 25-hydroxyvitamin D in nephrotic syndrome: studies in 26 patients, Ann. Intern. Med. **87**:664, 1977.
256. Hodsman, A.B., et al.: Vitamin-D-resistant osteomalacia in hemodialysis patients lacking secondary hyperparathyroidism, Ann. Intern. Med. **94**:629, 1981.
257. Jowsey, J., et al.: Microradiographic studies of bone in renal osteodystrophy, Arch. Intern. Med. **124**:539, 1969.
258. Kaehny, W.D., Hegg, A.P., and Alfrey, A.C.: Gastrointestinal absorption of aluminum from aluminum-containing antacids, N. Engl. J. Med. **296**:1389, 1977.
259. Kaehny, W.D., et al.: Aluminum transfer during hemodialysis, Kidney Int. **12**:361, 1977.
260. Korkor, A., et al.: Absence of metabolic bone disease in adult patients with nephrotic syndrome (NS) and normal renal function (NRF): proceedings from the thirteenth Annual Meeting of The American Society of Nephrology, Washington, D.C., 23A, 1980, Charles B. Slack, Inc.
261. Kovalchik, M.T., et al.: Aluminum transfer during hemodialysis, J. Lab. Clin. Med. **92**:712, 1978.
262. Krempien, B., Mehls, O., and Ritz, E.: Morphological studies on pathogenesis of epiphyseal slipping in uremic children, Virchows Arch. (Pathol. Anat.) **362**:129, 1974.
263. Llach, F., et al.: Skeletal resistance to endogenous parathyroid hormone in patients with early renal failure: a possible cause for secondary hyperparathyroidism, J. Clin. Endocrinol. Metab. **41**:339, 1975.
264. Mahony, J.F., et al.: Hypophosphatemic osteomalacia in patients receiving haemodialysis, Br. Med. J. **2**:142, 1976.
265. Malluche, H.H., et al.: Bone histology in incipient and advanced renal failure, Kidney Int. **9**:355, 1976.
266. Martin, K.J., et al.: The renal handling of parathyroid hormone: role of peritubular uptake and glomerular filtration, J. Clin. Invest. **60**:808, 1977.
267. Massry, S.G., et al.: Skeletal resistance to the calcemic action of parathyroid hormone in uremia: role of $1,25(OH)_2D_3$, Kidney Int. **9**:467, 1976.
268. Massry, S.G., et al.: Role of uremia in the skeletal resistance to the calcemic action of parathyroid hormone, Min. Electrolyte Metab. **1**:172, 1978.
269. Mehls, O., et al.: Skeletal changes and growth in experimental uremia, Nephron **18**:288, 1977.
270. Mehls, O., et al. Growth in renal failure, Nephron **21**:237, 1978.
271. Parkinson, I.S., et al.: Fracturing dialysis osteodystrophy and dialysis encephalopathy, Lancet **1**:406, 1979.

272. Pierides, A.M., Skillen, A.W., and Ellis, H.A.: Serum alkaline phosphatase in azotemic and hemodialysis osteodystrophy: a study of isoenzyme patterns, their correlation with bone histology, and their changes in response to treatment with 1α OHD_3 and $1,25(OH)_2D_3$, J. Lab. Clin. Med. **93**:899, 1979.
273. Reiss, E., Canterbury, J.M., and Kanter, A.: Circulating parathyroid hormone concentration in chronic renal insufficiency, Arch. Intern. Med. **124**:417, 1969.
274. Russell, J.E., Avioli, L.V., and Mechanic, G.: Short communications: the nature of the collagen cross-links in bone in the chronic uremic state, Biochem. J. **145**:119, 1975.
275. Rutherford, W.E., et al.: Phosphate control and 25-Hydroxycholecalciferol administration in preventing experimental renal osteodystrophy in the dog, J. Clin. Invest. **60**:332, 1977.
276. Schmidt-Gayk, H., et al.: 25-Hydroxy-vitamin-D in nephrotic syndrome, Lancet **2**:105, 1977.
277. Simmons, J.M., et al.: Relation of calorie deficiency to growth failure in children on hemodialysis and the growth response to calorie supplementation, N. Engl. J. Med. **285**:653, 1971.
278. Slatopolsky, E., et al.: On the pathogenesis of hyperparathyroidism in chronic experimental renal insufficiency in the dog, J. Clin. Invest. **50**:492, 1971.
279. Slatopolsky, E., et al.: The pathogenesis of secondary hyperparathyroidism in early renal failure. In Norman, A.W., et al., editors: Vitamin D: basic research and its clinical application, New York, 1979, Walter de Gruyter.
280. Stanbury, S.W.: Bony complications of renal disease. In Black, D.A.K., editor: Renal disease, ed. 2, Philadelphia, 1967, F.A. Davis Co.
281. Teitelbaum, S.L., et al.: Calcifediol in chronic renal insufficiency: skeletal response, J.A.M.A. **235**:164, 1976.
282. Teitelbaum, S.L., et al.: The relationship of biochemical and histometric determinants of uremic bone, Arch. Pathol. Lab. Med. **103**:228, 1979.
283. Teitelbaum, S.L., et al.: Do parathyroid hormone and 1,25-dihydroxyvitamin D modulate bone formation in uremia? J. Clin. Endocrinol. Metab. **51**:247, 1980.
284. Ward, M.K., et al.: Osteomalacia dialysis osteodystrophy: evidence for a water-borne aetiological agent, probably aluminum, Lancet **1**:841, 1978.
285. Ward, M.K., et al.: Newcastle bone disease. In Norman, A.W., et al., editors: Vitamin D: basic research and its clinical application, New York, 1979, Walter de Gruyter.
286. Weinberg, S.G., et al.: Myelofibrosis and renal osteodystrophy, Am. J. Med. **63**:755, 1977.
287. Weinstein, R.S.: Decreased mineralization in hemodialysis patients after subtotal parathyroidectomy, Calcif. Tissue Int. **34**:16, 1982.

Calcitonin

288. Baud, C.A., et al.: The effects of prolonged administration of thyrocalcitonin in human senile osteoporosis. In Taylor, S., and Foster, G., editors: Calcitonin—1969, New York, 1970, James H. Heineman, Inc.
289. Bauer, W.C., and Teitelbaum, S.L.: Thyrocalcitonin activity of particulate fractions of the thyroid gland, Lab. Invest. **15**:323, 1966.
290. Baylink, D., Morey, E., and Rich, C.: Effect of calcitonin on the rates of bone formation and resorption in the rat, Endocrinology **84**:26, 1969.
291. Bordier, P., Hioco, D., and Tun-Chot, S.: Calcitonin: acute effects upon serum calcium, urinary hydroxyproline excretion and osteoclasts in man. In Taylor, S., and Foster, G., editors: Calcitonin–1969, New York, 1970, James H. Heineman, Inc.
292. Boris, A., et al.: Inhibition of diphosphonate-blocked bone mineralization: evidence that calcitonin promotes mineralization, Acta Endocrinol. **91**:351, 1979.
293. Brand, J.S., and Raisz, L.G.: Effects of thyrocalcitonin and phosphate ion on the parathyroid hormone–stimulated resorption of bone, Endocrinology **90**:479, 1972.
294. Delling, G., Schafer, A., and Siegler, R.: The effect of calcitonin on fracture healing and ectopic bone formation in the rat. In Taylor, S., and Foster, G., editors; Calcitonin—1969, New York, 1970, James H. Heineman, Inc.
295. Fornasier, V.L., Stapleton, K., and Williams, C.C.: Histologic changes in Paget's disease treated with calcitonin, Hum. Pathol. **9**:455, 1978.
296. Haddad, J.G., Birge, S.J., and Avioli, L.V.: Effects of prolonged thyrocalcitonin administration on Paget's disease of bone, N. Engl. J. Med. **283**:549, 1970.
297. Jowsey, J., et al.: Effects of prolonged administration of porcine calcitonin in post-menopausal osteoporosis, J. Clin. Endocrinol. **33**:752, 1971.
298. Jowsey, J., et al.: Calcium and salmon calcitonin in treatment of osteoporosis, J. Clin. Endocrinol. Metab. **47**:633, 1978.
299. Krane, S.M., et al.: Acute effects of calcitonin on bone formation in man, Metabolism **22**:51, 1973.
300. Marx, S.J., Woodard, C.J., and Aurbach, G.D.: Calcitonin receptors of kidney and bone, Science **178**:999, 1972.
301. Melvin, K.E.W., Tashjian, A.H., and Bordier, P.: The metabolic significance of calcitonin-secreting thyroid carcinoma. In Frame, B., Parfitt, A.M., and Duncan, H., editors: Clinical aspects of metabolic bone disease, Int. Congr. Ser. No. 270, Amsterdam, 1973, Excerpta Medica Foundation.
302. Norimatsu, H., Vander Wiel, C.J., and Talmage, R.V.: Electron microscopic study of the effects of calcitonin on bone cells and their extracellular milieu, Clin. Orthop. **139**:250, 1979.
303. Schatzker, J., et al.: The effect of calcitonin on fracture healing, Clin. Orthop. **141**:303, 1979.
304. Talmage, R.V., et al.: Evidence for an important physiological role for calcitonin, Proc. Natl. Acad. Sci. U.S.A. **77**:609, 1980.
305. Tashjian, A.H., et al.: Immunoassay of human calcitonin: clinical measurement, relation to serum calcium, and studies in patients with medullary carcinoma, N. Engl. J. Med. **283**:890, 1970.
306. Wase, A.W., et al.: Action of thyrocalcitonin on bone, Nature **214**:388, 1967.
307. Whyte, M.P., et al.: Arrest and healing of osteolytic Paget's bone disease with synthetic human calcitonin therapy: radiographic documentation. In Pecile, A., editor: Calcitonin—1980, Amsterdam, 1980, Excerpta Medica.
308. Williams, C.P., Meachim, G., and Taylor, W.H.: Effect of calcitonin treatment on osteoclast counts in Paget's disease of bone, J. Clin. Pathol. **31**:1212, 1978.
309. Zichner, L.: The effect of calcitonin on bone cells in young rats: an electron microscopic study, Isr. J. Med. Sci. **7**:359, 1971.

Estrogens

Senile osteopenia

310. Albright, F., Bloomberg, E., and Smith, P.H.: Postmenopausal osteoporosis, Trans. Assoc. Am. Physicians **55**:298, 1940.
311. Alhava, E.M., and Puittinen, S.: Fractures of the upper end of the femur as an index of senile osteoporosis in Finland, Ann. Clin. Res. **5**:398, 1973.
312. Avioli, L.V., et al.: The biochemical and skeletal heterogeneity of "post-menopausal" osteoporosis. In Barzel, U.S., editor: Osteoporosis, vol. 2, New York, 1979, Grune & Stratton, Inc.
313. Barzel, U.S.: The effect of excessive acid feeding on bone, Calcif. Tissue Res. **4**:94, 1969.
314. Darby, A.J., and Meunier, P.J.: Mean wall thickness and formation periods of trabecular bone packets in idiopathic osteoporosis, Calcif. Tissue Int. **33**:199, 1981.
315. Gallagher, J.C., et al.: Intestinal calcium absorption and serum vitamin D metabolites in normal subjects and osteoporotic patients, J. Clin. Invest. **64**:729, 1979.
316. Gallagher, J.C., et al.: Effect of estrogen on calcium absorption and serum vitamin D metabolites in postmenopausal osteoporosis, J. Clin. Endocrinol. Metab. **51**:1359, 1980.
317. Gallagher, J.C., et al.: The effect of age on serum immunoreactive parathyroid hormone in normal and osteoporotic women, J. Lab. Clin. Med. **95**:373, 1980.
318. Gershon-Cohen, J., and Jowsey, J.: The relationship of dietary calcium to osteoporosis, Metabolism **13**:221, 1964.
319. Heaney, R.P., Recker, R.R., and Saville, P.D.: Menopausal changes in bone remodeling, J. Lab. Clin. Med. **92**:964, 1978.
320. Heaney, R.P., Recker, R.R., and Saville, P.D.: Menopausal changes in calcium balance performance, J. Lab. Clin. Med. **92**:953, 1978.

321. Iskrant, A.P., and Smith, R.W., Jr.: Osteoporosis in women 45 years and over related to subsequent fracture, Public Health Rep. **84**:33, 1969.
322. Jowsey, J.: Age changes in human bone, Clin. Orthop. **17**:210, 1960.
323. Jowsey, J., and Balasubramaniam, P.: Effect of phosphate supplements on soft tissue calcification and bone turnover, Clin. Sci. **42**:289, 1972.
324. Kelly, P.J., et al.: Relationship between serum phosphate concentration and bone resorption in osteoporosis, J. Lab. Clin. Med. **69**:110, 1967.
325. Meunier, P.J., et al.: Histological heterogeneity of apparently idiopathic osteoporosis. In DeLuca, H.F., et al., editors: Osteoporosis: recent advances in pathogenesis and treatment, Baltimore, 1980, University Park Press.
326. Newton-John, H.F., and Morgan, D.B.: The loss of bone with age, osteoporosis, and fractures, Clin. Orthop. **71**:229, 1970.
327. Riggs, B.L., et al.: Differential changes in bone mineral density of the appendicular and axial skeleton with aging, J. Clin. Invest. **67**:328, 1981.
328. Shamonki, I.M., et al.: Age-related changes of calcitonin secretion in females, J. Clin. Endocrinol. Metab. **50**:437, 1980.
329. Stevens, J., et al.: The incidence of osteoporosis in patients with femoral neck fracture, J. Bone Joint Surg. **44B**:520, 1962.
330. Teitelbaum, S.L., et al.: Histological studies of bone from normocalcemic post-menopausal osteoporotic patients with increased circulating parathyroid hormone, J. Clin. Endocrinol. Metab. **42**:537, 1976.
331. Teitelbaum, S.L., et al.: Failure of routine biochemical studies to predict the histological heterogeneity of untreated post-menopausal osteoporosis. In DeLuca, H.F., et al., editors: Osteoporosis: recent advances in pathogenesis and treatment, Baltimore, 1981, University Park Press.
332. Trotter, M., Bromar, G.E., and Peterson, R.R.: Densities of bones of white and Negro skeletons, J. Bone Joint Surg. **42A**:50, 1960.
333. Whyte, M.P., et al.: Postmenopausal osteoporosis: a heterogeneous disorder as assessed by histomorphometric analysis of iliac crest bone from untreated patients, Am. J. Med. **72**:193, 1982.

Ovarian dysgenesis

334. Ashby, J.P., et al.: Plasma cyclic-AMP response to parathyroid hormone in Turner's syndrome and Albright's hereditary osteodystrophy, Clin. Endocrinol. **10**:553, 1979.
335. Brown, D.M., Jowsey, J., and Bradford, D.S.: Osteoporosis in ovarian dysgenesis, J. Pediatr. **84**:816, 1974.
336. Finby, N., and Archibald, R.M.: Skeletal abnormalities associated with gonadal dysgenesis, Am. J. Roentgenol. **89**:1222, 1963.
337. Garn, S.M., Poznanski, A.K., and Nagy, J.M.: Bone measurement in the differential diagnosis of osteopenia and osteoporosis, Radiology **100**:509, 1971.
338. Preger, L., et al.: Roentgenographic abnormalities in phenotypic females with gonadal dysgenesis, Am. J. Roentgenol. **104**:899, 1968.
339. Riggs, B.L., et al.: Short- and long-term effects of estrogen and synthetic anabolic hormone in postmenopausal osteoporosis, J. Clin. Invest. **51**:1659, 1972.

Growth hormone

340. Aloia, J.F., and Yeh, J.K.: Growth hormone and intestinal calcium transport in the rat, Metab. Bone Dis. Rel. Res. **2**:251, 1980.
341. Aloia, J.F., et al.: Effects of growth hormone in osteoporosis, J. Clin. Endocrinol. Metab. **43**:992, 1976.
342. Bell, N.H., and Bartter, F.C.: Studies of ^{47}Ca metabolism in acromegaly, J. Clin. Endocrinol. **27**:178, 1967.
343. Daughaday, W.H., and Kipnis, D.M.: The growth-promoting and anti-insulin actions of somatotropin, Recent Prog. Horm. Res. **22**:49, 1966.
344. Delling, G.R., and Schulz, A.: Bone cells and remodelling surfaces in acromegaly, Calcif. Tissue Res. **22**(suppl.):255, 1977.
345. Fidler, M.W., and Brook, C.G.D.: Slipped upper femoral epiphyses following treatment with human growth hormone, J. Bone Joint Surg. **56A**:1719, 1974.
346. Grunt, G.A., and Reynolds, D.W.: Insulin, blood sugar, and growth hormone levels in an anencephalic infant before and after intravenous administration of glucose, J. Pediatr. **76A**:112, 1970.
347. Halse, J., and Haugen, H.N.: Calcium and phosphate metabolism in acromegaly, Acta Endocrinol. **94**:459, 1980.
348. Harris, W.H., and Heaney, R.P.: Effect of growth hormone on skeletal mass in adult dogs, Nature **223**:403, 1969.
349. Harris, W.H., et al.: Growth hormone: the effect of skeletal renewal in the adult dog. I. Morphometric studies, Calcif. Tissue Res. **10**:1, 1972.
350. Heins, J.N., Garland, J.T., and Daughaday, W.H.: Incorporation of ^{35}S-sulfate into rat cartilage explants in vitro: effects of aging on responsiveness to stimulation by sulfation factor, Endocrinology **87**:688, 1970.
351. Henneman, P.H., et al.: Effects of human growth hormone in man, J. Clin. Invest. **39**:1223, 1960.
352. Lung, B.J., et al.: High serum 1,25-$(OH)_2D$ in acromegaly: effect of bromocriptine treatment. In Norman, A.W., et al., editors: Vitamin D: basic research and its clinical application, New York, 1979, Walter de Gruyter.
353. Ramser, J.R., Frost, H., and Smith, R.: Tetracycline-based measurement of the tissue and cell dynamics in rib of a 25-year-old man with active acromegaly, Clin. Orthop. **49**:169, 1966.
354. Riggs, B.L., et al.: The nature of the metabolic bone disorder in acromegaly, J. Clin. Endocrinol. Metab. **34**:911, 1972.
355. Scott, C.I.: The genetics of short stature. In Steinberg, A.G., and Bearn, A.B., editors: Progress in medical genetics, New York, 1972, Grune & Stratton, Inc.
356. Urist, M.R.: Growth hormone and skeletal tissue metabolism. In Bourne, G.H., editor: The biochemistry and physiology of bone. Vol. 2, Physiology and pathology, ed. 2, New York, 1972, Academic Press, Inc.

Thyroid hormone

357. Adams, H.P., et al.: Effects of hyperthyroidism on bone and mineral metabolism in man, Q. J. Med. **36**:1, 1967.
358. Bordier, P., et al.: Bone changes in adult patients with abnormal thyroid function (with special reference to ^{45}Ca kinetics and quantitative histology), Proc. R. Soc. Med. **60**:1132, 1967.
359. Bouillon, R., and DeMoor, P.: Parathyroid function in patients with hyper- or hypothyroidism, J. Clin. Endocrinol. Metab. **38**:999, 1974.
360. Bouillon, R., Muls, E., and DeMoor, P.: Influence of thyroid function on the serum concentration of 1,25-dihydroxyvitamin D_3, J. Clin. Endocrinol. Metab. **51**:793, 1980.
361. Burkhart, J.M., and Jowsey, J.: Parathyroid and thyroid hormone in the development of immobilization osteoporosis, Endocrinology **81**:1053, 1967.
362. Castro, J.H., Genuth, S.M., and Klein, L.: Comparative response to parathyroid hormone in hyperthyroidism and hypothyroidism, Metabolism **24**:839, 1975.
363. Clarke, J.T.: Colorimetric determination and distribution of urinary creatinine and creatine, Clin. Chim. **7**:371, 1961.
364. Clerkin, E.P., et al.: Osteomalacia in thyrotoxicosis, Metabolism **13**:161, 1964.
365. Dearden, L.C., and Mosier, D.H.: Growth retardation and subsequent recovery of rat tibia, a histochemical, light, and electron microscopic study. I. After propylthiouracil treatment, Growth **38**:253, 1974.
366. Haldimann, B., et al.: Intestinal calcium absorption in patients with hyperthyroidism, J. Clin. Endocrinol. Metab. **51**:955, 1980.
367. High, W.B., Capen, C.C., and Black, H.E.: Effects of thyroxine on cortical bone remodeling in adult dogs: a histomorphometric study, Am. J. Pathol. **102**:438, 1981.
368. Jowsey, J., and Detenbeck, L.C.: Importance of thyroid hormones in bone metabolism and calcium homeostasis, Endocrinology **85**:87, 1969.
369. Lekkerkerker, J.F.F., and Doorenbos, H.: The influence of thyroid hormone on calcium absorption from the gut in relation to urinary calcium excretion, Acta Endocrinol. **73**:672, 1973.
370. Maxon, H.R., Apple, D.J., and Goldsmith, R.E.: Hypercalcemia in thyrotoxicosis, Surg. Gynecol. Obstet. **147**:694, 1978.

371. Melsen, F., and Mosekilde, L.: Dynamic studies of trabecular bone formation and osteoid maturation in normal and certain pathological conditions, Metab. Bone Dis. Rel. Res. **1**:45, 1978.
372. Meunier, P.J., et al.: Bony manifestations of thyrotoxicosis, Orthop. Clin. North Am. **3**:745, 1972.
373. Mundy, G.R., et al.: Direct stimulation of bone resorption by thyroid hormones, J. Clin. Invest. **58**:529, 1976.
374. Newman, R.J.: The effect of thyroid hormone on vitamin D–induced nephrocalcinosis, J. Pathol. **111**:13, 1973.
375. Parfitt, A.M., and Dent, C.E.: Hyperthyroidism and hypercalcemia, Q. J. Med. **39**:171, 1970.
376. Pavlovitch, H., Presle, V., and Balsani, S.: Decreased bone sensitivity of thyroidectomized rats to the calcaemic effects of 1,25-dihydroxycholecalciferol, Acta Endocrinol. **84**:774, 1977.
377. Ray, R.D., et al.: Growth and differentiation of the skeleton in thyroidectomized-hypophysectomized rats treated with thyroxine, growth hormone, and the combination, J. Bone Joint Surg. **36A**:94, 1954.
378. Wilkin, L.: Epiphyseal dysgenesis associated with hypothyroidism, Am. J. Dis. Child. **61**:13, 1941.

Adrenal corticosteroids

379. Avioli, L.V.: Osteoporosis: pathogenesis and therapy. In Avioli, L.V., and Krane, S.M., editors: Metabolic bone disease, vol. 1, New York, 1977, Academic Press, Inc.
380. Bernick, S., and Ershoff, B.H.: Histochemical study of bone in cortisone treated rats, J. Clin. Endocrinol. Metab. **72**:231, 1963.
381. Bressot, C., et al.: Histomorphometric profile, pathophysiology and reversibility of corticosteroid-induced osteoporosis, Metab. Bone Dis. Rel. Res. **1**:303, 1979.
382. Chen, T.L., and Feldman, D.: Glucocorticoid receptors and actions in subpopulations of cultured rat bone cells, J. Clin. Invest. **63**:750, 1979.
383. Curtiss, P.H., Clark, W.S., and Herndon, C.H.: Vertebral fractures resulting from prolonged cortisone and corticotrophin therapy, J.A.M.A. **156**:467, 1954.
384. Cushing, H.: The basophil adenomas of the pituitary body and their clinical manifestations, Bull. Johns Hopkins Hosp. **50**:137, 1932.
385. Dietrich, J.W., et al.: Effects of glucocorticoids on fetal rat bone collagen synthesis in vitro, Endocrinology **104**:715, 1979.
386. Duncan, H.: Bone histodynamic changes in the rheumatic diseases, Clin. Orthop. **49**:124, 1966.
387. Epker, B.N.: Studies on bone turnover and balance in the rabbit. I. Effects of hydrocortisone, Clin. Orthop. **72**:315, 1970.
388. Frantz, A.G., and Rabkin, M.T.: Human growth hormone: clinical measurement, response to hypoglycemia, and suppression by corticosteroids, N. Engl. J. Med. **271**:1375, 1964.
389. Friedman, M., and Strang, L.B.: Effect of long-term corticosteroids and corticotrophin on the growth of children, Lancet **1**:568, 1966.
390. Gallagher, H.C., et al.: Corticosteroid osteoporosis, Clin. Endocrinol. **2**:355, 1973.
391. Hahn, T.J., Halstead, L.R., and Baran, D.T.: Effects of short-term glucocorticoid administration on intestinal calcium absorption and circulating vitamin D metabolite concentrations in man, J. Clin. Endocrinol. Metab. **52**:111, 1981.
392. Hahn, T.J., et al.: Altered mineral metabolism in glucocorticoid-induced osteopenia: effect of 25-hydroxyvitamin D administration, J. Clin. Invest. **64**:655, 1979.
393. Hough, S., et al.: Isolated skeletal involvement in Cushing's syndrome: response to therapy, J. Clin. Endocrinol. Metab. **52**:1033, 1981.
394. Howland, W.J., Pugh, D.G., and Sprague, R.G.: Roentgenologic changes in the skeletal system in Cushing's syndrome, Radiology **71**:69, 1968.
395. Hulth, A., and Westerborn, O.: Effect of cortisone on epiphyseal cartilage: a histologic and autoradiographic study, Virchows Arch. (Pathol. Anat.) **336**:209, 1963.
396. Iannaccone, A., et al.: Osteoporosis in Cushing's syndrome, Ann. Intern. Med. **52**:570, 1960.
397. Jee, W.S.S., et al.: Interrelated effects of glucocorticoid and parathyroid hormone upon bone remodeling. In Talmage, R.V., and Munson, P.L., editors: Calcium, parathyroid hormone and the calcitonins, Amsterdam, 1972, Excerpta Medica Foundation.
398. Klein, M., Villanueva, A.R., and Frost, H.M.: A quantitative histological study of rib from eighteen patients treated with adrenal cortical steroids, Acta Orthop. Scand. **35**:171, 1965.
399. Maassen, A.P.: The effect of desoxycorticosterone acetate (Doca) on body-growth and ossification, Acta Endocrinol. **9**:291, 1952.
400. Manolagas, S.C., Anderson, D.C., and Lumb, G.A.: Glucocorticoids regulate the concentration of 1,25-dihydroxycholecalciferol receptors in bone, Nature **277**:314, 1979.
401. Ng, B., Hekkelman, J.W., and Heersche, J.N.M.: The effect of cortisol on the adenosine 3′5′-monophosphate response to parathyroid hormone of bone in vitro, Endocrinology **104**:1130, 1979.
402. Peck, W.A., Brandt, J., and Miller, I.: Hydrocortisone-induced inhibition of protein synthesis and uridine incorporation in isolated bone cells in vitro, Proc. Natl. Acad. Sci. U.S.A. **57**:1599,1967.
403. Raisz, L.G., et al.: Effect of glucocorticoids on bone resorption in tissue culture, Endocrinology **90**:961, 1972.
404. Ruder, H.J., Loriaux, D.L., and Lipsett, M.B.: Severe osteopenia in young adult associated with Cushing's syndrome due to micronodular adrenal disease, J. Clin. Endocrinol. Metab. **39**:1138, 1974.
405. Sisson, J.C., Kirchick, H., and Kothary, P.: Inhibition of glucosaminoglycans production in retrobulbar fibroblast cultures by ethacrynic acid and hydrocortisone, J. Clin. Endocrinol. Metab. **38**:777, 1974.
406. Sissons, H.A., and Hadfield, G.J.: The influence of cortisone on the structure and growth of bone, J. Anat. **89**:69, 1955.
407. Soffer, L.J., Iannaccone, A., and Gabrilove, J.L.: Cushing's syndrome: a study of fifty patients, Am. J. Med. **30**:129, 1961.
408. Solomon, I.L., and Schoen, E.J.: Juvenile Cushing syndrome manifested primarily by growth failure, Arch. Am. J. Dis. Child. **130**:200, 1976.
409. Strumpf, M., Kowalski, M.A., and Mundy, G.R.: Effects of glucocorticoids on osteoclast-activating factor, J. Lab. Clin. Med. **92**:772, 1978.
410. Teitelbaum, S.L., Malone, J.D., and Kahn, A.J.: Glucocorticoid enhancement of bone resorption by rat peritoneal macrophages in vitro, Endocrinology **108**:795, 1981.

Diabetes mellitus

411. Canalis, E.: Effect of insulin-like growth factor I on DNA and protein synthesis in cultured rat calvaria, J. Clin. Invest. **66**:709, 1980.
412. Dixit, P.K., and Ekstrom, R.A.: Decreased breaking strength of diabetic rat bone and its improvement by insulin treatment, Calcif. Tissue Int. **32**:195, 1980.
413. Frazer, T.E., et al.: Alterations in circulating vitamin D metabolites in the young insulin-dependent diabetic, J. Clin. Endocrinol. Metab. **53**:1154, 1981.
414. Hahn, T.J., Downing, S.J., and Phang, J.M.: Insulin effect on amino acid transport in bone: dependence on protein synthesis and Na^+, Am. J. Physiol. **220**:1717, 1971.
415. Heath, H., Melton, L.J., and Chu, C.-P.: Diabetes mellitus and risk of skeletal fracture, N. Engl. J. Med. **303**:567, 1980.
416. Hough, S., et al.: Correction of abnormal bone and mineral metabolism in chronic streptozotocin-induced diabetes mellitus in the rat by insulin therapy, Endocrinology **108**:2228, 1981.
417. Levin, M.E., Boisseau, V.C., and Avioli, L.V.: Effects of diabetes mellitus on bone mass in juvenile and adult-onset diabetes, N. Engl. J. Med. **294**:241, 1976.
418. McNair, P., et al.: Osteopenia in insulin-treated diabetes mellitus: its relation to age at onset, sex, and duration of disease, Diabetologia **15**:87, 1978.
419. Monnier, L., et al.: Intestinal and renal handling of calcium in human diabetes mellitus: influence of acute oral glucose loading and diabetic control, Eur. J. Clin. Invest. **8**:225, 1978.
420. Prasad, G.C., and Rajan, K.T.: Effect of insulin on bone in tissue culture, Acta Orthop. Scand. **51**:44, 1970.

421. Shires, R., et al.: The effect of streptozotocin-induced chronic diabetes mellitus on bone and mineral homeostasis in the rat, J. Lab. Clin. Med. **97**:231, 1981.
422. Smith, D.M., et al.: In vivo measurement of bone mass: its use in demineralized states such as osteoporosis, J.A.M.A. **219**:325, 1972.
423. Spencer, E.M., Khalil, M., and Tobiassen, O.: Experimental diabetes in the rat causes an insulin-reversible decrease in renal 25-hydroxyvitamin D_3-1 α-hydroxylase activity, Endocrinology **107**:300, 1980.
424. Weiss, R.E., and Reddi, A.H.: Influence of experimental diabetes and insulin on matrix-induced cartilage and bone differentiation, Am. J. Physiol. **238**:E200, 1980.
425. Wettenhall, R.E.H., Schwartz, P.L., and Bornstein, J.: Actions of insulin and growth hormone on collagen and chondroitin sulfate synthesis in bone organ cultures, Diabetes **18**:280, 1969.

Vitamin C

426. Bourne, G.H.: Some experiments on the possible relationship between vitamin D and calcification, J. Physiol. **102**:319, 1943.
427. Bourne, G.H.: The relative importance of periosteum and endosteum in bone healing and the relationship of vitamin C to their activities, Proc. R. Soc. Med. **37**:275, 1944.
428. Fernandez-Madrid, F.: Collagen biosynthesis: a review, Clin. Orthop. **68**:163, 1970.
429. Follis, R.H.: The pathology of nutritional diseases, Oxford, Eng., 1948, Blackwell Scientific Publications, Ltd.
430. Follis, R.H.: Histochemical studies on cartilage and bone. II. Ascorbic acid deficiency, Bull. Johns Hopkins Hosp. **89**:9,1951.
431. Hertz, J.: Studies on the healing of fractures, with special references to the significance of the vitamin content of the diet, Acta Pathol. Microbiol. Scand. **28**(suppl.): 134, 1936.
432. Hess, A.F.: Scurvy past and present, Philadelphia, 1920, J.B. Lippincott Co.
433. Kivirikko, K.I., and Prockop, D.J.: Parietal purification and characterization of protocollagen lysine hydroxylase from chick embryos, Biochim. Biophys. Acta **258**:366, 1972.
434. Murray, P.D.F., and Kodicek, E.: Bones, muscles and vitamin C. I. Effect of partial deficiency of vitamin C on repair of bone and muscle in guinea-pigs, J. Anat. **83**:158, 1949.
435. Murray, P.D.F., and Kodicek, E.: Bones, muscles and vitamin C. II. Partial deficiencies of vitamin C and mid-diaphyseal thickenings of the tibia and fistula in guinea pigs, J. Anat. **83**:205, 1949.
436. Murray, P.D.F., and Kodicek, E.: Bones, muscles and vitamin C. III. Repair of the effects of total deprivation of vitamin C at the proximal ends of tibia and fibula in guinea-pigs, J. Anat. **83**:285, 1949.
437. Patnaik, B.K.: Age related studies on ascorbic acid metabolism, Gerontologia **17**:122, 1971.
438. Peck, W.A., Birge, S.J., and Brandt, J.: Collagen synthesis by isolated bone cells: stimulation by ascorbic acid in vitro, Biochim. Biophys. Acta **142**:512, 1967.
439. Schwartz, E.R.: Effect of vitamins C and E on sulfated proteoglycan metabolism and sulfatase and phosphatase activities in organ cultures of human cartilage, Calcif. Tissue Int. **28**:201, 1979.
440. Schwartz, E.R., and Adamy, L.: Effect of ascorbic acid on arylsulfatase activities and sulfated proteoglycan metabolism in chondrocyte cultures, J. Clin. Invest. **60**:96, 1977.
441. Thornton, P.A.: Influence of exogenous ascorbic acid on calcium and phosphorus metabolism in the chick, J. Nutr. **100**:1479, 1970.
442. Wolbach, S.B., and Maddock, C.L.: Cortisone and matrix formation in experimental scorbutus and repair therefrom, with contributions to the pathology of experimental scorbutus, Arch. Pathol. **53**:54, 1952.

Vitamin A

443. Barnicot, N.A.: The local action of vitamin A on bone, J. Anat. **84**:374, 1950.
444. Caffey, J.: Chronic poisoning due to excess of vitamin A: description of the clinical and roentgen manifestations in seven infants and young children, Am. J. Roentgenol. **65**:12, 1951.
445. Fell, H.B., and Thomas, L.: Comparison of the effects of papain and vitamin A on cartilage. I. The effects on organ cultures of embryonic skeletal tissue, J. Exp. Med. **111**:719, 1960.
446. Frame, B., et al.: Hypercalcemia and skeletal effects in chronic hypervitaminosis A, Ann. Intern. Med. **80**:44, 1974.
447. Gerber, A., Raab, A.P., and Sobel, A.E.: Vitamin A poisoning in adults with description of a case, Am. J. Med. **16**:729, 1954.
448. Gerlings, P.G.: Clinical and histopathological investigations of the labyrinth in oxycephaly, Acta Otolaryngol. **35**:91, 1947.
449. Harris, S.S., and Navia, J.M.: Sulfate metabolism in rat calvaria cultured under vitamin A–deficient conditions, J. Nutr. **108**:1777, 1978.
450. Howard, L., et al.: Vitamin A deficiency from long-term parenteral nutrition, Ann. Intern. Med. **93**:576, 1980.
451. Kochkar, D.M.: Cellular basis of congenital limb deformity induced in mice by vitamin A, Birth Defects **13**:111,1977.
452. Kochkar, D.M., and Johnson, E.M.: Morphologic and autoradiographic studies of cleft palate induced in rat embryos by maternal hypervitaminosis A, J. Embryol. Exp. Morphol. **14**:223,1965.
453. Mahoney, C.P., et al.: Chronic vitamin A intoxication in infants fed chicken liver, Pediatrics **65**:893, 1980.
454. Mellanby, E.: Nutrition in relation to bone growth and the nervous system, Proc. R. Soc. London (Biol.) **132**:28, 1944.
455. Pease, C.N.: Focal retardation and arrestment of growth of bones due to vitamin A intoxication, J.A.M.A. **182**:980, 1962.
456. Persson, B., Tunell, R., and Ekengren, K.: Chronic vitamin A intoxication during the first half year of life: description of 5 cases, Acta Paediatr. Scand. **54**:49, 1965.
457. Rodahl, K.: Toxicity of polar bear liver, Nature **164**:530, 1949.
458. Ruby, L.K. and Mital, M.A.: Skeletal deformities following chronic hypervitaminosis A: a case report, J. Bone Joint Surg. **56**:1283,1974.
459. Sauer, G.J.R., and Evans, C.A.: Hypervitaminosis A and matrix alterations in maxillary explants from 16-day rat embryos, Teratology **21**:123, 1980.
460. Wolbach, S.B.: Vitamin D deficiency and excess in relation to skeletal growth, J. Bone Joint Surg. **29**:171, 1947.

Phosphorus

461. Barzel, U.S., and Jowsey, J.: The effects of chronic acid and alkali administration on bone turnover in adult rats, Clin. Sci. **36**:517, 1969.
462. Baylink, D.J., Wergedal, J., and Stouffer, M.: Formation, mineralization, and resorption of bone in hypophosphatemic rats, J. Clin. Invest. **50**:2519, 1971.
463. Chanard, J.M., et al.: A simplified technique for the measurement of intestinal absorption of calcium in the dog: effects of PO_4 depletion and 25 $(OH)D_3$ in uremia, Calcif. Tissue Int. **30**:199, 1980.
464. Cooke, N., Teitelbaum, S., and Avioli, L.V.: Antacid-induced osteomalacia and nephrolithiasis, Arch. Intern. Med. **138**:1007, 1978.
465. Dimuzio, M.T., and Veis, A.: Phosphophoryns—major noncollagenous proteins of rat incisor dentin, Calcif. Tissue Res. **25**:169, 1978.
466. Dominquez, J.H., Gray, R.W., and Lemann, J., Jr.: Dietary phosphate deprivation in women and men: effects of mineral and acid balances, parathyroid hormone and the metabolism of 25-OH-vitamin D, J. Clin. Endocrinol. Metab. **43**:1056, 1976.
467. Emmett, M., et al.: The pathophysiology of acid-base changes in chronically phosphate-depleted rats, J. Clin. Invest. **59**:291, 1977.
468. Feinblatt, J., Belanger, L.F., and Rasmussen, H.: Effect of phosphate infusion on bone metabolism and parathyroid hormone action, Am. J. Physiol. **28**:1624, 1970.
469. Glimcher, M.J., and Krane, S.M.: The incorporation of radioactive inorganic orthophosphate as organic phosphate by collagen fibrils in vitro, Biochemistry **3**:195, 1964.
470. Goldsmith, R.S., et al.: Effect of phosphate supplements in patients with fractures, Lancet **1**:688, 1967.
471. Haddad, J.G., and Avioli, L.V.: Comparative effects of phosphate and thyrocalcitonin on skeletal turnover, Endocrinology **87**:1245, 1970.

472. Hong, K.C., and Cruess, R.L.: Changes in organic matrix of bone and of bone and blood ATP in rats fed rachitogenic diets, Calcif. Tissue Res. **25**:241, 1978.

473. Knochel, J.P.: The pathophysiology and clinical characteristics of severe hypophosphatemia, Arch. Intern. Med. **137**:203, 1977.

474. Lee, D.B.N., et al.: Role of growth hormone in experimental phosphorus deprivation in the rat, Calcif. Tissue Int. **32**:105, 1980.

475. Lee, S.W., Russell, J.E., and Avioli, L.V.: 25-hydroxycholecalciferol: conversion impaired by systemic metabolic acidosis, Science **195**:994, 1977.

476. Lemann, J., Litzow, J.R., and Lennon, E.J.: The effects of chronic acid loads in normal man: further evidence for the participation of bone mineral in the defense against chronic metabolic acidosis, J. Clin. Invest. **45**:1608, 1966.

477. Martin, K.J., et al.: The effect of acute acidosis on the uptake of parathyroid hormone and the production of 3′-5′ cyclic adenosine monophosphate by isolated perfused bone, Endocrinology **106**:1607, 1980.

478. Matthews, J.L.: Ultrastructure of calcifying tissues, Am. J. Anat. **129**:451, 1970.

479. Matthews, J.L., and Martin, J.H.: Intracellular calcium in connective tissue cells, Int. Congr. Ser. No. 229, Amsterdam, 1970, Excerpta Medica Foundation.

480. Nollen, A., and Bijvoet, O.: The effect of phosphate on fracture healing in rabbits, Isr. J. Med. Sci. **7**:508, 1971.

481. Rasmussen, H.: Ionic and hormonal control of calcium homeostasis, Am. J. Med. **50**:567, 1971.

482. Russell, J.E., and Avioli, L.V.: Bone maturation in the vitamin D, phosphate deficient rat and the response to acid loading, Calcif. Tissue Int. **27**:233, 1979.

483. Tanaka, Y., Frank, H., and DeLuca, H.F.: Intestinal calcium transport: stimulation by low-phosphorus diets, Science **181**:564, 1973.

Hypophosphatemic osteomalacia

484. Choufoer, J.H., and Steendijk, R.: Distribution of the perilacunar hypomineralized areas in cortical bone from patients with familial hypophosphatemic (vitamin D–resistant) rickets, Calcif. Tissue Int. **27**:101, 1979.

485. Costa, T., et al.: X-linked hypophosphatemia: effect of calcitriol on renal handling of phosphate, serum phosphate, and bone mineralization, J. Clin. Endocrinol. Metab. **52**:463, 1981.

486. Cowgill, L.D., et al.: Evidence for an intrinsic renal tubular defect in mice with genetic hypophosphatemic rickets, J. Clin. Invest. **63**:1203, 1979.

487. Dent, C.E., and Harris, H.: Hereditary forms of rickets and osteomalacia, J. Bone Joint Surg. **38B**:204, 1956.

488. Drezner, M.K., and Feinglos, M.N.: Osteomalacia due to 1,25-dihydroxycholecalciferol deficiency, J. Clin. Invest. **60**:1046, 1977.

489. Drezner, M.K., et al.: Evaluation of a role for 1α,25-dihydroxyvitamin D_3 in the pathogenesis and treatment of x-linked hypophosphatemic rickets and osteomalacia, J. Clin. Invest. **66**:1020, 1980.

490. Engfeldt, B., Zetterstrom, R., and Winberg, T.: Primary vitamin D–resistant rickets. III. Biophysical studies of skeletal tissue, J. Bone Joint Surg. **38A**:1323, 1956.

491. Frost, H.M.: A unique histological feature of vitamin D–resistant rickets observed in four cases, Acta Orthop. Scand. **33**:220, 1963.

492. Frymoyer, J.W., and Hodgkin, W.: Adult-onset vitamin D–resistant hypophosphatemic osteomalacia, J. Bone Joint Surg. **59A**:101, 1977.

493. Fukumoto, Y., et al.: Tumor-induced vitamin D–resistant hypophosphatemic osteomalacia associated with proximal renal tubular dysfunction and 1,25-dihydroxyvitamin D deficiency, J. Clin. Endocrinol. Metab. **49**:873, 1979.

494. Glorieux, F.H., and Scriver, C.R.: Loss of a parathyroid hormone-sensitive component of phosphate transport in x-linked hypophosphatemia, Science **175**:997, 1972.

495. Glorieux, F.H., et al.: Bone response to phosphate salts, ergocalciferol, and calcitriol in hypophosphatemic vitamin D–resistant rickets, N. Engl. J. Med. **303**:1023, 1980.

496. Lyles, K.W., et al.: Hypophosphatemic osteomalacia: association with prostatic carcinoma, Ann. Intern. Med. **93**:275, 1980.

497. Marie, P.J., and Glorieux, F.H.: Histomorphometric study of bone remodeling in hypophosphatemic vitamin D–resistant rickets, Metab. Bone Dis. Rel. Res. **3**:31, 1981.

498. Marie, P.J., Travers, R., and Glorieux, F.H.: Healing of rickets with phosphate supplementation in the hypophosphatemic male mouse, J. Clin. Invest. **67**:911, 1981.

499. Meyer, R.A., Jr., Gray, R.W., and Meyer, M.H.: Abnormal vitamin D metabolism in the x-linked hypophosphatemic mouse, Endocrinology **107**:1577, 1980.

500. Perry, W., and Stamp, T.C.B.: Hereditary hypophosphataemic rickets with autosomal recessive inheritance and severe osteosclerosis, J. Bone Joint Surg. **60B**:430, 1978.

501. Wilson, D.R., et al.: Studies in hypophosphatemic vitamin D–refractory osteomalacia in adults: oral phosphate supplements as an adjunct to therapy, Medicine **44**:99, 1965.

502. Winters, R.W., et al.: A genetic study of familial hypophosphatemic and vitamin-D-resistant rickets with a review of the literature, Medicine **37**:97, 1958.

Fluoride

503. Azar, H.A., et al.: Skeletal fluorosis due to chronic fluoride intoxication: cases from an endemic area of fluorosis in the region of the Persian Gulf, Ann. Intern. Med. **55**:193, 1961.

504. Baud, C.A., et al.: Value of the bone biopsy in the diagnosis of industrial fluorosis, Virchows Arch. (Pathol. Anat.) **380**:283, 1978.

505. Baylink, D.J., and Bernstein, D.S.: The effects of fluoride therapy on metabolic bone disease, Clin. Orthop. **55**:51, 1967.

506. Belanger, L.F., et al.: Rachitomimetic effects of fluoride feeding on the skeletal tissue of growing pigs, Am. J. Pathol. **34**:25, 1958.

507. Bernstein, D.S., et al.: Prevalence of osteoporosis in high and low fluoride areas in North Dakota, J.A.M.A. **198**:499, 1966.

508. Cass, R.M., et al.: New bone formation in osteoporosis following treatment with sodium fluoride, Arch. Intern. Med. **118**:111, 1966.

509. Eanes, E.D., et al.: Small-angle x-ray diffraction and analysis of the effect of fluoride on human bone apatite, Arch. Oral Biol. **10**:161, 1965.

510. Faccini, J.M.: Fluoride and bone, Calcif. Tissue Res. **3**:1, 1969.

511. Faccini, J.M., and Teotia, S.P.S.: Histopathological assessment of endemic skeletal fluorosis, Calcif. Tissue Res. **16**:45, 1974.

512. Jowsey, J., Schenk, R.K., and Reutter, F.W.: Some results of the effect of fluoride on bone tissue in osteoporosis, J. Clin. Endocrinol. **28**:869, 1968.

513. Jowsey, J., et al.: Effect of combined therapy with sodium fluoride, vitamin D, and calcium in osteoporosis, Am. J. Med. **53**:43, 1972.

514. Lui, C.C., and Baylink, D.J.: Stimulation of bone formation and bone resorption by fluoride in thyroparathyroidectomized rats, J. Dent. Res. **56**:304, 1977.

515. Meunier, P.J., et al.: Radiological and histological evolution of post-menopausal osteoporosis treated with sodium fluoride-vitamin-D-calcium: preliminary results. In Couvoisier, B., Donath, A., and Bauer, E., editors: Fluoride and bone, Bern, 1978, Hans Huber.

516. Ramberg, C.F., et al.: Inhibition of calcium absorption and elevation of calcium removal rate from bone in fluoride-treated calves, J. Nutr. **100**:981, 1970.

517. Riggins, R.S., et al.: The effect of fluoride supplementation on the strength of osteopenic bone, Clin. Orthop. **114**:352, 1976.

518. Rosenquist, J.B.: Effects of supply and withdrawal of fluoride, Acta Pathol. Microbiol. Scand. **83**:628, 1975.

519. Spencer, G.R., Cohen, A.L., and Garner, G.E.: Effect of fluoride, calcium, and phosphorus on periosteal surface, Calcif. Tissue Res. **15**:111, 1974.

520. Stein, I.D., and Granik, G.: Human vertebral bone: relation of strength, porosity, and mineralization to fluoride content, Calcif. Tissue Int. **32**:189, 1980.

521. Teotia, S.P.S., and Teotia, M.: Secondary hyperparathyroidism in patients with endemic skeletal fluorosis, Br. Med. J. **1**:637, 1973.

522. Weatherell, J.A., and Weidmann, S.M.: The skeletal changes of chronic experimental fluorosis, J. Pathol. Bacteriol. **78**:233, 1959.

Hypophosphatasia

523. Bethune, J.E., and Dent, C.E.: Hypophosphatasia in the adult, Am. J. Med. **28**:615, 1960.
524. Fraser, D.: Hypophosphatasia, Am. J. Med. **22**:730, 1957.
525. Fraser, D., and Yendt, E.R.: Metabolic abnormalities in hypophosphatasia, Am. J. Dis. Child. **90**:552, 1955.
526. Fraser, D., Yendt, E.R., and Christie, F.H.E.: Metabolic abnormalities in hypophosphatasia, Lancet **1**:286, 1955.
527. Goldfischer, S., Johnson, A.B., and Morecki, R.: Hypophosphatasia: a cytochemical study of phosphate activities, Lab. Invest. **35**:55, 1976.
528. McCance, R.A., et al.: Genetic, clinical, biochemical and pathological features of hypophosphatasia, Q. J. Med. **25**:523, 1956.
529. Pimstone, B., Eisenberg, E., and Silverman, S.: Hypophosphatasia: genetic and dental studies, Ann. Intern. Med. **65**:722, 1966.
530. Rathburn, J.C.: Hypophosphatasia: a new developmental abnormality, Am. J. Dis. Child. **75**:822, 1948.
531. Weinstein, R.S., and Whyte, M.P.: Heterogeneity of adult hypophosphatasia: report of severe and mild cases, Arch. Intern. Med. **141**:727, 1981.

Immobilization osteopenia

532. Hantman, D.A., et al.: Attempts to prevent disuse osteoporosis by treatment with calcitonin, longitudinal compression, and supplementary calcium and phosphate, J. Clin. Endocrinol. Metab. **36**:845, 1973.
533. Heaney, R.P.: Radiocalcium metabolism in disuse osteoporosis in man, Am. J. Med. **33**:188, 1962.
534. Hulley, S.B., et al.: The effect of supplemental oral phosphate on the bone mineral changes during prolonged bed rest, J. Clin. Invest. **50**:2506, 1971.
535. Jaworski, Z.F.G., Leskova-Kiar, M., and Uhthoff, H.K.: Effect of long-term immobilisation on the pattern of bone loss in older dogs, J. Bone Joint Surg. **62B**:104, 1980.
536. Lerman, S., Canterbury, J.M., and Reiss, E.: Parathyroid hormone and the hypercalcemia of immobilization, J. Clin. Endocrinol. **45**:425, 1977.
537. Lindgren, J.U.: Studies on the calcium accretion rate of bone during immobilization in intact and thyroparathyroidectomized adult rats, Calcif. Tissue Res. **22**:41, 1976.
538. Lutwak, L., Whedon, G.D., and LaChance, P.A.: Mineral electrolyte and nitrogen balance studies of the Gemini-VII fourteen-dog orbital space flight, J. Clin. Endocrinol. Metab. **29**:1140, 1969.
539. Martin, R.B., and Gutman, W.: The effect of electric fields on osteoporosis of disuse, Calcif. Tissue Res. **25**:23, 1978.
540. Minaire, P., et al.: Quantitative histological data on disuse osteoporosis, Calcif. Tissue Res. **17**:57, 1974.
541. Morey, E.R., and Baylink, D.J.: Inhibition of bone formation during space flight, Science **201**:1138, 1978.
542. Nilsson, B.E.R.: Post-traumatic osteopenia: a quantitative study of the bone mineral mass in the femur following fracture of the tibia in man using americium-241 as a photon source, Acta Orthop. Scand. **37**:1, 1966.
543. Pennock, J.M., et al.: Hypoplasia of bone induced by immobilization, Br. J. Radiol. **45**:641, 1972.
544. Stinchfield, A.J., Reidy, J.A., and Barr, J.S.: Prediction of unequal growth of lower extremities in anterior poliomyelitis, J. Bone Joint Surg. **31A**:478, 1949.
545. Uhthoff, H.K., and Jaworski, Z.F.G.: Bone loss in response to long-term immobilization, J. Bone Joint Surg. **60B**:420, 1978.
546. Whedon, G.D., Lutwak, L., and Rambout, P.C.: Mineral and nitrogen balance observations: the second manned Skylab mission, Aviat. Space Environ. Med. **47**:391, 1976.

Osteitis deformans (Paget's disease)

547. Albright, F., Aub, J.C., and Bauer, W.: Hyperparathyroidism, a common and polymorphic condition, as illustrated by seventeen proven cases from one clinic, J.A.M.A. **102**:1276, 1934.
548. Allen, M.L., and John, R.L.: Osteitis deformans (Paget's disease): fissure fractures—their etiology and clinical significance, Am. J. Roentgenol. **38**:109, 1937.
549. Altman, R.D., et al.: Influence of disodium etidronate on clinical and laboratory manifestations of Paget's disease of bone (osteitis deformans), N. Engl. J. Med. **289**:1379, 1973.
550. Anderson, J.T., and Dehner, L.P.: Osteolytic form of Paget's disease: differential diagnosis and pathogenesis, J. Bone Joint Surg. **58A**:994, 1976.
551. Bijvoet, O.L.M., et al.: Treatment of Paget's disease with combined calcitonin and disphosphonate (EHDP), Metab. Bone Dis. Rel. Res. **1**:251, 1978.
552. Caffey, J.: Familial hyperphosphatasemia with ateliosis and hypermetabolism of growing membranous bone: review of the clinical, radiographic, and chemical features, Prog. Pediatr. Radiol. **4**:438, 1973.
553. Canfield, R., et al.: Diphosphonate therapy of Paget's disease of bone, J. Clin. Endocrinol. Metab. **44**:96, 1977.
554. Collins, D.H.: Paget's disease of bone: incidence and subclinical forms, Lancet **2**:51, 1956.
555. Edeiken, J., DePalma, A.F., and Hodes, P.J.: Paget's disease: osteitis deformans, Clin. Orthop. **46**:141, 1966.
556. Edholm, O.G., Howarth, S., and McMichael, J.: Heart failure and bone blood flow in osteitis deformans, Clin. Sci. **5**:249, 1945.
557. Franck, W.A., et al.: Rheumatic manifestations of Paget's disease, Am. J. Med. **56**:592, 1974.
558. Galbraith, H.J.B.: Familial Paget's disease of bone, Br. Med. J. **2**:29, 1954.
559. Harris, E.D., and Krane, S.M.: Paget's disease of bone, Bull. Rheum. Dis. **18**:506, 1968.
560. Jung, A., Bisaz, S., and Fleisch, H.: The binding of pyrophosphate and two diphosphonates by hydroxyapatite crystals, Calcif. Tissue Res. **11**:269, 1973.
561. Khairi, M.R.A., et al.: Paget's disease of bone (osteitis deformans): symptomatic lesions and bone scan, Ann. Intern. Med. **79**:348, 1973.
562. Lindsay, J.R., and Lehman, R.H.: Histopathology of the temporal bone in advanced Paget's disease, Laryngoscope **79**:213, 1969.
563. Meunier, P.J., et al.: Bone histomorphometry in Paget's disease: quantitative and dynamic analysis of Pagetic and nonpagetic bone tissue, Arthritis Rheum. **23**:1095, 1980.
564. Mills, B.G., et al.: Immunohistological demonstration of respiratory syncytial virus antigens in Paget's disease of bone, Proc. Natl. Acad. Sci. U.S.A. **78**:1209, 1981.
565. Nagant de Deuxchaisnes, C., and Krane, S.M.: Paget's disease of bone: clinical and metabolic observations, Medicine **43**:233, 1964.
566. Paget, J.: On a form of chronic inflammation of bones (osteitis deformans), Trans. Med. Chir. Soc. Lond. **60**:37, 1877.
567. Price, C.H.G.: The incidence of osteogenic sarcoma in southwest England, and its relationship to Paget's disease of bone, J. Bone Joint Surg. **44B**:366, 1962.
568. Rasmussen, H., and Bordier, P.: The physiological and cellular bases of metabolic bone disease, Baltimore, 1974, Williams & Wilkins Co.
569. Rebel, A., et al.: Osteoclast ultrastructure in Paget's disease, Calcif. Tissue Res. **20**:187, 1976.
570. Reynolds, J.J., et al.: The effect of two diphosphonates on the resorption of mouse calvaria in vitro, Calcif. Tissue Res. **10**:302, 1972.
571. Rhodes, B.A., et al.: Absence of anatomic arteriovenous shunts in Paget's disease of bone, N. Engl. J. Med. **287**:686, 1972.
572. Schenk, R., et al.: Effect of ethane-1-hydroxy-1, 1-diphosphonate (EHDP) and dichloromethylene diphosphonate ($C1_2MDP$) on the calcification and resorption of cartilage and bone in the tibial epiphysis and metaphysis of rats, Calcif. Tissue Res. **11**:196, 1973.
573. Schmorl, G.: Ueber osteitis deformans Paget, Virchows Arch (Pathol. Anat.) **283**:694, 1932.
574. Singer, F.R., and Mills, B.G.: The etiology of Paget's disease of bone, Clin. Orthop. **127**:37, 1977.

Skeletal dysplasia

Osteogenesis imperfecta

575. Eyre, D.R.: Collagen: molecular diversity in the body's protein scaffold, Science **207**:1315, 1980.
576. Falvo, K.A., Root, L., and Bullough, P.G.: Osteogenesis imperfecta: clinical evaluation and management, J. Bone Joint Surg. **56A**:783, 1974.
577. Fujii, K., and Tanzer, M.L.: Osteogenesis imperfecta: biochemical studies of bone collagen, Clin. Orthop. **124**:271, 1977.
578. Goldfarb, A.A., and Ford, D.: Osteogenesis imperfecta in connective siblings, J. Pediatr. **44**:264, 1954.
579. Jowsey, J., and Johnson, K.A.: Juvenile osteoporosis: bone findings in seven patients, J. Pediatr. **81**:511, 1972.
580. Lancaster, G., et al.; Dominantly inherited osteogenesis imperfecta in man: an examination of collagen biosynthesis, Pediatr. Res. **9**:83, 1975.
581. Pettinen, R.P., et al.: Abnormal collagen metabolism in cultured cells in osteogenesis imperfecta, Proc. Natl. Acad. Sci. U.S.A. **72**:586, 1975.
582. Rieseman, R.F., and Yates, W.M.: Osteogenesis imperfecta: its incidence and manifestations in seven families, Arch. Intern. Med. **67**:950, 1941.
583. Sillence, D.O., Senn, A., and Danks, D.M.: Genetic heterogeneity in osteogenesis imperfecta, J. Med. Genet. **16**:101, 1979.
584. Smith, R., Francis, M.J.O., and Bauze, R.J.: Osteogenesis imperfecta: a clinical and biochemical study of a generalized connective tissue disorder, Q. J. Med. **44**:555, 1975.
585. Sykes, B., Francis, M.J.O., and Smith, R.: Altered relation of two collagen types in osteogenesis imperfecta, N. Engl. J. Med. **296**:1200, 1977.
586. Teitelbaum, S.L., et al.: Bone collagen aggregation abnormalities in osteogenesis imperfecta, Calcif. Tissue Res. **17**:75, 1974.
587. Trelsted, R.L., Rubin, D., and Gross, J.: Osteogenesis imperfecta congenita: evidence for a generalized molecular disorder of collagen, Lab. Invest. **36**:501, 1977.

Osteopetrosis

588. Brown, D.M., and Dent, P.B.: Pathogenesis of osteopetrosis: a comparison of human and animal spectra, Pediatr. Res. **3**:181, 1971.
589. Dent, C.E., Smellie, J.M., and Watson, L.: Studies in osteopetrosis, Arch. Dis. Child. **40**:7, 1965.
590. Fraser, D., et al.: Congenital osteopetrosis: a failure of normal resorptive mechanisms of bone, Calcif. Tissue Res. **2**(suppl.):52, 1968.
591. Glorieux, F.H., et al.: Induction of bone resorption by parathyroid hormone in congenital malignant osteopetrosis, Metab. Bone Dis. Rel. Res. **3**:143, 1981.
592. Hoyt, C.S., and Fillson, F.A.: Visual loss in osteopetrosis, Am. J. Dis. Child. **133**:955, 1979.
593. Johnson, C.C., et al.: Osteopetrosis: a clinical, genetic, metabolic and morphologic study of the dominantly inherited, benign form, Medicine **47**:149, 1968.
594. Loria-Cortes, R., Quesada-Calvo, E., and Cordero-Chaverri, C.: Osteopetrosis in children, J. Pediatr. **91**:43, 1977.
595. Marks, S.C., Jr.: Studies of the cellular cure for osteopetrosis by transplanted cells: specificity of the cell type in *ia* rats, Am. J. Anat. **151**:131, 1978.
596. Reeves, J., et al.: The pathogenesis of infantile malignant osteopetrosis: bone mineral metabolism and complications in five infants, Metab. Bone Dis. Rel. Res. **3**:135, 1981.
597. Shapiro, F., et al.: Human osteopetrosis: a histological, ultrastructural, and biochemical study, J. Bone Joint Surg. **62A**:384, 1980.
598. Teitelbaum, S.L., et al: Malignant osteopetrosis: a disease of abnormal osteoclast proliferation, Metab. Bone Dis. Rel. Res. **3**:99, 1981.
599. Walker, D.G.: Congenital osteopetrosis in mice cured by parabiotic union with normal siblings, Endocrinology **91**:916, 1972.
600. Walker, D.G.: Experimental osteopetrosis, Clin. Orthop. **97**:158, 1973.
601. Walker, D.G.: Osteopetrosis cured by temporary parabiosis, Science **180**:875, 1973.
602. Walker, D.G.: Bone resorption restored in osteopetrotic mice by transplants of normal bone marrow and spleen cells. Science **190**:784, 1975.
603. Walker, D.G.: Spleen cells transmit osteopetrosis in mice, Science **190**:785, 1975.
604. Whyte, M.P., et al.: Osteopetrosis, renal tubular acidosis, and basal ganglia calcification in three sisters, Am. J. Med. **69**:64, 1980.

Achondroplasia

605. Cooper, R.R., Ponseti, I.V., and Maynard, J.A.: Pseudoachondroplastic dwarfism: a rough-surfaced endoplasmic reticulum storage disorder, J. Bone Joint Surg. **55A**:475, 1973.
606. Maynard, J.A., et al.: Histochemistry and ultrastructure of the growth plate in achondroplasia, J. Bone Joint Surg. **63A**:969, 1981.
607. McKusick, V.A., Kelley, T.E., and Dorst, J.P.: Observations suggesting allelism of the achondroplasia and hypochondroplasia genes, J. Med. Genet. **10**:11, 1973.
608. Nelson, M.A.: Spinal stenosis in achondroplasia, Proc. Soc. Med. **65**:1028, 1972.
609. Pedrini-Mille, A., and Pedrini, V.: Studies of human iliac crest cartilage. III. Protein polysaccharides in human achondroplasia, Calcif. Tissue Res. **8**:106, 1971.
610. Ponseti, I.V.: Skeletal growth in achondroplasia, J. Bone Joint Surg. **52A**:701, 1970.
611. Rimoin, D.L., et al.: Endochondral ossification in achondroplastic dwarfism, N. Engl. J. Med. **283**:728, 1970.
612. Rimoin, D.L., et al.: Histologic appearances of some types of congenital dwarfism, Prog. Pediatr. Radiol. **4**:68, 1973.
613. Scott, C.I.: Achondroplastic and hypochondroplastic dwarfism, Clin. Orthop. **114**:18, 1976.
614. Stanescu, V., Bona, C., and Ionescu, V.: The tibial growing cartilage biopsy in the study of growth disturbances, Acta Endocrinol. **64**:577, 1970.

Mucopolysaccharidoses

615. Anderson, C.E., et al.: Morquio's disease and dysplasia epiphysalis multiplex: a study of epiphyseal cartilage in seven cases, J. Bone Joint Surg. **44A**:295, 1962.
616. Bach, G., et al.: The defect in Hurler and Scheie syndromes: deficiency of -L-iduronidase, Proc. Natl. Acad. Sci. U.S.A. **69**:2048, 1972.
617. Bona, C., et al.: Histochemical and histoenzymological study of tibial growing cartilage in Hurler's syndrome, Acta Histochem. **23**:231, 1966.
618. Bona, C., et al.: Differential regional distribution of mucopolysaccharides in the human epiphyseal cartilage matrix in normal and pathological conditions, Virchows Arch. (Pathol. Anat.) **342**:274, 1967.
619. Caffey, J.: Gargoylism (Hunter-Hurler disease, dysostoses multiplex, lipochondrodystrophy): prenatal and neonatal bone lesions and their early postnatal evolution, Am. J. Roentgenol. **67**:715, 1952.
620. Dawson, I.M.P.: The histology and histochemistry of gargoylism, J. Pathol. **67**:587, 1954.
621. Dorfman, A., and Lorincz, A.E.: Occurrence of urinary acid mucopolysaccharides in the Hurler syndrome, Proc. Natl. Acad. Sci. U.S.A. **43**:443, 1957.
622. Einhorn, N.H., Moore, J.R., and Rowntree, L.G.: Osteochondrodystrophia deformans (Morquio's disease): observations at autopsy in one case, Am. J. Dis. Child. **72**:536, 1946.
623. Fratantoni, J.C., Hall, C.W., and Heufeld, E.F.: Hurler and Hunter syndromes: mutual correction of the defect in cultured fibroblasts, Science **162**:570, 1968.
624. Kaplan, D.: Classification of the mucopolysaccharidoses based on the pattern of mucopolysacchariduria, Am. J. Med. **47**:721, 1969.
625. Kresse, H., and Neufeld, E.F.: The Sanfilippo A corrective factor, purification and mode of action, J. Biol. Chem. **247**:2164, 1972.
626. Lindsay, S., et al.: Gargoylism: study of pathologic lesions and clinical review of twelve cases, Am. J. Dis. Child. **76**:239, 1948.

627. Maroteaux, P., et al.: Une nouvelle dysostose avec elimination urinaire de chondroitine-sulfate B, Press. Med. **71**:1849, 1963.
628. Matalon, R., and Dorfman, A.: Sanfilippo A syndrome: sulfamidase deficiency in cultured skin fibroblasts and liver, J. Clin. Invest. **54**:907, 1974.
629. McKusick, V.A.: Heritable disorders of connective tissues, ed. 4, St. Louis, 1972, The C.V. Mosby Co.
630. Pedrini, V., Lenuzzi, L., and Zambotti, V.: Isolation and identification of keratosulfate in urine of patients affected by Morquio-Ullrich disease, Proc. Soc. Exp. Biol. Med. **110**:847, 1962.
631. Sanfilippo, S.J., Yunis, J., and Worthen, H.G.: An unusual storage disease resembling the Hurler-Hunter syndrome (abstract), Am. J. Dis. Child. **104**:553, 1962.
632. Schenk, E.A., and Haggerty, J.: Morquio's disease: a radiologic and morphologic study, Pediatrics **34**:839, 1964.
633. Sengal, A., Stoebner, P., and Juif, J.: Les chondrocytes de la maladie de Morquio: vacuoles ergastroplasmiques a inclusions specifiques, J. Microsc. **10**:33, 1971.
634. Silberberg, R., et al.: Ultrastructure of cartilage in the Hurler and Sanfilippo syndromes, Arch. Pathol. **94**:500, 1972.
635. Zellwager, H., et al.: Morquio-Ullrich's disease: report of two cases, J. Pediatr. **59**:549, 1961.

Osteonecrosis

636. Boettcher, W.G., et al.: Non-traumatic necrosis of the femoral head. I. Relation of altered hemostasis to etiology, J. Bone Joint Surg. **52A**:312, 1970.
637. Cruess, R.L., Ross, D., and Crawshaw, E.: The etiology of steroid-induced avascular necrosis of bone, Clin. Orthop. **113**:178, 1975.
638. Ferguson, A.B.: The pathology of Legg-Perthes disease and its comparison with aseptic necrosis, Clin. Orthop. **106**:7, 1975.
639. Fisher, D.E., and Bickel, W.H.: Corticosteroid-induced avascular necrosis: a clinical study of seventy-seven patients, J. Bone Joint Surg. **53A**:859, 1971.
640. Garden, R.S.: Malreduction and avascular necrosis in sub-capital fractures of the femur, J. Bone Joint Surg. **53B**:183, 1971.
641. Glimcher, M.J., and Kenzora, J.E.: The biology of osteonecrosis of the human femoral head and its clinical implications. I. Tissue biology, Clin. Orthop. **138**:284, 1979.
642. Glimcher, M.J., and Kenzora, J.E.: The biology of osteonecrosis of the human femoral head and its clinical implications. II. The pathological changes in the femoral head as an organ and in the hip joint, Clin. Orthop. **139**:283, 1979.
643. Glimcher, M.J., and Kenzora, J.E.: The biology of osteonecrosis of the human femoral head and its clinical implications. III. Discussion of the etiology and genesis of the pathological sequelae: comments on treatment, Clin. Orthop. **140**:273, 1979.
644. Herndon, J.H., and Aufranc, O.E.: Avascular necrosis of the femoral head in the adult: a review of its incidence in a variety of conditions, Clin. Orthop. **86**:43, 1972.
645. Inoue, A., and Ono, K.: A histological study of idiopathic avascular necrosis of the head of the femur, J. Bone Joint Surg. **61B**:138, 1979.
646. Inoue, A., et al.: The pathogenesis of Perthes' disease, J. Bone Joint Surg. **58B**:453, 1976.
647. Jacobs, B.: Epidemiology of traumatic and nontraumatic osteonecrosis, Clin. Orthop. **130**:51, 1978.
648. Jaffe, W.L., et al.: The effect of cortisone on femoral and humeral heads in rabbits: an experimental study, Clin. Orthop. **82**:221, 1972.
649. Jones, J.P., and Engleman, E.P.: Avascular necrosis of bone in alcoholism, Arthritis Rheum. **10**:287, 1967.
650. Katz, J.F., and Siffert, R.S.: Capital necrosis, metaphyseal cyst, and subluxation in coxa plana, Clin. Orthop. **106**:75, 1975.
651. Laurent, J., et al.: Recherches sur la pathogenie des necroses aseptiques de la tete femorale, Nouv. Presse Med. **2**:1755, 1973.
652. McKibben, B., and Ralis, Z.: Pathological changes in a case of Perthes disease, J. Bone Joint Surg. **56B**:438, 1974.
653. Mielants, H., et al.: Avascular necrosis and its relation to lipid and purine metabolism, J. Rheumatol. **2**:430, 1975.
654. Norman, A., and Bullough, P.: The radiolucent crescent line—an early diagnostic sign of avascular necrosis of the femoral head, Bull. Hosp. Joint Dis. **24**:99, 1963.
655. Pierides, A.M., et al.: Avascular necrosis of bone following renal transplantation, Q. J. Med. **44**:459, 1975.
656. Ponseti, I.V., and Cotton, R.L.: Legg-Calvé-Perthes disease: pathogenesis and evolution, J. Bone Joint Surg. **43A**:261, 1961.
657. Snyder, C.R.: Legg-Perthes disease in the young hip: does it necessarily do well? J. Bone Joint Surg. **57A**:751, 1975.
658. Solomon, L.: Drug-induced arthropathy and necrosis of the femoral head, J. Bone Joint Surg. **55B**:246, 1973.
659. Wang, G.J., et al.: Fat-cell changes as a mechanism of avascular necrosis of the femoral head in cortisone-treated rabbits, J. Bone Joint Surg. **59**:729, 1977.

Osteomyelitis

Pyogenic osteomyelitis

660. Curtiss, P.H.: Some uncommon forms of osteomyelitis, J. Bone Joint Surg. **41B**:671, 1959.
661. Harris, N.H., and Kirkaldy-Willis, W.H.: Primary subacute pyogenic osteomyelitis, J. Bone Joint Surg. **47B**:526, 1965.
662. Kahn, D.S., and Pritzker, K.P.H.: The pathophysiology of bone infection, Clin. Orthop. **96**:12, 1973.
663. Kandel, S.N., and Mankin, H.J.: Pyogenic abscess of the long bones in children, Clin. Orthop. **96**:108, 1973.
664. Kelly, P.J.: Osteomyelitis in the adult, Orthop. Clin. North Am. **6**:983, 1975.
665. Kelly, P.J., Wilkowske, C.H., and Washington, J.A.: Comparison of Gram-negative bacillary and staphylococcal osteomyelitis of the femur and tibia, Clin. Orthop. **96**:70, 1973.
666. Kemp, H.B.S., et al.: Pyogenic infections occurring primarily in intervertebral discs, J. Bone Joint Surg. **55B**:698, 1973.
667. Kido, D., Bryan, D., and Halpern, M.: Hematogenous osteomyelitis in drug addicts, Am. J. Roentgenol. Radium Ther. Nucl. Med. **118**:356, 1973.
668. Meyers, B.R., Berson, B.L., and Gilbert, M.: Clinical patterns of osteomyelitis due to Gram-negative bacteria, Arch. Intern. Med. **131**:228, 1973.
669. Morrey, B.F., and Peterson, H.A.: Hematogenous pyogenic osteomyelitis in children, Orthop. Clin. North Am. **6**:935, 1975.
670. Trueta, J.: The three types of acute haematogenous osteomyelitis, J. Bone Joint Surg. **41B**:671, 1959.
671. Waldvogel, F.A., and Vasey, H.: Osteomyelitis: the past decade, N. Engl. J. Med. **303**:360, 1980.
672. Waldvogel, F.A., et al.: Osteomyelitis: a review of clinical features, therapeutic considerations, and unusual aspects, N. Engl. J. Med. **282**:198, 1970.
673. West, W.F., Kelly, P.J., and Martin, W.J.: Chronic osteomyelitis. I. Factors affecting the results of treatment in 186 patients, J.A.M.A. **213**:1837, 1970.
674. Winters, J.L., and Cahen, I.: Acute hematogenous osteomyelitis: a review of sixty-six cases, J. Bone Joint Surg. **42A**:691, 1960.

Skeletal tuberculosis

675. Davidson, P.T., and Horowitz, I.: Skeletal tuberculosis: a review with patient presentations and discussion, Am. J. Med. **48**:77, 1970.
676. Kelly, P.J., and Karlson, A.G.: Musculoskeletal tuberculosis, Mayo Clin. Proc. **44**:73, 1969.
677. O'Connor, B.T., Oswestry, W.M.S., and Sanders, R.: Disseminated bone tuberculosis, J. Bone Joint Surg. **52A**:1027, 1965.

CHAPTER 41 **Tumors and Tumorlike Conditions of Bone**

JUAN ROSAI

ETIOLOGY AND PREDISPOSING FACTORS

Bone tumors are the oldest form of neoplasia documented in paleopathology; they existed on earth long before human life appeared. In humans, bone neoplasms occur in all races and in all countries. The annual incidence of malignant bone tumors is approximately one case per 100,000 inhabitants.

There are various circumstances, including some benign diseases, that are seen associated with the appearance of bone neoplasms in a significant fashion. However, they account for only a minority of the cases even when considered as a group.

The possibility of trauma predisposing to the development of malignant tumors of bone has been suggested many times but never proved. Major trauma to the bone, such as that resulting from fracture, surgery (particularly amputation), and exodontia, has no statistical relation to bone sarcoma.[109] It is therefore difficult to believe that the relatively insignificant trauma that patients with bone tumors often cite could possibly have been the cause of the neoplasm.

It has been known for many years that various modalities of ionizing radiation can result in the appearance of bone sarcomas. One of the first demonstrations of this occurrence was the production by Lacassagne[89] of a tumor interpreted as fibrosarcoma of the tibia in a rabbit 36 months after irradiation of an abscess near the bone. Osteosarcomas in laboratory animals can be induced with intraperitoneal injections of ^{45}Ca or ^{89}Sr, local inoculation of ^{144}Ce,[42] or intravenous injection of ^{55}Fe.[91] Interestingly, radioactive calcium produces sarcomas chiefly in the spine and pelvis, whereas strontium induces them in the bones of the limb.[11,72]

The most dramatic series of radiation-induced bone sarcomas in humans was the one reported by Martland and Humphries (Fig. 41-1).[103] The victims were young women employed in the painting of clock dials with luminous paint made of zinc sulfide and 1 part in 40,000 of radium, mesothorium (an isotope of radium), and radiothorium. It was the custom of the workers to moisten the bristles of the brush between their lips, and this led to the ingestion of a certain amount of radioactive material. Of the 18 patients who died of radium poisoning, five had osteosarcomas.

A large number of osteosarcomas have been seen after the use of thorium in the treatment of tuberculosis and ankylosing spondylitis.[153] A few cases of osteosarcoma have been reported in patients who had undergone angiographic studies with Thorotrast during childhood.[151] Cases of bone sarcomas developing in apparent connection with the local administration of radiation for therapeutic purposes have been reported from several medical centers.[32,68] All bones are susceptible to this complication. The usual interval between the time of irradiation and the clinical appearance of the tumor is between 9 and 15 years. Approximately two thirds of the sarcomas have arisen in preexisting bone lesions, particularly giant cell tumor. The most common types of radiation-induced sarcoma of bone are osteosarcoma, malignant fibrous histiocytoma, and fibrosarcoma.[173]

The danger of this complication, although it is of extremely grave consequence, should be viewed in the proper perspective. In most reported cases, the dose of radiation has been 3000 rad or higher, and the patient has received repeated courses. The practical hazard of radiation-induced sarcoma appears to be very remote and should not be a contraindication to the treatment of carinomas; however, radiotherapy for benign bone tumors should probably be reserved for lesions not amenable to surgical therapy.

It has been well documented that Paget's disease predisposes to the development of bone tumors, especially in men. In extensive and advanced cases the rate of malignant transformation is about 10%[45] but the overall incidence is probably less than 1%. This malignant transformation has been attributed to the higher rate of bone turnover seen in Paget's disease, as indicated by the

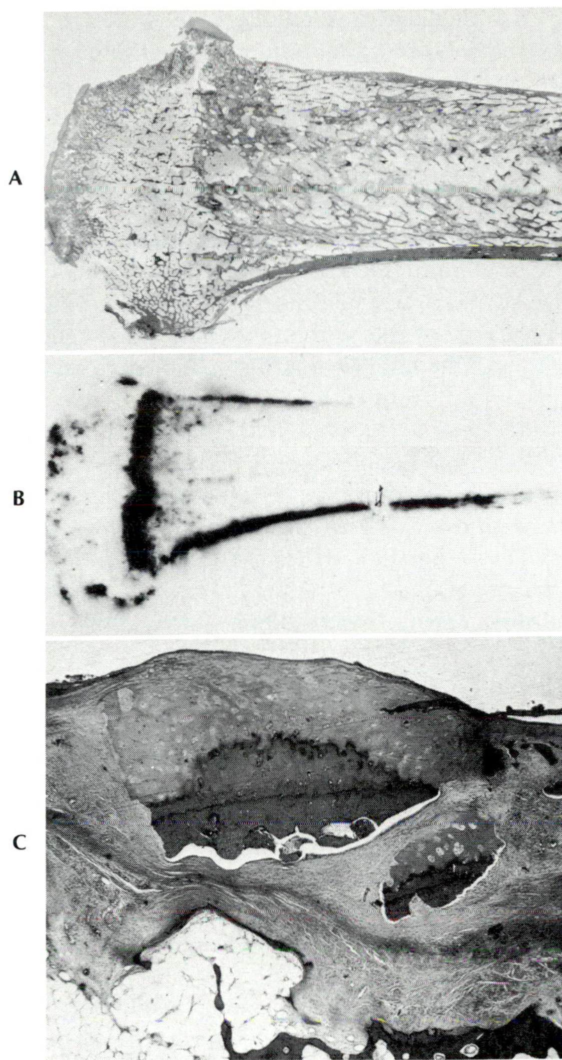

Fig. 41-1. Bone and cartilage changes caused by irradiation. Patient, 46-year-old woman, had worked as watch- and clock-dial painter for 3½ months when 16 years of age. Lower extremity was amputated because of sarcomatous change originating in diseased femur. Tumor was classified as fibrosarcoma. **A,** Large section of lower segment of femur showing necrosis. **B,** Autoradiogram made from section similar to specimen shown in **A.** Note evidence of intense radioactivity in region of metaphyseal end of diaphysis, which marks growth zone at time patient was exposed to radioactive material. **C,** As result of radiation injury, articular cartilage and subchondral bone have undergone necrosis and fragmentation.

marked resorptive and osteoblastic activity. Osteosarcomas predominate, but chondrosarcomas, fibrosarcomas, and giant cell tumors have also been reported.[74,175] The sarcoma developing in Paget's disease usually occurs in areas in which the process is most advanced. The bones involved by sarcoma in patients with Paget's disease, in order of frequency, are the pelvis, femur, humerus, tibia, skull and facial bones, and scapula. The prognosis for sarcoma arising in Paget's disease is extremely poor; almost 30% of the patients have metastatic disease at the time of diagnosis, and only 8% of the whole group survive for 5 years.[175]

Fibrous dysplasia may also be complicated with bone sarcoma, although the incidence is very low. Most of the cases of fibrous dysplasia in which this complication has supervened have been of the polyostotic type.[148] The tumor is usually an osteosarcoma, although fibrosarcoma and chondrosarcoma can also occur.[76]

Recently an increasing number of malignant bone tumors have been reported at the site of bone infarcts, such as those seen in caisson workers. The types were osteosarcoma, malignant fibrous histiocytoma, and fibrosarcoma.[59,108]

The malignant tumors associated with long-standing osteomyelitis usually take the form of squamous cell carcinoma arising from the draining sinuses. Rarely, fibrosarcoma or angiosarcoma may develop within the inflamed bone as well as in the surrounding soft tissue.

At least three cases of osteogenesis imperfecta associated with osteosarcoma have been reported.[45] In this condition, however, it is much more common to see an exuberant callus at a site of fracture that is confused roentgenographically and even microscopically with an osteosarcoma.

Two polyostotic bone disorders, of either a neoplastic or developmental nature, are associated with an increased occurrence of chondrosarcoma; these are enchondromatosis and osteochondromatosis and are discussed in the section of chondroblastic (cartilage-forming) tumors.

Claims of malignant transformation have been made in isolated cases of benign bone tumors, such as chondroblastoma, chondromyxoid fibroma, nonossifying fibroma, giant cell tumor, and osteoblastoma. Although some of these reports are probably authentic (especially for the last two tumors), it seems likely that many of these cases were initially misdiagnosed as benign or that they represent radiation-induced sarcomas.[167]

Fraumeni[57] made the intriguing observation that American youngsters under 18 years of age with osteosarcomas were significantly taller than those in a control group with nonosseous malignant tumors.

Osteosarcomas have been produced by viral inoculations into chickens, mice, and rats[55,117] and by the administration of chemical carcinogens, particularly beryllium salts, into rabbits.[162] There are several clinical and laboratory observations suggesting the possibility of a viral etiology for human osteosarcoma.[122] The concurrent development of tumors in members of the same family implicates either genetic or infectious factors. This has been documented for osteosarcoma, chondrosarcoma, and Ewing's sarcoma.[67,141] Unusual clustering of bone sarcomas has been seen in small communities.[58,166] Statistical differences in the incidence of osteosarcoma in genetically homogeneous populations depending on geographic location (and presumably caused by environmental factors) have been documented in Malaysia and Kenya. The possibility that human osteosarcomas may be produced by viruses is being seriously considered after the demonstration by immunologic techniques of a high incidence of antibodies to a common antigen of osteosarcoma in the sera of patients with this disease and in members of their immediate families.[111,152] This observation obviously suggests the association of an infectious agent with this neoplasm, which appears capable of infecting relatives and close associates of the patients.

Another experiment suggesting a viral etiology for human osteosarcoma was performed by Finkel and collaborators.[54] They were able to produce osteosarcomas, fibrosarcomas, and benign bone tumors in neonatal hamsters by injecting them with cell-free extracts of human osteosarcomas. These authors also demonstrated with immunofluorescence techniques a reactivity between the serum of human patients with osteosarcoma and sarcoma tissue from hamsters that had been induced with extracts of human osteosarcoma, suggesting the transmission of a virus in the inoculated extract.

Electron microscopic studies have also lent support to the viral hypothesis. Thin sections of human bone tumors and of pelleted extracts of these tumors have shown particles that could possibly be associated with viral deoxyribonucleic acid (DNA),[64] and viral particles of ribonucleic acid (RNA) nature (probably corresponding to an oncornavirus) have been detected in murine osteosarcoma.[114]

These studies strongly suggest a relation between a viral infectious agent and human osteosarcoma. However, the fundamental question as to whether this agent is directly related to the tumor etiology or is an incidental passenger remains unanswered.

CLASSIFICATION AND DISTRIBUTION

The presence of a large variety of tissues within the skeletal system, the rarity of bone neoplasms, and the uncertainty that still exists regarding their histogenesis have all contributed to the confusion in terminology and classification that for many years has plagued this field of tumor pathology. Fortunately, a satisfactory degree of uniformity in the nomenclature has now been reached. The main contributions for these achievements have been the pioneering work of H.L. Jaffe,[79] the fascicle "Tumors of Bone and Cartilage" of the *Atlas of Tumor Pathology* series (now in its second series),[155] and the manual by Schajowicz, Ackerman, and Sissons, published under the auspices of the World Health Organization as part of their *International Histological Classification of Tumours* series.[140]

The classification presented in this chapter is based largely on the last work and is of histogenetic character. Tumors are classified according to the tissue or cell type from which they are presumed to arise, which in turn is deduced mainly from the tissue that the tumor cells are able to manufacture. Thus a bone tumor composed of cells that produce osteoid or bone is presumed to originate from osteoblasts, a tumor composed of cells that produce cartilage (and only cartilage) is presumed to originate from chondroblasts, and so on. In other instances, the histogenetic presumption of origin is derived not from the identification of a manufactured product of the tumor cell but rather from the morphologic similarity of this cell to a given normal cell when studied by light microscopy, histochemistry, and electron microscopy. For instance, a malignant bone tumor composed of small round cells that morphologically resemble normal lymphocytes is presumed to arise from these cells and is therefore designated malignant lymphoma. Some terms that have very little histogenetic meaning have remained either to honor the scientist who first recognized them (for example, Ewing's sarcoma) or for no other reason than tradition (for example, myeloma).

It should be understood that the histogenetic classification of tumors in general, and of bone tumors in particular, is no more than a useful conceptual framework that might be even misleading if taken too literally. To mention just one example, it is entirely possible—and indeed likely—that osteosarcoma does not arise from preexisting well-differentiated osteoblasts but rather from primitive and multipotential mesenchymal cells that differentiate toward osteoblasts in the course of neoplastic transformation.

The reader who first scans a classification of bone neoplasms such as the one presented here is likely to wonder what its real practical significance is. This is understandable because there have been in the past (and are even now) classifications of tumors that describe minimal morphologic variations of a basic tumor pattern that have no clinical, surgical, or prognostic significance whatsoever. The reader may be assured that this is not the case with the classification of bone tumors presented here. Each of the entities listed has a personality of its own; its preference for a given bone, site within the bone, age of the patient, roentgenographic appearance, and behavior are distinctive and allow the clinician to suggest a specific diagnosis, plan therapy, and predict the evolution with a high degree of accuracy.

The basic information regarding these parameters is included in Table 41-1. The data concerning age, sex, bone, and bone site most commonly involved are generally not repeated in the text. For a proper understanding of this table, a brief recapitulation of some terms of normal bone anatomy might be helpful. *Medulla* (medullary cavity or marrow cavity) refers to the inner or central portion of the bone, composed of a network of cancellous (spongy, reticular) bone trabeculae that enclose bone

Table 41-1. Characteristics of most common primary bone tumors and tumorlike lesions*

Tumor or tumorlike lesion	Age (yr)	Sex M:F	Bones most commonly affected (in order of frequency)	Usual location within long bone	Behavior
Osteoma	40-50	2:1	Skull and facial bones	—	Benign
Osteoid osteoma	10-30	2:1	Femur, tibia, humerus, hands and feet, vertebrae, fibula	Cortex of metaphysis	Benign
Osteoblastoma	10-30	2:1	Vertebrae, tibia, femur, humerus, pelvis, ribs	Medulla of metaphysis	Benign
Osteosarcoma	10-25	3:2	Femur, tibia, humerus, pelvis, jaw, fibula	Medulla of metaphysis	Malignant; 20% to 40% 5-year survival rate
Juxtacortical (parosteal) osteosarcoma	30-60	1:1	Femur, tibia, humerus	Juxtacortical area of metaphysis	Malignant; 80% 5-year survival rate
Chondroma	10-40	1:1	Hands and feet, ribs, femur, humerus	Medulla of diaphysis	Benign
Osteochondroma	10-30	1:1	Femur, tibia, humerus, pelvis	Cortex of metaphysis	Benign
Chondroblastoma	10-25	2:1	Femur, humerus, tibia, feet, pelvis, scapula	Epiphysis, adjacent to cartilage plate	Practically always benign
Chondromyxoid fibroma	10-25	1:1	Tibia, femur, feet, pelvis	Metaphysis	Benign
Chondrosarcoma	30-60	3:1	Pelvis, ribs, femur, humerus, vertebrae	Central—medulla of diaphysis or metaphysis Peripheral—cortex or periosteum of metaphysis	Malignant; 5-year survival rate—low grade, 78%; moderate grade, 53%; high grade, 22%
Mesenchymal chondrosarcoma	20-60	1:1	Ribs, skull and jaw, vertebrae, pelvis, soft tissues	Medulla or cortex of diaphysis	Malignant; extremely poor prognosis
Giant cell tumor	20-40	4:5	Femur, tibia, radius	Epiphysis and metaphysis	Potentially malignant; 50% recur; 10% metastasize
Ewing's sarcoma	5-20	1:2	Femur, pelvis, tibia, humerus, ribs, fibula	Medulla of diaphysis or metaphysis	Highly malignant; 20%-30% 5-year survival rate in recent series
Malignant lymphoma, histiocytic (reticulum cell sarcoma) and mixed cell types	30-60	1:1	Femur, pelvis, vertebrae, tibia, humerus, jaw, skull, ribs	Medulla of diaphysis or metaphysis	Malignant; 22%-50% 5-year survival rate
Plasma cell myeloma	40-60	2:1	Vertebrae, pelvis, ribs, sternum, skull	Medulla of diaphysis, metaphysis, or epiphysis	Malignant; diffuse form always fatal; localized form often controlled with radiotherapy
Hemangioma	20-50	1:1	Skull, vertebrae, jaw	Medulla	Benign
Desmoplastic fibroma	20-30	1:1	Humerus, tibia, pelvis, jaw, femur, scapula	Metaphysis	Benign
Fibrosarcoma	20-60	1:1	Femur, tibia, jaw, humerus	Medulla of metaphysis	Malignant; 28% 5-year survival rate
Chordoma	40-60	2:1	Sacrococcygeal, spheno-occipital, cervical vertebrae	—	Malignant; slow course; locally invasive; 48% distant metastases
Solitary bone cyst	10-20	3:1	Humerus, femur	Medulla of metaphysis	Benign
Aneurysmal bone cyst	10-20	1:1	Vertebrae, flat bones, femur, tibia	Metaphysis	Benign; sometimes follows another bone lesion
Metaphyseal fibrous defect	10-20	1:1	Tibia, femur, fibula	Metaphysis	Benign
Fibrous dysplasia	10-30	3:2	Ribs, femur, tibia, jaw, skull	Medulla of diaphysis or metaphysis	Locally aggressive; rarely complicated by sarcoma
Eosinophilic granuloma	5-15	3:2	Skull, jaw, humerus, rib, femur	Metaphysis or diaphysis	Benign

Slightly modified from Rosai, J.: Ackerman's Surgical Pathology, ed. 6, St. Louis, 1981, The C.V. Mosby Co.

*It should be emphasized that these data correspond to the typical case and that they should not be taken in an absolute sense. Isolated exceptions to practically every one of these statements have occurred.

marrow hemopoietic elements, adipose tissue, blood and lymph vessels, and nerves. The *cortex*, composed of compact (dense) bone and essentially devoid of bone marrow and other soft tissue components, surrounds the medulla in a circumferential fashion. The *periosteum*, which covers the outer surface of the bone, consists of a thick external layer of fibrous connective tissue and a thin osteoblastic layer. Bone tumors in the region of the periosteum, and possibly arising from it, are often designated as periosteal, parosteal, or juxtacortical.

A typical adult long bone is composed of a *diaphysis*, which is the central cylindrical shaft; the *epiphyses*, which are two roughly spherical terminal regions covered by the articular cartilage; and the *metaphyses*, two intermediate conelike regions connecting the shaft and the articular ends (Fig. 41-2). The metaphysis is particularly important in bone pathology because in the growing person it is adjacent to a cartilaginous *epiphyseal plate*. The latter represents the area of most active bone growth and, perhaps as a result, is the most common site of occurrence of many bone neoplasms.

Definitions of normal bone histologic features that are important to remember in the context of the subject of this chapter include the following. *Osteoid* (preosseous tissue) is the extracellular material produced by the osteoblasts and composed of collagen fibers (largely of type I) and an amorphous protein-poysaccharide matrix.

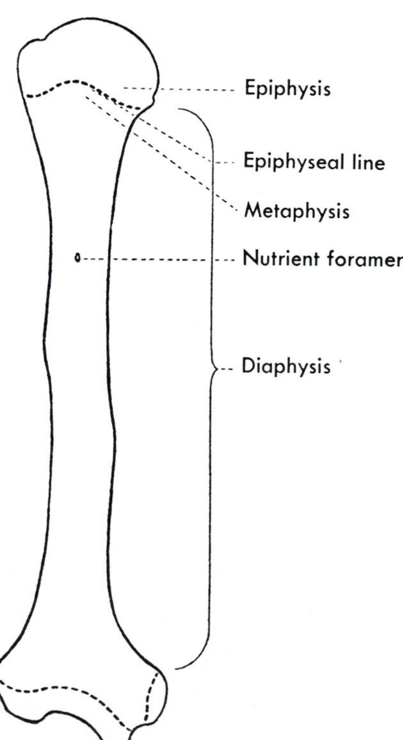

Fig. 41-2. Sketch of long bone (humerus) identifying different anatomic landmarks important for determining location of bone neoplasms.

Bone refers to the same tissue after calcium salts have been deposited on it. *Woven (membrane) bone* is the type of bone produced normally in the course of intramembranous ossification and abnormally in a fracture callus, fibrous dysplasia, and a variety of bone neoplasms; it is characterized by the haphazard placement of collagen fibers throughout the osteoid matrix. One can observe this particularly well with polarizing lenses. *Lamellar bone*, on the other hand, is laid down in concentric layers containing collagen in ordered parallel arrays.

The classification* that follows also includes a group of nonneoplastic conditions, mostly of obscure pathogenesis, that can closely resemble a bone neoplasm on roentgenographic and morphologic grounds.

A. Osteoblastic (bone-forming) tumors
   1. Benign
      a. Osteoma
      b. Osteoid osteoma and osteoblastoma
   2. Malignant
      a. Osteosarcoma
      b. Juxtacortical (parosteal) osteosarcoma
B. Chondroblastic (cartilage-forming) tumors
   1. Benign
      a. Chondroma
      b. Osteochondroma
      c. Chondroblastoma
      d. Chondromyxoid fibroma
   2. Malignant
      a. Chondrosarcoma
      b. Mesenchymal chondrosarcoma
C. Giant cell tumor (osteoclastoma)
D. Marrow tumors
   1. Ewing's sarcoma
   2. Malignant lymphoma
   3. Plasma cell myeloma
E. Vascular tumors
   1. Benign
      a. Hemangioma
      b. Lymphangioma
      c. Glomus tumor
      d. Hemangiopericytoma
   2. Borderline
      a. Hemangioendothelioma (histiocytoid or epithelioid)
   3. Malignant
      a. Angiosarcoma
      b. Hemangiopericytoma
F. Fibrous tissue tumors
   1. Benign
      a. Desmoplastic fibroma

*Modified from Schajowicz, F., Ackerman, L.V. and Sissons, H.A.: Histological typing of bone tumours, International Histological Classification of Tumours, No. 6, Geneva, 1972, World Health Organization.

2. Malignant
    a. Fibrosarcoma
G. Other primary tumors
    1. Chordoma
    2. "Adamantinoma" of long bones
    3. Tumors of peripheral nerves
    4. Tumors of adipose tissue
    5. Tumors of alleged histiocytic origin
    6. Tumors of smooth muscle
H. Metastatic tumors
I. Unclassified tumors
J. Tumorlike lesions
    1. Solitary bone cyst
    2. Aneurysmal bone cyst
    3. Ganglion cyst of bone
    4. Metaphyseal fibrous defect (nonossifying fibroma)
    5. Fibrous dysplasia
    6. Myositis ossificans
    7. Histiocytosis X (eosinophilic granuloma, Hand-Schüller-Christian disease, and Letterer-Siwe disease)

DIAGNOSIS, TREATMENT, AND PROGNOSIS

The diagnosis of bone tumors and tumorlike conditions should always be based on a combined clinical, roentgenographic, and pathologic evaluation. In some specific instances, biochemical and hematologic information is also of crucial importance. Laboratory data that are particularly important in this regard include serum levels of calcium, phosphorus, alkaline phosphatase, and acid phosphatase. The tumors and tumorlike conditions in which the knowledge of these data is essential are hyperparathyroidism, Paget's disease, plasma cell myeloma, and metastatic carcinoma. Bone marrow cytology and serum and urinary immunoglobulin determinations are important for the diagnosis of plasma cell myeloma; a thorough hematologic investigation is essential in the evaluation of malignant lymphoma and leukemia of bone; and urinary catecholamine determination is a useful adjunct for the diagnosis of metastatic neuroblastoma.

The most important clinical parameter is the patient's age. Most bone neoplasms show a definite preference for a given age range and are distinctly unusual in another. For instance, a diagnosis of giant cell tumor in a child or of Ewing's sarcoma in an octogenarian should be viewed with great skepticism. Along the same line, a malignant bone tumor composed of uniform small round cells in an infant is likely to be a metastatic neuroblastoma, in a child a Ewing's sarcoma, and in an adult a malignant lymphoma or a metastatic lung carcinoma. The sex of the patient, on the other hand, is of little importance in the differential diagnosis of bone tumors, except for some types of metastases.

Symptoms are of importance for the initial detection of the lesion, but are of little consequence in the differential diagnosis; on occasion, they may even be misleading. For instance, a bone tumefaction associated with local pain and redness, fever, and leukocytosis may lead the physician to a diagnosis of osteomyelitis, yet Ewing's sarcoma can result in an identical picture. In general, the larger and more destructive the tumor is, the more likely that it will be malignant. However, one of the largest and most spectacular masses that one can encounter is an aneurysmal bone cyst, which is perhaps not even neoplastic in nature.

The other important information regarding the clinical evaluation pertains to the presence of any of the conditions known to predispose to the appearance of bone tumors, such as Paget's disease, irradiation, bone infarcts, enchondromatosis (Ollier's disease), osteochondromatosis, and fibrous dysplasia.

Radiologic investigation is always of extreme importance. Routine roentgenograms in different views usually provide most of the necessary data for a proper evaluation, but in some cases tomograms, xeroradiograms, arteriograms, and the newly developed computed tomography (CT) scans may provide important additional information.[60] Roentgenographic techniques are also useful for guiding the performance of a percutaneous needle biopsy.

The roentgenographic data important for the diagnosis of a bone tumor are the bone involved, precise localization of the lesion (whether medullary, cortical, or juxtacortical and whether diaphyseal, metaphyseal, or epiphyseal if located in a long bone), indication as to whether the lesion has originated in bone or has extended to it from soft tissues, size and shape, margins (whether sharply or ill defined), nature of any changes in the surrounding bone, presence and type of so-called tumor matrix (calcified osteoid or cartilage), and presence and type of periosteal reaction.

On some occasions a tumor that is extensively involving a given bone can hardly be detected by roentgenographic examination. The explanation is that the tumor diffusely permeates the bone marrow spaces without destroying the bone trabeculae (so-called permeative and moth-eaten patterns).

Although a high degree of diagnostic accuracy can be reached on the basis of the roentgenographic examination of the lesion, the final diagnosis on which all prognostic and therapeutic considerations will be made should always be based on a careful pathologic study. I must also emphasize that the relevant clinical and roentgenographic information should always be available to the pathologist before a final diagnosis is made. This is important because lesions that have a totally different clinical and roentgenographic presentation and are therefore easily distinguished on this basis can have a very similar appearance under the microscope.

Histologic study of a bone tumor usually involves examination of a biopsy specimen, a procedure that should never be omitted when radical surgery, radiotherapy, or chemotherapy is contemplated. The specimen is obtained by either open surgical biopsy (incisional or excisional biopsy) or needle biopsy (aspiration or trochar biopsy).[43,142] Performance of an open surgical biopsy entails a small risk of tumor implantation in the soft tissue, especially in the case of cartilaginous tumors. However, the information obtained by the use of the biopsy far outweighs this potential risk and the procedure should never be omitted. If the tumor proves to be malignant and amenable to surgical ablation, the needle biopsy track is excised in continuity with the tumor mass to prevent a local implantation.

The majority of pathologic diagnoses are based on the examination of routinely processed material, that is, tissue that has been subjected to formalin fixation, decalcification if needed, paraffin embedding, and hematoxylin and eosin staining. On occasion, histochemical stains provide additional information of diagnostic significance, such as glycogen identification in Ewing's sarcoma, pyroninophilia of the cytoplasm in plasma cell myeloma, and intense alkaline phosphatase activity in osteosarcoma. Examination of smears of imprints can be useful for the identification of hemopoietic malignancies, such as malignant lymphoma and plasma cell myeloma. Immunohistochemical preparations may permit the precise identification of a cell product, such as factor VIII in endothelial cells, lysozyme (muramidase) in histiocytes, or immunoglobulins in plasma cells and their lymphoid precursors. Electron microscopic examination in selected instances has given support for a given diagnosis or has proved of value in elucidating the histogenesis of a neoplasm, as in the case of so-called adamantinoma of long bones.

The therapeutic approach to bone tumors varies according to their nature. The three main modalities are surgery, radiotherapy, and chemotherapy. The surgical approach, which is used for most neoplasms, generally consists of curettage (usually followed by packing with bone chips) for benign lesions, block excision for more aggressive but not fully malignant tumors, and radical operations (such as amputation or disarticulation) for highly malignant neoplasms. Radiotherapy and chemotherapy are particularly important for Ewing's sarcoma and malignant lymphoma.[160] In some instances the combination of these modalities offers better possibilities of cure than when they are given individually. An additional benefit of this approach is that the surgery can be less radical than when it is administered as the only therapy.[82]

From the point of view of behavior, most classifications (including the present one) divide bone neoplasms into a benign and a malignant category. This is done for orientation purposes, but it represents a gross oversimplification of the real situation. As is often the case in real life as compared with western movies, bone neoplasms cannot be sharply segregated into the "bad guys" and the "good guys." There is instead a whole range of intermediate characters between the perfectly innocuous tumor and the highly invasive and metastasizing neoplasm.

As a general rule the most benign tumors are well circumscribed, with sharply defined outlines, and are surrounded by an area of sclerosis (indicative of slow growth). They may be located within either the medulla or the cortex, and show no evidence of soft tissue extension or periosteal reaction. The most malignant bone tumors tend to be large and poorly circumscribed, often permeate the medullary cavity, extend into the soft tissues, elicit prominent new bone formation from the periosteum, and have the propensity to give distant metastases. The last property is the main criterion for including a bone tumor in the "malignant" category in the classification presented in this chapter. The majority of distant metastases of bone tumors are blood borne and appear in the lungs. Some bone sarcomas, such as Ewing's sarcoma and osteosarcoma, initially located within a single bone, have a tendency to show up later in other bones. Whether these foci represent metastases from the original lesion or multicentric foci of involvement is a moot point.[10] The rarest form of distant metastasis in bone sarcoma is the lymph-borne type. Although instances of lymph node metastases in osteosarcoma and other bone tumors have been reported, the incidence is so low that it can be disregarded when planning therapy.

One should understand that local recurrence of a tumor after conservative surgical therapy does not necessarily indicate that it is malignant. The reason for this should be obvious. The most common surgical approach to benign bone tumors consists of unroofing the lesion and removing it in bits with a sharp curette; the space thus formed is then packed with bone chips. No matter how thorough the curettage is, the possibility always exists that a small portion of tumor will remain in situ and provide the nidus for a recurrence.

OSTEOBLASTIC (BONE-FORMING) TUMORS

The common property of the osteoblastic group of bone tumors is the capacity of their constituent cells to produce osteoid or bone, or both, thus fulfilling the criterion of functional osteoblasts. For osteoid or bone formation to be important in this regard, it must be the direct product of the tumor cells. Reactive bone formation by osteoblasts at the periphery of a tumor or the endochondral ossification that neoplastic cartilage can undergo in the same fashion as normal cartilage does not necessarily indicate that the tumor with them is of osteoblastic origin.

Benign tumors

Osteoma

Osteoma is composed of well-differentiated compact bone of lamellar structure. It has an extremely slow growth rate. It is almost entirely restricted to the skull and facial bones, from which it may grow into the paranasal sinuses.[65] The roentgenographic appearance is that of a dense ivory-like mass. Osteomas can be seen as a component of Gardner's syndrome (intestinal polyposis and soft tissue tumors).[28] The behavior of osteomas is perfectly benign.

The bone lesion we call osteoma is probably not a true neoplasm and perhaps not even a uniform entity. Some cases seem to represent the site of a former traumatic injury, such as a subperiosteal hematoma or a localized inflammatory process; others appear to be hamartomas, that is, a type of malformation; still others probably result from osteochondroma or fibrous dysplasia.

Osteoid osteoma and osteoblastoma

Osteoid osteoma and osteoblastoma are so closely related that it is better to discuss them together.[145] Their common features include a benign behavior, a preference for children and young adults, and a microscopic

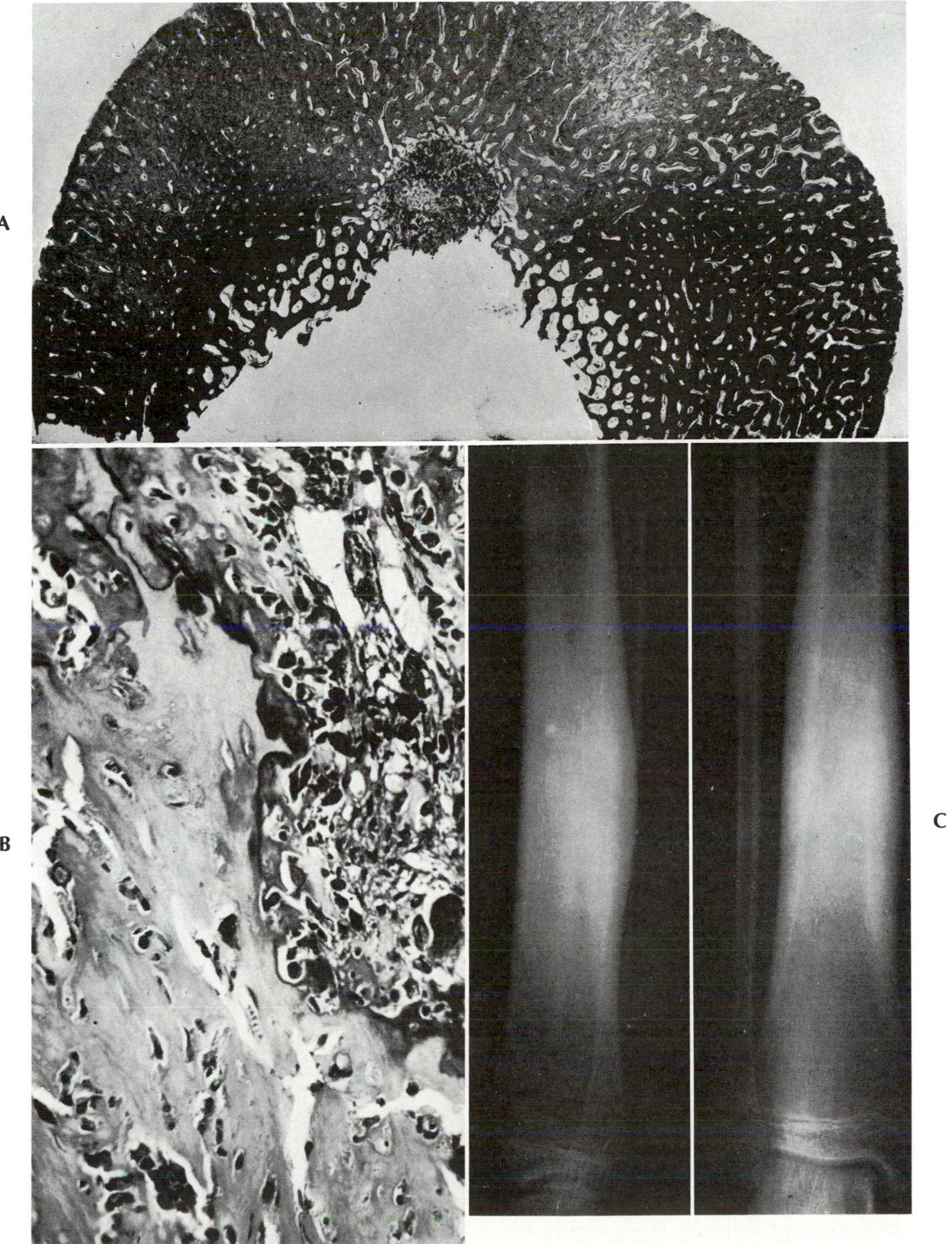

Fig. 41-3. Osteoid osteoma. **A,** Cross section through nidus. Note thickening and condensation of surrounding cortical bone. **B,** Boundary between highly cellular nidus *(upper right)* and surrounding sclerotized bone. **C,** Lateral and anteroposterior roentgenograms showing typical sclerosis associated with this lesion. Nidus is not well appreciated in this view. (**B,** 180×.)

appearance characterized by extremely active formation of osteoid and immature bone by plump osteoblasts situated in a highly vascularized stroma (Figs. 41-3 and 41-4). The differences between the two, which are not always clear cut in an individual case, refer to size, presence of pain, location of the lesion, and roentgenographic appearance. Osteoid osteoma is small (usually less than 1 cm), often located in the cortex of a long bone, painful, clearly demarcated, and surrounded by a zone of sclerotic reactive bone (Fig. 41-3).[99] Thus it appears radiographically as a small radiolucent area (the nidus), with or without a minute dense center, in an otherwise sclerotic mass. In the past, it was often confused with a chronic bone abscess or sclerosing osteomyelitis. Osteoblastoma

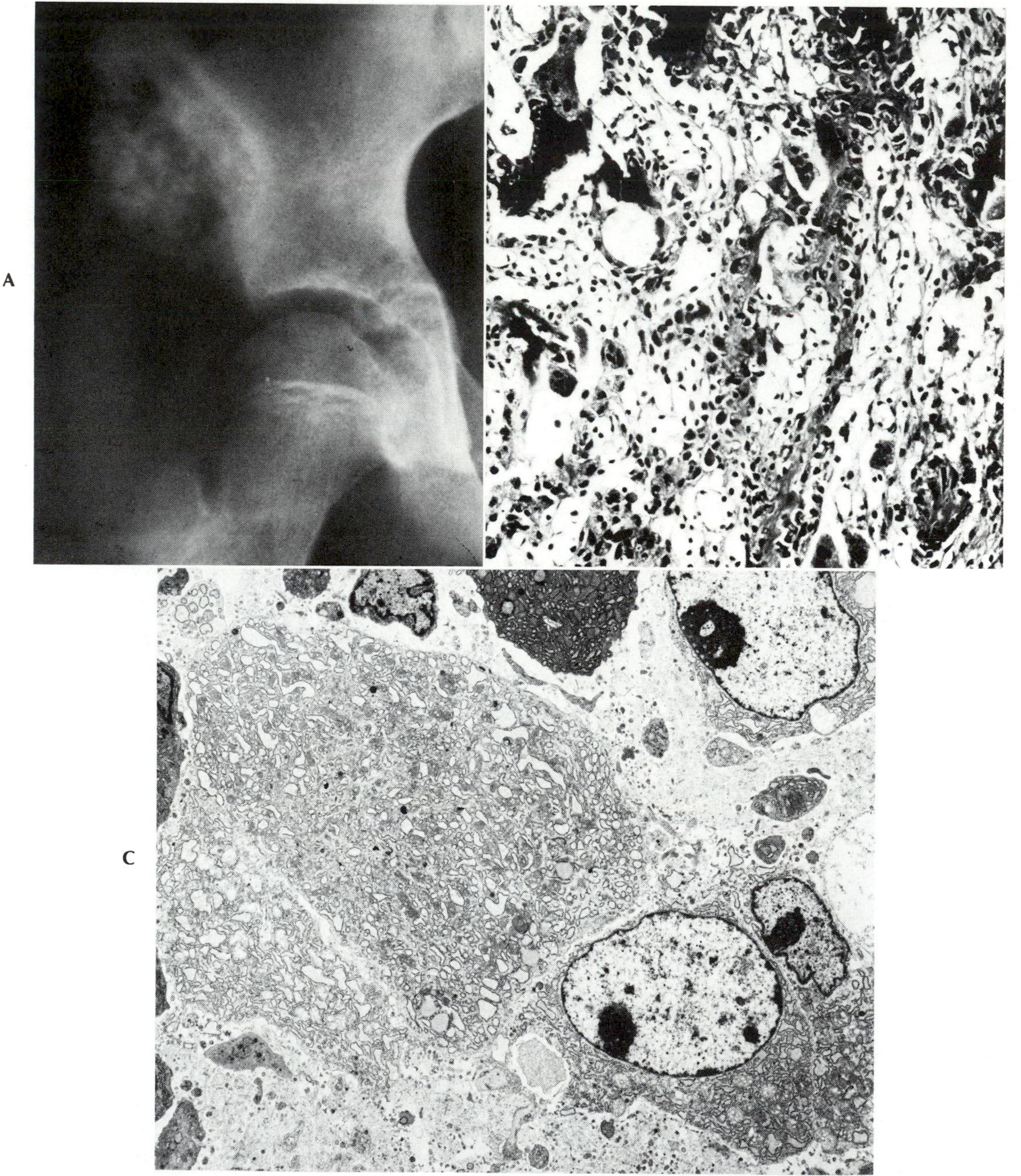

Fig. 41-4. Osteoblastoma. **A,** Roentgenogram showing well-circumscribed lesion in iliac bone, with thin sclerotic border and diffuse ossification. **B,** Microscopic appearance is that of active new osteoid formation by plump fibroblasts. Deposition of calcium salts is evident in upper portion. **C,** Ultrastructurally cells of osteoblastoma show extreme development of granular endoplasmic reticulum. Deposition of interstitial material consistent with osteoid is apparent. (**B,** 160×; **C,** 3950×.)

is larger (usually more than 1 cm), painless, located in the vertebrae, in the medulla of long bones, or in the iliac bone, and usually accompanied by a lesser degree of reactive bone formation (Fig. 41-4). It is possible that many of these differences are simply related to the respective sites of the two lesions when they involve a long bone: cortical for osteoid osteoma and medullary for osteoblastoma.[18,44] Examples of osteoid osteoma and osteoblastoma located in the parosteal (juxtacortical) region have been observed.

Osteoid osteomas and the large majority of osteoblastomas are benign. Occasional osteoblastomas behave in a locally aggressive fashion. They are referred to as aggressive osteoblastomas,[128] or malignant osteoblastomas.[146] They should be distinguished from both the ordinary osteoblastomas and the well-differentiated osteosarcomas, not always an easy task.

Malignant tumors

Osteosarcoma

Osteosarcoma is the primary malignant tumor of osteoblasts and is identified microscopically by the direct formation of osteoid or bone, or both, by the neoplastic cells. It is the most common primary malignant tumor of bone, and it is also known as osteogenic sarcoma.[21,37,50] Most cases appear in adolescents and young adults. Males are affected more often than females. Many osteosarcomas developing after middle age represent a complication of Paget's disease or irradiation therapy to the area (Fig. 41-5).[175] The classic site of occurrence is the medulla of the metaphysis of long bones, particularly the lower end of the femur, the upper end of the tibia, and the upper end of the humerus. In rare cases there are multiple independent foci throughout the skeleton.

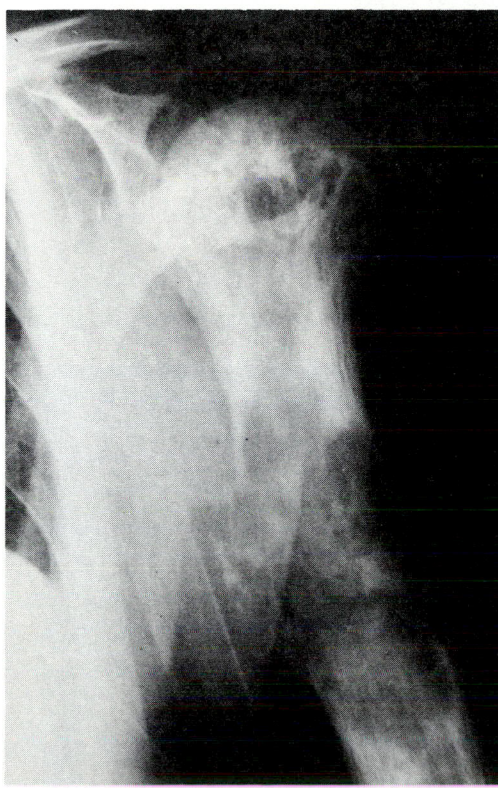

Fig. 41-5. Paget's disease complicated by osteosarcoma and pathologic fracture. Note thickening of bone resulting from Paget's disease and destructive lytic process in center of figure, corresponding to poorly differentiated osteosarcoma with scanty osteoid formation.

Osteosarcoma is a highly invasive neoplasm. It permeates the medullary cavity and can extend for a long distance from its site of inception (this being one of the causes for the stump recurrences often seen after amputations done too close to the tumor mass)[96]; it also breaks through the cortex, elevates the periosteum, and grows relentlessly into the soft tissues (Fig. 41-6). Only one tissue is able to stop, at least temporarily, the advance of this tumor; it is the cartilage of the epiphyseal plate (Fig. 41-7). Because of this, it is relatively uncommon for osteosarcomas in young persons (when the epiphyseal plate is present) to extend into the epiphyses; once the cartilage from the epiphyseal plate has disappeared, the tumor freely extends into the articular end of the bone and may even penetrate the joint cavity. This remarkable capacity of cartilage to resist the invasion by osteosarcoma cells is also evident in organ-cell culture systems and may be caused by the release of a collagenase inhibitor.[87]

Satellite nodules (known as "skip" metastases) may be found proximal to the primary lesion, either in the same bone or into another transarticularly.[51] Distant metastases are common and are the reason for the present high rate of failures in the treatment of this neoplasm. They are generally blood borne, and the lungs are the most common site of involvement (Fig. 41-8).

The roentgenographic appearance depends a great deal on the relative amount of bone produced in a particular tumor. A tumor that produces a large amount of osteoid matrix that calcifies will appear as a highly sclerotic lesion; a less-differentiated tumor that produces little or no recognizable bone will occur as a lytic lesion (Fig. 41-9).

The gross appearance of an osteosarcoma depends largely on the relative amounts of osteoid, bone, and cartilage being produced. Tumors with an abundance of these materials have a hard, partially calcified appearance, whereas more undifferentiated tumors are softer and whitish or pink, with frequent areas of necrosis and hemorrhage. Foci of cartilage formation appear as white, glistening, somewhat mucoid areas. Some osteosarcomas are accompanied by telangiectatic blood vessels that result in a multicystic appearance not unlike that of aneurysmal bone cyst.[104]

Osteosarcomas show a considerable variation in microscopic pattern.[41] The tumor cells may be small and more

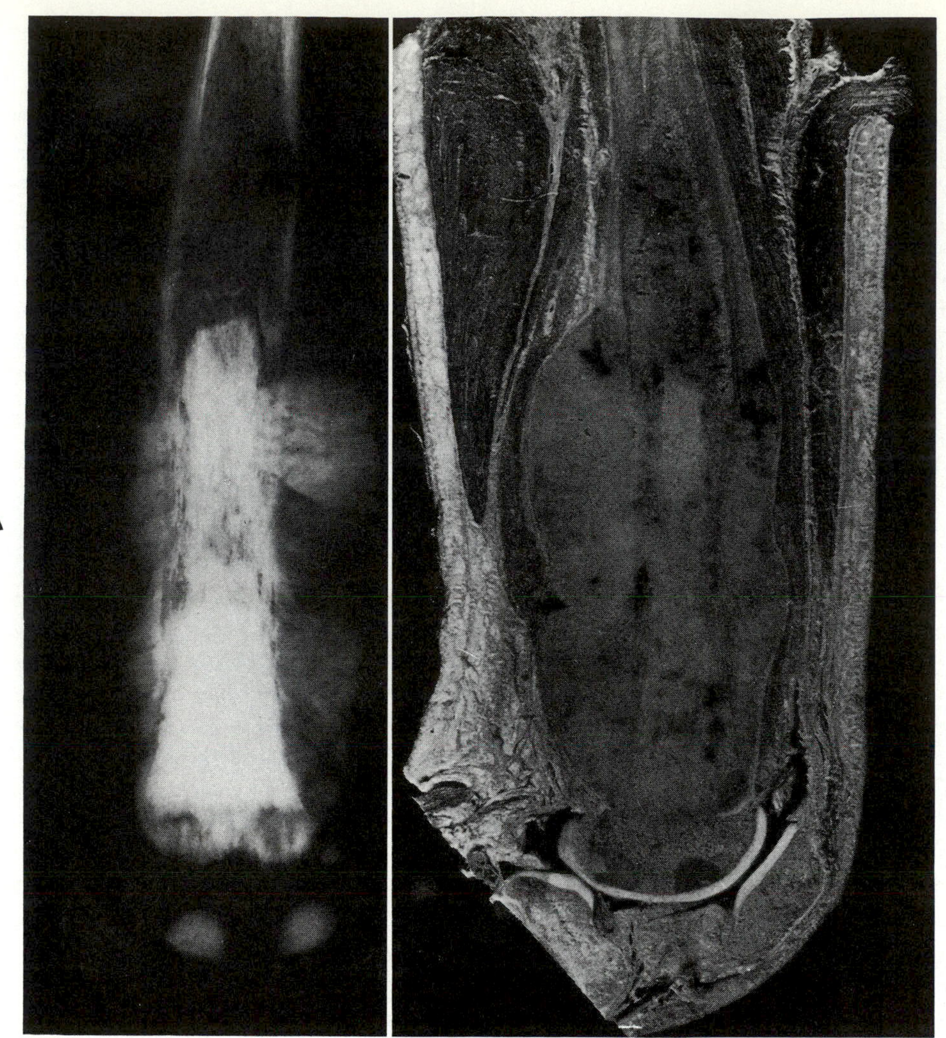

Fig. 41-6. Osteosarcoma. **A,** Roentgenogram of midsagittal slice of femur massively invaded by heavily ossified osteosarcoma. Note condensation and loss of architectural design of affected segment of femur and pronounced osseous tissue growth subperiosteally. **B,** Gross appearance of sectioned surface of sarcoma shown in **A.**

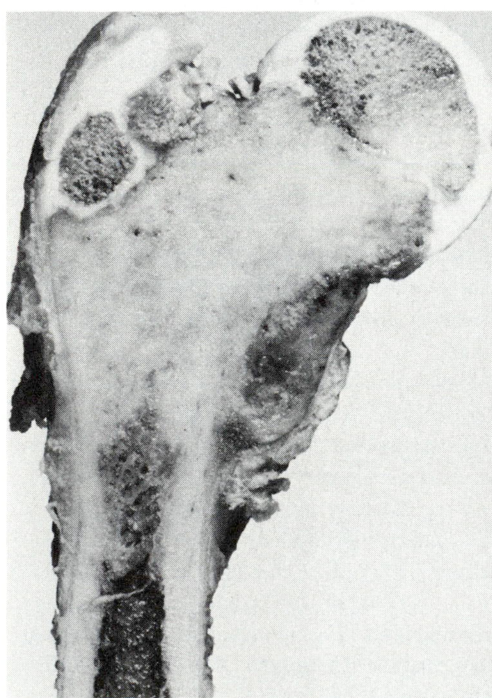

Fig. 41-7. Osteosarcoma of proximal femur in 10-year-old boy. There are extensive involvement of medullary cavity, invasion of cortex and soft tissues, and periosteal elevation. Note how tumor growth is restrained by epiphyseal cartilage.

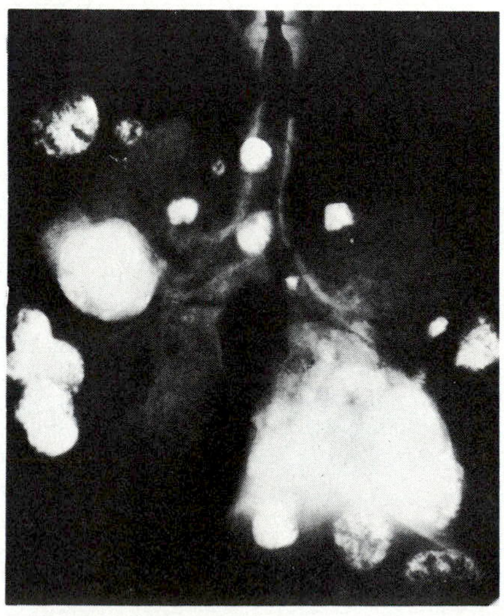

Fig. 41-8. Roentgenogram of lungs removed from patient who died of osteosarcoma. Metastases consist of bone that is heavily mineralized.

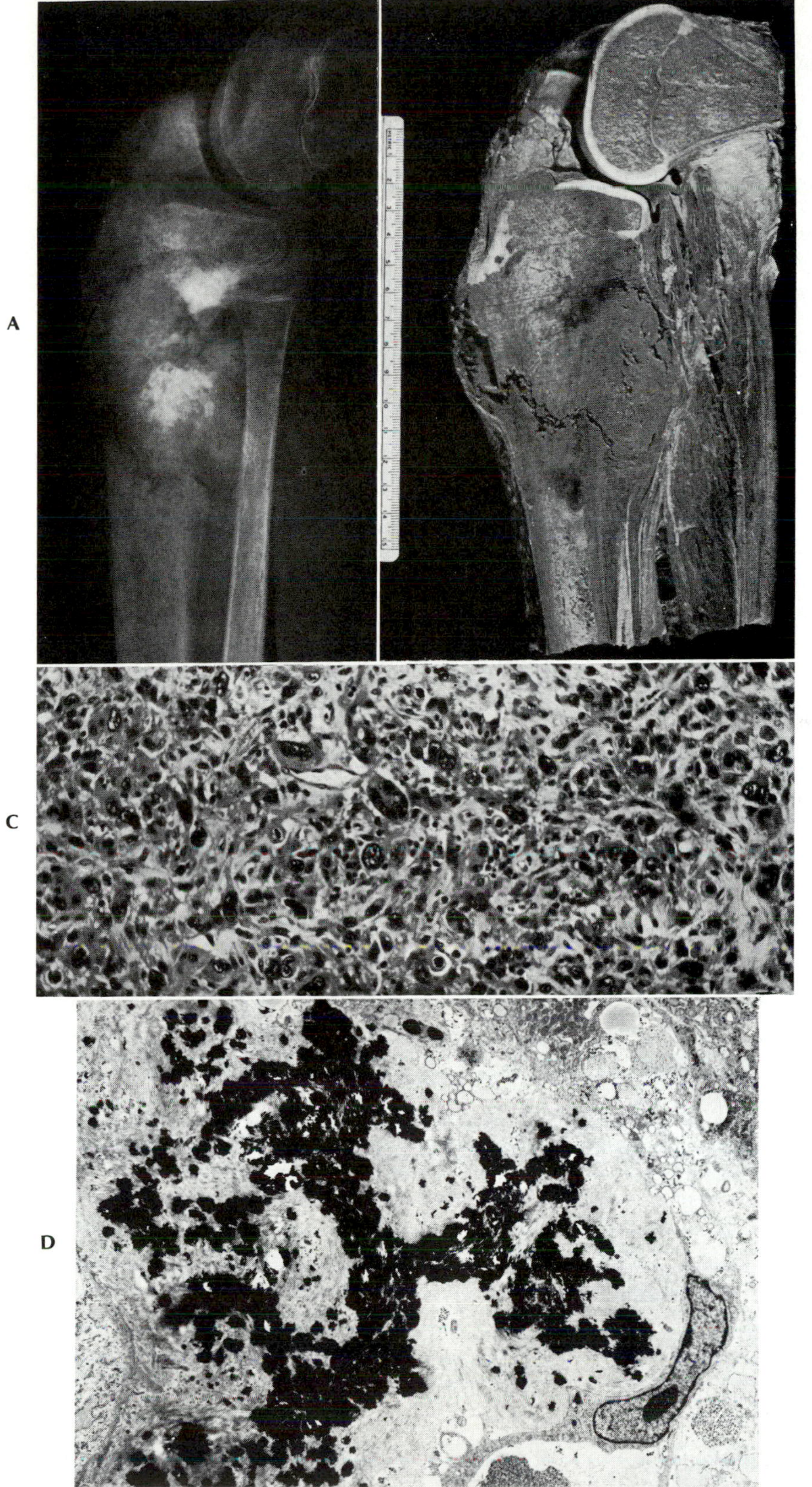

Fig. 41-9. Osteosarcoma. **A** and **B,** Destructive and rapidly growing tumor of tibia that has resulted in pathologic fracture. **C,** Variation in size and shape of cells, bizarre mitoses, and little or no evidence of bone matrix formation are noteworthy features in this lytic form of osteosarcoma. **D,** Electron microscopy shows heavy deposition of interstitial material composed of collagen and acid glycosaminoglycans (osteoid), which is becoming transformed into bone in center through precipitation of darkly staining calcium salts. (**C,** 165×; AFIP 73613; **D,** 3950×.)

or less uniform in size and shape or highly pleomorphic, with bizarre nuclear and cytoplasmic shapes and numerous mitoses (Figs. 41-9 and 41-10). Osteosarcomas predominantly composed of small round cells with little osteoid production can be confused with Ewing's sarcoma.[149] Other intraosseus osteosarcomas are so well differentiated as to simulate fibrous dysplasia.[171]

In addition to osteoid and bone, the tumor cells of osteosarcoma may produce cartilage, fibrous tissue, or myxoid tissue. In fact, in some tumors the production of cartilage or fibrous tissue is even greater than that of osteoid or bone. Other areas may have a totally undifferentiated appearance, without any type of intercellular material being deposited. However, I should emphasize that as long as a malignant bone tumor is producing osteoid or bone directly from the neoplastic cells, it should be designated as osteosarcoma regardless of how focal this production may be and regardless of how many other materials (cartilage, fibrous tissue) are being produced elsewhere by the tumor. Some authors have subclassified osteosarcomas into osteoblastic, chondroblastic, and fibroblastic on the basis of the relative amounts of osteoid, cartilage, and collagen they produce, but there is little if any relationship between these types and the prognosis.

The neoplastic osteoblasts have many of the attributes of their normal counterparts; they contain large amounts of enzymes of the alkaline phosphatase group, produce largely type I procollagen,[158] and have a greatly developed granular endoplasmic reticulum when examined under the electron microscope.[126]

As previously mentioned, most osteosarcomas arise within the medullary cavity. There is, on the other hand, a type of osteosarcoma that originates in a location extrinsic to the cortex, that is, in the periosteal or parosteal region. It is designated as juxtacortical or parosteal osteosarcoma (Fig. 41-11).[170] It is an osteosarcoma in the true sense of the word, in that it produces neoplastic osteoid and bone. However, it should be distinguished from the more common medullary variety because of its distinct form of presentation and better prognosis.[49] It occurs in an older age group, shows no sex predilection, grows relatively slowly, is circumscribed and sometimes lobulated, and is nearly always located in the lower end of the femur. Roentgenologic examination usually reveals a dense bony mass that, although firmly attached to the

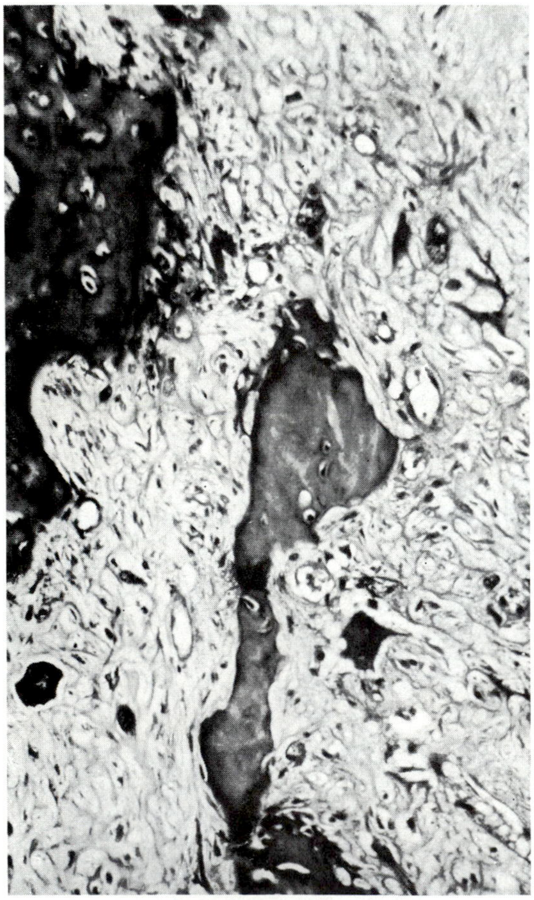

Fig. 41-10. Osteosarcoma. Bizarre cellular pattern and irregular ossification are shown. (230×; AFIP 63769.)

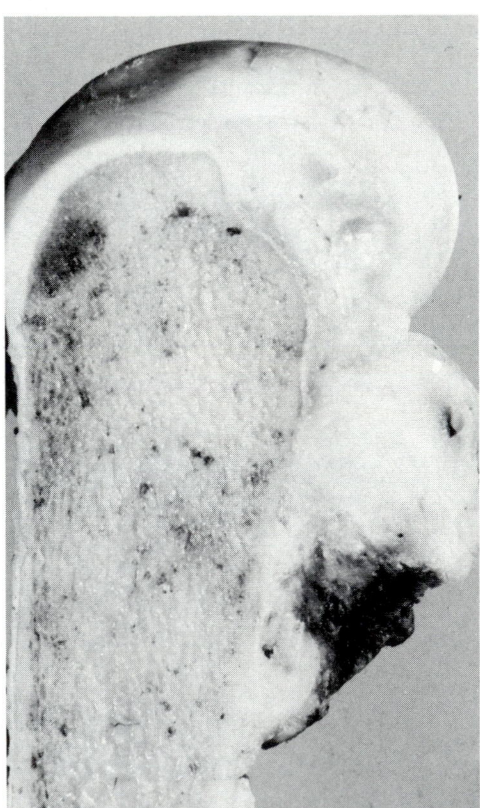

Fig. 41-11. Juxtacortical osteosarcoma in 57-year-old-man. Note periosteal location and lack of intraosseous involvement. Patient remains well over 10 years after amputation.

bone cortex over a wide base, tends to encircle the shaft as a bulky and heavily calcified growth (Fig. 41-12, *A*). Microscopically it usually shows a high degree of structural differentiation. It is composed of a mass of bone trabeculae, often mature and lamellar, which merge with the adjacent cortical bone (Fig. 41-12, *B*). As in the case of the medullary osteosarcoma, fibrous tissue and cartilage may also be present. The tumor cells are often well differentiated, with few mitoses and very little pleomorphism. The diagnosis is often difficult and usually requires a combined evaluation of roentgenographic and microscopic findings. Many of the cases are misdiagnosed as atypical osteochondromas or myositis ossificans. The prognosis is much better than that of the usual osteosarcoma as long as the microscopic pattern remains well differentiated. The rare parosteal osteosarcomas with highly malignant cytologic features behave in a correspondingly aggressive fashion.[9]

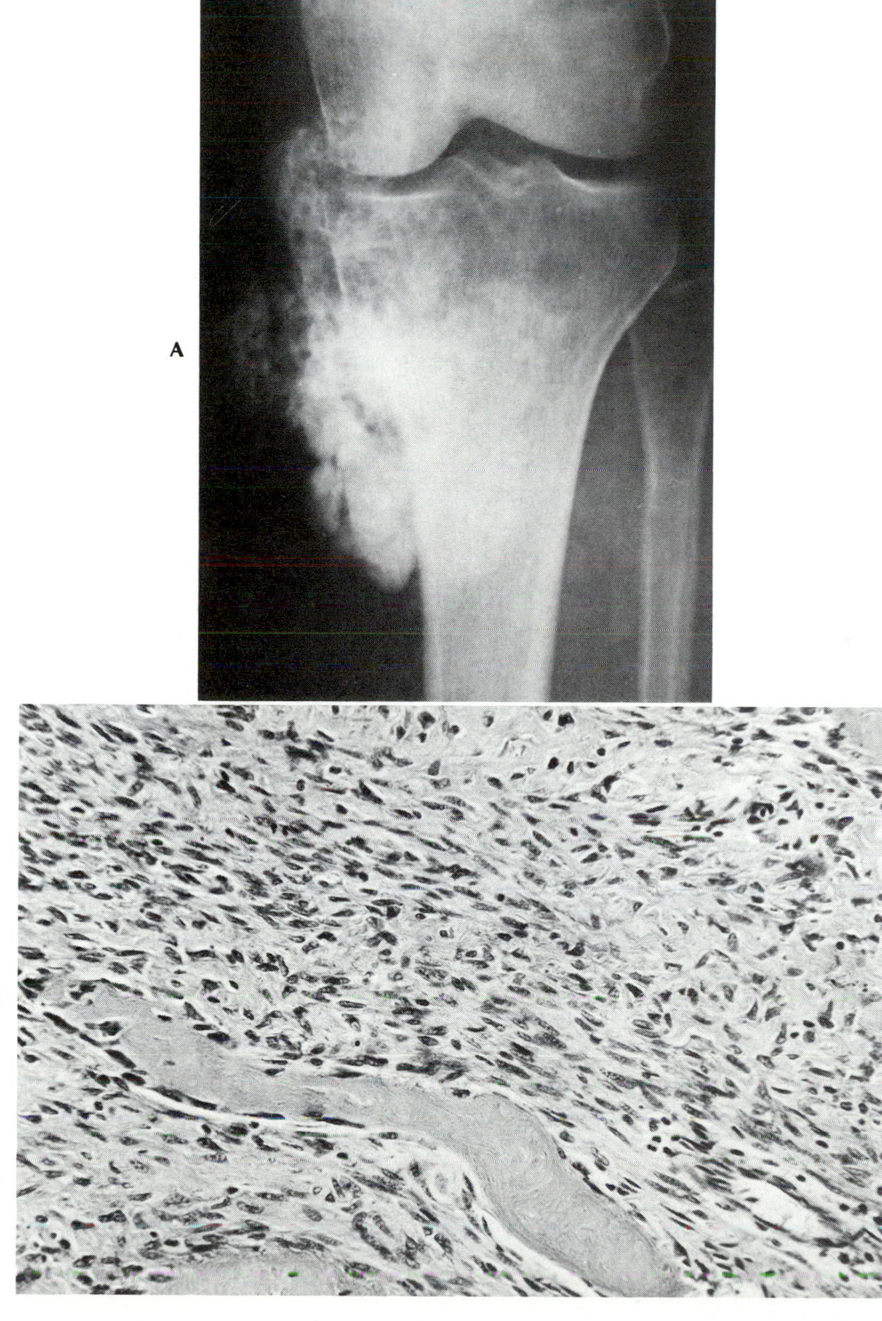

Fig. 41-12. A, Typical juxtacortical osteosarcoma in 40-year-old woman. Note large extracortical component. **B,** Same lesion shown in **A** demonstrating well-differentiated character of sarcomatous stroma. This lesion had been present for several years. (**B,** 250×.)

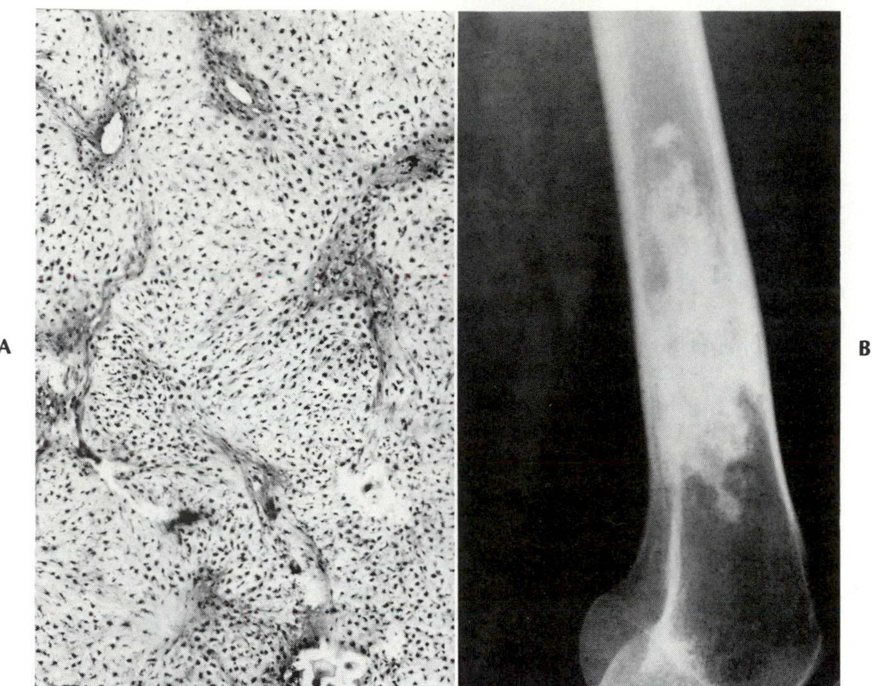

Fig. 41-13. Enchondroma. **A,** Large, benign, cartilaginous tumor of femur exhibiting massive calcification. Lesion was discovered accidentally in 42-year-old woman. It was easily detectable on bone scan because of presence of foci of bone production. **B,** Microscopic appearance of chondroma, showing mature hyaline cartilage growing in lobular arrangement. (**B,** 64×.)

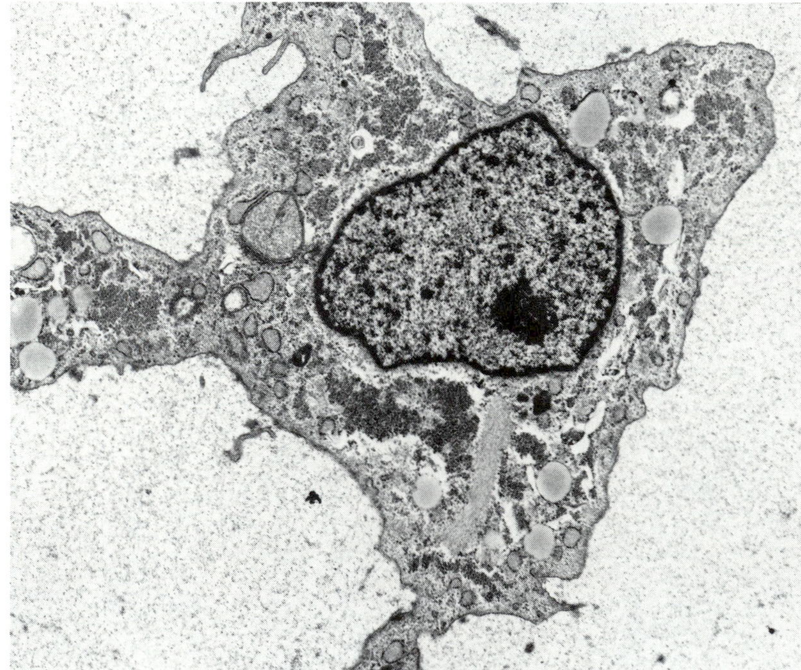

Fig. 41-14. Ultrastructural appearance of cartilaginous cell from patient with enchondroma associated with Maffucci's syndrome. Cytoplasm contains glycogen, lipid vacuoles, scanty mitochondria, and bundles of microfilaments. Cell is surrounded by abundant cartilaginous matrix. (8640×.)

Periosteal osteosarcoma (not to be confused with the just-described parosteal variety) is a high-grade tumor that grows on the bone surface (usually in the tibia or femur) and has a prominent cartilaginous component. It is probably the same lesion that other authors designate as juxtacortical chondrosarcoma.[139]

CHONDROBLASTIC (CARTILAGE-FORMING) TUMORS

Benign tumors

Chondroma

The chondroma is a relatively common tumor composed of the elements of mature hyaline cartilage. It typically involves the short tubular bones of the hands and feet and, less commonly, the ribs (particularly at the costochondral junction) and long bones.[161] Chondroma may be solitary or multiple; the latter condition, which is not familial, is referred to as multiple enchondromatosis. Cases of multiple enchondromatosis with an exclusive or predominant unilateral distribution are known as Ollier's disease, or dyschondroplasia. When multiple chondromas are accompanied by multiple soft tissue hemangiomas, the term *Maffucci's syndrome* is used.[95]

Most chondromas are located in the medullary portion of the diaphysis and are therefore referred to as enchondromas. They result in a well-circumscribed lytic lesion. Calcification, usually present in the form of small punctate areas, may be massive in some cases (Fig. 41-13, *A*). A less common variant of chondroma is seen outside the cortex and is referred to as juxtacortical or periosteal chondroma.[97]

Grossly and microscopically, chondromas recapitulate the appearance of normal adult hyaline cartilage, although their pattern of orientation is abnormal. They have a characteristic lobulated appearance and may undergo necrosis, calcification, endochondral ossification, and myxoid degeneration. The nuclei of the cartilaginous cells are small, single, and irregular; mitotic figures are absent (Fig. 41-13, *B*). The ultrastructural features are very similar to those of normal cartilaginous cells (Fig. 41-14). The behavior of both solitary and multiple chondromas is benign. However, chondrosarcomas develop in a small percentage of patients with multiple enchondromatosis.[31] Benign cartilaginous tumors of long and flat bones are very rare; any cartilaginous tumor in these locations should be viewed with suspicion, even if the microscopic features are those of a well-differentiated neoplasm.

Osteochondroma

The term *osteochondroma* refers to an exophytic mass protruding from the metaphyseal area of a long bone and invariably pointing in a direction opposite to the articular cavity. It is also referred to as an exostosis or osteocartilaginous exostosis in the orthopedic literature. It is probably the most common bone tumor. As in the case of the osteoma, it is doubtful that osteochondroma is a true neoplasm. It may represent instead a disorder of growth. It is usually solitary, although it may appear as part of a familial condition known as multiple hereditary exostoses (diaphyseal aclasis, hereditary deforming chondrodysplasia) (Fig. 41-15).

Grossly, osteochondromas may have either a broad or a narrow base that is continuous with the cortical bone (Fig. 41-16). Microscopically they are composed of a center of mature lamellar bone covered by a cartilaginous cap (Fig. 41-17). Active endochondral ossification is seen at the interphase between the two tissues. Eventually, all the cartilage is replaced by bone that contains bone marrow elements between its trabeculae.

It is not clear whether subungual exostosis is a type of osteochondroma or an independent entity; it is often painful and forms beneath the nail of the finger or toe, especially the great toe.[92]

Malignant transformation, usually in the form of chon-

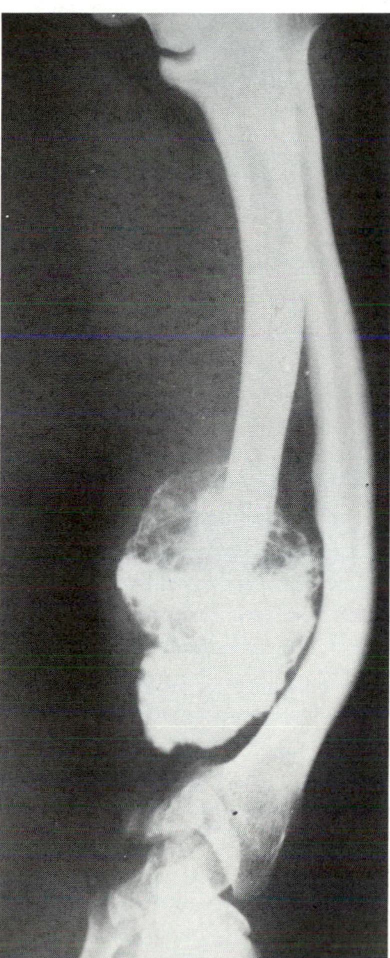

Fig. 41-15. Multiple osteochondromatosis. Large osteochondroma is seen involving distal end of ulna and deforming radius by compression.

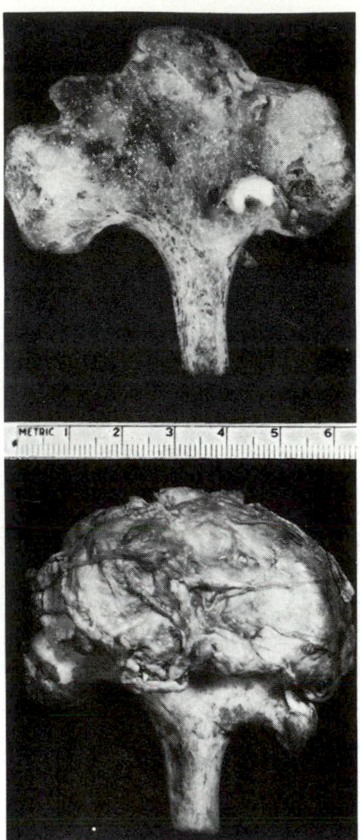

Fig. 41-16. Typical mushroom-shaped osteochondroma.

drosarcoma, is rare with the solitary osteochondroma but is seen with some frequency in patients with multiple hereditary exostoses.

Chondroblastoma

Chondroblastoma is a rare benign cartilaginous tumor that occurs almost exclusively in the epiphyseal ends of long bones, adjacent to the epiphyseal cartilage plate (Fig. 41-18).[143] Occasionally it extends into the adjacent metaphysis. The majority of the patients are under 25 years of age. The roentgenographic appearance is that of a well-circumscribed lytic lesion with multiple small foci of calcification.[77] The gross appearance is not distinctive. The tumor has a granular texture and a gray to whitish color. Microscopically the first impression is not that of a cartilaginous tumor. What one sees is a polymorphic, highly cellular lesion in which scattered multinucleated cells with the appearance of osteoclasts alternate with much more numerous, small, polygonal or round, mononuclear cells. Because of the numerous multinucleated giant cells, this lesion was originally misinterpreted as a variant of giant cell tumor. In this regard, it is important to remember that the mere presence of multinucleated giant cells in a bone tumor is by no means justification to label this neoplasm as a giant cell tumor. One should realize, instead, that giant cells are a common nonspecific accompaniment of a variety of benign and malignant bone tumors and tumorlike nonneoplastic conditions. The important cells are the smaller and more numerous mononuclear elements. In the case of chondroblastoma, these are chondroblasts, as evidenced by their electron microscopic appearance and the fact that a careful search under the light microscope invariably reveals the presence of small amounts of cartilaginous intercellular matrix with areas of focal calcification.[93] In some instances, typical areas of chondroblastoma alternate with large blood-filled vascular spaces reminiscent of aneurysmal bone cysts. These are referred to as cystic chondroblastomas.

The behavior of chondroblastoma is generally benign. Some tumors recur after curettage, and on occasion they extend into the articular space or the soft tissue.[129] Exceptionally, a tumor that has all the microscopic appearance of chondroblastoma has given rise to distant metastases.[83] This is so uncommon that for purposes of therapy chondroblastoma should be regarded as a benign neoplasm.

Chondromyxoid fibroma

A chondromyxoid fibroma is also a benign tumor of cartilaginous origin, despite its name, which suggests a primarily fibrous derivation. It often occurs in the metaphysis of long bones, and the upper end of the tibia is the single most common area of involvement.[125] The bones of the feet are another site of preferential involvement by this tumor. Roentgenographically, it appears as an eccentric, sharply outlined, radiolucent area that often causes expansion of the bone (Fig. 41-19, *A*).[144] Calcification within the lesion is not as common as with other cartilaginous tumors. A thin sclerotic inner border is usually present, as in most benign bone tumors. Grossly it is solid, often lobulated, and yellowish white or tan. Usually there is a quality of translucency, suggesting cartilaginous derivation. Microscopically a lobulated architecture can be readily observed with low-power examination. The lobules are separated by bands of fibrous tissue lined on the sides by a variable number of multinucleated giant cells with the appearance of osteoclasts (Fig. 41-19, *B*). The lobules themselves are composed of immature cartilage with a prominent myxoid pattern. Easily identifiable chondroblasts alternate with stellate myxoid cells and scattered large pleomorphic cells. The latter may result in an erroneous diagnosis of malignancy. Mitoses are uncommon. Rarely tumors representing hybrids between chondromyxoid fibroma and chondroblastoma are encountered.[35] This is not surprising in view of the close histogenetic relationship between these neoplasms.

Chondromyxoid fibroma is essentially a benign tumor, yet it may manifest a certain degree of aggressive behavior. The recurrence rate after curettage approaches 25%,

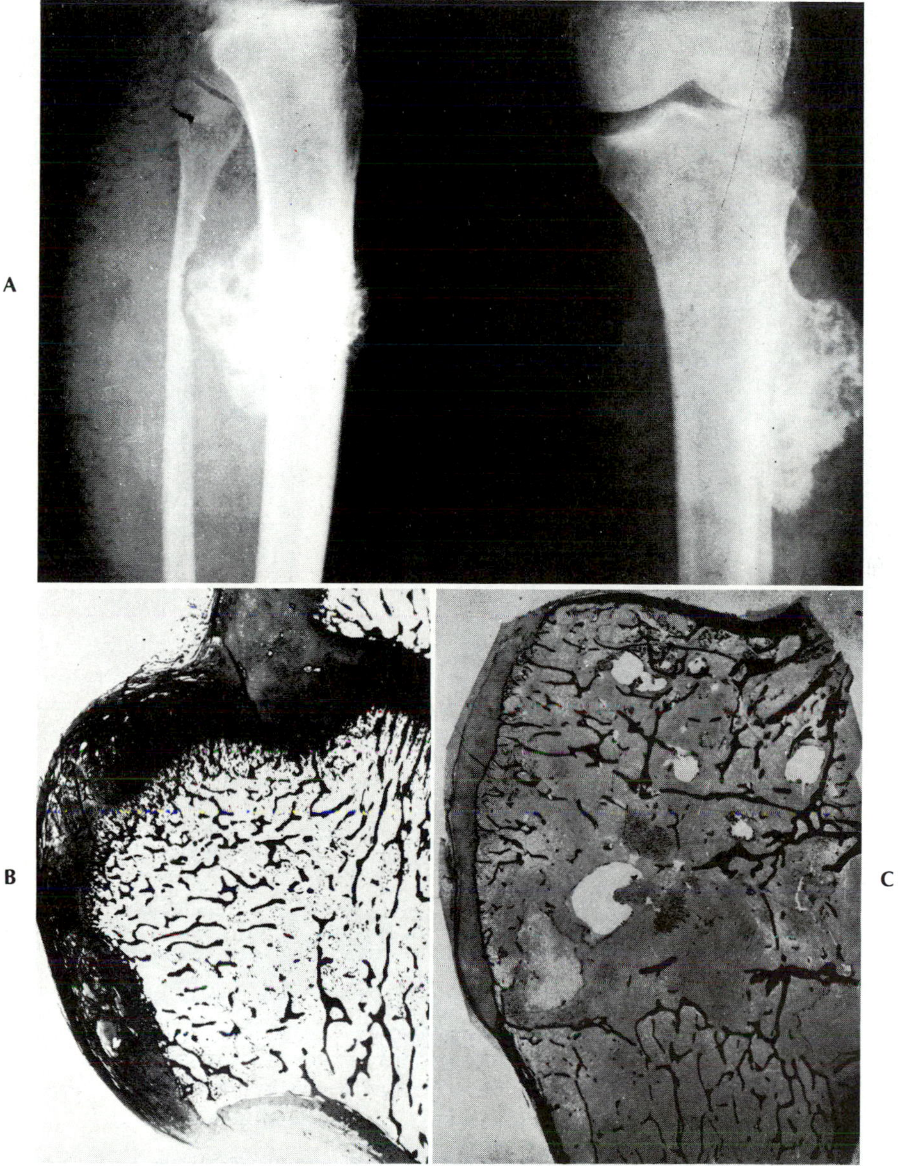

Fig. 41-17. Osteochondroma. **A,** Large, pedunculated osteochondroma of tibia. Direction of growth has been away from epiphyseal end of shaft. Pressure atrophy of fibula from contact with tumor is apparent in lateral view. **B,** Osteochondroma in early stage of development in young child. Section through junction of metaphyseal end of tibia *(lower three fourths)* and epiphysis *(upper right)*. Relation of tumor to perichondrium is apparent. **C,** Flat osteochondroma of upper end of femur. Note perichondrial layer, growing cartilage, and irregular trabecular bone that has resulted from imperfect endochondral ossification. (**A,** AFIP 77515.)

A

B

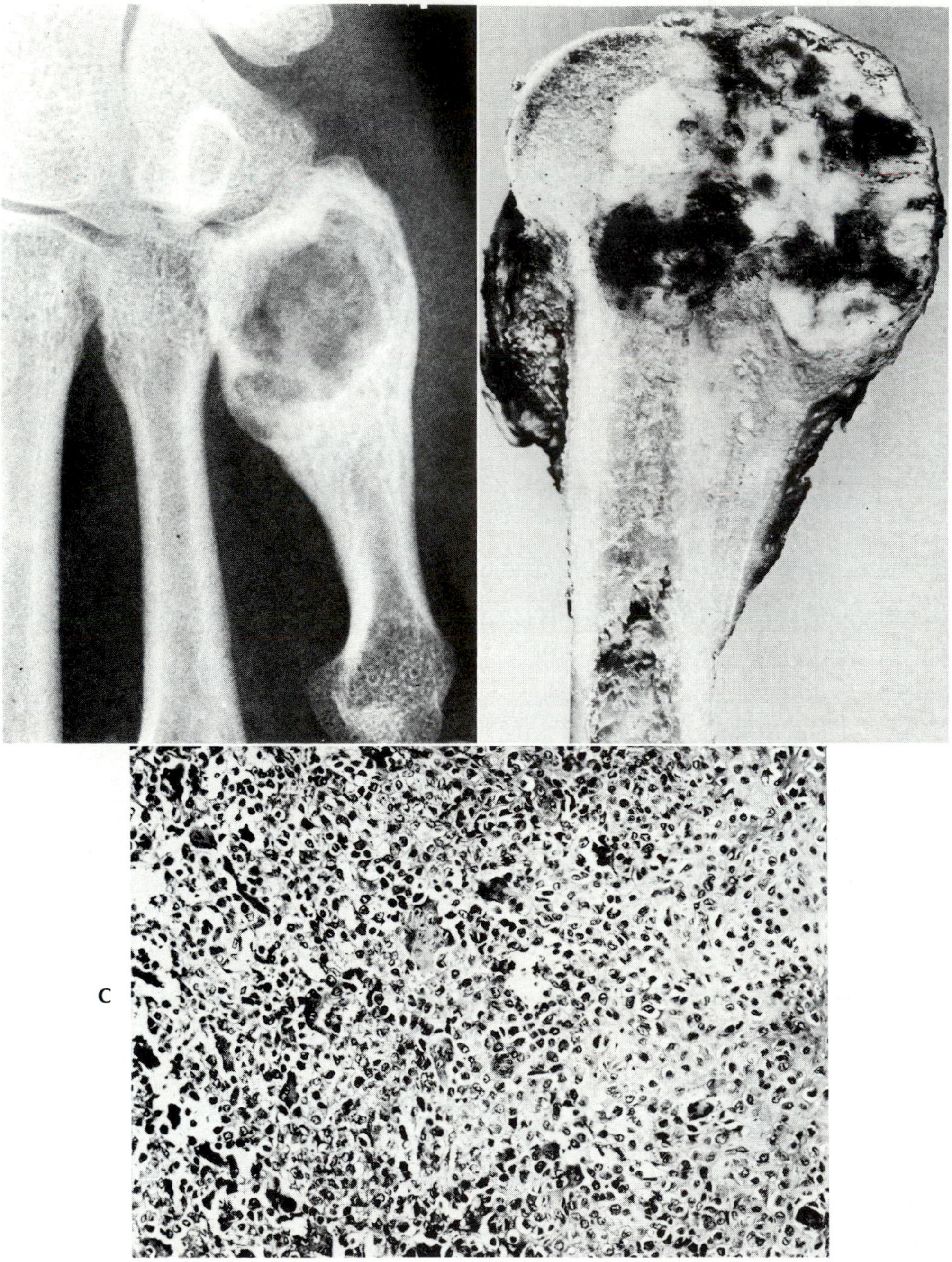

C

Fig. 41-18. Chondroblastoma. **A,** Roentgenogram shows tumor in proximal epiphysis of fifth metacarpal bone of 17-year-old girl. Lesion is well circumscribed and expansile with sclerotic border, and it exhibits minute foci of calcification. **B,** Gross appearance of well-outlined chondroblastoma involving epiphysis of humerus in young adult. **C,** Microscopic appearance of chondroblastoma is characterized by osteoclast-like giant cells separated by small polygonal cells representing chondroblasts. Deposition of cartilaginous matrix can be appreciated on right side of photograph. (160×.)

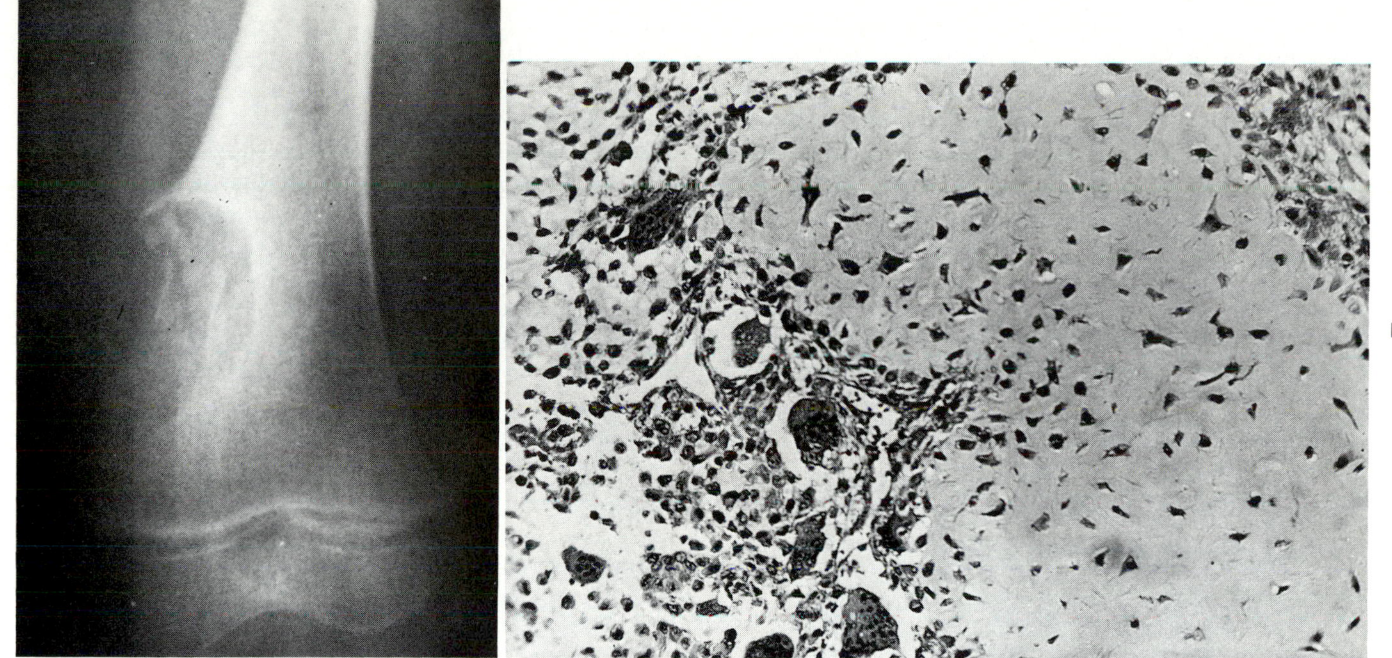

Fig. 41-19. Chondromyxoid fibroma. **A,** Roentgenogram shows involvement of lower femoral epiphysis by eccentrically located tumor with sharp and sclerotic borders. **B,** Microscopically there is alternation of giant cells, fibroma-like cellular areas, and cartilage. (**B,** 200×.)

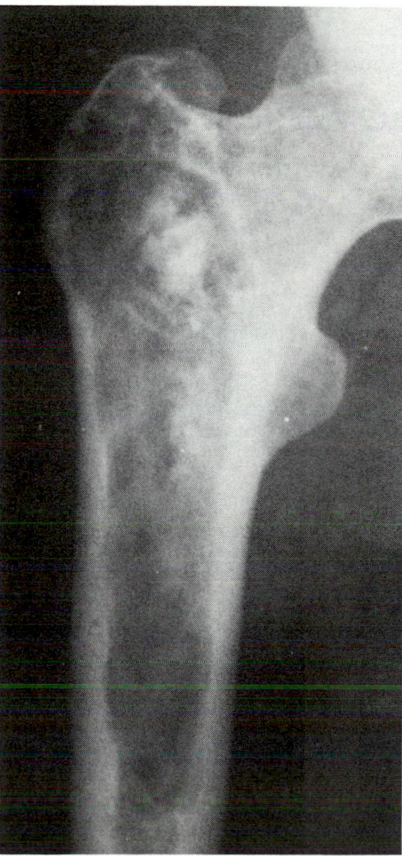

Fig. 41-20. Central chondrosarcoma involving upper metaphysis of femur. Note splotchy calcification, lobulated contour, and cortical destruction.

and because of this some orthopedic surgeons prefer to treat it with an en bloc excision. Extension or implantation into soft tissues has also been seen,[88] but distant metastases have not been encountered so far.

Malignant tumors

Chondrosarcoma

As the name indicates, chondrosarcoma is a malignant tumor of chondroblasts.[16,23] It usually develops in middle age or later. Two major varieties—the central and the peripheral—exist.[39] The central chondrosarcoma originates, presumably de novo, in the medullary cavity of the diaphysis or metaphysis. The typical roentgenographic appearance is an osteolytic lesion with splotchy calcification, ill-defined margins, fusiform thickening of the shaft, and perforation of the cortex (Fig. 41-20).[106] The peripheral form, which is cortical in location, can be primary or represent a malignant degeneration in the cartilage of an osteochondroma. Roentgenographically, it is a large tumor, with a heavily calcified center surrounded by a less dense periphery with splotchy calcification. A less common and somewhat controversial variety of chondrosarcoma arises in relation to the periosteum and is known as juxtacortical chondrosarcoma.[139]

The gross appearance of chondrosarcoma betrays its cartilaginous composition. The tumor is often extremely large and has a lobulated outline (especially in the peripheral variety), firm consistency, and a glistening white or bluish, translucent cut surface (Fig. 41-21). A gelatinous or myxoid quality is often evident. Calcification is often present and may be extreme. Foci of ossification may be encountered. The central chondrosarcoma may be seen pushing into the cortex and eventually reaching the periosteum and surrounding soft tissues.[118]

Microscopically the hallmark of chondrosarcoma is the presence of chondroblasts having atypical cytologic features, situated in a more or less organized cartilaginous matrix (Fig. 41-22). The cytologic signs of malignancy can be very obvious or quite subtle. In the well-differentiated examples the pathologist must rely on minimal morphologic deviations, such as plump nuclei, multinucleated chondroblasts, presence of multiple chondroblasts in a single lacuna, and strikingly accelerated growth activity at the margins of the individual lobules or nodules. In these cases evaluation of the clinical and roentgenographic features is of paramount importance. The just-mentioned minor microscopic characteristics, if present in an invasive tumor of the medullary cavity of a long bone, are diagnostic of chondrosarcoma but, if present in a small cartilaginous tumor of the hand, are usually of no significance.

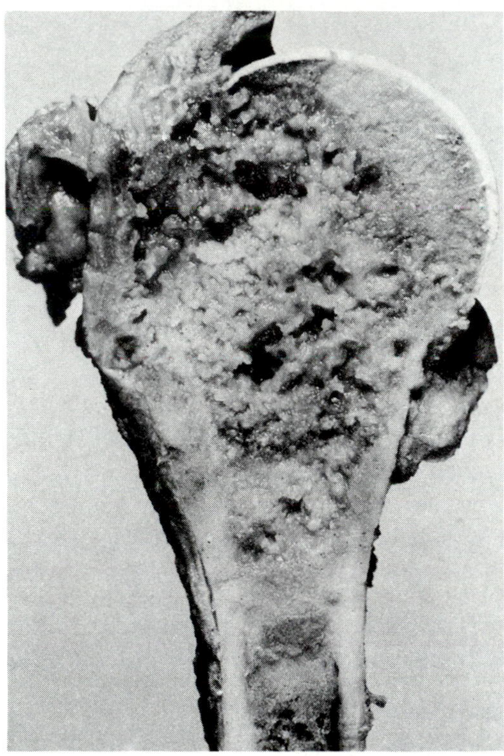

Fig. 41-21. Chondrosarcoma of head of humerus.

On occasion the tumor cells of a chondrosarcoma can have abundant clear cytoplasm, which may lead to confusion with metastatic carcinoma (particularly from the kidney) and chondroblastoma.

Neoplastic cartilage, like its normal counterpart, may be replaced by bone by a mechanism of endochondral ossification. In this process the cartilage is reabsorbed and new bone is laid down in its place by osteoblasts, that is, different cells from those that produced the cartilage. Presence of endochondral ossification in a neoplastic cartilage is not an indication that the tumor is an osteosarcoma or a reason to call the tumor an osteochondrosarcoma. It is only when the bone or osteoid is produced directly by the neoplastic cells, that is, without the interposition of a cartilaginous phase, that the term *osteosarcoma* should be used. Sometimes it is difficult to decide the nature of the bone present in a tumor that otherwise would qualify as chondrosarcoma; this probably explains why the same tumor is regarded as a juxtacortical chon-

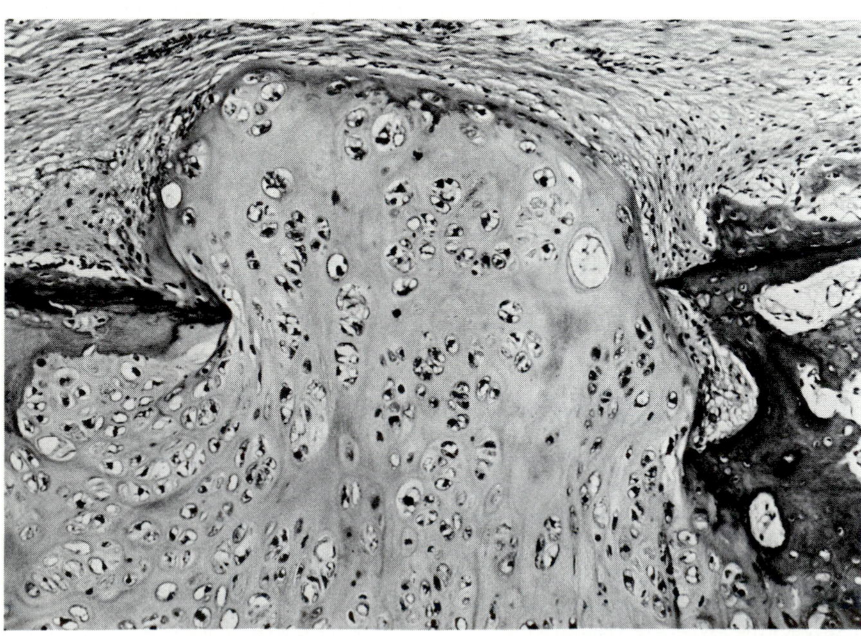

Fig. 41-22. Bizarre and plump nuclei in well-differentiated chondrosarcoma from pelvis. This histologic section also shows tumor protruding through cortical bone into surrounding soft tissues. This feature and lobular pattern seen grossly illustrate danger of enucleating these tumors, which leads almost inevitably to tumor recurrence. (125×.)

drosarcoma by some authors and a periosteal osteosarcoma by others.

Although both chondromas and osteochondromas (especially the generalized forms) can lead to chondrosarcoma development, it seems likely that the majority of chondrosarcomas are primary tumors.

The behavior of chondrosarcoma varies a great deal according to the degree of microscopic differentiation.[52,136] Well-differentiated ("low-grade") neoplasms grow slowly and rarely metastasize. Poorly differentiated ("high-grade") tumors invade quickly and are prone to distant metastases, particularly to the lungs. Occasionally, well-differentiated chondrosarcomas of long standing undergo focal dedifferentiation; these areas may resemble fibrosarcoma or osteosarcoma and are indicative of an aggressive clinical course and an accelerated tempo of the disease.[36] A peculiar feature of chondrosarcoma is its capacity to implant in soft tissues as a result of surgical manipulation. This property is probably attributable to the relatively low need for oxygen that cartilaginous tissue is known to have.[123] In some instances autopsy reveals a continuous intravascular growth of tumor, which may extend to the right side of the heart or even into the pulmonary arteries.

A variant of chondrosarcoma that deserves to be considered separately is the mesenchymal chondrosarcoma.[134] It is more malignant than the conventional variety and more often multicentric. In a significant percentage of cases it arises primarily in the soft tissues.[63] The distinctive microscopic appearance is provided by the alternate arangements of two greatly different patterns—one of relatively well-differentiated cartilage and the other of highly cellular and vascularized small cells of either round or spindle shape. Although the small cells have some morphologic resemblance to pericytes when viewed with the light microscope, their fine structural appearance and relationship with the other component of the tumor suggest that they are instead poorly differentiated chondroblasts. Jacobson[78] regards mesenchymal chondrosarcoma as the most conspicuous member of a family of neoplasms that arise from primitive multipotential cells; he designates these tumors as polyhistiomas.

GIANT CELL TUMOR (OSTEOCLASTOMA)

The giant cell tumor is a category by itself in most classifications of bone tumors, mainly because of the uncertainty that still exists regarding its histogenesis. Some investigators even doubt that it constitutes a valid entity. However, the elimination from the category of giant cell tumor of many neoplasms and tumorlike conditions that simulated it because of their high content of giant cells has resulted in the delineation of a lesion with quite definite clinicopathologic features (Fig. 41-23).[22,38,113]

Giant cell tumor is, by and large, a tumor of adults. Although well-documented cases have been recorded in children, one should always keep in mind that if a giant cell–containing lesion is found in a patient younger than 15 years of age, the chances are overwhelming that it will prove to be something other than a true giant cell tumor.

The giant cell tumor shares with chondroblastoma a predilection for epiphyseal involvement, although in the case of the former there is nearly always also some involvement of the metaphysis, from which the tumor perhaps arises.[22] It may be significative in this regard that the overwhelming number of giant cell tumors occurs after the epiphyses have closed. The lower end of the femur, upper end of the tibia, and lower end of the radius are the most common sites of involvement, in that order of frequency. Pain that is especially severe on weight bearing and motion is usually the first symptom. Later there may be noticeable swelling. A pathologic fracture may supervene. Roentgenographically, giant cell tumor appears as a somewhat lobulated lytic lesion, generally without sclerosis of the borders and usually located eccentrically within the epiphysis, in a condyle. On gross inspection it is well circumscribed and often has a granular hemorrhagic appearance. The expanded portion is partially or completely encased in a thin shell of bone. The neoplastic tissue is firm and friable. It is often grayish, with either a pinkish or a brownish tint. Focal areas of cystic degeneration, of yellow-brown color, and hemorrhagic areas that are red or dark brown, depending on the age of the hemorrhage, are usually present.

The microscopic hallmark of this neoplasm is the presence of a large number of multinucleated giant cells that are regularly scattered throughout the tumor mass. This spatial relationship between giant cells and other cellular components is important in the differential diagnosis with the diseases that simulate giant cell tumors; in giant cell tumors the giant cells are irregularly distributed, often in clumps or surrounding blood vessels, with large tumor areas being devoid of them.

The giant cells of this neoplasm have an abundant acidophilic cytoplasm and as many as 100 nuclei. Their light microscopic, enzymatic, histochemical, and fine structural features are similar to those of normal osteoclasts.[138] Thus acid phosphatase activity is very high and a large number of mitochondria are present in the cytoplasm.[157] Because of these similarities, giant cell tumor of bone is also known as osteoclastoma.

The second microscopic component of the giant cell tumor is often given the unassuming name *stromal cell*. Although far less spectacular than the giant cell when examined under the microscope, it is probably the basic tumor element. It is certainly more important numerically than the giant cell. The relative number and appearance of these stromal cells correlates with the clin-

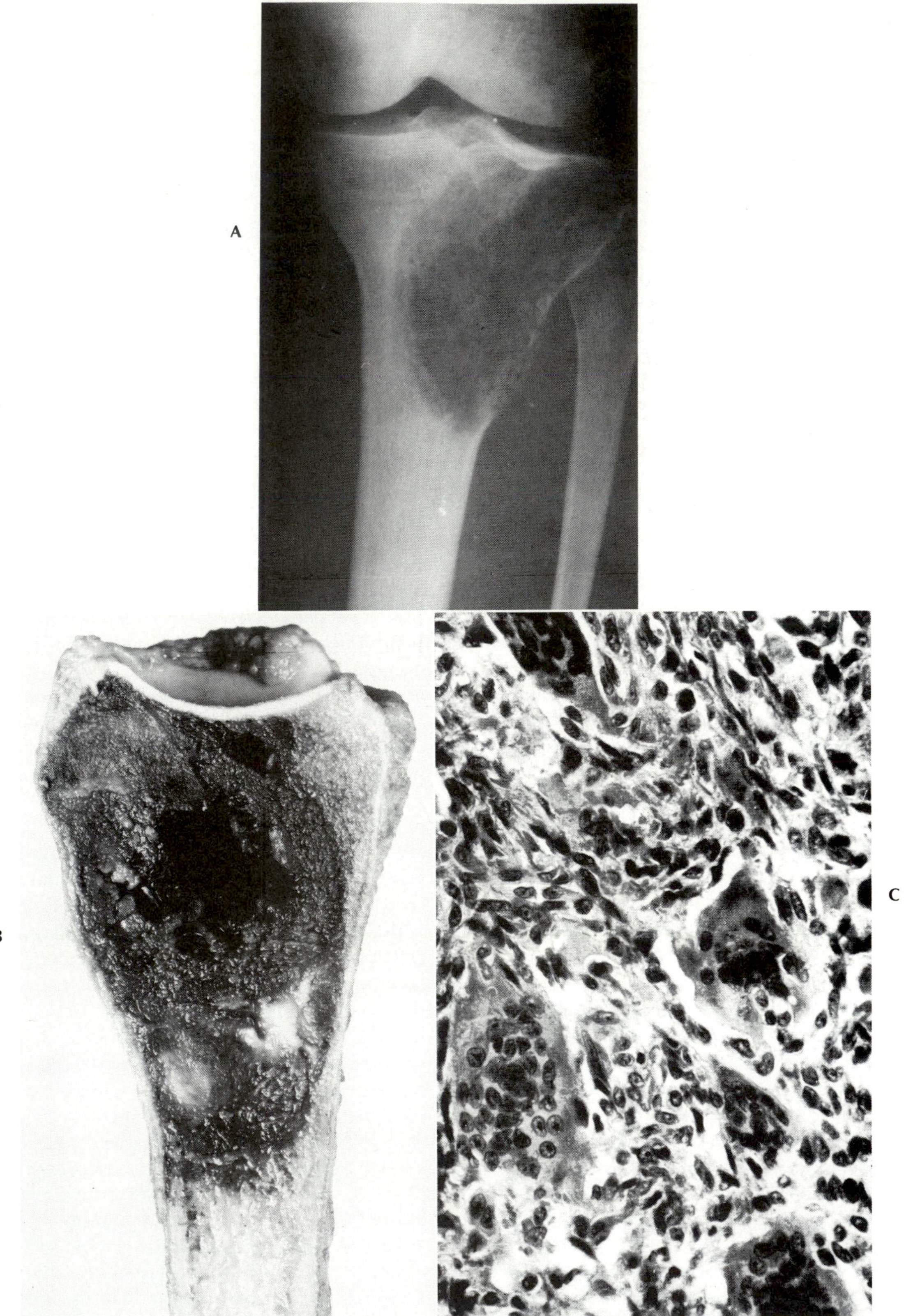

Fig. 41-23. Giant cell tumor. **A,** Typical roentgenographic appearance. Tumor involves upper tibial epiphysis and diaphysis. It is eccentrically located and shows little or no sclerosis of margins. **B,** Gross appearance of giant cell tumor involving upper epiphysis and metaphysis of tibia. Note granular hemorrhagic appearance and central cystic degeneration. Articular cartilage is intact. **C,** Microscopically, giant cells with features of osteoclasts are seen regularly scattered among smaller mononuclear cells. (**B,** 765×; AFIP 63505).

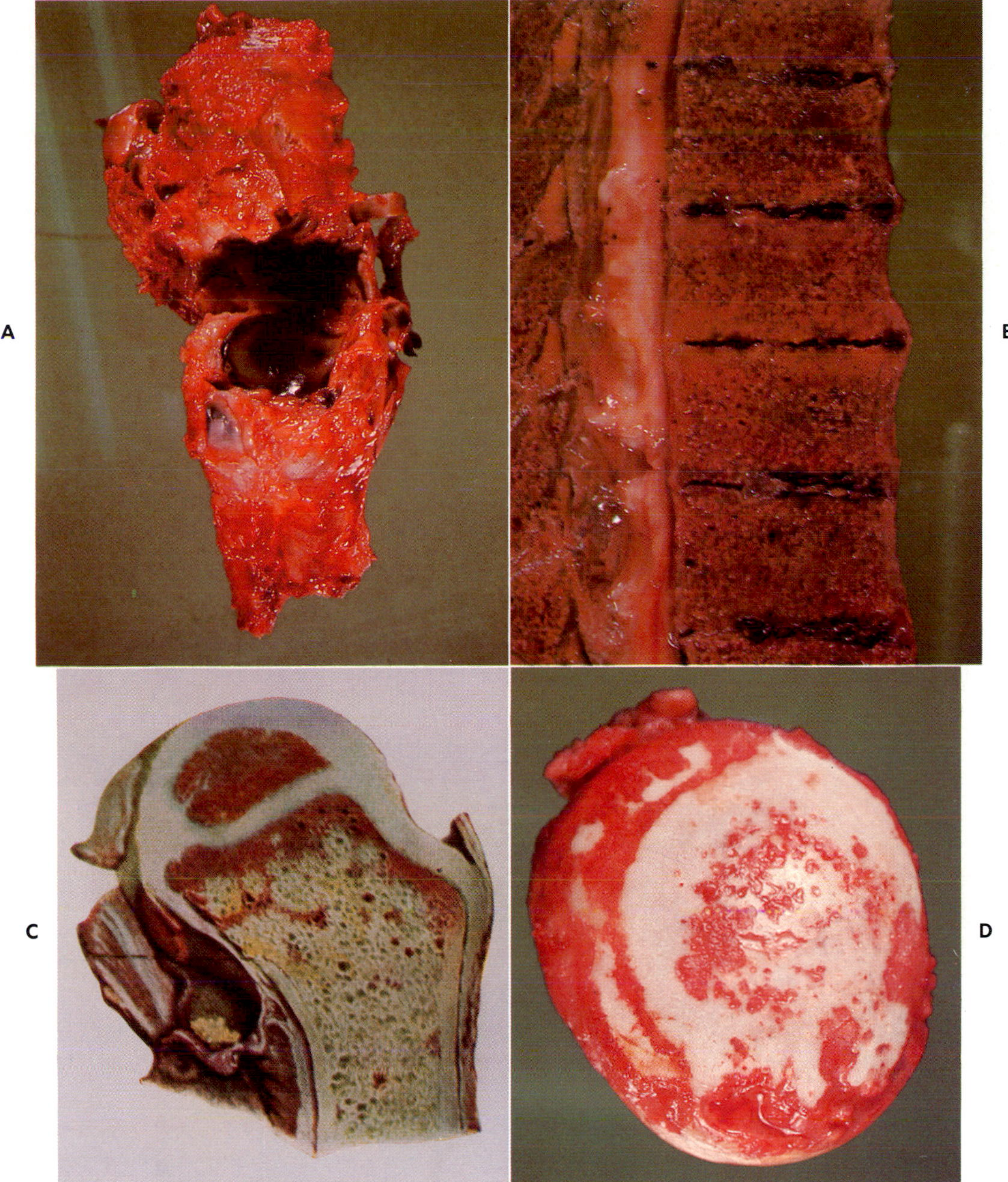

Plate 8

A, Ochronosis of knee joint. Intensely black stain of articular cartilage.

B, Ochronosis of intervertebral discs. Discs are stained deep black.

C, Purulent arthritis developing in course of staphylococcic osteomyelitis. Purulent exudate in both joint capsule *(E)* and bone marrow. *P,* Communication between bone marrow and joint space.

D, Osteoarthrosis of femoral head. Pronounced ulceration of articular cartilage and some marginal lipping.

(**A** and **B,** Courtesy Dr. Steven L. Teitelbaum, St. Louis, Mo.; **C,** from Henke, F., and Lubarsch, O., editors: Handbuch der pathologischen Anatomie und Histologie, New York, 1934, Springer-Verlag, vol. 9, chap. 2; **D,** BH 75-1635.)

ical evolution. In locally aggressive and metastasizing lesions, one often gets the impression that the stromal cell component has taken over the neoplasm. The stromal cells of a typical giant cell tumor are medium sized and oval or spindle shaped, with rather plump nuclei and ill-defined acidophilic cytoplasm. Mononuclear macrophages are also present in large numbers, but they probably are nonneoplastic and an expression of the host reaction to the tumor.[85] The stroma is richly vascularized and contains a small amount of collagen. In about a third of the cases, foci of osteoid or bone formation of reactive appearance are found. Under the electron microscope the stromal cells are seen to contain a well-developed granular endoplasmic reticulum. Their appearance is reminiscent of a fibroblast or an osteoblast.[66]

Giant cell tumors are aggressive lesions. As much as 60% recur after curettage, and about 10% result in distant metastases, usually to the lungs. Metastasis is almost always preceded by a history of repeated curettages and recurrences. Because of this, many authors recommend en bloc excision as the treatment of choice for this neoplasm. It has been suggested that radiotherapy may be influential in triggering the malignant transformation of this tumor.[173]

The microscopic grading systems proposed to allow prediction of the clinical behavior of this tumor have not proved satisfactory, and there is no agreement on specific histologic features that dependably indicate the likelihood of malignant behavior. However, it is safe to assume that the rare giant cell tumors that are cytologically malignant will behave in an aggressive fashion,[115] and that most metastasizing giant cell tumors will be histologically malignant.[135]

MARROW TUMORS

Ewing's sarcoma

Ewing's sarcoma, a highly malignant neoplasm first described by Ewing in 1921, usually occurs in patients between the ages of 5 and 20 years. Nearly all cases are in whites.[61] Typically the patient complains of pain in the affected area. Swelling may be present. The patient may have a slight fever, and the leukocyte count and erythrosedimentation rate may be slightly or moderately elevated. These signs and symptoms may lead to an erroneous diagnosis of osteomyelitis. Roentgenographically it is predominantly osteolytic. However, the bone destruction is often associated with patchy reactive periosteal bone formation, which may result in the pattern that radiologists call onion-skin appearance (Fig. 41-24, *A*). Grossly the tumor is white and exceedingly soft and friable; large areas of necrosis and hemorrhage are often encountered. The site of origin is the medullary canal of the diaphysis or metaphysis, from which the tumor permeates the cortex and invades the soft tissues. The bone marrow permeation can be quite extensive and still leave the bone trabeculae relatively undisturbed so that the tumor may be missed on roentgenographic examination. Distant metastases are common, particularly to the lung, the liver, other bones, and the central nervous system.[163]

Microscopically the tumor tissue has a rather uniform appearance. It is made up of densely packed small cells with round nuclei, frequent mitoses, scanty cytoplasm, and ill-defined cytoplasmic outlines (Fig. 41-24, *B*). The cytoplasm contains a moderate to large amount of glycogen granules, a feature of importance in the differential diagnosis (Fig. 41-24, *C*).[137] Fibrous septa divide the tumor tissue into irregular lobules. Areas of necrosis are frequent; these may be secondarily infiltrated with acute inflammatory cells. Vascularization is usually well developed. The tumor cells may be grouped around blood vessels, producing a false rosette. The fine structural appearance is that of primitive cells without signs of differentiation.[100] Focal new bone formation is usually encountered, but this is thought to be of reactive nature. In some cases of Ewing's sarcoma the tumor cells have larger nuclei, with more conspicuous nucleoli than in the usual variety.[116] Tumors morphologically indistinguishable from Ewing's sarcoma are occasionally seen in the soft tissues, particularly in the paravertebral region.[13]

The histogenesis is still disputed, although most investigators favor an origin from primitive bone marrow elements. Ultrastructural and immunohistochemical evidence suggesting early vascular differentiation has been detected in some cases.[158]

The microscopic differential diagnosis must be made primarily with other "small round cell tumors" of bone—malignant lymphoma, metastatic neuroblastoma, and osteosarcoma of small cell type. Malignant lymphoma affects an older age group, the cells are larger, the nuclei often have a vesicular or indented configuration, glycogen is absent, and reticulin is more prominent. In metastatic neuroblastoma the bone lesions are often multiple and the predilection is for children under 3 years of age. Glycogen is not as prominent and rosettes may be present. When grown in tissue culture, neurites form in 24 to 48 hours; levels of urinary catecholamine derivatives are almost always elevated. Osteosarcoma exhibits signs of osteoid formation by the tumor cells.

In the past the prognosis of Ewing's sarcoma was dismal. In most series the 5-year survival rate was less than 5%. This has changed dramatically in the last decade with the institution of an aggressive combined therapeutic regimen consisting of radiotherapy to the entire bone affected and systemic (and sometimes intrathecal) chemotherapy.[27,132] Even patients with advanced regional and metastatic disease can be saved.[121]

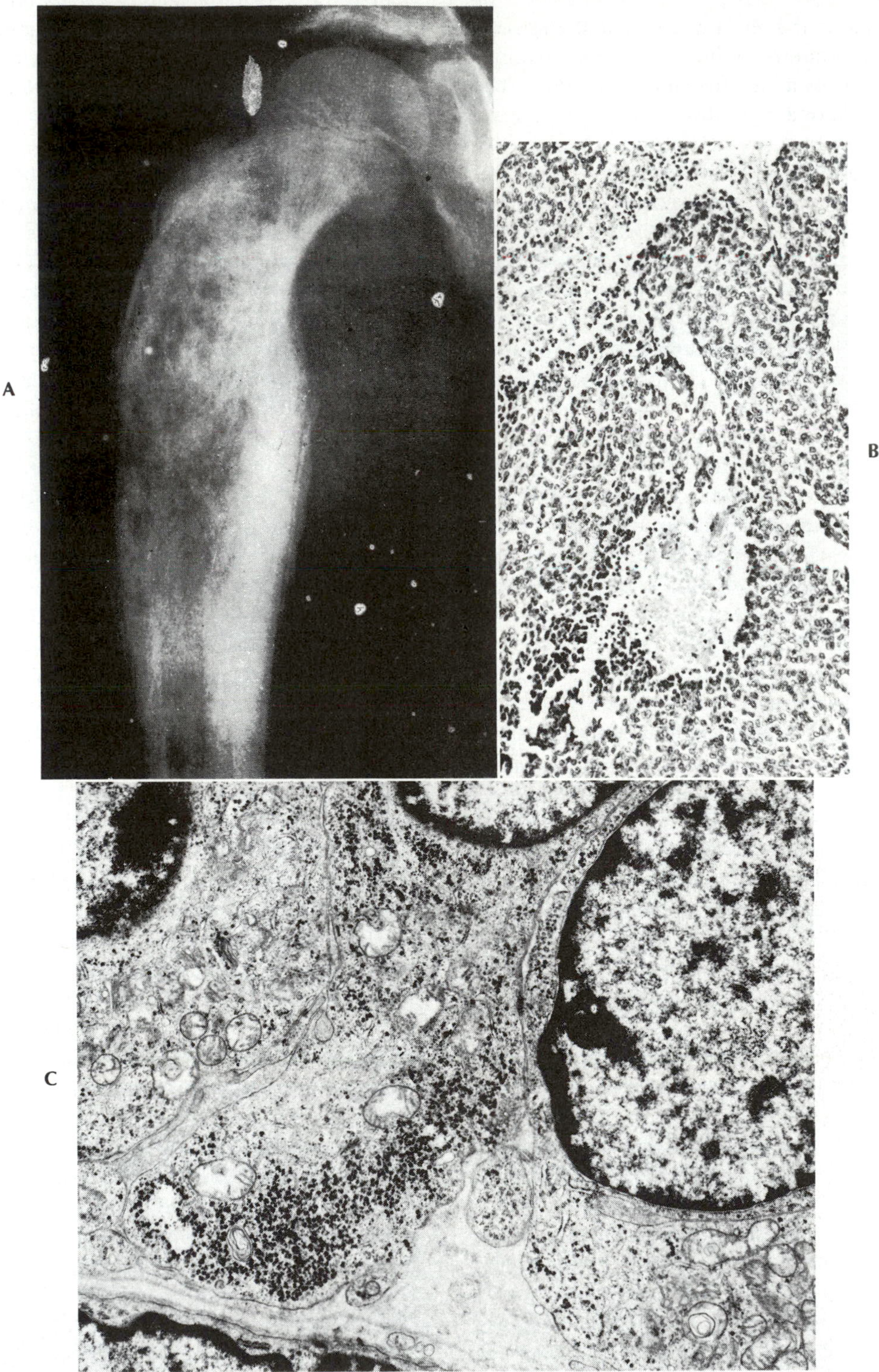

Fig. 41-24. Ewing's sarcoma. **A,** Roentgenographic appearance. Note irregular areas of bone destruction and production, loss of bone architecture, and multilayered periosteal new bone formation. **B,** Microscopic appearance is that of highly cellular tumor made up of small round or oval cells with scanty cytoplasm. Areas of necrosis are evident. **C,** Ultrastructure of Ewing's sarcoma is that of primitive cells without signs of differentiation. Numerous glycogen particles are seen in cytoplasm. There are several poorly developed cell junctions. Basal lamina in lower left corner belongs to capillary. (**B,** 160×; **C,** 232×.)

Malignant lymphoma

Any type of malignant lymphoma and leukemia can involve the skeletal system, either as an expression of systemic involvement or as the first manifestation of the disease.[25] Hodgkin's disease produces roentgenographically visible bone lesions in 15% of the cases.[71] The involvement is multifocal in 60%, and the bones most often affected are the vertebrae, pelvis, and ribs. In the vertebrae the lesions often have a striking osteoblastic appearance. Of the four microscopic types of Hodgkin's disease, mixed cellularity and lymphocyte depletion have the greatest tendency to involve bones.

Non-Hodgkin's malignant lymphoma primarily involving bones tends to occur in patients over the age of 30 years.[150] It involves the diaphysis or metaphysis of the bone, producing a roentgenographically ill-defined cortical and medullary destruction (Fig. 41-25, *A*). It has been observed that the affected patients may remain in good health, even when the tumor has reached a large size, and that dissemination is slow to occur.[17] Grossly the tumor is pinkish gray and granular. It frequently extends into the soft tissues and invades the muscle. Microscopically most bone lymphomas are composed of round cells with relatively large vesicular nuclei, often indented or horseshoe shaped, and prominent nucleoli. Cytoplasmic outlines tend to be well defined, and the cytoplasm is abundant and eosinophilic (Fig. 41-25, *B*). A rich reticulin framework surrounds individual cells.[101] In the traditional classification of malignant lymphoma this tumor would be classified as a reticulum cell sarcoma; in Rappaport's classification, most cases would be included in the histiocytic category. In the light of recent immunologic and immunohistochemical observations, it appears instead that, in the bone as well as in the lymphoid organs, most cases of lymphoma composed of large cells actually originate from cells of the lymphocytic line (B lymphocytes or null cells more often than T lymphocytes).[102] Accordingly, in recently proposed classifications of lymphomas, this type is designated as the large cell type and is further subdivided—if feasible—according to the criteria specified in Chapter 30. By using these guidelines, it was found that most lymphomas of bone belong to the group of large noncleaved cell lymphomas.[48]

A combination of surgery and radiotherapy is the treatment of choice for localized lesions; in cases with extraosseous involvement, chemotherapy is mandatory.[127]

Plasma cell myeloma

Plasma cell myeloma is a malignant tumor of plasma cells that can lead to a variety of clinicopathologic expressions (Fig. 41-26).[14] The most common form is generally known as multiple myeloma. It usually occurs between 40 and 60 years of age and is manifested by pain, weak-

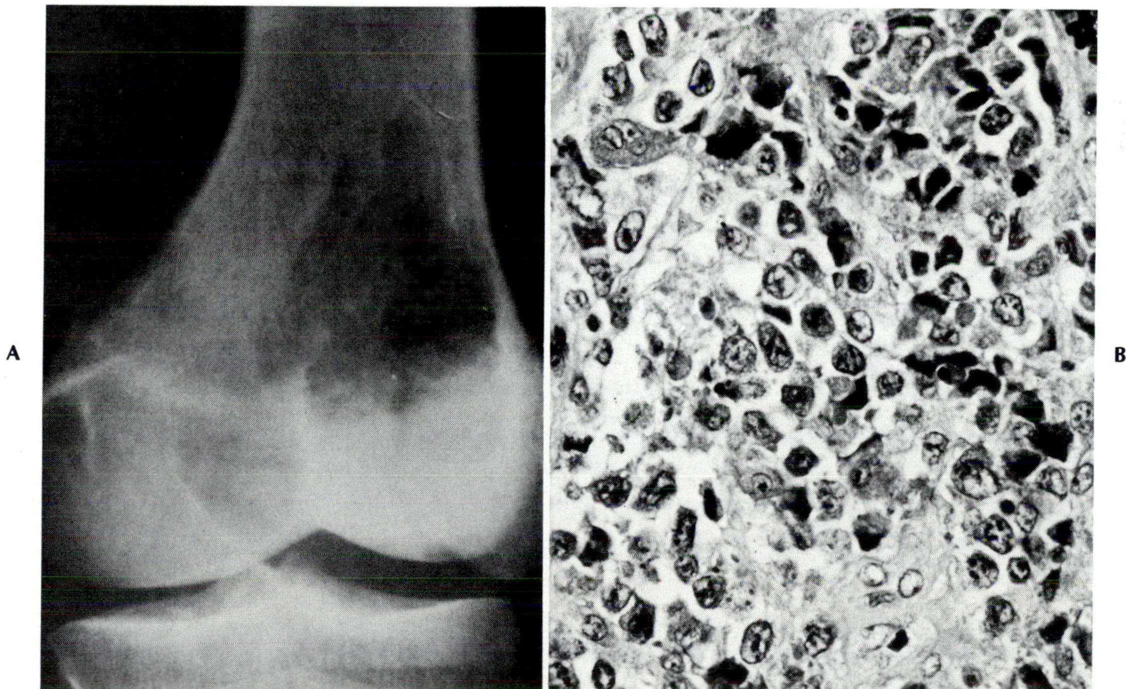

Fig. 41-25. Malignant lymphoma. **A,** Roentgenogram of distal femur showing lytic lesion with irregular outlines, lack of calcification, and absence of periosteal reaction. **B,** Microscopically, large lymphoid cells grow in diffuse fashion. There are associated fibrosis and a residual osteoclast. Tumor cells are larger than those in Ewing's sarcoma. (**B,** 400×.)

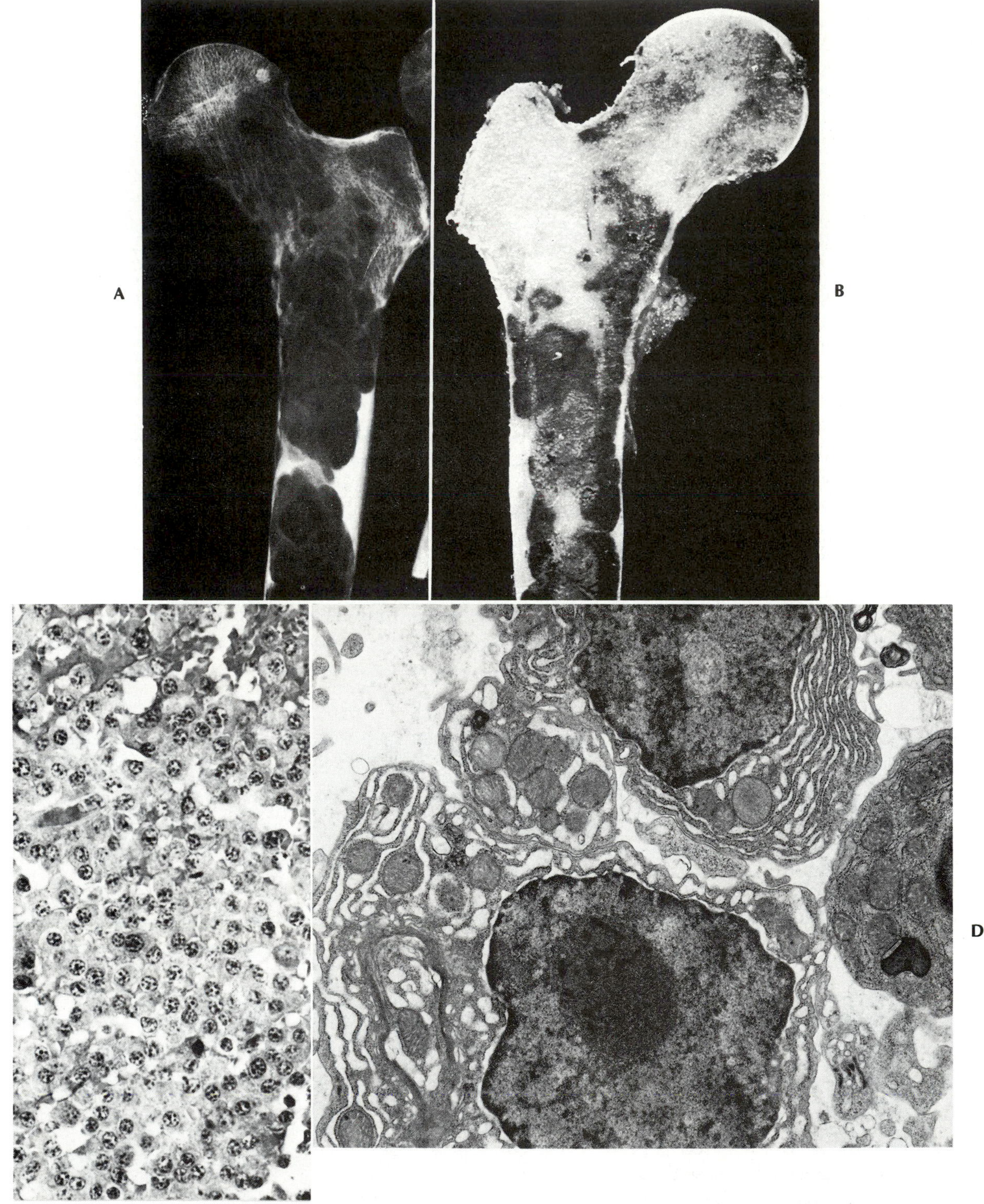

Fig. 41-26. Plasma cell myeloma. **A,** Roentgenogram of hemisection of femur showing extensive bone destruction caused by tumor. Note absence of reactive bone formation. **B,** Gross specimen from same patient. Myelomatous foci appear as dark granular areas with ill-defined borders. **C,** Microscopic section shows monotonous proliferation of immature plasma cells. Note clumped chromatin pattern and nuclear peripheralization. **D,** When viewed with electron microscope, neoplastic plasma cells are characterized by well-developed parallel stacks of granular endoplasmic reticulum and prominent Golgi apparatus. (**C,** 400×; **D,** 12,960×.)

ness, weight loss, and osteolytic lesions in the vertebrae, pelvis, rib, sternum, and skull. In rare cases the bone lesions have an osteoblastic roentgenographic appearance.[47] Signs and symptoms referable to pressure on the spinal cord or the spinal nerves may occur. Another complication of the disease is compression fractures of vertebrae or pathologic fractures of other involved bones. Some degree of anemia is usually noted, and examination of the blood often reveals excessive rouleau formation. Roentgenologic examination reveals multiple small and large areas of bone destruction. These have sharp borders ("punched-out" areas) and are unaccompanied by proliferative reactions at the margins unless a fracture has occurred. In advanced cases, extraskeletal spread may be seen, either in the soft tissues adjacent to involved bones or as distant involvement of lymph nodes, spleen, liver, and other organs.[120] Immunoglobulin abnormalities are very common (87% of the cases) and express the functional capability of the neoplastic plasma cells. In a series of 112 patients, increased serum IgG was found in 61%, IgA in 18%, and light chains only (Bence Jones protein) in 9%.[24] The most common finding in the urine of patients with myeloma is the presence of Bence Jones protein, which represents the light chain of the immunoglobulin molecule. Rarely, neoplastic plasma cells are detected in the peripheral circulation. The name *plasma cell leukemia* is sometimes used to designate this phase of plasma cell myeloma (see also p. 1338.)

The other major clinicopathologic form of plasma cell myeloma is represented by the appearance of a solitary tumor mass, either in a bone[30] or in the soft tissues (nasopharynx, nose, tonsil).[176] These are usually not accompanied by immunoglobulin abnormalities. Many of these localized lesions eventually become disseminated in bone, although this may occur many years later and even then may run a more indolent course than the form that is generalized from the beginning.

The gross and microscopic features of the disease are similar in the generalized and localized forms. Grossly the tissue is soft, friable, and hemorrhagic. The focal, slowly growing tumor may have a fairly well-defined border.

Microscopically there is a wide range of differentiation that the neoplastic cells may exhibit. On one extreme there is the tumor that is composed of plasma cells so well differentiated that a confusion with an inflammatory condition may arise; on the other, one sees a highly undifferentiated tumor with formation of tumor giant cells, in which the plasmacytic nature may be missed altogether. The characteristic features of plasma cells, which persist in all but the more undifferentiated neoplasms, include oval cytoplasm, eccentric nucleus with cartwheel distribution of the chromatin, and a distinct perinuclear clear halo. The high ribosomal content of the cytoplasm can be made evident with the methyl green–pyronine stain, which stains cytoplasmic and nucleolar RNA red (pyroninophilic) and nuclear DNA green. By electron microscopy, the most distinctive features are the presence of a highly developed granular endoplasmic reticulum, usually arranged in the form of parallel cisternae, and a prominent Golgi apparatus, the latter corresponding to the perinuclear clear halo of light microscopy.[56]

Osteomyelitis rich in plasma cells (so-called plasma cell osteomyelitis) can be distinguished from plasma cell myeloma by the absence of atypical nuclear forms; no or few binucleated plasma cells; presence of abundant Russell's bodies (intracytoplasmic round eosinophilic bodies that represent inspissated immunoglobulin and are of very rare occurrence in myeloma); presence of other inflammatory components, such as lymphocytes, eosinophils, and neutrophils; and a richer reticular and collagenous background.

In a certain percentage of myeloma cases a deposition of amyloid is observed in the tumor tissue or in other organs; in these cases the amyloid material is made up largely of the immunoglobulin produced by the neoplastic plasma cells.

VASCULAR TUMORS

The most common vascular tumor is the benign tumor of the blood vessel, that is, hemangioma.[168] It is usually of the cavernous variety, in the sense that it is composed of capillaries and venules with thin walls and greatly dilated lumina packed with red blood cells. The vascular spaces permeate the bone marrow and, if large enough, expand the bone and elicit periosteal new bone formation. In flat bones, particularly the skull, this results in a typical sunburst effect on roentgenographic examination. The most common locations of clinically significant hemangiomas are the skull, vertebrae, and jaw bones. Collections of dilated blood-filled vessels are commonly encountered in the vertebrae at autopsy, but they probably represent malformations rather than true neoplasms.

Bone hemangiomas can be multiple, especially in children; half of these multiple cases are associated with cutaneous, visceral, or soft tissue hemangiomas.[154]

Massive osteolysis (Gorham's disease) is a disease of unknown etiology and pathogenesis characterized by a progressive replacement of the bone structures by heavily vascularized fibrous tissue. This may lead eventually to resorption of a whole bone or several bones.[62]

Three other types of benign vascular tumors that in rare cases involve bone are lymphangioma, glomus tumor, and hemangiopericytoma. Lymphangioma is usually multiple and may be associated with similar lesions in soft tissues. Glomus tumor of bone is invariably located in a terminal phalanx.[98] Most reported cases of hemangiopericytoma of bone have been malignant; as with hemangiopericytomas in other locations, the diagnosis of this tumor type should be made only after excluding other tumors that may exhibit a similar vascular pattern.

Angiosarcomas are highly malignant tumors of endothelial cells. They most commonly occur in long bones and have a tendency for multicentricity. Grossly they are cellular, friable, hemorrhagic, and necrotic.[46,168] Microscopically the hallmark of the lesion is the formation of anastomosing vascular channels lined with atypical endothelial cells. These are often combined with solid, less-differentiated foci. Distant metastases, particularly to the lungs, are common. The differential microscopic diagnosis needs to be made with well-vascularized osteosarcoma and with metastatic carcinoma (particularly from the kidney).

There exists in the skeletal system a vascular tumor that is somewhat intermediate in behavior between the innocuous hemangioma and the highly malignant angiosarcoma. This is often referred to as hemangioendothelioma. In some series it has been grouped with the angiosarcoma, but I believe that it represents a distinct entity. A characteristic feature of this tumor is that the neoplastic endothelial cells have a plump, often grooved nucleus and an abundant acidophilic, sometimes vacuolated cytoplasm. The cells have a somewhat histiocytoid appearance, which has led to the proposal of the term *histiocytoid hemangioma* or *hemangioendothelioma* for these tumors.[130] They probably correspond to the grade I (and perhaps some grade II) hemangioendotheliomas described by other authors.[20] Their behavior, although sometimes locally aggressive, is usually benign; simple curettage cures most lesions.

FIBROUS TISSUE TUMORS

Desmoplastic fibroma

Desmoplastic fibroma is a nonmetastasizing but locally aggressive neoplasm that is characterized microscopically by the presence of mature fibroblasts separated by abundant collagen.[124] Ultrastructurally most of the tumor cells have features intermediate between those of fibroblasts and smooth muscle cells (so-called myofibroblasts).[90] The absence of pleomorphism, necrosis, and mitotic activity distinguishes this tumor from fibrosarcoma. Local recurrences are common. It is likely that desmoplastic fibroma represents the osseous counterpart of soft tissue fibromatosis (so-called desmoid tumor).

Fibrosarcoma is the malignant tumor of fibroblasts.[40] In one large series as many as 17% represented radiation-induced neoplasms.[173] Fibrosarcoma usually involves

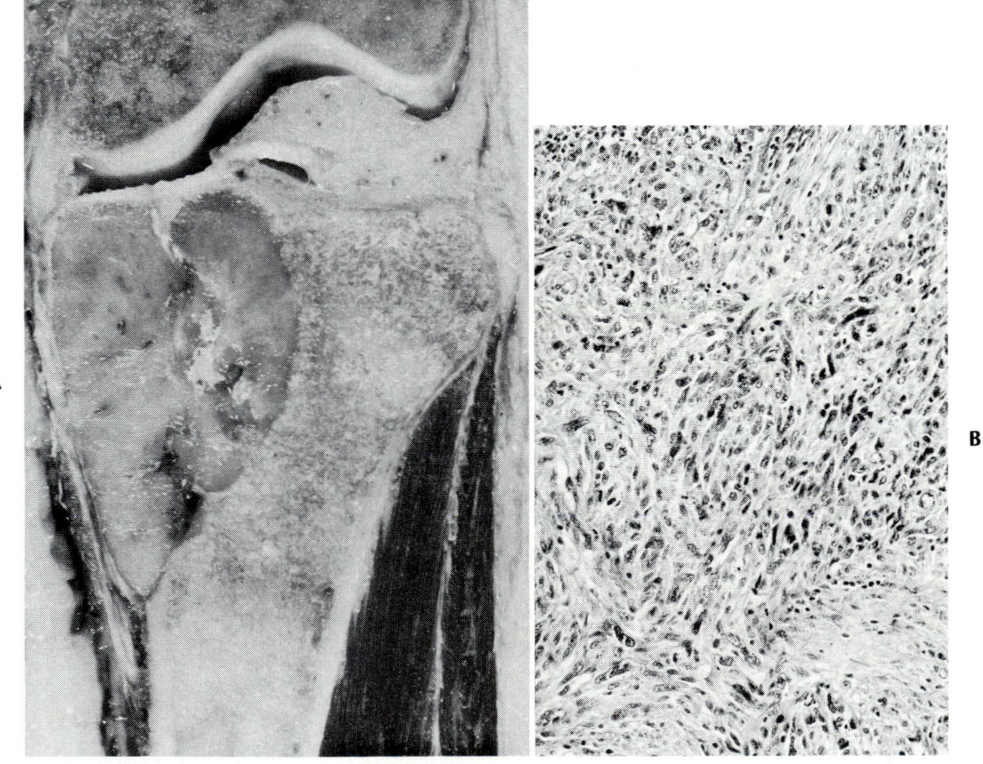

Fig. 41-27. Fibrosarcoma. **A**, Gross appearance of amputation specimen. Well-circumscribed lytic lesion involving epiphysis and metaphysis is seen. **B**, Microscopically a highly cellular proliferation of spindle tumor cells is seen. There is collagen deposition but no evidence of osteoid or bone production. (**B**, 160×.)

the metaphysis of long bones in adults. It appears roentgenographically as an osteolytic lesion with frequent extension into soft tissues.[75] Most cases arise within the medullary canal (endosteal or medullary fibrosarcomas),[34] but well-documented periosteal examples have also been reported. Grossly the tumor is whitish, firm, and homogeneous (Fig. 41-27, *A*). The microscopic appearance is similar to that of the more common fibrosarcoma of soft tissue and is characterized by atypical spindle cells that form interlacing bundles of collagen fibers *but no cartilage or bone* (Fig. 41-27, *B*). The latter feature is important in the differential diagnosis, because both osteosarcoma and chondrosarcoma can have similar spindle cell areas. Fibrosarcomas are less malignant as a group than are osteosarcomas.

OTHER PRIMARY TUMORS

Chordoma

Chordoma is believed to arise from developmental remnants of the notochord. The notochord is the original axial skeleton that is subsequently replaced by the spine; its remnants are represented by the nucleus pulposus of the intervertebral discs and small clumps of notochordal cells within the vertebral bodies. Because of their highly vacuolated cytoplasm, these cells are also known as physaliphorous (*physalis*, "bubble"; *phoros*, "bearing").

All true chordomas arise in the axial skeleton. The sacral and spheno-occipital regions are the most common sites,[69,70] with the intervening vertebrae being involved only rarely. Chordomas are slowly growing tumors. They infiltrate adjacent structures and stubbornly recur after excision. Distant metastases are rare and occur late in the course of the disease; skin and other bones are the most common sites.[26] Roentgenographically, chordomas appear as osteolytic or rarely osteoblastic processes. They may encroach on the spine and give rise to symptoms of spinal cord compression.[70] Grossly these tumors are gelatinous and soft and often contain areas of hemorrhage. Microscopically they are formed by cell cords and lobules separated by a variable but usually abundant amount of myxoid intercellular tissue (Fig. 41-28). The tumor cells are quite large, with vacuolated cytoplasm and prominent vesicular nuclei. The cytoplasm contains glycogen and mucosubstances but no fat. Areas of cartilage, bone, or fibrous tissue may be present. Some chordomas in the spheno-occipital region have an abundant cartilaginous component; they are known as chondroid chordomas and have a relatively good prognosis.[69]

Tumors microscopically resembling chordomas (and therefore sometimes known as chordoid sarcomas) are seen occasionally in the extra-axial skeleton or in soft tissues; they probably represent a morphologic variant of chondrosarcoma.

"Adamantinoma" of long bones

"Adamantinoma" of long bones, a mysterious neoplasm that shows a great predilection for the tibia, is so designated because of its microscopic resemblance to the adamantinoma (ameloblastoma) of jawbones (Fig. 41-29).[15,110] The origin of the latter tumor is the odontogenic tissue, but this can hardly be the case for its long bone counterpart. Three major tissues have been proposed as the origin: epithelial cells, blood vessels, and intraosseous synovial cells. The weight of the evidence favors

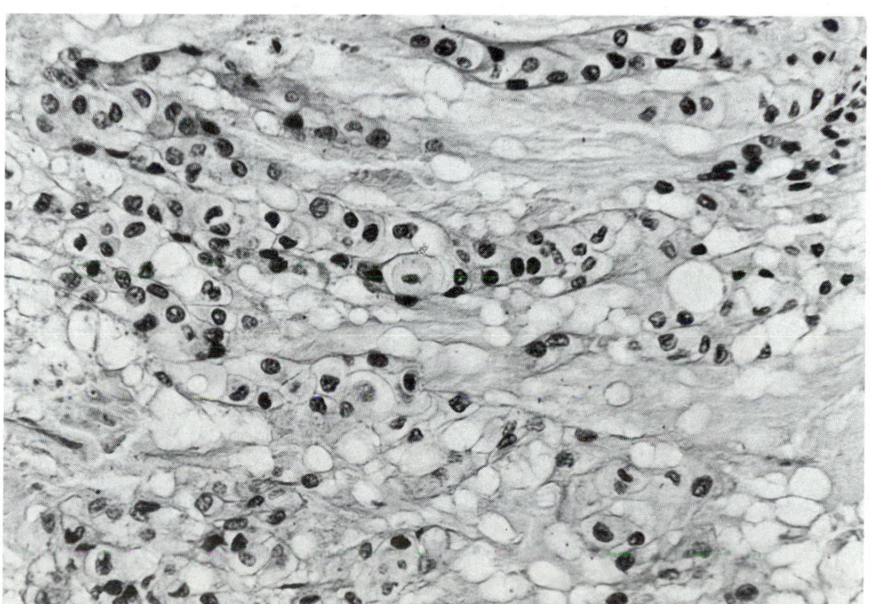

Fig. 41-28. Chordoma of spheno-occipital region. Cuboid and polyhedral cells with central nucleus form rows and nests among abundant myxoid matrix. (350×.)

the epithelial cells. The typical tumor has an obvious epithelial architecture, being formed by lobules with peripheral palisading and a central looser arrangement.[178] By electron microscopy the tumor cells contain tonofibrils and complex desmosomes, two well-known markers of epithelial cells.[178] Immunocytochemical studies have shown the presence of keratin, another well-known marker for epithelial cells.[131]

Naturally, the question arises as to how a primary epithelial tumor could arise within a long bone. Significative in this regard is that the most common location is the tibia, which is closer to the skin than any other long bone. Conceivably epithelial cells from the epidermis or its adnexa find their way beneath the periosteum, either as a result of traumatic inclusion or as an abnormality of development, and later undergo a neoplastic transformation. In support of this interpretation, there is a close morphologic similarity between "adamantinoma" of long bones and sweat gland carcinoma of the skin. It is also possible that this tumor could arise from primitive intraosseous mesenchymal cells that have retained the capacity to partially differentiate into epithelial tissue.[174]

Long bone "adamantinoma" produces rounded or oval, sometimes loculated areas of bone destruction that can be seen in roentgenograms and on gross examination. Occasionally it has a fibro-osseous component morphologically similar to that seen in fibrous dysplasia[29]; it is a malignant neoplasm, prone to local recurrence and sometimes leading to distant metastases.[169]

Tumors of peripheral nerves

Peripheral nerve tumors are rare and represented mainly by the benign neurilemoma (schwannoma), which is most often located in the mandible.[177] Although von Recklinghausen's disease is often accompanied by skeletal deformities, the occurrence of intraosseous neurofibromas is virtually nonexistent.[73]

Tumors of adipose tissue

Adipose tissue tumors are exceptional and basically represented by the benign lipoma. This is a small to

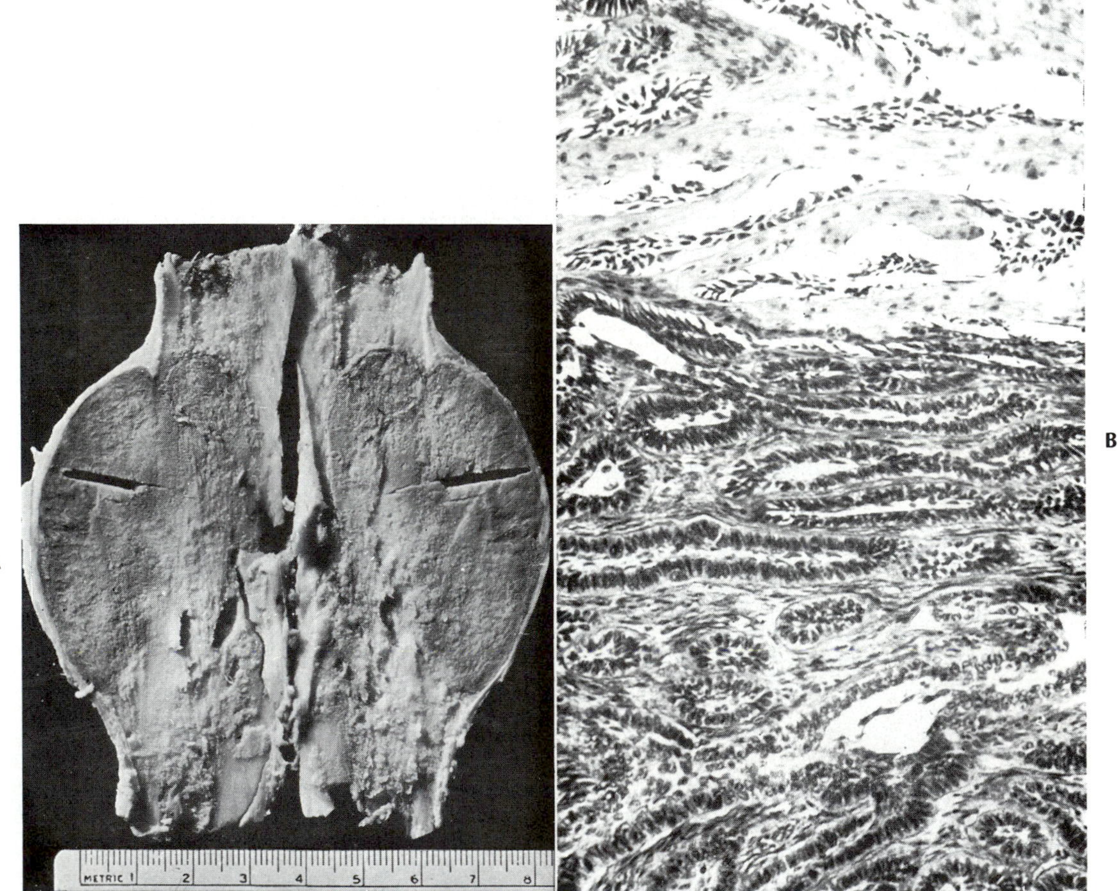

Fig. 41-29. Adamantinoma of tibia. **A,** Large, solitary tumor mass in midportion of tibia had led to sharply defined bone destruction. Neoplasm was dense but moderately cellular and friable. **B,** Alveolar arrangement of tall cylindrical cells with central fusiform and oval cells. Invasion of bone is evident at upper margin. (**B,** 145×.)

medium-sized nodule of mature fat tissue fairly well demarcated from bone marrow. Primary liposarcomas of bone exist but are rare. Most cases reported in the older literature would probably carry a different diagnosis today.

Tumors of alleged histiocytic origin

It is currently postulated that a relatively large number of soft tissue neoplasms arise from fixed histiocytes (as distinguished from the mobile histiocytes of lymphoid and hemopoietic organs),[53,86,119] or alternatively from primitive mesenchymal cells that differentiate toward histiocytes. These tumors are designated as histiocytomas and fibrous histiocytomas, the latter having in addition to the histiocytic elements a fibroblastic component, originating either from the histiocytes through a modulating process (facultative fibroblasts) or by divergent differentiation from the same primitive mesenchymal cell that gave rise to the cells with histiocytic features. Each category can be roughly subdivided into a benign and a malignant type. It is becoming evident that similar tumors exist in bone, although their frequency is certainly less than in soft tissue.[84,105] Benign histiocytomas often have a prominent component of fat-containing foamy macrophages (xanthoma cells) and are also referred to as xanthomas. The rib is the most common location. Malignant fibrous histiocytomas, also known as fibroxanthosarcomas and xanthosarcomas, predominate in long bones, where they tend to involve the medullary portion in the metaphyseal area. Roentgenographically, they appear as large lytic destructive lesions. The gross appearance is that of a variegated tumor with yellow foci alternating with areas of hemorrhage. Microscopically, spindle cells predominate. They are often arranged around a central point, producing radiating spokes grouped at right angles to each other, a pattern referred to as storiform. Foamy cells, hemosiderin-laden macrophages, and bizarre giant tumor cells are common.

Some cases of malignant fibrous histiocytomas have been reported as a late complication of bone infarcts.[108]

There is much controversy in the literature concerning the behavior to be expected from this tumor. In most series, however, the prognosis of this neoplasm has proved to be better than that of osteosarcoma.[105]

Tumors of smooth muscle

A few cases of primary leiomyosarcoma of bone have been described.[12] Most of these tumors have appeared in the lower end of the femur in adults.

METASTATIC TUMORS

Metastases to the skeletal system from neoplasms arising in other organs are the most frequent of all malignant

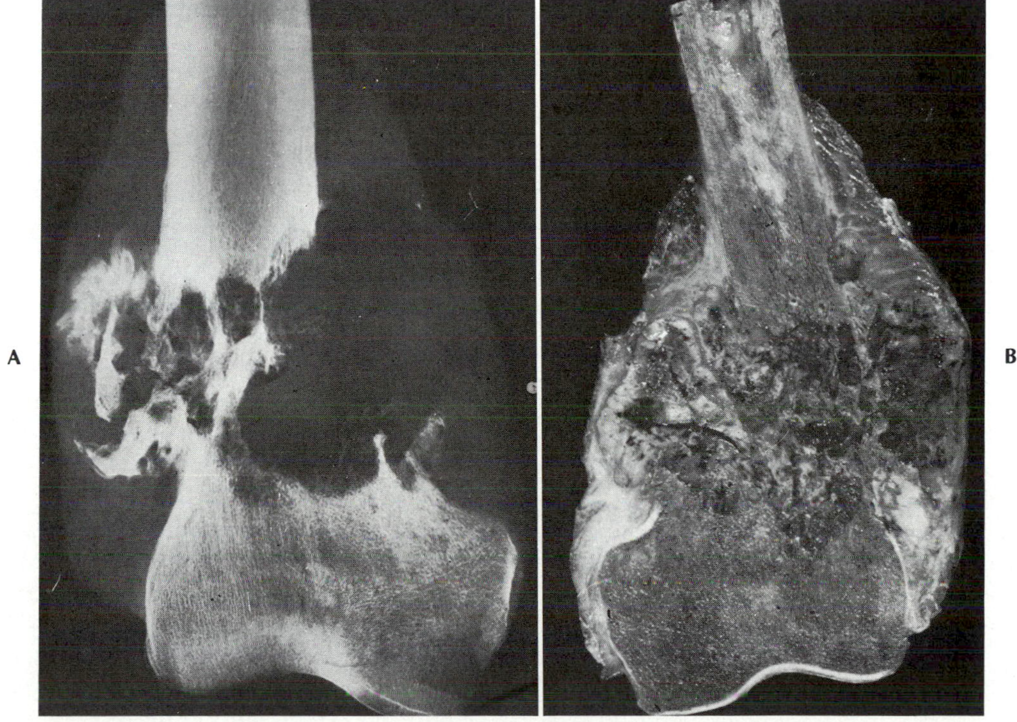

Fig. 41-30. Bone metastasis from renal cell carcinoma. **A,** Roentgenographic appearance of slice of femur showing large destructive lesion with pathologic fracture. **B,** Gross appearance of same specimen.

neoplasms of bone. Carcinomas greatly predominate over sarcomas. The most common types of carcinomas resulting in bone metastases are those that originate in the breast, prostate, lung, kidney, stomach, and thyroid. Cancers arising in other organs, such as the body and cervix of the uterus, bladder, and testicle, also may spread to bone. Melanomas and adrenal neuroblastomas sometimes give rise to extensive skeletal involvement.

The metastatic foci can be multiple or single. The latter are particularly common with thyroid and renal cancers. In order of frequency, the bones most commonly involved are the spine, pelvis, femur, skull, ribs, and humerus. Metastases to distal bones, such as the bones of forearm, wrist, hand, leg, ankle, and foot, are quite unusual. Roentgenographically, most metastases appear as destructive lytic lesions (Fig. 41-30). Others may be seen as a mixture of lytic and sclerotic changes, and still others may elicit such an exuberant osteoblastic reaction as to produce a roentgenographic sclerotic appearance. Tumors with a particular tendency to produce osteoblastic bone metastases are carcinoma of prostate, carcinoid tumor, and oat cell tumor of lung. Rarely, this feature is also seen with breast and stomach cancer.[112,164] The mechanism for the osteoblastic stimulation is not known. Metastases from renal and thyroid cancers may pulsate and give rise to an audible bruit because of their pronounced vascularity. Pathologic fracture is often the first evidence that metastasis to a bone has taken place.

The area of long bone most commonly involved by a metastatic process is the metaphysis, presumably by virtue of its greater vascularity.

As mentioned previously, sarcomas metastasize to the skeletal system only rarely. The outstanding exception is embryonal rhabdomyosarcoma of soft tissues, which is complicated by blood-borne osseous metastases in a large percentage of cases.[19] It should also be mentioned that, among primary bone tumors, Ewing's sarcoma and osteosarcoma have a certain propensity to metastasize to other regions of the skeletal system.

Skeletal metastases, when demonstrated in a patient with cancer, are obviously of great importance in determining prognosis and guiding treatment. Routinely taken bilateral core biopsy samples of the iliac crest are valuable for the early detection of bone metastases.[107] In general, the consequences of such lesions to the patient are pain that is frequently intolerable and disability to the point of complete invalidism until the patient dies of the disease.

TUMORLIKE LESIONS

Solitary bone cyst

Solitary bone cyst is a benign condition, also known as simple or unicameral bone cyst. It appears as a cavity filled with clear or blood-tinged fluid in the metaphysis of a long bone, particularly the upper ends of the humerus and femur (Fig. 41-31).[81] It may also develop in a short bone such as the calcaneus. Most cases occur in children and adolescents.[159] The pathogenesis is unknown. Microscopically the cavity is lined by a membrane of variable thickness that is formed by loose connective tissue with a scattering of osteoclasts and newly formed trabeculae of reactive nature (Fig. 41-31). Often a layer of organizing fibrin coats the inside of this membrane. Areas of recent or old hemorrhage and cholesterol clefts can sometimes be found, particularly after a fracture of the cyst. The latter is a common event. The treatment consists of curettage followed by packing of the cavity with bone chips.

Aneurysmal bone cyst

The aneurysmal bone cyst, which was often confused in the past with the giant cell tumor, is an expansile mass formed by blood-filled spaces of variable but often large size. Most cases occur in patients under 30 years of age and involve either the shaft of metaphysis of long bones or the vertebral column.[133] Pain and swelling are the main symptoms. The roentgenographic appearance is quite distinctive by virtue of the expansile nature of the mass, resulting in a ballooned-out distension of the periosteum (Fig. 41-32, *A*).[165] Grossly it forms a spongy hemorrhagic mass that may extend into the soft tissue and be covered by a thin shell of reactive bone. Microscopically most of the cysts are lined not by endothelial cells but rather by fibrous septa containing osteoid and numerous osteoclast-like multinucleated giant cells (Fig. 41-32, *B*). The pathogenesis is not clear. Some authors have postulated a persistent local alteration in hemodynamics leading to increased venous pressure and the subsequent development of a dilated and vascular bed within the transformed bone area.

Cystic changes, apparently secondary and closely resembling those of aneurysmal bone cyst, are occasionally found in chondroblastoma, fibrous dysplasia, giant cell tumor, osteosarcoma, and other lesions.[94] Therefore it is important to rule out these conditions by carefully examining the entire material when confronted with this situation.

Ganglion cyst of bone

Ganglion cyst is a common lesion of soft tissue, where it appears as a mucus-filled cystic mass in a periarticular location. Sometimes a lesion of similar appearance and pathogenesis is found within a bone, usually at the lower end of the tibia or humerus.[147] Roentgenographically, it appears as a well-defined osteolytic area with a surrounding zone of osteosclerosis, always close to the joint space. Grossly it is often multiloculated and has a gelatinous content. Microscopically it lacks synovial lining. It has

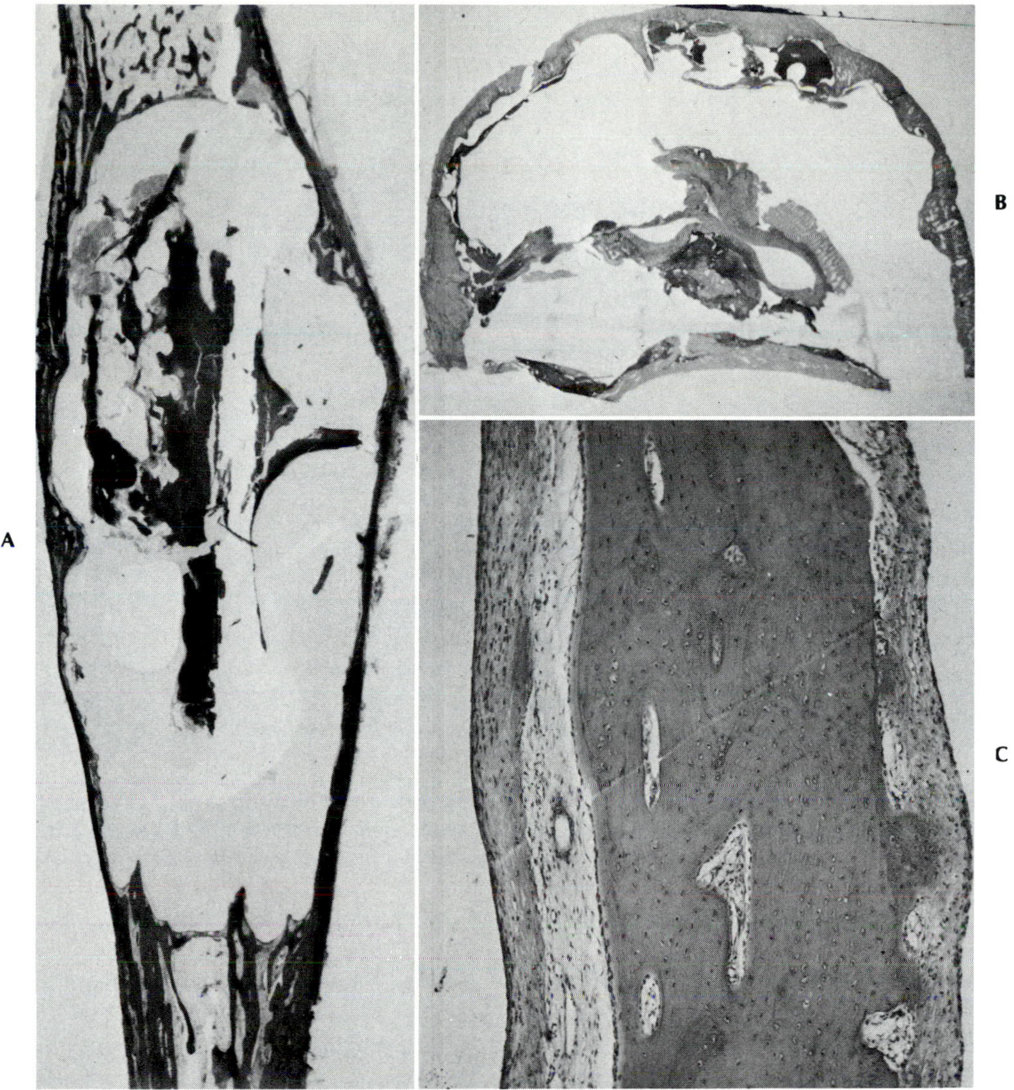

Fig. 41-31. Solitary bone cyst. **A,** Intact cyst included in longitudinal section of bone. Cortex is greatly reduced in thickness and bone shaft is widened. **B,** Cross section illustrating fibrous tissue septa that partially divide such cysts. **C,** Thin bony wall of cyst with fibrous connective tissue lining on left and proliferative changes in subperiosteal layer on exterior surface of expanded bone on right.

instead a flat fibrous lining, like its soft tissue counterpart.

Metaphyseal fibrous defect

The metaphyseal fibrous defect is a roentgenographically distinctive benign lesion occurring in the metaphyseal cortex of long bones in children (Fig. 41-33).[33] It is usually solitary but may appear as multiple or even bilaterally symmetric defects. The upper or lower tibia and the lower femur are the sites of predilection. Roentgenographically the lesion is eccentric, has sharply delimited borders, and is centered in the metaphysis. More extensive lesions, involving the medullary canal and resulting in a fusiform expansion of the bone, are sometimes referred to as nonossifying or nonosteogenic fibromas (Fig. 41-34).[80] The morphologic appearance of the two lesions is similar, suggesting that they are examples of the same entity.[156] Grossly the lesion is granular and brown or dark. Dense bone can be seen around it. Microscopically it consists of cellular masses of fibrous tissue with a storiform pattern of growth, accompanied by scattered osteoclast-like giant cells, hemosiderin-laden macrophages, and foamy cells. The lesion is often asymptomatic and is usually discovered incidentally in a roentgenogram taken for another reason.

The pathogenesis is unknown. The designation "de-

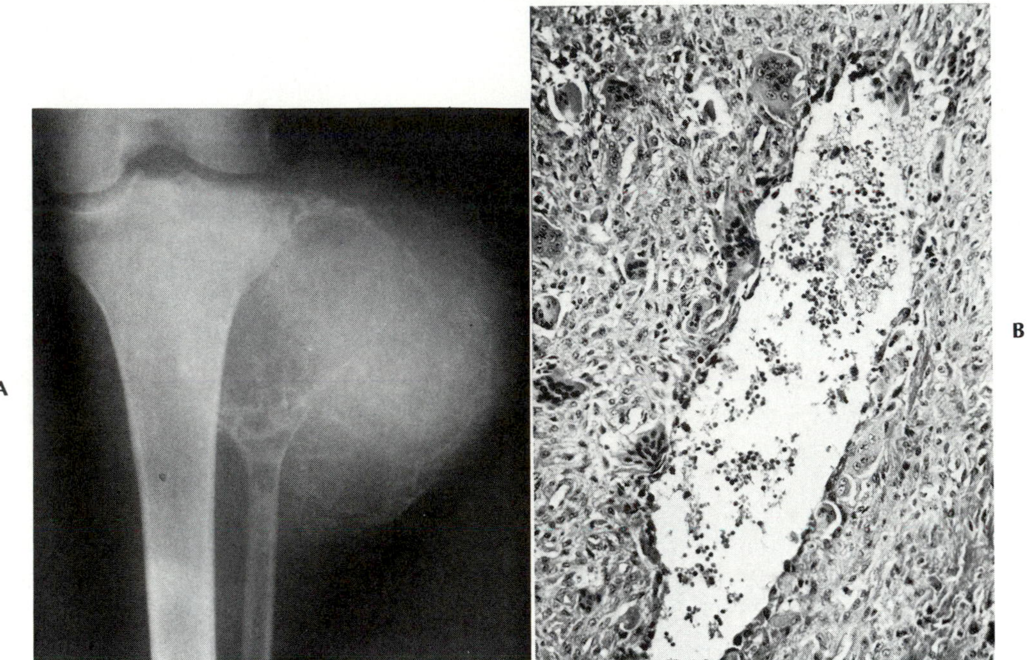

Fig. 41-32. Aneurysmal bone cyst. **A,** Roentgenogram shows ballooned-out expansile lesion of upper end of fibula. Lesion started in metaphysis but now involves entire end of bone. **B,** Microscopic hallmark of lesion is aneurysmal spaces filled with blood and partially lined by osteoclast-like giant cells. (**B,** 160×.)

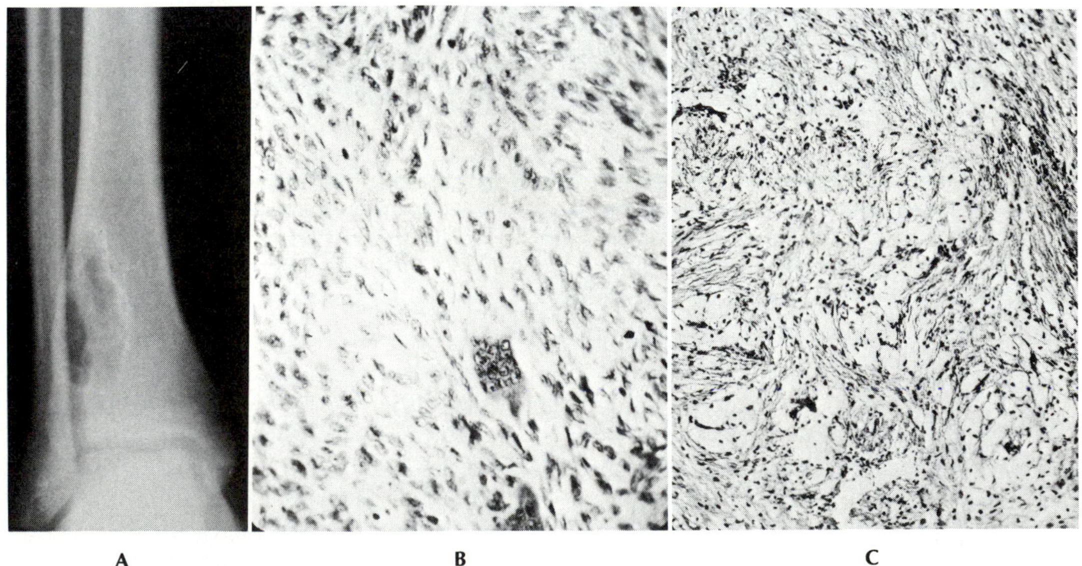

Fig. 41-33. Metaphyseal fibrous defect. **A,** Eccentric lytic area with sharply delimited sclerotic borders in metaphysis. **B,** Cellular lesion composed of plump fibroblasts and scattered giant cells. **C,** Clusters of lipid-laden histiocytes among spindle cells.

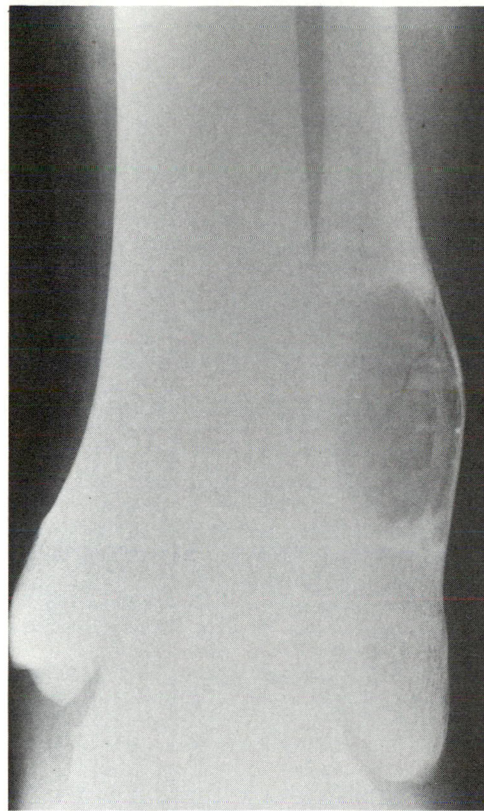

Fig. 41-34. Nonossifying fibroma with superimposed fracture. Lesion, which involves lower metaphysis of tibia, is distinguished from metaphyseal fibrous defect by virtue of its large size and presence of medullary involvement and bone expansion.

fect" implies that the lesion arises as the result of some developmental aberration at the epiphyseal plate. In favor of this interpretation is the fact that concomitant epiphyseal disorders are not infrequently present. Another possibility is that it belongs to the group of tumors described in the discussion of tumors of alleged histiocytic origin. The histologic resemblance to them is certainly pronounced.

REFERENCES

General

1. Dahlin, D.C.: Bone tumors, ed. 3, Springfield, Ill., 1978, Charles C Thomas, Publisher.
2. Huvos, A.G.: Bone tumors: diagnosis, treatment and prognosis, Philadelphia, 1979, W.B. Saunders Co.
3. Jaffe, H.L.: Tumors and tumorous conditions of the bones and joints, Philadelphia, 1958, Lea & Febiger.
4. Lichtenstein, L.: Bone tumors, ed. 5, St. Louis, 1977, The C.V. Mosby Co.
5. Mirra, J.M.: Bone tumors: diagnosis and treatment, Philadelphia, 1979, J.B. Lippincott Co.
6. Schajowicz, F.: Tumors and tumor-like lesions of bone and joints, New York, 1981, Springer-Verlag New York, Inc.
7. Schajowicz, F., Ackerman, L.V., and Sissons, H.A.: Histologic typing of bone tumours. In International Histological Classification of Tumours, No. 6, Geneva, 1972, World Health Organization.
8. Spjut, H.J., et al.: Tumors of bone and cartilage. In Atlas of tumor pathology, Section 2, Fascicle 5, Washington, D.C., 1971, Armed Forces Institute of Pathology.

Specific

9. Ahuja, S.C., et al.: Juxtacortical (parosteal) osteogenic sarcoma: histologic grading and prognosis, J. Bone Joint Surg. **59A:**632, 1977.
10. Amstutz, H.C.: Multiple osteogenic sarcomata—metastatic or multicentric? Report of two cases and review of literature, Cancer **24:**923, 1969.
11. Anderson, W.A.D., Zander, G.E., and Kuzma, J.F.: Cancerogenic effects of Ca^{45} and Sr^{89} on bones of CF_1 mice, Arch. Pathol. **62:**262, 1956.
12. Angervall, L., et al.: Primary leiomyosarcoma of bone: a study of five cases, Cancer **46:**1270, 1980.
13. Angervall, L., and Enzinger, F.M.: Extraskeletal neoplasm resembling Ewing's sarcoma, Cancer **36:**240, 1975.
14. Azar, H.A.: Plasma cell myelomatosis and other monoclonal gammopathies, Pathol. Annu. **7:**1, 1972.
15. Baker, P.L., Dockerty, M.B., and Coventry, M.B.: Adamantinoma (so-called) of the long bones, J. Bone Joint Surg. **36A:**704, 1954.
16. Barnes, R., and Catto, M.: Chondrosarcoma of bone, J. Bone Joint Surg. **48B:**729, 1966.
17. Boston, H.C., Jr., et al.: Malignant lymphoma (so-called reticulum cell sarcoma) of bone, Cancer **34:**1131, 1974.
18. Byers, P.D.: Solitary benign osteoblastic lesions of bone—osteoid osteoma and benign osteoblastoma, Cancer **22:**43, 1968.
19. Caffey, J., and Andersen, D.H.: Metastatic embryonal rhabdomyosarcoma in the growing skeleton: clinical, radiographic, and microscopic features, Am. J. Dis. Child. **95:**581, 1958.
20. Campanacci, M., Boriani, S., and Giunti, A.: Hemangioendothelioma of bone: a study of 29 cases, Cancer **46:**804, 1980.
21. Campanacci, M., and Cervellati, G.: Osteosarcoma: a review of 345 cases, Ital. J. Orthop. Traumatol. **1:**5, 1975.
22. Campanacci, M., Giunti, A. and Olmi, R.: Giant-cell tumours of bone: a study of 209 cases with long-term followup in 130, Ital. J. Orthop. Traumatol. **1:**249, 1975.
23. Campanacci, M., et al.: Chondrosarcoma: a study of 133 cases, 80 with long term follow up, Ital. J. Orthop. Traumatol. **1:**387, 1975.
24. Carbone, P.P., Kellerhouse, L.E., and Gehan, E.A.: Plasmacytic myeloma: a study of the relationship of survival to various clinical manifestations and anomalous protein type in 112 patients, Am. J. Med. **42:**937, 1967.
25. Chabner, B.A., Haskell, C.M., and Canellos, G.P.: Destructive bone lesions in chronic granulocytic leukemia, Medicine **48:**401, 1969.
26. Chambers, P.W. and Schwinn, C.P.: Chordoma: a clinicopathologic study of metastasis, Am. J. Clin. Pathol. **72:**765, 1979.
27. Chan, R.C., et al.: Management and results of localized Ewing's sarcoma, Cancer **43:**1001, 1979.
28. Chang, C.H.J., et al.: Bone abnormalities in Gardner's syndrome, Am. J. Roentgenol. Radium Ther. Nucl. Med. **103:**645, 1968.
29. Cohen, D.M., Dahlin, D.C., and Pugh, D.G.: Fibrous dysplasia associated with adamantinoma of the long bones, Cancer **15:**515, 1961.
30. Corwin, J., and Lindberg, R.D.: Solitary plasmacytoma of bone vs. extramedullary plasmacytoma and their relationship to multiple myeloma, Cancer **43:**1007, 1979.
31. Cowan, W.K.: Malignant change and multiple metastases in Ollier's disease, J. Clin. Pathol. **18:**650, 1965.
32. Cruz, M., Coley, B.C., and Stewart, F.W.: Postradiation bone sarcoma, Cancer **10:**72, 1957.
33. Cunningham, J.B., and Ackerman, L.V.: Metaphyseal fibrous defects, J. Bone Joint Surg. **38A:**797, 1956.
34. Cunningham, M.P., and Arlen, M.: Medullary fibrosarcoma of bone, Cancer **21:**31, 1968.
35. Dahlin, D.C.: Chondromyxoid fibroma of bone, with emphasis on its morphological relationship to benign chondroblastoma, Cancer **9:**195, 1956.

36. Dahlin, D.C., and Beabout, J.W.: Dedifferentiation of low-grade chondrosarcomas, Cancer **9**:461, 1971.
37. Dahlin, D.C., and Coventry, M.B.: Osteogenic sarcoma: a study of 600 cases, J. Bone Joint Surg. **49A**:101, 1967.
38. Dahlin, D.C., Cupps, R.E., and Johnson, E.W., Jr.: Giant-cell tumor: a study of 195 cases, Cancer **25**:1061, 1970.
39. Dahlin, D.C., and Henderson, E.D.: Chondrosarcoma, a surgical and pathological problem, J. Bone Joint Surg. **38A**:1025, 1956.
40. Dahlin, D.C., and Ivins, J.C.: Fibrosarcoma of bone: a study of 114 cases, Cancer **23**:35, 1969.
41. Dahlin, D.C., and Unni, K.K.: Osteosarcoma of bone and its important recognizable varieties, Am. J. Surg. Pathol. **1**:61, 1977.
42. Delbruck, H.G., et al.: Bone tumors induced in rats with radioactive cerium, Br. J. Cancer **41**:809, 1980.
43. DeSantos, L.A., Murray, J.A., and Ayala, A.G.: The value of percutaneous needle biopsy in the management of primary bone tumors, Cancer **43**:735, 1979.
44. de Souza Dias, L., and Frost, H.M.: Osteoid osteoma—osteoblastoma, Cancer **33**:1075, 1974.
45. Dorfman, H.D.: Malignant transformation of benign bone lesions. In Proceedings of the Seventh National Cancer Conference, vol. 7, Philadelphia, 1973, J.B. Lippincott Co.
46. Dorfman, H.D., Steiner, G.C.,and Jaffe, H.L.: Vascular tumors of bone, Hum. Pathol. **2**:349, 1971.
47. Driedger, H., and Pruzanski, W.: Plasma cell neoplasia with osteosclerotic lesions: a study of five cases and a review of the literature, Arch. Intern. Med. **139**:892, 1979.
48. Dumont, J., and Mazabraud, A.: Primary lymphomas of bone (so-called "Parker and Jackson's reticulum cell sarcoma"): histological review of 75 cases according to the new classifications of non Hodgkin's lymphomas, Biomedicine (Express) **31**:271, 1979.
49. Edeiken, J., et al.: Parosteal sarcoma, Am. J. Roentgenol. Radium Ther. Nucl. Med. **111**:579, 1971.
50. Enneking, W.F., editor: Osteosarcoma, Symposium Clin. Orthop. **111**:1, 1975.
51. Enneking, W.F., and Kagan, A.: "Skip" metastases in osteosarcoma, Cancer **36**:2192, 1975.
52. Evans, H.L., Ayala, A.G., and Romsdahl, M.M.: Prognostic factors in chondrosarcoma of bone: a clinicopathologic analysis with emphasis on histologic grading, Cancer **40**:818, 1977.
53. Feldman, F., and Norman, D.: Intra- and extraosseous malignant histiocytoma (malignant fibrous xanthoma), Radiology **104**:497, 1972.
54. Finkel, M.P., Biskis, B.O., and Farrell, C.: Osteosarcomas appearing in Syrian hamsters after treatment with extracts of human osteosarcomas, Proc. Natl. Acad. Sci. U.S.A. **60**:1223, 1968.
55. Finkel, M.P., Biskis, B.O., and Jinkins, P.B.: Virus induction of osteosarcoma in mice, Science **151**:698, 1966.
56. Fisher, E.R., and Zawadski, A.: Ultrastructural features of plasma cells in patients with paraproteinemias, Am. J. Clin. Pathol. **54**:779, 1970.
57. Fraumeni, J.F., Jr.: Stature and malignant tumors of bone in childhood and adolescence, Cancer **20**:967, 1967.
58. Frentzel-Beyme, R., and Wagner, G.: Malignant bone tumours: status of aetiological knowledge and needs of epidemiological research, Arch. Orthop. Trauma Surg. **94**:81, 1979.
59. Furey, J.G., Ferrer-Torells, M., and Reagan, J.W.: Fibrosarcoma arising at the site of bone infarcts: a report of two cases, J. Bone Joint Surg. **42A**:802, 1960.
60. Ginaldi, S., and de Santos, L.A.: Computed tomography in the evaluation of small round cell tumors of bone, Radiology **134**:441, 1980.
61. Glass, A.G., and Fraumeni, J.F., Jr.: Epidemiology of bone cancer in children, J. Natl. Cancer Inst. **44**:187, 1970.
62. Gorham, L.W., and Stout, A.P.: Massive osteolysis (acute spontaneous absorption of bone, phantom bone, disappearing bone): its relation to hemangiomatosis, J. Bone Joint Surg. **37A**:985, 1955.
63. Guccion, J.G., et al.: Extraskeletal mesenchymal chondrosarcoma, Arch. Pathol. **95**:336, 1973.
64. Gyorkey, F., Sinkovics, J.G., and Gyorkey, P.: Electron microscopic observations on structures resembling myxovirus in human sarcomas, Cancer **27**:1449, 1971.
65. Hallberg, O.E., and Begley, J.W., Jr.: Origin and treatment of osteomas of the paranasal sinuses, Arch. Otolaryngol. **51**:750, 1950.
66. Hanaoka, H., Friedman, B., and Mack, R.P.: Ultrastructure and histogenesis of giant cell tumor of bone, Cancer **25**:1408, 1970.
67. Harmon, T.P., and Morton, K.S.: Osteogenic sarcoma in four siblings, J. Bone Joint Surg. **48B**:493, 1966.
68. Hatcher, C.H.: The development of sarcoma in bone subjected to roentgen or radium irradiation, J. Bone Joint Surg. **27**:179, 1945.
69. Heffelfinger, M.J., et al.: Chordomas and cartilaginous tumors at the skull base, Cancer **32**:410, 1973.
70. Higinbotham, N.L., et al.: Chordoma: thirty-five-year study at Memorial Hospital, Cancer **20**:1841, 1967.
71. Horan, F.T.: Bone involvement in Hodgkin's disease, Br. J. Surg. **56**:277, 1969.
72. Howard, E.B., et al.: Strontium-90–induced bone tumors in miniature swine, Radiat. Res. **39**:594, 1969.
73. Hunt, J.C., and Pugh, D.G.: Skeletal lesions in neurofibromatosis, Radiology **76**:1, 1961.
74. Hutter, R.V.P., et al.: Giant cell tumors complicating Paget's disease of bone, Cancer **16**:1044, 1963.
75. Huvos, A.G., and Higinbotham, N.L.: Primary fibrosarcoma of bone: a clinicopathologic study of 130 patients, Cancer **35**:837, 1975.
76. Huvos, A.G., Higinbotham, N.L., and Miller, T.R.: Bone sarcomas arising in fibrous dysplasia, J. Bone Joint Surg. **54A**:1047, 1972.
77. Huvos, A.G., et al.: Chondroblastoma of bone: a clinico-pathologic and electron microscopic study, Cancer **29**:760, 1972.
78. Jacobson, S.A.: Polyhistioma: a malignant tumor of bone and extraskeletal tissues, Cancer **40**:2116, 1977.
79. Jaffe, H.L.: Tumors and tumorous conditions of the bones and joint, Philadelphia, 1958, Lea & Febiger.
80. Jaffe, H.L., and Lichtenstein, L.: Nonosteogenic fibroma of bone, Am. J. Pathol. **18**:205, 1942.
81. Jaffe, H.L., and Lichtenstein, L.: Solitary unicameral bone cyst, Arch. Surg. **44**:1004, 1942.
82. Jaffe, N., et al.: Local en bloc resection for limb preservation, Cancer Treat. Rep. **62**:217, 1978.
83. Kahn, L.B., Wood, F.M., and Ackerman, L.V.: Malignant chondroblastoma: report of two cases and review of the literature, Arch. Pathol. **88**:371, 1969.
84. Kahn, L.B., et al.: Malignant fibrous histiocytoma (malignant fibrous xanthoma: xanthosarcoma) of bone, Cancer **42**:640, 1978.
85. Kasahara, K., Yamamuro, T., and Kasahara, A.: Giant-cell tumour of bone: cytological studies, Br. J. Cancer **40**:201, 1979.
86. Kempson, R.L., and Kyriakos, M.: Fibroxanthosarcoma of the soft tissues: a type of malignant fibrous histiocytoma, Cancer **29**:961, 1972.
87. Kuettner, K.E., Pauli, B.E., and Soble, L.: Morphological studies on the resistance of cartilage to invasion by osteosarcoma cells in vitro and in vivo, Cancer Res. **38**:277, 1978.
88. Kyriakos, M.: Soft tissue implantation of chondromyxoid fibroma, Am. J. Surg. Pathol. 3:363, 1979.
89. Lacassagne, A.: Conditions dans lesquelles ont été obtenus, chez le lapin, des cancers par action des rayons x sur des foyers inflammatoires, C.R. Soc. Biol. **112**:562, 1933.
90. Lagacé, R., et al.: Desmoplastic fibroma of bone: an ultrastructural study, Am. J. Surg. Pathol. 3:423, 1979.
91. Laissue, J.A., et al.: Induction of osteosarcomas and hematopoietic neoplasms by ^{55}Fe in mice, Cancer Res. **37**:3545, 1977.
92. Landon, G.C., Johnson, K.A., and Dahlin, D.C.: Subungual exostoses, J. Bone Joint Surg. **61A**:256, 1979.
93. Levine, G.D., and Bensch, K.G.: Chondroblastoma—the nature of the basic cell: a study by means of histochemistry, tissue culture, electron microscopy, and autoradiography, Cancer **29**:1546, 1972.

94. Levy, W.M., et al.: Aneurysmal bone cyst secondary to other osseous lesions: report of 57 cases, Am. J. Clin. Pathol. **63**:1, 1975.
95. Lewis, R.J., and Ketcham, A.S.: Maffucci's syndrome: functional and neoplastic significance; case report and review of the literature, J. Bone Joint Surg. **55A**:1465, 1973.
96. Lewis, R.J., and Lotz, M.J.: Medullary extension of osteosarcoma: implications for rational therapy, Cancer **33**:371, 1974.
97. Lichtenstein, L., and Hall, J.E.: Periosteal chondroma: a distinctive benign cartilage tumor, J. Bone Joint Surg. **34**:691, 1952.
98. Mackenzie, D.H.: Intraosseous glomus: report of two cases, J. Bone Joint Surg. **44B**:648, 1962.
99. MacLennan, D.I., and Wilson, F.C., Jr.: Osteoid osteoma of the spine: a review of the literature and report of six new cases, J. Bone Joint Surg. **49A**:111, 1967.
100. Mahoney, J.P., and Alexander, R.W.: Ewing's sarcoma: a light and electron microscopic study of 21 cases, Am. J. Surg. Pathol. **2**:283, 1978.
101. Mahoney, J.P., and Alexander, R.W.: Primary histiocytic lymphoma of bone: a light and ultrastructural study of four cases, Am. J. Surg. Pathol. **4**:149, 1980.
102. Mann, R.B., Jaffe, E.S., and Berard, C.W.: Malignant lymphomas—a conceptual understanding of morphologic diversity: a review, Am. J. Pathol. **94**:105, 1979.
103. Martland, H.S., and Humphries, R.E.: Osteogenic sarcoma in dial painters using luminous paint, Arch. Pathol. **7**:406, 1929.
104. Matsuno, T.: Telangiectatic osteogenic sarcoma, Cancer **38**:2538, 1976.
105. McCarthy, E.F., Matsuno, T., and Dorfman, H.D.: Malignant fibrous histocytoma of bone: a study of 35 cases, Hum. Pathol. **10**:57, 1979.
106. McKenna, R.J., et al.: Sarcomata of the osteogenic series (osteosarcoma, fibrosarcoma, chondrosarcoma, parosteal osteogenic sarcoma, and sarcomata arising in abnormal bone), J. Bone Joint Surg. **48A**:1, 1966
107. Meinshausen, J., Choritz, H., and Georgii, A.: Frequency of skeletal metastases as revealed by routinely taken bone marrow biopsies, Virchows Arch. (Pathol. Anat.) **389**:409, 1980.
108. Mirra, J.M., et al.: Malignant fibrous histiocytoma and osteosarcoma in association with bone infarcts, J. Bone Joint Surg. **56A**:932, 1974.
109. Monkman, G.R., Orwoll, G., and Ivins, J.C.: Trauma and oncogenesis, Mayo Clin. Proc. **49**:157, 1974.
110. Moon, N.F.: Adamantinoma of the appendicular skeleton: a statistical review of reported cases and inclusion of 10 new cases, Clin. Orthop. **43**:189, 1965.
111. Morton, D.L., and Malmgren, R.A.: Human osteosarcomas: immunologic evidence suggesting an associated infectious agent, Science **162**:1279, 1968.
112. Muggia, F.M., and Hansen, H.H.: Osteoblastic metastases in small-cell (oat-cell) carcinoma of the lung, Cancer **30**:801, 1972.
113. Murphy, W.R., and Ackerman, L.V.: Benign and malignant giant-cell tumors of bone, Cancer **9**:317, 1956.
114. Nakata, Y., et al.: Identification of type A and type C virus particles in BF murine osteosarcoma, Cancer Res. **40**:127, 1980.
115. Nascimento, A.G., Huvos, A.G., and Marcove, R.C.: Primary malignant giant cell tumor of bone: a study of eight cases and review of the literature, Cancer **44**:1393, 1979.
116. Nascimento, A.G., et al.: A clinicopathologic study of 20 cases of large-cell (atypical) Ewing's sarcoma of bone, Am. J. Surg. Pathol. **4**:29, 1980.
117. Olson, H.M., and Capen, C.C.: Virus induced animal model of osteosarcoma in the rat, Am. J. Pathol. **86**:437, 1977.
118. O'Neal, L.W., and Ackerman, L.V.: Chondrosarcoma of bone, Cancer **5**:551, 1952.
119. Ozzello, L., Stout, A.P., and Murray, M.R.: Cultural characteristics of malignant histiocytomas and fibrous xanthomas, Cancer **16**:331, 1963.
120. Pasmantier, M.W., and Azar, H.A.: Extraskeletal spread in multiple plasma cell myeloma: a review of 57 autopsied cases, Cancer **23**:167, 1969.
121. Pilepich, M.V., et al.: Radiotherapy and combination chemotherapy in advanced Ewing's sarcoma—intergroup study, Cancer **47**:1930, 1981.
122. Pritchard, D.J., Finkel, M.P., and Reilly, C.A.: The etiology of osteosarcoma: a review of current considerations, Clin. Orthop. **111**:14, 1975.
123. Pritchard, D.J., et al.: Chondrosarcoma: a clinicopathologic and statistical analysis, Cancer **45**:149, 1980.
124. Rabhan, W.N., and Rosai, J.: Desmoplastic fibroma: report of ten cases and review of the literature, J. Bone Joint Surg. **50A**:487, 1968.
125. Rahimi, A., et al.: Chondromyxoid fibroma: a clinicopathologic study of 76 cases, Cancer **30**:726, 1972.
126. Reddick, R.L., et al.: Osteogenic sarcoma: a study of the ultrastructure, Cancer **45**:64, 1980.
127. Reimer, R.R., et al.: Lymphoma presenting in bone: results of histopathology, staging, and therapy, Ann. Intern. Med. **87**:50, 1977.
128. Revell, P.A., and Scholtz, C.L.: Aggressive osteoblastoma, J. Pathol. **127**:195, 1979.
129. Reyes, C.V., and Kathuria, S.: Recurrent and aggressive chondroblastoma of the pelvis with late malignant neoplastic changes, Am. J. Surg. Pathol. **3**:449, 1979.
130. Rosai, J., Gold, J., and Landy, R.: The histiocytoid hemangiomas: a unifying concept embracing several previously described entities of skin, soft tissue, large vessels, bone, and heart, Hum. Pathol. **10**:707, 1979.
131. Rosai, J., and Pinkus, G.S.: Immunocytochemical demonstration of epithelial differentiation in adamantinoma of the tibia, Am. J. Surg. Pathol. **6**:427, 1982.
132. Rosen, G., et al.: Ewing's sarcoma: ten-year experience with adjuvant chemotherapy, Cancer **47**:2204, 1981.
133. Ruiter, D.J., van Rijssel, T.G., and van der Velde, E.A.: Aneurysmal bone cysts: a clinicopathological study of 105 cases, Cancer **39**:2231, 1977.
134. Salvador, A.H., Beabout, J.W., and Dahlin, D.C.: Mesenchymal chondrosarcoma: observations on 30 new cases, Cancer **28**:605, 1971.
135. Sanerkin, N.G.: Malignancy, aggressiveness, and recurrence in giant cell tumor of bone, Cancer **46**:1641, 1980.
136. Sanerkin, N.G., and Gallagher, P.: A review of the behaviour of chondrosarcoma of bone, J. Bone Joint Surg. **61A**:395, 1979.
137. Schajowicz, F.: Ewing's sarcoma and reticulum-cell sarcoma of bone: with special reference to the histochemical demonstration of glycogen as an aid to differential diagnosis, J. Bone Joint Surg. **41A**:349, 1959.
138. Schajowicz, F.: Giant-cell tumors of bone (osteoclastoma): a pathological and histochemical study, J. Bone Joint Surg. **43A**:1, 1961.
139. Schajowicz, F.: Juxtacortical chondrosarcoma, J. Bone Joint Surg. **59A**:473, 1977.
140. Schajowicz, F., Ackerman, L.V., and Sissons, H.A.: Histologic typing of bone tumours. In International Histological Classification of Tumours, No. 6, Geneva, 1972, World Health Organization.
141. Schajowicz, F., and Bessone, J.E.: Chondrosarcoma in three brothers, J. Bone Joint Surg. **43A**:1, 1961.
142. Schajowicz, F., and Derqui, J.C.: Puncture biopsy in lesions of the locomotor system: review of results in 4,050 cases, including 941 vertebral punctures, Cancer **21**:531, 1968.
143. Schajowicz, F., and Gallardo, H.: Epiphysial chondroblastoma of bone: a clinico-pathological study of sixty-nine cases, J. Bone Joint Surg. **52B**:205, 1970.
144. Schajowicz, F., and Gallardo, H.: Chondromyxoid fibroma (fibromyxoid chondroma) of bone: a clinico-pathological study of thirty-two cases, J. Bone Joint Surg. **53B**:198, 1971.
145. Schajowicz, F., and Lemos, C.: Osteoid osteoma and osteoblastoma, Acta Orthop. Scand. **41**:272, 1970.
146. Schajowicz, F., and Lemos, C.: Malignant osteoblastoma, J. Bone Joint Surg. **58B**:202, 1976.
147. Schajowicz, F., Sainz, M.C., and Slullitel, J.A.: Juxta-articular bone cysts (intra-osseous ganglia), J. Bone Joint Surg. **61B**:107, 1979.
148. Schwartz, D.T., and Alpert, M.: The malignant transformation of fibrous dysplasia, Am. J. Med. Sci. **247**:1, 1964.

149. Scranton, P.E., et al.: Prognostic factors in osteosarcoma: a review of 20 years' experience at the University of Pittsburgh Health Center Hospitals, Cancer **36:**2179, 1975.
150. Shoji, H., and Miller, T.R.: Primary reticulum cell sarcoma of bone: significance of clinical features upon the prognosis, Cancer **28:**1234, 1971.
151. Sindelar, W.F., Costa, J., and Ketcham, A.S.: Osteosarcoma associated with Thorotrast administration, Cancer **42:**2604, 1978.
152. Singh, I., Tsang, K.Y., and Blakemore, W.S.: Immunologic studies in contacts of osteosarcoma in humans and animals, Nature **265:**541, 1977.
153. Spiess, H., Poppe, H., and Schoen, H.: Strahleninduzierte Knochentumoren nach Thorium X-Behandlung, Monatsschr. Kinderheilkd. **110:**198, 1962.
154. Spjut, H.J., and Lindbom, A.: Skeletal angiomatosis: report of two cases, Acta Pathol. Microbiol. Scand. **55:**49, 1962.
155. Spjut, H.J., et al.: Tumors of bone and cartilage. In Atlas of tumor pathology, Section II, Fascicle 5, Washington, D.C., 1971, Armed Forces Institute of Pathology.
156. Steiner, G.C.: Fibrous cortical defect and nonossifying fibroma of bone, Arch. Pathol. **97:**205, 1974.
157. Steiner, G.C., Ghosh, L., and Dorfman, H.D.: Ultrastructure of giant cell tumors of bone, Hum. Pathol. **3:**569, 1972.
158. Stern, R., et al.: Procollagens as markers for the cell of origin of human bone tumors, Cancer Res. **40:**325, 1980.
159. Stewart, M.J., and Hamel, H.A.: Solitary bone cyst, South. Med. J. **43:**926, 1950.
160. Suit, H.D.: Role of therapeutic radiology in cancer of bone, Cancer **35:**930, 1975.
161. Takigawa, K.: Chondroma of the bones of the hand, J. Bone Joint Surg. **53A:**1591, 1971.
162. Tapp, E.: Osteogenic sarcoma in rabbits following subperiosteal implantation of beryllium, Arch. Pathol. **88:**89, 1969.
163. Telles, N.C., Rabson, A.S., and Pomeroy, T.C.: Ewing's sarcoma: an autopsy study, Cancer **41:**2321, 1978.
164. Thomas, B.M.: Three unusual carcinoid tumours, with particular reference to osteoblastic bone metastases, Clin. Radiol. **19:**221, 1968.
165. Tillman, B.P., et al.: Aneurysmal bone cyst: an analysis of 95 cases, Mayo Clin. Proc. **43:**478, 1968.
166. Turner, R.C.: Unusual group of tumours among schoolgirls, Br. J. Cancer **21:**17, 1966.
167. Unni, K.K., and Dahlin, D.C.: Premalignant tumors and conditions of bone, Am. J. Surg. Pathol. **3:**47, 1979.
168. Unni, K.K., et al.: Hemangioma, hemangiopericytoma, and hemangioendothelioma (angiosarcoma) of bone, Cancer **27:**1403, 1971.
169. Unni, K.K., et al.: Adamantinomas of long bones, Cancer **34:**1796, 1974.
170. Unni, K.K., et al.: Parosteal osteogenic sarcoma, Cancer **37:**2466, 1976.
171. Unni, K.K., et al.: Intraosseous well-differentiated osteosarcoma, Cancer **40:**1337, 1977.
172. Varela-Duran, J., and Dehner, L.P.: Postirradiation osteosarcoma in childhood: a clinicopathologic study of three cases and review of the literature, Am. J. Pediatr. Hematol. Oncol. **2:**263, 1980.
173. Weatherby, R.P., Dahlin, D.C., and Ivins, J.C.: Postradiation sarcoma of bone: review of 78 Mayo Clinic cases, Mayo Clin. Proc. **56:**294, 1981.
174. Weiss, S.W., and Dorfman, H.D.: Adamantinoma of long bone: an analysis of nine new cases with emphasis on metastasizing lesions and fibrous dysplasia–like changes, Hum. Pathol. **8:**141, 1977.
175. Wick, M.R., et al.: Sarcomas of bone complicating osteitis deformans (Paget's disease): fifty years' experience, Am. J. Surg. Pathol. **5:**47, 1981.
176. Wiltshaw, E.: The natural history of extramedullary plasmacytoma and its relation to solitary myeloma of bone and myelomatosis, Medicine **55:**217, 1976.
177. Wirth, W.A., and Bray, C.B.: Intra-osseous neurilemoma: case report and review of thirty-one cases from the literature, J. Bone Joint Surg. **59A:**252, 1977,
178. Yoneyama, T., Winter, W.G., and Milsow, L.: Tibial adamantinoma: its histogenesis from ultrastructural studies, Cancer **40:**1138, 1977.

CHAPTER 42 Diseases of Joints

RUTH SILBERBERG

NORMAL JOINT STRUCTURE AND FUNCTION

Diarthrodial joints

The joints most commonly affected by disease are the diarthrodial or synovial joints. Unlike the serosal cavities of pleurae and peritoneum, joint spaces are not closed or lined by a continuous layer of mesothelial cells. Instead, they are open tissue spaces, communicating directly with the periarticular tissues.

The articulating ends of two bones are held together by the joint capsule, a tubular structure of dense connective tissue inserting at the outer surfaces of the bony shafts. The capsule has an abundant supply of sensory nerve fibers that are highly sensitive to stretching and twisting and that are primarily responsible for the intense pain accompanying many joint lesions. Ligaments and tendons insert at the outer surface of the capsule. The capsule is lined by the synovial membrane, or synovium, which also cover the soft structures within the joints, fat pads, and ligaments and which forms outpouchings (bursae). The bursae communicate with the joint space and are therefore likely to become involved in pathologic processes affecting the joints and vice versa. The articulating surfaces of the bones are covered by bluish glistening hyaline cartilage, which varies in thickness not only in different joints but also within the same joint, with weight-bearing areas usually having a thicker cartilage cover than non-weight-bearing areas. The cartilage is supported by a layer of cancellous bone.[94]

A small amount of free viscid fluid is present in the joint space and, by forming a thin layer over the cartilage, acts as a lubricant during joint motion.

Histologically and by electron microscopy, the surface of the articular cartilage is not smooth but shows innumerable roundish pits 20 to 30 μm in diameter, which correspond to the underlying most superficially located cartilage cells. The articular surface proper is entirely composed of matrix with cells. This architecture is of importance to the nutrition of the avascular articular cartilage, since it facilitates the flow of the synovial fluid into the cartilage. The chondrocytes vary in size, shape, and distribution. Three zones are usually distinguishable: a superficial zone characterized by spindle-shaped cells with their long axis oriented circumferentially; an intermediate or midzone of groups or small columns of polygonal cells, which are capable of multiplying and which are highly active metabolically; and the deepest, the pressure zone, possessing the largest cells, often in perpendicular orientation to the joint surface and separated from the underlying bone by a narrow layer of calcified matrix. By electron microscopy, articular chondrocytes have been shown to possess all the subcellular organelles of cells engaged in active synthesis and secretion—rough endoplasmic reticulum, free ribosomes, a Golgi apparatus, mitochondria, and so on. They produce the intercellular matrix and have been shown to respond readily to changes in the internal environment.[215]

The matrix of the articular cartilage is composed of an amorphous phase (the ground substance) and a fibrillar phase (collagen fibrils). The ground substance contains water, minerals, and a variety of protein-polysaccharides (glycosaminoglycans or proteoglycans), chiefly chondroitin sulfates A and C and keratan sulfate,[195] that are responsible for the elasticity of the cartilage. The collagen fibrils vary in thickness and distribution. Near the surface they are oriented in a circumferential direction, an arrangement that enables the cartilage to resist shearing forces; in the midzone they are meshlike in distribution; and in the deep zone, where they are thicker and more densely packed than elsewhere, they are often perpendicularly oriented to the joint surface. "Arcades," formed by fibers, presumably in conformity with mechanical stresses[23] and visualized at the tissue level, are not apparent on electron micrographs.

The synovial membrane is composed of an outer layer of loose vascular connective tissue and an inner discontinuous layer of specialized cells, the synoviocytes.[84]

Synoviocytes synthesize and secrete hyaluronate, which is given off into the joint space. Two morphologic types of synoviocytes have been described, one rich in endoplasmic reticulum (B cells) and the other with a prominent Golgi apparatus (A cells). It is likely that these two types represent different functional states of the same cell.

The articular cartilage is constantly exposed to mechanical stresses occurring during joint motion and as a result of static loading. The mechanical forces acting on a joint are those of tangential shear and of static pressure, forces that may act with sudden impact or in a protracted fashion. Static forces are brought about by weight and, more important, by the action of muscles and ligaments. A number of mechanisms protect the joints from damage by such forces: the elasticity and the surface architecture of the cartilage permit it to absorb some force; and the synovial fluid provides lubrication that is ideally adapted to maintain joint function.[225]

The synovial fluid or synovia, a term used first by Paracelsus, is a dialysate of plasma. It becomes viscid because of the discharge into it of protein hyaluronate, secreted by the synoviocytes. Under normal conditions the synovial fluid forms a thin film on the cartilaginous surfaces; the total amount of synovial fluid is small, about 3 ml in the adult knee joint. Its lubricating effect is enhanced by changes in viscosity with joint motion. At rest or at slow motion it is more viscid than at high rates of motion. Normal synovial fluid contains about 3.5 mg/g of hyaluronate bound to protein, plasma components, polymorphonuclear and mononuclear leukocytes, and some sloughed-off synoviocytes. The fluid acts not only as a lubricant but also as the main source of nutrients for the articular cartilage into which it penetrates because of a pumping effect created by joint motion.

The biomechanical mechanisms whereby joint lubrication is accomplished are still under discussion. The original concept of simple hydrodynamic action has been supplemented by the concepts of boundary lubrication and weeping lubrication. Boundary lubrication stresses the interaction of small irregularities in the articulating surfaces (as shown by scanning electron microscopy) with extremely thin layers of lubricating fluid in the lubricating process. The concept of weeping lubrication is based on the fact that cartilage acts like a sponge, from which tissue fluid is expressed during stresses on the joint and into which fluid is sucked after release of the stress.[260] Whatever the mechanisms of lubrication, a decrease in lubrication causes increasing friction between the articulating surfaces and leads to tissue damage.

Vertebral joints

The vertebrae possess two kinds of joints. (1) Small apophyseal joints link the spinal processes and are typically diarthrodial in architecture. Thus anatomic, physiologic, and pathologic principles governing these joints are the same as those applying to all other diarthrodial joints. (2) The articulations between the vertebral bodies are unique in so far as the free joint space is replaced by the intervertebral discs. These cushion the impact of mechanical forces on the vertebrae by virtue of their elasticity and their intrinsic pressure. The discs have a jellylike center, the nucleus pulposus, containing much water and a variety of mucopolysaccharides, and an outer coat of dense connective tissue, the anulus fibrosus. The anulus restrains the nucleus within its boundaries during motion; it inserts at the opposing "end-plates" of the vertebral bodies. These end-plates are the actual articulating surfaces of the vertebral bodies and are composed of stratified cartilage structured similar to that of the diarthrodial joints. In the course of time, this cartilage may be partly replaced by bone and the anulus becomes inserted into bone rather than into cartilage.

The joints commonly affected by disease are the diarthrodial or synovial joints. The normal functioning of these joints depends on a delicate balance of morphologic, physiologic, and biochemical conditions,* some of which are local but many of which are modifiable by extra-articular factors. By the same token, joint diseases may be purely local in character or may be manifestations of systemic disorders.

CONGENITAL MALFORMATIONS AND DEVELOPMENTAL DEFECTS OF JOINTS

Disregarding traumatic dislocation of joints during birth, congenital deformities occur in about 6% of newborns.[24] Such lesions may result from abnormalities in muscles or capsular connective tissue, or they may be primary in the osseous system.

Generalized joint rigidity, a rare condition, is seen in arthrogryphosis multiplex, which is characterized by clubfeet, clubhands, and contractures of the large joints.[240] The etiology of the disorder is unknown.

The opposite condition, joint flaccidity, is generalized in the Ehlers-Danlos syndrome, which is associated with hyperextensibility of joints; it results in loosening of the joint capsule. This abnormality is often the cause of congenital subluxation of the hip.[46] It is hereditary, transmitted as an autosomal recessive, and results from inadequate cross-linking of the collagen molecule. The basic defect is the inadequate hydroxylation of lysine.[186]

Clubfoot, a positional abnormality involving flexion of the ankle, inversion of the foot, and medial rotation of the tibia, has been attributed to intrauterine compression, a widely held but poorly substantiated point of view. The increased concordance of the lesion in monozygotic twins (32%) as compared with 2.9% in fraternal twins suggests the presence of a genetic factor.[114]

---

*References 23, 80, 84, 94, 118, 128, 149, 160, 200, 215, 221, 241, 260.

Defective development, dysplasia, of the acetabulum is difficult to diagnose in the newborn but becomes more distinct with increasing age. Inadequate ossification of the roof of the acetabulum prevents the formation of a close-fitting socket for the femoral head. Consequently the femoral head becomes dislocated cranially, posteriorly or laterally, with resulting complete luxation of the hip. Major developmental defects of the large joints have been noted in children born to mothers who had received thalidomide during pregnancy.[154]

NONINFLAMMATORY JOINT DISEASES

Joint disorders caused by physical injury

The term "traumatic arthritis," under which joint disorders caused by physical injury are usually classified, is a misnomer. Although physical injury may cause inflammatory changes, as implied in the term, the sequelae of physical injury are most often noninflammatory. All tissue components of the joints may be affected, and most repair processes correspond to those seen in other locations. However, disorders involving the articular cartilage have special significance. Although articular chondrocytes retain some growth potential into old age, the healing tendency of the cartilage is poor. Once the continuity of the surface has been disrupted, it is rarely if ever restored to normal, despite active proliferation and synthetic activity of many of the chondrocytes in the middle and deep layers of the articular covering. Defects that reach as deep as the subchondral bone are repaired by fibrous tissue growing into the defect from the bone marrow. Under the effects of friction and pressure during motion, this "scar" may be transformed into fibrocartilage.[44,145]

Injuries of the joints resulting from physical forces are of two main types: (1) acute injuries, which are usually produced by the action of a single violent force, and (2) chronic injuries, which occur after minor and frequently repeated inflictive forces.

Acute injuries

Any one of the component parts of a joint may be injured by physical force, particularly if the stress is applied suddenly. If a joint is twisted, hyperextended, hyperflexed, or otherwise forced to move beyond the limits permitted by the elasticity of its ligaments, a sprain, subluxation, or dislocation occurs. Such injuries represent varying degrees of a single type of damage. Thus, as the result of a twist, blow, or fall, the synovial tissues, the ligaments, or the capsule may be stretched, lacerated, or ruptured. In the knee, menisci may be displaced, detached, or torn. The articular cartilage may be compressed, split, or detached from the underlying bone. More severe injuries include lacerations of ligaments and joint capsules. Despite spontaneous or surgery-aided healing processes, such severely damaged joints may be permanently weakened, unstable, and predisposed to recurrent dislocation. With greater violence the articulating bones may be dislocated or fractured, and there may be a bloody effusion into the joint space.

Usually extravasated blood is completely absorbed. In some instances, however, the blood clot organizes, with the production of fibrous adhesions across the joint space. Portions of bone that are completely detached by the fracture become necrotic, although the cartilage survives. These detached fragments of cartilage and bone remain in the joint as loose bodies ("joint mice") and may cause pain or recurrent locking of the joint. Malalignment of the fracture fragments may cause an uneven joint surface and thus excessive friction. The relation of these factors to secondary osteoarthrosis is discussed in a later section of this chapter.

Open laceration of a joint capsule may lead to secondary infection. In addition, physical injury may trigger recurrence of, or reactivate, old quiescent lesion such as tuberculosis, gouty arthritis, or pyogenic infections.

Chronic injuries

Injuries from minor repeated forces are of many kinds and grades of severity. They include those incurred in daily activities, those sustained in recreational or occupational pursuits, and mechanical dysfunction induced by abnormal posture, disturbed locomotion, or skeletal deformities. The articular changes produced by chronic injury are varied in both kind and extent of involvement. In some instances the lesions are confined to periarticular structures, including ligaments, tendon sheaths, or bursae. More frequently the joint proper is the site of involvement. Effusions of fluid into the bursae, tendon sheaths, or articular cavities occasionally result. Loose bodies may be present within distended bursal or synovial cavities. Occasionally, calcification is found in tendons or bursal walls. Such changes are especially common in the shoulder region.[163]

Neuropathic joint disease (Charcot's joint)

The lesions of neuropathic joint disease, usually monarticular, are seen in patients with a variety of neurologic disorders. Originally described by Charcot in 1868, they were attributed chiefly to tabes or syringomyelia; they are now known to be associated with spina bifida, with amyloid infiltration in the course of multiple myeloma,[207] with diabetes mellitus,[219] and with chronic alcoholism.[243] The site of the neurologic lesion determines which joint is affected; with tabes, it is commonly a knee, with syringomyelia the shoulder, with spina bifida the hip, and with diabetes the small joints of the feet and ankles.

An initial nonspecific noninflammatory effusion within the joint space may subside without further damage. Subsequently there are increasing deterioration and erosion of the articular cartilage and sclerosis of the adjacent bone. Eventually the bone also undergoes necrosis and disintegrates, a condition leading to gross disfiguration or even disappearance of the involved epiphysis.

Anesthetization of the joint caused by the disrupted nerve supply has been incriminated as a main contributor to the lesion. The patient suffering no pain is not aware of a disease process and continues to traumatize the joint. However, factors other than purely neurologic dysfunction may be involved in the pathogenesis of some forms of Charcot's joints; diabetic neuropathy especially may be complicated by simultaneous vascular disease, and the disturbed glucose metabolism may directly alter the protein-polysaccharide composition of the cartilage matrix.

Amyloid arthropathy

Generalized amyloidosis can affect multiple joints with deposition of amyloid in the synovium, in cartilage, and in the joint cavity. The shoulder is a site of predilection, but elbows, hands, knees, and temporomandibular and sternoclavicular joints are also commonly involved. Large quantities of amyloid may be free in the joint cavity or deposited in the tissues.[169] Cartilage containing amyloid is whitish opaque, and infiltrated synovium is stiffened. By electron microscopy typical amyloid fibrils with a 75 to 100 Å diameter and a periodicity of two or three per 100 Å length are found extracellularly in the synovium. With special stains, amyloid may be identified as a thin layer on and slightly below the surface of the cartilage. The surface may be smooth or frayed, depending on whether there is associated degradation of the matrix. No amyloid is found within the chondrocytes.[39] The problem of how the amyloid reaches the joint cavity—whether by precipitation from the synovial fluid or by discharge of synovial deposits into the free joint space—is unresolved.

Arthropathy associated with ochronosis

The joint disease associated with ochronosis is caused by the intra-articular deposition of polymerized homogentisic acid, a black pigment. The homogentisic acid is the product of incomplete degradation of tyrosine and phenylalanine, occurring because of an inborn absence of the enzyme homogentisic acid oxidase. The joints involved are primarily those of the vertebral column, although later in the course of the disorder, hips, knees, and shoulder joints may become affected.

Grossly the large joints may be distended by effusion, which is usually noninflammatory. The cartilage is stained a deep black to various shades of gray and is fragmented and brittle (Plate 8, *A* and *B*). The synovium has hypertrophic folds that contain small fragments of detached deteriorated cartilage.

Microscopically, granular pigment is seen within chondrocytes and synovial lining cells. Calcium pyrophosphate crystals may be associated with the pigmentation.[204] The synovium may show evidence of acute or chronic inflammation. By electron microscopy, amorphous pigment particles have been demonstrated in both the chrondrocytes and the surrounding matrix.[133]

Arthropathy associated with hemochromatosis

Joint involvement is seen in about half the cases of primary hemochromatosis, and frequently there is associated chondrocalcinosis. The small joints of the hands are most conspicuously affected, but knees, hips, and the vertebral column also become involved.[40,59]

Grossly the synovium is brownish red. In the presence of chondrocalcinosis, multiple, whitish, chalklike deposits are present in the cartilage, especially in fissures and erosions that appear during the course of the disease.

Microscopically the synovium shows slight hyperplasia with proliferation of fibroblasts, perivascular deposits of hemosiderin in the deep layers, thickening of the vessel walls, occasional microaneurysms, and medial calcification. By electron microscopy the pigment can be demonstrated mainly in synoviocytes.[202] Inflammatory changes are negligible. The cartilage does not contain pigment, but calcium pyrophosphate crystals can be demonstrated together with the fibrillation and erosion characteristic of chondrocalcinosis.

The pathogenic mechanism leading to the joint changes is unknown. The deposition of hemosiderin as such is apparently not injurious, since the lesions do not occur in other conditions associated with iron deposition in joints. This raises the question of a possible role of the abnormal glucose metabolism of hemochromatosis.

Arthropathy associated with hemophilia

Adverse joint manifestations eventually develop in 80% to 90% of hemophiliacs because of hemorrhage into the articular cavities and periarticular tissues. A single hemorrhagic episode may be followed by complete resorption and restoration of normal conditions. Repeated hemorrhage, however, sets off a sequela of changes resulting in severe disfiguration and functional impairment of the involved joints.[106,226]

Grossly the synovium takes on a reddish brown color and becomes hypertrophic with polypous folds or diffuse mosslike thickening. With increasing duration of the condition, there is more fibrous thickening of the synovium, as well as of the subsynovial connective tissue, and development of fibrous adhesions between the opposing surfaces of the joint. The cartilage becomes eroded and cystic because of the focal necrosis. The subchondral bone responds with early sclerosis, which may give way to atrophy and breakdown with formation of cysts in the epiphyses. Such cysts enclose organizing blood clot and may communicate with the articular cavity.

Microscopically the synovium contains numerous hemosiderin-laden macrophages, especially in the near-surface layers. By electron microscopy hemosiderin has been found in the cytoplasm of some chondrocytes but not in the extracellular matrix.[110] The lining cells, particularly B cells, are hyperplastic, as are the fibroblasts of the deep layers. Especially near the insertion of ligaments, ingrowth of synovium into degenerating cartilage may be seen. In advanced cases the cartilage resembles that found in osteoarthrosis.[58,129]

Osteochondroses

Osteochondroses result from aseptic necrosis of the bone underlying the articular cartilage. Since the articular cartilage does not depend on blood vessels for its nutritional supply, the injury to the cartilage is not attributable to nutritional failure. Rather, it is the loss of mechanical support from the underlying bone that causes the cartilage to break down. The ensuing defects may initially be small, but there may be further deterioration of the articular covering and reactive chondrocyte proliferation, resulting in lesions similar to those of osteoarthrosis. Many syndromes associated with osteochondrosis have been described in various skeletal sites (see Chapter 40).

Osteochondrosis dissecans

The formerly used term "osteochondritis" is a misnomer that should be abandoned. The lesion has no inflammatory component, and therefore the suffix "-itis" is inappropriate. The characteristic gross findings in the joints are single or multiple loose or lightly attached bodies composed of cartilage and underlying bone. These bodies, termed "joint mice," are ovoid or roundish and measure 0.5 to 1.5 cm in diameter and several millimeters in thickness (Fig. 42-1). Often a groove in the articular surface indicates the site from which a body has been detached. Microscopically the grooves are covered with fibrous tissue. The cartilage of the fragments may be intact or show various degrees of fibrillation and foci of calcification. The attached bone is usually sclerotic with thickened trabeculae.

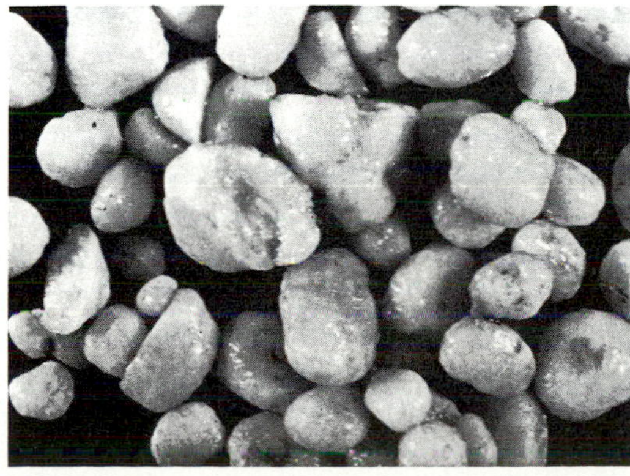

Fig. 42-1. Joint mice removed from shoulder joint. Synovial membrane was studded with small nodules composed of dense fibrous tissue and cartilage. Detachment of these tissue excrescences was apparent source of loose bodies.

The lesions are commonly found in children and adolescents, in boys more often than in girls, and usually involve the knee joint, especially the medial condyle of the femur. However, hip, shoulder, and elbow may also be affected.[189] Mechanical forces, acting on normal joint tissue or on local developmental defects, have been considered a major cause of the changes; the lesions also develop as a result of aseptic necrosis of subchondral bone.[222] Apparent familial aggregation has been reported.

Arthropathy associated with sickle cell disease

Sickling and thrombosis occur in small vessels of the articular tissues as in nonskeletal locations. Thrombi composed of dead cells, platelets, and red blood corpuscles occlude vascular lumina; the cartilage becomes involved secondarily because of avascular necrosis of the subchondral bone. Tissue destruction, which may become extensive, thus resembles that seen in aseptic avascular necrosis as well as, in advanced cases, that seen in aseptic necrosis. Microinfarcts may develop in the synovium. The vascular basement membranes are thickened, and perivascular fibrosis is present.[203] The synovium shows low-grade infiltration by mononuclear leukocytes. The joints most commonly involved are hip, shoulder, and knee in the order mentioned.

Hypertrophic osteoarthropathy

The clubbing of fingers and toes characteristic of hypertrophic osteoarthropathy is primarily attributable to periarticular and periosteal hyperemia and fibroblastic proliferation and to overgrowth of bone; joints may become involved, with an increase of synovial fluid that is rich in mucins but has fewer cells than would be present with an inflammatory lesion. The condition is found in association with circulatory failure as occurs in congenital heart disease, with a variety of digestive disorders, and chiefly with malignant or chronic benign pulmonary disease.

In addition to this secondary type of clubbing, there is a primary form of the disease, pachydermatoperiostosis, that is inherited as a sex-linked dominant trait.[191]

Aging of articular cartilage

The morphologic, biochemical, and physical properties of the articular cartilage change with age. These changes are important pathogenically because they render the cartilage more susceptible to injury.

The growth potential and the cellularity of the articular cartilage decrease progressively from birth to the end of the growth period, but some growth potential persists throughout life.[213] This fact is responsible for lifelong cell renewal, the gradual remodeling of the articular contour,[118] and the resumption of cell proliferation under pathologic conditions, such as osteoarthrosis of old age or of hyperpituitarism. During adulthood the decline in cellularity slows down, and in old age a slight increase in the number of cells may occur.[237] Associated with this increase in cell number is an increase in cellular activity, as indicated by increased uptake of radiosulfate by the articular chondrocytes.[51] An age-linked increase in intracellular lipid apparently does not interfere with the functioning of the chondrocytes.

The matrix likewise changes with advancing age. During growth the ratio of chondroitin-4-sulfate to chondroitin-6-sulfate decreases, and an increase in keratan sulfate is demonstrable in tissue sections and biochemically by a decrease in the galactosamine/glucosamine ratio. From early adulthood on, there is a net loss of water and total proteoglycans.[4,201,238] In many joints proteoglycan content becomes stabilized thereafter; however, proteoglycan molecules appear less aggregated than in the joints of young persons.[184] No further changes occur unless additional pathogenic factors become active.

As proteoglycans decrease, the collagen fibrils increase in thickness and become packed more tightly than in the young person.[232] Focal whorl-like aggregations of collagen fibrils develop at the sites of disintegrated cells (Fig. 42-2). Associated with these changes are impairment of tensile strength and elasticity and an increase in compliance of the articular cartilage.[8,128] The remaining chondrocytes, in an apparent attempt at repair, become temporarily overactive and after this are prematurely exhausted and die; thus a vicious circle is initiated resulting ultimately in osteoarthrosis. The age-linked progressive accumulation of lipid in the matrix results from disintegration of cell components but does not seem to influence subsequent disease processes.

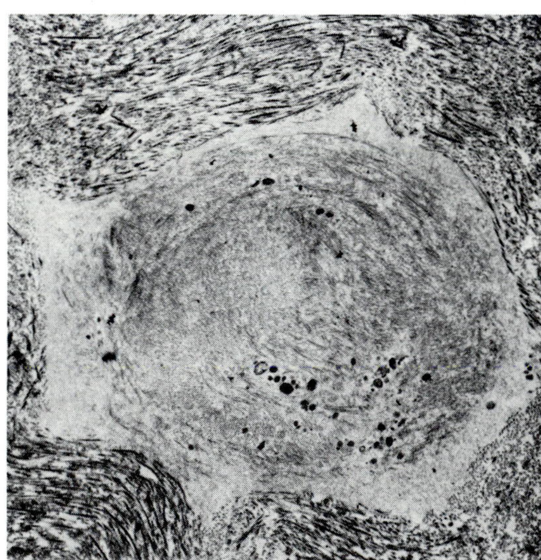

Fig. 42-2. Electron micrograph of "microscar" in aging human articular cartilage of hip joint. Whorls of collagen fibrils with intermingled electron-dense fat globules have replaced disintegrated chondrocyte. Scar is still surrounded by halo of relatively electron-lucent matrix, which surrounded former chondrocyte. There is regular matrix with collagen fibrils at periphery. (Courtesy Dr. Max Spycher, Zurich.)

Age changes in capsule, ligaments, and synovial membrane presumably are the same as those in connective tissue in other locations.[249]

Osteoarthrosis

Osteoarthrosis, a noninflammatory disorder of synovial joints, is characterized by regressive changes and proliferation of the articular cartilage and by overgrowth of subchondral and juxta-articular bone and intra-articular soft tissues. The disease is, so far as is known, a strictly skeletal disorder without accompanying changes in the biochemistry of body fluids or in nonskeletal tissues.

In view of the absence of inflammatory changes, synonyms such as osteoarthritis, hypertrophic arthritis, or arthritis deformans are misnomers. The term "degenerative joint disease" is correct only insofar as it denotes general deterioration of the joints; it does not take into account the prominent processes of growth occurring in the course of the disease, and furthermore, it disregards the fact that "degeneration" of articular tissues occurs in many other joint disorders.

Prevalance and distribution

Osteoarthrosis is one of the oldest and most widespread diseases known. The characteristic alterations have been observed in the skeletons of prehistoric animals, in many nonmammalian and mammalian species of present-day animals,[225] and in humans. The disease is age linked, starting as subtle biochemical, biophysical, and microscopic changes at the beginning of the third decade, becoming roentgenographically noticeable at the end of the fourth decade, and giving rise to clinical symptoms some time thereafter. Practically no aging human is spared the development of osteoarthrosis in one or several locations. Particularly severe or early clinical involvement of one joint may be so prominent as to make the disease appear monarticular, although commonly multiple joints are affected to a lesser degree. Pathologic involvement is thus more widespread than clinical symptoms would suggest, and localized monarticular osteoarthrosis should be considered a special occurrence rather than the rule. Reports of a higher incidence of clinical disease in women than in men are not borne out by autoptic and roentgenographic observations. In men the disease develops at least as often and at even earlier ages than in women; however, the advanced lesions of later ages seem to be more common in women than in men.[93,102,123,245]

Osteoarthrosis is most conspicuous in the large joints

of the lower extremity, knees, and hips, but the interphalangeal, shoulder, metacarpophalangeal, and sternoclavicular joints are commonly involved. The temporomandibular joints may also be affected by the disease.

Histogenesis

The early stages of the disease merge imperceptibly with the late aging changes.[17,20,156,157] Because of loss of mucopolysaccharides, which normally invest the collagen fibrils, the latter are unmasked and the cartilage appears fibrillated; the fibrils are held together less tightly than normal, and, if this process involves the surface layer, they change from the circumferential to a radial orientation as the articular surface becomes frayed and fissured (Fig. 42-3). The chondrocytes respond with proliferation and hypertrophy, followed by accelerated disintegration (Fig. 42-4). Changes in water content and in the amount and proportion of proteoglycans observed in osteoarthrotic cartilage[4,165] seem to be related to the presence of young chondrocytes and newly formed matrix and thus to be nonspecific. The same may be true for the appearance of type I collagen in osteoarthrotic cartilage.[82,173]

Once the continuity of the articular surface has been disrupted, the conditions for smooth joint motion and normal lubrication no longer exist, and mechanical forces

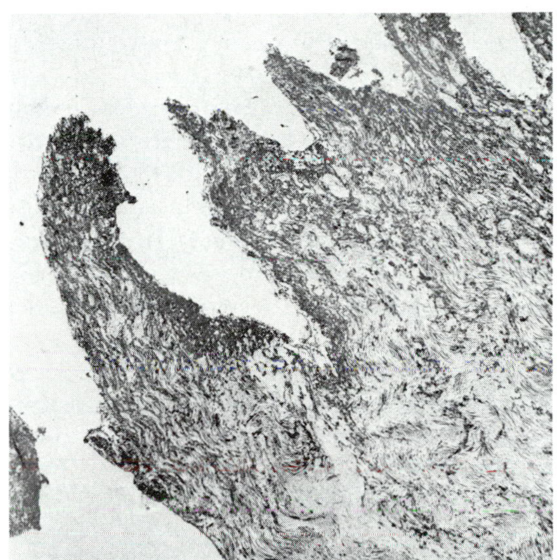

Fig. 42-3. Electron micrograph from osteoarthrotic ulcer at femoral head. Surface of lesion is frayed, and villous projections are composed of short, irregularly clustered collagen fibrils, mainly in radial orientation to joint surface. (Courtesy Dr. Max Spycher, Zurich.)

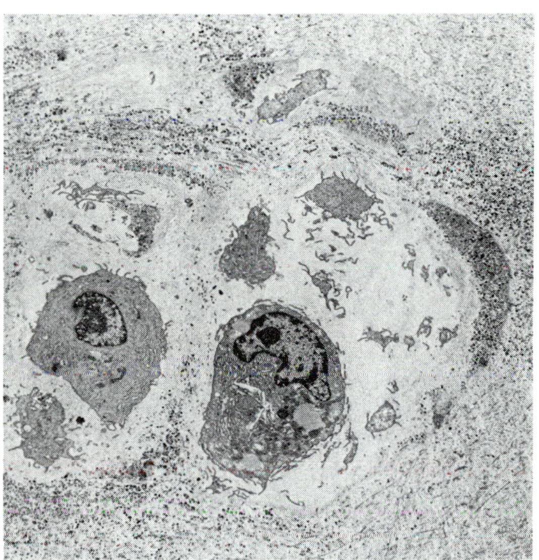

Fig. 42-4. Electron micrograph from osteoarthrotic femoral head. Cluster of chondrocytes indicates proliferation. Two chondrocytes are shown completely; others are sectioned tangentially and only partly shown. Numerous electron-dense granules—some scattered diffusely and others aggregated in crescents—represent lipid derived from disintegrated cells. (Courtesy Dr. Max Spycher, Zurich.)

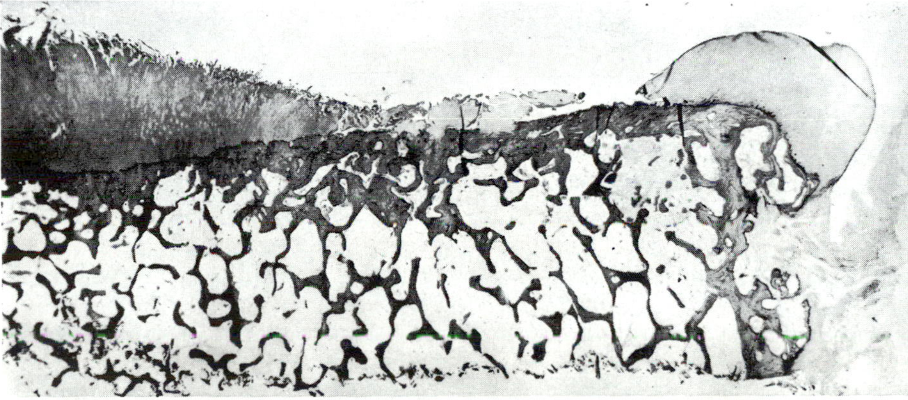

Fig. 42-5. Low-power photomicrograph of cartilage of patellar surface of femur: osteoarthrosis. Fibrillation and splitting of matrix are seen. Fragmentation and detachment of cartilage are evident toward right, where subchondral bone has been denuded. (10×; AFIP 67996.)

contribute to further erosion of the articular surface. The cartilage may show increased calcification, invasion by blood vessels, and progressive ulceration (Fig. 42-5 and Plate 8, *D*). The underlying bone is bared and reacts with osteosclerosis; the epiphyseal bone marrow often becomes fibrotic and occasionally cystic. The intra-articular soft tissues, synovial villi, and fat pads become hypertrophic, but unlike conditions in inflammatory joint disease, pannus does not develop. Fragments of cartilage may be detached into the joint cavity and persist and move about as free bodies. Although destructive processes are prominent in the center regions of the joints, the cartilage at the periphery proliferates, ossifies, and with new periosteal bone forms large, elevated, overhanging outgrowths (Figs. 42-6 and 42-7). This process, described as "lipping," results in further distortion of the articular surface, with considerable functional impairment. However, even in severely altered osteoarthrotic joints, complete immobilization rarely occurs.

Etiology and pathogenesis

Osteoarthrosis is now recognized as being of multifactorial origin, and the earlier simplistic concept of a "wear-and-tear disease" is outdated. From an etiologic point of view, primary and secondary osteoarthrosis may be distinguished, although morphologically the two types are indistinguishable. Secondary osteoarthrosis is posttraumatic in the broadest sense of the term, with trauma being related to (1) action of mechanical force on a joint, as by a single impact or presumably a series of repeated occupational insults (for example, those incurred by professional dancers or men working with pneumatic tools); (2) malalignment of joints attributable to congenital malformations, to incongruencies of the opposing articular surfaces, to metabolic or circulatory bone disease, or to superimposition on previous inflammatory disease associated with fibrosis and scarring of the joint capsule; or (3) deposition of extraneous injurious material within the articular tissues. Most experimental models are examples of secondary osteoarthrosis.

Osteoarthrosis is considered primary if none of the foregoing conditions applies. In the absence of unequivocal evidence as to the etiology of the disorder, a number of hypotheses have been advanced in the past, among which the "wear-and-tear" hypothesis was the most widely held. This concept maintained that the microtrauma of daily wear and tear was the basic etiologic factor in the disorder; accordingly, it was postulated that the greater the mechanical stress of weight bearing, the greater would be the propensity of a particular joint to become diseased. However, this concept did not clearly distinguish between the traumatic and the primary forms

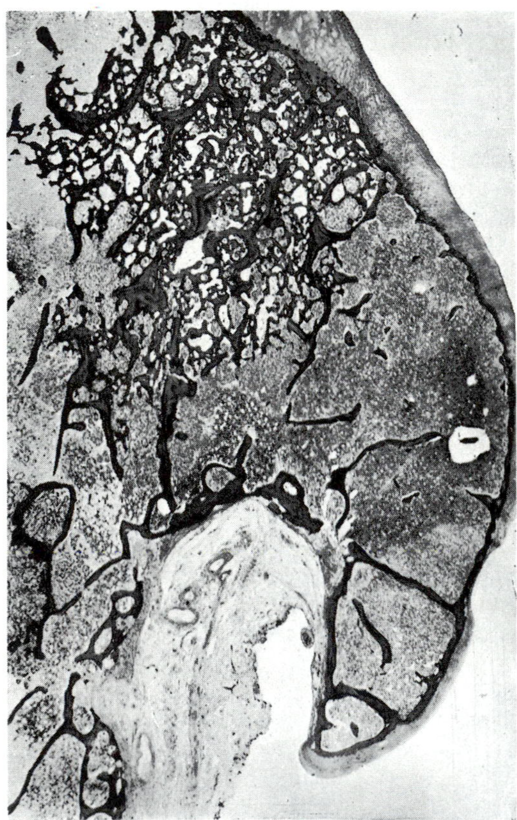

Fig. 42-6. Low-power photomicrograph of joint, showing extensive marginal lipping. "Lip" is extension of epiphyseal end of tubular bone. (AFIP 67998.)

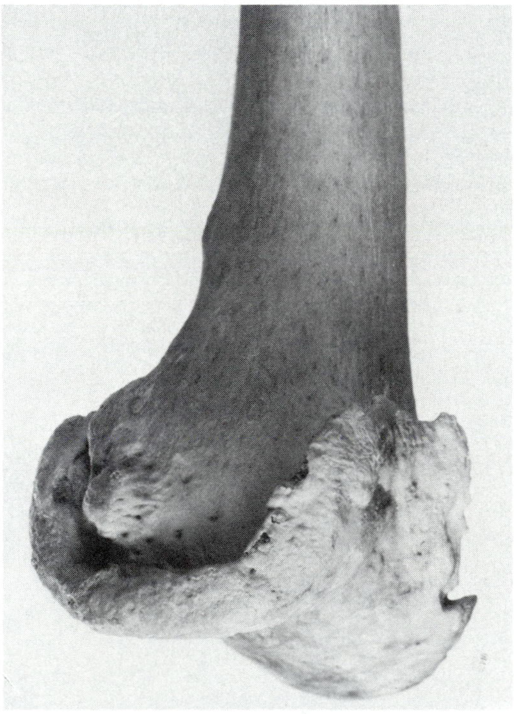

Fig. 42-7. Macerated specimen of lower femur. There is pronounced osteoarthrosis of femoral aspect of knee joint with extensive marginal lipping.

of the disease; nor did it account for the facts that osteoarthrosis is not increased in athletes,[2,188] that the disorder commonly involves non-weight-bearing joints,[214] and that particularly severe forms of the disease occur in such locations as the interphalangeal joints regardless of the amount of use to which these joints have been subjected before the onset of the disease. Furthermore, the "wear-and-tear" concept disregarded the fact that early changes can involve the non-weight-bearing rather than the weight-bearing areas of a joint.[35,156] The modern version of the wear-and-tear hypothesis introduces the concept of fatigue failure of the articular cartilage.[43] However, unlike metal, from which the analogy is derived, cartilage contains living cells, which support maintenance of the matrix and a turnover of proteoglycans and collagen (although turnover of collagen may be extremely slow).

Some of the problems of pathogenesis can be overcome by the concept of variability in tissue susceptibility, which may depend on variations in cellularity and in biochemical and biophysical properties of the matrix. In the presence of high tissue susceptibility, a comparatively low-grade extraneous influence suffices to produce a lesion, whereas more powerful stimuli are required to trigger disease if the tissue is comparatively resistant. The following factors have been shown to determine the susceptibility of the articular cartilage to becoming arthrotic:

1. *Genetic factors*. This is demonstrated by increased familial incidence of a special type of osteoarthrosis of the interphalangeal joints, Heberden's nodes,[235] and of polyarticular osteoarthrosis.[125]
2. *Hormonal factors*. This is indicated by the earlier onset and increased severity of osteoarthrosis associated with acromegaly and diabetes.[216]
3. *Nutritional factors*. This is shown by the frequent coexistence of osteoarthrosis and obesity. This coexistence is not fortuitous, nor is osteoarthrosis the consequence of the increased weight bearing associated with obesity[70,197] (as demonstrated by the finding that Heberden's nodes are as common in obese as in nonobese men). It appears more likely that both obesity and osteoarthrosis are related to a metabolic disorder involving lipid metabolism.
4. *Biologic age*. The articular changes occurring at a relatively early age are pacemakers for the disease. The rate at which they proceed is decisive for the subsequent pathologic events into which they gradually merge.[20,185]

In addition to these and possibly other systemic factors,[4] there may be local factors, that is, blood and nerve supply. The concept of multiple etiologic factors acting on the joints to produce osteoarthrosis is illustrated diagrammatically in Fig. 42-8.

Osteoarthrosis associated with acromegaly

In patients with acromegaly, joint lesions develop that are grossly indistinguishable from those of the usual type of osteoarthrosis.[9,216] Microscopically proliferation of chondrocytes may be more pronounced than that in senile osteoarthrosis, especially in the young acromegalic person[72,212]—a quantitative difference not sufficient to prove a specific nature of the arthropathy. The changes that distinguish the arthropathy of acromegaly from the age-linked disorder are associated with extra-articular skeletal manifestations of hyperpituitarism, particularly the resumption of osteogenesis at periosteal surfaces.

Kashin-Beck disease

Kashin-Beck disease is a special form of severe osteoarthrosis endemic to areas of Siberia. It occurs in young children and is associated with pronounced disturbances of skeletal growth. The joint lesions, typically those of osteoarthrosis, have been attributed to the presence of a fungus, *Fusarium sporotrichiella*, in grain used in the diet and to toxic effects of the fungus on cartilage.[171]

INFLAMMATORY JOINT DISEASES

Arthritis caused by infectious agents

Infectious arthritis is one of the possible complications of any infectious disease. Although the incidence of

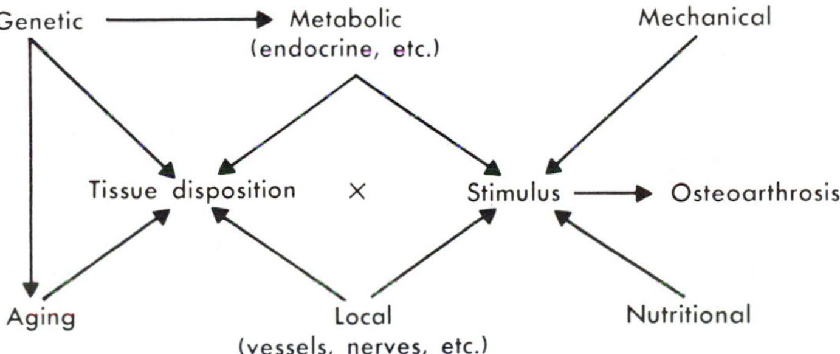

Fig. 42-8. Diagram illustrating the multifactorial etiology of osteoarthrosis. (From Silberberg, R., and Silberberg, M.: Pathol. Microbiol. **27:**447, 1964.)

infectious joint lesions has decreased with the advent of antibiotic therapy, the disorders still are of considerable clinical importance.

The histogenetic mechanisms active in the development of infectious arthritides are the same as those prevailing in other connective tissue spaces, modified by the special anatomic and physiologic conditions prevailing in joints. The infection may be attributable to direct contamination as in open wounds, to extension from the adjacent tissue, or to lymphatic spread, or it may be blood borne (Plate 8, *C*). The process begins acutely with hyperemia and swelling of the synovium, infiltration by polymorphonuclear and mononuclear leukocytes, and development of an effusion in the joint cavity. The exudate may be predominantly serous or fibrinous or purulent, depending on the severity of the infection, the resistance of the host, and the duration of the process. The synovium may be involved diffusely or focally. A predominantly serous effusion or comparatively small amounts of fibrin may disappear completely, the latter after fibrinolysis has occurred. With increasing amounts of fibrin and increasing duration of the infection, however, granulation tissue develops with formation of adhesions between the soft tissues of the joints and between opposing articular surfaces; synovium and subsynovial tissues become thickened and fibrotic. In pyogenic infections this is accompanied by abscess formation, which may involve the entire joint space or more or less isolated pockets. Even after successful surgical intervention, which usually is required to remove the exudate, the increase in fibrous tissue and the subsequent collagenization may result in permanent impairment of joint motion.

The characteristic feature of inflammatory arthritis is the involvement of the articular cartilage. The changes are degenerative rather than inflammatory, which is consistent with the fact that the cartilage contains no blood vessels. With the development of exudate in the joint cavity and granulation tissue in the synovium, the cartilage becomes frayed and eroded. In advanced cases it may disappear completely, and the underlying bones undergo osteosclerosis, or it may be thinned out and eroded by granulation tissue. This tissue may then invade the epiphyseal marrow cavity.

The injury to the cartilage is presumably brought about by lysosomal enzymes, such as cathepsins, collagenase, and hyaluronidase, which attack both the protein and the nonprotein moieties of the matrix. Since chondrocytes contain few lysosomes, it must be surmised that the degradative enzymes are chiefly derived from leukocytes of the exudate and the synovium. Yet enzymes produced by chondrocytes may contribute to the destruction of the matrix.[134,141,254,255]

The pathogenic organisms most commonly found in bacterial arthritis of adults are *Staphylococcus aureus*, hemolytic streptococci,[50,127] *Neisseria gonorrhoeae*,[109,182] and *Haemophilus influenzae*. *Haemophilus influenzae* arthritis in infants and children and *Serratia* arthritis in adults are seen with increasing frequency.[66,170] Pneumococci,[244] *Pseudomonas, Proteus, Salmonella, Enterobacter, Bacteroides, Escherichia*, and other intestinal organisms are among the rarer causes of bacterial arthritis (Plate 8, *C*).[126]

Joint involvement is monarticular more often than polyarticular. The large joints of the lower limbs, knee, and hip are usually affected. In the most instances, predisposing factors are demonstrable, such as oral or local corticosteroid administration, diabetes, or preexisting rheumatoid arthritis.[120]

Viral arthritis

Rubella, mumps, infectious mononucleosis, lymphogranuloma venereum, variola, and other generalized viral infections may be accompanied by episodes of acute arthritis,[62] yet reports of tissue changes are scanty. The findings in mumps-associated arthritis are probably characteristic of viral joint inflammations in general; synovial biopsies show edema, lymphocytic infiltration, and hyperplasia of synoviocytes. A patchy fibrinous exudate completes the picture of a nonspecific synovitis.[262]

With the use of immunohistochemical methods evidence for the presence of virus in synovial tissue can be obtained in arthritis after smallpox or rubella vaccination.[218]

Tuberculous arthritis

Approximately 1% of subjects with tuberculosis have skeletal involvement; in 30%, hips or knees are involved, and in 20% various other joints. Not uncommonly, the skeletal infection remains dormant and without clinical symptoms for many years. Almost invariably tuberculous arthritis results from hematogenous dissemination of the organisms. These may reach the synovial membrane directly or they may involve the joint secondarily, spreading from a focus of tuberculous osteomyelitis close to the articulation. Thus, in the knee of adults, the synovial membrane is frequently the primary site, whereas in children the secondary spread from a focus in the adjacent metaphyseal or epiphyseal bone is the more common occurrence. Regardless of the point of origin, the result of the infection is likely to be the same. The synovial membrane becomes hyperemic and edematous. A grayish yellow exudate is deposited on its surface, and occasionally tubercles can be recognized on gross inspection. In some cases the synovium is transformed into a necrotic mass mixed with a shaggy fibrinous exudate; the joint space contains grayish white bodies the size and shape of melon seeds and varying amounts of turbid or clear exudate. Occasionally an excessive amount of fluid distends the joint (tuberculous hydrops). The changes in the articular cartilage depend to a considerable extent on the duration of the infection. In early stages the cartilage may merely lose its glistening appearance, a change sometimes accompanied by the extension of tuberculous granulation tissue from the synovium over the cartilaginous surfaces. In more severely affected joints, fragments of cartilage are loosened and detached from the underlying bone, leaving an uneven granular ulcerated base of necrotic bone and exudate.

Microscopically the loosened fragments consist of necrotic cartilage with faintly staining matrix and devoid of cells. The involved areas of bone show caseous necrosis surrounded by tuberculous granulation tissue. The necrotic trabeculae undergo gradual resorption (caries). The synovial membrane contains numerous solitary or conglomerate tubercles.

Healing may occur, with the result depending on the extent of the lesion. If the lesion was confined to the synovial membrane, functional impairment may be limited; advanced involvement of cartilage and bone may result in total destruction of the articulation, with either fibrous or bony union of the articulating bones (ankylosis).

Syphilitic arthritis

The frequency with which joints are involved in syphilis is declining. Arthritis may, however, occur in congenital as well as in acquired forms of the disease.

In congenital syphilis varying degrees of involvement of the joint capsules and epiphyses may accompany the characteristic changes of osteochondritis and periostitis. Microscopically these joints show hyperemia, edema, lymphoid and plasma cell infiltration, and proliferation of fibroblasts. In addition, there may be small areas of necrosis in cartilage, bone, and capsular tissues.

In older children showing manifestations of congenital syphilis a peculiar form of arthritis, known as Clutton's joint,[49] may develop. One or both knees, and occasionally other joints, are swollen and lax and contain an excessive amount of fluid. The synovial membrane is thickened and appears gelatinous. Microscopically there are edema, diffuse infiltration with lymphocytes and plasma cells, and occasional gummas.[7]

Acquired syphilis

Pathologic investigations of joint tissues in secondary syphilis are notably lacking; however, inflammatory and vascular lesions resembling those found in skin and mucous membranes may produce an acute synovitis, sometimes associated with a transitory effusion. The knee joint is more often affected than other articulations, and the involvement is often bilateral.

In later stages of acquired syphilis the joints may be the site of gumma formation or of a diffuse chronic nonspecific synovitis with more or less pronounced effusion. Gummas may also be found in ligaments, cartilage, and adjacent bone. Conversely, gummas may spread by direct extension from the bone marrow and bone to neighboring joints.

As a nonspecific sequela of tabes dorsalis, neuropathic joint disease may ensue.

Arthritis of brucellosis

Arthritis occurs as a complication of *Brucella bovis* or *B. suis* infection in about 10% of affected individuals. Hips, sacroiliac, and the small joints of hands and feet may be the site of acute suppurative synovitis or of chronic synovitis and bursitis.[231] Involvement of the spine is prominent. Subacute osteomyelitis of the vertebral bodies with destruction of cancellous bone and microabscesses is associated with destruction of the endplates, separating the vertebral body from the intervertebral disc, and with breakdown of the discs. There is a tendency to repair, with production of granulomas. Although blood-borne infection of the intervertebral discs has been considered a primary event in the evolution of the lesion, it appears more logical, in the absence of clear-cut evidence, to assume that the process starts as an osteomyelitis and involves the discs secondarily as seen in other chronic infections.[143]

Fungal arthritis

A variety of fungal organisms may lodge in the synovium and give rise to suppurative or granulomatous lesions. The synovium may be the primary site of joint involvement, or the infection may spread from the marrow cavity to the subchondral bone and from there into the articular tissues.[16]

Arthritis associated with rheumatic fever

The arthritis that occurs in most patients with acute rheumatic fever is characteristically an acute, transient, migratory disorder, involving most commonly the large articulations such as knees, ankles, and wrists. A nonspecific synovitis involves the joint cavity proper as well as bursae and tendon sheaths. The effusion present in the joint cavity is always sterile; initially the inflammatory cells are predominantly polymorphonuclear leukocytes, with varying numbers of eosinophils; at later stages mononuclear cells may predominate. If the occlusive vasculitis characteristic of rheumatic fever is present in synovium or periarticularly, the diagnosis of rheumatic arthritis can be made. The arthritis usually subsides after a few weeks without residual changes.[167]

Rheumatic arthritis is often accompanied by the appearance of subcutaneous nodules in the vicinity of joints. These nodules resemble in some ways the subcutaneous nodules of rheumatoid arthritis on the one hand and the Aschoff bodies of the myocardium on the other. The nodules usually measure several millimeters in diameter. Microscopically they have an acellular center of eosinophilic material, much of which can be identified as swollen or disintegrated collagen, with an admixture of mucopolysaccharides and, more rarely, necrotic tissue elements. This center is surrounded by a rim of lymphocytes, large and small monocytes, multinucleated giant cells, and occasionally eosinophils. Typical rheumatic vasculitis is usually found in the immediate vicinity of the nodules.[19] The nodules may be completely resorbed after a few weeks of existence. Some of the features that distinguish the rheumatic from the rheumatoid nodules seem related to the time factor involved in their pathogenesis: nodules of rheumatic fever come and go quickly and fail to show the extensive necrosis and the granulomatous character of the rheumatoid nodules, which develop and regress in a more chronic fashion.

The pathogenesis of the arthritis of rheumatic fever is unknown, although it has been shown experimentally that streptolysin, injected into the joint cavity, will produce arthritis, probably by disrupting lysosomes and thus liberating enzymes.[255] The possibility that streptococcal debris might also call forth the synovial inflammation has not been ruled out.

Repeated attacks of rheumatic arthritis of the hands or feet may be followed by flexion deformities, particularly striking in metacarpophalangeal joints. The condition, described first by Jaccoud in 1869[115] and therefore termed Jaccoud's arthritis, is associated with pronounced ulnar deviation of the digits. However, the deformities seem to be attributable to fibrosis of fasciae and tendons rather than to synovitis.[37]

Rheumatoid arthritis

Rheumatoid arthritis (RA) is a chronic progressive inflammatory arthritis of unknown origin involving multiple joints and characterized by a tendency to spontaneous remissions and subsequent relapses.

Arthritis is the most prominent manifestation of rheumatoid disease, a generalized connective tissue disorder that may involve para-articular structures such as bursae, tendon sheaths, and tendons as well as extra-articular tissues such as the subcutis,[227] cardiovascular system, lungs, spleen, lymph nodes, skeletal muscle, central and peripheral nervous system, and eyes.[113]

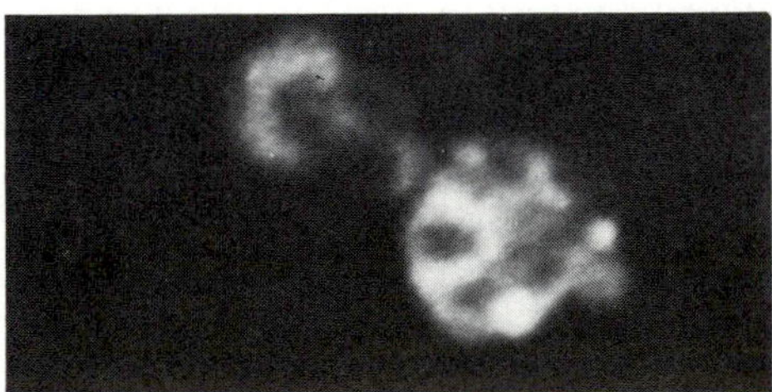

Fig. 42-9. Cell from synovial fluid of patient with rheumatoid arthritis. Cell was treated with serum containing antigammaglobulin. Brightly fluorescent globular inclusion suggests presence of rheumatoid factor (RF). (From Zucker-Franklin, D.: Arthritis Rheum. 9:24, 1966.)

Rheumatoid disease is often accompanied by characteristic immunoglobulin, called rheumatoid factors (RFs), in affected persons' serum. These factors are of considerable complexity; they are capable of acting as antiglobulins and of forming complexes with abnormal antigenic gamma globulins in vivo and in vitro. With appropriate techniques, such antigens or antibodies or their complexes can be demonstrated in serum, in synovial fluid, in leukocytes of blood and articular exudates, and in the synovial tissues (Fig. 42-9). Several tests have been developed to detect these immune bodies, using the agglutination of antibody on antigen-coated particles, such as red blood corpuscles,[136] bacteria,[251] or inert latex or bentonite particles.[32]

RF is present in 85% to 95% of subjects with rheumatoid arthritis, and a distinction is therefore made between seropositive and seronegative forms of the disease. On the other hand, RF may be found in 2% to 7% of patients with connective tissue diseases other than rheumatoid arthritis. Yet, the tests are considered useful for diagnostic and prognostic purposes, since there is a positive correlation between the level of the serum titers of RF and the severity of the clinical disease.

Distribution and prevalence

Young adults are frequently affected, but with increasing age an increase in prevalence has been reported.[246] Depending on the criteria used for diagnosis, women are 2½ to 5 times more often affected than men.[180,246] Familial aggregation seems safely established for the severe forms of seropositive disease, whereas no such aggregation is seen in seronegative or low-grade seropositive forms.[57,138] Geographic distribution, considered significant at one time, has recently been shown to be random.[36,138] A slightly increased incidence is seen in men engaged in occupations requiring physical work as compared with those in professional or managerial positions.[246] The small joints of hands and feet are usually the first and most common to be involved, with lesions of the large joints appearing later in the course of the disease.

Pathologic anatomy

The basic tissue changes of rheumatoid disease are similar, regardless of site. In different locations they are modified in accordance with the properties peculiar to the tissue in which they take place. None of the histologic changes is by itself specific; but in combination they give a fairly typical and diagnostically suggestive picture. Similar uncertainties exist in regard to the clinical diagnosis of rheumatoid arthritis.[194]

Several features characterize the rheumatoid lesion:

1. Diffuse or focal infiltration of the tissue by lymphocytes or plasma cells, or both, with development of lymphoid centers
2. Vasculitis with endothelial proliferation, narrowing or occlusion of the lumina, fibrinoid change or necrosis of the walls, and perivascular aggregation of lymphocytes and plasma cells
3. The rheumatoid granuloma, a focal lesion with an amorphous center composed of necrotic tissue,[265] fibrin, and immune complexes surrounded by a band of oblong histiocytes (often in palisade-like radial orientation) and an outer zone of granulation tissue containing a variety of mononuclear leukocytes, capillaries, and fibroblasts; with time the granuloma may undergo resorption or increasing fibrosis and collagenization

In the joints the early changes involve the synovium, which becomes congested, edematous, and infiltrated by small and large lymphocytes, plasma cells, plasmoblasts, and macrophages, indicating the presence of both humoral and cellular immune responses (Fig. 42-10).[264] There often are small areas of superficial necrosis of synovial lining cells with formation of superficial erosions covered by fibrinoid deposits; these deposits are composed of fibrin and small amounts of gamma globulin and complement components. An exudate containing polymorphonuclear leukocytes, many with ingested immune complexes, accumulates in the joint cavity. At later stages the synovitis is characterized by plasma cells, lymphoid centers, occasional multinucleated giant cells, and vasculitis. Granulation tissue composed of synovial fibroblasts and capillaries causes grossly recognizable villous thickening of the synovium, whose lining cells become hypertrophic and hyperplastic. In some of these lining

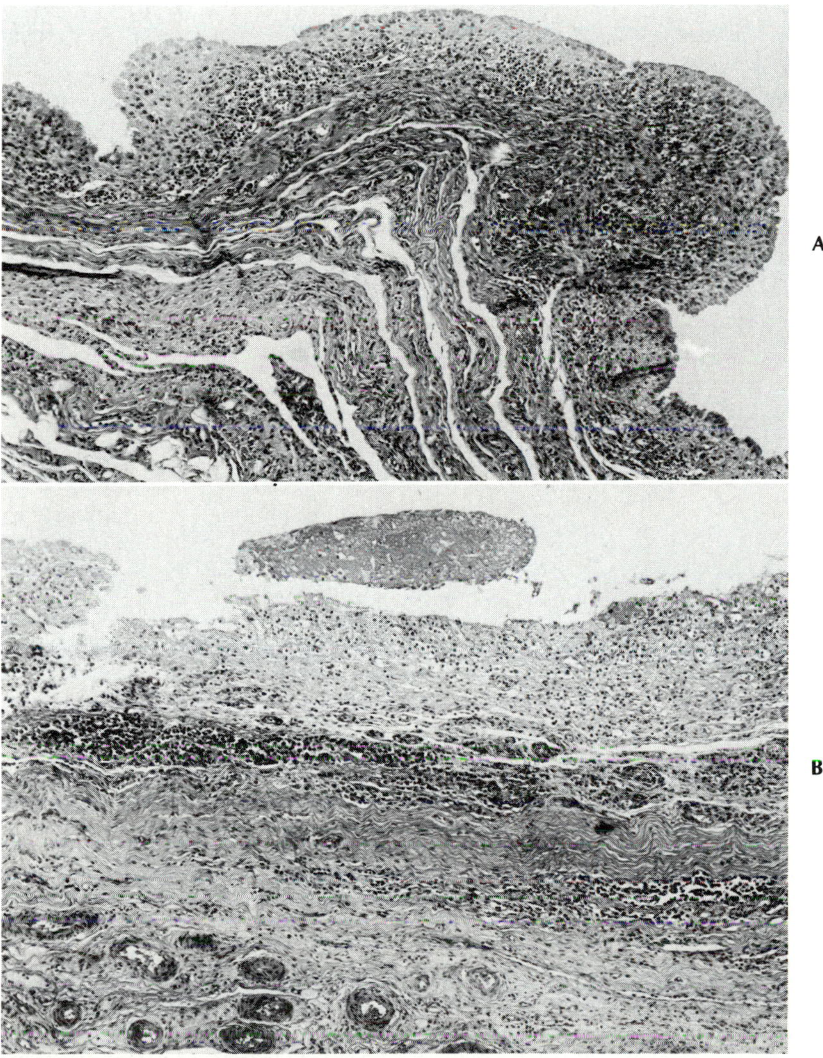

Fig. 42-10. Rheumatoid synovitis. **A,** There is infiltration of synovium by lymphocytes. **B,** Fibrinous exudate is superimposed on inflamed synovium. Superficial layer of synovium is necrotic, and subsynovial tissue is thickened and necrotic.

cells as well as in lymphocytes and plasma cells of the synovium and in leukocytes of the synovial fluid, rheumatoid factor, gamma globulins, and antigen-antibody complexes can be demonstrated after incubation of smears or of tissue sections with the proper fluorescein-conjugated antigens.[30,34,108] The granulation tissue does not remain localized to the synovium but spreads over the surface of the articular cartilage and produces adhesions between the opposing joint surfaces (Figs. 42-11 to 42-13). This pannus comes to be interposed between the cartilage and the lumen of the joint cavity and may interfere with the flow of synovial fluid into the cartilage. Thus malnutrition of the cartilage may contribute to its destruction, although most of the destruction is attributed to the action of hydrolytic enzymes released from lysosomes of neutrophils and cells of the pannus.[255] As the pannus ages, fibrosis and collagenization lead to shrinkage of the capsule, progressive narrowing of the joint space, and displacement or increasing approximation of the ends of the opposing bones. Closely apposing bones may become fused by bony bridges developing in the scar tissue, or they may be telescoped into each other, with complete elimination of the joint (Figs. 42-14 to 42-16). Disuse osteoporosis develops locally in the immobilized bones and becomes generalized in patients totally crippled by the disease and bedridden for long periods of time. The osteopenia may be compounded by prolonged corticosteroid therapy given to alleviate the arthritic symptoms.

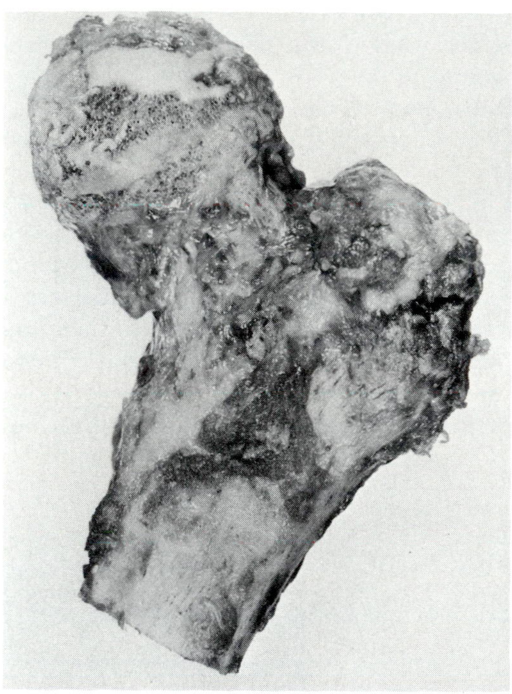

Fig. 42-11. Fresh specimen of proximal femur, showing rheumatoid arthritis with destruction of joint surface by pannus. (WU 49-5578.)

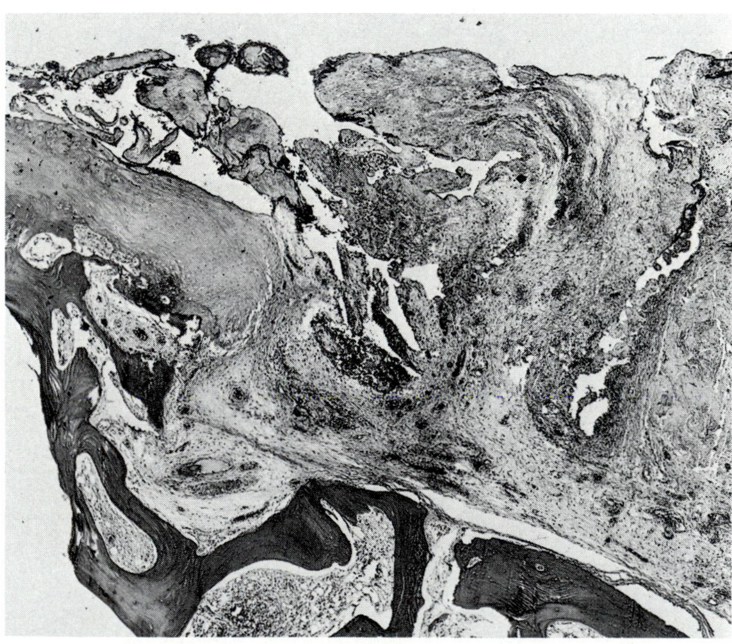

Fig. 42-12. Rheumatoid pannus. Exuberant granulation tissue replaces most of articular cartilage and forms hypertrophic villi projecting into joint space. Some preserved articular cartilage is seen at left.

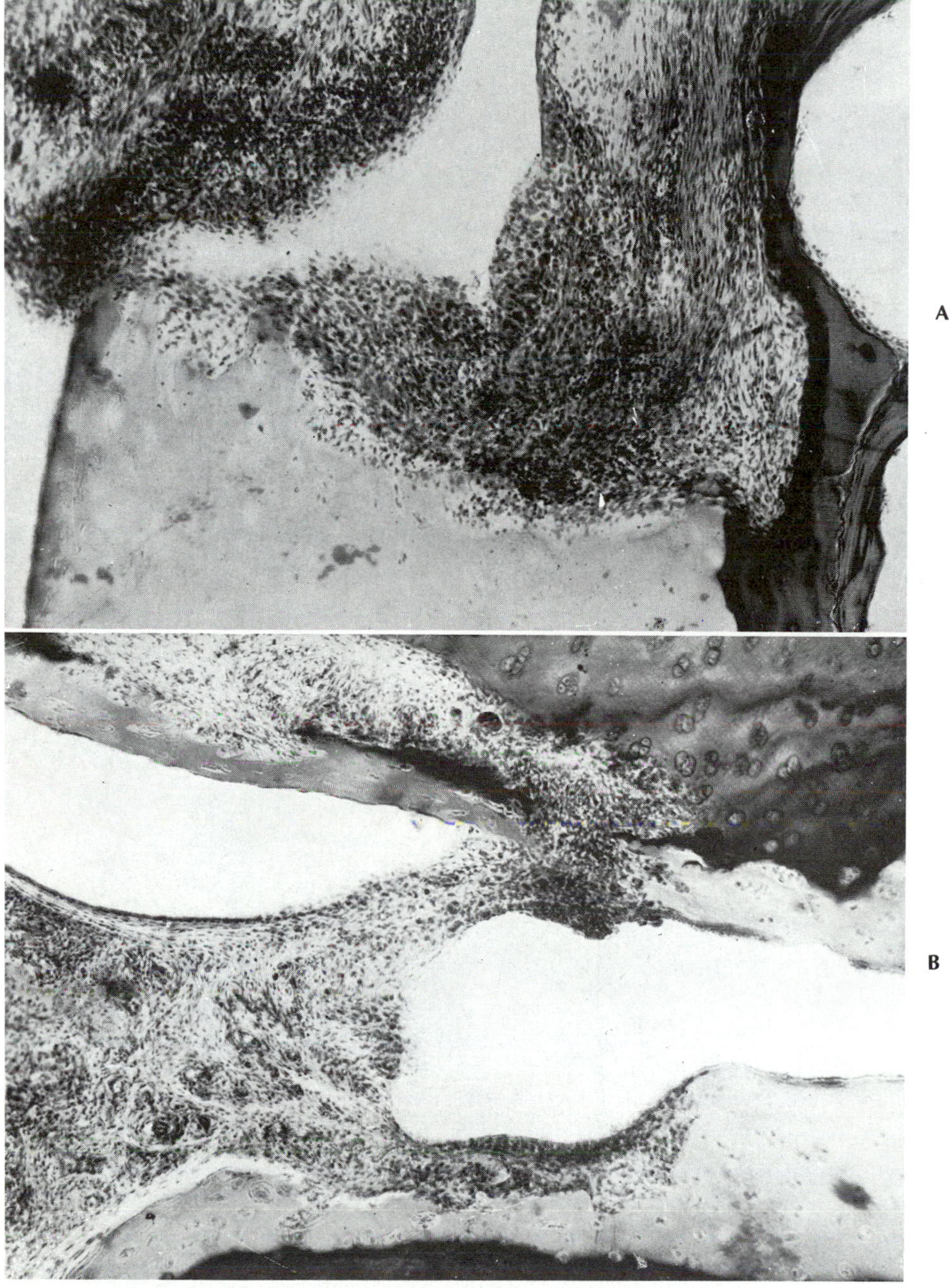

Fig. 42-13. Rheumatoid arthritis. **A,** Early stage of fibrous ankylosis. **B,** Granulation tissue projecting inward from margin of interphalangeal joint has formed adhesion across joint space. Nearly all articular cartilage has disappeared beneath pannus, which is clearly shown in lower half.

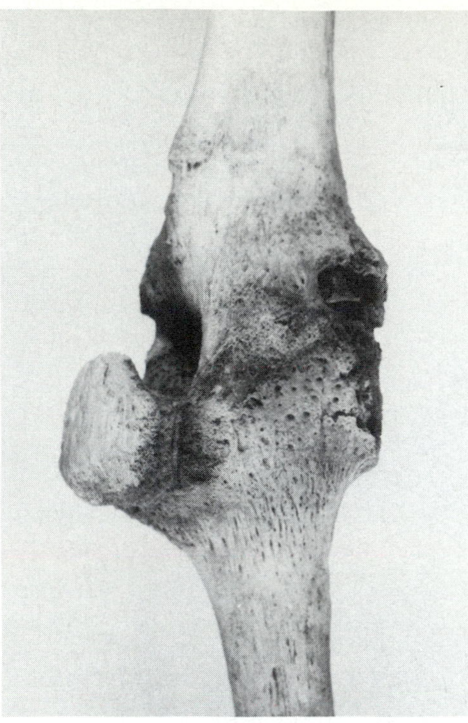

Fig. 42-14. Macerated specimen of knee joint. Advanced rheumatoid arthritis with bony fusion (ankylosis) of patella, femur, and tibia.

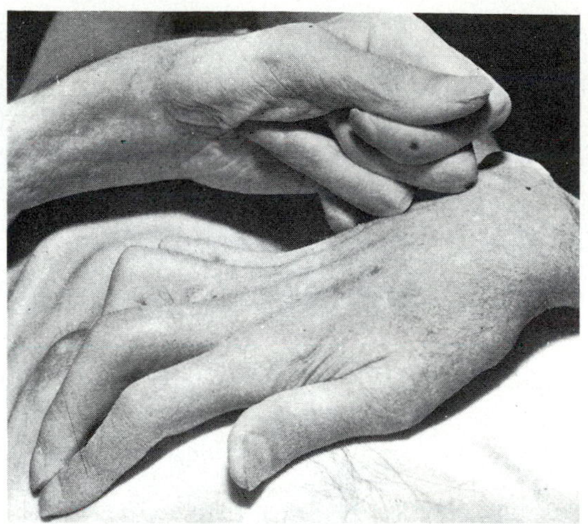

Fig. 42-15. Deformed and stiffened hands in chronic rheumatoid arthritis. Note evidence of muscular atrophy and smooth glossy skin.

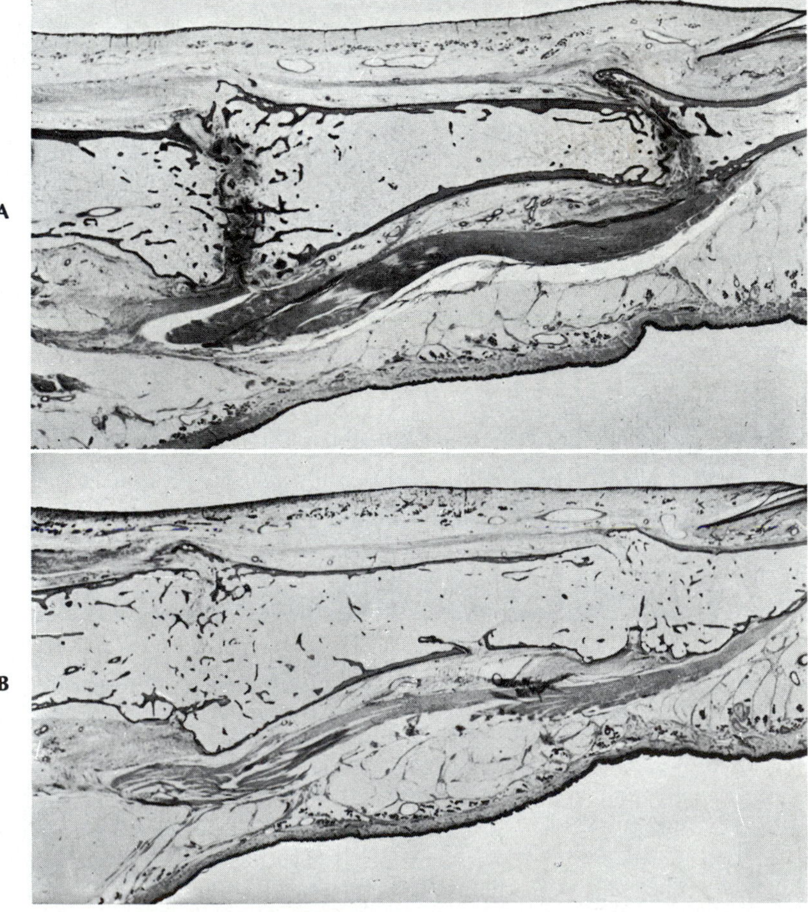

Fig. 42-16. Midline longitudinal sections of second and fourth digits. Atrophy of osseous and dermal tissues is evident in both **A** and **B.** Active chronic inflammation is shown in middle and terminal interphalangeal joints in **A.** All other joints have been destroyed, and bony ankylosis is evident.

Extra-articular rheumatoid disease

The most common extra-articular lesion is the subcutaneous nodule, a granuloma of a few millimeters to several centimeters in size, developing usually in areas close to the joints and subject to minor mechanical insults (Figs. 42-17 to 42-19).

Nodules are more common in seropositive patients and in those with high serum titers of RF than in seronegative persons with low titers of RF. An arteritis is often found close to a nodule and may contribute to the gradual expansion of the necrotic center of the granuloma. Nodules may also be found in bursae and tendon sheaths. In contradistinction to the similar but smaller nodules of rheumatic fever, the rheumatoid nodules develop and regress slowly and are less rich in hydroxyproline than are the former nodules.

Vasculitis associated with deposition of immune complexes in vessel walls is seen especially in patients with high serum titers of IgM-RF complex; occlusion of the vessel may result in ischemia and microinfarcts, charac-

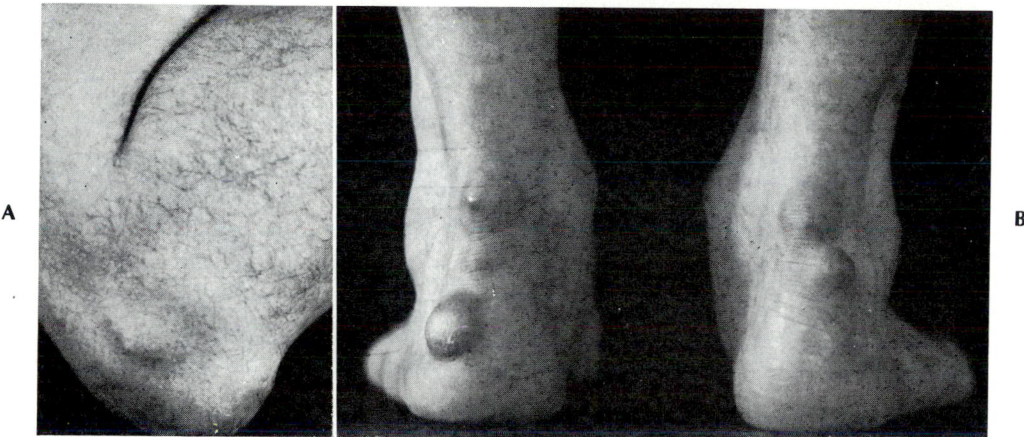

Fig. 42-17. Rheumatoid arthritis. **A,** Large subcutaneous nodule over olecranon process. **B,** Subcutaneous nodules of tendo achillis areas having typical morphologic features of nodule of rheumatoid arthritis. (Courtesy Dr. F.A. Chandler, Atlanta, Ga.)

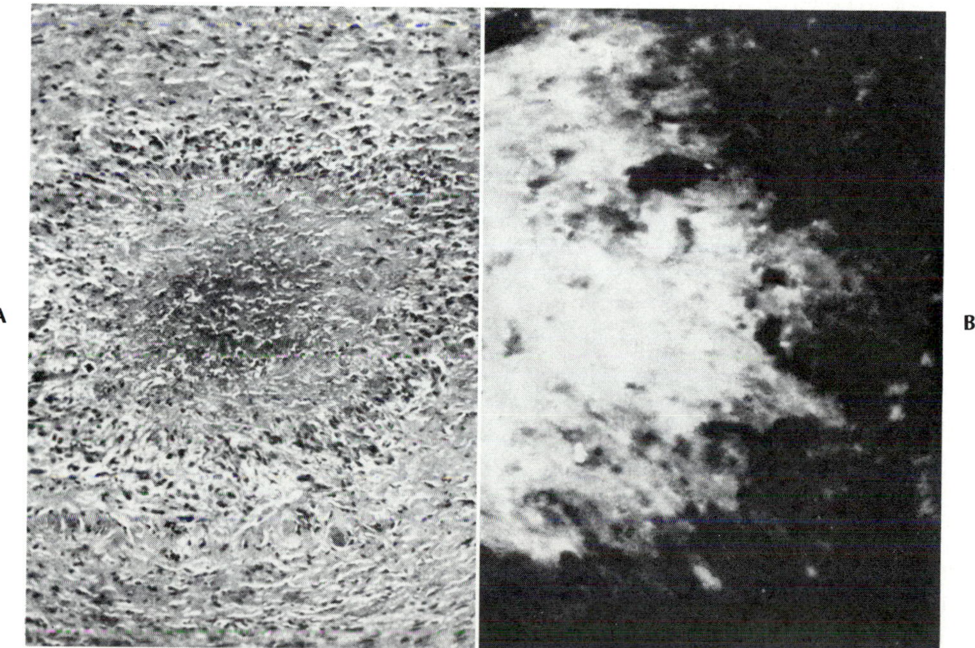

Fig. 42-18. Two consecutive microscopic sections of rheumatoid nodule. **A,** Hematoxylin and eosin stain shows center of fibrinoid necrosis and rim of macrophages with some palisading. **B,** Unstained section treated with fluorescein-conjugated antigammaglobulin. Large fluorescing area indicates presence of gamma globulin in nodule. (From Vazquez, J.J., and Dixon, F.J.: Lab. Invest. **6**:205, 1957.)

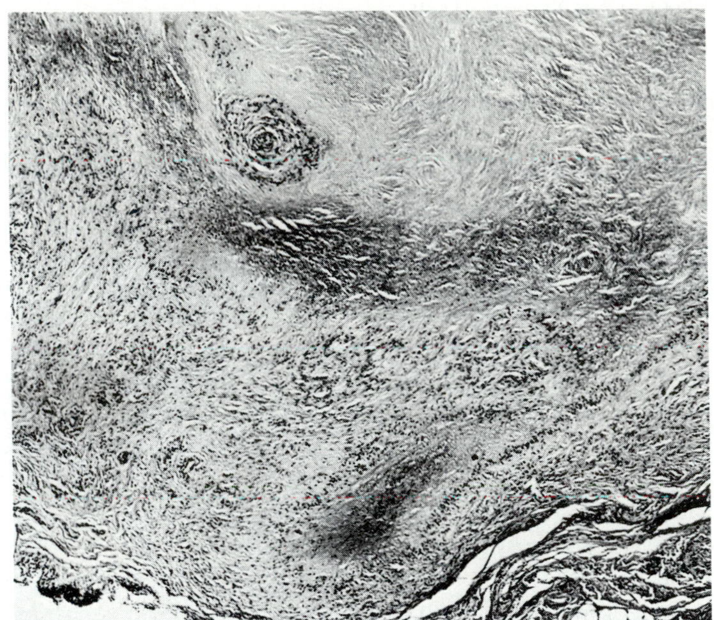

Fig. 42-19. Subcutaneous rheumatoid granuloma with occluded vessel at its periphery.

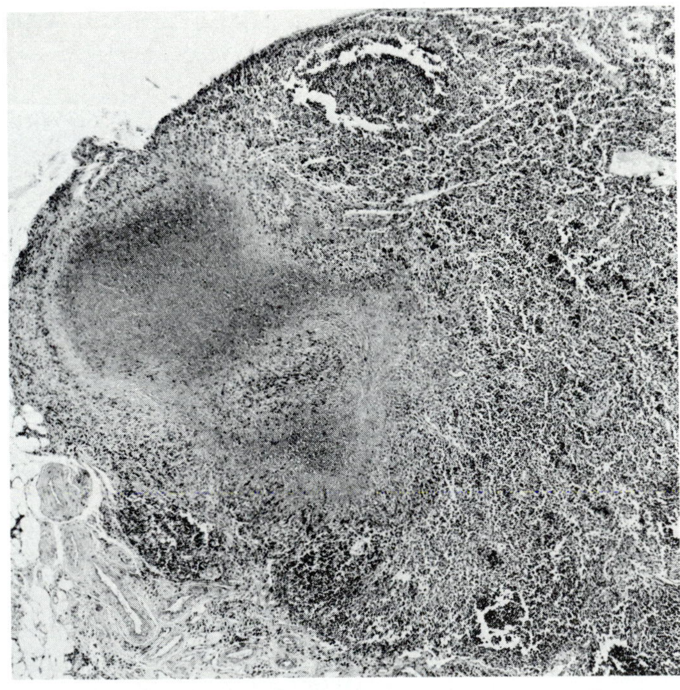

Fig. 42-20. Rheumatoid granuloma in lymph node.

teristically occurring along the nail beds. Occlusion of larger vessels can cause gangrene of the terminal phalanges of fingers and toes.

Cardiac lesions may involve the pericardium, myocardium, and endocardium, with focal accumulation of lymphocytes and plasma cells, vasculitis, granulomas, fibrosis, and amyloidosis.[113]

Pulmonary lesions may be focal and granulomatous or diffuse, interstitial, or intra-alveolar. The result is focal or diffuse fibrosis. In association with pneumoconiosis, especially of coal miners, rheumatoid pneumoconiosis develops (see Chapter 22).[45] Rheumatoid factor has been demonstrated in such lungs.[252] Both pleural effusions containing T lymphocytes and fibrous adhesions are common.

Lymph nodes, especially those draining the areas of involved joints show hyperplasia and, less commonly, granulomas (Fig. 42-20).

Several types of scleritis and retinopathy have been described in about 1% of patients with rheumatoid disease.[113]

Arteritis and granulomas or inflammatory processes extending from diseased joints nearby may involve the central and peripheral nervous systems. Characteristic complications are degenerative myelopathy resulting from subluxation of the atlanto-occipital joint and the "entrapment" syndromes resulting from pressure on peripheral nerves.[113]

Sjögren's syndrome, a combination of typical, but relatively mild, nondestructive rheumatoid arthritis with keratoconjunctivitis sicca, iridocyclitis, and parotitis, develops in 10% to 15% of patients with rheumatoid arthritis.[210,220]

The association of rheumatoid arthritis with splenomegaly and leukopenia is known as Felty's syndrome.[12,74,113]

Amyloidosis is a late complication of rheumatoid arthritis, with data on the frequency varying from 25% to 60%.[39,242]

Etiology and pathogenesis

Of the factors once believed to play a role in the etiology or pathogenesis of rheumatoid arthritis, several (such as allergy, endocrine imbalance, climate, and "collagen disease") have not withstood tests by strict standards; others (especially infections,[22,95] postinfectious immunopathology,[267] autoimmunity,[150] and heredity[138]) are still being actively investigated, as are the effects of psychophysiologic disorders that seem to be related to the onset of attacks.[76,158] No living organism has consistently been found in rheumatoid joints despite widespread search, which in years past was directed mainly toward streptococci[95] and more recently has centered on mycoplasma and diphtheroids.[117] The role of viruses remains controversial.[62,150] Yet infection—systemic or localized extra-articularly and often observed clinically some time before an attack[151]—may be responsible for initiating a sequence of immune processes that, in turn, seem involved in the pathogenesis of articular and extra-articular lesions. The absence of an inciting organism from the joint thus need not preclude infection as cause of the disease.

On the basis of available data, two concepts of the nature of rheumatoid arthritis have emerged:

1. A noxious foreign agent may be the primary trigger in the sequence of immunologic, biochemical, and histologic events—some of them specific and others nonspecific—that combine to produce the lesions. It is surmised that the responding immune system is basically normal and that potential changes in the reacting components result secondarily from the action of the invading organism.
2. The alternative hypothesis suggests a primary defect of the immune system, which reacts abnormally to agents that are readily handled and eliminated by a normal immune system. The abnormality may reside in any or several of the effector cells or mediators involved in the immune response.

Regardless of the nature of the primary cause of rheumatoid arthritis, its pathogenesis comprises processes common to other types of acute or chronic inflammation together with those that are characteristic of—although not necessarily specific for—the disease. The role of immune processes in the development of the rheumatoid lesions is indicated by a number of observations of patients with the disease:

1. The presence of gamma globulins (in particular, IgG and IgM) in synovial fluid[100,181] and leukocytes,[108] in synovial plasma cells,[247] lymphoid centers,[153] and lining cells,[130] and in subcutaneous nodules and vessel walls[267]; these gamma globulins are not a direct cause of rheumatoid disease, since the disease occurs in persons with agammaglobulinemia[87]
2. The presence of RF in synovial plasma cells and in synovial lining cells, which are capable of synthesizing RF[267]
3. The presence of antigen-antibody complexes (RF plus gamma globulin) in synovial plasma cells[30] and synoviocytes[130]
4. The presence in synovial leukocytes, interstitial connective tissue, and lining cells of complement components[34,267] associated with decreased complement titers in the synovial fluid[101]
5. The presence of IgG, IgA, IgM, and B_{1c} complement in the articular cartilage of patients with classic rheumatoid arthritis, in contradistinction to patients with first- or second-degree osteoarthrosis[52]
6. The presence of antinuclear factor (ANF) in the

serum of patients with advanced disease; this suggests a role of autoimmunity, if not as the primary cause then perhaps owing to the chronicity of rheumatoid arthritis[13]
7. The common association of rheumatoid arthritis with amyloidosis[42,242]

A role of heredity in rheumatoid arthritis is not inconsistent with that of abnormal immune mechanisms. The propensity to formation of abnormal gamma globulins or to abnormal tissue reactivity to all kinds of challenges may well be under genetic control.[85,135] The first mentioned possibility is strongly supported by clinical observations: some rheumatoid factors show familial aggregation regardless of the presence or absence of joint disease.[139] The association of rheumatoid arthritis and related disorders with HLA-DW4, HLA-B27, or other HLA antigens seems to provide a link between immune processes and genetics in relation to joint disease.[33]

Results of investigations into the role of heredity in rheumatoid arthritis differ with the methods of sampling. When strict criteria have been used (such as inclusion into the surveys of only those patients with severe erosive involvement of multiple joints), familial aggregation has been demonstrated.[138] This aggregation is apparently not attributable to the common environment shared by members of the same family: in pairs of monozygotic twins, rheumatoid arthritis occurred 33 times more often than in pairs of dizygotic twins. The dizygotic twins showed no higher propensity for the disease than would be expected from a sample of the general population.

On the basis of available histologic and immunologic data, a concept of the histogenesis of rheumatoid arthritis has evolved. An antigen, which could be extraneous (related to infection) or endogenous (related to abnormal gamma globulins), gains access to the joint cavity and elicits an immune reaction that is both humoral and cell mediated and in which polymorphonuclear leukocytes, T and B lymphocytes, and macrophages interact. (The histocompatibility between these cells, normally required for recognition and elimination of the antigen, and the potential lack of histocompatibility in disease stress the role of genetic factors in the pathogenesis of rheumatoid arthritis.) Complexes of various immunoglobulins, RF, and complement—some quite large and insoluble—are formed and phagocytosed by cells termed RA cells or rhagocytes[266]; thus the inflammatory process is set in motion, terminating in the formation of granulation tissue and scarring. Lysosomal enzymes from the cells of the exudate and from the pannus participate in the destruction of cartilaginous matrix by degrading both proteoglycans and collagen; they thus play a major role in the deterioration of the joint.

No plausible concept has yet been developed to explain the chronicity of the disease. There is no spontaneous animal analog of the disorder, and numerous attempts to create an animal model with consistent chronicity without the need for repeated challenge have failed[79] (which has reinforced the hypothesis that autoimmunity may be involved in this as well as in other aspects of rheumatoid arthritis).

SERONEGATIVE SPONDYLOARTHROPATHIES

Several arthritides, formerly considered to be variants of rheumatoid arthritis, have more recently been grouped as seronegative spondyloarthropathies. They differ from rheumatoid arthritis in various, especially immunologic, respects.[29,259] Patients with these types of joint diseases are—as the term implies—seronegative for rheumatoid factor; however, 90% or more of the patients possess HLA-B27 antigens, which show familial aggregation and, when present, multiply many times the risk of developing the disease. Spinal involvement is universally present, and there is male predominance. The group comprises the enteropathic arthropathies, Reiter's disease, Behçet's disease, psoriatic arthritis, Still's disease, ankylosing spondylitis, and possibly others.

Enteropathic arthritis

Included with enteropathic arthritis are the arthritides that are commonly associated with *Yersinia* infection,[3] ulcerative colitis, regional ileitis (Crohn's disease), and intestinal lipodystrophy (Whipple's disease).[29,60] First as well as recurring episodes follow bowel involvement. After surgical removal of the diseased segment of the intestine, arthritis does not recur. The lesions are usually monarticular; the knees are most commonly involved, with the ankle next in order of frequency.

For reasons discussed elsewhere (p. 1075), Whipple's disease is no longer considered to be a metabolic disorder; rather, it is now thought to be due to an infectious agent. The associated arthritis is a transient, migratory, nonspecific synovitis that subsides without residual changes.[47,126] The rodlike particles seen in large numbers in the intestinal laminae propriae have not been demonstrated in articular tissues.

Reiter's syndrome

Reiter's syndrome was originally described as a combination of conjunctivitis, urethritis, and arthritis. More recently keratoderma, oral ulcerations, and cardiovascular abnormalities have been added to the list of characteristic lesions. The arthritis is polyarticular and asymmetric, involving the knee and ankles and often starting at the heel. The usual subacute stage is characterized by a fibrinopurulent exudate. The synovium is hyperemic and infiltrated by polymorphonuclear leukocytes, lymphocytes, and a few plasma cells. Some extravasation of red blood corpuscles may occur and lead to deposition of small amounts of hemosiderin. Commonly there is no major residual change; a few lymphocytic foci in the synovium may be the only evidence of the earlier involvement.

More rarely the subacute process progresses with development of synovial hypertrophy and proliferation of synovial lining cells and fibroblasts. This pannus spreads over the cartilage and erodes it as well as the subchondral bone. Ultimately the appearance of the joints may be similar to that in rheumatoid arthritis.[132] However, a para-articular ossifying periostitis distinguishes these lesions of Reiter's syndrome from rheumatoid arthritis.

The spondylitis of Reiter's syndrome resembles roentgenographically that of psoriasis in the random distribution of osteophytic outgrowths.[155]

The etiology of Reiter's syndrome is unknown; a genetic background has been demonstrated, but its role in the pathogenesis of the disease has not been clarified.

Behçet's syndrome

Behçet's syndrome, a multisystem disorder causing ulcerations of skin, eyes, and mucous membranes, involves large and small joints with a nonspecific, self-limited synovitis in about 90% of patients.[177,248] The changes resemble those of rheumatoid arthritis but are milder and lead only rarely to shallow erosions of the articular cartilage.

Arthritis associated with psoriasis

The association of arthritis and psoriasis is more than coincidental but nevertheless occurs in only 5% to 7% of patients suffering from psoriasis. The lesions involve mainly the distal interphalangeal joints in an asymmetric fashion. Histologically the chronic fibrosing synovitis and subsequent destruction of the joint resemble those of rheumatoid arthritis. In advanced stages osteolysis of the tips (acra) of the phalanges occurs.[15,162] A characteristic finding is terminal convolutions of the nail capillaries in the vicinity of the affected joints, suggesting a role of decreased vascular supply in the necrotizing process involving the epiphyses of the phalanges. A triggering role has been attributed to mechanical injury. Spondylitis also occurs as a complication of psoriasis; the lesions resemble those of Reiter's syndrome.

Still's disease

Rheumatoid arthritis occurring before the age of 16 years has been termed juvenile rheumatoid arthritis (JRA) or Still's disease.[236] Morphologically the lesions are identical to those of the adult disorder, but clinically the disease differs from that in adults. Three clinical forms are distinguished depending on systemic involvement with fever, lymphadenopathy, skin rash, pleurisy, pericarditis, or iridocyclitis. Joint involvement may be polyarticular; lesions are found predominantly in the joints of the hands, or a few of the large joints (knees, ankles, and elbows) may be affected. This variability in the distribution of lesions, in their clinical course, and in the results of immunologic tests for rheumatoid and antinuclear factors has suggested to some investigators that JRA is not a single disease entity but a group of heterogeneous disorders.[198] Pairs of monozygotic twins show a high level of concordance for the disorder, whereas dizygotic twins do not.[6]

Ankylosing spondylitis

Ankylosing spondylitis is discussed in a later section with diseases of the spine (p. 1847).

Arthritis associated with viral hepatitis

Viral hepatitic arthritis occurs in the presence of high serum titers of hepatitis-associated antigen (HAA) and decreased serum levels of the C4 component of complement.[5,178] Although no immune complexes have yet been demonstrated in the articular tissues, it is believed that complexes of HAA, homologous antibody, and early components of complement are causes of the joint lesions.

Arthritis associated with familial Mediterranean fever

A genetic background has been demonstrated for arthritis of familial Mediterranean fever, which occurs mainly in populations of Mediterranean origin, Sephardic Jews, Arabs, and Armenians. The acute, subacute, or chronic synovitis may be accompanied by an effusion that is sterile on culture. After repeated attacks, changes of early osteoarthrosis may develop. One joint at a time is usually involved, but in the course of years, multiple joints may be affected.[199]

Arthritis associated with sarcoidosis

Acute or chronic nonspecific, often symmetric, synovitis can develop in the course of a sarcoid-associated arthritis.[230] Formation of granulomas in the synovium may be followed by erosion of the cartilage, advanced joint destruction, and osteophytic outgrowth at the joint margins. Ankle and knee joints are most commonly affected, but as a rule, joint involvement is less conspicuous than that of adjacent or distant bones.

Arthritis associated with connective tissue diseases

Acute transitory arthritides may be more or less prominent in serum sickness but are particularly common in association with lupus erythematosus, erythema nodosum, and various forms of vasculitis.[13,89] Familial aggregation and increased concordance in monozygotic twins suggest some genetic influences in the propensity of lupus patients to develop arthritis.[28]

Usually no permanent lesions ensue. An exception is the changes seen in progressive systemic sclerosis. In this disorder progressive resorption of the tufts of the terminal phalanges eventually involves the distal interphalangeal joints; because of occlusive disease of the afferent vessels, the subchondral bone and the overlying cartilage undergo avascular necrosis accompanied by fibrinous synovitis and progressive synovial fibrosis.[192,256]

CRYSTAL DEPOSITION DISEASES

Gout (crystal deposition disease, type I)

Gout is a disorder of purine metabolism directly related to serum levels of uric acid and characterized by deposition of monosodium urate monohydrate crystals in various connective tissues. A distinction is usually made between primary or idiopathic gout, developing on the basis of a primary abnormality of purine metabolism, and secondary gout, associated with diseases conducive to "secondary" hyperuricemia. There is no known difference in the tissue changes seen in the two forms of gout.

Historical background

Gout belongs to that group of diseases known and discussed through the ages.[88,97,193] From Hippocrates to Galen and physicians of the Renaissance, the disease was considered to be caused by bad humors, poisoning the body in association with excessive eating, drinking, and generally lecherous living. Paracelsus was the first to attribute the disease to the deposition of an abnormal substance, tartar, derived from food and subsequently altered to form stony material, especially when mixed with "synovia," an egg white–like substance contained in the joints. Sydenham still held onto the concept of ill humors but elaborated specifically on the connection between gout and stone formation and gave a classic description of the disease.

Modern thinking about gout seems to have originated in 1769 with the discovery by Scheele that kidney stones found in patients with gout were made up of an acid, which was also present in the urine. The identification of urates in tophi by Wollaston in 1797[257] and the discovery of hyperuricemia in patients suffering from gout by Garrod in 1848[81] created new directives for all subsequent work dealing with this disorder. Gout is distinctly familial in distribution, with both hereditary and environmental factors having been shown to be involved in the pathogenesis.[31,179,206,211]

Distribution and prevalence

The disease usually begins in the third decade. Men are affected more often and at an earlier age than women. The higher the serum level of uric acid, the greater is the likelihood that the disease will develop. Yet the number of persons with hyperuricemia who actually develop gouty arthritis is small, probably not exceeding 2% or 3%.[137,140] The mere presence of hyperuricemia at one time or another is a predisposing factor for local manifestations of gout to appear, regardless of the cause of hyperuricemia.

The joint most commonly involved is the metatarsophalangeal joint of the great toe, but knees and ankles, elbows and fingers, and spinal and sternoclavicular joints are commonly affected. Arthritis does not develop in all patients suffering from gout: lesions may be confined to periarticular tissues and extraskeletal sites, such as the outer ear, eyelids, scleras, kidneys, heart valves, blood vessels, and cartilages of the respiratory system.

Pathologic anatomy

The acute lesion is triggered by precipitation of needle-shaped crystals of monosodium urate from serum or synovial fluid. In the joints the crystals produce an acute synovitis accompanied by an effusion with numerous polymorphonuclear leukocytes. These leukocytes may take up as much as 95% of the urates into their cytoplasm or into phagosomes. There is hyperplasia of synoviocytes, some of which are being sloughed off into the effusion. Urate crystals are found in synoviocytes and interstitially in the synovial membrane, where they tend to form clusters.[263] By electron microscopy, crystals measure 10×0.5 nm and consist of dense globular bodies suspended in an electron-lucent matrix.[187]

With recurring attacks the lesions become chronic. The deposits enlarge, and urate crystals disposed radially around an amorphous proteinaceous matrix become the center of a foreign body granuloma with a rim of fibroblasts and multinucleated giant cells (Fig. 42-21). Immunoglobulins IgM, IgG, and IgA have been demonstrated in the granulomas by immunofluorescent techniques.[99] The granuloma is spoken of as tophus (Latin *tophus* or *tofus*, "porous stone"). Tophi vary in diameter from a few millimeters to several centimeters. If located subcutaneously, they occur as prominent nodules; if on the hands or feet, they may cause conspicuous disfiguration. More or less diffuse fibrosis may develop around tophi as the lesions age. Synovial granulomas may erode the articular cartilage, but crystals are also directly precipitated in the cartilage. Since articular cartilage is avascular, there is no inflammatory reaction to such deposits; urates at first occupy the superficial layers of the cartilage, which undergo necrosis and assume an opaque, whitish, chalky appearance. Incrustation of the deeper layers of the cartilage is seen in association with advanced regression, resembling the changes of early osteoarthrotis (Fig. 42-22).

Pathogenesis

Hyperuricemia may be primary or secondary; one form of primary hyperuricemia is the result of a deficiency of the enzyme hypoxanthine-guanine phosphoribosyltransferase (HGPRT), a defect that inhibits reconversion

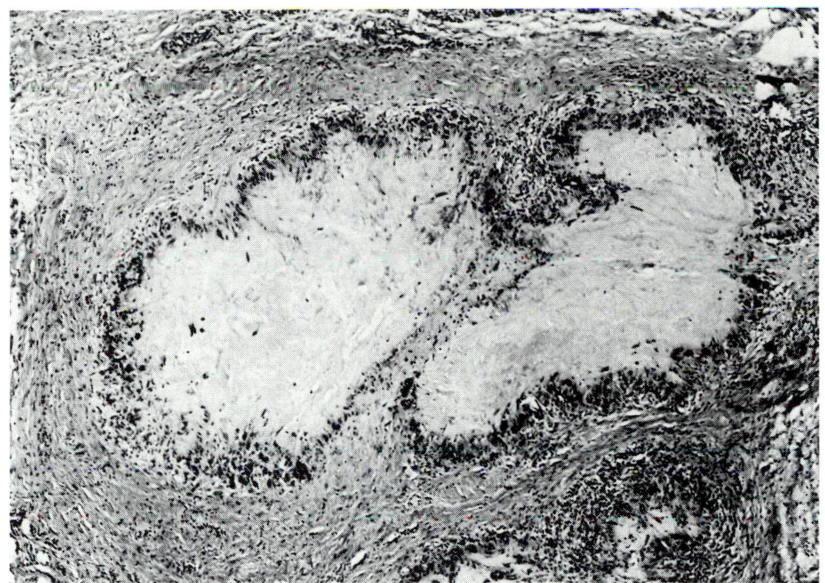

Fig. 42-21. Photomicrograph of portion of gouty tophus in periarticular tissue. Two of several aggregates of which tophus is composed. Urate crystals originally present have been dissolved in processing of tissue, and only proteinaceous matrix is preserved in centers. Latter are surrounded by corona of granulation tissue with numerous multinucleated giant cells. (BH 69-1754.)

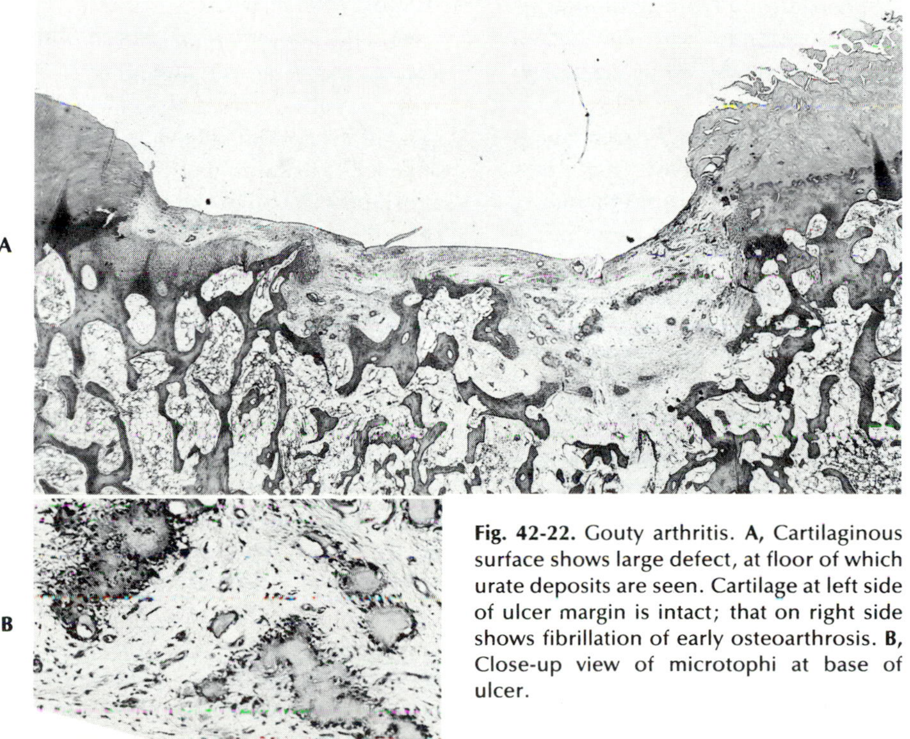

Fig. 42-22. Gouty arthritis. **A,** Cartilaginous surface shows large defect, at floor of which urate deposits are seen. Cartilage at left side of ulcer margin is intact; that on right side shows fibrillation of early osteoarthrosis. **B,** Close-up view of microtophi at base of ulcer.

of hypoxanthine to inosinic acid, one step in purine resynthesis. Consequently, hypoxanthine is further degraded to produce excessive quantities of uric acid.[18,91,103,122,261] In addition, overactivity of the enzyme 5-phosphoribosyl-1-pyrophosphate synthetase contributes to hyperuricemia.[105]

Secondary hyperuricemia is seen when excessive amounts of nuclear material are being degraded as in leukemia or polycythemia, or when renal excretion is impaired as in lead poisoning or renal calcification. Characteristically, in secondary hyperuricemia the pathways of purine degradation are normal.

The mechanism that causes deposition of urates in tissues is complex and is discussed in Chapter 3. Rapid fluctuations in uric acid serum levels as after excessive alcohol consumption, fasting, or the administration of uricosuric drugs[148] are likely to trigger an acute attack in persons predisposed to gout.

Tissues with low oxygen tension are particularly prone to becoming the site of urate precipitation. Moreover, the peak incidence of gouty arthritis coincides with the age at which age-linked loss of mucopolysaccharide from the cartilaginous matrix is maximal.

The irritating effect of urate crystals is attributable to their physical configuration and not to their chemical composition: a minor inflammatory response is observed after introduction of dissolved sodium urate into tissues, in contradistinction to the intense reaction to crystalline monosodium urate. Agents differing from sodium urate chemically, but similar in crystallinity, evoke an inflammatory reaction resembling that produced by crystalline sodium urate.[73]

A decrease in pH, as occurs in acute inflammation, promotes crystal deposition[209]; thus a vicious circle may be initiated that is responsible for self-perpetuation of the lesion. The importance of the Hageman factor in the inflammatory sequence of gout has been questioned, since crystals may provoke acute inflammation in the absence of the factor.[229] Similarly, the role played by kinins in the process has been doubted. Complement, however, is still considered to be involved.[121] The mechanism of action of polymorphonuclear leukocytes, by contrast, remains unexplained: in experimentally produced aleukocytosis no attack develops.[208] The role of prostaglandins is being investigated; some experimental evidence suggests that several of the prostaglandins promote urate crystal–induced inflammation.[61]

Pyrophosphate arthropathy

Among the other names for pyrophosphate arthropathy are pseudogout, articular calcinosis, and crystal deposition disease type II. This abnormality was recognized after demonstration of calcium pyrophosphate in the synovial fluid of certain inflamed joints. It is an example of crystal deposition disease, characterized by the presence of calcium pyrophosphate dihydrate crystals in articular cartilage, synovium, articular ligaments, and intervertebral discs. The crystals can be demonstrated by polarized light or by x-ray diffraction.[25,135] The disorder differs from true gout not only in the chemical nature of the crystals but also in distribution; in pseudogout the large joints such as knees, hips, and shoulders are preferentially involved rather than the small joints of hands and feet.

Pyrophosphate arthropathy occurs by itself or, more rarely, in association with other metabolic aberrations such as hyperparathyroidism, true gout, diabetes, and acromegaly.[55] The joints show an acute synovitis, often with a large effusion—changes that may subside without residual damage. With repeated recurrences, or insidiously without an acute phase, changes typical of osteoarthrosis develop, and deposits of calcium pyrophosphate are found in the articular cartilage. These deposits are composed of crystals or microspheroliths[25]; they are confined to the midzone of the cartilage and have no apparent relationship to chondrocytes.

Neither the etiology nor the pathogenic mechanism by which the lesions evolve is known. Occasional familial aggregation of persons with the disorder points to a genetic background.[250] No basic biochemical abnormalities have been found.

Apatite arthropathy

Needle-shaped crystals 75 × 250 Å have been identified as apatite in the sediment of joint effusions and in synovial cells of patients with acute arthritis. Injection of crystalline apatite into dog knees has produced similar lesions.[205] Besides apatite, other calcium phosphates are presumed to give rise to crystal-induced arthropathies.[64]

Relapsing polychondritis (chronic atrophic polychondritis)

Relapsing polychondritis, which occurs in both men and women, is characterized by degeneration and inflammation of any of the cartilages of the body.[65] The disintegration leads to gross deformities, such as floppy ears, saddle nose, and collapse of the trachea. Involvement of intervertebral discs may lead to spondylitis and, at late stages, to deformities of the spine. In the joints a picture resembling rheumatoid arthritis is seen. The synovium is infiltrated by lymphocytes and plasma cells, and there is an increase in both A and B cells. The cartilage matrix loses some of the acid mucopolysaccharides, resulting in decreased staining with Alcian blue and other cationic dyes. The cartilage is infiltrated by lymphocytes, and many chondrocytes disappear from their capsules. Electron microscopy shows that chondrocytes have peculiar bulbous bodies attached to or within the elongated cytoplasmic processes; the cells contain an unusual number of lysosomes and dense bodies, both signs of degeneration. In the cell vicinity, aggregates of granular material appear from which long spacing bodies are formed.[161] The nature of this material is unknown, but it seems related to degenerative processes in both cells and matrix. The etiology of the disorder is likewise unknown; repeated suggestions of a role played by autoimmune processes have not been substantiated.[104]

Diseases of bursae, tendons, and fasciae

Bursitis

Since bursae are synovial membrane-lined sacs, their reaction to injury may be expected to resemble that of the synovial lining of joints (Fig. 42-23). The common lesions are those following mechanical insults or infection.

Traumatic bursitis may result from a single injury, such as a blow to the elbow (olecranon bursa) or the knee (prepatellar bursa). More commonly, however, it is the repeated injuries from excessive pressure or bruises that initiate the inflammatory changes. This is exemplified by "housemaid's knee," in which the prepatellar bursa becomes enlarged and painful as the result of crawling on floors and closing drawers and doors with the knee.

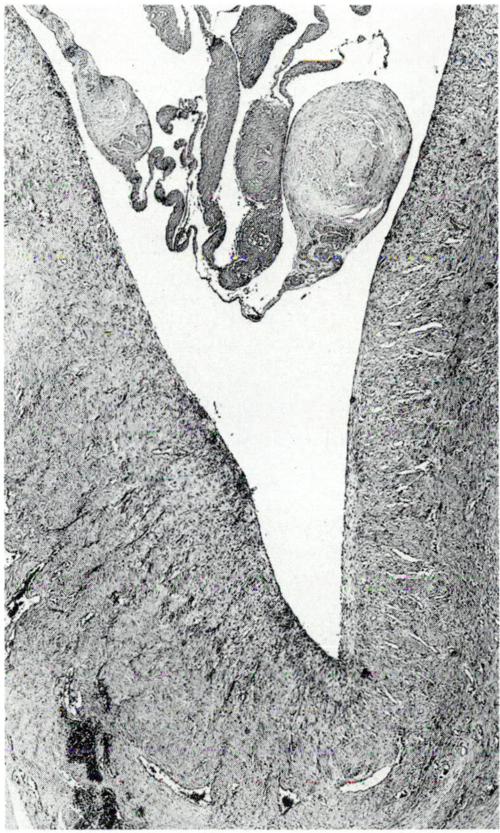

Fig. 42-23. Portion of wall of chronically inflamed bursa. Synovial lining has been replaced by layer of vascular fibrous tissue infiltrated by lymphocytes. Inspissated old exudate is present in bursal lumen.

Purulent inflammation of bursal cavities may be caused by pathogenic microorganisms. This may follow penetrating injuries, be an extension of infection from an adjacent cellulitis or abscess, or result from embolization of blood-borne organisms.

Tendinitis and tenovaginitis

Inflammation of tendons and tendon sheaths may follow chronic mechanical insults or direct or blood-borne infection. The lesions can assume any form of acute or chronic inflammation with or without effusion, with or without suppuration, or with development of diffuse granulation tissue or granulomas. A special type of involvement is known as stenosing tenovaginitis. This lesion develops preferably in places where tendons pass over bony prominences, especially at the wrist. The tendon sheath is narrowed because of annular fibrosis of the wall, which inhibits the free motion of the tendon. The tendon distal to the stenosis becomes thickened and at times locked in a certain position, from which it must be unlocked before normal motion is restored.

Dupuytren's contracture

Contracture of the digits of the hand, first observed by Plater in 1614, was recognized as due to changes in the palmar aponeurosis by Dupuytren[67] and more recently reported as also occurring in the plantar aponeurosis. The lesion results in permanent flexion contracture, with the fifth, fourth, and third digits being usually involved in this order of frequency. Men are more commonly affected than women, and in about half the patients the lesion is bilateral.

Grossly the involvement may be diffuse or nodular. Microscopically three developmental phases have been described[144]: (1) proliferation of fibroblasts, (2) decreasing cellularity and increasing collagenization, and (3) a residual stage, characterized by regression of the nodules, atrophy of the fibrous cords, and almost complete acellularity. The lesions extend into the adjacent subcutaneous fat tissue and into the corium, causing attachment of the aponeurosis to the skin. In the past, contraction of the excessive collagen was considered the principal pathogenic mechanism involved. However, the chemical composition of collagen and glycoproteins of the ground substance has been found to be normal.[112] Electron microscopic investigations have disclosed a cytoplasmic fibrillar system and other evidence of contractility in the cells of the lesion. The involved cells thus appear to be myofibroblasts, which have the ability to contract. This property is believed to play a role in the clinical contracture.

The etiology of the lesion is unknown. A more than coincidental association with diabetes has been observed,[63] and heredity may be involved in some cases.[142]

CYSTS OF JOINTS AND PARA-ARTICULAR TISSUES

Cysts of ganglion

The lesions are round or ovoid, movable, subcutaneous nodules that may be cystic or semicystic. They occur most commonly on the wrist but also on the dorsal surface of the foot, close to the ankle, or about the knee. They may or may not have a pedicle attachment to or communicate with a tendon sheath or a joint cavity. The cysts are filled with a clear mucinous fluid that by electron microscopy contains flakes or delicate filaments and disintegrated collagen. In some instances the cysts have a more or less continuous lining of cells resembling synovial cells. In others the lining is discontinuous or lacking altogether; the cyst wall then consists of dense connective tissue lined by necrotic cells, cell debris, and disintegrated collagen.[83] Other ganglia contain fragments of tissue resembling synovium incorporated in a loose edematous connective tissue mass.

The histogenesis of the lesion is disputed. Herniation of the synovium into the surrounding tissue, displacement of synovial tissue during embryogenesis, and posttraumatic degeneration of connective tissue have all been incriminated as causes.[228] More recently demonstrated aggregates of cytoplasmic filaments in lining cells have indicated a possible relationship to smooth muscle fibrils. It was therefore suggested that the lesions arise from proliferating pluripotential mesenchymal cells.

Cysts of semilunar cartilage

Cysts of the semilunar cartilages are usually located in the lateral meniscus near its anterior insertion. They contain a number of indistinct locules filled with mucinous or gelatinous fluid. Microscopic sections may reveal bits of synovial lining and diffuse fraying of the fibrocartilage of the meniscus. The fraying probably results from seepage of mucin-containing fluid into the interstices of the dense and relatively acellular tissue of the semilunar cartilage. These lesions have much in common with ganglia of tendon sheath origin and are probably formed in a similar manner.

Bursal cysts connected with the knee joint cavity are not uncommon, particularly in patients with rheumatoid arthritis. In some cases the cysts communicate with the articular space by a long and tortuous duct. The opening may become obliterated by cicatrization. These cysts are usually referred to as Baker's cysts, although Baker originally described cystic lesions in association with a variety of pathologic conditions of dissimilar etiology.[10,131]

Bursal cysts have a dense fibrous wall of variable thickness. The enclosed cavity often is divided partially or completely into two or more chambers by fibrous septa that project inward from the cyst wall. The lumen contains fluid that may be either clear or turbid and either watery or mucinous. At times the fluid is stained with blood pigment. Some cavities contain "melon seed" bodies originating from detached small excrescences or tips of villi projecting into the cavity.

Microscopically synovial membrane may be present, but more frequently the cyst is lined with dense fibrous connective tissue that contains focal and diffuse infiltrates of lymphocytes and hemosiderin-laden phagocytes.

TUMORS AND TUMORLIKE LESIONS OF JOINTS, BURSAE, TENDONS, AND TENDON SHEATHS

Any of the tissue components of the articulations, including bursae, tendons, and tendon sheaths, may give rise to benign or malignant neoplasms. Among the benign tumors are chondromas, osteochondromas, myxomas, angiomas, fibromas, and lipomas. These neoplasms and the malignant tumors derived from corresponding cell types are no different from tumors of the same histologic composition elsewhere in the body. Neoplasms whose origin and behavior are determined by the presence of specialized synovial lining cells, and which are thus peculiar to structures normally lined by such cells, may be benign or malignant.

Xanthofibroma

Included as synonyms for xanthofibroma are villonodular synovitis, giant cell tumor of tendon sheath, and benign synovioma.

Xanthogranulomas occur most commonly in young adults and are localized on fingers, wrists, ankles, feet, and knees. They grow slowly, with compression and displacement of the adjacent tissues. Where the tendons and other tissues are firmly anchored in bone, the tumors may cause surface erosions or deep rounded depressions in the bone from pressure atrophy.

The gross appearance of these tumors varies within wide limits. They measure from a few millimeters to several centimeters in greatest diameter. They have a dense fibrous covering formed by the compressed surrounding tissues. They are firm and only slightly elastic. Cut surfaces show a gray, dense, inelastic tissue and in many instances yellowish flecks or streaks, proportional to the amount of lipid contained within histiocytes. Because of the yellow color, these lesions have been named xanthomas or xanthofibromas.

Microscopically the tumors are characteristically composed of small oval or spindle-shaped cells, multinucleated giant cells, lipid-laden macrophages, and irregularly placed bundles of connective tissue. The ratio of these elements is exceedingly variable within the same and in different tumors. Some neoplasms are highly cellular and show active cell proliferation. Others are dense and fibrous with few cellular elements. Giant cells may be numerous or few. They contain many small oval nuclei that are usually crowded together in one portion of the cell. The cytoplasm may be scant or abundant, and the shape of the cells is equally variable. The number of lipid-laden phagocytes ("foam cells") is also variable; some tumors are composed chiefly of foam cells whereas others contain only small aggregates or scattered single such cells (Fig. 42-24).

Some tumors show irregular slitlike cavities lined by oval or flattened cells. Small tufts of these cells may project into the cavities. Cellular tumors with many clefts and tufts may be difficult to distinguish from synovial sarcoma.

The origin and histogenesis of xanthofibroma have been traced to the proliferation of synovial cells resembling histiocytes. These cells are transformed into multinucleated giant cells and macrophages laden with hemosiderin or lipid. The underlying tissue is infiltrated by lymphocytes, a finding of basic significance in support of the view that the nodules are of inflammatory rather than neoplastic origin. As the nodules age, collagenous and often hyalinized matrix is laid down between the cells. Doubt has been cast on the neoplastic character of the lesions, especially because similar changes may involve the synovium of joints, bursae, and tendon sheaths multifocally or diffusely. The term *villonodular synovitis* is being used to describe the diffuse lesion; benign giant cell tumor of the tendon sheath and villonodular synovitis have been considered to be manifestations of the same underlying process: a chronic granulomatous inflammation, of as yet unknown etiology.[116]

Osteochondromatosis

Osteochondromatosis may occur as an isolated lesion or in conjunction with other forms of joint disease. It is characterized by the development, in the synovial tissues, of cartilaginous nodules that tend to undergo secondary ossification. The synovial lining contains translucent masses of proliferating cartilage projecting from the surface or hanging from narrow pedicles into the joint space (Fig. 42-25). Many of the nodules become detached, and dozens or even hundreds of them float free in the joint fluid, where they may continue to grow or become inactive.[159] By electron microscopy, transition from regular synovial cells to chondrocytes producing cartilaginous matrix along with deposition of crystals

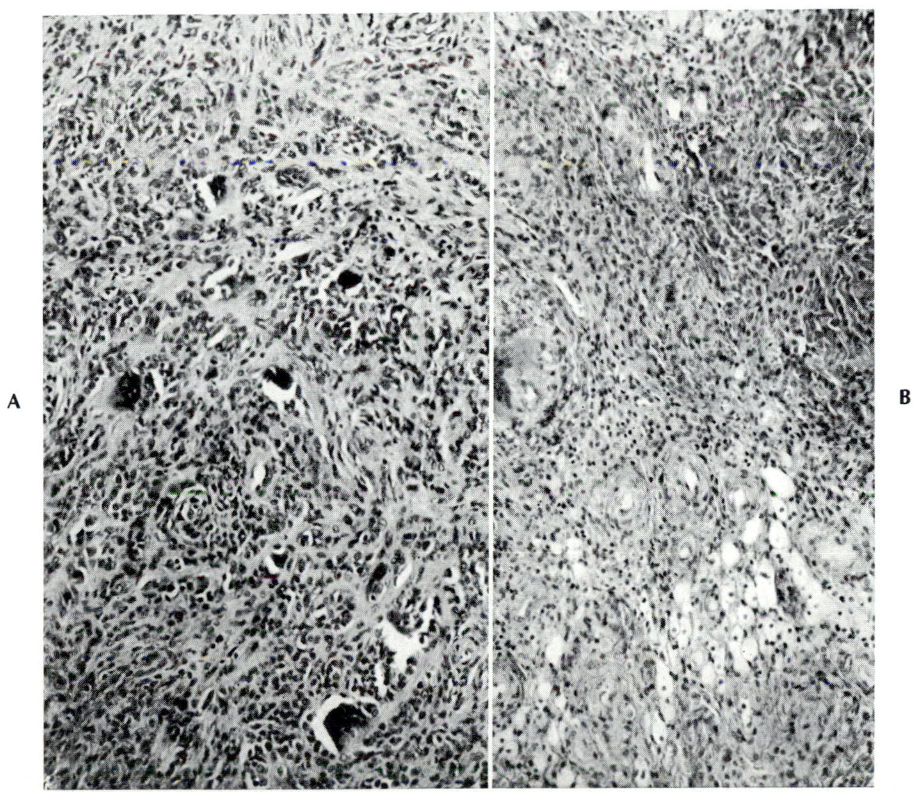

Fig. 42-24. Xanthofibromas of tendon sheath. **A,** Tumor composed of spindle-shaped fibroblasts and giant cells. **B,** Tumor containing many lipid-laden cells. (130×; **A,** AFIP 90662; **B,** AFIP 82251.)

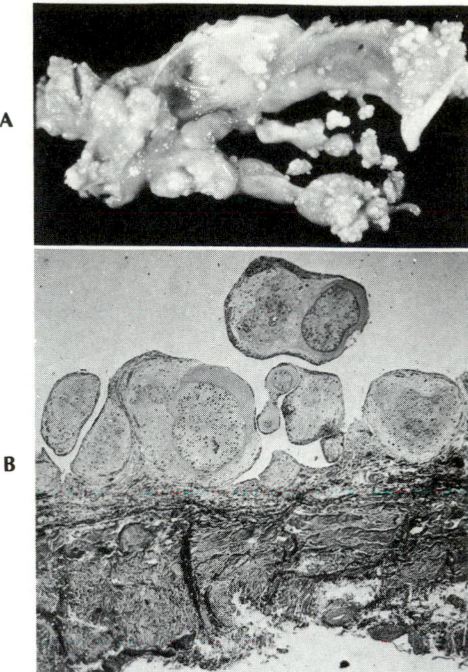

Fig. 42-25. Osteochondromatosis. **A,** Portions of synovial membrane showing numerous attached and superimposed cartilaginous nodules. **B,** Photomicrograph of synovial membrane showing ectopic cartilage forming numerous nodules projecting into joint cavity.

in the collagen fibrils of the matrix can be demonstrated.[53]

The etiology of the disorder is unknown. Although mechanical injury and inflammation have been implicated, the lesions can occur in the absence of either. Histogenetically two mechanisms must be considered: (1) metaplasia from regular elements of the synovium and (2) development from undifferentiated chondrogenic cells; such cells are to be expected, especially at the reflection of the synovium, where during embryogenesis cells develop into either synoviocytes or chondrocytes.[183]

An uncommon variant of osteochondromatosis has been described as *osteomatosis*. In this disorder multiple osseous bodies develop in the synovial tissue without previous formation of cartilage.[68,168]

Synovioma (synovial sarcoma)

The term *synovioma* was suggested to designate a group of rare malignant tumors involving the regions of diarthrodial joints and once believed to arise from the synovium.[223] However, only 10% of the tumors develop within the joint cavities; the rest arise in tissues close to the articulations and seem to involve the synovium secondarily.[239] The tumor is most often seen in young adults, and the sex ratio is 3:2 (males predominating). The knee joint is the most common site. The survival rate is low, and metastasis occurs more often by the bloodstream than by lymphatics.

Grossly the tumors are usually single, roughly ovoid, often lobulated, and vary from 1 to 18 cm in diameter.[41] They may be sharply delimited but may extend along fascial planes. Growing expansively, they are partially or completely surrounded by a pseudocapsule formed by the compressed or attenuated adjacent nontumorous tissue. On the cut surface the tumors may be firm, focally gritty, or spongy and friable. Homogeneous areas alternate with areas of fibrous, even whorl-like appearance, and hemorrhage, necrosis, or cysts may be present, the cysts containing gelatinous or mucinous material.

Microscopically the tumors are characterized by a biphasic cell pattern: (1) areas resembling fibrosarcoma, composed of fairly uniform spindle-shaped cells with hyperchromatic nuclei and densely packed in bands or sheets, and (2) cells resembling epithelium (synovioblastic cells), arranged in pseudoglandular structures, lining clefts in the fibrosarcomatous stroma or forming papillae (Figs. 42-26 and 42-27). These cells vary in shape from cuboid to tall columnar; they may secrete a mucopolysaccharide, probably hyaluronic acid, which is also found in the occasional cysts. The cell sheets are surrounded by abundant masses of reticulin, but no fibrils are found between the cells. In addition, there is nonfibrillar eosinophilic material that resembles osteoid and sometimes contains deposits of calcium. In the presence of an old hemorrhage, hemosiderin-laden macrophages or, more rarely, foreign body giant cells may be found. The number of mitoses varies from moderate to large. The tumor may invade adjacent tissues and blood vessels.

The biphasic pattern of the tumors has been confirmed by electron microscopy.[78,146] Stromal cells have folded nuclei with clumped chromatin at the membrane and prominent nucleoli; the cytoplasm is vesiculated. Endoplasmic reticulum, both rough and smooth, and microfilaments are more prominent than Golgi apparatus of mitochondria. The epithelium-like cells, by contrast, contain many mitochondria. The cells are always in contact with one another; the presence of desmosomes, other junctional zones, and a basement membrane at the junction of stromal and epithelioid cells indicates a comparatively advanced stage of differentiation of a tumor.[75]

The histogenesis of the neoplasm is obscure. The similarity of the cells to the two types found in normal synovium is suggestive of synovial origin. However, the extra-articular origin of the majority of the tumors, the presence of transitional cell types, and the behavior of the tumor cells in tissue culture are not consistent with this hypothesis. It seems more justified to consider a pluripotential undifferentiated mesenchymal cell as the true precursor of the neoplasm.

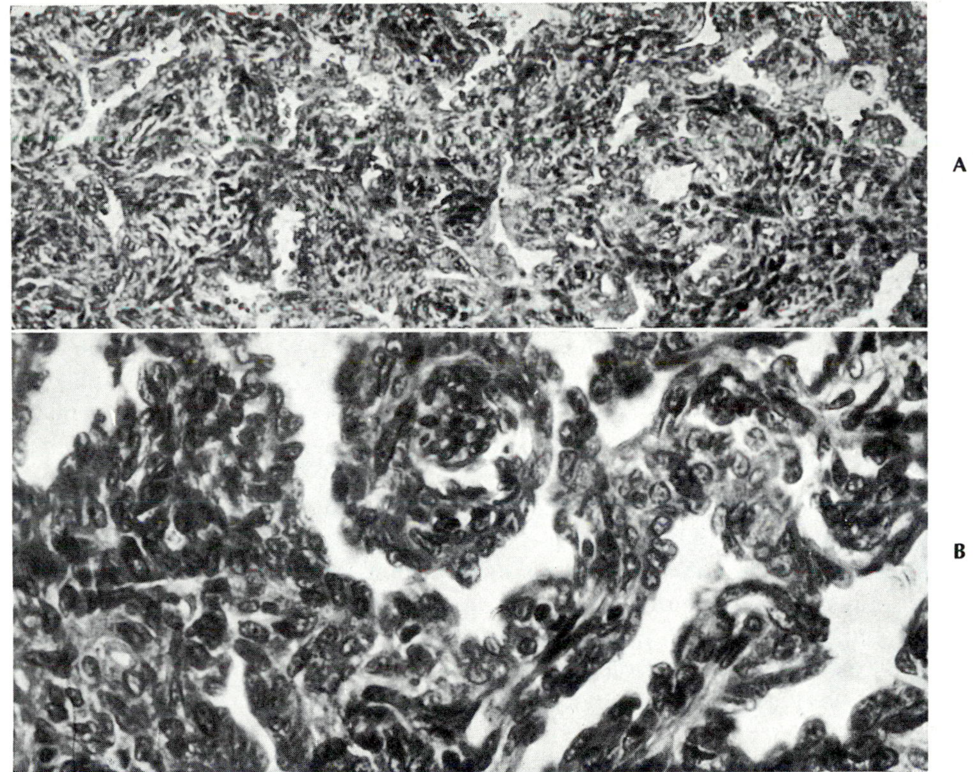

Fig. 42-26. Synovial sarcoma. **A,** Low-power view. **B,** High-power view. (**A** and **B,** AFIP 90623.)

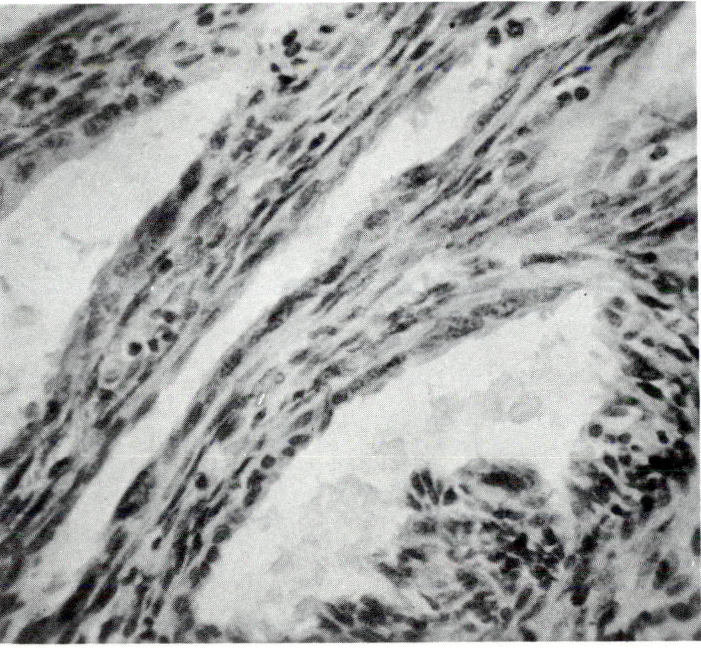

Fig. 42-27. Highly differentiated synovial sarcoma with epithelium-like cells forming surface lining of tissue clefts.

Clear cell sarcoma of tendon sheaths and aponeuroses

Clear cell sarcoma of tendon sheaths and aponeuroses has been recognized only recently.[27,71] It occurs most commonly in the region of the hands or feet. The spherical smooth or nodular tumors are attached to tendons or aponeuroses; on cut surface they are grayish white, solid, and sometimes gritty, with occasional foci of necrosis or cysts. Microscopically they are not biphasic like the synoviomas but consist of nests of pale, fusiform, epithelioid cells surrounded by delicate fibrous septa. The tumor cells have light-staining nuclei with contrasting prominent nucleoli and do not contain lipid. Multinucleated giant cells are common. By electron microscopy melanosomes have been found in such a tumor.[107]

Miscellaneous malignant lesions

Malignant giant cell tumor of the tendon sheath combines features of clear cell sarcoma and benign giant cell tumor of tendon sheaths. It differs from clear cell sarcoma in that there are transitions between the clear cells and foam cells and the multinucleated giant cells of osteoclastic or Touton type. The intercellular substance, which can be removed with bovine hyaluronidase, is closely related to the plasma membrane of the tumor cells, a finding that suggests secretion of the substance by the membrane.[119,175]

Chondrosarcoma of the joint is a rare and highly malignant neoplasm[86] that involves the joints diffusely, simulating benign chondromatosis at the early stages. The tumor may arise from the synovium directly or from previously present chondromatosis.[166] Histologically the neoplasm is characterized by large atypical cells with hyperchromatic nuclei and by large binucleated or multinucleated cells.

Multicentric histiocytic reticulosis may involve multiple or simple joints by development of granulomatous tissue in the synovium. As elsewhere in this disorder, the granulation tissue is characterized by the presence of numerous histiocytes, multinucleated giant cells, and forms transitional between the two. All these cells may characteristically have a foamy cytoplasm and, with special stains, can be shown to contain neutral fats and phospholipids.[14] More rarely, lipid may be absent from the cells.[69] The granulation tissue spreads aggressively, and with time there is extensive destruction of the articular cartilage and the adjacent bone, leading to partial or complete loss of joint function.

DISEASES OF THE VERTEBRAL COLUMN

Deformities

The significance of spinal deformities lies in their effects on motor activity, on the integrity of peripheral joints, and on the viscera (such as the heart and lungs, which depend on normal spatial relations for their proper functioning.)

Deformities of the spine may be caused by changes in the vertebral bodies (a topic outside the scope of this chapter) or by changes in the intervertebral discs. Three types of deformity involving large segments of the spine exist: (1) kyphosis, characterized by increased convexity in the anteroposterior direction; (2) lordosis, increased concavity in the anteroposterior direction; and (3) scoliosis, lateral deviation from the normal orientation. One of the most common deformities, kyphosis of old age (senile kyphosis), is caused by uneven distribution of degenerative processes in the discs that cause the discs to collapse anteriorly so the anterior portions of the vertebral bodies tilt toward each other.

Disc disease

Starting in late adolescence and progressing with increasing age, the intervertebral discs can deteriorate.[241] Water is lost from the nucleus, and there are loss of chondroitin sulfate, increase of keratan sulfate and collagen, and calcification. These changes lead to a decrease in intranuclear pressure and loss of elasticity. The anulus fibrosus likewise loses water, becomes fibrillated and fissured, and loses its tight attachment to the vertebral bone. It thus exerts less than normal restraints on the nucleus during mechanical stress. Sudden or, more commonly, chronic stretching and bending that produce mechanical strain may then force the nucleus out of the confines of the anulus into neighboring structures. If the prolapse occurs into the spinal canal, pressure on and potential damage to neural tissues ensue. Another site of predilection for prolapses is the terminal plates of the vertebrae; disc tissue may penetrate the bone marrow space of the vertebral body and there form globular masses. These structures are termed Schmorl's nodules; roentgenographically, they superficially resemble metastatic tumors. Prolapsed nuclei undergo further degeneration, such as hyalinization and sclerosis.

Spondylosis

Degenerating discs, even if they do not prolapse, may yet assume a role in the initiation of spondylosis deformans, although this disorder can also develop in the absence of disc disease. Spondylosis deformans, or hypertrophic spondylosis, is a disease peculiar to vertebral bodies and their articulating surfaces. It does not involve the small joints of the spinal processes, which are subject to osteoarthrosis like other large diarthrodial joints. Spondylosis deformans is an age-linked disorder having its steepest rise in incidence during the fourth to sixth decades, after which age nearly everyone is affected.[200] Men seem to be affected somewhat more severely and at an earlier age than women.[102] The increased inci-

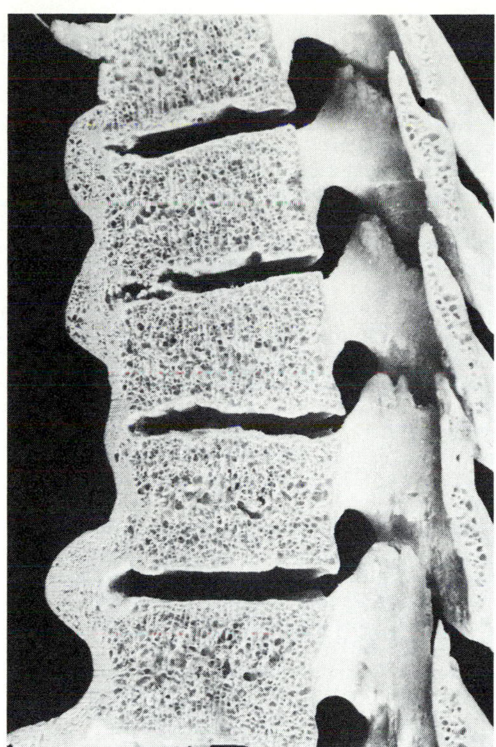

Fig. 42-28. Hyperostotic spondylosis. Anterior fusion of vertebral bodies by osseous bridges. (Courtesy Dr. Max Aufdermaur, Lucerne.)

dence of the disorder in miners as compared with that found in factory workers or craftsmen has suggested to some investigators an etiologic role of extraneous mechanical stresses.

The fully developed lesions of spondylosis are characterized by fraying, fibrillation, and chondrocyte proliferation of the cartilage of the terminal plates and by chondro-osseous outgrowths (osteophytes) at the vertebral margins. Osteophytes may bridge the narrowed intervertebral space and overlap the adjacent vertebral edge (Fig. 42-28). Two opposing osteophytes may fuse, causing immobilization of the joint. The origin of the osteophytes is disputed, but one should keep in mind that during development the edge of the vertebral body consists of a cartilaginous ring. Although this ring ossifies in time, the adjacent fibrous tissues still contain cells with a chondrogenic or osteogenic potential that is activated under the effect of stimulating factors. The age-linked loosening of the anulus fibrosus in association with the narrowing of the intervertebral space gives rise to friction, which has long been recognized as a cause of spondylosis. The frequent association with diabetes mellitus[216] indicates that metabolic factors may enter into the etiology of the disorder, either by acting on the vertebral end-plates directly or by first causing abnormalities in the intervertebral discs.

In ochronosis the intervertebral discs are discolored a deep black; they are softened or calcified and brittle, shrunken, and often prolapsed posteriorly into the spinal canal or anteriorly through the retaining ligaments. With shrinkage of the discs the intervertebral spaces are narrowed, and eventually the vertebral bodies touch and become fused by osseous links (Plate 8, *B*).

Ankylosing spondylitis (Marie-Strümpell-Bekhterev disease)

Ankylosing spondylitis is a chronic progressive inflammation of unknown origin involving primarily the small apophyseal and costovertebral joints of the spine, as well as the sacroiliac joints. The overall incidence of the disorder in the general population is less than 1%; men are affected nine times more frequently than women. The disease usually starts late in the second or in the third decade, progresses to involve several segments or the entire length of the spine, and terminates in ankylosis of individual joints with immobilization of the involved segments of the spine. The histologic changes are basically similar to those seen in rheumatoid arthritis: a nonspecific chronic synovitis with destruction of the cartilage by pannus, adhesions between the opposing surfaces of the joint, and thickening and fibrosis of the joint capsule. In contrast to the situation observed in spondylosis, the intervertebral spaces are not narrowed, but the discs may be partially or completely destroyed by granulation tissue, which undergoes fibrosis, calcification, and ossification.[54] The process may extend into ligaments and their insertion at the vertebral bodies[11]; consequently, adjacent vertebrae may become fused by osseous bridges that often protrude from under the longitudinal ligament and give rise to the gross appearance of the "bamboo spine."

Etiology

Despite their morphologic similarity, ankylosing spondylitis differs from rheumatoid arthritis. As a member of the group of spondyloarthropathies (see p. 1836), ankylosing spondylitis shares with the other members of that group an unknown etiology, a male preponderance, the absence of rheumatoid factors, and the positive association with HLA-B27 antigens, found in 90% of the patients with this disease. This association, however, varies in different populations.[33] Familial incidence is high, especially in fathers of probands who are HLA-B27 positive,[172] but identical twins are discordant for ankylosing spondylitis, an observation that points to an etiologic role by environmental factors.

REFERENCES

1. Acheson, R.M., and Collart, A.B.: New Haven survey of joint diseases. XVII. Relationship between some systemic characteristics and osteoarthrosis in a general population, Ann. Rheum. Dis. **34**:379, 1975.

2. Adams, I.I.: Osteoarthrosis and sport, Clin. Rheum. Dis. **2**:523, 1976.
3. Akoonen, P.: Human yersinosis in Finland, Ann. Clin. Res. **4**:30, 1977.
4. Ali, S.Y.: New knowledge of osteoarthrosis, J. Clin. Pathol. **31**(suppl. 12): 191, 1978.
5. Alpert, E., Isselbacher, K.J., and Schur, P.H.: The pathogenesis of arthritis associated with viral hepatitis, N. Engl. J. Med. **285**:185, 1971.
6. Ansell, B.M.: Chronic arthritis in childhood, Ann. Rheum. Dis. **37**:107, 1978.
7. Argen, R.J., and Dixon, A.S.: Clutton's joint with keratitis and periostitis, Arthritis Rheum. **6**:341, 1963.
8. Armstrong, C.G., Bahrani, A.S., and Gardner, D.L.: Alteration with age in compliance of human femoral head cartilage, Lancet **1**:1103, 1977.
9. Arnold, J.: Acromegalie, Pachyacrie oder Ostitis, Beitr. Pathol. Anat. **10**:1, 1891.
10. Baker, W.M.: On the formation of synovial cysts in the leg in connection with disease of the knee joint, St. Barth. Reports **13**:245, 1877.
11. Ball, J.: Articular pathology in ankylosing spondylitis, Clin. Orthop. **143**:30, 1979.
12. Barnes, C.G., Turnbull, A.L., and Vernon-Roberts, B.: Felty's syndrome, Ann. Rheum. Dis. **30**:359, 1971.
13. Barnett, E.V., et al.: Anti-nuclear factors in systemic lupus erythematosus and rheumatoid arthritis, Ann. Intern. Med. **63**:100, 1965.
14. Barrow, M.V., et al.: Identification of tissue lipids in lipid dermatoarthritis (multicentric reticulohistiocytosis), Am. J. Clin. Pathol. **47**:312, 1967.
15. Bauer, W., Bennett, G.A., and Zeller, J.W.: The pathology of joint lesions in patients with psoriasis and arthritis, Trans. Assoc. Am. Phys. **56**:349, 1941.
16. Bayer, A., et al.: Fungal arthritis. V, Semin. Arthr. Rheum. **9**:218, 1980.
17. Bayliss, M.J., and Ali, S.Y.: Isolation of proteoglycans from human articular cartilage, Biochem. J. **169**:123, 1978.
18. Becker, M.A., et al.: Purine overproduction in man associated with increased phosphoribosylpyrophosphate synthetase activity, Science **179**:1123, 1973.
19. Bennett, G.A.: Comparison of the pathology of rheumatic fever and rheumatoid arthritis, Ann. Intern. Med. **19**:111, 1943.
20. Bennett, G.A., Waine, H., and Bauer, W.: Changes in the knee joints at various ages with particular reference to the nature of degenerative joint disease, New York, 1942, Commonwealth Fund.
21. Bennett, G.A., Zeller, J.W., and Bauer, W.: Subcutaneous nodules of rheumatoid arthritis and rheumatic fever, Arch. Pathol. **30**:70, 1940.
22. Bennett, J.C.: The infectious etiology of rheumatoid arthritis, Arthritis Rheum. **21**:531, 1978.
23. Benninghoff, A.: Form und Bau der Gelenkknorpel in ihren Beziehungen zur Funktion, Z. Zellforsch. **2**:783, 1925.
24. Bick, E.M.: Congenital deformities of the musculoskeletal system noted in the newborn, Am. J. Dis. Child. **100**:861, 1960.
25. Bjelle, A.O.: Morphological study of articular cartilage in pyrophosphate arthropathy, Ann. Rheum. Dis. **31**:449, 1972.
26. Bjelle, A.O.: Glycosaminoglycans in human articular cartilage of the lower femoral epiphysis in osteoarthrosis, Scand. J. Rheumatol. **6**:37, 1977.
27. Bliss, B.O., and Reed, R.J.: Large cell sarcomas of tendon sheath, Am. J. Clin. Pathol. **49**:776, 1968.
28. Block, S.R., et al.: Studies of twins with systemic lupus erythematosus, Am. J. Med. **59**:533, 1975.
29. Bluestone, R.: Seronegative spondyloarthropathies (editorial), Clin. Orthop. **143**:2, 1979.
30. Bonomo, H., et al.: Immune complexes in rheumatoid syntovitis: a mixed staining immunofluorescence study, Immunology **18**:557, 1970.
31. Boyle, J.A., et al.: Relative role of genetic and environmental factors in the control of serum uric acid levels in normouricemic subjects, Ann. Rheum. Dis. **26**:234, 1967.
32. Bozicevich, J., et al.: Bentonite flocculation test for rheumatoid arthritis, Proc. Soc. Exp. Biol. Med. **97**:180, 1958.
33. Brewerton, D.A.: HLA system and rheumatic disease, J. Clin. Pathol. **31**(suppl. 12):117, 1978.
34. Britton, M.C., and Schur, P.H.: The complement system in rheumatoid synovitis. II. Intracytoplasmic inclusions of immunoglobulins and complement, Arthritis Rheum. **14**:87, 1971.
35. Bullough, P.G., Goodfellow, J., and O'Connor, J.: The relationship between degenerative changes and load bearing in the human hip, J. Bone Joint Surg. **55B**:746, 1973.
36. Bunim, J.J., Burch, T.A., and O'Brien, W.M.: Influence of genetic and environmental factors in the occurrence of rheumatoid arthritis and rheumatoid factors in American Indians, Bull. Rheum. Dis. **15**:349, 1964.
37. Bywaters, E.G.L.: The relation between heart and joint disease including "rheumatoid" heart disease and chronic posttraumatic arthritis (type Jaccoud), Br. Heart J. **12**:101, 1950.
38. Bywaters, E.G.L.: Pathologic aspects of juvenile chronic polyarthritis, Arthritis Rheum. **20**:271, 1977.
39. Bywaters, E.G.L., and Dorling, J.: Amyloid deposits in articular cartilage, Ann. Rheum. Dis. **30**:294, 1971.
40. Bywaters, E.G.L., and Hamilton, E.B.D.: The spine in idiopathic hemochromatosis, Ann. Rheum. Dis. **30**:457, 1971.
41. Cadman, N.L., Soule, E.H., and Kelly, P.J.: Synovial sarcoma: an analysis of 134 tumors, Cancer **18**:613, 1965.
42. Calkins, E., and Cohen, A.S.: Diagnosis of amyloidosis, Bull. Rheum. Dis. **10**:215, 1960.
43. Cameron, H.K., and Fornasier, V.L.: Trabecular stress fractures, Clin. Orthop. **111**:266, 1975.
44. Campbell, C.J.: The healing of cartilage defects, Clin. Orthop. **64**:45, 1969.
45. Caplan, A., Payne, R.B., and Whitey, J.L.: A broader concept of Caplan's syndrome related to rheumatoid factors, Thorax **17**:205, 1962.
46. Carter, C., and Wilkinson, J.: Persistent joint laxity and congenital dislocation of the hip, J. Bone Joint Surg. **46B**:40, 1964.
47. Caughey, D.E., and Bywaters, E.G.L.: The arthritis of Whipple's disease, Ann. Rheum. Dis. **22**:327, 1963.
48. Chung, S.M.K., and Ralston, E.L.: Necrosis of femoral head associated with sickle cell anemia and its genetic variant, J. Bone Joint Surg. **51A**:33, 1969.
49. Clutton, H.H.: Symmetrical synovitis of the knee in hereditary syphilis, Lancet **1**:391, 1866.
50. Cohen, A.S., and Kim, I.C.: Acute suppurative arthritis. In Hill, A.S., editor: Modern trends in rheumatology, London, 1966, Butterworth & Co. (Publishers), Ltd.
51. Collins, D.H., and McElligott, T.F.: Sulphate ($^{35}SO_4$) uptake by chondrocytes in relation to histological changes in osteoarthritic human cartilage, Ann. Rheum. Dis. **19**:318, 1960.
52. Cooke, T.D.V., et al.: Localization of antigen-antibody complexes in intraarticular collagenous tissues, Ann. N.Y. Acad. Sci. **256**:10, 1975.
53. Cotta, H., et al.: Elektronenoptische and biochemische Untersuchungen an der Gelenkchondromatose, Arch. Orthop. Unfallchir. **63**:73, 1968.
54. Cruickshank, B.: Lesions of cartilaginous joints in ankylosing spondylitis, J. Pathol. Bacteriol. **71**:73, 1956.
55. Currey, H.L.F.: Pyrophosphate arthropathy and calcific periarthritis, Clin. Orthop. **71**:70, 1970.
56. Davidson, P.T., and Horowitz, J.: Skeletal tuberculosis, Am. J. Med. **48**:77, 1970.
57. de Blécourt, J.J.: Hereditary factors in rheumatoid arthritis and ankylosing spondylitis. In Kellgren, J.H., Jeffrey, M.R., and Ball, J., editors: The epidemiology of chronic rheumatism, Philadelphia, 1963, F.A. Davis Co.
58. De Palma, A.F.: Hemophilic arthropathy, Clin. Orthop. **52**:145, 1967.
59. de Sèze, S., et al.: Joint and bone disorders and hyperparathyroidism in hemochromatosis, Semin. Arthritis Rheum. **2**:71, 1972.
60. Dekker-Saeys, B.J., et al.: Prevalence of peripheral arthritis, sacroileitis, and ankylosing spondylosis in patients suffering from inflammatory bowel disease, Ann. Rheum. Dis. **37**:33, 1978.

61. Denko, C.W.: Effect of prostaglandins in urate crystal inflammation, Pharmacology **12**:331, 1974.
62. Denman, A.M.: Rheumatoid arthritis—a virus disease? J. Clin. Pathol. **31**(suppl. 12):132, 1978.
63. Devach, M., and Cabilli, C.: Dupuytren's contracture and diabetes mellitus, Isr. J. Med. Sci. **8**:774, 1972.
64. Dieppe, P.: New knowledge of chondrocalcinosis, J. Clin. Pathol. **31**(suppl. 12):214, 1978.
65. Dolan, D.L., Lemmon, J.B., Jr., and Teitelbaum, S.L.: Relapsing polychondritis, Am. J. Med. **41**:285, 1966.
66. Donovan, T.L., et al.: Serratia arthritis, J. Bone Joint Surg. **58A**:1009, 1976.
67. Dupuytren, G.: Permanent retraction of the fingers produced by an affection of the palmar fascia. (Translation from original French: Lecons orales, Vol. 1, 1832.) Med. Class. **4**:142, 1939.
68. Ehalt, W., Ratzenhofer, M., and Gergen, M.: Die synoviale Osteochondromatose kombiniert mit paraartikulaerer cartilaginaerer Exostose und die Beziehungen zu einem seltenen Fall primaerer synovialer Osteomatose, Chirurg **40**:464, 1969.
69. Ehrlich, G.E., et al.: Multicentric reticulohistiocytosis (lipid dermatoarthritis): multisystem disorder, Am. J. Med. **52**:830, 1972.
70. Engel, A.: Osteoarthritis and body measurements, Series 11, no. 29, Washington, D.C., 1968, U.S. Public Health Service, National Center for Health Statistics.
71. Enzinger, F.M.: Clear cell sarcoma of tendons and aponeuroses, Cancer **18**:1163, 1965.
72. Erdheim, J.: Die Lebensvorgaenge im normalen Knorpel and seine Wucherung bei Akromegalie: Pathologie in Einzeldarstellungen, Berlin, 1931, Springer Verlag.
73. Faires, J.S., and McCarthy, D.J., Jr.: Acute synovitis in normal joints of man and dog produced by injections of microcrystalline sodium urate calcium oxalate, and corticosteroid esters, Arthritis Rheum. **5**:295, 1962.
74. Felty, A.R.: Chronic arthritis in the adult associated with splenomegaly and leucopenia, Bull. Johns Hopkins Hosp. **35**:16, 1924.
75. Fernandez, G.B., and Hernandez, F.J.: Poorly differentiated synovial sarcoma: a light and electron microscopic study, Arch. Pathol. Lab. Med. **100**:221, 1976.
76. Friedman, H.: Aspects psychosomatiques de la polyarthrite chronique évolutive (PCE) ou polyarthrite rhumatoide, Acta Psychiatr. Belg. **72**:117, 1972.
77. Gabbiani, G., and Majno, G.: Dupuytren's contracture: fibroblast contraction? An ultrastructural study, Am. J. Pathol. **66**:131, 1972.
78. Gabbiani, G., et al.: Synovial sarcoma: electron microscopic study of a typical case, Cancer **28**:1031, 1971.
79. Gardner, D.L.: The experimental production of arthritis, Ann. Rheum. Dis. **19**:297, 1960.
80. Gardner, E.: The nerve supply of muscles, joints, and other deep structures, Bull. Hosp. Joint Dis. **21**:153, 1960.
81. Garrod, A.B.: The nature and treatment of gout, London, 1859, Walton & Maberly.
82. Gay, S., Müller, P.K., and Lemmen, C.: Immunohistological study on collagen in cartilage-bone metamorphosis and degenerative osteoarthrosis, Klin. Wochenschr. **54**:969, 1976.
83. Ghadially, F.N., and Mehta, P.N.: Multifunctional mesenchymal cells resembling smooth muscle cells in ganglia of the wrist, Ann. Rheum. Dis. **30**:31, 1971.
84. Ghadially, F.N., and Roy, S.: Ultrastructure of synovial joints in health and disease, New York 1969, Appleton-Century-Crofts.
85. Glynn, L.E.: Pathogenesis and etiology of rheumatoid arthritis, Ann. Rheum. Dis. **31**:412, 1972.
86. Goldman, R.L., and Lichtenstein, L.: Synovial chondrosarcoma, Cancer **17**:1233, 1964.
87. Good, R.A., and Rotstein, J.: Rheumatoid arthritis and agammaglobulinemia, Bull. Rheum. Dis. **10**:203, 1960.
88. Graham, W., and Graham, K.M.: Martyrs to the gout, Metabolism **6**:209, 1966.
89. Grigor, R., et al.: Systemic lupus erythematosus, Ann. Rheum. Dis. **37**:121, 1978.
90. Gutman, A.B.: Renal mechanisms for regulation of uric acid excretion with special reference to normal and gouty man, Semin. Arthritis Rheum. **2**:1, 1972.
91. Gutman, A.B., and Yü, T.F.: Hyperglutamatemia in primary gout, Am. J. Med. **54**:713, 1973.
92. Haagensen, C.D., and Stout, A.P.: Synovial sarcoma, Ann. Surg. **120**:826, 1942.
93. Hagemann, R., and Rüttner, J.R.: Arthrosis of the sternoclavicular joint, Z. Rheumatol. **38**:27, 1979.
94. Ham, A.W., and Cormack, D.H.: Joints. In Histology, ed. 8, Philadelphia, 1979, J.B. Lippincott Co.
95. Hamerman, D.: Evidence for an infectious etiology of rheumatoid arthritis, Ann. N.Y. Acad. Sci. **256**:25, 1975.
96. Harris, E.D., Faulkner, C.S., and Brown, F.E.: Collagenolytic systems in rheumatoid arthritis, Clin. Orthop. **110**:303, 1975.
97. Hartung, E.F.: Historical considerations, Metabolism **6**:196, 1957.
98. Hass, J.: Congenital dislocation of the hip, Springfield, Ill., 1957, Charles C Thomas, Publisher.
99. Hasselbacher, P., and Schumacher, H.R.: Localization of immunoglobulins in gouty tophi by immunhistology and on the surface of monosodium urate crystals by immune agglutination, Arthritis Rheum. **19**:802, 1976.
100. Hay, F.C., et al.: Intraarticular and circulating immune complexes and antiglobulins (IgG and IgM) in rheumatoid arthritis: correlation with clinical features, Ann. Rheum. Dis. **38**:1, 1979.
101. Hedberg, H.: Studies on the depressed hemolytic complement activity of synovial fluid in adult rheumatoid arthritis, Acta Rheum. Scand. **9**:165, 1963.
102. Heine, J.: Ueber die Arthritis deformans, Virchows Arch. (Pathol. Anat.) **260**:521, 1926.
103. Henderson, J.F., et al.: Variations in purine metabolism of cultured skin fibroblasts from patients with gout, J. Clin. Invest. **47**:1511, 1968.
104. Herman, J.H., and Dennis, M.: Immunopathologic studies in relapsing polychondritis, J. Clin. Invest. **52**:549, 1973.
105. Hershfield, M.S., and Seegmiller, J.E.: Gout and the regulation of purine biosynthesis, Horiz. Biochem. Biophys. **2**:134, 1976.
106. Hilgartner, M.W.: Hemophilic arthropathy, Adv. Pediatr. **21**:139, 1974.
107. Hoffman, G.J., and Carter, D.: Clear cell sarcoma of tendons and aponeuroses with melanin, Arch. Pathol. **95**:22, 1973.
108. Hollander, J.L., et al.: Studies on the pathogenesis of rheumatoid joint inflammation. I. The RA cell and a working hypotheses, Ann. Intern. Med. **62**:271, 1965.
109. Holmes, K.K., Counts, G.W., and Beatty, H.N.: Disseminated gonococcal infection, Ann. Intern. Med. **74**:979, 1971.
110. Hough, A.J., Banfield, W.G., and Sokoloff, L.: Cartilage in hemophilic arthropathy, Arch. Pathol. **100**:91, 1976.
111. Howie, S., and Feldmann, M.: Cellular interaction in antibody production, Clin. Rheum. Dis. **4**:481, 1978.
112. Hunter, J.A.A., Ogden, C., and Norris, M.G.: Dupuytren's contracture. I. Chemical pathology, Br. J. Plast. Surg. **28**:10, 1975.
113. Hurd, E.R.: Extraarticular manifestations of rheumatoid arthritis, Semin. Arthritis Rheum. **8**:151, 1979.
114. Idelberger, K.: Die Ergebnisse der Zwillingsforschung beim angeborenen Klumpfuss, Verh. Dtsch. Ges. Orthop. **33**:272, 1939.
115. Jaccoud, F.S.: Leçons de clinique médicale faites a l'Hôpital de la Charité, ed. 2, Paris, 1869, Delahaye.
116. Jaffe, H.L., Lichtenstein, L., and Sutro, C.J.: Pigmented nodular synovitis, bursitis, and tenosynovitis, Arch. Pathol. **31**:731, 1941.
117. Jansson, E.: Isolation of fastidious mycoplasma from human sources, J. Clin. Pathol. **24**:53, 1971.
118. Johnson, L.C.: Morphologic analysis in pathology. In Frost, H.M., editor: Bone dynamics, Boston, 1964, Little, Brown & Co.
119. Kahn, L.B.: Malignant giant cell tumor of the tendon sheath: ultrastructural study and review of the literature, Arch. Pathol. **95**:203, 1973.
120. Karten, I.: Septic arthritis complicating rheumatoid arthritis, Ann. Intern. Med. **70**:1147, 1969.
121. Kellermeyer, R.W., and Naff, G.B.: Chemical mediators of inflammation in gout, Arthritis Rheum. **19**:765, 1975.

122. Kelley, W.N., et al.: Hypoxanthine guanine-phosphoribosyltransferase deficiency in gout, Ann. Intern. Med. **70**:155, 1969.
123. Kellgren, J.H.: Osteoarthrosis in patients and populations, Br. Med. J. **5243**:1, 1961.
124. Kellgren, J.H. In discussion of Lawrence, J.L., and Bier, F.: Nodal and non-nodal forms of generalized osteoarthrosis, Ann. Rheum. Dis. **23**:205, 1964.
125. Kellgren, J.H., Lawrence, J.S., and Bier, F.: Genetic factors in generalized osteo-arthrosis, Ann. Rheum. Dis. **22**:237, 1963.
126. Kelly, J.J., III, and Weisiger, B.B.: The arthritis of Whipple's disease, Arthritis Rheum. **6**:615, 1963.
127. Kelly, P.J., Martin, W.J., and Coventry, M.B.: Bacterial (suppurative) arthritis in the adult, J. Bone Joint Surg. **52A**:1595, 1970.
128. Kempson, G.E.: The tensile properties of articular cartilage and their relevance to osteoarthrosis, Orthop. Surg. Traumatol. **12**:44, 1973.
129. Key, J.A.: Hemophilic arthritis, Ann. Surg. **95**:198, 1932.
130. Kinsella, T.D., Baum, J., and Ziff, M.: Immunofluorescent demonstration of an IgG-B_1C complex in synovial lining cells of rheumatoid synovial membrane, Clin. Exp. Immunol. **4**:265, 1969.
131. Kogstad, O.: Baker's cyst, Acta Rheum. Scand. **11**:194, 1965.
132. Kulka, J.P.: The lesions of Reiter's syndrome, Arthritis Rheum. **5**:195, 1962.
133. Kutty, M.K., Iqbal, Q.M., and Eng-Chuan, T.: Ochronotic arthropathy, Arch. Pathol. **96**:100, 1973.
134. Lack, C.H.: Lysosomes in relation to arthritis. In Dingle, J.T., and Fell, H.B., editors: The lysosomes, vol. 1, New York, 1968, John Wiley & Sons, Inc.
135. Lagier, R., Baud, C.A., and Buchs, M.: Crystallographic identification of calcium deposits as regards their pathological nature with special reference to chondrocalcinosis. In Fleisch, H., Blackwood, H.J.J., and Owen, M., editors: Calcified tissues, New York, 1966, Springer Verlag New York.
136. Lamont-Havers, R.W.: Nature of serum factors causing agglutination of sensitized sheep cells and group A hemolytic streptococci, Proc. Soc. Exp. Biol. Med. **88**:35, 1955.
137. Lawee, D.: Uric acid: the clinical application of 1000 unsolicited determinations, Can. Med. Assoc. J. **100**:838, 1969.
138. Lawrence, J.S.: Rheumatoid arthritis—nature or nurture? (Heberden oration), Ann. Rheum. Dis. **29**:357, 1970.
139. Lawrence, J.S.: Rheumatoid factors in families, Semin. Arthritis **3**:177, 1973.
140. Lawrence. J.S., Hewitt, J.V., and Popert, A.J.: Gout and hyperuricemia in the United Kingdom. In Kellgren, J.H., et al., editors: The epidemiology of chronic rheumatism, Philadelphia, 1963, F.A. Davis Co.
141. Lazarus, G.S., et al.: Human granulocyte collagenase, Science **159**:1483, 1968.
142. Ling, R.S.M.: The genetic factor in Dupuytren's disease, J. Bone Joint Surg. **45B**:709, 1963.
143. Lowbeer, L.: Brucellosis osteomyelitis in man and animals, Am. J. Pathol. **24**:723, 1948.
144. Luck, V.: Dupuytren's contracture, J. Bone Joint Surg. **41A**:635, 1959.
145. Luck, V.: Articular cartilage: responses to destructive influence. In Bassett, C.E., editor: Cartilage, degradation and repair, Washington, D.C., 1967, National Research Council.
146. Luse, S.A.: A synovial sarcoma—studies by electron microscopy, Cancer **13**:321, 1960.
147. Mackenzie, M.D.: Synovial sarcoma, Cancer **19**:169, 1966.
148. MacLachlan, M.D., and Rodnan, G.P.: Effects of food, fast, and alcohol on serum uric acid and acute attacks of gout, Am. J. Med. **42**:38, 1967.
149. Mankin, H.J., and Radin, E.: Structure and function of joints. In McCarty, D.J., editor: Arthritis and allied diseases, Philadelphia, 1979, Lea & Febiger.
150. Marmion, B.P.: Infection, autoimmunity and rheumatoid arthritis, Clin. Rheum. Dis. **4**:565, 1978.
151. Martenis, T.W., Bland, J.H., and Phillips, C.A.: Rheumatoid arthritis after rubella, Arthritis Rheum. **11**:683, 1968.
152. Martens, M., et al.: Pigmented villonodular synovitis of joints, tendons, and bursae, Acta Orthop. Belg. **38**:233, 1972.
153. McCormick, J.N.: An immunofluorescence study of rheumatoid factor, Ann. Rheum. Dis. **22**:1, 1963.
154. McCredie, J.: Thalidomide and congenital "Charcot joints," Lancet **2**:1058, 1973.
155. McEwen, C., et al.: Ankylosing spondylitis accompanying colitis, regional ileitis and Reiter's disease, Arthritis Rheum. **14**:291, 1971.
156. Meachim, G.: Age changes in articular cartilage, Clin. Orthop. **64**:33, 1969.
157. Meachim, G., and Emery, I.H.: Cartilage fibrillation in shoulder and hip joints in Liverpool necropsies, J. Anat. **116**:161, 1973.
158. Meyerowitz, S.: The continuing investigation of psychosocial variables in rheumatoid arthritis, Mod. Trends Rheum. **2**:92, 1971.
159. Milgram, W.J.: Synovial osteochondromatosis: a histopathological study of 30 cases, J. Bone Joint Surg. **59A**:792, 1978.
160. Miller, E.J.: A review of biochemical studies on the genetically distinct collagens of the skeletal system, Clin. Orthop. **92**:260, 1973.
161. Mitchell, N., and Shepard, N.: Relapsing polychondritis: an electron microscopic study of synovium and articular cartilage, J. Bone Joint Surg. **54A**:1235, 1972.
162. Moll, J.H.M., and Wright, V.: Psoriatic arthritis, Semin. Arthritis Rheum. **3**:55, 1973.
163. Moseley, H.F.: Shoulder lesions, ed. 3, Baltimore, 1969, The Williams & Wilkins Co.
164. Mubarak, S.J., and Carroll, N.C.: Familial osteochondritis dissecans of the knee, Clin. Orthop. **140**:131, 1979.
165. Muir, H.: Molecular approach to the understanding of osteoarthrosis, Ann. Rheum. Dis. **36**:199, 1976.
166. Mullins, F., Berard, C.W., and Eisenberg, S.H.: Chondrosarcoma following synovial chondromatosis, Cancer **18**:1180, 1965.
167. Murphy, E.G.: The histopathology of rheumatic fever: a critical review. In Lewis, L.T., editor: Rheumatic fever, Minneapolis, 1952, University of Minnesota Press.
168. Murphy, F.P., Dahlin, D.C., and Sullivan, C.R.: Articular synovial chondromatosis, J. Bone Joint Surg. **44**:77, 1962.
169. Nashel, D.J., Widerlite, L.W., and Pekin, T.J.: IgD myeloma with amyloid arthropathy, Am. J. Med. **55**:426, 1973.
170. Nelson, J.A., and Koontz, W.C.: Septic arthritis in infants and children, Pediatrics **38**:966, 1966.
171. Nesterov, A.I.: The clinical course of Kashin-Beck disease, Arthritis Rheum. **7**:29, 1964.
172. Nichol, F.E., and Woodrow, J.C.: Genetics of ankylosing spondylitis. In Van der Korst, J.K., editor: Proceedings, 9th European Congress on Rheumatism, Wiesbaden, 1979, Bern, 1979, Hans Huber Verlag.
173. Nimni, M., and Dekmush, K.: Differences in collagen metabolism between normal and osteoarthritic human articular cartilage, Science **181**:751, 1973.
174. Nowoslawski, A.: Immunopathological features of rheumatoid and arthritis. In Mueller, W., Harwerth, H.G., and Fehr, K., editors: Rheumatoid arthritis, New York, 1971, Academic Press, Inc.
175. O'Brien, J.E., and Stout, A.P.: Malignant fibrous xanthomas, Cancer **17**:1445, 1964.
176. O'Brien, W.W.: Twin studies in rheumatic diseases, Arthritis Rheum. **11**:81, 1968.
177. O'Duffy, J.D., Carney, J.A., and Deodhar, S.: Behcet's disease: a report of 10 cases, three with new manifestations, Ann. Intern. Med. **75**:561, 1971.
178. Onion, D.K., Crumpacker, C.S., and Gilliland, B.C.: Arthritis of hepatitis associated with Australia antigen, Ann. Intern. Med. **75**:29, 1971.
179. O'Sullivan, J.B.: Gout in a New England town: a prevalence study in Sudbury, Mass., Ann. Rheum. Dis. **31**:166, 1972.
180. O'Sullivan, J.B., and Cathcart, E.S.: The prevalence of rheumatoid arthritis, Ann. Intern. Med. **76**:573, 1972.
181. Panush, R.S., Bianco, N.E., and Schur, P.H.: Serum and synovial fluid IgG, IgA, and IgM antigammaglobulins in rheumatoid arthritis, Arthritis Rheum. **14**:737, 1971.
182. Partain, J.O., Cathcart, E.S., and Cohen, A.S.: Arthritis associated with gonorrhea, Ann. Rheum. Dis. **27**:156, 1968.
183. Paul, G.R., and Leach, R.E.: Synovial chondromatosis of the shoulder joint, Clin. Orthop. **68**:130, 1970.

184. Perricone, E., Palmoski, M.J., and Brandt, K.D.: Failure of proteoglycans to form aggregates in morphologically normal aged human cartilage, Arthritis Rheum. **20**:1372, 1977.
185. Peyron, J.G.: Epidemiologic and etiologic approach to osteoarthritis, Semin. Arthritis Rheum. **8**:288, 1979.
186. Pinnell, S.R., et al.: A heritable disorder of connective tissue: hydroxylysine-deficient collagen disease, N. Engl. J. Med. **286**:1013, 1972.
187. Pritzker, K.P.H., et al.: The ultrastructure of urate crystals in gout, J. Rheumatol. **5**:1, 1978.
188. Puranen, J., et al.: Running and primary osteoarthrosis of the hip, Br. Med. J. **2**:424, 1975.
189. Reichelt, A.: Beitraege zur Aetiologie der Osteochondrosis dissecans des Hueftgelenkes, Arch. Orthop. Unfallchir. **65**:220, 1969.
190. Riddle, J.M., Bluhm, G.B., and Barnhart, M.J.: Ultrastructural study of leucocytes and urates in gouty arthritis, Ann. Rheum. Dis. **26**:389, 1967.
191. Rimoin, D.L.: Pachydermoperiostosis; genetic and physiologic considerations, N. Engl. J. Med. **222**:923, 1965.
192. Rodnan, G.P.: The nature of joint involvement in progressive systemic sclerosis (diffuse scleroderma); clinical study and pathologic examination of synovium in twenty-nine patients, Ann. Intern. Med. **56**:422, 1962.
193. Rodnan, G.P.: Early theories concerning etiology and pathogenesis of gout, Arthritis Rheum. **8**:599, 1965.
194. Ropes, M.W., Bennett, G.A., and Cobb, S.: Revision of diagnostic criteria for rheumatoid arthritis, Ann. Rheum. Dis. **18**:49, 1958.
195. Rosenberg, L.C.: Structure and function of proteoglycans. In McCarty, D.J., editor: Arthritis and allied diseases, Philadelphia, 1979, Lea & Febiger.
196. Ruettner, J.R., and Spycher, M.: Electron microscopic investigations on aging and osteoarthrotic human cartilage, Pathol. Microbiol. **31**:4, 1968.
197. Saville, P.D.: Age and weight in osteoarthrosis of the hip, Arthritis Rheum. **11**:635, 1968.
198. Schaller, J., and Wedgwood, R.J.: Juvenile rheumatoid arthritis: a review, Pediatrics **50**:940, 1967.
199. Schar, E., Pras, M., and Gafni, J.: Familial Mediterranean fever and its articular manifestations, Clin. Rheum. Dis. **1**:195, 1975.
200. Schmorl, G., and Junghanns, H.: The human spine in health and disease. (English translation by S.P. Wilkins and L.S. Coin.) New York, 1959, Grune & Stratton, Inc.
201. Schofield, J.D., and Weightman, B.: New knowledge of connective tissue aging, J. Clin. Pathol. **31**(suppl.12):174, 1978.
202. Schumacher, H.R., Jr.: Ultrastructure of the synovial membrane in idiopathic hemochromatosis, Ann. Rheum. Dis. **31**:465, 1972.
203. Schumacher, H.R., Jr., Andrews, R., and McLaughlin, G.: Arthropathy in sickle cell disease, Ann. Intern. Med. **78**:203, 1973.
204. Schumacher, H.R., Jr., and Holdsworth, D.E.: Ochronotic arthropathy. I. Clinico-pathologic aspects, Semin. Arthritis Rheum. **6**:207, 1977.
205. Schumacher, H.R., Jr., et al.: Arthritis associated with apatite crystals, Ann. Intern. Med. **87**:411, 1977.
206. Scott, J.T., and Pollard, A.C.: Uric acid excretion in the relatives of patients with gout, Ann. Rheum. Dis. **29**:397, 1970.
207. Scott, R.B., et al.: Neuropathic joint disease (Charcot joints) in Waldenstrom's macroglobulinemia with amyloidosis, Am. J. Med. **54**:535, 1973.
208. Seegmiller, J.E., Howell, R.R., and Malawista, S.E.: The inflammatory reaction to sodium urate, J.A.M.A. **180**:469, 1973.
209. Seegmiller, J.E., Laster, L., and Howell, R.R.: Biochemistry of uric acid and its relation to gout. III, N. Engl. J. Med. **268**:821, 1963.
210. Shearn, M.A.: Sjögren's syndrome, Philadelphia, 1971, W.B. Saunders Co.
211. Shirahama, T., and Cohen, A.S.: Ultrastructural evidence for leakage of lysosomal contents after phagocytosis of monosodium urate crystals, Am. J. Pathol. **76**:501, 1974.
212. Silberberg, M., and Silberberg, R.: The effects of endocrine secretions on articular tissues and their relation to the aging process. In Slocum, C.H., editor: Rheumatic diseases: Philadelphia, 1952, W.B. Saunders Co.
213. Silberberg, M., and Silberberg, R.: Ageing changes in cartilage and bone. In Bourne, G.H., editor: Structural aspects of ageing, London, 1961, Pitman Medical Publishers.
214. Silberberg, M., et al.: Aging and osteoarthrosis of the human sternoclavicular joint, Am. J. Pathol. **35**:831, 1959.
215. Silberberg, R.: Ultrastructure of articular cartilage in health and disease, Clin. Orthop. **57**:233, 1968.
216. Silberberg, R.: The pituitary in skeletal aging and disease. In Everitt, A.V., and Burgess, J.A., editors: Hypothalamus, pituitary, and aging, Springfield, Ill., 1976, Charles C. Thomas, Publisher.
217. Silberberg, R.: Obesity and osteoarthrosis. In Mancini, M., Lewis, B., and Contaldo, F., editors: Proceedings, International Conference on Clinical Complications of Obesity, Naples, March 1979, London, Academic Press.
218. Silby, H.M., et al.: Acute monoarticular arthritis after vaccination, Ann. Intern. Med. **62**:347, 1965.
219. Sinha, S., Munichovdappa, C.L., and Kozak, G.P.: Neuro-arthropathy (Charcot joints) in diabetes mellitus, Medicine **51**:191, 1966.
220. Sjögren, H.: Keratoconjunctivitis sicca and chronic polyarthritis, Acta Med. Scand. **130**:484, 1948.
221. Sledge, C.B.: Structure, development, and function of joints, Orthop. Clin. North Am. **6**:619, 1973.
222. Smillie, J.L.: Osteochondritis dissecans: loose bodies in joints; etiology, pathology, treatment, Edinburgh, 1960, E. & S. Livingstone, Ltd.
223. Smith, L.W.: Synoviomata, Am. J. Pathol. **3**:355, 1927.
224. Snyderman, R., and McCarty, G.A.: The role of macrophages in the rheumatic diseases, Clin. Rheum. Dis. **4**:499, 1978.
225. Sokoloff, L.: The biology of degenerative joint disease, Chicago, 1969, University of Chicago Press.
226. Sokoloff, L.: Biochemical and biophysical aspects of degenerative joint disease with special reference to hemophilic arthropathy, Ann. N.Y. Acad. Sci. **240**:285, 1975.
227. Sokoloff, L., McCluskey, R.T., and Bunim, J.J.: Vascularity of the early subcutaneous nodule of rheumatoid arthritis, Arch. Pathol. **55**:475, 1955.
228. Soren, A.: Pathogenesis and treatment of ganglion, Clin. Orthop. **48**:173, 1966.
229. Spilberg, J.: Current concepts of the mechanism of acute inflammation in gouty arthritis, Arthritis Rheum. **18**:129, 1975.
230. Spilberg, J., Silzbach, L.E., and McEwen, C.: The arthritis of sarcoidosis, Arthritis Rheum. **12**:126, 1969.
231. Spink, W.W.: The nature of brucellosis, Minneapolis, 1956, University of Minnesota Press.
232. Spycher, M., Moor, H., and Ruettner, J.R.: Electron microscopic investigation on aging and osteoarthrotic cartilage, Z. Zellforsch. **98**:512, 1969.
233. Statsny, P.: Immunogenic factors in rheumatoid arthritis, Clin. Rheum. Dis. **3**:315, 1977.
234. Statsny, P., et al.: Lymphokines in the rheumatoid joint, Arthritis Rheum. **18**:237, 1975.
235. Stecher, R.M.: Heberden's nodes: a clinical description of osteoarthritis of the finger joints (Heberden oration), Ann. Rheum. Dis. **14**:1, 1955.
236. Still, G.F.: On a form of chronic joint disease in children, Med. Chir. Trans. (Lond.) **80**:47, 1897.
237. Stockwell, R.A.: The cell density of human articular cartilage and costal cartilage, J. Anat. **101**:753, 1967.
238. Stockwell, R.A.: Changes in the acid glycosaminoglycan content of the matrix of aging human articular cartilage, Ann. Rheum. Dis. **29**:509, 1970.
239. Stout, A.P., and Lattes, R.: Tumors of soft tissues. In Atlas of tumor pathology, Series 2, Fascicle 1, Bethesda, Md., 1967, Armed Forces Institute of Pathology.
240. Swinyard, C.A., and Mayer, V.: Multiple congenital contractures (arthrogryphosis), J.A.M.A. **183**:23, 1963.

241. Sylvén, B., et al.: Biophysical and physiological investigations on cartilage and other mesenchymal tissues. II. The ultrastructure of bovine and human nuclei pulposi, J. Bone Joint Surg. **33A**:333, 1951.
242. Teilum, G., and Lindahl, A.: Frequency and significance of amyloid changes in rheumatoid arthritis, Acta Med. Scand. **149**:449, 1954.
243. Thornhill, H.L., et al.: Neuropathic arthropathy (Charcot forefeet) in alcoholics, Orthop. Clin. North Am. **4**:7, 1973.
244. Torres, J., Rathburn, H.K., and Greenough, W.B.: Pneumococcal arthritis: report of a case and review of the literature, Johns Hopkins Med. J. **132**:234, 1973.
245. U.S. National Center for Health Statistics: Prevalence of osteoarthritis in adults, 1961-1962. Series 11, No. 15, Washington, D.C., 1962, The Center.
246. U.S. National Health Service: Rheumatoid arthritis in adults. Series 11, no. 17, Washington, D.C., 1966, U.S. Public Health Service.
247. Vaughn, J.H., et al.: Intracytoplasmic inclusions of immunoglobulins in rheumatoid arthritis and other disorders, Arthritis Rheum. **11**:125, 1968.
248. Vernon-Roberts, B., Barnes, C.G., and Revell, R.A.: Synovial pathology in Behçet's syndrome, Ann. Rheum. Dis. **37**:139, 1978.
249. Verzar, F.: Aging of connective tissue, J. Gerontol. **12**:915, 1964.
250. Vlasik, J., Zitman, D., and Sitaj, S.: Articular chondrocalcinosis. II. Genetic study, Ann. Rheum. Dis. **22**:153, 1963.
251. Waaler, E.: The occurrence of a factor in human serum activating the specific agglutination of sheep blood corpuscles, Acta Pathol. Scand. **17**:173, 1940.
252. Wagner, J.C., and McCormick, J.N.: Immunological investigations of coal workers' disease, J. R. Coll. Phys. **2**:49, 1967.
253. Wayne, H., et al.: Association of osteoarthritis and diabetes, Tufts Folia Med. **7**:13, 1961.
254. Weissman, G.: Studies on lysosomes. VII. Acute and chronic arthritis produced in intraarticular injections of streptolysin S in rabbits, Am. J. Pathol. **46**:129, 1968.
255. Weissman, G., et al.: Mechanisms of lysosomal enzyme release from leucocytes exposed to immune complexes and other particles, J. Exp. Med. **134**:149s, 1971.
256. Wilde, A., Mankin, H.J., and Rodnan, G.P.: Avascular necrosis of the femoral head in scleroderma, Arthritis Rheum. **13**:445, 1970.
257. Wollaston, W.H.: On gouty and urinary concretions, Philos. Trans. R. Soc. Lond. **87**:388, 1797.
258. Wood, G.C., Pryce-Jones, R.H., and White, D.D.: Chondromucoprotein-degrading neutral protease activity in rheumatoid fluid, Ann. Rheum. Dis. **30**:73, 1971.
259. Wright, V.: Seronegative polyarthritis: a unified concept, Arthritis Rheum. **21**:619, 1978.
260. Wright, V., Dowson, D., and Kerr, J.: The structure of joints, Int. Rev. Connect. Tissue Res. **6**:105, 1973.
261. Wyngaarden, J.B.: The overproduction of uric acid in primary gout, Arthritis Rheum. **8**:648, 1965.
262. Yanex, J.E., et al.: Rubella arthritis, Ann. Intern. Med. **64**:772, 1966.
263. Zevely, H.A., et al.: Synovial specimens obtained by knee joint punch biopsy, Am. J. Med. **20**:510, 1956.
264. Ziff, M.: Relation of cellular infiltration of rheumatoid synovial membrane to its immune response, Arthritis Rheum. **17**:313, 1974.
265. Ziff, M., et al.: Studies on the composition of the fibrinoid material in the subcutaneous nodule of rheumatoid arthritis, J. Clin. Invest. **32**:1253, 1953.
266. Zucker-Franklin, D.: The phagosomes in rheumatoid synovial fluid leucocytes: a light, fluorescence, and electron microscopic study, Arthritis Rheum. **9**:24, 1966.
267. Zwaifler, M.: Immunopathology of joint inflammation in rheumatoid arthritis, Adv. Immunol. **16**:265, 1973.

CHAPTER 43

Diseases of Skeletal Muscle

A.R.W. CLIMIE

EMBRYOGENESIS AND STRUCTURE[1,4a,5,10]

An understanding of the embryogenesis of muscle is of value in the interpretation of histopathologic changes in certain diseases, since damaged or regenerating muscle fibers frequently resemble embryonic fibers at various stages of development. Myoblasts develop in the myotomes of the embryonic somites, in the limb buds, and in the mesenchyme of the branchial arches. Myoblasts initially multiply by mitotic division but later elongate and become multinucleated myocytes by fusion of adjacent cells. By the ninth week of fetal life each cell forms a long myotube with a row of central nuclei and scanty peripheral cytoplasm in which fine fibrils are randomly dispersed. Filaments of actin, 6 to 7 nm in diameter, are the first to form. Shortly thereafter thicker (10 nm) filaments composed of myosin appear, each of which is immediately surrounded by actin filaments forming a hexagonal pattern that is retained throughout adult life. The myosin-actin complexes initially become oriented in a linear fashion to form a nonstriated myofibril, but by the eleventh week cross striations can be detected; these become more apparent in subsequent weeks. Concurrent with these changes, the nuclei move to a peripheral position and the myofibrils toward the center. Longitudinal splitting of muscle fibers occurs during the twelfth to fourteenth weeks of embryogenesis, but thereafter no additional new fibers are formed. A gradual increase in the length and width of the fibers follows. Connective tissue develops simultaneously with the formation of myoblasts but does not penetrate between individual fibers until late in fetal life. Nerve fibers, present earlier in the connective tissue, reach the muscle fibers by the eleventh week of embryogenesis, and by the thirteenth week motor nerve endings are recognizable.

In adults skeletal muscle fibers are composed of long, multinucleated cells enclosed by an inner plasma membrane (sarcolemma) separated by a uniform space from the external basement membrane. The cytoplasm consists of myofibrils paralleling the long axis of the fiber and of sarcoplasm containing mitochondria, glycogen particles, lipid bodies, lysosomes, and an intermyofibrillary tubular complex composed of the sarcoplasmic (endoplasmic) reticulum and a transverse (T) tubular system. The latter is formed by periodic invaginations of the plasma membrane. The T system, the ends of which open on the surface of the fiber, is believed to conduct the depolarizing electrical impulse into the fiber, releasing calcium from the sarcoplasmic reticulum.

The free calcium ions indirectly activate myosin adenosine triphosphatase to hydrolyze ATP with a release of energy that is used to initiate contraction, which involves a sliding interaction of myosin and actin filaments. The cross striations, which are perpendicular to the long axis of the muscle fiber, are caused by the alignment of corresponding parts of adjacent myofibrils that have differing indices of refraction. With light microscopy, two bands are clearly visible—a darker, anisotropic (A) band and a lighter, isotropic (I) band. In the middle of the I band is a thin, darker zone, the Z* band or disc. With electron microscopy, an additional light zone, the H band, can be discerned in the center of the A band, and this in turn contains a central, darker M band. The structural unit of the muscle fiber, the sarcomere, extends between two anchoring Z bands (Fig. 43-1). The banded appearance of muscle fibers results from the intracellular arrangement of the two major proteins of muscle, actin and myosin. Thin actin fibrils are attached at right angles to the Z disc and interdigitate with thicker myosin fibers, which occupy the central portion of the sarcomere. The light I band is composed only of actin filaments on both sides of the Z disc. The darker A band consists of overlapping actin and myosin filaments, the intermediate H

*Other abbreviations are from German: Z, *Zwischenscheibe* (intermediate disc); H, *heller* (lighter, brighter); M, *Mittelscheibe* (middle disc).

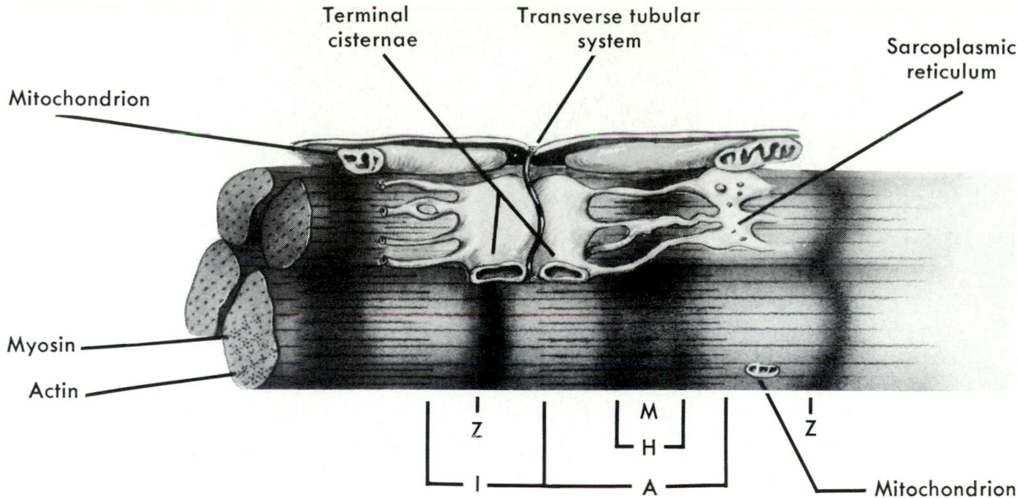

Fig. 43-1. Skeletal muscle fiber. Important components of sarcomere. See text for explanation of letters.

band of myosin filaments, and their central M band of so-called M substance. The width of all the bands except the Z disc varies with the state of contraction of the muscle. In normal muscle virtually all the nuclei are in a subsarcolemmal location, but internal nuclei may be seen near myotendinous junctions. A few nuclei are located between the plasma membrane and basement membrane. These belong to satellite cells or persisting myoblasts that have the capacity to proliferate with fiber injury and thus are a source of regenerative activity. The supporting connective tissue of the muscle is the endomysium, a thin sheath of fine reticulin fibers surrounding the basement membrane of each fiber. The endomysium extends into the perimysium, which surrounds varying numbers of fibers arranged in fascicles. The whole muscle, composed of numbers of fascicles, is enclosed by the epimysium, which forms the attachments to fascia and tendons. The arrangement of this supporting tissue is such as to permit normal contraction and relaxation and to prevent overstretching.

Each muscle is supplied by motor nerves originating from alpha motor neurons in the spinal cord or brainstem. Each axon divides into multiple branches, thereby innervating scattered fibers through motor end-plates located on the surface of each fiber. The number of muscle fibers innervated by a single motor neuron varies from 20 to 30 (for ocular muscles) to several hundreds (for limb muscles). In the motor end-plate the axon, devoid of myelin and covered by a Schwann cell coat, lies adjacent to synaptic folds of the sarcolemma. Terminal dilatations of the axon contain synaptic vesicles of acetylcholine, which is released in hundreds of quanta when reached by an action potential. These quanta traverse the synaptic space and attach to specific receptors on the tips of the folds of the postsynaptic membrane. Permeability of the membrane to sodium and potassium increases with resultant depolarization and initiation of muscular contraction. Cholinesterase from the postsynaptic and presynaptic membranes and Schwann cells then hydrolyzes the acetylcholine, and repolarization occurs as the muscle fiber relaxes. An alpha motor neuron, its axon, and the muscle fibers supplied by its branches form a motor unit. The muscular nerves contain 30% to 50% sensory fibers, many from muscle spindles in the perimysium between fascicles. Each spindle consists of small, central muscle fibers surrounded by a thick connective tissue capsule. The central (intrafusal) fibers penetrate the ends of the capsule, thereby becoming partially extrafusal in location. Specialized sensory nerve endings surround the intrafusal fibers and are responsible for measuring the tension of muscle.

The range of cross-sectional diameters of normal skeletal muscle fibers in the adult varies from 20 μm for the extraocular muscles to 100 μm for the gluteus maximus. In muscles from the limbs, from which biopsy samples are commonly obtained, the average diameter in men is 60 to 70 μm and in women 50 to 60 μm.[25,26] In children the average diameter shortly after birth is 15 μm, and there is a steady increment of 2 to 4 μm annually until adult size is reached at about 15 years of age.[26]

Human skeletal muscle is composed of a mixture of two major types of fibers identified by histochemical reactions.[27,62,78] Type I fibers contain numerous mitochondria and lipid droplets and are rich in oxidative enzymatic activity (for example, nicotinamide adenine dinucleotide dehydrogenase, succinic dehydrogenase)

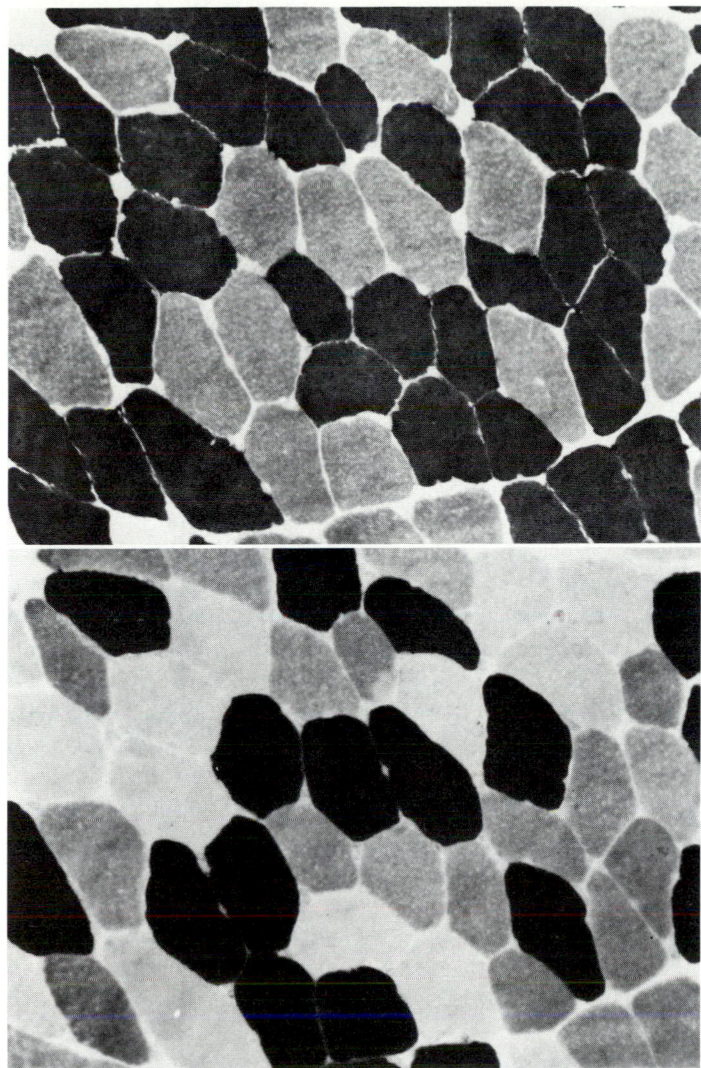

Fig. 43-2. Serial sections of normal skeletal muscle. Mosaic of type I and type II fibers. **A,** Myosin ATPase, pH 9.4: type I fibers light, type II fibers dark. **B,** Myosin ATPase, preincubated at pH 4.6: type I fibers dark, type IIA light, type IIB intermediate. (175×.)

and low in glycogen, myophosphorylase, and myofibrillar adenosine triphosphatase (myosin ATPase) activities. Type II fibers have fewer mitochondria, depend more on glycolysis for energy, and have reciprocal histochemical properties. Type I fibers correspond roughly to the slow-twitch, red muscles, and type II fibers to the fast-twitch, white muscles of certain animals. In humans, however, all muscles are mixed, with the two types of fibers randomly distributed in an approximate ratio of one third type I to two thirds type II. A cross section of muscle appropriately prepared appears as a mosaic of light and dark fibers (Fig. 43-2). In women the diameter of type II fibers is generally smaller than that of type I fibers, whereas the converse is true in men.[25,77] In general, there is more variability in the size of type II than of type I fibers, a factor of some importance in the diagnosis of certain types of atrophy. The myosin ATPase reaction is probably the most reliable for fiber typing and has the added advantage of being technically simple.[36] With this reaction at pH 9.4, type I fibers stain light and type II dark. Preincubation of sections at pH 4.6 reverses these staining qualities, revealing subtype fibers IIA and IIB in approximately equal numbers.[27] Type I fibers under these conditions stain dark, type IIA are almost unstained, and type IIB are of intermediate intensity.

It is clear from cross-innervation experiments in animals and from studying the results of reinnervation of previously denervated muscles in humans that the histochemical reactivity of a muscle fiber is not an intrinsic property of the fiber but is determined by the specific type of alpha motor neuron from which its nerve supply is derived.[62] Thus a denervated type I fiber takes on the biochemical and histochemical characteristics of a type II fiber if reinnervated by axonal sprouts from an intact type II alpha motor neuron.

MUSCLE BIOPSY[4,5a,33,36,61]

Muscle biopsy is valuable in diagnosis when properly performed. Care must be taken to select a muscle actively involved by the disease. It is important to obtain in advance a baseline estimation of serum creatine kinase, since its level may rise after the trauma of biopsy. Sites of prior intramuscular injection or electromyographic needling must be avoided because of the associated focal necrosis and reactive inflammation. Local anesthetic should not be injected into the specimen of muscle, which should measure approximately 2 cm in length and 1 cm in diameter with the muscle fibers oriented longitudinally. The contractile nature of muscle is such that formalin-fixed sections show many retraction and contraction artifacts that obscure minor pathologic changes. This difficulty is best avoided by flash-freezing of blocks of muscle in isopentane cooled to −160° C by liquid nitrogen and then by preparation of frozen sections for both routine stains and histochemical reactions. Tissue frozen at customary cryostat temperatures of −20° to −30° C contains artifacts because of the formation of ice crystals within muscle fibers. Frozen tissue remaining after sectioning can be preserved indefinitely for further sectioning or biochemical analysis if stored at −70° C in an airtight container.

Longitudinally oriented fresh fragments of muscle, 3 × 1 mm, may be fixed in glutaraldehyde for electron microscopic studies. Formalin-fixed, paraffin-embedded tissue is useful for identification of inflammatory cell types and for a permanent record. If material is limited, preference should be given to transverse sections of muscle from which more information can usually be obtained. As a minimum, serial, flash-frozen, transverse sections should be stained with hematoxylin and eosin, with a trichrome stain, and for myosin ATPase and NADH activities. Histochemical reactions for a variety of enzymes and stains for glycogen and lipid are of value in selected cases. Examination of muscle at autopsy has the advantage of offering widespread sampling. Although not always as well defined as in biopsy specimens during life, many histochemical reactions are of value for 48 hours after death.

PATHOLOGIC REACTIONS OF MUSCLE[4,7,111,112]

The histopathologic reactions of muscle fibers are limited. Those related to loss of motor nerve supply are considered in the section on denervation atrophy. An increase in lipid bodies may be noted in certain atrophic fibers; in the aged a slight increase in lipochrome pigment may develop in the sarcoplasm at the ends of the nuclei. Injury to muscle is followed by a relatively constant series of histopathologic changes. First to be noticed is swelling of the fiber with loss of staining qualities and blurring of the striations. Ultrastructurally this is attributable to swelling and disruption of Z discs, increase in the number and size of mitochondria, and formation of membranous structures derived from the sarcoplasmic reticulum or mitochondria.

Frank necrosis of fibers follows more prolonged or severe injury. The cytoplasm breaks up into small granules or larger, eosinophilic, flocculent masses, whereas the nuclei become pyknotic and may migrate centrally into the necrotic area. The plasma membrane and sarcoplasmic tubules rupture, as do the enlarged mitochondria. Z disc substance is the first to be lost, followed by the I bands and finally the entire myofibrillar substructure. The basement membrane may remain intact, thus forming a supporting structure for subsequent regenerative attempts by the satellite cells.

Inflammatory cells appear in the muscle within a few hours of injury. Neutrophils may be present transiently, but more striking is the perivascular accumulation of lymphocytes and the invasion of necrotic fibers by mononuclear macrophages, which phagocytose and remove sarcoplasmic debris. Fragments of sarcoplasm that contain nuclei, or the remaining intact portion of a fiber only segmentally necrotic, frequently undergo attempts at regeneration. Complete regeneration of muscle occurs only under certain circumstances. When the basement membrane remains intact and the necrotic segment is not too large, complete reconstitution of the original structure is possible. If the fiber has been completely sectioned and the distance between two regenerating ends is short, continuity may be reestablished but not necessarily with the original fiber. If the distance is greater or fibrous tissue intervenes, regeneration remains incomplete. With a focally necrotic fiber, regenerative activity is indicated when the adjacent sarcoplasm becomes deeply basophilic and the nuclei enlarge, become vesicular, develop prominent nucleoli, and migrate centrally into the fiber. Portions of fragmented fibers may develop into spindle-shaped cells or myoblasts, which may then fuse to form multinucleated sarcoblasts in which further nuclear division is amitotic. Genesis of myofibrils and other subcellular components proceeds in sarcoblasts much as in embryonic life, but the resulting cell is functionally deficient, for regeneration is limited and continuity of fibers usually is not achieved. The role of the nerve supply in regeneration of muscle is not well defined, but it is unlikely that complete functional reconstitution can occur in the absence of innervation.

Hypertrophy of muscle results from increased activity or workload and is frequently seen as a compensatory mechanism in cells adjacent to atrophic fibers. After birth individual fibers increase in diameter and length but not in numbers. This principle also applies in hypertrophy, but it is less clear whether the bulk of individual fibers is caused by an increase in the amount of sarcoplasm and the size of myofibrils or whether there may be neogenesis of myofibrils.

ATROPHY OF DISUSE AND STEROID THERAPY[62,81,95,109]

Prolonged disuse of normally innervated muscle causes a preponderant or exclusive atrophy of type II fibers. Similar changes may be seen in cachetic patients and in those undergoing long-term steroid therapy or with Cushing's syndrome. Except in cases of long duration, type I fibers remain of normal size whereas type II fibers are reduced in size, are angular in cross section, and often have concave rather than the normal, slightly convex borders (Fig. 43-3). In some patients type IIB fibers are predominantly affected. Sarcolemmal nuclei retain their peripheral location, but fiber necrosis and inflammatory changes are absent. Electron microscopic studies in type II atrophy show a preponderant loss of myofilaments from the peripheral portion of the fiber, with glycogen granules filling the empty spaces.[95] Mitochondria are decreased in number, and the sarcoplasmic reticulum is dilated. The plasma and basement membranes are widely separated, but the nuclei are normal. The findings are similar to those in denervation atrophy, possibly suggesting an alteration of a trophic neural influence on the fibers, particularly of type II. Type II fiber atrophy is reversible with appropriate exercise or discontinuation of steroid therapy. It should be stressed that a diagnosis of type II fiber atrophy cannot be made in the absence of fiber typing. At best, routine sections demonstrate scattered atrophic fibers indistinguishable from the pattern in many patients with early denervation. Care should be taken not to overdiagnose type II atrophy, since normal type II fibers vary considerably in size. This is especially important when examining biopsy specimens from women whose type II fibers are smaller than those of type I.

DENERVATION ATROPHY[4,5b,45,62]

Denervation (neurogenic) atrophy of muscle results from interruption of the motor nerve supply at any point from the motor nerve cell to its terminal axonal sprouts, which reach the motor end-plates. Both motor neuron disease and peripheral neuropathies (acute and chronic) cause denervation, but histopathologic distinction of one from the other is possible only in a limited number of cases.

The gross appearance of denervated muscle is not remarkable until late in the course of the disease when the atrophic muscle is largely replaced by fat and fibrous tissue. Microscopically it is convenient to divide the changes from denervation into early, advanced, and terminal stages. An early change detectable in cross section is the presence of scattered, small, angular fibers with concave margins (Fig. 43-4). The atrophic fibers sometimes occur in small groups surrounded by fibers of normal size and shape. Type I and type II fibers are usually equally affected. Compensatory hypertrophy of intact fibers may be seen. Sarcolemmal nuclei remain peripherally located, and cross striations are retained. A diagnostic feature not always present is the appearance of target fibers, which may represent either recently denervated[83] or recently reinnervated fibers.[4] This change is

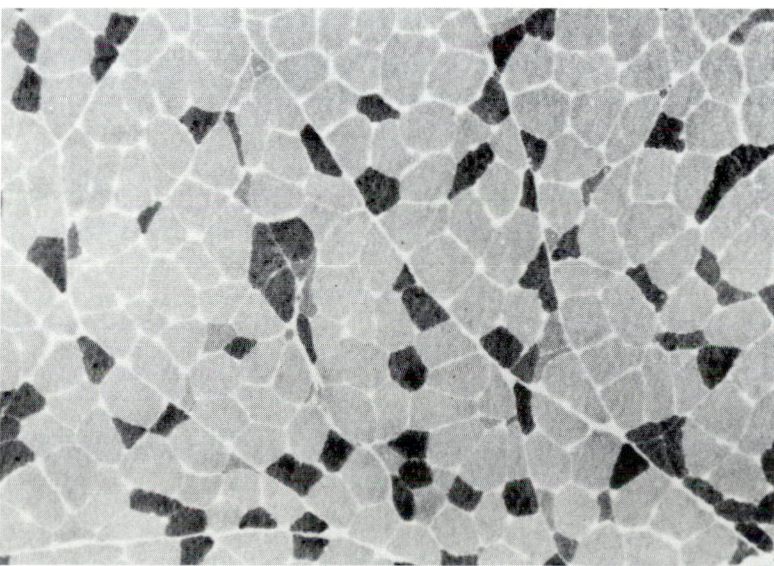

Fig. 43-3. Type II fiber atrophy. (Myosin ATPase, pH 9.4; 80×.)

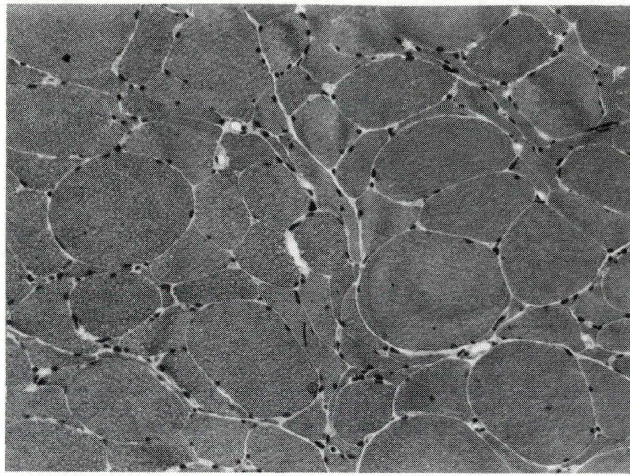

Fig. 43-4. Denervation atrophy. Angular, atrophic fibers are interspersed with normal and hypertrophied fibers. (Hematoxylin and eosin; 212×.)

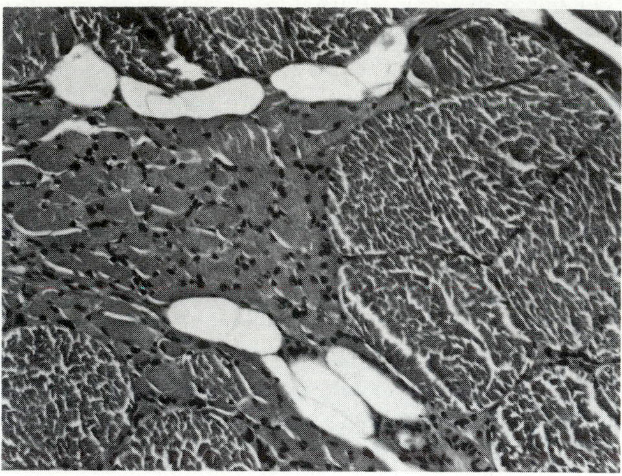

Fig. 43-5. Denervation atrophy affecting a large group of fibers. (Hematoxylin and eosin; 212×.)

usually restricted to type I fibers, which on myosin ATPase stains have a central zone devoid of reactivity, surrounded first by a zone of increased activity and then by a zone of normal activity. Fiber necrosis, regenerative changes and interstitial inflammation are rarely seen and probably indicate an abnormal susceptibility of denervated fibers to minor trauma. At a more advanced state of denervation, atrophy of large groups of fibers or of entire fascicles occurs (Fig. 43-5). Type grouping of fibers may also be seen in which the normal mosaic of type I and type II fibers is replaced by large clusters of fibers, all with like histochemical reactivity (Fig. 43-6). Type grouping is the result of reinnervation of fibers within a restricted zone by axonal sprouts from healthy motor neurons. It is most common in peripheral neuropathy, particularly if chronic. In longitudinal sections the loss of sarcoplasm results in a relative increase in the subsarcolemmal nuclei, which become pyknotic and are arranged in peripheral chains or clusters. In terminal stages many fibers have vanished, and those remaining measure only 10 to 15 μm in diameter and consist of little more than a sarcolemmal sheath containing clumped nuclei. Fat and fibrous tissue replace the muscle, but it is important to emphasize that this is a late occurrence when compared with similar changes in muscular dystrophy and severe polymyositis. Muscle spindles usually remain unaffected throughout and thus appear unusually prominent in the end stage of denervation atrophy. The alterations in fine structure in denervation atrophy are similar to those described for type II fiber atrophy in disuse. Infantile spinal muscular atrophy (Werdnig-Hoffmann disease) differs in appearance from the other denervation processes in two ways: the atrophic fibers remain rounded rather than angular, and there is a selective hypertrophy of type I fibers in certain fascicles.[45]

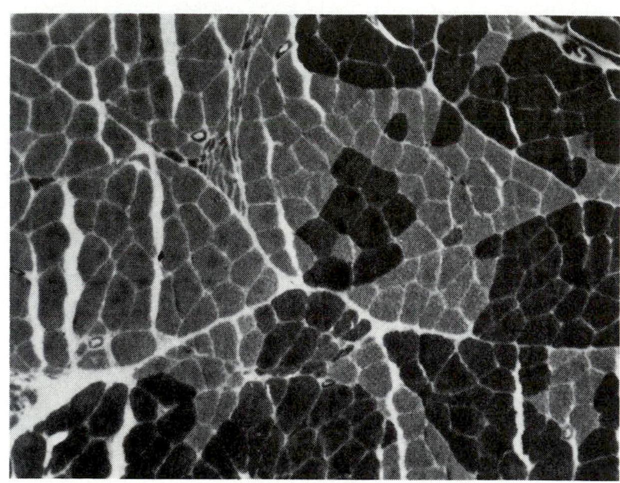

Fig. 43-6. Denervation atrophy with reinnervation. There is prominent fiber-type grouping of reinnervated fibers. Atrophic fibers of both types are also present. (Myosin ATPase, pH 9.4; 85×.)

MUSCULAR DYSTROPHY[11,68,69,117]

The muscular dystrophies comprise a group of hereditary and progressive disorders manifested clinically by muscle weakness and in some types by abnormalities of other organs. Numerous classifications of muscular dystrophy have been proposed of which the most practical remains that of Walton and Gardner-Medwin.[128] Based on the mode of inheritance and clinical features, it is presented in slightly modified form as follows:

1. Sex-linked inheritance
   a. Severe (Duchenne type)
   b. Benign (Becker type)
2. Autosomal recessive inheritance (limb-girdle type)

3. Autosomal dominant inheritance
   a. Facioscapulohumeral type
   b. Myotonic dystrophy
4. Miscellaneous dystrophies (distal, ocular, oculopharyngeal)

The etiology and pathogenesis of muscular dystrophy are unknown. The proteins specific to muscle are normal,[116] but recent studies have demonstrated morphologic[59,74,96] and biochemical[117] abnormalities in the plasma membranes of muscle and other cells, especially erythrocytes.[11,93,110,115] In Duchenne dystrophy ultrastructural defects in the sarcolemma of nonnecrotic muscle fibers may explain the early escape of intracellular enzymes into the blood.[96] Also in Duchenne dystrophy red cells examined by scanning electron microscopy are misshapen.[93,115] Red cell membranes, which can be harvested free from contaminating tissue components, have been used to demonstrate an increase in endogenous protein phosphorylation in Duchenne dystrophy and a decrease in myotonic dystrophy.[11] A variety of techniques have been used to show that cell membrane fluidity is altered in several types of dystrophy.[14,108] Genetically induced diseases are typically caused by a biochemical abnormality; the cell membrane defects demonstrated in a muscular dystrophy probably represent no more than detectable manifestations of such an aberration.

Clinical features

Duchenne muscular dystrophy is transmitted by a sex-linked recessive gene, although spontaneous mutations are relatively common. Only males are affected; females are carriers. Symptoms begin in childhood usually before the age of 4. Since the muscles of the pelvis are the first to be affected, the initial symptom is difficulty in walking, running, and rising from a sitting position. Other muscles, especially those of the shoulder girdle, are affected in relentless progression until the patient is confined to a wheelchair or bed, at which time contractures rapidly supervene. At some stage of the disease hypertrophy of muscles is usually noted, particularly in the calves. This change is probably attributable in part to true hypertrophy of unaffected muscle fibers and in part to a pseudohypertrophy produced by fatty infiltration of the muscle. The heart muscle is involved in virtually all cases. Death is caused by either respiratory or cardiac failure and usually occurs by the age of 20. Serum enzymes, especially creatine kinase (CK), are invariably elevated early, but the CK level drops rapidly after the age of 10.[98] Electromyographic findings are abnormal. Approximately 70% of female carriers also show elevation of the serum CK, although this is not constant and may be detected only after repeated measurement.[105,107] Carriers may also show myoglobinemia[8] and electromyographic abnormalities, and fiber necrosis may be found on muscle biopsy. By the combined use of the serum CK, serum myoglobin, electromyography, and biopsy, approximately 80% of carriers should be identified; thus genetic counseling is greatly aided.

Although serum CK is elevated at birth, determination of fetal CK levels has not so far proved reliable in distinguishing affected from unaffected infants among those genetically at risk.[50]

The Becker variety of sex-linked dystrophy comes to attention between the ages of 5 and 25 years.[24] Similar in other respects to the Duchenne variety, it has a much slower clinical course and is usually without cardiac involvement. Persons having the Becker type of dystrophy frequently survive to sexual maturity, and so transmission of the trait from affected males becomes possible.

Limb-girdle dystrophy, transmitted as an autosomal recessive trait, affects both sexes. Spontaneous mutations are not uncommon. Initial symptoms begin in early adult life and first affect muscles of the shoulder or pelvic girdle. Pseudohypertrophy of the calves occurs, but cardiac involvement is rare. The progress of the disease is variable, but few patients have a normal life span. Longevity is, however, considerably greater than that in Duchenne dystrophy.

Facioscapulohumeral dystrophy bears many resemblances to the limb-girdle variety. Major differences include autosomal dominant inheritance in most, the occurrence of weakness of facial muscles, the rarity of pseudohypertrophy, the occurrence of incomplete forms of the disease, and a normal life expectancy in all but the most rapidly progressive cases.

Myotonic dystrophy[74] (dystrophia myotonica, myotonia atrophica) is transmitted by an autosomal dominant gene, and its manifestations are not confined to skeletal muscle. Other lesions include cardiac involvement, frontal baldness, cataracts, gonadal atrophy, and mental deficiency. Symptoms usually begin in early adult life, and the muscles most commonly affected are those of the face, forearm, and lower legs. This distal pattern of involvement, together with the phenomenon of myotonia (inability to relax the muscles after contraction), distinguishes the disease from most of the other dystrophies, which predominantly affect proximal muscles.

The miscellaneous dystrophies (distal, ocular, oculopharyngeal) are too rare to justify separate attention. Some may have been confused with various rare, familial denervation diseases.

Elevation of the serum CK activity is a common finding in all varieties of dystrophy except the myotonic, in which it is variable. Levels are highest in Duchenne dystrophy and may even be normal at times in other varieties during quiescent periods. The elevation of the enzyme in the serum is probably related to the number of actively necrotic muscle fibers from which it leaks. The

CK can therefore be expected to be highest in the acute phases of muscle destruction and when the disease is rapidly progressive.

Pathologic features

Gross pathologic changes in muscular dystrophy are nonspecific. They consist of an early replacement by fat and fibrous tissue so that the muscle appears yellow or white and floats in the fixative solution. It is this infiltration that gives rise to the pseudohypertrophic appearance of certain muscles, although compensatory hypertrophy of intact individual fibers also occurs. Except for myotonic dystrophy, the histopathologic aspect of the various forms of muscular dystrophy varies only in minor respects (Fig. 43-7). The earliest change is the appearance of focally necrotic fibers infiltrated by macrophages but generally without an associated interstitial inflammatory infiltrate. Adjacent to the zone of necrosis are basophilia of sarcoplasm and internal migration of enlarged nuclei characteristic of regeneration. Continuity of necrotic fibers may be reestablished in the early stages of the disease, but regenerative activity decreases later, as the destructive process predominates. In dystrophy, atrophic fibers tend to retain a rounded cross-sectional appearance, differing in this respect from the angular, atrophic fibers of denervation. Uninvolved fibers commonly are hypertrophied so that a transverse section of muscle appears as a haphazard mosaic of small, normal-sized, and enlarged fibers. Internal migration of nuclei, longitudinal splitting of fibers, and ring fibers may all be prominent. Ring fibers, which may be seen in other diseases and occasionally in normal muscle, consist of a peripheral layer of myofibrils running at right angles to, or in spiral fashion about, a central core of longitudinally oriented myofibrils. Electron microscopic changes in fibers with early necrosis are nonspecific; they consist of streaming or fragmentation of the Z discs, shredding of myofibrils, dilatation of the sarcoplasmic reticulum, swelling and disruption of mitochondria, and accumulation of lipid vacuoles and myelin-like figures. As the dystrophic process advances, individual fibers are separated by ever-increasing amounts of endomysial fibrous tissue (Fig. 43-8). Histochemical typing is less reliable in dystrophic than in normal muscle. However, with care one can demonstrate that both fiber types are affected,

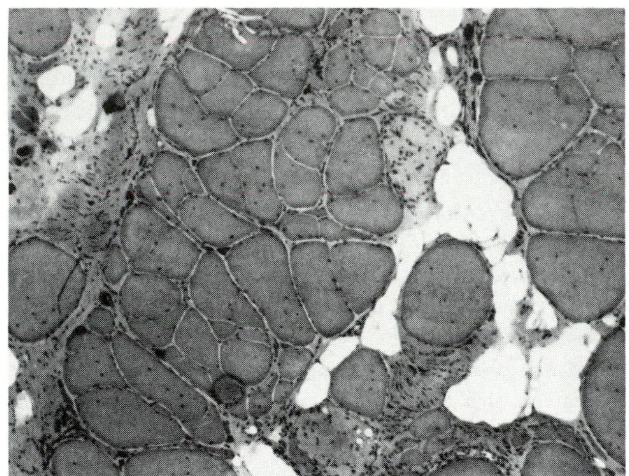

Fig. 43-7. Limb-girdle dystrophy. Note two necrotic fibers invaded by histiocytes, prominent fiber splitting, variation in fiber size, many internal nuclei, clumped nuclei in severely atrophic fibers, and ingrowth of fibrous tissue and fat. (Hematoxylin and eosin; 85×.)

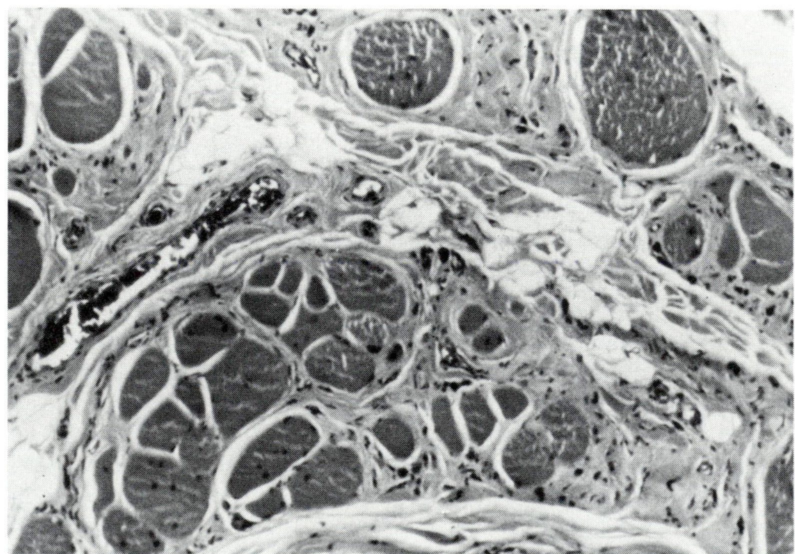

Fig. 43-8. Advanced muscular dystrophy. Haphazard atrophy of fibers with replacement by fat and fibrous tissue. (Hematoxylin and eosin; 175×.)

although the normal orderly relationship may be lacking.[12] In the terminal stages the muscle is replaced by fat and fibrous tissue in which rare surviving fibers can be seen together with muscle spindles, which are seldom affected. At this point histologic differentiation from end-stage denervation atrophy or polymyositis may not be possible. The histopathologic aspect of myotonic dystrophy differs from that of the other diseases in this group in several respects. Typical changes include atrophy of type I fibers, relatively little necrosis or phagocytosis, chains of central nuclei, ring fibers, and sarcoplasmic masses.

MYOSITIS

Inflammatory diseases of muscles are divisible into two major groups, those of known and those of unknown etiology. A practical classification is as follows:

A. Known etiology
   1. Bacteria
   2. Fungus
   3. Parasite
   4. Virus
   5. Mechanical, physical, and chemical agents
B. Unknown etiology
   1. Polymyositis (dermatomyositis)
      a. Acute
      b. Chronic
   2. Acute rhabdomyolysis
   3. Interstitial myositis
      a. Miscellaneous collagen diseases
      b. Polyarteritis nodosa
      c. Sarcoidosis

Bacterial myositis is uncommon and is almost always caused by direct implantation of the causative organism. The course of localized inflammation, necrosis, and abscess formation differs little from that seen in other tissues. The effectiveness of repair and regeneration after resolution of the inflammatory process depends on the extent of the destruction. In most cases regeneration is incomplete and a fibrous scar remains. Specific diseases such as gas gangrene, fungal and viral infections, and parasitic infestations have been considered previously under their appropriate designations. Heat, cold, and trauma result in nonspecific necrosis, degeneration, and regeneration of muscle.

Polymyositis[20,21,104,127]

Polymyositis is a disease of unknown etiology, but the frequent elevation of serum globulins, the association with "autoimmune" diseases of the collagen group, and the response to therapy with steroids have all suggested a relationship to an autoimmune phenomenon. There is some evidence of a cell-mediated immune reaction to skeletal muscle characterized by activation and infiltration of T lymphocytes.[20,42,104] It is therefore postulated that the infiltrating lymphocytes may have been sensitized to muscle in some manner and so are directly responsible for initiating necrosis of fibers. Viruslike inclusions have been described in a few cases of polymyositis,[92,125] but their pathogenic significance if any is unknown.

Polymyositis may occur at any age, but the peak incidence is in the fourth through sixth decades. It is twice as common in women as in men. A cutaneous rash is seen in 35% of cases, but the histopathologic changes in the muscles are identical with and without the rash. Dermal lesions are particularly common in children and in the 10% to 20% of cases of polymyositis with an associated internal malignancy, usually a carcinoma. The incidence of concomitant malignancy is much greater in patients whose disease begins after age 50.[15] Polymyositis may be associated with other collagen diseases, such as rheumatoid arthritis, lupus erythematosus, and scleroderma. Raynaud's phenomenon is not uncommon, and there is also an association with Sjögren's syndrome. A localized nodular form has been described, which may progress to typical polymyositis.[39]

The onset of polymyositis may be acute or gradual. When it is acute the patient experiences severe muscular weakness, myalgia, fever, malaise, and other constitutional symptoms. Death may occur from failure of the respiratory muscles. More often the onset of polymyositis is gradual, with the development of muscular weakness first affecting proximal limb muscles and then progressing to others. Muscular pain and tenderness are less common. When the dermal component of the disease is present, it typically takes the form of an erythematous rash seen especially on the face but also on the trunk and proximal limbs. Serum enzymes, especially CK, are elevated in proportion to the amount of muscle necrosis. Serial estimations of CK are useful in following the activity of the disease and its response to treatment.

In acute polymyositis there are atrophy, degeneration, and necrosis of muscle fibers. Both fiber types and muscle spindles are affected. The peripheral fibers of fascicles may atrophy disproportionately, especially early in the course and in children,[35] but later this selective pattern of involvement is often lost (Fig. 43-9). Muscle fibers show a complete spectrum of degeneration from vacuolar changes to frank necrosis. Segmental involvement of fibers is frequent. Regenerative attempts are prominent in the form of both isolated myoblasts and muscle giant cells and proliferating buds at the disrupted ends of fibers. Electron microscopic findings are nonspecific and generally are indistinguishable from those described for muscular dystrophy. The endomysium and perimysium are infiltrated by variable numbers of lymphocytes, plasma cells, and macrophages and lesser numbers of neutrophils (Fig. 43-10). There is little relationship between the amount of inflammatory exudate and the degree of muscle damage. As the necrotic muscle

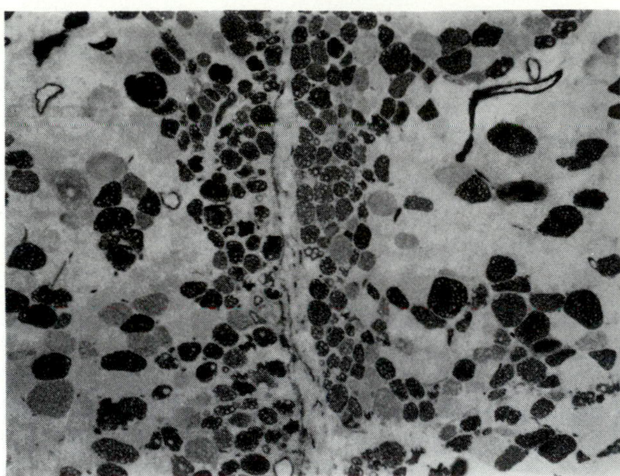

Fig. 43-9. Polymyositis. There is selective atrophy of fibers at periphery of fascicles. (Myosin ATPase, preincubated at pH 4.5; 85×.)

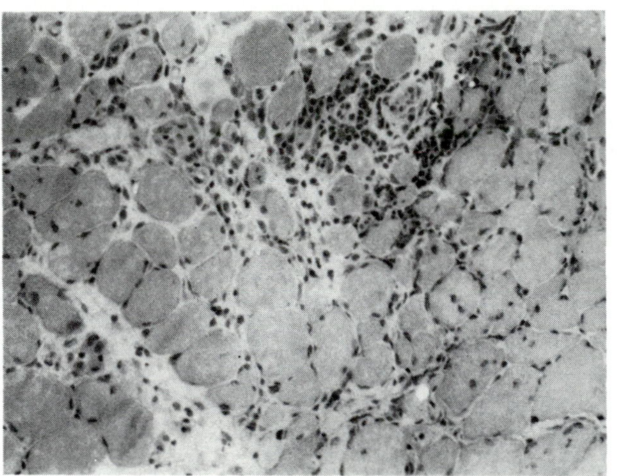

Fig. 43-10. Polymyositis. Atrophic and necrotic fibers, some internal nuclei, lymphocytic infiltrate, and early fibrosis are present. (Hematoxylin and eosin; 212×.)

is removed, it is replaced by connective tissue and fat, until in the terminal stage the appearance is nonspecific.

In chronic cases the histopathologic changes may be limited to isolated necrotic fibers and an associated minor inflammatory infiltrate. Since there is also variation in fiber size, the findings may be remarkably similar to those in early muscular dystrophy; thus they may pose a problem in differential diagnosis.

Acute rhabdomyolysis[118]

Acute rhabdomyolysis or paroxysmal myoglobinuria is characterized by attacks of muscle pain and cramps associated with severe weakness and, on occasion, with systemic symptoms. Half the cases occur after an episode of unaccustomed physical exertion,[43,121] and the remainder are related to trauma, viral infections,[17] excessive alcohol intake,[79] potassium deficiency,[32,82] or exposure to certain drugs and toxins.[48,76,91] Shortly after the onset of an attack, dark urine containing myoglobin is passed. In severe cases renal tubular necrosis may develop and be followed by oliguria and azotemia. It is important to analyze both serum and urine for myoglobin during the acute attack because plasma clearance is rapid and later specimens may be normal. Histologically there is a striking segmental necrosis of muscle fibers with concomitant attempts at regeneration from adjacent unaffected zones. Necrotic segments are infiltrated by macrophages, but there is little interstitial inflammatory infiltrate in relation to the amount of muscular damage. Regeneration is usually complete because the basement membrane and endomysium remain intact. If repeated attacks occur, there may be permanent muscular damage and weakness.

Interstitial myositis

Focal interstitial collections of inflammatory cells, especially lymphocytes, are found in a variety of diseases. Scattered necrosis of muscle fibers may also be noted but is not usually prominent. Lesions of this type are most common in the collagen group of diseases, especially rheumatoid arthritis, lupus erythematosus, scleroderma, and polymyalgia rheumatica.[28] The findings are nonspecific and should not be misinterpreted as polymyositis. Type II fiber atrophy may be present as the result of disuse, steroid therapy, or both.

Polyarteritis nodosa[9,38,103]

Polyarteritis nodosa affects skeletal muscle in over 50% of cases, although clinically it is not always apparent. It may also involve peripheral nerves with secondary denervation atrophy of muscles. In selection of a muscle for biopsy the chance of success in demonstrating the lesion is proportional to the local severity of pain or weakness. Most commonly the affected arteries lie in the perimysium, and the perivascular inflammatory infiltrate frequently extends into the peripheral zones of adjacent muscle fascicles. Necrosis and degeneration of muscle may be present, and should sections lack a typical arterial lesion, it may be impossible to distinguish the disease from polymyositis.

Sarcoidosis[46,114,123]

Sarcoidosis may affect skeletal muscle more commonly than is generally realized. Clinical evidence of muscular pain or weakness is uncommon, but biopsies have revealed typical noncaseous epithelioid cell granulomas in over 50% of patients. The granulomas are usually located in the perimysium, often adjacent to an artery or vein. More rarely a granuloma may develop in the endomysium, often associated with focal atrophy or necrosis of the adjacent muscle fibers. In the differential diagnosis it is important to consider that a granulomatous response can be seen adjacent to each *Trichinella* larva. Sarcoidosis involving peripheral motor nerves results in secondary denervation atrophy of muscle.

MYASTHENIA GRAVIS[47,49,73,88,126]

Myasthenia gravis is a disease of muscle characterized by excessive weakness and fatigue after repetitive movements or on sustained muscular contraction. Its prevalence approximates one per 20,000 population. Age at onset reaches a peak in the third decade for women and the sixth decade for men. The overall incidence is greater in women than in men in a ratio of 3:2. Although familial cases have been reported, there is no heritable pattern.[31] Onset is usually gradual, with manifestations restricted to ocular muscles in 20%; in another 50% ocular symptoms and mild or moderate generalized myasthenia are concomitant. In 10% weakness is severe, progressive, and generalized with involvement of the "bulbar" and respiratory muscles. Remissions occur in the early stages but become less common and of shorter duration as the disease progresses. Death is usually attributable to respiratory failure complicated by aspiration pneumonia that results from the severe dysphagia.

On muscle biopsy the classic (but not always present) lesion is a focal lymphocytic infiltrate (lymphorrhage), often perivascular but sometimes located in the endomysium, where it displaces adjacent muscle fibers. Necrosis is rare, but muscle atrophy occurs in the later stages. The most common finding is type II fiber atrophy related to disuse or steroid therapy. In long-standing cases, especially in patients over the age of 50, changes of denervation and sometimes of reinnervation may be seen.[30,37]

When an action potential reaches the distal end of an axon, it stimulates the release of quanta of acetylcholine, which cross the synaptic space and attach to specific receptors on the postsynaptic membrane, thus initiating ionic movements that result in muscle contraction. A cobra venom, alpha-bungarotoxin, binds specifically and irreversibly to acetylcholine receptors and can be quantitated by labeling it either with ^{125}I[63] or with peroxidase.[16] Quantitation in patients with myasthenia gravis indicates that the number of acetylcholine receptors is reduced to 36% of normal, and some of those remaining have antibody bound to them so that they may be blockaded or at least be rendered functionally inefficient.[89] Electron microscopic studies have not only demonstrated shortening and simplification of the postsynaptic membrane folds[58,120] but also have shown that the binding of peroxidase-labeled alpha-bungarotoxin to receptors is reduced or absent.[60]

Following the discovery that acetylcholine receptors can be isolated and purified from the electric organ of electric eels,[101] antibodies to receptor have been found in the serum of 90% of patients with myasthenia gravis.[90] Furthermore, an IgG antibody and the C3 component of complement are bound to receptor sites on the postsynaptic membrane.[56] These findings suggest that an autoimmune humoral mechanism is the basis for the loss of receptor substance. The mechanism by which the autoantibody destroys acetylcholine receptors is as yet unclear, but Engel and associates[60] have recently identified the C9 (lytic) component of complement on degraded fragments of postsynaptic membrane lying in the synaptic space, suggesting that a complement-mediated lytic process may damage the receptor sites. Support for the autoimmune pathogenesis of myasthenia gravis also comes from an extensive series of studies in which animal models were used. When rabbits or rats are injected with purified acetylcholine receptor, antibodies are formed, and experimental autoimmune myasthenia gravis develops.[101] This disease is characterized by an acute phase in which mononuclear cells invade the neuromuscular junction and the postsynaptic membrane separates from the muscle fiber. Simplification of the postsynaptic membrane, similar to that seen in human disease, develops in the chronic phase.[58] There is no counterpart in humans to the early inflammatory changes seen in animals, but in most other respects the diseases are similar.

The concept that myasthenia gravis may be an autoimmune disease predates the modern experimental findings by many years. The observation that myasthenia gravis is frequently associated with other autoimmune diseases (such as Hashimoto's thyroiditis, pernicious anemia, diabetes mellitus, rheumatoid arthritis, and polymyositis) first stimulated this belief.[124] Supportive laboratory evidence included the presence of serum autoantibodies of varying type and depression of serum complement levels. Finally, some infants born of mothers with myasthenia gravis were known to have a myasthenic syndrome, suggesting transplacental passage of a maternal autoantibody that was presumed to blockade or deplete the infant's acetylcholine receptor sites.

The role of the thymus in myasthenia gravis remains unknown. Thymomas are present in 10% to 15% of patients, the incidence increasing with the age of onset. In 65% of patients the thymus, although little if at all enlarged, appears hyperplastic because of the presence of active germinal centers and an increased number of lymphocytes and plasma cells.[86] Similar changes may be present in residual thymic tissue surrounding a thymoma. Antistriational antibodies, which react against both skeletal muscle and the "myoid" cell of the thymus, occur frequently in myasthenia gravis, especially in the presence of a thymoma.[113,126] Unfortunately, they also occur in other diseases, so their diagnostic significance is limited and any pathogenic relationship to the disease remains unproved. A thymectomy frequently results in clinical improvement,[100] which may be accompanied by a fall in receptor antibody titer.[85] It has therefore been postulated that deranged thymic function in the presence of a thymoma or hyperplasia may deplete a humoral factor that normally inhibits the production of autoantibodies.[49] The possibility of a viral infection as the initiating mechanism has been suggested.[41]

GLYCOGEN-STORAGE DISEASE[22,75]

The glycogen-storage diseases are inborn, heritable errors of metabolism characterized by an abnormal accumulation of glycogen in the tissues. The classification (Table 43-1) now includes eight types in which a specific enzymatic defect has been established. Additional isolated cases have been reported in which the defect has not been as well defined. Abnormal deposition of glycogen in skeletal muscle is found in all but types I and VI, although the amount present varies considerably with the different enzymatic defects. Only those affecting muscle are discussed here. Diagnosis depends on biochemical identification of the enzymatic abnormality, except for type II, in which the histologic appearance is characteristic, and type V, for which a reliable histochemical method is available. The less rare glycogenoses of muscle are types II, III, and V.

Type II glycogenosis (Pompe's disease) is transmitted by an autosomal recessive gene and becomes manifest at 3 to 4 months of age with muscular weakness, cyanosis, and cardiac and lingual enlargement. The muscular weakness correlates poorly with the firm, apparently well-developed muscles. Death usually occurs within the first year of life because of cardiac failure or pneumonia. The enzymatic defect is a deficiency in lysosomal alpha-1,4-glucosidase (acid maltase). At autopsy, massive accumulations of glycogen are found in a variety of organs, including skeletal, cardiac, and smooth muscle, liver, kidneys, and central nervous system. In muscle the glycogen appears as large vacuoles that are periodic acid–Schiff positive. Islands of myofibrillar substance remain as condensed masses often in a subsarcolemmal location. With electron microscopy the excess glycogen is seen to lie free, in membrane-bound structures and in autophagic vacuoles.[51] Glycogen in normal muscle is probably ingested by lysosomes and later degraded by the lysomal acid maltase. In the absence of the enzyme, glycogen accumulates and distends the lysosomes to such an extent that myofibrils are mechanically disrupted. The onset of symptoms in type II glycogenosis has occasionally been delayed until later childhood or adulthood.[44] Cardiac involvement has then been absent, and the disease may mimic muscular dystrophy. Heterozygous carriers can be detected by assay of muscle enzyme content.[54]

Type III glycogenosis (limit dextrinosis, debrancher enzyme defect, Forbes' disease, Cori's disease) is caused by a deficiency of amylo-1,6-glucosidase (debrancher enzyme). This enzyme is responsible for hydrolysis at the alpha-1,6 linkage and hence for the continuation of glycogenolysis after the initial breakdown of the straight outer chains of the molecule by phosphorylase. In the enzyme's absence an abnormal glycogen with short outer chains accumulates in the affected organs. Several subtypes are now recognized, depending on whether the enzyme is absent from liver, muscle, or both. The mode of inheritance is autosomal recessive. Symptoms begin in the neonatal period and may decrease with age. They are related more to involvement of the liver than to muscle, with hypoglycemia, hyperlipidemia, hepatomegaly, infections, and ketoacidosis. Muscle weakness when present may be mistaken for muscular dystrophy and in some patients may not become apparent until adult life. The excessive glycogen is subsarcolemmal, often in a semilunar vacuole. Electron microscopy reveals the glycogen to be free and membrane bound, both in intermyofibrillar spaces and beneath the sarcolemma.

The extremely rare type IV glycogenosis (Andersen's disease) is caused by a deficiency of amylo-1,4→1,6-transglucosylase (brancher enzyme). Transmission is autosomal recessive. Excess glycogen resembling amylopectin is found in many organs, including skeletal muscle. Symptoms are primarily related to hepatic damage.

Type V glycogenosis (McArdle's disease) is an autosomal recessive disease characterized by an absence of

Table 43-1. The glycogenoses*

Type		Enzymatic defect	Organ affected
I	(von Gierke's disease)	Glucose-6-phosphatase	Liver, kidney
II	(Pompe's disease)	Alpha-1,4-glucosidase (acid maltase)	Generalized; liver, muscle
III	(Cori's disease, Forbes' disease)	Amylo-1,6-glucosidase	Generalized; liver, muscle
IV	(Andersen's disease)	Amylo-1,4→1,6-transglucosylase	Generalized; liver
V	(McArdle's syndrome)	Muscle phosphorylase	Muscle
VI	(Hers' disease)	Hepatic phosphorylase	Liver, leukocytes
VII	(Tarui's disease)	Phosphofructokinase	Muscle, erythrocytes
VIII		Hepatic phosphorylase kinase	Liver

*Inheritance: VI, unknown; VIII, sex-linked recessive; all others, autosomal recessive.

phosphorylase from muscle but not from liver.[94] The enzymatic lack blocks the breakdown of glycogen to glucose-1-phosphate, and hence excess glycogen collects in the muscle. Muscular stiffness, weakness, and pain on exertion usually begin in childhood but may be delayed until adult life. Episodes of myoglobinuria are common. Exercise with ischemia results in contracture of the muscles, with inability to relax and electrical silence on electromyography. Failure of the blood lactate level to rise after a period of ischemic exercise should suggest the diagnosis. Histochemical examination of muscle reveals the complete absence of phosphorylase. Excess glycogen may or may not be detectable in muscle. When present, it is likely to be in subsarcolemmal blebs or in the intermyofibrillar spaces. Excess glycogen has also been described in enlarged mitochondria. Myopathic changes characterized by isolated fiber necrosis may be seen and thus simulate an early stage of muscular dystrophy.

Type VII glycogenosis is caused by a deficiency of phosphofructokinase. There may be an excess of glycogen in skeletal muscle, and the symptoms and laboratory findings resemble those of type V glycogenosis. Transmission is probably autosomal recessive.

A form of glycogenosis that results in decreased glycogen in both liver and muscle has also been described.[87] The disease is caused by a deficiency of UDGP-glycogen transglucosylase, probably transmitted by an autosomal recessive gene. Symptoms begin shortly after birth and are characterized by hypoglycemic convulsions. Mild ketonuria may be present. The fasting hypoglycemia is unresponsive to glucagon given intramuscularly.

PERIODIC PARALYSES[102]

The several forms of periodic paralyses are characterized by episodic attacks of flaccid paralysis. The primary or familial periodic paralyses can be divided into hypokalemic, normokalemic, and hyperkalemic varieties. Secondary periodic paralyses are associated with thyrotoxicosis, primary aldosteronism, and abnormalities of potassium metabolism in diabetic acidosis and renal tubular acidosis.

The most common primary periodic paralysis is the hypokalemic form, which is transmitted by an autosomal recessive gene but is three times more frequent in males than in females. Attacks of paralysis are characteristically nocturnal and occur after a period of vigorous exercise. Symptoms usually appear first in the second decade and tend to become less severe with age. The attack, which may last from a few hours to several days, affects the musculature of the limbs and trunk but spares the facial and respiratory muscles. Although associated with low levels of serum potassium, weakness may begin at potassium levels higher than those that would induce paralysis in a normal individual.

Histologic examination of muscle fibers reveals single or multiple, centrally located, intracellular vacuoles with displacement of the myofibrils to the periphery. Type I and type II fibers are equally affected. The vacuoles appear to begin as dilatations of the sarcoplasmic reticulum that are later surrounded by a membrane derived from the T tubular system, which connects the vacuoles with the extracellular fluid.[51] This form of periodic paralysis is believed to be related to an alteration in cellular polarization attributable either to defects in the sarcolemma or sarcoplasmic reticulum or to abnormal intracellular carbohydrate metabolism. Attacks may be aborted by the oral or intravenous administration of potassium.

Hyperkalemic and normokalemic periodic paralyses are rarer. In the hyperkalemic form, paralysis occurs typically by day during rest after a period of exercise and is often associated with myotonia. In the normokalemic form, the characteristic attacks are nocturnal and prolonged, often lasting for days or weeks. Vacuolar changes occur in the muscle fibers in both the hyperkalemic and hypokalemic types of periodic paralyses but are less constant and severe than in the hypokalemic form.

MISCELLANEOUS DISEASES

Two disorders of lipid metabolism may affect muscle. The first, carnitine deficiency, occurs in two forms: systemic and restricted to muscle.[22,34,52] In the systemic variety serum carnitine levels are significantly decreased, and hepatic insufficiency predominates. In the restricted form serum carnitine levels are minimally if at all decreased. In both, muscle weakness is prominent, and lipid droplets accumulate in muscle. The second lipid disturbance results from a deficiency of palmityl transferase in muscle.[13,22] Clinically there is muscle weakness on prolonged exercise, often with episodes of myoglobinuria. Lipid accumulation in muscle is rare.

A deficiency of muscle adenylate deaminase has been documented histochemically in young men, probably as a sex-linked recessive trait. The patients have muscular weakness or cramping after exercise.[65] Apart from the absence of adenylate deaminase, muscle biopsy findings appear to be normal.

Myopathic changes have been described in association with a number of endocrinopathies. Among them may be included the muscular weakness experienced by certain patients with hyperthyroidism, hypothyroidism, hyperparathyroidism, hyperaldosteronism, Addison's disease, Cushing's syndrome, and diabetes mellitus. Although electromyographic findings may be abnormal at some time in all, demonstrable abnormalities in muscle are either absent or nonspecific, although type II atrophy from disuse may be seen.

Myopathy is an uncommon complication of chronic alcoholism. When it does occur, proximal muscle weakness is usual, with isolated fiber necrosis, a vacuolar myopathy, and rarely rhabdomyolysis.[79,106] It has been suggested that these lesions may be secondary to chronic hypokalemia, but since denervation atrophy has also been reported, it is possible that the mucular weakness is the result of a concomitant peripheral neuropathy with secondary myopathic changes.[64]

Congenital myotonia (Thomsen's disease) is characterized by a delay in relaxation of muscle resulting in a tonic cramp and immobility. Patients with Thomsen's disease have difficulty initiating movement after a period of rest, but persistent and repetitive attempts usually result in normal freedom of response. Most cases are transmitted as an autosomal dominant trait, but 10% to 15% appear to be autosomal recessive. Symptoms usually begin in childhood but may be delayed until early adult life. No pathologic lesions are recognized in muscle other than striking hypertrophy of muscle fibers resulting from an increase in the number of myofibrils.

A number of congenital myopathies have been described and classified primarily on the basis of particular morphologic abnormalities within muscle fibers. The names given to these diseases (nemaline [rod],[99] centronuclear or myotubular,[18,23,97] central core,[71] multicore,[55] mitochondrial,[66] tubular aggregate,[62] reducing body,[29] fingerprint body[53] myopathies) reflect the most prominent histologic findings, but the rarity of the conditions precludes detailed discussion here.

Myositis (fibroplasia) ossificans progressiva is a rare disease characterized by the development of extraosseous connective tissue masses that eventually become ossified. The disease usually begins in childhood with the appearance of rubbery masses in the connective tissues of the neck or back and later in the limbs. The lesions may form in connective tissue or muscle and initially consist of proliferating fibroblasts devoid of inflammatory reaction. When muscle is affected, the fibers are fragmented and destroyed, and contractures develop as the nodule matures into collagen. Finally osteoid is formed either directly in the collagen or through an intermediate cartilaginous step. The result is progressive immobility because of ossification of many muscle groups. Pneumonia, the most common cause of death, follows involvement of the respiratory muscles. Although this has not been established with certainty, the disease is probably hereditary and may be transmitted by an autosomal dominant gene. Congenital abnormalities may occur, particularly microdactyly of the great toe or thumb. Cases have also been associated with polyostotic fibrous dysplasia, a finding that suggests that the basic defect is a disseminated dysplasia of connective tissue.[67] Recurrence is usually rapid if the ectopic bone is surgically removed, but administration of the diphosphonate disodium ethidronate before operation has been successful in preventing reossification.[119]

Arthrogryposis multiplex congenita[19,40] is a rare congenital condition characterized by deformities of the limbs and trunk. Mental retardation coexists in about half the cases. It appears that there may be multiple causes. Some cases are the result of maldevelopment of anterior horn cells in the spinal cord with consequent failure of innervation of specific muscles. Others represent a failure to recruit myoblasts from the primitive mesenchyme during fetal life or are examples of a congenital muscular dystrophy. In neurogenic arthrogryposis muscle fibers are extremely small, whereas in the myopathic forms there are variation in fiber size and increase in endomysial fibrous tissue.

The stiff-man syndrome[72,84] begins with intermittent pain and tightness of the muscles of the neck and trunk and later progresses to involve the limbs so that voluntary movement becomes increasingly difficult. Severe, painful spasms or cramps then develop and may be triggered by either physical or emotional stimuli. It is likely that other conditions with spasticity or rigidity have been confused with the stiff-man syndrome. The diagnosis should be restricted to cases in which electromyography shows constant tonic muscle contractions associated with continuous firing of nerve impulses. The abnormal electrical and contractile state is abolished by sleep, myoneural blocking agents, nerve block, and general anesthesia. The pathophysiology of the stiff-man syndrome is uncertain but probably involves a central mechanism. There are many similarities to tetanus, and there is probably more than one cause. Muscle biopsy shows only necrosis and other nonspecific changes explainable by trauma induced by the spasms.

TUMORS OF SKELETAL MUSCLE

Tumors and tumorlike lesions of skeletal muscle have been considered elsewhere (p. 1661).

REFERENCES

General

1. Adams, R.D.: Diseases of muscle: a study in pathology, ed. 3, Hagerstown, Md., 1975, Harper & Row, Publishers, Inc.
2. Bethlem, J.: Myopathies, Philadelphia, 1977, J.B. Lippincott Co.
3. Dubowitz, V.: Muscle disorders in childhood, Philadelphia, 1978, W.B. Saunders Co.
4. Dubowitz, V., and Brooke, M.H.: Muscle biopsy: a modern approach, Philadelphia, 1973, W.B. Saunders Co.

4a. Korényi-Both, A.L.: Muscle pathology in neuromuscular disease, Springfield, Ill., 1983, Charles C Thomas, Publisher.

4b. Mastaglia, F.L., and Walton, J., editors: Skeletal muscle pathology, New York, 1982, Churchill Livingstone.

5. Pearson, C.M., editor: The striated muscle, Baltimore, 1973, The Williams & Wilkins Co.

5a. Sarnat, H.B.: Muscle pathology and histochemistry, Chicago, 1983, American Society of Clinical Pathologists Press.

5b. Swash, M., and Schwartz, M.D.: Neuromuscular disease: a practical approach to diagnosis and management, New York, 1981, Springer-Verlag.

6. Walton, J.N., editor: Disorders of voluntary muscle, ed. 4, New York, 1981, Churchill Livingstone.

Specific

7. Adams, R.D., and Åstrom, K.E.: Pathological reactions of the skeletal muscle fibre in man. In Walton, J.N., editor: Disorders of voluntary muscle, ed. 4, New York, 1981, Churchill Livingstone.
8. Adornato, B.T., Kagen, L.J., and Engel, W.K.: Myoglobinaemia in Duchenne muscular dystrophy patients and carriers: a new adjunct to carrier detection, Lancet **2**:499, 1978.
9. Alarcon-Segonia, D.: The necrotizing vasculitides: a new pathogenetic classification, Med. Clin. North Am. **61**:241, 1977.
10. Allen, E.R.: Immunochemical and ultrastructural studies of myogenesis. In Pearson, C.M., editor: The striated muscle, Baltimore, 1973, The William & Wilkins Co.
11. Appel, S.H., and Rosen, A.D.: The muscular dystrophies. In Stanbury, J.B., et al., editors: The metabolic basis of inherited disease, ed. 5, New York, 1983, McGraw-Hill Book Co.
12. Baloh, R., and Cancilla, P.A.: An appraisal of histochemical fiber types in Duchenne muscular dystrophy, Neurology **22**:1243, 1972.
13. Bank, W.J., et al.: Disorder of muscle lipid metabolism and myoglobinuria: absence of carnitine palmityl transferase, N. Engl. J. Med. **292**:443, 1973.
14. Barchi, R.L.: Physical probes of biological membranes in studies of the muscular dystrophies, Muscle Nerve **3**:82, 1980.
15. Barnes, B.E.: Dermatomyositis and malignancy: a review of the literature, Ann. Intern. Med. **84**:68, 1976.
16. Bender, A.N., Ringel, S.P., and Engel, W.K.: Immunoperoxidase localization of alpha bungarotoxin: a new approach to myasthenia gravis, Ann. N.Y. Acad. Sci. **274**:20, 1976.
17. Berlin, B.S., Simon, N.M., and Bovner, R.N.: Myoglobinuria precipitated by viral infection, J.A.M.A. **227**:1414, 1976.
18. Bethlem, J., et al.: Centronuclear myopathy with type I fiber atrophy and "myotubes," Arch. Neurol. **23**:70, 1970.
19. Bharucha, E.P., Pandya, S.S., and Dastur, D.K.: Arthrogryposis multiplex congenita. I. Clinical and electromyographic aspects, J. Neurol. Neurosurg. Psychiatry **35**:425, 1972.
20. Bohan, A., and Peter, J.P.: Polymyositis and dermatomyositis (in two parts), N. Engl. J. Med. **292**:344, 403, 1975.
21. Bohan, A., et al.: A computer-assisted analysis of 153 patients with polymyositis and dermatomyositis, Medicine **56**:255, 1977.
22. Bosch, E.P., and Munsat, T.L.: Metabolic myopathies, Med. Clin. North Am. **63**:759, 1979.
23. Bradley, W.G., Price, D.L., and Watanabe, C.K.: Familial centronuclear myopathy, J. Neurol. Neurosurg. Psychiatry **33**:687, 1970.
24. Bradley, W.G., et al.: Becker-type muscular dystrophy, Muscle Nerve **1**:111, 1978.
25. Brooke, M.H., and Engel, W.K.: The histographic analysis of human muscle biopsies with regard to fiber type. I. Adult male and female, Neurology **19**:221, 1969.
26. Brooke, M.H., and Engel, W.K.: The histographic analysis of human muscle biopsies with regard to fiber types. IV. Children's biopsies, Neurology **19**:591, 1969.
27. Brooke, M.H., and Kaiser, K.K.: Muscle fiber types: how many and what kind, Arch. Neurol. **23**:369, 1970.
28. Brooke, M.H., and Kaplan, H.: Muscle pathology in rheumatoid arthritis, polymyalgia rheumatica, and polymyositis: a histochemical study, Arch. Pathol. **94**:101, 1972.
29. Brooke, M.H., and Neville, H.E.: Reducing body myopathy, Neurology **22**:829, 1972.
30. Brownell, B., Oppenheimer, D.R., and Spalding, J.M.K: Neurogenic muscle atrophy in myasthenia gravis, J. Neurol. Neurosurg. Psychiatry **35**:311, 1972.
31. Bundey, S.: A genetic study of infantile and juvenile myasthenia gravis, J. Neurol. Neurosurg. Psychiatry **35**:41, 1972.
32. Campion, D.S., Arias, J.M., and Carter, N.W.: Rhabdomyolysis and myoglobinuria: association with hypokalemia of renal tubular acidosis, J.A.M.A. **220**:967, 1972.
33. Cancilla, P.A.: Techniques of muscle biopsy and staining methods with particular emphasis on commonly encountered artifacts. In Pearson, C.M., editor: The striated muscle, Baltimore, 1973, The Williams & Wilkins Co.
34. Chapoy, P.R., et al.: Systemic carnitine deficiency: a treatable inherited lipid-storage disease presenting as Reye's syndrome, N. Engl. J. Med. **303**:1389, 1980.
35. Chou, S.M., and Miike, T.: Ultrastructural abnormalities and perifascicular atrophy in childhood dermatomyositis, Arch. Pathol. Lab. Med. **106**:76, 1981.
36. Climie, A.R.W.: Muscle biopsy: technic and interpretation, Am. J. Clin. Pathol. **60**:753, 1973.
37. Coërs, C., and Telerman-Toppet, N.: Morphological and histochemical changes of motor units in myasthenia, Ann. N.Y. Acad. Sci. **274**:6, 1976.
38. Cohen, R.H., Conn, D.L., and Illstrup, D.M.: Clinical features, prognosis, and response to treatment in polyarteritis, Mayo Clin. Proc. **55**:146, 1980.
39. Cumming, W.J.K., et al.: Localized nodular myositis: a clinical and pathological variant of polymyositis, Q. J. Med. **56**:531, 1977.
40. Dastur, D.K., Razzak, Z.A., and Bharucha, E.P.: Arthrogryposis multiplex congenita. II. Muscle pathology and pathogenesis, J. Neurol. Neurosurg. Psychiatry **35**:435, 1972.
41. Datta, S.K., and Schwartz, R.S.: Infection (?) myasthenia (editorial), N. Engl. J. Med. **291**:1304, 1974.
42. Dawkins, R.L., and Mastaglia, F.L.: Cell-mediated cytotoxicity to muscle in polymyositis: effect of immunosuppression, N. Engl. J. Med. **288**:434, 1973.
43. Demos, M.A., Gitin, E.L., and Kagen, L.J.: Exercise myoglobinemia and acute exertional rhabdomyolysis, Arch. Intern. Med. **134**:699, 1974.
44. DiMauro, S., et al.: Adult-onset acid maltase deficiency: a postmortem study, Muscle Nerve **1**:27, 1978.
45. Dorman, J.D.: The histopathology of neurogenic muscular atrophy. In Pearson, C.M., editor: The striated muscle, Baltimore, 1973, The Williams & Wilkins Co.
46. Douglas, A.C., MacLeod, J.G., and Mathews, J.D.: Symptomatic sarcoidosis of skeletal muscle, J. Neurol. Neurosurg. Psychiatry **36**:1034, 1973.
47. Drachman, D.B.: Myasthenia gravis, N. Engl. J. Med. **298**:136, 186, 1978.
48. Duane, D.D., and Engel, A.G.: Emetine myopathy, Neurology **20**:733, 1970.
49. Elias, S.B., and Appel, S.H.: Current concepts of pathogenesis and treatment of myasthenia gravis, Med. Clin. North Am. **63**:745, 1979.
50. Emery, A.E.H., et al.: Antenatal diagnosis of Duchenne muscular dystrophy, Lancet **1**:847, 1979.
51. Engel, A.G.: Vacuolar myopathies: multiple etiologies and sequential structural studies. In Pearson, C.M., editor: The striated muscle, Baltimore, 1973, The Williams & Wilkins Co.
52. Engel, A.G., and Angelini, C.: Carnitine deficiency of human skeletal muscle with associated lipid storage myopathy: a new syndrome, Science **179**:899, 1973.
53. Engel, A.G., Angelini, C., and Gomez, M.R.: Fingerprint body myopathy: a newly recognized congenital muscle disease, Mayo Clin. Proc. **47**:377, 1972.
54. Engel, A.G., and Gomez, M.R.: Acid maltase levels in muscle in heterozygous acid maltase deficiency and in non-weak and neuromuscular disease controls, J. Neurol. Neurosurg. Psychiatry **33**:801, 1970.
55. Engel, A.G., Gomez, M.R., and Groover, R.V.: Multicore disease: a recently recognized congenital myopathy associated with multifocal degeneration of muscle fibers, Mayo Clin. Proc. **46**:666, 1971.
56. Engel, A.G., Lambert, E.H., and Howard, F.M.: Immune complexes (IgG and C3) at the motor end plate in myasthenia gravis, Mayo Clin. Proc. **52**:267, 1977.
57. Engel, A.G., and Santa, T.: Histometric analysis of the ultrastructure of the neuromuscular junction in myasthenia gravis and in the myasthenic syndrome, Ann. N.Y. Acad. Sci. **183**:46, 1971.
58. Engel, A.G., et al.: The motor end plate in myasthenia gravis and in experimental autoimmune myasthenia gravis: a quantitative ultrastructural study, Ann. N.Y. Acad. Sci. **274**:60, 1976.
59. Engel, A.G., et al.: Ultrastructural clues in Duchenne dystrophy: pathogenesis of human muscular dystrophies, Amsterdam, 1977, Excerpta Medica.

60. Engel, A.G., et al.: The ultrastructural localization of the acetylcholine receptor, immunoglobulin G and the third and ninth complement components at the motor end plate and implications for the pathogenesis of myasthenia gravis. In Aguayo, A.J., et al., editors: Proceedings of the Fourth International Congress of Neuromuscular Diseases, Amsterdam, 1979, Excerpta Medica.
61. Engel, W.K.: Muscle biopsies in neuromuscular disease, Pediatr. Clin. North Am. **14**:963, 1967.
62. Engel, W.K.: Selective and non-selective susceptibility of muscle fiber types: a new approach to human neuromuscular diseases, Arch. Neurol. **22**:97, 1970.
63. Fambrough, D.M., Drachman, D.B., and Satyamurti, S.: Neuromuscular junction in myasthenia gravis: decreased acetylcholine receptors, Science **182**:293, 1973.
64. Faris, A.A., and Reyes, M.G.: Reappraisal of alcoholic myopathy, J. Neurol. Neurosurg. Psychiatry **34**:86, 1971.
65. Fishbein, W.N., Griffin, J.L., and Armbrustmacher, V.W.: Stain for skeletal muscle adenylate deaminase: an effective tetrazolium stain for frozen biopsy specimens, Arch. Pathol. Lab. Med. **104**:462, 1980.
66. Fisher, E.R., and Danowski, T.S.: Mitochondrial myopathy, Am. J. Clin. Pathol. **51**:619, 1969.
67. Frame, B., et al.: Polyostotic fibrous dysplasia and myositis ossificans progressiva, Am. J. Dis. Child. **124**:120, 1972.
68. Furukawa, T., and Peter, J.B.: The muscular dystrophies and related disorders. I. The muscular dystrophies, J.A.M.A. **239**:1537, 1978.
69. Furukawa, T., and Peter, J.B.: The muscular dystrophies and related disorders. II. Diseases simulating muscular dystrophies, J.A.M.A. **239**:1654, 1978.
70. Geller, S.A.: Extreme exertion rhabdomyolysis: a histopathologic study of 31 cases, Hum. Pathol. **4**:241, 1973.
71. Gonatas, N.K., et al.: Central "core" disease of skeletal muscle: ultrastructural and cytochemical investigations in two cases, Am. J. Pathol. **47**:503, 1965.
72. Gordon, E.E., Januszko, D.M., and Kaufman, L.: A critical survey of stiff-man syndrome, Am. J. Med. **42**:582, 1967.
73. Grob, D., editor: Myasthenia gravis (symposium), Ann. N.Y. Acad. Sci. **274**:1, 1976.
74. Harper, P.S.: Myotonic dystrophy, Philadelphia, 1979, W.B. Saunders Co.
75. Howell, R.R., and Williams, J.C.: The glycogen storage diseases. In Stanbury, J.B., et al., editors: The metabolic basis of inherited disease, ed. 5, New York, 1983, McGraw-Hill Book Co.
76. Itabashi, H.H., and Kokmen, E.: Chloroquine neuromyopathy: a reversible granulovacuolar myopathy, Arch. Pathol. **93**:209, 1972.
77. Jennekens, F.G.I., Tomlinson, B.E., and Walton, J.N.: The sizes of the two main histochemical fibre types in five limb muscles in man: an autopsy study, J. Neurol. Sci. **13**:281, 1971.
78. Jennekens, F.G.I., Tomlinson, B.E., and Walton, J.N.: Data on the distribution of fibre types in five human limb muscles: an autopsy study, J. Neurol. Sci. **14**:245, 1971.
79. Kahn, L.B., and Meyer, J.S.: Acute myopathy in chronic alcoholism: a study of 22 autopsy cases with ultrastructural observations, Am. J. Clin. Pathol. **53**:516, 1970.
80. Karpati, G.: A review of the morphologic features and consequences of muscle cell necrosis in Duchenne disease: clues to the pathogenesis. In den Hartog Jager, W.A., et al., editors: Neurology, Amsterdam, 1978, Excerpta Medica.
81. Klinkerfuss, G.H., and Haugh, M.J.: Disuse atrophy of muscle, Arch. Neurol. **22**:309, 1970.
82. Knochel, J.P.: Exertional rhabdomyolysis, N. Engl. J. Med. **287**:927, 1972.
83. Kovarsky, J., Schochet, S.S., and McCormick, W.F.: The significance of target fibers: a clinicopathologic review of 100 patients with neurogenic atrophy, Am. J. Clin. Pathol. **59**:790, 1973.
84. Layzer, R.B., and Rowland, L.P.: Cramps, N. Engl. J. Med. **285**:31, 1971.
85. Lefvert, A.K., et al.: Determination of acetylcholine receptor antibody in myasthenia gravis: clinical usefulness and pathogenetic implications, J. Neurol. Neurosurg. Psychiatry **41**:394, 1978.
86. Levine, G.D.: Pathology of the thymus in myasthenia gravis: current concepts. In Dau, P.C., editor: Plasmapheresis and the immunobiology of myasthenia gravis, Boston, 1979, Houghton-Mifflin Co.
87. Lewis, G.M., Spencer-Peet, J., and Stewart, K.M.: Infantile hypoglycemia due to inherited deficiency of glycogen synthetase in liver, Arch. Dis. Child. **38**:40, 1963.
88. Lindstrom, J., and Dau, P.: Biology of myasthenia gravis, Annu. Rev. Pharmacol. Toxicol. **20**:337, 1980.
89. Lindstrom, J.M., and Lambert, E.H.: Content of acetylcholine receptor and antibodies bound to receptor in myasthenia gravis, experimental autoimmune myasthenia gravis, and Eaton-Lambert syndrome, Neurology **28**:130, 1978.
90. Lindstrom, J.M., et al.: Antibody to acetylcholine receptor in myasthenia gravis: prevalence, clinical correlates, and diagnostic value, Neurology **26**:1054, 1976.
91. MacDonald, R.D., and Engel, A.G.: Experimental chloroquine myopathy, J. Neuropathol. Exp. Neurol. **29**:479, 1970.
92. Mastaglia, F.L., and Walton, J.N.: Coxsackie virus–like particles in skeletal muscle from a case of polymyositis, J. Neurol. Sci. **11**:593, 1970.
93. Matheson, D.W., and Howland, J.L.: Erythrocyte deformation in human muscular dystrophy, Science **184**:165, 1973.
94. McArdle, B.: Myopathy due to a defect in muscle glycogen breakdown, Clin. Sci. **10**:13, 1951.
95. Mendell, J.R., and Engel, W.K.: Fine structure of type II muscle fiber atrophy, Neurology **21**:358, 1971.
96. Mokri, B., and Engel, A.G.: Duchenne dystrophy: electron microscopic findings pointing to a basic or early abnormality in the plasma membrane of the muscle fiber, Neurology **25**:1111, 1975.
97. Munsat, T.L., Thompson, L.R., and Coleman, R.F.: Centronuclear (myotubular) myopathy, Arch. Neurol. **20**:120, 1969.
98. Munsat, T.L., et al.: Serum enzyme alterations in neuromuscular disorders, J.A.M.A. **226**:1536, 1973.
99. Neustein, H.B.: Nemaline myopathy, Arch. Pathol. **96**:192, 1973.
100. Papatestas, A.E., et al.: Thymectomy in myasthenia gravis: pathologic, clinical, and electrophysiologic correlations, Ann. N.Y. Acad. Sci. **274**:555, 1976.
101. Patrick, J.J., and Lindstrom, J.: Autoimmune response to acetylcholine receptor, Science **180**:871, 1973.
102. Pearson, C.M.: The pathologic features of the periodic paralyses. In Pearson, C.M., editor: The striated muscle, Baltimore, 1973, The Williams & Wilkins Co.
103. Pearson, C.M.: Muscular involvement in polyarteritis. In Walton, J.N., editor: Disorders of voluntary muscle, ed. 2, London, 1969, J. & A. Churchill.
104. Pearson, C.M., and Bohan, A.: The spectrum of polymyositis and dermatomyositis, Med. Clin. North Am. **61**:439, 1977.
105. Percy, M.E., et al.: Serum creatinine kinase and pyruvate kinase in Duchenne muscular dystrophy carrier detection, Muscle Nerve **2**:329, 1979.
106. Perkoff, G.T., Hardy, P., and Velez-Garcia, E.: Reversible acute muscular syndrome in chronic alcoholism, N. Engl. J. Med. **274**:1277, 1966.
107. Perry, T.B., and Frazer, F.C.: Variability of serum creatinine phosphokinase activity in normal women and carriers of the gene for Duchenne muscular dystrophy, Neurology **23**:1316, 1973.
108. Pickard, N.A., et al.: Systemic membrane defect in the proximal muscular dystrophies, N. Engl. J. Med. **299**:841, 1978.
109. Pleasure, D.E., Walsh, G.O., and Engel, W.K.: Atrophy of skeletal muscle in patients with Cushing's syndrome, Arch. Neurol. **22**:118, 1970.
110. Plishker, G.A., and Appel, S.H.: Red blood cell alterations in muscular dystrophy: the role of lipids, Muscle Nerve **3**:70, 1980.
111. Price, H.M.: Ultrastructural pathologic characteristics of the skeletal muscle fiber: an introductory survey. In Pearson, C.M., editor: The striated muscle, Baltimore, 1973, The Williams & Wilkins Co.
112. Reznik, M.: Current concepts of skeletal muscle regeneration. In Pearson, C.M., editor: The striated muscle, Baltimore, 1973, The Williams & Wilkins Co.

113. Rimmer, J.J.: Myoid cells and myasthenia gravis: a phylogenetic overview, Dev. Comp. Immunol. **4**:385, 1980.
114. Rosen, Y., et al.: Sarcoidosis from the pathologist's vantage point. In Sommers, S.C., and Rosen, P.P., editors: Pathology annual (part 1), New York, 1979, Appleton-Century-Crofts.
115. Roses, A.D., and Appel, S.H.: Muscular dystrophies, Lancet **2**:1400, 1974.
116. Rowland, L.P.: Pathogenesis of muscular dystrophies, Arch. Neurol. **33**:315, 1976.
117. Rowland, L.P.: Biochemistry of muscle membranes in Duchenne muscular dystrophy, Muscle Nerve **3**:3, 1980.
118. Rowland, L.P., and Penn, A.S.: Myoglobinuria, Med. Clin. North Am. **56**:1233, 1972.
119. Russell, R.G.G., et al.: Treatment of myositis ossificans progressiva with a diphosphonate, Lancet **1**:10, 1972.
120. Santa, T., Engel, A.C., and Lambert, E.H.: Histometric study of neuromuscular junction ultrastructure, Neurology **22**:71, 1972.
121. Schiff, H.B., MacSearraigh, E.T., and Kallmeyer, J.C.: Myoglobinuria, rhabdomyolysis, and marathon running, Q. J. Med. **188**:463, 1978.
122. Schotland, D.L., Bonilla, E., and Wakayama, Y.: Pathogenesis of muscle cell damage in the dystrophies: morphologic aspects including freeze fracture studies. In Aguayo, A.J., and Karpati, G. editors: Current topics in nerve and muscle research, Amsterdam, 1979, Excerpta Medica.
123. Silverstein, A., and Siltzbach, L.E.: Muscle involvement in sarcoidosis: asymptomatic, myositis, and myopathy, Arch. Neurol. **21**:235, 1969.
124. Simpson, J.A.: Myasthenia gravis: a personal view of pathogenesis and mechanism, Muscle Nerve **1**:45, 151, 1978.
125. Tang, T.T., et al.: Chronic myopathy associated with coxsackie virus type A9, N. Engl. J. Med. **292**:608, 1975.
126. Vincent, A.: Immunology of acetylcholine receptors in relation to myasthenia gravis, Physiol. Rev. **60**:756, 1980.
127. Walton, J.N.: Polymyositis and related disorders. In den Hartog Jager, W.A., et al., editors: Neurology, Amsterdam, 1978, Excerpta Medica.
128. Walton, J.N., and Gardner-Medwin, D.: Progressive muscular dystrophy and the myotonic disorders. In Walton, J.N., editor: Disorders of voluntary muscle, ed. 4, New York, 1981, Churchill Livingstone.

CHAPTER 44 Nervous System

JACOB L. CHASON

CENTRAL NERVOUS SYSTEM

The diseased nervous system offers an exceptional opportunity for the correlation of structure with function. Although the pathologic processes that affect the nervous system differ little from those occurring elsewhere in the body, the functional changes that result have both greater variability and greater uniformity. The variability of the effects on neurologic function is related to the anatomic localization of the disease. The uniformity of neurologic response, on the other hand, depends on several factors, among which are the following:

1. Fixed size of space enclosing the central nervous system (after fusion of the sutures of the skull)
2. Limited mobility of the nervous system within the space
3. Immobility of the dura and dural folds
4. Uniformity of structural change and progression of most lesions, that is, "the biologic behavior of the lesion" (Essential to the correlation of structure and function is an understanding of the reactions of the components of the nervous system to injury.)

Cell structure, function, and reaction to injury

Neuron

The nerve cell consists of a nucleus and a cell body, the perikaryon, with one or more processes known as dendrites and a single larger process, an axon. The perikaryon of the cell ranges in diameter from 5 μm in internal granular cells of the cerebellum to 80 μm or more in the Betz cells of the motor cortex.

The larger cells have a single, large, round to oval, usually vesicular nucleus with a well-defined nuclear membrane and a large nucleolus. With the exception of some cells of the hypothalamus, brainstem, and Clarke's column of the spinal cord, the nucleus is in a central portion in the perikaryon. The cytoplasm, except at the base of the axon, contains basophilic, granular to block-like material called Nissl substance. This material, as identified by electron microscopy, represents the ribosomes and the rough endoplasmic reticulum, which are the sites of protein metabolism. Nissl substance has the staining characteristics of the nucleolus, where it is believed to be formed and from which it spreads throughout the cytoplasm, appearing initially as a nuclear cap. In most large cells the Nissl substance is relatively evenly divided throughout the cytoplasm. In the cells normally having an eccentric nucleus, it is characteristic for the Nissl substance to be concentrated at the peripheral margins of the cell cytoplasm.

Many of the larger cells contain a brown, granular, intracytoplasmic lipochrome or lipofuscin pigment that increases with age.[1,6] This pigment has the same staining characteristics and significance as the lipofuscin in parenchymal cells elsewhere. A neuromelanin pigment, morphologically similar to that of melanin, is normally present in the cytoplasm of the perikaryon of the cells of the substantia nigra, the locus ceruleus, and some cells of the motor nuclei along the floor of the fourth ventricle and in melanophores in the posterior lobe of the pituitary gland. This pigment first appears in the cells of the locus ceruleus, microscopically visible at about the eighth intrauterine month and grossly visible by the eighth postnatal month. In the substantia nigra the pigment appears microscopically visible at approximately 1½ years of age and grossly visible at 3 years of age. Adult pigment levels are reached by the end of adolescence.

Dendrites and axons of variable lengths are cytoplasmic extensions of the neurons. The longest, the axons of the Betz cells, extend for almost 1 m. Coursing from a dendrite to the axon through the perikaryon are microtubules and neurofilaments (both types individually visible only with electron microscopy). It is believed that these structures help maintain the shape of the cell and are the pathways for the orderly transfer of materials from one part of the cell to the other. Aggregates of the neurofilaments or neurotubules characteristic of certain disease states can be seen more easily with special silver stains.

Other components of the nerve cells generally cannot be adequately demonstrated or studied either individually or in groups by light microscopy. Their presence and actual or potential activities sometimes can be demonstrated from the enzyme content. The acid phosphatase reaction is a marker for, and represents one of, the enzymatic actions of the lysosomes. Some of the oxidative enzyme reactions are used as markers for mitochondria and to demonstrate the type and relative amounts of the enzymes.

The specialized sites, or synapses, being forms of the contact of the nerve cells, require electron microscopy for study. The presynaptic terminally expanded axon contains mitochondria and vesicles with acetycholine, norepinephrine, or other transmitter substance. Release of the chemical at the synapse results in the transmission of the impulse to the receptor, usually the dendrite, or to the end button (synaptic knob, end foot, terminal bouton), cell body, or even axon, of the succeeding cell.

The recognition and separation of antemortem and postmortem changes in nerve cells are essential. Because minor degrees of structural variation within the cells may be associated with abnormalities of function, constant use of control sections is necessary for separation of the normal appearance from fixation artifacts, structural variations caused by disease, and autolytic change.

Shrinkage and increased staining of the entire cell with tortuosity of the cell processes constitute one of the most common of nerve cell changes (chronic neuronal disease). Although it has been described as an aging process in some cells and is a form of reaction to a variety of acute and chronic diseases, it is also commonly found in the second and third cortical layers, where it is attributable to the effects of fixation. Low-grade chronic injury to nerve cells is believed to result in an abnormal increase in the intracytoplasmic lipofuscin (lipochrome) pigment. This is known as pigmentary atrophy and more recently has been associated with the disease lipofuscinosis. The abnormal increase in this pigment, which is sudanophilic and sometimes acid fast, is believed to interfere with the normal cellular metabolic activity, perhaps by causing coating of the cell organelles. Cloudy swelling or, as it is known in the central nervous system, acute nerve cell change is characterized by cellular swelling and staining pallor of the perikaryon with loss of Nissl substance. This condition is considered to be reversible up to the point at which the cell processes are fragmented and separated from the cell body. It is a nonspecific response to a variety of injurious agents and is a well-known postmortem change. Ischemic change in the cell results from hypoxia, anoxia, and hypoglycemia or occurs after the ingestion of poisons that block the utilization of oxygen or glucose. With ischemia, there is early pronounced cytoplasmic eosinophilia accompanying the rapid destruction of the Nissl substance. The cell soon begins to swell, the cytoplasm becomes finely granular, and the nucleus becomes pyknotic. Shortly thereafter the eosinophilia begins to fade, the perikaryon shrinks, and the nucleus undergoes karyorrhexis with total cell disintegration. Central chromatolysis (retrograde or axonal degeneration) occurs after injury to the cell axon (only when near the perikaryon). In the affected cell the nucleus is displaced to one side of the swollen and rounded perikaryon, and the Nissl substance is lost first about the nucleus and later toward the periphery. With recovery the nucleolus enlarges, the Nissl substance reappears initially as a nuclear cap, later filling the perikaryon and dendrites, and the nucleus gradually resumes its normally central position. Complete structural recovery may take several months. By light microscopy this entire series of changes can be adequately studied only with the Nissl stain. Because cells with eccentrically placed nuclei and peripheral Nissl substance are normally present in certain portions of the central nervous system, adequate control must be used. Degeneration with swelling and fragmentation of the axon distal to the site of injury (wallerian degeneration) resembles that of the peripheral nervous system (p. 1931). The covering myelin formed by the oligodendrogliocytes simultaneously degenerates. Mononuclear inflammatory cells, attracted to the area, phagocytose the axonal fragments and the altered myelin, converting the myelin to neutral fats. The portion of the axon attached to the perikaryon may swell and have one or more fine silver-positive sprigs extending from it, but effective regeneration of the axon as in the peripheral nervous system does not occur. Since oligodendroglial cells may be the source of myelin for more than one axon, they degenerate only with loss of significant numbers of axons. Wallerian degeneration is grossly recognizable only after several months and only when a large and relatively compact tract is affected. The affected tract may gradually become whiter and more sharply demarcated from the surrounding tissue, especially when the degeneration is the result of a rapid and massive destruction of the axons. If the cause results in gradual axonal destruction, the affected tract may barely be discerned and then only by a decrease in its cross-sectional size. Other specific nerve cell changes are described in discussions of the diseases with which they are associated.

One should recognize that an oligodendroglial cell can be destroyed without structural damage to the surrounded axon. Conversely, destruction of the axon, either directly or indirectly (because of injury to the nerve cell), always results in destruction of the covering myelin sheath and sometimes of the oligodendrocyte. With the hematoxylin and eosin stain, one of the earliest reliable indications of myelin damage is the presence of myelin- or lipid-containing macrophages, first within the area of damage and later around adjacent blood vessels. Occasionally, one is able to recognize swelling of the axon and surrounding myelin by the presence of 20 to 25 μm, circular or cylindrical, eosinophilic masses in the white matter of the brain or spinal cord. The darker core of these eosinophilic structures indicates the swollen axon, and the lighter outer zone represents the altered myelin. Occurring simultaneously, but difficult to recognize, are shrinkage and further hyperchromatism of the oligodendroglial nucleus. These changes are more easily and adequately recognized with special stains for myelin and axons that demonstrate irregular swelling, pallor, and fragmentation of both structures well before the routine stains appear abnormal. Although slight staining pallor of the area may be recognizable with the routine stains after the loss or removal of myelin, the state is more easily appreciated with any of the variety of stains for myelin. The interfascicular oligodendrocytes of the white matter cover a single segment of one or more axons. The junction between the two cell membranes covering an axon is known as a node of Ranvier. With brain edema or swelling, the nonstaining halo of the interfascicular oligodendrocyte may become filled with a pink mucoid material (mucinous degeneration). The nonstaining halo seen around almost all of the oligodendroglial nuclei may increase in size as a part of the postmortem autolytic change. Oligodendrocytes also are found in the gray matter of the central nervous system, where they form satellite cells about the larger nerve cells. The satellite type of oligodendroglial cell has been considered by some to act both as a protector of the perikaryon and as a part of the route for the transport of nutrients to the cells. With the routine stains and at the usual 6 to 7 μm thickness of the sectioned tissue, one or occasionally two satellite cells may be found around one nerve cell body.

Neuroglia: neuroectodermally derived supporting cells of central nervous system

The astrocytes are the principal supporting cells of the central nervous system. Astrocytes supply structural support to the central nervous system, their foot processes form an important part of the blood-brain barrier, and they may be the route for transport of nutrients to nerve cells from blood vessels and for the reverse transport of metabolites. Astrocytic processes surround and isolate synapses. Finally, much like fibroblasts, they function in the reparative response to injury. With the routine hematoxylin and eosin stain, the only component of a normal astrocyte that ordinarily can be seen is the nucleus. It is 8 to 10 μm in diameter, round to oval, and vesicular with finely granular chromatin and has a definite nuclear membrane of uniform thickness. A nucleolus usually is not visible with light microscopy.

Astrocytes of two basic structural forms differing in their processes have been described. The more common fibrillar astrocyte located predominantly in the white matter and on the cortical surface has long, thin, and usually nonbranching fibrillary processes, of which one extends to the wall of a blood vessel and another may extend to the pial membrane. Protoplasmic astrocytes present in the gray matter have shorter, wider, and branching processes. Some astrocytes with both types of processes, as well as the ability to convert from one to the other, have been described. The structural distinction does not appear to indicate an essential functional or biologic difference. The reactive astrocyte, whatever the source type, may assume a fibrillar appearance. The Fañanás cell of the cerebellar cortex has some similarity to the protoplasmic astrocyte, whereas the Bergmann cell of the internal granular layer of the cerebellum has greater resemblance to the fibrous form.

The response of the astrocyte to injury can be recognized in a variety of ways. The presence of a slightly eosinophilic halo around the nucleus is one form of early reactive change visible with the hematoxylin and eosin stain. It is, however, also characteristic of many normal astrocytes in newborn infants and young children. When there is an abundant amount of eosinophilic cytoplasm, the astrocyte is of the gemistocytic type. This structural change can be seen within hours of injury. It is associated with the rapid formation of mitochondria and their enzymes. Another form of reactive change is indicated by the presence of nuclear pairs and sometimes tetrads. This, of course, is interpreted as representing cell multiplication supposedly by amitosis, because a reactive astrocyte in mitosis is seen very rarely. The increase in astrocytes is known as astrocytosis. In astrocytic gliosis, another type of response to injury, there is an increase in the fibrillar processes of the astrocytes. When the gliotic pattern follows the preexisting normal structure, it is called isomorphic gliosis; in anisomorphic gliosis the proliferation of processes has a haphazard arrangement. These are best seen with special stains, although they usually can be recognized with the routine stains. In chronic toxic states, either endogenous, as in uremia, liver disease with jaundice, and Wilson's disease, or exogenous, with a variety of toxins, some astrocytic nuclei may enlarge as a result of swelling and become more vesicular. The nucleus maintains a definite nuclear membrane with several infoldings, and one or more nucleoli may become evident. These are the Alzheimer's type II cells. In Wilson's disease, also known as hepatolenticular or hepatocerebral degeneration, transitions from type II cells to Alzheimer type I cells have been described. The type I cell has a large, darkly basophilic nucleus with a single darker nucleolus and a lighter basophilic, sometimes granular cytoplasm. Processes are not found extending from the bodies of these cells. Among the poorly understood changes occurring in astrocytes are the corpora amylacea. These are slightly eosinophilic to basophilic, sometimes concentrically laminated, periodic acid–Schiff–positive, 10 to 15 μm, spherical bodies. They are present in astrocytic processes in both the gray and white matter of the central nervous system; their numbers are larger in the aged and when there has been preexisting disease.

Myelin is a complex proteolipid formed by the winding of double layers of the cell membrane of the oligodendrocytes about the axons of most nerve cells of the central nervous system. Each layer (seen only by electron microscopy) is composed of double plasma membranes—the inner membrane surfaces have come together, displacing the cytoplasmic contents toward the nucleus of the cell. The sandwich of double plasma membrane, by differential growth of these approximated cell membranes, is believed to result in the spiral coating about the axon. The oligodendrocyte nucleus and cytoplasm are gradually displaced ahead of their newly formed plasma membrane in its spiral about the axon. Only the 5 to 7 μm, round, hyperchromatic nucleus of the oligodendrocytes stains with hematoxylin and eosin. The cytoplasm and plasma membrane remain as a clear, unstained halo around the nucleus.

The ependymal cells, cuboid to columnar, line the ventricles, the choroid plexuses, and the central canal of the spinal cord. Microscopic remnants of detached portions of ventricles, predominantly at the occipital and, to a lesser extent, the frontal poles of the lateral ventricles, and the ventriculus terminalis of the filum terminale also are lined. Some cells are ciliated, presumably to help propel the cerebrospinal fluid. The presence of blepharoplasts (best seen with the Mallory phosphotungstic acid–hematoxylin stain), which are small cytoplasmic hematoxylinophilic granules surrounded by a clear halo, can be of great help in the identification of cells of ependymal origin. These granules are believed to be remnants of the cilia whose portions outside the cell have disappeared. Reactions of the ependyma to injury are few. Ulceration of the ventricular lining may be seen during and after local inflammations and when there is pronounced dilatation of the ventricular system. The underlying reactive subependymal astrocytes may produce nodules of astrocytic fibers that occasionally surround trapped ependymal cells. This produces an irregularity of the ventricular surface and is known as granular ependymitis or ependymal granulations.

Microglia (mesodermal glia)

During the period of vascularization early in the development of the central nervous system, another type of "glial" cell makes its appearance. Of mesodermal origin, the microglial cells represent a portion of the reticuloendothelial system. These cells are scattered irregularly in both gray and white matter and among the astrocytes and oligodendrocytes. In the resting phase only the short, oval to kidney-shaped, hyperchromatic nuclei of these cells are stained with hematoxylin and eosin. Their scant cytoplasm and their relatively few processes (as compared with the astrocytes) are best demonstrated with the Hortega silver stain. Microglial cells react in response to injury with a great variety of structural change. Initially, they may proliferate locally about a small area of necrosis with the formation of a small group of cells, producing a so-called glial nodule. Their occurrence in a group phagocytosing a dead nerve cell is known as neuronophagia. Because of chemotactic influences, the cells may move toward the area damaged. In the process of movement their nuclei are enlarged and elongated. Because of the shape of the cells during such movement, they are known as rod cells. A microglial cell also may be transformed into a mononuclear (less often multinuclear) macrophage, during which its processes are lost and its cytoplasm becomes evident, in part because of the phagocytosed content of myelin, lipid, and so on. Such cells are then known as scavenger cells, gitter cells, compound granular corpuscles, lipophages, or myelinophages. Many of the cells so named, however, may have their origin from monocytes that reach the central nervous system through the bloodstream.

Vasculature

The blood vessels of the central nervous system, in addition to their usual functions, help through their contribution to the blood-brain barrier to maintain hemostasis and to aid in the return of interstitial fluid to the veins across the perivascular (Virchow-Robin) space. The blood-brain barrier is a physiologic phenomenon with which several structural features have been associated. Although the movement of water and lipid-soluble substances across this barrier is relatively unrestricted, the transfer of other substances such as glucose, amino acids, and inorganic ions is inhibited to varying degrees. It has been stated that the large size of some molecules and the nonutilization by the nervous system of many smaller molecules determine the degree of their exclusion by the blood-brain barrier. However, the mechanism for this barrier effect is unknown. It has been related to the properties of the capillary endothelium, the basement membrane, and the pericytes; to the astrocytic foot processes that almost completely surround the capillaries; and to the relative absence of an extracellular space (from early electron microscopic studies). The presence of tight junctions between the endothelial cells differentiates the central nervous system capillaries from those in many other parts of the body.

Except in the absence of endothelial pores and the presence of tight junctions, the structure of the capillaries of the central nervous system does not differ significantly from that of the capillaries in many parts of the body. Only approximately 85% of their circumference is covered by the astrocytic glial sheath. Moreover, the size of the extracellular space has not been settled.[99] Although no agreement has been reached between the estimates derived from chemical studies and those derived from electron microscopy, the space is now believed to be approximately 10% to 15% of the volume of the brain.

The perivascular or Virchow-Robin space lies between the adventitia and the pial membrane and is continuous with the subarachnoid space. Extending about the blood vessels only as far as the capillaries, it is believed to form a route for the return of subarachnoid fluids and cells to and through the subarachnoid space to the vascular system.

Developmental disorders

The nervous system begins as a longitudinal, middorsal, ectodermal thickening. Cellular proliferation with ventral grooving and dorsal fusion of the freed lateral margins results in the formation of the neural tube, which is separated from the adjacent neural crest and the overlying skin. Continued orderly development with cell proliferation, peripheral migration, growth, and maturation are paralleled by growth, closure, and fusion of surrounding bones.[9,128]

The long period of maturation of the central nervous system is an important factor in its involvement in approximately 10% to 20% of all developmental defects. The known or suspected teratogens that often act in conjunction with either monogenetic or polygenetic defects include the following:

1. Maternal infections (such as rubella)
2. Fetal infections
3. Fetal hypoxia
4. Irradiation
5. Nutritional deficiencies and excesses
6. Chemical agents
7. Mechanical forces

Each of these factors appears to be capable of producing its effect only at a particular time in the course of development of the embryo.[44,120] Since continued normal development depends on the preceding stage, the earlier the injury, the more serious the malformation.

Agenesis is the condition in which there is absence of the anlage of a structure. In anencephaly,[121] the most severe form of agenesis, most of the brain is absent and sometimes also the spinal cord (amyelia). There are usually associated failures of closure of the skull and vertebral arches (rachischisis). All of these changes appear to begin with early defective closure of the neural tube (dysrhaphism). When the calvaria remain intact, the skull is of normal size, and the brain is replaced by fluid (hydranencephaly), one should suspect paranatal injury rather than dysrhaphism and agenesis. Agenesis of specific portions of the brain, although uncommon, is well known. Many such defects are compatible with life and may be first recognized as incidental findings at postmortem examination. Among these are agenesis of the cerebellum and agenesis of all or only the caudal portion of the corpus callosum.[87,113,128] Absence of the cerebral pallium with failure of separation of the cerebral tissue (telencephalon impar) is accompanied by absence of the calvaria.

Holoprosencephaly is the result of varying degrees of failure of separation of the cerebral hemispheres, for example, alobar, semilobar, lobar. When accompanied by a single median eye (cyclopia) and by a supraorbital nasal trunk with arrhinencephaly, it is usually compatible with survival for only a few hours. Agenesis of a portion of the brain is usually bilateral and most often affects the parietal lobes. The underlying lateral ventricles at these sites are dilated and communicate with the subarachnoid space (porencephaly) (see p. 1878). Similar ventricular dilatation may be seen after occlusion of the arteries or veins supplying or draining these areas or after trauma or infection, all occurring early in embryonic development with failure of development of the affected portion of one or both cerebral hemispheres.

Errors of closure of the neural tube and fusion of the surrounding bony structures are common, particularly at the lumbosacral level of the spinal cord. When the defect is complete, the dorsal portion of the spinal cord is not formed and its lateral margins remain attached to the modified ectoderm (amyelocele). The most frequent developmental defect of the neural tube, however, is failure of complete closure of the vertebral arches (spina bifida). Herniation of only the meninges through this defect is known as a meningocele. When a portion of the cord also is included, the defect is called a meningomyelocele. A meningomyelocystocele includes the meninges, a portion of the cord, and a portion of the central canal. In spina bifida occulta the failure of fusion of the affected vertebral arches may result in dimpling of the overlying skin and separating fibrous tissue, but with no herniation of the cord or its coverings. Herniations of a portion of the brain and its covering during closure of the skull bones are far less frequent. These occur in the region of the glabella, at the occipital bone, and at the roof of the mouth. Like herniations of the spinal cord, they are known as meningocele, meningoencephalocele, and meningoencephalocystocele.

In the Arnold-Chiari malformation, there is caudal displacement of the medulla and vermis of the cerebellum below the level of the foramen magnum into the spinal canal. A notch frequently develops on the anterior surface of the cervical cord, where it is overridden by the

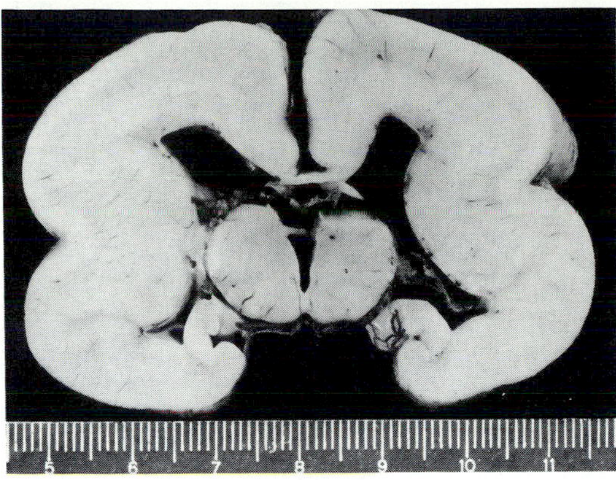

Fig. 44-1. Agyria (lissencephaly).

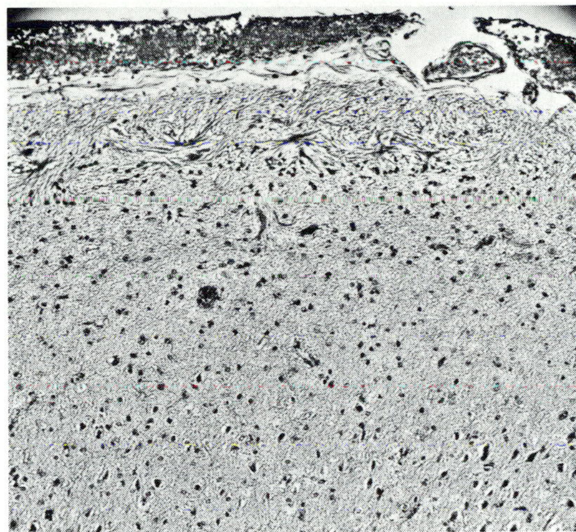

Fig. 44-2. Tuberous sclerosis with characteristic sheaflike astrocytic gliosis in first cortical layer. (Hematoxylin and eosin; 90×.)

displaced medulla. The malformation is associated with a small posterior fossa and flattening of the base of the skull (platybasia) and sometimes with internal hydrocephalus and a meningomyelocele. The association of internal hydrocephalus with the platybasia has suggested to some that the brain has been forced downward during development. Fixation of the spinal cord in the patients with a meningomyelocele, on the other hand, may have displaced the brainstem and spinal cord downward because of the greater growth of the vertebra as compared with the spinal cord. Both hypotheses have been refuted by evidence suggesting that the initial defect is failure of formation of the pontine flexure.

Defective cell migration and maturation result in faulty cell position (heterotopia) and abnormalities in the formation of the gyri. The absence of gyrus formation is known as lissencephaly (agyria) (Fig. 44-1).[31] It is often, but not always, associated with generalized hypoplasia of the brain (microcephaly) and with developmental hydrocephalus. Focal hypoplasias are uncommon. They usually involve the related nuclei of the pons, medulla, and cerebellum.

Conversely, an overly large brain, macrocephaly (megalocephaly), is due in part to hyperplasia and often in part to dysplastic development.

Tuberous sclerosis

Tuberous sclerosis is usually a heredofamilial, autosomally dominant disease that results in dysplastic development and heterotopia of the ectodermal cells of the central nervous system.[80] Often associated are a variety of developmental abnormalities of other organs of the body, including the skin—the adenoma sebaceum at the nasolabial folds and the subungual nodules, both of which are fibrovascular overgrowths, and shagreen skin *(peau de chagrin)* of the midlumbar skin of the back. Accompanying renal tumors, often bilateral, are either mixtures of blood vessels, fibrous tissue, fat, and smooth muscle (the angiomyolipofibromas) or tubular adenomas.[68] Nodular, gray-yellow, glycogen-filled myocardial tumors termed rhabdomyomas may be found in some patients who die early with the disease. Pulmonary fibrosis, cysts, and bronchial hamartomas also have been seen.

The brain is usually of normal size or small. Affected gyri are slightly to greatly enlarged, white, and hard, with poor demarcation between the cortex and the white matter. The first layer of the cortical tuber may have foci of thick astrocytic fibrillae in a characteristic sheaflike cluster (Fig. 44-2). The normal laminar arrangement of the cortical cells is considerably disturbed. In addition to the astrocytic gliosis, there are large globoid to spidery cells with both neuronal and astrocytic characteristics. Hard nodular areas, more easily felt than seen, may be found in the white matter and are composed of foci of astrocytic gliosis. Periventricular gray to white, hard, often mineralized tumors project into the lateral ventricles. These nodules are formed by partly mineralized clusters of large bizarre cells of astrocytic appearance (subependymal giant cell astrocytomas).[113] Retinal lesions, referred to as phakomas, are related tumors formed by the abnormally developed glial cells.

Aqueductal stenosis

Abnormal formation of the cerebral aqueduct in fetal life may be attributable either to an intrauterine inflammation with periaqueductal gliosis or to a disturbance in development. On rare occasions the aqueduct is developmentally small and may be double, the so-called forking of the aqueduct. The two channels are too small for adequate cerebrospinal fluid flow. Hydrocephalus resulting from any of the causes may be first manifest at

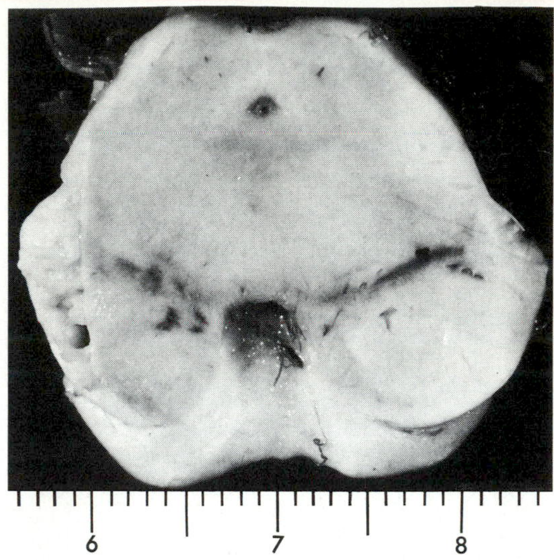

Fig. 44-3. Congenital aqueductal gliotic stenosis after intrauterine infection.

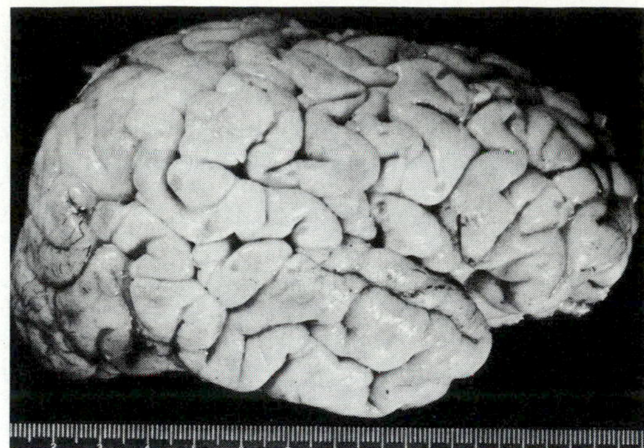

Fig. 44-4. Down's syndrome. Small superior temporal gyrus and blunted occipital lobe.

birth (congenital) or during infancy or early childhood, depending on the degree of stenosis. Accurate recognition of its cause (Fig. 44-3) requires a good history, multiple sections of the aqueduct taken at close intervals and at right angles to its path, and comparison with normal controls.

Down's syndrome[73]

At least two karyotypes of Down's syndrome have been reported. The more common form, characterized by an extra 21 chromosome, is the result of the failure of separation of one pair of these chromosomes in oogenesis and is more likely to occur in infants of older mothers. In the other type, unrelated to maternal age, the extra 21 chromosome is believed to have been translocated to the end of another large chromosome. Translocation Down's syndrome may arise de novo or be hereditary, particularly in the rare G21/G21. Of the remaining patients, one of the parents may be found to have the translocation, more commonly to chromosome 14, and only 45 chromosomes, or it may have arisen during gamete formation in normal parents.

A variety of structural abnormalities have been reported in the brains of these patients. The most characteristic is the blunting of the occipital portion of the brain and a small but nonspecific superior temporal gyrus (Fig. 44-4). The cerebellum may be small as well. No uniform microscopic changes have been described, although neuritic plaques and neurofibrillary tangles have been seen in those who live to or beyond the 30 years of age. Diagnosis, however, is based on the characteristic mongol facies with rounded head, prominent epicanthal folds, oblique palpebral fissures, dysplastic ears, high-arched palate, palm-print abnormalities, a palm with four finger lines, a curved fifth finger, a large space between the first and second toes, other nonspecific body changes, and occasional cardiac malformations.

Syringomyelia and syringobulbia[58]

Named for the characteristic irregular tubular cavity, syringomyelia is a disorder of the spinal cord ascribed to multiple causes. One form, sometimes associated with neurofibromatosis, is believed to be caused by a defect in closure of the alar plates of the spinal cord. On the other hand, the cavity or cavities may be the residua of a previous inflammation, infarct, or hemorrhage or a component of a glial neoplasm. Stenosis of the exits from the fourth ventricle that results in an increase in intraventricular pressure has been considered as another etiologic factor. Transmission of the increased pressure with dilatation of an open central canal of the spinal cord is known as hydromyelia. With continued enlargement there may be loss of some of the ependymal lining with replacement by astrocytes and their processes: hydrosyringomyelia. Syringomyelia follows when the entire wall is lined by astrocytes and their processes. A more recent suggestion as to cause includes an initial ring of adhesive arachnoiditis that directs the flow of cerebrospinal fluid at that level toward the central portion of the cord. Rupture of the fluid outside the Virchow-Robin space leads to a gradually enlarging cavity surrounded by a reactive astrocytosis and gliosis.

The cervical portion of the spinal cord is the most frequently affected and, when the lesions are multiple, usually contains the largest of the cavities. Each syrinx is filled with a watery to slightly xanthochromatic fluid. The lesion may begin anywhere within the cord; in the developmental form it is most often in the cervical cord, extending both longitudinally and laterally to involve the gray and white matter (Fig. 44-5). Its lining is formed by astrocytic processes (Fig. 44-6) except in areas in which there is residual ependyma of an included central canal. The cavity may extend for only a few segments or involve

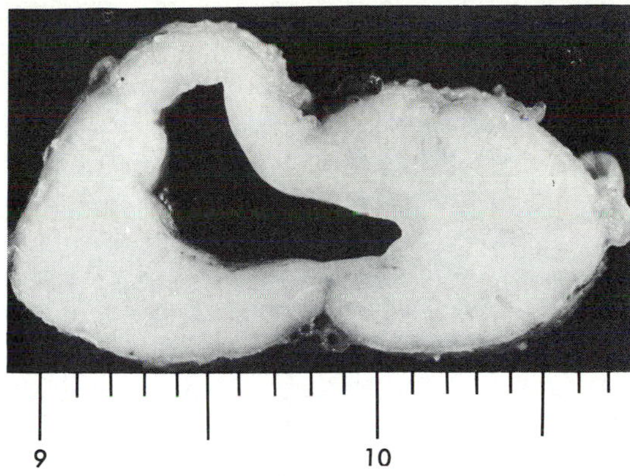

Fig. 44-5. Syringomyelia. Cervical portion of spinal cord.

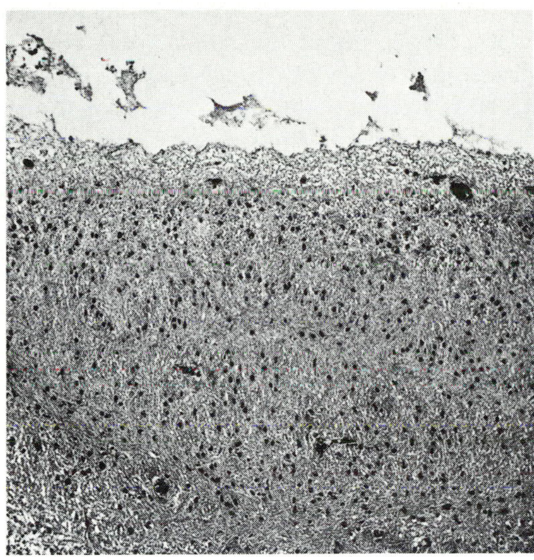

Fig. 44-6. Wall of syrinx with astrocytic proliferation. (Hematoxylin and eosin; 90×.)

the entire cord, or, as noted previously, there may be multiple cavities. The lateral extent of the cavity or cavities determines the site and degree of ascending and descending wallerian degeneration. Involvement of the medulla (syringobulbia) may occur separately or as an extension of a lesion in the cervical portion of the cord. In the medulla the cavity is a winglike, medial or dorsolateral slit. It may be unilateral or bilateral and roughly symmetric. Similar cavities have been described as occurring in the pons and even more rarely in the cerebral hemispheres, where they end in the head portion of either or both caudate nuclei.

Dilatation of the central canal (hydromyelia) is a frequent and asymptomatic finding seen at all levels of the spinal cord examined routinely at autopsy. Some consider it the mildest form of spinal dysrhaphism, that is, the mildest form of syringomyelia.

Hydrocephalus[111]

The descriptive term *hydrocephalus* is used to indicate an increased amount of cerebrospinal fluid in the ventricles, in the subarachnoid space about the brain, or in both. This is recognized from enlargement of these spaces rather than by measurement of the fluid. The condition is classified in several ways. When the increased fluid accumulation is limited to the dilated ventricular system, the hydrocephalus is called internal (Fig. 44-7). External hydrocephalus is the presence of excess fluid in the enlarged subarachnoid space over the brain. Separation of hydrocephalus into communicating and noncommunicating types is useful for the clinician. In the communicating type there is normal free flow of fluid between the ventricles and the subarachnoid space about the cauda equina. With obstruction or block of free flow between these two sites, the hydrocephalus is considered to be noncommunicating. Varying degrees, sites, and causes of flow impedance are causes for limitation of the value of this classification.

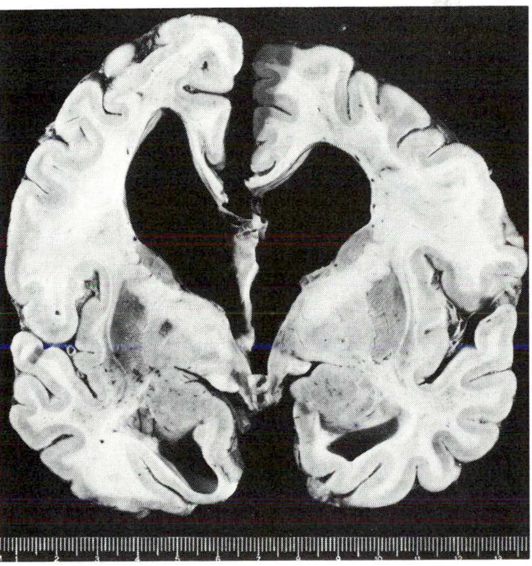

Fig. 44-7. Internal hydrocephalus of lateral and third ventricles caused by obstructive lesion in fourth ventricle (not illustrated).

The most useful classification is that described by Russell[111] and slightly modified here. To understand this classification, a limited knowledge of formation, flow, and removal of spinal fluid is essential. Cerebrospinal fluid is formed chiefly by the choroid plexuses of the lateral, third, and fourth ventricles. From the lateral ventricles, flow is directed into the third ventricle through the two interventricular foramina. The fluid then flows through the cerebral aqueduct into the fourth ventricle, from which it exits into the subarachnoid spaces through the two lateral recesses and the foramina of Luschka and through the middle foramen of Magendi. Most of the fluid is finally returned to the venous system through the arachnoid villi that lie in the several venous sinuses and to a lesser degree about the spinal rootlets. With this brief description as a background, hydrocephalus can be considered to have arisen from an imbalance or derangement of one or more of these factors.

Hydrocephalus resulting from the overproduction of cerebrospinal fluid is the least common. Proven instances of overproduction (that is, caused by hypertrophy or neoplasms of choroid plexuses) are medical curiosities. Obstruction of the great vein of Galen, previously considered a cause of fluid overproduction, has not been confirmed.

Decreased outflow (or absorption) of fluid through the arachnoidal lining cells or through narrowed or closed pores in the arachnoid villi offers another possible mechanism.[45] Direct and adequate examination of these pores is possible only by means of electron microscopy, and this has not been described. Moreover, there is some question whether such pores actually exist. The mechanism of decreased outflow, however, has been used, probably correctly, to explain the hydrocephalus seen with fibrosis covering the arachnoid granulations and with thrombosis of the superior sagittal sinus.

Obstruction to the flow of fluid is a common cause of internal hydrocephalus. The obstructing lesion may be developmental, inflammatory, mechanical, or neoplastic and may be almost anywhere in the flow tract. The pattern of ventricular enlargement frequently can be used as a guide to determine the site of the obstructing lesion. Ventricular dilatation is limited to that portion proximal to the obstruction (Fig. 44-7). Dilated ventricles with subependymal petechiae are diagnostic of an acute obstructive hydrocephalus (Fig. 44-8). The petechiae result from venous compression with continued subependymal arteriolar flow.

Two other mechanisms must also be considered in the production of hydrocephalus. Once the fontanels are closed and growth has ceased, the skull encloses an intracranial space of fixed size. Loss of brain tissue for any reason must therefore be accompanied by increase in fluid and enlargement of the subarachnoid or ventricular spaces. This is known as compensatory hydrocephalus (hydrocephalus ex vacuo). It is the most common form of hydrocephalus, although in most instances it is not clinically symptomatic. A less frequent cause of hydrocephalus and one that often is not considered is failure in development of all or a portion of the brain. Although the ventricles are small in such instances, they are relatively large when compared with the overall size of the brain. This is developmental hydrocephalus.

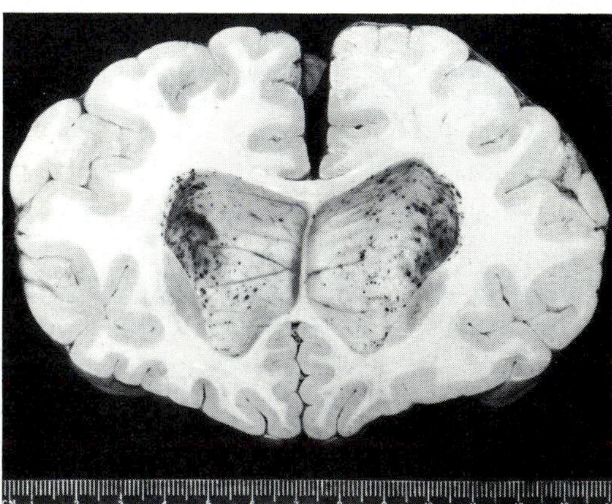

Fig. 44-8. Acute internal hydrocephalus with numerous subependymal petechiae caused by obstructive lesion in fourth ventricle (not illustrated).

Porencephaly is a related condition. The term originally was meant to designate an abnormal cavity that connected the ventricular and subarachnoid spaces through a defect in the cerebrum. With this definition the cause was attributable to the failure of development of a portion of the primitive ependymal lining in the line of the primary fissure. The defect was usually bilateral and symmetric. Much of this meaning has been lost, for most observers now use the term to describe any large intracerebral cavity, usually with an opening into an adjacent ventricle.

Vascular diseases

Hypoxic encephalopathy (anoxic encephalopathy)

Despite the many variables that could be expected to alter the pattern of damage to the central nervous system subjected to hypoxia, there is an unusual degree of uniformity of histologic change. The increased susceptibility of the central nervous system to oxygen deprivation is the result of a combination of factors, each of which is of critical importance. Almost all of the central nervous system function is subserved by energy derived from aerobic metabolism of carbohydrates. This 2% of the body utilizes 20% of the oxygen and 20% of the cardiac output in the resting state. Because of the lack of significant oxygen and carbohydrate reserves within the central nervous system, a constant resupply of both is required. The structural changes depend on the degree and duration of the hypoxia, on length of survival, and, when present, on a preceding period of a lesser degree of hypoxia. Antecedent asymptomatic or mild hypoxia depletes the affected cells of enzymes that promote individual cell destruction. Lindenberg[86] believes that a preceding mild hypoxia is therefore desirable in that structural and functional recovery are then more likely to occur. Gross structural changes generally are not striking with hypoxia except when associated with severe venous engorgement that produces duskiness of the entire central nervous system, sometimes with petechial hemorrhages. When the cause is ischemia, there is mild to pronounced pallor. The brain is slightly to greatly swollen with some blurring of the margins between the cortex and the underlying white matter; occasionally there are petechiae around the third ventricle and in the floor of the fourth ventricle.

Although the first microscopic changes may be seen after survival of only 4 hours, they usually are not discernible until after survival of at least 8 to 12 hours. With general hypoxia (as with cardiac failure, respiratory disease, and anemia, or resulting from thromboemboli), the most susceptible cells, including their processes, are those in Sommer's sector in the hippocampal portion of the temporal lobe, the Purkinje cells of the cerebellum, and the cells of the third, fourth, and fifth cortical layers of the cerebral hemispheres. The earliest microscopic changes consist of slight cell enlargement and cytoplasmic eosinophilia with loss of the Nissl substance. Affected cells occur singly or in clusters and may be separated by cells with a normal appearance. The hypoxic cells and adjoining blood vessels are surrounded by edematous zones that stain less eosinophilic than the normal.

Later the affected cells become irregularly shrunken and their nuclei eccentric, small, and hyperchromatic. Eventually the cells and their processes that are injured beyond recovery disappear. Petechiae that occur without other tissue damage disappear without remnants; with necrosis, the area becomes organized and recognizable because of the residual hemosiderophages.

Infarcts

A localized area of necrosis caused by circulatory insufficiency is known as an infarct. Large infarcts may be associated with atherosclerosis with or without thrombosis, with emboli in large arteries, with veno-occlusive disease, in prolonged hypoglycemia, and rarely with a dissecting hematoma that compresses the lumen of the affected artery.[8,18,35] Small infarcts occur with disease of small arteries and arterioles (usually related to hypertension) and sometimes because of emboli in these vessels. With adequate collateral channels, particularly through the circle of Willis and leptomeningeal vessels, gradual occlusion of even a large artery may not result in an infarct. Conversely, the gradual narrowing of a small artery can, in the absence of an adequate collateral, cause infarction. Infarcts are classified as pale (anemic) or red (hemorrhagic), depending on the amount of blood in the necrotic area (Fig. 44-9). They also are divided into those that are recent (usually under 3 weeks), old (3 to 6 weeks), and remote (over 6 weeks).

Anemic infarcts most frequently are associated with atherosclerosis with or without thrombosis. In the absence of a thrombus there is often a preceding episode of hypotension or hypoxia or both. These infarcts are more likely to occur in normotensive or hypotensive states and in the presence of disseminated vascular disease that impairs the limited collateral circulation. Initially an anemic infarct is dusky because of continued deoxygenation of the retained intravascular blood. Shortly afterward, the infarct begins to enlarge in volume because of the influx of fluid from adjacent functioning blood vessels and tissues. The increasing volume of the infarct within the fixed intracranial space compresses the contained vessels. By forcing the sludged intravascular blood away into the draining venous channels, the infarct becomes pale. There is a simultaneous and progressive decrease in size of the adjacent spaces (subarachnoid and ventricular). In some, the rapid increase in volume of a large infarct may produce brain displacement, with herniations and even resulting pressure hemorrhages in the brainstem. The initial microscopic changes are similar to those described under hypoxic encephalopathy but with more diffuse and severe involvement. The outermost cortical layer usually remains intact with a reactive astrocytosis and gliosis.

An infarct of the third and usually also the fourth and fifth layers of the cerebral cortex, regularly in the depth of a convolution, is known as a laminar (or pseudolaminar) infarct. When more severe, the infarct extends to involve the cortex toward the crest of the gyri and the second and deeper cortical layers and may even extend into the underlying white matter. As noted previously, the intact first cortical layer regularly is noted to have an astrocytosis and gliosis. The laminar infarct occurs more frequently in the so-called watershed zones of the parieto-occipital convexities but may be found in all parts of the cerebral cortex and in the cerebellum. This type of infarct frequently is found in a patient after a period of prolonged shock as may occur with gastrointestinal bleeding, hypoglycemia, myocardial infarction, temporary cardiac arrest, and so on.

In the following description of the natural history of infarcts, one should recognize that the time sequences are approximations. The rates and degrees of reaction are dependent on many variables existing among individuals

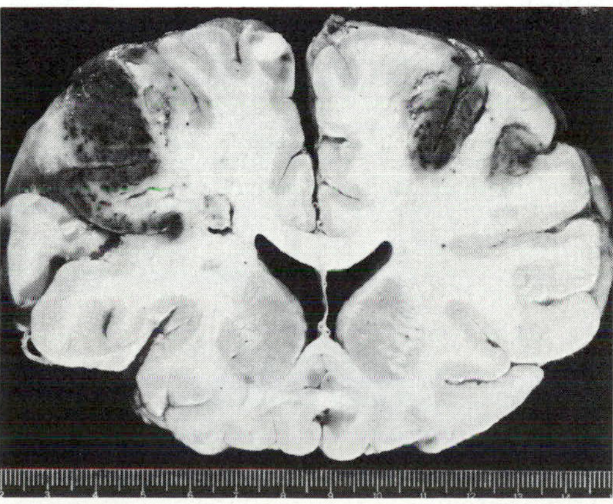

Fig. 44-9. Recent mixed hemorrhagic and anemic infarcts resulting from emboli in middle cerebral arteries.

and in the same patient with differing conditions. In addition, various portions of a single large lesion often become infarcted at different times.

In all anemic infarcts the cytoplasm of the nerve cell initially becomes eosinophilic and its nucleus shrunken and hyperchromatic. All the other components also become necrotic except for some of the blood vessels, whose endothelial cells often hypertrophy. With the influx of fluid, the infarcted tissue progressively becomes more pale staining (Fig. 44-10) except the intact first cortical layer, in which only a reactive astrocytosis occurs. The first reactive cells, usually between the eighteenth and twenty-fourth hour of the infarct, are neutrophils. These cells, usually in small numbers, are found in the walls of blood vessels within the infarct and the immediately adjacent necrotic tissue near the infarct periphery. They may reach the adjacent subarachnoid space. Activation of the surrounding microglial cells and the appearance of perivascular lymphocytes and monocytes at the edges of the infarct may be seen by the second day but most frequently are not found until the third. During the following 2 weeks, the infarct continues to enlarge and soften, with progressive liquefaction (Fig. 44-11). Beginning by the fourth day and increasing thereafter, it becomes filled with the mononuclear cells, many of which have become lipophages. The blood vessels within the infarct are gradually reopened by the flow of blood from the collateral channels. Reactive astrocytes in the brain immediately surrounding the infarct, first seen during the third day, become easily evident by the fifth day. The volume of the anemic infarct is greatest during the second week. Thereafter its gradual decrease in volume is associated with the decrease in lipophages and loss of fluid. At the end of the third week, its volume approximates that of the original tissue. Continued removal of the necrotic material and fluid gradually transforms the infarct by the sixth week into a pale spongelike cavity traversed by a network of small blood vessels, some of which are newly formed (Fig. 44-12). A few lipophages within the infarct and a narrow wall of reactive astrocytes remain for the life of the individual. The presence of an intact (but abnormal) first cortical layer aids in the differentiation of an infarct from a contusion or laceration (Fig. 44-11). The spaces adjacent to

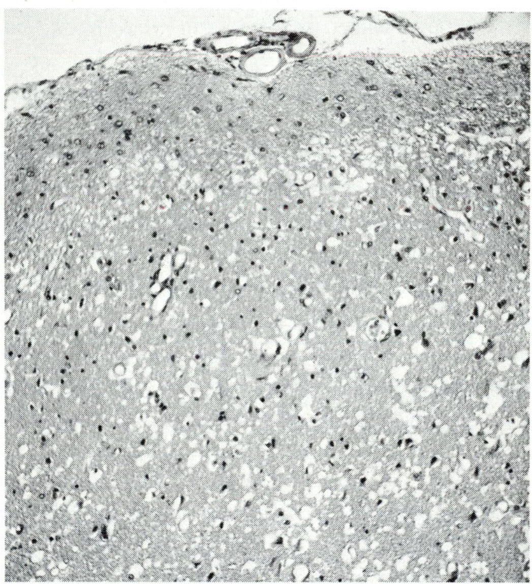

Fig. 44-10. Recent anemic infarct. There is intact outer cortical layer with reactive astrocytosis. Pallor, cellular pyknosis, and microcavitation result from edema in deeper cortical layers. (Hematoxylin and eosin; 90×.)

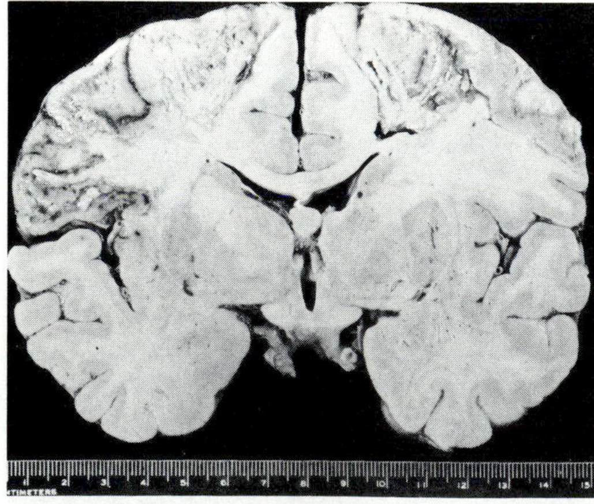

Fig. 44-11. Liquefaction of recent anemic infarcts with beginning gross cavitation (end of second week), resulting from emboli in branches of middle cerebral arteries.

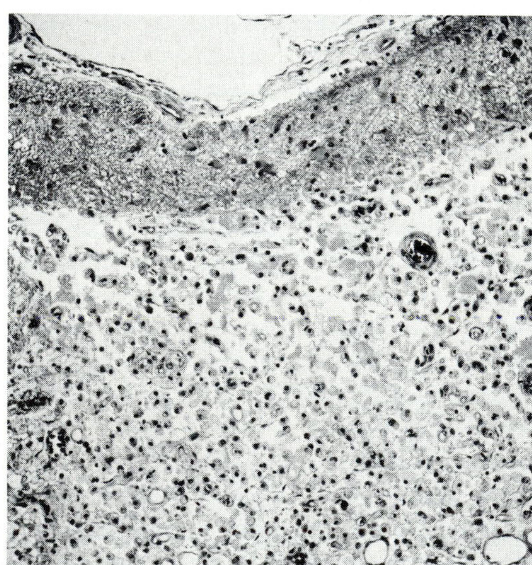

Fig. 44-12. Remote anemic infarct. There is intact outer cortical layer with reactive astrocytosis. Note scattered macrophages and newly formed capillaries in cavity. (Hematoxylin and eosin; 135×.)

the infarct, first narrowed and compressed, enlarge (compensatory hydrocephalus) as the infarct volume decreases.

Hemorrhagic infarcts are associated with hypertension, with emboli, and with venous occlusion and may occur in patients with a bleeding tendency. The duskiness of the early hemorrhagic infarct becomes dark red because of the inflow of blood into the necrotic tissue from reopening of the occluded vessel or from collateral channels, or because the initial lesion was the result of a venous occlusion. In comparison with the anemic infarct, the hemorrhagic infarct enlarges more rapidly and to a greater degree and retains its increased volume for a longer period. Hemosiderophages, found with difficulty before the third or fourth day, become progressively more prominent thereafter, and, along with lipophages, some remain locally for the life of the individual. Reactive astrocytes forming the infarct wall sometimes contain hemosiderin granules. The brown color of the remote lesion (after 6 weeks), attributable to hemosiderin and hematoidin, distinguishes it from an anemic infarct, and the bridging blood vessels separate it from a massive hemorrhage. Compensatory hydrocephalus, external or internal, may also be associated with the larger hemorrhagic infarcts.

Mixed anemic and hemorrhagic infarcts (Fig. 44-9) are not rare. The hemorrhagic component is always in the gray matter, whereas the anemic component can involve both white and gray matter.

Infarcts, anemic and hemorrhagic, from 1 mm to 1 cm in size (lacunar) are common in the putamina and thalami (Fig. 44-13) and to a lesser degree in the base of the pons and in the other central gray masses of the cerebral hemispheres in patients with a long history of hypertension.[66] Bilateral lesions are almost limited to patients with long-standing hypertension. Slightly larger infarcts in the central white matter of the cerebral hemispheres are equally characteristic of long-standing hypertension, especially when the infarcts are hemorrhagic or have more than the expected amount of connective tissue about the blood vessels within them (Fig. 44-14). Small, subcortical areas of necrosis usually have been considered as infarcts resulting from severe arteriolosclerosis in patients with hypertension. Recently, however, these have been described as the end stages of recurrent or severe local edema associated with hypertensive encephalopathy.[47] The associated clinical state is known as Binswanger's disease.[47]

Hemorrhage

Hemorrhage into the central nervous system may result from any of the diseases that destroy the integrity of the blood vessels or decrease the coagulability of the blood.[22,90,100] Petechial hemorrhages, especially those in the floor and walls of the third ventricle and floor of the fourth ventricle, are most often the result of hypoxia from respiratory failure in which the heart has continued to beat for a short time.

Hemorrhages may be the result of mechanical trauma to the head, fat embolism, chemical toxins such as the arsenical compounds, intrinsic disorders of the hemopoi-

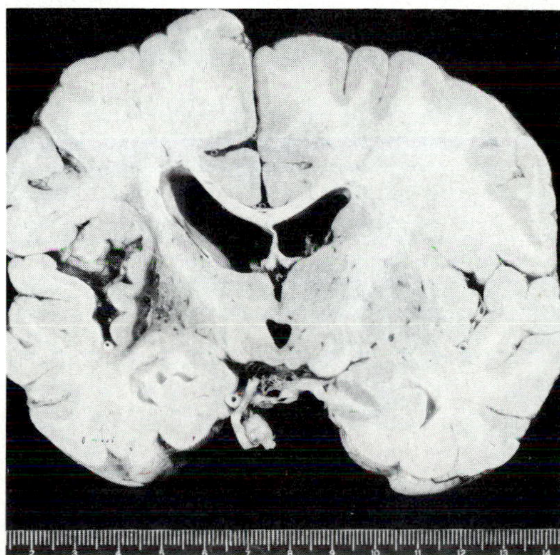

Fig. 44-13. Remote anemic and hemorrhagic infarcts in putamina and caudate nuclei. Patient had long-standing hypertension. There are compensatory internal hydrocephalus and severe segmental atherosclerosis.

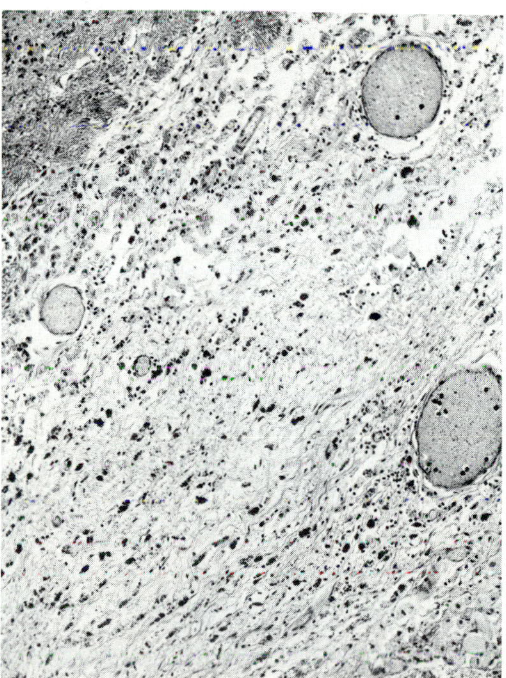

Fig. 44-14. Remote hemorrhagic infarct containing newly formed capillaries, hemosiderin-laden macrophages, and fibrous tissue. Patient was hypertensive. (Hematoxylin and eosin; 90×.)

etic system that have a tendency toward bleeding, anticoagulant therapy, endogenous toxic conditions such as uremia, and diseases of the blood vessels. In most instances there are multiple causative agents that act synergistically. A recent petechial hemorrhage, often confused with an engorged blood vessel, may be recognized because it is usually significantly larger than the otherwise normal but dilated vessels in the area, is slightly irregular, has a less sharp margin than that seen with an engorged blood vessel, and, with semitangential lighting, has a convex meniscus rather than the concave meniscus of blood within a vessel. When not completely resorbed, the petechial hemorrhages are brown to yellow and slightly depressed. This is the result of the conversion of the hemoglobin to hemosiderin and hematoidin by the macrophages accompanied by some tissue loss and mild reactive astrocytosis. Massive hemorrhages (3 cm or more in the cerebrum, 1.5 cm or more in the brainstem and cerebellum) may be ascribed to any of the aforementioned causes. Under these circumstances (not associated with hypertension), the hemorrhages are frequently multiple and sharply demarcated, with petechiae peripherally and often with no swelling or edema of the adjacent brain. Although these hemorrhages may sometimes extend through the cortex into the subarachnoid space, these nonhypertensive hemorrhages rarely rupture into an adjoining ventricle.

Massive brain hemorrhages have been a common cause of death in patients with inadequately treated or uncontrolled hypertension.[49] About 70% of the hemorrhages are in the lateral or medial ganglionic regions of the cerebral hemispheres (lenticular nuclei, thalami, and internal capsules; Fig. 44-15).[22,49] From these regions the hemorrhages often rupture into the adjacent ventricle; this may be preceded by extension of the hemorrhage along the nerve tracts to the midbrain and even to the pons or into the adjacent frontal or parietal lobes. The cerebral hemispheres are equally affected. About 20% of the hemorrhages begin initially in the midbrain, pons, or white matter of the cerebellum (Fig. 44-16). The remaining 10% begin in any of the remaining portions of the cerebral hemispheres. The medulla is never the primary site of this type of hemorrhage and is rarely involved by extension. The hemorrhages in fatal cases almost always have ruptured into the adjacent ventricle and from there have followed the cerebrospinal flow to reach the subarachnoid space. Relatively few rupture directly into the overlying subarachnoid space, and very rarely have the hemorrhages ruptured simultaneously or successively into both. Less than 1% of these massive hemorrhages are multiple. Death occurs in over 90% of these patients, usually within 96 hours (except in patients maintained by respirator for longer periods). On postmortem examination the brain is pale and swollen and asymmetric, usually with asymmetric subarachnoid hemorrhage at the base (Fig. 44-17). In the asymmetrically swollen brain the larger hemisphere contains the hemorrhage. It usually is covered by a lesser degree of subarachnoid blood because of greater compression of the space by the more swollen gyri. Brain displacement with herniations and resulting brainstem hemorrhage are common. The occurrence and localization of these secondary changes are dependent on the site and size of the massive hemorrhage.

The brain immediately surrounding the hemorrhage is greatly swollen and edematous and often has many petechiae in one or more areas immediately about the hemorrhage. The absence of brain tissue within the hemorrhage and the presence of blood not limited to the region

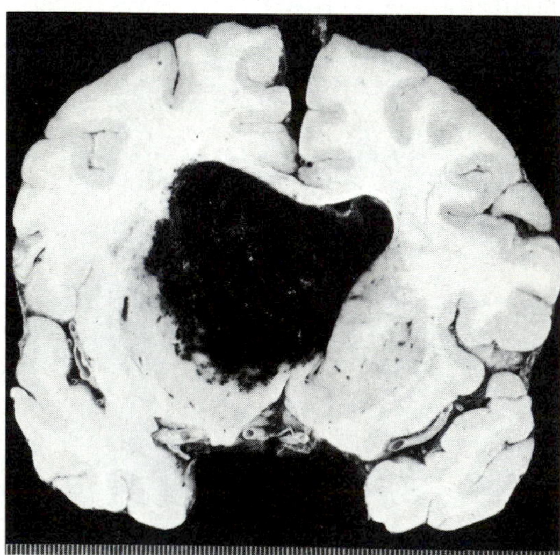

Fig. 44-15. Recent massive hemorrhage in inner striate area, with rupture into lateral ventricle in patient with hypertension. There are remote lacunar infarcts in putamina.

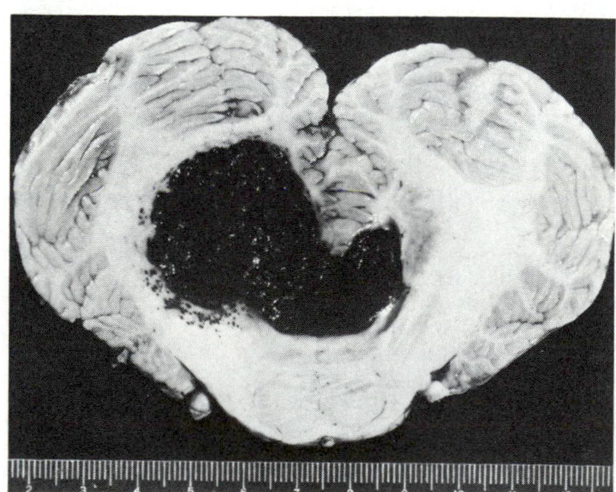

Fig. 44-16. Recent massive cerebellar hemorrhage with petechiae in wall and rupture into fourth ventricle in patient with hypertension.

supplied by an artery or drained by a vein serves to distinguish macroscopically the hemorrhage from a hemorrhagic infarct. On microscopic examination a characteristic structural pattern usually can be recognized. Within the hemorrhage, only a rare remnant of the original tissue can be found among the blood cells. The immediately surrounding swollen and edematous brain contains numerous severely sclerotic small arteries and arterioles and capillaries and venules. In the regions with petechiae, there usually are necrotic arterioles, venules, and capillaries infiltrated and surrounded by red blood cells and sometimes a few neutrophils. When the routine examination includes only a single or, at most, several sections through this region, infrequent aneurysmally dilated arterioles and small arteries are to be found (Fig. 44-18). Serial sections through these zones often result in a significant increase in their yield, but they are never frequent. The zone immediately peripheral to the petechial hemorrhages contains hyalinized, thick-walled blood vessels surrounded by large lakes of fluid high in protein content. There is a moderate degree of brain swelling and edema in this area, but this is less than in the portion of the brain immediately adjacent to the hemorrhage. In the remainder of the brain, there are arterioles and small arteries that exhibit varying degrees of arteriolosclerosis. Frequently, many of the infarcts previously described as occurring in patients with hypertension are also present. In hypertensive patients in whom no petechial hemorrhages are to be found in the walls of the massive hemorrhage, there is a different structural stratification. At one edge of the hemorrhage, there may occasionally be evidence of a preexisting or almost simultaneously occurring anemic or hemorrhagic infarct. The other portions of its wall are similar to those seen in the other hemorrhages, with brain swelling, edema, and arteriolosclerosis of moderate to pronounced degree.

These findings have stimulated at least three hypotheses as to the pathogenesis of the massive hemorrhages[22,27,28]:

1. Necrotizing arteriolitis with rupture of many arterioles
2. Arteriolosclerosis with a few or many arterioles undergoing necrosis, microaneurysm formation, and rupture (Fig. 44-18)
3. Massive hemorrhage in an area of earlier infarct

In 5% to 10% of the hypertensive patients with a massive hemorrhage, the lesion is not fatal. Although survival may occur with the larger cerebral hemorrhage that has not ruptured into a ventricle, it is more frequently seen with the smaller ganglionic hemorrhages and those in the less characteristic sites that have neither extended nor ruptured into the ventricular or subarachnoid spaces. In these, only the outer 1 to 2 mm of the hemorrhage is organized, with conversion of the hemoglobin to hemosiderin and hematoidin. A mild reactive astrocytic proliferation is present in the immediately surrounding brain. The blood in the interior of the hemorrhage becomes dark (chocolate red) and remains semiliquid

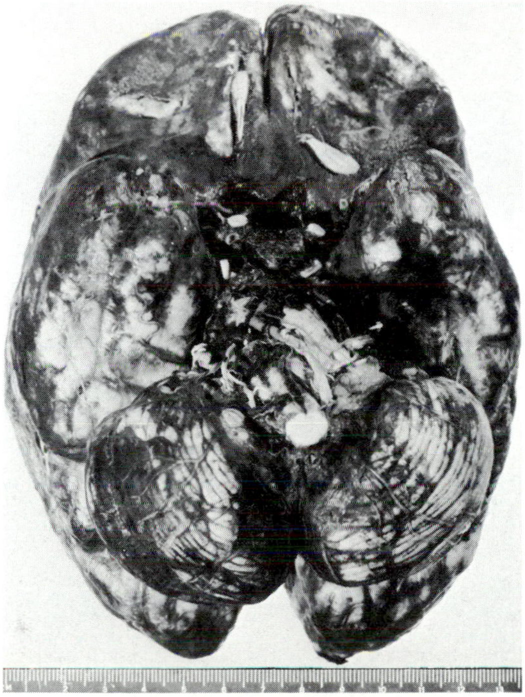

Fig. 44-17. Recent diffuse subarachnoid hemorrhage in patient with massive intracerebral hemorrhage.

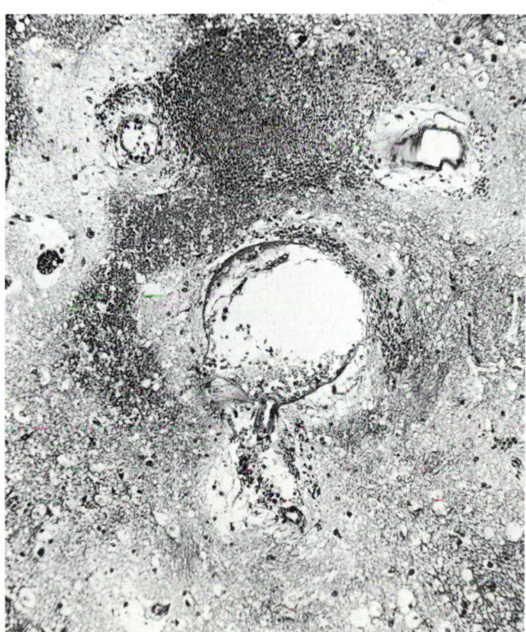

Fig. 44-18. Microaneurysm in wall of massive recent hypertensive hemorrhage. (Hematoxylin and eosin; 90×.)

and unorganized. When the blood is manually evacuated, a brown smooth-walled cavity not traversed by blood vessels remains.

Hypertensive encephalopathy characterized by recurrent attacks of sudden and severe headaches with vomiting, mental confusion, and visual, sensory, or motor disturbances is common in patients with untreated or inadequately treated hypertension.[130] Although one of these attacks may precede the appearance of a massive hemorrhage, death during an uncomplicated attack is rare. The mechanism of the syndrome is unknown, although arteriolar spasm and arteriolar and capillary thrombi have been suggested. The changes in the brain are neither characteristic nor uniform. Brain swelling with pallor and scattered petechiae has been described. In other cases, however, no gross abnormalities have been recognized. On microscopic examination there are usually varying degrees of arteriolosclerosis. In some there is arteriolar necrosis with surrounding petechiae. Identical changes may be seen in hypertensive patients dying of chronic uremia. The relationship of hypertensive encephalopathy to the small and larger hemorrhages and to the areas of necrosis in patients with hypertension is not known, although there has been much speculation.

Intraventricular hemorrhage is a frequent cause of death in the immature newborn. It occurs predominantly in infants between the twenty-fifth and thirty-second weeks of gestational age and in those weighing less than 1500 g. These subependymal matrix hemorrhages are most frequent in the caudate nucleus facing the interventricular foramen but can occur in any part of the subependymal germinal matrix. They are thought to be due to compression of the thalamostriate vein as it curves through the foramen, with rupture of its venules and capillaries. The hemorrhages may be bilateral. The ventricles are filled with a cast of clotted blood that can reach the subarachnoid space. When not fatal, the hemorrhage may resolve or be associated with varying degrees of neurologic deficit.

Aneurysms

Aneurysms of the arteries of the circle of Willis have been classified as berry (so-called congenital), atherosclerotic, inflammatory (mycotic), traumatic, and developmental. Of this group, only the first is of frequent clinical importance. The traumatic lesion usually is an arteriovenous fistula rather than an aneurysm. True developmental aneurysms are exceptionally rare.

Berry aneurysms.[20,28] The most common of this group of blood vessel lesions, berry aneurysms are found in 5% to 6% of all adults at postmortem examination.[20] Most occur in the bifurcation pockets of the arteries forming (Fig. 44-19) or extending from the circle of Willis (Fig. 44-20). The initial defect is considered by many to be a developmental deficiency or absence of the medial smooth muscle in the crotch of the bifurcation. Similar aneurysms not in these pockets are said to occur after

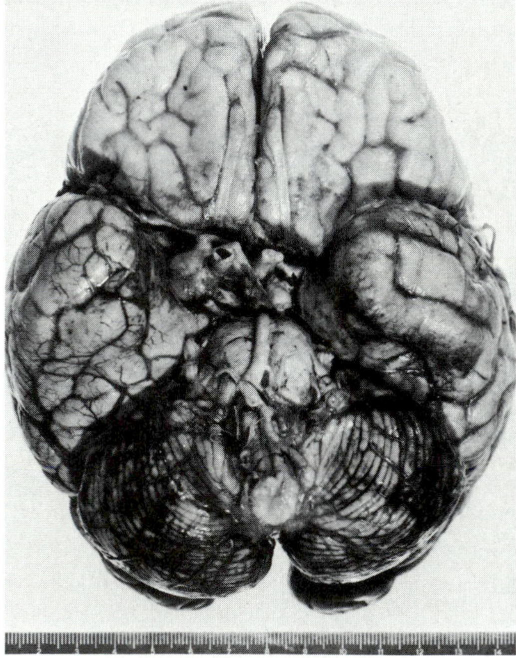

Fig. 44-19. Berry aneurysm at junction of right internal carotid and posterior communicating arteries. Pons is slightly widened and foreshortened, and there is cerebellomedullary herniation—both caused by rupture of aneurysm with intracerebral and intraventricular extension of hemorrhage that has reached cerebellar subarachnoid space through ventricular system.

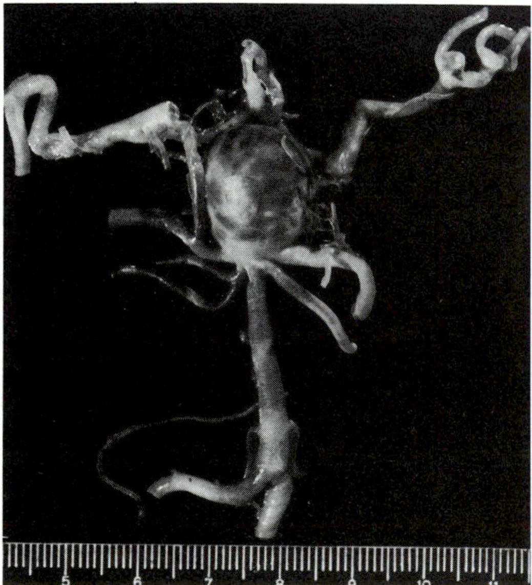

Fig. 44-20. Unruptured berry aneurysms. Larger aneurysm is at terminal portion of basilar artery. Smaller aneurysm is in bifurcation angle of middle cerebral artery on right.

incomplete resorption of unused embryonic arteries. The aneurysms form later after damage of the internal elastic lamina, probably because of a preceding focal atherosclerotic change. Some, however, have incorrectly considered this damage to be caused by disease of the vasa vasorum of these vessels. The normal thin adventitia of the arteries of the circle of Willis contributes significantly to the lack of adequate resistance to the intravascular pressure.

The aneurysms are, for reasons unknown, twice as common in women as in men. Only about 40% found at necropsy show evidence of bleeding or rupture. About 30% are multiple, and of these, two thirds are bilateral. Association with polycystic renal disease and with coarctation of the aorta can usually be related to the coexistent hypertension. Hypertension is present in 80% of those who have these aneurysms (with and without bleeding). The average age at the time of fatal rupture is between 50 and 55 years. The mortality of the first rupture is between 25% and 50%, and it is believed to be even higher with each succeeding rupture. In those with fatal ruptures, death occurs within 24 hours in almost 50%, many within the first hour, and in 95% within 2 weeks. The arteries forming the anterior half of the circle are involved about six times more frequently than those of the posterior half.[20] The sides of the circle are affected equally.

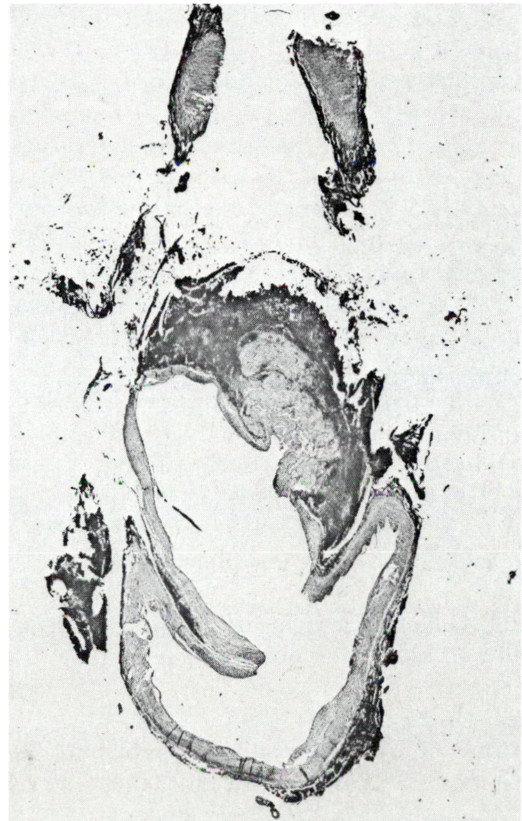

Fig. 44-21. Recently ruptured berry aneurysm. There is thrombus in fundus at site of rupture. (Hematoxylin and eosin; 8×.)

Although some aneurysms are cylindrical, most are berry shaped. They have narrowed necks of variable lengths. The mouth of the aneurysm internally often is constricted by an encircling endothelial fibrous cushion covering the frayed ends of the internal elastic lamina (Fig. 44-21).[112] The wall of the aneurysm is formed by a few layers of connective tissue devoid of the elastic lamina. It becomes progressively thinner toward the fundus, where rupture is most likely to occur (Fig. 44-21).[20] An electron microscopic study of these aneurysms has suggested the presence of smooth muscle cells within the wall of the aneurysm.[84] The occasional presence of a few neutrophils in the wall immediately adjacent to sites of leakage or rupture is due to their attraction by the necrotic aneurysm wall.

In over two thirds of the patients with fatal rupture, the asymmetric subarachnoid hemorrhage is only one of the complications.[20,29] Extension of the hemorrhage into the adjacent brain and often into a ventricle is common. Subdural hemorrhage occurs but is infrequent. Cerebral infarcts occurring with or after rupture are frequent. Some are caused by emboli and some by severe and prolonged local vasospasm. Brain displacement, herniation, and brainstem hemorrhage also are frequent secondary complications.

Atherosclerotic aneurysms. Atherosclerotic aneurysms are usually manifest as elongated cylindrical dilatations affecting the terminal portions of the internal carotid arteries and the basilar artery. Although rupture is rare, the carotid aneurysms often compress either or both of the optic nerves, sometimes with recognizable and characteristic narrowing of the visual fields. The wall of the atherosclerotic aneurysm has an intima variably thickened by lipophages, cholesterol esters, and fibrous tissue, a fragmented internal elastic lamina, a thinned media with little or no smooth muscle, and a thin adventitia.

Inflammatory aneurysms. An inflammatory (mycotic) aneurysm occurs at the site of attachment of an infected embolus whose usual source is a vegetation from a left-sided heart valve or pulmonary infection. These aneurysms are more frequent in the first and second major bifurcations of either middle cerebral artery. They are sometimes associated with a purulent leptomeningitis, a brain abscess, or a cerebral infarct. Leakage or rupture of the aneurysm into the subarachnoid space is frequent.

Arteriovenous fistula (internal carotid artery–cavernous sinus fistula). Before entering the intracranial cavity, the internal carotid arteries pass through the lumina of the cavernous sinuses. Disruption of the internal carotid artery at this level often is associated with a blow to the frontal area of the head, sometimes with fracture of one of the bones of the paranasal sinus. In some cases a history of antecedent injury is not obtained. The presence of significant concomitant degenerative disease of the carotid artery has not received adequate attention, since this region has not been routinely examined at necropsy. Rupture of the artery results in severe distension of the cavernous sinus and of the veins draining into it.

Developmental (true congenital) aneurysms.[117] Developmental aneurysms are exceedingly rare lesions. They are seen as a dilatation of an arterial wall not occurring at a bifurcation. There is no change in the intima, the internal elastic lamina is absent, the media is loose and contains only a few cells with the characteristics of smooth muscle, and the adventitia is thin.

Trauma

The effects of mechanical forces, either direct or indirect, on the central nervous system, although varied, are frequently predictable.[32] A systematic approach to the structural changes resulting from mechanical forces causing injury, usually begins with lesions of the dura, followed by the lesions that are produced at successively deeper levels.

Epidural hematoma

The dura mater covering the brain is represented by a fused dura and periosteum of the skull. Below the level of the foramen magnum, the two layers are separated by adipose tissue, blood vessels, and nodular accumulation of lymphocytes, sometimes with follicle formation. Epidural hematomas from blunt traumatic forces are almost limited to the region of the skull (Fig. 44-22).[90] They usually are associated with a recent skull fracture that frees the dura and, in crossing the groove of the middle meningeal artery, tears that artery and often the accompanying vein as well. Rarely the hematoma may be attributable to a tear in the anterior or posterior meningeal artery or in a vein between the skull and dura. Because of its position, the lesion also can be considered as a subperiosteal hematoma.

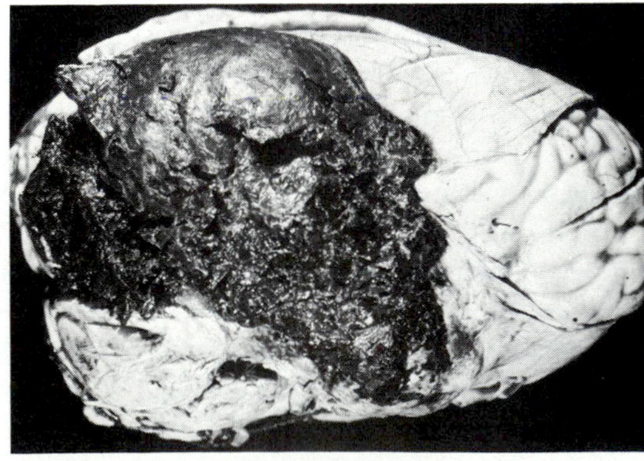

Fig. 44-22. Acute epidural hematoma resulting from skull fracture with tear of middle meningeal artery and vein.

These hematomas rarely organize or resolve without surgical intervention. The usual amount of blood found at autopsy in untreated persons varies between 75 and 125 g. This amount is in the same range found in fatal acute subdural hematomas and intracerebral hypertensive hemorrhages. Death is caused by the effects of brain compression, with brain displacement, herniation, secondary brainstem hemorrhages, and neurogenic pulmonary edema.

Subdural hematoma

Subdural hematomas usually result from blunt injury to the skull without fracture. They can, however, occur without direct injury to the skull. This is particularly true in older persons with brain atrophy in whom sudden anterior or posterior movement of the head, as from stumbling, may easily tear one of the bridging veins. On rare occasions, arterial bleeding may be the cause of the hematoma.

With the acute subdural hematoma, blood accumulates rapidly after a tear of a bridging vein at the point where the vessel leaves the subdural space (a potential space) to enter the dura. Because most veins cross the subdural space in the vicinity of the superior sagittal sinus, most hematomas begin parasagittally. The reason they remain as tumorous collections in this region rather than form a diffuse hematoma is unknown. Some believe that it is because of the pressure exerted by the brain at the rim of the hematoma. There is little or no evidence of early organization of the acute subdural hematoma on its dural surface or at its margins, nor is there any evidence of organization of the hematoma from the arachnoid membrane except when this membrane is torn.

Organization of subdural blood in the formation of a chronic subdural hematoma begins within the first week and is evident after 2 weeks. The hematoma is encapsulated by highly vascular granulation tissue originating from the overlying dura, with the dura at the edges of the hematoma, and from blood monocytes that migrate to its inner rim where a fibrin layer has formed contributing to the formation of the granulation tissue that separates the blood from the underlying arachnoid membrane (Fig. 44-23). The granulation tissue on the dural surface is known as the outer membrane, and that on the undersurface of the hematoma, the inner membrane (Fig. 44-24).

Others believe that some chronic subdural hematomas result from the tearing of a bridging vein as it crosses between the outer and inner layers of the meningeal dura.

Whatever the original site of the hemorrhage, the granulation tissue that surrounds the hematoma contains large, thin-walled vessels that act as semipermeable membranes (Fig. 44-24). The negative intracranial pressure when the patient is upright is believed to attract fluid from the surrounding sinusoidally dilated, thin-walled capillaries. This results in enlargement of the hematoma, with stretching, tearing, and hemorrhage from the vessels at the margins. Repetition of these processes leads to continued gradual and steplike enlargement of the hematoma. These hematomas regularly are associated with brain displacement, herniations, and, when fatal, brainstem hemorrhages and neurogenic pulmonary edema. Clinical classification of subdural hematomas with acute, subacute, and chronic types is related more to the time of development of signs and symptoms and their duration than to the structural characteristics.

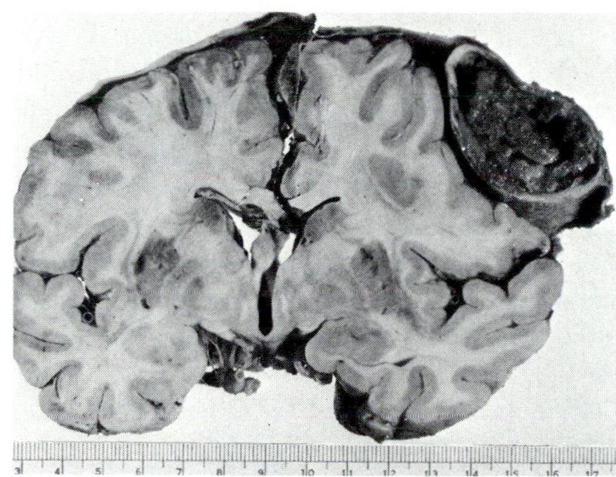

Fig. 44-23. Chronic subdural hematoma with compression of underlying brain and lateral ventricle. Note bone formation in falx and uncal herniation on side of hematoma.

A history of trauma is not obtained in every patient with a chronic subdural hematoma, even in those capable of giving reliable histories. This is attributable, in part, to the occasional long interval between the causative event and the first signs and symptoms. In some, the episode may have been ignored or forgotten, since the trauma appeared to be trivial or was to another part of the body (such as a fall on the buttocks or a jerking of the entire body on stumbling). Individuals undergoing anticoagulant therapy, particularly those who are older and have vascular disease, are more susceptible.

Organized subdural hemorrhages recognized grossly as rusty discoloration of the inner dural layer are frequent when the autopsy population has a high proportion of alcoholics and other adult groups with an unusual incidence of minor head trauma. In these the hemoglobin has been converted to hemosiderin and hematoidin. Occasionally a small recent hemorrhage is found, suggesting a new injury or the beginning of the cycle toward the formation of a hematoma.

A localized subdural collection of a yellow fluid with a high protein content is known as a subdural hygroma. It is an uncommon lesion believed to occur following a valvelike tear of the arachnoid that permits only the outward flow of subarachnoid fluid into the subdural space. Origin from a chronic subdural hematoma has been suggested for the encapsulated hygroma whose wall is a rusty brown. In these, organization has resulted in the gradual removal of the cellular elements but the reten-

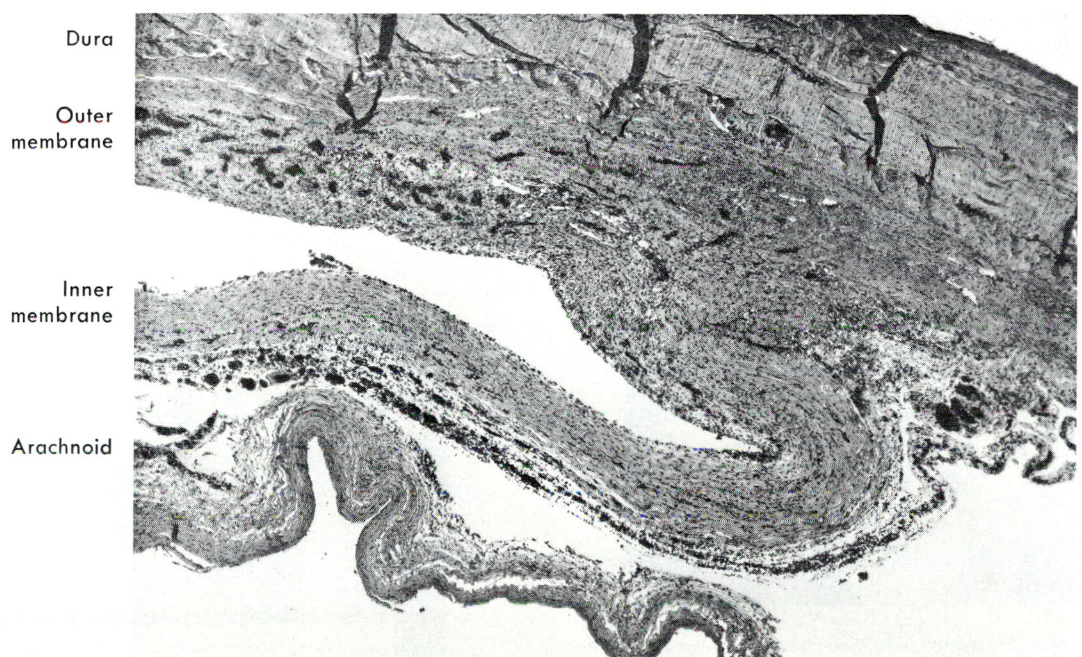

Fig. 44-24. Wall of chronic subdural hematoma at junction of inner and outer membranes. (Hematoxylin and eosin; 30×.)

tion of fluid stained to variable degrees by residual hemosiderin and hematoidin.

Subarachnoid hemorrhage

Bleeding into the subarachnoid space has many causes, one of the more common of which is blunt trauma to the skull with or without fracture. Although bleeding can be the sole result of trauma (at least clinically), at postmortem examination the hemorrhages often are associated with other lesions (for example, contusions and lacerations). With small hemorrhages the blood may be completely removed by following the cerebrospinal fluid flow into the draining sinuses. In some individuals, particularly those with other traumatic brain lesions, the blood may be trapped by adhesions and then converted to hemosiderin and hematoidin.

Contusion

Contusions of the brain are caused by blunt head trauma. The effects are transmitted to the brain by the deformation of the skull and by the inertia of the brain. Coup lesions occur at the point of impact and contrecoup lesions at a point away from the impact site. Contrecoup lesions are generally at or near the diametrically opposite side of the skull from the impact. The exact point depends on the skull curvature, direction of impact, and so on. The energy transferred to the brain—either positive (coup) or negative (contrecoup)—is accentuated by the inertia of the brain and the inbending at the point of impact and outbending of the deformed skull at the contrecoup site, combined with shearing rotational movements of this lacerated brain. Damage is diminished by the shape of the skull and the falx and tentorium.

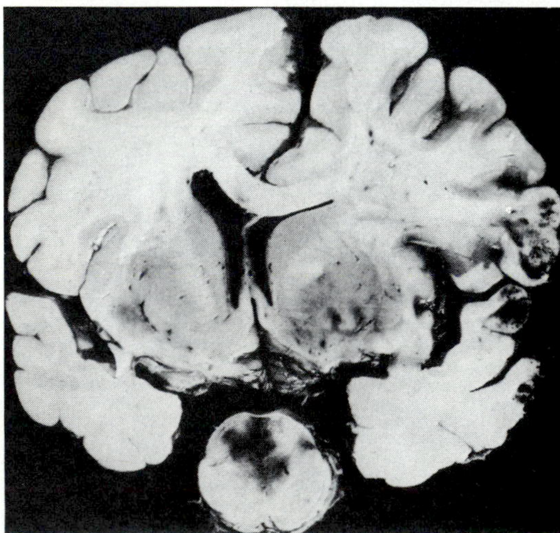

Fig. 44-25. Recent contusions of frontal and temporal lobes. There is displacement of cingulate gyrus and lateral ventricles. Secondary hemorrhages have occurred in lower midbrain and upper pons.

Most contusions are sustained by the impact of the moving head against a fixed or relatively stationary object. The contrecoup lesion with these deceleration injuries is usually larger than the coup lesion and is the result of the negative pressure. The coup and contrecoup lesions are roughly conical, with the base of the cone directed toward the arachnoid surface at the apex of one or more convolutions (Fig. 44-25). All tissues, including the surface cortical layer (therefore, all contusions are lacerations as well), are destroyed or damaged for varying depths. Initially the lesions are filled with necrotic cells and focal or diffuse collections of fresh blood from torn blood vessels. There is a variable degree of edema and swelling of the adjacent tissue. Early and transiently, a few neutrophils may be found in the walls of an occasional vessel at the margin of a contusion. Perivascular mononuclear cells appear during the second and third days, and reactive astrocytes are seen in the adjoining brain at about the same time. Organization proceeds with the formation of lipophages and the conversion of the blood to hemosiderin and hematoidin, much of which remains within the lesion. Thereafter the contusion-laceration is represented by an orange-brown, depressed, wedge-shaped region with a flattened apex (Fig. 44-26). The lesion, widest at the crest of a gyrus or gyri, often is covered by a leptomeningeal-cortical scar.

Contusion-lacerations are most frequent at the tips and orbital portions of the frontal lobes and tips and lateral portions of the temporal lobes. Other areas of involvement are the tips of the occipital lobes, the corpus callosum (from damage by the free margin of the falx), the cerebellum, and base of the pons.

Stretch (tension) tears

The corpus callosum and brainstem are the usual sites of stretch (tension) tears of fiber tracts. These occur with severe head injuries that result in marked transient deformation of the skull.

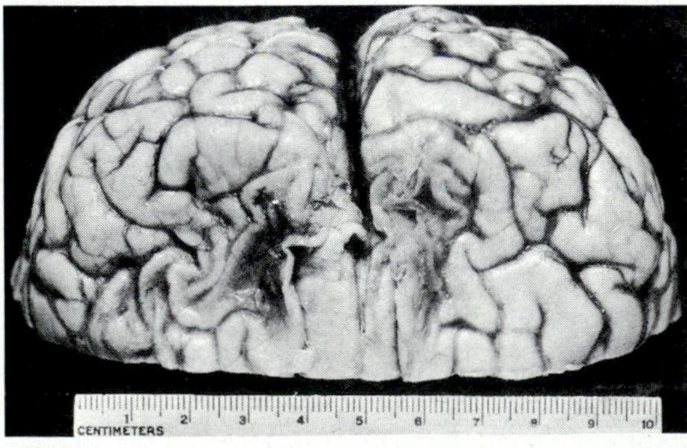

Fig. 44-26. Remote contusions of orbital gyri and olfactory bulbs.

Intracerebral hematoma

Intracerebral hematomas occurring after nonpenetrating trauma to the skull are presumably the result of shearing stresses on intracerebral vessels. The rupture of one or more large vessels may lead to a large hematoma or to several (Fig. 44-27). They are more likely to occur in the frontal lobes but may be found in other portions of the brain, including the cerebellum, midbrain, pons, and very rarely the medulla.

Multiple small hemorrhages, primarily in the white matter of the brain after nonpenetrating skull trauma, are more likely the result of hypoxia or fat embolism. Although the hemorrhages of fat embolism are far more frequent in the white matter (Fig. 44-28), fat emboli are more frequent in the adjoining gray matter. Fat emboli are more usual in the central nervous system in patients with injuries to long bones with or without fractures; they are also seen after burns or mechanical damage to large areas of subcutaneous fat, in sickle cell crisis, in patients with severe fatty change in the liver, and in patients with active pancreatitis. Fat emboli need not be accompanied by petechial hemorrhages. The fat obstructs many arterioles and capillaries throughout the brain. The petechiae result from vascular stasis with anoxia and endothelial damage of the vessels in the white matter; they are rare in the gray matter owing to the many capillary anastomoses that protect these vessels.

Concussion

Concussion is the sudden loss of neurologic function immediately after blunt injury, usually to the head. Much has been written concerning the definition of this entity, the mechanism of injury, and the physical principles involved in the transmission of force, as well as the structural changes, if any.

Uncomplicated concussion in humans is rarely fatal. Among those who have reported experimental observations, there is agreement that structural changes at the light microscopic level do occur. These changes consist of central chromatolysis of variable numbers of cells in the reticular substance of the brainstem with similar but lesser involvement of cells in the cerebral cortex.[24,25] Some believe that these changes are a result of damage to axons in the ventral portion of the upper cervical portion of the spinal cord, whereas others are of the opinion that the changes are caused by shear stresses in the cerebrum at the junction of the gray and white matter or directly on the affected cells.

Penetrating injuries to brain

The brain and spinal cord may be penetrated by bullets and fragments of metal and bone sometimes covered by scalp, hair, and other contaminated foreign material. The damage in high-velocity bullet injuries is generalized as well as local. Its effects are caused by the sudden increase in intracranial pressure, the shearing and tearing of the tissue, and the intense local heat. There is extensive necrosis and hemorrhage in and about the tract of the missile. In low-velocity injuries the damage is limited to the penetrated area.

Posttraumatic brain swelling and edema

Occasionally in children (rarely in adults), a minor degree of head trauma is associated with generalized and progressive swelling and edema of the brain. Other traumatic lesions are usually absent. The brain is enlarged and symmetric. The convolutions are flattened, the sulci narrowed, and the ventricles small. The white matter is prominent—bulging and dry in the swollen areas, depressed and wet in the edematous sites. Fluid high in protein content may be found about the blood vessels and in the Virchow-Robin space and tissue in brain edema (Fig. 44-29). The myelin sheaths are irregularly swollen and pale with enlarged clear spaces about the oligodendroglial nuclei in the areas of swelling. Increasing amounts of eosinophilic cytoplasm of the involved astro-

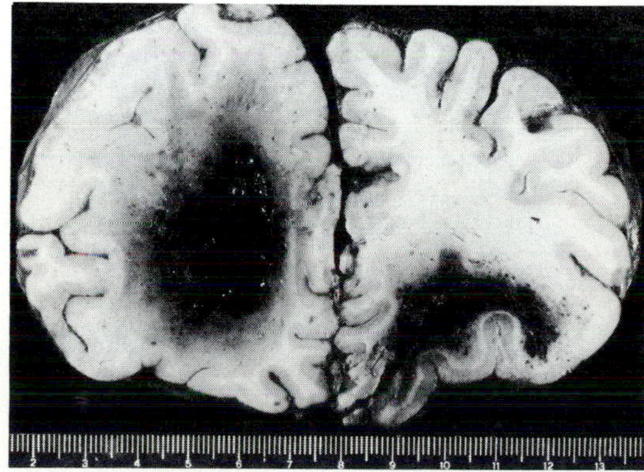

Fig. 44-27. Recent hematomas in frontal lobes, resulting from trauma.

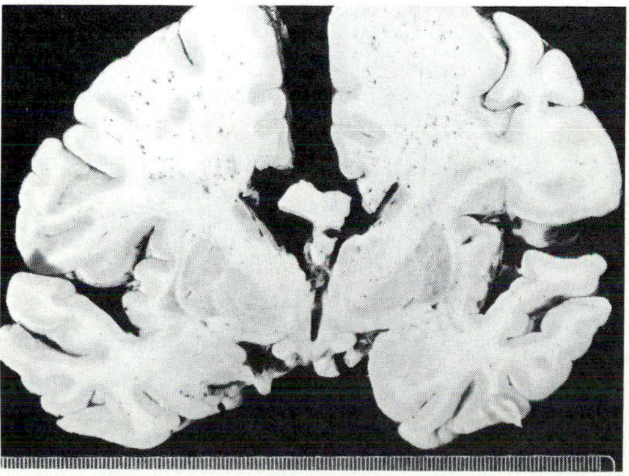

Fig. 44-28. Petechial hemorrhages in white matter in posttraumatic fat embolism.

cytes become visible by the end of the first day. Death usually is associated with hypoxia and neurogenic pulmonary edema.

Trauma of spinal cord

The spinal cord of the newborn infant can be injured in breech deliveries by the exertion of too great an extractile force with the hyperextended head. The overstretched cord, usually at the cervicothoracic level, has an hourglass narrowing (Fig. 44-30).

Hematomyelia with necrosis of the cord is usually caused by fractures or dislocations of the vertebrae with compression of the cord. In some cases the lesion appears to follow extreme degrees of hyperextension (Fig. 44-30) and hyperflexion at the cervical level with fracture or dislocation. The cord appears to be slightly to moderately narrowed at the level of compression, with bulging and softening above and below caused by necrosis with hemorrhage into the gray matter (Fig. 44-31). This may extend for several levels to either side of the point of initial injury.

The spinal cord may be compressed on its ventral surface by a herniated intervertebral disc (Fig. 44-32) or by osteophytic lipping of the vertebral bodies.[65,88] The former is more likely to affect the lumbar portion and the latter the cervical portion of the cord. There are, however, many exceptions. The spinal cord, stabilized by the denticulate ligaments, is injured by direct compression locally. Less often, the changes are from compression of the anterior spinal artery.

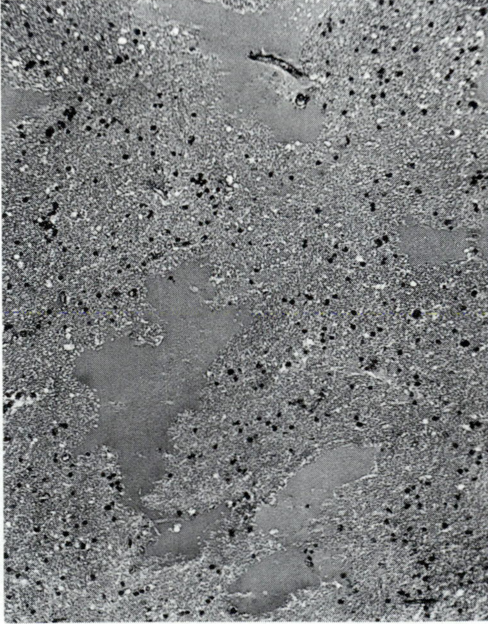

Fig. 44-29. Brain edema. Intercellular lakes of high protein content fluid. (Hematoxylin and eosin; 90×.)

Cerebral birth injury[119]

Cerebral birth injury (cerebral palsy, Little's disease, spastic diplegia) is a disorder of paranatal origin characterized clinically by disturbances of movement, sometimes associated with mental retardation. The disorder may be hereditary or caused by mechanical forces, anoxia, maternal infection, metabolic disease, or vascular disease, with the morphologic lesions spanning almost the entire range of neuropathologic disease. Each of the lesions should be evaluated separately.

Degenerative diseases

Brain atrophies[97,118,127]

Continuous loss of nerve cells and their processes and of the surrounding myelin and intercellular fluid regularly accompanies aging. The cell and fluid loss results in a compensatory hydrocephalus. There may also be slight focal fibrotic thickening of the leptomeninges.

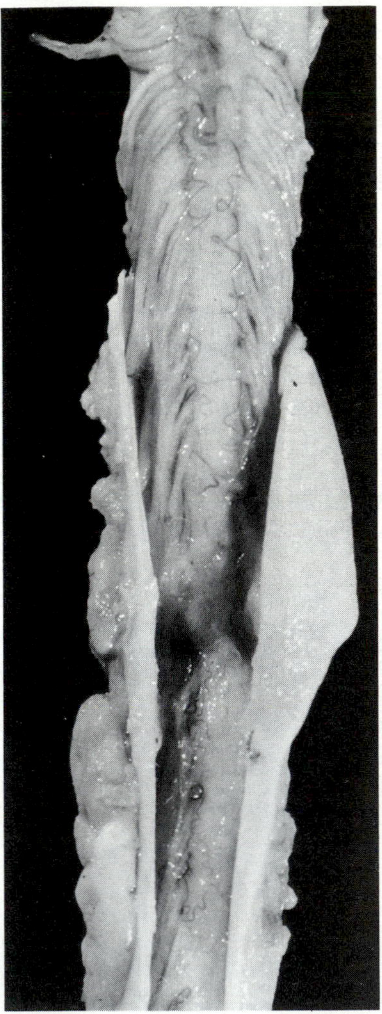

Fig. 44-30. Destruction of lower cervical portion of spinal cord of infant, attributed to stretching during breech delivery.

On microscopic examination the nerve cell loss may be recognizable within the cortex and the central gray matter by the presence of patchy areas devoid of cells. Many of the remaining, often shrunken, nerve cells contain excessive amounts of intracytoplasmic lipofuscin pigment. A mild to moderate reactive astrocytic gliosis is present and is most easily recognized in the outermost layers of the cortex. Hyaline congophilic thickening of the capillary walls in the occipital cortex frequently accompanies the aging process. Corpora amylacea are often prominent.

In the aging brain the loss of nerve cells and their processes may lead to a temporary condensation of the interfascicular oligodendrocytes and the eventual loss of white matter. In some individuals the process of aging is so severe that it produces varying degrees of dementia.

Alzheimer's disease

Formerly considered to be a disease whose clinical onset preceded the sixth decade, Alzheimer's disease is now recognized as a pathologic entity whose cause is unknown and whose clinical onset is most frequent in the fourth to sixth decades. With onset after the age of 65

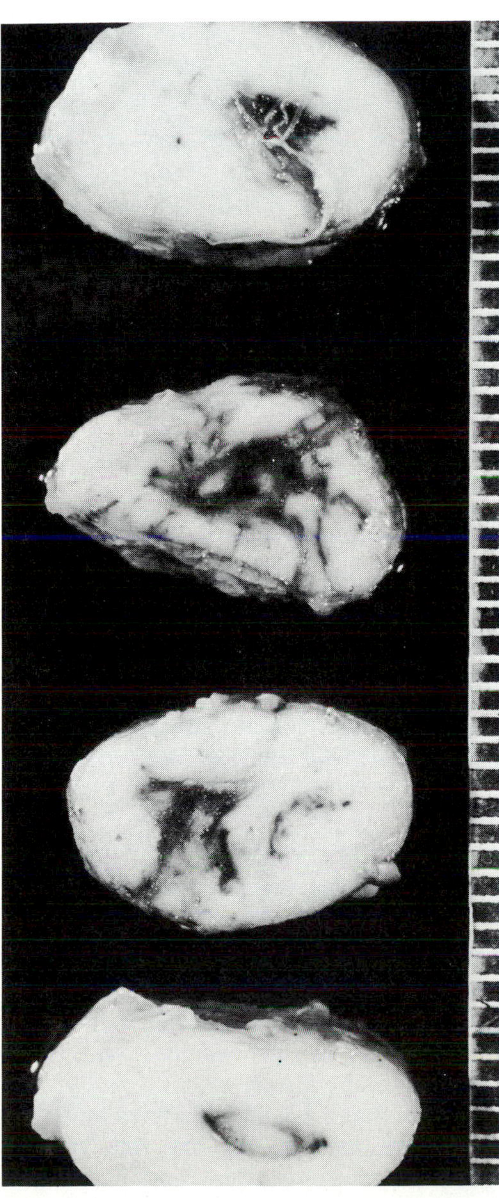

Fig. 44-31. Recent contusion and hemorrhage in cervical portion of spinal cord (hematomyelia) after dislocation of cervical vertebra.

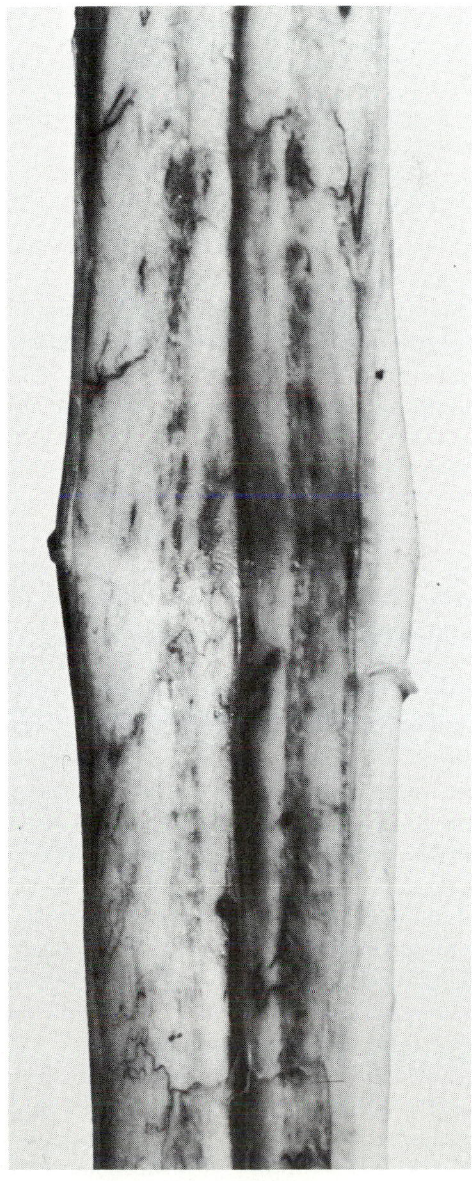

Fig. 44-32. Compression of cervical portion of spinal cord by ruptured disc. Patient was asymptomatic.

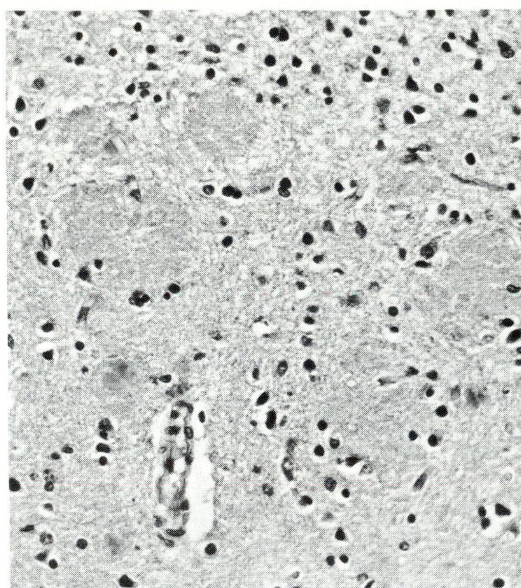

Fig. 44-33. Neuritic (senile) plaques in Alzheimer's disease. (Hematoxylin and eosin; 280×.)

years the condition is known as senile dementia, Alzheimer type (SDAT).

The brain is diffusely atrophic with a compensatory hydrocephalus. All the microscopic characteristics of the aging brain are present in great profusion. In addition there are neuritic (senile) plaques, Alzheimer's neurofibrillary tangles, and granulovacuolar changes in certain of the nerve cells. Neuritic plaques (Fig. 44-33) are irregularly distributed in the neuropil in all parts of the cerebral cortex, and when profuse in the neocortex along with neurofibrillary tangles, correlate well with dementia. Neuritic plaques are also found in the mamillary bodies, uncommonly in other gray matter, rarely in white matter, and in familial cases in the Purkinje layer of the cerebellum. The hematoxylin and eosin stain shows plaques to be eosinophilic fibrillar spheres 15 to 125 μm in diameter. The fibrils are either haphazardly arranged or radiate from a central hyaline eosinophilic core; at the periphery of the latter plaque there may be a deeply eosinophilic rim. Plaques are, however, more easily seen with silver stains (Fig. 44-34); the central cores stain as amyloid and with electron microscopy have the characteristics of amyloid. Variable numbers of reactive astrocytes surround the plaques. Alzheimer's neurofibrillary tangles occur in the perikaryon of many of the larger cortical nerve cells and, although recognizable with hematoxylin and eosin, they are best seen with special silver stains or by electron microscopy. These argyrophilic fibrillar tangles are formed by the condensation and twisting of the neurotubules with simultaneous displacement of the other cytoplasmic contents (Fig. 44-34). Granulovacuolar changes occur primarily in the larger cells of the hippocampus; the cells contain hematoxylinophilic and argyrophilic cytoplasmic granules, each within a nonstaining vacuole. Recent studies have suggested that the earliest lesions begin in the diagonal band of Broca and involve the cells of the nucleus basalis of Meynert.

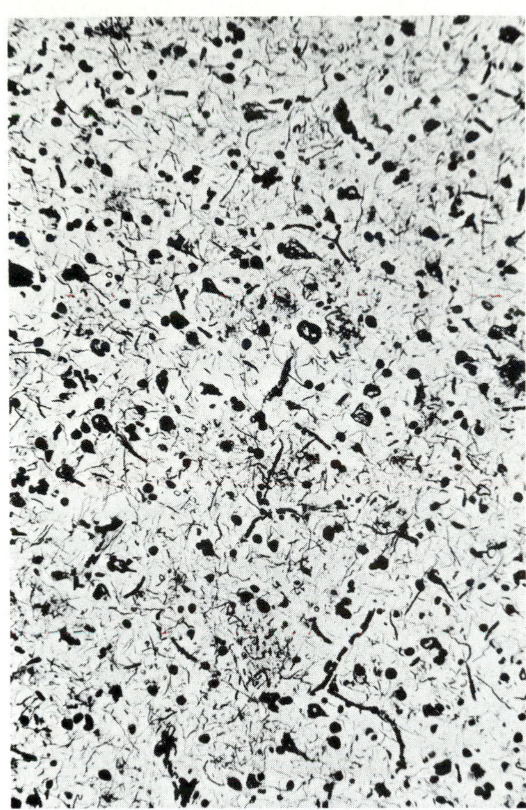

Fig. 44-34. Neuritic (senile) plaques and neurofibrillary tangles in Alzheimer's disease. (Hortega silver carbonate; 135×.)

Pick's disease (lobar sclerosis, circumscribed cortical atrophy)

Pick's disease[125] is an uncommon, sometimes familial disease of unknown cause. Although patients usually become symptomatic during the sixth and seventh decades, onset in the third decade and in the tenth decade has been recorded. Women are affected more often than men. The disease characteristically is fatal in 5 to 10 years.

The lobar atrophy, from which one of the names of the disease is derived, is most noticeable in the temporal and frontal lobes with the formation of the "saber gyri" (Fig. 44-35). The atrophy is usually symmetric and may extend to involve the insular cortex. Compensatory hydrocephalus is pronounced. The atrophy is primarily the result of the severe loss of nerve cells in the outer three cortical layers, frequently leaving a vacuolated appearance. Some of the residual degenerating nerve cells are swol-

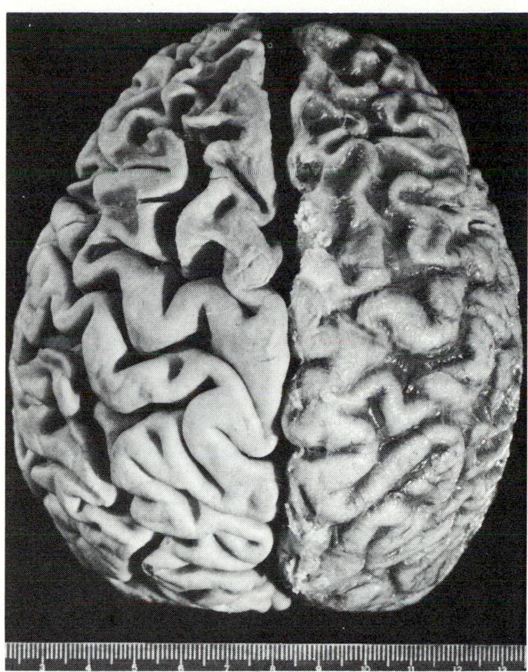

Fig. 44-35. Pick's disease. Pronounced atrophy of rostral frontal lobes with compensatory external hydrocephalus.

len with peripheral displacement of their nuclei. These abnormal cells, Pick's cells, contain intracytoplasmic, amphophilic (with hematoxylin and eosin), argyrophilic, and granular material. An astrocytic gliosis, sometimes very pronounced, in the outer cortical layers of the atrophic gyri is regularly present.

Spinocerebellar degenerations[79]

The spinocerebellar degenerations are an overlapping group of related diseases affecting the portions of the central nervous system that control coordination. The systems of cells involved are developmentally, functionally, and anatomically related. Although many of the diseases are hereditary (either dominant or recessive), previous infections, alcoholism, and the remote effects of cancer also have been implicated.

The disorders are first apparent clinically and structurally in the most peripheral portion of the processes of the affected cells, with retrograde progression toward the perikaryon. For ease of understanding, these disorders have been divided into (1) primarily spinal, (2) primarily cerebellar, and (3) mixed types.

Primarily spinal atrophies. The most common of the degenerations that are primarily spinal are Friedreich's ataxia and peroneal muscular atrophy.

Friedreich's ataxia. Friedreich's ataxia (hereditary spinal ataxia) is a rare progressive disease whose usual onset occurs during the first two decades of life. The sexes are affected equally, and the average life span after clinical onset is approximately 15 years. The cerebrum, brainstem, and cerebellum are normal. On the other hand, the spinal cord, its posterior roots, and the spinal ganglia are small at the time of death. This is attributed at first to demyelination and later to loss of axons in the posterior half of the cord.

Initially the fasciculi graciles are affected. With progression the disease in turn affects the fasciculi cuneati, the posterior roots, and the dorsal and then the ventral spinocerebellar tracts. In far-advanced disease, the lateral and later the anterior corticospinal tracts also may be involved. The cells of Clarke's columns with loss of Nissl substance become small, and finally many cells may disappear. At the time of death about half the patients have myocardial lesions: hypertrophy, fatty infiltration, focal myocarditis, and fibrosis, in any combination.

Peroneal muscular atrophy. Peroneal muscular atrophy (Charcot-Marie-Tooth disease; progressive neural muscular atrophy) is a hereditary disease usually dominant. It may occur in families in which other members have Friedreich's ataxia. The lesions are characterized by demyelination followed by axon loss beginning in the most distal portions of the peroneal nerves, initially involving the fibers supplying the small muscles of the feet. With progression the lesions ascend the nerves to involve the anterior horn cells and the cells of the spinal ganglia. In others there is a reactive Schwann cell proliferation about residual axons of the peripheral nerves, producing an onion-skin appearance. There may be degeneration of the posterior columns as well.

The rarer primary spinal atrophies include hereditary areflexic dystaxia (Roussy-Levy syndrome) and heredopathia atactica polyneuritiformis (Refsum's disease).

Primarily cerebellar atrophies. The degenerations that are primarily cerebellar include lamellar atrophy of Purkinje's cells, moderate decrease or loss of the internal granular layer, focal cerebellar sclerosis, and olivopontocerebellar atrophy. In this group of disorders, in contrast to the spinal forms, there are a later clinical onset, a more common involvement of the extrapyramidal tracts, and less commonly, extraneural signs.

Lamellar atrophy of Purkinje's cells. Lamellar atrophy of Purkinje's cells is a disorder of adults, more often past the age of 40 years. It usually is not hereditary. Some instances have been associated with alcoholism. Other suggested causes have included a variety of toxins, infections, and premature aging.

The cerebellum grossly appears normal or is only slightly decreased in size. Microscopically there is a sharp loss of Purkinje's cells (Fig. 44-36) that may be complete in the superior and anterior portions of the cerebellar vermis. There is a lesser loss of cells in the hemispheres. The molecular layer of the cerebellum is unaltered. A mild loss of the internal granular cells is sometimes noted.

Subacute cerebellar degeneration. Diffuse loss of Pur-

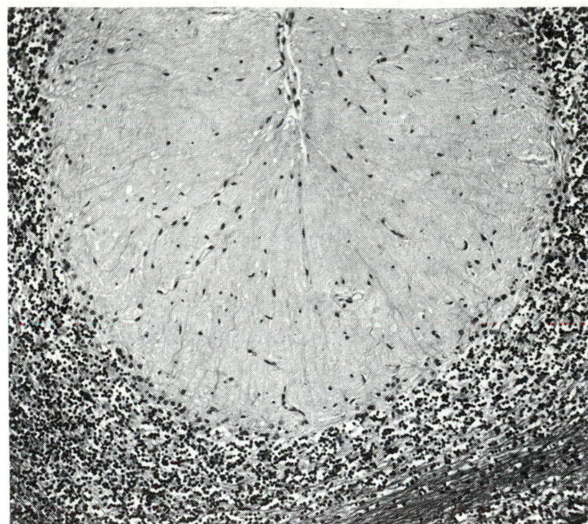

Fig. 44-36. Lamellar atrophy of Purkinje cells. (Hematoxylin and eosin; 90×.)

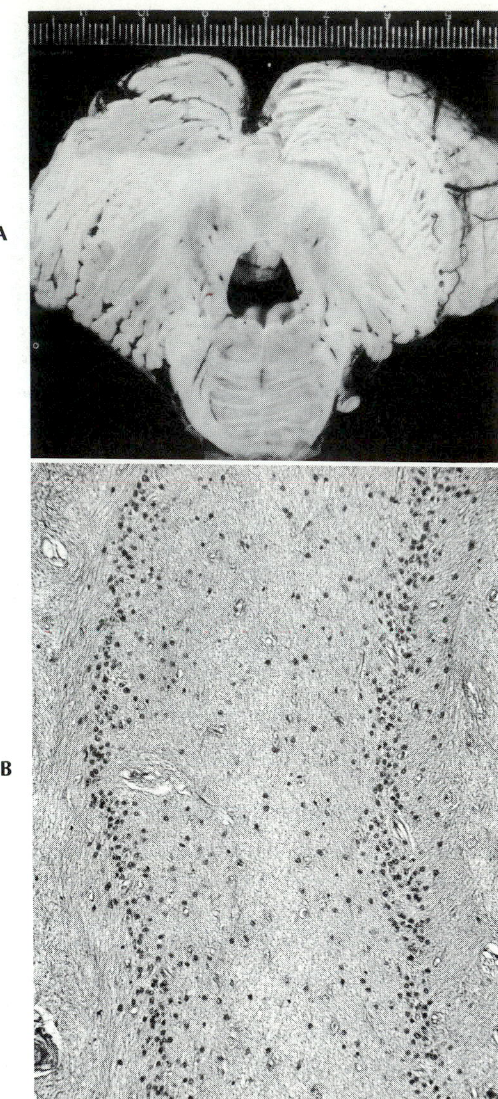

Fig. 44-37. Focal cerebellar sclerosis. **A,** Involvement of several cerebellar folia. **B,** Focus of loss of Purkinje and most internal granular cells. There is reactive astrocytic gliosis. (Hematoxylin and eosin; 90×.)

kinje cells (subacute cerebellar degeneration) has been ascribed to the remote effects of cancer. The great sensitivity of these cells to hypoxia, hyperthermia, a variety of chemical toxins, heavy metals, and possibly alcohol obscures the significance of cancer as the only cause of this change.

Degeneration of internal granular layer. Degeneration of the internal granular layer with either partial or complete loss of the cells is a common postmortem finding. It occurs regularly as an autolytic change in the so-called respirator brain and is seen in a great variety of disorders frequently associated with hyperthermia, as well as in alcoholism. Familial cases with onset in the first year of life associated with mental deficiency and ataxia also have been described. The cerebellum may be normal in size or slightly smaller than normal. The degree of internal granular cell loss is variable. Purkinje's cells are far less involved and occasionally may be displaced into the molecular or granular layers. The presence of a mild to moderate reactive astrocytosis in some cases suggests an extrinsic cause rather than a developmental lesion.

Focal cerebellar sclerosis (circumscribed atrophy of cerebellar cortex). In focal cerebellar sclerosis there is focal and severe degeneration of all three cerebellar layers and a marked reactive proliferation of Bergmann cells (Fig. 44-37). The superior and inferior semilunar and simplex lobules are most frequently involved. The cause of this usually clinically inapparent disease is unknown.

Olivopontocerebellar atrophies. The olivopontocerebellar atrophies are a group of related disorders characterized by the loss of nerve cells in the cerebellar cortex, the base of the pons, and the inferior olives (Fig. 44-38). Separation into five types has been based on their hereditary background, their clinical and pathologic characteristics, and involvement of other portions of the central nervous system. All but one are dominantly inherited. The life span after clinical onset is usually less than 10 years.

The great atrophy of the cerebellum (usually sparing the vermis), base of pons, and inferior olives is diagnostic and basic to all five types. This is caused by the loss of internal granular and Purkinje's cells with an astrocytosis in the cerebellum and loss of neurons in the base of the pons, the inferior olives, and in some cases the substantia nigra. Type 1 additionally exhibits degeneration of the middle cerebellar peduncles and the spinocerebellar tracts and posterior columns of the spinal cord with a decrease in cells in the anterior and posterior horns.

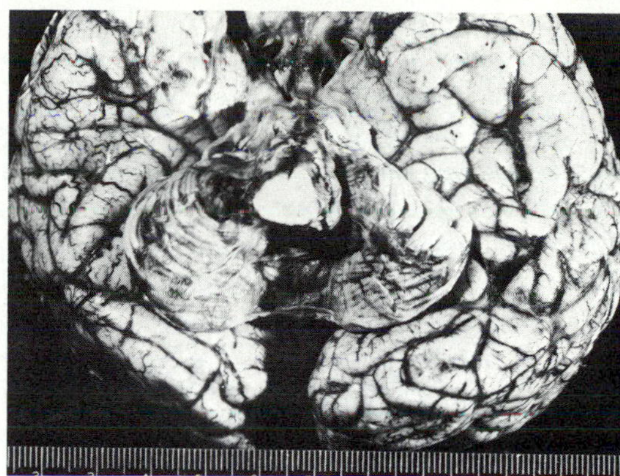

Fig. 44-38. Olivopontocerebellar atrophy. There is pronounced atrophy of cerebellum, pons, and inferior olives.

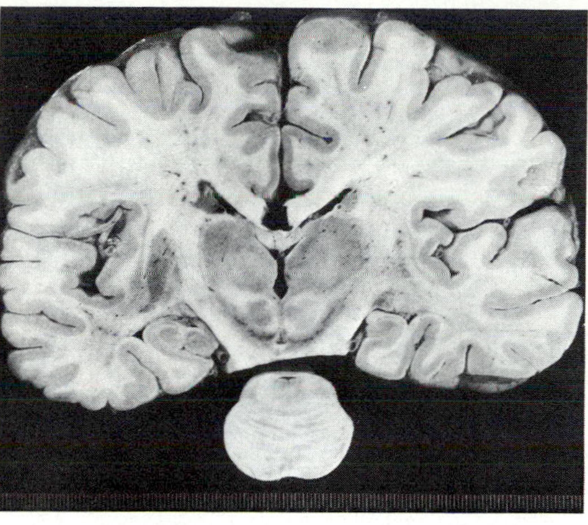

Fig. 44-39. Brain of patient who exhibited idiopathic parkinsonism shows partial loss of pigment in substantia nigra and complete loss in locus ceruleus, both bilaterally.

Type 2, recessively inherited, is without spinal cord involvement and with a variable cell loss in the substantia nigra. In type 3, the changes are those of type 1 with added retinal degeneration. Degeneration of cells of the vagus and hypoglossal nuclei superimposed on the basic changes is seen in type 4. In type 5 there is also loss of cells in the cerebral cortex, caudate and lenticular nuclei, and the third cranial nerve.

Parkinsonism

Formerly considered a disease, parkinsonism is now regarded as a symptom complex most frequently of idiopathic or viral origin.[34,42] Other causes are local vascular disease with infarction, anoxia caused by carbon monoxide, toxins, and drugs (manganese and the phenothiazines), metastatic lesions, and local physical injury. The term *paralysis agitans* usually is reserved for the idiopathic variety.

In most patients, in addition to a mild to moderate degree of generalized brain atrophy, the characteristic lesions are confined to pigmented cells of the brainstem such as those of the substantia nigra, locus ceruleus, and dorsal nucleus of the vagus. The grossly visible loss of pigment in these areas (Fig. 44-39) is the result of destruction of the cells with phagocytosis and removal of the cell products and specific pigment—neuromelanin. Many of the remaining cells are shrunken, and some are vacuolated. In other cells of these nuclei, including the hypothalamus, a coarse thickening of the neurofibrils (neurofibrillary tangles) may be visible with the routine hematoxylin and eosin stain (Fig. 44-40) and with Congo red and polarized light. Some cells may contain single or multiple cytoplasmic, spherical, hyaline, eosinophilic inclusions with dark centers; these are Lewy bodies (Fig. 44-41). Mild to moderate degrees of reactive astrocytosis often are present in the affected regions. In patients younger than 60 years the presence of general brain atrophy and Lewy bodies is more characteristic of the idiopathic type (paralysis agitans), whereas Alzheimer's neurofibrillary changes and disseminated focal astrocytic scars are more suggestive of the inflammatory variety. These distinctions are far less clear in older patients.[42]

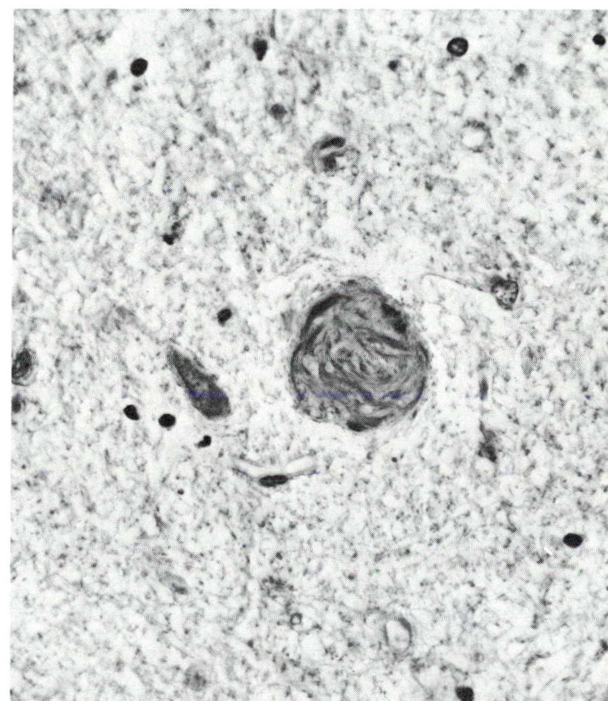

Fig. 44-40. Neurofibrillary change in cell of locus ceruleus in patient with parkinsonism. (Hematoxylin and eosin; 600×.)

Other lesions, not generally accepted, have been described in patients with either type of parkinsonism.[34] These include loss of the large cells of the caudate nuclei and putamina and "perivascular degeneration" of the outer segments of the globus pallidus with pallor from loss of myelinated fibers.

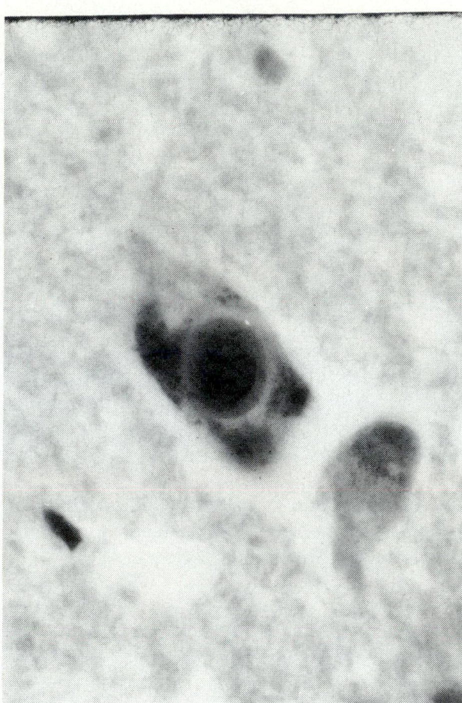

Fig. 44-41. Lewy body in cell of substantia nigra in patient with parkinsonism. (Hematoxylin and eosin; 1100×.)

In patients with parkinsonism from other causes, the lesions are generally widespread with the additional involvement of the substantia nigra.

Among the Chamorros in the Mariana Islands, parkinsonism often is associated with dementia or amyotrophic lateral sclerosis or both. These patients have a loss of pigmented cells, no Lewy bodies, many neurofibrillary tangles, frontal and temporal lobe atrophy, and, in some, microscopic changes characteristic of motor neuron disease. The disease may be the result of a "slow virus" infection.

Motor neuron disease (amyotrophic lateral sclerosis)[12,16,62,85]

The motor neuron diseases primarily if not exclusively affect the pyramidal (motor) system. Their clinical and structural variants are dependent on the motor level initially and predominantly involved. Although amyotrophic lateral sclerosis denotes the entire group, it also has been used to describe the variant in which the principal level of involvement is of the cells of the motor cortex and anterior horn cells of the spinal cord. In progressive bulbar palsy the most significant lesions are in the motor cranial nuclei. The anterior horn cells are primarily affected in the type known as progressive (spinal) muscular atrophy. When the lesions are confined to the lateral and anterior corticospinal tracts with little or no recognizable change in the motor cortex, the disease is considered by some to represent primary lateral sclerosis. One of the many causes of the "floppy infant" is infantile progressive spinal muscular atrophy (Werdnig-Hoffmann disease, amyotonia congenita, Oppenheim's disease). It has the microscopic atrophy and progressive bulbar palsy.

The unitarian concept of this group of diseases is suggested by the simultaneous involvement, often clinically and regularly at microscopy, of two or more levels of the motor system. Motor neuron disease has been classified among the abiotrophic conditions of the central nervous system. These are diseases in which genetic factors are considered to result in the gradual and premature death of the cells ordinarily destined to live many more years. This may account for the approximately 6% to 10% familial incidence of the adult form of this disease and the generally accepted autosomal recessive heredity of the infantile form. The initial degenerative change occurs in the most peripheral part of the longest cell process. With progression there is retrograde deterioration toward the cell body. It recently has been suggested that the disease may be caused by a slow virus, that is, one with an incubation period of years. It is assumed that the effect of the as yet unidentified virus is to gradually produce a change in the cell identical to that of the abiotrophic state. Previous suggestions of a host of other causes of motor neuron disease such as toxins, syphilis, and trauma have not been substantiated.

The gross appearance of the brain and spinal cord is usually not helpful for diagnosis. In a few cases there may be slight to moderate atrophy of the motor cortex, gray-white change in the lateral corticospinal tracts, or a decrease in size of the ventral roots at the lumbar and cervical levels of the spinal cord. The last is difficult to evalute because of the normally great variation in size of these roots.

Amyotrophic lateral sclerosis, the most common of the motor neuron diseases, is usually most easily recognized on microscopic examination (with special stains for axons and myelin) by the presence of axonal and myelin degeneration symmetrically affecting the motor tracts. This change is seen at all levels of the spinal cord and may be traced upward in the pyramidal system, usually easily as far as the pons and sometimes as far as the internal capsule. Degeneration of the myelin and axons in the internal capsule is recognizable in less than one third of the patients. Only an occasional lipid-containing macrophage and a few perivascular lymphocytes are found at any level. This suggests the very gradual progression of the disease rather than its inactivity. Neuronophagia of the cells of the motor cortex usually is not prominent and often may go unnoticed. There is simultaneous and similar involvement of the anterior horn cells and their processes.

With progressive bulbar palsy, there are degeneration, neuronophagia, and loss of the cells of the cranial motor nuclei with a reactive astrocytosis in these areas. The nuclei most frequently and severely affected, in descending order, are the hypoglossal nuclei, the nuclei ambigui, and the motor nuclei of the seventh and fifth nerves.

In spinal muscular atrophy there are severe loss of anterior horn cells and usually much reactive astrocytosis. Neuronophagia is not prominent, probably because the disease at this level is most prolonged. Axonal degeneration, evident in the ventral rootlets, corresponds to the anterior horn cells involved. Neurogenic atrophy is seen in the muscles innervated by the affected anterior horn cells.

The lesions in infantile progressive muscular atrophy involve loss or absence of the cells of the anterior horns of the spinal cord and the cranial motor nerve nuclei. The affected muscles have small fibers of the "fetal" or atrophic types.

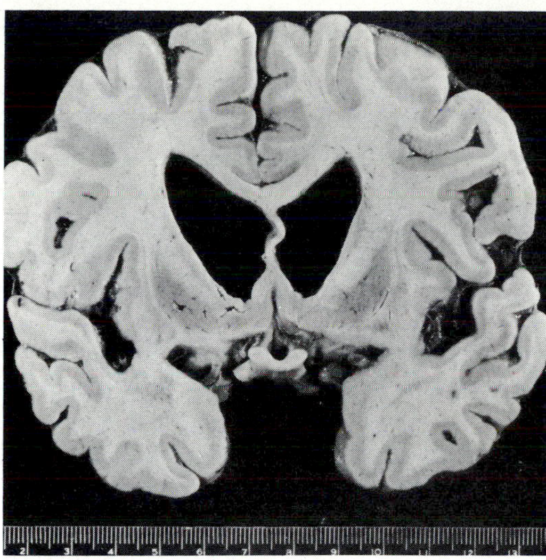

Fig. 44-42. Huntington's disease. Atrophy of caudate nuclei and putamina is diagnostic. Cortical atrophy is moderate. There is compensatory internal and external hydrocephalus.

Huntington's disease

Huntington's disease is a disorder with dominant inheritance. Its late clinical onset, rare before the end of the second decade, allows the patient to have a large family before there is significant mental deterioration or choreiform movements. The disease is slowly progressive with a long period of dementia.

The brain is moderately to greatly atrophic, particularly the frontal and temporal gyri. There is a sharp decrease in size of the caudate nuclei and the putamina and some decrease in size of the corpus callosum (Fig. 44-42). Compensatory internal and external hydrocephalus is characteristic. The changes in the caudate nuclei and putamina are caused by a great loss of their small nerve cells, usually with a pronounced reactive astrocytosis.[5] In the atrophic cerebral cortex the nerve cell loss and the reactive astrocytosis are more prominent in the third cortical layer.

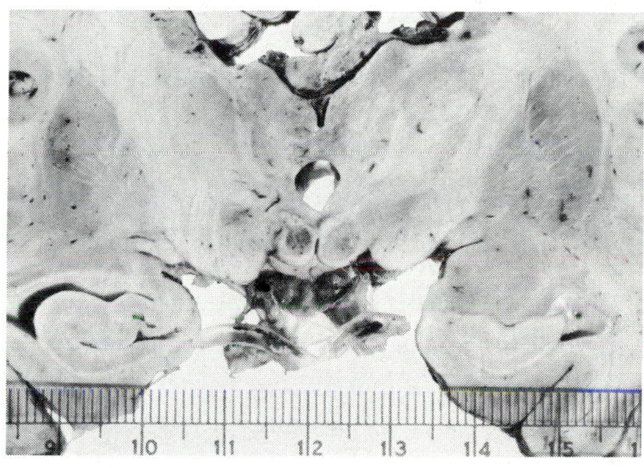

Fig. 44-43. Acute Wernicke's disease with involvement of mamillary bodies, hypothalami, and thalami.

Deficiency diseases

Wernicke's polioencephalopathy[109]

Like beriberi, Wernicke's syndrome is caused by a deficiency of vitamin B_1. Characteristically occurring in chronic alcoholics, it also has been found in persons with a variety of debilitating diseases in whom the diet consisted primarily of carbohydrates. The principal lesions, in decreasing order of frequency, involve the mamillary bodies, the gray matter of the hypothalami and thalami immediately surrounding the third ventricle (Fig. 44-43), the periaqueductal gray matter, and the floor and sometimes the roof of the fourth ventricle. Petechial hemorrhages in these regions, and from which the disease derived its original name (polioencephalitis hemorrhagica superior and inferior), may be absent or insignificant and are more likely the result than the cause of the initial lesions.

The early lesion is accompanied by decreased eosinophilia and granularity of the intercellular substance with loss of oligodendroglia and myelin in the affected sites. There is activation of the microglia with the formation of lipophages. The resultant vascular dilatation leads to engorgement, some endothelial hypertrophy and hyperplasia, and variable numbers of petechiae. A mild reactive astrocytosis is seen in the older lesions. Neurons in the affected regions are surprisingly little altered. A few may be shrunken, and a few may show eosinophilic homogenization. If death does not occur and therapy is adequate, the lesions become inactive. The areas affected, particularly the mamillary bodies, collapse and become browner than normal. At this stage, which is associated with the clinical state known as Korsakoff's syndrome, there are staining pallor, loosening of the tissues, increased lipofuscin in the nerve cells, and occasionally a few hemosiderophages.

Subacute necrotizing encephalomyelopathy (Leigh's disease)[46,57]

First described as limited to infants, subacute necrotizing encephalomyelopathy has also been reported in children and adults.[34,115] The necrotic lesions with a pronounced infiltration of lipophages are characteristically bilaterally symmetric. They involve the hypothalamus, the periaqueductal gray matter, the tegmental portion of the pons, and infrequently the mamillary bodies. The medulla and spinal cord sometimes are also involved.

The disease is presumed to be a genetically controlled metabolic defect. Because of the structural similarity to Wernicke's encephalopathy, it has been suggested that this defect involves the utilization of thiamin or a derivative.

Pellagra

Inadequate amounts of nicotinic acid in the diet can result in pellagra. The characteristic light-sensitive dermatitis and diarrhea may be accompanied or, as is more usual, followed by disorders of mentation and even of movement.

There are usually no gross changes in the central nervous system. Microscopically, many neurons at all levels of the central nervous system have the appearance characteristic of central chromatolysis with some increase in lipofuscin. There is little recognizable degeneration of the axons.

Posterolateral sclerosis (subacute combined degeneration of spinal cord)[108]

Pernicious anemia of the addisonian type and its neurologic associations are caused by a deficiency of vitamin B_{12}. The anemia may be accompanied, followed, or preceded by changes in the posterior and lateral columns of the spinal cord. The spinal cord lesions can also be seen in patients with sprue, with gastric cancer, after gastrectomy, or with folate deficiency. The spinal cord, usually of normal size, may be slightly small in circumference, with pallor and softening of the posterior columns. On microscopic examination, there is loss of myelin and oligodendroglia and of axons in the posterior and lateral columns. The early lesions may contain many lipophages. The later lesions are characteristically spongy, with almost complete absence of a reactive astrocytosis (Fig. 44-44). Moderate loss of nerve cells in the cerebral cortex with areas of degeneration of the white matter has been described.

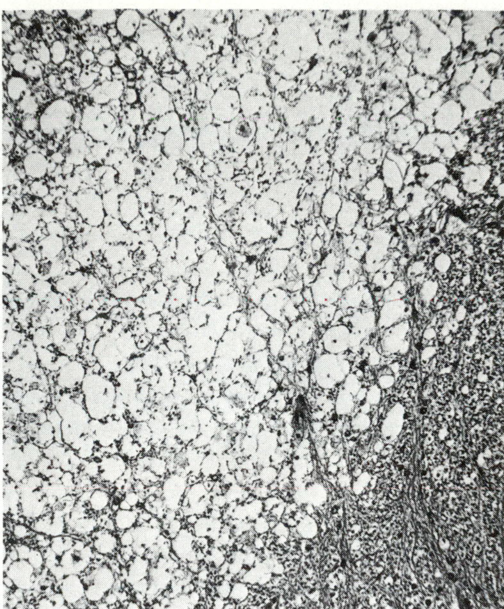

Fig. 44-44. Vacuolated appearance of fasciculus gracilis in patient with vitamin B_{12} deficiency. (Hematoxylin and eosin; 90×.)

Neuronal lipid-storage diseases[11,125]

The neuronal lipid-storage diseases are a group of rare disturbances of lipid metabolism caused by enzyme deficiencies that sometimes can be diagnosed ante mortem because of nerve cell involvement seen on brain, rectal, jejunal, or muscle biopsy and by enzyme assays of circulating leukocytes, serum, cultured fibroblasts, or amniotic cells obtained by amniocentesis,[98] and by examination of the urine.[36] The group includes Tay-Sachs disease, Batten's disease, Sandhoff's disease, Gaucher's disease, Niemann-Pick disease, Fabry's disease, and others.

Amaurotic familial idiocy

Tay-Sachs disease, the best known of this group, is a rare autosomally recessive disorder manifested by the intraneuronal accumulation of GM_2 ganglioside resulting from the deficiency of hexosaminidase A. Small amounts of the ganglioside without morphologic change in the cells can be found in other organs.

Because of slight enzymatic differences there are several variations of amaurotic familial idiocy. Most instances are of the infantile form (Tay-Sachs disease), with congenital, late infantile, juvenile, and adult forms having been described.

Early enlargement of the brain is followed by a decrease in size as the disease progresses. The larger nerve cells at all levels, including Purkinje's cells and the anterior horn cells of the spinal cord, are distended with Oil red positive, GM_2 ganglioside. As the intracytoplasmic material accumulates, the Nissl substance is gradu-

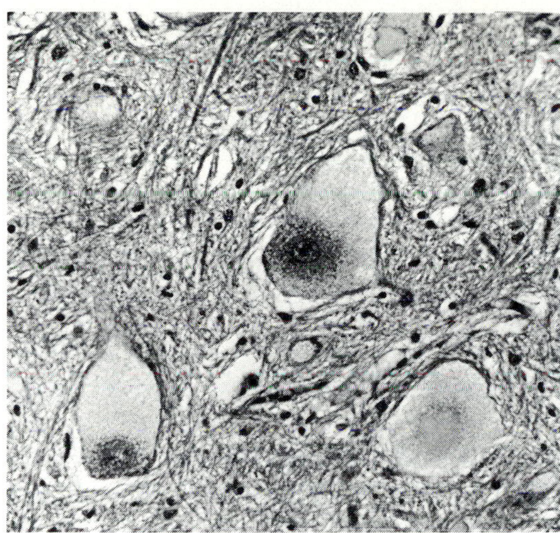

Fig. 44-45. Anterior horn cells in Tay-Sachs disease. Displacement of nucleus and Nissl substance are attributed to accumulation of ganglioside. (Hematoxylin and eosin; 280×.)

ally displaced to a small zone around the nucleus (Fig. 44-45). The material also is to be found enlarging the cell processes. Nonspecific lipid-containing macrophages can be found in the affected central nervous system and in the leptomeninges. There is a moderate reactive astrocytosis in the older lesions.

With electron microscopy, the accumulated lipid is represented by concentrically laminated ovoid bodies (membranous cytoplasmic bodies). These bodies, because of their marked acid phosphatase content, are thought to be derived from lysosomes. Membranous cytoplasmic bodies are present in Sandhoff's disease (hexosaminidase A and B deficiency) and in generalized gangliosidosis (beta-galactosidase deficency).

Since none of the morphologic changes is specific, it is essential that the enzyme deficiency be ascertained.

Niemann-Pick disease

In Niemann-Pick disease, nerve cells and the cells of the reticuloendothelial system and liver are distended with sphingomyelin. The similarity between nerve cells bloated with this stored material and nerve cells in the other lipid-storage diseases makes structural separation impossible. Although involvement of the liver and the reticuloendothelial system is helpful in differentiation, the absence of the enzyme sphingomyelinase is definitive (see p. 1261).

Ceroid lipofuscinosis

A morphologically similar but unrelated disease is ceroid lipofuscinosis. Here the materials that accumulate are ceroid and lipofuscin in varying amounts. With electron microscopy, these resemble fingerprints. The enzyme deficiency is unknown.

Gaucher's disease

The accumulation of a cerebroside (protein-bound glycolipid) is regularly seen in the perikaryon of nerve cells in patients with Gaucher's disease. The enzymatic defect is of beta-glucocerebrosidase. The material is periodic acid–Schiff positive. With routine stains the nerve cells appear vacuolated. Involvement of the reticuloendothelial system is described elsewhere (p. 1260).

Mucopolysaccharidoses

The mucopolysaccharidoses are a group of diseases characterized by the accumulation of various mucopolysaccharides in many nerve cells and tissues and cells of the reticuloendothelial system and by the urinary excretion of the affected mucopolysaccharides.

In gargoylism the material that accumulates in many nerve cells, in reticuloendothelial macrophages, and in bone and cartilage cells is a mucopolysaccharide. The mucopolysaccharidoses are either sex linked (Hunter's syndrome) or autosomally inherited (Hurler's syndrome, Sanfilippo's syndrome, Morquio's syndrome, Scheie's syndrome, Maroteaux-Lamy syndrome), and are attributable to the absence of one or more of a group of enzymes that degrade mucopolysaccharides (see p. 1758).

Accumulation of the material in the leptomeninges, the cause of their cloudy appearance, may also be the reason for the occasional occurrence of hydrocephalus. As with the lipoidoses, the material that accumulates distends the nerve cells with displacement of their nuclei and Nissl substance. The presence of zebra bodies and of membranous cytoplasmic bodies as detected by electron microscopy are again not specific. Since the same mucopolysaccharide may be present in several of the mucopolysaccharidoses and because the enzyme deficiencies are not known to occur in all, the entire constellation of chemical, biochemical, and morphologic characteristics is necessary before an accurate evaluation is possible.

Metabolic disturbances

Wilson's disease (hepatolenticular degeneration)

Wilson's disease is believed to be caused, at least in part, by an absence or insufficiency of the serum alpha globulin ceruloplasmin, which binds the serum copper. As a result, the bound and total serum copper levels are low, and free copper is deposited in the putamina and striate bodies, in Descemet's membrane of the eye, and in the liver. There is often an aminoaciduria, presumably as a result of renal tubular disease. In over half the patients, the disease is apparently inherited through a rare recessive gene (see p. 1164).

The brain is usually atrophic. There may be no grossly visible changes. In some cases there is softening with brown discoloration of the striate areas. On microscopic examination there is often a pronounced astrocytosis with type I and II Alzheimer's astrocytes in the central gray matter of the cerebral hemispheres. Large oval cells with small nuclei, the Opalski cells, sometimes are found in these same areas. The patients have a nodular cirrhosis and the brown Kayser-Fleischer rings of deposited copper at the margins of the corneas.

Amino acid disturbances

Several rare disorders of amino acid metabolism have been described. Among these is phenylketonuria (phenylpyruvic oligophrenia) caused by the lack of phenylalanine hydrolase, an enzyme that converts phenylalanine to tyrosine. Consequently, phenylalanine accumulates in the tissues, blood, and cerebrospinal fluid while phenylpyruvic acid, the deaminated by-product of phenylalanine, is excreted in the urine. Characteristic structural changes in the central nervous system have not been described in this recessively inherited condition. Hartnup disease is ascribed to a defect in the conversion of tryptophan to nicotinic acid. The central nervous system changes in this familial disease resemble those of pellagra (see p. 1898). Large amounts of 3-indolylacetic acid and indolylacetyl glutamine are excreted in the urine. Affected children have a pellagra-like skin rash, cerebellar ataxia, nystagmus, and sometimes dementia. Maple syrup urine disease is ascribed to an enzymatic deficiency that results in the accumulation in the tissues of the branched-chain alpha-keto acid derivatives of isoleucine, leucine, and valine; their excretion in the urine imparts the characteristic odor. The disease is familial. Structural changes in the nervous system have not been recorded.

Kernicterus (nuclear jaundice)[60]

Abnormally high concentrations of lipid-soluble, indirect-reacting bile pigments may discolor the globi pallidi, subthalamic nuclei, hippocampi, dentate nuclei, and inferior olivary nuclei in the newborn, especially when immature. The cerebral and cerebellar cortices and cochlear nuclei are less regularly affected. The high concentrations of bile pigment are most frequently attributed to severe hemolytic disease of the infant resulting from the presence of maternal antibodies, usually anti-D, but sometimes to an ABO incompatibility or to structural defects in erythrocytes leading to increased hemolysis. A further increase in the serum level of the indirect-reacting bile pigment in the immature infant is attributed, in part, to an initial liver deficiency of glucuronyl transferase. The presence of a low serum level of albumin, to which the indirect-reacting pigment ordinarily forms a loose attachment, permits the pigment to enter the tissues more easily. Although a serum level of indirect-reacting bile pigment of 18 to 20 mg/dl is considered critical, all factors must be considered. Nuclear jaundice has also been recorded in congenital familial nonhemolytic jaundice of the Crigler-Najjar type. Localization of the pigment deposits in the nuclear areas has been ascribed to focal immaturity of the blood-brain barrier and to previous hypoxic damage to the nerve cells in these areas; structural changes are variable. In many of the pigmented areas (subthalamic nucleus, globus pallidus, and hippocampus), the affected nerve cells have undergone severe ischemic changes and mineralization of their Golgi apparatus; the stained cells of the dentate nuclei and inferior olives may show little change.

Some surviving children, although actively treated, later manifest signs and symptoms resulting from damage and loss of many cells in the affected nuclei (see also p. 1156).

Epilepsy

Epilepsy is an abnormal functional state of the central nervous system that is characterized by uncontrolled outbursts of nerve cell activity and clinically by convulsive seizures with or without loss of consciousness or by their equivalents. In the idiopathic (primary or essential) form, the only structural changes are those related to hypoxia, which accompanies the attacks. The secondary (symptomatic) form of epilepsy has been associated with a great variety of diseases that affect the central nervous system. Loss of cells in Sommer's sector of the hippocampus with a reactive astrocytosis may be seen in both forms and in patients without epilepsy. In severe epilepsy with repeated and frequent attacks, there is usually other evidence of anoxic changes, including laminar cell loss in the cerebral cortex (third through fifth layers), especially in the cortex that lies in the depths of the sulci. Loss of Purkinje's cells, especially in the depths of the folia, is a common structural evidence of any hypoxic state, including that which accompanies epileptic seizures.

A special form of epilepsy, myoclonus (inclusion body) epilepsy, is a rare disease of unknown cause in which spherical intracytoplasmic basophilic inclusions (Lafora bodies) are found in the larger nerve cells of the cerebral cortex and the subcortical gray matter, the brainstem, and the subcortical nuclei of the cerebellum, as well as in myocardial fibers and liver cells (particularly those at the periphery of the lobules).

Inflammation

Inflammations of the brain and spinal cord generally are complications of similar inflammations elsewhere in the body. Normally the central nervous system is afforded great protection by the surrounding covering structures and by the actions of the blood-brain barrier. Once these defenses are breached, the resistance to infection is less than in most other organs of the body. There are four general routes by which pathogenic organisms may reach the central nervous system:

1. The most frequently utilized route is that of the blood vessels. Most intravascular spread to the central nervous system is by way of the arteries, the organisms usually having first produced disease of the lungs or heart valves. Less often, organisms reach the central nervous system through emissary or diploic veins as a component of a retrograde thrombophlebitis or embolus draining adjacent infections, or from distant structures. The paravertebral venous system is rarely implicated.
2. Infections of the mastoid sinuses, middle ears, paranasal sinuses, skull, and vertebra may extend directly to involve the brain or spinal cord or their coverings.
3. Organisms, chemical toxins, or even particulate materials may be directly implanted on the coverings or within the central nervous system as a result of gunshot wounds, mechanical trauma, or medical procedures, including surgery and lumbar puncture.
4. Certain viruses, including rabies and possibly herpes simplex and zoster, once implanted within the axoplasm of a peripheral nerve, can, by centripetal movement within the cell cytoplasm and perhaps through the neurotubules, reach the perikaryon within the spinal ganglia, spinal cord, or brain.

Once within the central nervous system, further dissemination of the infection may proceed by direct continuity or by way of the fluid within the ventricular, subarachnoid, or Virchow-Robin spaces in the usual direction of flow, retrograde, or both.

Inflammations of the central nervous system are classified according to the site of involvement and the type of exudate.

Meningeal infections

Meningeal infections may be separated into those affecting the dura mater and those affecting the pia-arachnoid.

Pachymeningitis. Purulent infections of the dura are most frequently from *Streptococcus pneumoniae*, *Staphylococcus aureus*, and beta-hemolytic streptococci. These infections are characterized as external (epidural or extradural) when the inflammation involves the outer surface and internal (subdural) when the inner surface is affected.

In the skull, most instances of epidural infection are the result of extension from an adjacent infection of the paranasal or mastoid sinuses with the formation of a small epidural (subperiosteal) abscess. Over the spinal cord, these abscesses are usually a result of infections of the vertebra. Less frequently, they may follow retroperitoneal or retropleural infections with extension to the epidural space through an intervertebral foramen. The epidural abscess of the spinal cord tends to become larger than that of the skull because the spinal dura is separate from the periosteum and the intervening tissues offer little mechanical resistance to spread. The prognosis is good in either of the abscesses only if the lesion is treated early and adequately.

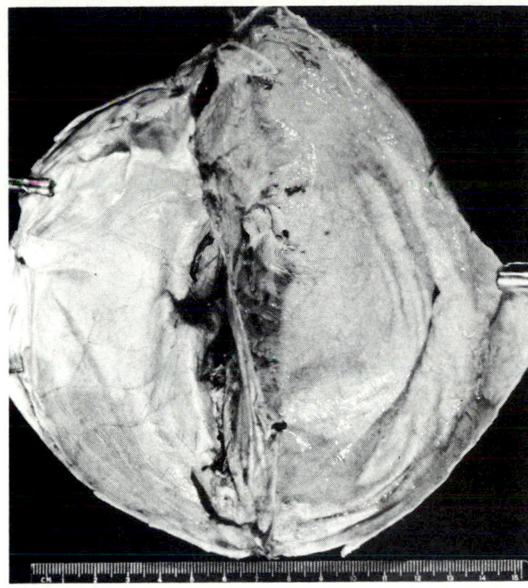

Fig. 44-46. Unilateral acute subdural empyema resulting from frontal sinusitis.

Purulent subdural infections (subdural empyema, subdural abscess) (Fig. 44-46), like their epidural counterparts, are most often complications of adjacent infections and occur with or without epidural infections. The organisms may bypass the external dura by extending through a dural sinus and bridging vein into the subdural space or may be spread there by eroding the dura locally, or it may be a complication of an infection in the subarachnoid space. Once in the subdural space, continued spread over the brain unilaterally is rapid, and it frequently becomes bilateral. The rare purulent spinal subdural infection is most likely to lie over the lower portion of the spinal cord and cauda equina. Reaction to the infection at both levels, at least initially, is from the vascular inner portion of the dura. There is no contribution from the arachnoid. Attempts to localize the infection by the formation of vascular pyogenic granulation tissue are late and generally inadequate. The tendency of the exudate and organisms to disseminate widely through the subdural space, to compress the underlying nervous system, and to spread to the subarachnoid space contributes to the high mortality in this condition.

Leptomeningitis. Purulent infections of the leptomeninges (leptomeningitis, meningitis) are seen with an ever-increasing variety of bacteria. At present, the most common in adults are *Streptococcus pneumoniae, Staphylococcus aureus,* beta-hemolytic streptococci, and meningococcus *(Neisseria meningitidis),* whereas in children the most common causative organisms are *Haemophilus influenzae* and *Escherichia coli*. Almost all of the routes of invasion described earlier are utilized. The bacteria may reach the subarachnoid space through the arteries by exiting from the small thin-walled arteries in the subarachnoid space or indirectly after exiting from the choroid plexuses into the ventricles. Contiguous paranasal and sinus infections are frequent sources. In any leptomeningitis, the source should be identified and that lesion treated as well as the infection of the central nervous system.

Early, the brain is variably swollen and its vessels are engorged. When the patient has died quickly, as some do with a fulminant meningococcemia, little or no exudate may be visible macroscopically. The earliest exudate that can be seen is recognizable first as thin gray streaks paralleling the lateral margins of superficial veins that lie over the sulci. The exudate soon becomes more diffuse, thick, gray, and often slightly green. Initially, it fills the sulci and later overlies and obscures the gyri (Fig. 44-47); finally the cisterns become filled. Later the exudate tends to concentrate in the subarachnoid space to either side of the superior sagittal sinus, with lesser amounts toward the base of the brain. Over the spinal cord, the exudate covering the posterior aspect is greatest in amount at the thoracic level, probably because of gravity in the relatively immobile patient lying recumbent.

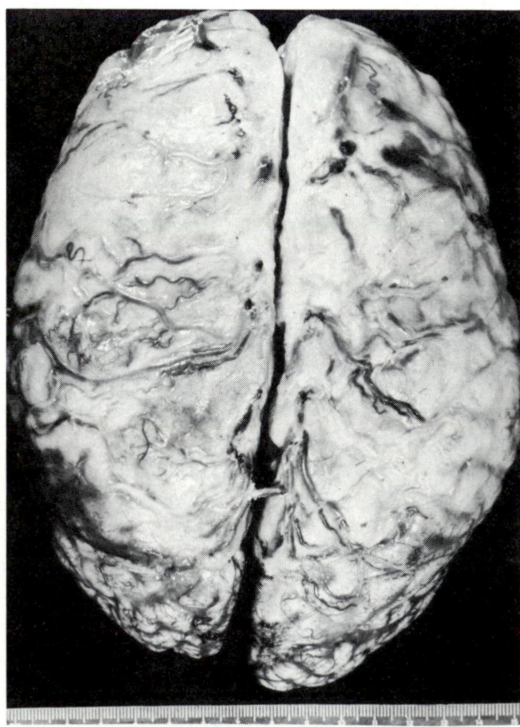

Fig. 44-47. Severe acute purulent leptomeningitis with thrombophlebitis.

When there has been little or no visible exudate macroscopically, sections from multiple areas or of rolls of leptomeninges covering all or portions of a hemisphere may contain only a few neutrophils, usually in small clusters. In the usual fatal case in which the infection had been present for 24 hours or more, the exudate is characterized initially by an extensive neutrophilic infiltration concentrated about the blood vessels (Fig. 44-48). The exudate later becomes more diffuse and is accompanied by increasing amounts of fibrin. With a Gram stain, both free and phagocytosed organisms may be found. As the disease progresses and there is evidence of response to therapy, the exudate gradually changes to one in which the predominant cell types are lymphocytes, monocytes, and, finally, mononuclear macrophages. In the fatal cases and, presumably to a lesser extent, in patients who recover, toxic effects of the leptomeningeal disease result in a reactive astrocytosis in the molecular layer (first layer) of the cortex with shrinkage and hyperchromatism of some of the superficial nerve cells in the second and third cortical layers. With uncomplicated recovery the exudate disappears, apparently by exiting into the dural venous sinuses through the arachnoid villi and, possibly, by entering some of the thinner-walled leptomeningeal veins. No structural residua may be seen in patients treated early and adequately. In most, however, organization of the exudate goes on to fibrosis, patchy or diffuse.

Thrombophlebitis involving several or many veins,

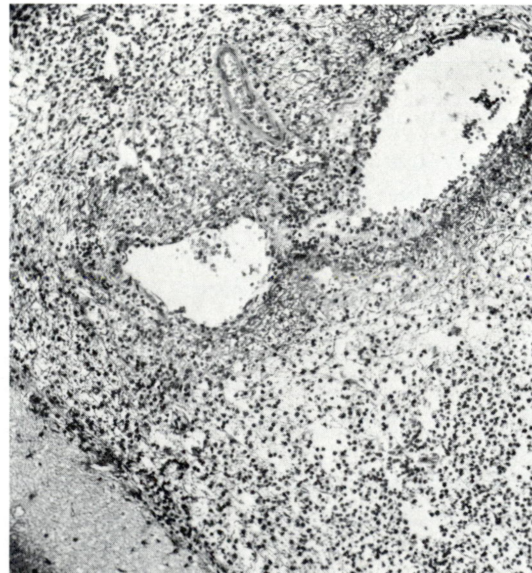

Fig. 44-48. Acute fibrinopurulent leptomeningitis with numerous neutrophils and some fibrin. (Hematoxylin and eosin; 90×.)

particularly those draining the parasagittal portions of the cerebral hemispheres, occurs in some patients. The occurrence of an arteritis or thromboarteritis is less common. Small cortical and subcortical hemorrhagic or anemic infarcts are the usual sequelae of these vascular complications. When the infarcts are of significant number and size and are situated at functionally important sites, they are manifest by a variety of clinical complications. In some patients the subarachnoid infection may extend into the brain along the Virchow-Robin spaces or in veins as a retrograde thrombophlebitis and result in the formation of one or more brain abscesses. Retrograde extension from the subarachnoid space through the lateral recesses of the fourth ventricle reaching the ventricular system then produces an inflammation of the ependyma and choroid plexus, initially of the fourth and later of the other ventricles. In these, the fibrinopurulent exudate covers the surfaces with areas of ependymal ulceration. Perivascular lymphocytic cuffs in the subependymal cell plate and of edema are evidence of further reaction to the inflammation. Not infrequently in children but rarely in adults, a unilateral or bilateral serous subdural effusion may overlie the purulent meningitis. A subdural empyema is now an infrequent complication.

As noted previously, small patches of leptomeningeal fibrosis frequently have been attributed to preexisting infections of the leptomeninges in which the exudate has been organized with the formation of a fibrous scar. These scars are significant when they are extensive or occur at critical areas in the path of cerebrospinal flow. An adhesive or constrictive band of scar tissue (adhesive or constrictive arachnoiditis) may be formed. Contraction of the scar can irritate the adjoining cells or destroy the encircled nervous system, including cranial nerves and spinal cord. A saclike leptomeningeal scar, by permitting the ingress of fluid and impeding its egress, can form the pocket for an enlarging subarachnoid cystic collection of fluid that compresses the underlying brain or spinal cord.

Brain abscess

As with the purulent leptomeningitides, the organisms producing an abscess can reach the brain through any of the routes previously described (see p. 1901) or as a complication of a purulent meningitis. Abscesses occurring after septic emboli are usually multiple and occur most frequently in the distribution areas of the middle cerebral arteries. When they are in the white matter, early there is sparing of the subcortical arcuate fibers. Both cerebral hemispheres are affected equally. An abscess whose source is a contiguous infection is usually single and more often involves the adjacent portion of the brain. Extension from the middle ear is to the ventrocaudal portion of the ipsilateral temporal lobe, whereas the abscess of mastoid origin is usually in the ipsilateral cerebellar hemisphere. Rarely, any of these infections may extend as a thrombophlebitis of a dural sinus to enter the brain at some point other than that adjacent to the original infection.

In its earliest stages, before abscess formation, the area is congested, edematous, soft, and with numerous petechiae; it is diffusely infiltrated with neutrophils. This is the stage known to clinicians as cerebritis. More intense neutrophilic infiltration with liquefaction necrosis rapidly ensues. Variable numbers of bacteria may lie free in the abscess or in neutrophils or in both. Without adequate therapy, there is continued enlargement and coalescence of abscesses, often with extension into the subarachnoid or ventricular cavities.

Adequate medical therapy decreases the local spread and the surrounding edema and swelling. Usually, inadequate amounts of vascular granulation tissue form about the abscess. The source of the granulation tissue is the mesenchymal cells in the walls of the blood vessels within the brain and adjoining leptomeninges and possibly the microglia. With treatment the neutrophils within the abscess gradually are replaced by lymphocytes, monocytes, and macrophages. The surrounding granulation and fibrous tissue remains thin and is surrounded by a narrow zone of reactive astrocytes and more peripherally by a moderately edematous and swollen brain in which there are perivascular lymphocytic cuffs. Although specific and intensive antibiotic therapy may have been given, a portion of the wall of almost every abscess, however chronic, shows evidence of continued enlargement with necrosis and often with the formation of satellite lesions (Fig. 44-49).

Granulomatous infections

Tuberculosis. The decreasing incidence of pulmonary tuberculosis, coupled with more adequate therapy, has made tuberculosis of the central nervous system relative-

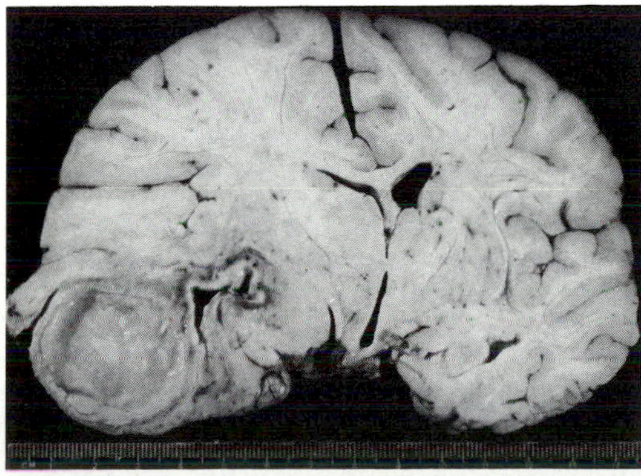

Fig. 44-49. Chronic brain abscesses in temporal lobe and insula. Surrounding brain shows swelling and edema. There are compression and displacement of lateral and third ventricles. Cingulate gyrus and uncal herniations are also present.

ly uncommon. Extension of a tuberculous infection from a vertebra to the epidural and subdural spaces is rare. A tuberculous leptomeningitis in children is most often a part of a generalized miliary infection. In adults the usual association is with pulmonary tuberculosis. The early report that a tuberculous leptomeningitis represents extension from an adjacent focus in the brain in at least 90% of the patients has not been substantiated. Many now believe that, as with purulent inflammations, the organisms enter the central nervous system from infections elsewhere in the body by way of the choroid plexuses or through the walls of the leptomeningeal vessels.

Early in tuberculous leptomeningitis, the exudate is usually scant, diffuse, and gray-white, sometimes with a faint green tinge. Later, 1 to 3 mm, discrete, gray nodules may be found, particularly along the course of the leptomeningeal blood vessels (Fig. 44-50). In patients with a relatively long history of tuberculous leptomeningitis, as with most granulomatous infections of the meninges, the exudate is more prominent at the base of the brain. The initial diffuse exudate is formed by lymphocytes, large mononuclear cells, serum and fibrin with small foci of caseation, and occasional neutrophils at sites of recent extension. The discrete nodules seen macroscopically consist of foci of caseation necrosis with fibrin surrounded by varying numbers of lymphocytes, plasma cells, and large mononuclear cells. Giant cells of Langhans' type are less frequent here than in other tissues (Fig. 44-51). Acid-fast bacilli may be numerous or rare. As with pyogenic infections, there may be spread along the ventricular system and into the brain along the Virchow-Robin spaces. Blood vessels within the leptomeningeal exudate have lymphocytes in their walls. They may exhibit a reactive, endothelial hypertrophy and hyperplasia, sometimes with thrombosis, leading to small anemic infarcts in the adjacent brain and spinal cord.

Early chemotherapy modifies the response and decreases the degree of fibrous tissue scarring. Because the exudate and the scars are more abundant at the base of the brain, they may significantly impede the flow of cerebrospinal fluid and thereby produce an obstructive internal hydrocephalus, and constriction of the scar may impair the function of one or more cranial nerves.

A tuberculous encephalitis usually is seen in one of two structural forms. In one there may be multiple granulomas all of about the same size (usually up to 1 cm). In the other there are a few (or one) that may reach a diameter of 5 to 6 cm, are solid, and have "growth rings" formed by the successive addition of layers of granulation tissue. The larger lesions are more common in the cerebellum.

Cryptococcosis. Cryptococcosis (caused by *Cryptococcus neoformans*, formerly *C. hominis*) of the central nervous system is a worldwide disease of increasing incidence. It is seen in patients with diabetes, in those who have undergone cardiac surgery, and in those who have received immunosuppressive treatment for a variety of diseases. The central nervous system disease is associated with infection of other organs, particularly the lungs, spleen, bone marrow, liver, and kidneys (see p. 390).

The leptomeninges and brain usually are involved simultaneously. The leptomeningeal exudate is variable in amount, clear to turbid, watery to gelatinous, and usually more prominent at the base of the brain and over the dorsal aspect of the thoracic portion of the spinal cord. Within the brain, especially in the gray matter, there may be many smooth-walled cavities from less than 1 mm to as much as 1 cm in diameter (Fig. 44-52). These are filled with fluid identical to that seen in the subarachnoid space. The ventricular system, particularly in the region

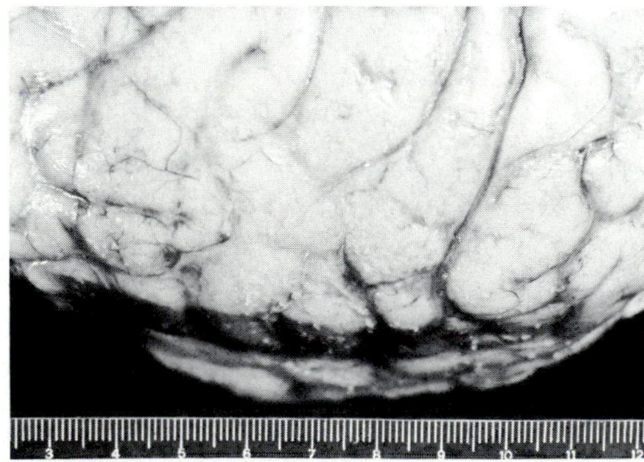

Fig. 44-50. Tuberculous leptomeningitis with numerous leptomeningeal tubercles.

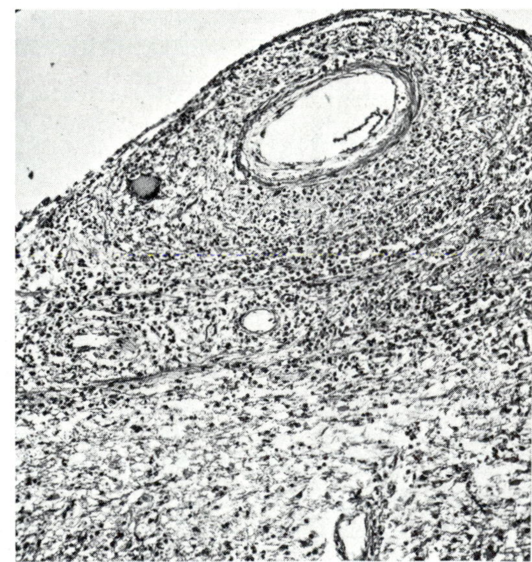

Fig. 44-51. Tuberculous leptomeningitis. Presence of Langhans' type of giant cell is unusual. (Hematoxylin and eosin; 90×.)

of the choroid plexuses, may contain the same type of exudate. The degree of cellular response is variable. In some areas, organisms may be present free in the subarachnoid and ventricular spaces or in the cystic cavities with almost no cell response. In other areas, particularly when the lesions have been present for a long time, there may be many lymphocytes, large mononuclear macrophages, some neutrophils and fibrin, and giant cells of both foreign body and Langhans' types. Characteristic organisms are usually easily found in all areas and in the lumbar cerebrospinal fluid. Mixed infections are sometimes seen.

Coccidioidomycosis. Coccidioidomycosis (caused by *Coccidioides immitis*) is an endemic disease of the southwestern United States. The central nervous system infection is always a complication of a disseminated disease, particularly that originating from an initial pulmonary infection (see p. 389).

The leptomeningeal exudate, although similar in many respects to that of tuberculosis, is usually more diffuse, more tenacious, and more abundant. The granulomas have a greater degree of central liquefaction. The infiltrates consist of mixtures of lymphocytes, neutrophils, plasma cells, large mononuclear cells, and giant cells of Langhans' type. Typical organisms are found in these cells as well as in the tissues.

Histoplasmosis and blastomycosis. Histoplasmosis (caused by *Histoplasma capsulatum*) and blastomycosis (caused by *Blastomyces dermatitidis*) are similar in that their involvement in the brain and spinal cord resembles tuberculosis. Both are associated with primary infection elsewhere in the body, most frequently of the respiratory tract.

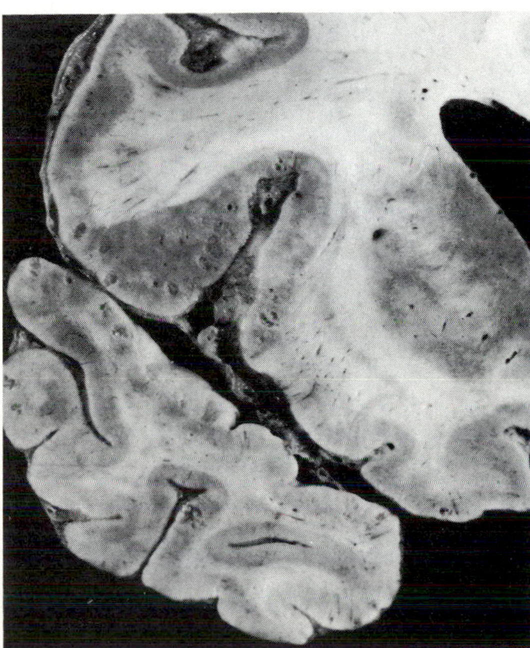

Fig. 44-52. Cryptococcosis with thin watery leptomeningeal exudate and many cortical cavities.

With histoplasmosis there is usually diffuse involvement of the reticuloendothelial system. In blastomycosis the skin and bones also are involved. In both the leptomeningeal exudate may be diffuse and gray with or without well-defined, firm, gray nodules. Similar nodules often are seen within the brain. The diffuse exudate consists of lymphocytes, large mononuclear cells, some plasma cells, and neutrophils embedded in a moderate amount of fibrin. The nodules are formed by lymphocytes and epithelioid and giant cells of both Langhans' and foreign body types, all surrounding a central core of necrotic debris. The organisms are found both free and in the large mononuclear and giant cells. Distinction between the two is sometimes difficult unless cultural studies are done (see pp. 387 and 394).

Actinomycosis. Actinomycotic infections of the central nervous system are rare. When they do occur, they are more likely caused by the acid-fast aerobe than by the non-acid-fast anaerobe. As with the other fungi, the central nervous system infection (usually abscess) is most frequently a complication of pulmonary disease and less frequently an extension from an adjacent infection. The cellular response is identical to that seen elsewhere in the body (see p. 382).

Neurosyphilis

The decreased incidence of syphilis of the central nervous system is the consequence of better control and of more adequate treatment during the early stages of the disease. Involvement of the central nervous system by the spirochete occurs during the secondary or the latent stage of the disease, always within the first 2 or 3 years of the infection.

Since syphilis may become inactive ("burned out") even without treatment both before and after meningeal spread, and because early meningeal involvement may be asymptomatic, the spinal fluid must be repeatedly examined for cells (lymphocytes), increase in proteins (globulin), and abnormal serologic findings. The symptomatic phase may resolve spontaneously or with treatment or may progress to a more advanced stage of neurosyphilis (see p. 1406).

Meningovascular syphilis. In the early stages of meningovascular syphilis there may be a cloudy gray exudate within the leptomeninges, usually more prominent at the base of the brain and, to a lesser extent, along the blood vessels over the cerebral convexities. Occasionally the cloudiness may be in patches or more diffuse. The characteristic exudate is composed primarily of lymphocytes, plasma cells, and large mononuclear cells, all with a tendency toward adventitial and perivascular concentration (Fig. 44-53). It is said that in about 5% of patients the disease begins as a severe acute meningitis.

In these the exudate is more abundant and the characteristic cellular infiltrate also contains neutrophils and fibrin. After adequate therapy and possibly spontaneously, the exudate becomes organized with patches or even extensive areas of fibrosis.

A significant part of the leptomeningeal infection is the accompanying involvement of the smaller arteries. In the more severe infections the inflammatory cells migrate into the media, separate the muscle fibers, split the internal elastic lamina, and stimulate a reactive intimal hyperplasia and endothelial hypertrophy (Heubner's endarteritis and panarteritis). These vascular changes, depending on the number of vessels and the degree and rapidity of involvement, can produce numerous small or large anemic infarcts.

General paresis (paretic dementia). General paresis is a form of progressive syphilitic meningoencephalitis. Adequate therapy only halts its progression. With the early or minimal lesion, no gross abnormalities may be recognized. Usually, however, there are patchy or diffuse thickening of the leptomeninges and cortical atrophy, often more noticeable over the frontal lobes. There may be a characteristic but nondiagnostic granularity of the ependyma lining the moderately enlarged ventricles. The floor of the fourth ventricle may have a thickened, gray appearance because of a highly characteristic, diffuse, astrocytic, glial proliferation.

The meningeal exudate is identical to that seen in syphilitic meningitis and usually is accompanied by the typical vasculitis. Within the brain, the lesions are more concentrated in the cerebral cortex and in the central gray matter than in the white matter. The intensity of the reactions roughly parallels the degree of overlying leptomeningeal involvement. The vessels within these areas and, to a lesser degree, those of the underlying white matter are surrounded by lymphocytes, plasma cells, and a few large mononuclear cells. Their walls are greatly thickened and their lumina narrowed because of endothelial hyperplasia and hypertrophy. As a result, many nerve cells are lost or in varying stages of ischemic change, and there are proliferation and rodlike elongation of the surrounding microglial cells. As the lesions undergo resolution and organization, they resemble microscopic infarcts with loss of cells, leading to focal collapse of the cortex, and distortion of the normal layering of the residual cells. There is a pronounced reactive astrocytosis. Iron-containing pigment in macrophages and in the walls of cortical blood vessels is highly characteristic of general paresis. In Lissauer's type of general paresis, there is an associated spongy destruction of the upper cortical layers and chromatolytic changes in some nerve cells of the fifth and sixth layers. In the untreated person, spirochetes may be found singly and in clusters about the blood vessels and in the cortex.

With treatment, demonstrable spirochetes rapidly disappear. The cellular exudate and the vascular changes decrease far more slowly. Leptomeningeal scars, the disseminated focal cortical atrophy and characteristic cortical disorganization, the ependymal granularity, the gliosis of the floor of the fourth ventricle, and the iron gran-

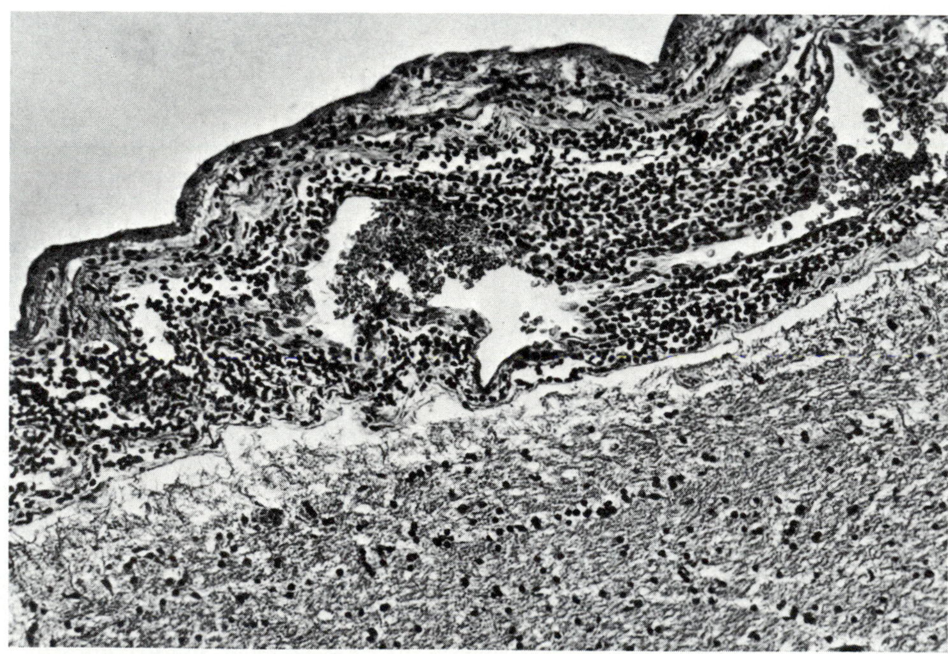

Fig. 44-53. Meningovascular syphilis. Lymphocytes and plasma cells are present in leptomeninges. (Hematoxylin and eosin; 180×.)

ules in macrophages and walls of the cortical blood vessels are the unalterable structural remnants of the disease.

Tabes dorsalis. The spinal cord in the patient with syphilis may be involved separately or in combination with the brain. Of the several patterns of spinal cord involvement, tabes dorsalis has been the most frequent. The exact site of syphilitic inflammation that results in degeneration of the fasciculi graciles and sometimes of the fasciculi cuneati and of the dorsal roots in unknown. One hypothesis suggests localization of the toxic effects of the spirochetes on the dorsal rootlets as they pass through the Obersteiner-Redlich area. The second assumes that there is involvement of the cells of the spinal ganglia and the fibers from these cells entering the spinal cord. In both hypotheses the caudalmost portion of the spinal cord is affected earliest and to the greatest degree.

The gross appearance of the spinal cord is characteristic but not diagnostic. The posterior columns are smaller than normal, often with dorsal concavity rather than convexity. Special stains reveal the absence of axons and myelin sheaths in the affected tracts. With tabes dorsalis the optic nerves are often similarly involved. The exact site of the lesion that produces the Argyll Robertson pupil seen in this disease is unknown.

The spinal cord may be affected in a variety of patterns that are less frequent and less characteristic of syphilis. These are attributed to differing localizations of lesions that extend into the cord from the leptomeninges and from variations in the sites of the vasculitis.

Toxoplasmosis[48,53]

A disease with worldwide distribution, toxoplasmosis is most often recognized in infants. It may, however, be the cause of a febrile or unsuspected disease in adults. The causative agent is the protozoan *Toxoplasma gondii*. The infant is infected in utero during the short period of parasitemia in the early stages of the disease in the mother, who may be asymptomatic. Fetal infection and damage are highest when maternal infection occurs during the first and second trimesters of pregnancy. Serologic test results become positive after the period of infectivity. Infections and clinical disease are increasing in incidence in adults treated with immunosuppressive drugs. Cats are considered to be the animal host.

The inflammatory aqueductal stenosis in infants results in an obstructive hydrocephalus (Fig. 44-54); microcephaly has been described in some newborns. There may be necrotic paraventricular basal ganglionic lesions that lead to mineralization often visible by x-ray examination. In adults there are multiple small areas of necrosis within the central portions of the brain. Involvement of the surface of the brain is associated with a focal chronic (lymphocytic) leptomeningitis. The ovoid organisms, which are 4 to 6 μm long and 2 μm wide, usually are found in clusters in the cytoplasm of a mononuclear macrophage. This is known as the pseudocyst (Fig. 44-55). The areas of necrosis in which the organisms are found and from which they may be cultured are surrounded by varying degrees of mononuclear cells and reactive astrocytosis.

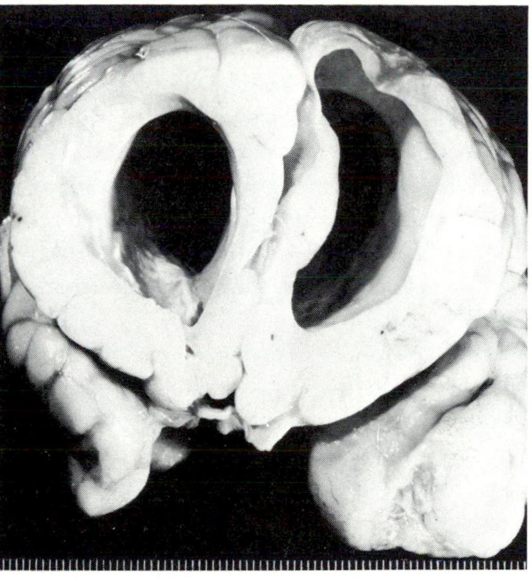

Fig. 44-54. Toxoplasmosis in 2-year-old child. There is conspicuous internal obstructive hydrocephalus with numerous subependymal calcifications.

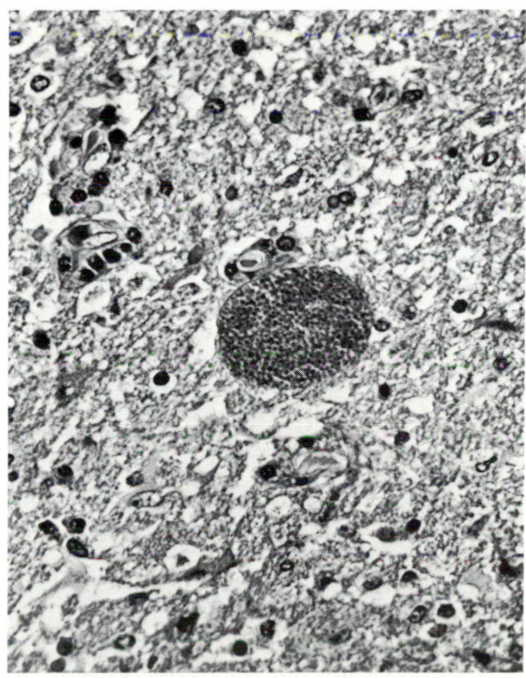

Fig. 44-55. Toxoplasmosis in adult with multiple myeloma. "Cyst" formation contains many organisms. (Hematoxylin and eosin; 370×.)

In infants other organs such as the eye or the myocardium often are affected as well. In adults the lungs and lymph nodes usually are involved.

Rickettsial encephalitides

Focal collections of a few neutrophils with lymphocytes and mononuclear macrophages in and about the walls of the smaller blood vessels in the brain are known as typhus nodules and are the characteristic but not diagnostic lesions in the rickettsial diseases (Fig. 44-56). Hypertrophy and hyperplasia of the endothelial cells result from the intraendothelial multiplication of the rickettsias. These are the lesions characteristic of typhus fever caused by *Rickettsia prowazekii* (see p. 340).

In Rocky Mountain spotted fever caused by *R. rickettsii*, the inflammatory and vascular changes are usually more severe, whereas in scrub typhus caused by *R. orientalis*, the vascular lesions are fewer and less severe.

Viral infections[40,52,61,71]

Human viral infections were expected to almost disappear with the use of the poliomyelitis vaccines. This has not occurred. Increased numbers of mild, severe, and fatal encephalitides caused by other viruses are now recognized. The basic similarities of the structural changes in the central nervous system in all viral diseases are ascribed to the obligate intracellular position of the viruses.

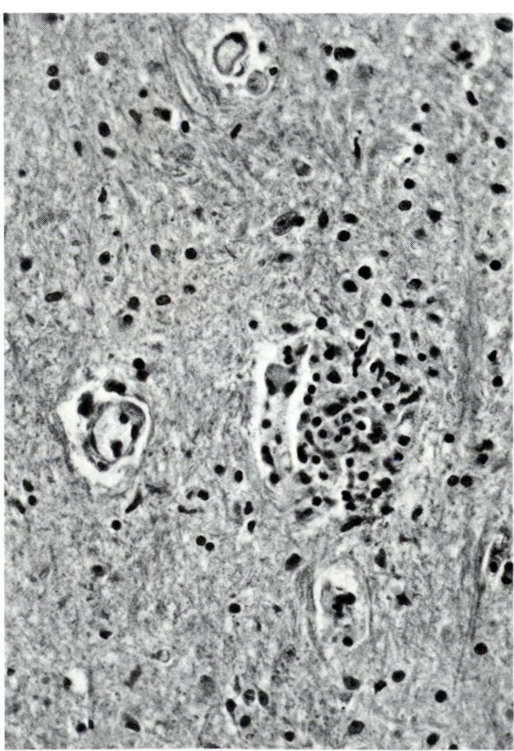

Fig. 44-56. Nodule of lymphocytes and mononuclear cells about wall of capillary in patient with scrub typhus. (Hematoxylin and eosin; 280×.)

When the injury is recent or mild, the infected nerve cells become slightly swollen, later to undergo shrinkage with neuronophagia by surrounding mononuclear cells. The later changes are accompanied by a perivascular inflammatory cell infiltrate, which initially and transiently may be neutrophilic. Later and more characteristically the cellular infiltrates are composed of lymphocytes, some plasma cells, and large mononuclear cells and macrophages (Fig. 44-57). Variations in this pattern depend on the locations of the cells, including glial as well as nerve cells, that are affected and the degree of necrosis of cells and surrounding tissues. In some of the viral infections, intranuclear or intracytoplasmic inclusion bodies may be formed within nerve and glial cells. Cowdry type A intranuclear inclusions (Fig. 44-58) may be found in the encephalitides caused by the measles virus, herpes simplex, cytomegalic inclusion disease, and herpes zoster. The relationship of Cowdry type B inclusion bodies to viral diseases is uncertain.

When the infection is limited to nerve cells, the central nervous system grossly may appear unchanged or focally or diffusely engorged. With a necrotizing encephalitis that includes destruction of white and gray matter, the nervous system early is enlarged, swollen, and engorged. The areas of necrosis that follow may be small and scattered or large, extending beyond the boundaries of an area supplied by a single or several blood vessels. In addition to the usual cellular infiltrate, there may be a pronounced reactive astrocytosis and a lesser gliosis.

Acute poliomyelitis (infantile paralysis). The sharp decrease in incidence of acute poliomyelitis in the past several years is one of the triumphs of medicine. Poliomyelitis is considered here because it is a prototype of the viral diseases. Formerly, it occurred both sporadically and more frequently in epidemics during the summer and autumn. The enterovirus enters the body through the gastrointestinal tract, from which, by way of the

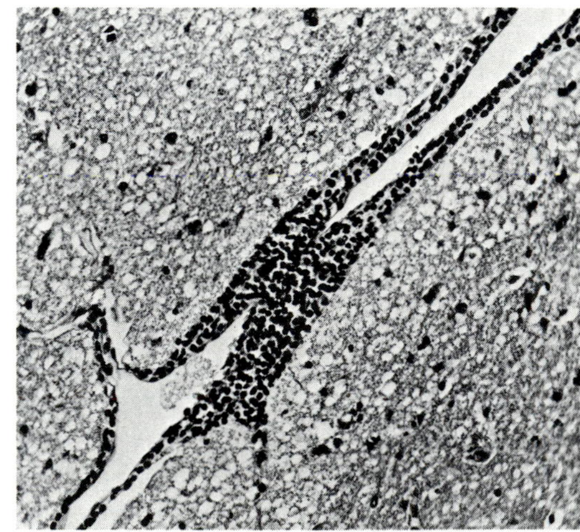

Fig. 44-57. Chronic encephalitis, viral type. (Hematoxylin and eosin; 90×.)

bloodstream, it spreads to involve the central nervous system. The incubation period is 7 to 10 days (see p. 356).

Alterations in the central nervous system vary with the intensity and duration of the illness. The nerve cells characteristically involved are the large anterior horn cells of the spinal cord, particularly those at the cervical and lumbar enlargements. With a more severe and usually fatal disease, the large nerve cells of the brainstem motor nuclei are involved (bulbar poliomyelitis), and in the most severe forms the large nerve cells of the motor cortex are involved, as well as cells in the thalamus, hypothalamus, and brainstem. It has never been clear why only some cells in each area are involved. Because of the similarity of change at all levels, it has been assumed that the cells were infected at one time.

The gross and microscopic appearances are those previously described for the nonnecrotizing encephalomyelitis. In the early and rapidly fatal disease there is vascular engorgement of the affected areas. There may be a few neutrophils in the leptomeninges and about some vessels within the affected areas. These are soon replaced by a considerable amount of perivascular lymphocytic infiltrate. The early swollen nerve cells rapidly undergo neuronophagia by large mononuclear cells. Loss of nerve cells is followed by degeneration of the axons and their sheaths with neurogenic atrophy of the muscles they innervate. The healed lesion is represented by a selective loss of nerve cells, collapse of the area, and focal astrocytic gliosis.

Other enteroviral encephalomyelitides. Other enteroviruses are often the cause of infections of the central nervous system. These include a large group of coxsackieviruses and the echovirus. One, the coxsackievirus type A7, is known to produce a disease that is structurally indistinguishable from that produced by the poliomyelitis viruses. The usual illness, however, is nonparalytic and generalized, sometimes with a myalgia or encephalalgia.

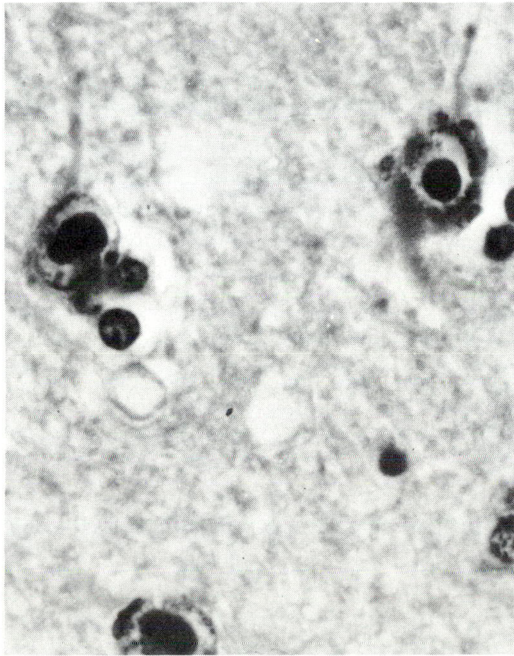

Fig. 44-58. Viral encephalitis. There are Cowdry type A intranuclear inclusions in nerve cells. (Hematoxylin and eosin; 1100×.)

Epidemic encephalitides. The epidemic encephalitides are a group of diseases that occur in epidemics and are presumed to be of viral origin. Among these is the lethargic encephalitis of von Economo, which may be ascribed to several different viruses. Others in this group are St. Louis encephalitis and equine encephalitis.

The localization of the pathologic changes varies greatly. In the von Economo type the lesions characteristically affect the brainstem most severely; the parkinsonian state may occur after an interval of weeks to years. The microscopic changes include nerve cell degeneration and adventitial infiltrates composed of lymphocytes, plasma cells, and large mononuclear cells; a few may persist for years after the onset of the disease.

Necrotizing and sclerosing encephalitides. The necrotizing encephalitides have been reported under a variety of names, including Dawson's inclusion body encephalitis, von Bogaert's subacute sclerosing leukoencephalitis, and Pette-Döring panencephalitis. These diseases are currently designated as subacute sclerosing panencephalitis.[15,69,70,74] Although these encephalitides were formerly considered to be caused by the herpes simplex virus, recent evidence strongly suggests that an incomplete or atypical measles virus is the cause.* The virus is believed to lie dormant in the individual, usually a child, for a period, sometimes years, after which it is reactivated. It characteristically destroys cortical nerve cells and supporting glia and may involve the cells of the central gray matter, pons, and cerebellum. The disease is gradually progressive, with death in months to a few years. Cowdry type A intranuclear inclusions may be found in involved nerve cells and glia with a perivascular, usually mononuclear infiltration containing macrophages. A reactive astrocytosis in the affected areas is prominent.

The increasingly frequent necrotizing encephalitis caused by the herpes simplex virus is characterized by extensive necrosis with some hemorrhage in the "limbic lobe" of the brain (Fig. 44-59).[67] The active portions of the disease exhibit the usual mixed mononuclear perivascular infiltrates. Cowdry type A inclusion bodies may be seen and are more likely to be found in oligodendrocytes than in the rapidly destroyed neurons (Fig. 44-58). There is a moderate, loose reactive astrocytosis. The early lesion is characterized by few or no inflammatory cells but by ischemic nerve cells, thereby simulating a recent

*References 15, 61, 69, 70, 74, 107.

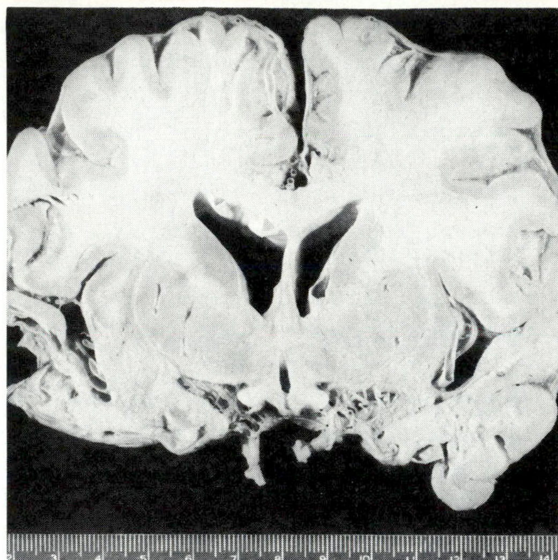

Fig. 44-59. Chronic necrotizing encephalitis caused by herpes simplex. There is necrosis of temporal lobes, insula, and cingulate gyri.

infarct. The diagnosis can be made by using the recently developed ABC-PAP technique. Cytomegalic inclusion disease[124] is caused by the cytomegalovirus, a large DNA virus of the herpes subgroup. In the brain are areas of necrosis that are predominantly periventricular, frequently with mineralization (calcification). There is little cellular response. The Cowdry type A intranuclear inclusions are exceedingly large and prominent; intracytoplasmic inclusions are also to be found. The disease may be generalized, acute, and fulminant. Although the infection occurs most frequently in newborn infants infected by their asymptomatic mothers, it has been recognized in adults whose immune response is impaired.

Lymphocytic choriomeningitis. The virus of lymphocytic choriomeningitis produces moderate lymphocytic infiltrations in the leptomeninges, choroid plexuses, and vessels beneath the ependyma. It appears to be transmitted to humans through the urine of infected mice that act as the host reservoir. The disease, rarely fatal in humans, also has been called benign lymphocytic meningitis. Diagnosis usually is based on the presence of a rising titer of specific neutralizing antibodies.

Progressive multifocal leukoencephalopathy.[4,129] Progressive multifocal leukoencephalopathy is an uncommon disease. Initially described as occurring particularly in patients with neoplastic diseases of the reticuloendothelial system, especially chronic lymphatic leukemia, and in sarcoidosis, it has now been seen in association with a variety of diseases, including "senility." The etiologic agents identified have been the SV40 and JC viruses, so-called slow viruses belonging to the polyoma group.

In the fixed specimen the islandlike multiple lesions affecting the brain and spinal cord have a granular gray

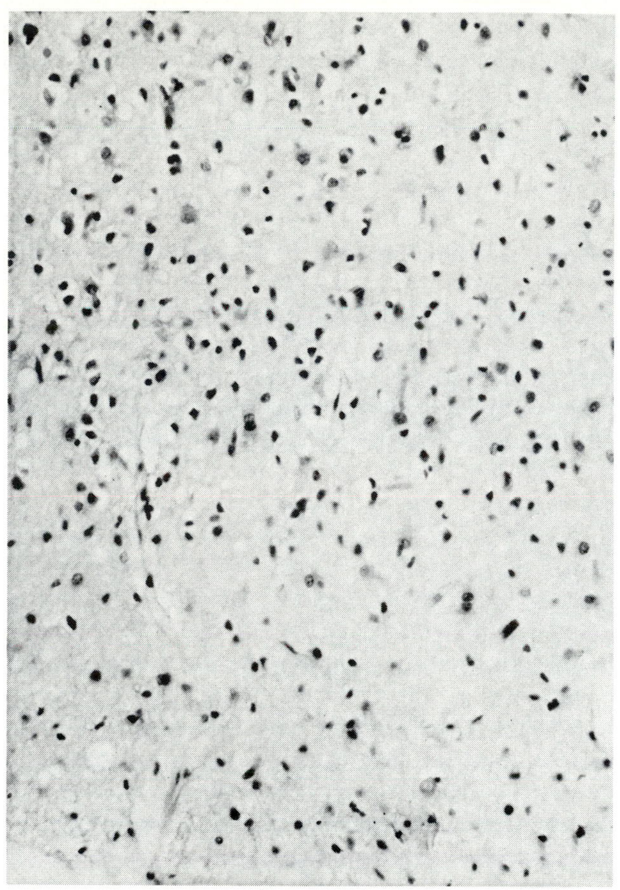

Fig. 44-60. Creutzfeldt-Jakob disease. There are spongioform changes in cerebral cortex and loss of nerve cells with mild reactive astrocytosis. (Hematoxylin and eosin; 157×.)

appearance. In only half of the reported cases are there perivascular cellular infiltrates consisting of lymphocytes and plasma cells. The viruses destroy the oligodendrocytes within the lesion while those at the periphery may contain an eosinophilic intranuclear inclusion. The nuclei of many of the surrounding astrocytes are enlarged, bizarre, irregular, and hyperchromatic, highly suggestive of an early stage of neoplastic transformation.

Creutzfeldt-Jakob disease. Creutzfeldt-Jakob disease is a spongioform encephalopathy whose cause is currently considered to be an unconventional viral agent. Although the incubation period is long, progression is characteristically rapid once clinical disease is apparent. The prolonged incubation period has been demonstrated in both primates and nonprimates. An increasing number of patients worldwide have been reported. The brain may appear normal or slightly atrophic with compensatory hydrocephalus. Microscopic examination of the involved areas (the disease is not diffuse) reveals many round to oval vacuoles throughout the involved cortex, generally in greater numbers in the deeper layers with an apparent decrease in nerve cells. A reactive astrocytic gliosis is greater in the later stages. No inflammatory cell response occurs (Fig. 44-60). With electron microscopy the vacuoles are found to be within the perikaryon and processes of neurons and astrocytes; this is accompanied by loss of dendrites of the pyramidal neurons. In some patients with involvement of the cerebellum there are burrlike eosinophilic plaques (kuru plaques) with amyloid similar to those seen in Alzheimer's disease. The causative agent is not destroyed by formalin fixation or by the usual methods of sterilization.[51,54,81,83,91]

Diseases of myelin

Myelin diseases are a group of disorders of the oligodendrocytes in which the effects are more apparent on myelin, the cell membrane. The surrounded axons are completely or relatively spared; when they are affected, their involvement follows that of the myelin. Neither clinical nor etiologic classifications have been satisfactory because of overlapping clinical appearances and because the causes are either unknown or in dispute. The diseases have been categorized as demyelinating (that is, myelinoclastic) or dysmyelinating (disorders of myelin formation, such as leukodystrophy).[104]

Demyelinating diseases[14]

Multiple sclerosis (disseminated sclerosis, insular sclerosis). Multiple sclerosis is the most common of the demyelinating diseases. It is characteristically chronic and relapsing, although acute and unremittent forms occur. Of the innumerable theories concerning its cause, those associated with disorders of blood vessels, with developmental defects of the glia, and with a great variety of toxic agents are no longer seriously considered. Currently the theories most supported are those related to a viral infection followed by an autoimmune reaction to the altered myelin. The increased prevalence in the colder latitudes and in families in which a member has the disease and the exacerbations and remissions, often years apart, have defied explanation. Seen at all ages after childhood, onset is most common between the ages of 20 and 40 years. Both sexes are affected, women more frequently and at an earlier age. The mean duration of the disease is over 20 years.

In the chronic relapsing form the gross appearance of the central nervous system is usually diagnostic. The brain is either normal in size or slightly atrophic, and the spinal cord is variably small. Lesions in the white matter are, on the cut surface, slightly depressed, gray to gray-pink, and sharply demarcated. Although these lesions (plaques) are more easily seen in the white matter, they extend to involve gray matter in almost every patient (Fig. 44-61). Plaques vary in size, shape, number, and position. In almost all patients, however, some plaques are seen with their bases at the angles of the lateral ventricles and with their apices toward the cortex. Plaques are frequent in the central and convolutional white matter of the brain and in the brainstem, cerebellum, and spinal cord.

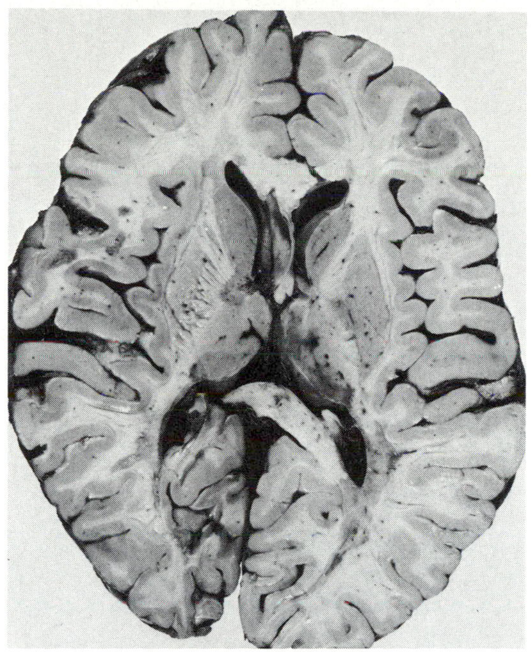

Fig. 44-61. Multiple sclerosis of chronic relapsing type with numerous plaques. Plaques occur in all characteristic areas. Cortex and arcuate fibers are involved in several areas.

All stages of the plaque development may be found in the patient in relapse. Perivascular lymphocytes and plasma cells (Fig. 44-62) characterize the acute lesions, with spillover of the cells into the leptomeninges in some instances. The degree and stages of oligodendroglial injury with myelin destruction and loss are seen with routine as well as with special stains (Fig. 44-63). In the slightly older and active lesions, there is a decrease in the myelin staining with swollen myelin. Here, in addition to the usual inflammatory cells, are macrophages with fragments of myelin or granules that are metachromatic or with neutral fat. The older and inactive lesions are sharply demarcated regions of myelin loss without inflammatory cells. Although the plaques are devoid of oligodendroglia, variable numbers of axons remain and are surrounded by a mild to moderate increase in astrocytes whose fibrillary processes follow the original axonal pattern (isomorphic gliosis).

Diffuse sclerosis (Schilder's disease, cerebral sclerosis, encephalitis periaxialis diffusa). In contrast to multiple sclerosis, in almost half of the patients with diffuse sclerosis the onset of disease occurs before the age of 10 years, with the mean duration of life being 6 years. The disease has been described in older adults. Bilateral but

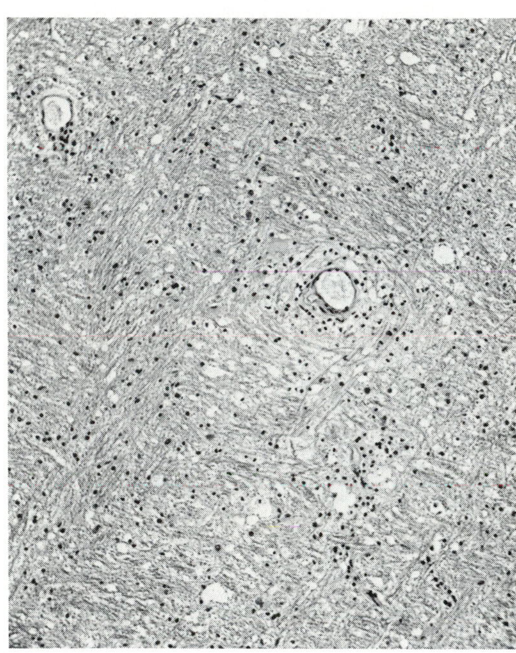

Fig. 44-62. Plaque of multiple sclerosis. This is active lesion with perivascular lymphocytes. Slightly lighter staining area in lower half of section is plaque. (Hematoxylin and eosin; 90×.)

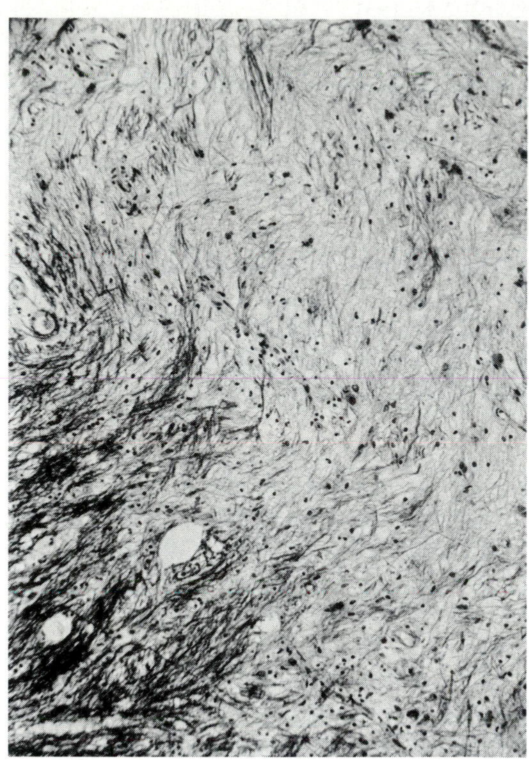

Fig. 44-63. Older plaque of multiple sclerosis with loss of myelin and retention of some axons in lighter-staining area. (Luxol-fast blue–silver nitrate; 135×.)

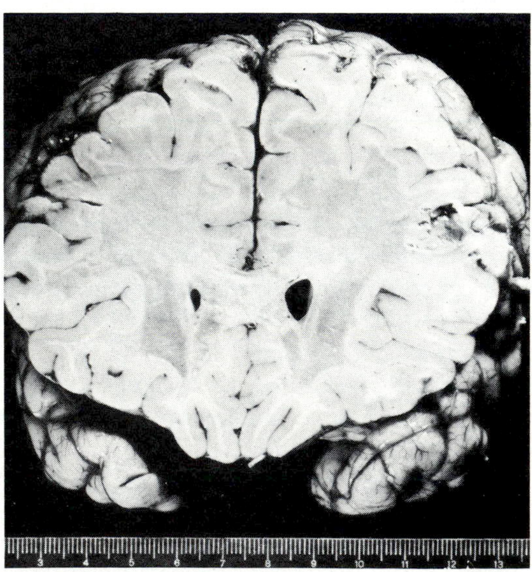

Fig. 44-64. Diffuse sclerosis. There is extensive loss of myelin in both frontal lobes.

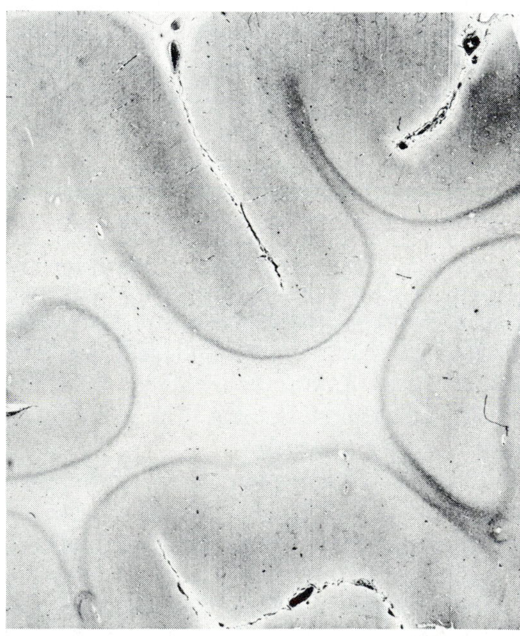

Fig. 44-65. Diffuse sclerosis. Arcuate fibers are partially retained. (Mahon stain; 8×.)

not necessarily symmetric involvement of the white matter of the cerebral hemispheres, especially of the occipital lobes, is usual (Fig. 44-64). The lesions are large and sharply demarcated, often spare the subcortical arcuate fibers (Fig. 44-65), and unite with each other across the corpus callosum. The older and larger lesions often are cavitated. The cellular response with destruction of oligodendrocytes and their myelin follows the same pattern as that seen in multiple sclerosis. Many axons are swollen, fragmented, and destroyed, whereas others are preserved. Reactive astrocytes are usually fibrillary, but many are gemistocytic and some are multinucleate. Axonal degeneration resulting from severe injury to the axons may be seen.

Neuromyelitis optica (Devic's disease, neuro-ophthalmomyelitis). The spinal cord (Fig. 44-66) and the optic nerves and chiasm are the principal sites of clinical and anatomic involvement in neuromyelitis optica. Like diffuse sclerosis, the disease is more common in the young and occurs to a lesser degree in older individuals. Although it is usually unremitting and progressive, it may become stationary for long periods or have remissions. The anatomic findings support an intermediate or transitional position of this disease between diffuse sclerosis on the one hand and multiple sclerosis on the other.

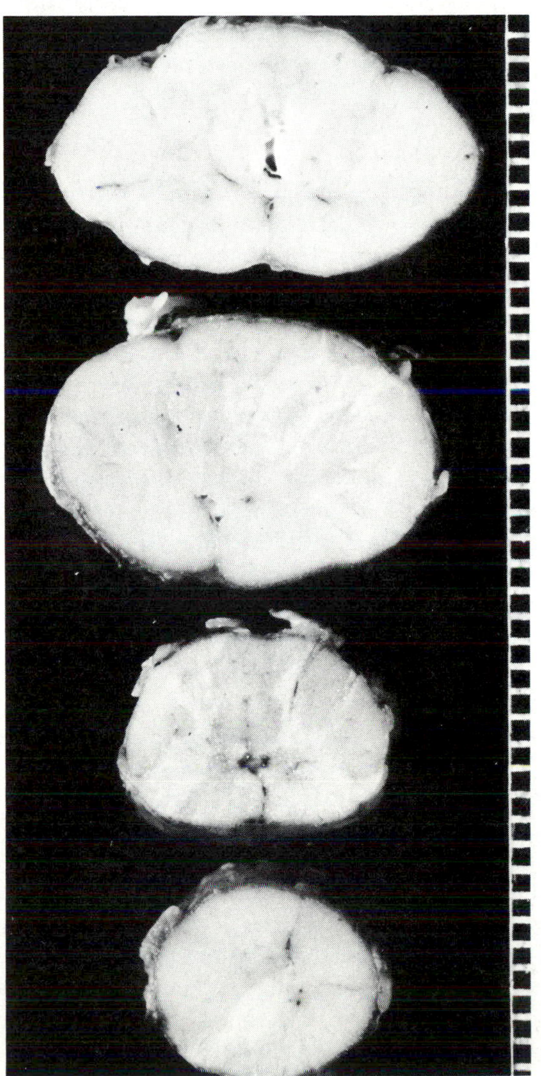

Fig. 44-66. Spinal cord in neuromyelitis optica.

The spinal cord is usually involved at one or more levels. Early, the affected white matter is swollen, soft, and slightly pink. Older lesions are depressed and gray, and some that are large may be cavitated. The optic nerves and chiasm are similarly involved, usually without cavitation. Both portions of the nervous system may be at the same stage or in different stages of involvement and may be affected equally, or, as is more usual, unequally. In some patients there may be lesions in other parts of the brain identical to those of multiple sclerosis.

The microscopic changes in the typical patient vary from the characteristic plaques of multiple sclerosis in all of its stages to those of diffuse sclerosis with areas of necrosis, cavitation, and axonal degeneration.

Acute perivenous encephalomyelitis (postvaccinal encephalomyelitis, postexanthematous encephalomyelitis). A disseminated infectious or postvaccinal encephalomyelitis may appear during the course of or shortly after recovery from several exanthems, such as chickenpox, German measles, or smallpox, and, rarely, after inoculations against smallpox, rabies, and typhoid. Although most of these illnesses are caused by viruses, none has, as yet, been identified in patients with postvaccinal encephalomyelitis.

The clinical and pathologic similarities of the involvement of the central nervous system and the uniform structural change have suggested an autoimmune response on the part of the central nervous system or the activation of a latent virus. In the fatal case the central nervous system is hyperemic, slightly swollen, and with occasional petechiae. Microscopically the lesions appear to be confined mainly to the white matter. Early, the congested vessels are surrounded by a few neutrophils that are soon replaced by lymphocytes and plasma cells. Macrophages, some containing lipid, occur during the later stages of the disease. The loss of myelin about the veins and the relatively undamaged axons usually can be recognized only with special stains. The disease is not progressive.

Acute necrotizing hemorrhagic encephalitis (acute hemorrhagic leukoencephalitis, acute hemorrhagic leukoencephalopathy). Acute necrotizing hemorrhagic encephalitis is a rare, usually rapidly fatal disorder with a sudden, severe, devastating onset and cause. It is often preceded by a nondescript infection, characteristically respiratory, from which the patient is recovering or has recovered. The brain is congested and swollen, with many isolated and confluent petechiae in the white matter involving one portion of the brain to a greater degree (Fig. 44-67).

On microscopic examination the walls of the small vessels are necrotic, with edema of the surrounding brain. Early, there are variable numbers of neutrophils and fibrin in the necrotic vessel walls. Lymphocytes and plasma cells later replace the neutrophils as the surrounding edematous and hemorrhagic brain undergoes necrosis. Death often supervenes before macrophages are to be found. This condition may represent a severe form of perivenous encephalomyelitis.

Central pontine myelinolysis.[21,82,130] Described first in 1959, central pontine myelinolysis has been associated with alcoholism, malnutrition, disturbances of electrolyte and water balance, extraneural infections, local venous obstruction, and unidentified agents. The lesion occurs in the central portion of the base of the pons, with its greatest transverse diameter at the level of the external origins of the trigeminal nerves (Fig. 44-68). Rostrally, the plaque may reach almost into the midbrain. Its caudal extent generally spares the lowermost pons. The well-formed lesion is granular, gray, well demarcated, and depressed.

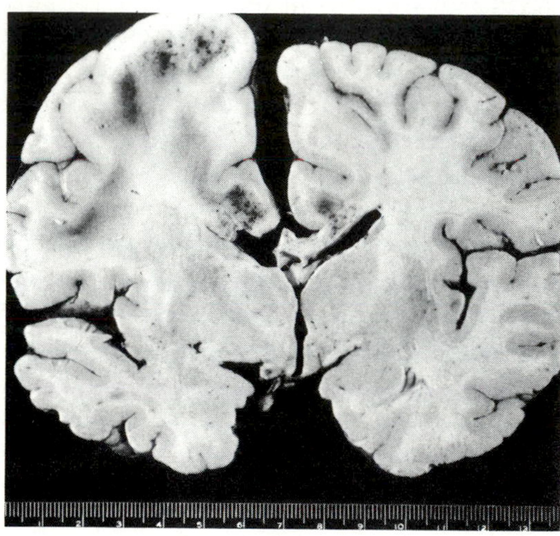

Fig. 44-67. Acute hemorrhagic leukoencephalitis, predominantly unilateral. (Courtesy Dr. J. Langston; from Chason, J.L.: Brain, meninges and spinal cord. In Saphir, O., editor: A text on systemic pathology, vol. 2, New York, 1958, Grune & Stratton, Inc.; by permission.)

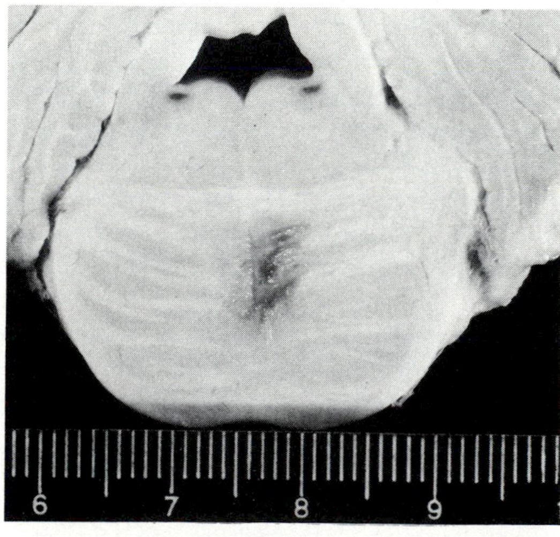

Fig. 44-68. Central pontine myelinolysis.

On coronal section it is diamond shaped, triangular with its base dorsal, or cylindrical. In some cases, only a poorly defined gray change is noted at the appropriate level. The area is pale with the routine hematoxylin and eosin stain, and there are occasional lipophages in the early and active lesions. Special stains disclose loss of myelin and retention of most or all of the axons. Metachromatic granular material may be seen early. In some plaques the myelin going in one direction may be lost, with sparing of the myelin sheathing fibers running in another direction. Oligodendrocytes are decreased or absent in the lesion. Reactive astrocytosis and gliosis are usually minimal.

Leukodystrophies

The leukodystrophies are metabolic diseases characterized by a disturbance in the formation of myelin (dysmyelinating diseases). They have been considered to be genetically determined and are often familial. Some are similar to the lipidoses. The leukodystrophies differ from the demyelinating diseases in that the lesions are likely to be bilateral and symmetric, involve more of the nervous system, and occur in younger individuals. The subcortical arcuate fibers are regularly spared, and the axons usually are destroyed. The biochemical criteria for this group of diseases are an increase in hexosamine content of the affected area and the absence of an enzyme. Whereas the leukodystrophies are similar in appearance grossly, they have characteristic microscopic features that permit their separation into subgroups. Only those that are generally accepted and are more common are described below.

Metachromatic leukodystrophy (sulfatide lipidosis).[56,64,72,102] Metachromatic leukodystrophy is a disease of both children and adults. The basic defect in myelin metabolism is a deficiency of the enzyme arylsulfatase A. The involved areas of the white matter contain large amounts of a sulfatide that exhibits brown gamma metachromasia with the von Hirsch–Pfeiffer cresyl violet–acetic acid stain. A relationship to the lipidosis has been suggested because the abnormal material also has been found in tissues other than the central nervous system, including the cells of the liver and kidneys, the white blood cells, and cells of the gallbladder. Schwann cells of the peripheral nerves and the cells of nerve plexuses also are involved. The anatomic diagnosis often can be made by biopsy examination of a peripheral nerve (usually sural) or of the nerve plexuses (rectal). The specific stain done on frozen sections with the presence of gamma metachromasia as described is diagnostic. Analysis of the more easily available urine, leukocytes, or fibroblasts in tissue cultures for the enzyme deficiency is a safer and more reasonable approach for diagnosis.

Globoid cell leukodystrophy (Krabbe's disease, globoid sclerosis). Globoid cell leukodystrophy is a disease that affects only the central nervous system of children. The accumulation of an abnormal periodic acid–Schiff–positive material, possibly a cerebroside of the kerasin type, leads to the formation of large epithelioid and multinucleated giant cells (the globoid cells) (Fig. 44-69). The mononuclear cells are found in clusters of varying sizes about blood vessels, whereas the multinucleated cells occur more frequently in the affected white matter. Galactosyl ceramide-beta-galactosyl hydrolase and other enzyme deficiencies have been described.[2]

Neutral fat leukodystrophy (sudanophilic leukodystrophy). Although neutral fat leukodystrophy resembles diffuse sclerosis, significant differences have suggested its inclusion with the dysmyelinating diseases. These include genetic background with a family history and increase in hexosamine in the affected area.

Adrenoleukodystrophy. Adrenoleukodystrophy is a rare, sex-linked recessive disorder usually occurring in children, although adults with the disease and symptomatic mothers have been recognized. The illness is slowly progressive and accompanied by adrenal insufficiency. The demyelinated areas have a marked cellular reaction including bizarre astrocytes. In addition, the atrophic adrenal cortices contain vacuolated and ballooned cells. Linear cytoplasmic inclusion in central nervous system macrophages, adrenocortical cells, and testicular Leydig cells seen with electron microscopy have been reported.

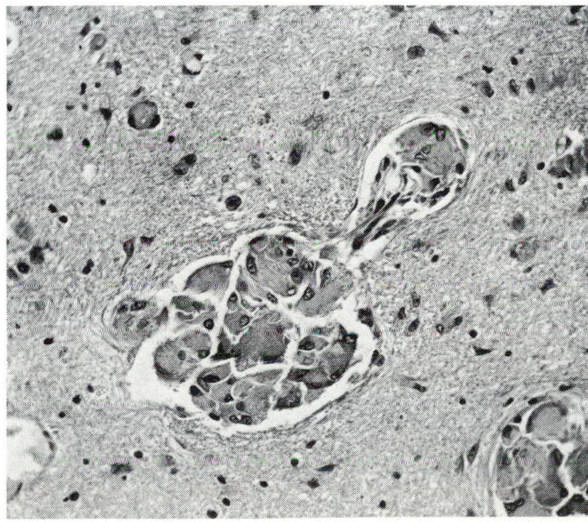

Fig. 44-69. Globoid sclerosis (Krabbe's disease). (Hematoxylin and eosin; 135×.)

Neoplasms

No accurate statistics reporting the frequency of neoplasms of the central nervous system are available. Estimates based on a variety of observations often include granulomas and are biased by the character of the hospital or clinic and by the interests of the clinician and pathologist. The estimate that 9% of all primary tumors (excluding those of the skin) are primary in the central nervous system is, at present, most reasonable.

Theories concerning the development of neoplasms elsewhere in the body are similar to those concerning the nervous system. Early tumor classifications were based on the cell rest theory of Cohnheim, in which neoplasms were believed to originate from activation of aberrant immature cells.[7] Cytologic similarities of neoplastic cells to those at different stages of maturation reinforced the opinions. Later classifications were based on the belief that fully mature cells could be stimulated to reproduce and to undergo anaplasia.[77] Experimental production of central nervous system lesions has not resolved these differences. The issues have become even more debatable by evidence that the structure of these neoplasms may be related to their position within the nervous system and that there is often a mixture of glial elements. Most modern classifications make use of both theories.

Gliomas

Tumors classified as gliomas should be limited to those neoplasms whose origin is the ectodermal supporting tissues (neuroglia) of the central nervous system. It has been customary, however, to include also the medulloblastomas and the pineal neoplasms. The classification proposed in 1926 by Bailey and Cushing[7] was based on the then current theories of histogenesis of the nervous system. The more recent classification proposed by Kernohan and associates[77] is, for the most part, adopted here. It is based on the assumption that some gliomas arise by anaplasia of adult cells. Stains for glial fibrillary acidic protein are often helpful in identifying the cells in this group of neoplasms.

Astrocytic series

Astrocytoma, grade I. Among the grade I astrocytomas, which constitute about 15% of all gliomas, are the fibrillary, protoplasmic, and pilocytic types. Although these types differ as to the amount of visible cytoplasm and degree of production of neuroglial fibers, they have, in general, the same biologic behavior. They are relatively slow growing, with an average survival of more than 3 years after the onset of symptoms. They may be found in any part of the central nervous system.

In adults these neoplasms are usually in one of the cerebral hemispheres. In young adults and in children the tumors are more frequent in the pons and cerebellum.[13] Those occurring in the cerebrum and pons are solid, gray, and firm, with poorly defined borders. Small cystic areas sometimes may be found in the tumors of the cerebrum. The cerebellar neoplasms more often are cystic. The cyst walls are surrounded by neoplastic cells in 60%, whereas in 40% only a mural nodule composed of neoplastic astrocytes is found.[13] The cavity contains a clear amber fluid high in protein. Similar but smaller lesions also occur in the spinal cord (Fig. 44-70).

The microscopic recognition of these neoplasms may be exceedingly difficult, particularly at biopsy, because of the following:

1. Astrocytes forming the tumors are within the cytologic limits of normality.
2. Mitoses are not found.
3. There is no area of necrosis or hemorrhage (except operative).
4. In the diffuse forms, normal-appearing nerve cells often are included within the lesion.
5. There are no changes of the blood vessels (see following) except an occasional perivascular scant lymphocytic cuff.

Diagnosis by biopsy depends on an evaluation of the history and the presence of increased numbers of astrocytes in the absence of an apparent cause for their increase.

The boundaries of the neoplasms that are solid or diffuse are difficult to demarcate by microscopic study. The reasons are the very gradual centrifugal decrease in numbers of astrocytes and the absence of evidence of compression or destruction of the surrounding brain. In occasional neoplasms examined in detail, there are nests of enlarged and sometimes pleomorphic astrocytes and recognizable increases in blood vessels, some with proliferation of the endothelial and adventitial layers. These are interpreted as evidence of increased anaplasia and biologic activity.

Occasionally a tumor of the cerebral hemispheres may be composed either entirely (less commonly) or in part by well-differentiated astrocytes with abundant eosinophilic cytoplasm. These are gemistocytic astrocytes. The biologic behavior of gemistocytic astrocytomas usually differs from those just described. These neoplasms rapidly undergo malignant change usually to grade III astrocytoma (glioblastoma multiforme). Because of this, it has been my practice to empirically add one cytologic grade to the neoplasm when large clusters of these cells are found.

Astrocytoma grade II. Grade II astrocytoma has also been called astroblastoma because of the resemblance of many of its constitutent cells to astroblasts. It represents approximately 1% of all gliomas. More common in young adults than in children, these neoplasms are solid and gray-white to white. The macroscopically discernible apparent borders sometimes give rise to a false impression of sharp demarcation because of compression of the surrounding brain.

Microscopically the tumor is more cellular than the lower-grade astrocytoma. The cells are generally larger, and in many there are cells with one or more plump cell processes that radiate about the walls of the moderately increased numbers of blood vessels. Mitoses and areas of necrosis are rare. When the lesions are examined to include the gross line of demarcation, neoplastic cells singly and in groups can be found to extend well beyond this point.

The average postoperative survival of patients with grade II astrocytomas is approximately 2 years.

Astrocytoma grade III and grade IV. Grade III and IV astrocytomas include glioblastoma multiforme, spongioblastoma multiforme, polar spongioblastoma, monstrocellular or gigantocellular glioblastoma, and so forth. These highly malignant and uniformly fatal neoplasms constitute 50% to 60% of all gliomas. They are more common in adults and in the cerebral hemispheres. Beginning more often in white matter, they often appear to be well demarcated because the surrounding brain is compressed, swollen, and edematous. The neoplasm is usu-

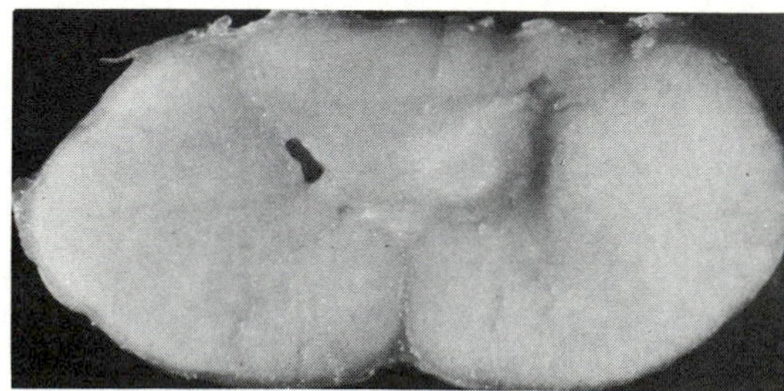

Fig. 44-70. Grade I astrocytoma (cytic) in cervical cord.

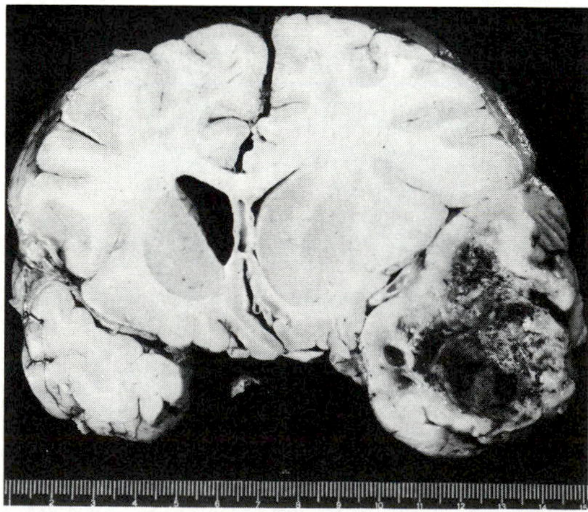

Fig. 44-71. Grade III astrocytoma in temporal lobe. There is brain displacement with cingulate gyrus herniation and compression of lateral ventricle.

ally slightly firmer than the adjacent tissue. Its surface has a variegated gray, white, yellow (necrotic), and reddish brown (hemorrhagic) appearance (Fig. 44-71). The tumors frequently extend into and across the corpus callosum into the opposite hemisphere. Multicentric origin (that is, two or more separate neoplasms) has been described in 15% of the cases. However, on microscopic study, I have frequently found neoplastic cells connecting the grossly separate tumors. It is my experience that multicentric origin does not exceed 5%.

The microscopic appearance of these lesions is characterized by profuse numbers of pleomorphic and frequently bizarre cells (Fig. 44-72). Among these are many cells with enlarged and irregular nuclei. Some cells can be identified by their processes as being of astrocytic origin. Other cells may be small with oval, hyperchromatic nuclei resembling the undifferentiated small cells of a bronchogenic carcinoma. In other areas there may be large cells with irregular large, vesicular nuclei and with an abundant eosinophilic cytoplasm suggesting an origin from gemistocytic astrocytes. In many areas within the neoplasm, one may find bizarre, multinucleate cells with abundant cytoplasm resembling strap cells of rhabdomyosarcomas. Mitoses, often abnormal, are usually easily found either in clusters or spread fairly regularly throughout the neoplasm. In many regions within the neoplasm are large and small areas of necrosis, often with a garland of small cell nuclei at the periphery (Fig. 44-73). Blood vessels are greatly increased in number and usually show endothelial or adventitial hypertrophy and hyperplasia. Occasionally, vessels with these changes are found well beyond the apparent microscopic limits of the neoplasm.

Despite the apparent sharp gross demarcation, neoplastic cells extend far beyond these borders because of the infiltration from the tumor and perhaps also because of the continued dedifferentiation of the surrounding cells. A sudden increase in signs and symptoms in patients with these neoplasms usually can be correlated with the occurrence of large areas of necrosis caused by the vascular changes, often with superimposed thromboses. Massive hemorrhages within the neoplasms less frequently cause rapid tumor enlargement and clinical deterioration.

Cells of any of the astrocytic neoplasms, but particularly those that are more malignant, may reach the subarachnoid or the ventricular spaces. From this point they may spread by way of the ventricular and subarachnoid cerebrospinal fluid and implant in other portions of the central nervous system. The presence of free neoplastic cells recognized on cytologic examination of cerebrospinal fluid does not necessarily indicate metastasis. Extracranial metastasis, although rare, is more apt to occur after operative removal of a portion of the neoplasm.

Most of the patients with a grade III astrocytoma live less than 18 months after diagnosis. More extensive surgical therapy has increased only the survival time—not the rate of cure.

Between 5% and 8% of these neoplasms are complicated by the development of a fibrosarcoma.[93] This is more common in the temporal lobe and with dural attachment, although neither is necessary. The fibrosarcoma is thought to arise from the walls of the reactive, hyperplastic vessels characteristic of the high-grade astrocytomas. The neoplasms are of leathery consistency, are well demarcated, and may obscure the presence of the preceding astrocytomas both from the gross appearance and microscopically by the replacement of the antecedent neoplastic astrocytes by the cells forming the fibrosarcoma.

In the rare cerebrospinal glioblastomatosis (gliomatosis cerebri), there may be no grossly visibly neoplasm or

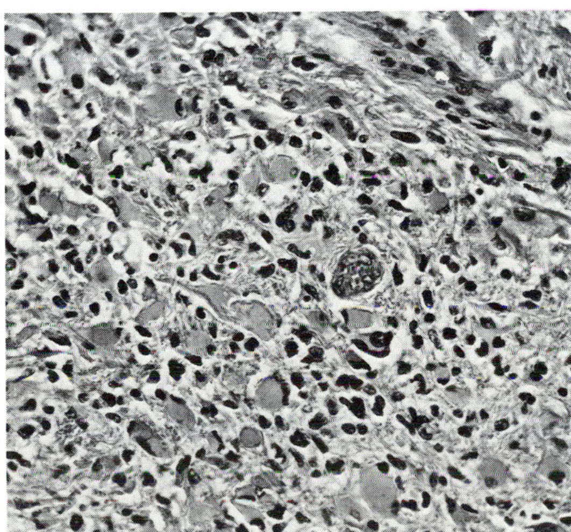

Fig. 44-72. Grade III astrocytoma. Note gemistocytic astrocytes and multinucleate cells. (Hematoxylin and eosin; 280×.)

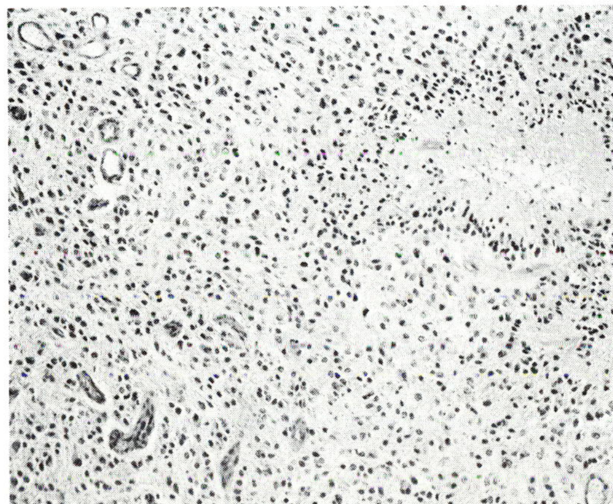

Fig. 44-73. Grade III astrocytoma. There is area of necrosis with garland formation in upper right. Note vascular proliferation. (Hematoxylin and eosin; 135×.)

at most one or two poorly defined areas of enlargement usually within the brain and less often in the spinal cord. On microscopic examination, multiple areas in the brain and spinal cord are composed of bizarre, neoplastic astrocytes of the type seen in the grade III astrocytomas. Most are so remote from possible implantation sites as to suggest that the lesions are multicentric in origin.

Ependymoma.[89] Approximately 5% of the intracranial gliomas are ependymomas, with 60% of the latter arising in the posterior fossa. In the spinal cord, 60% of the gliomas are of the ependymal group. Intracranial ependymomas have their origin from cells lining the ventricles and the choroid plexuses, and from cells of ependymal streaks that represent obliterated portions of the ventricles. In the spinal cord they arise from the ependymal cells lining the central canal or its remnants and from the cells of the ventriculus terminalis in the filum terminale. It is also possible that some may arise (usually mixed with other glial cells) from the cells of the subependymal plate.

These neoplasms are gray, moderately firm, and well demarcated from the adjoining compressed tissues (Fig. 44-74). Those in the fourth ventricle are usually solid, whereas those in the cerebral hemispheres and in the spinal cord are frequently cystic. Neoplasms of the choroid plexuses are gray-pink, fungating, and papillary. Ependymomas of the filum terminale are thinly encapsulated and cystic. The capsule may be breached in the larger lesions.

Their microscopic appearances are exceedingly variable among the tumors as a group and in different areas of the same tumor. Except for the choroid plexus papilloma, the most characteristic pattern of growth is the epithelial type whose cells form "rosettes" by lining tubular or ventricle-like spaces (Fig. 44-75). The lining cells are cuboid to columnar, with the appearance of ependymal cells. In some areas the cells line what has been interpreted as representative of a small portion of a poorly formed space, a partial rosette. Blepharoplasts are structures that represent the cytoplasmic residua of cilia. They may be found in some cells when stained with Mallory's phosphotungstic acid–hematoxylin and examined under high magnification. Blepharoplasts are small, circular or rod-shaped structures surrounded by a narrow unstained halo. They lie in that portion of the cell cytoplasm that is directed toward the lumen of the rosette. In other areas of the neoplasm and in other ependymomas, the tumors are formed by a diffuse proliferation of polygonal cells without a characteristic pattern, except for occasional cells whose processes radiate about a blood vessel (Fig. 44-76).

There are two varieties of papillary ependymomas: choroid plexus type and myxopapillary type. These tumors are formed by cuboid to columnar cells lining a central core of connective tissue containing a capillary. In the choroid plexus papilloma, the structure is very similar to that of a normal choroid plexus except that the epithelial cells are taller and larger than those of the normal plexus (Fig. 44-77). When the cellular anaplasia is marked, the neoplasm is considered to be a choroid plexus carcinoma.[39] Portions of either neoplasm may be separate from the tumor, be carried by the cerebrospinal fluid, and become implanted and grow anywhere in the ventricular cavity or subarachnoid space. The myxopapillary type can occur throughout the cerebrospinal axis and even in the hollow of the sacrum, but it is far more frequent at the level of the cauda equina. The vascular and connective tissue cores of the papillae have undergone a great degree of myxoid change.

In approximately one third of the ependymomas, there are nests of cells with the appearance of oligodendrocytes.

Histologic grading of this group of neoplasms was developed by Kernohan and Uihlein[77] using the same

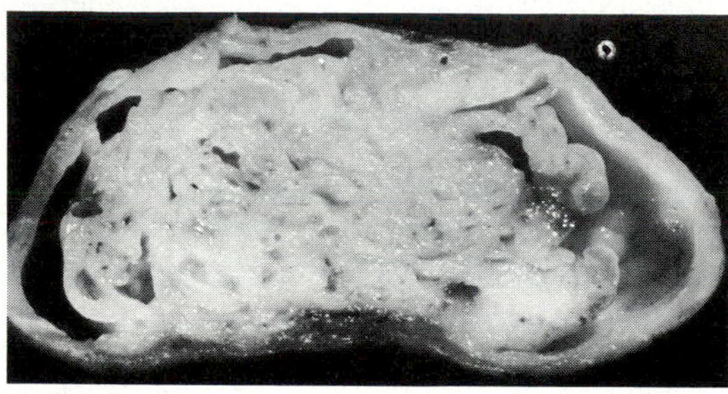

Fig. 44-74. Ependymoma of cervical portion of spinal cord. Residual spinal cord is represented by peripheral rim of tissue.

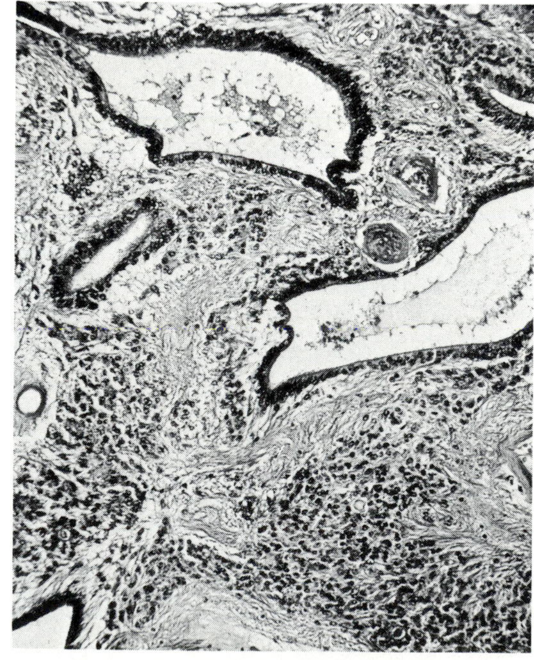

Fig. 44-75. Epithelial type of ependymoma with many rosettes. Tissue is from that in Fig. 44-74. (Hematoxylin and eosin; 90×.)

general criteria described for the astrocytoma group. The prognosis, however, is more dependent on the site of origin than on the histologic dedifferentiation, and therefore these neoplasms are usually not graded.

Medulloepitheliomas are rare neoplasms that are believed to originate from residual cells of the embryonic medullary canal. Their structural similarities to the ependymomas make their separation difficult, if not impossible.

Oligodendrogliomas.[123] Like the ependymomas, the oligodendrogliomas constitute about 5% of all gliomas. They are slow-growing tumors that are found in the white matter of a cerebral hemisphere of an adult, most frequently during the fourth or fifth decade of life. The tumors are gray-pink, well demarcated, and soft and frequently extend into the leptomeninges locally. About 20% are cystic, and in most the neoplastic tissue entirely surrounds the cyst. Areas of necrosis, hemorrhage, and mineralization are common in the larger lesions (Fig. 44-78). Mineralization (calcification) in the walls of the blood vessels and in larger confluent masses is visible on x-ray films in some 40% and is found on microscopic examination in 70%.

The usually described neoplastic cell has a lymphocyte-like nucleus surrounded by a clear, nonstaining halo with a definite cell membrane (Fig. 44-79). Groups of these cells produce the characteristic honeycombing. However, this appearance may be obscured in the bet-

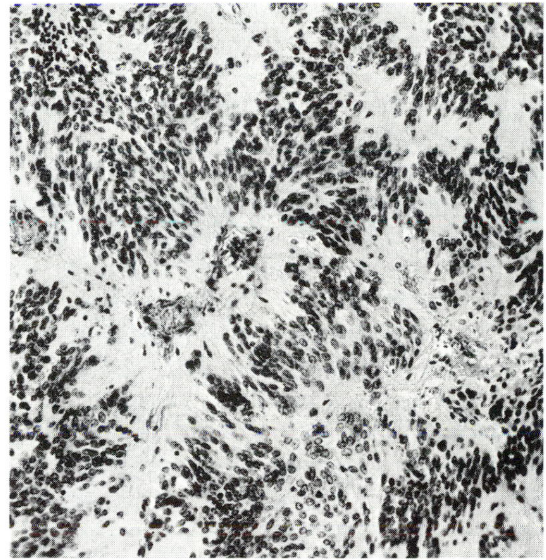

Fig. 44-76. Ependymoma, cellular type, with characteristic perivascular arrangement. (Hematoxylin and eosin; 90×.)

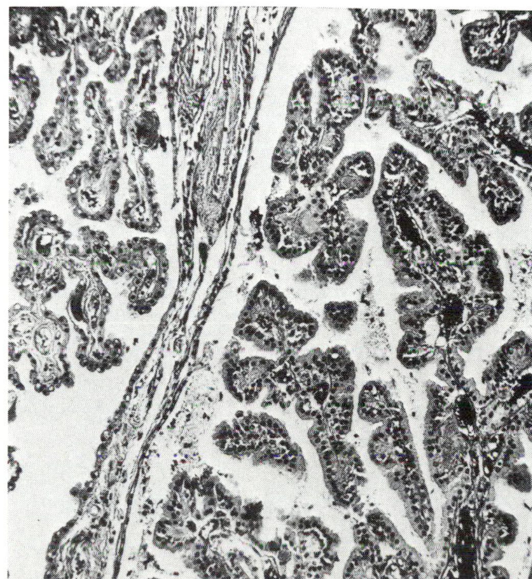

Fig. 44-77. Ependymoma, choroid plexus papilloma type. Larger papillary projections to right of lining represent neoplasm. Lesion was in left cerebellopontine angle. (Hematoxylin and eosin; 90×.)

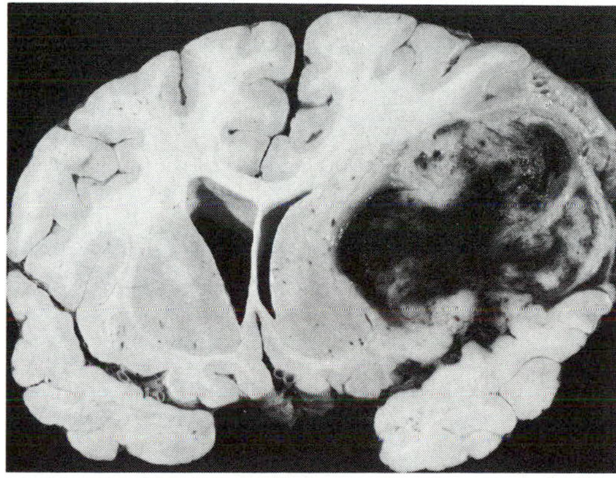

Fig. 44-78. Oligodendroglioma with operative hemorrhage. There is ventricular displacement and cingulate gyrus herniation.

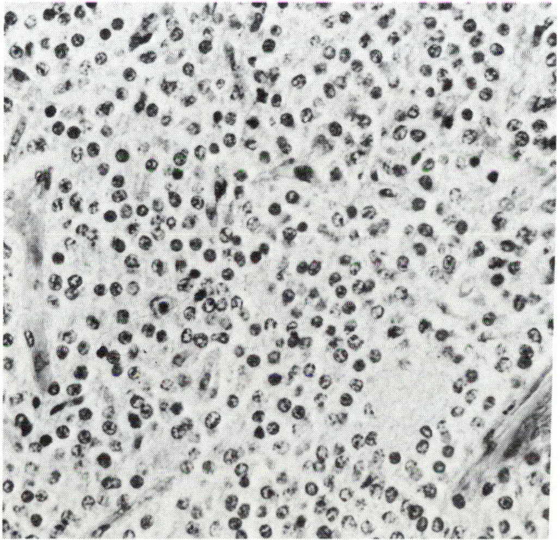

Fig. 44-79. Oligodendroglioma. Cells are compartmentalized by blood vessels. Some cells have nonstaining halos. (Hematoxylin and eosin; 280×.)

ter-preserved areas of the neoplasm by the staining of the finely granular, slightly hematoxylinophilic cytoplasm. Compartmentalization of groups of tumor cells by blood vessels is commonly present and is characteristic. The border zones of the neoplasms are relatively narrow but less well defined than the gross demarcation would suggest. Mitoses are rare. Their presence, sometimes in large numbers, in neoplasms containing cells with large pleomorphic nuclei has led some to classify the latter group as oligodendroblastomas.

Prognosis is related neither to the degree of mineralization nor to the cytologic appearance. Most patients live more than 4 years after clinical onset. Evidence of leptomeningeal spread is commonly found at necropsy and may be related to previous operative treatment.

Astrocytes frequently are found within these neoplasms, predominantly about blood vessels, perhaps serving as stromal support. In almost one third there are nests of ependyma-like cells.

***Medulloblastoma** (neuroblastoma, granuloblastoma).*[26,73,110] Medulloblastomas are highly malignant and heretofore uniformly fatal neoplasms whose origin is restricted to the cerebellum. Representing approximately 8% of all neuroglial neoplasms, they occur predominantly in children. The greatest incidence is in those 5 to 9 years of age, with another increase in incidence occurring between the ages of 20 to 24 years. Males are affected more than twice as frequently as females. Familial occurrences, including tumors in identical twins, have been described. In children most of the tumors originate in the region of the cerebellar vermis, possibly from microscopic remnants of the external granular layer of the cerebellum. In older patients the tumors may arise from one of the hemispheres.

Medulloblastomas are gray-pink to red, soft, friable, and often hemorrhagic and necrotic. Demarcation from the adjacent cerebellum is usually sharp. Because of the sites of origin, the fourth ventricle is almost regularly filled by the rapidly growing neoplasm, often with extensions of the tissue into and through the lateral recesses, the posterior roof of the fourth ventricle, the cerebral aqueduct, and the tissues of the floor and walls of the fourth ventricle. Nodules and sheets of implanted neoplastic cells are frequent in the lateral and third ventricles and in the subarachnoid space, particularly in the regions of the cauda equina because of spread via the cerebrospinal fluid (Fig. 44-80). These highly cellular neoplasms are composed of cells with small, round to oval, usually hyperchromatic nuclei. There is little visible cytoplasm (Fig. 44-81). The numbers of mitoses are variable. Although the neoplastic cells tend to grow

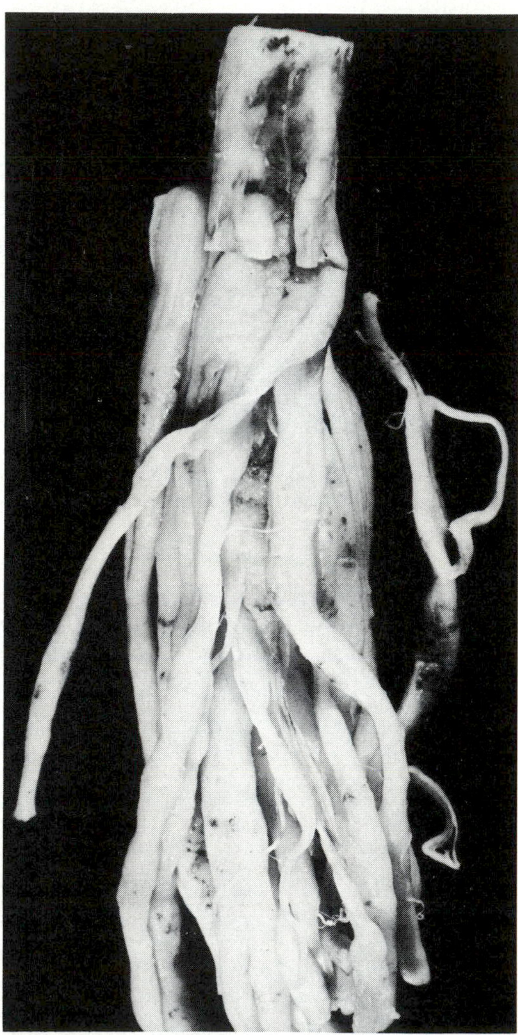

Fig. 44-80. Diffuse subarachnoid implants of medulloblastoma onto filaments of cauda equina. Every filament is covered with the implants; they are up to 20 times thicker than normal.

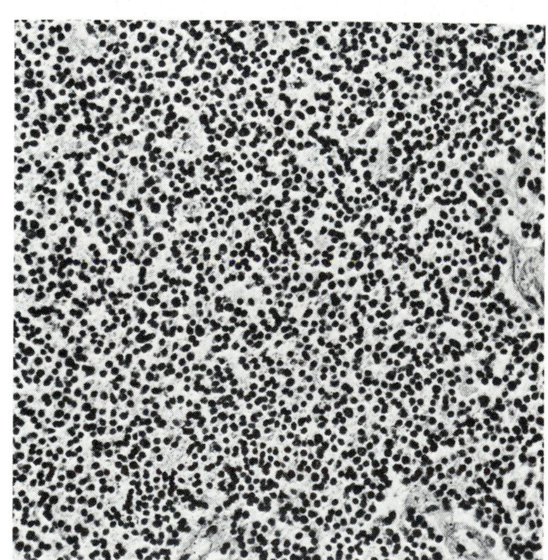

Fig. 44-81. Medulloblastoma originating in vermis of cerebellum. (Hematoxylin and eosin; 280×.)

about the blood vessels with necrosis at a distance, in most there is no special histologic pattern. Rosettes and a perivascular arrangement (pseudorosette) have been described, and evidence of continued maturation of some cells toward nerve cells and glial cells, although rare, may be seen.

Differences in the cytologic appearance and the histogenic pattern have led some to the opinion that neoplasms that lie predominantly in the leptomeninges are cerebellar sarcomas. Others have concluded that the atypical features are attributable to a spread and desmoplastic response following growth of cells of a medulloblastoma within the confines of the subarachnoid space.

Neoplasms of the pineal gland.[3,43] There are many classifications and interpretations of the 0.5% of all primary intracranial neoplasms that originate in and about the pineal gland. The cysts (epidermoid and dermoid) and the various gliomas should be so identified and designated. The very small group of remaining neoplasms are those of pineal parenchymal and germ cell origin.

Those of parenchymal origin include the pineocytoma and the pineoblastoma. The pineocytoma is generally circumscribed and formed by clusters of mature-appearing pineal cells of varying sizes and shapes, which is helpful in diagnosis. Pineoblastomas are gelatinous and invasive. These highly cellular neoplasms are composed of small cells with hyperchromatic round nuclei and little cytoplasm, thereby resembling the medulloblastomas including the formation of "rosettes" with central argyrophilic fibers. In some cases transitions between the pineocytoma and pineoblastoma have been described.

Among the teratomatous neoplasms, the germinoma is the most common (Fig. 44-82). Indistinguishable from the seminoma (or dysgerminoma), its component cells are of two types. The neoplastic cells are large, pale, polyhedral to spheroid, and separated into lobules by vascular connective tissue trabeculae next to which are small nests of lymphocytes (Fig. 44-83). The teratomas, as elsewhere in the body, have evidence of origin from multiple germ layers with varying degrees of differentiation. They may be benign or malignant, solid or cystic. Among the benign type are the epidermoid, dermoid, and differentiated teratomas. The malignant types include the teratocarcinomas, the embryonal carcinoma (endodermal sinus tumor), and some with foci of germinoma.

Mixed gliomas.[59] Gliomas of more than one cell type are common. However, the predominance of one cell type usually permits classification into one of the groups previously described. There are other gliomas that arise from cells of the subependymal cell plate.[10,17,50] These neoplasms are usually small, frequently multiple, and asymptomatic unless so strategically placed as to impede or obstruct the flow of cerebrospinal fluid. Although they are more common in the fourth ventricle (Fig. 44-84), identical neoplasms have been found about all parts of the ventricular system and about the central canal of the

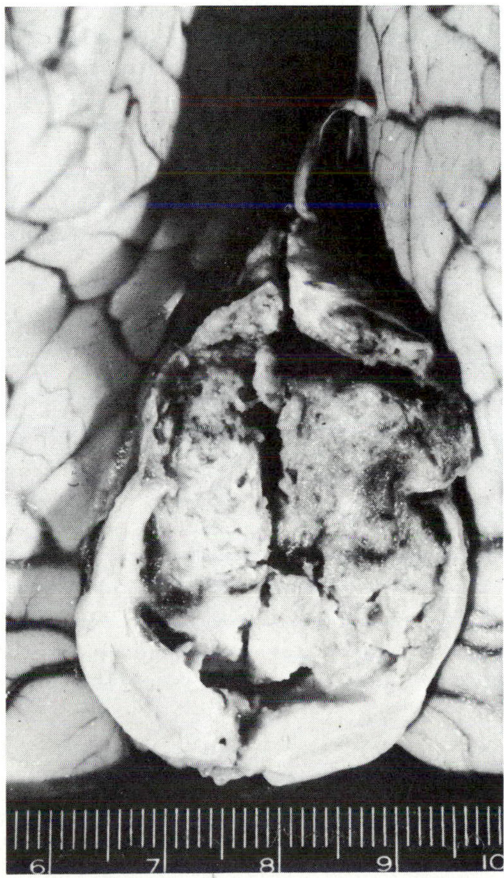

Fig. 44-82. Germinoma of pineal gland. There is gross compression of midbrain.

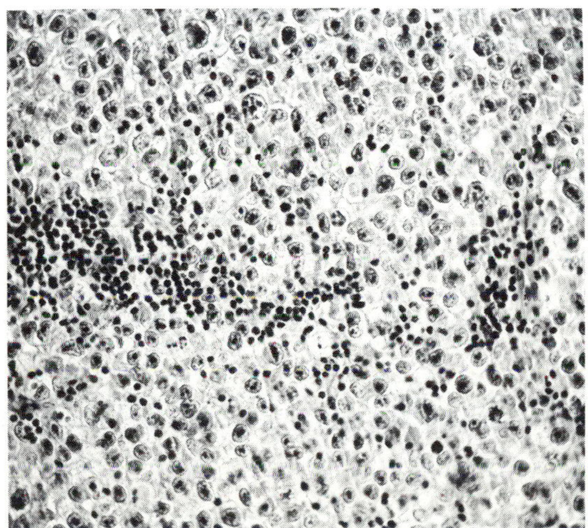

Fig. 44-83. Germinoma of pineal gland. (Hematoxylin and eosin; 135×.)

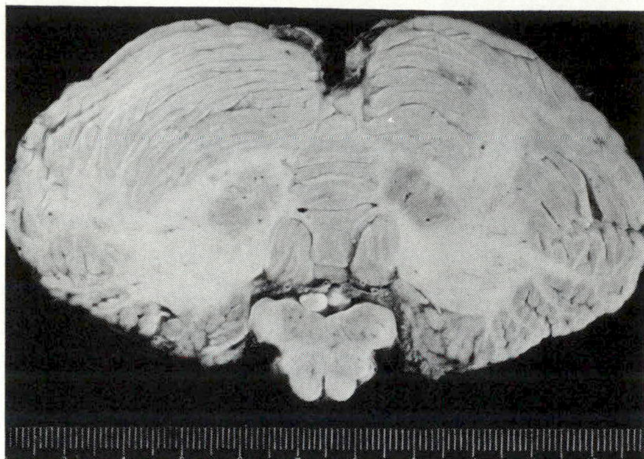

Fig. 44-84. Subependymal mixed gliomas arising in roof of fourth ventricle.

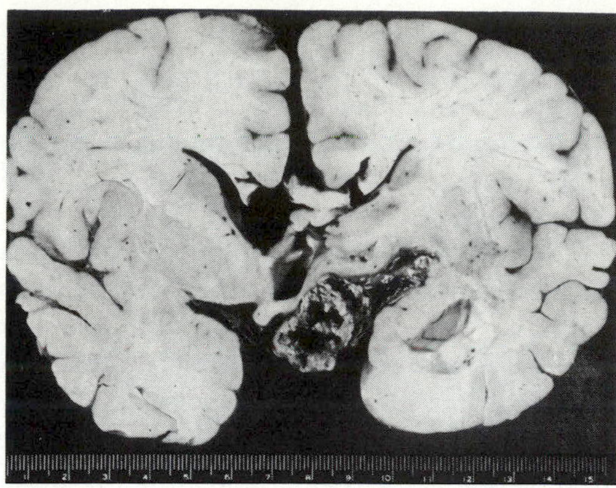

Fig. 44-85. Craniopharyngioma displacing floor of third ventricle and hypothalamus.

spinal cord. The tumors are solid, gray-white, well demarcated, firm, and sometimes mineralized. The larger neoplasms appear to be formed by the coalescence of smaller nodules of similar appearance. They are composed of plump spindle cells, some of which are in small clusters. Blepharoplasts have been demonstrated in some of the cells within the clusters. Although rosettes have been described, the usual arrangement is more like that of the obliterated central canal of the spinal cord. Surrounding these cell clusters, but also separate, are tight nodules of astrocytes with many fibrillary processes. These neoplasms have been classified as subependymal glomerate astrocytomas, as mixed subependymal gliomas, and as subependymomas. Why most have occurred in adult males is unexplained.

Ganglioglioma. Gangliogliomas are rare, usually slow-growing neoplasms that are composed of a mixture of neoplastic nerve cells most commonly with astrocytes. The structural criteria necessary for their diagnosis require the definite identification of neoplastic nerve cells rather than included normal cells. For this, it is generally required that binucleate and multinucleate nerve cells be present in addition to the neoplastic astrocytes and less often, oligodendrocytes.

Craniopharyngioma (Rathke's pouch tumor, suprasellular or epidermoid cyst)

Craniopharyngiomas form approximately 3% of all intracranial neoplasms. They appear to arise from squamous cell remnants of Rathke's pouch (Erdheim cell rests). These are cell nests that can be found at any level from the nasopharynx to the arachnoid membrane covering the mamillary bodies. Although craniopharyngiomas may be seen at most ages, there are three peaks of age incidence—childhood, early adulthood, and the fifth decade.

The encapsulated tumor has a smooth, usually lobulated, gray surface. The sectioned surface is pale gray in the solid portions with one or more cysts filled with an amber to brown fluid containing cholesterol or grumous yellow-gray material, or both (Fig. 44-85). In almost two thirds (more usual in childhood), areas of mineralization or ossification can be found scattered throughout the solid portions of the tumor. Compression of the pituitary gland, optic chiasm, nerves, and tracts and elevation of the floor of the third ventricle are common.

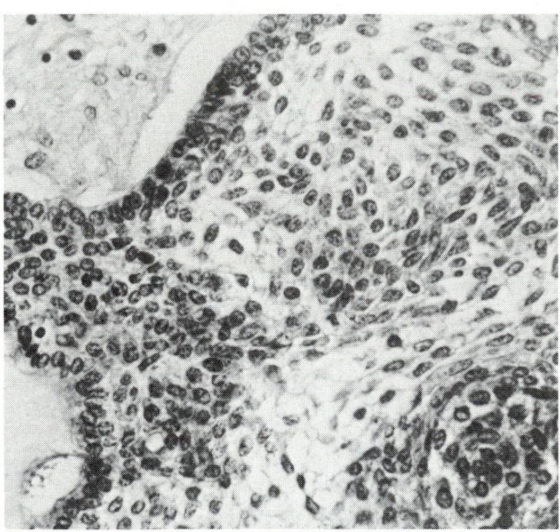

Fig. 44-86. Craniopharyngioma. Interior of islands have stellate cells with cuboid to columnar cells adjacent to stroma.

The solid portions of the neoplasm are formed by a thin layer of dense connective tissue containing a mosaic of anastomosing sheets and cords of squamous cells. The inner portions of the epithelial structures are often loose and vacuolated, whereas the outer layers of cells are usually cuboid to cylindrical. Liquefaction of the epithelial structure leads to the formation of the cystic spaces lined by stratified squamous epithelium (Fig. 44-86).

Dermoid and epidermoid cysts

It is generally conceded that the midline cysts of the dermoid and epidermoid varieties result from defects of closure of the neural tube with the heterotopic inclusion

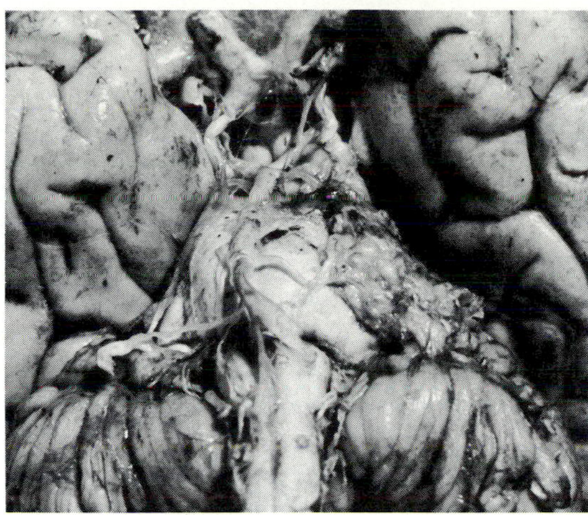

Fig. 44-87. Dermoid cyst. "Pearly" tumor is on left of the ventral surface of pons near cerebellopontine angle.

of the skin, sometimes with accessory skin structures. The cysts usually are found at or near the midline of the posterior fossa (Fig. 44-87), near the vermis, or in the fourth ventricle. The small group of epidermoid cysts in lateral positions and sometimes midline at the base of the brain are believed to represent portions of the metaplastic linings of the sinuses trapped intracranially during closure of the bones of the skull.

The cysts are rounded and circumscribed, with an outer thin connective tissue wall and with an inner cavity filled with a thick, sticky, yellow material. A stratified squamous layer with keratohyaline granules and intercellular bridges lines the cavities of the epidermoid cyst. In the dermoid cyst (Fig. 44-88), the walls also contain sweat glands, sebaceous glands, or hair follicles or all three. Spread of the contents, usually postoperative, leads to the formation of multiple small nodules formed by keratin-containing foreign body giant cells.

This entire group of cysts comprises less than 1% of all primary intracranial neoplasms.

Colloid cyst (paraphyseal cyst)[63]

According to a recent study, there are two types of ependyma-lined cysts. Both are limited to the roof of the third ventricle. The more frequent type arises after closure of an ependymal pouch whose cuboid to columnar cells contain blepharoplasts or cilia. The second type, also lined by cuboid or columnar cells without blepharoplasts or cilia, is believed to arise because of persistence of the embryonic paraphyseal pouch. The cysts are spherical masses attached to the most rostral portion of the roof of the third ventricle midway between the interventricular foramina (Fig. 44-89).

Whatever the origin of these cysts, their content is usually gray and gelatinous. When brown, the color is the result of preceding hemorrhage. The inner lining of either type of cyst wall is formed by a single layer of cuboid to columnar cells. These cells are the source of the amorphous, eosinophilic, periodic acid–Schiff–positive contents in which a few desquamated cells may be present. The outer cyst wall is formed by a thin fibrous connective tissue capsule that extends to the tela choroidea of the third ventricle. The autopsy incidence of about 2% of all intracranial tumors exceeds the clinical incidence of 0.5%, since only about one fourth of these neoplasms reach the clinically significant size of 1 cm.

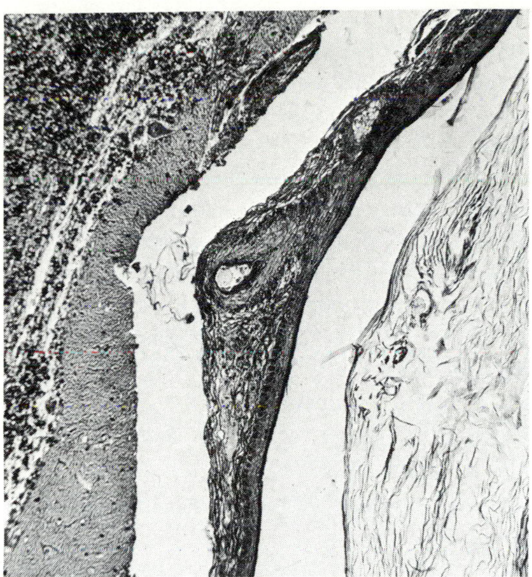

Fig. 44-88. Dermoid cyst. Stratified squamous epithelial lining of cyst contains hair follicle. Cyst lumen is filled with keratin. (Hematoxylin and eosin; 90×.)

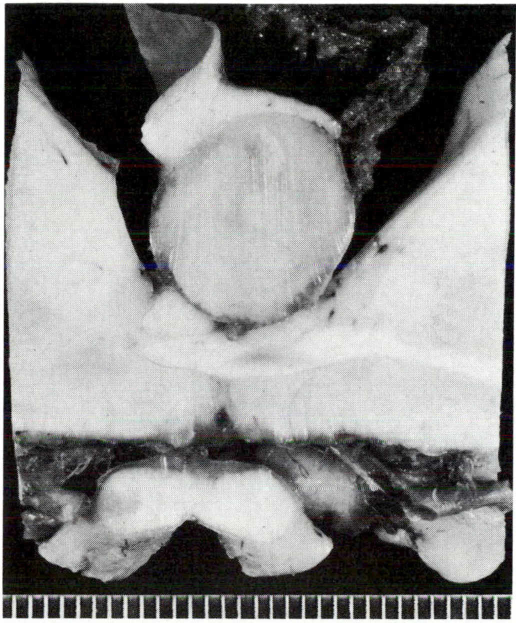

Fig. 44-89. Colloid cyst of third ventricle. Narrowed foramina of Monro are on either side of cyst.

Meningioma

Among all symptom-producing intracranial neoplasms, approximately 15% are classified as belonging to the meningiomas. This is a broad group of miscellaneous neoplasms with a variety of cells of origin.[30] Most have a dural attachment and are relatively slow growing. They are slightly more common in women and in the fifth decade. In decreasing order of frequency, the meningiomas occur parasagittally (Fig. 44-90) over the cerebral convexities, laterally over the sphenoid ridges, medially in the olfactory grooves, and in the posterior fossa (cerebellopontine angle).

Based as the classification has been on the anatomic site of origin of the tumor rather than on its cytologic origin, it is surprising that reasonably accurate generalizations as to biologic behavior are possible. Only one cell type, the arachnoid cap cell (meningocyte or meningothelial cell) is found solely in the leptomeninges. The remaining cells are those associated with the supporting tissues and blood vessels. Tumors arising from these cells have the appearance, both gross and microscopic, of similar tumors occurring elsewhere—such as fibroma, hemangioma, osteoma, chondroma, and lipoma (Fig. 44-91)—and therefore need no further description. The unencapsulated lipoma may represent a maldevelopment. About 90% to 95% of the meningiomas encountered are meningothelial, fibromatous, or inseparable mixtures of the two.

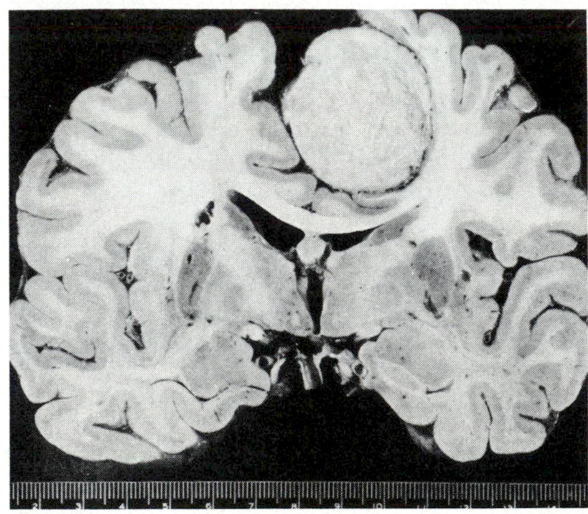

Fig. 44-90. Parasagittal meningioma, fibrous type. There are small, remote anemic infarcts in internal capsules and left putamen.

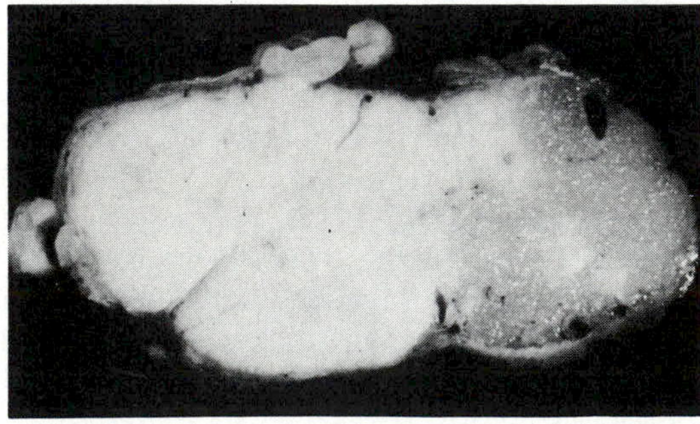

Fig. 44-91. Lipoma in leptomeninges of lumbar spinal cord. Lack of capsule on side of spinal cord is evident.

The meningothelial (meningocytic) meningioma is a thinly encapsulated, flat to spherical, moderately firm, yellow-gray, solid neoplasm usually firmly adherent at some point to the dura. The cell forming this type of neoplasm is polygonal, with poorly defined cell boundaries. Its centrally placed nucleus is relatively large and round and contains finely divided chromatin without an evident nucleolus. In some tumors the cells are arranged in onion-skin-like whorls or in sheets of varying sizes (Fig. 44-92). In the centers of many of the whorls and at the edges or within the sheets are capillaries or slightly larger blood vessels. Connective and elastic tissue and reticulin are confined to the blood vessel walls and act as a stroma supporting the neoplasm. Calcospheres (psammoma bodies) in varying numbers may be found in these neoplasms. They apparently represent a degenerative change with mineralization within the walls of blood vessels or tumor cells. When they predominate, the meningothelial meningioma is considered by some to be of the psammomatous type. This is a common occurrence at the spinal level, where it is associated with a long history and very slow progression of signs and symptoms.

Although these neoplasms are classified as benign, there may be recurrence even after the entire tumor appears to have been removed. Multiple tumors are

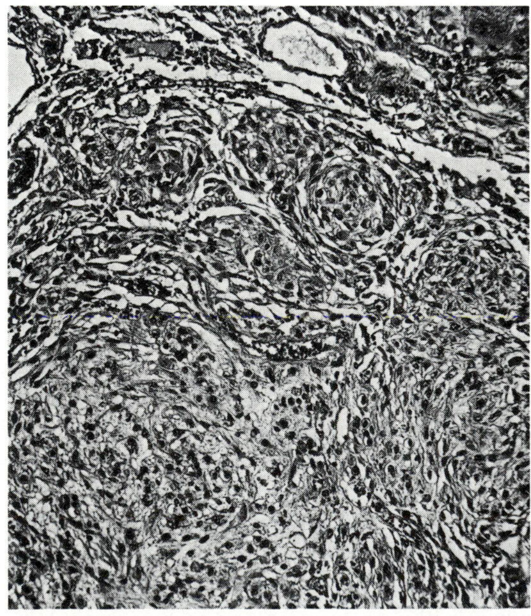

Fig. 44-92. Meningothelial meningioma with typical whorls. (Hematoxylin and eosin; 90×.)

infrequent. In addition, they have the propensity for growing into the adjacent dura, dural sinus, and skull, as do arachnoid granulations. Metastasis, on the other hand, is extremely rare. Cytologic and histologic criteria suggesting malignancy, such as nuclear enlargement, irregularity, hyperchromatism, and growth beyond the capsule, occur in about 10% of the surgically removed meningothelial meningiomas. This is, however, far in excess of any malignant biologic activity.

Extension of the neoplasm through the dura with reaction of the overlying bone may be helpful in determining the rate of growth of the tumor. Benign and slow-growing meningiomas often are associated with destruction of the inner table of the skull with a "sunburst" type of bone production of the outer table. More rapidly growing tumors destroy both tables without reactive bone formation.

"Incidental" asymptomatic, small meningiomas, usually of the meningothelial and fibromatous types, are a frequent finding at postmortem examination. Their numbers exceed those that have produced clinical symptoms and signs.

Schwannoma (neurilemoma, neurofibroma)

Schwannomas, neoplasms arising from the Schwann cells of peripheral nerves, comprise 8% of all intracranial neoplasms. They originate most commonly from the vestibular portion of the eighth nerve in the region of the internal acoustic meatus (Fig. 44-93) and grow into the cerebellopontine angle. They may arise from any of the cranial nerves having a Schwann sheath; the other cranial nerves of origin in decreasing order of frequency are the ninth, seventh, eleventh, fifth, and fourth.

The intracranial tumors are most often clinically apparent during the fourth through sixth decades and are two to three times more common in women than in men. The neoplasms are usually single; when multiple, they may be a manifestation of von Recklinghausen's disease (Fig. 44-94).

The intracranial tumors are encapsulated, firm, and gray-white and are attached to or appear as part of the cranial nerve, which is then stretched about or within the mass. The larger lesions often have an irregular lobulated surface with yellow, softened, and sometimes hemorrhagic areas internally. Among the several characteristic microscopic features of these neoplasms are the following:

1. The capsule is relatively thick (as compared with the meningioma).
2. The larger lesions are divided into compact, solid areas that are relatively highly cellular (Antoni type A) and areas that are loose, reticular, and less cellular (Antoni type B).
3. The cells of the more cellular areas are spindle shaped with long processes and nuclei that are long and narrow with finely granular chromatin.

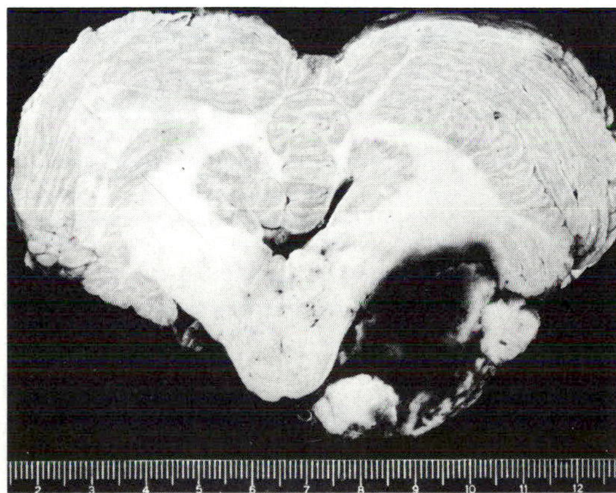

Fig. 44-93. Right cerebellopontine angle schwannoma with recent operative hemorrhage. Pons, cerebellum, and fourth ventricle are compressed and displaced.

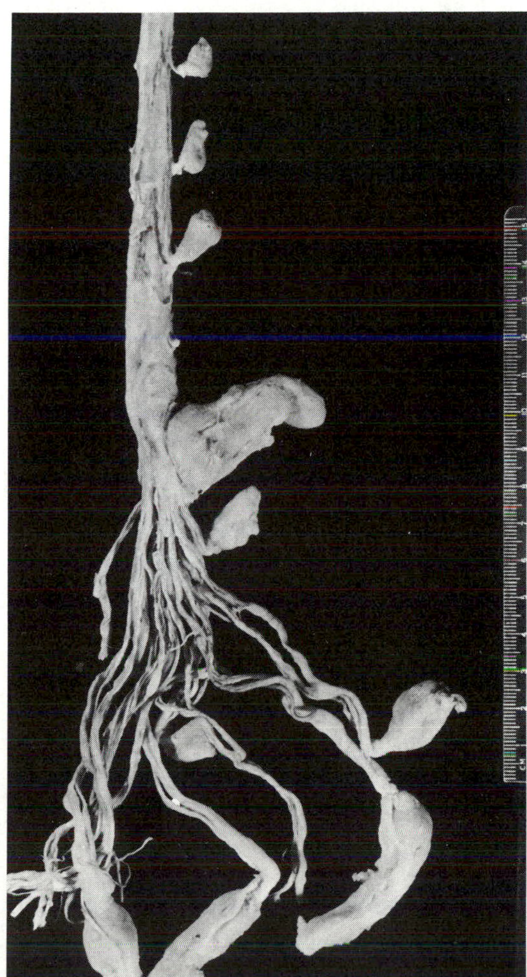

Fig. 44-94. Neurofibromatosis involving cauda equina and spinal ganglia in patient with von Recklinghausen's disease.

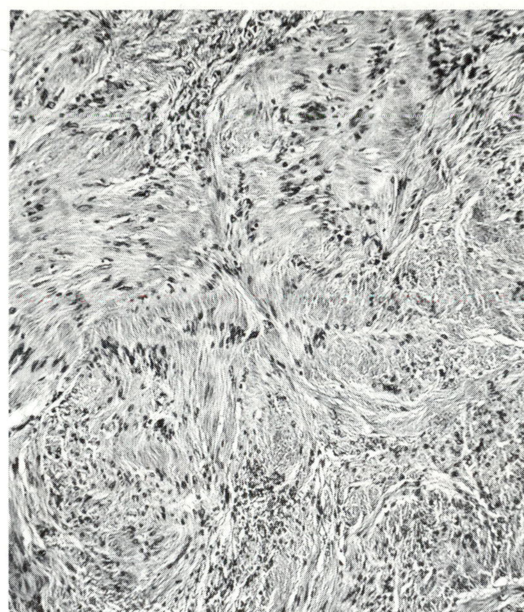

Fig. 44-95. Schwannoma. Portion with interlacing fascicular pattern. (Hematoxylin and eosin; 90×.)

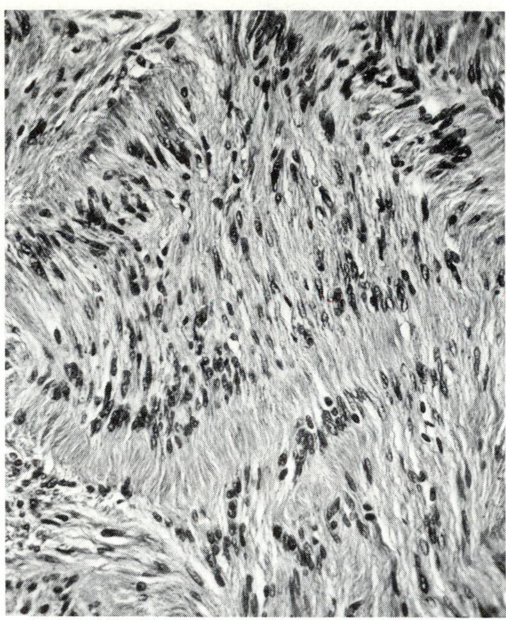

Fig. 44-96. Schwannoma. Palisading of nuclei. (Hematoxylin and eosin; 185×.)

4. A portion of the tumor regularly has cells with an interlacing fascicular pattern (Fig. 44-95).
5. In some areas the nuclei tend to align as palisades (Fig. 44-96).
6. An occasional whorl-like arrangement simulates a tactile end organ (Verocay body).
7. In the Antoni type B areas the neoplastic cells are more plump and more varied in appearance.
8. Pronounced hyalinization with thickening of the walls of the blood vessels is characteristic; it often leads to necrosis and hemorrhage, sometimes with thrombosis.
9. The cystic areas containing numerous lipid and hemosiderin-laden macrophages may be organized, with the formation of granulation tissue.

The intracranial schwannomas are histologically benign lesions, although they frequently recur if incompletely removed. Rarely do they undergo malignant transformation.

Almost one third of spinal tumors are schwannomas. They are always attached to a nerve root and occur at all levels, including the cauda equina (Fig. 44-97). In most cases the involved nerve root lies between the spinal cord and the dura. Of the remaining, an equal number involve the nerve root as it traverses the dura or lie outside the dura. The spinal schwannomas are smaller than the schwannomas of the eighth cranial nerve and, although they have the usual gross and microscopic features, the Antoni type A appearance is by far the more frequent.

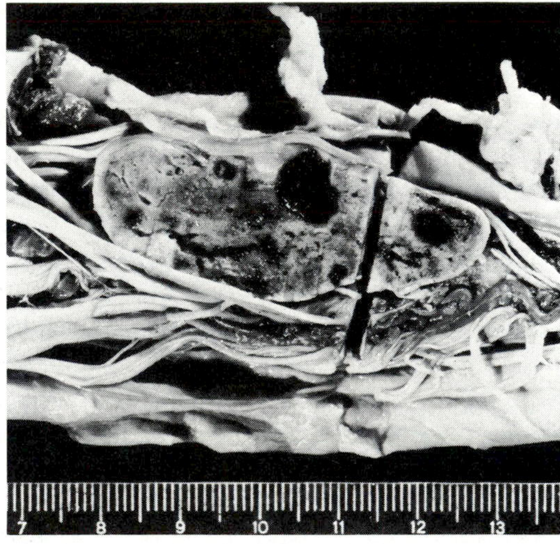

Fig. 44-97. Schwannoma originating in filament of cauda equina.

Vascular malformations and neoplasms

Vascular malformations in the central nervous system are frequent. During a 5-year period when the brain at postmortem examination was routinely sectioned at 2 to 3 mm intervals, vascular malformations were found in over 5%. In the majority the lesions were incidental. No classification satisfactorily encompasses the range of their structural appearances.[92] When thorough analyses are made of the lesions, frequently portions are found to have features of more than one type of lesion.

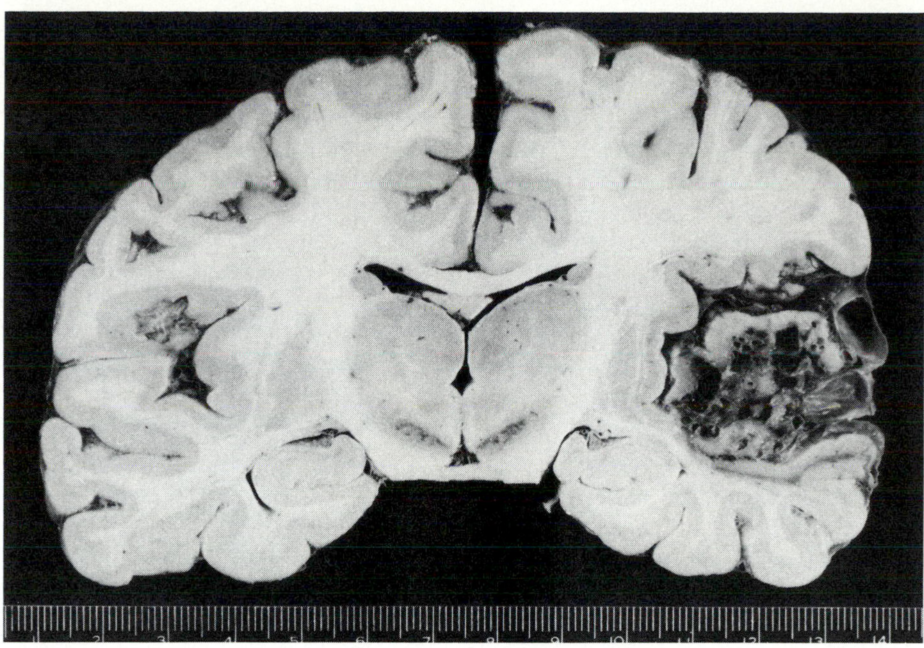

Fig. 44-98. Vascular malformation in superior temporal gyrus with large draining vein.

Telangiectasia (capillary telangiectasis, capillary angioma). Telangiectasia is the most frequent of the vascular malformations. They are found in adults of both sexes and in all portions of the brain. Because of their small size (usually less than 1 cm) and because they are usually single, they often are missed on the routine sectioning of the brain. They appear as well-circumscribed but nonencapsulated dark red areas in which there is a fine stippling caused by the engorged blood vessels. One portion or the entire area on occasion may have an orange-brown appearance because of remote bleeding.

Microscopically the lesion is composed of capillaries with some variation in size. In the usual small lesion, intervening brain tissue separates the capillaries. In the larger lesions this is noted only at the periphery, since the center contains larger capillary vessels with no intervening nerve tissue. These lesions occasionally lead to a small local hemorrhage. Their recognition in the wall of a massive hemorrhage, sometimes extending into the ventricular or subarachnoid spaces, is difficult. To adequately investigate such an instance, one should strain the blood obtained from the lesion through several layers of gauze as it is being washed, with the residual tissue retained by the gauze being examined for the presence of the vascular lesion.

Arteriovenous malformations. Although less frequent than the telangiectasia, arteriovenous malformations involve the brain (Fig. 44-98) and spinal cord. Based on the appearance of the vessel wall, traditional divisions of these lesions have been made to include arteriovenous and venous types.

The arteriovenous malformation is composed of a complex tangle of enlarged dilated arteries and veins without intervening identifiable capillaries. The lesions appear to be more common in men and are often in the area of the middle cerebral artery. On microscopic examination there is irregular fibrous thickening of the arterial intima, often with fraying, reduplication or the destruction of the internal elastic lamina, and variable thickening of the media. The thinner-walled veins usually have undergone varying degrees of hyalinization of their media and intimal fibrosis so that they resemble arteries. Although these lesions may be in the brain or in the leptomeninges, the malformation often enlarges sufficiently to involve both. Occasionally only venous types of vessels are recognized. These lesions may be asymptomatic or, with rupture, may be associated with the signs and symptoms of intraventricular or subarachnoid hemorrhage. In most, with their continued enlargement and some with minor bleeding as well, there is a surrounding astrocytic gliosis and gray matter atrophy; the resulting symptoms depend on the site of the malformation.

Sturge-Weber-Dimitri disease (cephalic neurocutaneous angiomatosis). Sturge-Weber-Dimitri disease is a rare developmental disturbance of blood vessels involving both the skin and the brain. It has been found in families and has been associated in some cases with mental retardation.

In this disease occurring in the leptomeninges and in atrophic portions of the brain (mainly the occipital and parietal lobes) including the cortex and white matter, there is a striking increase in blood vessels with collagenization of many. Mineralization is generally limited to the cortex and, when pronounced, produces a characteristic x-ray pattern. Cortical atrophy is accompanied by a reactive astrocytic gliosis and focal compensatory hydrocephalus. The associated skin lesion is a ipsilateral facial nevus flammeus (port-wine stain) in the distribution of one or more branches of the trigeminal nerve. Other developmental lesions have been associated in a few instances.

Capillary hemangioblastomas (hemangioendothelioma, angioblastic meningioma).[75,95,107] Hemangioblastomas are red to yellow-gray, firm neoplasms of varying size. Although found in all portions of the central nervous system, they are more common in the cerebellum. In the posterior fossa they comprise 7% of all primary tumors. The cerebral lesions are usually solid, but the cerebellar lesions are more characteristically cystic with a mural nodule. The neoplasm may be single or multiple but always has a leptomeningeal attachment.

The tumor is composed of well-formed capillaries with prominent endothelial cells (Fig. 44-99) in an abundant reticulin network extending radially from or concentrically about the capillaries (Fig. 44-100). Large lipid-containing macrophages are found scattered throughout the tumor, often imparting a yellow background to the usual red-gray gross appearance. The nuclei of the cells are usually large and uniform. Although variation in nuclear size may be found (Fig. 44-99), this is not indicative of malignant transformation.

The cerebellar lesion is usually single and near the midline, but exceptions to both have been described. With less than 10% of the cerebellar lesions, there is a similar tumor in the retina, vascular malformation of the spinal cord, cysts of the pancreas and liver, or cysts or tumors of the kidney (adenocarcinoma). This combination, known as von Hippel-Lindau disease, is more likely to occur with multiple cerebellar tumors. Familial occurrences and associations with erythremia and pheochromocytomas have been reported.

Sarcomas[76,101]

Sarcomas of the central nervous system originate from the multipotential cells in the walls of the blood vessels within the substance of the brain and spinal cord. Although almost any type of mesodermal tumor can develop from these cells, the most common primary lesions are those that resemble one of the malignant lymphomas. In my experience almost all are B cell type. They appear to arise from neoplastic cells formed elsewhere and escape destruction by the immune system. Having entered the central nervous system, they appear to be protected by the blood-brain barrier. Although similar lesions may be found elsewhere in the reticuloendothelial system, this is uncommon, even at postmortem examination. The response of sarcomas to treatment, even when they are multicentric in the central nervous system, is generally good (Fig. 44-101). The position of the "cerebellar sarcoma" as previously described is under active debate. At the present time, the evidence suggests that this is a form of medulloblastoma with extension into the leptomeninges.

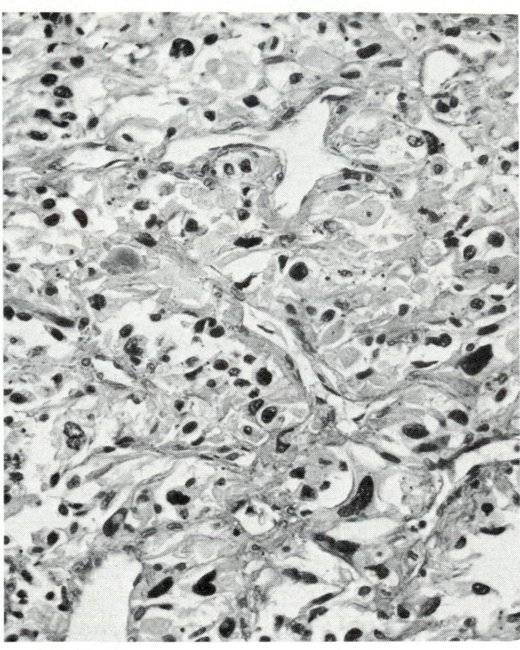

Fig. 44-99. Capillary hemangioblastoma in cerebellum. (Hematoxylin and eosin; 135×.)

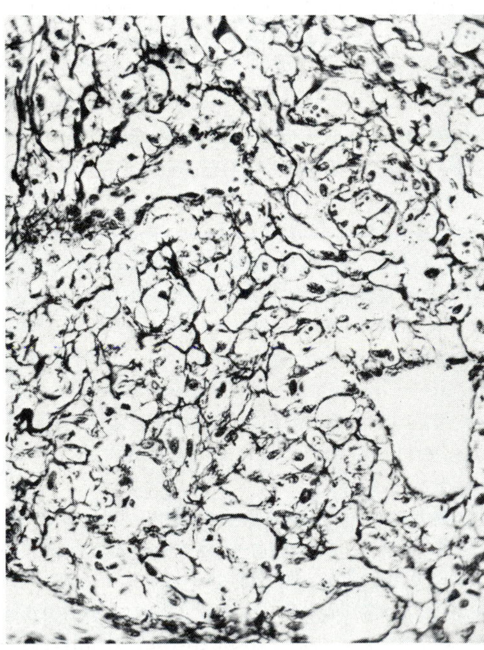

Fig. 44-100. Capillary hemangioblastoma in cerebellum. (Reticulin stain; 90×.)

Metastatic neoplasms[23]

It has been suggested that metastatic neoplasms comprise up to 30% of all intracranial tumors. The great variation in the estimated frequency is ascribed to inadequate and biased sampling. Metastatic tumors are well demarcated and multiple in over 80% of cases (Fig. 44-102). Those under 1 cm in size are usually solid. Larger lesions are cystic because of central necrosis, often with a 1 to 2 mm rim of neoplasm. Extension of the neoplasm into the subarachnoid space is common. Smaller metastases are often found in the white matter just beneath the arcuate fibers.

The primary sources, in order of frequency, are the lungs, breasts, kidneys, skin (melanoma), gastrointestinal tract, and prostate. Neoplastic cell emboli reach the nervous system almost exclusively by way of the arteries with preceding involvement of the lungs. Sole localization within the leptomeninges (primary meningeal carcinomatosis, carcinomatous meningitis) is uncommon. In 2% of those with brain metastases, the spinal cord or cauda equina or both (Fig. 44-103) are also involved.

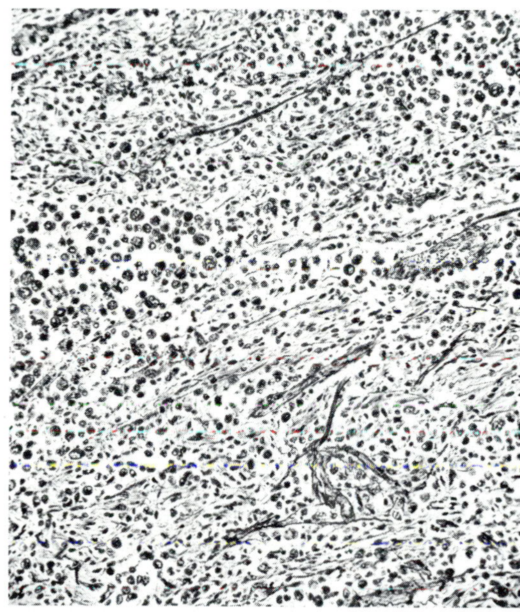

Fig. 44-101. Malignant lymphoma, histiocytic type (reticulum cell sarcoma) in brain. (Hematoxylin and eosin; 90×.)

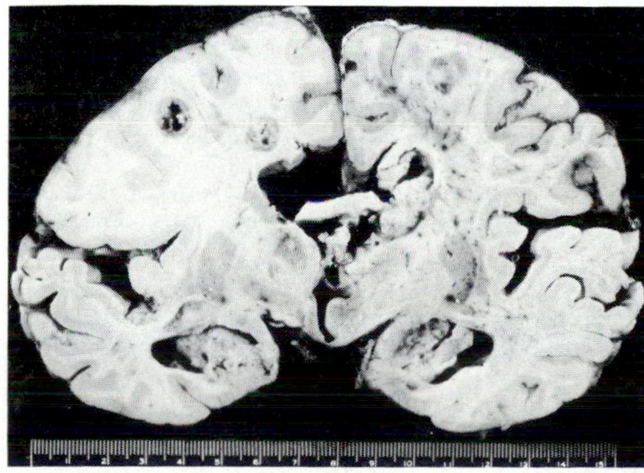

Fig. 44-102. Multiple metastases to brain and ependyma from carcinoma of lung.

Brain swelling and edema[121]

Enlargement of the brain resulting from the intracellular accumulation of colloidally bound fluid is known as brain swelling, or dry brain. Enlargement resulting from the presence of an increased amount of intercellular fluid is known as brain edema or wet brain. Both have been related to many causes, including trauma, neoplasms, toxic states, hypoxia, and inflammations. Swelling is of cytogenic origin, whereas edema is vasogenic. Brain swelling is much more common and usually precedes brain edema. The enlarged and swollen brain is heavy, with a decrease in size of the subarachnoid and ventric-

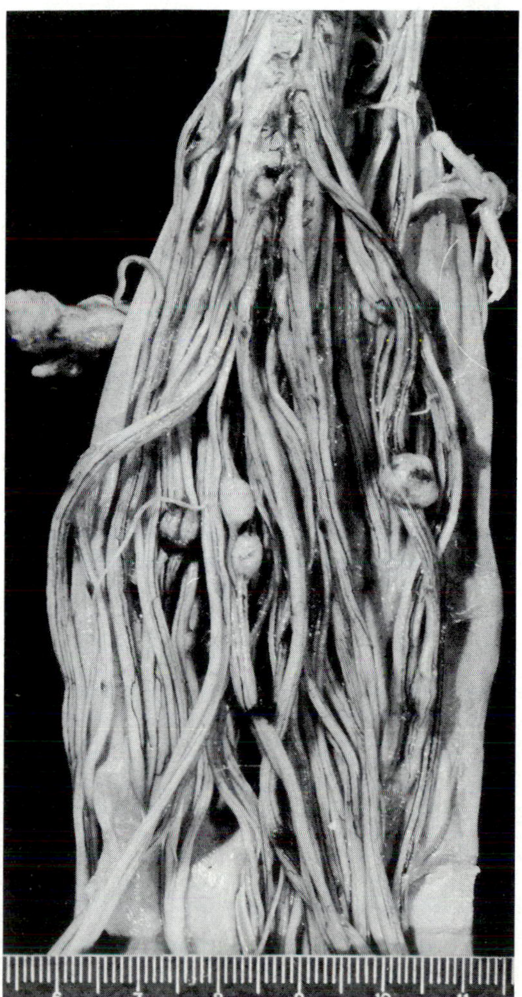

Fig. 44-103. Metastatic carcinoma onto filaments of cauda equina.

ular spaces. The cerebral convolutions are large, and their crests are flat with compression of the sulci. The sectioned surface of the brain is pale and dry and bulges slightly. The increase in size is attributable entirely to the increase in size of the central white matter. Despite the obvious gross changes, with routine stains the microscopic changes are minimal.

An accompanying edema can be recognized by depression and wetness of the cut surface. This is the result of the separation of the cell processes and myelin sheaths by the accumulation of fluid between them and about the blood vessels. When the fluid is high in protein content and is eosinophilic, recognition is easy. Separation of the microscopic changes from postmortem and processing artifacts is difficult when the fluid is low in protein and only enlargement of the spaces is to be seen.

Persistence of the edematous state is accompanied by a reactive astrocytosis characterized by cytoplasmic eosinophilia, focal enlargement and fragmentation of axons, loss of myelin, and occasional macrophages.

Brain displacement and herniation[78]

An expanding intracranial mass often combined with brain swelling and edema is frequently associated with brain displacement and herniation. The more slowly the expansion occurs, the greater the changes that may follow. When the lesion is in the midline and frontal or if both hemispheres are generally and equally affected, the cerebral hemispheres and portions of the midbrain are displaced downward through the incisura of the tentorium. As a result the midbrain is elongated and the unci become notched by the free margins of the tentorium. The structures occupying the posterior fossa may simultaneously be displaced downward, with impaction of the medulla and cerebellar tonsils into the funnel-shaped foramen magnum (Fig. 44-104). With this downward displacement the cerebellar tonsils become elongated and notched and the ventral surface of the medulla becomes flattened, sometimes even notched. The displaced pons simultaneously becomes foreshortened and widened. Each downward displacement produces a degree of obstruction of the flow of cerebrospinal fluid.

An expanding lateral or eccentrically placed cerebral mass may produce asymmetric brain displacement and herniation. When the displacement is toward the opposite hemisphere, the cingulate gyrus is forced across the midline beneath the free margin of the falx. Downward displacement to the side ipsilateral to the mass produces an ipsilateral uncal groove (Fig. 44-105), compression of the ipsilateral third nerve, and sometimes a notching of the ipsilateral cerebral peduncle by the free margin of the tentorium. With this caudal displacement, the free margin of the tentorium compresses the overriding ipsilateral posterior cerebral artery. The occlusion can, in turn, result in the production of an anemic and, on release, a hemorrhagic infarct in the area supplied (Fig. 44-105). The combination of downward and contralateral displacement produces another combination of herniations. More frequently, there is compression of the uncus on the ipsilateral side, and contralateral compression of the cerebral peduncle and posterior cerebral artery occurs.

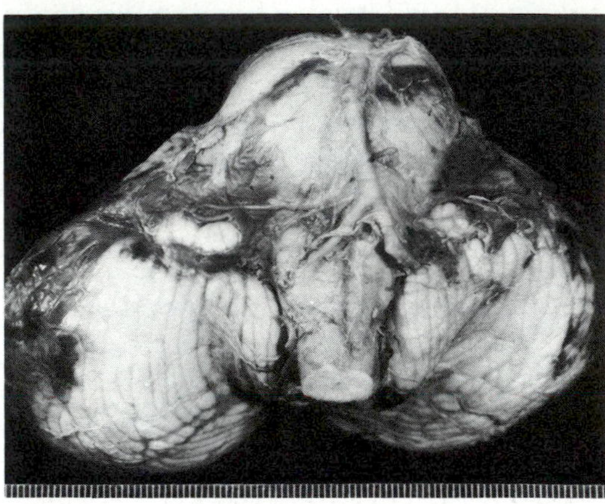

Fig. 44-104. Foreshortening and widening of pons with cerebellomedullary herniation resulting from cerebral mass lesion with brain swelling, edema, and displacement.

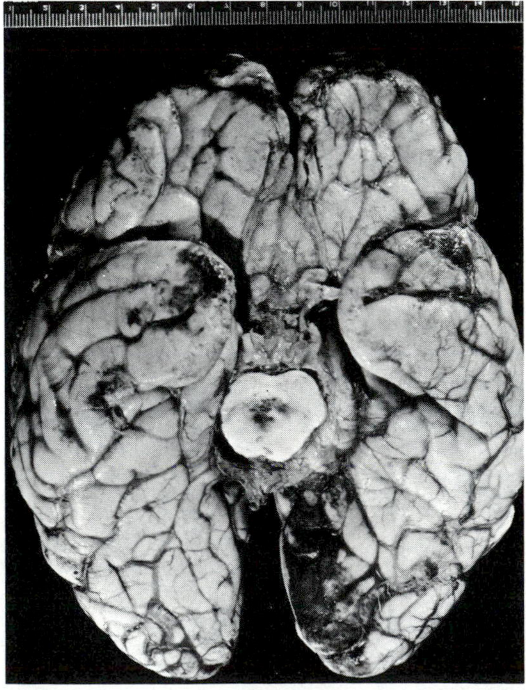

Fig. 44-105. Brain displacement with large right uncal herniation. There is compression of right posterior cerebral artery with hemorrhagic infarct of medial portion of occipital lobe and with overlying subarachnoid hemorrhage. Secondary hemorrhages are in lower midbrain.

Tumors of the posterior fossa are associated with downward displacement and notching of the medulla and cerebellar tonsils. There may be notching of the superior surface of the cerebellum if either or both hemispheres of the cerebellum are displaced upward. Downward displacements can be accentuated by the injudicious use of lumbar puncture.

The brain also may herniate through dural defects and irregularities such as the points of entrance or exit of the blood vessels. A large dural defect such as may be produced after operation can permit a large local herniation, fungus cerebri.

The microscopic appearances with each of the herniations are characteristic of focal ischemia and sometimes with small areas of necrosis.

Midbrain, pontine, and sometimes thalamic hemorrhages are common fatal secondary effects produced by supratentorial expanding masses. The mechanism causing these hemorrhages is unknown.[78] They appear to be related to the downward displacement of the brain without the simultaneous displacement of the basilar artery and its branches and to the dorsoventral stretching of these branches. These produce angulation, compression, and tearing of the vessels within the brainstem.

PERIPHERAL NERVOUS SYSTEM

Structure and function

Because much of the peripheral nervous system has been covered in the description of diseases of the various organs, this discussion is limited to the nervous system supplying the limbs. This portion includes the sensory fibers whose unipolar cell bodies are in the spinal ganglia, whose dendritic processes extend from the limbs, and whose axons reach to the spinal cord or brainstem. The motor fibers begin as peripheral nerves in the motor nerve root area of the spinal cord and brainstem. At the nerve root the myelin sheath, on both the sensory and motor sides, is abruptly changed from that formed by oligodendrocytes centrally to that formed by Schwann cells peripherally. This occurs at a node of Ranvier, and the portion of the nerve proximal to this change is in the Obersteiner-Redlich zone of the subarachnoid space. The site of change is easily recognizable with the hematoxylin and eosin stain because of the lighter staining of the central portion and the darker staining of the peripheral nervous system portion. Sensory, motor, and mixed nerves have the same general organizational pattern. Individual axons are surrounded by Schwann cells in a linear series separated at the junctions of Schwann cells, Ranvier's nodes. The basement membrane and a thin, fibrous layer, the endoneurium, surround the covering Schwann cells. Fascicular groups of fibers are surrounded by a more easily seen and thicker layer of connective tissue, the perineurium. The epineurium surrounds the entire nerve and extends to the surrounding connective tissues. The perikaryons of the cells of the spinal ganglia are large and spherical. They are surrounded by a single layer of flattened cuboid cap cells. These cells are considered to be the counterpart of Schwann cells peripherally and of the oligodendrocytes centrally. Unmyelinated fibers are covered by an infolded portion of a Schwann cell membrane. The linear series of these cells have tight male-female junctions.

Degenerations

Degenerative changes of the spinal ganglia cells and their reactions are similar to those of the large nerve cells elsewhere. Aging is associated with cell loss and the progressive accumulation of lipofuscin, a yellow to brown granular pigment, either about or to one side of the nucleus in the remaining cells. Cell shrinkage is associated with irregularities of shape, pyknosis of the nucleus, and proliferation of the surrounding cap cells. The changes of central and peripheral chromatolysis are identical to those in the cells of the central nervous system. Cell death is accompanied initially by proliferation of and, later, phagocytosis by the cap cells. Nageotte clusters represent a residual whorled arrangement of cap cells after the loss of a ganglion cell. Cell counts have demonstrated that there is a gradual and continuous loss of spinal ganglion cells with increasing age.

Disintegration of the axons may follow damage to the cell body or may be the result of local injury. With the latter, the change progresses centrally only as far as the next Ranvier's node. The axons may become focally swollen with varicosities or generally swollen and fragmented and later demonstrate increasing granularity. Myelin beading, swelling, and fragmentation accompany the changes in the axons. Chemical changes in the myelin sheath, demonstrable by special stains, first appear 8 to 10 days after the initial injury and probably are related to the formation of cholesterol esters. Stainable neutral fats appear soon afterward and are slowly removed by macrophages and Schwann cells. Regeneration is possible when the damage to the nerve cells of the spinal ganglia is minimal or is limited to the peripheral axon. Concurrently with the degenerative changes, Schwann cells begin to proliferate forming the so-called neurolemmal tubules. Multiple fibrillary outgrowths from the central end of the damaged axon make their initial appearance at the end of the first week in myelinated nerves and after the second week in the unmyelinated fibers. The downgrowing fibers enter the proximal ends of the neurolemmal tubules, sometimes before there is complete degeneration and removal of the injured tissues. It is assumed that there is an influence that governs the pattern of regeneration. There is, however, always some degree of loss of the normal relationships so that not all fibers reach and grow into the correct neurolemmal tubule. The degree of disorganization is more pronounced in the presence of foreign material and with the formation of scar tissue. The factor that determines which of the fiber branches continues to grow downward into the tubule and which disappears is not known. It is believed that those fibers that have entered improper tubules (that is, sensory fibers in a motor area) do not achieve function and eventually degenerate. Initially, all regenerated fibers are nonmyelinated. Myelination about some fibers proceeds distally from the central end, making its proximal appearance about 1 month after injury.

When these structures are examined routinely at autopsy, it can be seen that the spinal ganglia and peripheral nerves participate in many so-called nonneurologic diseases that affect the individual.

The causes of damage to a peripheral nerve are many, and the initial locus of damage is equally varied. Nerve biopsy is not common in these conditions, and the early changes usually are inferred from those found at autopsy or are found in the course of examination for other diseases. The limited response on the part of the peripheral nerve, however, places many disorders in relatively uniform categories of structural change. In all of these nonneoplastic disorders, the changes in the axons and myelin sheaths are swelling and fragmentation and eventual loss of the myelin sheath at that level. A mild to moderate reactive fibrosis is part of the response about the affected fibers. With continued injury the degenerative changes may progress toward the perikaryon. Early, one may find a mononuclear response with lipid-containing phagocytes in the areas of damage. With the most severe states of sensory nerve involvement, axonal degeneration may be seen in the cells of the spinal ganglia (central chromatolysis), with accompanying satellitosis and even neuronophagia.

Cysts of spinal ganglia[38]

Although of frequent occurrence, cysts of the spinal ganglia are rarely symptomatic. It has been assumed that they result from the cerebrospinal fluid pressure exerted on the sleeves of pia-arachnoid that accompany the nerves as they exit toward the intervertebral spaces. When the fine porous openings in the pia-arachnoid through which the nerve fibers course become narrowed, perhaps as a result of scarring, the cerebrospinal fluid pressure, increased by the long periods of upright position in humans, becomes more effective in bulging the walls of this funnel-like space. This results in the formation of a cyst whose distal outer wall often is in the proximal portion of the spinal ganglion. When clinically symptomatic, it is believed to be attributable to the effect of the pressure on the included nerve fibers.

Metastatic cancer to spinal ganglia and peripheral nerves

The spinal ganglia, like all living tissue of the body, can be expected to be the site for metastatic disease (Fig. 44-106). In a prospective postmortem study, the spinal ganglia were involved in 2% of all patients with carcinoma that had separately metastasized to the central nervous system as well.[23] It was recognized that this must have represented a minimal involvement, since usually only one ganglion and rarely more than two ganglia were examined in this study.

Involvement of the peripheral nerve by metastatic cancer has been reported on many occasions. This is particularly true with certain cancers, such as those of the prostate, urinary bladder, and cervix, where their mode of spread is believed to be through the perineural lymphatic spaces.

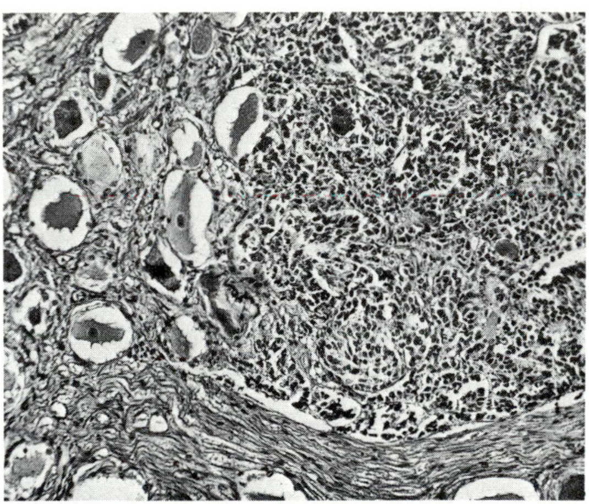

Fig. 44-106. Spinal ganglion with metastatic carcinoma from prostate. (Hematoxylin and eosin; 135×.)

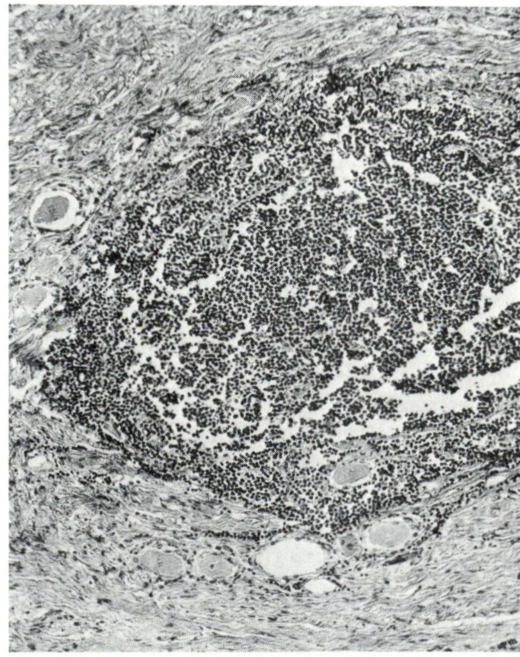

Fig. 44-107. Infiltrate of chronic granulocytic leukemia in spinal ganglion. (Hematoxylin and eosin; 90×.)

Spinal ganglia and peripheral nerves frequently are involved in patients with a lymphoma, leukemia (Fig. 44-107), or multiple myeloma.[37] The lack of clinical recognition, as with the carcinoma, is probably related to the more pressing and more symptomatic involvement of other tissues.

Amyloidosis

Amyloidosis, with the exception of familial cases, is a late and uncommon complication of diseases with which generalized amyloid deposition is to be expected. It is characterized by hyaline eosinophilic balls between nerve fibers in the spinal ganglia (Fig. 44-108) and in the peripheral nerves (Fig. 44-109). A relation to blood vessel walls is not always apparent. Typical deposition in the walls of smaller blood vessels also is seen. Familial cases of amyloidosis have been described as occurring in certain Portuguese families, possibly from genetic causes.

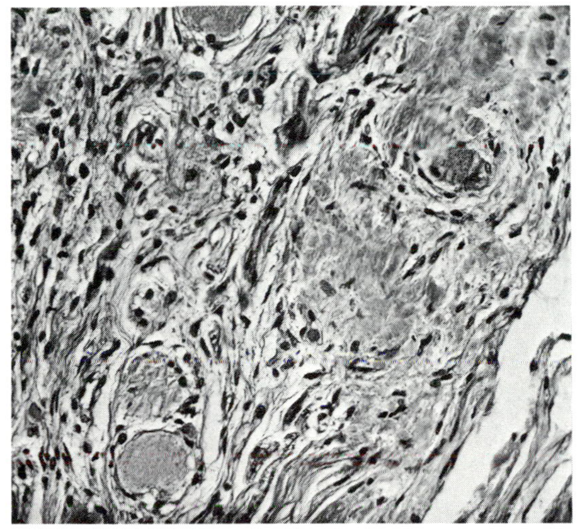

Fig. 44-108. Amyloidosis of spinal ganglion. (Hematoxylin and eosin; 280×.)

Hemorrhage

Hemorrhage into the proximal half of the dorsal root ganglion is not uncommon. Most frequently, it represents extension of subarachnoid hemorrhage in the pia-arachnoid sleeve that surrounds the peripheral rootlets. In most instances the blood appears to finally escape along the usual channels of cerebrospinal fluid flow. In some the blood becomes locally organized. The hemoglobin is converted to hemosiderin and hematoidin, and there is a moderate degree of reactive fibrosis. In our autopsy material, none of the hemorrhages had been recognized as symptomatic.

Inflammation

Nonspecific inflammatory changes in the spinal ganglia and peripheral nerves are not uncommon (Fig. 44-110). These changes are characterized by cellular infiltrates, predominantly lymphocytic, and sometimes by degenerative changes in the axons and in the myelin sheaths. Abnormalities of this type were seen in approximately 5% of routine autopsies in a general city hospital.[19] The lesions appear to be nonspecific and related more to a general state of the body than to a disease specifically affecting the nervous system. In most instances there was no clinical recognition of such involvement. When changes are severe and limited to the rootlets, sometimes with involvement of the spinal

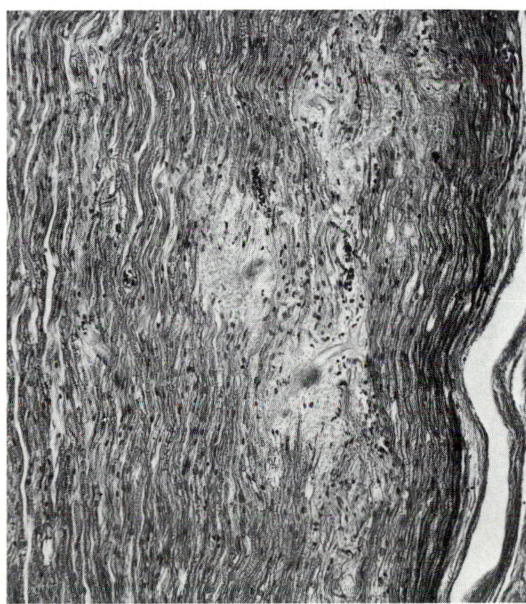

Fig. 44-109. Amyloidosis of peripheral nerve. (Hematoxylin and eosin; 90×.)

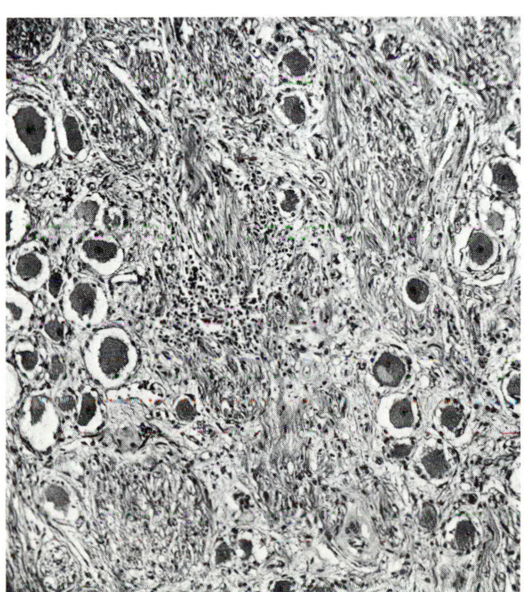

Fig. 44-110. Lumbar spinal ganglion with nonspecific focal chronic inflammation. (Hematoxylin and eosin; 90×.)

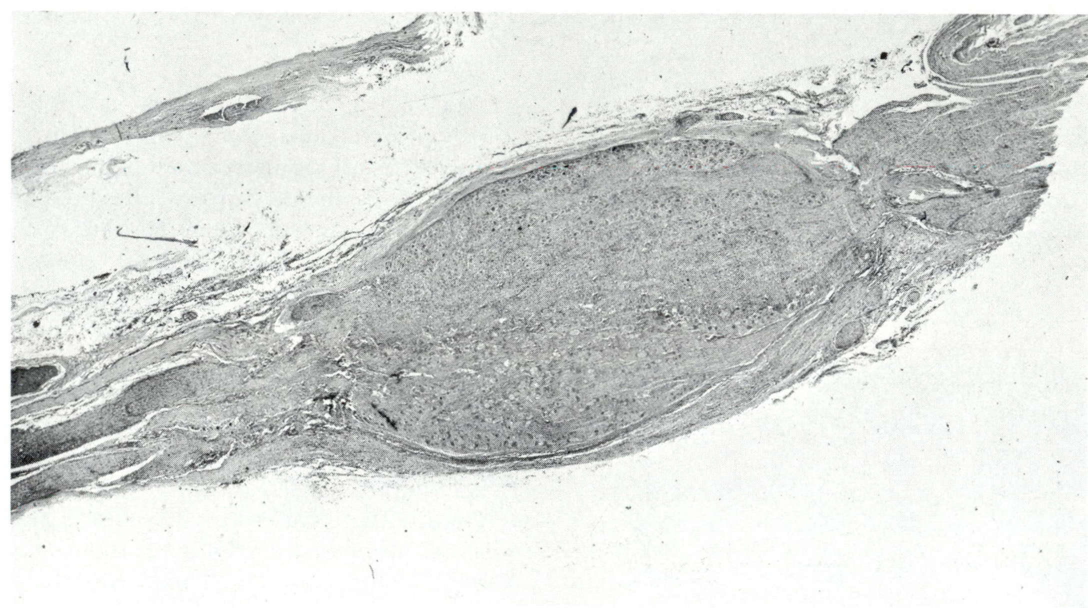

Fig. 44-111. Herpes zoster. There is necrosis of upper half of spinal ganglion. (Hematoxylin and eosin; 8×.)

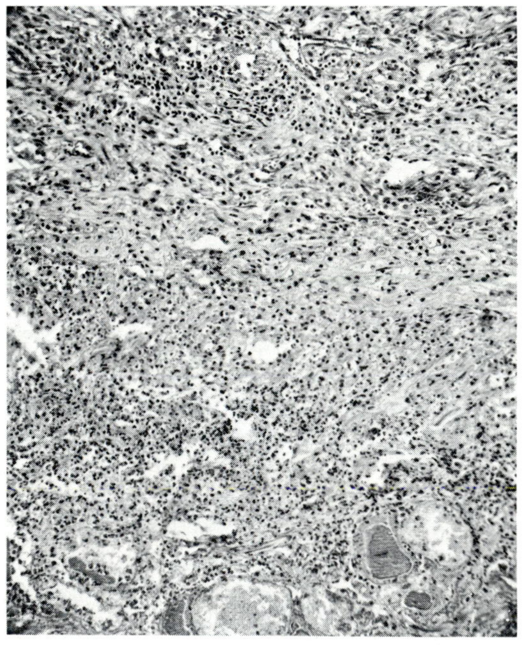

Fig. 44-112. Herpes zoster. There is necrosis of upper half of spinal ganglion. (Hematoxylin and eosin; 90×.)

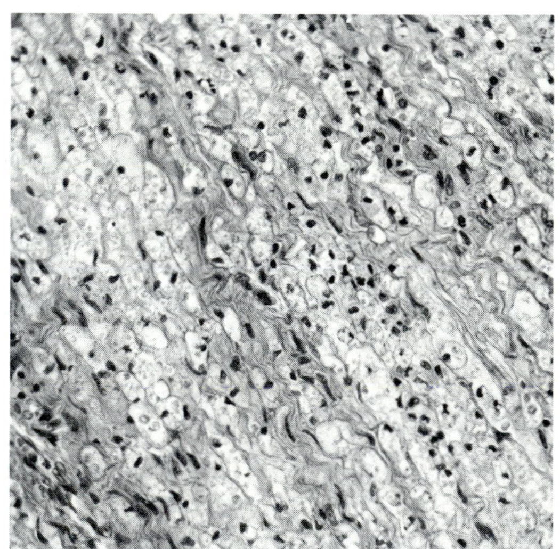

Fig. 44-113. Peripheral neuritis occurring after vincristine therapy. There are fragmentation and loss of axons and destruction of myelin. (Hematoxylin and eosin; 280×.)

cord, the Landry-Guillain-Barré syndrome results.

In herpes zoster infection the changes and the inflammatory responses are striking. The affected spinal ganglia may be swollen and red because of the considerable necrosis with hemorrhage, which simulates a hemorrhagic infarct (Figs. 44-111 and 44-112). Cowdry type A inclusions may be seen in the nerve cells and their capsule cells. Changes in the motor component result in damage to the motor neurons with satellitosis and neuronophagia of the anterior horn cells at that level.

The peripheral nervous system can be involved in all varieties of inflammatory disease, including the purulent, granulomatous, and viral diseases and the collagen diseases and sometimes after chemotherapy (Fig. 44-113).[55,94]

Vascular disease

Degenerative vascular disease such as that seen in patients with atherosclerosis or diabetes frequently affects the peripheral nervous system. Infarction of the spinal ganglia must be exceedingly rare, never having been recognized in our series of over 10,000 ganglia. Involvement of both sensory and motor nerves is, however, very common, particularly in the lower limbs of diabetic patients.[105]

A neuropathy from focal areas of degeneration in the peripheral nervous system has been seen in 16% of patients with diabetes mellitus in the fifth decade of life and in 37% of those in the seventh decade. The clinical and structural appearance of pseudotabes from wallerian degeneration as a result of changes in the peripheral nervous system also has been described in diabetic patients. Involvement of the peripheral nerves and perhaps also the intermediolateral columns of the spinal cord is probably an important factor in the development of the Charcot joints in patients with diabetes.

Pressure

Constant and prolonged pressure on the peripheral nerve can lead to structural as well as functional changes. The larger fibers are the most susceptible. The myelin sheaths are damaged first, followed by changes in the axon. Initially there is fragmentation of the myelin sheaths, followed by the chemical changes characteristic of myelin destruction. When the axons are damaged, they become swollen and fragmented. Both are removed by macrophages. Wallerian degeneration follows. Recovery is related to the reconstitution of the axons followed by the formation of the surrounding myelin. Depending on the degree of damage and fibrosis, recovery may take weeks or months.

Nutritional deficiencies

A peripheral neuropathy related to vitamin B_1 deficiency has been described frequently. The changes affect the distalmost portion of the fibers first, with a progressive dying back of the central portion of the neuron. The nerve cells appear to remain intact. The axons and myelin sheaths undergo swelling and fragmentation, followed by phagocytosis and removal. Recovery takes the pattern previously described for nerve fiber regeneration.

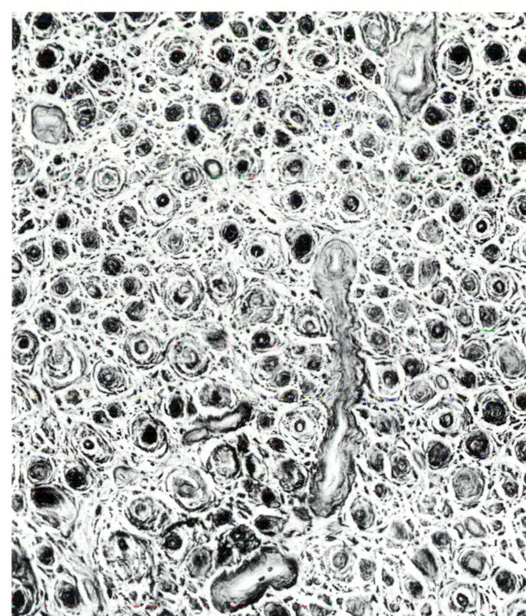

Fig. 44-114. "Onion-bulb" neuropathy. (Hematoxylin and eosin; 90×.)

Toxic disorders

Segmental demyelination involving both sensory and motor nerves has been described in the peripheral nervous system in patients with diphtheria, heavy metal poisoning (lead and arsenic), and porphyria.

"Onion-bulb" neuropathies (Déjérine-Sottas disease, hypertrophic interstitial radiculoneuropathy, Refsum's disease)*

The "onion-bulb" neuropathies are a group of conditions related only in that they are represented by a concentric-ring proliferation of Schwann cells and connective tissue about a peripheral axon. This reactive change can occur in almost any chronic peripheral neuropathy that is characterized by recurrent episodes of demyelination and remyelination.

Hypertrophic interstitial neuropathy of Déjérine-Sottas is a rare disorder resulting in enlargement of the sensory and motor nerves. It is characterized microscopically by the presence of concentric rings of connective tissue forming an onion-skin-like layering about the peripheral axon (Fig. 44-114). This was formerly considered to be a specific reaction, but at the present time it is not

*References 33, 41, 96, 103, 116, 122.

known if the proliferation of the connective tissue represents a genetic response or is evidence of excessive regeneration. As previously discussed, similar changes may be seen in one form of peroneal muscular atrophy (Charcot-Marie-Tooth disease).

Neoplasms

Neoplasms of the peripheral nervous system, except those of the eighth cranial nerve, are unusual. They are seen more commonly in patients with von Recklinghausen's disease, in whom neurilemomas, neurofibromas, or diffuse hyperplasias of a portion of the peripheral nervous system (usually confined to a limb) are seen. The appearance of these tumors is identical to that described for the peripheral nerves attached to the brain and spinal cord.

REFERENCES

1. Andrew, W.: Structural alterations with aging in the nervous system, J. Chronic Dis. **3**:575, 1956.
2. Andrews, J.M., et al.: Globoid cell leukodystrophy (Krabbe's disease): morphological and biochemical studies, Neurology **21**:337, 1971.
3. Arita, M., et al.: Embryonal carcinoma with teratomatous elements in the region of the pineal gland, Surg. Neurol. **9**:198, 1978.
4. Astrom, K.E., Mancall, E.L., and Richardson, E.P., Jr.: Progressive multifocal leuko-encephalopathy: a hitherto unrecognized complication of chronic lymphatic leukaemia and Hodgkin's disease, Brain **81**:93, 1958.
5. Averback, P.: Histopathology of acute cell loss in Huntington's chorea brain, J. Pathol. **132**:55, 1980.
6. Bailey, A.A.: Changes with age in the spinal cord, Arch. Neurol. Psychiatry **70**:299, 1953.
7. Bailey, P., and Cushing, H: A classification of the tumors of the glioma group on a histogenetic basis with a correlated study of prognosis, Philadelphia, 1926, J.B. Lippincott Co.
8. Barnett, H.J.M., and Hyland, H.H.: Noninfective intracranial venous thrombosis, Brain **76**:36, 1953.
9. Benda, C.E.: Developmental disorders of mentation and cerebral palsies, New York, 1952, Grune & Stratton, Inc.
10. Boykin, F.C., et al.: Subependymal glomerate astrocytomas, J. Neuropathol. Exp. Neurol. **13**:30, 1954.
11. Brady, R.D.: The lipid storage diseases: new concepts and control, Ann. Intern. Med. **82**:257, 1975.
12. Brownell, B., Oppenheimer, D.R., and Hughes, J.T.: The central nervous system in motor neurone disease, J. Neurol. Neurosurg. Psychiatry **33**:338, 1970.
13. Bucy, P.C., and Thieman, P.W.: Astrocytomas of the cerebellum: a study of a series of patients operated upon over 28 years ago, Arch. Neurol. **18**:14, 1968.
14. Burger, P.C., and Vogel, F.S.: Degenerative and demyelinating diseases, Am. J. Pathol. **99**:479, 1980.
15. Cape, C.C., et al.: Adult onset of subacute sclerosing panencephalitis, Arch. Neurol. **28**:124, 1973.
16. Carpenter, S.: Proximal axonal enlargement in motor neuron disease, Neurology **18**:841, 1968.
17. Chason, J.L.: Subependymal mixed gliomas, J. Neuropathol. Exp. Neurol. **15**:461, 1956.
18. Chason, J.L.: Cerebral infarction secondary to occlusive arterial disease, Radiology **70**:811, 1958.
19. Chason, J.L., and Dickenman, R.C.: Unpublished data on inflammations of spinal ganglia, 1959.
20. Chason, J.L., and Hindman, W.M.: Berry aneurysms of the circle of Willis: results of a planned autopsy study, Neurology **8**:41, 1958.
21. Chason, J.L., Landers, J.W., and Gonzalez, J.E.: Central pontine myelinolysis, J. Neurol. Neurosurg. Psychiatry **27**:317, 1964.
22. Chason, J.L., Mahoney, W.F., and Landers, J.W.: Massive intracerebral hemorrhage, Minn. Med. **49**:27, 1966.
23. Chason, J.L., Walker, F.B., and Landers, J.W.: Metastatic carcinoma of the central nervous system and dorsal root ganglia: a prospective autopsy study, Cancer **16**:781, 1963.
24. Chason, J.L., et al.: Alterations in cell structure of the brain associated with experimental concussion, J. Neurosurg. **15**:135, 1958.
25. Chason, J.L., et al.: Experimental brain concussion: morphologic findings and a new cytologic hypothesis, J. Trauma **6**:767, 1966.
26. Chatty, E.M., and Earle, K.M.: Medulloblastoma: a report of 201 cases with emphasis on the relationship of histological variants to survival, Cancer **28**:927, 1971.
27. Cole, F.M., and Yates, P.: Intracerebral microaneurysms and small cerebrovascular lesions, Brain **90**:759, 1967.
28. Cole, F.M., and Yates, P.O.: Pseudo-aneurysms in relationship to massive cerebral hemorrhage, J. Neurology Neurosurg. Psychiatry **30**:61, 1967.
29. Crowell, R.M., and Zervas, N.T.: Management of intracranial aneurysm, Med. Clin. North Am. **63**:695, 1979.
30. Cushing, H., and Eisenhardt, L.: Meningiomas: their classification, regional behaviour, life history and surgical end results, Springfield, Ill., 1938, Charles C Thomas, Publisher.
31. Daube, J.R., and Chou, S.M.: Lissencephaly: two cases, Neurology **16**:179, 1966.
32. Dawson, S.L., et al.: The contrecoup phenomenon: reappraisal of a classic problem, Hum. Pathol. **11**:155, 1980.
33. de los Reyes, R.A., et al.: Hypertrophic neurofibrosis with onion bulb formation in an isolated element of the brachial plexus, Neurosurgery **8**:397, 1981.
34. Denny-Brown, D.: The basal ganglia and their relation to disorders of movements, London, 1962, Oxford University Press.
35. DeReuck, J., Chattha, A.S., and Richardson, E.P., Jr.: Pathogenesis and evolution of periventricular leukomalacia in infancy, Arch. Neurol. **27**:229, 1972.
36. Desnick, R.J., et al.: Diagnosis of glycosphingolipidoses by urinary sediment analysis, N. Eng. J. Med. **284**:739, 1971.
37. Dickenman, R.C., and Chason, J.L.: Alterations in the dorsal root ganglia and adjacent nerves in the leukemias, lymphomas and multiple myeloma, Am. J. Pathol. **34**:349, 1958.
38. Dickenman, R.C., and Chason, J.L.: Cysts of dorsal root ganglia, Arch. Pathol. **77**:366, 1964.
39. Dohrmann, G.J., and Collias, J.C.: Choroid plexus carcinoma: case report, J. Neurosurg. **43**:225, 1975.
40. Dorfman, L.J.: Cytomegalovirus encephalitis in adults, Neurology **23**:136, 1973.
41. Dyck, P.J., and Gomez, M.R.: Segmental demyelinization in Dejerine-Sottas disease: light, phase-contrast and electron microscopic studies, Mayo Clin. Proc. **43**:289, 1968.
42. Earle, K.M.: Studies on Parkinson's disease including x ray fluorescent spectroscopy of formalin fixed brain tissue, J. Neuropathol. Exp. Neurol. **27**:1, 1968.
43. Eberts, T.J., and Ransburg, R.C.: Primary intracranial sinus tumor, J. Neurosurg. **50**:246, 1979.
44. Elizan, T.S., et al.: Viral infection in pregnancy and congenital CNS malformations in man, Arch. Neurol. **20**:115, 1969.
45. Ellington, E., and Margolis, G.: Block of arachnoid villus by subarachnoid hemorrhage, J. Neurosurg. **30**:651, 1969.
46. Feigin, I., and Goebel, H.: "Infantile" subacute necrotizing encephalopathy in the adult, Neurology **19**:749, 1969.
47. Feigin, I., and Popoff, N.: Neuropathological changes late in cerebral edema: the relationship to trauma, hypertensive disease and Binswanger's encephalopathy, J. Neuropathol. Exp. Neurol. **22**:500, 1963.
48. Frenkel, J.K.: Toxoplasmosis. In Minckler, J., editor: Pathology of the nervous system, vol. III, New York, 1972, McGraw-Hill Book Co.
49. Freytag, E.: Fatal hypertensive intracerebral haematomas: a survey of the pathological anatomy of 393 cases, J. Neurol. Neurosurg. Psychiatry **31**:616, 1968.

50. Fu, Y.-S., et al.: Is subependymoma (subependymal glomerate astrocytoma) an astrocytoma or ependymoma? Cancer **34**:1992, 1974.
51. Gajdusek, D.C., et al.: Precautions in medical care of, and in handling materials from patients with transmissible virus dementia (Creutzfeldt-Jakob disease), N. Engl. J. Med. **297**:1253, 1977.
52. Gerna, G., McCloud, J., and Chambers, R.W.: Immunoperoxidase technique for detection of antibodies to human cytomegalovirus, J. Clin. Microbiol. **3**:364, 1976.
53. Ghatak, N.R., Poon, T.P., and Zimmerman, H.M.: Toxoplasmosis of the central nervous system, Arch. Pathol. **89**:337, 1970.
54. Gibbs, C.J., Jr., et al.: Oral transmission of kuru, Creutzfeldt-Jakob disease, and scrapie to nonhuman primates, J. Infect. Dis. **142**:205, 1980.
55. Gottschalk, P.G., Dyck, P.J., and Kiely, J.M.: Vinca alkaloid neuropathy: nerve biopsy studies in rats and in man, Neurology **19**:875, 1968.
56. Greene, H.L., Hug, G., and Schubert, W.K.: Metachromatic leukodystrophy: treatment with arylsulfatase A, Arch. Neurol. **20**:147, 1969.
57. Greenhouse, A.H., and Schneck, S.A.: Subacute necrotizing encephalomyelopathy: a reappraisal of the thiamine deficiency hypothesis, Neurology **18**:1, 1968.
58. Hankinson, J.: The surgical treatment of syringomyelia. In Krayenbühl, H., editor: Advances and technical standards in neurosurgery, vol. 5, New York, 1978, Springer-Verlag New York, Inc.
59. Hart, M.M., Petito, C.K., and Earle, K.M.: Mixed gliomas, Cancer **33**:134, 1979.
60. Haymaker, W., et al.: Kernicterus and its importance in cerebral palsy, Springfield, Ill., 1961, Charles C Thomas, Publisher.
61. Herndon, R.M., and Rubinstein, L.J.: Light and electron microscopic observations on the development of viral particles in the inclusions of Dawson's encephalitis (subacute sclerosing panencephalitis), Neurology **18**:8, 1968.
62. Hirano, A.: Progress in the pathology of motor neuron disease, Prog. Neuropathol. **2**:181, 1973.
63. Hirano, A., and Ghatak, N.R.: The fine structure of colloid cysts of the third ventricle, J. Neuropathol. Exp. Neurol. **33**:333, 1974.
64. Hirose, G., and Bass, N.H.: Metachromatic leukodystrophy in the adult, Neurology **22**:312, 1972.
65. Hughes, J.T., and Brownell, B.: Cervical spondylosis complicated by anterior spinal artery thrombosis, Neurology **14**:1073, 1964.
66. Hughes, W.: Origin of lacunes, Lancet **2**:19, 1965.
67. Illis, L.S., and Gostling, J.V.T.: Herpes simplex encephalitis, Bristol, 1972, Scientechnica (Publishers) Ltd.
68. Inglis, K.: The relations of the renal lesions to the cerebral lesions in the tuberous sclerosis complex, Am. J. Pathol. **30**:739, 1954.
69. Jenis, E.H., et al.: Subacute sclerosing panencephalitis: immunoultrastructural localization of measles virus antigen, Arch. Pathol. **95**:81, 1973.
70. Johnson, K.P., Byington, D.P., and Gaddis, L.: Subacute sclerosing panencephalitis. In Thompson, R.A., and Green, J.R., editors: Infectious disease of the central nervous system, New York, 1974, Raven Press.
71. Johnson, R.T., and Mims, C.A.: Pathogenesis of viral infections of the central nervous system, N. Engl. J. Med. **278**:23, 84, 1968.
72. Julius, R., et al.: Diagnostic techniques in metachromatic leukodystrophy, Neurology **21**:15, 1971.
73. Kallen, B., and Levan, A.: Chromosomes in man, with special reference to neuropathological disorders. In Tedeschi, C.G., editor: Neuropathology methods and diagnosis, Boston, 1970, Little, Brown & Co.
74. Katz, M., et al.: Transmission of an encephalitogenic agent from brains of patients with subacute sclerosing panencephalitis to ferrets, N. Engl. J. Med. **279**:793, 1968.
75. Kawamura, J., Garcia, J.H., and Kamijyo, Y.: Cerebellar hemangioblastoma: histogenesis of stroma cells, Cancer **31**:1528, 1973.
76. Kernohan, J.W., and Uihlein, A.: Sarcomas of the brain, Springfield, Ill., 1962, Charles C Thomas, Publisher.
77. Kernohan, J.W., et al.: A simplified classification of the gliomas, Mayo Clin. Proc. **24**:71, 1949.
78. Klintworth, G.K.: Paratentorial grooving of human brains with particular reference to transtentorial hermiation and the pathogenesis of secondary brain-stem hemorrhages, Am. J. Pathol. **53**:391, 1968.
79. Konigsmark, B.W., and Weiner, L.P.: The olivopontocerebellar atrophies: a review, Medicine **49**:227, 1970.
80. Lagos, J.C., and Gomez, M.R.: Tuberous sclerosis: reappraisal of a clinical entity, Mayo Clinic. Proc. **42**:26, 1967.
81. Lampert, P.W., Gajdusek, D.C., and Gibbs, C.J., Jr.: Pathology of dendrites in subacute spongioform virus encephalopathies, Adv. Neurol. **12**:465, 1975.
82. Landers, J.W., Chason, J.L., and Samuel, V.N.: Central pontine myelinolysis: a pathogenetic hypothesis, Neurology **15**:968, 1965.
83. Landis, D.M.D.: Case records of the Massachusetts General Hospital, N. Engl. J. Med. **303**:1162, 1980.
84. Lang, E.R., and Kidd, M.: Electron microscopy of human cerebral aneurysms, J. Neurosurg. **22**:554, 1965.
85. Lawyer, T., Jr., and Netzky, M.G.: Amyotrophic lateral sclerosis: a clinicoanatomic study of fifty-three cases, Arch. Neurol. Psychiatry **69**:171, 1953.
86. Lindenberg, R.: Anoxia does not produce brain damage, Jpn. J. Legal Med. **36**:38, 1982.
87. Loeser, J.D., and Alvord, E.C., Jr.: Agenesis of the corpus callosum, Brain **91**:553, 1968.
88. Mair, W.G.P., and Druckman, R.: The pathology of spinal cord lesions and their relation to the clinical feature in protrusions of cervical intervertebral discs: a report of four cases, Brain **76**:70, 1953.
89. Mark, S.J., and Løken, A.C.: Ependymoma: a follow-up study of 101 cases, Cancer **40**:907, 1977.
90. Markham, J.W., Lynge, H.N., and Stahlman, G.E.B.: The syndromes of spontaneous epidural hematoma: report of three cases, J. Neurosurg. **26**:334, 1967.
91. Masters, C.L., et al.: Creutzfeldt-Jakob disease: patterns of worldwide occurrence and the significance of familial and sporadic clustering, Ann. Neurol. **5**:177, 1979.
92. McCormick, W.F., Hardman, J.M., and Boulter, T.R.: Vascular malformations ("angiomas") of the brain, with special reference to those occurring in the posterior fossa, J. Neurosurg. **28**:241, 1968.
93. Morantz, R.A., Feigin, I., and Ransohoff, J.: Clinical and pathological study of 24 cases of gliosarcoma, J. Neurosurg. **45**:398, 1976.
94. Moress, G.R., D'Agostino, A.N., and Jarcho, L.W.: Neuropathy with lymphoblastic leukemia treated with vincristine, Arch. Neurol. **16**:377, 1967.
95. Nibbelink, D.W., Peters, B.H., and McCormick, W.F.: On the association of pheochromocytoma and cerebellar hemangioblastoma, Neurology **19**:455, 1968.
96. Nichols, P.C., Dyck, P.J., and Miller, D.R.: Experimental hypertrophic neuropathy: change in fascicular area and fiber spectrum after acute crush injury, Mayo Clin. Proc. **43**:297, 1968.
97. Nikaido, T., et al.: Studies in ageing of the brain. II. Microchemical analyses of the nervous system in Alzheimer patients, Arch. Neurol. **27**:549, 1972.
98. Noonan, S.M., Weiss, L., and Riddle, J.M.: Ultrastructural observations of cytoplasmic inclusions in Tay-Sachs lymphocytes, Arch. Pathol. Lab. Med. **100**:595, 1976.
99. Oldendorf, W.H., and Davson, H.: Brain extracellular space and the sink action of cerebrospinal fluid: measurement of rabbit brain extracellular space using sucrose labeled with carbon 14, Arch. Neurol. **17**:196, 1967.
100. Paulson, O.B.: Cerebral apoplexy (stroke): pathogenesis and therapy as illustrated by regional blood flow measurements in the brain, Stroke **2**:327, 1971.
101. Peison, B.: Microglial glioma of brain with extracerebral involvement, Cancer **20**:983, 1967.

102. Pilz, H.: Late onset metachromatic leukodystrophy: arylsulfatase A activity of leukocytes in two families, Arch. Neurol. **27**:87, 1972.
103. Pleasure, D.E., and Towfighi, J.: Onion-bulb neuropathies, Arch. Neurol. **26**:289, 1972.
104. Poser, C.M.: In Minckler, J. editor: Pathology of nervous system, New York, 1968, McGraw-Hill Book Co.
105. Raff, M.C., Sangalang, V., and Asbury, A.K.: Ischemic mononeuropathy multiplex associated with diabetes mellitus, Arch. Neurol. **18**:487, 1968.
106. Resnick, J.S., Engel, W.K., and Sever, J.L.: Subacute sclerosing panencephalitis: spontaneous improvement in a patient with elevated measles antibody in blood and spinal fluid, N. Engl. J. Med. **279**:126, 1968.
107. Rivera, E., and Chason, J.L.: Cerebral hemangioblastoma: case report, J. Neurosurg. **25**:452, 1966.
108. Robertson, D.M., Dinsdale, H.B., and Campbell, R.J.: Subacute combined degeneration of the spinal cord: no association with vitamin B-12 deficiency, Arch. Neurol. **24**:203, 1971.
109. Rosenblum, W.I., and Feigin, I.: The hemorrhagic component of Wernicke's encephalopathy, Arch. Neurol. **13**:627, 1965.
110. Rubinstein, L.J., and Northfield, D.W.C.: The medulloblastoma and the so-called "arachnoidal cerebellar sarcoma": a critical reexamination of a nosological problem, Brain **87**:379, 1964.
111. Russell, D.S.: Observations on the pathology of hydrocephalus, Medical Research Council Special Report Series (London) No. 265, 1966.
112. Sahs, A.L.: Observations on the pathology of saccular aneurysms, J. Neurosurg. **24**:792, 1966.
113. Shaw, C.M., and Alvord, E.C., Jr.: Cava septi pellucidi et vergae: their normal and pathological states, Brain **92**:213, 1969.
114. Sima, A.A.F., and Robertson, D.M.: Subependymal giant-cell astrocytoma, J. Neurosurg. **50**:240, 1979.
115. Sipe, J.C.: Leigh's syndrome: the adult form of subacute necrotizing encephalomyelopathy with prediliction for the brainstem, Neurology **23**:1030, 1973.
116. Snyder, M., Cancilla, P.A., and Batzdorf, U.: Hypertrophic neuropathy simulating a neoplasm of the brachial plexus, Surg. Neurol. **7**:131, 1977.
117. Thompson, R.A., and Pribram, H.F.W.: Infantile cerebral aneurysm associated with ophthalmoplegia and quadriparesis, Neurology **19**:785, 1969.
118. Torack, R.M.: Adult dementia: history, biopsy, pathology, Neurosurgery **4**:434, 1979.
119. Towbin, A.: Pathology of cerebral palsy, Springfield, Ill., 1960, Charles C Thomas, Publisher.
120. Vogel, F.S., and McClenahan, J.L.: Anomalies of major cerebral arteries associated with congenital malformations of the brain with special reference to the pathogenesis of anencephaly, Am. J. Pathol. **28**:701, 1952.
121. Wasterlain, C.G., and Torack, R.M.: Cerebral edema in water intoxication. II. An ultrastructural study, Arch. Neurol. **19**:79, 1968.
122. Webster, H. deF., et al.: The role of Schwann cells in the formation of "onion bulbs" found in chronic neuropathies, J. Neuropathol. Exp. Neurol. **25**:276, 1967.
123. Weir, B., and Elvidge, A.R.: Oligodendrogliomas: an analysis of 63 cases, J. Neurosurg. **29**:500, 1968.
124. Weller, T.H.: The cytomegalovirus: ubiquitous agents with protean clinical manifestations, N. Engl. J. Med. **285**:203, 267, 1971.
125. West, H.H.: The sphingolipidoses: an overview, Postgrad. Med. **61**:90, 1977.
126. Wisneiwski, H., Coblentz, J.M., and Terry, R.T.: Pick's disease: a clinical and ultrastructural study, Arch. Neurol. **26**:97, 1972.
127. Wisniewski, H., Terry, R.D., and Hirano, A.: Neurofibrillary pathology, J. Neuropathol. Exp. Neurol. **29**:163, 1970.
128. Wolstenholme, G.E.W., and O'Connor, C.M., editors: Ciba Foundation Symposium on congenital malformations, Boston, 1960, Little, Brown & Co.
129. Woolsey, R.M., and Nelsen, J.S.: Progressive multifocal leukoencephalopathy, Neurology **15**:662, 1965.
130. Wright, D.G., Laurino, R., and Victor, M.: Pontine and extrapontine myelinolysis, Brain **102**:361, 1979.
131. Ziegler, D.D., Zosa, A., and Zileli, T.: Hypertensive encephalopathy, Arch. Neurol. **12**:472, 1965.

Index

Page numbers in *italics* indicate illustrations.
Page numbers followed by *t* indicate tables.

B

I

M

N

Q

R

S